Principles and Practice of

ASSISTED REPRODUCTIVE TECHNOLOGY

Principles and Practice of ASSISTED REPRODUCTIVE TECHNOLOGY

VOLUME 1

INFERTILITY

Third Edition

Editor

Kamini A Rao
MBBS DGO MCh FRCOG FNAMS FICOG PGDMLE
Chief Mentor
Former Founder and Medical Director
Milann Group of Fertility Centers
Bengaluru, Karnataka, India

Co-Editors

Vyshnavi A Rao
MBBS MS (OBG) FRM
Senior Consultant Reproductive Medicine
Milann Fertility and Birthing Center
Bengaluru, Karnataka, India

Devi R
MBBS MS (OBG) Fellowship in Reproductive Medicine
Clinical Head and Fertility Specialist
Oasis Fertility, Banashankari
Bengaluru, Karnataka, India

Foreword

Geeta Nargund

JAYPEE

JAYPEE BROTHERS MEDICAL PUBLISHERS
The Health Sciences Publisher
New Delhi | London

Jaypee Brothers Medical Publishers (P) Ltd.

Headquarters
EMCA House, 23/23-B
Ansari Road, Daryaganj
New Delhi 110 002, India
Landline: +91-11-23272143, +91-11-23272703
+91-11-23282021, +91-11-23245672
e-mail: jaypee@jaypeebrothers.com

Corporate Office
4838/24, Ansari Road, Daryaganj
New Delhi 110 002, India
Phone: +91-11-43574357
Fax: +91-11-43574314
e-mail: jaypee@jaypeebrothers.com

Overseas Office
JP Medical Ltd.
83, Victoria Street, London
SW1H 0HW (UK)
Phone: +44-20 3170 8910
e-mail: info@jpmedpub.com

EU GPSR Authorised Representative
Logos Europe, 9 rue Nicolas Poussin
17000, La Rochelle, France
Phone: +33 (0) 6 67 93 73 78
e-mail: contact@logoseurope.eu

Website: www.jaypeebrothers.com
Website: www.jaypeedigital.com

Inquiries for bulk sales may be solicited at: jaypee@jaypeebrothers.com

Principles and Practice of Assisted Reproductive Technology—Vol. 1 (Infertility)

First Edition: 2014
Second Edition: 2019
Third Edition: 2023, *Reprint: 2024, 2025,* **2026**

ISBN: 978-93-5696-037-4

Printed at: Samrat Offset Pvt. Ltd.

Dedicated to

To all my students and patients who taught me.

Contributors

Abha Bhat MBBS DGO MRCOG
Consultant Reproductive Endocrinologist
Herts and Essex Fertility Center, UK
Cheshunt, United Kingdom

Abha Majumdar MS MBBS FICS
Director and Head
Departments of Obstetrics and Gynecology
Radiology and Ultrasound
Center of IVF and Human Reproduction
Sir Ganga Ram Hospital
New Delhi, India

Abhishek Shah BHMS
Regional Head
Department of Embryology
Oasis Fertility
Vadodara, Gujarat, India

Aditi M Kunte MS
Consultant (Ob-Gyn)
Patki Hospital and Post Graduate Institute
Kolhapur, Maharashtra, India

Adrija Kumar Datta MD FRCOG
IVF Consultant
ISMAAR Research Coordinator
Department of Reproductive Medicine
St Bartholomew's Hospital
London, United Kingdom

Ajitabh Shukla MD DNB FNB
IVF Consultant
Department of Obstetrics
and Gynecology
Genome The Fertility Center
Kolkata, West Bengal, India

Akanksha Gautam Allahbadia MS
Consultant Reproductive
Endocrinology and IVF
Sumitra Hospital
Noida, Uttar Pradesh, India

Alex C Varghese MSc PhD
Group Scientific Director
Fertility Associates
Remuera, Auckland, New Zealand
and Scientific Director
Sunfert International Fertility Center
(FA Group)
Kuala Lumpur, Malaysia

Ameya Rangnath Sangle
Senior Resident
Department of Urology
MS Ramaiah Medical College
Bengaluru, Karnataka India

Amit J Upadhyay FNB
(Reproductive Medicine) DNB (Obstetrics
and Gynecology) FCPS (Obstetrics and
Gynecology) DGO MBBS
Director and IVF Consultant
Chaturthi Hospitals LLP
Mumbai, Maharashtra, India

Amr Wahba MRCOG MD
Head
Department of Obstetrics and Gynecology
Cairo University
Cairo, Egypt

Ana Cobo PHD
Director of the Cryobiology Unit in the IVF lab
at IVI Valencia
Valencia, Spain

Aneesha Grover MBBS GAGE DNB
(OBG) MNAMS MSc (Clinical Embryology and
Preimplantation Genetics) Diploma
in Clinical ART
Infertility Specialist
Nova Southend IVF and Fertility
Gurugram, Haryana, India

Anindita Thakker MD(OBG) FRM
Junior Consultant
Milann Fertility
Bengaluru, Karnataka, India

Anitha S Kumari K BSc MSc PhD (AM)
Former Consultant Embryologist
Milann – The Fertility Center
Bengaluru, Karnataka, India

Anjali Sharma MS DNB FNB MRCOG
Center Head
Indira IVF
Prayagraj, Uttar Pradesh, India

Anshu Dhar MBBS MD (Obs & Gyne)
FNB Reproductive Medicine
Milann Hospital
Bengaluru, Karnataka, India

Anu Kottur MBBS MD (Medicine)
Senior IVF Coordinator and Consultant
Milann Fertility
Bengaluru, Karnataka, India

Anubhuti Patel MS FNB Reproductive
Medicine
Assistant Professor
IMS and SUM Hospital
Bhubaneswar, Odisha, India

Anuja Kamath MSc
Head
Nova Academy of Clinical Embryology Training
Nova IVF Fertility
Bengaluru, Karnataka, India

Anupama Deenadayal Mettler MD PhD
Scientific Head of the IVF Lab
University Reproductive Medical Unit at
Universitäres Kinderwunschzentrum, UKSH
Campus Kiel, Kiel, Germany

Anupama Patil MS (OBG) FRM FMAS
Advanced Diploma in ART (Germany)
Consultant
Kritu Fertility Center
Gadag, Karnataka, India

Anuradha Kumari MS OBG FMAS
Junior Consultant
Milann Fertility Center
Indiranagar, Bengaluru
Milann Fertility Center
Bengaluru, Karnataka, India

Arati R Rao MBBS MD DNB MNAMS MRCOG
Senior Consultant and Lead Clinician
Department of Fetal Medicine and
Fertility Units at Milann Whitefield Hospital
Bengaluru, Karnataka, India

Arjun N MBBS MS MCh
Associate Professor
Department of Urology
Sapthagiri Medical College
Bengaluru, Karnataka, India

Arnav Pai MBBS MS
Obstetrics and Gynecology Resident
Dr DY Patil, Hospital and Research Center
Navi Mumbai, Maharashtra, India

Arunima Halder MBBS MS (OB&GYN) DNB (OB&GYN) FNB (Reproductive Medicine)
Consultant Reproductive Medicine
Manipal Hospital, Whitefield
Bengaluru, Karnataka, India

Arveen Vohra MBBS MS (OBG) FRM
Medical Director and Senior Reproductive Medicine Consultant
Anaahita Fertility Clinic
Bengaluru, Karnataka, India

Arya Rajendran MBBS MD (OG) DNB (OG) FNB (Reproductive Medicine)
Consultant
Reproductive Medicine
Nova IVF Fertility
Palakkad, Kerala, India

Ashish S Reddy MBBS MD DM
Consultant Endocrinologist
Department of Endocrinology
Yashoda Hospitals, Secunderabad
Hyderabad, Telangana, India.

Ashwini Mohandas DM (Medical & Hemato-Oncology)
Superspeciality Resident
Regional Cancer Center Thiruvananthapuram
Thiruvananthapuram, Kerala, India

Ashwini Sidhmalswamy G MBBS MS (Obstetrics & Gynecology), Dip USG MRCOG PGDMLE
IVF Specialist
Department of Obstetrics and Gynecology
Motherhood Hospital – Hebbal
Bengaluru, Karnataka, India

Aswathy Kumaran
MBBS DGO MS DNB FNB
Consultant
Reproductive Medicine
Aster MIMS Kottakkal
Kerala, India

Ayesha Gupta MBBS MD (Obstetrics and Gynecology) MPH FRM
Consultant
Infertility Specialist
Department of Obstetrics and Gynecologist
Clinical Fellow in Reproductive Medicine
Milann Fertility Center
Bengaluru, Karnataka, India

Baiju Pookilath FNB (Reproductive Medicine)
Consultant
Department of Reproductive Endocrinology and Fertility
Ncare IVF Center Kannur and Parappanangadi
Kozhikode , Kerala, India

Bezar Ghan VV PhD ESHRE ASCP FAGE R-Immunology
Chief Clinical Embryologist and HCLD
Craft Fertility Center
Gunasheela IVF Center
Hamad Medical Corporation KMC, YMC, Milann
Qatar, India, Sweden

Bharti Jain DNB
IVF and Infertility Specialist
KJIVF and Laparoscopy Center
New Delhi, India

Bindu Chimote MSc MPhil PhD (Biochemistry) MSc (Clinical Embryology) Leeds UK
IVF Scientist and Sr Embryologist
Department of Embryology Reproductive Endocrinology
Vaunshdhara Fertility Center
Nagpur, Maharashtra , India

Chaitanya Nagori MD DGO
Consultant and Director
Dr Nagori's Institute for Infertility and IVF
Ahmedabad, Gujarat, India

Chaitra Narayan Nayak
MBBS MS (OBG) FNB (REP MED)
Consultant Reproductive Medicine
Cloud Nine Hospitals
Bengaluru, Karnataka, India

Chandana C MBBS MS DNB (Obs & Gyne)
Professor
The Oxford Medical College
Hospital and Research Center
Bengaluru, Karnataka, India

Chandrika Kulkarni MBBS MD (Obstetrics & Gynecology) Fellowship in Reproductive Medicine DNB - Obstetrics and Gynecology
Reproductive Endocrinologist (Infertility)
Gynecologist, Obstetrician, Infertility Specialist
Cloudnine Fertility - IVF Center
Bengaluru, Karnataka, India

CV Kannaki Uthraraj MD DGO
Director
Thamarai Fertility Center
Sivameds Hospital
Barathi Street
Pollachi, Tamil Nadu, India

D Ramesh Raja
MBBS PGDCE Fellowship in Clinical Andrology FCSM (Sexual Medicine)
Senior Consultant in Clinical Embryology and Andrology
Nakshatra Men, Women and Fertility Clinic
Chennai, Tamil Nadu, India

Deepak Modi PhD FNASc
Scientist F
ICMR-National Institute for Research in Reproductive and Child Health
Mumbai, Maharashtra, India

Deepti Sharma
FNB (Reproductive Medicine) MS (OBGY)
Infertility and IVF consultant
Rohilkhand Infertility and IVF Center
Bareilly, Uttar Pradesh, India

Devi R
MBBS MS (OBG) Fellowship in Reproductive Medicine
Clinical Head and Fertility Specialist
Oasis Fertility, Banashankari
Bengaluru, Karnataka, India

Dhiraj Gada MD DGO DFP FICMCH
Director
Shalby Gadalife ART Center
Shalby Hospital and Research Center
Indore, Madhya Pradesh, India

Dileep Kumar R MBBS MD DNB MRCP (UK)
Internal Medicine Specialist
Dr Mehta's Hospitals
Chennai, Tamil Nadu, India

Dipti Das MD ((Obs & Gyn)
Fellow in Reproductive Medicine
BACC Healthcare
Bengaluru, Karnataka, India

Divya Sardana MD (OBG) DNB (OBG) FNB (Reproductive Medicine)
Senior Consultant (IVF)
Cloudnine Hospital
Gurugram, Haryana, India

Divyashree PS MBBS DNB (OBG) FNB (Reproductive Medicine) PGDMLE
Medical Director and Consultant
Reproductive Medicine
Genea Fertility Center
Bengaluru, Karnataka, India

Dorothy Dessa MBBS(Gold Medalist) MS (G&O) Fellowship in Reproductive Medicine, Milann
Bengaluru, Karnataka, India
RMO-cum Clinical Tutor
Department of Obstetrics and Gynecology
Medical College Hospital
Kolkata, West Bengal, India

Durga G Rao
MBBS DGO MRCOG(UK)
Medical Director
Infertility Specialist
Laparoscopic Surgeon (Obs & Gyn)
Reproductive Endocrinologist (Infertility)
Oasis Center for Reproductive Medicine
Hyderabad, Telangana, India

Duru Shah
MD FRCOG FCPS FICS FICOG DGO DFP FICMCH
Scientific Director
Gynaecworld, the Center for Womens Health and Fertility
Mumbai, Maharashtra, India

Erika Patel MBBS MS(Obs & Gyn) MCh (Reproductive Medicine and Surgery)
Infertility Specialist
ART Fertility Clinics
Chennai, Tamil Nadu, India

Fahim L Rajwate
MBBS MS (General Surgery) MCH (Urology)
Consultant Microsurgical Andrologist and Urologist
Department of Reproductive Medicine
Ankur Healthcare
Bengaluru, Karnataka, India

Gaurav Majumdar MCE PhD
Chief Embryologist and Lab Director
Center of IVF and Human Reproduction
Sir Ganga Ram Hospital
New Delhi, India

Gautam Allahbadia
MD DNB FNAMS FCPS DGO DFP FICOG FICMU
Consultant Reproductive Endocrinology and IVF
Millennium Medical Center
MMC IVF, DHCC, Dubai and Bourn Hall IVF Jumeirah
Dubai, United Arab Emirates

Gautam Khastgir MD FRCS FRCOG
Medical Director and Consultant in Reproductive Medicine and Surgery
Bengal Infertility and Reproductive Therapy Hospital
Kolkata, West Bengal, India

Gautham T Pranesh MBBS MD DNB
Research Development Consultant at MitoPower LLC
Bengaluru, Karnataka, India

Geeta Nargund MBBS FRCOG (London)
Founder/Medical Director
Department of Reproductive Medicine
St George's Hospital
London, United Kingdom

Goral Gandhi MSc
Founder and Scientific Director
Global Fertility Solutions
Mumbai, Maharashtra, India

Gotte Jhansi MBBS DGO
Reproductive Medicine
Milann Hospital
Peddapalli, Telangana, India

Gowri Rapaka MD
Senior Resident
Department of Obstetrics and Gynecology
All India Institute of Medical Sciences
New Delhi, India

Guruprasad Kalthur MSc PhD
Professor and Head
Kasturba Medical College, Manipal
Division of Reproductive Biology
Department of Reproductive Science
Kasturba Medical College, Manipal
Manipal Academy of Higher Education
Manipal, Karnataka, India

Haritha Mannem
MBBS MS (OBGY) FRM (RGUHS) FMAS
Consultant Reproductive Medicine
Nova Southend Fertility Center
Ghaziabad, Uttar Pradesh, India

Harmi Thakkar MSc (Biotechnology)
Research Associate
Akanksha Hospital and Research Institute, Lambhvel
Anand, Gujarat, India

Harpreet Kaur MBBS MD DNB FNB (Rep. Medicine) MRCOG (UK)
Associate Professor
All India Institute of Medical Sciences
Bilaspur, Himachal Pradesh, India

Harsha K Bhadarka PhD
IVF Lab Director
Akanksha Hospital and Research Institute, Lambhvel
Anand, Gujarat, India

Hemanth Kumar MA
MBBS DNB (General Surgery)
Consultant
Fortis Flt Lt Rajan Dhall Hospital
New Delhi, India

Himanshu Singhal MBBS MD FRM
Consultant
Cloudnine Fertility
Bengaluru, Karnataka, India

HK Nagaraj MBBS MS MCh FICS
Professor
Department of Urology
Sapthagiri Medical College
Bengaluru, Karnataka, India

Hrishikesh Pai MD FRCOG (HON) FCPS FICOG MSc (USA)
Scientific Director and Co-Founder
Bloom IVF
Scientific Director and Co-Founder
BAUFICI Genetics
President Elect, FOGSI
Director Corporate Affairs, IFFS
Past President, ISAR, IAGE, MOGS and MSR
Founder Chair, Indian SIG ASRM

Jaideep Malhotra
MD FICMCH FICOG FRCOG FRCPI FMAS
Managing Director
ART Rainbow IVF and MNMH (P) Ltd and Ujala Cygnus Rainbow Hospital
Agra, Uttar Pradesh, India
President, SAFOM/ISPAT
Past President, IMS/ISAR/FOGSI/ASPIRE

Jampana Pallavi MBBS MS DNB
Fellow in Reproductive Medicine
Milann Fertility Center
Andhra Pradesh, India

Jana EJ Pittman BMedRes
School of Medicine
Western Sydney University
Campbelltown, New South Wales, Australia

JB Sharma MD FRCOG FAMS PhD
Professor
Department of Obstetrics and Gynecology
All India Institute of Medical Sciences
New Delhi, India

José María de los Santos PhD
IVF Lab Department Director
Valencia, Spain

Josep Lluís Romero MD
IVF Lab II Department Director
Valencia, Spain

Jwal Banker MD
Obstetrician and Gynecologist
Infertility Specialist
Nova IVI Fertility
Ahmedabad, Gujarat, India

Jyoti Mhatre MD DGO DFP
Consultant
Kedar Hospital
Mumbai, Maharashtra, India

K Aruna Saradha MBBS M S (OBG)
Fellow in Reproductive Medicine
Milann Group of Fertility Centers
Bengaluru, Karnataka, India

Kamini A Rao MBBS DGO MCh FRCOG FNAMS FICOG PGDMLE
Chief Mentor
Former Founder and Medical Director
Milann Group of Fertility Centers
Bengaluru, Karnataka, India

Kannamannadiar Jayaprakasan
MD DNB FRCOG PhD
Honorary Associate Professor and Subspecialist in Reproductive Medicine and Surgery
Royal Derby Hospital
Derby, United Kingdom

Kenichiro Hiraoka PhD
ART Laboratory Manager
Kameda IVF Clinic Makuhari
Chiba, Japan

Kinjal Shah DNB (OBG) DFP (Gold Medalist)
FNB (Reproductive Medicine)
Consultant Gynecologist and
Infertility Specialist
Bloom IVF—Lilavati Hospital
Mumbai, Maharashtra, India

Korula George MD MRACOG
Former Head of the Department
Department of Reproductive
Medicine and Surgery
Christian Medical College
Vellore, Tamil Nadu, India

Krishna Chaitanya M MBBS PGDHOM
Graduate Diploma in Reproductive
Health Sciences, Masters of Clinical Embryology
Scientific Head and Clinical Embryologist
Oasis Fertility
Hyderabad, Telangana, India

KS Mangayarkarasi PhD (Fenetics)
Lab director
Thamarai Fertility Services
Sivameds Hospital, Barathi Street
Pollachi, Tamil Nadu, India

Kuldeep Jain
MD Fellowship in ART (Singapore)
Managing Director and IVF and Fertility
Specialist
KJIVF and Laparoscopy Center
Delhi, India

Maansi Jain MS (Obst & Gyne) Diploma
Clinical ART Fellowship in Reproductive Medicine
and Reproductive Surgery (Singapore)
Consultant ART and Laparoscopic Surgeon at
KJIVF and Laparoscopy Center
Delhi, India

Madhuri Milind Patil
MD DGO FCPS DFP FICOG (Mumbai)
Infertility Specialist
Reproductive Endocrinologist (Infertility),
Gynecologist
Dr Patil's Fertility and Endoscopy Clinic
Bengaluru, Karnataka, India

Mahendra V Javali MD DM (Neurology)
Professor of Neurology
MS Ramaiah Medical College and Hospitals
Bengaluru, Karnataka, India

Mahesh Koregol MBBS MS (Obstetrics
and Gynaecology) Fellowship in Reproductive
Medicine
Infertility Specialist
Nova IVF Fertility
Bengaluru, Karnataka, India

Mala Arora MBBS Fellow of Royal College of
Obstetricians and Gynecologists FRCOG (London)
Consultant
Department of Obstetrician and Gynecologist
Fortis la femme
New Delhi, India

Mamta Dighe
Director
Xenith Advanced Fertility Center

Mandeep Kaur
MBBS MD FNB (Reproductive Medicine)
Medical Director
Star Fertility
Jalandhar, Punjab, India

Manish Banker MD FICOG
Infertility Specialist
Laparoscopic Surgeon (Obs & Gyn)
Medical Director
Nova IVI Fertility
Ahmedabad, Gujarat, India

Manishi Mittal MD (OBG) Fellow
Reproductive Medicine
Consultant OBG
Mittal Maternity and Superspeciality Hospital
Yamunanagar, Haryana, India

Manjunath C Swamy MBBS MS (Obstetrics
and Gynecology) FGE (Fellowship in Gynec
Endoscopy)
Gynecologist and Infertility Specialist
Apollo Spectra
Bengaluru, Karnataka, India

Marcos Meseguer
PHD (Obstetrics and Gynecoloy)
Scientific Supervisor and Senior Embryologist
IVI Valencia
Valencia, Spain

Mats Brännström MD PhD
Department of Obstetrics and Gynecology
University of Gothenburg
Sahlgrenska University Hospital
Göteborg, Sweden

Mir Jaffar PhD
Scientific Director and Chief Embryologist
Valley Fertility Center
Srinagar, Jammu and Kashmir, India

Mirudhubashini Govindarajan
FRCS (Canada) FICOG
Clinical Director
Womens Center and Hospitals
Coimbatore, Tamil Nadu, India

Mohammed Ashraf C PhD
Associate Director and Senior Embryologist
Milann Fertility Centre
Bengaluru, Karnataka, India

Mohan S Kamath MS (AFMC) DNB Fellow
(Reproductive Medicine) (CMC, Vellore)
Commonwealth Fellow (Reproductive
Medicine) (UK)
Professor and Head
Department of Reproductive
Medicine and Surgery
Christian Medical College
Vellore, Tamil Nadu, India

Molina N Patel MD (Obs & Gyn)
IVF Consultant and Aesthetic Gynecologist
Akanksha Hospital and
Research Institute, Lambhvel
Anand, Gujarat, India

Muthukumar K MD
Associate Research Officer
Reproductive Medicine Unit
Christian Medical College
Vellore, Tamil Nadu, India

N Pandiyan MBBS DGO MD (OG) MNAMS
Professor Emeritus
The Tamil Nadu Dr MGR Medical University
Retired Chief Consultant and HOD
Department of Andrology and
Reproductive Medicine
Chettinad Super Specialty Hospital
Chettinad Health City, Kelambakkam
Rajiv Gandhi Salai
Chennai, Tamil Nadu, India

Nalini Mahajan
MD MMed Sci (ART) (UK) FICOG
Director Mother and Child Hospital
New Delhi, India

Nandita Palshetkar
MD FRCOG FICOG FCPS
Professor in Obstetrics and Gynecology
DY Patil Medical College Navi Mumbai
Director at NINE BLOOM IVF Centers
Mumbai, Maharashtra, India

Narendra Malhotra
MD FICMCH FICOG FRCOG FICS FMAS FIAP
Managing Director
Global Rainbow Health Care and MNMH
and Ujala Cygnus Rainbow Hospital
Agra, Uttar Pradesh, India
Professor, Sarajevo School of Science and
Technology, Croatia
Past President, FOGSI/IFUMB/ISPAT/ISAR,
INSARG
Vice President, WAPM/SAFOG
Director, International IAN Donald School
and SAFOG

Natchandra Chimote PhD (Clinical
Embryology)
Consultant Embryologist Vaunshdhara
Fertility Center
Nagpur, Maharashtra, India

Navina Singh
FRM MS Dip (Medicolegal System)
Lilavati, Jaslok and AMP; Sir HN Reliance Foundation Hospital and Research Center
Mumbai, Maharashtra, India

Navya N MBBS MS(OBG)
Consultant Fetal Medicine
Ovum Hospital, Banashankari
Bengaluru, Karnataka, India

Navya V MBBS MS (OBG) FRM (Fellowship in Reproductive Medicine)
Consultant
Department of Reproductive Medicine Tirupati
Andhra Pradesh, India

Nayana H Patel MD (Obs & Gyn)
Medical Director and Infertility Specialist
Akanksha Hospital and Research Institute, Lambhvel
Anand, Gujarat, India

Neelima Gupta
MBBS DGO DNB FNB (Reproductive Medicine)
Senior Consultant IVF
Milann—The Fertility Center
New Delhi, India

Neeti Tiwari MD (OBG) FICOG
Consultant Center of IVF and Human Reproduction
Sir Ganga Ram Hospital
New Delhi, India

Neha Tyagi MBBS DNB (OBG) FRM
Infertility Specialist
Milann—The Fertility Center
Bengaluru, Karnataka, India

Neharika Malhotra MD (Gold Medalist)
DRM (Germany) FICMCH Fellow ICOG (Rep Med) ICOG (USG)
Director and Consultant
ART Rainbow IVF and MNMH (P) Ltd and Ujala Cygnus Rainbow Hospital
Agra, Uttar Pradesh, India
Joint Secretary, FOGSI Chair
YTP Committee, FOGSI

Nidhi Shah Gandhi DNB DGO
Consultant Obstetrician and AMP
Gynecologist Women's Care Clinic
Mumbai, Maharashtra, India

Niket H Patel MD (Obs & Gyn)
Director
Endoscopic Surgeon and IVF Consultant
Akanksha Hospital and Research Institute, Lambhvel
Anand, Gujarat, India

Nisha Singh MBBS MS (OBG) DNB (OBG) FNB (Reproductive Medicine)
Infertility Specialist Milann—The Fertility Center
Bengaluru, Karnataka, India

Nitin Laxmikant Lad FICOG MD (BOM)
DGO DFP MNAMS MCE (Singapore) MMC
Accredited Speaker Director and Consultant ART Dr Lad's Navjeevan Hospital
Nasik, Maharashtra, India

Nivedita Ananth DNB FRM
Fellow
Craft Hospital
Kerala, India

Nivedita Shetty MD (OBG) FRCOG (UK)
Fellowship in Reproductive Medicine (National Board, New Delhi)
Director of the ART Unit
Manipal Hospital
Mysore, Karnataka , India

Nivita Gugnani MSc (Reproductive Biology and Clinical Embryology)
Embryologist
Milann Fertility and Birthing Hospital
Delhi, India

Nupur Garg MBBS MS FRM (BACC)
Consultant SCI IVF Center Noida
Ghaziabad, Uttar Pradesh, India

Nutan Jain MD
Director
Vardhman Trauma and Laparoscopy Center
Muzaffarnagar, Uttar Pradesh, India

Osama Shawki MD
Emeritus Professor
Cairo University
Cairo, Egypt

Padma Rekha Jirge MRCOG (UK)
FICOG MBA (Health Care Management)
PG DMLE (Med Law & Ethics)
IVF Specialist, Scientific Director
Shreyas Hospital and Sushrut Assisted Conception Clinic
Kolhapur, Maharashtra, India

Pankaj Talwar MBBS MD
Director
Assisted Reproductive Technologies Center
Army Hospital (R & R)
New Delhi, India

Parimala Chinta MS Post Doc Fellow (Reproductive Medicine)
Assistant Professor
Department of Reproductive Medicine and Surgery
Christian Medical College
Vellore, Tamil Nadu, India

Parul Arora MD DNB
Associate Gynecologist
Nova IVF Fertility
Ahmedabad, Gujarat, India

Petra De Sutter MD PhD
Professor
Department of Reproductive Medicine
University Hospital
Ghent , Belgium

Pooja Awasthi MSc (Biochemistry)
Embryologist Origin IVF and Fertility Center
Ghaziabad, Uttar Pradesh, India

Prashant Puranik MCh (Plastic Surgery) DNB (Plastic Surgery) Fellowship in Reconstructive Oncology Consultant
Department of Plastic Surgeon Health Care
Global Hospital
Bengaluru, Karnataka, India

Pratap Kumar MD DGO FICS FICOG
Professor
Kasturba Medical College Manipal
Karnataka, India

Prathap Tharyan
DGO MD FICOG FICS FICMCH
Professor
Kasturba Medical College and Hospital
Manipal, Karnataka, India

Prathima Tholeti BSc MSc
Lecturer
Department of Reproductive Science
Kasturba Medical College
Manipal, Karnataka, India

Pratibha Saran Malik MBBS MD (OBG)
DNB (OBG) MNAMS FNB (Reproductive Medicine National Board) MRCOG (UK)
Senior Consultant IVF and Infertility Specialist
Cloudnine Hospital
Gurugram, Haryana, India

Pravin Mhatre MD FCPS DGO DFP
Professor Emeritus
Seth GS Medical College
KEM and Wadia Hospital
Mumbai, Maharashtra, India

Priya Kannan MBBS MMed MCE
Embryologist
Garbba Rakshambigai Fertility Center
Chennai, Tamil Nadu, India

R Suchindra MBBS MD (OBG) FRM
Consultant
Department of Reproductive Medicine
Milann—The Fertility Center
Bengaluru, Karnataka, India

Radha Pandiyan MBBS DGO MD (OG)
Retired Senior Consultant
Department of Andrology and
Reproductive Medicine
Chettinad Super Specialty Hospital
Chettinad Health City
Kelambakkam, Rajiv Gandhi Salai
Chennai, Tamil Nadu, India

Rajvi H Mehta PhD
Director Academics
Research and Training Trivector Origio
Mumbai, Maharashtra, India

Ramya Jayaram MBBS MS (OB&GYN)
Consultant
Reproductive Medicine and
Endo-Gynec Surgery
Motherhood Women and Children's Hospital
Coimbatore, Tamil Nadu, India

Ranjana Mangoli MSc PhD
Senior Embryologist Fertility Clinic
and IVF Center
Mumbai, Maharashtra, India

Ravi Kumar IR MBBS MD
Senior Consultant Anesthesiologist
Milann—The Fertility Center
Bengaluru, Karnataka, India

Revathi S Rajan MBBS DGO DNB (OBG)
Fellowship in Fetomaternal Medicine (RGUHS)
Chief Consultant
Department of Maternal Fetal Medicine
Managing Director
Mirror Health
Bengaluru, Karnataka, India

Richa Sharma MBBS MS FNBE FRM MRCOG
IVF Consultant Private Practitioner
Mumbai, Maharashtra, India

Rishma Dhillon Pai
MD DNB DGO FCPS FICOG
Consultant
Gynecologist and IVF Expert
Lilavati and Jaslok Hospitals
Mumbai, Maharashtra, India
Past President, Indian Society of Assisted
Reproduction
Past President, IAGE
Past President, FOGSI, President, Mumbai
Obstetrics and Gynecological Society

Ritu Gada MSc (Clinical Embryology)
Researcher/Student University of Oxford
Embryologist, Bloom IVF
Mumbai, Maharashtra, India

RK Sharma (Brig.)
Director and Head
Institute of Reproductive Medicine
and IVF Center
Primus Super Speciality Hospital, New Delhi
Ex-Professor and Head
Department of Obstetrics and Gynecology and
ART Center Army Hospital (R&R), New Delhi
and Command Hospital (SC) Armed Forces
Medical College
Pune, Maharashtra, India

Rohan Palshetkar MS (OBG)
Assistant Professor
DY Patil IVF Center Navi Mumbai
Navi Mumbai, Maharashtra, India

Rohit Gutgutia MBBS DGO
Medical Director
NOVA IVF Fertility East
Kolkata, West Bengal, India

Roopini Sathiasai Kumar MD
Embryologist
Manipal Hospitals
Whitefield
Bengaluru, Karnataka, India

Ruchi Narula MSc (Bioinformatics) ISAR
Certificate Course in Clinical Embryology
Regional Head and Senior Embryologist
Oasis Fertility
Ranchi, Jharkhand, India

Rutvij Dalal MBBS DGO DNB FNB
REPRODUCTIVE MEDICINE
IVF Specialist
Janini IVF
New Delhi, India

S Sowbarnika BDS PGDCE MSc
Clinical Embryologist
Department of Andrology and
Reproductive Medicine,
Chettinad Super Speciality Hospital
Chettinad Health City
Kelambakkam, Rajiv Gandhi Salai
Chennai, Tamil Nadu, India

Sabahat Rasool MD MRCOG DNB
MNAMS FMAS
Fertility Consultant and Reproductive
Medicine Specialist
Gynaecworld Fertility Center
Kemps Corner
Mumbai, Maharashtra, India

Sandhya Krishnan
DNB FNB (Reproductive Medicine) PGDMLE
Senior consultant
N-CARE IVF
Calicut, Kerala, India

Sandhya Kumari MSc PhD
Assistant Professor
Kasturba Medical College, Manipal
Division of Reproductive Biology
Department of Reproductive Science
Kasturba Medical College, Manipal
Manipal Academy of Higher Education
Manipal, Karnataka, India

Sangita Sharma MD DNB FNB
(Reproductive Medicine) MNAMS
Unit Head and Consultant
Manipal Fertility
Jaipur, Rajasthan, India

Sanjay Shukla MSc PhD (Life Sciences)
Laboratory Director
Shivani Fertility and IVF Center
Jaipur, Rajasthan, India

Sankalp Singh MS DNB MRCOG FRM DRM
Director
Yaami Fertility and IVF Center
Indore, Madhya Pradesh, India

Santosh Kumar Jena MS FNB
(Reproductive Medicine)
Consultant
NOVA IVF Fertility
Kolkata, West Bengal, India

Sathya Balasubramanyam
MD DNB FNB FRCOG
Clinical Director Cloudnine Fertility, Chennai
Kids Clinic India, Athipet
Chennai, Tamil Nadu, India

Satish Kumar Adiga MSc PhD
Professor and Head
Kasturba Medical College
Manipal, Karnataka, India

Satish Patki MD
Medical Director and IVF Consultant
Patki Hospital and Post Graduate Institute
Kolhapur, Maharashtra, India

Selva Karthick M M BTech (Biotechnology)
QC Manager
Oasis Fertility
Hyderabad, India

Shailaja Gada Saxena
MBBS MSc Genetics (UK) PhD
Head
Molecular Medicine Reliance Life
Sciences (RLS)
Dhirubhai Ambani Life Sciences Center
Navi Mumbai, Maharashtra, India

Shayari Jain MS
Research Fellow
Vardhman Trauma and Laparoscopy Center Pvt. Ltd.
Muzaffarnagar, Uttar Pradesh, India

Sherin Theresa Mathew M Medsci ART
Embryologist
Oasis Fertility
Chennai, Tamil Nadu, India

Shraddha Pol MBBS MS (OBGY) DNB OBGY
Fellowship in Reproductive Medicine
Consultant Infertility Specialist, Gynecologist
Milann
Bengaluru, Karnataka, India

Shrey Balani MBBS MD DNB, Fellowship in Reproductive Medicine
Consultant and Founder
Shree Jeevan IVF Center
Jodhpur, Rajasthan, India

Shweta Patki MS
IVF Consultant
Patki Hospital and Post Graduate Institute
Kolhapur, Maharashtra, India

Smitha AP MBBS DNB FFM
Consultant
Cloudnine Hospital
Bengaluru, Karnataka, India

Snehal Dhobale Kohale MS DNB (OBGY)
MRCOG (UK) Fellowship in Reproductive Medicine
Consultant Fertility Specialist and Clinical Director
Ova Fertility and Women Care
Thane, Maharashtra, India

Sona Dharmendra PhD Scholar
Department of Obstetrics and Gynecology
All India Institute of Medical Sciences
New Delhi, India

Sonal Agarwal
MBBS MS DNB FNB (Rep Med) FMAS PGDLME
Senior Infertility Specialist
Creations world IVF Center
Noida, Uttar Pradesh, India

Sonal Panchal MD
Consultant
Dr Nagori's Institute for Infertility and IVF
Ahmedabad, India

Sonia Malik
Programme Director
Southend Fertility and IVF, Delhi
President Indian Fertility Society
Chairperson, FOGSI Infertility Committee

Soumya Mahesh Koregol
MBBS MS (OBG)
Consultant Gynecologist
Shreshtha Women/S Care Clinic
Bangalore, India

Srividhya GK MS Fellowship in Fetal Medicine
Consultant
Department of Fetal Medicine
Milann Hospital
Bengaluru, Karnataka, India

Stacy Colaco PhD
DHR Young Scientist
ICMR-National Institute for Research in Reproductive and Child Health
Mumbai, Maharashtra, India

Stuart Campbell
DSc (Lond) FRCP (Edin) FRCOG
Director
Department of Ultrasound CREATE Fertility
London, United Kingdom

Sudeepa Chaparala MBBS MS (OBG)
Fellowship in Reproductive Medicine
Milann
Krishna, Andhra Pradesh, India

Surbhi Gupta MBBS MS (OBG)
DNB FNB (Reproductive Medicine)
Associate Consultant
Cloudnine Hospital
Gurugram, Haryana, India

Surhud S Patki MS
Endoscopy Surgeon
Patki Hospital and Post Graduate Institute
Kolhapur, Maharashtra, India

Sushma Baxi MBBS MD (OBGYN)
Clinical Head and Fertility Specialist
Oasis Fertility
Vadodara, Gujarat, India

Sushma Madhuprakash DGO FFM
Consultant
Milann—The Fertility Center
Bengaluru, Karnataka, India

Suvarna Rathor Zirpe
MBBS MS (OBGY) DNB FRM
Consultant
Department of Reproductive Medicine
Babysure Fertility Center
Pune, Maharashtra, India

Swati Gautam Allahbadia MD DGO
Consultant Reproductive Endocrinology and IVF
Rotunda—The Center for Human Reproduction
Mumbai, Maharashtra, India

Swati Singh MD DNB FRM DRM
Senior Consultant
Yaami Fertility and IVF Center
Vijay Nagar, Indore, India

Syed Waseem Andrabi PhD
Associate Director—Embryology
Milann Fertility and Birthing Center
New Delhi, India

Tania G Singh MS
Research Fellow
Vardhman Trauma and Laparoscopy Center
Muzaffarnagar, Uttar Pradesh, India

Tarun Dilip Javali MBBS MS MCh
Associate Professor
Department of Urology
Andrology and Renal Transplant
MS Ramaiah Hospital
Bengaluru, Karnataka, India

Taswin Kaur MBBS DGO FRM FMAS
Scientific Director
Maatrikas Fertility Center
Anantapur, Andhra Pradesh, India

Thamara Viloria PhD
Senior Clinical Embryologist
IVIRMA, Medical Laboratory in Valencia
Valencia, Spain

Tity Chacko MD DNB FNB
Reproductive Medicine Consultant
Lakshmi Hospital
Ernakulam, India

Ujjwala Patki MBBS MD
IVF Consultant
Patki Hospital and Research Foundation
Kolhapur, Maharashtra, India

Utpala Sen MD
Consultant in Reproductive Medicine
Bengal Infertility and Reproductive Therapy Hospital
Kolkata, West Bengal, India

Vandana Jain MS
Director
Vardhman Trauma and Laparoscopy Center
Muzaffarnagar, Uttar Pradesh, India

Varsha Patil MBBS DGO DNB (OBG)
Fellowship in Reproductive Medicine
Milann
Bengaluru, Karnataka, India

Varsha Samson Roy
MBBS MD (O&G) MCE (S'pore)
Scientific Director
Advanced Fertility Center
Bengaluru, Karnataka, India

Varun Huilgol MD
Senior Resident
Vardhaman Mahaveer Medical College and Safdarjung Hospital
New Delhi, India

Vasan SS DNB (Surgery) DNB (Urology)
Fellowship in Andrology and Incontinence (Singapore), FICS
Chairman
Manipal Fertility
Bengaluru, Karnataka, India

Veena Gangaraju MSc (Zoology)
Embryologist Milann—The Fertility Center
Bengaluru, Karnataka, India

Veronica Irene Yuel
MD DNB FRM FICOG
ART Consultant/Gynec Laparoscopic Surgeon/
Obstetrician and Gynecologist
NH - MMI Superspeciality Hospital
Raipur, Chhattisgarh, India

Vijay Mangoli PhD
IVF Laboratory Director
Fertility Clinic and IVF Center
Vasant Vihar
Thane, Maharashtra, India

Vinay Kumar MBBS MD (Obs and Gyne) FRM (Fellowship Reproductive Medicine) FMAS DMAS (Fellowship and Diploma Minimal Access Surgery)
Consultant
Obstetrician and Gynecologist J and K Health Services
Jammu and Kashmir, India

Vyshnavi A Rao MBBS MS (OBG) FRM
Senior Consultant Reproductive Medicine
Milann Fertility and Birthing Center
Bengaluru, Karataka, India

Yalavarthi Pavan Ganesh MBBS MS
Senior Resident – Department of Urology
Ramaiah Medical College and Hospital
Bengaluru, Karnataka, India

Yehia Shawki
RCOG Member, AAGL Elected Member
Director, Endoplanet
Center of Excellence for Uterine Surgery
Cairo, Egypt

Yuvraj D Jadeja MBBS MD (Obs) Fellowship in Reproductive Endocrinology
Medical Director
Nimaaya Center for Womens Health
Self-Employed
Nimaaya Center for Womens Health
Vadodara, Gujarat, India

Zakiya Ahmed MBBS MD
Fellowship in Reproductive Medicine
Milann, JP Nagar
Prestige Falcon City
Konanakunte Cross
Bengaluru, Karnataka, India

Foreword

Infertility today is an international health problem. It concerns all social classes and races. Advances in assisted reproductive technologies over the years, have provided greater possibilities for successful infertility treatment. Generally, however, over the past forty years or so, emphasis has been mainly on how to "improve" results of infertility treatment, not on how to strike a balance between success, risks and costs. The time has now come to shift focus and trade off the efficacy of treatment against its quality and safety. The essence of infertility treatment in general is to provide infertile couples with a single healthy baby, with a minimum of complications at a reasonable cost. The end of treatment does not come with a positive pregnancy test, but with a liveborn healthy child who has a potential to grow up as a healthy adult. It is the duty of the infertility specialist to guide patients not only through the procedure, but also about the risks associated with it.

Over 44 years since the birth of the first IVF baby, reproductive medicine has expanded much. A noble attempt to keep ourselves updated about the advances in this specialty and passing on the light to those who seek knowledge is the need of the hour. Dr Kamini Rao and her team have managed to put out a very comprehensive book which can be considered one of the greatest works in reproductive medicine of all times. The beauty of this book is that it covers all the aspects of infertility starting from basics to the most recent advances in this field. It is a unique compilation where each topic is written by experts who have relevant experience in that field. Hence in each chapter the reader will not only get a bird's eye view on the topic, but also opportunities for a deep dive into the same. Approaching the most relevant topics in a very practical manner is a highlight of this book.

The previous 2 editions of "the principles and practice of assisted reproductive technology" speak for themselves. They are widely read and cherished. The third edition has not only managed to keep up with the high standards of the previous editions, but also brings a fresh perspective to many socially relevant topics like addressing the fertility issues with gender transformation, fertility options in the LGBTQ community and the like. The book stays at the top of the game by having new chapters on every new advance in reproductive medicine like rejuvenation therapy. It is indeed very thoughtful of the team to include a chapter on the COVID-19 pandemic as well. At the time of the release of this book there are major shifts happening in the field of assisted reproduction in India through new rules and regulations. It is quite commendable that they have managed to put together the latest information on these regulations.

This gigantic work should be a must read and a companion to any professional who is associated with fertility medicine including gynecologists, reproductive medicine specialists, embryologists and medical students. It will remain treasured by students of reproductive medicine for years to come. Such a gigantic, yet comprehensive treasury is a valuable asset to the entire fraternity of reproductive medicine specialists and each one of us will proudly own, nourish and cherish this noble work.

Geeta Nargund
Founder and Medical Director
CREATE Fertility and abc IVF, UK
Senior Consultant Gynecologist and Lead Consultant
Reproductive Medicine Services
St George's Hospital
London, United Kingdom

Preface to the Third Edition

"If hope is what keeps us alive, I owe my life to all those wonderful humans who kept their hopes alive!"

Reproduction is the basic instinct of all living forms and not being able to have a progeny is perceived as an irreplaceable loss. Human reproduction is on the decline. 10 to 15 percent of the population across the globe finds it difficult to conceive. Reproductive medicine is a field which is evolving at a rapid pace. It has been 44 years since the first IVF baby was born. Over these years we have seen tremendous advances in fertility treatments and lab techniques. We started with purified gonadotropin preparations, basic IVF and manual monitoring in labs. We upgraded ourselves to recombinant drugs, ICSI and automated systems, hence achieving excellent quality control in labs and reasonably good pregnancy and live birth rates. Newer protocols targeting personalized controlled ovarian hyperstimulation, more physiological and patient friendly medications targeting different patient groups, improving sperm selection by using magnification, magnetic field or physiology, putting the quality monitoring on a cloud, using artificial intelligence, genetic testing of embryos for aneuploidies or known genetic disorders, personalizing embryo transfers using the power of gene expression testing and doing the most atraumatic embryo transfers using ultrasound guidance have been some of the advances that we accustomed ourselves to in our urge to strive toward excellence. Even in this 21st century implantation is something which still keeps us baffled. We still droop our heads when it comes to dropping oocyte numbers and quality. We are at a stage where we are still trying to battle it out with the new weapons in our armory—endometrial and ovarian rejuvenation. Stem cell therapy is the new kid in the block whom we all look upon with hopes. This book is coming out at a time when 3rd party reproduction is coming under unreasonable scrutiny in the light of new laws.

Assisted reproduction has evolved significantly since the last edition of this textbook came out. Old information had to go away paving the way for newer advances. We saw the need for bringing out a new edition of this book where we had to not only update existing chapters with all the recent advances, but also remove old and outdated parts of the same. We had to keep up with the astonishing pace at which science is growing. So, we had to add a whole lot of new chapters. New chapters on endometrial and ovarian rejuvenation are examples. Medicolegal aspects of fertility and the new ART laws had to be addressed through new chapters. Nowadays we see many women coming to us at an advanced age attempting a pregnancy. Addressing ART in women with chronic medical disorders was the need of the hour. Similarly an honest attempt was made to discuss male infertility also in detail. The new chapters on varicocele and fertility issues in males with spinal cord injuries were refreshing additions in this regard. No book will be complete in this century if we did not discuss COVID and its effects on fertility. Last but not the least we understood the welcoming changes in the society towards sexuality, thus including new chapters on gender transformations and fertility options in the LGBTQ community.

This book is meant to be a companion for all professionals involved in ART: Clinicians, aspiring students, Embryologists and paramedical personnel working in an Infertility unit. It will serve as a ready reckoner covering all the important topics in reproductive medicine. It allows the readers a deep dive into the subject with an opportunity to go down many rabbit holes as well if they choose to do so.

I am grateful that students and clinicians have nurtured the previous 2 editions of this book. Participating with colleagues to collate this 3rd Edition of the Principles & Practice of ART has been a thoroughly enjoyable experience, but could not have been completed to a high standard without the dedication and precious time and skills of my coeditors. I am deeply honored to be their colleague and thankful for all the efforts they have put in.

Kamini A Rao

Preface to the First Edition

Infertility is a fast-emerging global disease. The speed, at which the incidence of infertility is rising, has been matched equally by the growth of our understanding of the disease and the pace of emerging new technologies. Thirty-five years after the birth of Louise Brown, the first child to be conceived by assisted reproductive technology (ART), the treatment options are mind-boggling. The use of medical interventions for fertility preservation has reached new heights. We are now able to cryopreserve embryos, spermatozoa and oocytes as well as ovarian tissue. The breakthrough technology of vitrification has ensured that egg banking is appropriate for women who wish to defer family building into later years when ovarian function may decline, or for women facing treatment such as cancer therapy that may diminish ovarian function or lead to menopause. With increasingly complex modalities, available for treatment, come the need for a clear, concise and practical textbook, which can serve as a ready-reckoner for healthcare providers.

The book has been divided into three volumes to adequately cover the enormity of the diverse field of reproductive medicine. The objective of the book is to present important and cutting-edge topics relevant to fertility and make it accessible to all ART specialists and gynecologists involved in treating infertile couples. All the chapters have been written by acknowledged pioneers and experts in their own respective areas with special emphasis on evidence-based medicine. Notwithstanding the limitations of our published literature, we have endeavored to provide a balanced view of existing information that is clinically relevant for the evolving areas of our specialty. The text is directed at a broad reader base and will be of immense value to clinicians, embryologists, andrologists, and ultrasonographers from all spheres, be they laboratory technicians, postgraduates, postdoctoral fellow students, private practitioners or researchers.

Volume 1: Infertility

This well-illustrated volume provides concise yet comprehensive practical information on the modern-day approach to the diagnosis and treatment of infertility. It starts from basic principles of reproductive physiology, before moving on to the evaluation and management of the infertile couple and then describes and explains the full armory of ART from ovulation induction and its complications to the outcome following ART. We have also introduced a section highlighting the dilemmas frequently encountered in the field of reproductive medicine in which contrasting points of view are presented. Some recent advances, such as cryopreservation of ovarian tissue and oocytes, have generated great excitement, because of the prospect of fertility preservation prior to cancer therapy which has been covered in-depth. Future clinical applications, such as endometrial stem cells and reproduction, are also dealt with in a separate section.

Volume 2: IVF and Laboratory Aspects of Andrology

The set-up of an in vitro fertilization (IVF) laboratory and the equipment that is used during the IVF process must provide an optimum environment for embryos while they are growing in the laboratory. The personnel should be adequately trained in reproductive research techniques as well as have the necessary technical and administrative skills to manage these laboratories. The text of this volume deals with the laboratory aspects of ART with an emphasis on practical information through which one can readily translate theory into clinical practice. It covers the whole of andrology and embryology dealing with it in four separate sections. The section on andrology deals with all aspects starting from semen examination and interpretation of reports to its cryopreservation. The techniques of intracytoplasmic sperm injection (ICSI), assisted hatching and polar body biopsy have been dealt with a special focus on practicalities. Recent newer techniques, such as intracytoplasmic morphologically selected sperm injection (IMSI), polarization microscopy and omics, have also been well covered. Laboratory management deserves utmost importance with all aspects of quality control and quality management playing a vital role in the success rates of an ART clinic. Practitioners wishing for a greater understanding of the intricacies of how a sperm meets an egg will find this volume especially useful in their clinical practice.

Volume 3: Atlas of Human Embryology

To complement the two volumes, we have designed a high-quality comprehensive Atlas of Human Embryology which offers an exciting, pictorial glimpse into oocytes and embryos at various stages of development. The text here is limited to a brief description of the images. Owing to sophisticated computer technology that is currently on hand, we have made great efforts to capture all the photographs on digital films and digital videotapes. This volume serves as a handbook and ready-reckoner for all embryologists who, when in doubt, can get a sneak peek of the images when working in the laboratory.

Throughout the book, the aim has been to explain issues clearly, simply and directly in such a way that it will be understood by gynecologists, infertility specialists as well as scientists and laboratory personnel. The end aim of the book is to help in optimizing results and generate ART treatment of high quality and we are confident that it works towards this end and that all our readers will appreciate the book's distinctiveness and merit.

Kamini A Rao
Howard Carp
Robert Fischer

Acknowledgments

We would like to express our gratitude to all the expert contributors, for their valuable time, humongous efforts and dedication to passing on the light to the seekers of knowledge.

A book of this magnitude and quality could never have been achieved without the singular efforts of the entire Milann team and the publication team of Shri Jitendar P Vij (Group Chairman) and Mr Ankit Vij (Managing Director) of M/s Jaypee Brothers Medical Publishers (P) Ltd, New Delhi, India, whose untiring work ensured that the book was released on time. A special mention of gratitude to Kritika Dua (Senior Development Editor) at Jaypee brothers for working with us tirelessly.

We will always remain indebted to Dr Shantala Kumari R for being there with us day and night through the mayhem of our final proof readings. Without your support, it would not have been possible to release this book on time.

We are deeply indebted to Kala Diwakar for the extra time and effort that she put into coordinating and corresponding with authors, constantly following up with them and the publishers was a mammoth of a task which she has gracefully managed to complete on time.

We are grateful to our families for being supportive through this tough journey. This success is fueled by your love and faith in us.

Contents

VOLUME 1: INFERTILITY

SECTION 1: ANATOMY AND PHYSIOLOGY

SECTION 2: REPRODUCTIVE ENDOCRINOLOGY

SECTION 6: INTRAUTERINE INSEMINATION

SECTION 10: THIRD PARTY REPRODUCTION

SECTION 11: OUTCOME FOLLOWING ASSISTED REPRODUCTIVE TECHNIQUE

VOLUME 2: LABORATORY ASPECTS OF IVF AND ANDROLOGY

SECTION 14: ANDROLOGY

SECTION

1 Anatomy and Physiology

CHAPTER 1

Anatomy of the Reproductive System

Sonal Agarwal, Mir Jaffar

INTRODUCTION

The reproductive system or genital system is a system of organs working together for the purpose of reproduction. The two important functions of the female reproductive system are to produce female gamete and to nourish the developing offspring until birth. The male reproductive system has the primary function of generation of male gamete (sperm) and deposition of the same inside the female reproductive tract for the fertilization of female gamete (ovum).

FEMALE REPRODUCTIVE SYSTEM

The female internal genital organs include:

- Ovaries
- Uterine tubes
- Uterus
- Vagina.

Embryology

Origin

From the outer part of the intermediate mesoderm **(Fig. 1)**.

Development of Internal Reproductive Organs in Females

Paramesonephric ducts persist in females.[1] The internal portion of the genital cord undergoes fusion and forms uterus and vagina. This begins early in the third month of fetal life.

Medial walls fuse forming septum, which undergoes resorption from below upward. Fallopian tubes are formed from parts outside the cord. At about the fifth month, the uterocervical junction is marked by a ring-like constriction and at the sixth month, thickening of uterine walls begins. Future vaginal fornix is formed from ring-like outgrowth at

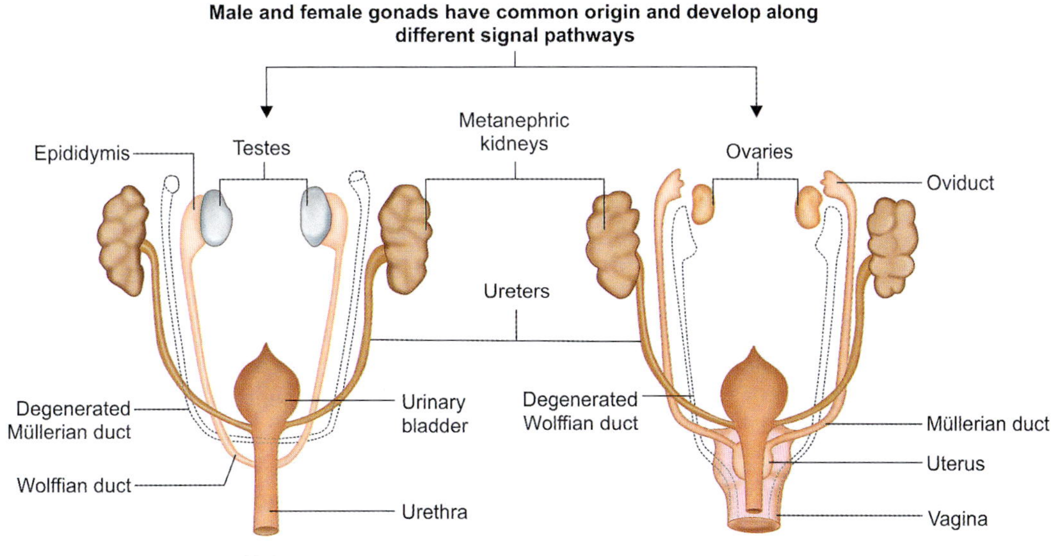

Fig. 1: Embryological development of gonads.

the lower end of the uterus. Simultaneously, the lumen of the vagina is formed by the breakage of central epithelial cells. The hymen is formed from the remnant of sinus tubercle.

Atrophy in Female

In the female, atrophy of paramesonephric bodies and ducts occurs. Epoophoron and paroophoron represent nonfunctional remains of the mesonephric ducts along with rudimentary blind tubules, situated in the mesosalpinx.

Remnants

The lower part of the mesonephric duct disappears, while the upper part persists as epoophoron, also called Gartner's duct. Suspensory ligaments of the ovary are remnants of the mesonephric duct too.

Gonads

Gonads start development initially from the mesothelial layer of peritoneum.

The ovary is covered by the surface layer named germinal epithelium. Immature ova originate from the cells of the dorsal endoderm of yolk sac. In ridge, they are called oogonia. A layer of connective tissue cells, called pregranulosa cells, surround oogonia. The embryological origin of granulosa cells is controversial. As in males, females also have gubernaculum, which pulls the ovary downward but is not as developed as in males. Later, this divides into ovarian and round ligament of uterus **(Fig. 2)**.

Skene's glands in female urethra are homologous to prostatic glands in males. Epithelial lining of the urogenital sinus has diverticula, which correspond to Bartholin's glands.

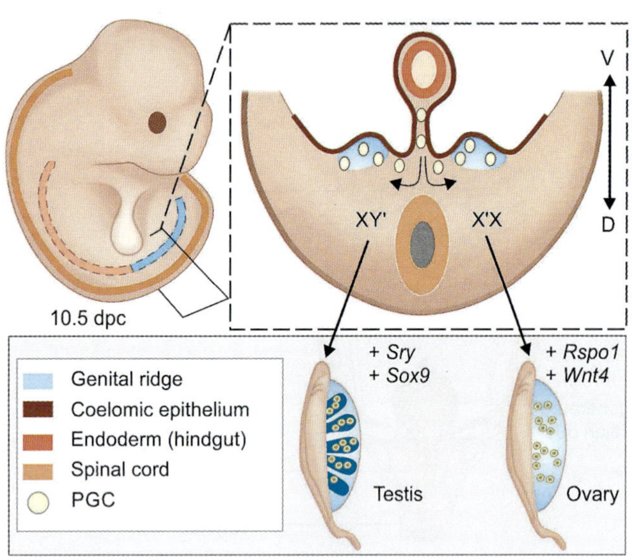

Fig. 2: Development of gonads through gonadal ridge. (PGC: primordial germ cells)

Development of External Genitalia

Until about the ninth week of gestation, the external genitalia of both sexes look the same because they follow a common path of development. The genital tubercle develops with a dorsal membrane, which covers urogenital opening. There is a development of labioscrotal fold, which forms the labioscrotal swelling. The urogenital fold evolves into labia minora and the labioscrotal swelling forms the labia majora.

Initially, the cloacal membrane comprises endoderm and ectoderm, which separates cloaca from the exterior. The separation of the rectum from the dorsal part of the cloaca occurs and the ventral part of the cloacal membrane contributes to the urogenital membrane. The primordial phallus is formed from the tubercle, which is the first rudiment of clitoris.

The corpus cavernosum of clitoris arises from the mesodermal tissue in phallus with cavernous vascular tissue in it. The prepuce is formed as ectodermal growth into the superficial part of the phallus; a horseshoe shape is seen on the coronal section. The ectodermal plate is divided centrally into two lamellae. This results in a cutaneous folding named as prepuce. It forms a hood over the glans. The sides of it grow dorsal and forward as the labioscrotal folds form labia majora. Labia minora arise from the lips of groove on the undersurface of phallus and the remaining part of the phallus forms clitoral glans.

Anatomy

Ovaries

The almond-shaped ovaries are the female gonads in which the germ cells develop. Endocrine function is also carried by female gonads. The support of the ovary is mesovarium, which is a short peritoneal fold. In prepubertal females, the ovary has a capsule called tunica albuginea and the surface is covered with a single cuboidal layer of germinal epithelium. The surface of the ovary is dull, has a grayish appearance, and is continuous with shiny peritoneal mesovarium. At puberty, repeated follicle rupture and ovulation start, which lead to distortion and scarring of the ovarian surface. Scarring is less in women on oral contraceptive pills. Lymphatics, vascular branches, and nerves pass through the suspensory ligament and cross pelvic brim and continue into mesovarium of the broad ligament. Due to lack of peritoneum, the oocyte is expelled into the peritoneal cavity at ovulation. Fimbriae of the infundibulum part of the fallopian tube trap the oocyte and peristaltic movement of the tube carries it to ampulla for fertilization.

During embryonic development, the germ cells are differentiated into oogonia, which divide mitotically and enter the first phase of meiotic division and get arrested at the diplotene stage of prophase-one stage without completing it. During fetal life, the primary oocytes are surrounded by a spindle-shaped single layer of squamous cells—primordial follicle. Before puberty, the cortex contains only primordial follicle. Beginning at puberty under the influence of pituitary hormones [follicle-stimulating hormone (FSH)], the primordial follicles grow and enlarge to become primary, secondary, and the large mature follicles which can occupy the part of medulla also. Postpubertal ovary has follicles in different stages of development. In addition to the follicles, the ovary may contain a large corpus luteum of an ovulated follicle or corpus albicans of a degenerated corpus luteum. At birth, the cortex contains about 1–2 million primordial follicles. Most of the follicles degenerate before puberty by the process of apoptosis (programmed cell death). About 40,000 follicles persist at puberty and exhibit periodic changes during the rest of the reproductive life. Out of these, about 5–10 follicles undergo a process of maturation in each menstrual cycle. Mostly one follicle from any one of the two ovaries fully matures, ruptures, and discharges a secondary oocyte in the peritoneal cavity and is subsequently picked up by the respective fimbriae. Thus on an average, about 400 follicles attain such maturity during the reproductive life of a woman.

Ovary is mainly supplied by the ovarian artery branch of abdominal aorta and partly by uterine artery branches. Veins from the pampiniform plexus join to form one vein in the suspensory ligament of the ovary. The right ovarian vein ascends at an acute angle to drain into inferior vena cava and the left ovarian vein drains almost at the right angle into the left renal vein.[2]

Uterine Tubes

The uterine tubes (formerly called oviducts or fallopian tubes) are the channel through which the oocyte is carried from the periovarian peritoneal cavity to the uterine cavity. The uterine tubes lie in the mesosalpinx, forming the free anterosuperior edges of the broad ligaments. Tubes are in posterolateral location of lateral pelvic walls and arch anterosuperiorly to ovaries. In "immotile cilia syndrome", the transport of ova takes place only by peristalsis if at all carried by the tube to the uterine cavity. When an ovary does ovulate and release the oocyte, it is swept into the lumen of the uterine tube by the fimbriae which is further facilitated by the longitudinal grooves on the inner aspect of these fimbria, suction created by the ciliary beats of the tube and also by the peristalsis of the tubal musculature. During ovulation, the uterine tubes literally come close to the ovary to pick up the oocyte which may be hormoneregulated. Each tube presents two openings: (1) Uterine ostium which is 1 mm in diameter and opens into the superolateral angle of the uterus and (2) the other, pelvic (abdominal) ostium which is 3 mm in diameter and opens at the bottom of infundibulum near the corresponding ovary. The uterine tubes have four parts from lateral to medial end:

1. *Infundibulum:* The funnel-shaped distal end of the tube, closest to the ovary and about 1 cm long, opens into the peritoneal cavity through the abdominal ostium, the circumference of which is provided with the fimbria. One of the fimbriae is longer (ovarian fimbria) than the rest.
2. *Ampulla:* The widest and longest part (5 cm) is thin-walled, dilated, and tortuous. Fertilization of the ova usually takes place in the ampulla.
3. *Isthmus:* It is rounded and cord like because the walls are thicker than the lumen and resembles the spermatic cord in men. It joins the uterine tube to the uterus. The length of the isthmus measures about 3 cm. The exceedingly narrow lumen suggests the existence of an anatomical sphincter, which prevents the entrance of exogenous microorganisms from vagina to the peritoneal cavity.
4. *Uterine (interstitial/intramural/parts of uterine tube):* It is about 1 cm long, and traverses the thick musculature of the uterus at the junction of the fundus and the uterus to open into the uterine cavity via the uterine ostium **(Fig. 3)**.

Innervation of ovaries and uterine Tubes: Innervation is via both ovarian and uterine plexus. Afferent pain fibers along with descending sympathetic fibers of lumbar splanchnic nerves and ovarian plexus merge into cell bodies in T11–L1 sensory spinal ganglia. Inferior hypogastric plexuses and pelvic splanchnic nerves merge into cell bodies in the S2–S4 sensory ganglia.

Uterus

The uterus (womb) is pear shaped, has thick walls, and is a hollow muscular organ. The nongravid uterus is located in the lesser pelvis with cervix between the urinary bladder and the rectum. The normal position of the uterus is that of anteversion and anteflexion. The average size of a nongravid uterus is 7.5 × 5 × 2 cm and weight is about 90 g. Its dimensions change rapidly dramatically during pregnancy. At birth, the uterus is relatively large and has a body:cervix ratio of 2:1 because of maternal hormone influence in intrauterine life. Several weeks after birth, childhood dimensions and proportions are obtained. The body:cervix ratio becomes 1:1.

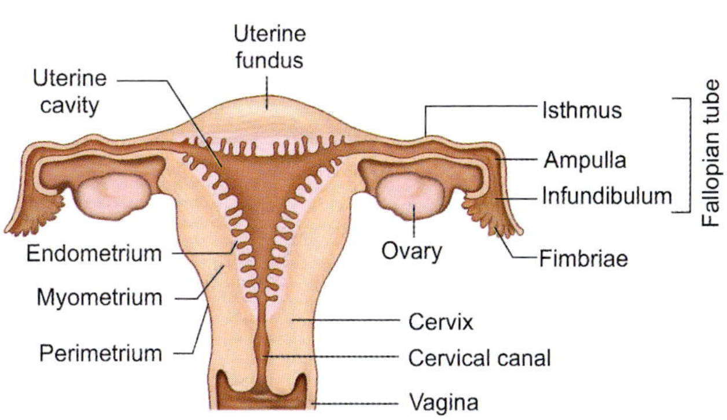

Fig. 3: Female reproductive system.

Because of the small size of the pelvic cavity, it remains in the abdomen and descends down afterward and becomes pelvic organ. Typical angulation between the uterus and vagina is not established. During puberty, the uterus (especially the body) grows rapidly in size thereby again assuming adult proportions because of hormonal exposure.

Axes of Uterus

Normally, the adult uterus is anteverted and anteflexed.

Anteversion: The angle between the cervices relative to the axis of the vagina measures about 90°, provided that the bladder and the rectum are empty. The anteversion is maintained by the forward pull on the uterine fundus by the traction of the round ligaments of the uterus, backward pull on the cervix by the traction of the uterosacral ligaments, and the intrinsic growth of the uterine musculature. Maintenance of the anteversion angle is an important prerequisite to prevent the prolapse of the uterus **(Figs. 4A and B)**.

Anteflexion: It is the forward angle between the body and cervix at the isthmus, creating the angle of flexion measuring about 125° so that the main bulk of the uterus rests on the bladder for better support. On an empty bladder, the uterus is in transverse plane.

Flexion of the uterus takes place at the transverse plane of the internal orifice (os). Normally, the uterus rotates forward around this axis known as anteflexion. When it rotates backward (reverse direction), it is referred to as retroflexion. It is usually found in the cases of disrupted perineal body or weak pelvic floor muscles and ligaments.

Usually, the uterus lies in the median plane and is twisted to the right or left side. Sometimes, the fundus is tilted more to the right pelvic wall known as dextrorotation of the fundus. In such situations, the right uterine tube comes in more close contact with the lateral pelvic wall and may be related to the pelvic type of the vermiform appendix.

Consequently, the cervix is tilted more to the left side known as levorotation of the cervix.

The uterus is divided into body and cervix. The body lies between the layers of the broad ligament and is freely movable. It has two vesical and intestinal surfaces. The body is demarcated from the cervix by the isthmus of the uterus, a constricted segment, 1 cm long. The cervix of the uterus is 2.5 cm in length and cylindrical in the adult nonpregnant woman. The part between the isthmus and the vagina is called supravaginal part and the vaginal part protrudes in the superior most part of the anterior vaginal wall. The rounded vaginal part surrounds the external os of the uterus and is surrounded in turn by a narrow recess, the vaginal fornix. The supravaginal part is separated from the bladder anteriorly by loose connective tissue and from the rectum posteriorly by the rectouterine pouch. The slit-like uterine cavity is 6 cm in length from the external os to the wall of fundus. The uterine cavity continues inferiorly as the cervical canal. The uterine body has three coats: (1) Perimetrium which is the outer serous coat of the peritoneum with a thin layer of connective tissue; (2) myometrium which is the middle coat of smooth muscle with the main branches of vascular and nerve supply traversing through it; and (3) endometrium, which is the innermost coat with firm adherence to myometrium. Endometrium attains different histopathology during all the phases of the menstrual cycle. The endometrium or mucous membrane of the body of the uterus consists of surface epithelium and lamina propria of variable thickness depending on the stage of menstrual cycle. Before puberty, the surface is lined by the ciliated columnar cells; during the reproductive period, it is lined by the simple columnar epithelium because cilia cannot grow due to repeated destruction of the superficial part of the endometrium. Functionally, the endometrium consists of an outer basal layer and an inner functional layer. In a nonpregnant female, the inner functional layer with the uterine glands and blood vessels is sloughed off or shed during menstruation, leaving

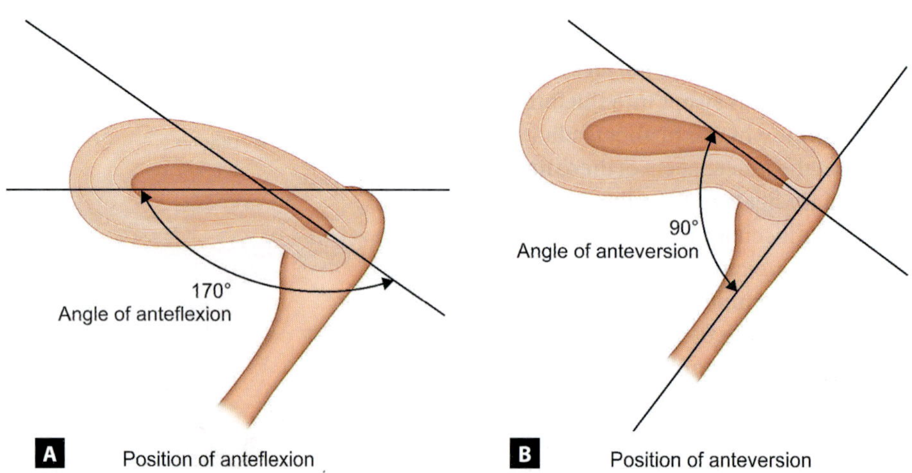

Figs. 4A and B: Uterine axis.

intact the deeper basalis layer with the basal remnants of the uterine glands—the source of cells for regeneration of new functional layer. The basal layer is supplied by the straight basal arteries, whereas the functional layer is supplied by the spiral arteries which are highly sensitive to the hormonal changes in the blood and undergo vasoconstriction before menstruation with eventual casting of the endometrium due to ischemic necrosis followed by the hemorrhage.

Menstruation occurs only in primates and in mankind who possess the spiral arteries of the endometrium. Fundus and body are developed by the fusion of the intermediate parts of the two paramesonephric (Müllerian) ducts. While the cervix is developed from the upper part of the uterovaginal canal, which in turn is formed by the fusion of the lower vertical parts of the two paramesonephric ducts, the lower part of the uterovaginal canal forms the major portion of the vagina.

The principal supports of the uterus are both passive and active. Pelvic diaphragm acts as an active support. Change in tone is due to changes in intra-abdominal pressure conditions transmitted through the surrounding pelvic organs and the endopelvic fascia in which they are embedded. Passive support of the uterus is provided by its position. When intra-abdominal pressure is increased, the uterus is pressed against the bladder. The cervix has the least mobility due to condensed endopelvic fascia attached to it.

Arterial and Venous Supply of Uterus

The uterus is supplied by the uterine arteries mainly and collateral supply is through the ovarian arteries. Uterine plexus veins drain in internal iliac veins. Lymphatics from the fundus drain along the ovarian vessels to lumbar (caval/aortic) lymph nodes. The isthmic part of tubes and round ligament attachments drain into superficial inguinal lymph nodes.

Vagina

The vagina is a musculomembranous tube (7–9 cm long), extending from the cervix to the vaginal orifice. All vestibular glands have their opening in the vaginal vestibule. The vagina plays the role of a canal for menstrual bleeding, receives the penis and ejaculate during sexual intercourse, and communicates superiorly with cervix and inferiorly with vestibule of the vagina. The vagina does not have any glands in its wall. Mucous produced by cells in the cervical glands lubricate the vaginal lumen. In a nulliparous adult, the vagina is H-shaped in section with transverse folds called vaginal rugae which render the vagina highly distensible. Before puberty, rugae are absent. In the elderly, the vagina becomes less elastic and appears pale and smooth due to loss of rugae. Vagina is closely related to many pelvic floor muscles which provide support and act as potential sphincters for the vagina. All these muscles rhythmically contract during the orgasm.[3]

The vaginal epithelium exhibits minimal changes during the menstrual cycle. During the proliferative (follicular) phase of the menstrual cycle, under the influence of high estrogen secretion, the vaginal epithelium increases in thickness and stimulates the vaginal cells to synthesize and accumulate an increased amount of glycogen as these cells migrate toward the vaginal lumen into which they are shed off. The fermentative action of Doderlein's bacillus on glycogen-rich desquamated cellular debris (glycogen is converted to lactic acid) renders the vaginal fluid acidic which inhibits the growth of microorganisms or pathogenic invasion. Hence, the vaginal infections are more common after menopause as the glycogen content becomes lesser. Arterial supply is from tributaries of uterine artery and internal pudendal artery. The uterovaginal venous plexus drains into the internal iliac veins through the uterine vein. Lymphatic vessels from the superior part of the vagina drain to internal and external iliac lymph nodes, middle part to internal iliac nodes, and inferior part to sacral and common iliac nodes. External os drains into the superficial lymph nodes.

Innervation of the Uterus and the Vagina

Somatic supply is present in the inferior, one fifth to a quarter of the vagina in the form of deep perineal nerve. Sensations of touch and temperature are present. The upper portion of the vagina and uterus has visceral innervation by hypogastric and thoracolumbar spinal ganglia.

Applied Anatomy

- During childbirth, myometrial contractions are mediated hormonally at decreasing length intervals so as to dilate the lower segment of the uterus. During menses, myometrial contractions are responsible for cramping pain.
- Infections of the female genital tract can lead to peritoneal infections due to direct communication and vice versa. A major cause of tubal factor infertility is salpingitis.
- Patency of tubes can be checked by hysterocontrast salpingography (HyCoSy), ultrasound, and endoscopy.
- Ligation of uterine tubes is a surgical method of birth control. It can be done by either abdominal or laparoscopic route.
- Ectopic tubal pregnancy is the most common ectopic gestation occurring in approximately 1 in every 250 pregnancies. Late diagnosis can result in rupture of ectopic gestation which can lead to severe hemorrhage into the abdominopelvic cavity. It should be differentially diagnosed from appendix pathology and acute abdomen.
- Congenital anomalies such as unicornuate uterus, bicornuate uterus, doubled uterine cavities, and uterus didelphys are seen.
- Persistence of remnants of mesonephric ducts in the form of epoophoron can enlarge and result in cyst formation and torsion.

- Female brain has hermunculus in the clitoral cortex which on stimulation is associated with intercourse frequency. Research is being focused on this region in women with vaginismus and decreased libido.
- Increased intra-abdominal pressure can result in increased flexion and version. Damaged ligaments and weak supports of the uterus can cause uterovaginal prolapse and retroversion.
- *Infection of greater vestibular glands:* Palpable when infected. Occlusion can predispose to bartholinitis and cyst formation. It can lead to vulvar adenocarcinomas.
- Emphasis on prepartum classes (Kegel exercises) should be present to reduce the muscular obstruction to passage for fetus and decrease the chances of perineal muscle damage.
- Levator ani muscles are closely related to the vagina on its lateral side, and any pathology to these muscles is significantly responsible for either the painful intercourse or orgasm. From our clinical experience, we have noticed many patients, especially those suffering from coccydynia (tailbone pain) in which the levator ani muscle is mostly tender on rectal examination and surprisingly the same mechanism is seen in the males as well.
- Recent 3D organoid technology is developed for the study of female reproductive tract that mimics ovaries, fallopian tubes, endometrium, and cervix, as well as placental trophoblast. These 3D models help in further studies about the biology and physiology of the female genital system.[4]

Histology

The ovary has cuboidal germinal epithelium continuous with peritoneal mesothelium. Beneath it is a fibrous tunica albuginea capsule. Oviduct has mucosa, muscularis layer, and serosa with connective tissue.[5]

The uterus has mucosa, endometrium, myometrium, and peritoneal layer serosa. Endometrium consists of simple columnar epithelium (ciliated cells and secretory cells) and an underlying thick connective tissue stroma. Vagina has mucosa, muscularis, and adventitia.

MALE REPRODUCTIVE SYSTEM

Introduction

The male reproductive axis of hormones and organs is a well-efficient biological system. It is responsible for reproductive tract formation and development, pubertal maturation, and maintenance of fertility. Understanding the basis of male infertility is becoming a growing trend among infertility specialists because of the progressive decrease in semen parameters over recent years. To understand the basic pathophysiology and the cause of male infertility, it is imperative to have knowledge about the anatomy, physiology, development, and hormonal control of the male genital and duct system for the effective evaluation and treatment of male infertility.

Embryology

As urinary and genital systems are located closely and overlap each other, development of them is described as the development of urinary and reproductive systems together. Intermediate mesoderm forms the reproductive organs embryonically. These embryonic structures are the mesonephric ducts (Wolffian ducts) in males and the paramesonephric ducts (Müllerian ducts) in females.

Origin

Under the ectoderm in the outer intermediate mesoderm, there is C5–T3 vertebral segment, which is a series of short evaginations extending caudally from dorsal growth and fuses successively from before backward to form pronephric duct. It grows caudally to open into the ventral part of cloaca to form a mesonephric duct, which remains after the atrophy of pronephros duct.

Development of Internal Reproductive Organs in Male

In males, duct persists to form tube of epididymis, vas deferens, and ejaculatory duct. Seminal vesicles arise during the third month of fetal life from hinder part. A large part of the head of mesonephros atrophies leaving anterior efferent ducts of testicle and posterior ductuli aberrantes and paradidymis.

Paramesonephric Ducts

After the formation of mesonephric ducts, paramesonephric ducts develop. Each arises on the lateral aspect of the corresponding mesonephric duct as tubular invagination of cells lining the abdominal cavity. Ducts pass backward lateral to the mesonephric ducts, but toward the posterior end of the embryo they cross medially and lie side to side leading to the formation of the common genital cord. The mesonephric ducts end in an epithelial elevation and the sinus tubercle on the ventral part of the cloaca between the orifices of the mesonephric ducts. Sinus tubercle connects paramesonephric ducts with cloaca.

Atrophy in Males

Paramesonephric ducts atrophy and only traces of anterior ends form the appendix of testis of male, while terminal fused portions form the prostatic utricle in the floor of the prostatic urethra. This is due to production of anti-Müllerian hormone (AMH) by Sertoli cells of testes.

Gonads

Gonads initially develop from the mesothelial layer of peritoneum. Testis periphery is converted into tunica albuginea. The cords of the central mass form a network to become rete testis and seminiferous tubules. Via the rete testis, the seminiferous tubules become connected with efferent ducts of the testis. Descent of testes occurs followed by the development of gubernaculum.[6] Failure in this process leads to indirect hernia or infantile hydrocele.

The rectum gets separated from the dorsal part of cloaca and the ventral part becomes primary urogenital sinus. Sinus divides into superficial definitive urogenital sinus and deeper anterior vesicourethral portion. Vesicourethral portion is the deepest portion continuous with allantois. It absorbs ends of mesonephric ducts and associated ends of renal diverticula and gives rise to trigone of urinary bladder and prostatic urethra part. Remainder forms the body of the bladder and part of the prostatic urethra; its apex is prolonged to umbilicus as a narrow canal called urachus, which is obliterated in later life to form the median umbilical ligament in adults.

Prostate

A series of diverticular buds arise from the epithelial lining of the urogenital sinus and vesicourethral part of the cloaca, between the third and fourth months. These buds become tubular and form glandular substance of two lobes which fuse behind urethra and extend onto ventral aspect. The median lobe of prostate is formed as an extension of the lateral lobes between the common ejaculatory ducts and bladder.

Bulbourethral glands also arise as diverticula from the epithelial lining of urogenital sinus.

Development of External Genitalia

The urogenital fold evolves into shaft of the penis and labioscrotal swelling evolves into the scrotum. Genital tubercle develops into primordial phallus, the first rudiment of penis. Corpus cavernosum penis and corpus spongiosum penis arise from phallus with the development of cavernous spaces in it later on. The prepuce is formed by the growth of a solid plate of ectoderm, which is horseshoe shaped on the coronal section. A cutaneous fold of prepuce forms a hood over the glans. The pelvic portion of the cloaca undergoes more development, pushing phallic portion. The labioscrotal folds extend around to form scrotal area. During descent, along with testis, the scrotal area is drawn out to form scrotal sacs. The penis is developed from the phallus. The urogenital membrane undergoes absorption, forming a channel on the undersurface of the phallus; this channel extends only as far forward as the corona glandis. The longer urethra is formed by the greater growth of the pelvic portion of cloaca. Later, this opening, which is located on the dorsal side of the penis closes from behind forward. The urethral plate of the glans breaks and forms a median groove continuous with the primitive ostium. Groove closes leaving a small pipelike opening in between. Thus, the urogenital opening is shifted forward to the end of glans.[7]

Anatomy

During embryonic development, the male genital tract is a straight duct system with the developing testes high up inside the abdomen and the ejaculatory organ (penis) outside the body. Since testes need 1–2°C temperature lower than the normal body temperature to function normally, they descend down in the scrotum normally during birth outside the body forming a loop of duct system. Vasa deferentia run parallel to the urethra but in the opposite direction. The initial secretory part of the duct begins outside the body (scrotum), the middle part intra-abdominal, and the terminal ejaculatory part ends outside. The male internal genital organs include the testes, epididymides, ductus deferens, seminal glands, ejaculatory ducts, prostate, and bulbourethral glands.[8]

Testis is suspended in the scrotum by the spermatic cord which starts at deep inguinal ring lateral to inferior epigastric vessels, passes in inguinal canal, and comes out of superficial inguinal ring, ending at scrotum. The coverings of the spermatic cord include the following: Internal spermatic fascia, cremasteric fascia and muscle, and external spermatic fascia. It contains vas deferens, testicular artery, cremasteric artery, artery of ductus deferens, pampiniform venous and lymphatic plexus, sympathetic nerve fibers, and processus vaginalis. The cremaster muscle is responsible for the cold reflex which draws testis superiorly. Warm reflex is opposite to it. These occur to regulate temperature of testis for regulating spermatogenesis (1°C below core temperature).

The genital branch of the genitofemoral nerve (L1 and L2) innervates the cremaster striated muscle, while dartos is a smooth muscle innervated by the autonomic nerves **(Fig. 5)**.

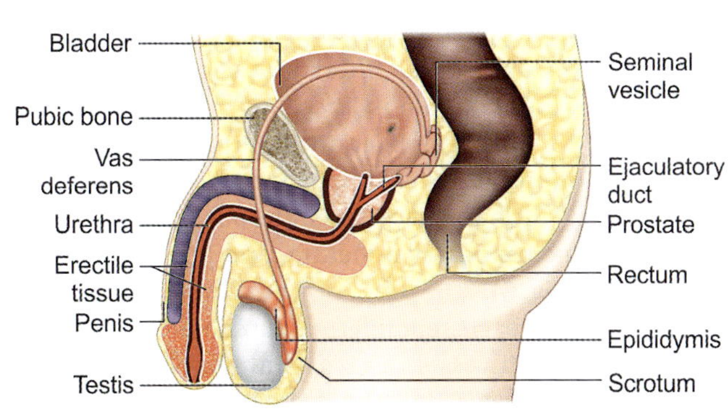

Fig. 5: Male reproductive tract.

Scrotum

The scrotum is the saccular part consisting of two layers—(1) heavily pigmented skin and (2) a fat-free dartos fascial layer along with smooth muscle fibers giving rugose appearance to scrotum. In cold conditions, contraction of the dartos muscle causes thickening of the integumentary layer as it is attached to the skin, and reduces scrotal surface area overall, thus reducing heat loss.

The scrotum is divided by scrotal raphe. It marks the line of fusion for embryonic labioscrotal swellings. Fascia does not contain fat. The arterial supply of scrotum is from the perineal artery (branch of the internal pudendal artery), deep external pudendal artery, and cremasteric artery. Scrotal veins accompany arteries. Superficial inguinal lymph nodes drain it. Innervation is by the genital branch of the genitofemoral nerve (L1, L2), ilioinguinal nerve (L1), posterior scrotal branches of the pudendal nerve (S2–S4), and perineal branches of the posterior cutaneous nerve of the thigh (S2, S3).

Testes

Testes are the male gonads suspended in the scrotum by the spermatic cords, with the left testis inferior to the right testis. Each has a volume of 15 mL or more and measures around 5 cm in length. The surface is covered by the visceral layer of the tunica vaginalis, except at attachment to epididymis and spermatic cord. Fluid separates visceral and parietal layers for free movement in scrotum. The testes have a tough fibrous outer surface, the tunica albuginea that thickens into a ridge on its internal and posterior aspects as the mediastinum of the testis. It has little distensibility; thus, any condition leading to edema can cause ischemic damage to the testis. Beneath tunica albuginea is a vascular layer called tunica vasculosa, which contains blood vessels with numerous mast cells.[9] A thin connective tissue septum extends from the mediastinum testis anteriorly and subdivides each testis into about 250 incomplete compartments or testicular lobules, each containing one to four coiled seminiferous tubules. The mediastinum contains a network of channels known as the rete testis, which receives the terminal segments of the seminiferous tubules (straight tubules) in which the sperms are produced.

Each testicular lobule contains tightly packed seminiferous tubules and sparse interstitial connective tissue. Each seminiferous tubule is lined by stratified germinal epithelium, containing proliferative spermatogenic (germ) cells and nonproliferating supporting (sustentacular) or Sertoli cells.[10] It is in these seminiferous tubules where spermatogenic cells divide, mature, and are transformed into sperms **(Fig. 6)**.

Surrounding each seminiferous tubule are connective tissue cells, blood vessels, nerves and lymphatic vessels, steroid-secreting cells, and the interstitial cells of Leydig-producing testosterone. Seminiferous tubules comprise 95% of testicular volume and are devoted to the production of spermatozoa. There are approximately 500 tubules per testis. The tubules are divided by fibrous septae and surrounded by the tough tunica albuginea.

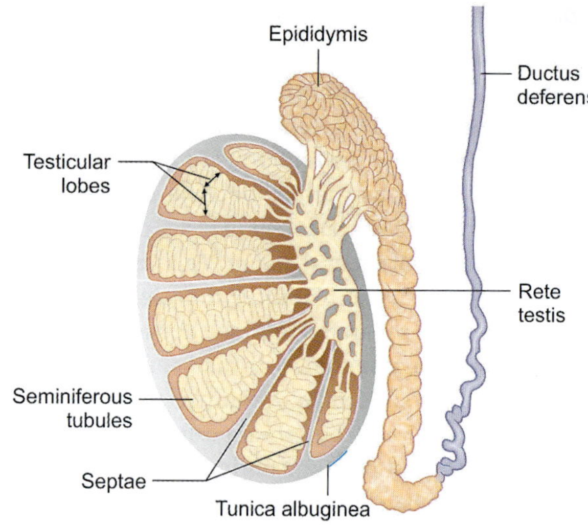

Fig. 6: Macroscopic structure of testes.

Each tubule is 30–70 cm long and 200–300 μm in diameter. Tight convolutions can result in incomplete obstruction. As the tubule reaches the mediastinum, convolutions decrease and ultimately straighten out to form tubuli recti (straight ducts), which connect to the developmentally different set of network of tubules called rete testes. Sperm produced by the seminiferous tubules passes out of the testis into the ductal system, beginning with the rete testis to the epididymis and then to the vas deferens. Sperm in the vas deferens is joined by the seminal vesicle secretions as they pass through the prostate via the ejaculatory ducts into the urethra.

The long testicular arteries arise from the abdominal aorta just inferior to the renal arteries. Pampiniform plexus converge, forming the right testicular vein, which enters inferior vena cava, and the left testicular vein, which enters left renal vein and surrounds the testicular artery in the spermatic cord. It provides thermoregulation. The lymphatics drain into bilateral lumbar and preaortic lymph nodes. The autonomic nerves contain vagal parasympathetic and visceral afferent fibers and sympathetic fibers from T10 to T11 segment.

Epididymis

The epididymis is an elongated structure on the posterior surface of the testis, which receives sperms from efferent ductules through rete testis. It has convolutions and appears solid. The epididymis has three parts: (1) head, which is the superior extended part composed of lobules of coiled ends of 12–14 efferent ductules; (2) body, which is major part consisting of the tightly convoluted duct of the epididymis; and (3) tail, which is tapering continuation with the ductus deferens.[11] It is made up of tightly packed convoluted tubules with little supporting loose connective tissue. These efferent ductuli are very fine and lined by highly ciliated columnar epithelium for maximum absorption of water, both to increase the concentration of sperms as well as to transport the sperms from testes to epididymis by creating the suction effect. The walls have myoid cells, which undergo frequent contractions to enhance the absorption of fluid as well as the mobilization of sperms.

All these minute ductules of the head of the epididymis join together and form one single duct, which coils on itself called the canal of epididymis or epididymal duct. It forms most of the body and tail of the epididymis and lies alongside the posterolateral border of the testis. The epididymal duct is approximately 6 m in length. The duct is lined by pseudostratified columnar epithelium with nonmotile stereocilia due to the absence of axoneme. The passage of sperms across the epididymis takes 7–10 days. However, the transit time is dependent on the amount of sperms produced; the higher the sperm production, the lesser the transit time it takes. From head to tail, it moves by spontaneous peristaltic movements during which sperms attain their maturity, motility, and fertilization capacity. The tail of the epididymis is evolved as the sperm storage organ only in animals forced to wait for female ovulation. Maturation of sperms is dependent on the luminal flow of testosterone. Prominent dilatation of the epididymal head is known as "Bayle's sign", which is palpable in case of epididymal obstruction or absent vas deferens in men.

Ductus Deferens

The ductus deferens, a primary component of the spermatic cord, has thick muscular walls and a minute lumen, giving it a cord-like firmness. It begins in the tail of the epididymis, runs via the inguinal canal, and ends by joining the duct of seminal gland to form ejaculatory duct. The relationship of ductus deferens to ureter is similar to that of uterine artery to ureter in the female but is of lesser significance.

In adults, vas measures about 25 cm in length and can be palpated as a 3–5 mm thick string on both sides of the scrotum. The ductus deferens enlarges and forms ampulla of ductus deferens (2 cm in length) before its termination. Ampulla also serves as the storage for the sperms prior to the ejaculation but is controversial because of the temperature issues. Because of the long and complicated course of the duct, absence of the duct, or multiple blocks in the duct, surgical retrieval followed by the assisted reproductive technology (ART) is preferred over corrective surgeries.

The vas has three robust layers of smooth muscles: Outer and inner longitudinal and middle circular layers. These muscles are under the sympathetic stimulation and show mass contraction when stimulated which transport spermatozoa from the epididymis tail to the prostatic urethra within a second.

Artery to ductus deferens supplies ductus deferens. Veins drain into testicular vein including distal pampiniform plexus.

Seminal Glands

Each seminal gland (vesicle) is an elongated structure lying between the fundus of the bladder and rectum, 5 cm long approximately. Seminal glands do not store sperms as believed earlier. They secrete a thick alkaline fluid mixed with fructose and coagulating agent that mixes with sperms as they pass into ejaculatory ducts and urethra.

Inferior vesical and middle rectal arteries supply it. Veins accompany it. The secretion of the gland is viscid, yellowish-white alkaline fluid and forms the bulk of the semen which is rich in fructose, prostaglandin, and a coagulating enzyme—vesiculase. The activity of the mucous membrane is regulated by the secretion of the androgen (testosterone). Fructose is believed to serve as an energy source of sperms. The seminal glands contain 40 million times higher concentrations of prostaglandins than the blood. In cases of absent vas deferens, the seminal glands are also absent in most of such cases as they have the same developmental origin (Wolffian duct system) **(Fig. 7)**.

Ejaculatory Ducts

The ejaculatory ducts arise by the union of the ducts of the seminal glands with the ductus deferentes approximately 2.5 cm long. The ejaculatory ducts converge to open on seminal colliculus by tiny, slit-like apertures on, or just within the opening of the prostatic utricle. Ducts traverse the glandular prostate but secretions from prostate gland do not join seminal fluid till ejaculatory ducts terminate in the prostatic urethra. Ejaculatory ducts have the same blood supply as ductus deferens. The veins join the prostatic and vesical venous plexuses.

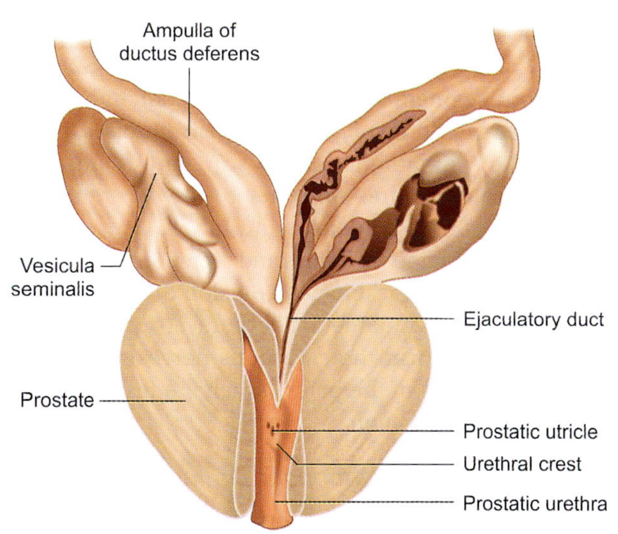

Fig. 7: Seminal glands.

Prostate

Prostate is a firm and walnut-shaped gland with a size of approximately 4 × 3 × 2 cm and is the largest accessory gland of the male reproductive system surrounding the prostatic urethra. Two-third part is glandular and one-third is fibromuscular. Capsule is fibrous and neurovascular, incorporating the prostatic plexuses of veins and nerves.[12]

The prostatic ducts are 20–30 in number opening chiefly on the posterior wall of the urethra through sinuses. Prostatic fluid is acidic and milky fluid forming 20% of the semen volume and is biochemically very active. Prostatic secretions contain a large amount of enzymes that play a role in both semen clotting and liquefaction. The enzyme vesiculase induces clotting and a number of proteases, peptidases, and hyaluronidase, which cause the breakdown of the clot.

Inorganic elements such as zinc, magnesium, and calcium are also present. Zinc is known to provide protection of spermatozoa against spermiophagic cells in the female genital tract and acts as a chelating agent by protecting free sulfhydryl groups present on protamines so as to prevent "superstabilization" of the condensed chromatin of sperm.

The prostatic arteries are mainly branches of inferior vesical, internal pudendal, and middle rectal arteries. The prostatic venous plexus drains into internal iliac veins. It is continuous with the vesical venous plexus and the internal vertebral venous plexus.

Bulbourethral Glands

Bulbourethral glands are also known as Cowper's glands. They are pea sized. Ducts open in spongy urethra in bulb of penis. Their mucus-like secretion enters the urethra during sexual arousal.

Innervation of Male Pelvis

The ductus deferens, seminal glands, ejaculatory ducts, and prostate are richly innervated by sympathetic nerve fibers with presynaptic cell bodies in the intermediolateral cell column of T12–L2 (or L3) spinal cord segments.

Presynaptic parasympathetic fibers from S2 to S3 spinal cord segments traverse pelvic splanchnic nerves and join the inferior hypogastric or pelvic plexuses. During orgasm, the sympathetic system stimulates contraction of the internal urethral sphincter to prevent retrograde ejaculation. Simultaneous stimulation causes rapid peristaltic contractions of ductus and secretion from seminal and prostate glands results in expulsion of semen during ejaculation. Parasympathetic fibers traverse the prostatic nerve plexus to form the cavernous nerves that pass to the erectile bodies of the penis, which are responsible for producing penile erection.

Vascular Supply and Lymphatic Drainage

The arterial supply of the scrotum is from the perineal artery (branch of the internal pudendal artery), deep external pudendal artery, and cremasteric artery. Scrotal veins accompany the arteries. Lymphatic drainage is by superficial inguinal lymph nodes. The long testicular arteries arise from the abdominal aorta just inferior to the renal arteries. Pampiniform plexus converges into right and left testicular veins. The lymphatics of testis drain into preaortic and lumbar lymph nodes. The artery to ductus deferens is the arterial supply of ductus deferens. Veins drain into the testicular vein, including the distal pampiniform plexus. Inferior vesical and middle rectal arteries supply seminal vesicles. Veins accompany it. The arteries to ductus deferens supply the ejaculatory ducts. The veins follow prostatic and vesical venous plexuses. Prostatic arteries are mainly the branches of inferior vesical arteries, internal pudendal, and middle rectal arteries. Prostatic venous plexus drains into internal iliac veins. It is continuous with the vesical venous plexus and the internal vertebral venous plexus.

Applied Anatomy

- The common method of sterilizing males is vasectomy. Ductus deferens is ligated through an incision in the superior scrotum. No scalpel vasectomy is done these days. Reversal of vasectomy is successful in young patients of less than 30 years of age and having <7 years of postoperative time. An operating microscope-aided reattachment of ends of sectioned ductus is done.
- Seminal gland enlargement and abscesses can be palpated during a rectal examination. For microscopic examination, seminal glands are massaged to release secretions to detect the organism for gonococci infection.
- Prostate hypertrophy is common after middle age affecting urination by distorting the prostatic urethra and causing dysuria, urgency, nocturia, cystitis, and kidney damage. Examination can be done by digital rectal examination.[13]
- Prostate-specific antigen (PSA) is secreted by prostate, clinically used as a clinical marker in suspected cases of carcinomas.
- Ejaculatory duct obstruction can be suspected in fructose-negative cases which can be resected through transurethral resection of duct (TURD).
- Men with premature ejaculation are advised to practice training voluntary muscles.
- Horizontal testes are more prone to torsion injuries.
- Small size testis is indicative of damage to the seminiferous epithelium which forms the major portion of the testicular volume. It can be measured by an orchidometer.
- Small and firm testes, usually <3 mL in volume, are found in men with Klinefelter syndrome.
- Patients with hypogonadotropic hypogonadism have small testes, but size usually measures between 5 and 12 mL.

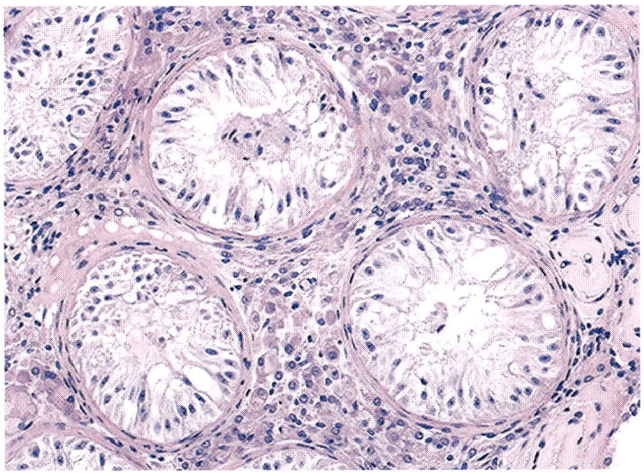

Fig. 8: Sertoli cell-only syndrome—histological section.

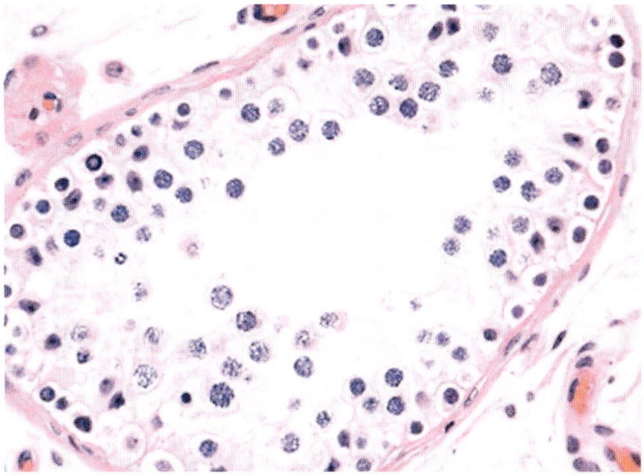

Fig. 9: Histological section of maturation arrest syndrome.

- Microdeletions in Y chromosome are found in higher rates in infertile men than in fertile controls. Azoospermia factor (AZF) focus at Yq11 has partial deletion of AZFa, AZFb, and AZFc with Sertoli cell-only syndrome **(Fig. 8)**, maturation arrest **(Fig. 9)**, and occasional spermatogenesis, respectively.
- *Anesthesia for sperm retrieval techniques*: Local anesthesia in percutaneous epididymal sperm aspiration (PESA) or testicular or epididymal sperm aspiration (TESA) can be achieved by injecting 10 mL of 1% lignocaine solution along sides of vas deferens near external inguinal ring. This is called spermatic cord block. Only in apprehensive patients, intravenous sedation can be given as backup. For microsurgical procedures, general anesthesia is preferred.

Penis

The penis is the male copulatory organ and provides a common outlet for urine and semen. It consists of glans, body, and root. It is composed of three cylindrical cavernous bodies of erectile tissue: the paired corpora cavernosa and single corpus spongiosum. Penis is in anatomical position when erect and its dorsum is anterior in flaccid condition. The skin of the penis is thin, darkly pigmented relative to adjacent skin, and connected to the tunica albuginea by loose connective tissue. At the neck of the glans, the skin and fascia of the penis are prolonged as a double layer of skin, the prepuce (foreskin) which in uncircumcised males covers the glans penis mostly.

Penis is supplied by the dorsal artery of penis, deep artery, and artery of bulb of penis. Cavernous space blood is drained through prostatic venous plexus.

Innervation of penis: The nerves derive from the S2–S4 spinal cord segments and spinal ganglia, passing through the pelvic splanchnic and pudendal nerves, respectively. Sensory and sympathetic innervation is provided primarily by the dorsal nerve of the penis.

Erection, emission, ejaculation, and remission: When a male is stimulated erotically, arteriovenous anastomoses are closed and smooth muscles relax due to parasympathetic stimulation. This results in increased blood flow to cavernous spaces in corpora of penis. The bulbospongiosus and ischiocavernosus muscles compress veins impeding venous flow return. As a result, engorgement of erectile bodies occurs resulting in erection.

Emission (expression of secretions into the urethra) is a sympathetic response (L1–L2 nerves). During ejaculation, expulsion of semen occurs through the external urethral orifice due to closure of internal urethral sphincter (sympathetic) and contraction of urethral and bulbospongiosus muscle (parasympathetic). After ejaculation, the penis becomes flaccid due to relaxation of muscles allowing blood to drain from cavernosa to deep dorsal vein.

The first part of the semen comes from the cauda of the epididymis suspended in prostatic fluid. Spermatozoa in zinc-rich prostate fluid preserve motility, vitality, and the stability of their nuclear chromatin. The second part is mainly composed of a fluid from the seminal glands, which is rich in fructose and prostaglandin. The first part of the ejaculate is deposited on to the cervical mucus comprising spermatozoa in prostatic fluid and the second part of the semen mainly from seminal glands forms the plug to prevent backflow of the first part of the ejaculate. Semen collected in a predetermined sequence is known as a "split ejaculate".

Semen

Semen is a grey opalescent fluid. Testes have 5% contribution to ejaculate and seminal vesicles and prostate make up to 90%. The remaining 5% of the ejaculatory volume is formed by the bulbourethral and urethral glands. These volumes are outlined in **Table 1**.[12] Secretions have an important role. Minor changes also in consistency of fluid have a profound effect. Reproductive failure can be the result of pathology in one of the accessory glands rather than the result of any abnormality of sperm production.

TABLE 1: Contribution of secretions of each gland to make up seminal fluid.[12]

Source of secretion	*Ejaculate (%)*
Testes and efferent ducts	5
Prostate	13–33
Seminal gland	46–80
Bulbourethral glands	2–5

After ejaculation, mixing of components takes place and thus loss of any part of the semen sample during ejaculation can result in a false-positive abnormality in semen analysis.

Testicular Contribution

No major contribution is there toward volume so after vasectomy, semen volume does not change. The fluid from testis enters efferent ductules and is known as rete testis fluid. This fluid is rich in testosterone which is bound to androgen-binding protein (ABP) secreted by the Sertoli cells. Rete testis fluid also contains inhibin, ceruloplasmin, and transferrin.

Reduction in their concentration is seen in men with epididymal obstruction and Sertoli cell dysfunction.

Lactate dehydrogenase C4 is an enzyme released when sperms die or break up. Its presence may indicate damage of sperm during passage through the epididymal duct. L-carnitine and glycerophosphorylcholine are added through the passage in the epididymal duct.

Seminal Vesicles and their Secretions

Seminal vesicle secretions make 40–60% of the total ejaculatory volume. They have a major effect on the functions of sperm and physical properties of seminal plasma. The secretion is alkaline and contains fructose, prostaglandins, and fibrinogen-like substrate on which the enzyme vesiculase acts to induce clotting. The fructose component is absent in some mammals such as dogs and horses. Prostaglandins may act as calcium ionophores.

Prostatic fluid is biologically active and contains enzymes involved in semen clotting and liquefaction. It also contains protease, peptidase, and hyaluronidase. The prostatic secretions also contain the bacteriostatic amine called spermine, acid phosphatase, citrate, calcium, zinc, and magnesium. Crystallization may be seen when a semen sample is left for some time and pH of the seminal plasma is allowed to fall.

Secretions of the bulbourethral and urethral glands have little significance. Immunoglobulin G present in it is responsible for antisperm antibodies.

Endocrinology of the Testis

Leydig cells secrete testosterone and Sertoli cells secrete inhibin and ABP and follistatin in the testis. This is controlled by pituitary gonadotropins—luteinizing hormone (LH) and FSH which in turn are under control of the hypothalamic hormone, gonadotropin-releasing hormone (GnRH). LH acts on Leydig cells and FSH acts on Sertoli cells. A concentration gradient for testosterone thus exists between the interstitial tissue and the interior of the Sertoli cell. ABP testosterone complex is formed within the Sertoli cell and provides androgen for spermatogenesis. This ABP testosterone complex enters the lumen of the seminiferous tubules by exocytosis. Testosterone has a negative paracrine feedback action for LH on the pituitary–hypothalamic axis. Inhibin acts as negative feedback for FSH secretion. It is produced in two forms known as b-A and b-B. The subunit b-B is present only in male serum.

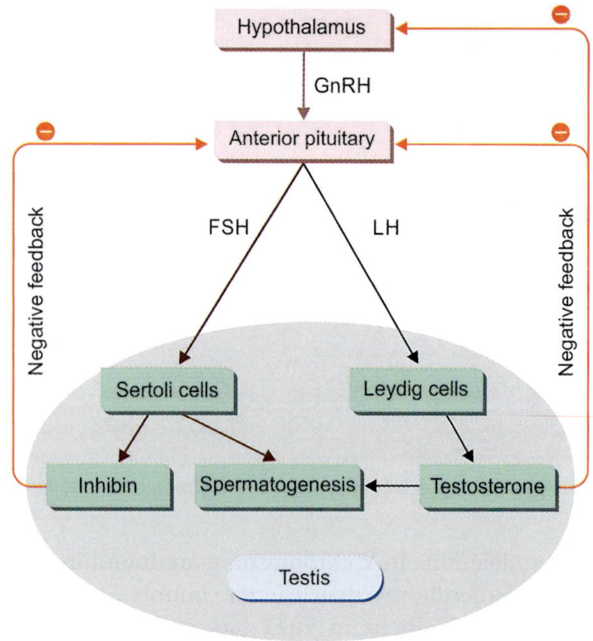

Fig. 10: Hormonal circuit for male reproduction.
(FSH: follicle-stimulating hormone; GnRH: gonadotropin-releasing hormone; LH: luteinizing hormone)

There is an inverse relationship between inhibin B and FSH in male sera, but no such relationship exists between inhibin A and FSH levels in the serum of male patients. Damage to the Sertoli cell reduces inhibin B production and therefore will cause an increase in FSH secretion. Activin stimulates FSH production.[14]

Follistatin also suppresses FSH secretion, but it is much less potent than inhibin. Sertoli cells also produce modulating substance to act on Leydig cells. Thus, it is a complex interrelationship between cells and axis **(Fig. 10)**.

Histology

Interstitial tissue is interspersed with convoluted tubules and has tunica vasculosa testis tissue beneath tunica albuginea.

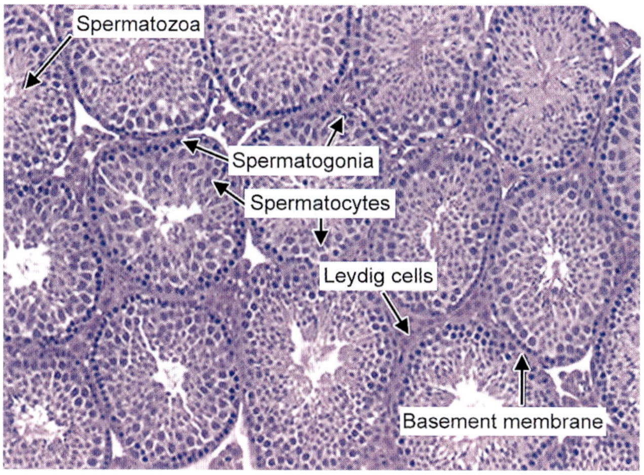

Fig. 11: Normal histology of testes.

Tubules are surrounded by three to four layers of smooth muscle cells or myoid cells **(Fig. 11)**.

Primary spermatocytes are visible in cross sections of seminiferous tubules. Incomplete cell divisions result in syncytium of cells with bridges of cytoplasm in between. Spermatids lie in the lumina of seminiferous epithelium. They are small with nucleus in eccentric position. During condensation, the nucleus becomes smaller and stains darker.

The nucleus of Sertoli cells is ovoid or angular and contains a large nucleolus. The nuclear membrane fold is characteristic of Sertoli cells, but not always visible in a light microscope. Tight junctions form a blood-testis barrier.

Spermatozoa pass through tubuli recti having low columnar epithelium and rete testis having flattened or cuboidal epithelium into a number of ductuli efferentes, containing both absorptive and ciliated cells.

The ductuli efferentes are lined by tall pseudostratified columnar epithelium. Toward the basal lamina are present a number of small nuclei, belonging to basal cells of the ductus epididymidis. These cells regenerate the epithelium.

The vas deferens is lined by pseudostratified columnar epithelium with long stereocilia.

Simple columnar epithelium of prostatic secretory ducts changes into transitional type near openings of ducts. Corpora amylacea in secretory alveoli are the characteristic features of prostate with round eosinophilic bodies.

Seminal vesicles mucosa is branched into anastomosing folds of honeycomb-like structure with columnar or pseudostratified lining. Lumen is filled with acidophilic secretion.

CONCLUSION

Within the milieu of producing progeny, female reproductive system has four major functions i.e. to produce egg, transport and sustain cells, to produce hormones and nurture developing embryo. These functions are carried through ovaries, fallopian tubes, uterus and accessory organs. Like that of female, male reproductive system also has a role in formation of a new individual i.e. to fulfil reproduction. Male reproductive system has one pair testes, excretory ducts network, glands like prostate, seminal vesicles, bulbourethral glands and penis.

KEY POINTS

- The human reproductive system is a complex arrangement of specialized organs.
- These organs function efficiently under the influence of neural and hormonal signals together with each other to produce a new life.

REFERENCES

1. Moore KL, Persaud TVN. The Developing Human: Clinically Oriented Embryology, 8th edition. Philadelphia, PA: Saunders; 2008.
2. Gray H, Williams PL, Bannister LH. Gray's Anatomy: The Anatomical Basis of Medicine and Surgery, 38th edition. New York: Churchill Livingstone; 1995.
3. Datta AK. Essentials of Human Anatomy (Thorax and abdomen), 8th edition. India, Kolkata: Current Books International; 2008.
4. Alzamil L, Nikolakopoulou K, Turco MY. Organoid systems to study the human female reproductive tract and pregnancy. Cell Death Differ. 2021;28:35-51.
5. Eroschenko VP. diFiore's Atlas of Histology with Functional Correlations, 11th edition. Philadelphia, PA: Lippincott Williams & Wilkins; 2008.
6. Backhouse KM. The gubernaculum testis Hunteri: testicular descent and maldescent. Ann R Coll Surg Engl. 1964; 35(1):15-33.
7. Keith L Moore, TVN Persaud, Mark G Torchia. The Developing Human: Clinically Oriented Embryology 10th Ed. Elsevier Health Sciences, 2016 ISBN 978-0323313483, pp. 267-9.
8. Moore KL, Dalley AF, Agur AMR. Clinically Oriented Anatomy, 6th edition. Philadelphia, PA: Lippincott Williams & Wilkins; 2010.
9. Dym M, Fawcett DW. The blood-testis barrier in the rat and the physiological compartmentation of the seminiferous epithelium. Biol Reprod. 1970;3(3):308-26.
10. Clermont Y. The cycle of the seminiferous epithelium in man. Am J Anat. 1963;112(1):35-51.
11. Glover TD, Nicander L. Some aspects of structure and function in the mammalian epididymis. J Reprod Fertil Suppl. 1971;13(Suppl. 13):39-50.
12. Aumuller G. Morphologic and regulatory aspects of prostatic function. Anat Embryol (Berl). 1989;179(6):519-31.
13. Myers RP, Cahill DR, Devine RM, King BF. Anatomy of radical prostatectomy as defined by magnetic resonance imaging. J Urol. 1998;159(6):2148-58.
14. Brooks DE. Epididymal functions and their hormonal regulation. Aust J Biol Sci. 1983;36(3):205-21.

CHAPTER 2

Regulation and Physiology of Menstrual Cycle

Arveen Vohra

INTRODUCTION

The normal menstrual cycle is one of the most complex, elegant, and yet one of the simplest physiologic processes. It is mandatory for a clinician and infertility consultant to completely understand the menstrual cycle. The menstrual cycle, under the control of the endocrine system, is necessary for reproduction. It is the cycle of changes that occurs in the ovary and uterus for the purpose of sexual reproduction, being essential for the production of eggs and for the preparation of the uterus for pregnancy. The normal menstrual cycle is the orderly cyclic hormone production and parallel proliferation of the uterine lining in preparation for implantation of the embryo failing, which it prepares for the next cycle.

Menstruation is defined as the cyclic, orderly sloughing of the uterine lining in response to the interactions of hormones produced by the hypothalamus, pituitary, and ovaries. Menarche is typically followed by 5–7 years of relatively long cycles that gradually decrease in length and become regular. Variations in cycle length reflect differences in the length of the follicular phase, as the luteal phase is fairly consistent.

In humans, the menstrual cycle is a monthly cycle that averages 28 days per cycle. It varies in different women and even in the same woman during various cycles. Menstrual cycle is counted from the first day of menstrual bleeding. Each menstrual cycle can be divided into three phases based on the following ovarian and endometrial events:

1. *Ovarian cycle (events in the ovary):* It consists of the follicular phase, ovulation, and luteal phase along with the luteal–follicular transition phase.
2. *Uterine cycle (events in the uterus):* It consists of menstruation, proliferative phase, and secretory phase.

This chapter encompasses in detail the neuroendocrinology and physiology of menstrual cycle, which in synchrony are responsible for the regulation of the menstrual cycle in women. The genomic profiling, which has now highlighted the various hormonal and the hormone receptor polymorphisms, is also discussed along with newer concepts in primordial follicle activation.

REPRODUCTIVE NEUROENDOCRINOLOGY

Introduction

The female and male reproductive systems function as an orchestra in harmony with a set of reproductive hormones under the influence of regulatory hormones secreted by the hypothalamus and pituitary gland. Initially, the pituitary gland was considered as the master of the endocrine orchestra, but recently, the hypothalamus has equitably replaced this status. The hypothalamus exerts its influence via neurotransmitters transported to the pituitary gland by means of a portal vessel network in response to both peripheral and central nervous system signals.

The hypothalamus and the pituitary are essential for the operation of the menstrual cycle, in synchrony with the endocrine feedback by the ovary on the anterior pituitary that leads to ovulation. The physiology of the menstrual cycle is dependent on signaling whereby the "ovarian clock" modulates hypothalamic–pituitary function as well as endometrial proliferation and secretion.

The predominant hormones involved in the menstrual cycle are gonadotropin-releasing hormone (GnRH), follicle-stimulating hormone (FSH), luteinizing hormone (LH), estrogen, and progesterone. GnRH is secreted by the hypothalamus, the gonadotropins FSH and LH are secreted by the anterior pituitary gland, and estrogen and progestins are secreted at the level of the ovary. GnRH stimulates the release of FSH and LH from the anterior pituitary, which in turn stimulate the release of estrogen and progestin at the level of the ovary.

Hypothalamo-hypophyseal Portal Circulation

Hypothalamus

The hypothalamus is a small, cone-shaped neural structure situated at the base of the brain above the optic chiasma

TABLE 1: Pituitary releasing factors from the hypothalamus.

Hypothalamic hormone	*Action*
Gonadotropin-releasing hormone (GnRH)	Controls the secretion of luteinizing hormone (LH) and follicle-stimulating hormone (FSH)
Corticotropin-releasing hormone (CRH)	Controls the release of adrenocorticotropic hormone (ACTH)
Growth hormone-releasing hormone (GHRH)	Regulates the release of growth hormone (GH)
Thyrotropin-releasing hormone (TRH)	Regulates the secretion of thyroid-stimulating hormone (TSH)

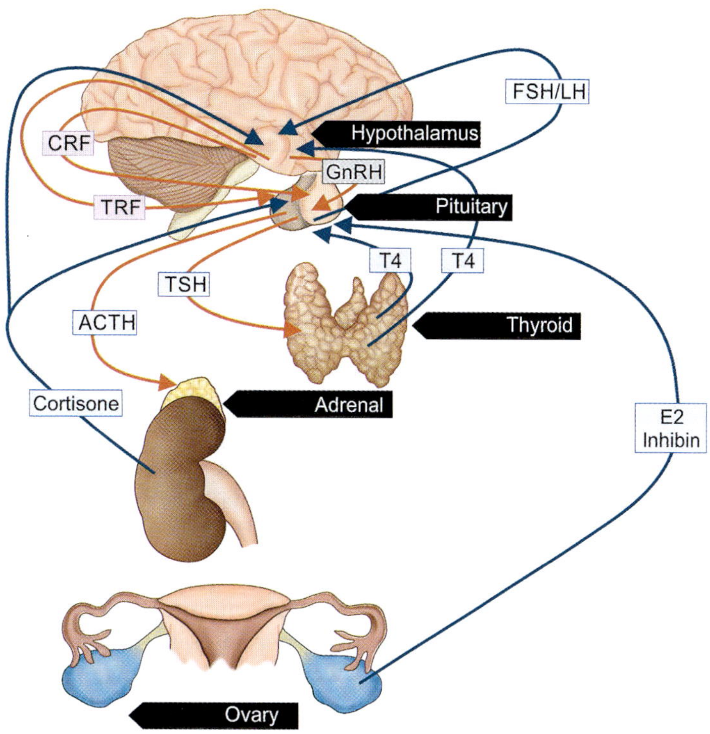

Fig. 1: Pituitary-releasing factors that control the endocrine function of the ovaries, thyroid, and adrenal glands. Note the feedback from the target hormones (marked in blue lines).
(ACTH: adrenocorticotropic hormone; CRF: corticotropin-releasing factor; E2: estradiol; FSH: follicle-stimulating hormone; GnRH: gonadotropin-releasing factor; LH: luteinizing hormone; TRF: thyrotropin-releasing factor; TSH: thyroid-stimulating hormone; T4: thyroxine)

and below the third ventricle forming the lower part of diencephalon. It is connected directly to the pituitary gland and is the source of many pituitary secretions.

The hypothalamus has peptidergic neural cells that secrete releasing and inhibiting hormones. These cells resemble both neurons and endocrine gland cells and respond to signals in the bloodstream as well as to neurotransmitters within the brain in a process known as *neurosecretion*. These neurotransmitters are secreted at the nerve terminal. Neuroendocrine agents originating in the hypothalamus have positive stimulatory effects on growth hormone (GH), thyroid-stimulating hormone (TSH), adrenocorticotropic hormone (ACTH), and the gonadotropins **(Table 1 and Fig. 1)**.

Several levels of feedback to the hypothalamus exist and are known as the long, short, and ultrashort feedback loops **(Flowchart 1)**. The long feedback loop is composed of endocrine input from circulating hormones, just as feedback

Flowchart 1: Hypothalamic–pituitary–ovary feedback loop mechanisms.

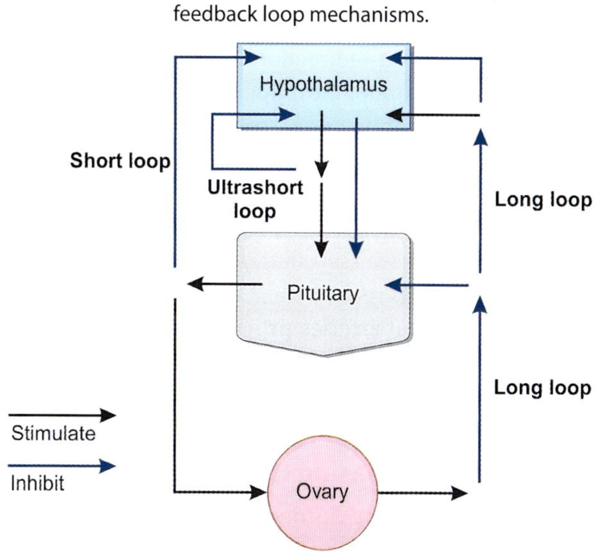

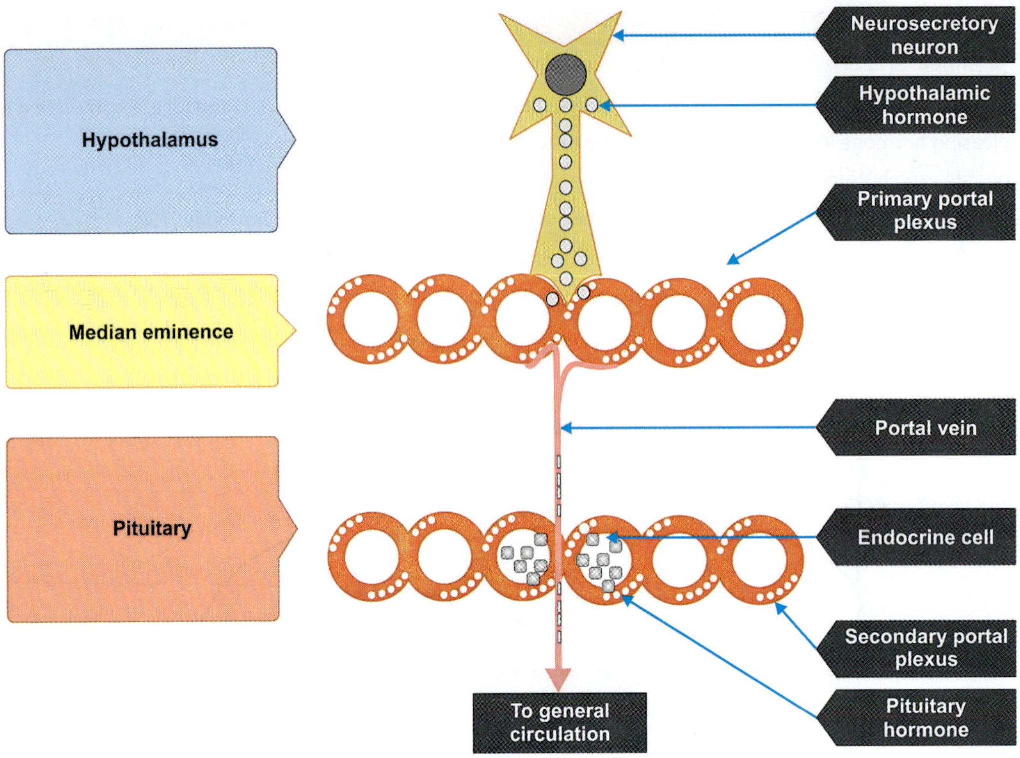

Fig. 2: Hypothalamic–pituitary axis with the portal system.

of androgens and estrogens on to steroid receptors is present in the hypothalamus. In short-loop feedback, pituitary hormones send feedback to the hypothalamus and serve important regulatory functions. Hypothalamic secretions may directly feedback to the hypothalamus itself in an ultrashort feedback loop.[1,2]

Pituitary

The pituitary consists of two lobes—anterior (adenohypophysis) and posterior (neurohypophysis), which are structurally different. The unique fenestrated capillaries in this region eliminate the blood-brain barrier in the median eminence and permit bidirectional feedback control. The anterior pituitary is under the influence of the hypothalamus by means of neurohormones released into this portal circulation. There also exists retrograde flow so that pituitary hormones can be delivered directly to the hypothalamus, creating the opportunity for pituitary feedback on the hypothalamus. Short vessels that originate in the posterior pituitary that in turn receive their arterial supply from the inferior hypophyseal arteries provide an additional blood supply **(Fig. 2)**.

HORMONES IN FEMALE REPRODUCTION

Gonadotropin-releasing Hormone

Gonadotropin-releasing hormone (also called luteinizing hormone-releasing hormone or LHRH) is the controlling factor for gonadotropin secretion. There is a single neurohormone (GnRH) for both FSH and LH. It is a decapeptide with the gene located on chromosome 8p and works through its own receptor, encoded on chromosome 4q. It is produced by neurons with cell bodies primarily in the arcuate nucleus of the hypothalamus and in many extrapituitary tissues, such as the ovarian follicle and the placenta. GnRH has autocrine-paracrine functions throughout the body **(Fig. 3)**.

Pulsatile secretion of GnRH: The half-life of GnRH is only 2–4 minutes. A prominent feature of the reproductive system is the absolute requirement for pulsatile secretion of GnRH from the arcuate nucleus of the hypothalamus into the pituitary portal system for normal gonadotropin secretion. The increase in the GnRH pulses marks the onset of puberty. GnRH is unique as it regulates the secretion of two hormones—FSH and LH—and must be secreted in a pulsatile fashion within a critical range in frequency and amplitude. Knobil et al. showed that in hypothalamic-lesioned monkeys receiving GnRH, intermittent stimulation of the pituitary results in secretion of LH and FSH, whereas constant GnRH stimulation leads to suppression of gonadotropin levels.[3]

The frequency of GnRH secretion is once per 90 minutes in the early follicular phase, which increases to once per 60–70 minutes in the late-follicular phase. Lower GnRH pulse frequencies favor FSH secretion and higher frequencies favor LH secretion. Pulsatile GnRH secretion is more frequent but lower in amplitude during the follicular phase.

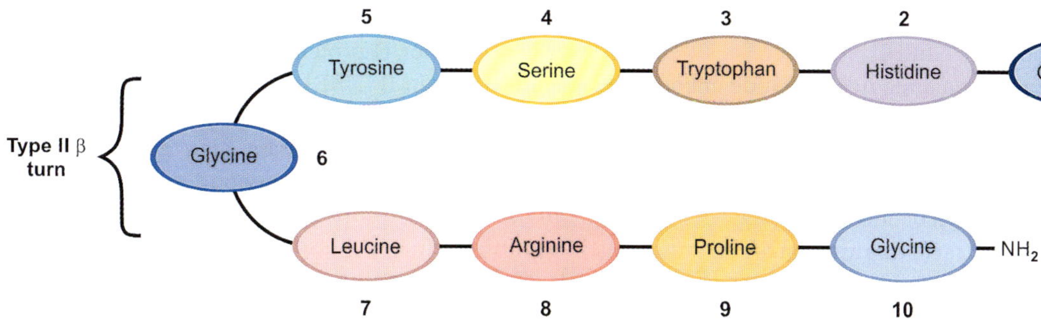

Fig. 3: Structure of gonadotropin-releasing hormone molecule.

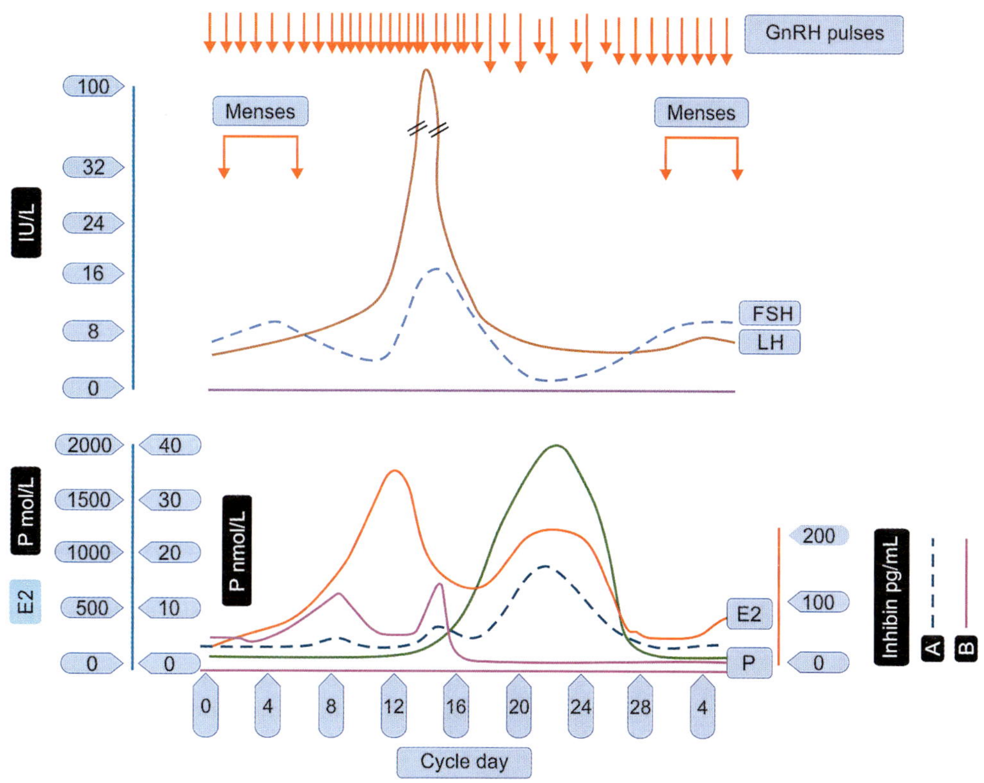

Fig. 4: Gonadotropin-releasing hormone (GnRH) pulsatility affecting gonadotropin and steroid release during menstrual cycle. (E2: estradiol; FSH: follicle-stimulating hormone; LH: luteinizing hormone; P: progesterone)

An increase in frequency and amplitude during mid-cycle favors LH surge necessary for ovulation. Slowing of pulse frequency in the late-luteal phase favors FSH synthesis and allows the rise in FSH essential for the next cycle **(Fig. 4)**.

Control of GnRH pulses: Catecholamines such as norepinephrine, dopamine, and serotonin, and transmitters, such as opiates and prostaglandins, also appear to influence the secretion of GnRH from the hypothalamus. Norepinephrine seems to stimulate GnRH release, whereas dopamine, serotonin, endogenous opioids, and corticotropin-releasing hormone (CRH) appear capable of inhibiting or suppressing GnRH, as witnessed by the association of stress with hypothalamic amenorrhea in some women. Biogenic catecholamines modulate GnRH pulsatile release by influencing the frequency (and perhaps the amplitude) of GnRH discharge **(Flowchart 2)**.

The *dopamine* tuberoinfundibular tract arising within the medial basal hypothalamus and terminating in the median eminence provides the dopaminergic effect on the pituitary. Dopamine is directly secreted into the portal blood, thus behaving like a neurohormone. It directly suppresses GnRH activity and is transported via the portal system to directly and specifically suppress pituitary prolactin secretion.

Neuropeptide Y (NPY), a polypeptide, stimulates appetite, decreases heat production, and increases insulin and cortisol secretion. The secretion and gene expression of NPY in hypothalamus are regulated by gonadal steroids.

It stimulates pulsatile release of GnRH and potentiates gonadotropin response to GnRH.[4]

Kisspeptin is a hypothalamic neuropeptide encoded by the gene *Kiss1*, which has recently emerged as a key central regulator of gonadotropin secretion. The kisspeptin neurons have estrogen and progesterone receptors and are essential for the normal development of puberty.[5]

Kisspeptins and their receptors are expressed by neurons in the arcuate and anteroventral periventricular nuclei of the hypothalamus. **Figure 5** shows structure of kisspeptin.

Puberty is regulated by the maturation of kisspeptin neurons as well as by interactions between kisspeptins and leptin.[6]

The obligatory kisspeptin signaling for normal puberty is evidenced by a failure to progress through puberty in individuals with mutations in genes encoding kisspeptin and its receptor, G-protein coupled receptor 54 (GPR54).[7]

Flowchart 2: Control of catecholamines and dopamine on gonadotropins.

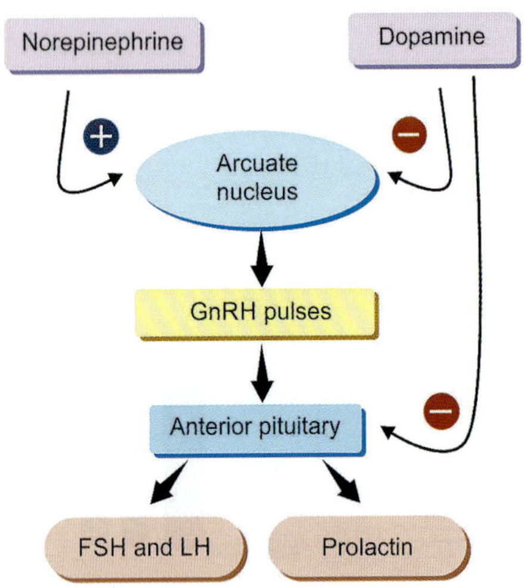

(FSH: follicle-stimulating hormone; GnRH: gonadotropin-releasing hormone; LH: luteinizing hormone)

Neurokinin B (NKB) and dynorphin (Dyn) are cotransmitters of kisspeptin signaling **(Figs. 6A to D)**.[6]

Sex steroids can regulate *Kiss1* gene expression both positively and negatively, depending on the physiological environment. Some studies have demonstrated that administration of kisspeptin, as the longer kisspeptin fragment kisspeptin-54 (Kp54), stimulates gonadotropin secretion in healthy women and in women with hypothalamic amenorrhea. However, another study suggested that kisspeptin-10 does not stimulate gonadotropin secretion in women.[8]

Various studies have shown that intravenous infusion of kisspeptin-10 can stimulate LH pulse frequency in men. This is, however, still a controversial area where more research is needed.[9] Assessment of gonadotropin response to the administration of exogenous kisspeptin provides a novel investigative tool to assess GnRH neuronal function in vivo in reproductive health medicine **(Figs. 7A to C)**.

Kisspeptin agonists may be used to localize lesions causing hypothalamic–pituitary–gonadal axis dysfunction and evaluate the gonadotrophic potential of subfertile individuals. Kisspeptin antagonists may be used as contraceptives in women through the prevention of premature luteinization during in vitro fertilization and also in the treatment of sex steroid-dependent diseases and metastatic cancers.

The role of kisspeptins as ovulation triggers is also being studied extensively.

KISS1R/Kiss1r is desensitized with continuous kisspeptin exposure. In animals, intermittent kisspeptin administration can raise LH levels. However, LH gets suppressed after continuous administration of kisspeptin, as it induced long-lasting depolarization in GnRH neurons, followed by

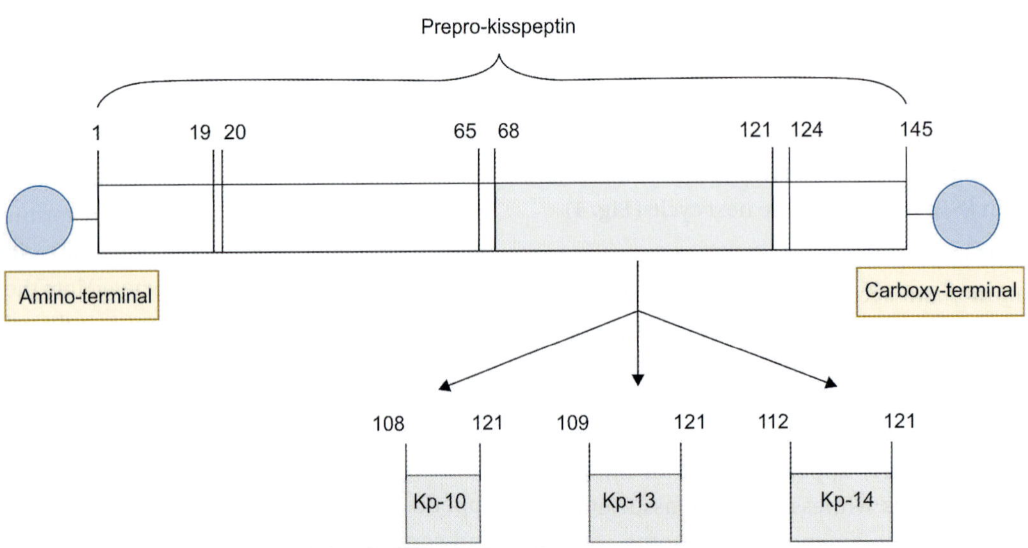

Fig. 5: Structure of kisspeptin (Kp) protein.

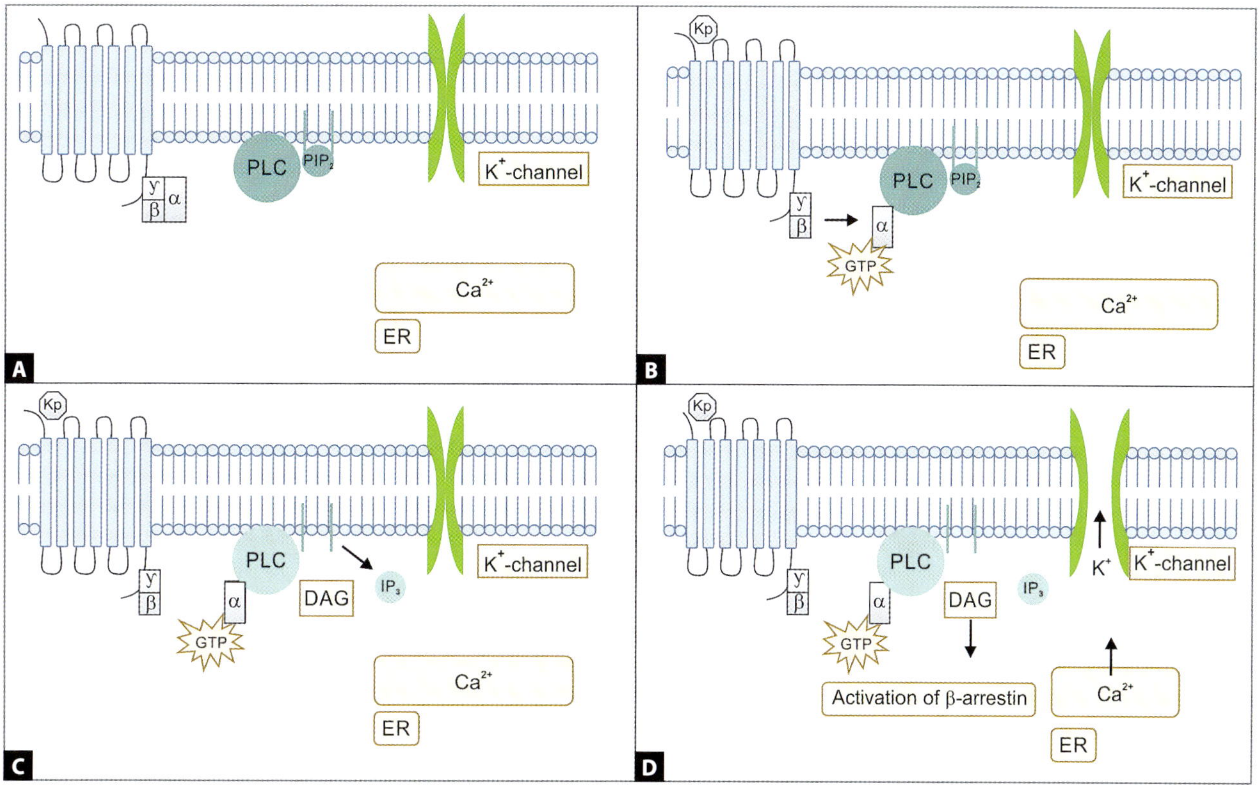

Figs. 6A to D: (A) KISS1R in the dormant state; (B) kisspeptin ligand (Kp) binding activating the G protein subunit, Gq/11α, and subsequently phospholipase C (PLC); (C) PLC activation leading to the formation of inositol-1,4,5-triphosphate (IP_3) and diacylglycerol (DAG); (D) IP_3 causing the release of intracellular calcium (Ca^{2+}) from the endoplasmic reticulum (ER). PLC-independent mechanisms open the potassium (K^+) channels. These events depolarize the kisspeptin neuron. (GTP: guanosine triphosphate; PIP_2: phosphatidyl inositol bisphosphate)[6]

desensitization. This desensitization is not due to GnRH depletion but due to clathrin-mediated internalization of arrestin and KISS1R in internalized vesicles after kisspeptin activation.[6]

Activins, Inhibins, and Follistatins

Intrapituitary cytokines and growth factors provide an autocrine-paracrine system for regulating pituitary cell development and replication as well as pituitary hormone synthesis and secretion. Activins and inhibins are peptide members of the transforming growth factor-beta (TGF-β) superfamily.

Inhibins are secreted by granulosa cells. FSH stimulates secretion of inhibin, and inhibin suppresses FSH secretion. Inhibin blocks synthesis and secretion of FSH, prevents upregulation of GnRH receptors, and at high levels, may also promote degradation of gonadotropins.

The inhibins, named for their inhibitory control of FSH, are composed of two dissimilar peptides linked by disulfide bonds. There are two forms of inhibin that are composed of one of the two inhibin β subunits and a closely related α subunit to form inhibin A or inhibin B. Inhibin B, peaking in mid-follicular phase, amplifies the withdrawal of FSH from other follicles allowing emergence of the dominant follicle. After appearance of LH receptors and formation of corpus luteum (CL), it comes under control of LH and inhibin A dominates. Inhibin has little or no effect on GH, ACTH, and prolactin production.[10,11] Inhibin blocks the synthesis and secretion of FSH, prevents the upregulation of GnRH receptors, and at high levels, may also promote degradation of gonadotropins.

Activins are derived from granulosa cells and pituitary gonadotrophs. They are composed of two subunits identical to the β subunits of inhibin A and B. They augment FSH secretion but inhibit prolactin, ACTH, and GH responses.[11-13] Marked increase in activin tone helps in FSH-dependent follicle selection. Activin increases pituitary response to GnRH by enhancing GnRH receptor formation. The effects of activin are blocked by inhibin and follistatin.[14,15]

Follistatin, also called the FSH-suppressing protein, is a glycopeptide secreted by a variety of pituitary cells, including the gonadotrophs. Its main action is inhibiting FSH synthesis, secretion, and the FSH response to GnRH, probably by binding to and decreasing activity of activin.[16,17] Activin stimulates follistatin production and inhibin prevents this response.

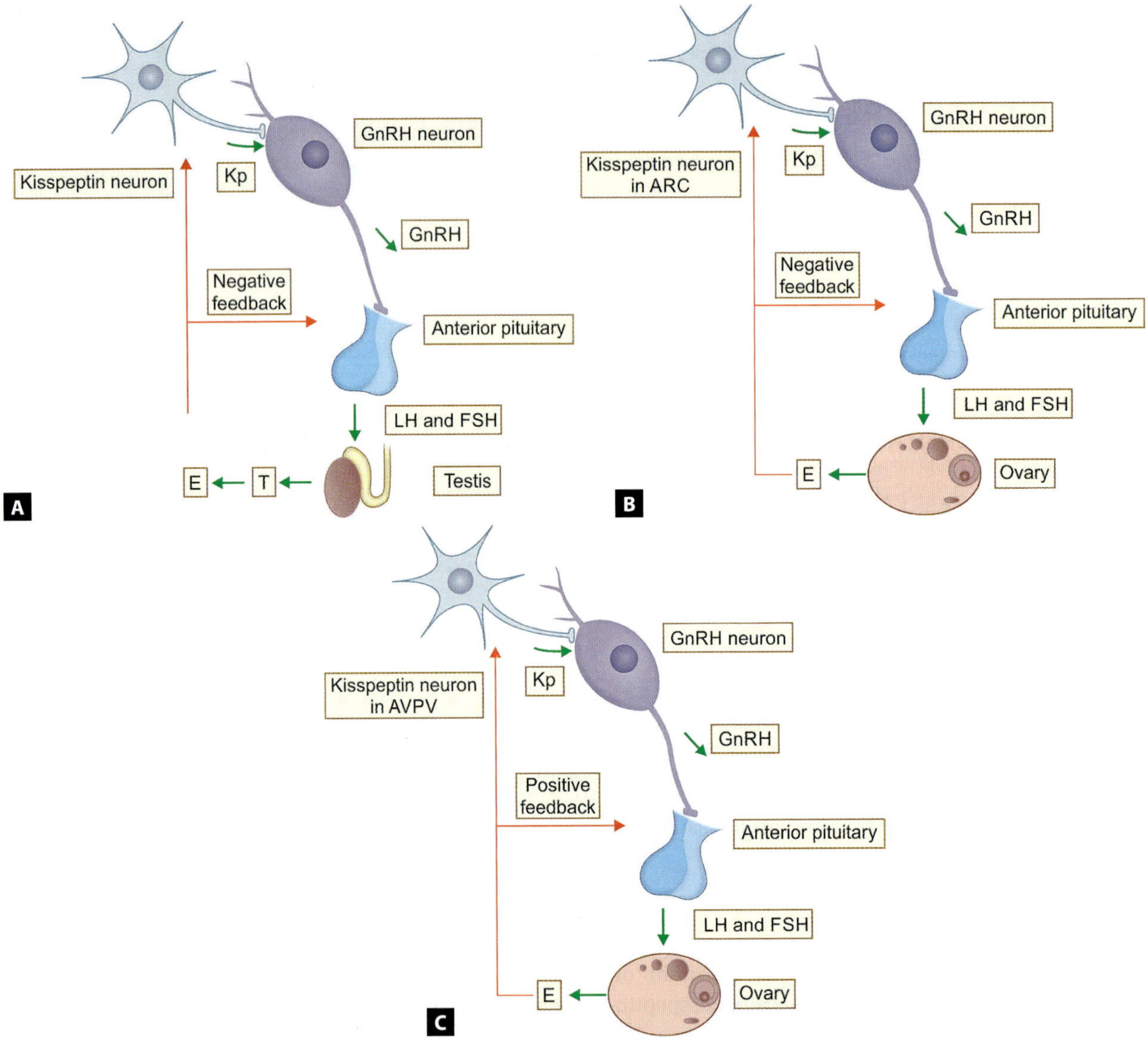

Figs. 7A to C: The diagram shows that (A) kisspeptin (Kp) stimulates gonadotropin-releasing hormone (GnRH) secretion and subsequent gonadotropin release. Testosterone (T) is aromatized to estrogen (E), which exerts negative feedback on the anterior pituitary gland and hypothalamus. (B) E exerts negative feedback on GnRH via Kp neurons in the arcuate nucleus (ARC). (C) E exerts positive feedback on GnRH via Kp neurons in the anteroventral periventricular nucleus (AVPV).
(FSH: follicle-stimulating hormone; LH: luteinizing hormone)

Endogenous Opioids and Effects on Gonadotropin-releasing Hormone

The endogenous opioids are three related families of naturally occurring substances produced in the CNS that represent the natural ligands for the opioid receptors.[18-20] They exert their effects by binding to the G protein-coupled receptors, delta opioid receptor (DOR), kappa opioid receptor (KOR), and mu opioid receptor (MOR). These include:

- *Endorphins* (α, β, γ) are produced in the hypothalamus from the precursor proopiomelanocortin (POMC) with morphine-like activity and help in regulation of temperature, appetite, mood, and behavior.
- *Enkephalins* are most widely distributed opioid peptides in the brain and function primarily in regulation of the autonomic nervous system. Proenkephalin A is the precursor for the two enkephalins of primary importance: Methionine-enkephalin and leucine-enkephalin.
- *Dynorphins* are produced from the precursor prodynorphin that serves a function similar to that of the endorphins, producing behavioral effects and exhibiting high analgesic potency.

Endorphins appear to inhibit GnRH release within the hypothalamus, resulting in inhibition of gonadotropin secretion but have no effect on the pituitary response to GnRH.[21] The principal endogenous opiates affecting GnRH release are β-endorphin and Dyn, probably by modulation of the catecholamine pathway, principally norepinephrine. β-endorphins are 5–10 times more potent than morphine. Ovarian sex steroids can increase the secretion of central endorphins, further depressing gonadotropin levels.[22] Endorphin levels vary significantly throughout the menstrual cycle, with peak levels in the luteal phase and a nadir during menses.[23] The dysphoria experienced by some women in the premenstrual phase of the cycle may be related to a withdrawal of endogenous opiates.

The emerging evidence indicates the participation of opioid peptides in the regulation of reproductive function through a direct local action within reproductive tissues, mainly the endometrium. Various studies have reported the role of these peptides in different phases of endometrial development and implantation; however, more research is needed.[24]

Prolactin

Prolactin is a 198 amino acid polypeptide, with the gene expression occurring in the lactotrophs of the anterior pituitary gland, decidualized endometrium, and the myometrium. The prolactin secreted in these various sites is identical, but differences in messenger ribonucleic acid (mRNA) indicate differences in gene regulation. Three types of prolactin have been identified based on size and structural modifications that are the result of glycosylation, phosphorylation, additions and deletions—little, big, and big-big prolactin.

Prolactin secretion is under tonic inhibitory control by the hypothalamic secretion of dopamine. The dopamine action in the pituitary is mediated by receptors coupled to inhibition of adenylate cyclase. Among the five forms of the dopamine receptor divided into two functional groups, D1 and D2, the D2 type is the predominant receptor in the anterior pituitary gland. Prolactin secretion follows a circadian rhythm, with the maximum secretion 5–8 hours after the onset of sleep. The release is pulsatile with the frequency of pulses reaching maximum in the mid-cycle and then declining in the luteal phase.

Prolactin homeostasis is regulated mainly by prolactin itself, feeding back on the dopamine-releasing neurons. Prolactin gene transcription is principally stimulated by estrogen, thyroid-releasing hormone (TRH), breast manipulation, drugs, stress, exercise, hormones including TRH (explaining the hyperprolactinemia seen with TRH elevation in hypothyroidism), vasopressin, γ-aminobutyric acid (GABA), β-endorphin, vasoactive intestinal peptide, epidermal growth factor (EGF), angiotensin II, and possibly GnRH.[25,26]

It has a direct action on the ovaries, which is responsible for the menstrual irregularities associated with hyperprolactinemia **(Box 1)**.

BOX 1: Effects of hyperprolactinemia on female reproductive function.

- Disrupts normal follicular development
- Inhibits aromatase enzyme
- Premature destruction of the corpus luteum
- Atresia of the dominant follicle
- Inhibits progesterone synthesis by the corpus luteum
- Induces uterine adenomyosis

Other Factors

Prostaglandins and catechol estrogens possibly act as neuromodulators by altering the function of catecholamines through inhibition of tyrosine hydroxylase and competing for the enzyme catechol-O-methyltransferase.

Leptin induces weight loss due to decreased appetite and food consumption and an increase in heat production and activity, associated with a decrease in the NPY expression. The *Lep* gene in humans is located on chromosome 7q31 and leptin receptor gene is located on chromosome 1. Fasting and exercise decrease leptin secretion and increase NPY in the arcuate nucleus. The NPY neurons stimulate feeding and inhibit heat production by inhibiting sympathetic nervous activity.[27]

Ghrelin is a complex hormone that stimulates the release of GH and is secreted mainly in the stomach, intestine, pituitary, hypothalamus, kidney, ovary, testes, and placenta. It is the only hormone known that stimulates food intake. The regulation of food intake occurs via the NPY pathway, with ghrelin and leptin having opposing actions. It is reduced with food intake and increased with fasting.

Differential Control of Follicle-stimulating Hormone and Luteinizing Hormone Secretion

The anterior pituitary secretes the major hormone releasing factors—FSH, LH, TSH, and ACTH along with GH and prolactin. FSH and LH are both glycoproteins that share identical α subunits along with TSH and placental human chorionic gonadotropin (hCG) and differ only in the structure of their β subunits, which confers receptor specificity.

Although secreted from common gonadotrophs, FSH and LH have markedly different functions in the control of ovarian physiology. The divergent control of FSH and LH is achieved through a combination of differential control of their synthesis and secretion by GnRH. The preferential control of FSH synthesis is by the activin/follistatin system, and differential feedback by ovarian steroids and inhibins **(Flowchart 3)**.

Follicle-stimulating Hormone

Follicle-stimulating hormone is essential for follicular growth. It induces estrogen and progesterone secretion at the level of the ovary by activating aromatase and p450 enzymes and exerts negative feedback on GnRH secretion.

Flowchart 3: Role of follicle-stimulating hormone (FSH) and inhibin in controlling ovarian function.

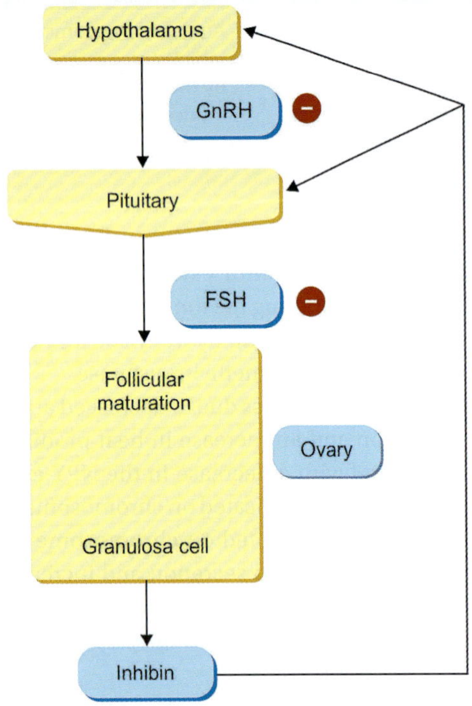

(GnRH: gonadotropin-releasing hormone)

BOX 2: Functions of follicle-stimulating hormone (FSH) in menstrual cycle.

- Selection and maturation of dominant follicle
- Proliferation of granulosa cells
- Aromatization within granulosa cells
- Induction of FSH and LH receptors on granulosa cells
- Production of autocrine–paracrine factors—activin and inhibin
- FSH surge helps in ovulation
- Prevents germ cells from atresia in luteal–follicular transition

(LH: luteinizing hormone)

FSH further induces the proliferation of granulosa cells and expression of FSH and LH receptors on granulosa cells. The rise in FSH during the LH surge helps in ovulation by stimulating plasminogen activator activity **(Box 2)**.

Luteinizing Hormone

Luteinizing hormone is secreted by the anterior pituitary gland and is required for both growth of preovulatory follicles, and ovulation and luteinization of the dominant follicle. During the follicular phase of the menstrual cycle, LH induces androgen synthesis by theca cells that is essential for robust steroidogenesis; stimulates proliferation, differentiation, and secretion of follicular thecal cells; and increases LH receptors on granulosa cells. The preovulatory LH surge drives the oocyte into the first meiotic division and initiates luteinization of thecal and granulosa cells. The resulting CL produces high levels of progesterone and some estrogen.

TABLE 2: Impact of different concentrations of luteinizing hormone (LH) on the menstrual cycle.

Effects below LH threshold	***Effects within LH window***	***Effects above LH ceiling***
Absent paracrine signaling between granulosa and theca	Normal follicular growth and development	Suppression of granulosa proliferation
Inadequate androgen and estrogen synthesis	Adequate granulosa proliferation and functional maturation	Follicular premature luteinization
Compromised oocyte maturation	Normal estrogen and androgen biosynthesis	Compromised oocyte development
	Optimum oocyte maturation	

The LH-dependent phase of preovulatory follicular development proceeds normally only if LH is present at concentrations within the *LH window*, which is over the threshold level and beneath the ceiling value **(Table 2)**.

Pharmacogenomics—Follicle-stimulating Hormone and Luteinizing Hormone Polymorphisms

Response to hormones depends on variations in the gene sequence of the receptor or the ligand. Association studies assess whether a gene variant is present more often than expected in a population and evaluate whether a medical condition or a phenotype is associated with a gene variant. Gene variants may consist of insertions or deletions of one or more bases, or may be single-base changes, known as single-nucleotide polymorphisms (SNPs). A genetic variant is considered a polymorphism when it reaches a frequency higher than 1% in a sample population; otherwise, it is considered a gene mutation.

With the advent of pharmacogenomics, various polymorphisms have been identified that may lead to impaired responses to various hormones (FSH and LH) and steroids (estrogen and progesterone). The effects of variations in different biochemical pathways involved in estrogen production and action (aromatase and estrogen receptor genes), folliculogenesis [bone morphogenetic protein 15 (BMP15), growth differentiation factor-9 (GDF-9), and anti-Müllerian hormone (AMH)], and other areas have been observed. These variations may alter the response to controlled ovarian stimulation (COS). In this chapter, we will discuss about the common variations in FSH and LH hormones and their receptors.

Follicle-stimulating Hormone Polymorphism

With advancements in the pharmacogenomics, various polymorphisms have been identified that attribute to altered function and efficacy of FSH.

Follicle-stimulating hormone works by binding to its specific receptor, the follicle-stimulating hormone receptor (*FSHR*, gene ID: 2492, location: 2p21-p16, OMIM: 136435). Research now highlights the role of common genetic variants of *FSHR* and FSH beta subunit (*FSHB*, gene ID: 14308, location: 11p13, OMIM: 136530) in the determination of individual serum hormone levels and target organ response. However, controversies exist concerning the impact of genetic polymorphisms of these genes on gonadotropin treatment and some contradictory findings have been published, necessitating further research.[28]

The current evidence suggests that the combination of *FSHR* and *FSHB* genotypes is predicted to have a much stronger impact than either one alone, on both male and female gonadal function. This is because about 20% of people are carriers of the allele combinations associated with lower serum FSH levels and lower *FSHR* expression or activity. The advent of powerful, sensitive, and inexpensive techniques assessing several SNPs simultaneously will be very helpful in the identification of the patients at infertility risk.[29]

The *FSHR* gene is located at chromosome region 2p21 and consists of 10 exons. A large number of SNPs in the gene have been identified (1,488 SNPs). The most common and well-studied SNPs in *FSHR* are Thr307Ala (rs6165) and Asn680Ser (rs6166). Both polymorphisms are located within exon 10, where Thr307Ala is located in the extracellular domain of the protein (the hormone-binding area) and Asn680Ser is located in the intracellular domain. These two polymorphisms are in near complete linkage disequilibrium.

The *FSHR* 680Ser variant is usually associated with elevated basal levels of FSH and elevated gonadotropin requirements during COS. A29 polymorphism reduces expression of *FSHR*. S680 is a "resistance factor" to FSH stimulation determining a higher ovarian threshold of the gonadotropin and reflecting a different pattern of ovarian secretion during the cycle transition phase. Another *FSHR* polymorphism, G/A, located in the promoter region at position 29, could modulate ovarian response to FSH and may require higher gonadotropin doses for COS.

The Asn680 allele has been found to be a risk factor and predictor of severity of symptoms for ovarian hyperstimulation syndrome (OHSS).[29]

Luteinizing Hormone Polymorphism

Luteinizing hormone beta (LHB) polypeptide encodes the beta subunit of the hormone and determines the specificity of binding to luteinizing hormone/choriogonadotropin receptor (LHCGR). LH has a key role in steroidogenesis and folliculogenesis (with FSH), ovulation, and luteinization.

The *LHB* gene is located at chromosome region 11p13 and has three exons. A number of polymorphisms in the gene have been identified (179 SNPs). Three polymorphisms in the coding area have been found to lead to decreased LH activity: Polymorphisms Trp8Arg and Ile15Thr have been associated with slightly suppressed fertility, menstrual irregularities causing infertility and recurrent pregnancy loss, and the Gly102Ser SNP has been associated with infertility and menstrual disorders.[29]

Luteinizing hormone receptor: LH exerts its actions by binding to its cell surface receptor, *LHR* (also known as LHCGR, as LH and hCG bind to the same receptor). The *LHR* gene is located at chromosome region 2p21, consisting of 11 exons, and several common polymorphisms have been identified (over 520 SNPs). Polymorphisms 18insLeuGln, Asn291Ser, and Ser312Asn in the *LHR* gene are associated with increased receptor activity, and their possible effects in steroid hormone-related diseases have been suggested, though still not established.[29]

Hypothalamic–Pituitary–Ovarian Axis

In the presence of a GnRH pulse, the pituitary and ovarian hormones exert mutual control over the circulating levels of one another. The complex interactions between pituitary and ovarian hormones involve forward control, positive feedback, and negative feedback mechanisms and serve to sustain a self-perpetuating monthly endocrine cycle **(Fig. 8)**.

Ovarian Feedback on the Hypothalamus and Pituitary

Estrogen

Estrogen produced at the level of the ovary is crucial for the development of the antrum and maturation of the

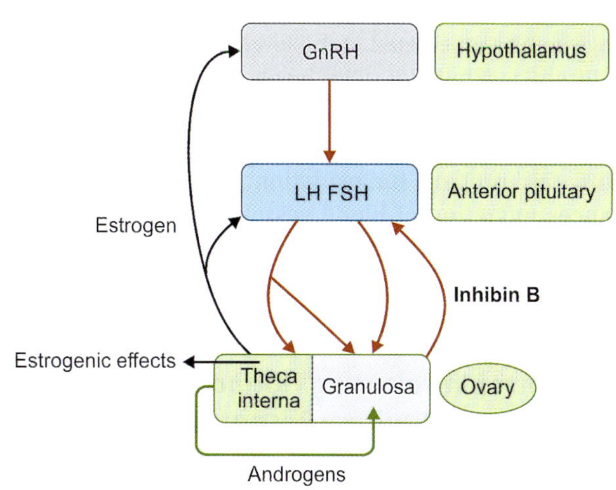

Fig. 8: Hypothalamic–pituitary–ovarian axis.
(FSH: follicle-stimulating hormone; GnRH: gonadotropin-releasing hormone; LH: luteinizing hormone)

Flowchart 4: Hypothalamic and ovarian control of pituitary secretions.

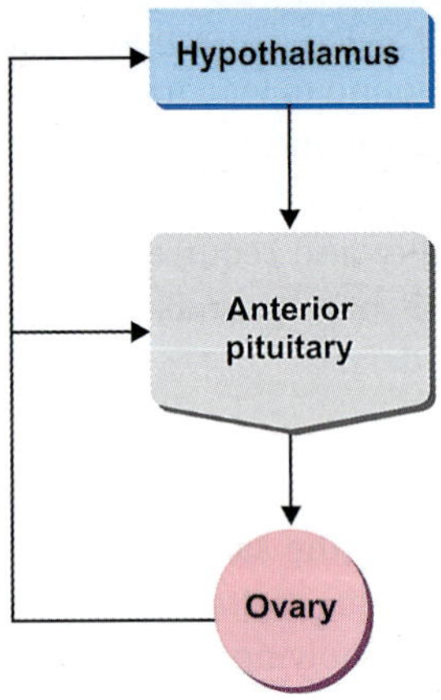

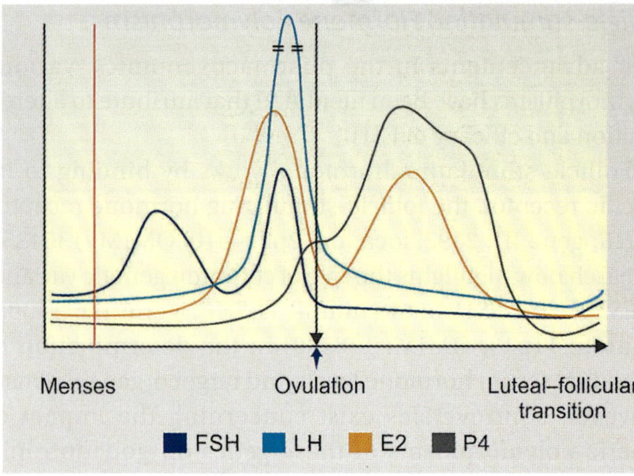

Fig. 9: Pituitary and ovarian hormonal interrelationships during the menstrual cycle.
(E2: estradiol; FSH: follicle-stimulating hormone; LH: luteinizing hormone; P4: progesterone)

Graafian follicle. Estrogen is predominant at the end of the follicular phase, directly preceding ovulation. Estradiol, the most potent and abundant estrogen, is primarily derived from androgens produced by thecal cells. The androgens migrate from the theca cells to the granulosa cells, where they are converted into estradiol by aromatase enzyme. The actions of estradiol include induction of FSH receptors on granulosa cells, proliferation and secretion of follicular and thecal cells, induction of LH receptors on granulosa cells, and proliferation of endometrial stromal and epithelial cells. At low circulating levels, estrogens exert negative feedback on FSH and LH secretion, and at very high levels, estrogens exert positive feedback on LH secretion.[30] Estrogen further induces proliferation of estrogen-converting granulosa cells and synthesis of estrogen receptors, establishing a positive feedback loop on itself. In the endometrial cycle, estrogen induces proliferation of the endometrial glands **(Flowchart 4)**.

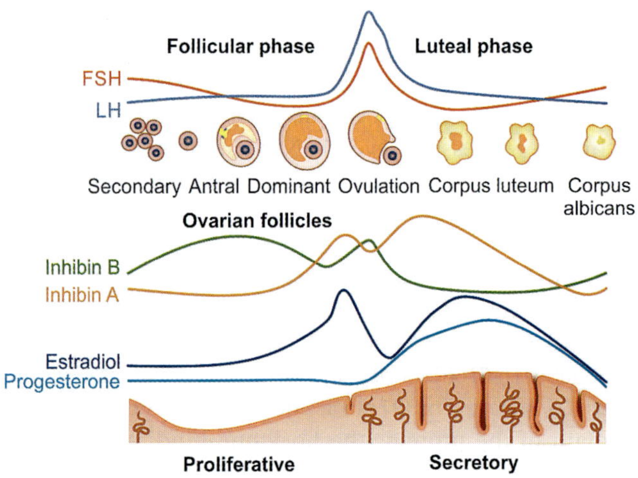

Fig. 10: Overview of hormonal and peptide variations in the menstrual cycle.
(FSH: follicle-stimulating hormone; LH: luteinizing hormone)

Progesterone

Progesterone is secreted at the level of the ovary, primarily by luteinized follicles. The levels increase just prior to ovulation and peak 5–7 days postovulation. It stimulates the release of proteolytic enzymes from thecal cells that ultimately prepare for ovulation. Progesterone further induces migration of blood vessels into the follicle wall and stimulates prostaglandin secretion in follicular tissues. During the luteal phase, progesterone induces swelling and increased secretion of the endometrium **(Flowchart 4)**.

Gonadotropin-releasing Hormone Dynamics and Pituitary Responsiveness

The interplay between pituitary and ovarian hormones gives rise to a stereotyped pattern of hormone levels during the menstrual cycle. The graph shows relative hormone trends in an average 28-day cycle **(Fig. 9)**.

Physiology of Menstrual Cycle

Following the exhaustive discussion about the neuroendocrinological control and the hypothalamic–pituitary–ovarian (HPO) axis, the understanding of the physiology of menstrual cycle becomes comprehensive. The menstrual cycle is divided into four phases based on the ovarian cycle as described below **(Fig. 10)**.

1. Follicular phase (further classified into early- and late-follicular phases)
2. Ovulatory phase
3. Luteal phase
4. Luteal–follicular transition phase.

Based on the uterine cycle, it may be divided into:

- Proliferative phase
- Secretory phase
- Menstruation

Ovarian Cycle

The menstrual cycle is divided into four phases based on the ovarian cycle.

Follicular Phase

The follicular phase of the menstrual cycle spans from the first day of menstruation until ovulation. The primary goal is to develop a viable follicle capable of undergoing ovulation. The early events of the follicular phase are initiated by a rise in FSH levels at the luteal–follicular transition attributed to a decrease in progesterone, estrogen, and inhibin levels at the end of the previous cycle and the subsequent removal of inhibition of FSH. Rise of FSH rescues a cohort of preantral follicles from apoptosis—a phenomenon called recruitment, which requires a certain minimum concentration of FSH called *FSH threshold*. The time frame for which this threshold surpasses the level of FSH needs to be maintained for follicular recruitment and growth. This is called *FSH window* **(Fig. 11)**.

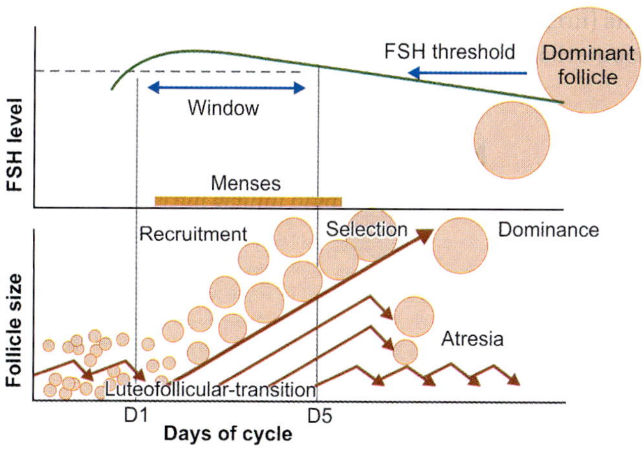

Fig. 11: Concept of follicle-stimulating hormone (FSH) window and threshold.

This requires an orderly sequence of events and a series of sequential actions of hormones and autocrine-paracrine peptides on the follicle, through a period of initial growth from a primordial follicle through the stages of the preantral, antral, and preovulatory follicle.[31,32] As folliculogenesis has already been described in another chapter, this chapter only discusses the physiological attributes of the ovarian events **(Fig. 12)**.

Primordial Follicle

The primordial germ cells originate in the endoderm of the yolk sac, allantois, and hindgut of the embryo and by 5–6 weeks of gestation, they have migrated to the genital ridge. A rapid mitotic multiplication of germ cells begins at 6–8 weeks of pregnancy, and by 16–20 weeks, the maximum number of oocytes reaches to a total of 6–7 millions in both ovaries.[33] The primordial follicle is nongrowing and consists of an oocyte, arrested in the diplotene stage of meiotic prophase, surrounded by a single layer of spindle- shaped granulosa cells.

Until the follicle numbers are exhausted, some grow while some undergo atresia, uninterrupted by even pregnancy, ovulation, or periods of anovulation, continuing through infancy and up to menopause. The rate of decrease in follicle number is proportional to the total number present, implying that the most rapid decrease occurs before birth resulting in 2 million oocytes at birth and 300,000 at puberty. Out of these, about 400 follicles will ovulate during a woman's reproductive years[33] **(Fig. 13)**.

Intrafollicle signaling regulating primordial follicle activation: The phosphatidylinositol 3-kinase (PI3K) pathway, the mechanistic target of rapamycin complex 1 (mTORC1) pathway, the p27Kip1 (p27) cyclin-dependent kinase (CDK) system, and several oocyte-specific transcription factors have been shown to play roles in regulating the activation of dormant oocytes in the mammalian ovary.

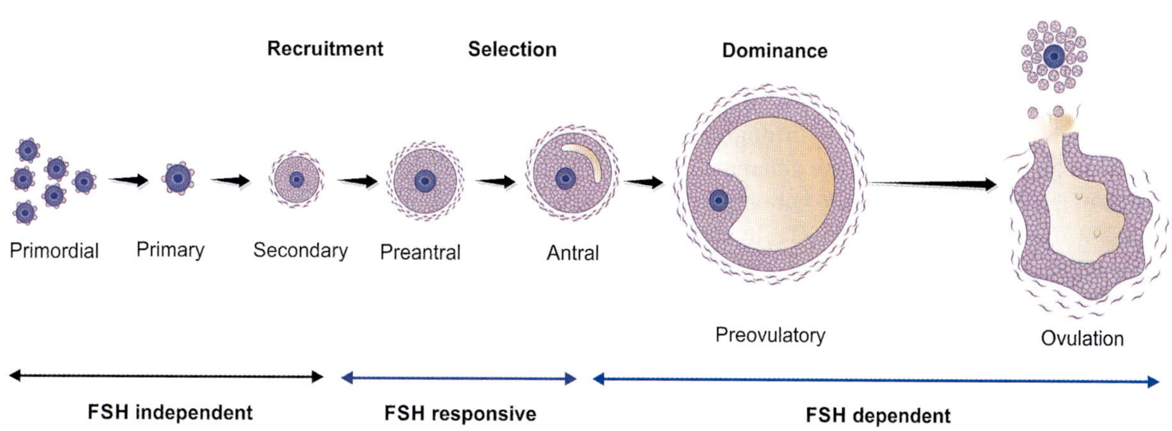

Fig. 12: Stages of follicular growth. (FSH: follicle-stimulation hormone)

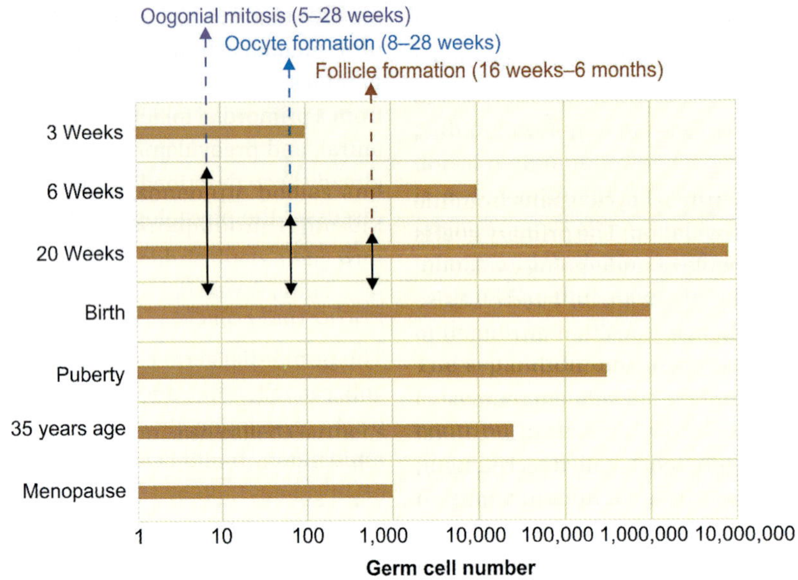

Fig. 13: Changes in germ cell numbers in relation to age.

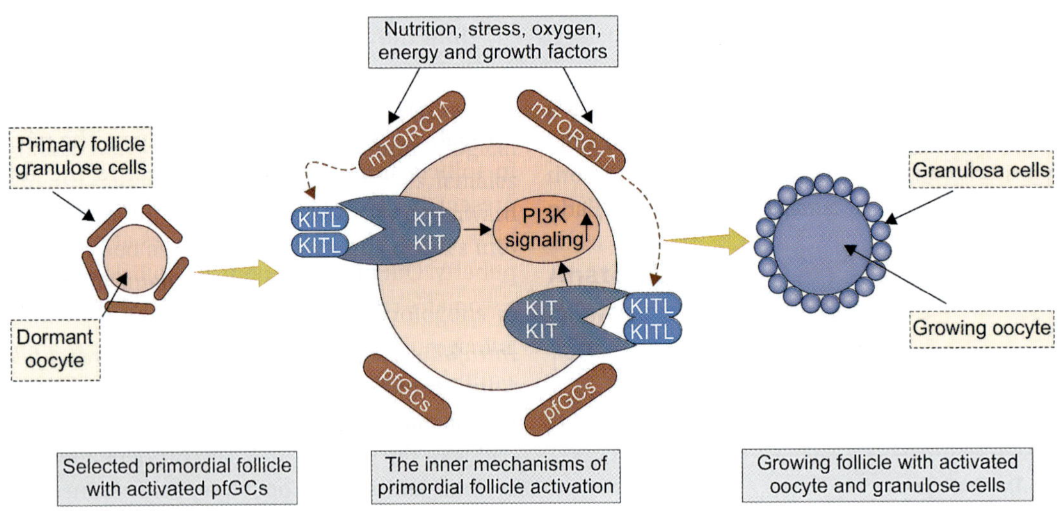

Fig. 14: Primordial follicle activation model for the mammalian ovary.
(KITL: KIT ligand; mTORC1: mechanistic target of rapamycin complex 1; pfGCs: primordial follicle granulosa cells; PI3K: phosphatidylinositol 3-kinase)

Recent evidence suggests that the somatic primordial follicle granulosa cells (pfGCs) play an important role in initiating the activation of primordial follicles in the adult ovary. It is primarily achieved through mTORC1 activation in pfGCs, which mediates the differentiation and proliferation of the flattened pfGCs into cuboidal granulosa cells and simultaneously promotes KIT ligand (KITL) expression. KITL secreted from the pfGCs subsequently binds to the KIT receptor on the oocyte surface, resulting in the phosphorylation of KIT Y719, which then activates intraoocyte PI3K signaling. The PI3K signaling in the dormant oocytes is then responsible for triggering the events that awaken the oocyte from its quiescence into a robust developmental state.[34]

In the adult mammalian ovary, only a small proportion of dormant primordial follicles are awakened to move on to further developmental stages. In response to stimulation by nutrition and other factors, the mTORC1 signaling is activated in the pfGCs of selected primordial follicles, leading to their differentiation and proliferation. The activated mTORC1 signaling in pfGCs also stimulates an upregulation of KITL secretion. KITL binds to KIT on the surface of the dormant oocyte, which leads to activation of PI3K signaling. Activated PI3K signaling in oocytes awakens the dormant oocytes and stimulates their growth **(Fig. 14)**.

The application of this understanding of primordial follicle activation could be beneficial for women with low ovarian reserve and for cancer survivors.

Primary Follicle

With multiplication of the cuboidal granulosa cells, the primordial follicle becomes a primary follicle. The granulosa cell layer gets separated from the stromal cells by a basement membrane called the basal lamina. The stromal cells are further subdivided into theca interna and theca externa.

Rescue from atresia: The early growth of follicles occurs over the time span of several menstrual cycles, approximately 85 days. The follicle destined to ovulate is one of a cohort that is recruited at the luteal-follicular transition.[35] Until a late stage, the growth is independent of hormonal regulation.[36] Eventually, this cohort of follicles reaches a stage where unless recruited or rescued by FSH, it is doomed toward apoptosis, a programmed physiologic cell death.[37]

Recruitment is the process by which the cohort of follicles responding to FSH at the beginning of the cycle gets rescued from apoptosis and competes for the selection of the dominant follicle.

Early signs of follicular development are an increase in the size of the oocyte, cuboidal pattern of granulosa cells—a change from their original squamous shape and the appearance of gap junctions between the granulosa cells and the oocyte, essential for nutritional, metabolite, and signal interchange **(Fig. 15)**.

Follicular atresia is regulated by endocrine factors, such as FSH and LH, and by paracrine factors, including insulin-like growth factor 1 (IGF-1), EGF, basic fibroblast growth factor (bFGF), tumor necrosis factor-alpha (TNF-α), interleukin 6 (IL-6), and others.

Preantral Follicle

With accelerated growth promoted by the gonadotropins, the granulosa cells undergo a multicellular proliferation leading to an increased production of not only estrogen but also other steroids, such as androgens and progestins. The oocyte also enlarges and is surrounded by zona pellucida, an acellular glycoprotein membrane. FSH receptors are acquired through which FSH aromatizes androgens to estrogens, generating an *estrogenic microenvironment.*[38] Together, FSH and estrogen synergistically promote a rapid accumulation of FSH receptors, allowing the follicle to respond to relatively low concentrations of FSH **(Fig. 15)**.

Androgens have a complex role in early follicular development. At low concentrations, androgens serve as a substrate for FSH-induced aromatization to the extent of even enhancing the enzyme. But, in androgen-rich environment, the limited capacity of aromatization is overwhelmed and the preantral granulosa cells instead favor the conversion of androgens to more potent 5α-reduced androgens.[39] These androgens inhibit aromatase activity and FSH-induced LH receptor formation as they cannot convert to estrogen leading the follicle toward atresia.[40,41] Hence, the fate of the preantral follicle is in delicate balance depending on the ability to convert an androgen-dominant microenvironment to an estrogen-dominated microenvironment for survival **(Box 3)**.

Formation of gap junctions: Oocytes are unable to use glucose, as an energy source to support meiotic maturation, cannot transport certain amino acids, and lack both the enzymes

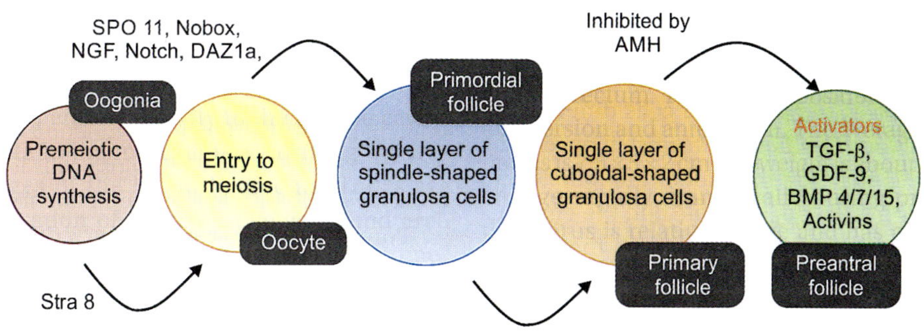

Activators	Inhibitors
Kit ligand	AMH
GDF-9	Foxl2
FGF-2	PTEN
BMP-4/7/15	p27
C-kit	
LIF	

Fig. 15: Series of events in follicular development. Note the genes involved in early stages of folliculogenesis.
[AMH: anti-Müllerian hormone; BMP: bone morphogenetic protein; DNA: deoxyribonucleic acid; FGF-2: basic fibroblast growth factor; GDF-9: growth differentiation factor-9; LIF: leukemia inhibitory factor; NGF: nerve growth factor; Nobox (expressed in germ cells): newborn ovary homeobox; PTEN: tumor suppressor gene (phosphatase and tensin homolog deleted on chromosome 10); TGF-β, transforming growth factor-β]

BOX 3: Role of androgens.

- Substrate for aromatization into estrogens within granulosa cells at low levels—estrogenic microenvironment
- Enhance atresia of less mature follicles
- Systemic effect of stimulating libido periovulation

necessary for cholesterol synthesis and the receptors for its uptake. This is overcome by the presence of gap junctions that link the oocytes to the granulosa cells. Their role is to allow passage of small molecules such as ions (e.g., calcium), metabolites (e.g., pyruvate, nucleic acids, and inositol), amino acids (e.g., L-alanine), cholesterol, and intracellular signaling molecules [e.g., cyclic adenosine monophosphate (cAMP)] between granulosa cells and oocytes. In mice, targeted deletions of gap junction proteins (known as connexins) disrupt follicular and oocyte development.

Consequently, oocytes are dependent on adjacent granulosa cells for growth and multiplication of the granulosa cells and for nutrition, metabolism, transport, and regulation of oocyte development.[42,43] In turn, oocytes stimulate glycolysis, amino acid transport, and cholesterol synthesis in granulosa cells via paracrine and juxtacrine signals to meet their demands. Connexin expression in ovarian follicles is upregulated by FSH and downregulated by LH.[44] In addition, FSH maintains an open channel in the gap junctions, a pathway that is closed by LH.[45] After ovulation, the gap junctions are important in the CL, where their function is regulated by locally produced oxytocin.[46]

The bulk of oocyte growth occurs in preantral follicles, where the oocyte is closely associated with relatively undifferentiated granulosa cells. Upon follicular antrum formation, which approximately corresponds to the end of the oocyte growth phase, the granulosa cells differentiate into two anatomically and functionally distinct lineages: The mural granulosa cells that line the wall of the follicle and that have principally a steroidogenic role and the cumulus cells (CCs) form an intimate association with the oocyte. CCs possess highly specialized transzonal cytoplasmic projections that penetrate through the zona pellucida and form gap junctions at their tips with the oocyte, forming an elaborate structure called the cumulus-oocyte complex (COC).

Antral Follicle

Follicular fluid accumulated in the intercellular spaces of the granulosa eventually coalesces into a cavity—the antrum. This fluid being rich in hormones, growth factors, and cytokines, nurtures the oocyte. The granulosa cells surrounding the oocyte form the cumulus oophorus. LH is normally not present in the fluid until the mid-cycle. Antral follicles with the lowest androgen/estrogen ratios are most likely to house a healthy oocyte.[47] The synthesis of steroids is functionally compartmentalized within the follicle as the two-cell system.

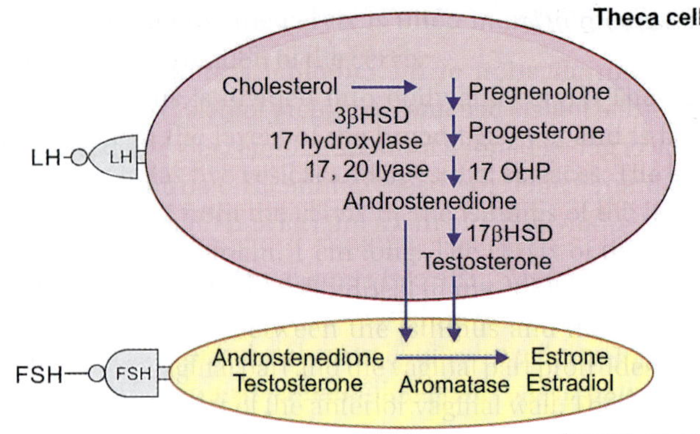

Fig. 16: Two-cell, two-gonadotropin concept.
(FSH: follicle-stimulating hormone; HSD: hydroxysteroid dehydrogenase; LH: luteinizing hormone; OHP: hydroxyprogesterone)

Two-cell, two-gonadotropin concept in follicle selection: FSH receptors are present only on the granulosa cells. LH receptors are present only on theca cells.[48] LH optimizes final stages of maturation. FSH-stimulated estrogen production from the granulosa cells is dependent on LH-stimulated androgen production by the theca cells. This is not fully functional until the later part of antral development. Theca cells are characterized by expression of LH receptors, 3β-hydroxysteroid dehydrogenase, and cyp-P450c 17, which are essential for internalizing low-density lipoprotein (LDL) cholesterol into mitochondria and thereby converting 21 carbons to androgens.[49] Granulosa cells lack these receptors and in fact express FSH receptors and cyp-450 aromatase to convert androgen substrate from theca into estrogens. Increased expression of aromatase indicates increased follicular maturity. Exclusive function of P450c 17 in theca cells and aromatase in granulosa cells is the basic principle of the two-cell, two-gonadotropin theory.[50]

Pure FSH treatment causes early development of follicles, but estradiol production is limited.[51,52] Some aromatization occurs from the androgens of adrenal glands, but robust steroidogenesis is not possible. Only a follicle with more number of FSH receptors, higher aromatase activity, and robust steroidogenesis is selected as dominant follicle **(Fig. 16)**.

Selection of the dominant follicle: The successful conversion to an estrogen-dominant follicle marks the selection of a follicle destined to ovulate. This process is attributed to a few of the estrogen actions, namely positive influence of estrogen on FSH within the maturing follicle and a negative feedback relationship with FSH at the hypothalamic-pituitary level serving to withdraw gonadotropin support. The dominant follicle, with its high concentration of FSH receptors, continues to acquire more FSH even as FSH levels decrease. The remaining, poorly FSH receptor-endowed follicles ultimately show reduced aromatase activity, granulosa proliferation, and function and hence undergo an irreversible atretic change.

The dominant follicle matures and secretes increasing amounts of estradiol, which is essential for its complete maturation. At this critical moment, estrogen exerts positive feedback on LH, generating a dramatic preovulatory LH surge.

Tumor necrosis factor-α, which is produced in the granulosa cells, inhibits FSH stimulation of estradiol secretion, except in the dominant follicle.[53]

Selection of the dominant follicle is established during days 5–7, and consequently, peripheral levels of estradiol begin to rise significantly by day 7 of the cycle.[54] The dominant follicle has two significant advantages, mainly its acquisition of a greater content of FSH receptors due to a rate of granulosa proliferation that surpasses the proliferation of its cohorts and the enhancement of FSH action because of its high intrafollicular estrogen concentration, a consequence of local autocrine–paracrine molecules. Thus, the dominant follicle is more sensitive to FSH, and as long as a critical duration of FSH exposure is initially present, the dominant follicle continues to develop.[55] Improved theca vascularity allowing a preferential delivery of gonadotropins to the dominant follicle also contributes.[54]

In order to respond to LH surge and become a CL, granulosa cells must acquire LH receptors. With increasing concentrations of estrogen, FSH changes its focus of action from upregulation of FSH receptors to upregulation of LH receptors.[56] Moreover, LH can induce development of its own receptors in FSH-primed granulosa cells. LH plays a critical role in the final stages of follicular development, providing support for final follicular maturation.[57,58]

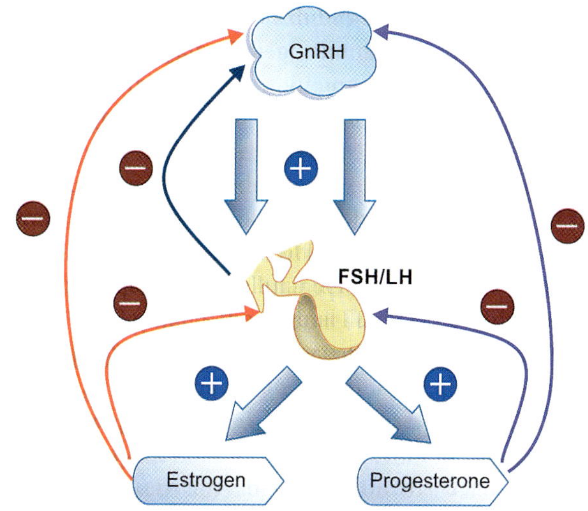

Fig. 17: Feedback mechanism.
(FSH: follicle-stimulating hormone; GnRH: gonadotropin-releasing hormone; LH: luteinizing hormone)

TABLE 3: Role of mid-cycle surge of gonadotropins.

LH surge	***FSH surge***
Resumption of meiosis in the oocyte	Frees the oocyte from follicular attachments → free floating oocyte in the antral fluid
Luteinization of granulosa cells to secrete progesterone	LH receptors on granulosa cells → adequate luteal function
Cumulus expansion	Cumulus expansion
Prostaglandin and eicosanoid synthesis → follicular rupture	Plasminogen → plasmin: Follicular rupture
LDL cholesterol internalization → corpus luteum steroidogenesis	

(FSH: follicle-stimulating hormone; LDL: low-density lipoprotein; LH: luteinizing hormone)

Feedback System

The FSH secretion is very sensitive to the negative inhibitory effects of estrogen at low levels, and at higher levels, this effect of estrogen is supplemented by inhibin. In contrast, the transition from suppression to stimulation of LH release occurs as estradiol fulfills two critical events—estradiol concentration rising above 200 pg/mL and sustained for about 50 hours, usually occurring when the dominant follicle reaches 15 mm in diameter[59,60] **(Fig. 17)**.

Preovulatory Follicle

The preovulatory follicle gets a hyperemic appearance with the granulosa cells enlarging and acquiring lipid inclusions and the theca cells getting vacuolated and vascular. The oocyte also proceeds in meiosis, approaching completion of its reduction division. Approaching maturity, the preovulatory follicle, produces increasing amounts of estrogen, peaking at 24–36 hours prior to ovulation.[61] The onset of LH surge occurs when peak levels of estradiol are reached. In providing the ovulatory stimulus to the selected follicle, the LH surge seals the fate of the remaining follicles, with their lower estrogen and FSH content, by further increasing the androgen superiority.

Luteinizing hormone promotes luteinization of the granulosa in the dominant follicle producing progesterone, which via its own receptors and only after adequate estrogen priming facilitates the positive feedback of estrogen on LH. If administered before the estrogen stimulus or in doses high enough to achieve a blood level >2 ng/mL, progesterone blocks the mid-cycle LH surge. Hence, appropriate low levels of progesterone derived from the maturing follicle contribute to the precise synchronization of the mid-cycle LH and the FSH surge **(Table 3)**.

With the smaller follicles undergoing atresia, theca cells form the stromal tissue, enhancing androgen production to enhance libido and accelerate atresia.

Role of inhibin, activin, follistatin, and growth factors: The actions of these factors come together as described here.

Inhibin and activin regulate androgen synthesis in theca cells.[62] Inhibin enhances and activin suppresses the stimulatory action of LH and/or IGF-1 on thecal androgen synthesis, and inhibin can overcome the inhibitory action of activin. In the granulosa cells of immature follicles in the early follicular phase, activin enhances FSH activities, including FSH receptor expression, aromatization, and LH receptor expression, while simultaneously suppressing theca androgen synthesis to allow estrogen microenvironment.[63] Inhibin B reaching a peak in the mid-follicular phase amplifies the withdrawal of FSH from other follicles allowing the emergence of the dominant follicle. In the late-follicular phase, rise in levels of inhibin B and reduced activin promote androgen synthesis in the theca in response to LH and IGF-2 to provide substrate for even greater estrogen production in the granulosa, which will act to trigger LH surge.

In the mature granulosa of the dominant preovulatory follicle, activin serves to prevent premature luteinization and progesterone production. Activin further peaks at menses allowing FSH to rise appropriately at the time of luteal-follicular transition.

Insulin-like growth factors and binding proteins help in folliculogenesis. Binding proteins help in function of growth factors. Insulin-like growth factor-binding protein 4 (IGFBP-4) decreases the availability of IGF-1 and dominant follicles have IGFBP-4 protease and increased availability of growth factors. Role of IGF-2 is clearer in folliculogenesis, as in Laron-type dwarfism, there is a deficiency of IGF-1 but normal folliculogenesis.[64] IGF-2, being the most abundant IGF in human ovarian follicles, has a vital role in stimulating estrogen production and granulosa cell mitosis.[65] It facilitates the action of FSH on the granulosa cells and the action of LH on the theca cells.

Ovulation

Ovulation is the phase of menstrual cycle in which a mature egg is released from the ovarian follicle into the fallopian tube. In humans, ovulation occurs about midway through the menstrual cycle, after the follicular phase. The few days surrounding ovulation (from approximately days 10 to 18 of a 28-day cycle) constitute the most fertile phase.

Ovulation occurs in the morning in springs and in the evening in autumn and winter. It occurs 55% of the time from the right ovary. Oocytes from the right ovary are said to have a higher potential for pregnancy.[66] Contralateral ovulation favors pregnancy more than ipsilateral ovulation, while ipsilateral ovulation occurs more with advancing age.[67]

The underlying physiology of ovulation is complex. The pulsatile GnRH secretion forms an important prerequisite for normal pituitary secretion. However, the feedback responses regulating gonadotropin levels are controlled primarily by ovarian steroid feedback on the anterior pituitary cells.

The inhibiting tone of endogenous opiates is reduced at the time of the ovulatory surge, allowing a release from suppression. This is probably a response to estrogen-induced decrease in opioid receptor binding and subsequent opioid release.

The primary oocyte is in a state of arrest in the late prophase of meiosis I.[33] Until ovulation, high cAMP levels inhibit resumption of meiosis of the oocyte. During the surge, LH blocks cAMP transport into the oocyte, thus removing inhibition of meiosis and allowing meiosis to resume. Meiosis suppression by oocyte maturation inhibitor and luteinization inhibitor is also removed.[68] LH surge causes disruption of gap junctions, and the transport of cAMP from granulosa cells to oocytes is halted. Gap junction integrity in the oocyte is also contributed by nitric oxide (NO). NO resists resumption of meiosis and breakdown of gap junctions until a massive LH surge overcomes this resistance.

The LH surge also induces release of proteolytic enzymes in association with FSH rise, which degrade the cells at the surface of the follicle, and stimulates angiogenesis in the follicular wall and prostaglandin secretion. These effects of LH cause the follicle to swell and rupture. LH surge also causes luteinization of granulosa cells, progesterone production, expansion of cumulus, and production of prostaglandins.

At ovulation, the secondary oocyte (arrested until fertilization in the metaphase of meiosis II) and its surrounding corona radiata are expelled into the peritoneal cavity. The oocyte adheres to the ovary and the muscular contractions of the fallopian tube bring the oocyte into contact with the tubal epithelium to initiate migration through the oviduct.

The onset of the LH surge appears to be the most reliable indicator of impending ovulation, occurring 34–36 hours prior to follicle rupture.[69] The LH surge usually lasts for 48–50 hours.[69] Threshold concentration of LH must be maintained for 14–27 hours for full maturation of oocytes to occur.[70] Ovulation occurs 10–12 hours after LH peak and 24–36 hours after estradiol peak.[71,72]

The LH surge tends to occur at around 3:00 AM, beginning between midnight and 8:00 AM in over two-third of women.[60] LH may be detectable in the urine by evening.

Progesterone rise increases the distensibility of the follicular wall and promotes proteolytic activity to digest collagen in the follicular wall, making it thin and stretched out, facilitating rupture. It also acts to terminate the LH surge by exerting a negative feedback effect at higher concentrations.

Escape of ovum is associated with thinning and degeneration of collagen in the follicular wall. Plasminogen activators release plasmin and generate collagenase to disrupt follicular wall.

Plasminogen inhibitory system active before and after ovulation prevents inappropriate disruption of follicular wall. Ovulation is the result of proteolytic digestion of follicular apex called stigma.

Prostaglandins, mainly prostaglandin E2 (PGE2) but also prostaglandin F2 alpha (PGF2α), and other eicosanoids, such as hydroxyeicosatetraenoic acid (HETE), are increased markedly in preovulatory follicular fluid in response to LH surge.[73-75] Cyclooxygenase-2 (COX- 2) inhibitors block follicular rupture without affecting luteinization and oocyte maturation.[76,77] Prostaglandins act to free proteolytic enzymes from the follicular wall and may promote angiogenesis and hyperemia. They also help to contract smooth muscle, aiding extrusion of oocyte cumulus mass.

The FSH surge, a result of preovulatory progesterone rise, expands and disperses the CCs allowing the oocyte–CC mass to become free-floating in the antral fluid just before follicular rupture. Also, FSH peak promotes plasminogen activator production and an adequate LH receptor concentration, ensuring adequate luteal phase functioning. This explains why GnRH agonist ovulation trigger is more physiological as it causes both LH and FSH surges **(Flowchart 5)**.

Decline of LH surge: Within hours after LH rise, there is a precipitous drop in plasma estrogens. This LH fall may be due to loss of the positive stimulating action of estradiol or to an increasing negative feedback of progesterone. High levels of progesterone inhibit pituitary secretion of gonadotropins by inhibiting GnRH pulses at the level of the hypothalamus. In addition, high levels of progesterone can antagonize pituitary response to GnRH by interfering with estrogen action.

The abrupt decline in LH may also reflect exhaustion of pituitary LH stores due to downregulation of GnRH receptors.[78,79]

Activity of a nonsteroidal ovarian substance, named gonadotropin surge-attenuating factor (GnSAF), is hypothesized to regulate the amplitude of the endogenous LH surge at mid-cycle, by antagonizing the sensitizing effect of estradiol on the pituitary.[80] It is produced by the granulosa cells and has a role in prevention of premature luteinization. All these events lead to shutdown of LH surge.

Luteal Phase

Normal luteal function requires optimal preovulatory follicle development. Granulosa and theca lutein cells continue to enlarge and accumulate yellow pigment lutein. For successful steroidogenesis and supply of adequate LDL cholesterol substrate, good vascularization is required. Rapid vascularization is mediated by vascular endothelial growth factor (VEGF).[81] By day 8 or 9 after ovulation, a peak of vascularization is reached, associated with peak levels of progesterone and estradiol in the blood. CL has highest blood flow per unit mass of body and spontaneous bleeding can occur specially in anticoagulated patients.

The luteal phase is defined by the luteinization of the follicles forming CL initiated by the LH surge. The major

Flowchart 5: Key events leading to ovulation.

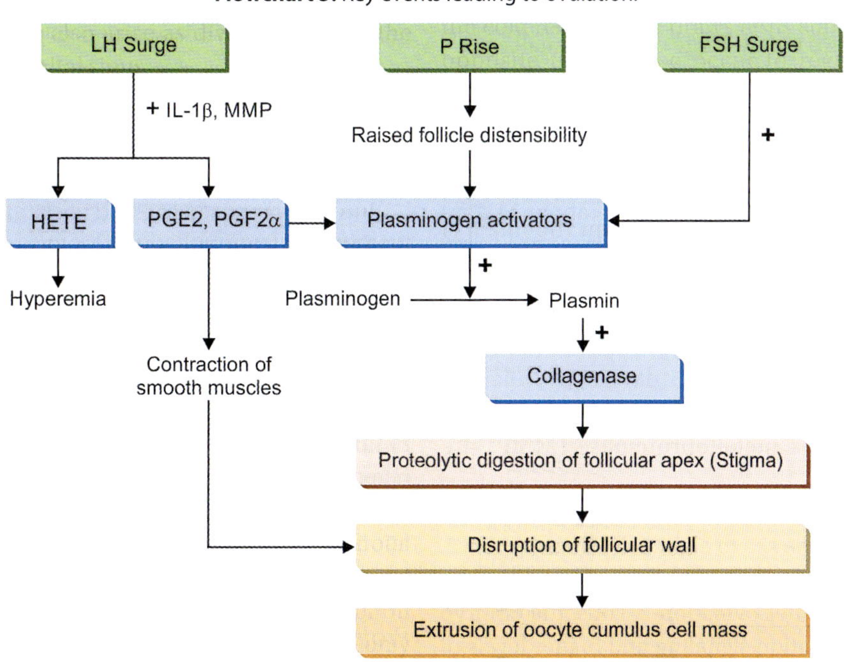

(FSH: follicle-stimulating hormone; HETE: hydroxyeicosatetraenoic acid; IL-1β: interleukin-1β; LH: luteinizing hormone; MMP: matrix metalloproteinase; P: progesterone; PGE2: prostaglandin E2; PGF2: prostaglandin F2)

effects of the LH surge are the conversion of granulosa cells from predominantly androgen-converting cells to predominantly progesterone-synthesizing cells and the expression of new LH receptors that foster increased progesterone synthesis with some estrogen secretion. LH regulates LDL receptor binding, internalization, and processing.[82] Induction of LDL receptors in granulosa cells occurs in response to LH surge. Progesterone secretion by the CL peaks between 5 and 7 days postovulation. High progesterone levels exert negative feedback on GnRH, and subsequently, GnRH pulse frequency decreases, leading to reduced FSH and LH secretion. The CL further loses its FSH and LH receptors. Lacking stimulation by FSH and LH, after 14 days CL undergoes atresia. With the decline in both estrogen and progesterone levels, an important negative feedback control on FSH is removed, and FSH levels rise once again to initiate the next menstrual cycle.

If fertilization and subsequent implantation of the blastocyst do not occur, the CL undergoes apoptosis and becomes the corpus albicans, a white scar. Luteal apoptosis involves a loss of LH-binding receptors and is mediated by prostaglandins.

The life span of CL depends on tonic LH secretion as evident by prompt luteolysis occurring when GnRH antagonist or agonist is continued in the cycles. Estrogen and progesterone production by CL is under control of LH. High levels of estrogen, progesterone, and inhibin A suppress new follicular growth.

The CL is not homogenous as it is composed of luteal cells, endothelial cells, leukocytes, and fibroblasts.[83] Nonsteroidogenic cells form 70% of the cells. Endothelial cells (35%) contribute to the vasoactive compounds.[84]

Luteal cells are of two types—large cells and small cells.[83] Large cells formed from granulosa cells are the sites of steroidogenesis, whereas small cells formed from theca cells contain receptors and provide a stimulus for large cells to function.[85]

The LH surge to menses is on an average about 14 days ranging from 11 to 17 days, with short luteal phase occurring in about 5–6% of women.[86]

Luteal phase cannot be extended for long despite continuous LH stimulation, suggesting an active luteolytic mechanism. CL rapidly declines 9–11 days after ovulation. NO, prostaglandin F2α, endothelin-1, TNF-α, and proteolytic enzymes such as matrix metalloproteinase (MMP) are involved in luteolysis.[87]

Emerging hCG from pregnancy rescues the CL. mRNA for hCG can be detected in the six- to eight-cell human embryo, i.e., even before implantation, and it can be detected in the mother about 6–7 days after ovulation.[88] Thus, the embryo is capable of preimplantation signaling and higher levels of estradiol and progesterone can be measured in the maternal circulation even before maternal hCG is detectable.

Luteal–Follicular Transition

The luteal–follicular transition is a period of selective increase in FSH beginning about 2 days before the onset of menses.[89]

It occurs due to:

- Demise of CL results in nadir in circulating levels of estradiol, progesterone, and inhibin.
- Decrease in negative feedback effect of luteal steroids and inhibin (particularly inhibin A).
- Change in pulsatile GnRH secretion toward an increasing pulse frequency which favors predominant FSH secretion.[90]

The increase in FSH is instrumental in rescuing approximately a 70-day cohort of follicles from atresia, allowing a dominant follicle to begin its emergence **(Fig. 18)**.

Uterine Endometrial Cycle

The uterus is a dynamic structure, responding in a sensitive fashion to classic hormonal signals (the endocrine events of the menstrual cycle) **(*see* Fig. 10)**. Cyclical changes in the endometrium prepare for implantation in the event of fertilization and necessitate menstruation in the absence of fertilization. The integrated evolutionary cycle of endometrial growth and regression is described in four phases:

1. Proliferative or follicular phase
2. Secretory or luteal phase
3. Preparatory phase for implantation
4. Menstrual phase or the phase of endometrial breakdown.

Morphologically, the endometrium consists of an upper two-third "functionalis/functionale" layer, which is the site of proliferation and secretion meant for blastocyst implantation, and a lower one-third "basalis" layer serving as the source of regenerative endometrium after menstrual breakdown.[91]

The functionalis layer is subdivided further into two parts:

1. *Stratum compactum:* A superficial layer closer to the lumen, composed of gland necks and dense stromal cells.
2. *Stratum spongiosum:* The deeper functionale layer adjacent to the underlying basale layer contains predominantly endometrial glands, increased interstitial tissue, and less dense stroma.

The functionalis undergoes changes throughout the menstrual cycle and is shed during menstruation, while the basalis remains constant during the menstrual cycle and regenerates the functionalis each month. Almost two-third of the functioning endometrium is shed out during menstruation. The residue is a stable, basalis component and a small, variable amount of residual stratum spongiosum **(Fig. 19)**.

Proliferative or Follicular Phase

The proliferative or follicular phase spans from the end of the menstruation until ovulation. As estrogen secretion

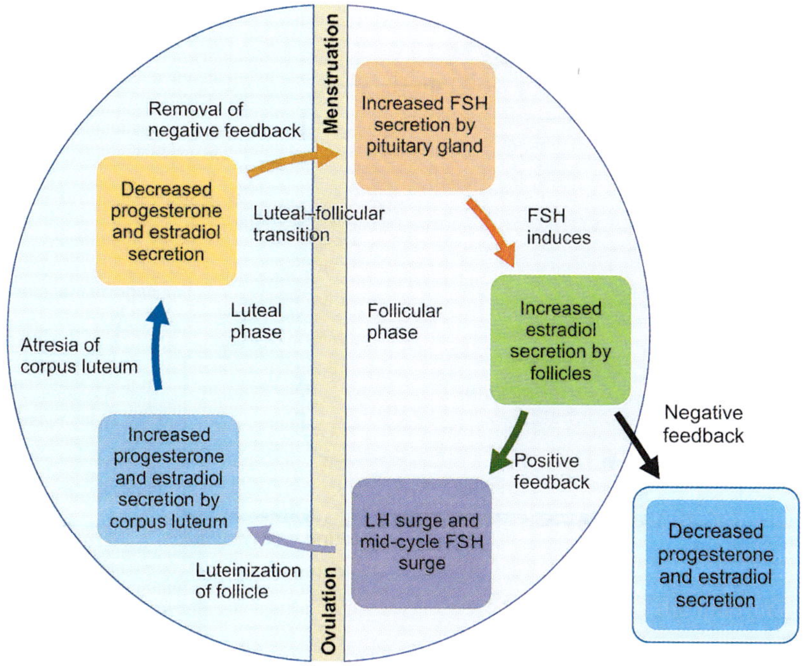

Fig. 18: Summary of ovarian events in menstrual cycle.
(FSH: follicle-stimulating hormone; LH: luteinizing hormone)

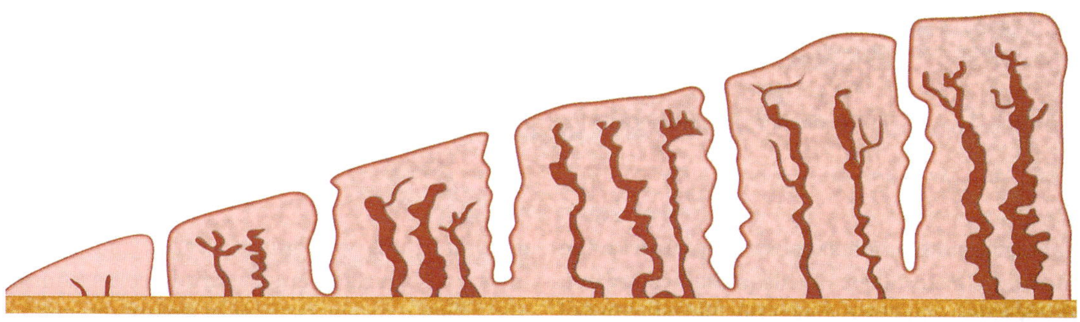

Proliferative functions	Secretory functions		
Cellular proliferation	**Early secretory**	**Mid secretory**	**Late secretory**
Cellular differentiation	Metabolism	Metabolism	Extracellular matrix degradation
Extracellular matrix remodeling	Transport	Glandular secretion	Inflammatory response
Angiogenesis and vasculogenesis	Proliferation inhibition	Cell differentiation	Apoptosis
DNA synthesis	Mitosis inhibition	Cell communication	
Adhesion		Innate immune response	
Ion channels		Response to stress, injury	
		Adhesion	
		Proteolysis regulation	

Fig. 19: Biological functions of endometrium in different stages of uterine cycle. (DNA: deoxyribonucleic acid)

occurs, mitosis and pseudostratification predominate. Rapid re-epithelialization and proliferation of cells from the stumps of glands in the basalis layer, especially in the isthmic and tubal ostial sites, is initiated within 24–48 hours. By days 5–6, there is onset of stromal growth. There is proliferation of all elements slowly at first but later at a rapid pace. Ovarian follicular phase corresponds to proliferative phase.

By the mid-follicular phase, increasing levels of estrogen from the growing follicle induce proliferation of the functionalis from stem cells of the basalis, proliferation of endometrial glands, and proliferation of stromal connective tissue. Endometrial glands are elongated with narrow lumens and their epithelial cells contain some glycogen. Glycogen, however, is not secreted during the follicular phase. As the

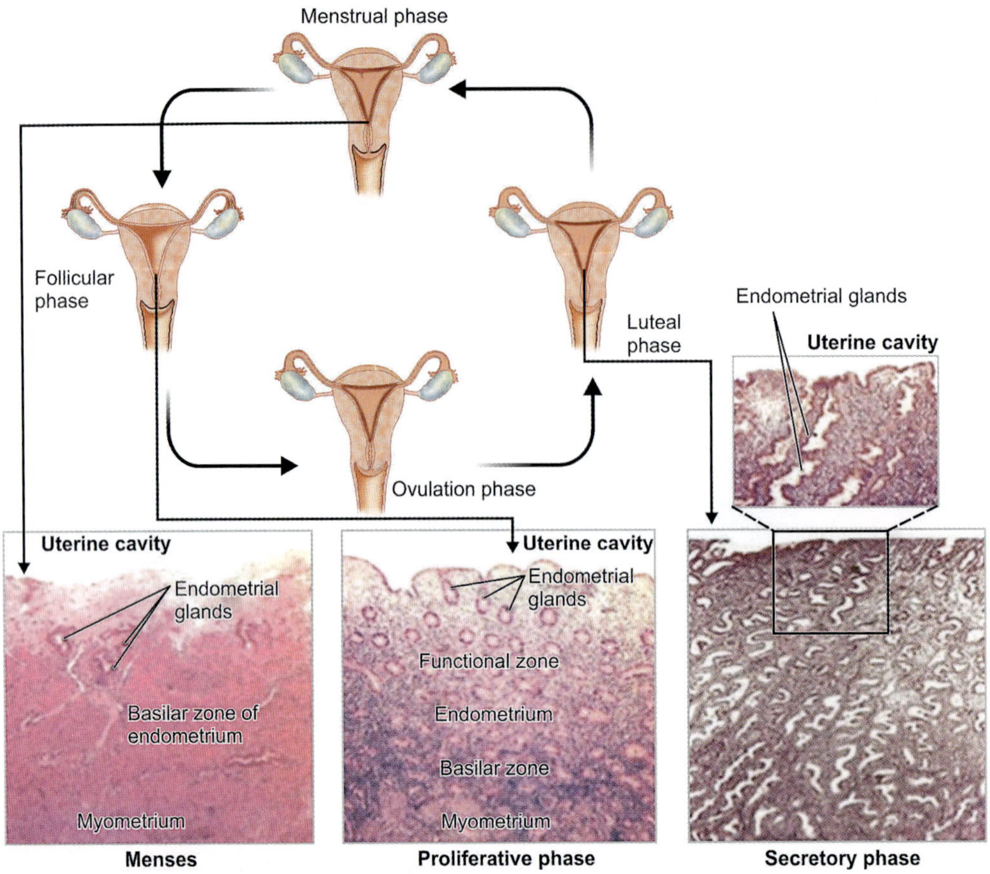

Fig. 20: Changes in endometrial histology in different stages of uterine cycle.

glands get tubular, epithelium becomes columnar with the nuclei placed at the base. Stromal cells, initially compact, evolve through subepithelial congestion. Spiral arteries elongate and span the length of the endometrium but remain unbranched **(Fig. 20)**.

Proliferation peaks on days 8–10 of the cycle reflecting peak estrogen receptors and concentration.[92] The thickness of the endometrium measures about 4–6 mm in the mid-follicular phase, and by the end of the proliferative phase, the mean endometrial thickness on ultrasound increases to "trilaminar pattern" of 12 mm. Pseudostratification of the cells lining the glandular epithelium also peaks immediately before ovulation.

Secretory or Luteal Phase

The secretory or luteal phase begins at ovulation and lasts until the menstrual phase of the next cycle. In the early luteal phase, progesterone induces the endometrial glands to secrete glycogen, mucus, and other substances. These glands become tortuous and have large lumens due to increased secretory activity. The spiral arteries extend into the superficial layer of the endometrium. Due to the effects of progesterone from the CL on an estrogen-primed endometrium, proliferation ceases, and there is a decline in mitosis. Surface epithelium becomes more columnar and ciliated at places. Glands enlarge to get a cork-screw shape. Subnuclear glycogen vacuolation is an evidence of progesterone effect but does not confirm ovulation. Blood vessels undergo marked spiraling. Endometrial trilaminar pattern is lost, and there is an increased and uniform echogenicity of the endometrium **(*see* Fig. 20)**.

Implantation Phase

Around the 7th–13th postovulation day (days 21–22 of the cycle), the distended tortuous secretory glands are prominent with some intervening stroma. The endometrium has three distinct zones—basal, middle lace- like edematous stratum spongiosum, and superficial stratum compactum. Engorged vessels, intense infiltration of leukocytes, synthesis of prostaglandins and growth factors, decidualization of stromal cells, and a complex array of peptides and cytokines mark this phase meant to receive and nurture the blastocyst. It is discussed in detail in the chapter on implantation.

The mid- to late-secretory endometrial glands become increasingly tortuous, and the stroma becomes edematous and vascular. If implantation of the blastocyst into the endometrium does not occur and hCG is not present, the glands begin to fragment and collapse in the late-luteal phase. In the absence of fertilization by day 23 of the menstrual cycle, the CL begins to degenerate and consequently ovarian hormone levels decrease. As estrogen and progesterone levels decrease, the endometrium undergoes involution. On days 25–26 of the menstrual cycle, endothelin and thromboxane begin to mediate vasoconstriction of the spiral arteries. The resulting ischemia may cause some early menstrual cramps. By day 28 of the menstrual cycle, intense vasoconstriction and subsequent ischemia cause mass apoptosis of the functionalis **(*see* Fig. 20)**.

Flowchart 6: Key events leading to endometrial breakdown.

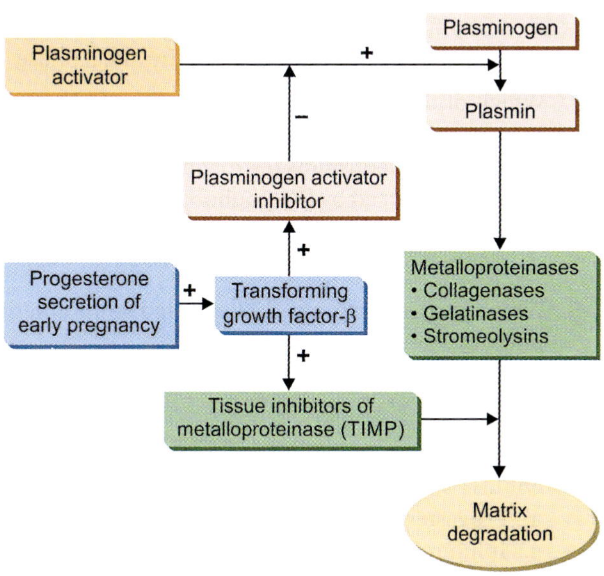

Menstrual Phase or Phase of Endometrial Breakdown

In the event of nonestablishment of pregnancy, the fixed life span of the CL gets completed and the waning levels of estrogen and progesterone initiate important endometrial events. These events include blood stasis, arteriolar spasm, tissue necrosis, ischemia, and eventually enzymatic autodigestion caused by release of lysosomal proteolytic enzymes.[93]

The menstrual phase begins as the spiral arteries rupture secondary to ischemia, releasing blood into the uterus, and the apoptosed endometrium is sloughed off and usually lasts 4 days. Menstruation begins in different areas of the endometrium at different times. Sloughing of the endometrium occurs predominantly in the fundus and

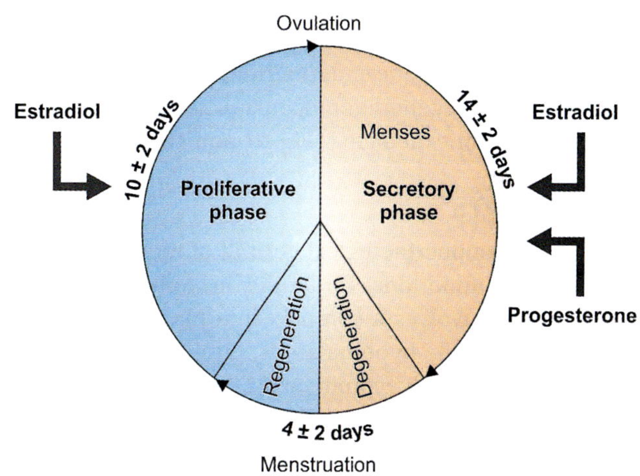

Fig. 21: Summary of endometrial events in menstrual cycle.

TABLE 4: Summary of ovarian and uterine events in a 28-day menstrual cycle with hormonal dynamics.

Days	*Ovarian events*	*Endometrial events*	*Hormonal dynamics*
1–4	*Recruitment:* Cohort of follicles start growing	Endometrial lining sloughs	• E2 and P4 are low • FSH and LH are released from inhibition
5–7	*Selection:* A single follicle is destined to ovulate. No surrogate follicle	Endometrium proliferates	Plasma E2 rises due to secretion from selected dominant follicle
8–12	*Dominance:* • Atresia of all other follicles except dominant follicle • Dominant follicle thrives uniquely, despite the suppressive milieu	Increased E2 stimulates the growth of glands and stroma	Increased E2 and inhibin will inhibit FSH
13–15	*Ovulation:* • Mediated by follicular enzymes and prostaglandins • Oocyte is induced to complete its first meiotic division	Transition from proliferative to secretory endometrium	LH surge induced by high plasma E2 (positive feedback)
15–25	Corpus luteum forms	Secretory endometrium develops	• P4 and E2 are secreted • FSH and LH secretion is inhibited, so no new follicle develops
25–28	*Luteolysis:* • Corpus luteum degenerates • Recruitment of new follicles for next cycle	Endometrium begins to slough due to withdrawal of progesterone support	• Plasma E2 and P4 decrease release of hypothalamus and pituitary from negative feedback • FSH begins to rise

(E2: estradiol; FSH: follicle-stimulating hormone; LH: luteinizing hormone; P4: progesterone)

minimally in the isthmus or cornual regions, and the natural cleavage point is between basalis and spongiosum. Autolysis with subsequent desquamation of the stratum functionale layer begins. The bleeding occurs from broken arteries, veins and capillaries, and stromal hematoma. Arterial and venous blood, remnants of endometrial stroma and glands, leukocytes, and red blood cells are all present in the menstrual flow. Blood along with the superficial functional layer is shed into the uterine cavity **(Flowchart 6)**.

Cessation of menstruation occurs due to a combined effect of prolonged vasoconstriction, myometrial contraction, and local aggregation of platelets with fibrin deposition. Resumption of estrogen secretion leads to repair of endometrium from the basalis layer. Regeneration of the endometrium begins 36 hours after menses onset at the isthmic recesses and the cornual region even as endometrial shedding continues in other areas of the uterus. Bleeding usually ceases by cycle day 5 after complete re-epithelialization of the endometrium is accomplished.

Endometrial regeneration occurs in response to injury and is not hormone mediated **(Fig. 21 and Table 4)**.

KEY POINTS

- The neuroendocrinological control of menstrual cycle is of prime importance for fertility in women. As clearly evident, it involves a complex interplay of hormones produced by the hypothalamus, pituitary, and ovaries during the monthly reproductive cycle.
- The hormonal regulation of the reproductive system is complex and imperative for the proper functioning of the gonads (oogenesis and spermatogenesis), thus maintaining the vital menstrual function in females along with fertility in both genders.
- The developments in the field of pharmacogenomics have improved the understanding of infertility and the variable patient response to COS. With the understanding of mechanism of primordial follicle activation, infertility treatment could be advanced especially in women with low ovarian reserve.
- Although more research should be performed, the use of existing primordial follicles as a source for obtaining fertilizable oocytes as a new treatment for female infertility is just around the corner.
- Hence, the clinicians and specifically the infertility specialists need to have an in-depth understanding of the underlying physiology and neuroendocrinology for better patient care in their day-to-day practice.

MULTIPLE CHOICE QUESTIONS WITH ANSWERS

1. Shortly before menstruation:
   a. Blood levels of estrogen and progesterone decrease
   b. Blood levels of estrogen and progesterone increase
   c. Blood levels of FSH stabilize
   d. The CL secretes progesterone
2. During the menstrual cycle:
   a. LH stimulates estrogen production by follicles
   b. FSH stimulates growth of the ovarian follicles
   c. LH stimulates the formation of a CL from the collapsed follicle
   d. All of the above
3. Which of the following is true?
   a. Endorphins stimulate GnRH release within the hypothalamus
   b. α-Endorphin is 10 times more potent than morphine
   c. β-Endorphin is 10 times more potent than morphine
   d. Endorphin levels are lowest in the luteal phase
4. Which of the following is associated with the CL of menstruation, not the CL of pregnancy?
   a. Ovarian luteotropins (estrogens, IGF-I, IGF-II)
   b. hCG produced by the trophoblast of the chorion
   c. LH and prolactin
   d. Corpus albicans
5. Which are the hormones NOT secreted by the anterior pituitary?
   a. FSH b. LH
   c. GnRH d. TSH
6. Which of the following specifically inhibits FSH, but not LH?
   a. Progesterone b. Estradiol
   c. Inhibin d. Androgen
7. Chronic high levels of which of the following lead to a positive feedback loop in the HPO axis?
   a. Dopamine b. Estrogen
   c. Inhibin d. Progesterone
8. Theca cells produce androgens (e.g., testosterone) that diffuse into granulosa cells under the influence of:
   a. Estradiol b. Testosterone
   c. LH d. FSH
9. Which of the following statements about prolactin is false?
   a. Prolactin secretion is under tonic inhibitory control of dopamine
   b. Prolactin secretion follows a circadian rhythm
   c. Prolactin has a direct action on the ovaries
   d. Prolactin secretion is under tonic inhibitory control of TSH
10. A 19-year-old woman presents with complaints of no periods for the past 7 months. During this time, she started college and felt that her stress level had increased. The patient also changed her eating habits, which led to a weight decrease from 66 to 45 kg. She

has noted no other changes in her health. Which of the following tests should be ordered initially?

a. TSH, prolactin
b. Testosterone, β-hCG
c. FSH, β-hCG
d. Prolactin, β-hCG, dehydroepiandrosterone sulfate (DHEAS)

ANSWERS

1. a	2. d	3. c	4. d	5. c
6. c	7. b	8. c	9. d	10. a

REFERENCES

1. Simerly RB, Chang C, Muramatsu M, Swanson LW. Distribution of androgen and estrogen receptor mRNA-containing cells in the rat brain: an in situ hybridization study. J Comp Neurol. 1990;294(1):76-95.
2. Brown TJ, Hochberg RB, Naftolin F, MacLusky NJ. Pubertal development of estrogen receptors in the rat brain. Mol Cell Neurosci. 1994;5(5):475-83.
3. Belchetz PE, Plant TM, Nakai Y, Keogh EJ, Knobil E. Hypophysial responses to continuous and intermittent delivery of hypopthalamic gonadotropin-releasing hormone. Science. 1978;202(4368):631-3.
4. Pau KY, Berria M, Hess DL, Spies HG. Hypothalamic site-dependent effects of neuropeptide Y on gonadotropin-releasing hormone secretion in rhesus macaques. J Neuroendocrinol. 1995;7(1):63-7.
5. Rance NE. Menopause and the human hypothalamus: evidence for the role of kisspeptin/neurokinin B neurons in the regulation of estrogen negative feedback. Peptides. 2009;30(1):111-22.
6. Tng EL. Kisspeptin signalling and its roles in humans. Singapore Med J. 2015; 56(12):649-56.
7. Oakley AE, Clifton DK, Steiner RA. Kisspeptin signaling in the brain. Endocr Rev. 2009;30(6):713-43.
8. Jayasena CN, Nijher GMK, Comninos AN, Abbara A, Januszewki A, Vaal ML, et al. The effects of kisspeptin-10 on reproductive hormone release show sexual dimorphism in humans. J Clin Endocrinol Metab. 2011;96(12):E1963-72.
9. George JT, Veldhuis JD, Roseweir AK, Newton CL, Faccenda E, Millar RP, et al. Kisspeptin-10 is a potent stimulator of LH and increases pulse frequency in men. J Clin Endocrinol Metab. 2011;96(8):E1228-36.
10. Bauer-Dantoin AC, Wess J, Jameson JL. Roles of estrogen, progesterone, and gonadotropin-releasing hormone (GnRH) in the control of pituitary GnRH receptor gene expression at the time of the preovulatory gonadotropin surges. Endocrinology. 1995;136(3):1014-9.
11. Blumenfeld Z. Response of human fetal pituitary cells to activin, inhibin, hypophysiotropic and neuroregulatory factors in vitro. Early Pregnancy. 2001;5(1):41-2.
12. Billestrup N, Gonzalez-Manchon C, Potter E, Vale W. Inhibition of somatotroph growth and growth hormone biosynthesis by activin in vitro. Mol Endocrinol. 1990;4(2):356-62.
13. Corrigan AZ, Bilezikjian LM, Carroll RS, Bald LN, Schmelzer CH, Fendly BM, et al. Evidence for an autocrine role of activin B within rat anterior pituitary cultures. Endocrinology. 1991;128(3):1682-4.
14. Kaiser UB, Conn PM, Chin WW. Studies of gonadotropin-releasing hormone (GnRH) action using GnRH receptor-expressing pituitary cell lines. Endocr Rev. 1997;18(1):46-70.
15. Norwitz ER, Xu S, Jeong KH, Bédécarrats GY, Winebrenner LD, Chin WW, et al. Activin A augments GnRH-mediated transcriptional activation of the mouse GnRH receptor gene. Endocrinology. 2002;143(3):985-97.
16. Kogawa K, Nakamura T, Sugino K, Takio K, Titani K, Sugino H. Activin-binding protein is present in pituitary. Endocrinology. 1991;128(3):1434-40.
17. Welt C, Sidis Y, Keutmann H, Schneyer A. Activins, inhibins, and follistatins: from endocrinology to signaling. A paradigm for the new millennium. Exp Biol Med (Maywood). 2002; 227(9):724-52.
18. Hughes J, Smith TW, Kosterlitz WH, Fothergill LA, Morgan BA, Morris HR. Identification of two related pentapeptides from the brain with potent opiate agonist activity. Nature. 1975;258(5536):577-80.
19. Howlett TA, Rees LH. Endogenous opioid peptides and hypothalamo-pituitary function. Annu Rev Physiol. 1986; 48:527-36.
20. Facchinetti F, Petraglia P, Genazzani AR. Localization and expression of the three opioid systems. Semin Reprod Endocrinol. 1987;5:103.
21. Grossman A. Opioid peptides and reproductive function. Semin Reprod Endocrinol. 1987;5:115-24.
22. Reid RL, Hoff JD, Yen SS, Li CH. Effects of exogenous beta h-endorphin on pituitary hormone secretion and its disappearance rate in normal human subjects. J Clin Endocrinol Metab. 1981;52(6):1179-84.
23. Yen SSC. The hypothalamic control of pituitary hormone secretion. In: Yen SSC, Jaffe RB (Eds). Reproductive Endocrinology, 3rd edition. Philadelphia, PA, USA: WB Saunders; 1991. pp. 65-104.
24. Totorikaguena L, Olabarrieta E, Matorras R, Alonso E, Agirregoitia E, Agirregoitia N. Mu opioid receptor in the human endometrium: dynamics of its expression and localization during the menstrual cycle. Fertil Steril. 2017; 107(4):1070-7.e1.
25. Matsushita N, Kato Y, Shimatsu A, Katakami H, Yanaihara N, Imura H. Effects of VIP, TRH, GABA and dopamine on prolactin release from superfused rat anterior pituitary cells. Life Sci. 1983;32(11):1263-9.
26. Burrow GN. The thyroid gland and reproduction. In: Yen SSC, Jaffe RB (Eds). Reproductive Endocrinology, 3rd edition. Philadelphia, PA, USA: WB Saunders; 1991. pp. 555-75.
27. Bohler H, Mokshagundam S, Winters SJ. Adipose tissue and reproduction in women. Fertil Steril. 2010;94(3):795-825.
28. Simoni M, Casarini L. Mechanisms in endocrinology: genetics of FSH action: a 2014-and-beyond view. Eur J Endocrinol. 2014;170(3):R91-107.
29. Altmae S, Hovatta O, Stavreus-Evers A, Salumets A. Genetic predictors of controlled ovarian hyperstimulation: where do we stand today? Hum Reprod Update. 2011;17(6):813-28.
30. Menon M, Peegel H, Katta V. Estradiol potentiation of gonadotropin-releasing hormone responsiveness in the anterior pituitary is mediated by an increase in gonadotropin-releasing hormone receptors. Am J Obstet Gynecol. 1985; 151(4):534-40.
31. Hirshfield AN. Development of follicles in mammalian ovary. Int Rev Cytol. 1991;124:43-101.
32. Gougeon A. Dynamics of follicular growth in the human: a model from preliminary results. Hum Reprod. 1986;1(2):81-7.
33. Baker TG. A quantitative and cytological study of germ cells in human ovaries. Proc R Soc Lond B Biol Sci. 1963;158:417-33.

34. Zhang H, Liu K. Cellular and molecular regulation of the activation of mammalian primordial follicles: somatic cells initiate follicle activation in adulthood. Hum Reprod Update. 2015;21(6):779-86.
35. Gougeon A. Regulation of ovarian follicular development in primates: facts and hypotheses. Endocr Rev. 1996;17(2):121-55.
36. Oktay K, Newton H, Mullan J, Gosden RG. Development of human primordial follicles to antral stages in SCID/hpg mice stimulated with follicle stimulating hormone. Hum Reprod. 1998;13(5):1133-8.
37. Hsueh AJW, Eisenhauer K, Chun SY, Hsu SY, Billig H. Gonadal cell apoptosis. Recent Prog Horm Res. 1996;51:433-55.
38. McNatty KP, Makris A, DeGrazia C, Osathanondh R, Ryan KJ. The production of progesterone, androgens, and estrogens by granulosa cells, thecal tissue, and stromal tissue from human ovaries in vitro. J Clin Endocrinol Metab. 1979;49(5):687-99.
39. McNatty KP, Makris A, Reinhold VN, De Grazia C, Osathanondh R, Ryan KJ. Metabolism of androstenedione by human ovarian tissues in vitro with particular reference to reductase and aromatase activity. Steroids. 1979;34(4):429-43.
40. Hillier SG, van den Boogaard AM, Reichert Jr LE, van Hall EV. Intraovarian sex steroid hormone interactions and the regulation of follicular maturation: aromatization of androgens by human granulosa cells in vitro. J Clin Endocrinol Metab. 1980;50(4):640-7.
41. Jia X-C, Kessel B, Welsh Jr TH, Hsueh AJ. Androgen inhibition of follicle-stimulating hormone-stimulated luteinizing hormone receptor formation in cultured rat granulosa cells. Endocrinology. 1985;117(1):13-22.
42. Su YQ, Sugiura K, Eppig JJ. Mouse oocyte control of granulosa cell development and function: paracrine regulation of cumulus cell metabolism. Seminars Reprod Med. 2009;27(1):32-42.
43. Ackert CL, Gittens JE, O'Brien MJ, Eppig JJ, Kidder GM. Intercellular communication via connexin43 gap junctions is required for ovarian folliculogenesis in the mouse. Dev Biol. 2001;233(2):258-70.
44. Granot I, Dekel N. Developmental expression and regulation of the gap junction protein and transcription in rat ovaries. Mol Reprod Dev. 1997;47(3):231-9.
45. Granot I, Dekel N. The ovarian gap junction protein connexin43: regulation by gonadotropins. Trends Endocrinol Metab. 2002;13(7):310-3.
46. Khan-Dawood FS. Oxytocin in intercellular communication in the corpus luteum. Semin Reprod Endocrinol. 1997;15(4):395-407.
47. Andersen CY. Characteristics of human follicular fluid associated with successful conception after in vitro fertilization. J Clin Endocrinol Metab. 1993;77(5):1227-34.
48. Kobayashi M, Nakano R, Ooshima A. Immunohistochemical localization of pituitary gonadotrophins and gonadal steroids confirms the 'two-cell, two-gonadotrophin' hypothesis of steroidogenesis in the human ovary. J Endocrinol. 1990;126(3):483-8.
49. Magoffin DA. Regulation of differentiated functions in ovarian theca cells. Semin Reprod Endocrinol. 1991;9(4):321-31.
50. Sasano H. Functional pathology of human ovarian steroidogenesis: normal cycling ovary and steroid-producing neoplasms. Endocr Pathol. 1994;5(2):81-9.
51. Schoot DC, Coelingh-Bennink HJT, Mannaerts BM, Lamberts SW, Bouchard P, Fauser BC. Human recombinant follicle-stimulating hormone induces growth of preovulatory follicles without concomitant increase in androgen and estrogen biosynthesis in a woman with isolated gonadotropin deficiency. J Clin Endocrinol Metab. 1992;74(6):1471-3.
52. Shoham Z, Mannaerts B, Insler V, Coelingh-Bennink H. Induction of follicular growth using recombinant human follicle-stimulating hormone in two volunteer women with hypogonadotropic hypogonadism. Fertil Steril. 1993;59(4):738-42.
53. Montgomery Rice V, Limback SD, Roby KF, Terranova PF. Differential responses of granulosa cells from small and large follicles to follicle stimulating hormone (FSH) during the menstrual cycle and acyclicity: effects of tumour necrosis factor-α. Hum Reprod. 1998;13(5):1285-91.
54. Zeleznik AJ, Schuler HM, Reichert Jr LE. Gonadotropin-binding sites in the rhesus monkey ovary: role of the vasculature in the selective distribution of human chorionic gonadotropin to the preovulatory follicle. Endocrinology. 1981;109(2):356-62.
55. Schipper I, Hop WC, Fauser BC. The follicle-stimulating hormone (FSH) threshold/window concept examined by different interventions with exogenous FSH during the follicular phase of the normal menstrual cycle: duration, rather than magnitude, of FSH increase affects follicle development. J Clin Endocrinol Metab. 1998;83(4):1292-8.
56. Richards JS, Jahnsen T, Hedin L, Lifka J, Ratoosh S, Durica JM, et al. Ovarian follicular development: from physiology to molecular biology. Recent Prog Horm Res. 1987;43:231-76.
57. The European Recombinant Human LH Study Group. Recombinant human luteinizing hormone (LH) to support recombinant human follicle-stimulating hormone (FSH) induced follicular development in LH- and FSH-deficient anovulatory women: a dose finding study. J Clin Endocrinol Metab. 1998;83(5):1507-14.
58. Filicori M, Cognigni GE, Tabarelli C, Pocognoli P, Taraborrelli S, Spettoli D, et al. Stimulation and growth of antral ovarian follicles by selective LH activity administration in women. J Clin Endocrinol Metab. 2002;87(3):1156-61.
59. Young JR, Jaffe RB. Strength-duration characteristics of estrogen effects on gonadotropin response to gonadotropin-releasing hormone in women. II. Effects of varying concentrations of estradiol. J Clin Endocrinol Metab. 1976;42(3):432-42.
60. Cahill DJ, Wardle PG, Harlow CR, Hull MG. Onset of the preovulatory luteinizing hormone surge: diurnal timing and critical follicular prerequisites. Fertil Steril. 1998;70(1):56-9.
61. Pauerstein CJ, Eddy CA, Croxatto HD, Hess R, Siler-Khodr TM, Croxatto HB. Temporal relationships of estrogen, progesterone, and luteinizing hormone levels to ovulation in women and infrahuman primates. Am J Obstet Gynecol. 1978;130(8):876-86.
62. Hillier SG, Yong EL, Illingworth PJ, Baird DT, Schwall RH, Mason AJ. Effect of recombinant inhibin on androgen synthesis in cultured human thecal cells. Mol Cell Endocrinol. 1991;75(2):R1-6.
63. Xiao S, Robertson DM, Findlay JK. Effects of activin and follicle stimulating hormone (FSH)-suppressing protein/follistatin on FSH receptors and differentiation of cultured rat granulosa cells. Endocrinology. 1992;131(3):1009-16.
64. Dor J, Ben-Shlomo I, Lunenfeld B, Pariente C, Levran D, Karasik A, et al. Insulin-like growth factor-I (IGF-I) may not be essential for ovarian follicular development: evidence from IGF-I deficiency. J Clin Endocrinol Metab. 1992;74(3):539-42.
65. el-Roeiy A, Chen X, Roberts VJ, LeRoith D, Roberts Jr CT, Yen SS. Expression of insulin-like growth factor-I (IGF-I) and IGF-II and the IGF-I, IGF-II, and insulin receptor genes and

localization of the gene products in the human ovary. J Clin Endocrinol Metab. 1993;77(5):1411-8.
66. Fukuda M, Fukuda K, Andersen CY, Byskov AG. Right-sided ovulation favours pregnancy than left-sided ovulation. Hum Reprod. 2000;15(9):1921-6.
67. Fukuda M, Fukuda K, Andersen CY, Byskov AG. Characteristics of human ovulation in natural cycles correlated with age and achievement of pregnancy. Hum Reprod. 2001;16(12): 2501-7.
68. Zelinski-Wooten MB, Hess DL, Baughman WL, Molskness TA, Wolf DP, Stouffer RL. Administration of an aromatase inhibitor during the late follicular phase of gonadotropin-treated cycles in Rhesus monkeys: effects on follicle development, oocyte maturational, and subsequent luteal function. J Clin Endocrinol Metab. 1993;76(4):988-95.
69. Hoff JD, Quigley ME, Yen SS. Hormonal dynamics at midcycle: a reevaluation. J Clin Endocrinol Metab. 1983;57(4):792-6.
70. Zelinski-Wooten MB, Hutchison JS, Chandrasekher YA, Wolf DP, Stouffer RL. Administration of human luteinizing hormone (hLH) to Macaques after follicular development: further titration of LH surge requirements for ovulatory changes in primate follicles. J Clin Endocrinol Metab. 1992;75(2):502-7.
71. Fritz MA, McLachlan RI, Cohen NL, Dahl KD, Bremner WJ, Soules MR. Onset and characteristics of the midcycle surge in bio active and immunoactive luteinizing hormone secretion in normal women: influence of physiological variations in periovulatory ovarian steroid hormone secretion. J Clin Endocrinol Metab. 1992;75(2):489-93.
72. Temporal relationships between ovulation and defined changes in the concentration of plasma estradiol-17β, luteinizing hormone, follicle-stimulating hormone, and progesterone. I. Probit analysis. World Health Organization, Task Force on Methods for the Determination of the Fertile Period, Special Programme of Research, Development and Research Training in Human Reproduction. Am J Obstet Gynecol. 1980;138(4):383-90.
73. Lumsden MA, Kelly RW, Templeton AA, Van Look PF, Swanston IA, Baird DT. Changes in the concentrations of prostaglandins in preovulatory human follicles after administration of hCG. J Reprod Fertil. 1986;77(1):119-24.
74. Espey LL, Tanaka N, Adams RF, Okamura H. Ovarian hydroxy-eicosatetraenoic acids compared with prostanoids and steroids during ovulation in rats. Am J Physiol. 1991;260(2 Pt 1): E163-9.
75. Duffy DM, Dozier BL, Seachord CL. Prostaglandin dehydrogenase and prostaglandin levels in periovulatory follicles: implications for control of primate ovulation by prostaglandin E2. J Clin Endocrinol Metab. 2005;90(2): 1021-7.
76. O'Grady JP, Caldwell BV, Auletta FJ, Speroff L. The effects of an inhibitor of prostaglandin synthesis (indomethacin) on ovulation, pregnancy, and pseudopregnancy in the rabbit. Prostaglandins. 1972;1(2):97-106.
77. Killick S, Elstein M. Pharmacologic production of luteinized unruptured follicles by prostaglandin synthetase inhibitors. Fertil Steril. 1987;47(5):773-7.
78. Katt JA, Duncan JA, Herbon L, Barkan A, Marshall JC. The frequency of gonadotropin-releasing hormone stimulation determines the number of pituitary gonadotropin releasing hormone receptors. Endocrinology. 1985;116(5):2113-5.
79. Adams JM, Taylor AE, Schoenfeld DA, Crowley Jr WF, Hall JE. The midcycle gonadotropin surge in normal women occurs in the face of an unchanging gonadotropin releasing hormone pulse frequency. J Clin Endocrinol Metab. 1994;79(3):858-64.
80. de Koning J. Gonadotrophin surge-inhibiting/attenuating factor governs luteinizing hormone secretion during the ovarian cycle: physiology and pathology. Hum Reprod. 1995;10(11):2854-61.
81. Christenson LK, Stouffer RL. Follicle-stimulating hormone and luteinizing hormone/chorionic gonadotropin stimulation of vascular endothelial factor production by macaque granulosa cells from pre- and periovulatory follicles. J Clin Endocrinol Metab. 1997;82(7):2135-42.
82. Golos TG, Soto EA, Tureck RW, Strauss 3rd JF. Human chorionic gonadotropin and 8-bromo-adenosine 3',5'-monophosphate stimulate [125I] low density lipoprotein uptake and metabolism by luteinized human granulosa cells in culture. J Clin Endocrinol Metab. 1985;61(4):633-8.
83. Retamales I, Carrasco I, Troncoso JL, Las Heras J, Devoto L, Vega M. Morpho-functional study of human luteal cell subpopulations. Hum Reprod. 1994;9(4):591-6.
84. Lei ZM, Chegini N, Rao CV. Quantitative cell composition of human bovine corpora lutea from various reproductive states. Biol Reprod. 1991;44(6):1148-56.
85. Brannian JD, Stouffer RL. Progesterone production by monkey luteal cell subpopulations at different stages of the menstrual cycle: changes in agonist responsiveness. Biol Reprod. 1991;44(1):141-9.
86. Lenton EA, Landgren BM, Sexton L, Harper R. Normal variation in the length of the follicular phase of the menstrual cycle: effect of chronological age. Br J Obstet Gynaecol. 1984; 91(7):681-4.
87. Speroff L, Fritz MA. Regulation of the menstrual cycle. In: Speroff L, Fritz MA (Eds). Clinical Gynecologic Endocrinology and Infertility, 8th edition. Philadelphia, PA, USA: Lippincott Williams and Wilkins; 2011. pp. 199-242.
88. Bonduelle M, Dodd R, Liebaers I, Van Steirteghem A, Williamson R, Akhurst R. Chorionic gonadotropin-β mRNA, a trophoblast marker, is expressed in human 8-cell embryos derived from tripronucleate zygotes. Hum Reprod. 1988;3(7):909-14.
89. Roseff SJ, Bangah ML, Kettel LM, Vale W, Rivier J, Burger HG, et al. Dynamic changes in circulating inhibin levels during the luteal–follicular transition of the human menstrual cycle. J Clin Endocrinol Metab. 1989;69(5):1033-9.
90. Hall JE, Schoenfeld DA, Martin KA, Crowley Jr WF. Hypothalamic gonadotropin-releasing hormone secretion and follicle-stimulating hormone dynamics during the luteal follicular transition. J Clin Endocrinol Metab. 1992;74(3):600-7.
91. Chan RWS, Schwab KE, Gargett CE. Clonogenicity of human endometrial epithelial and stromal cells. Biol Reprod. 2004;70(6):1738-50.
92. Bergeron C, Ferenczy A, Shyamala G. Distribution of estrogen receptors in various cell types of normal, hyperplastic, and neoplastic human endometrial tissues. Lab Invest. 1988; 58(3):338-45.
93. Fata JE, Ho AT, Leco KJ, Moorehead RA, Khokha R. Cellular turnover and extracellular matrix remodelling in female reproductive tissues: functions of metalloproteinases and the inhibitors. Cell Mol Life Sci. 2000;57(1):77-95.

CHAPTER 3

Oogenesis and Folliculogenesis

Suvarna Rathor Zirpe

INTRODUCTION

The ovary plays a dual role, reproductive as well as endocrine, in the female body. It acts as a reproductive organ by production and periodical release of the female gamete—oocyte. Regnier de Graaf was one of the first to recognize ovary as a producer of egg.[1] Earlier scientists believed that follicle itself was egg. The discovery that oocyte was enclosed within the follicle was made by Karl Ernst von Baer in 1827.[2] The ovary acts as an endocrine organ by producing hormones such as estrogen, progesterone, and testosterone, which are responsible for pubertal growth and menstrual cycle.

In this chapter, we review and understand the process of oogenesis and folliculogenesis, various stages of development, and the role of different factors involved in this process. This will help us to understand the clinical implications of the process.

FORMATION OF FEMALE GONADS

If the indifferent gonad is destined to become testis, differentiation will occur at 6–9 weeks. In the absence of SRY (sex-determining region on Y chromosome), ovary formation is initiated. Both ovary and testis formation require dominantly acting genes. SRY causes testis development via upregulation of *SOX9* (SRY-related HMG box gene). Overexpression in either *DAX1* (dosage-sensitive sex reversal, adrenal hypoplasia critical region, on chromosome X, gene 1) or *WNT4* (member of wingless family of genes)/ *RSPO1* (R-spondin-1) antagonizes testis formation and promotes the development of ovary. Also *FOXL2* (forkhead box protein L2) inhibits the upregulation of *SOX9* and promotes the formation of ovary **(Flowchart 1)**.

Flowchart 1: Formation of female gonads.

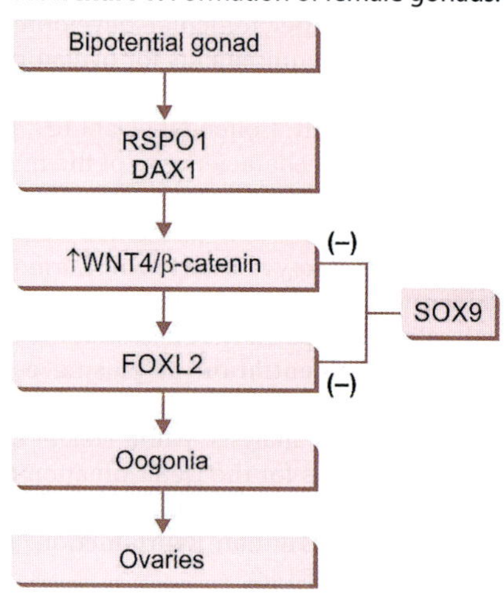

Primordial germ cells (PGCs) appear first in the dorsal wall endoderm of yolk sac near the allantois as a cluster of 100 cells by 3–4 weeks of gestation.[3] PGCs migrate to the hindgut and dorsal mesentery by fourth and fifth weeks of gestation, respectively.[3] Gonadal tissue colonization by germ cells is completed by 7 weeks of gestation. Germ cells are essential for the formation and maintenance of the ovary. In the absence of germ cells, the gonad degenerates into cord-like structures.[4] The migration of germ cells to the gonadal ridge happens as shown in **Figures 1A and B**.

Oogenesis: It is a process of developing a mature oocyte from an oogonium.

Folliculogenesis: It is the maturation of the ovarian follicle (densely packed shell of somatic cells containing the oocyte) from primordial follicle into a large preovulatory follicle.

STAGES OF OOGENESIS

Oogenesis starts in *prenatal life* as early as 4 weeks of gestation. During the process of oogenesis, all primary oocytes get arrested at the diplotene stage of prophase I of the first meiotic division, until puberty. In *postnatal life* after puberty, there is reinitiation of further development of primary oocyte to form a mature oocyte. The different stages of development in oogenesis are as follows:

- Primordial germ cell
- Oogonia

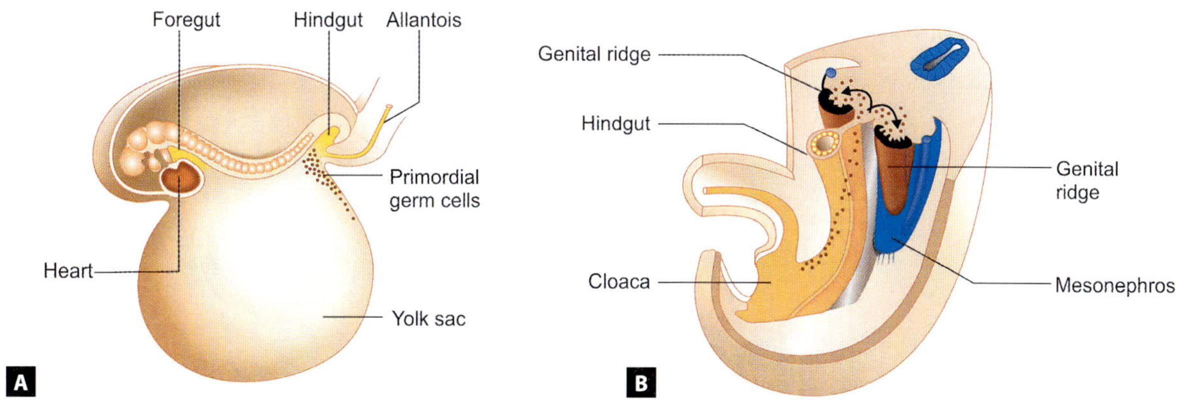

Figs. 1A and B: Primordial germ cell migration.

- Primary oocyte
- Secondary oocyte
- Oocyte maturation
- Oocyte activation.

Primordial Germ Cells

Primordial germ cells reach gonads by 7 weeks of gestation. They undergo rapid proliferation and increase from merely 10,000 at 6 weeks of gestation to 6 lakhs at the 8th week, and to 6 million at the 20th week of gestation. Then the rate of oogonial mitosis slowly decreases and mitosis stops at 28 weeks of gestation. Simultaneously, there is onset of oogonial atresia at around 8 weeks which is maximum around 20 weeks of gestation. At birth, around 1 million germ cells exist in the ovary of which only 3–4 lakhs will remain till puberty due to atresia. Around 1% (300) manage to grow till the ovulatory state before menopause.[5]

Oogonia

Primordial germ cells on reaching gonads are called oogonia. They have high mitotic activity and undergo rapid mitosis and multiplication before the onset of meiosis. This mitotic activity ceases by 28 weeks of gestation. Formed oogonia are bound together in cellular bridges forming syncytium (clusters of cell). In these connected oogonia, there is synchronous onset of the subsequent meiosis. Mitosis and the simultaneously occurring oogonial atresia determine the final ovarian reserve.

Primary Oocyte

After the onset of meiosis, oogonia are called primary oocytes. Oogonia enter meiosis around 8–13 weeks of gestation. Gene *Stra8* is crucial for meiosis as DNA synthesis fails to occur in *Stra8* null mice.[6] Meiosis begins with a prophase stage, which is further divided into five stages: (1) Leptotene, (2) zygotene, (3) pachytene, (4) diplotene, and (5) diakinesis. On entering into the diplotene stage of prophase, oocytes go into a protracted resting phase called dictyate. The primary oocyte gets arrested at the first meiotic prophase stage, dictyate. Chromatin in the meiotically arrested oocytes is encapsulated by a nuclear structure and is called the *germinal vesicle (GV)*. GV oocytes are present in the primordial follicles. Recommencement of meiosis occurs in postnatal life just prior to ovulation.

It was believed that the number of primary oocytes is predetermined and cannot be increased beyond those indigenously laid down when the ovary was formed.[7,8] But few recent studies have shown oocyte regeneration from putative germ cells in bone marrow and peripheral blood.[9,10] In a recent study, oocytes and offspring were generated from female germ stem cells (FGSC) in mice.[11] These findings have significant implications for human reproduction, preservation of the fertility, and prevention of some health problems.

The remaining stages of development in oogenesis, i.e., secondary oocyte, oocyte maturation, and activation (all occurring in postnatal life after puberty), will be described after the stages of folliculogenesis.

STAGES OF FOLLICULOGENESIS

Oogonia are surrounded by somatic cells from the primitive gonads to form a follicle. The primary function of a follicle is to support the oocyte growth. Vascularization of ovarian cortex marks the beginning of folliculogenesis, which starts around the fourth month of gestation.

Different stages of development in folliculogenesis are shown in **Figure 2**.

- Primordial follicle
- Primary follicle
- Secondary/preantral follicle
- Antral follicle
- Selection and dominance of follicle
- Graafian/preovulatory/mature follicle.

Most of the growing follicles progress till antral stage and then undergo atresia. But after puberty, gonadotropins rescue few of the antral follicles and they continue to grow; out of these, one dominant follicle is formed every month,

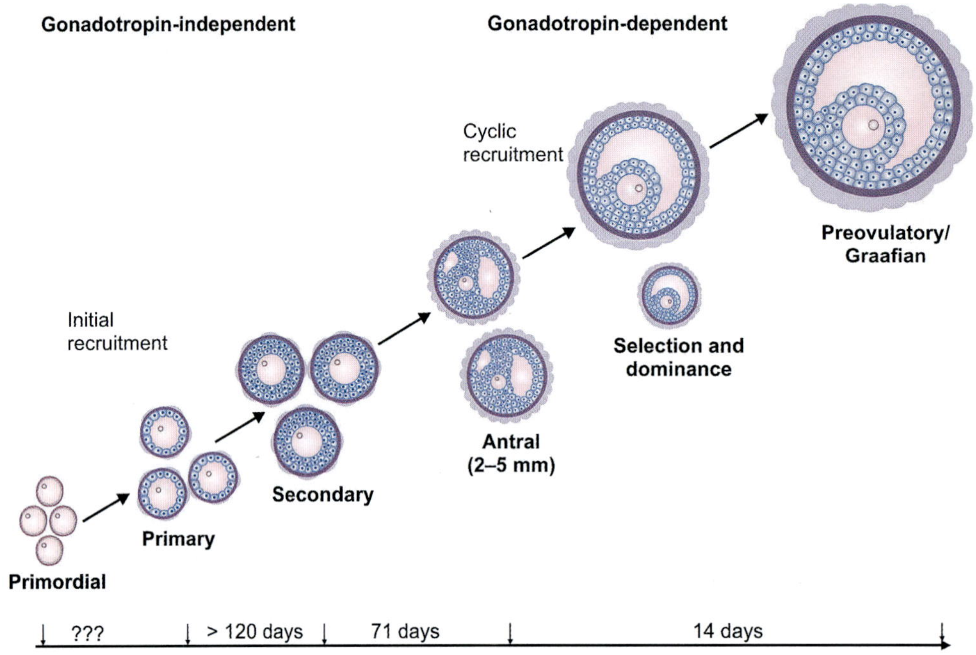

Fig. 2: Stages of folliculogenesis.

which ovulates. It takes 14 days to form a Graafian/dominant follicle from the antral follicle, but >85 days for a secondary follicle to grow into a Graafian follicle[12] **(Fig. 2)**. Moreover, it is estimated that >120 days might be required for the formation of secondary follicle from primary follicle and even longer for the formation of primary follicle from primordial follicle[12] **(Fig. 2)**. Thus, the whole growth phase of a follicle is greater than eight menstrual cycles or 220 days.

Primordial Follicle

Primordial follicle (30–60 μm) contains primary oocyte encircled by flattened pregranulosa cells. Its formation starts in the intrauterine life by the 15th week and is completed 6 months after birth. Various genes involved in its formation are transcription factors, meiosis-specific enzymes, zona proteins, and nerve growth factors. The total number of primordial follicles in the ovary ascertains the reproductive life span of a female. The process by which primordial follicles undergo further development is called "initial recruitment." Initial recruitment is moderated by various stimulatory and inhibitory hormones and locally produced growth factors.

Primary Follicle

Primary follicle (60 μm) has primary oocyte encircled by zona pellucida and granulosa cells which have become cuboidal from flattened state. Certain growth factors and extracellular matrix components having autocrine and paracrine effects act as stimulators and inhibitors **(Table 1)** in the transition of primordial to primary follicles.[13-15]

TABLE 1: Factors acting as stimulators and inhibitors in the formation of primary follicle from primordial follicle.

Stimulators	*Inhibitors*
• Kit ligand FGF-2 (basic fibroblast growth factor) – Keratinocyte growth factor – Leukemia inhibitory factor – BMP4/7/15 (bone morphogenetic protein) – Growth differentiation factor 9	• PTEN tumor suppressor gene (phosphatase and tensin homolog deleted on chromosome 10) – Tsc1/mTORC1 (tumor suppressor Tsc1) • Foxo3a (forkhead transcription factor) – P27 (cyclin-dependent kinase inhibitor 1B) – Foxl2 (winged-helix transcription factor) – Anti-Müllerian hormone

Inhibitory signals keep primordial follicles in the resting state (mice studies). Premature activation of the primordial follicle happens if there is loss of function of any of the inhibitory molecules.

FOXL2 has a crucial role in the transition of pregranulosa cells to granulosa cells. *FOXL2 mutation* has been associated with premature ovarian failure (POF) in humans[16] and also causes blepharophimosis, ptosis, and epicanthus inversus syndrome in humans.[17]

In polycystic ovaries, there is increased accumulation of primary follicles which is termed stockpiling. The explanation for stockpiling is either a slower rate of loss by atresia or higher initial population of primordial follicles in polycystic ovaries.[18]

Significance of anti-Müllerian hormone (AMH): It is a dimeric glycoprotein belonging to transforming growth factor beta (TGF-β) family. AMH is manufactured by the granulosa cells of primary, preantral, and small antral follicles from 36 weeks of intrauterine life. It is a detector of ovarian reserve having least inter- and intracycle variability. At puberty, AMH levels are at its peak and become obscure after menopause.[19] AMH inhibits the recruitment of primordial follicles. Thus in the absence of AMH, there is increased recruitment of primordial follicles leading to follicular depletion from the ovaries. Also AMH reduces follicle responsiveness to follicle-stimulating hormone (FSH) and acts as a negative regulator of follicle selection.[20] It is also a predictor of response to ovarian stimulation. The cutoff range for poor responders is 0.5–1.1 ng/mL (≤3.6–7.8 pmol/L) and for hyperresponders is >3.5 ng/mL (25 pmol/L).

Anti-Müllerian hormone is secreted from small- and medium-sized antral follicles, which are typically increased in polycystic ovaries; thus, significantly higher levels of AMH are seen in this population. Similarly, with the increasing age, there is a simultaneous decrease in small- and medium-sized follicles due to continuous atresia responsible for lower AMH levels in this population.

Recruitment of follicles: It includes initial and cyclic recruitment of follicles. As shown in **Figure 2**, in *initial recruitment*, the dormant primordial follicles are continuously recruited for further development. It starts immediately after the follicle formation and continues throughout life. After the initial recruitment, the follicle grows but the oocyte still remains arrested in the stage of prophase of meiosis I and the nonrecruited follicles remain dormant. As functional gonadotropin receptors are not developed in primordial follicles, FSH and luteinizing hormone (LH) are unlikely to have a role in the initial recruitment.[21] The above-mentioned stimulators and inhibitors may have a role in the initial recruitment. *Cyclic recruitment* occurs after puberty and is due to increase in FSH in the circulation that rescues a cohort of antral follicles (2–5 mm in diameter) from atresia in every cycle. Oocyte in these follicles is competent of resuming meiosis. Out of this cohort, one becomes the dominant follicle and the rest undergo apoptosis.

Atresia of oocytes: It is a continuous and ongoing process. It starts as early as 8 weeks of gestation. Oocytes which are not encircled by the granulosa cells for the formation of primordial follicle are lost by apoptosis. On entering the initial recruitment, the follicle progresses till the antral stage; after that, it automatically undergoes atresia. It is only after puberty that few antral follicles are conserved from atresia by cyclic recruitment, developing into mature Graafian follicle and ovulation. It is still not well understood why millions of germ cells are wastefully lost while only few [300–400 (1%)] reach the ovulatory stage. It has been proposed that factors such as age, pregnancy, lactation, hypophysectomy, unilateral ovariectomy, hormones, nutrition, ischemia, grafting, and X irradiations may influence follicular atresia.

Secondary/Preantral Follicle

Secondary follicle (120–150 μm) contains primary oocyte, zona pellucida, multiple layers of granulosa cells, and basal lamina surrounded by theca cells. An intricate network of capillary vessels is formed between the layers of theca cells. Although FSH receptors may be expressed on preantral follicles, the role of FSH in its development is debated. Members of TGF superfamily produced from granulosa and theca cells, activins from granulosa cells, GDF-9, oocyte-derived bone morphogenetic protein 15 (BMP15), and thecal cell-derived BMP-4/7 play a significant role in the growth of secondary follicle.

Granulosa cells do not have their own blood supply. Blood–follicle barrier is formed by the basal lamina. Between the granulosa cells, there exists an extensive network of gap junctions formed by connexin proteins. These gap junctions are extremely important in follicle development. They form an effective conveyance among the granulosa cells and also with the oocyte. In mice deficient for connexin 43 and 37, follicles do not grow beyond primary and preantral stages, respectively.[22,23]

Antral Follicle

There is further multiplication of granulosa and theca cells, increased vascularization, growth of oocyte, and formation of fluid-filled spaces which merge and form a cavity called antrum. These antral follicles are around 2–5 mm in diameter and can be seen on ultrasonography. Day 2 antral follicle count (AFC) is a crucial indicator of ovarian reserve. On the antral follicles, FSH and LH receptors are present on granulosa cells and theca cells, respectively. At this stage, follicles are dependent on FSH and LH for further development and are rescued from atresia by *cyclic recruitment* **(Fig. 2)**. The selective rise in serum FSH beyond a critical "threshold" level during the luteal follicular transition is a potent stimulus for the recruitment and growth of follicle. Rise in FSH also leads to maturation of granulosa cells, induction of LH receptors on it, stimulation of aromatase activity, and inhibin biosynthesis by granulosa cells. All these together lead to selection and dominance of only one follicle in natural cycle.

Following are the important concepts to be understood in folliculogenesis:

- *Follicle-stimulating hormone threshold:* According to this concept, FSH concentrations need to transcend a distinct level to stimulate ovarian follicle growth.
- *Follicle-stimulating hormone window/gate:* It is the period for which the elevated level of FSH above the threshold

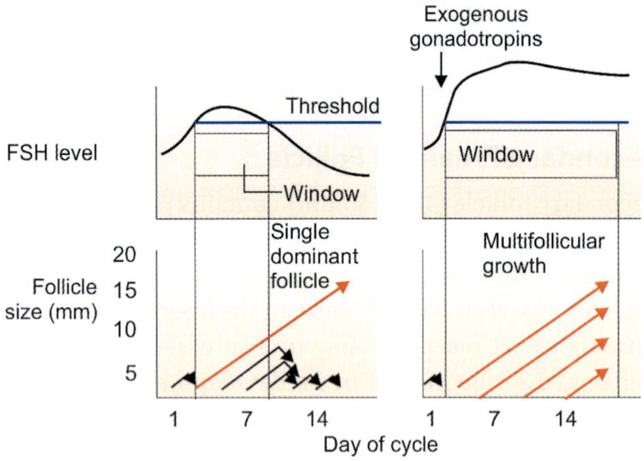

Fig. 3: Concept of FSH threshold and FSH window.
(FSH: follicle-stimulating hormone)

needs to be maintained for follicular recruitment and growth.

- *Luteinizing hormone window:* This indicates the concentration of LH essential for follicular growth and selection of dominant follicle. A *threshold* and *ceiling* level for LH (therapeutic window) is proposed, below the threshold estrogen production is inadequate, and beyond the ceiling level LH may be deleterious to follicular growth.
- *Luteinizing hormone surge:* It is the rise in LH that stimulates the series of events leading to ovulation.

Follicle-stimulating hormone threshold and window concept **(Fig. 3)** help us to understand the monofollicular growth in a natural cycle. FSH on rising beyond the threshold stimulates recruitment and growth of follicles. FSH falls below the threshold due to the rising estrogen level which maintains the FSH window in natural cycle leading to monofollicular development.

It also forms the basis for multifollicular growth in stimulated cycles. The FSH window is extended by giving FSH externally above the threshold which leads to recruitment and continuous growth of many follicles leading to multifollicular development.

Flowchart 2: Selection and growth of dominant follicle in a natural cycle.

Rise of FSH beyond certain threshold during luteal follicular transition

↓

Follicular recruitment (cyclic recruitment)

↓

Selection of dominant follicle—follicle with GC (granulosa cell) most responsive to FSH (lowest FSH threshold), secrete estrogens

↓

Negative feedback to hypothalamo-pituitary axis (HPA)

↓

Suppress FSH secretion

↓

FSH insufficient to sustain development of other follicles with higher FSH threshold

↓

Other follicles undergo atresia while dominant follicle continues to grow and secrete estrogen

↓

Dominant follicle

↓

Increased synthesis of estrogen with increased expression of LH receptors on GC which are adequately stimulated by FSH

↓

LH sustains preovulatory follicular endocrine activity induced by FSH

↓

LH plays primary role in complete maturation of follicle and development of oocyte competence

↓

Mid cycle LH surge

↓

Disrupts GC contacts in cumulus oophorus and induces oocyte maturation

↓

Follicle rupture (ovulation) followed by induction of GC luteinization

(FSH: follicle-stimulating hormone; LH: luteinizing hormone)

Selection and Dominance of Single Follicle

Changes occurring in the granulosa and theca cells in response to FSH and LH explain the selection and dominance process. The follicle whose granulosa cells are most responsive to FSH (lowest FSH threshold) becomes first in the cohort to secrete estrogen and inhibin. Increasing estrogen and inhibin levels send feedback to the hypothalamic-pituitary axis (HPA) and begin to suppress pituitary FSH secretion. Decreasing FSH concentrations are inadequate to maintain the growth of other follicles that have higher FSH threshold leading to the growth of a single follicle having the lowest threshold. Induction of LH receptors on the maturing follicle reduces its dependence solely on FSH. This follicle distinctively responds to both FSH and LH and continues to grow and secrete estrogen in spite of decreasing concentration of circulating FSH **(Flowchart 2)**.

Thus, both FSH and LH are essential for normal follicular growth. FSH plays a crucial part in recruitment, selection, and dominance, while LH contributes to dominance, final maturation, and ovulation. LH has a crucial role in steroidogenesis. So in hypogonadotropic hypogonadism, both FSH and LH supplementation are required to ensure normal follicular development.

In anovulatory polycystic ovary syndrome (PCOS), there is arrested development of follicle and failure to develop a single dominant follicle due to FSH levels below the required threshold.[18] Also LH at inappropriately high concentration leads to follicular atresia or prematurely luteinization.

Graafian/Preovulatory/Mature Follicle

Graafian follicle or preovulatory follicle is a stage after the completion of the first meiotic division but before the ovulation. It contains a 2N haploid secondary oocyte located eccentrically surrounded by zona pellucida, corona radiata, cumulus oophorus, large antral cavity, granulosa cells, basal lamina, and theca (interna and externa) cells. The preovulatory follicle is around 16–29 mm and grows at a rate of 1–4 mm/day.[2] A dominant follicle having least FSH threshold, increased aromatase activity, and LH receptors on granulosa cells produces >90% of estrogen in the preovulatory period.[24] The estradiol level on reaching 200 pg/mL for >48 hours stimulates LH surge by providing positive feedback signal to the hypothalamus and pituitary which is needed for inducing ovulation. After the preovulatory estradiol peak, the serum progesterone level starts rising indicating the onset of follicular luteinization.[2] This midcycle progesterone rise may be responsible for FSH surge prior to ovulation. The growth and development of dominant follicle is explained in **Flowchart 2**.

The remaining stages of development of oogenesis are described in the following text.

Secondary Oocyte

Just before the ovulation, the arrested primary oocyte resumes meiosis I and the division is completed by the formation of a haploid secondary oocyte and first polar body.

Maintenance of primary oocyte in meiotic arrest: Primary oocytes are arrested in meiosis I till the LH surge; after puberty, meiosis I resumes. As shown in **Figure 4**, granulosa cells produce cyclic adenosine monophosphate (cAMP) and cyclic guanosine monophosphate (cGMP), which reach the oocyte via gap junctions.[20] Protein kinase A (PkA) is activated by cAMP which inhibits oocyte maturation and maintains meiotic arrest.

Resumption of meiosis: LH peak and various autocrine and paracrine signals are involved in the resumption of meiosis as shown in **Figure 5**. LH peaking leads to dispersion of cumulus cells and thus disruption of gap junction. This causes a fall in intra-oocyte cAMP and reinitiation of meiosis I. Also, LH peak causes influx of calcium which activates protein kinase C (PkC) which help to initiate meiosis I. Immediately after meiosis I, the secondary oocyte begins meiosis II and again gets arrested in metaphase of meiosis II (*called MII oocyte*). Meiosis II is complete only if fertilization occurs.

Understanding the importance of LH surge, it is to be administered in stimulated cycles as a trigger for the final maturation. Human chorionic gonadotropin (hCG) which acts as a surrogate for LH by binding to the same receptor (i.e., LH/hCG receptor) or gonadotropin-releasing hormone (GnRH) agonists which release FSH and LH from the pituitary are the different triggers used in stimulated cycles.

Various cascades of events occurring in oogenesis and folliculogenesis are shown in **Figure 6**.

Oocyte Maturation

Oocyte maturation includes resumption of meiosis I and nuclear and cytoplasmic maturation of the oocyte. LH surge initiates resumption of meiosis I. Once the oocytes begin to mature, their nuclei (i.e., GV) break down and chromosome condenses [i.e., GV breakdown (GVBD)]. Chromosomes are then arranged in metaphase I (MI) stage which is followed by anaphase I to telophase I completing meiosis I. Then oocyte enters meiosis II and gets arrested in metaphase called MII oocytes.[25] Cytoplasmic maturity of an oocyte includes

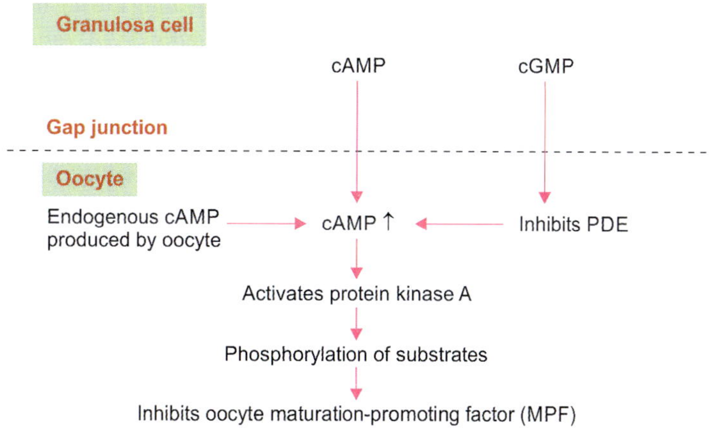

Fig. 4: Maintenance of primary oocyte in meiotic arrest.
(cAMP: cyclic adenosine monophosphate; cGMP: cyclic guanosine monophosphate; PDE: phosphodiesterase)

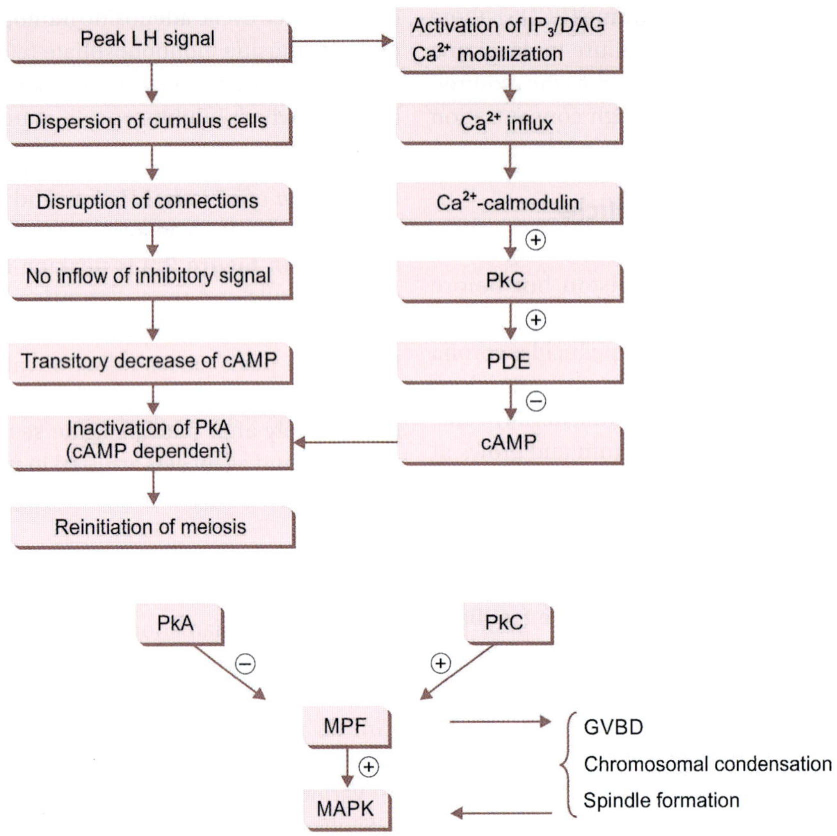

Fig. 5: Resumption of oocyte meiosis I.
(cAMP: cyclic adenosine monophosphate; DAG: diacylglycerol; GVBD: germinal vesicle breakdown; IP3: inositol-1,4,5-triphosphate; LH: luteinizing hormone; MAPK: mitogen-activated protein kinase; MPF: maturation-promoting factor; PDE: phosphodiesterase; PkA: protein kinase A; PkC: protein kinase C)

various events such as correct placement of organelles, post-translational modifications of mRNAs, synthesis of proteins, change in the number and morphology of mitochondria, ultrastructural modifications of Golgi complex, and accumulation of ribosomes. Then the mature oocyte is ovulated and is ready for fertilization.

Clinical implication: Retrieval of oocytes is done before ovulation in in vitro fertilization (IVF) or intracytoplasmic sperm injection (ICSI). These oocytes are not fully mature, although the first polar body is released and MII oocyte is seen.[26,27] There is asynchrony between the nuclear and cytoplasmic maturity in the stimulated cycles.[28,29] Thus cytoplasmic maturity may be induced by incubation of oocytes postretrieval, before IVF or ICSI, which eventually improves the fertilization and pregnancy rates.

Clinical significance of GV, MI, and MII oocytes: IVF or ICSI is performed on a fully mature MII oocyte. Collected GV or MI oocytes have to undergo in vitro maturation (IVM) before undergoing the IVF or ICSI procedure. The IVM procedure is beneficial and is indicated in a selected group of patients having polycystic ovaries, history of ovarian hyperstimulation, for fertility preservation (e.g., cancer patients), etc. In rare instances, there can be failure to complete meiosis in all the collected oocytes called oocyte maturation failure. Very few cases have been reported in the literature where all oocytes collected in GV or MI stage failed to resume meiosis when cultured in vitro.

Errors in meiosis: Gametes undergo meiosis for the maintenance of ploidy in the species. Meiotic dysfunctions are mistakes happening during meiosis.

- *Errors during DNA replication:* This occurs during DNA synthesis called S phase of meiosis. Errors while copying DNA cause alteration in the gene and can lead to mutations. Examples of diseases due to genetic mutation are sickle cell anemia, color blindness, etc.
- *Errors during recombination:* This occurs during meiosis I and II and can lead to alteration in the structure of chromosome. Mistakes while swapping of genetic material between paired chromosomes lead to errors such as duplication, deletion, inversion, and translocation (reciprocal and Robertsonian) of chromosome. Charcot-Marie-Tooth disease, Duchenne muscular dystrophy, hemophilia A, leukemia, etc., are examples of disorders caused due to recombination errors.

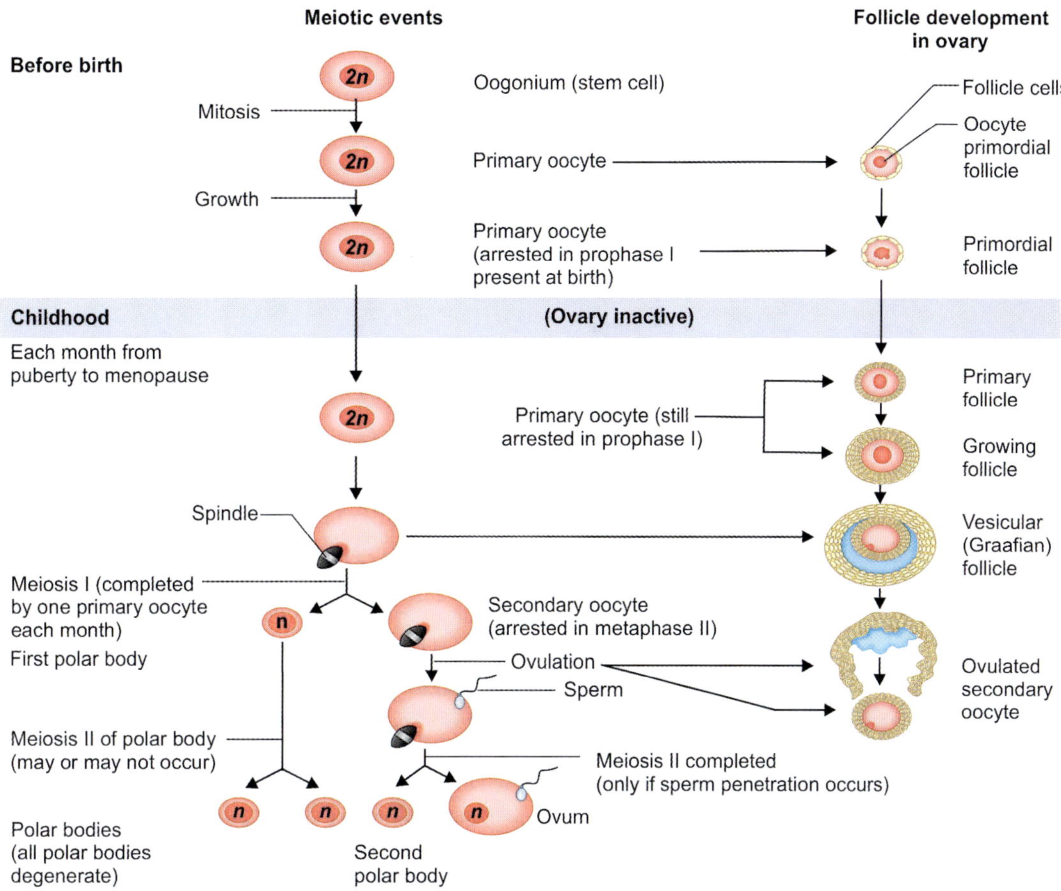

Fig. 6: Events occurring in oogenesis and folliculogenesis.

- *Errors during segregation:* This occurs during meiosis I and II due to nondisjunction of chromosomes. Prolonged arrest in the dictyate stage predisposes the oocytes for segregation errors resulting in aneuploid embryos leading to monosomies and trisomies (e.g., Turner and Down syndrome).

Ovulation

Ovulation is the process of release of female gamete from the ovary. It includes a series of changes occurring in the collagenous wall of the follicle to release the cumulus-oocyte complex. Ovulation occurs 10–12 hours after the LH peak and 24–36 hours after the estradiol peak. Roles of different hormones in ovulation are shown in **Figure 7**. All these hormones act together to breach the follicular wall and release the oocyte **(Fig. 8)**.

Cyclo-oxygenase (COX) inhibitors cause block in the synthesis of prostaglandins without an effect on LH-induced action on maturation and luteinization. Thus, nonsteroidal anti-inflammatory drugs (NSAIDs) taken near ovulation prevent rupture of follicle and may lead to luteinized unruptured follicle (LUF).

PREVENTION OF PREMATURE LUTEINIZATION

With continued cell proliferation and follicle growth, it is essential to prevent premature luteinization of growing follicles. Oocyte-derived BMP6, BMP15, and GDF9 prevent premature luteinization and control progesterone rise by suppressing gonadotropin-driven progesterone rise.[30] The effect of these luteinization inhibitors vanishes after ovulation, and luteinization will commence.

TWO-CELL, TWO-GONADOTROPIN THEORY

This theory explains the endocrine regulation of estrogen synthesis in a growing follicle. The gene *CYP17* encoding 17-hydroxylase/C-17-20-lyase activity is pivotal in androgen synthesis and is present only in theca cells. The role of FSH in a growing follicle is to increase FSH receptors on granulosa cells, LH receptors on theca cells, and granulosa cell aromatase activity. LH stimulates theca cells to produce androgens. Androstenedione produced by theca cells diffuse into granulosa cells and is converted to estradiol by aromatase (CYP19A1) activity **(Fig. 9)**. Androgens also play a role in follicle selection and dominance. Androgens

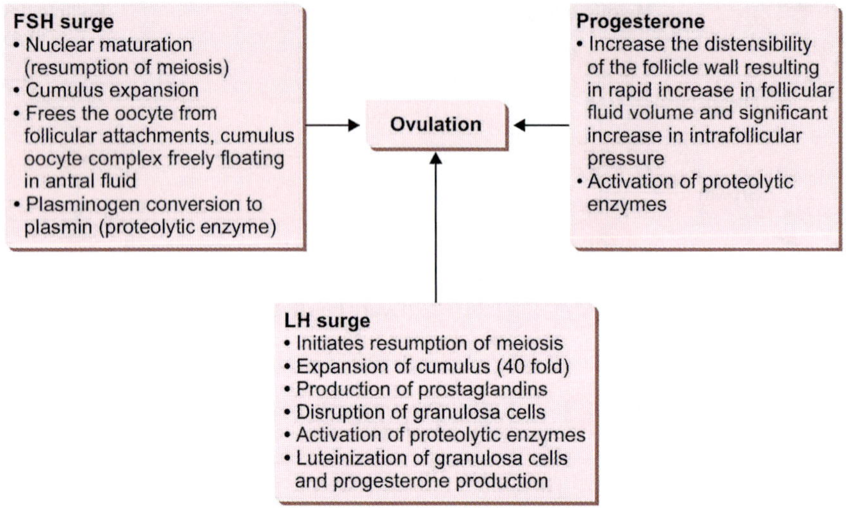

Fig. 7: Role of hormones in ovulation.
(FSH: follicle-stimulating hormone; LH: luteinizing hormone)

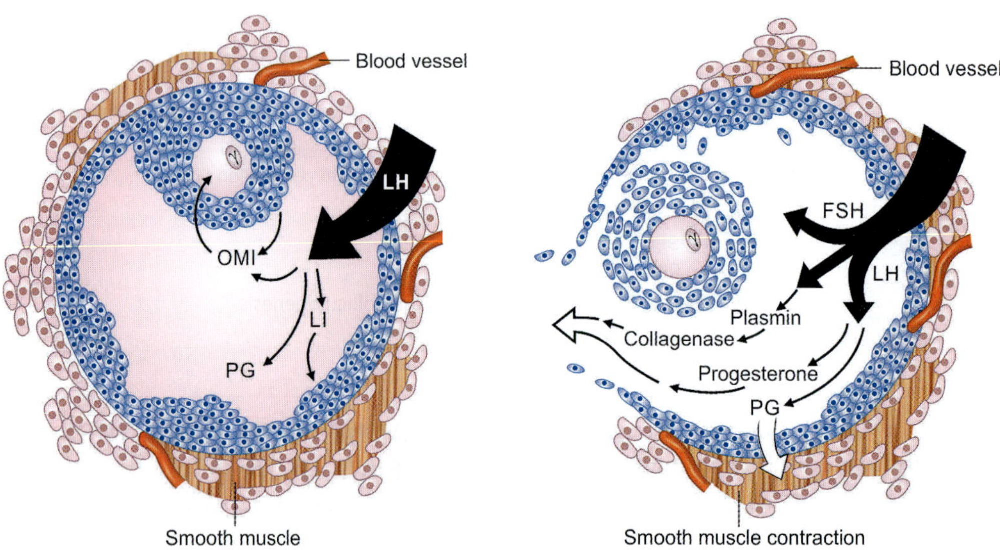

Fig. 8: Process of ovulation.
(FSH: follicle-stimulating hormone; LH: luteinizing hormone; LI; leukotriene; OMI: oocyte maturation inhibitor; PG: prostaglandin)

at low concentrations serve as a substrate for and enhance aromatase activity forming estrogen. At high concentration, androgens inhibit aromatase activity and FSH-induced LH receptor formation. Thus in hypothalamic hypogonadism, stimulation with FSH alone is not effective. Although it leads to the development of follicular size, estradiol production remains low and hence the occurrence of fertilization and pregnancy is low. These findings highlight the significance of both FSH and LH in follicle development **(Fig. 9)**.

CLINICAL IMPLICATIONS

Analysis of basics of oogenesis and folliculogenesis has important clinical implications.

- Multifollicular ovarian stimulation and development of different ovarian stimulation protocols
- Advancement of assisted reproductive techniques for the treatment of subfertile couples
- Preservation of fertility in individuals at risk of depleting ovarian reserve such as advancing age, any cancer, exposure to gonadotoxic agents, POF, and surgical menopause.

Understanding the basics has also answered some interesting queries like:

- *Does early menarche lead to early menopause*?
  All primordial follicles are destined to be subjected to apoptosis if not salvaged by FSH; thus, initial recruitment is responsible for follicular pool depletion rather than the cyclic recruitment. This indicates that even before the onset of puberty, follicles are lost from the pool by initial recruitment. Early menarche due to nutritional,

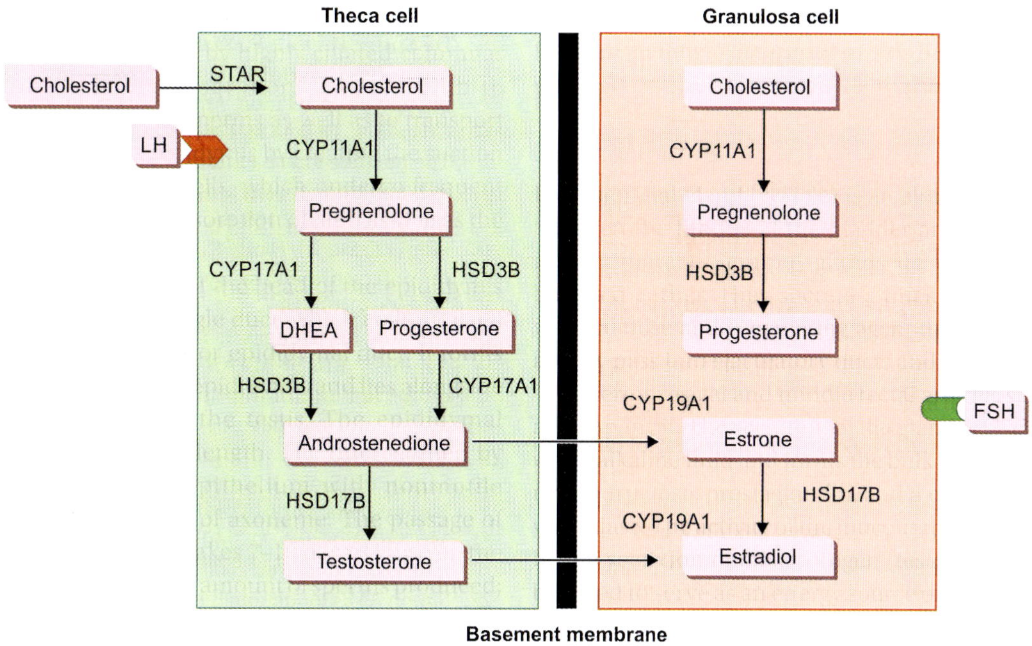

Fig. 9: Two-cell, two-gonadotropin theory. Cholesterol is internalized into the mitochondria via the steroidogenic acute regulatory protein (STAR). It is then converted to pregnenolone in the mitochondria via cytochrome-P450 cholesterol side-chain cleavage (CYP11A1). Pregnenolone then diffuses out of the mitochondria and is transported to the smooth endoplasmic reticulum where it is converted to progesterone or dehydroepiandrosterone (DHEA) via 3β-hydroxysteroid dehydrogenase (HSD3B) or 17α-hydroxylase-17,20-desmolase (CYP17A1), respectively. Progesterone and DHEA are then converted to the androgen androstenedione again via CYP17A1 or HSD3B, respectively. Androstenedione can then be converted to either testosterone or estrone via 17β-hydroxysteroid dehydrogenase (HSD17B) or aromatase (CYP19A1), respectively. Testosterone and estrone are then converted to the most potent estrogen, estradiol, via CYP19A1 (aromatase) or HSD17B, respectively.
(FSH: follicle-stimulating hormone; LH: luteinizing hormone)

environmental, or pathophysiological factors leads to early onset of cyclic recruitment, which should not affect the timing of follicle pool depletion and menopause.

- *Does unilateral ovariectomy or chemotherapy affect the age of menopause?*
  Unilateral ovariectomy or chemotherapy diminishes the pool of resting follicles, which is an important determining factor of ovarian aging. So it leads to early onset of menopause.
- *Does steroidal contraception delay menopause?*
  It mainly affects the surge of gonadotropins and thus prevents ovulation. It does not affect the initial or cyclic recruitment and so probably has no effect on age of menopause. But few epidemiological studies suggest that the age of menopause might be somewhat delayed; hence, more detailed studies are needed to prove its effects.
- *Whether increased parity delays menopause?*
  During pregnancy, progesterone in the circulation is elevated which might suppress initial follicular recruitment maintaining a greater follicle pool size. So, increased parity may lead to late onset of menopause.
- *Does repeated ovarian stimulation with gonadotropins lead to early onset of menopause?*
  Probably no, as the gonadotropins mainly act on antral follicles to promote cyclic recruitment. Gonadotropins may not have a role in initial recruitment, but it is uncertain whether repeated exogenous gonadotropin might increase follicle loss by an indirect action mediated through gonadotropin-responsive preantral follicles. Well-designed studies in egg donors need to be conducted to prove the effects of repeated ovarian stimulation on the age of menopause.

CONCLUSION

Remarkable progress is achieved in understanding the process of folliculogenesis and oogenesis, the gonadotropin-independent and -dependent phases, and various factors that act as stimulators and inhibitors in this process. Understanding the role of individual gonadotropins and the accessibility of recombinant preparations of FSH, LH, and hCG have opened the way to a more sophisticated and individualized approach to ovarian stimulation. Also, knowing the hormonal details of recruitment, follicular atresia, follicular maturation, and ovulation will facilitate to device new methods of contraception, to make improvements in culture conditions, and to treat subfertility associated with abnormal follicle development. May be in future we could extend the female reproductive life span and delay the age of menopause if we are able to formulate regimens that will suppress the initial recruitment of the follicles.

REFERENCES

1. Cobb M. Generation: The Seventeenth Century Scientists Who Unraveled the Secrets of Sex, Life and Growth. New York: Bloomsbury Publishing; 2006.
2. Baerwald AR, Adams GP, Pierson RA. Ovarian antral folliculogenesis during the human menstrual cycle: a review. Hum Reprod Update. 2012;18(1):73-91.
3. McKay DG, Hertig AT, Adams EC, Danziger S. Histochemical observations on the germ cells of human embryos. Anat Rec. 1953;2:201-19.
4. Merchant-Larios H, Centeno B. Morphogenesis of the ovary from the sterile W/Wv mouse. Prog Clin Biol Res. 1981; 59B:383-92.
5. Oktem O, Oktay K. The ovary: anatomy and function throughout human life. Ann NY Acad Sci. 2008;1127:1-9.
6. Baltus AE, Menke DB, Hu YC, Goodheart ML, Carpenter AE, de Rooij DG, et al. In germ cell of mouse embryonic ovaries, the decision to enter meiosis precedes premeiotic DNA replication. Nat Genet. 2006;38(12):1430-4.
7. Waldeyer W. Eierstock und Ei. Leipzig: Verlag von Wilhelm Engelmann; 1870.
8. Zuckerman S. The number of oocytes in the mature ovary. Recent Prog Horm Res. 1951;6:63-109.
9. Johnson J, Bagley J, Skaznik-Wikiel M, Lee H-J, Adams GB, Niikura Y, et al. Oocyte generation in adult mammalian ovaries by putative germ cells in bone marrow and peripheral blood. Cell. 2005;2:303-15.
10. Lee HJ, Selesniemi K, Niikura Y, Niikura T, Klein R, Dombkowski DM, et al. Bone marrow transplantation generates immature oocytes and rescues long-term fertility in a preclinical mouse model of chemotherapy-induced premature ovarian failure. J Clin Oncol. 2007;22:3198-204.
11. Zou K, Yuan Z, Yang Z, Luo H, Sun K, Zhou L, et al. Production of offspring from a germline stem cell line derived from neonatal ovaries. Nat Cell Biol. 2009;5:631-6.
12. Gougeon A. Regulation of ovarian follicular development in primates: facts and hypotheses. Endocr Rev. 1996;17:121-55.
13. Oktay K, Briggs D, Gosden RG. Ontogeny of follicle-stimulating hormone receptor gene expression in isolated human ovarian follicles. J Clin Endocrinol Metab. 1997;11:3748-51.
14. Eppig JJ. Oocyte control of ovarian follicular development and function in mammals. Reproduction. 2001;6:829-38.
15. Skinner MK. Regulation of primordial follicle assembly and development. Hum Reprod Update. 2005;5:461-71.
16. De Baere E, Beysen D, Oley C, Lorenz B, Cocquet J, De Sutter P, et al. FOXL2 and BPES: mutational hotspots, phenotypic variability, and revision of the genotype-phenotype correlation. Am J Hum Genet. 2003;2:478-87.
17. Crisponi L, Deiana M, Loi A, Chiappe F, Uda M, Amati P, et al. The putative forkhead transcription factor FOXL2 is mutated in blepharophimosis/ptosis/epicanthus inversus syndrome. Nat Genet. 2001;2:159-66.
18. Franks S, Stark J, Hardy K. Follicle dynamics and anovulation in polycystic ovary syndrome. Hum Reprod Update. 2008;14(4):367-78.
19. Hudson PL, Dougas I, Donahoe PK, Cate RL, Epstein J, Pepinsky RB, et al. An immunoassay to detect human mullerian inhibiting substance in males and females during normal development. J Clin Endocrinol Metab. 1990;1:16-22.
20. Sánchez F, Smitz J. Molecular control of oogenesis. Biochim Biophys Acta. 2012;1822:1896-912.
21. McGee EA, Hsueh AJ. Initial and cyclic recruitment of ovarian follicles. Endocr Rev. 2000;21(2):200-14.
22. Simon AM, Goodenough DA, Li E, Paul DL. Female infertility in mice lacking connexin 37. Nature. 1997;6616:525-9.
23. Juneja SC, Barr KJ, Enders GC, Kidder GM. Defects in the germ line and gonads of mice lacking connexin43. Biol Reprod. 1999;5:1263-70.
24. Baird D, Fraser I. Blood production and ovarian secretion rates of estradiol and estrone in women throughout the menstrual cycle. J Clin Endocrinol Metab. 1974;38:1009-17.
25. Trounson A, Anderiesz C, Jones G. Maturation of human oocytes in vitro and their developmental competence. Reproduction. 2001;121:51-75.
26. Kubiak JZ. Mouse oocytes gradually develop the capacity for activation during the metaphase II arrest. Dev Biol. 1989;136(2):537-45.
27. Balakier H, Sojecki A, Motamedi G, Librach C. Time dependent capability of human oocytes for activation and pronuclear formation during metaphase II arrest. Hum Reprod. 2004;19(4):982-87.
28. Eppig JJ, Schultz RM, O'Brien M, Chesnel F. Relationship between the developmental programs controlling nuclear and cytoplasmic maturation of mouse oocytes. Dev Biol. 1994;164(1):1-9.
29. Sundstorm P, Nilsson BO. Meiotic and cytoplasmic maturation of oocytes collected in stimulated cycles is asynchronous. Hum Reprod. 1988;3(5):613-9.
30. Otsuka F, Moore RK, Lemura S, Ueno N, Shimasaki S. Follistatin inhibits the function of the oocyte derived factor BMP-15. Biochem Biophys Res Commun. 2001;5:961-6.

CHAPTER 4

Spermatogenesis

Manishi Mittal

INTRODUCTION

The sperm is a unique cell produced in the mammalian male. Its specialized ability to move enables it to migrate through the female genital tract and fertilize the oocyte in vivo or in vitro. Its basic function is to carry the 23 male chromosomes to the egg at fertilization, and form the zygote. Also, the sperm centrosome provides the mechanism for cell division enabling mitosis and further development of the embryo.

GONADOGENESIS

The gonads develop in the gonadal ridge, by multiplication of primordial germ cells that originate in the extraembryonic mesoderm posterior to the primitive streak and thereafter cross the dorsal mesentery. This process is complete by 6 weeks of intrauterine life.[1] The developing gonad cannot be differentiated into male or female at this stage. Identification of gender starts after another 7–10 days.[2]

As opposed to females where oogenesis starts in utero; in males, meiosis is initiated with the onset of puberty. However, the foundation is laid during fetal development and any disturbance at this time may affect adult spermatogenesis.[3] The first cells to differentiate are the Sertoli cells (SC), which coordinate the development of the testis. The SC surround the germ cells (GC), which are further surrounded by the peritubular myoid cells to form the seminiferous cords which subsequently elongate to form the seminiferous tubules.[4]

THE SEMINIFEROUS TUBULES

The testis comprises an extensive tubular network which functions as the site for spermatogenesis. The tubules are lined by the seminiferous epithelium and contain a fluid-filled lumen, into which fully formed spermatozoa are released. Interstitial tissue lying between the tubules is formed of layers of myoid cells, fibrocyte-like adventitial cells, and collagen matrix. It contains blood vessels, lymphocytes, plasma cells, and Leydig cells. Peritubular myoid cells have properties similar to both fibroblasts and muscle cells. They provide support to the SC and drive testicular fluid, containing immotile spermatozoa, toward the *rete testis*. In addition, myoid cells help in paracrine control of SC function and preservation of the blood-testis barrier. It is believed that myoid cells secrete proinflammatory cytokines like tumor necrosis factor alpha (TNFα), escalation of which may cause peritubular wall remodeling and hence infertility.[5] Underneath the seminiferous tubules, there is a basement membrane, which lies on a connective tissue layer, the tunica propria.

Leydig cells are positioned in clusters between the blood vessels and seminiferous tubules. They are the main site of testosterone secretion in males. In humans, differentiation of these cells occurs in waves corresponding to the triphasic production of testosterone during fetal maturation. The first wave transpires between 8 and 18 weeks of gestation causing differentiation of male secondary sexual characteristics.[6] This is followed by the second wave in the first few months after birth, and the final wave during puberty.

The spermatogenic epithelium, including SC, is extremely susceptible to damage from toxins and ischemia. This damage may be partial, focal or complete, leading to abnormal sperm counts. The Leydig cells generally remain functional. Severe damage may cause complete destruction and hyalinization of the tubules, wherein they eventually get replaced by fibrous tissue.

Two main cell types are found in the seminiferous tubules:

1. *Sertoli cells:* They surround the GC and their cytoplasm extends through the entire height of the epithelium. Sertoli cells take up 17–20% of the adult spermatogenic epithelium and their number is directly proportional to the number of GC produced.[7] They are connected to each other by tight junctions. Structure of SC transforms continuously, helping in migration of developing GC toward the tubular lumen. One SC can sustain around 30–50 GCs at various points of differentiation.[8]

    Sertoli cells provide nutrition to the developing GC by transferring carbohydrates, amino acids, vitamins, lipids, and metal ions. Furthermore, SC secrete numerous compounds that help in spermatogenesis, e.g., androgen-binding protein (ABP), proteases, vasoactive peptides, transferrin, vitamin transporters, lactate, acetate, extracellular matrix components, glial cell-derived neurotrophic factor (GNDF), TGF-a, TGF-b and interleukins.[9] They also deposit collagen and laminin along with forming junctions to maintain the seminiferous epithelium. Additionally, they provide immunoprotection and physical support. Alteration in any of these actions can cause infertility.

Sertoli cells multiply antenatally, in the neonatal period and just before attaining puberty. Different factors affect their growth; predominantly testosterone in the fetal and postnatal period and follicle-stimulating hormone (FSH) prior to puberty.[10] Multiplication of SC during any of these periods can be impaired by different environmental agents, thus limiting the production of GC leading to oligospermia. Functioning of SC is affected by presence of insulin, especially formation of lactate during carbohydrate metabolism. Moreover, lactate is a primary energy source for developing GC. Lactate production is decreased in absence of insulin, partly explaining adverse effect of diabetes on spermatogenesis.

2. *Germ cells:* They divide and migrate from the basement membrane vicinity, crossing the tight junctional complexes of adjacent SC to be ultimately discharged into the lumen as full-grown sperms. Any cross section of a normal seminiferous tubule shows four or five distinct generations of GC; earlier ones seen near the basement membrane, and the more mature ones toward the lumen **(Fig. 1)**. However, a single cross section does not simultaneously show all the stages.

The various GC seen in the cross section of seminiferous tubules (in ascending order of maturation) are as follows:[11]

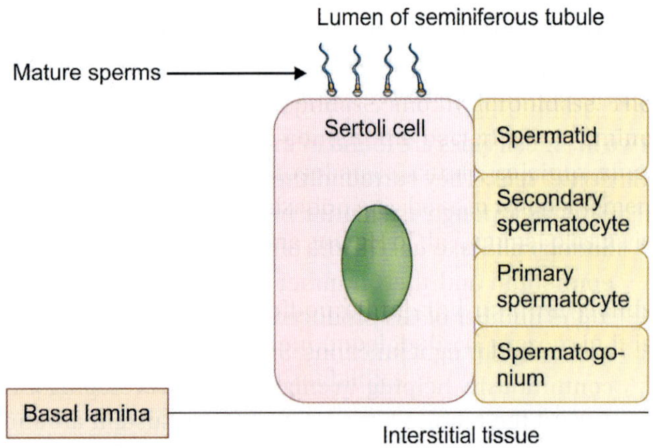

Fig. 1: Schematic of cross-section of seminiferous tubules showing various stages of spermatogenesis, with late spermatids in the lumen attached to tip of Sertoli cells.

- *Progenitor A dark (Ad)/A0 spermatogonia:* They provide a continuous supply of stem cells for spermatogenesis. They can divide into both type Ad and type Ap cells. They are located near the basement membrane.
- *Progenitor and committed A pale (Ap)/A1 spermatogonia:* Progenitor and committed cells have similar morphology but the committed ones go through repeated mitosis to form a clone of cells—type B spermatogonia. They are joined together by cytoplasmic bridges for synchronized development.
- *B spermatogonia:* Their division produces the first cell of the second phase, the diploid preleptotene spermatocyte, which crosses through the tight junctions between SC.
- Preleptotene (young primary spermatocytes), leptotene, zygotene, pachytene, and diplotene spermatocytes: These are the different stages seen during meiosis that progressively move toward the adluminal compartment.
- Secondary spermatocytes
- *Spermatids:* These are seen attached to the tip of SC. They are subdivided into Sa, Sb, Sc, Sd1, and Sd2 types.
- Spermatozoa.

SPERMATOGENESIS

Most mammals need 30–40 days to form mature spermatozoa, though in humans a mean interval of 74 days was observed between commitment of the Ap spermatogonium and extrusion of mature spermatozoon.[12] However, recent research has established a range of 42–76 days for total time required in formation of mature sperm in humans.[13] The number of sperms generated in a single male is thought to be approximately 150–275 million spermatozoa per day.[14] As opposed to the somewhat quiescent oocytes, spermatozoa are continuously produced by the testes and go through constant cell reproduction, meiosis, and spermiogenesis. Moreover, due to lack of recombination repair, male gametes are at a greater risk of damage to nuclear deoxyribonucleic acid (DNA).

Primordial GC form gonocytes, which stay in arrest in G0 phase till birth. Development of primordial GC and gonocytes is affected by products such as stem cell factor, stromal cell-derived factor 1, activator protein-2, growth and differentiation factor 3 (GDF3), estradiol, retinoic acid, and methylated DNA. Hence, these may be antecedent to various causes of infertility and some testicular tumors.[15] After birth, gonocytes develop into spermatogonia, which are inactive till 5–7 years age, subsequently undergoing mitosis. Ensuing puberty, further development starts.[16]

Spermatogenesis follows a rigid time scale. Ap spermatogonia simultaneously become committed at circumscribed areas within each seminiferous tubule. Hence, growing cells form clusters, which develop at intervals (16 days), specific for that location.[14] As a single spermatogonium develops, its progeny stay joined together by cytoplasmic bridges until the late spermatid stage. The approximate number of spermatids developing from one spermatogonium is 512.[17] Multiple clusters are seen simultaneously, as the total duration of sperm formation is greater than the interim between commitment of spermatogonia at a particular position (74 vs. 16 days), forming *layers* or *generations*, with the earliest near the basement membrane. The multiple cohorts (six in humans) developing synchronously at a circumscribed area are called *cellular associations*.[12,14] Anomalous cellular associations may be seen in males with poor sperm formation, because of absent GC or mixing of different cohorts.

Spermatogenesis can be divided into four interdependent parts that are coordinated by factors emitted from the SC, peritubular cells, Leydig cells, and the vasculature:
1. Proliferation (spermatocytogenesis)
2. Meiosis
3. Differentiation (spermiogenesis)
4. Spermiation.

The phases of spermatogenesis transform with time as well as along the length of the tubular loop. The sequential change of cycle stage along the length is called the *wave* of the spermatogenic epithelium. The lesser stages are located near the middle of the loop and the advanced ones near the rete testis.[18]

Proliferation

The proliferation of the interphase GC begins at puberty. An estimated 500 spermatozoa per second are formed per gram of testis in the adult mammal.[19] Proliferation involves mitosis for regeneration of progenitor Ad and Ap spermatogonia, formation of B-spermatogonia from committed cells and their further development to preleptotene spermatocytes **(Flowchart 1)**. Any defect in proliferation can seriously affect the resulting sperm number.

Sertoli cells secrete factors that cause the spermatogonia to renew, differentiate or become apoptotic, a mechanism to control the SC/GC ratio. These factors include GNDF (promotes self-renewal), SCF, bone morphogenetic protein 4 (BMP4), retinoic acid, notch1/jagged 2 signaling system and many micro-RNAs.[20] The transition of Ad to Ap spermatogonia is regulated by pulses of retinoic acid which are staggered at regular intervals along the seminiferous tubules leading to asynchronous sperm formation. Any deviation in retinoic acid pulses may affect spermatogenesis.[21] Apoptosis is promoted by Bcl-2, Bax, and TNF-α acting thorough FaS/FaSL system. Any disruption in these mechanisms can cause infertility.

Inability of spermatogonia to evolve further causes eventual azoospermia. The pattern seen on histopathology is known as Sertoli cell only syndrome (SCO). SCO type 1 occurs due to abnormal migration of primordial GC from the yolk sac and is characterized by complete absence of GC. SCO type 2 occurs due to subsequent problems and shows occasional foci of spermatogenesis. In these cases, sperms may be retrieved with help of microdissection.

Meiosis

The primary spermatocytes are arrested in prophase of the first meiotic division until puberty (preleptotene spermatocytes). At puberty, these develop by meiosis into haploid secondary spermatocytes **(Flowchart 2)**. Prophase may last for nearly 3 weeks.[22] The pachytene stage is imperative to human evolution as it involves DNA recombination. Hence, there are many checkpoints during this stage as well as metaphase and anaphase. Recombination failure has been seen in around 10% of men with nonobstructive azoospermia (NOA),[23] and sperm aneuploidy may be the cause of 45% cases of recurrent miscarriage.[24] *TEX11* is a gene on the X chromosome that controls homologous chromosome

Flowchart 1: Different stages of germ cells seen during spermatogenesis.

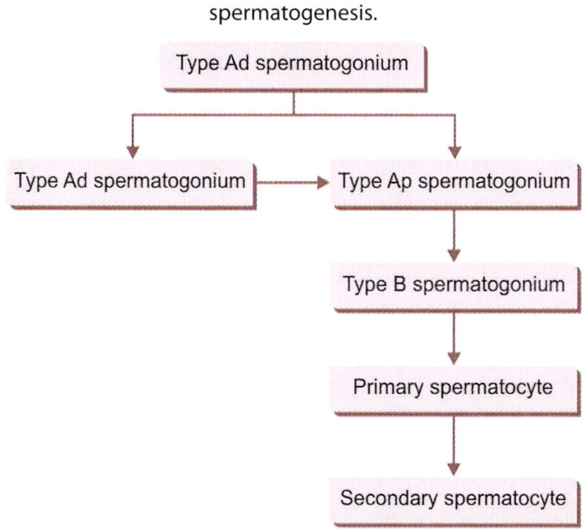

(Ad: progenitor A dark; Ap: progenitor and committed A pale)

Flowchart 2: Effect of mitosis and meiosis on chromosomal number.

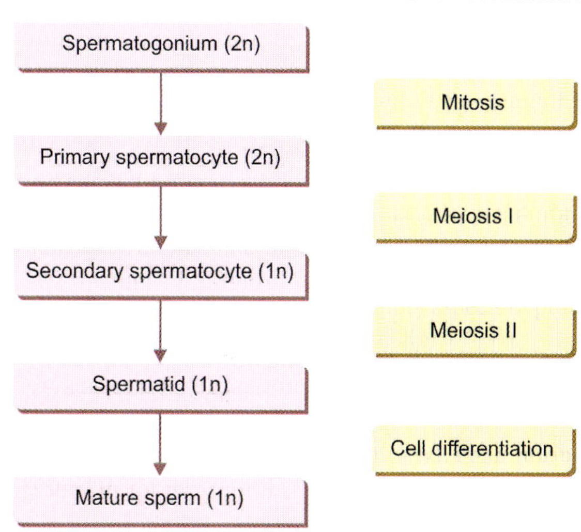

(n: set of chromosomes; 1n: haploid; 2n: diploid)

synapses and double-strand DNA break repair. Its mutation was seen in 2.4% of men with "idiopathic infertility".[25] Early maturation arrest, or arrest seen in meiosis affects around 10% of men with NOA. This is seen more often during meiosis 1 as quality control is more extensive in this stage. These men can have focal areas of normal spermatogenesis and show a 20–40% sperm retrieval rate with microdissection.[26]

Secondary spermatocytes have the shortest life span—1.1–1.7 days.[27] They undergo meiosis II, eventually forming haploid spermatids. The autosomes in the spermatid nucleus sustain production of small amounts of ribosomal and messenger RNA and proteins, so that they can enter into a protracted stage of terminal differentiation or spermiogenesis.

Differentiation

This process refers to the morphological differentiation of round spermatids to elongated cells with a species-specific shape. Duration of spermiogenesis is roughly 14 days in most species, wherein there are 16–18 delineated stages.[28]

There are three major modifications:
1. The nucleus elongates and chromatin condenses into a very dark staining structure, forming the head of the sperm.
2. The Golgi apparatus produces a lysosomal-like granule that spreads over the nucleus, with help of perinuclear theca, to form the future acrosome, which is rich in enzymes required for oocyte penetration and fertilization.
3. Reorganization of the cytoplasm leads to formation of the tail and the midpiece. The midpiece contains the mitochondria and related control mechanisms required for mobility.

The sperm cell needs to be compacted; therefore the DNA is condensed to below 10% of volume of a somatic cell. The solenoid structure is replaced by toroids which are further supercoiled into toroidal loops. Deoxyribonucleic acid is at first packaged with histones; subsequently, at secondary spermatocyte stage, histones are replaced by transition proteins followed by protamines. Compaction is achieved by disulfide bonding between DNA and protamines. Other factors helping to package sperm DNA include histone modifications, chromatin-binding proteins, and noncoding RNAs.[29] Protamines make up roughly 85%, and histones around 15% of proteins in mature sperm.[30] Underprotamination causes defective chromatin packaging, seen as presence of endogenous nicks in ejaculated spermatozoa.[31] The extent of protamine replacement reflects the fertilizing capacity of the sperm. Low H4 hyperacetylation has been associated with maturation arrest.[32] Remaining histone-bound DNA content is important for proper sperm function and early embryo evolution. Proportion of different protamine types also influences fertility. Males with lower P1/P2 ratio were seen to have higher DNA fragmentation index (DFI).[33]

Deoxyribonucleic acid packaging has multiple purposes, which are as follows:
- Reducing volume of the spermatozoa for easy travel through the genital tract.
- Attenuating exogenous damage before fertilization.
- Keeping the genome transcriptionally dormant.

Anomalous formation of acrosome affects the shape of sperm head, a condition known as globozoospermia. It is a rare ailment wherein round headed sperms are seen, which cannot penetrate or activate oocytes. Hence, to achieve good results in assisted reproduction techniques (ART), conventional ICSI needs to be combined with assisted oocyte activation.[34]

Reorganization of the cytoplasm causes elongation of the sperm. Extra cytoplasm is discarded as the cytoplasmic lobe that eventually gets phagocytosed by the SC as the residual body. Intercellular bridges connect residual bodies, resulting from incomplete division during spermatogenesis. Appearance of residual body indicates final maturation.[1] The mitochondria are organized around the microtubules in the tail and provide energy for motion. The mitochondria have been observed to perform indispensable function in the GC including energy production and apoptosis. Moreover, they are imperative for proliferation and mitotic regulation. Mutations in mitochondrial genome are recognized in infertile patients especially those with asthenospermia. Aging, obesity, and metabolic disorders affect mitochondrial action on fertility.[35]

When sperms are near the last stages of spermiogenesis, their ribosomes have almost disappeared, and the endoplasmic reticulum is absent. Since now, no mechanism remains for protein synthesis; hence, sperms have to acquire factors needed for further transport from external environment, or store them beforehand.

Six stages of differentiation are as follows:
1. *Sa1 and Sa2:* They contain well-differentiated Golgi complex and mitochondria. The acrosome vesicle, proximal centriole, and axial filaments appear. The chromatin body appears in one pole opposite to the acrosome vesicle.
2. *Sb1 and Sb2:* The formation of acrosome and intermediate piece is completed.
3. *Sc1 and Sc2:* Tail development is completed.

Arrest of spermiogenesis at the early spermatid phase (dark round nuclei) is known as late maturation arrest, which is less common then early maturation arrest (arrest at spermatogonia/spermatocyte stage). These sperms may still be used in ART after using microdissection techniques like microTESE. Better sperm retrieval rate is seen in late arrest (50–80%). Arrest during late spermiogeneisis (condensed oval spermatids) is known as hypospermatogenesis and has best sperm retrieval rate (80–90%) among all causes of NOA.[36]

If the male pronucleus has obvious flaws such as compromised genomic integrity, aneuploidy, or misestablished epigenetic information, the effects may become obvious only after fertilization.[37] Apoptosis of defective GC helps to prevent transmission of such defects. On the other hand, increase in apoptosis by stimuli such as hormonal irregularity, ionizing radiation, chemotherapy, cell injury and cell stress, can lead to abnormal fall in number of GC.[7]

Intracytoplasmic sperm injection (ICSI) is a procedure that can use testicular sperms for the management of azoospermic males. However, these sperms may be defective and not yet have undergone apoptosis. These may fertilize the oocyte but the embryos would have poor reproductive outcome. Few studies have identified molecular markers that assess the protein and ribonucleic acid (RNA) content of spermatozoa prior to their use in assisted ART.[37] Further research in this area will help to improve results.

In spite of extensive defense systems, both developing and mature sperms can suffer DNA breakage, leading to subfertility. This damage is assessed with the help of DNA fragmentation index (DFI). A rise in sperm double-stranded DNA breaks has been seen with increasing age of the human male, along with a fall in regulatory sperm apoptosis. This indicates that the system of selection of healthy sperms declines with age.[38] High DFI is observed in diabetics, which can be attributed to increased oxidative stress because of advanced glycation end products.[39]

Spermiation

This process involves the extrusion of the elongated spermatid from the SC into the tubular lumen. Residual bodies remain embedded in the epithelium. The stalk connecting it to the spermatid breaks, resulting in formation of proximal cytoplasmic droplet in neck region of the spermatozoon. The embedded residual bodies are phagocytosed and protoplasm is recycled. Degenerated GC are also phagocytosed. Follicle-stimulating hormone and testosterone act synergistically to aid spermiation as seen by dysfunction in disengagement of spermatids from SC after suppression of both these hormones, in animal studies.[40]

Epigenetic State during Spermatogenesis

Epigenetic changes during spermatogenesis **(Fig. 2)** are significant as they aid in the following:

- Silencing of transposable elements
- Paternal imprinting
- Chromatin remodeling
- Sex chromosome inactivation
- DNA compaction.

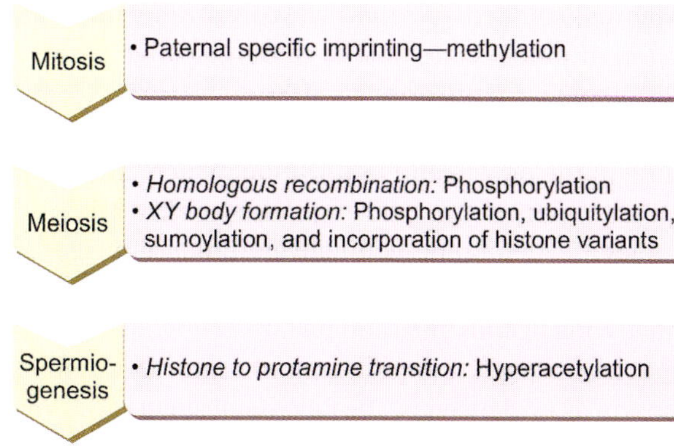

Fig. 2: Epigenetic changes during different stages of spermatogenesis.

Paternally imprinted genes are methylated, hence silenced in male GC so that expression is from maternal gene. Paternal imprinting starts in the gonocytes and is carried through remaining spermatogenesis.

Clinical implications include the following:

- Defective methylation may lead to oligospermia.[41]
    - Use of such sperm for intracytoplasmic sperm injection (ICSI) may cause transmission of epigenetic defects to subsequent generations.
- If genomic imprinting is not finished at the round spermatid stage, it could be completed after round spermatid enters the ooplasm, as DNA methylation has been demonstrated at the blastocyst stage and early embryonic development.[42]

Researchers have tried to generate elongated spermatids from surgically removed testicular spermatogenic GC, for use in ICSI for azoospermic men with maturation arrest.[43] However, it is not sure if imprinting can be successfully completed in vitro, hence leading to tumor susceptibility or other imprinting disorders after fertilization. Some conditions such as obesity and environmental exposure are postulated to affect spermatogenesis through epigenetic mechanisms, though further evidence is required in this field.[44]

Epididymal Maturation

Spermatozoa gain the ability to fertilize oocytes by various changes in the epididymis, collectively known as epididymal maturation, e.g., an increase in net negative charge of the sperm head, which facilitates attachment to the zona pellucida. Sperms undergo various complex biochemical, biophysical, and ultrastructural molecular changes, such as, loss of protein, cyclic adenosine monophosphate (cAMP), modification in energy metabolism, and changes in lipoprotein content, size, shape, and structure of acrosome. There are no obvious changes in the sperm tail though the cytoplasmic droplet seen around the neck is gradually lost.

Sperms aspirated from the distal corpus, after undergoing maturation process, are able to undergo capacitation and fertilization, hence preferred for ICSI.

The testis synthesizes many antigens required for binding to the oocyte and fertilization, which are activated when the sperms pass through the epididymis. A few examples are membrane-bound hyaluronidase (PH20/2B1), fertilin, proacrosin, 1, 4-galactosyl transferase (GalTase), and putative zona ligands sp56 and p95.[45]

Passage through the epididymis also provides motility to the sperm as evidenced by the fact that testicular spermatozoa are immotile even though flagellar morphological structures are acquired during spermiogenesis. Motility is possibly regulated at the level of the plasma membrane which alters progressively as sperm passes through the epididymis since the osmolality and chemical composition of the epididymal fluid differs in each segment.[46] During maturation, sperms use up the endogenous energy reserves and become dependent on external fructose.

In the human male, spermatozoa travel from the seminiferous tubules to the rete testis, further via the ductuli efferentia, finally into the caput epididymis. Testicular fluid gets resorbed in the proximal epididymis leading to concentration of the spermatozoa up to 10–100 times. Sperms negotiate the epididymis in 2–14 days and subsequently are stored in the cauda, vas, seminal vesicles, and ampullae before ejaculation. However, the viability of sperms is affected with increased duration of storage; therefore, for accurate semen analysis, sample should not be taken >5–7 days after ejaculation.

Abnormality at any of the stages of epididymal maturation may result in different pathologies, including azoospermia. The tubular lumen is highly sensitive to toxins and any damage results in altered sperm counts. Reactive oxygen species (ROS), in spite of being important for sperm capacitation, can themselves induce peroxidative damage and subsequently decreased sperm motility. Hence, supplementation with antioxidants helps to improve asthenospermia. However, care should be taken not to overload as even the normal action of reactive oxygen species (ROS) may be lost.

Blood–Testis Barrier

The testicular circulation is separated from the general circulation by a "blood-testis barrier" composed of tight junctions between adjacent SC **(Fig. 3)**. The main function of this barrier is to control passage of large molecules from the interstitial tissue and the basal compartment of the seminiferous tubule to the lumen and surrounding area. However, steroids can cross this barrier easily. Moreover, some proteins may also travel from SC to Leydig cells and vice versa in a paracrine manner.

Movement of developing GC from the basal compartment to the lumen is seen to occur without disruption of the barrier by progressive breakdown of the tight junctions above the GC, and concomitant formation of new tight junctions below them.

The blood–testis barrier is responsible for a particular composition of the luminal fluid of the tubule. The fluid is rich in androgens, estrogens, K^+, inositol, and glutamic and aspartic acids, with traces of protein and glucose. An osmotic gradient is created that promotes fluid entry into the lumen. Another important function of the barrier is to protect the developing spermatozoa from blood-borne toxins. It also prevents antigenic products of spermatogenesis from entering the circulation and generating an autoimmune

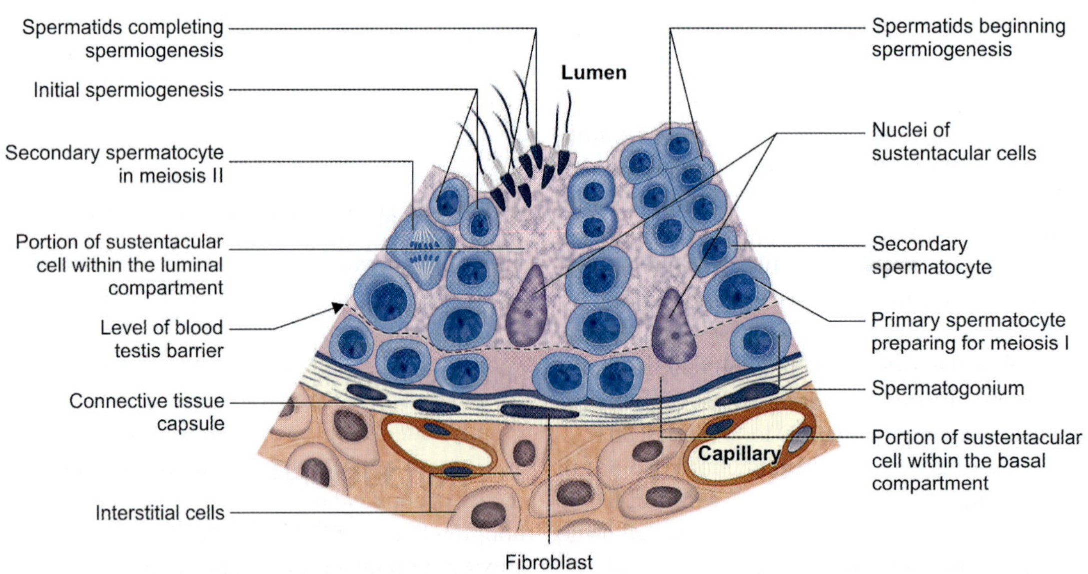

Fig. 3: Tight junctions between adjacent Sertoli cells form the blood-testis barrier.

Flowchart 3: Endocrine control of spermatogenesis.

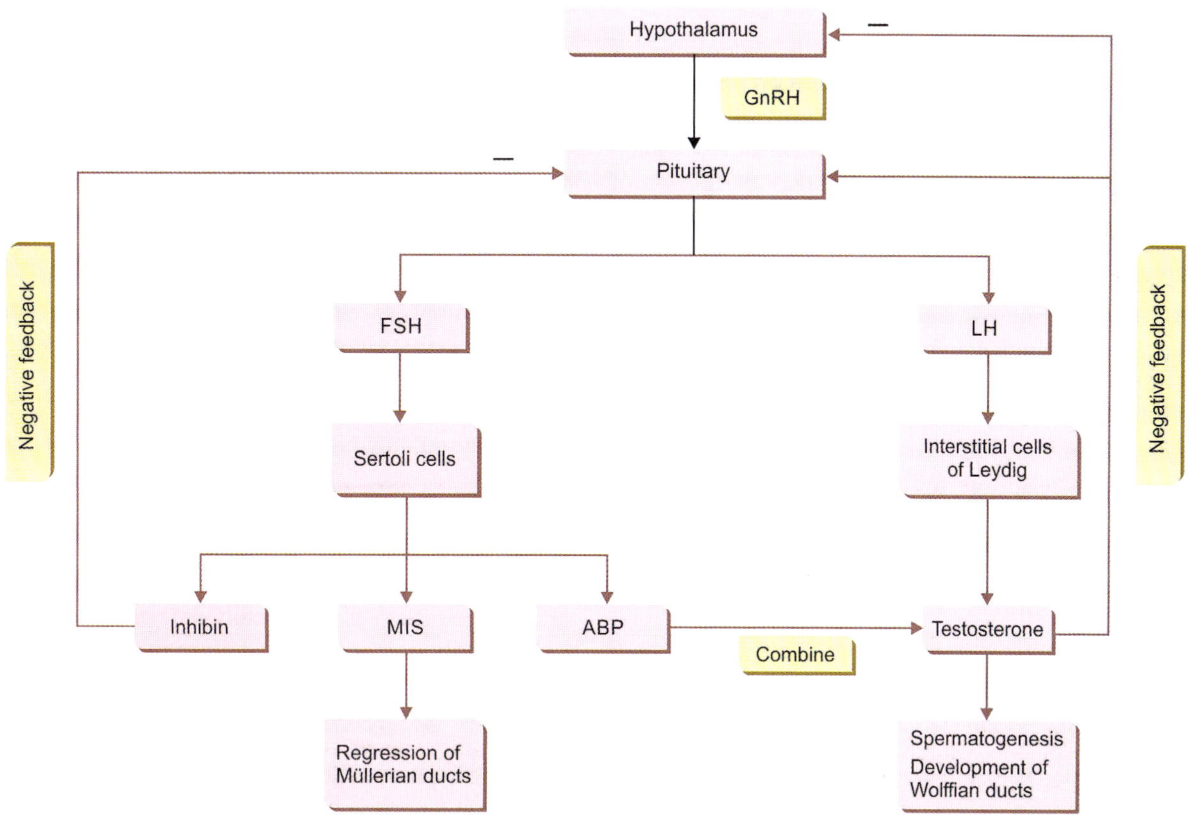

(GnRH: gonadotropin-releasing hormone; MIS: Müllerian inhibiting substance; ABP: androgen binding protein; LH: luteinizing hormone; FSH: follicle stimulating hormone)

response. Diseases like diabetes mellitus affect proper functioning of the blood–testis barrier causing male infertility.

Endocrine Control

The hypothalamic-pituitary-gonadal axis is a complex system of feedback and feed forward loops responsible for spermatogenesis and appearance of secondary sexual characteristics **(Flowchart 3)**. The hypothalamus releases various gonadotropin-releasing hormones that regulate the secretion of gonadotropins from the pituitary, which further act on the gonads. Therefore, hypothalamic disease leads to atrophy of the testes and loss of their function.

Gonadotropins released from the pituitary are FSH and luteinizing hormone (LH). FSH acts on the SC to produce ABP. LH stimulates the interstitial cells of Leydig to produce testosterone. Testosterone, in turn, combines with ABP in the seminiferous tubules, and controls LH secretion by negative feedback to the hypothalamus and pituitary. Interaction between these hormones is responsible for normal spermatogenesis. Novel research has shown that FSH may not be crucial for spermatogenesis as shown by the fact that spermatogenesis persisted in men with poor FSH production or FSH receptor mutation, though it was adversely affected.[47] Estimation of blood levels of FSH, LH, and testosterone is necessary to evaluate males with abnormal semen parameters as enumerated in **Table 1**.

TABLE 1: Endocrine profile in azoospermia.

	Endocrine profile			
Category	***LH***	***FSH***	***Testo***	***Diagnosis***
Eugonadotropic azoospermia	N	N	N	• Local factors—obstruction, maturation arrest • Sexual dysfunction
Hypergonadotropic azoospermia	↑	↑	↓	Testicular dysgenesis
Hypogonadotropic azoospermia	↓	↓	↓	Central defect—hypothalamus and pituitary

(FSH: follicle-stimulating hormone; LH: luteinizing hormone; Testo: testosterone; N: normal)

Androgen-binding protein (ABP) is responsible for sustaining high androgen concentration in testis and epididymis, by controlling their bioavailability, decreasing metabolism and improving their uptake.[48] High intratesticular testosterone is necessary for normal sperm development; low levels cause spermatogonial apoptosis and defective spermiogenesis.

Different stages of spermatogenesis are under different endocrine control, for example, proliferation and meiosis appear to be androgen-independent. However, differentiation depends on androgens acting on the SC, where the developing spermatozoa are embedded. Final stages of spermatid maturation are expedited by FSH action on SC. Androgen receptors are located in the SC, Leydig cells, peritubular muscle cells, and vascular smooth muscle cells; but not in GC.[49] Testosterone regulates LH secretion by negative feedback on the hypothalamus and pituitary and Leydig cell action through an ultrashort loop negative feedback.[50]

Development of gonocytes is affected by activin A, follistatin, and inhibin. FSH promotes inhibin and follistatin secretion from SC, thus indirectly affecting gonocyte maturation.[51] Moreover, FSH decreases degeneration of spermatogonia and promotes their entry into meiosis along with testosterone. Inhibin B is a glycoprotein hormone that controls FSH secretion, and partly LH secretion, through negative feedback on the pituitary. The α subunit of inhibin B is located primarily in the SC, whereas, the β subunit is located predominantly in GC.[52] Hence, SC and GC must cooperate for formation of inhibin B, which further acts in a paracrine and autocrine manner to regulate SC and Leydig cell function. Damage to SC affects inhibin production, in turn raising serum FSH.

Exogenous use of androgenic steroids decreases secretion of LH from the pituitary. This decreases intratesticular testosterone, thereby inhibiting spermatogenesis. However, this suppression is temporary and is reversed after stopping steroid use.[53] This effect has been seen in athletes who take steroids; and is also used for male contraception.

Another important hormone required for development of male characteristics is the Müllerian inhibiting substance (MIS) or Müllerian regression factor. Secreted by SC, MIS reaches average plasma concentration of 48 ng/mL by the age of 1–2 years. Thereafter, it declines to low levels by puberty and remains at low but detectable levels throughout life. The interplay between MIS and testosterone is an important determinant for male sexual development. While these two hormones act unilaterally on the internal genitalia, the action on external genitalia is opposite. Main function of MIS is to promote regression of the Müllerian ducts by apoptosis, whereas, testosterone stimulates the development of the vas deferens and related structures from the Wolffian ducts. The testosterone metabolite dihydrotestosterone is responsible for formation of male external genitalia and secondary sex characteristics.

Sertoli cells do not synthesize androgens, but they contain aromatase (CYP19), that produce estrogen from androgens. The local interaction between androgens and estrogen is necessary to maintain normal spermatogenesis. It has been seen that low seminal testosterone/estradiol ratio and high seminal estradiol levels can be used to predict rate of surgical retrieval of sperms from testes of males with NOA.[54] Estrogen promotes germ cell functions such as movement and substrate metabolism. It also helps in vitro survival of sperms.[55] On the other hand, estrogens have a negative impact as they disturb development of interstitial cells antenatally. They also disrupt multiplication and differentiation of gonocytes and spermatogonia.[56] Extrinsic estrogen use causes apoptosis of GC. A useful function of the female hormone is seen in the rete testis where concentration of semen occurs. Here, the fluid has high estrogen levels, and the walls contain numerous ERα receptors. Defective working of the rete testis results in dilution of the semen entering the epididymis resulting in infertility.

Genetic Control

Thousands of genes have been identified as affecting sperm production. Abnormalities in any of these should affect spermatogenesis. Still, practically only a few have till now been identified as related to failure of spermatogenesis. Mutations in genes related to meiosis lead to either GC arrest or formation of abnormal gametes **(Table 2)**. Even though more and more genes are being identified as related to male infertility, their use as part of diagnostic workup is limited.

Normal spermatogenesis is under the control of azoospermia factor (AZF) region located on the euchromatin zone of long arm of Y chromosome. There are around 14 protein encoding genes divided into three groups—*AZFa*, *AZFb*, and *AZFc*.

- Microdeletions in any of these regions can lead to infertility though incidence and phenotype varies geographically and ethnically.[57]
- Microdeletions are seen in 10% of men with NOA and 5% of those with severe oligospermia.
- AZFc deletion is more frequently responsible.

Screening for Yq microdeletions is commonly used in males with severe oligospermia or azoospermia. Further analysis of the effects of genetic variants on sperm production is under research.

Klinefelter syndrome is the most common genetic cause of male infertility. The prevalence is 5% in severe oligospermia and 10% in NOA.[58] Though karyotype is

TABLE 2: Genetic abnormalities affecting spermatogenesis.[76]

Genetic abnormality	*Examples*
Numerical and structural chromosomal abnormalities	Klinefelter syndrome (XXY), reciprocal translocations, and pericentric inversions
Y chromosome deletions	AZFa, P5/proximal P1 (AZFb), P5/distal P1, b2/b4 (AZFc), and gr/gr deletions
Monogenic disorders	Endocrine defects, e.g., Kallmann syndrome and Noonan syndrome

mainly 47,XXY, around 20% show mosaic patterns such as 46,XY/47,XXY, 48XXXY, or 48 XXYY.[59] The process of inactivation of extra X chromosome is disturbed in Klinefelter syndrome affecting androgen production and spermatogenesis.

Micro-RNAs are short (20–23 nucleotides) single-stranded noncoding nucleotides. These are abundantly found in GC, many being stored in the chromatoid body. Newer studies have observed their effect on apoptosis, proliferation and differentiation. This post-transcriptional action is important because of silencing of GC during few stages of spermatogenesis. Anomalous expression of micro-RNA may adversely affect spermatogenesis leading to "idiopathic" infertility.[60]

Effect of Environment and Lifestyle (Flowchart 4)

Temperature

- Spermatogenesis requires the temperature of the testes to be lesser than in the interior of the body (about 32°C).[61]
- It is theorized that cooler conditions are due to air circulating around the scrotum and a countercurrent heat exchange between the spermatic vessels.
- Exposure to higher temperature can lead to degeneration of the spermatogenic epithelium, leading to infertility, for example, as seen in cryptorchidism.
- Evidence suggests that hot baths (43–45°C for 30 min/day) and insulated athletic supporters can reduce the sperm count, sometimes by 90%.[62]
- A seasonal effect has also been propounded, with higher sperm counts in winter regardless of the temperature to which the scrotum is exposed.
- Temperature can also be affected by viral fevers like influenza, or occupation like in bakers or foundry workers.
- High temperature can lead to hypoxia and oxidative stress in the developing sperms.
- Regarding this, much speculation has been made about the increasing use of laptops and smartphones. However, studies done on males who spend long time in sitting position or use laptops have not shown a direct correlation between time spent and poor semen parameters.[63] Still, they may exacerbate the action of other adverse environmental factors.
- Varicocele (dilated spermatic cord veins) affect spermatogenesis by raising the scrotal temperature. Moreover, it also causes oxidative stress through testicular hypoxia and disruption of blood-testis barrier.

Obesity

- Obesity is related to both female and male infertility.
- High body mass index (BMI) (>25 kg/m^2) in males has been seen to decrease sperm count and motility by 25%.[64]
- Rise in BMI is directly proportional to fall in testosterone levels, affecting spermatogenesis.[65]
- Higher peripheral conversion to estrogens can alter T/E2 ratio.
- Fat may get deposited near scrotal vasculature affecting cooling.

Smoking and Alcohol

- Lifestyle problems such as smoking and chronic alcohol consumption affect sperm counts significantly, especially in combination.[3,66]
- Maternal smoking during pregnancy can impair spermatogenesis in male fetus.[67]
- Smoking causes hypoxic damage while alcoholism can lower testosterone values.

Flowchart 4: Environmental factors affecting spermatogenesis—at adult stage and during antenatal period.

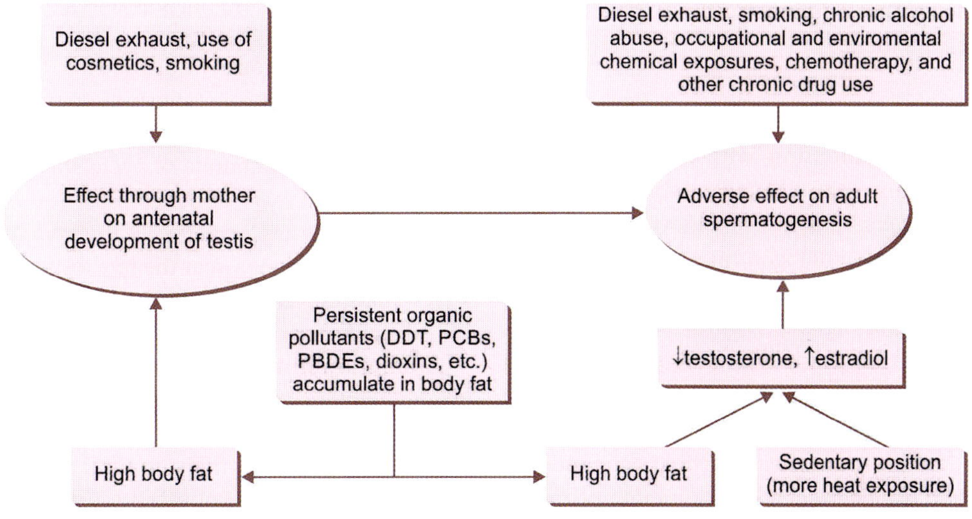

(DDT: dichlorodiphenyltrichloroethane; PCBs: polychlorinated biphenyls; PBDEs: polybrominated diphenyl ethers)

Effect of Drugs

- Chemotherapy (cyclophosphamide, etc.)[68] and radiotherapy are well known to hamper spermatogenesis. Hence, before starting this treatment, any male desiring future fertility should be advised to freeze semen.
- Chronic use of some medicines can alter spermatogenesis and cause infertility, e.g., sulfasalazine (used in irritable bowel syndrome),[69] H1 receptor antagonists (for allergies), antiepileptics, antibiotics and H2 receptor antagonists (cimetidine).[70]

Occupational Exposure

- Few occupations have been associated with male infertility due to chemical exposure, such as dibromochloropropane (nematocide used on crops), glycol ethers (solvents in various procedures), heavy metals (lead, cadmium, and mercury), metal welding fumes and carbon disulphide.[3]
- Heavy metals like lead may also affect general population due to exposure from paints, petrol and diesel fumes, and consumption of fish in which metals get concentrated.
- Farmers in India are a high-risk group due to excessive use of pesticides without adequate protective gear. Chronic exposure to pesticides such as dichlorodiphenyltrichloroethane (DDT) and organophosphates is associated with poor semen parameters, altered hormonal status, and sperm chromatin damage, leading to infertility.[71] In vitro sperm quality is also decreased, affecting assisted reproductive technique success rates.[72] Use of multiple pesticides can have additive effect.
- Few pesticides persist in the crops, affecting the consumers.

Many environmental factors affecting the adult sperm producing capacity may affect a male fetus through maternal exposure too. They can exacerbate the effect on adult.[3] More research is necessary in environmental factors affecting spermatogenesis so that eliminating the exposures may decrease infertility incidence.

In Vitro Spermatogenesis

Researchers are experimenting with new approaches to improve fertility potential of men unable to produce functional sperm or for fertility preservation. Animal trials have been performed with autologous methods such as stem cell transplantation, de novo morphogenesis, and testicular tissue grafting. Xenografting and in vitro spermatogenesis are other methods.[73] All these approaches have shown some promise. The only method that has been tried in human males is autologous spermatogonial stem cell transplantation,[74] but the outcomes have not been reported, though the method has been successfully used in primates. Another possibility is autologous testicular tissue grafting which has been successfully used in primates, though no human trials have yet been done.[75]

In vitro spermatogenesis, if successfully replicated, will have an advantage in not risking malignant reintroduction or retroviral infection (as possible in testicular tissue grafting and xenografting). Complete in vitro spermatogenenesis has been performed in mice, but the results could not be reproduced in primates or humans. Human testicular tissue has been cultured up to haploid round spermatid stage but epigenetic/genetic normality and fertilization capacity is still elusive. Better appraisal of fertility potential of these cells in primates is necessary before human trials.

A better knowledge of basic human physiology will help us to improve ART procedures affecting the clinical outcome. Knowledge about factors affecting spermatogenesis is also important to improve reproductive health of males.

KEY POINTS

- Primordial germ cells arise just behind the primitive streak in the extraembryonic mesoderm. They migrate through the dorsal mesentery, and finally colonize the gonadal ridge.
- As opposed to females, where oogenesis starts in utero; in males, meiosis is initiated with the onset of puberty.
- The site for spermatogenesis is seminiferous tubules of testis.
- Sertoli cells are an important component of spermatogenesis. Their number is directly proportional to the number of GC produced.
- Germ cells divide and move from the basement membrane region, through tight junctional complexes of adjacent SC to be finally released into the lumen as mature sperms. The younger ones are at the basement membrane, and the more mature ones are located near the lumen.
- Mean interval of 74 days has been observed between commitment of the Ap spermatogonium and extrusion of mature spermatozoon.
- Spermatogenesis can be divided into four interdependent parts: proliferation (spermatocytogenesis), meiosis, differentiation (spermiogenesis), and spermiation.
- The sequential change of cycle stage along the length is called the wave of the seminiferous epithelium. The lesser stages are located near the middle of the loop and the advanced ones near the rete testis.
- Proliferation involves mitosis for renewal of progenitor Ad and Ap spermatogonia, formation of B-spermatogonia from committed cells, and their further division to preleptotene spermatocytes.
- The primary spermatocytes are arrested in prophase of the first meiotic division until puberty (preleptotene spermatocytes). At puberty these develop by meiosis into haploid secondary spermatocytes.

- *Differentiation:* Round spermatids are differentiated morphologically into elongated cells with a condensed nucleus and a flagellum.
- Epigenetic changes during spermatogenesis are significant as they aid in silencing of transposable elements, paternal imprinting, chromatin remodeling, sex chromosome inactivation, and DNA compaction.
- *Epididymal maturation:* Sperms undergo various complex biochemical, biophysical, and ultrastructural molecular changes such as loss of protein, cyclic adenosine monophosphate (cAMP), modification in energy metabolism, changes in lipoprotein content, size, shape, and structure of acrosome.
- Luteinizing hormone stimulates the interstitial cells of Leydig to produce testosterone.
- Testosterone combines with ABP in the seminiferous tubules, and controls LH secretion by negative feedback to the hypothalamus and pituitary.
- High intratesticular testosterone is necessary for normal spermatogenesis.
- Screening for Yq microdeletions remains the only genetic test commonly used in males with severe oligospermia or azoospermia.
- Various environmental factors such as high temperature, obesity, drugs, and occupational exposure have been seen to adversely affect spermatogenesis.
- In vitro spermatogenesis, if successfully replicated, will have an advantage in not risking malignant reintroduction or retroviral infection.

REFERENCES

1. Hafez ESE, Hafez SD. Atlas of Clinical Andrology, 1st edition. London: Taylor and Francis; 2005.
2. Johnson M. Essential Reproduction, 6th edition. Oxford: Blackwell Scientific Publications; 2007.
3. Sharpe RM. Environmental/lifestyle effects on spermatogenesis. Philos Trans R Soc Lond B Biol Sci. 2010;365(1546):1697-712.
4. Brennan J, Capel B. One tissue, two fates: molecular genetic events that underlie testis versus ovary development. Nat Rev Genet. 2004;5(7):509-21.
5. Schell C, Albrecht M, Mayer C, Schwarzer JU, Frungieri MB, Mayerhofer A. Exploring human testicular peritubular cells: identification of secretory products and regulation by tumor necrosis factor-alpha. Endocrinology. 2008;149(4):1678-86.
6. Prince FP. The triphasic nature of Leydig cell development in humans, and comments on nomenclature, J. Endocrinol. 2001;168(2):213-6.
7. Dimitriadis F, Tsiampali C, Chaliasos N, Tsounapi P, Takenaka A, Sofikitis N. The Sertoli cell as the orchestra conductor of spermatogenesis: spermatogenic cells dance to the tune of testosterone. Hormones (Athens). 2015;14(4):479-503.
8. Cheng CY, Wong EW, Yan HH, Mruk DD. Regulation of spermatogenesis in the microenvironment of the seminiferous epithelium: new insights and advances. Molecular and cellular endocrinology. 2010;315(1-2):49-56.
9. Rato L, Alves MG, Socorro S, Duarte AI, Cavaco JE, Oliveira PF. Metabolic regulation is important for spermatogenesis. Nature Reviews Urology. 2012;9(6):330-8.
10. Sharpe RM, McKinnell C, Kivlin C, Fisher JS. Proliferation and functional maturation of Sertoli cells, and their relevance to disorders of testis function in adulthood. Reproduction. 2003;125(6):769-84.
11. Ehmcke J, Wistuba J, Schlatt S. Spermatogonial stem cells: questions, models and perspectives. Hum Reprod Update. 2006;12(3):275-82.
12. Clermont Y. Kinetics of Spermatogenesis in mammals: seminiferous epithelium cycle and spermatogonial renewal. Physiol Rev. 1972;52(1):198-236.
13. Misell LM, Holochwost D, Boban D, Santi N, Shefi S, Hellerstein MK, et al. A stable isotope-mass spectrometric method for measuring human spermatogenesis kinetics in vivo. J Urol. 2006;175(1):242-6.
14. Amann RP. The cycle of the seminiferous epithelium in humans: a need to revisit? J Androl. 2008;29(5):469-87.
15. de Rooij DG, van Dissel-Emiliani FM. 9-Regulation of proliferation and differentiation of stem cells in the male germ line. Stem cells. 1997;283-313.
16. Paniagua RI, Nistal MA. Morphological and histometric study of human spermatogonia from birth to the onset of puberty. J Anat. 1984;139(Pt 3)(Pt 3):535-52.
17. Hess RA. Spermatogenesis, overview and morphology. In: Knobil E, Neill JD (Eds). Encyclopedia of Reproduction. California: Academic Press; 1998.
18. Sadler TW. Langman's Medical Embryology, 12th edition. Philadelphia: Lippincott Williams and Wilkins; 2011.
19. Boron WF, Boulpaep EL (Eds). Medical Physiology. Philadelphia: Saunders; 2003.
20. van den Driesche S, Sharpe RM, Saunders PT, Mitchell RT. Regulation of the germ stem cell niche as the foundation for adult spermatogenesis: a role for miRNAs? Semin Cell Dev Biol. 2014;29:76-83.
21. Griswold MD. Spermatogenesis: The Commitment to Meiosis. Physiol Rev. 2016;96(1):1-17.
22. Sharpe R. Regulation of Spermatogenesis. In: Knobil E, Neill JD (Eds). The Physiology of Reproduction. New York: Raven Press; 1994.
23. Gonsalves J, Sun F, Schlegel PN, Turek PJ, Hopps CV, Greene C, et al. Defective recombination in infertile men. Hum Mol Genet. 2004;13(22):2875-83.
24. Ramasamy R, Scovell JM, Kovac JR, Cook PJ, Lamb DJ, Lipshultz LI. Fluorescence in situ hybridization detects increased sperm aneuploidy in men with recurrent pregnancy loss. Fertil Steril. 2015;103(4):906-9.e1.
25. Yatsenko AN, Georgiadis AP, Röpke A, Berman AJ, Jaffe T, Olszewska M, et al. X-linked TEX11 mutations, meiotic arrest, and azoospermia in infertile men. N Engl J Med. 2015;372(22):2097-107.
26. Bernie AM, Shah K, Halpern JA, Scovell J, Ramasamy R, Robinson B, et al. Outcomes of microdissection testicular sperm extraction in men with nonobstructive azoospermia due to maturation arrest. Fertil Steril. 2015;104(3):569-73.e1.
27. Barrett KE, Brooks H, Barman SM, Boitano S. Ganong's Review of Medical Physiology, 24th edition. US: McGraw Hill Professional; 2012.

28. Elder K, Dale B (Eds). In Vitro Fertilization, 3rd edition. Cambridge: Cambridge University Press; 2011.
29. Turner JM. Meiotic sex chromosome inactivation. Development. 2007;134(10):1823-31.
30. Jones R. Spermiogenesis and sperm maturation in relation to development of fertilizing capacity. In: Lauria A (Ed). Gametes: Development and function; 1998.
31. Sailer BL, Jost LK, Evenson DP. Mammalian sperm DNA susceptibility to in situ denaturation associated with the presence of DNA strand breaks as measured by the terminal deoxynucleotidyl transferase assay. J Androl. 1995;16(1):80-7.
32. Sonnack V, Failing K, Bergmann M, Steger K. Expression of hyperacetylated histone H4 during normal and impaired human spermatogenesis. Andrologia. 2002;34(6):384-90.
33. Gardiner-Garden M, Ballesteros M, Gordon M, Tam PP. Histone-and protamine-DNA association: conservation of different patterns within the β-globin domain in human sperm. Molecular and cellular biology. 1998 Jun 1;18(6):3350-6.
34. Kuentz P, Vanden Meerschaut F, Elinati E, Nasr-Esfahani MH, Gurgan T, Iqbal N, et al. Assisted oocyte activation overcomes fertilization failure in globozoospermic patients regardless of the DPY19L2 status. Human reproduction. 2013;28(4):1054-61.
35. Rajender S, Rahul P, Mahdi AA. Mitochondria, spermatogenesis and male infertility. Mitochondrion. 2010;10(5):419-28.
36. Raheem AA, Garaffa G, Rushwan N, De Luca F, Zacharakis E, Abdel Raheem T, et al. Testicular histopathology as a predictor of a positive sperm retrieval in men with non-obstructive azoospermia. BJU international. 2013;111(3):492-9.
37. Wu TF, Chu DS. Epigenetic processes implemented during spermatogenesis distinguish the paternal pronucleus in the embryo. Reprod BioMed Online. 2008;16(1):13-22.
38. Singh NP, Muller CH, Berger RE. Effects of age on DNA double-strand breaks and apoptosis in human sperm. Fertil Steril. 2003;80(6):1420-30.
39. Karimi J, Goodarzi MT, Tavilani H, Khodadadi I, Amiri I. Relationship between advanced glycation end products and increased lipid peroxidation in semen of diabetic men. Diabetes Res Clin Pract. 2011;91(1):61-6.
40. Saito K, O'Donnell L, McLachlan RI, Robertson DM. Spermiation failure is a major contributor to early spermatogenic suppression caused by hormone withdrawal in adult rats. Endocrinology. 2000;141(8):2779-85.
41. Kobayashi H, Sato A, Otsu E, Hiura H, Tomatsu C, Utsunomiya T, et al. Aberrant DNA methylation of imprinted loci in sperm from oligospermic patients. Hum Mol Genet. 2007;16(21):2542-51.
42. Fishel S, Aslam I, Tesarik J. Spermatid conception: a stage too early, or a time too soon? Hum Reprod. 1996;11(7):1371-5.
43. Sofikitis N, Pappas E, Kawatani A, Baltogiannis D, Loutradis D, Kanakas N, et al. Efforts to create an artificial testis: culture systems of male germ cells under biochemical conditions resembling the seminiferous tubular biochemical environment. Hum Reprod Update. 2005;11(3):229-59.
44. Stuppia L, Franzago M, Ballerini P, Gatta V, Antonucci I. Epigenetics and male reproduction: the consequences of paternal lifestyle on fertility, embryo development, and children lifetime health. Clinical epigenetics. 2015;7:120.
45. Moore HDM. The influence of the epididymis on human and animal sperm maturation and storage. Hum Reprod. 1996;11:103-10.
46. Kirchhoff C, Osterhoff C, Pera I, et al. Function of human epididymal proteins in sperm maturation. Andrologia. 1998;30(4-5):225-32.
47. Walker WH, Cheng J. FSH and testosterone signaling in Sertoli cells. Reproduction. 2005;130(1):15-28.
48. Santiemma V, Rosati P, Guerzoni C, Mariani S, Beligotti F, Magnanti M, et al. Human Sertoli cells in vitro: morphological features and androgen-binding protein secretion. J Steroid Biochem Mol Biol. 1992;43(5):423-9.
49. De Gendt K, Swinnen JV, Saunders PT, Schoonjans L, Dewerchin M, Devos A, et al. A Sertoli cell-selective knockout of the androgen receptor causes spermatogenic arrest in meiosis. Proc Natl Acad Sci USA. 2004;101(5):1327-32.
50. Purvis K, Clausen OP, Hansson V. Androgen effects on rat Leydig cells. Biol Reprod. 1979;20(2):304-9.
51. Meehan T, Schlatt S, O'Bryan MK, de Kretser DM, Loveland KL. Regulation of germ cell and Sertoli cell development by activin, follistatin, and FSH. Dev Biol. 2000;220(2):225-37.
52. Marchetti C, Hamdane M, Mitchell V, Mayo K, Devisme L, Rigot JM, et al. Immunolocalization of inhibin and activin alpha and betaB subunits and expression of corresponding messenger RNAs in the human adult testis. Biol Reprod. 2003;68(1):230-5.
53. Knuth UA, Maniera H, Nieschlag E. Anabolic steroids and semen parameters in bodybuilders. Fertil Steril. 1989;52(6):1041-7.
54. Zhang Q, Bai Q, Yuan Y, Liu P, Qiao J. Assessment of seminal estradiol and testosterone levels as predictors of human spermatogenesis. J Androl. 2010;31(2):215-20.
55. Pentikainen V, Erkkila K, Suomalainen L, Parvinen M, Dunkel L. Estradiol acts as a germ cell survival factor in the human testis in vitro. J Clin Endocrinol Metab. 2000;85(5):2057-67.
56. O'Donnell L, Robertson KM, Jones ME, Simpson ER. Estrogen and spermatogenesis. Endocr Rev. 2001;22(3):289-318.
57. Sen S, Pasi AR, Dada R, Shamsi MB, Modi D. Y chromosome microdeletions in infertile men: prevalence, phenotypes and screening markers for the Indian population. J Assist Reprod Genet. 2013;30(3):413-22.
58. Abramsky L, Chapple J. 47,XXY (Klinefelter syndrome) and 47,XYY: estimated rates of and indication for postnatal diagnosis with implications for prenatal counselling. Prenat Diagn. 1997;17(4):363-8.
59. Foresta C, Galeazzi C, Bettella A, Stella M, Scandellari C. High incidence of sperm sex chromosomes aneuploidies in two patients with Klinefelter's syndrome. J Clin Endocrinol Metab. 1998;83(1):203-5.
60. Lian J, Zhang X, Tian H, Liang N, Wang Y, Liang C, et al. Altered microRNA expression in patients with non-obstructive azoospermia. Reprod Biol Endocrinol. 2009;7(1):13.
61. Hall JE. Guyton and Hall Textbook of Medical Physiology, 12th edition. Philadelphia: Saunders; 2010.
62. Mieusset R, Bujan L. Testicular heating and its possible contributions to male infertility: a review. Int J Androl. 1995;18(4):169-84.
63. Støy J, Hjøllund NH, Mortensen JT, Burr H, Bonde JP. Semen quality and sedentary work position. Int J Androl. 2004;27(1):5-11.
64. Kort HI, Massey JB, Elsner CW, Mitchell-Leef D, Shapiro DB, Witt MA, et al. Impact of body mass index values on sperm quantity and quality. J Androl. 2006;27(3):450-2.

65. Gould DC, Kirby RS, Amoroso P. Hypoandrogen-metabolic syndrome: a potentially common and underdiagnosed condition in men. Int J Clin Pract. 2007;61(2):341-4.
66. Harlev A, Agarwal A, Gunes SO, Shetty A, du Plessis SS. Smoking and Male Infertility: An Evidence-Based Review. World J Mens Health. 2015;33(3):143-60.
67. Ramlau-Hansen CH, Thulstrup AM, Storgaard L, Toft G, Olsen J, Bonde JP. Is prenatal exposure to tobacco smoking a cause of poor semen quality? A follow-up study. Am J Epidemiol. 2007;165(12):1372-9.
68. Nudell DM, Monoski MM, Lipshultz LI. Common medications and drugs: how they affect male fertility. Urol Clin North Am. 2002;29(4):965-73.
69. O'Morian C, Smethurst P, Dore CJ, Levui AJ. Reversible male infertility due to sulphasalazine: studies in man and rat. Gut. 1984;25(10):1078-84.
70. Hayashi T, Miyata A, Yamada T. The impact of commonly prescribed drugs on male fertility. Hum Fertil (Camb). 2008;11(3):191-6.
71. Jamal F, Haque QS, Singh S, et al. The influence of organo-phosphate and carbamate on sperm chromatin and reproductive hormones among pesticide sprayers. Toxicol Ind Health. 2016;32(8):1527-36.
72. Sengupta P, Banerjee R. Environmental toxins: alarming impacts of pesticides on male fertility. Hum Exp Toxicol. 2014;33(10):1017-39.
73. Pelzman DL, Orwig KE, Hwang K. Progress in translational reproductive science: testicular tissue transplantation and in vitro spermatogenesis. Fertil Steril. 2020;113(3):500-9.
74. Radford J. Restoration of fertility after treatment for cancer. Horm Res 2003;59(Suppl 1):21-3.
75. Fayomi AP, Peters K, Sukhwani M, Valli-Pulaski H, Shetty G, Meistrich ML, et al. Autologous grafting of cryopreserved prepubertal rhesus testis produces sperm and offspring. Science. 2019;363(6433):1314-9.
76. Visser L, Repping S. Unravelling the genetics of spermatogenic failure. Reproduction. 2010;139(2):303-7.

CHAPTER 5

Fertilization and Embryogenesis

Divya Sardana

INTRODUCTION

The spontaneous fusion of the sperm and the egg forms the zygote, the first cell of a baby through the process of fertilization. Fertilization is a complex sequence of coordinated molecular events beginning after the contact between a sperm and an oocyte. This is followed by intermingling of the parental chromosomes (of mother and father) and restoring the genetic constitution of the normal human being.[1] The zygote may die if there is any defect at any stage in the sequence of these events.

EGG TRANSPORT

The usual site of fertilization is the ampullary portion of the fallopian tube which is also the longest and the widest part.

At the time of ovulation, the secondary oocyte which is expelled from the ovarian follicle is swept into the funnel-shaped infundibulum of the fallopian tube. A picture of mature metaphase oocyte is shown in **Figure 1**.

This sweeping action is the result of the peristaltic movement of cilia on the mucosal cells of the fimbriae. With this movement, the oocyte reaches the ampulla of the tube.[2]

While the fertilization and dispersal of the cumulus cells occurs in the ampulla at its junction with the isthmus.

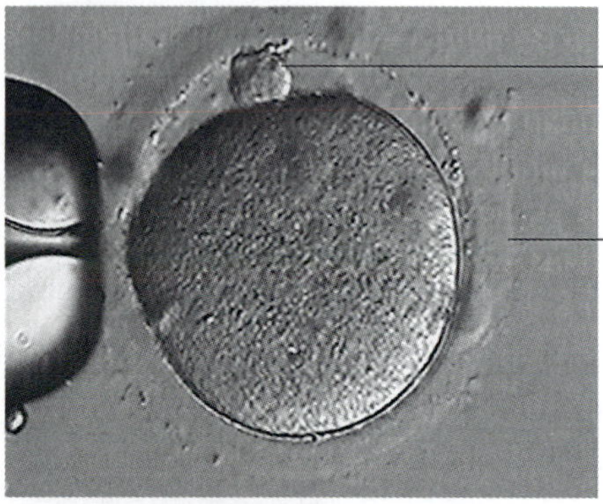

Fig. 1: Metaphase II oocyte (secondary oocyte) after denudation of the cumulus cells. The extruded first polar body can be seen at the top.

The transport of the fertilized oocyte through the tube requires about 3 days.[3] By this time, the endometrium becomes receptive for implantation.[4,5]

SPERM TRANSPORT

Following the deposition of semen through ejaculation, prostatic enzymes in the semen cause liquefaction. This takes around 20–30 minutes.

There is a transient protection of sperm from the acidic pH of vagina due to the alkaline pH of semen. The motile sperm enters into the cervical folds. Those that remain in vagina are immobilized within 2 hours.[6] The entry of the sperm into the cervical mucus is also aided by the contractions of the female reproductive tract. Cervix acts as a reservoir, and can provide sperm supply for up to 3 days. The sperms actively push their way through the cervical mucus.[7] This is enabled in part by the interaction between properties of the sperm head and the mucus.[8] Abnormal morphology of the sperm head can also result in poor penetration of cervical mucus.[9,10] The cervical mucus in turn has a filtering action on the less motile and less capable sperm.[11]

Throughout the sperm transport from vagina to the fallopian tube, there is substantial reduction in the number of sperms. The sperms are lost in vagina with semen expulsion from the introitus, digested by vaginal enzymes and by phagocytosis during the journey through the uterine cavity.

VIABILITY OF GAMETES

The human oocyte is known to survive for 12–24 hours after ovulation. After 24 hours, it degenerates whereas human sperms probably survive for 48 hours in the female genital tract. Some sperms remain in the cervical mucosal folds and are gradually released into the uterus up to 72 hours of coitus. Hence, there are maximum chances of conception when coitus happens within the 3-day-interval just before ovulation.[12,13]

CAPACITATION

Sperms which are freshly ejaculated cannot fertilize oocytes. They must undergo some cellular changes in the female reproductive tract, collectively called capacitation or physiological priming, to be able to fertilize the oocyte. This includes:

- The ability for acrosomal reaction
- Binding ability to the zona pellucida
- Hypermotility (hyperactivated motility).

In this capacitation, the seminal proteins and the glycoproteins are removed from the acrosome of the sperm and their surface charge is altered. Bicarbonate ion ($HCO3^-$) is present in various secretions of female reproductive tract. Bicarbonate influx in sperm leads to increased intracellular pH which causes plasma membrane collapse. Further, albumin present in female reproductive tract secretions causes cholesterol efflux from sperm plasma membrane making it more fluidic which in turn facilitates acrosome reaction. This process takes around 7 hours and happens in the uterus or tubes by substances secreted by these parts of the female reproductive tract.

When such sperms reach near the oocyte or follicular fluid, there is a breakdown of these plasma membrane and outer acrosomal membrane which is called the *acrosomal reaction.*[14] With the breakdown of the outer acrosomal membrane, there is release of the acrosomal enzymes namely—hyaluronidase, neuraminidase-like factor, cumulus-dispensing enzyme, and acrosin which probably play role in sperm penetration through the investments of the egg and digestion of zona pellucida.

Moreover, the capacitation results in increased velocity of the sperm and increased flagellar beat amplitude (hyperactivity) which helps in the penetration of zona pellucida. This process of capacitation is the result of influx of calcium ions in the sperm, in turn induced by progesterone. Increased intracellular calcium causes redox reactions in the sperm cell and the resulting changes in the sperm membrane.[15,16]

PROCESS OF FERTILIZATION

The sequence of events in the process of fertilization involves:

- *Sperm penetration through the corona radiata:* The capacitated sperms are guided to the oocyte by the chemical signals (attractants), secreted by the oocyte and the surrounding follicular cells. Oocyte factors especially growth differentiation factor 9 (GDF-9) and bone morphogenetic protein 15 (BMP-15) are important for cumulus differentiation and expansion. Preovulatory expansion of cumulus oophorus increases the chances of encounter with the sperm. The follicular cells are dispersed from the oocyte by the action of enzyme hyaluronidase from the sperm acrosome and also possibly by the enzymes from tubal mucosa.[17] Abnormal secretion of oocyte factors may impair sperm transit or sperm capacitation.
- *Penetration of zona pellucida:* This is an important step in fertilization. Zona pellucida is a glycoprotein layer that surrounds the oocyte and is made up of four proteins namely, ZP1, ZP2, ZP3, and ZP4. The acellular zona surrounding the egg is penetrated by the sperm with the help of acrosomal enzymes mainly—acrosin, esterase, and neuraminidase, as well as by sperm motility.[18,19]

  The zona pellucida has species-specific receptors for the sperm. The zona pellucida glycoprotein-3 (ZP3) is the main sperm ligand.[20] Once the sperm binds to ZP3, the acrosome reaction is triggered. This requires receptors on the sperm head also, e.g., tyrosine kinase, protein kinase C, and G-protein signaling system.[21-25] Once activated, there is:
  - Calcium influx
  - Efflux of hydrogen ions
  - Increase in pH
  - Fusion of sperm plasma membrane with outer acrosomal membrane leading to exocytosis of enzymes on the inner acrosomal membrane.
- Zona pellucida glycoprotein binding to sperm occurs after the acrosome reaction and this triggers *zona reaction* in which zona pellucida becomes impermeable to other sperms once the fertilizing sperm penetrates it. This is a protective mechanism to prevent polyploidy.[26] This zona reaction is a result of the action of lysosomal enzymes released by cortical granules near oocyte plasma membrane. When these granules discharge these enzymes into the perivitelline space, changes in the plasma membrane occur (rapid depolarization, hardening by cross-linking structural proteins, and inactivation of sperm ligands) which makes it impermeable to sperms.[27]
- *Fusion of plasma membranes of oocyte and sperm:* Sperm enters perivitelline space at an angle and then there is fusion of egg and sperm membranes. This is again mediated by specific proteins (ligands) on sperm head—PH-20 binds with zona pellucida; PH-30 (fertilin), and vitronectin help in fusion with oocyte.[28-30] Oolemma microvilli, CD-9-associated proteins, and glycosylphosphatidylinositol (GPI) proteins are thought to play role in fusion. The sperm nucleus enters the cytoplasm of the oocyte while the plasma membrane remains behind.
- *Completion of second meiotic division of oocyte and formation of female pronucleus (PN):* Human oocytes remain arrested at the metaphase stage of second meiotic division. This arrest is released and the development proceeds by a process called *"oocyte activation"*. This activation involves:
  - Release from meiotic arrest (after approximately 3 hours)[31]

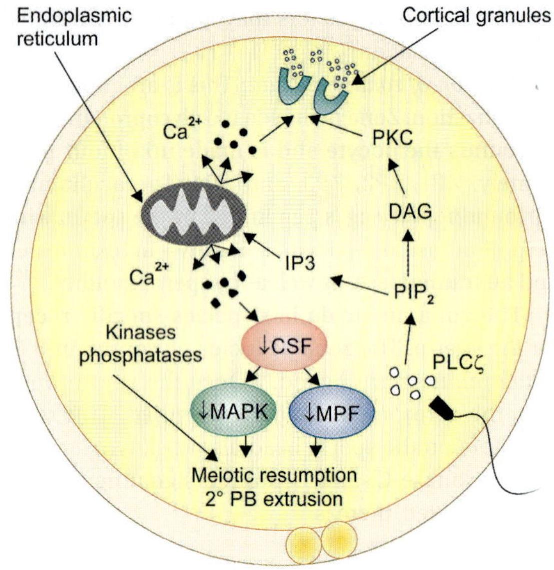

Fig. 2: Molecular mechanism of oocyte activation.

(CSF: cytostatic factor; DAG: diacylglycerol; PB: polar body; MAPK: mitogen-activated protein kinase; MPF: maturation-promoting factor; PKC: protein kinase C; PLCζ: phospholipase C zeta)

- Extrusion of second polar body
- Exocytosis of cortical granules
- Formation of female PN.[32-36]

This is the result of repeated oscillations of free cytosolic calcium. Though the precise mechanism of these oscillations is unclear, it is now widely believed to be the result of a soluble "sperm factor",[37-41] namely phospholipase C zeta (PLCζ)[42] localized to the equatorial region of the sperm head **(Fig. 2)**.[43]

The major cause of fertilization failure, or abnormally low fertilization after intracytoplasmic sperm injection (ICSI) is a deficiency in the process of oocyte activation during the process of *in vitro* fertilization (IVF).[44,45]

- *Formation of male pronucleus:* Nucleus of the sperm enlarges to form male PN within the oocyte cytoplasm. Tail of the sperm degenerates. Male PN forms slightly earlier or simultaneously with female PN (which forms adjacent to second polar body). This is the stage of fertilized egg (oocyte containing two haploid pronuclei) **(Fig. 3)**.
- *Zygote formation:* The pronuclei migrate toward each other via sperm aster microtubules, their opposing membranes break down, and their chromosomes get arranged on a spindle. There is restoration of the normal diploid number of chromosomes (46) in the zygote. Crossing over of chromosomes shuffles the genes and produces a unique recombination of the maternal and paternal genes.[46]

The sex of the embryo is determined by the genetic kind of sperm (X or Y) that fertilizes the oocyte. Fertilization by X-bearing sperm produces 46, XX zygote and by Y-bearing sperm produces XY zygote which develops into a female.

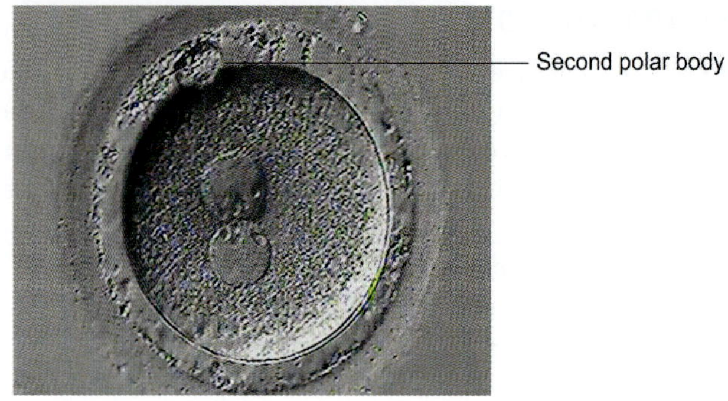

Fig. 3: Two pronuclei stage where pronuclei from male and female gametes are closely opposed. Second polar body can also be seen at the top.

Flowchart 1: Sequence of events during the process of fertilization.

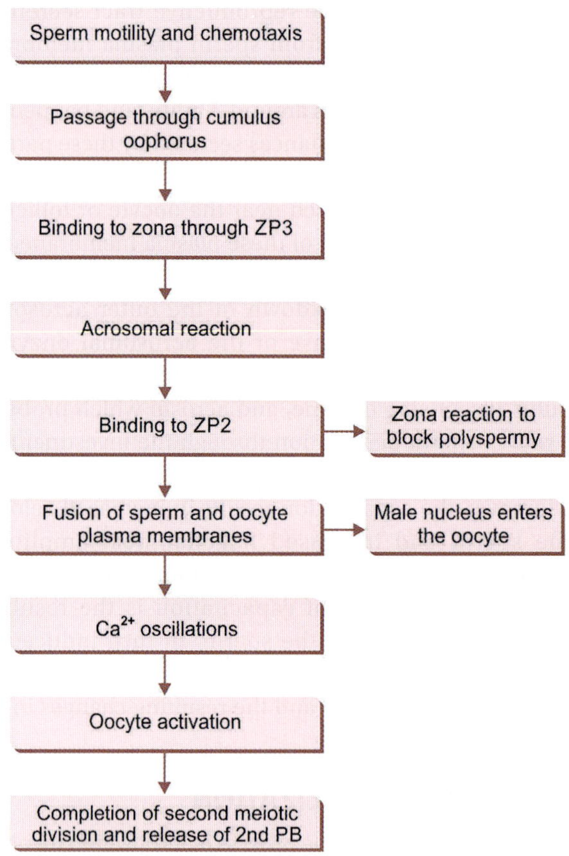

(PB: polar body; ZP3: zona pellucida glycoprotein-3)

This sequence of steps in the process of fertilization is shown in **Flowchart 1**.

EMBRYOGENESIS

The thick zona pellucida is present around the zygote during cleavage. Zygote starts dividing into blastomeres about 30 hours after fertilization, first forming the two-cell stage

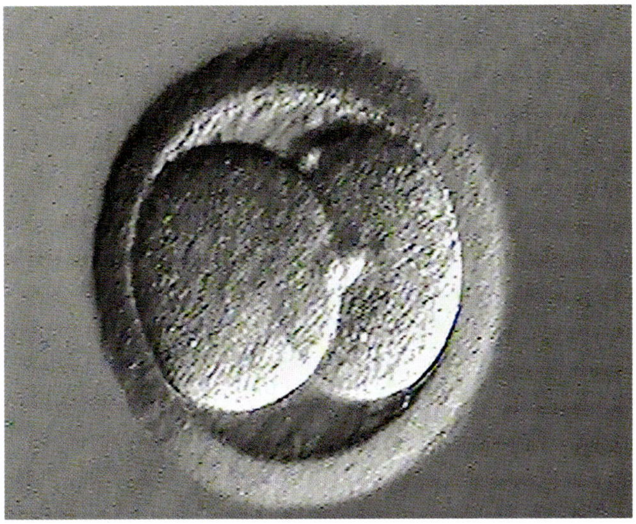

Fig. 4: Two-cell stage of the embryo (after the first cleavage of the zygote).

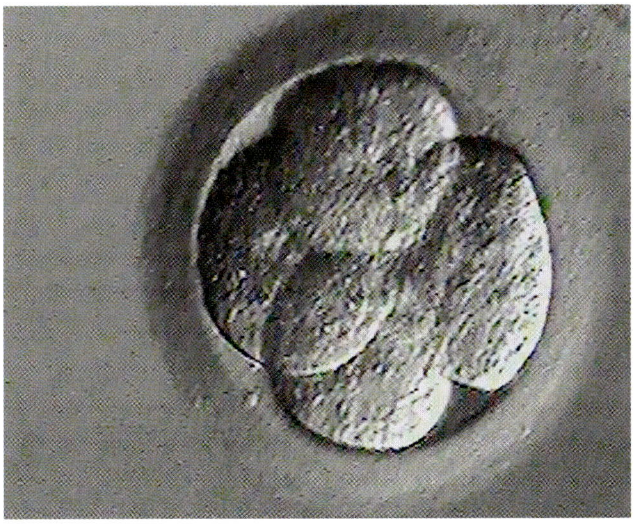

Fig. 5: Four-cell stage of the embryo.

(Fig. 4), and then the four-cell **(Fig. 5)**, and the eight-cell stage **(Fig. 6)**.

The zygote undergoes repeated mitotic divisions and there is a rapid increase in number of cells. The embryonic cells (blastomeres) gradually become smaller with each division.

There is a marked increase in ribonucleic acid (RNA) and protein synthesis, and change in patterns of phospholipid synthesis. These blastomeres which were originally round and loosely adherent, begin to flatten, increase cell-to-cell contact and align themselves tightly against each other to form a compact ball of cells. This process of compaction is mediated by cell surface adhesion glycoproteins. This allows greater cell-to-cell interaction and is important for segregation of internal cells that form inner cell mass (ICM) or embryoblast of future blastocyst.

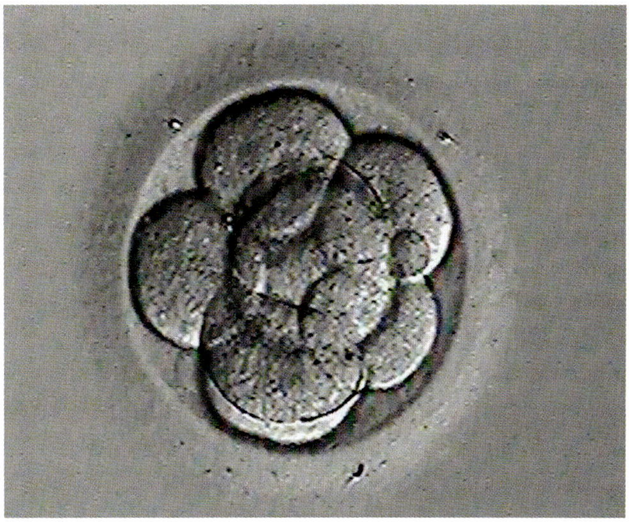

Fig. 6: Eight-cell stage of the embryo.

GENOME ACTIVATION

During its development, the oocyte accumulates reserves of messenger RNA (mRNA), proteins, organelles, etc. to support the early development. The zygote initially depends on stored maternal mRNA during its first cleavage divisions. Then there is critical transition to zygotic genomic activation during the four-to eight-cell stage in humans. Maternal mRNA rapidly disappears and further development is directed by the new embryonic genome. The mammalian embryo fails to develop further if the zygotic genome activation does not occur. There is modification in protein synthesis and nucleolar organizing region (NOR) also.

The compacted stage with 12–32 blastomeres is called a morula; this forms about 3 days after fertilization **(Fig. 7)**. The boundaries between membranes are not clearly distinguishable.

Cleavage of zygote and morula formation occurs during the passage of the dividing zygote through the fallopian tube. The spherical morula enters the uterus and blastocyst formation generally occurs in the uterus.

In spite of the increase in number of cells, there is no increase in size of developing embryo until the zona pellucida degenerates.[47]

BLASTOCYST FORMATION

About 4 days after fertilization, the embryo at the stage of morula enters the uterus and a fluid-filled space called blastocele appears inside it. This is the effect of activation of Na-K-ATPase system resulting in energy-dependent active transport of Na into the center of embryo, followed by osmotically driven movement of water inside.

Gradually, the fluid increases and it separates the blastomeres into an outer thin layer called the trophoblast and the central blastomere collection called the ICM

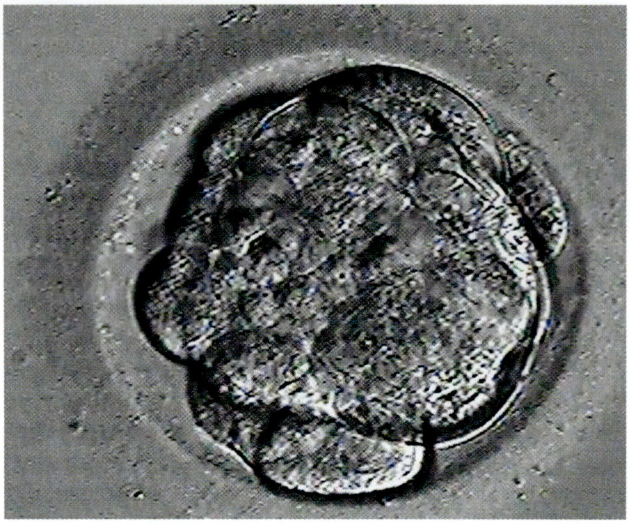

Fig. 7: Stage of morula with compacted cluster of cells formed by repeated division of the zygote. Till this stage the embryo travels through the fallopian tube.

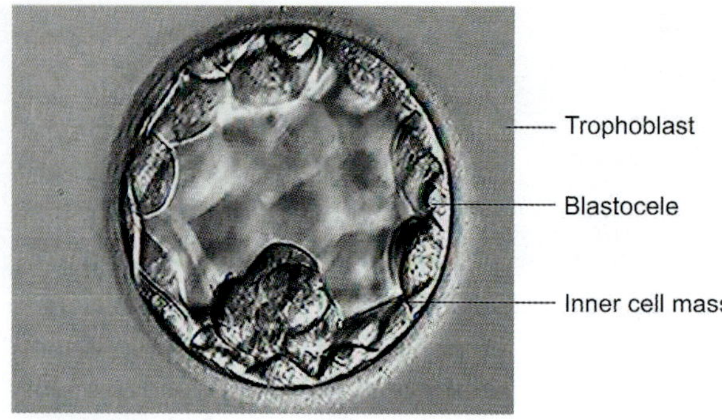

Fig. 8: Blastocyst stage with degenerating zona pellucida. The size of the blastocyst has increased and the cavity is filled with fluid (blastocele) separating the blastomeres into outer trophoblast and the inner cell mass. This generally develops in the uterine cavity.

(***see* Fig. 8**). While the blastomeres at previous stages are totipotent, at compaction the cells polarize radially and divide into the following:

- Outer polar cells with surface microvilli and these cells form trophectoderm
- Inner apolar cells with tight junctions having basal nuclei, which then form ICM.

The trophoblast later forms the placenta while the ICM forms the embryo proper (hence called the embryoblast).[47,48] At this stage, the conceptus is called the blastocyst. Initially, there is no increase in size (day 4/5) but subsequently blastocyst expands over next 1 or 2 days (day 5/6) by more fluid accumulation inside.

After 2 days, the zona pellucida gradually thins out and the blastocyst "hatches" (***see* Fig. 9**). This zona shedding allows the hatched blastocyst to rapidly increase in its size. This blastocyst then attaches to the endometrium, generally adjacent to the embryonic pole. At that time, the trophoblast rapidly divides and differentiates into outer syncytiotrophoblast (multinucleated mass with no cell boundaries) and inner cytotrophoblast. At about 6 days after fertilization (around day 20 of a 28-day cycle), syncytiotrophoblast extends its finger-like processes into the connective tissue beneath the endometrium.

Blastocyst thus, superficially implants in the endometrium by the end of the first week. The complete process of "implantation" is dealt with separately in another chapter.

CLINICAL APPLICATION IN ASSISTED REPRODUCTIVE TECHNOLOGY

- *Intracytoplasmic sperm injection:* It is an advanced assisted reproductive technology especially for male infertility, where the entire spermatozoon is inserted into the oocyte with the help of a fine injection pipette under micromanipulator (ICSI machine). It is different from natural fertilization as normally sperm plasma membrane and acrosomal contents never enter the oocyte, but in ICSI, the whole of the sperm and a small amount of extracellular medium are deposited in the oocyte.
- *Total fertilization failure (TFF):* This refers to failure of fertilization in all the mature oocytes. TFF is seen in 5–10% of IVF cycles and 1–3% of ICSI cycles.[49,50] TFF can happen due to failure of sperm penetration of cumulus, acrosome reaction, zona binding, gamete fusion, or oocyte activation. Assisted oocyte activation using strontium chloride, calcium ionophores, or electrical stimulus can be useful in certain cases of TFF.
- *Blastocyst culture:* Success rate of IVF has considerably improved with blastocyst transfer than transfer of day 2 or day 3 embryos as it is more in synchronization with the physiology that embryo reaches uterus at blastocyst

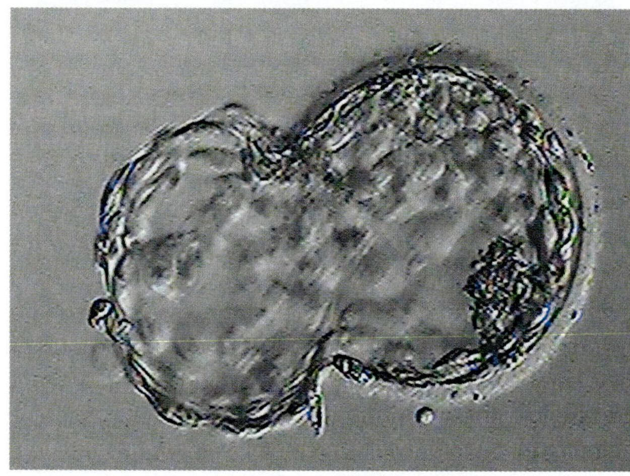

Fig. 9: The hatching blastocyst stage. Zona pellucida has degenerated and the embryo is escaping out.

stage and then implants there. This allows the possibility of single embryo transfer also with decent success rate in IVF and avoids the complications of multiple pregnancies.

REFERENCES

1. Sathananthan AH. Human Fertilization CD-ROM. Tokyo, Japan; 2003.
2. Lyons RA, Djahanbakhch O, Mahmood T, Saridogan E, Sattar S, Sheaff MT, et al. Fallopian tube ciliary beat frequency in relation to the stage of menstrual cycle and anatomical site. Hum Reprod. 2002;17(3):584-8.
3. Croxatto HB, Ortiz MS. Egg transport in the fallopian tube. Gynecol Invest. 1975;6(3-4):215-25.
4. Adams CE. Consequences of accelerated ovum transport, including a re-evaluation of Estes' operation. J Reprod Fertil. 1979;55(1):239-46.
5. Rosenwaks Z. Donor eggs: their application in modern reproductive technologies. Fertil Steril. 1987;47(6):895-909.
6. Devroey P, Liu J, Nagy Z, Tournaye H, Silber SJ, Van Steirteghem AC. Normal fertilization of human oocytes after testicular sperm extraction and intracytoplasmic sperm injection. Fertil Steril. 1994;62(3):639-41.
7. Yudin AI, Hanson FW, Katz DF. Human cervical mucus and its interaction with sperm: a fine-structural view. Biol Reprod. 1989;40(3):661-71.
8. Wang C, Baker HWG, Jennings MG, Burger HG, Lutjen P. Interaction between human cervical mucus and sperm surface antibodies. Fertil Steril. 1985;44(4):484-8.
9. Morales P, Katz DF, Overstreet JW, Samuels SJ, Chang RJ. The relationship between the motility and morphology of spermatozoa in human semen. J Androl. 1988;9(4):241-7.
10. Katz DF, Morales P, Samuels SJ, Overstreet JW. Mechanisms of filtration of morphologically abnormal human sperm by cervical mucus. Fertil Steril. 1990;54(3):513-6.
11. Krzanowska H. The passage of abnormal spermatozoa through the uterotubal junction of the mouse. J Reprod Fertil. 1974;38(1):81-90.
12. France JT, Graham FM, Gosling L, Hair P, Knox BS. Characteristics of natural conceptual cycles occurring in a prospective study of sex preselection: fertility awareness symptoms, hormone levels, sperm survival, and pregnancy outcome. Int J Fertil. 1992;37(4):244-55.
13. Wilcox AJ, Weinberg CR, Baird DD. Timing of sexual intercourse in relation to ovulation. Effects on the probability of conception, survival of the pregnancy, and sex of the baby. N Engl J Med. 1995;333(23):1517-21.
14. Yanagimachi R. Capacitation and the acrosome reaction. In: Asch R, Balmaceda JP, Johnston I (Eds). Gamete Physiology. Norwell, Massachusetts: Serono Symposia; 1990. pp. 31-42.
15. Aitken RJ. Molecular mechanisms regulating human sperm function. Mol Hum Reprod. 1997;3(3):169-73.
16. De Lamirande E, Leclerc P, Gagnon C. Capacitation as a regulatory event that primes spermatozoa for the acrosome reaction and fertilization. Mol Hum Reprod. 1997;3(3):175-94.
17. Guraya SS. Cellular and molecular biology of capacitation and acrosome reaction in spermatozoa. Int Rev Cytol. 2000;199:1-64.
18. Zaneveld LJD, Polakoski KL, Williams WL. Properties of a proteolytic enzyme from rabbit sperm acrosomes. Biol Reprod. 1972;6:30-9.
19. Jones R. Identification and functions of mammalian sperm-egg recognition molecules during fertilization. J Reprod Fertil Suppl. 1990;42:89-105.
20. Wassarman PM. Mouse gamete adhesion molecules. Biol Reprod. 1992;46(2):186-91.
21. Leyton L, Le Guen P, Bunch D, Saling PM. Regulation of mouse gamete interaction by a sperm tyrosine kinase. Proc Natl Acad Sci U S A. 1992;89(24):11692-5.
22. Burks DJ, Carballada R, Moore HD, Saling PM. Interaction of a tyrosine kinase from human sperm with the zona pellucida at fertilization. Science. 1995;269(5220):83-6.
23. Florman HM, Tombes RM, First NL, Babcock DF. An adhesion-associated agonist from the zona pellucida activates G protein-promoted elevations of internal Ca^{2+} and pH that mediate mammalian sperm acrosomal exocytosis. Dev Biol. 1989;135(1):133-46.
24. Ward CR, Storey BT, Kopf GS. Selective activation of Gi1 and Gi2 in mouse sperm by the zona pellucida, the egg's extracellular matrix. J Biol Chem. 1994;269(18):13254-8.
25. O'Toole CMB, Roldan ER, Fraser LR. Protein kinase C activation during progesterone-stimulated acrosomal exocytosis in human spermatozoa. Mol Hum Reprod. 1996;2(12):921-7.
26. Hartmann JF, Gwatkin RB. Alteration of sites on the mammalian sperm surface following capacitation. Nature. 1971;234(5330):479-81.
27. Barros C, Yanagimachi R. Induction of zona reaction in golden hamster eggs by cortical granule material. Nature. 1971;233(5317):268-9.
28. Lathrop WF, Carmichael EP, Myles DG, Primakoff P. cDNA cloning reveals the molecular structure of a sperm surface protein, PH-20, involved in sperm-egg adhesion and the wide distribution of its gene among mammals. J Cell Biol. 1990;111:2939-49.
29. Blobel CP, Wolfsberg TG, Turck CW, Myles DG, Primakoff P, White JM. A potential fusion peptide and an integrin ligand domain in a protein active in sperm-egg fusion. Nature. 1992;356:248-52.
30. Fusi FM, Bernocchi N, Ferrari A, Bronson RA. Is vitronectin the velcro that binds the gametes together? Mol Hum Reprod. 1996;2(11):859-66.
31. Lopata A, Sathananthan AH, McBain JC, Johnston WIH, Speirs AL. The ultrastructure of preovulatory human eggs fertilized *in vitro*. Fertil Steril. 1980;33(1):12-20.
32. Kline D, Kline JT. Repetitive calcium transients and the role of calcium in exocytosis and cell cycle activation in the mouse egg. Dev Biol. 1992;149(1):80-9.
33. Swann K, Ozil JP. Dynamics of the calcium signal that triggers mammalian egg activation. Int Rev Cytol.1994;152:183-222.
34. Miyazaki S, Ito M. Calcium signals for egg activation in mammals. J Pharmacol Sci. 2006;100(5):545-52.
35. Publicover S, Harper CV, Barratt C. $[Ca^{2+}]i$ signalling in sperm—making the most of what you've got. Nat Cell Biol. 2007;9(3):235-42.
36. Swann K, Yu Y. The dynamics of calcium oscillations that activate mammalian eggs. Int J Dev Biol. 2008;52:585-94.

37. Jones KT, Soeller C, Cannell MB. The passage of Ca^{2+} and fluorescent markers between the sperm and egg after fusion in the mouse. Development. 1998;125(23):4627-35.
38. Parrington J, Jones KT, Lai A, Swann K. The soluble sperm factor that causes Ca^{2+} release from sea-urchin (Lytechinus pictus) egg homogenates also triggers Ca^{2+} oscillations after injection into mouse eggs. Biochem J. 1999;341:1-4.
39. Jones KT, Matsuda M, Parrington J, Katan M, Swann K. Different Ca^{2+}-releasing abilities of sperm extracts compared with tissue extracts and phospholipase C isoforms in sea urchin egg homogenate and mouse eggs. Biochem J. 2000;346 Pt 3:743-9.
40. Rice A, Parrington J, Jones KT, Swann K. Mammalian sperm contain a $Ca^{(2+)}$-sensitive phospholipase C activity that can generate InsP(3) from PIP(2) associated with intracellular organelles. Dev Biol. 2000;228:125-35.
41. Parrington J, Lai FA, Swann K. The soluble mammalian sperm factor protein that triggers Ca^{2+} oscillations in eggs: evidence for expression of mRNA(s) coding for sperm factor protein(s) in spermatogenic cells. Biol Cell. 2000;92:267-75.
42. Saunders CM, Larman MG, Parrington J, Cox LJ, Royse J, Blayney LM, et al. PLC zeta: a sperm-specific trigger of Ca^{2+} oscillations in eggs and embryo development. Development. 2002;129(15):3533-44.
43. Swain JE, Pool TB. ART failure: oocyte contributors to unsuccessful fertilization. Hum Reprod Update. 2008;14(5):431-46.
44. Sousa M, Tesarik J. Ultrastructural analysis of fertilization failure after intracytoplasmic sperm injection. Hum Reprod. 1994;9:2374-80.
45. Heindryckx B, De Gheselle S, Gerris J, Dhont M, De Sutter P. Efficiency of assisted oocyte activation as a solution for failed intracytoplasmic sperm injection. Reprod Biomed Online. 2008;17:662-8.
46. Latham KE. Mechanisms and control of embryonic genome activation in mammalian embryos. Int Rev Cytol. 1999;193:71-124.
47. Rock J, Hertig AT. The human conceptus during the first two weeks of gestation. Am J Obstet Gynecol. 1948;55(1):6-17.
48. Sjoberg NO, Hamberger L. Blastocyst development and early implantation. Hum Reprod. 2000;15(Suppl 6).
49. Flaherty SP, Payne D, Swann NJ, Mattews CD. Aetiology of failed and abnormal fertilization after intracytoplasmic sperm injection. Hum Reprod. 1995;10(10):2623-9.
50. Mahutte NG, Arici A. Failed fertilization: is it predictable? Curr Opin Obstet Gynecol. 2003;15(3):211-8.

CHAPTER 6

Implantation

Nisha Singh, Divyashree PS

INTRODUCTION

Implantation is the process by which the blastocyst comes into intimate physical and physiological contact with the uterine endometrium. It requires:

- Competent embryo
- Receptive endometrium
- Synchrony between development of embryo and conditioning of the uterus **(Flowchart 1)**
- Factors involved in regulation of blastocyst implantation are incompletely understood. Human chorionic gonadotropin (hCG), growth factors and cytokines, steroid hormones, and other mediators produced either by the embryo, by the mother, or by both, during the periimplantation period dictate changes in the endometrium, in the immunological system of the mother, and in embryo metabolism which enables the embryo to implant.
- Successful implantation requires a synchronous development of a blastocyst competent to implant and an endometrium able to respond to the signals from the blastocyst.[1] Implantation is a complex process involving spatiotemporally regulated endocrine, paracrine, autocrine, and juxtacrine modulators that span cell-cell and cell-matrix interactions.[2]
- Despite experimental success in initiating embryonic development outside the uterus and in identifying numerous molecules involved in the embryo-uterine dialogue, there is a yet to be filled significant knowledge gap in understanding the in vivo events of implantation. Furthermore, the implantation process varies among species, thus precluding the formulation of a unified theme. In addition, ethical restrictions and experimental difficulties prevent direct analysis of embryo-uterine interactions during human implantation. This chapter is focused on the mechanisms of implantation, embryo-maternal cross talk, and immunotolerance of the fetus to accomplish implantation.

PREIMPLANTATION EMBRYO DEVELOPMENT AND GENOMIC ACTIVATION

Following successful fertilization, in most mammals the zygote starts a 4-5-day journey from the ampulla portion of the fallopian tube toward the uterus, developing to the morula stage by an increase in cell number. Whereas the

Flowchart 1: Contributors of implantation.

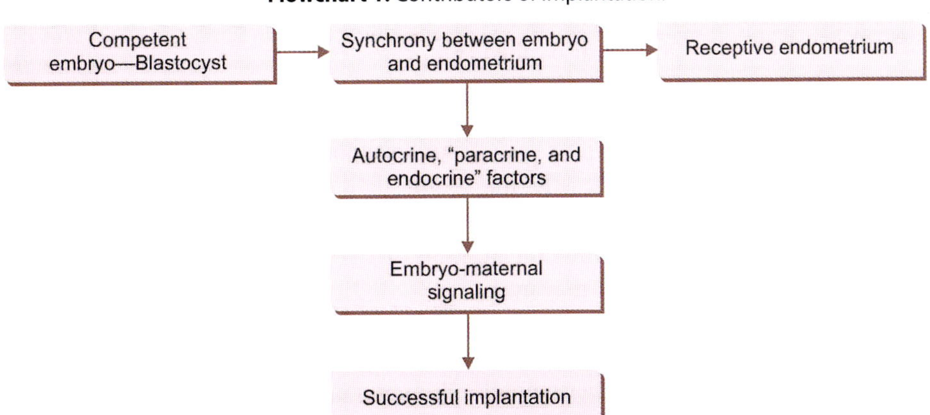

Flowchart 2: Preimplantation events.

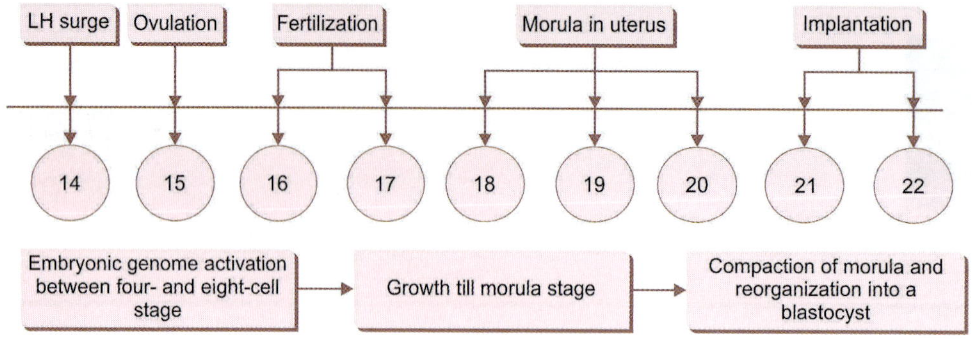

(LH: luteinizing hormone)

overall amount of cytoplasm in the embryo remains constant, the number of nuclei and the amount of deoxyribonucleic acid (DNA) increase exponentially. During this period, messenger ribonucleic acid (mRNA) and proteins are maternally driven and embryonic genome is transcriptionally activated only at later cell cycles.[3]

Timeline for Implantation

The maternal zygotic transition occurs at four- to eight-cell stage in humans.[3] Embryo enters into the uterine cavity, on average 3 days postovulation, the morula undergoes reorganization processes at the cellular level, compaction, and becomes "activated" to progress to the blastocyst stage **(Flowchart 2)**. This activation involves the expression and transcription of over 500 dormant genes. However, this embryonic (gene) activation might be delayed during which the embryo remains in a state, what is known as diapause, which causes delayed implantation.[4,5]

During the transition from eight-cell to blastocyst, several genes have been identified that are crucial for lineage segregations; some of the important ones include *OCT4*, *SOX2*, *NANOG*, *CDX*, *LEFTY*, and eomesodermin (*EOMES*) **(Fig. 1 and Table 1)**.[6]

The appearance of the inner cavity within the mass of cells is a sign of initiation of the formation of the blastocyst. The differentiated and expanded blastocyst is composed of two distinct types of cells: (1) The outer cell mass, also called the trophectoderm (TE) and (2) the inner cell mass (ICM).

Trophectoderm gives rise to trophoblast and extra-embryonic structures such as placenta, while ICM gives rise to the embryo.[14] On entry into the uterine cavity, the embryo will be relatively inactive for the embryo-maternal interaction until it hatches from its zona pellucida at 6 days postovulation.[15] This coincides with and may even induce the window of implantation (WOI). Preimplantation embryo development normally occurs within the zona pellucida. However, zona removal by various experimental manipulations does not deter embryonic development in vitro suggesting that this glycoprotein barrier is not essential for development to progress. The nonadhesive nature of the zona pellucida probably preventing implantation within the oviduct is thought to facilitate the journey of embryos through oviduct to uterus.[15]

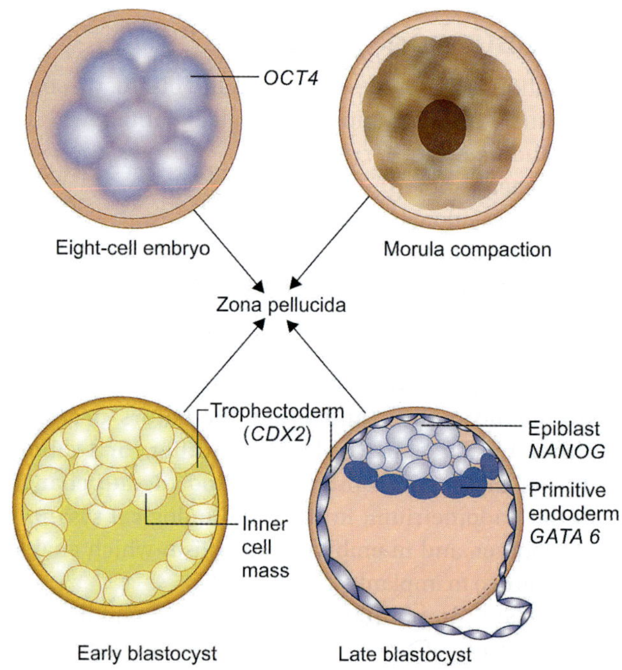

Fig. 1: Lineage differentiation during eight-cell to blastocyst transition and gene expression patterns during blastocyst formation. *OCT4* is expressed throughout the embryo before late morula and is crucial for the formation of inner cell mass. The expression of *NANOG* is induced in the inside cells of late morula. *CDX2* is expressed in trophectoderm. *GATA6* is expressed in the primitive endoderm of the late blastocyst.
Source: Adapted from Guzeloglu-Kayisli O et al.[13]

HATCHING OF BLASTOCYST

Hatching occurs in vitro as well, suggesting this process does not need a uterine environment,[16] albeit at lower rates than in vivo. Sathananthan has described electron

TABLE 1: Function of transcription factors known to be important for the fate of trophectoderm (TE) and the inner cell mass (ICM).

Gene	*Function*	*Reference*
OCT4	Restricted to ICM upon blastocyst formation, preventing TE formation	Kirchhof et al.[7]
SOX2	Similar to *OCT4*, prevents trophoblast specification	Avilion et al.[8]
NANOG	Sustaining the self-renewal capacity of embryonal stem cells and inhibiting their differentiation, ICM formation, and visceral parietal endoderm formation	Mitsui et al.[9]
CDX2	Segregating ICM and TE lineages, by suppressing *OCT4* and *SOX2*	Niwa et al.[10]
EOMES	Required for TE proliferation and differentiation at the blastocyst stage	Simmons and Cross[11]
LEFTY	Determining left–right axis in mouse embryos	Takaoka et al.[12]

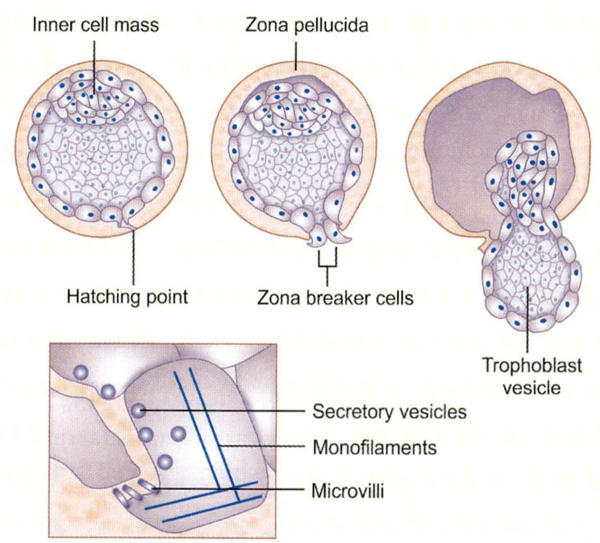

Fig. 2: Hatching of blastocyst.
Source: Adapted from Hoozemans DA et al.[48]

microscopical observations in the hatching process wherein both mechanical and chemical factors seem to be involved.[15] Hatching usually occurs on the opposite site of the embryonic pole. Specialized trophoblast cells called "zona breaker" cells have secretory vesicles that seem to facilitate opening the zona pellucida at the hatching point. Possibly the vesicles contain proteolytic enzymes, which help in the dissolution of the zona. Microvilli and contractile monofilaments make the embryo hatch out *mechanically* **(Fig. 2)**.[15]

Hatching failure in assisted reproduction possibly derives from hardening of the zona pellucida or general blastocystic inactivity.[15] To treat this hatching failure, assisted hatching procedures by means of laser, enzymes, or zona drilling have been attempted to rescue blastocysts.[17] The hatching of the blastocyst from its zona pellucida occurs approximately 72 hours after entry into the uterus.

The hatching process exposes the trophoblast cells, which express different molecules on their cell surface such as leukemia inhibitory factor (LIF), colony-stimulating factor (CSF), heparin-binding epidermal growth factor

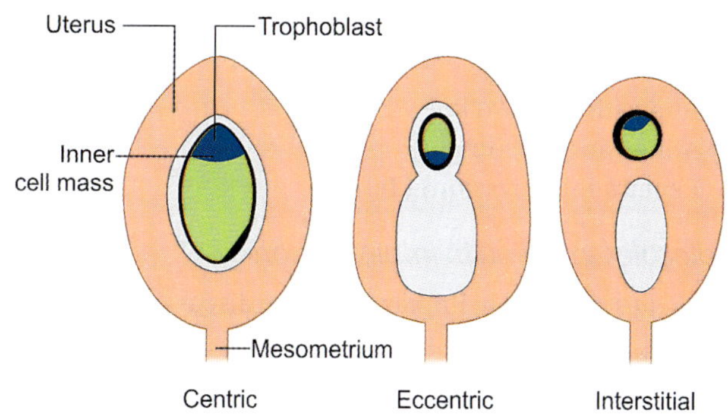

Fig. 3: Types of implantation.

(HB-EGF) receptors, L-selectin and integrins, and releases chemical messengers such as interleukin-1β (IL-1β). With the exposure of the trophoblast cells, their signal, and attachment molecules to the uterine environment, implantation begins approximately 7 days postovulation. The initial apposition of the hatched (and chromosomally normal) embryo has to take place at this time, since the WOI is open only for a limited period of 48 hours.

Based on the different types of blastocyst uterine cell interactions, implantation has been classified into three broad categories: (1) Centric, (2) eccentric, and (3) interstitial (Wimsatt, 1975) **(Fig. 3)**.

1. *Centric implantation* occurs when the blastocyst is able to grow large and form ample surface contact to fuse with the luminal epithelium without penetrating through it. Rabbits, dogs, domestic animals (cows, pigs, and sheep), and many marsupials have centric implantation.
2. In *eccentric implantation*, the luminal epithelium forms an invagination to surround the trophoblast. Mice, rats, and hamsters have eccentric implantation.
3. The third type of implantation is *interstitial*, in which the trophoblast passes through the luminal epithelium to invade the endometrial stroma and become embedded in the wall of the uterus. Implantation in humans and guinea pigs has been classified into this category (Wimsatt, 1975).[127,18]

EMBRYO-ENDOMETRIAL INTERACTION DURING IMPLANTATION

Embryo-endometrial interaction during implantation takes place through three ways:

1. Molecules and pathways known to initiate embryo apposition and attachment
2. Embryo invasion into stroma and mechanisms that safeguard quality implantation
3. Blastocyst regulation of implantation

Molecules and Pathways known to Initiate Embryo Apposition and Attachment

Enders and Schlafke have classified the process of implantation into three stages:[19]

1. Apposition and rolling
2. Adhesion (attachment)
3. Penetration (invasion) **(Table 2)**

Molecules Involved in Implantation

Molecules involved in implantation are discussed in **Table 3.**

Comparative model:

Embryonic implantation versus leukocyte transendothelial migration ***(Flowchart 3):*** A parallelism between the different steps in human embryo-endometrial apposition/adhesion/invasion and leukocyte (LK) endothelium rolling/adhesion/extravasation has been observed.[39] A cascade of multiple events that take place during both processes show similarities, although some details with respect to time scale, size of cells, identity of involved molecules, and others are different **(Fig. 7 and Flowchart 3)**.

Once the blastocyst enters the uterine cavity, free-floating sphere "rolls" on the surface and encounters the epithelial glycocalyx. The trophoectoderm of hatched human blastocyst expresses L-selectin, which recognizes specific sialylated or sulfated sugars, which are carried by certain mucins such as Mucin 1 (MUC-1) on apical surface of the endometrium. This initial weak adhesion locates embryo to a specific site and activates other molecules to establish further attachment. The ability of attaching embryo to remove the mucin barrier is the health test on the embryo.[46]

Human endometrium undergoes a complex series of organized proliferative and secretory changes in each menstrual cycle.[47] When implantation does not occur, there is a deliberate and timely destruction of the fully developed endometrium, which leads to menstruation, only for the same cycle of events to be repeated once again to prepare for the next-generation blastocyst.[47]

Embryo Invasion into Stroma and Mechanisms that Safeguard Quality Implantation

Factors Influencing Implantation[48-50]

- *Ovarian hormones*:
  - Estrogen
  - Progesterone
  - Relaxin
- *Endometrium*:
  - *Cytokines*: LIF, CSF, and IL-1
  - *Growth factors*: Insulin-like growth factor-1 (IGF-1), HB-EGF, transforming growth factor-beta (TGF-β) (inhibins and activins), and vascular endothelial growth factor (VEGF)
  - *Genes*: *HOXA10* and *HOXA11*, *BMP2*, and *WNT4*
  - *Proteins*: Glycodelin, matrix metalloproteinase-2 (MMP-2), and MMP-9, signal transducer, and activator of transcription 3 (STAT3) protein
- *Embryo*:
  - IL-1
  - VEGF
  - IGF-2
  - Chorionic gonadotropin (CG)
- *Peripheral*: Cyclooxygenase-2 (COX-2) signaling
- *Endocrine*:
  - Corticotropin-releasing hormone (CRH)
  - Leptin

Ovarian hormones and endometrium:

Estrogen and progesterone: Ovarian steroids, estrogen, and progesterone are the major factors that prepare the uterus for implantation. They initiate a cascade of paracrine and autocrine signal transduction which, via cell adhesion processes, will lead to attachment and the subsequent invasion of the embryo into the endometrium.

Estrogen causes:

- Upregulation of P4 receptors
- Also upregulates VEGF, IGF-1, L-selectin, and HB-EGF. Progesterone receptor is upregulated by estrogen.

Therefore, the highest concentration of progesterone receptors is found in the periovulatory region, and maturation disorders in the secretory phase might also have their origin in an inadequate proliferative phase. After ovulation, estrogen receptors and progesterone type B receptor vanish from the stroma.

Progesterone causes:

- Morphological changes in the endometrium
- Upregulates pinopode formation
- Upregulates CSF, LIF, IL-1, prostaglandin (PG), VEGF, glycodelin, fibronectin, MUC-1, and L-selectin
- Downregulation of LIF and beta3 integrin
- Downregulation of estrogen receptors

Relaxin: Relaxin is an ovarian peptide hormone of the IGF family. Its receptors are expressed in the endometrium spatiotemporally.

- Increases the production of glycodelin and VEGF secretion[51]

TABLE 2: Morphological steps of implantation.

S. No.	*Stages*	*Physiology*	*Mediators involved*	*Figure*
1.	Apposition (unstable adhesion of blastocyst to endometrial surface) **(Figs. 4A to C)**	• Once embryo reaches uterus via tapis roulant of mucin (MUC) flow, which is continuous toward cervix • Apposition is progressively increasing intimacy of contact between trophoblast and uterine epithelium • Characterized by: – Enlargement of embryo – Edema of endometrium – Decrease in uterine fluid volume – Obliteration of uterine lumen by closer apposition of apical end of endometrial and trophoblastic cells – Appearance of pinopodes	• MUC-1 • Chemokines: – Alpha (CXC chemokines) – Beta (CC chemokines)	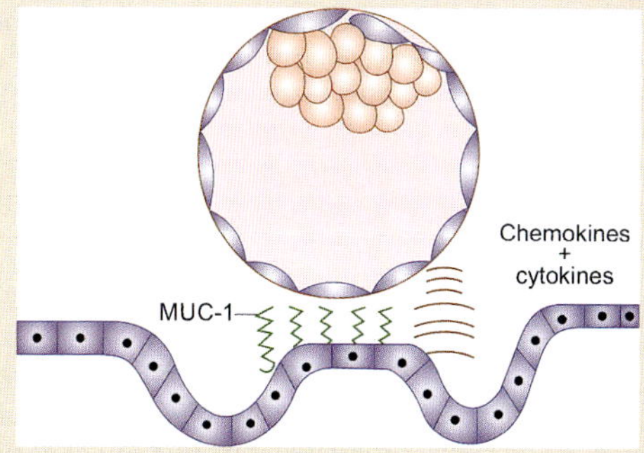 **Fig. 4A**
2.	Rolling over	Blastocyst enters the uterus and roll over the endometrium freely **(Figs. 4B and 5)**	L-selectin	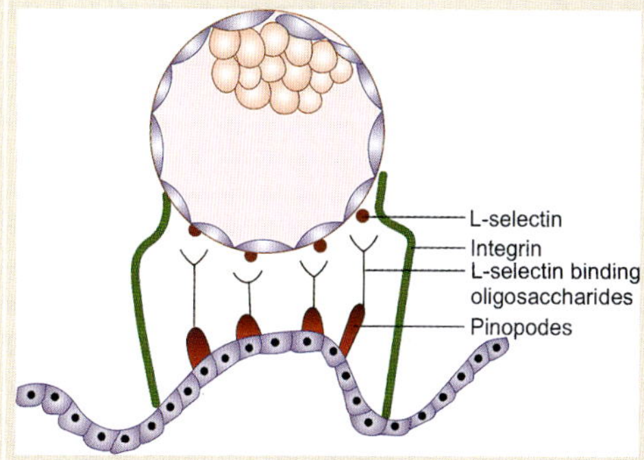 **Fig. 4B**
3.	Adhesion **(Fig. 4C)**	• Direct contact occurs between the maternal endometrial epithelium cell (EEC) and the embryonic trophectoderm (TE) • The first sign of attachment reaction occurs on days 20–21 in humans and coincides with a localized increase in the stromal vascular permeability at the site of blastocyst attachment[20,21] • Endometrium and embryo now express extracellular matrix (ECM) component which helps to mediate adhesion through adhesion molecules, e.g., integrins and selectin	• Cellular adhesion molecules: – Integrins – Heparin-binding epidermal growth factor (HB-EGF) – Cadherins – Immunoglobulin – Fibronectin and laminin	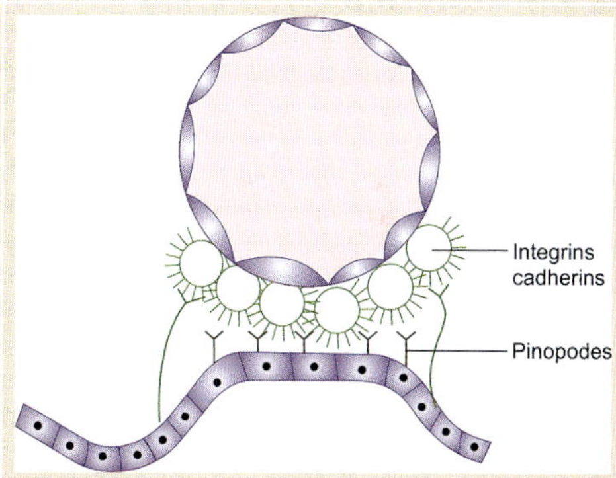 **Fig. 4C**
4.	Invasion	• Finally, in the invasion phase, the embryonic trophoblast breaches the basement membrane and invades the endometrial stroma up to the uterine vessels **(Fig. 4D)**. Three types of interaction occur between implanting trophoblast and uterine epithelium: • Trophectoderm cells from the blastocyst migrate between the epithelial cells, displacing them and penetrating as far as the basement membrane[21] • Epithelial cells lift off the basement membranes, an action that allows trophoblast to insinuate underneath the epithelium • Fusion of trophoblast with uterine epithelial cells	• Chemokines • Matrix metalloproteinase-2 (MMP-2)/MMP-9 • Vascular endothelial growth factor (VEGF) • Collagenases • Plasminogen activators • Selectins • Integrins	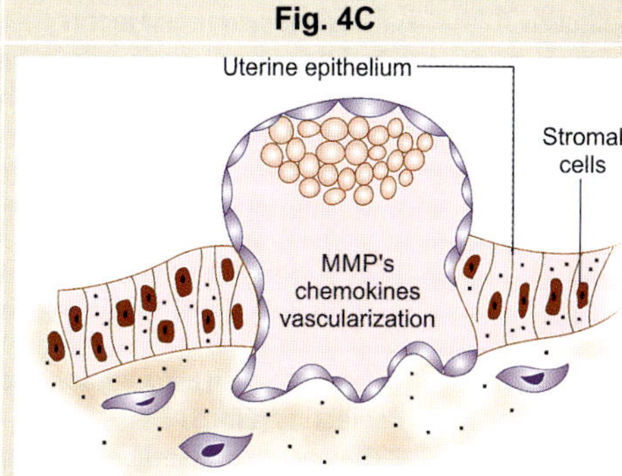 **Fig. 4D**

TABLE 3: Molecules involved in implantation.

Molecule	*Function*	*Relation to fertility*
Mucin-1 (MUC-1)	• Glycoprotein which is found on luminal surface of the epithelium • Mainly MUC-1, MUC-6 • First molecule that blastocyst encounters on the endometrial wall before implantation • Expression is highest in luteal phase and implantation period[22] • When highly expressed on a cell surface, MUC-1 produces a steric hindrance phenomenon interfering with cellular adhesion • Cell–cell and cell–matrix adhesions are inhibited in direct correlation to the length of the MUC-1 ectodomain • It repels and guides the blastocyst to find the correct place for implantation • There is a local loss of MUC-1 at the site of embryo attachment and in the immediate vicinity, whereas its expression is increased at a distance farther away from the implantation site[23,24] • Tumor necrosis factor-alpha (TNF-α) (proinflammatory cytokine) and sheddases[25] bring proteolysis of MUC-1 at the site of implantation	In women with recurrent implantation failure (RIF) and recurrent pregnancy loss (RPL), studies have shown reduced midsecretory phase levels of MUC-1 and its epitopes[26,27]
Chemokines	• Chemokines (short for chemoattractant cytokines) are a family of small polypeptides (70–80 amino acids) specialized in the attraction of specific leukocytes (LKs) • Interleukin-8 (IL-8) (α-chemokine) is a potent chemoattractant and activator of neutrophils and T lymphocytes	Chemokines act on a range of LK subsets, which in turn release proteases and mediators, which facilitate embryo apposition and invasion
	• Monocyte chemoattractant protein-1 (MCP-1), β-chemokine subfamily, is a potent chemoattractant and activator of monocytes, macrophages, T cells, basophils, mast cells, and natural killer (NK) cells • The β-chemokine regulated upon activation of normal T cell expressed and secreted (RANTES) is a chemoattractant of monocytes, eosinophils, and basophils, and is localized in eutopic endometrium and ectopic endometriotic implants • Chemokine receptors are G protein-coupled receptors (GPCRs) and are localized in the plasma membrane and trigger chemotactic response in many immune cells • During the apposition phase, there is a specific LK subset infiltration into the endometrium from blood vessels and neighboring tissues • Immunohistochemical localization demonstrated that IL-8, MCP-1, and the three receptors *CXCR1*, *CCR2B*, and *CCR5* were mainly expressed in glandular and luminal epithelium and endothelial cells, whereas RANTES staining was localized mainly in the stromal and perivascular cells of blood vessels[28] • After previous estradiol priming, progesterone upregulates endometrial epithelium cell (EEC) IL-8 and MCP1 messenger ribonucleic acid (mRNA) in the secretory phase of the menstrual cycle • The human embryo does not secrete IL-8, MCP-1, or RANTES, but curiously, it expresses some of these chemokine receptors, CCR2B (MCP-1 receptor) and CCR5 (RANTES receptor)	
Selectins	• *Most important:* L-selectin • Tether and rollover mechanism over the endometrial surface • L-selectin is expressed by the hatched embryo and selectin oligosaccharide-based ligand, MECA-79, is upregulated during the window of implantation (WOI) **(Fig. 5)** • Embryo is slowed down by integrin interactions • It facilitates the apposition of blastocyst to the endometrial epithelium[29]	It has been shown that lack of expression of the L-selectin ligand MECA-79 in midluteal endometrial biopsies were indicative of low or no chances of pregnancy[30]
Integrins	• Family of transmembrane glycoproteins • Formed by the interaction of two different, noncovalently linked alpha and beta subunits[25] • They establish a firmer adhesion after the appositioning process is initiated by selectins **(Fig. 5)** • They are expressed both by the endometrium and blastocyst • Alpha 5 beta 3 (αvβ3) integrin and its ligand osteopontin first interact with trophoblast • The expression of the αvβ3 integrin in the endometrial stroma has been shown to be stimulated by IL-α, IL-β, and tumor necrosis factor-α (TNF-α) • Integrins have been proposed as markers for endometrial receptivity, particularly the αvβ3 glycoprotein	• Blockage of αvβ3 integrin lowers the implantation rates in mice[31] • In humans, lower or absent concentrations of integrins (mainly αvβ3) in midluteal endometrial biopsy have been observed in unexplained infertility, polycystic ovarian syndrome (PCOS), and endometriosis[32-35]

Contd...

Contd...

Molecule	***Function***	***Relation to fertility***
Cadherins	• Cadherins are a group of glycoproteins responsible for calcium-dependent cell-to-cell adhesion through homotypic binding • In regard to implantation, E-cadherin represents the most studied subclass	• Genetic variants on the E-cadherin gene may be involved in endometriosis-related infertility • Potential role of *HOXA10* and E-cadherin in the implantation processes and altered expression in women with reproductive failure
	• E-cadherin possesses a dual function. In the preliminary phases, its expression at the cell surface is required to ensure adhesiveness. Subsequently in the luteal phase, E-cadherin may be downregulated to enable epithelial cells dissociation and blastocyst invasion. Interestingly, calcitonin (CT) expression is induced by progesterone leading to increased intracellular calcium which then suppresses E-cadherin expression **(Figs. 6A and B)**[36] • Calcitonin receptors have been identified in embryos between the eight-cell and blastocyst stage	
Immunoglobulins	• Among the cell adhesion molecules (CAMs) family, the immunoglobulins superfamily is the most extensive • Intercellular adhesion molecule-1 (ICAM1) or CD54 is a transmembrane glycoprotein, which is constitutively expressed on the cell surface of a variety of cell types, such as fibroblasts, LKs, macrophages, T lymphocytes, granulocytes, and endothelial and epithelial cells of the endometrium • This molecule is upregulated at the transcriptional level by both inflammatory and noninflammatory cytokines	• ICAM1 adhesive interactions are essential for the transendothelial migration of LKs and for various immunological functions • Decreased expression in women with implantation failures
Fibronectin and laminin	• They are ECM proteins abundantly secreted by decidualized endometrial stroma and are under progesterone control. They interact with integrins as signal-transducing ligands resulting in changes in the trophoblast invasiveness • Laminin expression is higher in the secretory phase of the menstrual cycle and increases with implantation and in early pregnancy37 • Laminin facilitates trophoblast invasion, probably via lowering of insulin-like growth factor-binding protein-1 (IGFBP-1) and prolactin, which are the two major secretory proteins of decidualized stromal cells • Fibronectin interacts with integrins expressed by trophoblast, and this integration inhibits trophoblast invasiveness	Fibronectin is increased in patients with fetal growth retardation and hypertensive disorders in comparison with controls. Total plasma fibronectin concentrations might predict the maternal restraint on the invading trophoblast before and during implantation and placentation[38]

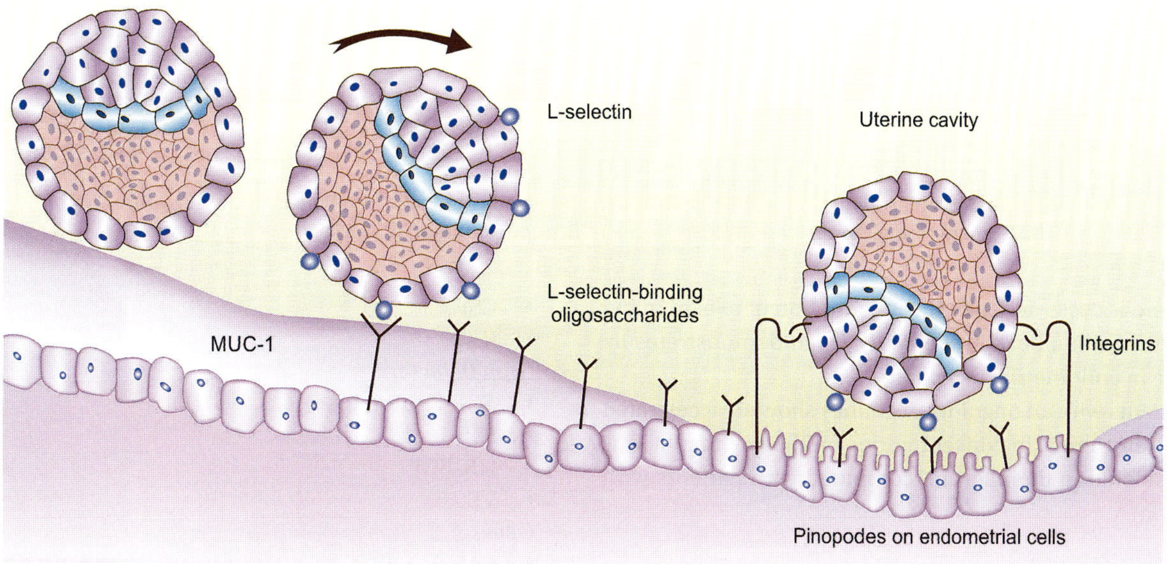

Fig. 5: The embryo at the implantation site via a "tapis roulant" of mucin flow. It is captured by L-selectin-ligand interaction; integrin attachment molecules provide adhesion at the implantation site. (MUC-1: Mucin-1)
Source: Adapted from Chaouat G et al.[20]

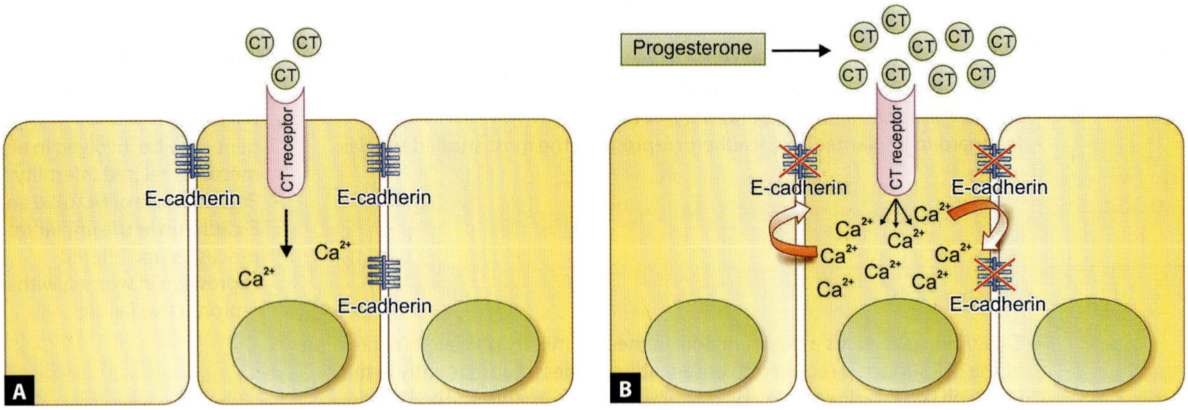

Figs. 6A and B: (A) Epithelial cell adhesiveness by E-cadherin is controlled by intracellular calcium; (B) Rising progesterone levels induce calcitonin (CT) expression and thus increase the concentration of intracellular calcium, which then suppresses E-cadherin expression at cellular contact sites facilitating blastocyst invasion.
Source: Adapted from Kumar S et al.[36]

Flowchart 3: Comparative model: Embryonic implantation versus leukocyte transendothelial migration.

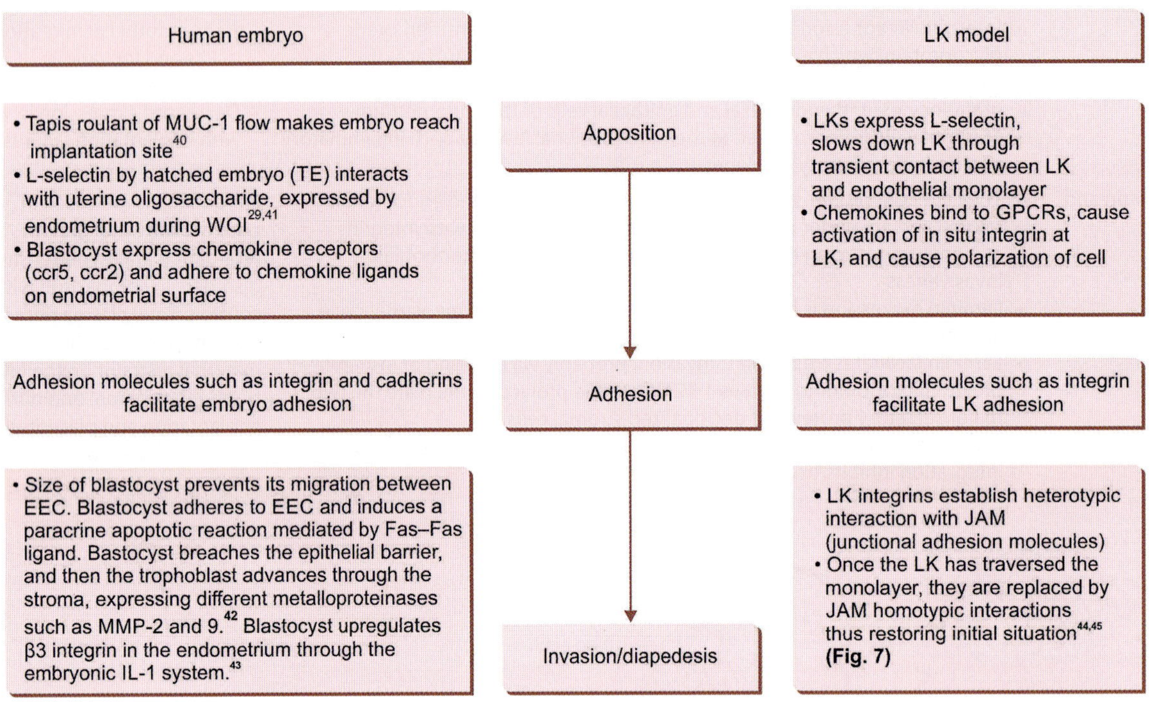

(EEC: endometrial epithelium cell; GPCR: G protein-coupled receptor; IL-1: interleukin-1; LK: leukocyte; MMP: matrix metalloproteinase; MUC-1: Mucin-1; TE: trophectoderm; WOI: window of implantation)

- There is cycle-dependent concentration of relaxin in the serum with a peak at the WOI, which demonstrates its role in endometrial receptivity.[52]

Patients with an ongoing pregnancy show an accelerated rise in serum relaxin concentrations on the day that hCG is first detected in their serum, compared with patients with abortion.[53]

Endometrium:

- *Cytokines*:
  - LIF
  - CSF
  - IL-1
- *Growth factors*:
  - TGF-β (inhibins and activins)
  - IGF-1
  - HB-EGF
  - VEGF
- *Genes*:
  - HOXA
  - BMP
  - WNT4

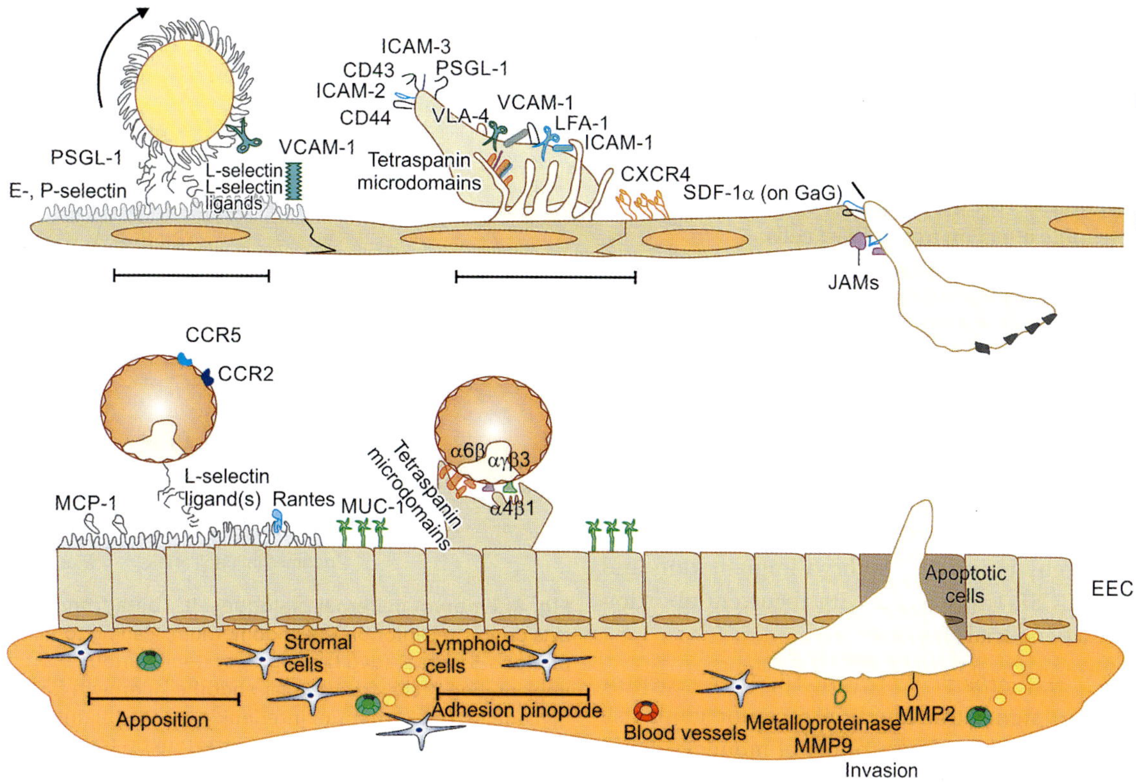

Fig. 7: Comparison of the sequential adhesion steps involved in LK transmigration and embryonic implantation and their molecular players. LK rolling, via the interaction of selectins with their carbohydrate ligands, slows down the LK and facilitates the binding of chemokines to their G protein-coupled receptors (GPCRs). Chemokines induce the high-affinity conformation of LK integrins, which bind to intercellular adhesion molecule-1 (ICAM-1) and vascular cellular adhesion molecule-1 (VCAM-1), included into tetraspanin microdomains and anchored to the cortical actin cytoskeleton on the apical surface of endothelial cells. Upon LK adhesion, endothelial cells develop a three-dimensional docking structure that prevents the detachment of the adhered LK, allowing it to proceed to diapedesis. During diapedesis, LK integrins interact with endothelial junctional adhesion molecules (JAMs) that reseal the junction by homophilic interactions once the LK has traversed the monolayer. In embryonic implantation, chemokines are implicated in embryonic apposition. Blastocyst presents CCR5 and CCR2 receptors on its surface, whereas chemokine ligands adhere to glycosaminoglycans in the endometrial epithelium. In the final invasion phase, the blastocyst breaches the epithelial barrier and advances through the stroma, expressing the metalloproteinases.[39] (EC: endothelial cell; EEC: endometrial epithelium cell; LFA-1: lymphocyte function-associated antigen-1; LK: leukocyte; MCP-1: monocyte chemoattractant protein-1; MMP: matrix metalloproteinase; MUC-1: Mucin-1; PSGL-1: P-selectin glycoprotein ligand-1)
Source: Adapted from Domniguez F et al.[39]

- *Protein signaling pathways*:
  - Glycodelin
  - MMP
  - Janus kinase (JAK)-STAT signaling

Leukemia inhibitory factor: LIF, a member of IL-6 type family, behaves as a pleotropic glycoprotein. LIF seems to be regulated by progesterone and some locally produced factors. LIF acts on cells by interacting with LIF receptor (LIFR), which exists as LIFR and gp130 and is expressed on TE and luminal and glandular epithelium.

Roles in implantation are as follows:

- In humans, LIF acts on cytotrophoblast (CTB), causing them to differentiate into anchoring phenotype, which is achieved by increased synthesis of fibronectin and decreased production of hCG protein, while inducing secretion of oncofetal fibronectin.
- In human endometrium, LIF is expressed in a cycle-dependent manner as well with secretory endometrium showing the maximum expression, more precisely in the WOI. In the endometrium of fertile women, LIF mRNA is expressed on days 18–28 of the menstrual cycle, suggesting a role in uterine receptivity.[54]

In a proven LIF-producing endometrial coculture, embryo quality and development are significantly higher compared with conventional media and a trend was seen in the subsequent pregnancy rates.[55] Being more assessable clinically, was also traced in endometrial cultures of women with unexplained infertility. Recently, recombinant human LIF has been developed for clinical use in assisted reproduction.

Colony-stimulating factor: CSF-1 or macrophage CSF is a hematopoietic growth factor inducing the proliferation and differentiation of cells belonging to mononuclear phagocytic lineage. Increased production of CSF-1 is found at fetomaternal interface during conception and pregnancy. Pollard et al.[56] was the first to describe the role of macrophages in the production of cytokines that regulate the process of implantation.

Roles in implantation are as follows:

- It has a trophic effect on trophoblast cells.
- Responsible for decidual function and placental growth. Progesterone regulates CSF production and CSF enhances macrophage growth and development. Production of CSF-1 in humans takes place in endometrial glands from the mid-proliferative phase to the mid-secretory phase.

There is no direct evidence to correlate the role of CSF in human implantation and pregnancy maintenance. Although low CSF-1 concentration is described in both preconception and conception in women with unexplained recurrent abortions, thereby promoting embryo implantation and substitution of CSF-1 in women with recurrent abortion seem to have a beneficial effect.[57]

Interleukin-1 and others: IL-1α, IL-1β, IL-1 receptor antagonist, and signal transduction receptor comprise the IL-1 family. IL-1, a known product of monocytes and macrophages, fine-tunes cell proliferation and differentiation, and is also present in both endometrium and embryo. Endometrial levels of IL-1α and IL-1β are under progesterone control. Only the type 1 receptor is functional in human endometrium. IL-1 and its receptors are localized on human oocyte and embryo. Embryo is the major source for IL-1β.

Role in implantation is as follows:

- IL-1β produced from embryo acts on IL-1RT-1 (receptor type-1) on the endometrium and upregulates integrin (alpha 5 beta 3) cascade and plays a role in adhesion **(Fig. 8)**.

Growth factors: Endometrium growth factors are presented in **Table 4**.

Genes:

- *HOXA (homeobox genes)*: They are transcription factors and regulators of embryonic morphogenesis and differentiation (Krumlauf, 1994).[66]
  HOXA10 and *HOXA11* are upregulated during WOI, and play a role in implantation. Also responsible for the upregulation of IGF-binding protein-1 (IGFBP-1), pinopodes, and beta3 integrin.[67] There is a reduced expression in hydrosalpinx, endometriosis, and polycystic ovarian syndrome (PCOS) leading to reduced implantation.[68]
- *WNT4 gene*: Once WNT protein binds to its ligands, *WNT* gene is activated and leads to transcription of target genes by either beta-catenin signaling or beta-catenin-independent pathway (noncanonical). WNT/β-catenin signaling is transiently and strictly induced at the prospective site of embryo attachment immediately before implantation.[69] It plays a role in:
  - Cell-cell adhesion in apposition phase
  - Morula to blastocyst transition
    - Embryo spacing via induction of evenly spaced bands in smooth muscle of uterus
    - Decidualization of uterus
- *BMP2 gene: BMP2* is a major player in decidualization, the levels of which increase during WOI.[70]

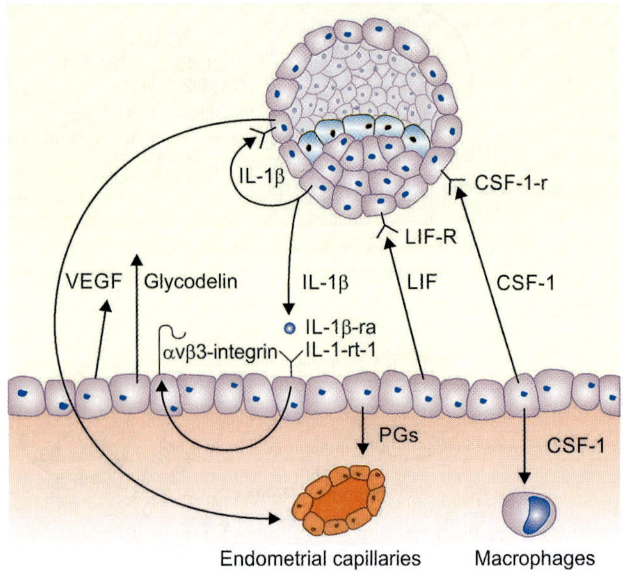

Fig. 8: Embryo–maternal dialogue—IL-1beta from the embryo acts on IL-1 receptor on the endometrium, leading to upregulation of alpha 5 beta 3 (αvβ3) integrin system. Various players in the implantation orchestra: Vascular endothelial growth factor (VEGF), glycodelin, αvβ3-integrin, interleukin-1β (IL-1β), interleukin-1β-receptor-antagonist (IL-1β-ra), interleukin-1-receptor-type-1 (IL-1-rt-1), prostaglandins (PG), leukemia inhibitory factor (LIF), LIF-receptor (LIF-R), and colony-stimulating factor type 1 (CSF-1).
Source: Hoozemans DA et al.[48]

Proteins:

Glycodelin: Glycodelin-A, also known as placental protein 14 (PP-14) or progesterone-associated endometrial protein (PEP), is the most abundantly secreted and consistently upregulated glycoprotein in late secretory endometrium and gestational decidua.[71]

Roles in implantation are as follows:

- Glycodelin has immunosuppressive role, suppresses the activity of natural killer (NK) cells, and protects the embryo from maternal immune rejection,[72] thus opens the WOI for developing blastocyst. Progesterone, hCG, and relaxin seem to be the regulatory pathways for glycodelin production.
- Glycodelin concentrations from cycle day 18 reach maximum in luteal phase and increases if conception occurs. Concentrations in uterine flushing (and not in

TABLE 4: Endometrium growth factors and their roles in implantation.

	Growth factor	*Role in implantation*	*Evidences*
1	HB-EGF	• Maximal expression during late secretory phase, at the sites of active blastocyst displaying ErbB4 • This induction is followed by expression of betacellulin, epiregulin, neuregulin-1, and COX2 at the time of attachment	Das et al.[58]
2	IGF	• Insulin-like growth factor system comprises IGF-1 and IGF-2 • All IGF participate in regulation of cellular growth and differentiation and have metabolic, antiapoptotic, and angiogenic effects, via increase in VEGF • In cycling human endometrium, IGF expression is restricted to stromal cells • IGF-2 dominates in secretory endometrium, expressed by trophoblast, while IGFBP is mainly by decidual cells • IGFBP-1 regulates the invading trophoblast, by modulating MMP-2 and MMP-9 levels • High IGFBP-1 levels in the decidua prevent deeper invasion and can lead to defective placentation • Within the EEM, IGFBP-3 binds IGF, but IGFBP-3 has a low affinity toward IGF, so making it available around EEM, to provide a free supply for embryo	Larsen et al.[59]
3	TGF-beta	• Inhibin and activin belong to TGF-beta subfamily[60] • Inhibin A and activin A levels increase during WOI[61] • Modulates maternal immune tolerance during implantation • TGF-beta signaling is associated with the onset of uterine receptivity and embryo-attachment reaction, whereas it diminishes when trophoblast invasion starts • Serum concentrations in the first trimester of pregnancy can possibly discriminate between a viable pregnancy and an abortion. This is mainly due to rescue of corpus luteal function by inhibin A[62]	Leung et al.[60]
4	VEGF	• VEGF is a major modulator of vascular growth and remodeling and it increases vascular permeability in the endometrium • It increases vascular permeability in the endometrium at implantation site, making it receptive to implantation	Risau[63] and Smith et al.[64,65]

(EEM: extraembryonic matrix; HB-EGF: heparin-binding epidermal growth factor; IGF: insulin-like growth factor; IGFBP: insulin-like growth factor-binding protein; MMP: matrix metalloproteinase; TGF-β: transforming growth factor-beta; VEGF: vascular endothelial growth factor; WOI: window of implantation)

serum), on the contrary, are higher in fertile patients than in patients with recurrent abortion.

Matrix metalloproteinase-2 and -9: Tissue remodeling and angiogenesis are hallmark events during implantation and decidualization. MMP and tissue inhibitors of metalloproteinase (TIMP) are thought to be key mediators for matrix degradation during implantation. There is evidence that a balance between a select set of MMP and TIMP is important for implantation.

Progesterone, growth factors, and cytokines including the EGF and TGF-β family members and LIF have been shown to modulate MMP and TIMP.[73]

Janus kinase-signal transducers and activators of transcription: In human endometrial stromal cells, STAT3 protein production is regulated by progesterone, LIF, and IL-11.[74] Furthermore, a role of STAT3 activity in trophoblast invasiveness has also been proposed.[75]

Blastocyst Regulation of Implantation

Embryo

Interleukin-1: Interleukin-1β is the major form produced by the preimplantation embryo. It acts on IL-1 receptor on the maternal side (epithelial and stromal) and causes endometrial transformation via integrin cascade, which is known to initiate NK cell differentiation.[76]

Interleukin-1 regulates the expression of several molecules in the endometrium, including IL-6, IL-8, LIF, CSF tumor necrosis factor alpha (TNF-α), COX-2, prostaglandin E2 (PGE2), prostaglandin F2-alpha (PGF2-alpha), MMP-1 and -9, and TIMP-1 and -3.

Vascular endothelial growth factor: In the developing embryo, release of IL-1β upregulates VEGF production from embryo **(Fig. 9)**. Both VEGF and its functional receptor are expressed by the trophoblast, most notably by the invasive first-trimester extravillous cytotrophoblast, suggesting that VEGF participates in regulating the proliferation, migration/invasion, and metabolic activity of the trophoblast in an autocrine fashion.[77]

The VEGF-A is the dominant subtype in the endometrium and VEGF-R1 and VEGF-R2 have been described as the main subtypes involved in implantation.

Insulin-like growth factor-2:

- Insulin-like growth factor-2 dominates in secretory endometrium, released by trophoblast, while IGFBP-1 is secreted by decidua.

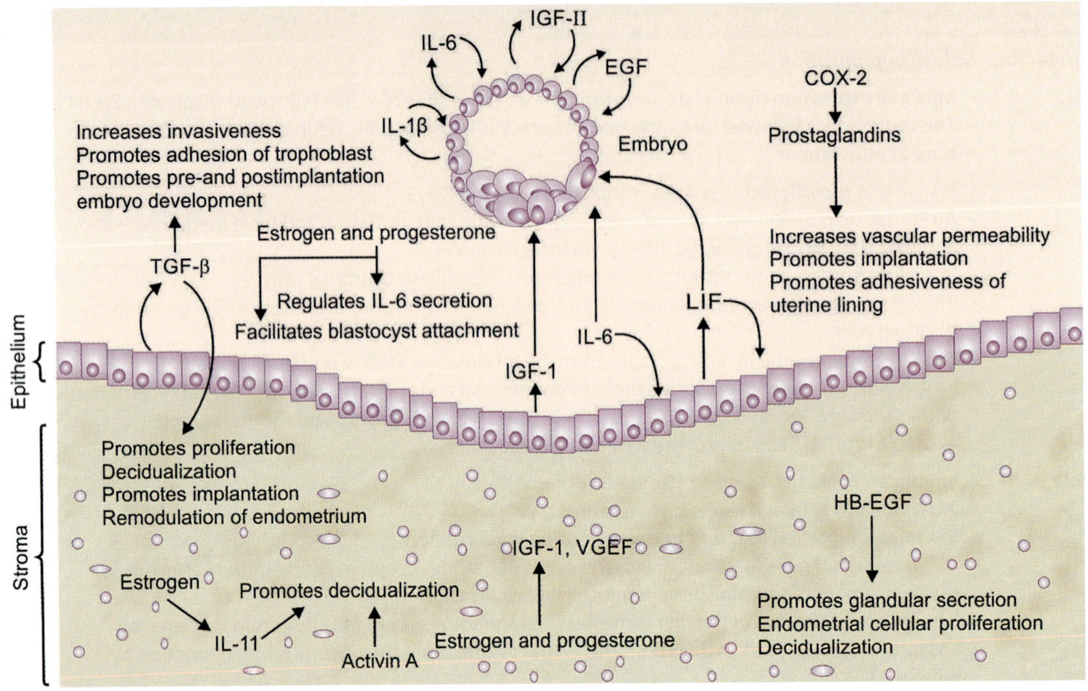

Fig. 9: Various players are ovarian hormones (E2 and P4): PR beta receptors in postovulation facilitate pinopode formation, upregulate MUC-1, L-selectin, LIF-CSF, IL-1, IL-6, PG, VEGF, IGF-II, and CRH. Embryo: Secretes IL-1beta (levels high during WOI), acts on IL-1-rt-1 on endometrium, plays a role in paracrine signaling via upregulation of integrin cascade. IL-1beta upregulates VEGF levels, which causes CTB proliferation, migration/invasion of trophoblast, and angiogenesis. IGF-II is secreted by trophoblast and mediates angiogenic effects via increase in VEGF. IGFBP-1 regulates trophoblast invasion, while IGFBP-3 makes more IGF-II available. Endometrium: IL-1 regulates the expression of several molecules in the endometrium, including IL-6, IL-8, LIF, CSF TNF alpha, COX-2, PGE2, PGF2 alpha, MMP-1 and -9, and TIMP-1 and-3. LIF makes CTB anchoring phenotype, and CSF helps in implantation. TGF-beta acts on both embryo and endometrium and helps in implantation and decidualization. Others: PG promotes vascular permeability and adhesiveness of uterus at site of implantation, HOXA, WNT4, and BMP-2 all are markers of receptivity. (CRH: corticotropin-releasing hormone; CTB: cytotrophoblast; E2: estradiol; IGF-II: insulin-like growth factor-II; IGFBP-1: insulin-like growth factor binding protein-1; IL: interleukin; IL-1-rt-1: interleukin-1-receptor-type-1; LIF-CSF: leukemia inhibitory factor-colony-stimulating factor; MUC-1: Mucin-1; P4: progesterone; PG: prostaglandin; TGF-beta: transforming growth factor-beta; TNF: tumor necrosis factor, VEGF: vascular endothelial growth factor; WOI: window of implantation)
Source: Adapted from Hoozemans DA et al.[48]

- All IGFs participate in the regulation of cellular growth and differentiation and have metabolic, antiapoptotic, and angiogenic effects, via increase in VEGF.
- Within the extraembryonic matrix (EEM), IGFBP-3 binds IGF, but IGFBP-3 has a low affinity toward IGF, so making it available around EEM to provide a free supply for embryo.

Chorionic gonadotropin: See in embryo maternal signaling section.

Peripheral: Cyclooxygenase-2 signaling: Progesterone influences the PG level in the human menstrual cycle. PGE2 and PGF2-alpha peak in midluteal phase, where WOI is situated, helps in implantation by increasing vascular permeability and bringing decidualization of the endometrium. In early pregnancy, two processes concerning PG take place. They are thought to be initiated by embryo, and the extent of endometrial reaction is due to endocrine effect (either progesterone or hCG by embryo).

1. The decidual PG levels drop remarkably low as compared to nonpregnant levels.
2. Increased local production of PG at the implantation site

The implanting embryo seems to be capable of triggering this mechanism as well, possibly by its own PG production.

Endocrine signals

Corticotropin-releasing hormone: Corticotropin-releasing hormone has been localized in endometrial glands and decidual stroma as well as trophoblast. Progesterone upregulates CRH production, which causes decidualization.[78] Also upregulates IL-1, IL-6, and PGE2.[79-81]

Corticotropin-releasing hormone participates in local inflammatory phenomena, which takes place at the implantation site, rendering the endometrial surface adhesive for the implanting blastocyst.[79] Indeed, CRH induces the synthesis of proapoptotic Fas ligand (FasL) on human invasive extravillous trophoblast and maternal decidual cells. Therefore, it potentiates the ability of these cells to induce apoptosis of surrounding activated maternal T cells bearing the Fas receptor (FasR) on their surface and facilitating trophoblast invasion.[82]

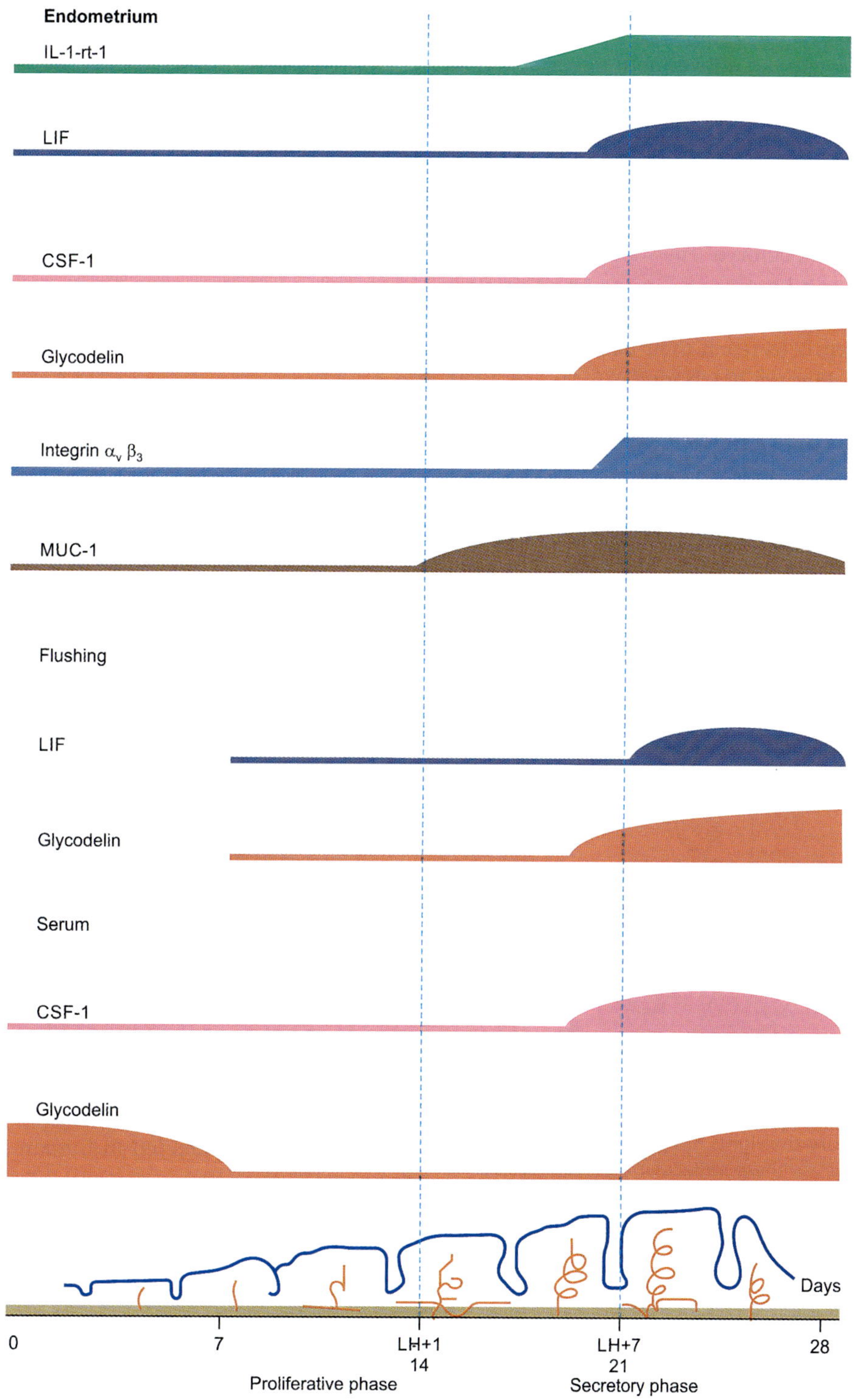

Fig. 10: Profiles across the menstrual cycle of factors of importance to the interaction between human blastocyst and endometrium. (CSF-1: colony-stimulating factor-1; IL: interleukin; IL-1-rt-1: interleukin-1-receptor-type-1; LH: luteinizing hormone; LIF: leukemia inhibitory factor; MUC-1: Mucin-1)

Leptin: Leptin is a product of the *OB* gene. Its receptors are found in the endometrium with maximal expression in the late luteal phase.[29] Additionally, leptin has also been shown to increase integrin β3 expression, which is essential for endometrial receptivity and implantation.[83]

Summary of Players in Implantation Orchestra

Summary of players in implantation orchestra has been shown in **Figures 9 and 10**.

EMBRYO–MATERNAL CROSS-DIALOGUE

As we have seen through the above-mentioned facts that both partners, the mother and the embryo, play equal roles in the embryo–maternal dialogue. For successful achievement of pregnancy, both the processes of implantation and trophoblast invasion play a crucial rule.

The EEM and zona pellucida represents the interface between the mother and embryo. The start of full embryo–maternal signaling can be expected to occur at around day 6 following the luteinizing hormone (LH) peak and have to pass this matrix to reach their destination, since the human embryo does not hatch till day 6. Hence, EEM of preimplantation embryos acts as a mailbox, through which signals traverse from embryo to mother or vice versa **(Fig. 11)**.

Herrler et al.[84] noticed through their animal experiments, investigating rabbit (rab) and horse embryos, which, like human embryos, remain surrounded by their EEM until shortly before adhesion to the endometrium.

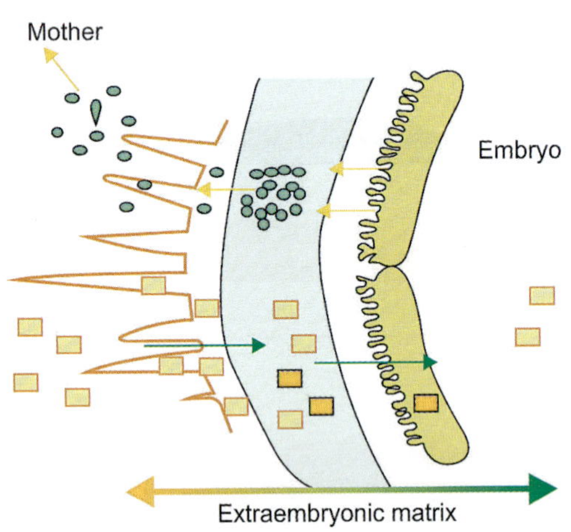

Fig. 11: Extraembryonic matrices surround most embryos until shortly before implantation. Maternal (from the left) as well as embryonic signals (from the right) have to pass them to reach their destination. However, these molecular messages are stored and modulated as generally in other extracellular matrices. Such extraembryonic matrices may serve as a mailbox in embryo maternal signaling before implantation.[82]

Only a few embryonic signals, which are clearly directed toward the mother during the preimplantation period are known; the most well-known is hCG.

Human Chorionic Gonadotropin: Classical Signal (Flowchart 4)

Like other gonadotropins, its secretion is regulated by gonadotropin-releasing hormone (GnRH), synthesized by the early blastocyst itself.[85] hCG mRNA is detectable as early as in the two-cell stage and detectable concentrations of hCG are already produced before implantation.[86,87] The critical days of the establishment of pregnancy are days 6–10 after the LH peak, which relates to the time of increasing hCG plasma concentrations.[88]

Preimplantation embryos of primates release CG under the control of GnRH from blastocyst, as the studies by Seshagiri et al.[85] have shown.

Sherwin et al.[89] concentrate on CG, which has long been thought to be secreted by the early blast, playing a major role in rescue of corpus luteum, moved to more attention in the role of CG in embryo implantation.

Embryonic action via hCG on the endometrium is through two effects:

1. An indirect, endocrine effect via rescue of the corpus luteum and subsequent progesterone release
2. A direct, paracrine effect on the *endometrium* **(Fig. 12)**. The luteotrophic activity of hCG is well documented. Progesterone controls endometrial function by increasing LIF secretion, mediated via IL-4, which originates from T cells.[90,91]

Chorionic Gonadotropin Receptor and Signal Transduction Pathways

Multiple mRNA transcripts for CG/LH receptor (CG/LH-R) have been detected in human gonadal tissues. In the human ovary, 8.0-, 7.0-, and 4.5-kb transcripts were seen with the 4.5-kb being predominant.[92] Extragonadal CG/LH-R expression has been reported in reproductive

Flowchart 4: Signaling pathways of chorionic gonadotropin.

Signaling pathways

Ovarian/conventional
CG acts onto GPCR (G protein-coupled receptor) increase in cAMP-adenylyl cyclase activation increase in the intracellular calcium through inositol triphosphate (IP3)/phospholipase A2 (PLA A2) pathway. Possible activation of protein kinase C through diacylglycerol (DAG) has also been suggested

↔

Extragonadal tissues
CG increases phosphorylation-dependent pathways, e.g., extracellular signal-regulated kinases (ERK1 and ERK2) and cyclooxygenase 2-independent PK-A pathways

(cAMP: cyclic adenosine monophosphate; CG: chorionic gonadotropin; PK-A: protein kinase)

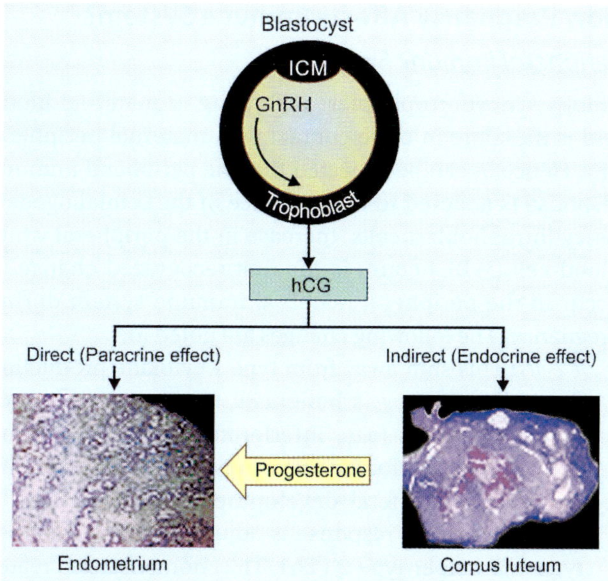

Fig. 12: The effects of hCG on the endometrium.
(GnRH: gonadotropin-releasing hormone; hCG: human chorionic gonadotropin; ICM: inner cell mass)
Source: Adapted from Herrler A et al.[84]

(uterus, placenta, and decidua) and several nonreproductive organs.

The existence of these LH/CG receptors within the endometrium is still debatable. However, these receptors are functional based on in vivo experiments in baboons[93] and in vitro studies with human endometrial cell lines.[94] CG/LH-R is a member of the subfamily of glycoprotein hormone receptors within the superfamily of G protein-coupled/seven transmembrane domain receptors (GPCR).

So, CG has a unique signal transduction pathway in the endometrium. Extracellular signal-regulated kinase 1/2 (ERK1/2) may be an important signal regulating these CG-mediated events in the endometrium.[95] The human endometrium exhibits high basal adenylyl cyclase (AC) activity and it possesses the capacity for cyclic adenosine monophosphate (cAMP) production in response to PGE2, PGF2, forskolin, and isoproterenol. In addition, endometrial AC has been shown to be upregulated by ovarian steroids.[96] Although evidence for a direct action of CG on uterine tissues is strong, characterization of the various isoforms of the CG/LH-R and their role in activating alternate signal transduction pathways remain to be elucidated.

Human CG directly causes endometrial differentiation, decidualization, and embryo invasion by **(Fig. 13)**:

- Modulating the endometrial activity through several proteins such as LIF, VEGF, IGFBP-1, monocyte CSF (MCSF), and MMP-9.[97] These paracrine factors are known to be associated with decidualization, angiogenesis, immunomodulation, and matrix remodeling, thereby promoting embryonic implantation.

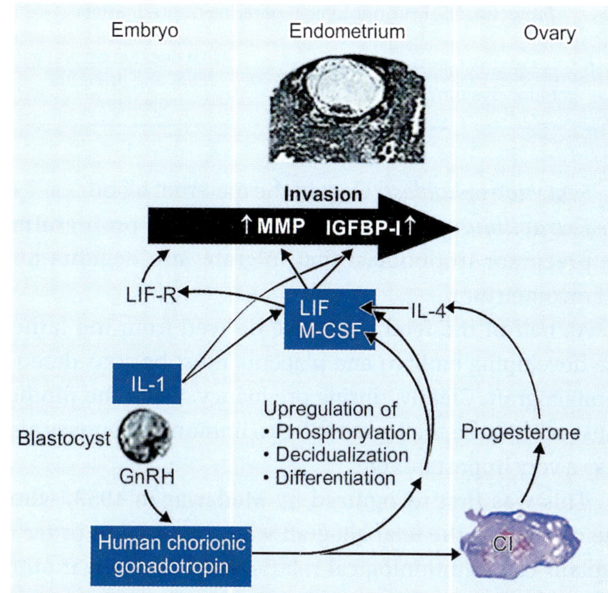

Fig. 13: Effects of human chorionic gonadotropin shown synoptically in three compartments (embryo, endometrium, and ovary) finally influencing endometrial differentiation, decidualization, phosphorylation, and embryonic invasion.
(GnRH: gonadotropin-releasing hormone; IGFBP-1: insulin-like growth factor-binding protein-1; IL: interleukin; LIF-R: leukemia inhibitory factor-receptor; M-CSF: macrophage colony-stimulating factor; MMP: matrix metalloproteinase)
Source: Adapted from Herrler A et al.[84]

- hCG interaction in synergy with IL-1β to induce IGFBP is well known. hCG inhibits apoptosis in steroid-treated stromal cells and enhances differentiation by IGFBP-1 expression.
- Srisuparp noticed through his studies on baboons, the observation of decidual plaque reaction and increase of glandular secretion following CG. The primary effect of CG on stromal fibroblast is induction of alpha-smooth muscle actin,[95,98] as a consequence of integrin upregulation by CG binding to extracellular matrix (ECM) proteins.[98] This leads to transformation of glandular epithelium and appearance of pinopodes.
- It has been shown that in vitro, hCG can stimulate monocytes to promote embryo invasion.[99]

IMMUNE ACCEPTANCE OF PREGNANCY

Fetal–Maternal Contact

Placenta plays a crucial role in establishing intimate contact of fetus with maternal uterine tissue. Since the trophoblast cells are the most important fetal cells coming in contact with maternal cells, and three different trophoblast populations that are exposed to different maternal elements can be distinguished.

1. *Villous cytotrophoblast*: Actively dividing trophoblast cells in the villi

Flowchart 5: Immunological paradox of pregnancy.

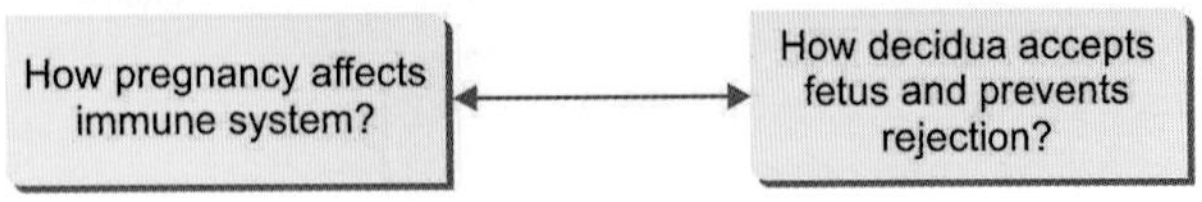
How pregnancy affects immune system?
How decidua accepts fetus and prevents rejection?

2. *Syncytiotrophoblast:* Float in the maternal blood
3. *Extravillous cytotrophoblast*: These are proliferating precursor trophoblast that migrate into decidua and myometrium.

As half of the fetal genes are derived from the father, the developing embryo and placenta must be considered a semiallograft. Clearly, during pregnancy, when the mother must accept a semiallogeneic fetus, immune responses also play a very important role.

This was first recognized by Medawar in 1953, when the concept of the fetal allograft was presented in order to explain the immunological relationship between mother and fetus.[100] He suggested that the fetus escapes rejection because the immunological interaction between the mother and fetus is suppressed. Medawar proposed that this was due to a lack of fetal antigen expression, resulting from an anatomical separation between the mother and the fetus, or from a functional suppression of maternal lymphocytes.

Immune Paradox of Pregnancy

To understand the concept of immunological paradox of pregnancy, we need to focus on two processes as mentioned in **Flowchart 5**.

Effect of Pregnancy on Immune System

Peripheral Immune System

- T cells
- Peripheral NK cells
- Monocytes, granulocytes, and dendritic cells (DCs)

Immune System in Decidua

- Uterine NK (uNK) cells
- Decidual T cells
- Macrophages

Mechanism to Escape Rejection by Fetus

- Major histocompatibility complex (MHC) expression by trophoblast
- *Uterine modulators*:
    - Haptoglobin
    - Uteroglobin
- *Downregulation of T-cell activity*:
    - Induction of T-cell anergy
    - Fas-Fas ligand

How Pregnancy Affects Immune System?

Peripheral Immune System

Villous syncytiotrophoblast is floating in maternal blood and is therefore in close contact with maternal peripheral LKs. Hence, it can be expected that the peripheral immune response is adapted to the presence of the semiallogeneic syncytiotrophoblast cells. Increase in the peripheral white blood cell (WBC) count is the first recognized change to occur in the peripheral maternal immune system during pregnancy. The following changes are noted in:

- *T cells:* This shift away from type 1 cytokine production during pregnancy is beneficial for pregnancy, since type 1 cytokines [e.g., interferon gamma (IFNγ) and TNF-α) are harmful for pregnancy because they inhibit embryonic and fetal development **(Flowchart 6)**.[101] Uterine immune response is adjusted so that T-helper type 1/T-helper type 2 (Th1/Th2) homeostasis creates an optimal environment fostering implantation **(Flowchart 7)**.
- *Peripheral natural killer cells*: The number of peripheral NK cells is decreased in pregnant women as compared with nonpregnant women. These changes in NK cell number and activity during pregnancy are also consistent with a shift from a cellular to a humoral immune response during pregnancy.
- *Monocytes and granulocytes and dendritic cells*: Sacks et al. in 1998 noticed the activation of innate immune response in pregnancy. The main factors for activation are the pregnancy hormones as well as the soluble mediators of placenta, which are released into maternal circulation. DCs may be involved in the regulation of type 1/type 2 cytokine balance.[102]

Immune System in the Decidua

The decidua is the maternal part of the placenta in which there is a close contact between maternal and fetal cells. Consequently, the decidual cells may play an important role in acceptance of the fetus and the control of trophoblast invasion. Hence, the decidua contains a diverse population of cells, including decidualized stroma cells, lymphocytes, uNK cells, monocytes, and epithelial cells. Bulmer et al. found that the proportion of LKs in the decidua is cycle dependent, from <10% in early proliferative phase to 20% in the late secretory, to >40% in early pregnancy. This is mainly due to increase in uNK cells, which comprise 60% of LKs.[103]

Uterine natural killer cells: The uNK cells have an NK cell-like function, but they are specific for the uterus. The presence of uNK cells in the decidua may be explained by two mechanisms.

1. The *first mechanism* is that peripheral blood uNK cells are selectively homing to the uterine mucosa, because they

Flowchart 6: Role of T cells in immune regulation.

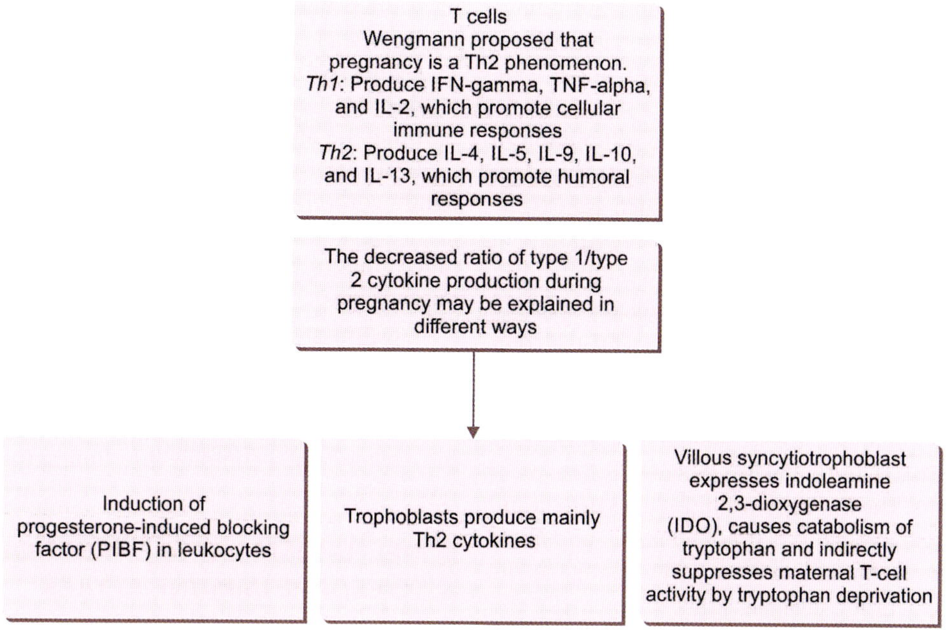

(IFN: interferon; IL: interleukin; Th2: T-helper type 2; Th1: T-helper type 1; TNF: tumor necrosis factor)

Flowchart 7: Immunomodulation during pregnancy.

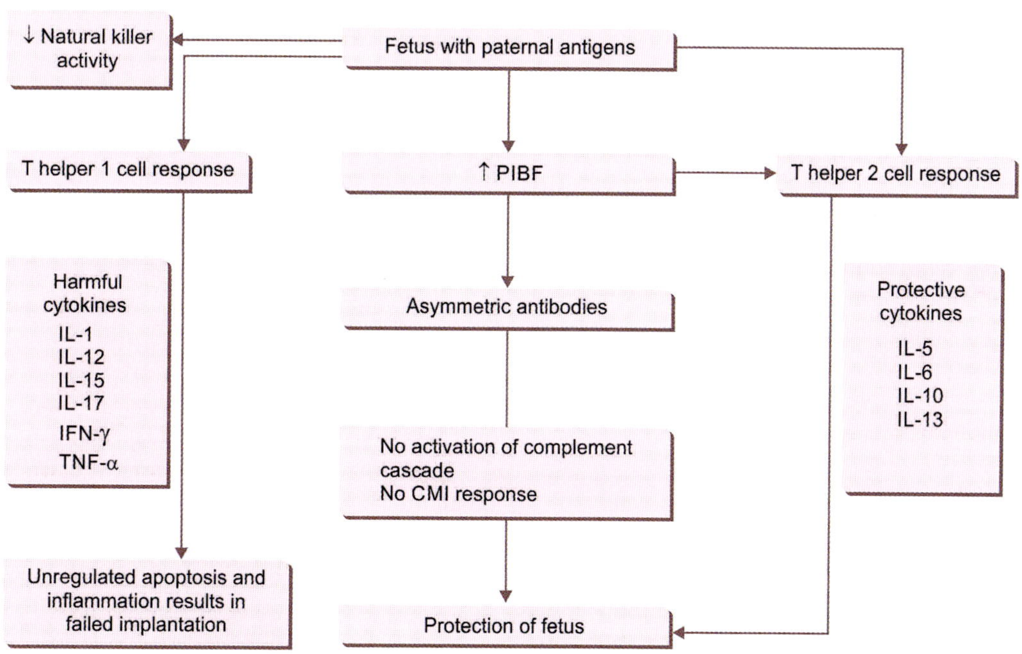

(CMI: cell-mediated immunity; IFN-γ: interferon-γ; IL: interleukin; PIBF: progesterone-induced blocking factor; TNF-α: tumor necrosis factor-α)

can interact with adhesion molecules on the decidual blood vessels.

2. *Second mechanism* is that uNK cells are actively dividing. Their proliferation can be stimulated either by cytokines produced by other decidual cells or by (steroid) hormones.

Uterine NK cells are different to mature circulating NK cells, yet phenotypically resemble the smaller unique NK cell subset, which is CD56/CD16/CD3 and has low direct cytotoxicity. Since they do not share all the membrane expression markers, it is not clear whether these cell types have same function.

Natural killer cells have been shown to be essential for implantation, as NK cell-deficient mice repeatedly have pregnancy failures.[104] Their uNK cell-derived cytokines, e.g., granulocyte-CSF (G-CSF), M-CSF, GC-MSF, and LIF are crucial for normal implantation.[105]

Proliferation of uNK cells is through the production of IL-15 by placental macrophages, expression of IL-15 receptor on $CD56^+$ uNK cells, and embryonic signals such as hCG.[106]

These $CD56^+$ NK cells and $CD8^+$ T cells accumulate at the decidua parietalis and trophoblast invasion front[107] and facilitate deep invasion of cytotrophoblasts into the myometrial segments thereby promoting spiral artery remodeling and angiogenesis.

Although the uNK cells are present in the decidua in large amounts, they do not attack the semiallogeneic nonvillous cytotrophoblast. This is due to the fact that uNK cells express inhibitory receptors. These receptors bind to the MHC-Ia and b [human leukocyte antigen-C (HLA-C), HLA-E, and HLA-G)] on trophoblast, by binding to these MHC-I antigens, the inhibitory receptors inhibit the lytic activity of the uNK cells. The types of inhibitory receptors on uNK cells are namely immunoglobulin (Ig)-like killer cell inhibitory receptor (KIR) (e.g., KIR2D, KIR2DL4) and lectin-like KIRs (CD94/NKG2A). But interaction with killer activating receptor (KAR) stimulates the production of trophic cytokines and angiogenic factors.[20,84]

Also consistent with a role for uNK cells in implantation and placentation were the findings that high preconceptional NK activity was associated with significantly higher rates of miscarriage[108] and infertility,[109] since these cells through Th1 cytokines can damage trophoblast and can cause fetal death.

Decidual T lymphocytes: Similar to the peripheral blood, the most accepted theory is the dominance of Th2 response over Th1. Th2 cells, placental (mostly), and decidual cells secrete Th2 cytokines (IL-5, IL-6, IL-10, and IL-13), which controls the Th1 responses, promote allograft tolerance, and may improve fetal survival.[110]

Macrophages (Flowchart 8)

In humans, macrophages are spread through the pregnant uterus, including the decidua[111] and are also associated with trophoblast cells of the placenta and extraplacental membranes.[103] In the decidua, macrophages constitute about 20–30% of all LKs. Factors responsible for increased invasion of macrophages into decidua are:

- *Pregnancy hormones*: Estrogen[112]
- *Cytotrophoblast*: Can attract macrophages into the decidua by producing monocytes inflammatory protein-1 alpha[113]

However, the number of uterine macrophages must be tightly controlled, since in preimplantation endometrium of patients with recurrent miscarriage significantly more macrophages were seen than in patients without these miscarriages.[114]

The present observations suggest that at the maternal and fetal interface, a balanced production of cytokines by various immune cells (T lymphocytes, uNK cells, and macrophages) is needed for a successful pregnancy, which in turn suggests the existence of a complex fine-tuning system for cytokine production.[115]

MECHANISMS AT THE TROPHOBLAST TO ESCAPE IMMUNE ATTACK

Human embryos are able to modulate the LK subtype composition and in consequence the corresponding cytokine pattern within the invaded decidual tissue. This results in modulation of maternal immunotolerance, allowing trophoblast invasion, while at the invasion front activated T cells control the depth of implantation **(Flowchart 9)**.

Major Histocompatibility Complex Expression by Trophoblast[116]

It is clear from the previous sections that immune cells are in close contact with the trophoblast cells but do not attack it, despite being activated. The highly polymorphic MHC is responsible for the distinction of the immune system between self and nonself. The MHC can be divided into three classes:

1. Class Ia (HLA-A, HLA-B, and HLA-C)
2. Class II (HLA-DP, HLA-DQ, and HLA-DR)
3. Class Ib (HLA-E, HLA-F, and HLA-G)

Major histocompatibility complex class Ia is expressed on all nucleated cells—present antigen to cytotoxic T cells,

Flowchart 8: Role of macrophages.

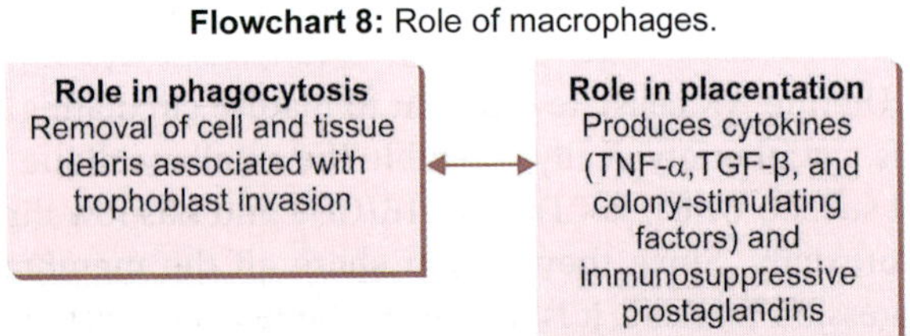

(TNF-α: tumor necrosis factor-α; TGF-β: transforming growth factor-β)

Flowchart 9: Mechanism to evade maternal immune response.

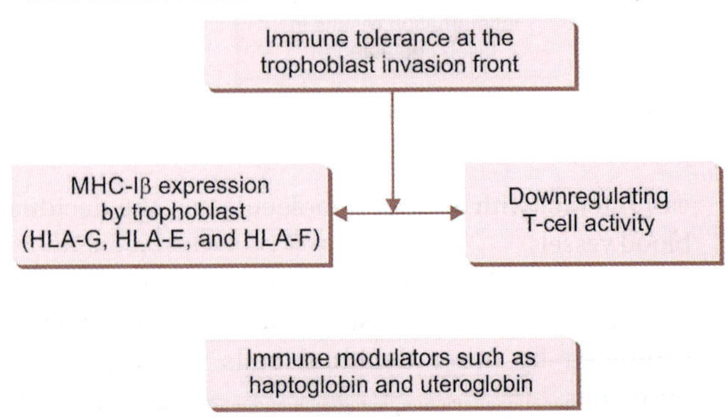

(HLA: human leukocyte antigen; MHC: major histocompatibility complex)

and play a role in the inhibition and activation of NK cells via inhibitory NK-cell receptors (KIR) and activating NK-cell receptors (KAR). Foreign cells, expressing nonself MHC-Ia, can be directly recognized by T-cell lymphocytes and killed.

Major histocompatibility complex class II expressed by B lymphocytes, antigen-presenting cell (APC), and present antigen to T-helper cells. MHC class Ib have a role in immunoacceptance of fetus.

Major histocompatibility complex-Ia is not expressed in trophoblasts. However, some authors have demonstrated the expression of HLA-C, which belongs to the MHC-Ia molecules, by nonvillous cytotrophoblast.

The trophoblast cells express a unique pattern of MHC nonclassic class I molecules, namely HA-Ib (HLA-G and HLA-E). Since they lack expression of most MHC-Ia molecules; they cannot be recognized as foreign by maternal T cells, though this lack of MHC-Ia may place the nonvillous trophoblast at risk of lysis by uNK cells, which dominate in the decidua. Therefore, nonvillous cytotrophoblast cells express MHC-Ib molecules such as HLA-G and HLA-E, both of which may be important at the maternal fetal interface by inhibiting lysis of nonvillous cytotrophoblast by uNK cells, via direct binding with inhibitory receptors on the uNK cells. Maternal T cells recognize placental MHC class I and secrete cytokines mostly CSF, IL-3, and MCSF, which act as growth factors on trophoblast.[106]

Haptoglobin and Uteroglobin as Immune Modulators

Haptoglobin

Haptoglobin is widely known as an "acute phase" protein, strongly binding to hemoglobin. The embryo does not express haptoglobin mRNA. In contrast, embryos accumulate considerable amounts of maternal haptoglobin within the embryonic coats and blastocyst fluid. Its secretion increases during the midluteal phase and peaks at the implantation window.[117]

Since it is concentrated within the embryonic coats, it is known to reduce LK activity by competitive binding to CD11b/CD18[118,119] and serve as early protection against maternal immune cells. Haptoglobin continuously released during trophoblast invasion may further induce immunological tolerance. This is in agreement with the recent findings of Bottini et al.,[120] who have shown that women carrying the haptoglobin alpha 1, alpha 1 isoform have slightly higher natural fertility than women with alpha 2 isoforms. In concordance with this, haptoglobin alpha1 has a significantly higher antiadhesion activity.

Uteroglobin

Another maternal protein taken up and accumulated within the blastocyst fluid is uteroglobin. Its secretion increases during the midluteal phase and peaks at the "implantation window."[117]

Embryo takes up the maternal uteroglobin and releases it following hatching, directed toward the endometrium and acts on maternal immune cells. It also reduces NK cell adhesion/invasion to ECMs.[121]

Another blastocyst fluid component, PGE, has been shown to decrease cytotoxic NK cell activity.[122]

Downregulation of T-cell Activity

As it has been shown in the above-mentioned text that immune competent cells play an important part in the embryo–maternal dialogue. Embryonic signals like hCG, through induction of MMP and IGFBP-1 via LIF, trigger monocyte capability to promote embryonic invasion.

Also, NK cells, the predominant intrauterine LK subpopulation, have been shown to be essential for regular implantation, as NK cell-deficient mice repeatedly have pregnancy failures. These NK cells as well as T cells accumulate at the trophoblast invasion front.[107] Therefore, it can be suggested that the invading trophoblast cells modulate the LK pattern in the invaded tissue as a result of the embryo–maternal dialogue. The physiological lack of NK cells in the endosalpinx and consequently the lack of their cytokines may be a significant reason for the pathological trophoblast over invasion of the tubal wall in tubal pregnancy. At the site of implantation front, specific pattern of LK subtypes within different areas of decidual tissue gets expressed, which regulate cytotoxic T-cell activity.

There are different pathways to downregulate T-cell activity, which are as follows:

- *Induction of anergy*: NK cells activate T cells and monocytes as well as induce trophoblast apoptosis via IFNγ at the invasion front. Afterward, macrophages present peptides from phagocytosed apoptotic trophoblast cells to Th1 cells.[123,124] This induces anergy of the T cells, as the costimulation signal CD86 is missing.[125,126]
- *Fas ligand system-induced apoptosis*: Another mechanism by which the trophoblast may escape attack by maternal immune cells is via the expression of apoptosis-inducing ligands. Induction of apoptosis by FasL in invading lymphocytes acts as a mechanism of immune privilege and is important in graft rejection. Increased FasR expression leads to increased susceptibility of the T cells for induction of apoptosis, called "activation-induced cell death (AICD)." Apoptosis may be induced either by FasL expressing LKs or by FasL-positive invading trophoblast cells **(Figs. 14 and 15)**.[81]
- Consequently, the precise balance between cytotoxic T-cell activity, controlling the amount of trophoblast invasion, and AICD or anergy induction of T cells, supporting trophoblast invasion via their cytokines, is necessary for an implantation process which is beneficial

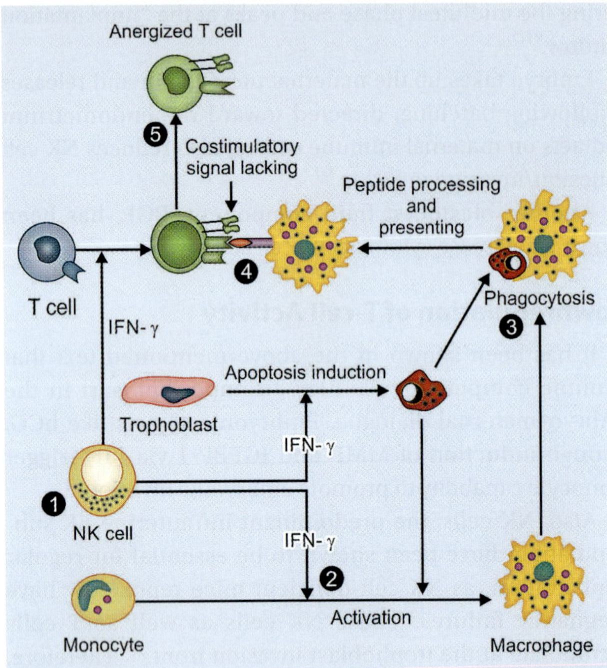

Fig. 14: Induction of T-cell anergy. (1) NK cells recognize trophoblast cells as "nonself" and induce apoptosis; (2) via IFN-γ secretion, NK cells activate macrophages and T cells; (3) phagocytosis of apoptotic bodies by macrophages leads to peptide presentation without (4) costimulatory signal; and (5) if this signal is missing, T cells which recognize the presented peptide are anergized. (NK: natural killer; IFN-γ: interferon-γ)

Source: Adapted from Herrler A et al.[84]

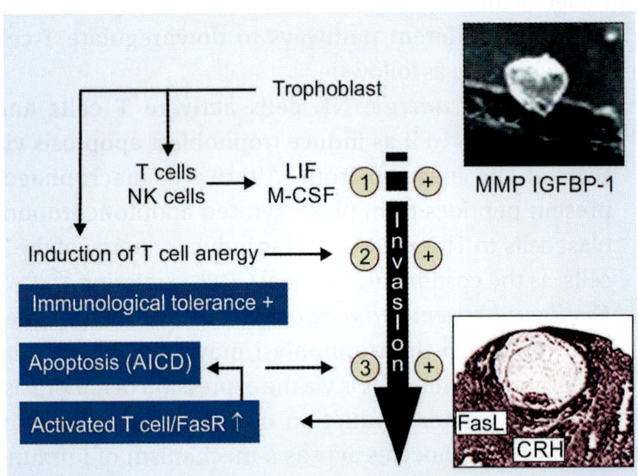

Fig. 15: Synopsis of immune tolerance at the trophoblast invasion front.

(AICD: activation-induced cell death; CRH: corticotropin-releasing hormone; FasL: Fas ligand; FasR: Fas receptor; IGFBP-1: insulin-like growth factor-binding protein-1; LIF: leukemia inhibitory factor; M-CSF: macrophage colony-stimulating factor; MMP: matrix metalloproteinase; NK: natural killer)

for the embryo and not detrimental to the mother. These data provide evidence for a tight interaction between embryo and maternal cells to establish a maternal immunological status that allows adequate trophoblast invasion.

However, addressing the establishment of pregnancy merely as a Th2 phenomenon is an oversimplification, because NK cells and inflammatory cytokines also seem to be important in this complex regulation.

CONCLUSION

Embryonic implantation thus involves the following:

- Anchoring of the conceptus in the maternal uterine wall
- Embryo maternal cross talk involving various growth factors, cytokines, and hormones
- Trophoblast migration and differentiation
- Establishment of vascular supply
- LK influx and activation
- Promotion of tolerance of fetal alloantigens encoded by paternal gene

KEY POINTS

- Blastocyst implantation requires a competent embryo and its ability to cross talk with a receptive endometrium, and the dialogue must talk about immunity and angiogenesis.
- The uterus is tailored to tolerate the fetal allograft and to allow controlled invasiveness of trophoblast only during the WOI, ensuring the success of the intricate cascade of implantation. It still remains an enigmatic process with many unknown factors and interactions.
- The embryonic metabolome is a source of multiple factors that may influence implantation.
- The data also suggest that measurement of blastocyst-derived factors, including micro-RNA, may be useful to identify blastocyst destined to implant and may also serve as useful targets to regulate their implantation.
- A better understanding of the process will improve not only the pregnancy rate of assisted reproductive technologies, but also will assist the understanding of several other pathophysiological processes such as tumor development, angiogenesis, and tumor metastasis. Future research should focus on further evaluation of this process.

REFERENCES

1. Nardo LG, Li TC, Edwards RG. Introduction: human embryo implantation failure and recurrent miscarriage: basic science and clinical practice. Reprod Biomed Online. 2006;13(1):11-2.
2. Dey SK, Lim H, Das SK, Reese J, Paria BC, Daikoku T, et al. Molecular cues to implantation. Endocr Rev. 2004;25(3):341-73.
3. Bettegowda A, Smith GW. Mechanisms of maternal mRNA regulation: implications for mammalian early embryonic development. Front Biosci. 2007;12:3713-26.
4. Edwards RG. Human uterine endocrinology and the implantation window. Ann N Y Acad Sci. 1988;541:445-54.

5. Hamatani T, Daikoku T, Wang H, Matsumoto H, Carter MG, Ko MSH, et al. Global gene expression analysis identifies molecular pathways distinguishing blastocyst dormancy and activation. Proc Natl Acad Sci U S A. 2004;101(28):10326-31.
6. Johnson MH, McConnell JM. Lineage allocation and cell polarity during mouse embryogenesis. Semin Cell Dev Biol. 2004;15(5):583-97.
7. Kirchhof N, Carnwath JW, Lemme E, Anastassiadis K, Schöler H, Niemann H. Expression pattern of Oct-4 in preimplantation embryos of different species. Biol Reprod. 2000;63(6):1698-705.
8. Avilion AA, Nicolis SK, Pevny LH, Perez L, Vivian N, Lovell-Badge R. Multipotent cell lineages in early mouse development depend on SOX2 function. Genes Dev. 2003;17(1):126-40.
9. Mitsui K, Tokuzawa Y, Itoh H, Segawa K, Murakami M, Takahashi K, et al. The homeoprotein Nanog is required for maintenance of pluripotency in mouse epiblast and ES cells. Cell. 2003;113(5):631-42.
10. Niwa H, Toyooka Y, Shimosato D, Strumpf D, Takahashi K, Yagi R, et al. Interaction between Oct3/4 and Cdx2 determines trophectoderm differentiation. Cell. 2005;123(5):917-29.
11. Simmons DG, Cross JC. Determinants of trophoblast lineage and cell subtype specification in the mouse placenta. Dev Biol. 2005;284(1):12-24.
12. Takaoka K, Yamamoto M, Shiratori H, Meno C, Rossant J, Saijoh Y, et al. The mouse embryo autonomously acquires anterior-posterior polarity at implantation. Dev Cell. 2006;10(4):451-9.
13. Guzeloglu-Kayisli O, Basar M, Arici A. Basic aspects of implantation. Reprod Biomed Online. 2007;15(6):728-39.
14. Kodaman PH, Taylor HS. Hormonal regulation of implantation. Obstet Gynecol Clin North Am. 2004;31(4):745-66.
15. Sathananthan H, Menezes J, Gunasheela S. Mechanics of human blastocyst hatching in vitro. Reprod Biomed Online. 2003;7(2):228-34.
16. Harlow GM, Quinn P. Development of preimplantation mouse embryos in vivo and in vitro. Aust J Biol Sci. 1982; 35(2):187-93.
17. Fong CY, Bongso A, Sathananthan H, Ho J, Ng SC. Ultrastructural observations of enzymatically treated human blastocysts: zona-free blastocyst transfer and rescue of blastocysts with hatching difficulties. Hum Reprod. 2001;16(3):540-6.
18. Lee KY, DeMayo FJ. Animal models of implantation. Reproduction. 2004;128(6):679-95.
19. Enders AC, Schlafke S. Cytological aspects of trophoblast-uterine interaction in early implantation. Am J Anat. 1969;125(1):1-29.
20. Chaouat G, Zourbas S, Ostoijc S, Lapprée-Delage G, Dubanchet S, Ledée N, et al. New insights into maternal-fetal interactions at implantation. Reprod Biomed Online. 2001;2(3):198-203.
21. Sharkey AM, Smith SK. The endometrium as a cause of implantation failure. Best Pract Res Clin Obstet Gynaecol. 2003;17(2):289-307.
22. Hey NA, Graham RA, Seif MW, Aplin JD. The polymorphic epithelial mucin MUC1 in human endometrium is regulated with maximal expression in the implantation phase. J Clin Endocrinol Metab. 1994;78(2):337-42.
23. Meseguer M, Aplin JD, Caballero-Campo P, O'Connor JE, Martín JC, Remohí J, et al. Human endometrial mucin MUC1 is up-regulated by progesterone and down-regulated in vitro by the human blastocyst. Biol Reprod. 2001;64(2):590-601.
24. Carson DD, Lagow E, Thathiah A, Al-Shami R, Farach-Carson MC, Vernon M, et al. Changes in gene expression during the early to mid-luteal (receptive phase) transition in human endometrium detected by high-density microarray screening. Mol Hum Reprod. 2002;8(9):871-9.
25. Achache H, Revel A. Endometrial receptivity markers, the journey to successful embryo implantation. Hum Reprod Update. 2006;12(6):731-46.
26. Aplin JD. Embryo implantation: the molecular mechanism remains elusive. Reprod Biomed Online. 2006;13(6):833-9.
27. Domínguez F, Remohí J, Pellicer A, Simón C. Human endometrial receptivity: a genomic approach. Reprod Biomed Online. 2003;6:332-5.
28. Dominguez F, Galan A, Martin JJ, Remohi J, Pellicer A, Simón C. Hormonal and embryonic regulation of chemokine receptors CXCR1, CXCR4, CCR5 and CCR2B in the human endometrium and the human blastocyst. Mol Hum Reprod. 2003;9(4):189-98.
29. Genbacev OD, Prakobphol A, Foulk RA, Krtolica AR, Ilic D, Singer MS, et al. Trophoblast L-selectin-mediated adhesion at the maternal-fetal interface. Science. 2003;299(5605):405-8.
30. Foulk RA, Zdravkovic T, Genbacev O, Prakobphol A. Expression of L-selectin ligand MECA-79 as a predictive marker of human uterine receptivity. J Assist Reprod Genet. 2007;24(7):316-21.
31. Illera MJ, Cullinan E, Gui Y, Yuan L, Beyler SA, Lessey BA. Blockade of the αvβ3 integrin adversely affects implantation in the mouse. Biol Reprod. 2000;62(5):1285-90.
32. Lessey BA, Castelbaum AJ, Sawin SW, Sun J. Integrins as markers of uterine receptivity in women with primary unexplained infertility. Fertil Steril. 1995;63(3):535-42.
33. Lessey BA. Endometrial receptivity and the window of implantation. Baillieres Best Pract Res Clin Obstet Gynaecol. 2000;14(5):775-88.
34. Lessey BA, Castelbaum AJ, Sawin SW, Buck CA, Schinnar R, Bilker W, et al. Aberrant integrin expression in the endometrium of women with endometriosis. J Clin Endocrinol Metabol. 1994;79(2):643-9.
35. Meyer WR, Castelbaum AJ, Somkuti S, Sagoskin AW, Doyle M, Harris JE, et al. Hydrosalpinges adversely affect markers of endometrial receptivity. Hum Reprod. 1997;12(7):1393-8.
36. Kumar S, Zhu LJ, Polihronis M, Cameron ST, Baird DT, Schatz F, et al. Progesterone induces calcitonin gene expression in human endometrium within the putative window of implantation. J Clin Endocrinol Metab. 1998;83(12):4443-50.
37. Brar AK, Frank GR, Richards RG, Meyer AJ, Kessler CA, Cedars MI, et al. Laminin decreases PRL and IGFBP-1 expression during in vitro decidualization of human endometrial stromal cells. J Cell Physiol. 1995;163(1):30-7.
38. Giudice LC. Potential biochemical markers of uterine receptivity. Human Reprod. 1999;14(Suppl 2):3-16.
39. Dominguez F, Yáñez-Mó M, Sanchez-Madrid F, Simón C. Embryonic implantation and leukocyte transendothelial migration: different processes with similar players? FASEB J. 2005;19(9):1056-60.

40. Paria BC, Reese J, Das SK, Dey SK. Deciphering the cross-talk of implantation: advances and challenges. Science. 2002;296(5576):2185-8.
41. Moser B, Loetscher P. Lymphocyte traffic control by chemokines. Nat Immunol. 2001;2(2):123-8.
42. Galán A, Herrer R, Remohí J, Pellicer A, Simón C. Embryonic regulation of endometrial epithelial apoptosis during human implantation. Hum Reprod. 2000;15(Suppl 6):74-80.
43. Alon R, Feigelson S. From rolling to arrest on blood vessels: leukocyte tap dancing on endothelial integrin ligands and chemokines at sub-second contacts. Semin Immunol. 2002;14(2):93-104.
44. Luscinskas FW, Ma S, Nusrat A, Parkos CA, Shaw SK. The role of endothelial cell lateral junctions during leukocyte trafficking. Immunol Rev. 2002;186(1):57-67.
45. Vestweber D. Regulation of endothelial cell contacts during leukocyte extravasation. Curr Opin Cell Biol. 2002;14(5):587-93.
46. Aplin JD, Ruane PT. Embryo-epithelium interactions during implantation at a glance. J Cell Sci. 2017;130:15-22.
47. Strowitzki T, Germeyer A, Popovici R, von Wolff M. The human endometrium as a fertility-determining factor. Hum Reprod Update. 2006;12(5):617-30.
48. Hoozemans DA, Schats R, Lambalk CB, Homburg R, Hompes PGA. Human embryo implantation: current knowledge and clinical implications in assisted reproductive technology. Reprod Biomed Online. 2004;9(6):692-715.
49. Wang H, Critchley HO, Kelly RW, Shen D, Baird DT. Progesterone receptor subtype B is differentially regulated in human endometrial stroma. Mol Hum Reprod. 1998; 4(4):407-12.
50. Bergeron C. Morphological changes and protein secretion induced by progesterone in the endometrium during the luteal phase in preparation for nidation. Hum Reprod. 2000;15(Suppl 1):119-28.
51. Unemori EN, Erikson ME, Rocco SE, Sutherland KM, Parsell DA, Mak J, et al. Relaxin stimulates expression of vascular endothelial growth factor in normal human endometrial cells in vitro and is associated with menometrorrhagia in women. Hum Reprod. 1999;14(3):800-6.
52. Einspanier A, Nubbemeyer R, Schlote S, Schumacher M, Ivell R, Fuhrmann K, et al. Relaxin in the marmoset monkey: secretion pattern in the ovarian cycle and early pregnancy. Biol Reprod. 1999;61(2):512-20.
53. Stewart DR, Celniker AC, Taylor Jr CA, Cragun JR, Overstreet JW, Lasley BL. Relaxin in the peri-implantation period. J Clin Endocrinol Metabol. 1990;70(6):1771-3.
54. Chen DB, Hilsenrath R, Yang ZM, Le SP, Kim SR, Chuong CJ, et al. Leukaemia inhibitory factor in human endometrium during the menstrual cycle: cellular origin and action on production of glandular epithelial cell prostaglandin in vitro. Hum Reprod. 1995;10(4):911-8.
55. Spandorfer SD, Navarro J, Levy D, Black AR, Liu HC, Veeck L, et al. Autologous endometrial coculture in patients with in vitro-fertilization (IVF) failure: correlations of outcome with leukemia inhibiting factor (LIF) production. Am J Reprod Immunol. 2001;46(6):375-80.
56. Pollard JW, Hunt JS, Wiktor-Jedrzejczak W, Stanley ER. A pregnancy defect in the osteopetrotic (op/op) mouse demonstrates the requirement for CSF-1 in female fertility. Dev Biol. 1991;148(1):273-83.
57. Scarpellini F, Sbracia M. Effectiveness of GM-CSF 1 in the treatment of habitual abortion in a controlled study. Fertil Steril. 2003;80(Suppl 3):S288.
58. Das SK, Wang XN, Paria BC, Damm D, Abraham JA, Klagsburn M, et al. Heparin-binding EGF-like growth factor gene is induced in the mouse uterus temporally by the blastocyst solely at the site of its apposition: a possible ligand for interaction with blastocyst EGF-receptor in implantation. Development. 1994;120(5):1071-83.
59. Larsen WF, DiAugustine R, Walmer DK, Klotz DM. Insulin-like growth factor-1 regulates VEGF expression in primary human uterine epithelial cells. Fertil Steril. 2003;80(Suppl 3):S269-70.
60. Leung PH, Salamonsen LA, Findlay JK. Immunolocalization of inhibin and activin subunits in human endometrium across the menstrual cycle. Hum Reprod. 1998;13(12):3469-77.
61. Godkin JD, Dore JJ. Transforming growth factor beta and the endometrium. Rev Reprod. 1998;3(1):1-6.
62. Treetampinich C, O'Connor AE, MacLachlan V, Groome NP, de Kretser DM. Maternal serum inhibin A concentrations in early pregnancy after IVF and embryo transfer reflect the corpus luteum contribution and pregnancy outcome. Hum Reprod. 2000;15(9):2028-32.
63. Risau W. Mechanisms of angiogenesis. Nature. 1997;386:671-4.
64. Smith SK. Angiogenesis, vascular endothelial growth factor and the endometrium. Hum Reprod Update. 1998;4(5):509-19.
65. Smith SK. Angiogenesis and implantation. Hum Reprod. 2000;15(Suppl 6):59-66.
66. Lim H, Song H, Paria BC, Reese J, Das SK, Dey SK. Molecules in blastocyst implantation: uterine and embryonic perspectives. Vitam Horm. 2002;64:43-76.
67. Daftary GS, Taylor HS. Molecular markers of implantation: clinical implications. Curr Opin Obstet Gynecol. 2001;13:269-74.
68. Hsieh-Li HM, Witte DP, Weinstein M, Branford W, Li H, Small K, et al. Hoxa 11 structure, extensive antisense transcription, and function in male and female fertility. Development. 1995;121(5):1373-85.
69. Mohamed OA, Jonnaert M, Labelle-Dumais C, Kuroda K, Clarke HJ, Dufort D. Uterine Wnt/beta-catenin signaling is required for implantation. Proc Natl Acad Sci U S A. 2005;102(24):8579-84.
70. Paria BC, Ma W, Tan J, Raja S, Das SK, Dey SK, et al. Cellular and molecular responses of the uterus to embryo implantation can be elicited by locally applied growth factors. Proc Natl Acad Sci U S A. 2001;98(3):1047-52.
71. Seppala M, Bohn H, Tatarinov Y. Glycodelins. Tumour Biol. 1998;19:213-20.
72. Okamoto N, Uchida A, Takakura K, Kariya Y, Kanzaki H, Riittinen L, et al. Suppression by human placental protein 14 of natural killer cell activity. Am J Reprod Immunol. 1991;26(4):137-42.
73. Vu TH, Werb Z. Matrix metalloproteinases: effectors of development and normal physiology. Genes Dev. 2000; 14(17):2123-33.
74. Dimitriadis E, Robb L, Liu Y-X, Enders AC, Martin H, Stoikos C, et al. IL-11 and IL-11Rα immunolocalisation at primate implantation sites supports a role for IL-11 in placentation and fetal development. Reprod Biol Endocrinol. 2003;1:34.
75. Corvinus FM, Fitzgerald JS, Friedrich K, Markert UR. Evidence for a correlation between trophoblast invasiveness and STAT3 activity. Am J Reprod Immunol. 2003;50(4):316-21.

76. Simón C, Valbuena D, Krüssel J, Bernal A, Murphy CR, Shaw T, et al. Interleukin-1 receptor antagonist prevents embryonic implantation by a direct effect on the endometrial epithelium. Fertil Steril. 1998;70(5):896-906.
77. Daniel Y, Geva E, Lerner-Geva L, Eshed-Englender T, Gamzu R, Lessing JB, et al. Levels of vascular endothelial growth factor are elevated in patients with ectopic pregnancy: is this a novel marker? Fertil Steril. 1999;72:1013-7.
78. Dautzenberg FM, Hauger RL. The CRF peptide family and their receptors: yet more partners discovered. Trends Pharmacol Sci. 2002;23(2):71-7.
79. Makrigiannakis A, Zoumakis E, Kalantaridou S, Coutifaris C, Margioris AN, Coukos G, et al. Corticotropin-releasing hormone promotes blastocyst implantation and early maternal tolerance. Nat Immunol. 2001;2(11):1018-24.
80. Makrigiannakis A, Margioris AN, Chatzaki E, Zoumakis E, Chrousos GP, Gravanis A. The decidualizing effect of progesterone may involve direct transcriptional activation of corticotrophin-releasing hormone from human endometrial stromal cells. Mol Hum Reprod. 1999;5(9):789-96.
81. Zoumakis E, Margioris AN, Stournaras C, Dermitzaki E, Angelakis E, Makrigiannakis A, et al. Corticotrophin-releasing hormone (CRH) interacts with inflammatory prostaglandins and interleukins and affects the decidualization of human endometrial stroma. Mol Hum Reprod. 2000;6(4):344-51.
82. Bamberger AM, Minas V, Kalantaridou SN, Radde J, Sadeghian H, Löning T, et al. Corticotropin-releasing hormone modulates human trophoblast invasion through carcinoembryonic antigen-related cell adhesion molecule-1 regulation. Am J Pathol. 2006;168(1):141-50.
83. Cervero A, Horcajadas JA, Martin J, Pellicer A, Simón C. The leptin system during human endometrial receptivity and preimplantation development. J Clin Endocrinol Metab. 2004; 89(5):2442-51.
84. Herrler A, von Rango U, Beier HM. Embryo-maternal signalling: how the embryo starts talking to its mother to accomplish implantation. Reprod Biomed Online. 2002; 6(2):244-56.
85. Seshagiri PB, Terasawa E, Hearn JP. The secretion of gonadotrophin-releasing hormone by peri-implantation embryos of the rhesus monkey: comparison with the secretion of chorionic gonadotrophin. Hum Reprod. 1994;9(7):1300-7.
86. Woodward BJ, Lenton EA, Turner K. Human chorionic gonadotrophin: embryonic secretion is a time-dependent phenomenon. Hum Reprod. 1993;8(9):1463-8.
87. Hearn JP, Hodges JK, Gems S. Early secretion of chorionic gonadotrophin by marmoset embryos in vivo and in vitro. J Endocrinol. 1988;119(2):249-55.
88. Ware CB, Horowitz MC, Renshaw BR, Hunt JS, Liggitt D, Koblar SA, et al. Targeted disruption of the low-affinity leukemia inhibitory factor receptor gene causes placental, skeletal, neural and metabolic defects and results in perinatal death. Development. 1995;121:1283-99.
89. Sherwin JR, Sharkey AM, Cameo P, Mavrogianis PM, Catalano RD, Edassery S, et al. Identification of novel genes regulated by chorionic gonadotropin in baboon endometrium during the window of implantation. Endocrinology. 2007;148(2):618-26.
90. Piccinni MP, Scaletti C, Mavilia C, Lazzeri E, Romagnani P, Natali I, et al. Production of IL-4 and leukemia inhibitory factor by T cells of the cumulus oophorus: a favorable microenvironment for pre-implantation embryo development. Eur J Immunol. 2001;31(8):2431-7.
91. Piccinni MP, Scaletti C, Vultaggio A, Maggi E, Romagnani S. Defective production of LIF, M-CSF and Th2-type cytokines by T cells at fetomaternal interface is associated with pregnancy loss. J Reprod Immunol. 2001;52(1-2):35-43.
92. Cameo P, Srisuparp S, Strakova Z, Fazleabas AT. Chorionic gonadotropin and uterine dialogue in the primate. Reprod Biol Endocrinol. 2004;2:50.
93. Nishimori K, Dunkel L, Hsueh AJ, Yamoto M, Nakano R. Expression of luteinizing hormone and chorionic gonadotropin receptor messenger ribonucleic acid in human corpora lutea during menstrual cycle and pregnancy. J Clin Endocrinol Metab. 1995;80(4):1444-8.
94. Fazleabas AT, Donnelly KM, Srinivasan S, Fortman JD, Miller JB. Modulation of the baboon (Papio anubis) uterine endometrium by chorionic gonadotrophin during the period of uterine receptivity. Proc Natl Acad Sci U S A. 1999;96(5):2543-8.
95. Srisuparp S, Strakova Z, Brudney A, Mukherjee S, Reierstad S, Hunzicker-Dunn M, et al. Signal transduction pathways activated by chorionic gonadotropin in the primate endometrial epithelial cells. Biol Reprod. 2003;68(2):457-64.
96. Bernardini L, Moretti-Rojas I, Brush M, Rojas FJ, Balmaceda JP. Changes in expression of adenyl cyclase activity in human endometrium during hormone replacement therapy and ovarian stimulation. Mol Hum Reprod. 1999;5(10):955-60.
97. Lim H, Paria BC, Das SK, Dinchuk JE, Langenbach R, Trzaskos JM, et al. Multiple female reproductive failures in cyclooxygenase 2-deficient mice. Cell. 1997;91:197-208.
98. Fazleabas AT, Bell SC, Fleming S, Sun J, Lessey BA. Distribution of integrins and the extracellular matrix proteins in the baboon endometrium during the menstrual cycle and early pregnancy. Biol Reprod. 1997;56(2):348-56.
99. Peng X, Kim JJ, Fazleabas AT. Apoptosis and differentiation in baboon stromal cells: a role for chorionic gonadotropin (CG)? Biol Reprod. 2000;62:307-8.
100. Medawar PB. Some immunological and endocrinological problems raised by the evolution of viviparity in vertebrates. Symp Soc Exp Biol. 1953;7:320-38.
101. Chaouat G, Menu E, Clark DA, Dy M, Minkowski M, Wegmann TG. Control of fetal survival in CBA x DBA/2 mice by lymphokine therapy. J Reprod Fertil. 1990;89(2):447-58.
102. Nishioka Y, Nishimura N, Suzuki Y, Sone S. Human monocyte-derived and CD83+ blood dendritic cells enhance NK cell-mediated cytotoxicity. Eur J Immunol. 2001;31(9):2633-41.
103. Bulmer JN, Johnson PM. Macrophage populations in the human placenta and amniochorion. Clin Exp Immunol. 1984;57(2):393-403.
104. Guimond MJ, Wang B, Croy BA. Engraftment of bone marrow from severe combined immunodeficient (SCID) mice reverses the reproductive deficits in natural killer cell-deficient tgε26 mice. J Exp Med. 1998;187(2):217-23.
105. Savion S, Zeldich E, Orenstein H, Shepshelovich J, Torchinsky A, Carp H, et al. Cytokine expression in the uterus of mice with pregnancy loss: effect of maternal immunopotentiation with GM-CSF. Reproduction. 2002;123(3):399-409.
106. Nakayama T, Fujiwara H, Maeda M, Inoue T, Yoshioka S, Mori T, et al. Human peripheral blood mononuclear cells (PBMC) in early pregnancy promote embryo invasion in vitro: HCG enhances the effects of PBMC. Hum Reprod. 2002;17(1):207-12.

107. von Rango U, Classen-Linke I, Kertschanska S, Kemp B, Beier HM. Effects of trophoblast invasion on the distribution of leukocytes in uterine and tubal implantation sites. Fertil Steril. 2001;76(1):116-24.
108. Aoki K, Kajiura S, Matsumoto Y, Ogasawara M, Okada S, Yagami Y, et al. Preconceptional natural-killer-cell activity as a predictor of miscarriage. Lancet. 1995;345(8961):1340-2.
109. Matsubayashi H, Hosaka T, Sugiyama Y, Suzuki T, Arai T, Kondo A, et al. Increased natural killer-cell activity is associated with infertile women. Am J Reprod Immunol. 2001;46(5):318-22.
110. Krishnan L, Guilbert LJ, Russel AS, Wegmann TG, Mosmann TR, Belosevic M. Pregnancy impairs resistance of C57BL/6 mice to Leishmania major infection and causes decreased antigen-specific IFN-gamma response and increased production of T helper 2 cytokines. J Immunol. 1996;156(2):644-52.
111. Khong TY. Immunohistologic study of the leukocytic infiltrate in maternal uterine tissues in normal and preeclamptic pregnancies at term. Am J Reprod Immunol Microbiol. 1987;15:1-8.
112. Zheng Y, Zhou ZZ, Lyttle CR, Teuscher C. Immunohistochemical characterization of the estrogen-stimulated leukocyte influx in the immature rat uterus. J Leukoc Biol. 1988;44:27-32.
113. Drake PM, Gunn MD, Charo IF, Tsou CL, Zhou Y, Huang L, et al. Human placental cytotrophoblasts attract monocytes and CD56(bright) natural killer cells via the actions of monocyte inflammatory protein 1α. J Exp Med. 2001;193:1199-212.
114. Quenby S, Bates M, Doig T, Brewster J, Lewis-Jones DI, Johnson PM, et al. Pre-implantation endometrial leukocytes in women with recurrent miscarriage. Hum Reprod. 1999;14:2386-91.
115. Chaouat G, Zourbas S, Ostojic S, Lappree-Delage G, Dubanchet S, Ledee N, et al. A brief review of recent data on some cytokine expressions at the materno-foetal interface which might challenge the classical Th1/Th2 dichotomy. J Reprod Immunol. 2002;53:241-56.
116. Veenstra van Nieuwenhoven AL, Heineman MJ, Faas MM. The immunology of successful pregnancy. Hum Reprod Update. 2003;9(4):347-57.
117. Müller-Schöttle F, Classen-Linke I, Beier-Hellwig K, Sterzik K, Beier HM. Uteroglobin expression and release in the human endometrium. Ann N Y Acad Sci. 2000;923:332-5.
118. El Ghmati SM, Van Hoeyveld EM, Van Strijp JG, Ceuppens JL, Stevens EA. Identification of haptoglobin as an alternative ligand for CD11b/CD18. J Immunol. 1996;156(7):2542-52.
119. Dobryszycka W. Biological functions of haptoglobin—new pieces to an old puzzle. Eur J Clin Chem Clin Biochem. 1997;35(9):647-54.
120. Bottini N, Gimelfarb A, Gloria-Bottini F, La Torre M, Lucarelli P, Lucarini N. Haptoglobin genotype and natural fertility in humans. Fertil Steril. 1999;72:293-6.
121. Nauta U, Beier HM, Herrler A. Haptoglobin in extracellular matrices reduce the adhesion/invasion of NK (CD11b+) cells. Reprod Abstracts Series. 2002;29:21.
122. Bergeron D, Ouellette MJ, Lambert RD. PGE2, but not TGFβ2, in rabbit blastocoelic fluid regulates the cytotoxic activities of NK and LAK cells. J Reprod Immunol. 1997;33:203-19.
123. von Rango U, Classen-Linke I, Raven G, Brocken F, Beier HM. Cytokine microenvironments in human first trimester decidua are dependent on trophoblast cells. Fertil Steril. 2003;79(5):1176-86.
124. Kadyrov M, Kaufmann P, Huppertz B. Expression of a cytokeratin 18 neo-epitope is a specific marker for trophoblast apoptosis in human placenta. Placenta. 2001;22(1):44-8.
125. Levine JS, Koh JS. The role of apoptosis in autoimmunity: immunogen, antigen, and accelerant. Semin Nephrol. 1999;19(1):34-47.
126. Steinman RM, Turley S, Mellman I, Inaba K. The induction of tolerance by dendritic cells that have captured apoptotic cells. J Exp Med. 2000;191(3):411-6.
127. Wimsatt WA. Some comparative aspects of implantation. Biol Reprod. 1975;12(1):1-40. doi: 10.1095/biolreprod12.1.1. PMID: 806310.

CHAPTER 7

Embryo-Endometrial Crosstalk and Endometrial Receptivity

Nalini Mahajan, Anshu Dhar

INTRODUCTION

The endometrium undergoes cyclical changes in response to ovarian hormones in its preparation for embryo implantation. During the window of implantation (WOI), many processes occur simultaneously and sequentially within the endometrium to allow changes at a morphological and molecular level for successful implantation. Some of the important transformations are cell cycle regulation, immune modulation of implantation, angiogenesis, growth factor actions, steroid hormone action and metabolism, production of extracellular matrix proteins, cell surface glycoproteins, and a variety of transcription factors.[1] Recent advances in genome sequencing which include the introduction of next-generation sequencing and bioinformatics analyses have made it possible to understand the omics involved in endometrial maturation and embryo-endometrial crosstalk. This information allows a better understanding of implantation failure and may help to improve infertility management.

IMPLANTATION

The process by which the blastocyst trophectoderm adheres to the endometrium of the uterus is called implantation. The three phases of implantation—apposition, adhesion, and invasion involve an intricate interplay of hormones, genes, and cytokine expression. During apposition and adhesion, the blastocyst establishes a firm contact with the epithelial lining, while invasion encompasses penetration of the endometrium by trophectoderm cells. The trophectoderm invades by displacing the endometrial cells in its attempt to establish contact with blood vessels and this process is aided by genes involved in tissue remodeling.[2] In response to this invasion, the endometrial stromal cells and extracellular matrix undergo decidualization essential for the sustainability of the pregnancy. The endometrial epithelial cells (EECs) undergo specific structural and functional changes. At a morphological level, there are changes in the plasma membrane and cytoskeleton (Murphy, 2000; Martın et al. 2000) leading to the formation of pinopods also known as uterodomes which are proposed to aid embryo adhesion by their various functions including endocytosis, exocytosis, and expression of adhesion molecules.[3] A delicate balance between trophoblastic invasion and decidual resistance ensures proper placentation. The prime players in the implantation process include a viable embryo, an endometrium that has undergone the necessary molecular and structural changes to accept the embryo, and the host immune system which must protect this semi-allograft. Embryo-endometrial crosstalk is a prerequisite for successful implantation. Though significant progress has been made in the identification of the molecular mechanisms involved, intricate details of the process still elude us. Implantation failure thus remains a major bottleneck in the success of assisted reproduction technologies.

Endometrial Receptivity

Endometrial receptivity (ER) defines the short window of time within which a zona-free blastocyst must attach, invade, and derive sustenance from the endometrium. Progesterone secretion is integral to this process as it brings about the necessary secretory changes in an estrogen-primed endometrium. It is also essential for the maintenance of pregnancy. The WOI or window of ER opens 4–5 days after progesterone secretion and lasts 30–36 hours depending on the patient. It occurs at luteinizing hormone (LH) + 6 to LH + 9 in natural cycles or P + 4 to P + 9 in hormone replacement therapy (HRT) cycles.[4] ER is a dynamic process that involves a series of changes within the endometrium at the morphological, biochemical, molecular, and immunological level in response to embryonic signaling. The systemic and local alterations that occur constitute is termed as "the maternal recognition of pregnancy".[5] Progesterone and estrogen are considered the key modulators of endometrial maturation and have a multifaceted role. Hormonal activity depends not only on the levels of progesterone, estrogen,

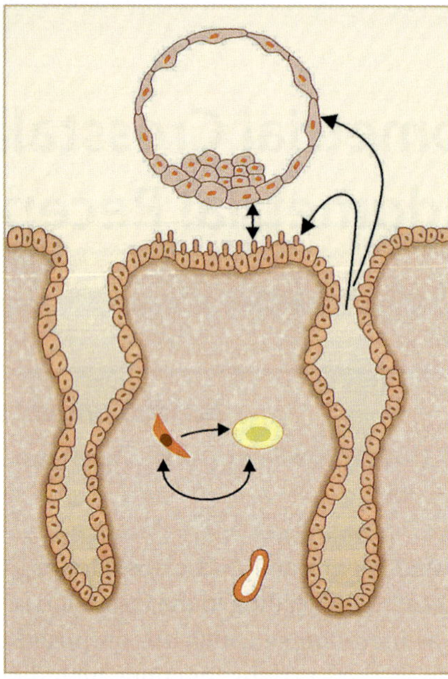

Location	Factors
Trophoblast	• Adhesion moleculus • Cytokine and chemokine receptors • Proteases
Luminal epithelium	• Glycocalyx components • Adhesion molecules • Cytokines/chemokines • Proteases • Calcium regulators
Glands	• Cytokines/chemokines • Growth factors • Nutrients
Extracellular matrix	• Hyaluronan • Collagens • Degradative enzymes/inhibitors
Decidualizing stroma	• Prostaglandins • Cytokines/chemokines • Growth factors • Proteases

Fig. 1: Factors involved in endometrial maturation.
(*Source:* Diedrich K, Fauser BC, Devroey P, Griesinger G, Evian Annual Reproduction (EVAR) Workshop Group. The role of the endometrium and embryo in human implantation. Hum Reprod Update. 2007;13(4):365-77).

and their receptors, but is also influenced by the coactivators, repressors, and paracrine signaling **(Fig. 1)**.[6]

Endometrium during "the Window of Implantation"

Changes in the endometrium occurring during this phase result from a well-coordinated action between autocrine, paracrine, and endocrine factors. At a *histological level*, increasing progesterone levels herald a secretory transformation—subnuclear vacuolation, stromal edema, increase in glands, and capillary permeability in the endometrium.[7,8] Pinopods or cytoplasmic projections of the luminal epithelium that facilitate blastocyst adhesion appear 6 days after ovulation and are retained for approximately 24 hours **(Box 1)**.[9,10]

BOX 1: Window of implantation.

LH + 6–LH + 9
- Phases: Signaling, apposition, attachment, and invasion
- Key findings in a receptive endometrium:
  - Luminal epithelial pinopods formation
  - Expression of adhesion molecules
  - Novel cytokines profile
  - Immune protection
  - Appropriate gene expression

Steroid Receptors during Window of Implantation

During the WOI, progesterone (P) acts more via paracrine and autocrine factors, this transition from direct or endocrine action to an indirect one is important for successful implantation. Epithelial estrogen receptor-alpha (ESR1) is downregulated and there is a shift of progesterone receptors (PR) from the epithelium to the stromal compartment. The persistence of ESR1 and PR in the glandular epithelium is associated with infertility and implantation defects. The action of estrogen (E) is also limited by progesterone (P) through induction of 17β-hydroxysteroid dehydrogenase type 2 (HSD17β2) in the endometrium that converts E2 to the less active estrone.[11]

Molecular Changes

At the molecular level, the pre-receptive early secretory phase is characterized by increased metabolic activity in preparation for implantation. This leads to a predominance of cellular metabolic products (fatty acids, eicosanoids, amino alcohols, and lipids), greater expression of transporters of biological molecules, and facilitation of sperm migration.[12] There is an inhibition of mitosis during this phase as suggested by the downregulation of several growth factors. In the receptive phase, there is an upregulation of gene expression. Apart from increased metabolic and secretory activity, there is an upregulation of genes involved in the activation of the immune response.[13] During the late secretory phase, the WOI closes and in this phase genes related to immune response—both cellular and humoral, blood coagulation, steroid biosynthesis, and prostaglandin metabolism are regulated.[14]

Estrogen, progesterone, and embryonic chorionic gonadotropin regulate the secretion of growth factors and cytokines which are the mediators of the embryo-maternal dialogue and initiation of decidualization.[15,16] A large number of molecular mediators that are important for ER have been identified. The ones extensively researched are integrins, leukemia inhibitory factor (LIF), homeobox A10, mucin 1, calcitonin, and cyclooxygenase 2.[17] *Integrins* are cell adhesion molecules that are involved in cell-to-cell and cell to extracellular matrix interaction facilitating signal transduction. The co-expression of αVβ3 and α4β1 during the WOI has been well-documented.[18-20] *Mucin 1* (MUC1), a glycoprotein and an antiadhesive molecule is localized to the luminal surface epithelium but is excluded from cells with pinopods allowing the blastocyst to preferentially attach to these specialized structures on the apical surface.[15] *Cytokines* are glycoproteins produced by the trophoblastic and endometrial cells that act via specific cell surface receptors. They are involved in intercellular signaling and regulate the embryo-maternal interactions. Their production is interlinked with the arrival of the blastocyst into the endometrial cavity. *LIF* expressed during the WOI appears to be important for the embryo-endometrial crosstalk.[21] It has been hypothesized that LIF plays a role in the adhesive and invasive phases of implantation because of its anchoring effect on the trophoblast.[22] Other factors such as the heparin-binding growth factor, epidermal growth factor, and insulin-like growth factor also seem to have a role in implantation as their expression is found during the WOI. *HOX* genes are upregulated by estrogen and progesterone and are essential for endometrial growth, differentiation, and receptivity. HOXA10 and HOXA11 messenger ribonucleic acid (mRNA) are expressed in endometrial epithelial and stromal cells, their expression being higher in the mid-and late secretory phase and decidua of early pregnancy.[23-25] *HOX* genes regulate many molecular and morphological markers specific to the WOI, e.g., pinopods, β3 integrin, and insulin-like growth factor-binding protein-1 (IGFBP-1). Women having decreased expression of HOXA10 or 11 during the secretory phase have been seen to have lower implantation rates. Expression of these genes is reduced in disorders such as endometriosis, polycystic ovary syndrome (PCOS), hydrosalpinx, and fibroids.[26,27] Calcitonin, L-selectin, and L-selectin ligand are also secreted by the EECs during the mid-secretory phase of the menstrual cycle. Prostaglandins and aromatase play an essential role in implantation. Ion channels in the endometrium are also emerging as important players in regulating ER and embryo implantation. Abnormal expression or function of ion channels in the endometrium may lead to impaired ER and/or implantation failure.[28]

Immunological Response

The maternal immune response is intricately linked to successful implantation though the exact mechanism is unclear. The results from transcriptome studies during the preimplantation phase suggest that instead of general suppression of the maternal immune system, there is a fine-tuned regulation of immune cells.[29] Immune cells in blood circulation regulate corpus luteum function and endometrial differentiation to promote subsequent embryo implantation.[30]

The balance between T-helper 1 and T-helper 2 cytokines: An existing paradigm suggests that for successful implantation, a balance between *T-helper 1 (Th1) and T-helper 2 (Th2) produced cytokines* is mandatory. A shift in the ratio toward Th1 cells leads to increased production of proinflammatory cytokines such as interferon-gamma (IFN-γ), interleukin-2 (IL-2), and tumor necrosis factor-alpha (TNF-α) resulting in a cytotoxic cell-mediated immune response and increased phagocytosis and inflammation. In contrast, Th2 cells produce a range of interleukins involved in the humoral immune response and inhibit several functions of phagocytosis which together represent an anti-inflammatory response. Several observational studies have reported an increased expression of proinflammatory cytokines in women with a history of recurrent pregnancy loss.

Natural killer cells: Despite the tremendous progress in the field of immunology, the origin of uterine natural killer (uNK) cells is still not clear. It has been hypothesized that hematopoietic precursor cells (HPCs), hosting in endometrium differentiate into uNK cells.[31] On the other hand, another hypothesis suggests that uNK cells are derived from differentiated peripheral blood NK cells, that are attracted to the endometrium by locally secreted cytokines and chemokines.

A disrupted population of *peripheral and/or uNK* cells has been implicated in implantation failure and early pregnancy loss. After ovulation, uNK cells become the dominant immune cells accounting for >30% of immune cells. In early gestation, the uNK cells expand in number and are thought to play an important role in maintaining a balance between the normal and excessive invasion of the trophoblast accounting for as much as 70% of the leukocyte population. As opposed to the peripheral NK cells, uNK cells express a unique pattern of surface markers being $CD45^+$ $CD56^{bright}$, $CD16^+$, and $CD9^+$ cells. They are characterized by a lower level of cytotoxic activity but produce abundant cytokines which are responsible for their varied actions. It is believed that during implantation, these cells communicate with the extravillous trophoblast cells (EVTs), recognizing the human leukocyte antigens G (HLA-G) via the killer cell immunoglobulin-like receptors (KIRs). These interactions cause immunological acceptance of the semi-allogeneic fetus, by the mother and trigger uNK cells to secrete several cytokines and growth hormones that promote trophoblast invasion. In addition, uNK cells secrete several matrix metalloproteinases (MMPs) and angiogenic factors, such as vascular endothelial growth factor (VEGF), that contribute to the remodeling of the spiral arteries. Successful orchestration of these events is essential to ensure invasion, acceptance, and further growth of fetus and maintenance of pregnancy.[32] Peripheral blood NK cells play an important part in the innate immune system and are not thought to play a role in endometrial function. *Human leukocyte antigen (HLA)* dissimilarity is crucial at early implantation and the similarity of HLA in the partners may interfere with implantation.[33]

The prognostic value of uNK cells is however unclear due to a lack of standardization in the techniques of measurement and defined cut-off values; as concluded by various systematic reviews.[34,35] The lack of good quality studies elucidating the role of the same also contributes to the confusion. At present, the testing for uNK cells and the provision of immunotherapy for correction of the same should be considered only within the realm of experimental medicine.

Role of human chorionic gonadotropin: Studies on mice suggest that the maternal immune system undergoes functional changes by recognizing the developing embryos in a stepwise manner from before fertilization to after embryo implantation. A novel concept has been proposed by Fujiwara et al. in 2016.[36] They hypothesize that immune cells receive information about the presence of a developing embryo in the female genital tract via the human chorionic gonadotropin (hCG) secreted by the embryo and transmit this information through blood circulation to the uterus. This induces endometrial changes that further facilitate embryo implantation. hCG has several immunological properties regulating not only the number of local immune cells but also making these cells adopt a unique phenotype to support and protect the fetus. It is also believed to upregulate the number of endometrial NK cells via the mannose receptor thereby positively influencing embryo implantation.[37]

Global profiling of genes in the endometrium, decidua, and trophoblast-decidual interface has provided significant insight into endometrial maturation and implantation.[38,39] Microarray technology has revealed an upregulation of >200 genes in the WOI and downregulation of 60.[40] Microarrays are now being replaced by next-generation sequencing.

Role of endometrial microbiota: The recognition of the existence of endometrial microbiota, as opposed to the previously believed concept of a sterile endometrial cavity, has opened a new field for research and analysis. In the study by Moreno et al, it was shown that the presence of non-*Lactobacillus* dominated microbiota, defined as the presence of *Lactobacillus* spp. <90% determined by next-generation sequencing of endometrial fluid samples was associated with a negative impact on endometrial function and has been considered as an emerging cause of implantation failure. Also, it was demonstrated that the levels of microbiota remain stable throughout the cycle, independent of hormonal regulation.[41] The mechanism for implantation failures associated with the same has been implicated to be the endometrial inflammation caused by the bacteria. Some other mechanisms associated with the direct production of microbial metabolites and/or enzymes, producing relevant substances that can induce key cellular pathways in the endometrium have also been considered. The commercially available tests Endometrial Microbiome Metagenomic Analysis (EMMA®) and Analysis of Infectious Chronic Endometritis (ALICE®) analyze the endometrial microbiome to help identify abnormalities associated with a poor reproductive prognosis. EMMA indicates the endometrial microbiome balance, providing information on the proportions of all endometrial bacteria, including those linked to higher pregnancy rates (PRs). EMMA also includes ALICE, which detects pathogenic bacteria that can cause chronic endometritis.

Markers of Endometrial Receptivity

Over the years, attempts have been made to develop tests for ER, especially in the context of improving in vitro fertilization (IVF) results. The markers of ER include:

- *Histological markers:* Histological dating of endometrial using the Noyes criteria is no longer considered a valid method for the diagnosis of luteal phase deficiency nor can it guide clinical management of infertility. Improvement in histological diagnosis of ER was sought by the use of electron microscopy which identified the formation of pinopods considered to be an important histological change that heralds implantation. However, apart from not having universal availability, pinopods are no longer considered to be accurate makers of ER.
- *Ultrasound:* It is the only clinically applicable marker of ER. Endometrial pattern, thickness, and blood flow have been used to determine ER. Unfortunately, these parameters are prognostic and not confirmatory.
- *Biochemical and molecular:* Assessment of many of the cytokines and growth factors evaluated (Integrins, LIF, VEGF, and interleukins) have not yielded definitive results.

Endometrial Transcriptomics

Transcriptomics is the study of "transcriptome", i.e., the complete set of RNA transcripts produced by the genome under specific circumstances or in a specific cell using high throughput methods. The use of microarray technology has now given way to evaluation using next-generation sequencing. Molecular studies have identified the endometrial transcriptomic signature of the WOI allowing identification of the displaced WOI which may contribute to recurrent implantation failure (RIF). It is believed that in approximately 30% of IVF cycles, the WOI may be displaced leading to embryo-endometrial desynchrony. Two such tests—endometrial receptivity array (ERA) and integrity are commercially available. ERA analyzes the expression levels of 238 genes linked to the status of ER using RNA sequencing taken from the endometrial tissue. Following analysis, a specific computational predictor classifies the samples according to their expression profile as receptive or nonreceptive (NR). The NR endometrium is further classified as pre- or post-receptive meaning that the endometrium has not reached the receptive phase yet or has passed it, respectively.[42,43]

In a recent randomized controlled trial, which is also the first of its kind, the authors concluded that the ERA test did not show any benefit in the intention to treat analysis, other than a statistically significant increase in clinical pregnancy rate (CPR) when compared to frozen embryo transfer (FET) and fresh embryo transfer. However, the per-protocol analysis showed a significant increase in PRs at the first and cumulative PRs up to 12 months, and implantation rates at the first attempt highlighting the potential usefulness of ERA. Hence, the authors emphasized the need to confirm the findings in larger controlled trials.[44]

Concept of Selectivity and Receptivity

Endometrial receptivity suggests that the endometrial changes in the mid-luteal phase ensure adequate embryo-endometrial crosstalk ensuring implantation and growth of the embryo. A new concept of selectivity suggests a key role for the decidua in directing the maternal response to the implanting embryo. If *selectivity of the endometrium is suboptimal and receptivity is increased*, then the biosensor function may be disrupted allowing implantation of poorly viable embryos to establish a clinical pregnancy which may end up in miscarriage. On the other hand, *excessive selectivity or reduced receptivity of the endometrium* would decrease the likelihood of implantation or may lead to RIF after IVF.[45]

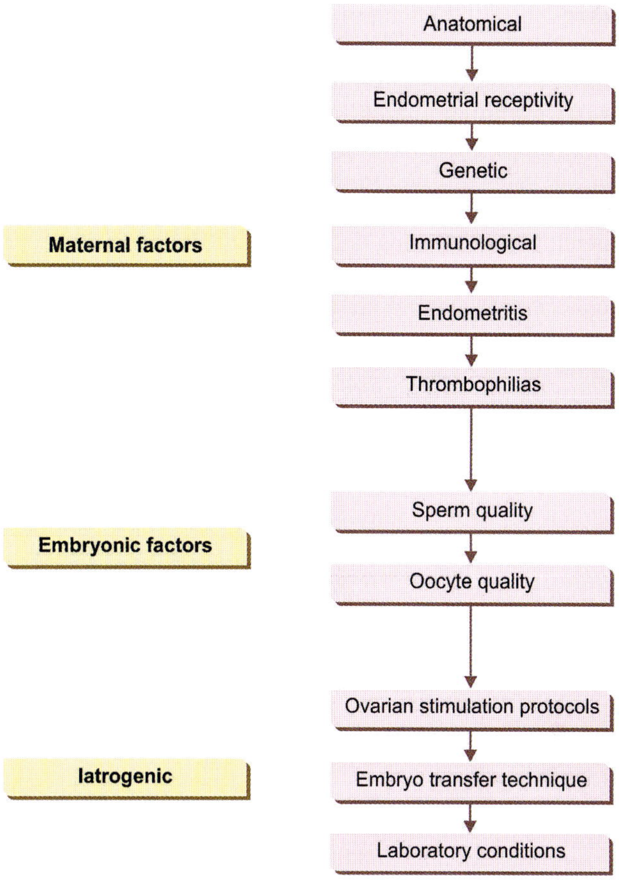

Fig. 2: Factors affecting implantation.

FACTORS AFFECTING IMPLANTATION

The major factors affecting implantation are listed in **Figure 2**.

Anatomical Factors

Congenital uterine anomalies—result mainly from fusion or canalization defects of the Müllerian ducts. Mutations of *HOXA10* and *HOXA11* genes that regulate Müllerian duct development have been implicated[46] in the adverse reproductive outcomes as the same genes are known to play an important role in decidualization and implantation.[47] The most common anomaly that leads to adverse reproductive outcomes is the septate uterus. It is suggested that it may also contribute to RIF and improvement in pregnancy outcome is seen after surgical correction.[48] Practice Committee of the American Society for Reproductive Medicine (ASRM) suggests that hysteroscopic septum excision might be associated with improved CPRs in women with infertility.[49]

Acquired Uterine Conditions

Fibroids, polyps, intrauterine adhesions, adenomyosis, and hydrosalpinx have all been considered as potential causes of implantation failure. These disorders lead to a mechanical obstruction, increased contractility, impaired vascularity, or altered ER. Most of them are easy to investigate and amenable to treatment. Studies in patients with RIF show that intracavity lesions and intrauterine adhesions may be found during routine hysteroscopy in 25–50% and 8.5% of patients, respectively.[50,51] Role of noncavity distorting intramural fibroids remains controversial and myomectomy does not improve PRs. According to the ASRM Practice Committee 2017, in asymptomatic women with cavity-distorting myomas (intramural with a submucosal component or submucosal), myomectomy (open or laparoscopic or hysteroscopic) may be considered to improve PRs.[52] Implantation failure in hydrosalpinx results from a mechanical washout effect of the hydro salpingeal fluid and an alteration in ER. Removal of hydrosalpinx by salpingectomy or clipping before IVF almost doubles the PRs and reduces the miscarriage rate to half.[53]

Adenomyosis is an acquired condition that may lead to alteration in ER, embryo-endometrial crosstalk, uterine contractility, and defective decidualization thereby affecting implantation.[54-56] ER studies have identified defects in the expression of important implantation factors such as LIF, HOXA10, and integrins that may play a role in the implantation failure associated with adenomyosis.[57] The role of the immune system in implantation failure is acknowledged though the exact mechanisms involved are yet to be defined. An increase in macrophages and NK cells has been demonstrated in women with adenomyosis.[58] producing inflammatory mediators and reactive oxygen species which may harm the embryo. Increased production of nitric oxide with abnormal expression of protein molecules has also been implicated. Long downregulation with gonadotropin releasing hormone (GnRH) agonist improves endometrial milieu and implantation.[59] Surgery could be beneficial for women with large focal adenomyosis who have experienced IVF treatment failures.

Thin endometrium: Endometrial thickness <7 mm is associated with implantation failure. The causes of thin endometrium could be either acute or chronic infections that lead to the destruction of the basal layer of the endometrium. Genital Kochs is an important cause of thin endometrium in developing nations; it may lead to extensive destruction of the basal layer. Iatrogenic causes include repeated or vigorous curettage, myomectomy and polypectomy, drugs such as clomiphene citrate, and individual uterine architecture or the intrinsic properties of endometrium that affect its growth.[60]

KEY POINTS

- The process of implantation is initiated with a dialogue between the hatched blastocyst and the endometrium. Paracrine signaling between the two, aids blastocyst adhesion and invasion.
- Since the endometrium becomes refractory in a short period, blastocyst entry must coordinate precisely with the period of ER.
- Cytokines and growth factors regulated by ovarian steroids and chorionic gonadotropin from the blastocyst play a crucial role in embryonic signaling.
- Implantation thus is a finely tuned, well-coordinated event involving a multitude of factors and a cascade of interactions.
- Precise identification of the factors involved and the spatial organization of events may bring us closer to a better understanding of the event and consequently improve assisted reproductive technology (ART) results.

REFERENCES

1. Giudice LC. Microarray expression profiling reveals candidate genes for human uterine receptivity. Am J Pharmacogenomics. 2004;4(5):299-312.
2. Mcgowen MR, Erez O, Romero R, et al. The evolution of embryo implantation. Int J Dev Biol. 2014;58(2-4):155-61.
3. Quinn KE, Matson BC, Wetendorf M, Caron KM. Pinopodes: recent advancements, current perspectives, and future directions. Mol Cell Endocrinol. 2020;501:110644.
4. Ruiz-Alonso M, Valbuena D, Gomez C, Cuzzi J, Simon C. Endometrial receptivity analysis (ERA): data versus opinions. Hum Reprod Open. 2021;2021(2):hoab011.
5. Duc-Goiran P, Mignot TM, Bourgeois C, Ferré F. Embryo-maternal interactions at the implantation site: a delicate equilibrium. Eur J Obstet Gynecol Reprod Biol. 1999;83(1):85-100.
6. Diedrich K, Fauser BC, Devroey P, G Griesinger, Evian Annual Reproduction (EVAR) Workshop Group. The role of the endometrium and embryo in human implantation. Hum Reprod Update. 2007;13(4):365-77.
7. Noyes RW, Hertig AT, Rock J. Dating the endometrial biopsy. Am J Obstet Gynecol. 1975;122(2):262-3.
8. Johannisson E, Landgren BM, Rohr HP, Diczfalusy E. Endometrial morphology and peripheral hormone levels in women regular menstrual cycles. Fertil Steril. 1987;48(3):401-8.
9. Edwards RG. The physiological and molecular aspects of implantation. Hum Reprod. 1995;10(suppl 2):1-13.
10. Nikas G. Cell-surface morphological events relevant to human implantation. Hum Reprod. 1999;14 (Suppl 2):37-44.
11. Fox C, Morin S, Jeong JW, Scott RT Jr, Lessey BA. Local and systemic factors and implantation: what is the evidence? Fertil Steril. 2016;105(4):873-84.
12. Díaz-Gimeno P, Ruíz-Alonso M, Blesa D, Simón C. Transcriptomics of the human endometrium. Int J Dev Biol. 2014;58(2-4):127-37.
13. Talbi S, Hamilton AE, Vo KC, Tulac S, Overgaard MT, Dosiou C, et al. Molecular phenotyping of human endometrium distinguishes menstrual cycle phases and underlying biological processes in normo-ovulatory women. Endocrinology. 2006;147(3):1097-121.
14. Critchley HO, Kelly RW, Brenner RM, Baird DT. The endocrinology of menstruation–a role for the immune system. Clin Endocrinol (Oxf). 2001;55(6):701-10.
15. Carson DD, Bagchi I, Dey SK, Enders AC, Fazleabas AT, Lessey BA, et al. Embryo implantation. Dev Biol. 2000;223(2):217-37.
16. Banerjee P, Fazleabas AT. Endometrial responses to embryonic signals in the primate. Int J Dev Biol. 2010;54(2-3):295-302.
17. Cavagna M, Mantese JC. Biomarkers of endometrial receptivity–a review. Placenta. 2003;24(Suppl B):S39-47.
18. Lessey BA, Damjanovich L, Coutfaris C, Castelbaum A, Albelda SM, Buck CA. Integrin adhesion molecules in the human endometrium: correlation with the normal and abnormal menstrual cycle. J Clin Invest. 1992;90(1):188-95.
19. Lessey BA, Castelbaum AJ, Buck CA, Lei Y, Yowell CW, Sun J. Further characterization of endometrial integrins during the menstrual cycle and in pregnancy. Fertil Steril. 1994;62(3):497-506.
20. Tabibzadeh S, Kong QF, Babaknia A. Expression of adhesion molecules in human endometrial vasculature throughout the menstrual cycle. J Clin Endocrinol Metab. 1994;79(4):1024-32.
21. Franasiak J, Holoch K, Yuan L, Schammel DP, Young SL, Lessey BA, et al. Prospective assessment of midsecretory endometrial leukemia inhibitor factor expression versus $\alpha v\beta 3$ testing in women with unexplained infertility. Fertil Steril. 2014;101(6):1724-31.
22. Dimitriadis E, Nie G, Hannan NJ, Paiva P, Salamonsen LA. Local regulation of implantation at the human fetal-maternal interface. Int J Dev Biol. 2010;54(2-3):313-22.
23. Sarno JL, Kliman HJ, Taylor HS. HOXA10, Pbx2, and Meis1 protein expression in the human endometrium: formation of multimeric complexes on HOXA10 target genes. J Clin Endocrinol Metab. 2005;90(1):522-8.
24. Taylor HS, Arici A, Olive D, Igarashi P. HOXA10 is expressed in response to sex steroids at the time of implantation in the human endometrium. J Clin Invest. 1998;101(7):1379-84.

25. Taylor HS, Igarashi P, Olive DL, Arici A. Sex steroids mediate HOXA11 expression in the human peri-implantation endometrium. J Clin Endocrinol Metab. 1999;84(3):1129-35.
26. Cakmak H, Taylor HS. Implantation failure: molecular mechanisms and clinical treatment. Hum Reprod Update. 2011;17(2):242-53.
27. Rackow BW, Taylor HS. Submucosal uterine leiomyomas have a global effect on molecular determinants of endometrial receptivity. Fertil Steril. 2010;93(6):2027-34.
28. Ruan YC, Chen H, Chan HC. Ion channels in the endometrium: regulation of endometrial receptivity and embryo implantation. Hum Reprod Update. 2014;20(4): 517-29.
29. Bauersachs S, Wolf E. Immune aspects of embryo-maternal cross-talk in the bovine uterus. J Reprod Immunol. 2013;97(1):20-6.
30. Fujiwara H. Immune cells contribute to systemic cross-talk between the embryo and mother during early pregnancy in cooperation with the endocrine system. Reprod Med Biol. 2006;5:19-29.
31. Vacca P, Vitale C, Montaldo E, Conte R, Cantoni C, Fulcheri E, et al. $CD34^+$ hematopoietic precursors are present in human decidua and differentiate into natural killer cells upon interaction with stromal cells. Proc Natl Acad Sci USA. 2011;108:2402-7.
32. Sfakianoudis K, Rapani A, Grigoriadis S, Pantou A, Maziotis E, Kokkini G, et al. The Role of Uterine Natural Killer Cells on Recurrent Miscarriage and Recurrent Implantation Failure: From Pathophysiology to Treatment. Biomedicines. 2021;9(10):1425
33. Hviid MM, Macklon N. Immune modulation treatments—where is the evidence? Fertil Steril. 2017;107(6):1284-93.
34. Tang AW, Alfirevic Z, Quenby S. Natural killer cells and pregnancy outcomes in women with recurrent miscarriage and infertility: a systematic review. Hum Reprod. 2011;26: 1971-80.
35. Seshadri S, Sunkara SK. Natural killer cells in female infertility and recurrent miscarriage: a systematic review and meta-analysis. Hum Reprod Update. 2014;20:429-38.
36. Fujiwara H, Araki Y, Imakawa K, Saito S, Daikoku T, Shigeta M, et al. Dual positive regulation of embryo implantation by endocrine and immune systems—step-by-step maternal recognition of the developing embryo. Am J Reprod Immunol. 2016;75(3):281-9.
37. Kane N, Kelly R, Saunders PT, Critchley HO. Proliferation of uterine natural killer cells is induced by human chorionic gonadotropin and mediated via the mannose receptor. Endocrinol. 2009;150:2882-8.
38. Carson DD, Lagow E, Thathiah A, Al-Shami R, Farach-Carson M, Vernon M, et al. Changes in gene expression during the early to mid-luteal (receptive phase) transition in human endometrium detected by high-density microarray screening. Mol Hum Reprod. 2002;8(9):871-9.
39. Borthwick JM, Charnock-Jones DS, Tom BD, Hull ML, Teirney R, Phillips SC, et al. Determination of the transcript profile of human endometrium. Mol Hum Reprod. 2003;9(1):19-33.
40. Riesewijk A, Martín J, van Os R, Horcajadas JA, Polman J, Pellicer A, et al. Gene expression profiling of human endometrial receptivity on days LH+2 versus LH+7 by microarray technology. Hum Reprod. 2003;9(5):253-64.
41. Moreno I, Codoñer FM, Vilella F, Valbuena D, Martinez-Blanch JF, Jimenez-Almazán J, et al. Evidence that the endometrial microbiota has an effect on implantation success or failure. Am J Obstet Gynecol. 2016;215(6):684-703.
42. Mahajan N. Endometrial receptivity array: clinical application. J Hum Reprod Sci. 2015;8(3):121-9.
43. Ruiz-Alonso M, Blesa D, Díaz-Gimeno P, Gómez E, Fernández-Sánchez M, Carranza F, et al. The endometrial receptivity array for diagnosis and personalized embryo transfer as a treatment for patients with repeated implantation failure. Fertil Steril. 2013;100(3):818-24.
44. Simo'n C, Go'mez C, Cabanillas S, Vladimirov L, Castillo'n G, Giles J, et al. A 5-year multicenter randomized controlled trial comparing personalized, frozen and fresh blastocyst transfer in IVF. Reprod Biomed Online. 2020;41:402-15.
45. Macklon NS, Brosens JJ. The human endometrium as a sensor of embryo quality. Biol Reprod. 2014;91(4):98.
46. Coughlan C, Ledger W, Wang Q, Liu F, Demirol A, Gurgan T, et al. Recurrent implantation failure: definition and management. Reprod BioMed Online. 2014;28(1):14-38.
47. He B, Ni ZL, Kong SB, Lu JH, Wang HB. Homeobox genes for embryo implantation: From mouse to human. Animal Models and Experimental Medicine. 2018;1(1):14-22.
48. Pabuccu R, Gomel V. Reproductive outcome after hysteroscopic metroplasty in women with septate uterus and otherwise unexplained infertility. Fertil Steril. 2004;81(6):1675-8.
49. Practice Committee of the American Society for Reproductive Medicine. Uterine septum: a guideline. Fertil Steril. 2016; 106(3):530-40.
50. Makrakis E, Pantos K. The outcomes of hysteroscopy in women with implantation failures after in vitro fertilization: findings and effect on subsequent pregnancy rates. Curr Opin Obstet Gynecol. 2010;22(4):339-43.
51. Demirol A, Gurgan T. Effect of treatment of intrauterine pathologies with office hysteroscopy in patients with recurrent IVF failure. Reprod Biomed Online. 2004;8(5): 590-4.
52. Practice Committee of the American Society for Reproductive Medicine. Removal of myomas in asymptomatic patients to improve fertility and/or reduce miscarriage rate: a guideline. Fertil Steril. 2017;108(3):416-25.
53. Strandell A, Lindhard A, Waldenstrom U, Thorburn J, Janson PO, Hamberger L. Hydrosalpinx and IVF outcome: a prospective, randomized multicentre trial in Scandinavia on salpingectomy prior to IVF. Hum Reprod. 1999;14(11):2762-9.
54. Campo S, Campo V, Benagiano G. Infertility and adenomyosis. Obstet Gynecol Int. 2012;2012:1-8.
55. Kissler S, Hamscho N, Zangos S, Wiegratz I, Schlichter S, Menzel C, et al. Uterotubal transport disorder in adenomyosis and endometriosis—a cause for infertility. BJOG. 2006;113(8):902-8.
56. Jiang Y, Jiang R, Cheng X, Zhang Q, Hu Y, Zhang H, et al. Decreased expression of NR4A nuclear receptors in adenomyosis impairs endometrial decidualization. Mol Hum Reprod. 2016;22(9):655-68.
57. Taylor HS, Bagot C, Kardana A, Olive D, Arici A, et al. HOX gene expression is altered in the endometrium of women with endometriosis. Hum Reprod. 1999;14(5):1328-31.
58. Tremellen KP, Russell P. The distribution of immune cells and macrophages in the endometrium of women with recurrent reproductive failure. II: adenomyosis and macrophages. J Reprod Immunol. 2012;93(1):58-63.
59. Lan J, Wu Y, Wu Z, Wu Y, Yang R, Liu Y, et al. Ultra-Long GnRH agonist protocol during IVF/ICSI improves pregnancy outcomes in women with adenomyosis: a retrospective cohort study. Front Endocrinol. 2021;12: 609771.
60. Mahajan N, Sharma S. The endometrium in assisted reproductive technology: How thin is thin? J Hum Reprod Sci. 2016;9(1):3-8.

SECTION

2 Reproductive Endocrinology

CHAPTER 8

Synthesis and Metabolism of Steroid Hormones

R Suchindra

INTRODUCTION

Steroid hormones, the lipophilic molecules, are synthesized from cholesterol which in turn is formed from acetate.[1] Plasma low-density lipoproteins derived from diet contribute to the major part of cholesterol. Cholesterol produced in the liver circulates in the form of high-density lipoprotein and low-density lipoprotein. Major sites of steroid synthesis include the adrenals, testes, ovaries, and placenta. Recently, neurosteroids have been discovered in the central nervous system and they have mainly "autocrine" or "paracrine" functions.

STEROID HORMONE SYNTHESIS

The four major types of steroid hormones are progestins, androgens, estrogens, and corticoids, which contain 21, 19, 18, and 21 carbons, respectively.[2] Steroid hormones are synthesized by dehydrogenases and cytochrome P450 enzymes from cholestane, a common cholesterol precursor through hydroxylation and dehydroxylation-oxidation reactions.

Cytochromes P450 are membrane-bound oxidative enzymes present in either the endoplasmic reticulum or inner mitochondrial membranes of steroidogenic cells.[3] Six cytochrome P450 enzymes are involved in the steroidogenesis.

The rate-limiting step for the synthesis of all steroid hormones is cleavage of the side chain from cholesterol (C27) to yield pregnenolone (C21) which is catalyzed by P450 cholesterol side-chain cleavage enzyme (P450scc). The anterior pituitary trophic hormones such as follicle-stimulating hormone (FSH), luteinizing hormone (LH), and adrenocorticotropic hormone (ACTH) regulate the synthesis and secretion of steroid hormones (adrenal and gonadal) through negative feedback mechanisms.

Angiotensin II and ion concentrations in the circulation regulate the mineralocorticoids synthesis.

Synthesis of Progesterone

Pregnenolone is the principal precursor for the synthesis of all the other steroid hormones by the testes, ovary, and adrenals. The rate-limiting step for the progesterone synthesis is side-chain cleavage of cholesterol by the enzyme cytochrome P450scc to yield pregnenolone. 3β-hydroxysteroid dehydrogenase (3β-HSD) converts pregnenolone into progesterone.

Progesterone produced during folliculogenesis serves as an intermediate for synthesis of androgen and estrogen. Whereas in the periovulatory and luteal phases, progesterone serves as a primary secretory hormone from the ovary. During the early stages of folliculogenesis, the synthesis of P4 is under the control of FSH and later in the ovarian cycle LH plays a role due to acquisition of LH receptors in the growing follicle. In early pregnancy, the increasing levels of human chorionic gonadotropin (hCG) stimulates the corpus luteum to synthesize and secrete progesterone. During pregnancy, the placenta secretes high levels of progesterone by a different isoenzyme of 3β-HSD (i.e., type I).

Synthesis of Androgen

The primary sites of androgen synthesis and secretion are the Leydig cells of the testes, theca cells of the ovary, and cells in the reticularis region of the adrenals. In the testis, LH stimulates the synthesis of testosterone by upregulating the levels of 17α-hydroxylase and C17,20-lyase. It is a rate-limiting enzyme for the conversion of C21 steroids into androgens. Testosterone is the predominant circulating androgen in the body. The circulating testosterone taken up by the target issues is reduced by 5α-reductase to an active metabolite 5α-dihydrotestosterone (5α-DHT). By a process of aromatization, the aromatase enzyme converts testosterone and androstenedione into estrogens such as 17β-estradiol (E2) or estrone. It is present in the granulosa cells of the ovary, Leydig cells of the testes, and other tissues including the pituitary, brain, placenta, liver, and adipose tissue. The testosterone exerts its effects on the target tissues mainly after conversion into either 5α-DHT or E2 within the tissues.

Synthesis of Estrogen

The predominant estrogen and progestin hormones (estradiol and progesterone) are synthesized primarily by maturing follicles of the ovary, corpus luteum, and the placenta. During folliculogenesis, androstenedione and testosterone are synthesized in the theca cells under the influence of LH. These hormones are subsequently aromatized in the granulosa cells to estrone and E2, respectively.

The production of estrogens and aromatase activity in the granulosa cells is under the control of FSH during midfollicular phases. Later in the cycle, E2 production is regulated by LH through the expression of greater number of LH receptors in the follicle and corpora lutea. During pregnancy, the placenta secretes large amounts of E2 by utilizing androgen precursors from the fetal adrenal gland.

Steroidogenesis in the Adrenal Cortex

The adrenal cortex is divided into three zones: (1) zona glomerulosa (outer zone), (2) zona fasciculata (intermediate), and (3) central zona reticularis. Each zone synthesizes a specific steroid hormone, the mineralocorticoids, glucocorticoids, and androgens, respectively. ACTH regulates mainly glucocorticoid production and weak androgen production via the cyclic adenosine monophosphate (cAMP)-mediated protein kinase A pathway that activates factors such as steroidogenic acute regulatory protein (StAR) and steroidogenic factor-1. Angiotensin II and potassium increases mineralocorticoid synthesis via the inositol triphosphate or diacylglycerol-mediated protein kinase C pathway.

Glucocorticoids play an important role in glucose homeostasis, stress response, fetal lung development, immune modulation, and maintenance of normal function of the tissues. Mineralocorticoids regulate the Na^+/K^+ balance in extracellular fluids.

In the adrenal cortex, the enzyme 21-hydroxylase (CYP21) plays an important role in the biosynthesis of mineralocorticoids and glucocorticoids. It is present in the smooth endoplasmic reticulum of all three zones and converts progesterone and 17α-hydroxyprogesterone to 11-deoxycorticosterone (mineralocorticoid) and 11-deoxycortisol (glucocorticoid) **(Flowchart 1)**.

These precursor hormones are in turn converted to the biologically active hormones aldosterone and cortisol by the two unique mitochondrial enzymes in the adrenal cortex, aldosterone synthase (CYP11B2) and steroid 11β-hydroxylase

Flowchart 1: Adrenal steroidogenesis pathway.

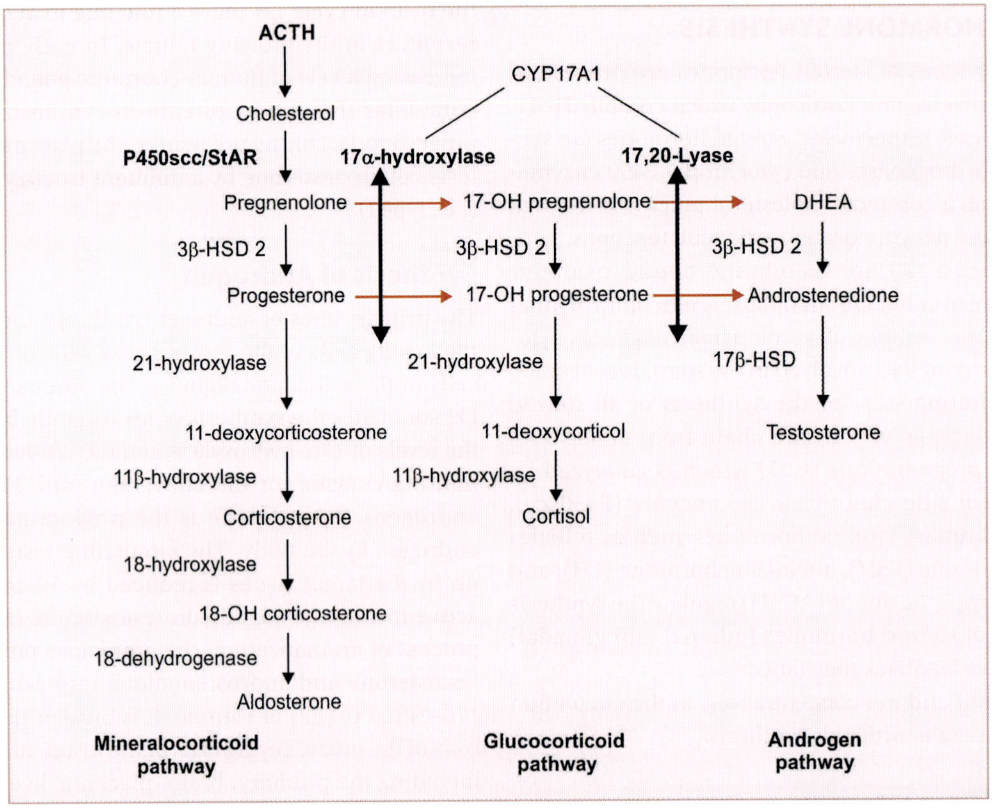

(ACTH: adrenocorticotropic hormone; DHEA: dehydroepiandrosterone; OH: hydroxylase; P450scc: P450 cholesterol side-chain cleavage enzyme; StAR: steroidogenic acute regulatory protein; 3β-HSD: 3β-hydroxysteroid dehydrogenase; 17β-HSD: 17β-hydroxysteroid dehydrogenase)

(CYP11B1). CYP11B1 seen in the zona fasciculata and reticularis has got only 11β-hydroxylase activity. CYP17, a single enzyme with both 17α-hydroxylase and 17,20-lyase activities, helps in the formation of adrenal androgens. CYP17 is also found in other steroidogenic tissues like ovary and testis but absent in human placenta.

The enzyme CYP17 has two distinct catalytic sites and it is expressed in the smooth endoplasmic reticulum. CYP17 hydroxylates pregnenolone and progesterone to form 17α-hydroxypregnenolone and 17α-hydroxyprogesterone. This process of hydroxylation occurs in the zona reticularis and fasciculata but not in the zona glomerulosa. So in the zona glomerulosa, from the C21-deoxysteroids, the mineralocorticoid aldosterone is produced as the final product.

In the zona fasciculata, where CYP17 hydroxylase activity is present but lyase is absent, C21, 17-hydroxysteroids are produced, and the main product formed is the glucocorticoid cortisol.[4] Where both the activities are seen in the zona reticularis, the 17α-hydroxylated steroids (17α-hydroxy-pregnenolone and 17α-hydroxyprogesterone) are converted to the weak androgens dehydroepiandrosterone (DHEA) and androstenedione, respectively.

Human Ovarian Steroidogenesis

The ovaries play an important role in the oogenesis and steroid hormone production. The two pituitary gonadotropins, FSH and LH are essential for the growth and development of the follicles. In the early antral follicles, FSH stimulates growth and differentiation of granulosa cells, steroidogenesis, and induces LH receptors expression on the follicles and transforming growth factor-β (TGF-β)-related growth factors.

The dominant follicle in the natural cycle continues to grow and synthesize hormone with decline in FSH concentrations, through increased LH sensitivity.[5,6] The follicular growth and estrogen secretion is mediated by FSH and LH through cAMP.

Follicle-stimulating hormone and LH receptors stimulation on granulosa cells activate the various intracellular and extracellular signaling pathways, such as protein kinase C, adenylate cyclase, and mitogen-activated protein kinase (MAP).[7] There are no known signaling pathways in human theca cells. However, bovine studies have shown that LH action on the theca cells is mediated via the MAP kinase signaling pathway.[8]

Granulosa Cells Responsiveness to Luteinizing Hormone

In the natural cycle, during early follicular phase the granulosa cells show low sensitivity to LH. As the follicles grow sensitivity to LH increases and they show reduced sensitivity toward FSH.[6] In the granulosa cells, LH receptor activation increases the protein production of cholesterol side-chain cleavage and aromatase (steroidogenic enzymes).

A study by Yong et al. has shown that both FSH and LH needed for maximal P450scc mRNA expression and biosynthesis of progesterone.[9] During follicular maturation, LH plays a key role in the steroid biosynthesis through supply of the androgen substrate for aromatase and the regulation of the enzyme activity.

Ovarian Steroidogenesis

The rate-limiting step in steroidogenic pathway is the conversion of cholesterol to pregnenolone which is catalyzed by **(Flowchart 2)**[4,10] cytochrome P450scc enzyme (mitochondrial enzyme) encoded by the *CYP11A* gene. There exists three metabolic pathways for the resulting pregnenolone. Two of which seen in the ovary are shown in **Flowchart 2**. One of the metabolic pathway is via the Δ5 (delta 5) pathway **(Flowchart 2)** in which the initial two steps are catalyzed by CYP17. This enzyme complex (17-hydroxylase/17,20-lyase) exhibits both hydroxylase and lyase activity.

Flowchart 2: Ovarian steroidogenesis in humans.

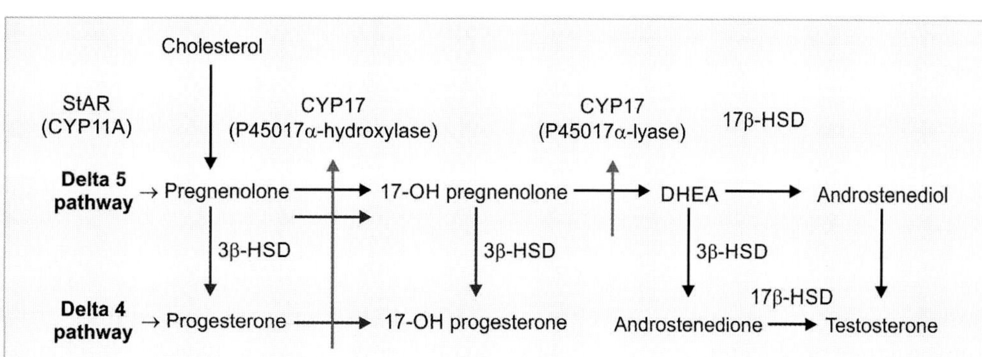

(CYP11A: gene encodes cytochrome P450 side-chain cleavage enzyme; CYP17: gene encodes the enzyme complex 17-hydroxylase/17-lyase; DHEA: dehydroepiandrosterone; StAR: steroidogenic acute regulatory protein; OH: hydroxylase; 3β-HSD: 3β-hydroxysteroid dehydrogenase; 17β-HSD: 17β-hydroxysteroid dehydrogenase)

Pregnenolone is hydroxylated to yield 17-hydroxypregnenolone and further removal of the acetyl group forms DHEA. The enzyme CYP17 is seen in thecal or interstitial cells exclusively,[11] whereas the aromatase enzyme (CYP19) is present only in the granulosa cells.[12] Thus, the androgens required to get converted to estrogens by the granulosa cells of the developing follicles is provided by the theca cells.[13]

Pregnenolone metabolism via the delta 5 pathway is shown by black arrows. An alternative route of metabolism of progesterone via delta 4 pathway is shown in blue arrows. In this pathway, the enzyme 3β-HSD converts pregnenolone to progesterone.

The second route of pregnenolone metabolism in the ovary **(Flowchart 2)** is mediated by the action of 3β-HSD which converts pregnenolone to progesterone. The enzyme CYP17 through the D4 pathway converts the resulting progesterone to 17-hydroxyprogesterone (17-OH progesterone). 17-OH progesterone produced in this pathway cannot be further metabolized in humans due to the species-specific differences in the lyase activity of CYP17.[14] Thus in humans CYP17 acts exclusively on 17-hydroxypregnenolone to form DHEA. But, only very little 17-OH progesterone can be converted to androstenedione.

Thus, pregnenolone metabolized through delta 4 pathway to progesterone and/or 17-OH progesterone serves as the end products in the granulosa cells. In humans, the only route for estradiol synthesis is through the delta 5 pathway. The third pathway for pregnenolone metabolism, which forms aldosterone, takes place in the adrenals.

CYP17 Activity

Factors which Regulate CYP17 Activity

Follicle-stimulating hormone is an important regulator of CYP17 activity in theca cells. Insulin and insulin-like growth factors (IGF-1 and IGF-2) stimulate human theca cells to produce androstenedione *in vitro*, and inhibin produced in the granulosa cells, also induces theca cell androgen synthesis.[15] Inhibitory factors include fibroblast growth factor, epidermal growth factor, TGF-β, growth differentiation factor-9 and activin.[14,16-18]

Implications of CYP17 Activity

The changes in enzyme activity of CYP17 will alter the relative contribution of progesterone from granulosa and theca cells. In theca cells, CYP17 activity mediates the pregnenolone metabolism to estradiol via the delta 5 pathway. This leads to the reduced pregnenolone substrate for 3β-HSD for progesterone production. When the follicle grows, the sensitivity of granulosa cells to LH increases and contributes to the increased proportion of progesterone from the granulosa cells.

Regulation of Other Steroidogenic Enzymes

CYP11A (P450scc)

The StAR protein, which facilitates cholesterol influx into mitochondria, exerts acute regulation on *CYP11A*.

Expression of StAR protein is enhanced by cAMP and by FSH and LH/hCG through granulosa cell stimulation. Chronic regulation is mediated through *CYP11A* gene transcription.

3β-hydroxysteroid Dehydrogenase

The dehydrogenase enzyme 3β-HSD expressed in both theca and granulosa cells is essential for synthesis of all other steroid hormones. The pregnenolone metabolism is determined by the relative levels of activity of the two enzymes (CYP17 and 3β-HSD). Pregnenolone metabolized via the delta 5 pathway leads to production of estrogen and the metabolism via delta 4 pathway leads to progesterone and 17-OH progesterone production. The expression of 3β-HSD is augmented by LH in the theca cells and FSH in the granulosa cells.[19]

Folliculogenesis and Steroids

During folliculogenesis, the general pattern of steroidogenic activity is that small follicles of <6 mm diameter are androgenic and larger follicles are estrogenic and become "progestogenic" in preovulatory stage. Both increased steroidogenic activity and increased LH sensitivity in the granulosa cells contribute to the change in the steroidogenic state in the follicles.[20]

Steroidogenesis in the Testes

Testosterone is the most important androgen produced by the testis. Testosterone plays a crucial role in the development of male secondary sexual characteristics at puberty, maintains adult sexual behavior and function, and necessary for the spermatogenesis in the late stages.[21] The most potent endogenous androgen DHT is formed from testosterone by the enzymatic action of 5α-reductase. This reaction is predominant in the epididymis and prostate where DHT plays an important role in maintaining sexual function. It is also expressed in other peripheral tissues such as skin and liver.

During fetal development, testosterone is essential for Wolffian duct differentiation into epididymides, vasa deferentia, and seminal vesicles and DHT for the development of external male urogenital system. Deficiency of 5α-reductase in men leads to male pseudohermaphroditism with the normal development of internal genital structures.[22]

Leydig cells of the testis secrete testosterone and E2 into seminiferous tubules, gonadal lymphatics, and venules. During intrauterine life, the peak testosterone secretion occurs at 12–14 weeks of gestation under the influence of maternal hCG on the fetal Leydig cells. This peak testosterone secretion is essential for the development of male urogenital system. Thereafter fetal Leydig cells start degenerating leading to decline in the testosterone production.

A second peak of androgen production occurs postnatally at 2–3 months due to proliferation of Leydig cells in the neonatal period and augmented pulsatile secretion of LH. The immature Leydig cells in the testis secrete 3α- and 5α-reduced androgens, whereas the mature ones seen in puberty secrete large amounts of testosterone. Testosterone concentrations decline with increased abdominal obesity and ageing.[23,24] The decrease in testosterone levels is by 0.6–1.1% annually. The decline begins in adulthood and progresses thereafter which results in a net decline of 35–50% from the young adult.

Testosterone synthesis from cholesterol is catalyzed by cytochrome P450 enzyme complexes. Five major enzymes involved are:

1. Cholesterol side-chain cleavage enzyme
2. 3β-hydroxysteroid dehydrogenase
3. 17α-hydroxylase
4. C17,20-lyase (enzyme complex)
5. 17β-HSD type III **(Flowchart 3)**.

The rate-limiting step in steroidogenesis is catalyzed by cytochrome P450scc which converts cholesterol to pregnenolone. However, the StAR protein regulates the delivery of cholesterol to the inner mitochondrial membrane and this StAR protein[25] in turn is activated by LH during steroidogenesis. Any defect in the steroidogenic pathway will result in male pseudohermaphroditism.

Pregnenolone is converted to progesterone under the enzymatic action of 3β-HSD. Pregnenolone (or its metabolite, progesterone) through cleavage and hydroxylation reactions catalyzed by enzyme complex C17,20-lyase and 17α-hydroxylase form androstenedione. Androstenedione is then converted to the potent androgen testosterone by the enzyme 17β-HSD type III.

Testicular steroidogenesis contributes to >95% of testosterone production in men, and only 5% is produced by the adrenal gland and extraglandular conversion of DHEA and androstenedione to testosterone. The average testosterone production in young men ranges from 4 to 9 mg/day.

The aromatase enzyme expressed in Leydig, Sertoli, and germ cells further converts testosterone produced from the Leydig cells into estradiol which is necessary for the initiation of spermatogenesis and mitosis of spermatogonia.[26]

STEROIDS AND PATHOPHYSIOLOGY

Steroid-related disorders include cancers that occur in the steroid target tissues such as breast, uterus, and prostate and steroid insensitivity syndromes resulting from defective steroid synthesis or function and receptor defect.

Disorders Resulting from Defective Synthesis of Steroids

- *Congenital adrenal hyperplasia (CAH):* This syndrome occurs due to deficiency of 21-hydroxylase with inadequate adrenal steroids secretion. It is associated with increased secretion of adrenal androgens following hyperstimulation by ACTH and partial virilization in

Flowchart 3: Testicular steroidogenesis. The principal delta 5 pathway takes place in humans.

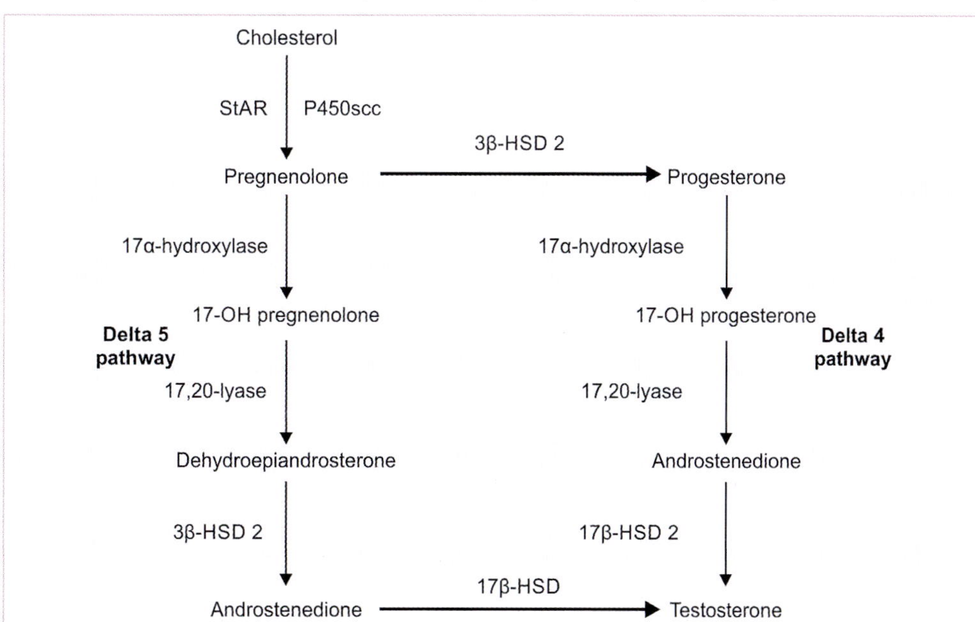

[P450scc: cytochrome P450 cholesterol side-chain-cleavage enzyme (CYP11A); P450c17: C17,20-lyase/17α-hydroxylase (CYP17A); P450arom: aromatase (CYP19); StAR: steroidogenic acute regulatory protein]

girls.[27] Occurrence of CAH due to enzyme deficiencies such as 17-hydroxylase or 18-hydroxylase is less common.

- *Male pseudohermaphroditism:* Defective androgen synthesis in the testis due to the deficiency of 17,20-lyase or 17β-HSD can lead to male pseudohermaphroditism. However, in 80% of the individuals it results from androgen action abnormalities at the target cell level due to 5α-reductase deficiency.

Disorders Resulting from Defects in Target Tissue Metabolism

Deficiency of 5α-reductase type 2 results in male pseudohermaphroditism. It is an autosomal recessive disorder with defective conversion of testosterone to 5α-DHT in the target tissues. In these individuals, Wolffian duct structures develop normally under the influence of normal levels of testosterone with varying degrees of feminization of the external genitalia.

This androgen resistance syndrome with female phenotype usually presents with masculinization due to the high levels of testosterone and/or amenorrhea during puberty. In individuals with complete feminization, inguinal, and labial testes have to be removed due to increase in the incidence of cancer in the gonads.

Estrogen Receptor Polymorphism

The gonadotropins (FSH and LH) and the steroid hormones (androgen and estrogen) play a fundamental role in folliculogenesis. Estrogens synthesized by growing follicles increase both FSH and estrogen receptors (ERs), promote granulosa cell growth and differentiation and prevents apoptosis of the cells. Estrogen affects the oocyte maturation and estrogen levels determine the quality of an oocyte and embryo.[28]

Estrogen exerts its action on various tissues through two subtypes of ERs (ERα and ERβ). The genes *ESR1* and *ESR2* located on the chromosomes 6 and 14 encode the receptors ERα and ERβ, respectively. ERα, the most abundant one plays an important role in reproduction. ER gene polymorphisms have been associated with a variety of disorders including infertility (male and female), endometriosis, breast cancer, cardiovascular disorders, and osteoporosis.

The *ESR1* gene is highly polymorphic. *PvuII* and *XbaI are the two most common single nucleotide polymorphisms (SNPs) in ESR1 gene.*[29] These two SNPs have been associated with the risk of infertility.[30]

Both the ERs are present in testicular germ cells at different stages of spermatogenesis, and play an important role in male reproduction. The receptors show variable expression in *ESR1 (PvuII* and *XbaI*) and *ESR2* (*RsaI* and *AluI*) genes in different ethnic groups. There is a significant risk of association of *ESR1 Pvu*II and *ESR2 RsaI* polymorphisms with male infertility. Asian male population shows a decreased risk for these polymorphisms, while the Caucasians show increased susceptibility to male infertility.[31]

The estrogen receptors (ERα and ERβ) mediate various effects of estrogen such as folliculogenesis, oogenesis, and endometrial preparation for successful implantation of an embryo. SNPs of various reproduction-related genes have been associated with recurrent implantation failure (RIF). These genes include *TP63*, *VEGFA*, *MMP2*, *ESR1*, and *ESR2* genes and *LIF* gene.

A study by LD Vagnini et al. in 2019 has shown that there is a stronger association between *ESR1* and *LIF* gene polymorphisms and RIF with an increase in the chance of women (7.9-fold) presenting with RIF when compared with women who became pregnant on their first cycle of *in vitro* fertilization/intracytoplasmic sperm injection (IVF/ICSI) treatment.[32]

Estrogen receptor-α gene polymorphisms affect male gamete maturation. Prevalence of p and x alleles in ER-α gene *PvuII* and *XbaI* polymorphisms was more among fertile men. Presence of P and X alleles was associated with increased incidence of male infertility (oligoasthenoteratozoospermia) for genotypes PP, XX than the genotypes pp and xx.[33]

Metabolism of Steroid Hormones

- The peripheral inactivation and catabolism of steroids mainly occur in the liver, but some metabolic activity also takes place in the kidneys and adipose tissue. Once inactivated, steroids are eliminated from the body as urinary excretion products after conversion to hydrophilic compounds (conjugated metabolites). The following reactions may be involved in the metabolism of steroid based on its structure:[34,35]
- Reduction
- Oxidation
- Hydroxylations of the steroid nucleus at different positions
- Conjugation (glucuronide and/or sulfate).

Steroid Excretion Products

Steroid excretion products have been shown in **Table 1**.

KEY POINTS

- Steroid hormones, the lipophilic molecules are derived from cholesterol.
- Dehydrogenases and cytochrome P450 enzymes are essential for the steroid hormone synthesis through hydroxylation and dehydroxylation-oxidation reactions.
- The rate-limiting step for the synthesis of all steroid hormones is cleavage of the side-chain from cholesterol to yield pregnenolone.
- Pregnenolone serves as a principal precursor for the synthesis of all the other steroid hormones by the gonads or adrenals

TABLE 1: Steroid excretion products.

Steroid class	*Starting steroid*	*Excretion product*	*Type of conjugate*
Progestins	Progesterone	Pregnanediol	Glucuronide
	17α-OH progesterone	Pregnanetriol	Glucuronide
Androgens	Testosterone	• Androsterone • Etiocholanolone	Glucuronide and/or sulfate
Glucocorticoids	Cortisol	11β-hydroxyandrosterone, allotetrahydrocortisone	Glucuronide

- Pregnenolone metabolism through the delta 5 pathway in the human ovary serves as the only route for estradiol synthesis
- The most potent endogenous androgen is DHT and is predominantly seen in epididymis and prostate.
- Defective adrenal steroid synthesis results in various disorders including CAH and male pseudohermaphroditism
- Estrogen receptor gene polymorphisms (*ESR1* and *ESR2*) have been associated with a variety of disorders including infertility (male and female), endometriosis, RIF, breast cancer, cardiovascular disorders, osteoporosis, etc.

REFERENCES

1. Mason JI, Rainey WE. Steroidogenesis in the human fetal adrenal: a role for cholesterol synthesized de novo. J Clin Endocrinol Metab. 1987;64(1):140-7.
2. Henley DV, Lindzey J, Korach KS. Steroid Hormones. In: Melmed S, Conn PM (Eds). Endocrinology: Basic and Clinical Principles. Totowa, New Jersey: Humana Press.
3. Gonzalez FJ. The molecular biology of cytochrome P450s. Pharmacol Rev. 1988;40(4):243-88.
4. Miller WL. Steroidogenic enzymes. Endocr Dev. 2008; 13:1-18.
5. Sullivan MW, Stewart-Akers A, Krasnow JS, Berga SL, Zeleznik AJ. Ovarian responses in women to recombinant follicle-stimulating hormone and luteinizing hormone (LH): a role for LH in the final stages of follicular maturation. J Clin Endocrinol Metab. 1999;84(1):228-32.
6. Jeppesen JV, Kristensen SG, Nielsen ME, Humaidan P, Dal Canto M, Fadini R, et al. LH-receptor gene expression in human granulosa and cumulus cells from antral and preovulatory follicles. J Clin Endocrinol Metab. 2012;97(8): E1524-31.
7. Conti M. Specificity of the cyclic adenosine 3′,5′-monophosphate signal in granulosa cell function. Biol Reprod. 2002;67(6):1653-61.
8. Fukuda S, Orisaka M, Tajima K, Hattori K, Kotsuji F. Luteinizing hormone-induced Akt phosphorylation and androgen production are modulated by MAP Kinase in bovine theca cells. J Ovarian Res. 2009;2(1):17.
9. Yong EL, Hillier SG, Turner M, Baird DT, Ng SC, Bongso A, et al. Differential regulation of cholesterol side-chain cleavage (P450scc) and aromatase (P450arom) enzyme mRNA expression by gonadotrophins and cyclic AMP in human granulosa cells. J Mol Endocrinol. 1994;12(2):239-49.
10. Wickenheisser JK, Nelson-DeGrave VL, McAllister JM. Human ovarian theca cells in culture. Trends Endocrinol Metab. 2006;17:65-71.
11. Smyth CD, Miró F, Whitelaw PF, Howles CM, Hillier SG. Ovarian thecal/interstitial androgen synthesis is enhanced by a follicle- stimulating hormone-stimulated paracrine mechanism. Endocrinology. 1993;133:1532-8.
12. Whitelaw PF, Smyth CD, Howles CM, Hillier SG. Cell-specific expression of aromatase and LH receptor mRNAs in rat ovary. J Mol Endocrinol. 1992;9:309-12.
13. Young JM, McNeilly AS. Theca: the forgotten cell of the ovarian follicle. Reproduction. 2010;140:489-504.
14. Filicori M, Cognigni GE, Taraborrelli S, Spettoli D, Ciampaglia W, de Fatis CT, et al. Luteinizing hormone activity supplementation enhances follicle-stimulating hormone efficacy and improves ovulation induction outcome. J Clin Endocrinol Metab. 1999;84(8):2659-63.
15. Nahum R, Thong KJ, Hillier SG. Metabolic regulation of androgen production by human thecal cells in vitro. Hum Reprod. 1995;10:75-81.
16. McAllister JM, Byrd W, Simpson ER. The effects of growth factors and phorbol esters on steroid biosynthesis in isolated human theca interna and granulosa-lutein cells in long term culture. J Clin Endocrinol Metab. 1994;79:106-2.
17. Spicer LJ, Aad PY, Allen DT, Mazerbourg S, Payne AH, Hsueh AJ. Growth differentiation factor 9 (GDF9) stimulates proliferation and inhibits steroidogenesis by bovine theca cells: influence of follicle size on responses to GDF9. Biol Reprod. 2008;78:243-53.
18. Fournet N, Weitsman SR, Zachow RJ, Magoffin DA. Transforming growth factor-beta inhibits ovarian 17 alpha-hydroxylase activity by a direct noncompetitive mechanism. Endocrinology. 1996;137(1):166-74.
19. Payne AH, Hales DB. Overview of steroidogenic enzymes in the pathway from cholesterol to active steroid hormones. Endocr Rev. 2004;25(6):947-70.
20. Westergaard L, Christensen IJ, McNatty KP. Steroid levels in ovarian follicular fluid related to follicle size and health status during the normal menstrual cycle in women. Hum Reprod. 1986;1:227-32.
21. Walker WH. Testosterone signaling and the regulation of spermatogenesis. Spermatogenesis. 2011;1(2):116-20.
22. Peterson RE, Imperato-McGinley J, Gautier T, Sturla E. Male pseudohermaphroditism due to steroid 5-alpha-reductase deficiency. Am J Med. 1977;62(2):170-91.
23. Derby CA, Zilber S, Brambilla D, Morales KH, McKinlay JB. Body mass index, waist circumference and waist to hip ratio and change in sex steroid hormones: the Massachusetts Male Ageing Study. Clin Endocrinol (Oxf). 2006;65(1):125-31.
24. Golan R, Scovell JM, Ramasamy R. Age-related testosterone decline is due to waning of both testicular and hypothalamic-pituitary function. Aging Male. 2015;18(3):201-4.

25. Strauss JF, Kallen CB, Christenson LK, Watari H, Devoto L, Arakane F, et al. The steroidogenic acute regulatory protein (StAR): a window into the complexities of intracellular cholesterol trafficking. Recent Prog Horm Res. 1999;54: 369-94; discussion 394-5.
26. Carreau S, Bouraima-Lelong H, Delalande C. Role of estrogens in spermatogenesis. Front Biosci (Elite Ed). 2012;4:1-11.
27. Griffin JE, Ojeda SR (Eds). Textbook of Endocrine Physiology. New York: Oxford University Press; 1988.
28. Loutradis D, Drakakis P, Kallianidis K, Milingos S, Dendrinos S, Michalas S. Oocyte morphology correlates with embryo quality and pregnancy rate after intracytoplasmic sperm injection. Fertil Steril. 1999;72(2):240-4.
29. Sundermann EE, Maki PM, Bishop JR. A review of estrogen receptor alpha gene (ESR1) polymorphisms, mood, and cognition. Menopause. 2010;17:874-86.
30. Ayvaz OU, Ekmekçi A, Baltaci V, Onen HI, Unsal E. Evaluation of in vitro fertilization parameters and estrogen receptor alpha gene polymorphisms for women with unexplained infertility. J Assist Reprod Genet. 2009;26(9-10):503-10.
31. Corbo RM, Ulizzi L, Piombo L, Martinez-Labarga C, De Stefano GF, Scacchi R. Estrogen receptor alpha polymorphisms and fertility in populations with different reproductive patterns. Mol Hum Reprod. 2007;13(8):537-40.
32. Vagnini LD, Renzi A, Petersen B, Canas MDCT, Petersen CG, Mauri AL, et al. Association between estrogen receptor 1 (ESR1) and leukemia inhibitory factor (LIF) polymorphisms can help in the prediction of recurrent implantation failure. Fertil Steril. 2019;111:527-34.
33. Zalata A, Abdalla HA, El-Bayoumy Y, Mostafa T. Oestrogen receptor alpha gene polymorphisms relationship with semen variables in infertile men. Andrologia. 2014;46(6):618-24.
34. Gower DB. Steroid Hormones: Croom Helm biology in medicine series. London: Croom Helm; 1979.
35. Norman AW, Litwack G (Eds). Hormones. Orlando: Academic Press; 1987.

CHAPTER 9

Puberty and Aberrations

Pratibha Saran Malik

INTRODUCTION

The term *puberty* is used to indicate the maturity of the reproductive axis, appearance of secondary sex characteristics, and the ability to reproduce. Puberty is a dynamic process which is brought about by a sequence of events resulting in the episodic secretion of gonadotropin-releasing hormone (GnRH) from hypothalamus.[1] This process is finely regulated by genetic, neuronal, environmental, and metabolic factors.

HYPOTHALAMIC–PITUITARY–GONADAL AXIS

Pulsatile secretion of GnRH into the hypophyseal portal venous system is critical for normal gonadotropin secretion and proper functioning of the reproductive system. The innate GnRH signaling from the hypothalamus to the anterior pituitary occurs episodically (every 1–4 hours). The GnRH hormone is a decapeptide secreted by GnRH neurons which attaches to its special receptors present on the gonadotrope cells of the anterior pituitary. GnRH is also known as luteinizing hormone-releasing hormone (LHRH) as it induces the release of both follicle-stimulating hormone (FSH) and luteinizing hormone (LH) by the anterior pituitary. This occurs in a synchronous manner which is vital for the proper functioning of gonads and normal menstrual cycle.

Onset of puberty occurs by the activation and maturation of the hypothalamic–pituitary–gonadal (HPG) axis and can be described in six phases **(Table 1)**:

1. *Fetal period:* During embryogenesis, the olfactory placode is the place of origin of the GnRH neurons from where they move to their definite destination in the medial basal hypothalamus between 6 and 9 weeks of pregnancy.[2] The development of the hypophyseal portal venous system starts at 6–10 weeks of pregnancy and is accomplished by 19–20 weeks.[3] The axons of the GnRH neurons establish contact with the blood vessels of the portal venous system in the floor of the hypothalamus. The GnRH neurons begin pulsatile secretion into the hypophyseal portal venous system.

   In response to the pulsatile GnRH secretion, the anterior pituitary starts to produce FSH and LH in the circulation of the fetus by the end of 12 weeks,[4] rising steadily to reach a peak at 20–24 weeks and then their levels gradually fall over the last 10 weeks of pregnancy.[5-7] Thus, the HPG axis is active in early intrauterine life.
2. *Function in infancy:* Soon after birth, there is temporary arousal of the newborn's HPG axis. During this phase, sometimes called as *minipuberty*, the FSH rises more in girls and LH rises more in boys. Gonadotropin and gonadal steroid levels escalate to maximum levels at 3–6 months in males and around 12–18 months in females, after which they fall continuously.[7]

   It was initially proposed that minipuberty occurred due to fall in placental steroid levels and the abrupt escape of the hypothalamic–pituitary–ovarian (HPO) axis from their negative feedback effect. But it was later found that the duration of this resurgence in gonadotropin levels is greater in preterm as compared to full-term born infants, hinting toward the fact that it is more of a function of a development of the HPG axis than its mere escape.

TABLE 1: Phases of onset of puberty.

1. In utero	*2. At birth*	*3. Neonatal period*	*4. Juvenile pause*	*5. Reactivation*	*6. Puberty*
HPG axis active in early intrauterine life	Brief activation of HPG axis	Peak at different times in boys and girls	Juvenile pause	HPG axis reactivates	HPG axis active
Axis inactive by birth	Minipuberty	Axis shuts down	FSH > LH	LH > FSH	Onset of pubertal changes

(FSH: follicle-stimulating hormone; HPG: hypothalamic-pituitary-gonadal; LH: luteinizing hormone)

3. *Gradual fall in activity of HPG axis:* The gonadotropin concentrations fall to low levels by 9–12 months in males and 24–36 months in females. The reproductive axis is again shut down and remains hypoactive until puberty.
4. *Juvenile pause:* Between the phases of infancy and puberty, known as *juvenile pause*, the HPG axis lies dormant. During childhood, the GnRH neurons generate pulses irregularly at reduced amplitude, although their activity is not completely abolished. Low amplitude LH pulses are detectable even in children aged 5 years, mostly during sleep. FSH levels rise more than LH levels, but there is no detectable increase in steroid hormone concentrations in blood.

   Gonadostat theory: It was postulated that the phase known as the juvenile pause occurs as there is very small amount of sex steroids in peripheral circulation, which block the gonadotropin secretion since there is increased sensitivity to the sex steroids and their negative feedback effect. However, even children with dysgenesis of gonads have comparable and often excessive biphasic patterns of gonadotropin secretion—first increase at infancy and secondly at puberty too. This proves that anterior pituitary and gonads are not the limiting factors for reactivation of HPG axis. Thus, this theory was discarded. Typical biphasic pattern of secretion of gonadotropins from birth to puberty is by changing levels of central suppression of pulsatile release of GnRH.
5. *Reactivation at night:* During adolescence, the HPG axis reawakens for a third and final time, and the GnRH neurons begin secretion in pulsatile form.

   Luteinizing hormone levels rise nocturnally in the early stages of puberty **(Fig. 1)**. LH increases in amplitude though not in frequency. Peak amplitude of LH rises 20–30 times while peak amplitude of FSH rises only twofold.[8]
6. *Puberty:* As puberty advances, LH rises even during day time but at a lower amplitude.

   Increasing gonadotropin (LH) levels lead to an increase in basal estradiol (E2) and the activation of gonads or *gonadarche*. This is followed by the development of secondary sexual characters in girls[9] and hence breast development known as *thelarche*. Sustained raised basal E2 levels continuously for 1 year heralds the onset of *menarche*. Regular ovulatory cycles start after 1 year of onset of menarche. Regular ovulation gives rise to regular menstrual cycles.

MENSTRUAL CYCLE: A RECAP OF EVENTS

During each menstrual cycle, there is a synchronized interplay of multiple hormones. In the follicular phase, pulsatile release of GnRH stimulates the secretion of FSH and LH, which results in the maturation of the ovarian follicle. The steadily increasing estrogen levels during late follicular phase lead to a positive feedback effect where it causes pulsatile secretion of GnRH with increased frequency. The pituitary has increased sensitivity to GnRH and this triggers the midcycle LH surge that causes ovulation. In the luteal phase, the corpus luteum secretes progesterone which is pivotal to support the implantation of the embryo. If implantation fails, the corpus luteum is involuted by apoptosis, causing fall in progesterone and estrogen levels resulting in menstrual bleeding.

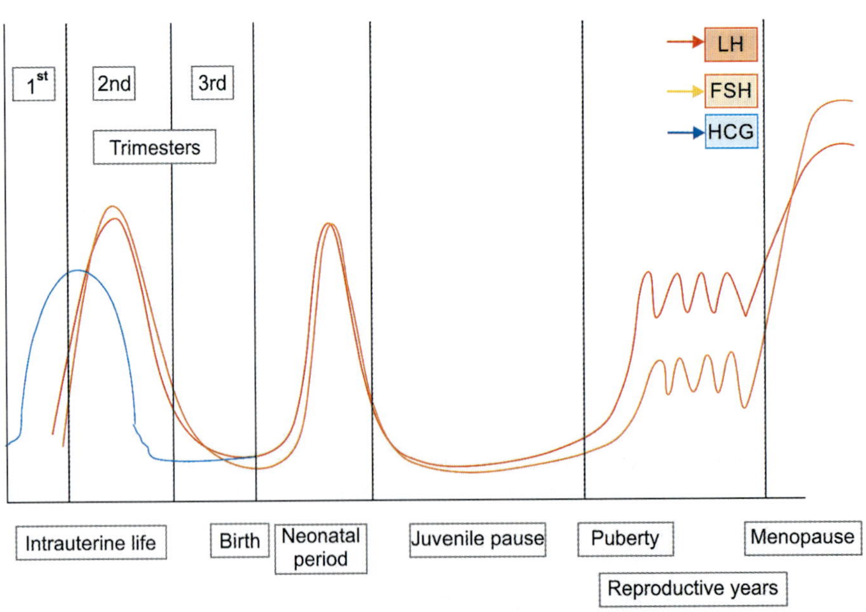

Fig. 1: Gonadotropin levels during various stages of life.

ONSET OF PUBERTY: NEUROENDOCRINE CONTROL

Two pathways are proposed:

1. *Central control mechanism:*
   a. *Gamma-aminobutyric acid (GABA):* GABA is a major neurotransmitter secreted by neurons of median eminence of hypothalamus. It has an inhibitory role on the GnRH pulse generation. Experiments in monkeys have demonstrated a fall in GABA content in the median eminence around puberty.
      i. *Clinical aspect:* Chronic administration of bicuculline, a GABA-A receptor antagonist, activates GnRH release and induces early menarche and precocious puberty in rhesus monkeys.[10]
   b. *Glutamate:* It is a neurotransmitter that stimulates GnRH release via *N*-methyl-d-aspartate (NMDA) receptors. Glutamate concentrations are found to be increased in hypothalamus at puberty.
      i. *Clinical aspect*: Prolonged intermittent NMDA stimulation of hypothalamus activates HPG axis and stimulates puberty in juvenile male monkeys.
   c. Makorin ring-finger protein 3 (*MKRN3*) gene inhibits the secretion of GnRH. Loss of function mutations in this gene leads to central precocious puberty (CPP).
   d. *Neuropeptide Y (NPY):* It is a peptide secreted by the hypothalamus which helps to regulate food intake and reproductive functions. GnRH secretion is inversely proportional to NPY gene activity.
   e. *Kisspeptins:* Exogenous kisspeptin administration switches on the dormant GnRH neurons in juvenile male monkeys.
2. *Peripheral signaling—leptin, insulin, ghrelin, peptide, and free fatty acids:*
   a. *Leptin,* a peptide produced by adipocytes, has receptors in the brain around the arcuate nucleus and ventromedial hypothalamus. Leptin acts to decrease appetite and increases energy expenditure, probably by decreasing the expression of NPY. Around puberty, leptin may play a permissive role by upregulating kisspeptin release.
   b. *Ghrelin* is a gut hormone, which operates as a signal of energy homeostasis. Its function is opposite to leptin. It is also a neuropeptide secreted in the human brain and inhibits the secretion of GnRH. It plays a physiological role in the regulation of pubertal onset and gonadal function.

GENETIC FACTORS CONTROLLING PUBERTAL ONSET

Technology of omics showed that many genes increase in expression at the age of puberty of which the *KISS1* gene is the most important. Furthermore, epigenetic mechanisms have been shown to influence pubertal onset. Imprinting disorders have been associated with CPP. Likewise, many other genetic disorders can affect the pubertal onset.

Kisspeptin System

The kisspeptin system has a paramount role in puberty. The beginning of puberty parallels the maturation of kisspeptin neurons. These neurons, also called kisspeptin/neurokinin B (NKB)/dynorphin (Dyn)/kisspeptin, neurokinin B, and dynorphin (KNDy) neurons, are present in the preoptic and infundibular region of hypothalamus. The kisspeptin axons project to GnRH neurons which express KISS1R, where they signal GnRH secretion. Thus, kisspeptin neurons regulate GnRH neurons.

The *KISS1 gene* on the long arm of chromosome 1 (1q32) encodes the neuropeptide kisspeptin and is secreted by the kisspeptin neurons of the hypothalamus.[11] The kisspeptin neurons also secrete neuropeptides NKB (TAC3 in humans) and Dyn A.

Neurokinin B acts on kisspeptin neuron to cause its stimulation, whereas Dyn A causes inhibition of kisspeptin release; thus, both are autocrine regulators of kisspeptin neurons **(Fig. 2)**.[12] Kisspeptin released from KNDy neurons acts directly on GnRH neurons. An increase in *KISS1* messenger ribonucleic acid (mRNA) expression occurs during pubertal maturation. Arousal of kisspeptin system activates the secretion of GnRH in a regular and pulsatile manner, bringing about the release of predominantly LH hormone from anterior pituitary. This leads to the reawakening of the reproductive axis and lifting the breaks leading to the pubertal switch.

It was shown in some patients with isolated hypogonadotropic hypogonadism (HH) that absent pubertal development was due to "loss of function" mutations of kisspeptin receptor *KISS1R* and *KISS1* gene.[13] Simultaneously, it was shown that an activating mutation in *KISS1R* and *KISS1* gene lead to CPP in girls.[14] Thus, kisspeptin system is an important regulator of HPG axis.[15,16]

Menstrual Cycle and Kisspeptin Neurons

Estrogen and testosterone are unable to act directly on GnRH neurons as the latter lacks receptors for the same.

Kisspeptin neurons express estrogen receptor alpha (ERα), progesterone receptors (PRs), and androgen receptors (ARs). Kisspeptin neurons act as intermediaries as they receive signals from sex steroids and relay it to the GnRH neuron. Therefore, the kisspeptin system has a vital role in the modulation of HPG axis and particularly in the timing of onset of puberty.

Kisspeptin neurons mediate both excitatory and inhibitory feedback of sex steroids on the hypothalamus.

- In the follicular phase of the menstrual cycle, estrogen secreted from the growing follicle acts on the receptors on kisspeptin neurons to decrease kisspeptin and NKB

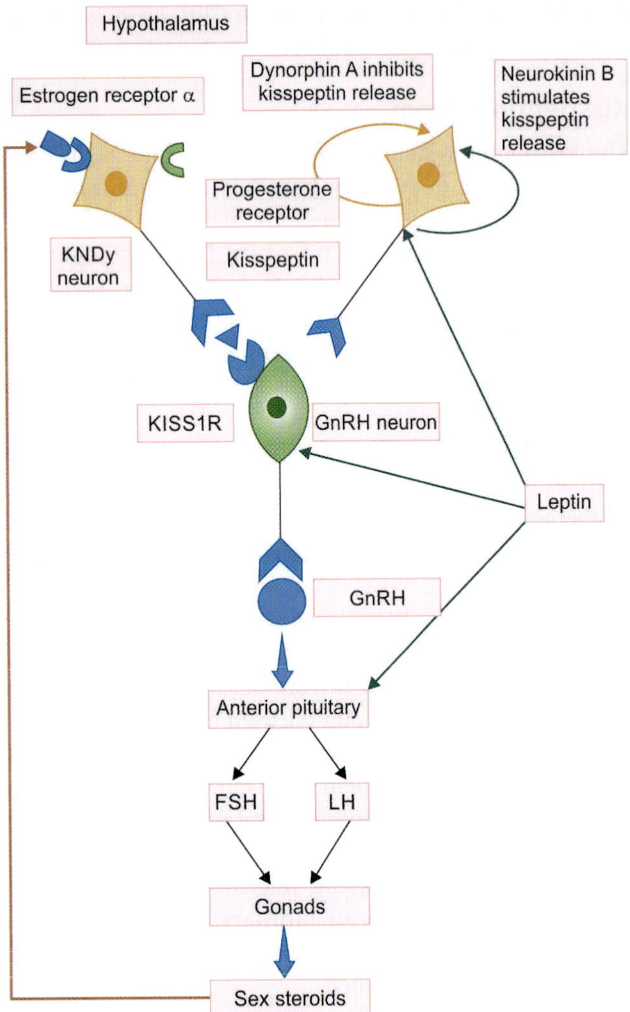

Fig. 2: The kisspeptin pathway.
(FSH: follicle stimulating hormone; GnRH: gonadotropin-releasing hormone; KNDy: kisspeptin, neurokinin B, and dynorphin; LH: luteinizing hormone)

release and increase the Dyn release.[17] Dyn inhibits the pulse frequency of GnRH release from hypothalamus to cause decrease in level of gonadotropin, which causes a dominant follicle to emerge and suppresses other growing follicles. This is the *negative feedback* effect.

- In the late follicular phase, sustained high estrogen levels mediate the release of kisspeptin, which increase the pulsatility of GnRH neurons and lead to an increased LH output from the anterior pituitary. This switch from negative to *positive feedback* of sex steroids induces the midcycle LH surge, which results in ovulation.[18]

Various experiments have successfully demonstrated that administration of kisspeptin induces LH secretion much more than FSH secretion in men and women, although the response is different.[19] The use of kisspeptin as a trigger for inducing final oocyte maturation during controlled ovarian stimulation (COS) is being explored as an innovative way to avoid ovarian hyperstimulation syndrome (OHSS) in high-risk in vitro fertilization (IVF) patients.

NUTRITIONAL FACTORS DETERMINING ONSET OF PUBERTY

Excessive eating of processed high-fat food, physical inactivity, and childhood obesity is consistently associated with early onset of puberty in girls with resultant slightly decreased adult height. Various epidemiological studies across all ethnic groups indicate a trend in relation to earlier onset of puberty, especially in girls, than in the previous century, probably as a result of better nutritional status.

One hypothesis stated that only after attaining a total body fat concentration of about 17% could puberty be triggered in girls.[20] The brain tracks the somatic cues and thus is thought of as the somatometer. In girls, higher body fat is correlated with early puberty.[21] One postulated mechanism of triggering puberty in overweight girls may be due to increased levels of leptin. Increased leptin levels are postulated to induce the release of kisspeptin. Other proposed mechanisms linking obesity to early onset of puberty are elevated insulin-like growth factor 1 (IGF-1), adiponectin, and C-reactive protein levels, insulin resistance as well as decreased levels of sex hormone-binding globulin (SHBG), thus increasing the bioavailable sex steroid levels. Recent studies also point toward vitamin D deficiency to early puberty in girls.

The relation between obesity and pubertal onset in boys is controversial and not yet proven. Few studies indicate that higher animal protein intake such as meat and milk consumption during childhood may be associated with the early puberty. It is thought that animal foods and dairy products cause stimulation of IGF-1 secretion, increased levels of which have been correlated with an earlier onset of puberty.[22,23] Animal foods are rich sources of many other nutrients, such as essential micronutrients and fatty acids, which may lead to an earlier sexual maturation.

Humans are abundantly exposed to environmental endocrine-disruptive chemicals (EDCs), which may lead to premature puberty.[24] EDCs hamper the endocrine system as they may have multiple modes of action, which may be cumulative. Examples include phthalate esters in plasticizers, polychlorinated biphenyls (PCBs) in fish from adulterated water, lead, bisphenol A, and plant-derived phytoestrogens used in packaging of food and beverage. Exposure to EDCs is proposed to increase the kisspeptin secretion. Their estrogenic content may be responsible for the early breast development in girls.

STAGES OF PUBERTAL DEVELOPMENT

The sequence and tempo of the events of puberty greatly varies in different children due to genetic factors accounting for 50–80%. Maternal and paternal pubertal timing is directly correlated with the age of onset of puberty in their children. The variables that may influence pubertal development are genetics, gender, nutrition, endocrine factors, physical inactivity, race, and many comorbid conditions.

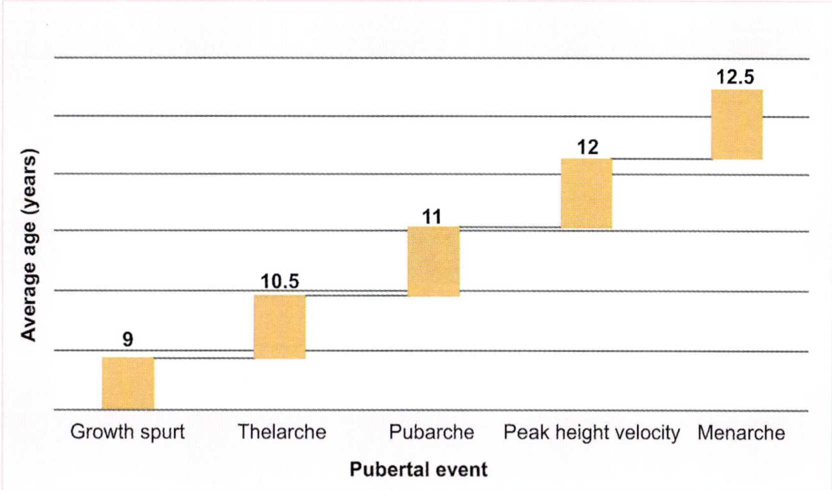

Fig. 3: Pubertal milestones in girls.

Adrenarche denotes adrenal cortex activation and secretion of adrenal androgens, namely dehydroepiandrosterone (DHEA), dehydroepiandrosterone sulfate (DHEAS), and androstenedione. Androgens stimulate the development of axillary and pubic hair, which is termed *pubarche*. Adrenarche occurs independently of onset of puberty.

Gonadarche denotes the activation of the gonads, gonadal sex steroid production, and initiation of gametogenesis. Gonadarche is recognized clinically by breast development or *thelarche* and finally *menarche* in girls and by testicular enlargement and virilization in boys.

In Girls (Fig. 3)

- *Adrenarche:* It starts around 6 years of age. Androgens secreted from the zona reticularis of adrenal cortex increase. Serum level of DHEAS reaches >40 μg/dL, which serves as the biochemical indicator of adrenarche.[25] The HPO axis generally activates 2–3 years after the attainment of adrenarche.
- *Pubertal growth spurt:* Approximately 15–20% of adult height is contributed by pubertal growth, which occurs before epiphyseal closure.

There is an increase primarily in height as well as weight which begins at early or mid-puberty at around 9–10 years in girls and 11–12 years in boys. Acceleration in height is the first sign of pubertal onset in girls. Both the peak growth rate and duration are higher for boys accounting for a difference of 11–13 cm in their final adult heights. Peak growth velocity is a part of pubertal growth spurt and occurs at 11–12 years in girls.

Increase in height is due to elongation of bones due to chondrogenesis at the epiphyseal plate, which is known as the growth plate. Estrogen enhances growth hormone (GH) levels early in puberty. GH stimulates the secretion of IGF-1 from liver and locally at the epiphyseal plate, which enhances longitudinal bone growth.[26] Prolonged high levels of estrogen ultimately result in epiphyseal plate closure, which halts further growth of bones.

Clinically, bone age or skeletal age is found by comparing X-ray of the wrist bones of the left hand to a standard. The Bayley-Pinneau tables in combination with the Greulich-Pyle atlas are used as a standard of reference. Bone age changes as age advances until the epiphysis fuses.

Typically bone age equals chronological age. In those with delayed puberty, bone age is delayed, while bone age is accelerated in precocious puberty.

Insulin is also essential for proper pubertal growth. Besides this, normal levels of thyroid hormones are essential for proper skeletal growth.

- *Thelarche* (breast budding): The first stage of breast development. Average age is 10–11 years.
- *Pubarche:* The appearance of pubic hair. Average age is 11 years.
- *Menarche:* The initiation of menses. Average age is 12.5 years.

In Boys (Fig. 4)

The first sign of puberty in males is *growth and enlargement of the testes* (Tanner stage 2 testicular length >2.5 cm or volume >4 mL), occurring around 11.5 years. In boys, testicular enlargement is followed by growth of pubic hair 2 years later. Axillary hair appears 2 years after pubic hair growth.

Rising testosterone levels lead to voice cracking or deepening and increased muscle mass. Testosterone is converted to the more potent dihydrotestosterone (DHT) by 5α-reductase, which leads to growth of the penis and scrotum, enlargement of prostate, and pubic hair. DHT leads to facial hair growth and is responsible for recession of the scalp temporal hairline.

The *growth spurt* is initiated when testicular volume reaches about 10–12 mL. Boys attain peak height velocity usually at 13–14 years.

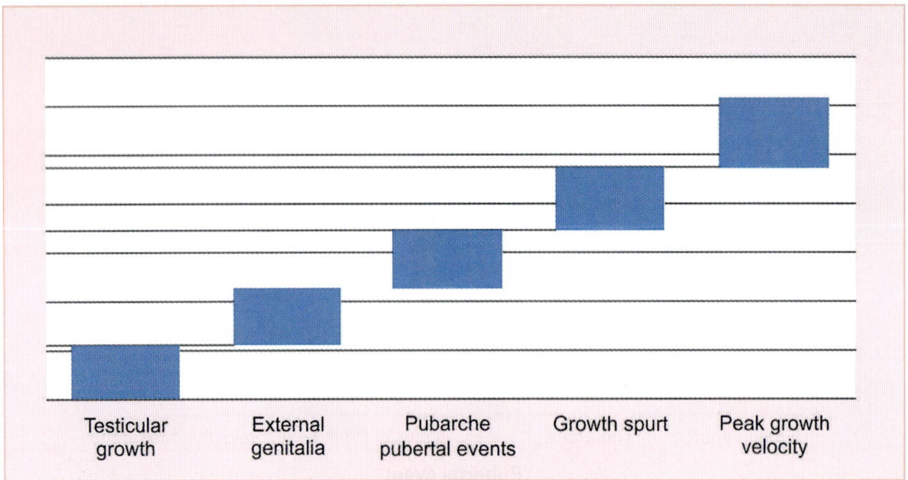

Fig. 4: Pubertal milestones in boys.

TABLE 2: Tanner stages of puberty.

Stage	Breast	Pubic hair in boys and girls	Male genitalia
1	Prepubertal	Prepubertal	Prepubertal. Testicular size <4 cc in volume and <2.5 cm in longest dimension
2	Breast buds (thelarche), growth of both breast and nipple as a small mound, slight increase in diameter of areola. Average age 11 years	Lightly pigmented hairs grow at the base of penis in boys and the mons/labia majora in girls	Growth of scrotum and testes—scrotal skin is thin and red, growth of testis to >4 cc or >2.5 cm, penis remains prepubertal
3	Further enlargement of both breast and areola with same contours. Average age 12.5 years	Darkening, curling, and coarsening of hair, extending over the pubic symphysis	Increase in length of penis. Further growth of testes and scrotum
4	Areola and nipple form a secondary mound which projects above the contour of the breast. Average age 13–14 years	Adult in appearance and extend to the suprapubic area	Further enlargement of the penis in width and length with enlargement of the glans. Further pigmentation of the scrotal skin
5	Adult shape. Areola and nipple merge with the contour of the breast. Average age 15 years	Spread to the medial thighs. May spread to the lower abdomen in boys	Testes, scrotum, and penis are adult in size and shape

Tanner stages refer to developmental milestones that occur during puberty. Changes in the development of breasts, growth as well as pattern of pubic hair, growth of male and female external genitalia are described conventionally in five stages as shown in **Table 2**.[27]

NORMAL VARIANTS OF PUBERTY

In *constitutional delay* puberty (pubertas tarda), puberty starts >2 standard deviations (SDs) later than the normal mean age of onset.

In *constitutional acceleration* puberty, puberty occurs >2 SDs earlier than the normal mean age of onset but not before age 8 in girls or before age 9 in boys.

Premature thelarche is an isolated form of breast development without any other signs of pubertal changes. Follow-up is needed at 6 monthly intervals to differentiate it from CPP. Premature thelarche is benign and may occur due to exposure to EDCs as elaborated above.

DISORDERS OF PUBERTY

Classification of Pubertal Disorders

Pubertal disorders can be due to either precocious (early) or delayed onset. Abnormal pubertal development can cause a huge distress to the child and family members. Failure in early recognition and treatment can lead to adverse outcomes such as decrease in adult height. In some cases, it could be a sign of underlying organic pathology (e.g., tumors).

Precocious Puberty

Precocious puberty results from increased sex hormone production and has been defined as development of secondary sexual characters before 8 years in girls and before 9 years in boys.[28] Precocious puberty may occur due to abnormal gonadotropin stimulation (central cause) or intrinsic disease of the ovary or adrenals (peripheral cause)

BOX 1: Causes of precocious puberty.

- *Gonadotropin-dependent or central or true precocious puberty*:
  - Idiopathic (familial/nonfamilial)
  - Central nervous system (CNS) tumors or lesions:
    - Hypothalamic hamartoma
    - Pituitary microadenoma
    - Craniopharyngioma
    - Ependymoma
    - Pinealomas
    - Optic astrocytoma
    - Optic glioma
    - Abscess, encephalitis, trauma
    - Hydrocephalus
    - Arachnoid cyst
    - Hydrocephalus
    - Encephalocele
    - Neurofibromatosis
    - CNS vascular malformation
    - CNS infections
  - Other miscellaneous cause:
    - Genetic causes
    - Cranial radiation
    - Chemotherapy
    - Primary hypothyroidism
    - Endocrine-disrupting chemical
    - Obesity
- *Gonadotropin-independent or pseudo or peripheral precocious puberty*:
  - Gonadal:
    - Ovarian cysts
    - Ovarian tumors (granulosa cell tumor, theca cell tumor, germ cell tumors)
    - McCune–Albright syndrome
    - Familial testotoxicosis [activating mutation of luteinizing hormone (LH) receptor]
    - Leydig cell tumor
  - Adrenal:
    - Congenital adrenal hyperplasia
    - Adrenal functional tumor
    - Familial glucocorticoid resistance
  - Human chorionic gonadotropin-producing tumors:
    - Choriocarcinoma
  - Others:
    - Familial male-limited precocious puberty (FMPP)
    - Exogenous hormone exposure

(Box 1 and Flowchart 1). The incidence of precocious puberty is almost 10 times more common in girls than in boys.[29] Central causes of precocious puberty are more common than peripheral causes.

Precocious puberty can be further categorized as either isosexual (where there are secondary sexual characteristics that are appropriate for the child's sex) or heterosexual/contrasexual (where secondary sexual characteristics are contrary to the phenotypic sex, i.e., there is virilization in girls). CPP is always isosexual, whereas peripheral precocious puberty (PPP) can be isosexual or heterosexual.

Clinically, the progression from Tanner stage 1 to another in 6 months along with increase in height velocity makes it a progressive condition. It is recognized as early breast development in females and increased testicular volume (>4 mL) in boys. Follow-up of the early signs of sexual development is important. If these signs are stationary at follow-up, then it could be assigned as a normal variant.

Due to early sex steroid secretion, there is accelerated bone development with advanced bone age on X-ray. Thus, there is early tall stature, but due to early epiphyseal closure, there is reduced final adult height. Although there is early physical sexual maturation, psychosexual maturation is lagging, which places these children at risk of sexual abuse, alcohol abuse, smoking, illicit drug intake, teenage pregnancy, sexually transmitted infections, and behavioral abnormalities such as aggressive behavior and poor academic performance. Thus, counseling is important. Early puberty is also associated with a higher risk of diabetes, obesity, and breast cancer in later life.

Central precocious puberty: Gonadotropin-releasing hormone-dependent or CPP is caused by premature activation of the HPG axis, pulsatile secretion of GnRH, gonadotropin secretion, and subsequent activation of the gonads. In most cases of CPP, no cause can be found on magnetic resonance imaging (MRI) of central nervous system (CNS), thus termed idiopathic. The prevalence of CPP is around 1 in 5,000–10,000 children, with a higher prevalence of idiopathic CPP in girls. Several cerebral disorders can cause CPP such as congenital malformations, tumors, or trauma, and such organic causes of CPP are common in boys **(Box 1)**. Among CNS lesions, hypothalamic hamartomas are most commonly associated with CPP.

Among familial causes of CPP is an imprinting disorder due to loss of functional mutations in the *MKRN3* gene. The gene for MKRN3 is present on chromosome 15 near the gene for Prader–Willi syndrome. Only the paternal allele is expressed, the maternal MKRN3 allele is imprinted or silenced, and thus inheritance is from fathers.[30] The average age of presentation of CPP in children with this genetic defect is usually around 6–8 years.

A recent systematic review suggests that small fetuses at birth which includes intrauterine growth restriction (IUGR), small for gestational age (SGA), and low birth weight (LBW) babies are associated with early onset of menarche and puberty in girls.[31]

In primary hypothyroidism, thyroid-stimulating hormone (TSH) is elevated in addition to elevated gonadotropins. Prolactin may also be increased, and galactorrhea may also occur.

Approach to the patient: The evaluation of CPP should include imaging of the CNS (high-resolution MRI of cranium and pituitary) to search for organic causes

Flowchart 1: Precocious puberty.

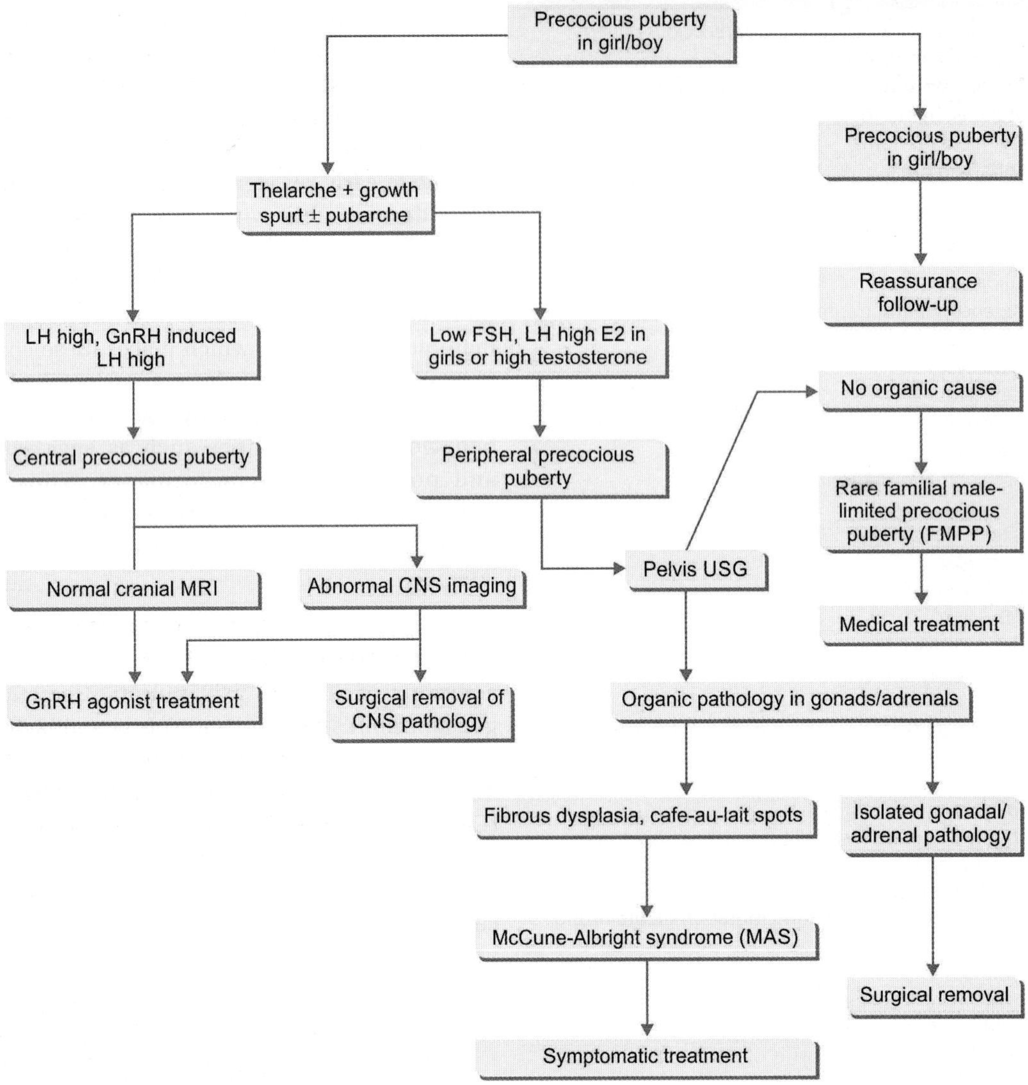

(CNS: central nervous system: E2: estradiol; FSH: follicle-stimulating hormone; GnRH: gonadotropin-releasing hormone; LH: luteinizing hormone; MRI: magnetic resonance imaging; USG: ultrasonography)

(Box 2), particularly in girls <6 years of age, all boys, and in those with neurological symptoms. A funduscopic examination should be performed to check visual fields and to detect papilledema.

Initial workup should include baseline FSH, LH, and sex steroids (testosterone and E2). LH level <0.1 mIU/L by a sensitive assay indicates prepubertal stage. Elevated E2 with low LH may suggest an estrogen-secreting tumor.

Biochemical diagnostic criteria for CPP include **(Box 3)**:

- Baseline LH >0.3 mIU/mL—most reliable laboratory finding for CPP.
- A serum LH concentration >5 mIU/L after GnRH agonist administration (GnRH stimulation test) once a child is 3 years old (specificity of 77%, and sensitivity of 95%).[32]

Bone age estimation by X-ray of the left wrist as advanced bone age (>2 SD) than the chronological age points in favor of progressive CPP and requires further testing.

Pelvic ultrasound for dimensions of uterus and ovaries should be done. Progressive precocious puberty is likely with increase in uterine length >35 mm, thickening of endometrium, and change in shape of uterus from prepubertal to pearl-like shape **(Box 3)**.

Treatment: While some CNS lesions will need surgical treatment, the majority of remaining causes of true precocious puberty (i.e., idiopathic) respond to GnRH analogs including GnRH hamartomas.[33] GnRH analogs should be used only in progressive cases of idiopathic CPP when it presents before 6 years of age. In cases of nonprogressive CPP, only follow-up every 3–6 months is needed. Counseling is important to deal with associated psychosocial problems. Decrease in adult height is a major concern with CPP, and early treatment is successful in preserving final adult height. A recent meta-analysis suggests that GnRH agonist treatment

BOX 2: Evaluation of precocious puberty.

History:
- Age of starting, order, and development of pubertal stages
- Family history in parents and siblings: Timing of puberty in them
- Personal history of any neurological symptoms (headache, seizures, cognitive, and visual changes)
- Steroid exposure in food, drugs, or cosmetics
- Social history

Clinical examination:
- Growth velocity (cm/year)
- Body mass index
- Pubertal Tanner staging
- Neurological examination including visual fields and fundoscopy
- Skin lesions
- Abdominal examination
- Examination of external genitalia
- Signs of virilization

Biochemical investigations:
- Serum LH and FSH level
- GnRH stimulation test
- Estradiol/testosterone levels
- Adrenal steroids
- Adrenocorticotropic hormone stimulation test
- Free thyroxine and thyroid-stimulating hormone
- Serum prolactin levels

Imaging:
- Bone age—X-ray of left wrist joint, bone scans for skeletal survey
- Head magnetic resonance imaging (MRI)/computed tomography (CT)
- CT adrenals
- Pelvic ultrasound

(FSH: follicle-stimulating hormone; GnRH: gonadotropin-releasing hormone; LH: luteinizing hormone)

BOX 3: Criteria to identify girls with progressive precocious puberty.

- Progression of pubertal staging in <3–6 months
- Growth velocity >6 cm/year
- Bone age advancement of >2 SD
- Uterine volume >2.0 mL, long diameter >35 mm, presence of thickened endometrium
- Ovarian volume >2–3 mL
- Peak LH >5.0 mIU/L at GnRH test, peak LH/FSH ratio >0.66
- Basal LH >0.3 mIU/mL, detectable basal estradiol

(FSH: follicle-stimulating hormone; GnRH: gonadotropin-releasing hormone; LH: luteinizing hormone; SD: standard deviation)

has significant improvement in final adult height in girls presenting early before 6 years with CPP, while it points toward the need for additional studies to prove the role of adding GH to this therapy.[34]

Long-acting GnRH analogs are the gold standard of treatment for patients with idiopathic CPP. GnRH analogs are utilized to suppress the HPG axis, pause pubertal development, retard bone maturation, and stop early fusion of growth plates, thus preserving height potential. Leuprolide acetate acts as an agonist at GnRH receptors. It causes prolonged desensitization and inhibits the release of FSH and LH from anterior pituitary, thus causing drastic reduction in output of sex steroids from gonads.

Leuprolide acetate depot is given at a starting dose of 3.75 mg intramuscularly or subcutaneously every 28 days in a child above 20 kg to continually suppress the gonadotropin output. Monitoring of pubertal stages, velocity of growth, and skeletal maturation is done during follow-up. Dose may be increased to 7.5 mg when there are progressive pubertal signs at subsequent visits.

Treatment with GnRH has been associated with a significant increase in final adult height of up to 5 cm, especially when it is initiated in cases presenting before the age of 6 years. The HPG axis restarts again within 3 months after discontinuation of the GnRH analog. Gonadal function is restored promptly after completion of treatment. GnRH analog treatment for CPP does not have negative impact on bone mineral density (BMD) when evaluation is done at least 2 years after stopping treatment.

Newer advances in the treatment of CPP include subdermal histrelin 50 mg implant for long-term treatment over 1 year.[35] Recently, extended-release leuprolide acetate injections of 11.25 mg used once in 3 months have been given in CPP, which has shown to clinically suppress signs of puberty, although it may not provide full biochemical suppression in CPP.[36]

Peripheral precocious puberty: In PPP, sex hormones are usually derived from the gonads or adrenals (autonomous production) or from exogenous sources (pharmacological or environmental). It occurs in girls with a frequency of about 1:400–1,000. Pelvic ultrasonography (USG) aids in confirming the source of the endogenous hormones. The hormone estrogen is secreted most commonly from ovarian follicular cysts. Other causes are gonadal and adrenal tumors **(Box 1)**. Overall, PPP is rarer than CPP.

Congenital or genetic causes include McCune–Albright syndrome (MAS), familial male-limited precocious puberty (FMPP), and congenital adrenal hyperplasia (CAH).

McCune–Albright syndrome is a rare genetic disorder that has a triad of café au lait spots, polyostotic fibrous dysplasia, and precocious puberty. MAS results from activating mutations in *GNAS1* gene, which is involved in intracellular cyclic adenosine monophosphate (cAMP) production, which is present in many tissues.[37] The café au lait spots in MAS have jagged borders known as "coast of marine" and do not cross the body's midline. Precocious puberty in girls with MAC is due to functioning ovarian cysts autonomously producing E2. Long bone X-rays usually depict fibrous dysplasia, although bone age may be normal at presentation. Fibrous dysplasia along with precocious puberty contributes to decreased adult stature.

Other endocrinopathies like hyperthyroidism, GH excess may also be associated. Diagnosis of MAC is primarily clinical. Laboratory tests show elevated E2 with low gonadotropins. Other rare causes are human chorionic gonadotropin (hCG)-secreting tumors and Leydig cell tumors in boys.

Familial male-limited precocious puberty or testotoxicosis in boys is due to activating mutations of LH receptor gene.[38] It is autosomal dominant sex-limited in inheritance. Presentation is with early pubertal development before the age of 4 years, along with rapid growth, minimal testicular enlargement, and pubic hair. This condition is heterogeneous and may present with varying degrees of severity. Laboratories reveal increased testosterone with suppressed gonadotropins. All the above-mentioned causes lead to isosexual or same sex precocious puberty.

In patients with PPP, the sexual characteristics can be appropriate for the child's sex (isosexual) or inappropriate, with virilization of girls or feminization of boys (contrasexual). CAH can result in heterosexual precocious puberty in girls.

Recently, it has been shown that girls with polycystic ovarian syndrome (PCOS) may show precocious puberty. The underlying pathology is ovarian hyperandrogenism and hyperinsulinemia. There may be LBW and IUGR in these girls, and so they are also at risk of metabolic syndrome in later life and need long-term follow-up.

Treatment: Treatment is directed toward the underlying causes. Surgical removal is advised for gonadal and adrenal tumors. Glucocorticoids are used for treatment of children with CAH. In primary hypothyroidism, thyroxine supplementation causes fast recovery.

McCune-Albright syndrome treatment is a challenge due to its heterogeneous nature of presentation. Cyproterone acetate (CPA) and medroxyprogesterone acetate (MPA) are two agents most commonly used in medical management of vaginal bleeding. A combination of anastrozole with leuprorelin has shown to improve predicted adult height (PAH) in girls with MAS.[39]

Various other agents like third-generation aromatase inhibitors like letrozole and selective estrogen receptor modulators (SERMs) like tamoxifen have been tried in MAS to block the estrogen synthesis with limited long-term benefits. Spironolactone (a weak androgen antagonist), testolactone (aromatase inhibitor), and ketoconazole have been shown to normalize growth rate and bone maturation and to improve PAH in boys with FMPP when used over a long period of time. Orthopedic treatment is required for bon deformities.

Delayed Puberty

Delayed puberty is the absence of secondary sexual characteristics by age 13 years in girls (absent breast development) or by age 14 years in boys (no testicular enlargement to at least 4 mL or 2.5 cm in length). In girls with some pubertal changes, the absence of menarche by 15 years demands evaluation. The prevalence of delayed puberty is estimated to be around 3% and is more common in boys. Constitutional delay of puberty (CDP) is the most common cause of delayed puberty (60%) when healthy teenagers spontaneously develop puberty after the upper age limit.

The absence or incomplete development of secondary sexual characteristics by age 18 years in both sexes is classified as hypogonadism **(Box 4)**.

BOX 4: Delayed puberty.

Constitutional delay:

With positive family history, short stature and normal fertility:
- Chronic disease
- Malnutrition
- Anorexia nervosa
- Type 1 diabetes mellitus
- Hypothyroidism

Hypergonadotropic hypogonadism:
- Premature ovarian failure—oophoritis
- Idiopathic testicular failure—orchitis
- Anorchia
- Chemotherapy for malignancy
- Turner syndrome
- Klinefelter syndrome

Hypogonadotropic hypogonadism:

Hypothalamic and pituitary causes of primary amenorrhea:

Inherited:
- Kallmann syndrome (with anosmia)
- Laurence–Moon–Biedl syndrome

Acquired:
- Anorexia nervosa
- Severe underweight
- Intense exercise
- Intracranial tumors, e.g., craniopharyngioma, prolactinoma
- Head injury
- Central nervous system (CNS) infections, e.g., encephalitis, meningitis
- Radiotherapy

Normogonadotropic eugonadism:

Uterine causes:
- Müllerian agenesis
- Testicular feminization syndrome
- Imperforate hymen
- Polycystic ovarian syndrome

Delay in puberty can have major psychological impact both on the individual and their parents. Concerns that need to be addressed are any associated pathology, short final adult height, decision for treatment and its duration, and long-term impact on fertility.

Approach to the patient: Family history of delay in pubertal milestones in older siblings and parents, anosmia points toward familial causes. Personal history of chronic medical illness (fatigue, pain, abnormal stools) suggests underlying metabolic disorder (inflammatory bowel disease), endocrine, or autoimmune disorders.

Flowchart 2: Delayed puberty.

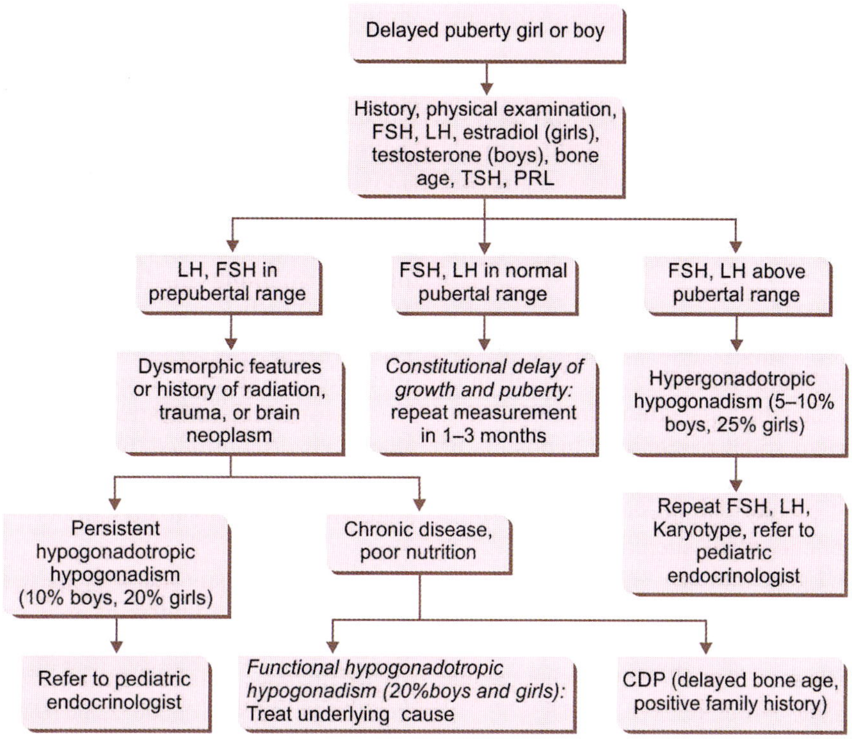

(CDP: constitutional delay of puberty; FSH: follicle-stimulating hormone; LH: luteinizing hormone; PRL: prolactin; TSH: thyroid-stimulating hormone)

Physical examination may show the presence of small penis and/or undescended testis, which go more in favor of congenital hypogonadotropic hypogonadism (CHH). Other features found in syndromic forms of CHH, such as Kallmann syndrome, are anosmia, cleft lip, cleft palate, sensorineural deafness, eunuchoid body proportions (arm span exceeds height by ≥5 cm), and coloboma of eyes. In girls, features of Turner syndrome may be seen, such as short height, webbed neck, shield chest, and cubitus valgus.

Tests such as X-ray of wrist joints may show delayed bone age which goes in favor of CDP.

Basal levels of FSH, LH, and sex steroids are low in CDP and HH, while FSH and LH levels are high in gonadal failure **(Flowchart 2)**. TSH and prolactin levels also need to be done.

Gonadotropin-releasing hormone-induced maximal LH levels (cutoff 4.3 mIU/L) are more in CDP than CHH.[40] Testicular size >2.5 cm indicates the child onset of puberty. Lower testicular volumes (<1.1 mL) are more associated with CHH.[40]

Apart from this, growth velocity should be charted. A slow growth velocity of <3 cm/year goes more in favor of CHH than a functional delay in boys but not so much in girls.[40] Differentiating between CDP and CHH is challenging. Newer investigations include 36-hour LHRH tests, anti-Müllerian hormone, and inhibin B, but they still require further evaluation.

Pelvic USG may reveal the absence of uterus. MRI is helpful for diagnosing dysgenetic or absent gonads and intracranial pathologies.

Karyotype will reveal chromosomal disorders such as Turner syndrome and Klinefelter syndrome. Genetic analysis may be done when karyotype is normal to diagnose rare genetic causes of HH.

Hypergonadotropic hypogonadism is more common in girls of which Turner syndrome is the prototype. Turner syndrome (45X0) is a chromosomal disorder with an incidence of 1:2,500 in live-born girls caused by the loss of an entire X chromosome, loss of a portion of the X chromosome, or complex rearrangements of the X chromosome.[41] Prenatal diagnosis can be done by the combined test in first trimester. A positive screening test can be confirmed by diagnostic tests such as chorionic villus sampling (CVS) in the first trimester and amniocentesis in the second trimester. A karyotype confirms the diagnosis. Postnatally, the girls show classical stigmata of short stature, ovarian failure secondary to gonadal dysgenesis, cardiac anomalies, renal anomalies, skeletal malformations, and autoimmune disorders. Treatment includes GH, estrogen, and progesterone for increase in height and induction of puberty, respectively.[42] Oocyte donation and IVF are indicated for the management of infertility, with caution as coarctation of aorta and other structural cardiac defects, along with many systemic disorders, place the patient in a high-risk obstetric category.

Thus, surrogacy is a better option.[43] Klinefelter syndrome (47XXY) is the most common cause of hypergonadotropic hypogonadism in males.

Premature ovarian insufficiency (POI) is the loss of ovarian activity before the age of 40 years. Although POI in adolescents traditionally is associated with primary amenorrhea and delayed puberty, a proportion of girls will present with irregular bleeding that may be mistaken for expected menstrual disturbances of puberty, thus delaying the diagnosis.[44]

Congenital hypogonadotropic hypogonadism occurs due to congenital deficiency of production of GnRH hormone. When it occurs due to abnormal embryonic migration of GnRH neurons from olfactory placode to forebrain and associated with deficient smell perception, hyposmia or anosmia, it is known as Kallmann syndrome. Kallmann syndrome is four times more common in boys. Anosmia suggests strongly a genetic cause, such as a *KAL1, KAL2, KAL3, NELF,* and *CHD7* gene mutation (all associated with different forms of Kallmann syndrome).[45] HH is considered idiopathic (IHH) when there is an isolated GnRH secretion deficiency in individuals over 18 years of age. Other genetic causes of HH could be due to mutations in *KISS1R.*

Treatment: Correctable causes must be addressed first, such as thyroid hormone therapy for hypothyroidism, dopamine agonist therapy for hyperprolactinemia, and excision of a craniopharyngioma or other operable central lesion. During infancy, cryptorchidism must be surgically corrected at 6–12 months.

A healthy lifestyle should be adopted to maintain normal body weight, recommended daily intake of calcium, vitamin D, and vitamin A.

In girls with Turner syndrome, GH therapy should be initiated early around 4 years of age.[46] Recombinant GH (rGH) is administered at a dose of 0.35–0.375 mg/kg/week given by daily subcutaneous injections at night.[47] Side effects of rGH are glucose intolerance, pancreatitis, slipped capital femoral epiphysis, and intracranial hypertension. Monitoring is done by measuring serum IGF-1 levels yearly with an aim to keep its level below 2 SD above the mean for age. Those girls who are older than 10 years with a decreased PAH with rGH therapy may be treated with additional oxandrolone, an anabolic steroid, at a dose of 0.03–0.05 mg/kg/day.[48] Virilization, enlargement of clitoris, and acne are its side effects. Puberty should be induced with low-dose transdermal 17β-E2 (TDE) at a dose of 3–7 μg/day at 11–12 years of age. Cyclic progestins should be started after at least 2 years of estrogen or when breakthrough bleeding occurs. Hormone replacement therapy (HRT) should be given throughout the reproductive life.

In gonadal failure, long-term sex hormone replacement is the only option, and gamete donation is for addressing the issue of fertility.

In girls with gonadal failure, estrogen is used to stimulate epiphyseal growth. Low-dose conjugated estrogens (0.3 mg) or E2 (0.5 mg) administered daily are effective in hypogonadal individuals.

In practice for delayed puberty, treatment with sex hormone replacement is often initiated in girls older than 13 years and boys older than 14 years as it causes significant psychological stress and low self-esteem. Goal of treatment is induction of virilization or estrogenization, promotion of growth, bone health, libido, psychological, and emotional well-being. In some cases (10–20%), pubertal onset is reported spontaneously, commonly by increase in testicular volume after the initiation of sex steroid treatment which indicates reversal and thus CDP. When therapy is discontinued, pubertal development continues in CDP. Monthly follow-up is needed. As soon as bone age and chronological age match, hormone intake should be stopped.

In CHH, sex steroids may be used for induction and maintenance of puberty as it is cheaper compared to gonadotropins. Gonadotropins result in testicular growth and spermatogenesis and their use is thus more physiological. hCG may be given at 1,500–2,000 IU intramuscularly at twice weekly intervals. hCG is costly and requires more frequent doses as compared to steroids. Serum testosterone levels are done to monitor response and preferably kept in the low normal range. Choice of treatment may be guided by physician and patient preference as well as cost.

Sex hormone replacement is the main available treatment for delayed puberty. Oral testosterone (undecanoate) has a short half-life and thus is not used for pubertal induction. In boys, long-acting injectable testosterone is started at low doses (e.g., 50–100 mg testosterone enanthate or cypionate intramuscularly every month) for 3–6 months. This is done to mimic the natural progression of puberty by gradually increasing the circulating testosterone levels. Monitoring is done by measuring serum testosterone levels 1 week after the injection to maintain testosterone levels in the mid-normal range.[49] In girls, overnight transdermal E2 (6.25 μg) for 3–6 months is initiated. Dose escalation should be individualized. Absence of pubertal progression within 3–6 months is an indication for referral to pediatric endocrinologist.

In CHH, genetic counseling is also indicated. When patients with CHH reach adulthood and fertility is desired, then treatment with gonadotropins is indicated.

GROWTH PROBLEMS IN NORMAL ADOLESCENTS

Growth in the height of humans can be divided into four phases:

1. Intrauterine—governed by maternal factors, placental factors, metabolic factors, genetic, and nutritional factors

2. Infancy—first 2–3 years are governed by nutritional factors and contribute to 30–35 cm in length
3. Childhood phase—governed by GH and thyroid hormone with a rate of 5–7 cm/year
4. Pubertal phase—governed by GH, sex steroids, and thyroid hormone. Peak height velocity is a penultimate part of pubertal growth spurt, which is around 8–14 cm/year.
   Predicted adult height in a prepubertal child can be assessed by taking an X-ray of the left wrist to know the bone age. Bayley–Pinneau tables, along with Greulich–Pyle atlas, can aid to predict the adult height.

Short Stature

Idiopathic short stature is defined as height falling <2 SDs below mean height for children of the same age and gender with no identifiable cause including heredity.

Treatment

- Support and reassurance
- A systematic review analyzing the use of rGH showed an increase in final height up to 3–7 cm with no serious adverse effects.

A recent meta-analysis showed that the use of rGH in children and adolescents showed an increase in the height of up to 4 cm.[50] Drawbacks are the response to therapy with rGH is highly variable, rGH treatment is very costly, has to be injected daily subcutaneously, and the increment in final height is small and modest.

Aromatase inhibitors prevent the conversion of testosterone to E2 and thus may aid in halting the epiphyseal closure brought about by E2.

Use of aromatase inhibitors in prepubertal boys with idiopathic short stature was studied in a systematic review which stated that it may be of some benefit, although 45% of boys reported with mild abnormalities of vertebrae as a side effect of letrozole.[51]

Tall Stature

Idiopathic tall stature is defined as height falling >2 SDs above the mean height for children of the same age and gender with no identifiable cause.

For boys, parents rarely seek treatment. Parents of girls may seek treatment when the PAH is >6 feet or >2.5 SDs above the mean.

Treatment

The most accepted way of treatment is inducing puberty early by utilizing testosterone in boys and estrogen in girls.

Treatment may start as early as 8 or 9 years of age and continue till epiphyses are fused.

Ethinyl E2, 50–100 μg, is started in girls. High doses of synthetic estrogens—ethinyl E2 has adverse effects such as weight gain, headache, nausea, vomiting, hypertension, deep vein thrombosis (DVT), risk of melanoma, migraine, and coagulation defects. Long-term risks on future fertility and risks of carcinoma breast are still not known. If such high doses are producing unpleasant symptoms, then the dose can be reduced or switched to 0.625–1.25 mg conjugated estrogens or 1–2 mg E2 (17β-E2).

In boys, testosterone enanthate 500 mg by intramuscular route is given at 2 weekly intervals.

Surgical method of height reduction by pediatric orthopedic surgery of the growth plates of femur, tibia, or fibula is used rarely.[52]

CONCLUSION

Puberty is a essential stage of life in humans. There can be aberrations and deviations from normal in some individuals. Timely identification and appropriate treatment can pave the way toward a normal transition to adulthood.

KEY POINTS

- Activation of the HPG axis is essential for puberty to develop normally.
- Kisspeptin system plays an important role in pubertal development.
- Central precocious puberty is treatable by GnRH analogs in idiopathic cases.
- In delayed puberty sex hormone replacement may be tried in idiopathic cases.

REFERENCES

1. Abreu AP, Kaiser UB. Pubertal development and regulation. Lancet Diabetes Endocrinol. 2016;4(3):254-64.
2. Schwanzel-Fukuda M, Crossin KL, Pfaff DW, Bouloux PM, Hardelin JP, Petit C. Migration of luteinizing hormone-releasing hormone (LHRH) neurons in early human embryos. J Comp Neurol. 1996;366:547-57.
3. Park SJ, Goldsmith LT, Weiss G. Age-related changes in the regulation of luteinizing hormone secretion by estrogen in women. Exp Biol Med (Maywood). 2002;227:455-64.
4. Kaplan SL, Grumbach MM. Pituitary and placental gonadotrophins and sex steroids in the human and sub-human primate fetus. Clin Endocrinol Metab. 1978;7:487-511.
5. DiVall SA, Radovick S. Pubertal development and menarche. Ann N Y Acad Sci. 2008;1135:19-28.
6. Styne DM. Physiology of puberty. Horm Res. 1994;41 (Suppl. 2):3-6.
7. Grumbach MM. The neuroendocrinology of human puberty revisited. Horm Res. 2002;57(Suppl. 2):2-14.
8. Mitamura R, Yano K, Suzuki N, Ito Y, Makita Y, Okuno A. Diurnal rhythms of luteinizing hormone, follicle-stimulating hormone, testosterone, and estradiol secretion before the onset of female puberty in short children. J Clin Endocrinol Metab. 2000;85:1074-80.
9. Oerter KE, Uriarte MM, Rose SR, Barnes KM, Cutler Jr GB. Gonadotropin secretory dynamics during puberty in normal girls and boys. J Clin Endocrinol Metab. 1990;71:1251-8.

10. Terasawa E, Fernandez DL. Neurobiological mechanisms of the onset of puberty in primates. Endocr Rev. 2001;22:111-51.
11. Roth CL, Mastronardi C, Lomniczi A, Wright H, Cabrera R, Mungenast AE, et al. Expression of a tumor-related gene network increases in the mammalian hypothalamus at the time of female puberty. Endocrinology. 2007;148:5147-61.
12. Skorupskaite K, George JT, Anderson RA. The kisspeptin-GnRH pathway in human reproductive health and disease. Hum Reprod Update. 2014;20(4):485-500.
13. de Roux N, Genin E, Carel JC, Matsuda F, Chaussain JL, Milgrom E. Hypogonadotropic hypogonadism due to loss of function of the KiSS1-derived peptide receptor GPR54. Proc Natl Acad Sci U S A. 2003;100(19):10972-6.
14. Teles MG, Bianco SD, Brito VN, Trarbach EB, Kuohung W, Xu S, et al. A GPR54-activating mutation in a patient with central precocious puberty. N Engl J Med. 2008;358:709-15.
15. Topaloglu AK, Tello JA, Kotan LD, Ozbek MN, Yilmaz MB, Erdogan S, et al. Inactivating KISS1 mutation and hypogonadotropic hypogonadism. N Engl J Med. 2012;366:629-35.
16. Silveira LG, Noel SD, Silveira-Neto AP, Abreu AP, Brito VN, Santos MG, et al. Mutations of the KISS1 gene in disorders of puberty. J Clin Endocrinol Metab. 2010;95:2276-80.
17. Navarro VM. Interactions between kisspeptins and neurokinin B. Adv Exp Med Biol. 2013;784:325-47.
18. Adachi S, Yamada S, Takatsu Y, Matsui H, Kinoshita M, Takase K, et al. Involvement of anteroventral periventricular metastin/kisspeptin neurons in estrogen positive feedback action on luteinizing hormone release in female rats. J Reprod Dev. 2007;53:367-78.
19. Jayasena CN, Comninos AN, Veldhuis JD, Misra S, Abbara A, Izzi-Engbeaya C, et al. A single injection of kisspeptin-54 temporarily increases luteinizing hormone pulsatility in healthy women. Clin Endocrinol (Oxf). 2013;79(4):558-63.
20. Frisch RE. Fatness of girls from menarche to age 18 years, with a nomogram. Hum Biol. 1976;48:353-9.
21. Lee JM, Appugliese D, Kaciroti N, Corwyn RF, Bradley RH, Lumeng JC. Weight status in young girls and the onset of puberty. Pediatrics. 2007;119:e624-30.
22. Kerver JM, Gardiner JC, Dorgan JF, Rosen CJ, Velie EM. Dietary predictors of the insulin-like growth factor system in adolescent females: results from the Dietary Intervention Study in Children (DISC). Am J Clin Nutr. 2010;91:643-50.
23. Thankamony A, Ong KK, Ahmed ML, Ness AR, Holly JM, Dunger DB. Higher levels of IGF-I and adrenal androgens at age 8 years are associated with earlier age at menarche in girls. J Clin Endocrinol Metab. 2012;97:E786-90.
24. Chen CY, Chou YY, Wu YM, Lin CC, Lin SJ, Lee CC. Phthalates may promote female puberty by increasing kisspeptin activity. Hum Reprod. 2013;28(10):2765-73.
25. Rich BH, Rosenfield RL, Lucky AW, Helke JC, Otto P. Adrenarche: changing adrenal response to adrenocorticotropin. J Clin Endocrinol Metab. 1981;52:1129-36.
26. Herrington J, Carter-Su C. Signaling pathways activated by the growth hormone receptor. Trends Endocrinol Metab. 2001;12:252-7.
27. Tanner JM. Growth at Adolescence. Springfield, IL: Charles C Thomas; 1962.
28. Berberoglu M. Precocious puberty and normal variant puberty: definition, etiology, diagnosis and current management. J Clin Res Pediatr Endocrinol. 2009;1(4):164-74.
29. Teilmann G, Pedersen CB, Jensen TK, Skakkebaek NE, Juul A. Prevalence and incidence of precocious pubertal development in Denmark: an epidemiologic study based on national registries. Pediatrics. 2005;116:1323-8.
30. Abreu AP, Dauber A, Macedo DB, Noel SD, Brito VN, Gill JC, et al. Central precocious puberty caused by mutations in the imprinted gene MKRN3. N Engl J Med. 2013;368:2467-75.
31. Deng X, Li W, Luo Y, Liu S, Wen Y, Liu Q. Association between small fetuses and puberty timing: a systematic review and meta-analysis. Int J Environ Res Public Health. 2017;14(11):1377.
32. Giabicani E, Allali S, Durand A, Sommet J, Couto-Silva AC, Brauner R. Presentation of 493 consecutive girls with idiopathic central precocious puberty: a single-center study. PLoS One. 2013;8:e70931.
33. de Brito VN, Latronico AC, Arnhold IJ, Lo LS, Domenice S, Albano MC, et al. Treatment of gonadotropin-dependent precocious puberty due to hypothalamic hamartoma with gonadotropin-releasing hormone agonist depot. Arch Dis Child. 1999;80:231-4.
34. Li P, Li Y, Yang CL. Gonadotropin-releasing hormone agonist treatment to increase final stature in children with precocious puberty: a meta-analysis. Medicine (Baltimore). 2014;93(27):e260.
35. Eugster EA, Clarke W, Kletter GB, Lee PA, Neely EK, Reiter EO, et al. Efficacy and safety of histrelin subdermal implant in children with central precocious puberty: a multicenter trial. J Clin Endocrinol Metab. 2007;92:1967-704.
36. Lee PA, Klein K, Mauras N, Neely EK, Bloch CA, Larsen L, et al. Efficacy and safety of leuprolide acetate 3-month depot 11.25 milligrams or 30 milligrams for the treatment of central precocious puberty. J Clin Endocrinol Metab. 2012;97:1572-80.
37. Lo FS, Chen TL, Chiou CC. Detection of rare somatic GNAS mutation in McCune-Albright syndrome using a novel peptide nucleic acid probe in a single tube. Molecules. 2017;22(11):1874.
38. Papadimitriou DT, Dermitzaki E, Papagianni M, Papaioannou G, Papaevangelou V, Papadimitriou A. Anastrozole plus leuprorelin in early maturing girls with compromised growth: the "GAIL" study. J Endocrinol Invest. 2016;39(4):439-46.
39. Schoelwer M, Eugster EA. Treatment of peripheral precocious puberty. Endocr Dev. 2016;29:230-9.
40. Varimo T, Miettinen PJ, Känsäkoski J, Raivio T, Hero M. Congenital hypogonadotropic hypogonadism, functional hypogonadotropism or constitutional delay of growth and puberty? An analysis of a large patient series from a single tertiary center. Hum Reprod. 2017;32(1):147-53.
41. Stochholm K, Juul S, Juel K, Naeraa RW, Gravholt CH. Prevalence, incidence, diagnostic delay, and mortality in Turner syndrome. J Clin Endocrinol Metab. 2006;91:3897-902.
42. Davenport ML. Approach to the patient with Turner syndrome. J Clin Endocrinol Metab. 2010;95:1487-95.
43. Practice Committee of American Society for Reproductive Medicine. Increased maternal cardiovascular mortality associated with pregnancy in women with Turner syndrome. Fertil Steril. 2012;97:282-4.
44. Webber L, Davies M, Anderson R, Bartlett J, Braat D, Cartwright B, et al. European Society for Human Reproduction and Embryology (ESHRE) Guideline Group on POI. ESHRE

guideline: management of women with premature ovarian insufficiency. Hum Reprod. 2016;31(5):926-37.
45. ESHRE Capri Workshop Group. Genetic aspects of female reproduction. Hum Reprod Update. 2008;14(4):293-307.
46. Gonzalez L, Witchel SF. The patient with Turner syndrome: puberty and medical management concerns. Fertil Steril. 2012;98(4):780-6.
47. Bryant J, Baxter L, Cave CB, Milne R. Recombinant growth hormone for idiopathic short stature in children and adolescents. Cochrane Database Syst Rev. 2007;(3):CD004440.
48. Sas TC, Gault EJ, Bardsley MZ, Menke LA, Freriks K, Perry RJ, et al. Safety and efficacy of oxandrolone in growth hormone-treated girls with Turner syndrome: evidence from recent studies and recommendations for use. Horm Res Paediatr. 2014;81(5):289-97.
49. Soliman AT, De Sanctis V. An approach to constitutional delay of growth and puberty. Indian J Endocrinol Metab. 2012;16(5):698-705.
50. Deodati A, Cianfarani S. Impact of growth hormone therapy on adult height of children with idiopathic short stature: systematic review. BMJ. 2011;342:c7157.
51. McGrath N, O'Grady MJ. Aromatase inhibitors for short stature in male children and adolescents. Cochrane Database Syst Rev. 2015;(10):CD010888.
52. Hannema SE, Sävendahl L. The evaluation and management of tall stature. Horm Res Paediatr. 2016;85:347-52.

CHAPTER

10 Amenorrhea

Abha Majumdar, Neeti Tiwari

INTRODUCTION

Amenorrhea is the absence of menses in a young girl till a particular age or in a woman of reproductive age for a defined period. This is categorized into two types: Primary and secondary amenorrhea. Primary amenorrhea is diagnosed if a girl fails to menstruate by the age of 15 years in the presence of secondary sexual characteristics or by the age of 13 years in absence of secondary sexual characteristics.[1] Secondary amenorrhea, on the other hand, is defined as cessation of menses in otherwise regularly menstruating women for a length of time equivalent to her three menstrual cycles or for 6 months.[2]

PHYSIOLOGY OF MENSTRUATION (FLOWCHART 1)

The normal menstrual flow requires a patent outflow tract between internal genital organs and perineum, i.e., patency and continuity of the uterine cavity with the cervical canal and vaginal canal to the perineal area. To achieve menstruation, the uterine cavity has to be lined with endometrium which must develop under the influence of steroidal hormones secreted by the ovary. These steroidal hormones are estrogen and progesterone; estrogen causes the proliferation of the endometrium and primes it to the effect of progesterone which in turn leads to secretory changes within this estrogen-primed endometrium. Withdrawal of progesterone secretion stops to support endometrial growth and brings about shedding of this carefully designed endometrium, thus resulting in menstruation.

The ovarian steroid production is orchestrated by the higher centers of the brain comprising the pituitary gland and the hypothalamus. The principal pituitary hormones are follicle-stimulating hormone (FSH) and luteinizing hormone (LH) secreted from its anterior lobe, which influence cyclical ovarian steroid production. Hypothalamus regulates the pituitary by secreting pulsatile gonadotropin-releasing hormone (GnRH), which reaches the pituitary via the portal vessels of the pituitary stalk, and thus a hypothalamic–pituitary–ovarian (HPO) axis is established. Environmental factors such as stress, excessive weight loss or gain, and certain drugs can influence the menstrual pattern through the hypothalamus and central nervous system. The ovarian hormones estrogen and progesterone also provide feedback signals to the anterior pituitary and hypothalamus to control their secretions.

Flowchart 1: Hypothalamo–pituitary–ovarian axis.

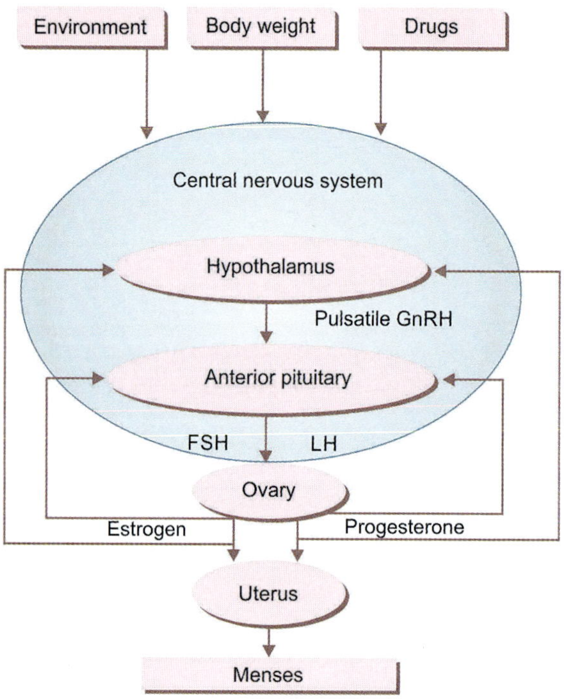

(FSH: follicle-stimulating hormone; GnRH: gonadotropin-releasing hormone; LH: luteinizing hormone)

CLASSIFICATION OF AMENORRHEA (ACCORDING TO THE ETIOLOGY LIST OF CONDITIONS) (BOX 1)

Menstruation is regulated by a complex interaction of the hormonal signals and disturbance at any level can result in

BOX 1: Classification of amenorrhea.

Anatomic or end-organ defects
- Müllerian agenesis
- Complete AIS
- Endometrial hypoplasia or aplasia
- Cervical agenesis
- Transverse vaginal septum
- Imperforate hymen
- Intrauterine synechiae (Asherman's syndrome)

Primary ovarian failure
- *Abnormal karyotype:*
  - 45, XO Turner's or mosaic Turner's syndrome (gonadal agenesis)
  - 46XY AIS and Swyer syndrome (gonadal dysgenesis)
- *Normal karyotype:*
  - 46XX pure gonadal agenesis
- Metabolic disorder: Galactosemia
- Enzymatic deficiency (17α-hydroxylase, 17,20-lyase, aromatase)
- Premature ovarian failure—injury or idiopathic or resistant ovary
- Fragile X syndrome

Pituitary causes
- Tumors—prolactinoma and pituitary adenoma
- Hyperprolactinemia—idiopathic and drug induced
- Necrosis—Sheehan's syndrome or panhypopituitarism
- Space-occupying lesions—empty sella and arterial aneurysm
- Mutation of FSH or LH receptor
- Autoimmune disease

Hypothalamic causes
- Dysfunctional—stress, exercise, and nutrition related
- Isolated gonadotropin deficiency—Kallmann's syndrome and hypogonadotropic hypogonadism
- Infections (tuberculosis, syphilis, and encephalitis)
- Inflammatory or infiltrative—sarcoidosis and hemochromatosis
- Chronic debilitating diseases
- Tumors—craniopharyngioma and hamartoma

Other endocrine gland disorders
- Adrenal—adult-onset adrenal hyperplasia and Cushing's syndrome
- Thyroid—hypothyroidism and hyperthyroidism
- Ovarian tumors—granulosa—theca cell tumor, Brenner tumor, cystic teratomas
- Multifactorial—polycystic ovary syndrome

(AIS: androgen insensitivity syndrome; FSH: follicle-stimulating hormone; LH: luteinizing hormone)

amenorrhea. There are three important areas involved in the causation of amenorrhea. Firstly, it could be the passage to reveal menstruation, i.e., the uterovaginal canal may be absent or obstructed; secondly, the failure of ovarian steroid production which is the endocrine organ responsible for making the endometrial layer to be shed during menstruation, and lastly, there could be reduced or absent stimulus from the anterior pituitary or the hypothalamus to the ovary owing to dysfunction of the HPO axis resulting in amenorrhea. In women presenting with secondary amenorrhea, 66% are either due to hypothalamic-pituitary causes or due to polycystic ovarian syndrome (PCOS), which is multifactorial in origin with dysfunction at all three levels of the HPO axis. Hyperprolactinemia and ovarian failure are further responsible for 13 and 12% of cases of secondary amenorrhea, respectively. In the remaining cases who present as secondary amenorrhea, end-organ failure is responsible for 7% of cases whereas 2% are due to hyperandrogenic states such as ovarian tumor or nonclassic congenital adrenal hyperplasia (CAH).[3]

In cases presenting with primary amenorrhea, gonadal agenesis and dysgenesis leading to primary ovarian failure alone account for 40% of cases. Out of the remaining cases of primary amenorrhea, 22% of the girls have normal secondary sex characteristics such as adequate breast development but have end-organ pathologies. In this group, Müllerian agenesis is seen in 10% of cases, androgen insensitivity syndrome (AIS) in 9%, and other obstructive pathologies in 3%. Hypothalamo-pituitary causes are responsible for approximately 20% of cases with primary amenorrhea. The remaining 18% of the girls have constitutional delay in attaining menarche.[3]

EVALUATION OF AMENORRHEA

In many instances, diagnosis can be clinched based on detailed history and physical examination only. Hence, it is important to keep in mind the common causes while evaluating the patient for the first time.

HISTORY AND EXAMINATION

Primary Amenorrhea

The history of pubertal development is important in terms of breasts, axillary, and pubic hair growth, the absence of which suggests primary ovarian or pituitary failure. If the patient is remarkably short as compared to other family members, Turner's syndrome should be considered. It is pertinent to seek the history of significant stress or change in diet, exercise, and weight to rule out hypothalamo-pituitary causes. The history of severe headaches, fatigue, and visual field defects also points toward hypothalamo-pituitary tumors. If secondary sex characteristics are well developed along with symptoms and signs of hirsutism or virilization, one needs to consider PCOS, CAH, and androgen-secreting ovarian or adrenal tumors as one of the underlying causes. The presence of the Y chromosome, absent uterus, or obstruction of menstrual flow generally presents with adequate development of secondary sexual characteristics. It is worthwhile to take detailed drug history as many drugs such as antidepressants and antipsychotics lead to hyperprolactinemia which can also result in primary amenorrhea. Constitutional delay is a diagnosis of exclusion and is generally accompanied by a family history of delayed puberty.

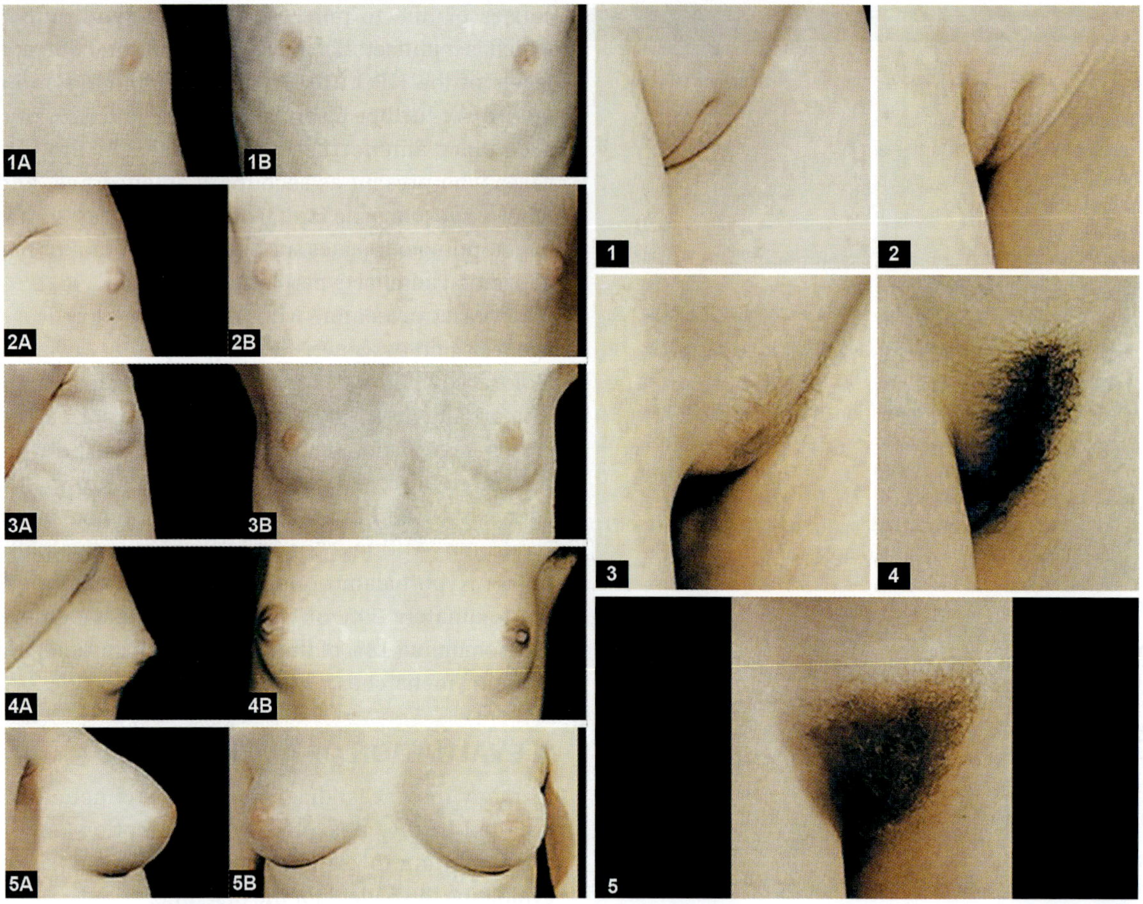

Fig. 1: Tanner stages of pubertal development in female.
Source: Reprinted with permission from Roede MJ, van Wieringen JC. Growth diagrams 1980: Netherlands third nationwide survey. Tijdschr Soc Gezondheidsz. 1985;63:1-34.

Examination of a patient with primary amenorrhea should always be done in the presence of mother or guardian, especially if she is a minor. Evaluation of pubertal changes, i.e., height, weight, and growth charting and Tanner staging of breasts and pubic hair is important in a girl with primary amenorrhea **(Fig. 1)**. We need to carefully look for signs of hirsutism, acne, striae, and acanthosis nigricans. A patient with Turner's syndrome can present with typical stigmata on examination, i.e., short height, webbed neck, low hairline, shield chest, and widely spaced nipples or may have a normal physical appearance. A gentle pelvic examination is required to establish patency of the outflow tract, i.e., hymenal opening, depth of vagina, and the presence and size of cervix and uterus. Fifteen percent of the patients with primary amenorrhea have blind or absent vagina. Clitoromegaly may be found in patients with virilizing disorders such as CAH.

Secondary Amenorrhea

History of significant change in diet and exercise, loss of weight, acute stress, or chronic illness suggests functional hypothalamic amenorrhea. On the other hand, severe headaches, visual disturbances, polyuria, and polydipsia can be due to hypothalamic or pituitary tumors. History of severe obstetric hemorrhage followed by failure of lactation and secondary amenorrhea implies the possibility of Sheehan's syndrome. History of repeated curettage after delivery or abortion or a surgical procedure such as myomectomy or even uterine artery embolization for conservative management of fibroids may be followed by amenorrhea with the development of Asherman's syndrome.[4] This syndrome leads to the destruction of endometrial lining, which can also occur after genital Koch's or long-standing endometritis. Significant weight gain with acne and hirsutism is a feature of PCOS, whereas the sudden onset of virilization with deepening of voice indicates adrenal or androgen-secreting ovarian tumor. Symptoms of estrogen deficiency, e.g., hot flashes, vaginal dryness, and decreased libido along with secondary amenorrhea, could be present due to premature ovarian failure (POF). History of milk discharge from breast makes it pertinent to obtain a drug intake history as mentioned before.

While examining a patient with amenorrhea apart from making a note of weight and body mass index, one must also look for signs of hirsutism, acne, acanthosis nigricans, and striae. Any thyroid enlargement or discharge from breasts should be noted. Pelvic examination is done to look for the presence of vaginal dryness, size of the uterus, and adnexal masses.

INVESTIGATIONS FOR PRIMARY AND SECONDARY AMENORRHEA

- Rule out pregnancy
- Pelvic ultrasound: 2D pelvic ultrasound is done to look for the presence and size of the uterus, endometrial thickness, ovarian volume, and antral follicle count and to rule out adnexal masses or tumors
- Serum prolactin and thyroid profile
- *Hormonal tests:* Serum FSH, LH, estradiol (E_2), and anti-Müllerian hormone (AMH).
    - Low serum FSH, LH, and E_2 levels with normal or low AMH indicate hypogonadotropic hypogonadism and one must look for hypothalamic and pituitary causes in these women.
    - Normal FSH and E_2 with normal or high LH and AMH are generally associated with PCOS and all three hormones in the normal range are mostly associated with obstructive amenorrhea.
    - High serum levels of FSH and LH with low serum E_2 imply ovarian failure.
- Serum prolactin two and a half times higher than the normal limit on two occasions without any history of drug intake may be considered as a cause for oligomenorrhea or amenorrhea.
- Thyroid profile which includes the estimation of T3, T4, and thyroid-stimulating hormone (TSH) should be done for women with amenorrhea as 40% of patients with hypothyroidism can have simultaneous hyperprolactinemia. Low serum level of T4 in primary hypothyroidism leads to increased secretion of thyrotropin-releasing hormone (TRH). This results in increased stimulation of both thyrotropes and lactotrophs, thereby increasing both TSH and prolactin.[5] This can manifest as galactorrhea and/or as amenorrhea.
- *Progestin challenge test* **(Flowchart 2)**: This test is a simple way to assess ovarian function. If a patient gets withdrawal bleeding after progestin treatment, it implies normal circulating estrogen levels and a patent outflow tract. For conducting this test, tablet medroxyprogesterone acetate (MPA) is given in doses of 10 mg once a day, or sustained release micronized progesterone 300 mg orally once a day for 5 days, or a single dose of 200 mg injectable progesterone in oil is given to initiate a withdrawal bleed which occurs usually within 7 days (range of 5–10 days) after the conclusion of progestin treatment.[5] If very little bleeding or spotting occurs, it generally indicates marginal levels of circulating estrogen. Endometrial thickness on ultrasound correlates well with estrogen levels as well as with the progestin challenge test; endometrial thickness of 6 mm or more predicts withdrawal bleeding with 95% accuracy. It is important to note that there is a subset of patients who may not have withdrawal bleeding after progestin treatment despite adequate circulating estrogen levels and endometrial thickness; this is due

Flowchart 2: Progestin challenge test.

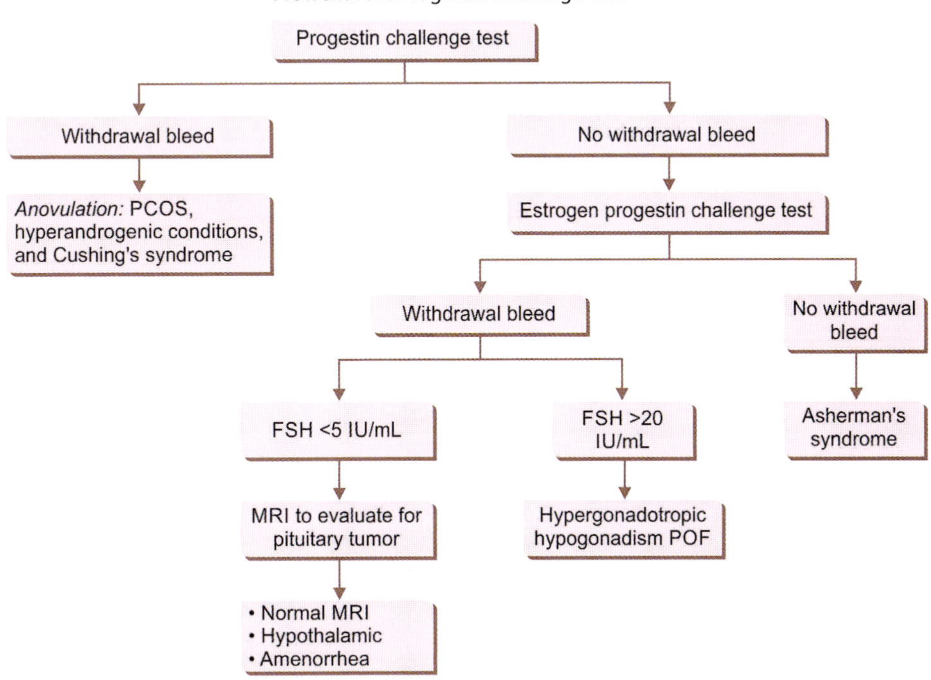

(FSH: follicle-stimulating hormone; MRI: magnetic resonance imaging; PCOS: polycystic ovary syndrome; POF: premature ovarian failure)

to decidualization of endometrium in response to high androgen levels as sometimes seen in women with PCOS with hyperandrogenemia.[6]

- *Magnetic resonance imaging (MRI) of head:* In patients with hypogonadotropic hypogonadism where there is suspicion of hypothalamic or pituitary masses, an MRI of the head is mandatory.
- *Chromosomal analysis:* Karyotype helps to clinch the diagnosis in patients with primary amenorrhea with chromosomal abnormalities; deletion of one X chromosome is associated with Turner's syndrome, (46, XO) or the presence of Y chromosome in a female phenotype is either due to AIS, also called testicular feminization syndrome, or due to Swyer syndrome. Chromosomal analysis is also desirable in patients of secondary amenorrhea with POF to rule out mosaic variants of Turner's syndrome.

EVALUATION OF SPECIFIC CONDITIONS IN AMENORRHEA

- *Primary amenorrhea with blind vagina* **(Flowchart 3)**: The presence of cyclical pain may suggest the possibility of imperforate hymen or transverse vaginal septum which can be diagnosed by local vaginal examination as well as confirmed by ultrasound examination by seeing collected blood in the vagina. If a girl with blind vagina is asymptomatic and has scant pubic hair consider the possibility of AIS, whereas if she has normal secondary sex characteristics the diagnosis of Müllerian agenesis is to be considered [also known as Mayer–Rokitansky–Küster–Hauser (MRKH) syndrome]. Both AIS and MRKH syndromes are characterized by congenital absence of uterus and vagina. A karyotype will help to finally differentiate between the two as it will be normal 46XX in Müllerian agenesis while in AIS it will be 46XY.
- *Secondary amenorrhea with hyperandrogenism:* Women presenting with the absence of menses with clinical symptoms and signs of raised circulating androgen levels, e.g., acne, hirsutism, male pattern baldness, and in severe cases signs of virilization which include features of clitoromegaly, can be attributed to one of the following probable causes:
  - *Ovarian:* PCOS and ovarian neoplasm
  - *Adrenal:* Late-onset CAH, Cushing's syndrome, and adrenal neoplasm.

To identify the underlying cause, one needs to assess serum testosterone, serum dehydroepiandrosterone sulfate (DHEA-S), and serum 17α-hydroxyprogesterone and then interpret the results to arrive at a diagnosis according to **Table 1**.

TABLE 1: Evaluation of secondary amenorrhea and hyperandrogenism.

Hormone	*Level*	*Indication*
Testosterone	≤200 ng/dL	PCOS
	>200 ng/dL	Evaluate for adrenal or ovarian tumor
DHEA-S	≤700 µg/dL	PCOS
	≤700 µg/dL	Evaluate for adrenal or ovarian tumor
17α-Hydroxypro-gesterone	>200 ng/dL	Consider ACTH stimulation test to diagnose CAH

(ACTH: adrenocorticotropic hormone; CAH: congenital adrenal hyperplasia; DHEA-S: dehydroepiandrosterone sulfate; PCOS: polycystic ovarian syndrome)

Flowchart 3: Evaluation of blind or absent vagina.

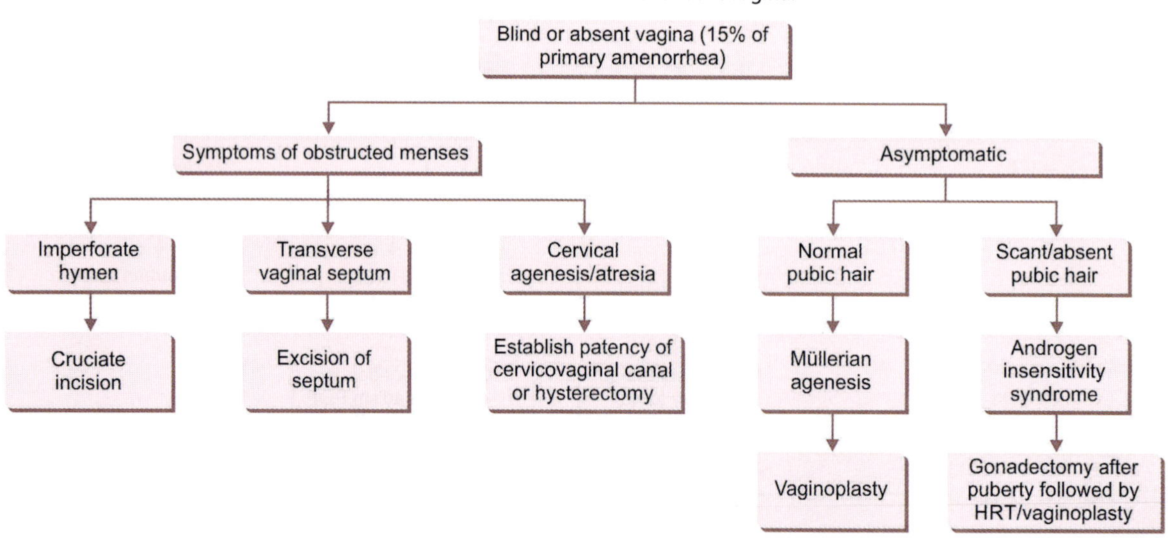

(HRT: hormone replacement therapy)

- *Secondary amenorrhea with POF:* The diagnosis of POF is made if a persistently high serum FSH with low E_2 is seen in women with secondary amenorrhea. The history of surgical intervention on ovaries, e.g., cystectomy or ovarian irradiation or chemotherapy, should be looked for in such cases. POF can also be encountered in chronic smokers; women with obesity; carriers of hepatitis B, C, or HIV; or those who have had chronic pelvic inflammatory diseases and genial tuberculosis. A family history of premature menopause should be sought for. In absence of these, it is important to identify the underlying pathology for which the following tests are recommended:
  - *Karyotype:* Turner mosaics can have normal cycles for a few years before they get amenorrheic.
  - *FMR 1 gene mutation:* 10–20% of carriers of Fragile X syndrome have POF.[7] Screening for Fragile X syndrome should always be considered in women with POF with a family history of premature menopause.
  - *Screening for autoimmune disorders:* POF may be associated with autoimmune disorders such as Addison's disease, autoimmune thyroid disease, and type 1 diabetes. All patients with POF should have an oral glucose tolerance test, thyroid profile, and anti-thyroid peroxidase antibodies. If symptoms warrant, Addison's disease should be ruled out with adrenal antibody titer (titer <1:10 is normal) or adrenocorticotropic hormone stimulation test.[8]

Galactosemia is a rare, inherited autosomal recessive disorder associated with POF. The deficiency of galactose-1-uridyl transferase leads to the accumulation of toxic metabolites, which can lead to reduced initial oocyte pool, increased follicular atresia during maturation, and perhaps reduced maturation of primordial follicles. These girls usually have impaired growth and development and can present as primary amenorrhea, secondary amenorrhea, or oligomenorrhea.[9]

- *Hypogonadotropic hypogonadism:* Both primary and secondary amenorrhea can be a manifestation of hypogonadotropic hypogonadism which is diagnosed by low serum FSH, LH, and estradiol levels. It is pertinent to look for an underlying cause to correct and treat or reverse the disorder effectively. The following conditions should be looked for:
  - *Severe weight loss:* Significant weight loss due to severe exercise, extreme nutritional deficiency or restriction, anorexia nervosa, bulimia, or wasting due to chronic illnesses can lead to an abnormal pattern of GnRH secretion causing disruption of the HPO axis and hence amenorrhea. This response of higher centers in the brain is considered vital, which aims to suppress reproductive function as a protective reaction to stressful situations in the body.[10]
  - *Hyperprolactinemia:* High serum prolactin levels may lead to hypogonadotropic hypogonadism which is one of the common causes of secondary amenorrhea. If it affects a girl before menarche, it can also present as delayed puberty with primary amenorrhea. A woman with increasing levels of prolactin usually progresses from luteal phase defect to anovulation, amenorrhea, and finally frank features of hypoestrogenism.[11] Only one third of the patients with hyperprolactinemia will present with galactorrhea. If serum prolactin levels are >100 ng/mL, an MRI of the brain is recommended to rule out prolactinoma or other adenomas of the pituitary gland.
  - *Sheehan's syndrome:* History of severe hemorrhage associated with cardiovascular collapse following delivery, with failure of lactation to occur and secondary amenorrhea, suggests postpartum pituitary gland necrosis. Immense hypertrophy and hyperplasia of lactotrophs during pregnancy lead to enlargement of the anterior pituitary without a corresponding increase in blood supply; hence, hypovolemic shock due to acute blood loss quite often may cause ischemic necrosis of the gland and deficient secretion of gonadotropins eventually.[12]
  - *Kallmann's syndrome:* This condition is characterized by a congenital deficiency in the pulsatile release of GnRH which is typically associated with a loss of sense of smell, also known as anosmia. Inheritance can be sex linked or autosomal dominant or recessive; therefore, obtaining a family history is important.[13]
  - *Idiopathic hypogonadotropic hypogonadism (IHH):* This condition is characterized by decreased secretion of gonadotropins and thus of sex steroids with intact uterus resulting in amenorrhea with poorly developed secondary sex characteristics. The pathogenesis is the failure of GnRH neurons to develop or differentiate from the hypothalamus for which many genetic mutations have been studied. It is different from Kallmann's syndrome by the fact that patients with IHH have an intact sense of smell.[14]

MANAGEMENT OF AMENORRHEA

Amenorrhea if left untreated may lead to many complications. On one side, it could be associated with poorly developed secondary sex characteristics along with other hypoestrogenic symptoms such as hot flashes, vaginal dryness, and high risk for osteoporosis owing to deficient mineralization of bones, stroke, and heart disease and on the other side, it may also be associated with unopposed estrogen exposure leading to endometrial hyperplasia and sometimes also to endometrial cancers. Thus, the objectives of management of amenorrhea are as follows:

- To treat the underlying disease

- To achieve resumption of menstruation and fertility, when desired
- To prevent complications of amenorrhea.

MANAGEMENT OF END-ORGAN DISORDERS

- *Imperforate hymen:* This condition requires a simple surgical procedure of cruciate incision and drainage.
- *Transverse vaginal septum:* A pelvic ultrasound or pelvic MRI should be done to rule out hematometra and hematosalpinges. Excision of the septum and primary anastomosis of the upper and lower vagina over the defect are done. If the defect is large, the application of graft may be required.
- *Cervical atresia:* This is a rare condition which is difficult to treat as it is difficult to make a sustainable passage between the vagina and uterus. Cervicovaginoplasty can be attempted, but hysterectomy is often required in these girls. Young girls with cervical atresia and severe dysmenorrhea can be treated with hormones to stop menstruation till surgery is undertaken.
- *Müllerian agenesis:* Development of normal secondary sexual characters along with history and local examination showing an absent or small but blind vagina clinches the diagnosis of MRKH. However, final confirmation can be done by a pelvic ultrasound and the presence of a normal 46XX karyotype. An ultrasound should be done to rule out associated renal anomalies. The primary goal of the treatment is to create a functional vagina which can be done by either of the following procedures:
  - *Frank's vaginal dilators* are used to gradually deepen the vaginal dimple.
  - *McIndoe procedure:* In this procedure, neovagina is created by dissection in the rectovesical space. This is followed by skin graft from the inner side of the thigh, buccal mucosa, oxidized cellulose, or amniotic membrane to cover the raw area created.
  - *Vecchietti operation:* This procedure is originated in Italy, and it involves surgical traction to dilate the rudimentary vaginal canal. It was earlier described as an open procedure, but then laparoscopic Vecchietti became more popular due to a surgeon's ease and patient's comfort. An ellipsoid bead or olive is placed on the vaginal dimple outside with inward traction applied through two sutures, one at each end. These sutures are taken inside through the peritoneal cavity and then taken out extraperitoneally to be attached to a traction device placed on the abdominal wall. Postoperatively, the traction is increased every day in such a way that the vaginal cavity is created at the rate of 1 cm/day; hence, by the end of 7 days, a 7 cm vagina is created.[15] In these patients, fertility is possible only with the help of surrogacy.
  - *Laparoscopic Davydov's vaginoplasty:* In this procedure, abdomen and vagina are approached simultaneously. Dissection of rectovesical space is done at the blind vaginal summit from below and then from above laparoscopically a transverse incision is made at the summit of blind vagina, the peritoneum is mobilized and it is pulled down to cover the neovagina and is stitched to the edges of the incised vaginal mucosa. The apex of the neovagina is then closed by a purse-string suture laparoscopically.
  - However, advocates feel that one must delay this reconstructive surgery until children are old enough to decide for themselves, and only if they choose to have it, one of the techniques described above can be used.
- *AIS:* Women with AIS are phenotypically tall and usually pretty, but their chromosomal analysis reveals a 46XY or male karyotype. These women have the presence of testis within their abdomen which produces both testosterone and AMH which on the one hand leads to either increased or normal serum testosterone or dihydrotestosterone (DHT) levels and on the other hand secretion of AMH prevents the development of the uterus and upper vagina. Imaging studies, such as pelvic ultrasound, confirm the absence of fallopian tubes and uterus due to the AMH secreted by these testes. The testes usually remain in the abdomen or occasionally move into the inguinal canals. The testes make enough testosterone, but no androgenic sexual differentiation occurs, and internal male genital ducts fail to form because of the lack of testosterone receptors. Puberty tends to begin slightly later as some of the testosterone is converted to estradiol, inducing normal breast development. Little or no pubic hair or other androgenic hair appears, and acne is rare but the most conspicuous feature of AIS is the absence of vagina. The length of the vagina may vary from a dimple at the perineum to almost normal length but is always blind ending.
  - Genetically in these cases of AIS the androgen receptor is rendered insensitive to the action of androgens secreted from the testes because of the presence of mutation of androgen receptor gene, which is situated on the X arm of the male sex chromosome. There could be complete or partial gene deletions, point mutations, or small insertions or deletions of the affected area on the X chromosome. DNA tests can be done for mutation analysis for androgen receptor gene on X chromosome.[16]
  - Developmental arrest of fetal germ cells in AIS can lead to the development of carcinoma in situ in the gonocytes which can further progress into malignant germ cell tumors, i.e., gonadoblastoma, seminoma,

teratoma, and embryonal tumors. Benign tumors such as hamartomas, Sertoli cell adenomas, and rarely Leydig cell tumors have also been reported in association with AIS. Gonadectomy is thus essential after these girls achieve puberty due to >30% risk of tumors in these dysgenetic gonads in adulthood.[17] This allows spontaneous pubertal development under the effect of estrogen produced from the aromatization of the high levels of testosterone in blood. However, there is a tendency to do gonadectomy as soon as the diagnosis is confirmed in childhood and these girls then need to take estrogen replacement for pubertal development. In addition, many women with AIS require vaginal lengthening procedures. These patients require both donor oocyte and surrogacy when fertility is desired.

- *Asherman's syndrome:* Intrauterine adhesions can occur due to endometrial infections such as genital tuberculosis or due to iatrogenic causes such as repeated curettage, especially of a pregnant uterus or following operative hysteroscopic procedure such as intrauterine polypectomy and myomectomy. This condition was first described in 1894 by Heinrich Fritsch[18] and further characterized by Israeli gynecologist Joseph Asherman in 1948.[19] It is also known as Fritsch syndrome, or Fritsch–Asherman syndrome. This syndrome is diagnosed when the cause of amenorrhea or hypomenorrhea is adhesions or synechiae within the endometrial cavity. These synechiae can be picked up quite often at 3D ultrasound and further confirmed by hysterosalpingography or saline sonohysterography. Hysteroscopic division of intrauterine synechiae is considered the standard procedure for this disorder. Generally, synechiolysis is followed by a high dose of exogenous estrogen given to the woman for 2–3 weeks followed by progesterone withdrawal. A study done on menstrual outcomes after surgical intervention in Asherman's syndrome over a period of 10 years in the Netherlands showed resumption of normal menses in 95% of the patients, though recurrence was reported in 27% of them.[20] Follow-up assessment of uterine cavity is recommended preferably with hysteroscopy after treatment of intrauterine adhesions.[21]

MANAGEMENT OF POLYCYSTIC OVARIAN SYNDROME WITH AMENORRHEA

The role of lifestyle modification should be emphasized in detail to women with PCOS, especially those who are overweight and obese. Women with PCOS with weight loss of even 5% of initial weight have reported spontaneous resumption of menses. The lifestyle changes include aerobic exercise for 150 minutes per week and a hypocaloric diet which could be started as a 500-calorie daily deficit in diet.[22] Periodic treatment with progestin is given to these women to induce regular menses and protect them from endometrial hyperplasia. The most commonly used regime is tablet MPA 10 mg twice daily for 5–7 days every month or alternate months. In women desiring contraception or those suffering from acne and hirsutism, combined oral contraceptive pills are recommended. Pills containing cyproterone acetate as progestogen are preferred as they not only ensure regular cycles but also reduce circulating androgen levels too. When fertility is desired ovulation induction is the way to it, which can be done by ovulation-inducing agents such as clomiphene citrate, letrozole, or tamoxifen and if they fail to induce ovulation then second-line drugs in the form of injectable gonadotropins are recommended to induce ovulation and attain fertility.

MANAGEMENT OF GONADAL AGENESIS AND DYSGENESIS

Turner's syndrome (46, XO): It is one of the common causes of primary amenorrhea and mosaics can present with POF. It is imperative to look for associated medical conditions which are additional features of Turner's syndrome; hence, echocardiography, audiometry, thyroid profile, blood sugar profile, liver and renal function tests, and ultrasonography should be done. These girls need estrogen replacement therapy which must be started as soon as the diagnosis of primary amenorrhea is confirmed, preferably before 15 years of age, so that they can attain adult height. Estrogen is started at a low dose (0.25–0.5 mg micronized estradiol) and increased every 6 months till sexual maturation is achieved. After 1–2 years of continuous estrogen, progestin is added to induce withdrawal bleeding. Fertility is possible with donor oocytes only Turner's syndrome: In classic Turner's syndrome, fertility is possible with donor oocytes only. Most of the mosaic variants also present with POF and require donor oocytes though spontaneous pregnancy has also been reported.

Swyer syndrome and AIS (46XY): AIS has been discussed in end-organ disorders. In Swyer syndrome, SRY region on Y chromosome is missing so testes fail to develop and there are only streak gonads present. In the absence of testicular development there is neither testosterone nor AMH secreted which leads to failure of the development of male secondary sexual characteristics, hence the female phenotype. In addition, in the absence of AMH, the Müllerian system develops in these girls resulting in functional uterus and vagina, which responds to hormones. Menstruation follows sequential hormone replacement therapy (HRT) with estrogen and progesterone in these girls as well as the development of endometrium, to support a pregnancy through a donated oocyte or embryo by in vitro fertilization (IVF). In Swyer syndrome, unlike AIS, gonadectomy is recommended as soon as the diagnosis is made to avoid the high risk of malignant transformation in these nonfunctional gonads as hormonal replacement for the development of secondary sex characters is mandatory.

MANAGEMENT OF PREMATURE OVARIAN FAILURE

These women require HRT, both estrogen and progestin, either in a continuous or cyclic manner. They should also take calcium and vitamin D_3 supplementation and exercise regularly to protect their bones. In case fertility is desired, IVF with donor oocytes is the only option to have children.

MANAGEMENT OF HYPOGONADOTROPIC HYPOGONADISM

In case of anorexia nervosa or severe malnutrition, behavioral and nutritional therapy alone can bring back the menstrual pattern once an optimal weight gain is achieved. If the condition is due to stressful situations, they must be treated by a psychiatrist to reverse the condition. Women with hyperprolactinemia are treated with dopamine agonists (cabergoline or bromocriptine) and ovulation and menses are resumed after 2–3 months of therapy. Women with hyperprolactinemia who are experiencing hypoestrogenic symptoms can be prescribed HRT also. Women with hypogonadotropic hypogonadism need to undergo ovulation induction with gonadotropins which contain both FSH and LH or human menopausal gonadotropin (HMG) when desirous of conception. Otherwise, HRT should be offered to prevent adverse sequel of the absence of ovarian steroid hormones in the body.

KEY POINTS

- Amenorrhea can occur as a natural part of life, such as during pregnancy or breastfeeding, or it can be a sign of a health problem; hence, it is pertinent to know the underlying reasons to decide on the appropriate treatment. However, in some cases leading to amenorrhea, it may not be possible to induce menstruation, as for those who do not have a uterus, as in MRKH syndrome, or AIS, or for girls with cervical atresia where hysterectomy needs to be undertaken to relieve her from cyclical pain.
- We also need to identify the subset of women who may not desire treatment for the resumption of menses as far as they have no health consequences such as those with end-organ failure or Asherman's syndrome.
- For all causes of amenorrhea which root from hypothalamus or pituitary, lifelong HRT is advisable till conception is desired.
- Amenorrhea stemming from the ovary has the most diverse management strategies; dysgenic gonads as those with XY karyotype need to be removed and HRT instituted, and ovarian agenesis or failure requires HRT lifelong during the reproductive years with oocyte donation and IVF for reproduction.
- Amenorrhea associated with androgen excess conditions, such as PCOS, needs to be managed as per the presenting features and health issues.
- Ovulation induction in this group of women is the best method to attain fertility. The key to the management of women with amenorrhea is to make a correct diagnosis, especially in young girls.
- Irregular menses can be managed with oral contraceptive pills, especially if hirsutism is a prominent feature, but a progesterone withdrawal may be sufficient to regularize menstruation. However, fertility issues are best addressed by induction of ovulation.
- Primary amenorrhea is a very emotionally draining concern, not only for the girl but also for the family, and counseling is an integral part of the management of all such cases.

REFERENCES

1. Hermen-Giddens ME, Slora EJ, Wasserman RC, Bourdony CJ, Bhapkar MV, Koch GG, et al. Secondary sexual characteristics and menses in young girls seen in office practice: a study from pediatric research in office setting network. Pediatrics. 1997;90:505-12.
2. Speroff L, Fritz MA (Eds). Clinical Gynecological Endocrinology and Infertility, 7th edition. New York: Lippincott Williams & Wilkins; 2005. p. 402.
3. Practice Committee of American Society for Reproductive Medicine. Current evaluation of amenorrhea. Fertil Steril. 2008;90:S219-25.
4. Gambadauro P, Gudmundsson J, Torrejon R. Intrauterine adhesions following conservative management of uterine fibroids. Obstet Gynecol Int. 2012;2012:853269.
5. Speroff L, Fritz MA (Eds). Clinical Gynecological Endocrinology and Infertility, 7th edition. New York: Lippincott Williams and Wilkins; 2005. p. 405.
6. Speroff L, Fritz MA (Eds). Clinical Gynecological Endocrinology and Infertility, 7th edition. New York: Lippincott Williams and Wilkins; 2005. p. 406.
7. Mallolas J, Duran M, Sanchez A, Jiménez D, Castellví-Bel S, Rifé M, et al. Implications of FMR 1 gene in menopause: study of 147 Spanish women. Menopause. 2001;8:106-10.
8. Lebovic DI. Premature ovarian failure: think autoimmune disorder. Sexual Reprod Menopause. 2004;2(4):230-3.
9. Fridovich-Kiel JL, Gubbles CS, Spencer JB, Sanders RD, Land JA, Rubio-Gozalbo E. Ovarian function in girls and women with GALT-deficiency galactosemia. J Inherit Metab Dis. 2011;34(2):357-66.
10. Berga SL. Behaviorally induced reproductive compromise in women and men. Semin Reprod Endocrinol. 1997;15:47.
11. Speroff L, Fritz MA (Eds). Clinical Gynecological Endocrinology and Infertility, 7th edition. New York: Lippincott Williams and Wilkins; 2005. p. 467.

12. Laway BA, Mir SA. Pregnancy and pituitary disorders: challenges in diagnosis and management. Indian J Endocrinol Metab. 2013;17(6):996-1004.
13. Dode C, Hardelin JP. Kallmann syndrome. Eur J Hum Genet. 2009;17(2):139-46.
14. Seminara SB, Hayes FJ, Crowley WF. Gonadotropin-releasing hormone deficiency in human (Kallmann's syndrome and idiopathic hypogonadotropic hypogonadism): pathophysiological and genetic considerations. Endocr Rev. 1998;19(5):521-39.
15. Harmanli OH, Grody MHT. Laparoscopic Vecchietti procedure: improving on an indispensable method. Novel variations on an essential technique may benefit surgeons and their patients. Am J Obstet Gynecol. 2008;199(6):713.e1-2.
16. Mendoza N, Rodriguez-Alcala C, Motos MA, Salamanca A. Androgen insensitivity syndrome: an update on the management in adolescents and young people. J Adolesc Pediatr Gynecol. 2017;30(1):2-8.
17. Hughes IA, Davies JD, Bunch TI, Pasterski V, Mastroyannopoulou K, MacDougall J. Androgen insensitivity syndrome. Lancet. 2012;380:1419-28.
18. Fritsch H, von volligem EF. Schwund der Gebormutterhohle nach Auskratzung. Zentralbl Gynaekol. 1894;18:1337-42.
19. Asherman JG. Traumatic intra-uterine adhesions. J Obstet Gynaecol Br Em. 1950;57(6):892-6.
20. Hanstede MM, van der Meij E, Goedemans L, Emanuel MH. Results of centralized Asherman surgery, 2003–2013. Fertil Steril. 2015;104:1561-8.
21. AAGL Elevating Gynecologic Surgery. AAGL practice report: practice guidelines on intrauterine adhesions developed in collaboration with European Society of Gynaecological Endoscopy (ESGE). Gynaecol Surg. 2017;14(1):6.
22. Karkanaki A, Kalogiannidis I, Panidis D. Effects of lifestyle modification on pregnancy success in obese and overweight women with PCOS. J Women's Health Care. 2013;2:125.

CHAPTER 11

Endocrine Disorders Affecting Reproduction

Chaitra Narayan Nayak

INTRODUCTION

Reproduction is affected by various factors, including, among others, nutrition, exposure to infections, and the hormonal milieu of the individual. Endocrine disorders have a profound impact on reproduction, and in women, polycystic ovarian syndrome (PCOS) is the most common endocrine syndromic disorder affecting reproduction.[1] The regulation of the hypothalamic–pituitary–gonadal axis is covered in Chapter 1, and the physiology of steroids and their regulations are covered in Chapter 2.

In this chapter, we will be discussing abnormalities of the hypothalamus, pituitary, adrenals, and thyroid and their effect on reproduction.

HYPOTHALAMUS–PITUITARY UNIT

For long known as the "master gland", the pituitary was thought to regulate almost all essential functions of the body, including growth, response to stress, functioning of thyroid, and reproduction to name a few.[2] In recent years, it has been found that the pituitary largely acts as a relay, transporting the regulatory hormones released by the hypothalamus. The pituitary is anatomically and embryologically divided into the anterior and posterior pituitary. Details of the same are covered elsewhere.

Unique Features of the Hypothalamus–Pituitary System[3]

- The neurosecretory cells of the hypothalamus secrete regulating factors in a pulsatile manner and control the functioning of the pituitary.
- The inhibitory and releasing factors are transported by a portal system through the pituitary stalk to the anterior pituitary.
- The posterior pituitary hormones, oxytocin, and vasopressin are secreted and regulated by the hypothalamus.
- Diurnal variation has an important impact on the functioning of the hypothalamus and, in turn, the pituitary.
- Most of the peptides secreted act as releasing hormones, except for prolactin, which is under inhibitory control.
- A strict feedback system from the end organs regulates the secretions of both the hypothalamus and the pituitary.

Only the most important endocrine abnormalities known to affect reproduction are discussed here.

Prolactin

Prolactin is a polypeptide of 198 amino acids, 23 kDa coded on a single gene on chromosome 6. Initially found to be secreted in a pulsatile manner from the lactotrophs of the anterior pituitary, prolactin has been isolated in other areas of the hypothalamus, placenta, and mammary glands. Dopamine through the pituitary portal system tonically suppresses prolactin. Estrogen, antidopaminergics, epidermal growth factor, and thyrotropin-releasing hormone are known to increase prolactin.[4]

While the majority (85%) of prolactin exists as the 23 kDa molecule, variants occur due to proteolytic cleavage, alternative splicing, or modifications post-translation. Covalently bound dimer (big prolactin) and polymeric dimer (big big prolactin) cause macroprolactinemia, where asymptomatic patients have incidental hyperprolactinemia. Delayed renal clearance of macroprolactin causes a false elevation in prolactin levels. It is detected by *polyethylene glycol precipitation* of the serum. If the only cause of hyperprolactinemia is confirmed to be macroprolactinemia, no further treatment is required.[5]

A single measurement of serum prolactin is recommended, and dynamic testing for prolactin is to be avoided. The serum sample can be taken at any time of the day, provided minimal venepuncture is done. Normal prolactin levels are <25 µg/L in women and lower in men. Prolactin levels of >500 µg/L are indicative of macroprolactinoma.

Most people with prolactin >250 µg/L should be evaluated for pituitary tumors.[5]

If a large pituitary tumor is found with mildly elevated prolactin levels, serial dilution of serum must be done to test for the "hook effect". High serum prolactin causes saturation of antibodies in the two-site immunometric assay. This results in direct binding of prolactin to signaling (second) antibody and less availability of the latter to bind to prolactin-bound coupling (first) antibody. It is recommended to either repeat the assay with 1:100 dilution or wash out the sample before adding the signaling antibody to prevent the hook effect.[5]

EPIDEMIOLOGY

Biochemical hyperprolactinemia is seen in about 0.4% of the general population, 9–17% in infertile patients, and is one of the most common disorders of the pituitary. Females have a higher incidence as compared to males, with peak prevalence at 25–34 years.

Women with galactorrhea, amenorrhea, oligomenorrhea, or infertility and men with hypogonadism, infertility, or impotence need the evaluation of prolactin levels.

About 10% of women with amenorrhea, 25% of women with galactorrhea, and 70% of women with both amenorrhea and galactorrhea are found to have high prolactin.

About 5% of men with either impotence or infertility have high prolactin. Impotence is not responsive to testosterone supplementation and is associated with reduced body hair, low muscle mass, and osteoporosis.

Hyperprolactinemia has also been called World Health Organization (WHO) type 4 anovulation due to the hypogonadism caused by high prolactin levels.

Causes of Hyperprolactinemia

Causes of symptomatic nonphysiological hyperprolactinemia would include medications, renal failure, parasellar tumors, and hypothyroidism **(Table 1)**.[6]

Drugs Causing Hyperprolactinemia[6]

- Medications are the most common cause of nontumoral hyperprolactinemia, with most patients having prolactin between 25 and 100 µg/L.
- Neuroleptics, antipsychotics, anticonvulsants, antihistamines, opiates, and antidepressants can all cause hyperprolactinemia.
- About 40–90% of patients on antipsychotics and 50–100% of patients on risperidone have hyperprolactinemia.
- Women present with amenorrhea and galactorrhea; men exhibit low libido or erectile dysfunction.
- In suspected symptomatic patients with hyperprolactinemia, it is recommended to discontinue or substitute the medicines for 3 days and reassess prolactin levels.
- Antipsychotics should be either modified or discontinued only after consulting the psychiatrist if found to cause hyperprolactinemia.
- Antipsychotics, such as aripiprazole, which has both dopamine agonistic and antagonistic properties or similar alternatives, are advisable where applicable.
- Dopaminergic drugs may worsen the psychosis in patients with hyperprolactinemia due to antipsychotics.

Delayed breakdown or clearance of prolactin causes hyperprolactinemia in one-third of patients with chronic *renal failure*. Dialysis is ineffective and only renal transplant normalizes the levels of prolactin.

Tumors of Pituitary

- Both functional and nonfunctional tumors of the pituitary can cause hyperprolactinemia.
- Most patients with prolactin >250 µg/L will have prolactinomas.
- Prolactinomas can be microadenomas (<10 mm) or macroadenomas (>10 mm).
- Stalk compression by intracranial tumors, parasellar tumors, and inflammation may also cause hyperprolactinemia by preventing the transport of inhibitory signals to the pituitary.

Common Presentations of Hyperprolactinemia

Common presentations are shown in **Table 2**.[4]

Management (Evidence-Based Guidelines)

Goals of treatment in hyperprolactinemia are mentioned in **Box 1**.

TABLE 1: Causes of hyperprolactinemia.

Physiological	*Pituitary*	*Central nervous system disorders*	*Systemic disease*
• Pregnancy • Lactation • Stress • Nipple stimulation • Sleep • Coitus • Exercise	• Prolactinoma • Hypothyroidism • Nonsecretory adenomas • Acromegaly • Cushing's disease • Empty sella turcica	• Tumors • Vascular malformations • Granulomatous autoimmune disease • Metastasis	• Chronic renal failure • Severe hypothyroidism • Cirrhosis • Cranial radiation • Chest wall trauma • Herpes zoster

Note: Pharmacological causes of hyperprolactinemia are discussed in the text.

TABLE 2: Common presentations of hyperprolactinemia.

Female (prolactin levels)	*Male*
• >100 ng/mL: Hypogonadism, galactorrhea, amenorrhea • 51–75 ng/mL: Oligomenorrhea • 31–50 ng/mL: Luteal phase defect, decreased libido, infertility • Osteopenia	Decreased libido, impotence, infertility, oligospermia, retrograde ejaculation gynecomastia

BOX 1: Goals of treatment in hyperprolactinemia.

- Restoration of normal gonadal function
- Restoring fertility
- Avoiding osteoporosis

Medical Management of Hyperprolactinemia

- Dopaminergic drugs are the first line of treatment in all cases of hyperprolactinemia and reduce tumor size, lower prolactin levels, and reestablish normal gonadal functions.
- Both bromocriptine (2.5–40 mg/day) and cabergoline (0.125–1 mg twice weekly) may be used.
- Cabergoline is highly efficacious and causes better shrinkage of tumors when compared to bromocriptine.
- Bromocriptine has been used for a longer duration. Nausea, giddiness, and nasal stuffiness are common side effects of the drug. The dosage is gradually increased until the serum levels of prolactin are normalized, which may take about 10 days.
- Cabergoline is used in bromocriptine resistance or intolerance.
- Men on 0.5–1 mg twice weekly cabergoline had normalization of semen parameters and prolactin levels after 6 months of treatment. 80% of men on dopamine agonists for micro- or macroadenoma respond to treatment.
- Patients on antidopaminergics need to have prolactin levels checked about 1 month after starting therapy to adjust the dosage. Repeat magnetic resonance imaging (MRI) after 1 year for microadenoma and 3 months for macroadenoma is done to look for tumor shrinkage.
- Dopamine agonists can be stopped after 2 years of achieving normal prolactin or no tumor residue on MRI.

Despite therapy, about 10% of patients with microprolactinomas and 18% with macroprolactinomas will continue to have high blood levels of the hormone. Newer drugs such as kisspeptin for hyperprolactinemia are under trial and results are awaited.

Drug-induced asymptomatic hyperprolactinemia needs no treatment other than discontinuation of the drug or substitution. Hypogonadism from prolonged drug-induced hyperprolactinemia is treated with estrogen or testosterone supplements.

Surgery

Surgery is reserved for nonfunctional tumors causing visual defects or stalk effect, and in those patients where *medical therapy has failed* or is not tolerated. Transsphenoidal resection is to be done with extreme caution in a center well versed in handling such cases. Recurrence of 20–50% has been reported with higher cure rates for microprolactinomas compared to macroprolactinomas. Such patients may ultimately require radiation if symptoms persist.

Hyperprolactinemia and Pregnancy[5]

- Women with prolactinoma on dopaminergic agonists should stop after discovering pregnancy.
- Patients with macroadenoma and visual symptoms with no prior radiotherapy or surgery may continue bromocriptine.
- Testing of prolactin in pregnancy is not recommended.
- Routine MRI of the pituitary in pregnancy in patients with macro- or microadenomas is to be avoided and must be done only if new symptoms, such as changes in the visual field, occur.
- Women with macroprolactinomas resistant to or intolerant to dopamine agonists must be strongly counseled for surgery before attempting pregnancy.
- Pregnant women with prolactinoma presenting with visual changes or severe headaches should have a formal assessment of the visual field and a noncontrast MRI.
- Bromocriptine is the drug of choice in pregnant women with symptomatic prolactinomas.

OTHER DISORDERS OF PITUITARY

Acromegaly

Acromegaly is a rare disorder occurring due to the hypersecretion of growth hormone (GH) or insulin-like growth factor 1 (IGF1) due to somatotropinomas or GH-releasing hormone tumors.[7] Changes in the bone and soft tissues along with easy fatigability, headache, excessive sweating, carpal tunnel syndrome, and sleep apnea may also occur. Gigantism occurs in children and has similar etiopathology to acromegaly but is identified earlier due to its florid manifestations.

Overexpression of the *GPR101* gene on the X chromosome has been found in patients with acromegaly or gigantism. Affected individuals have an insidious onset with most patients being diagnosed late. Acromegaly causes impaired fertility due to numerous factors, including stalk compression, hyperprolactinemia, mass effect, and direct excess GH.

Preconceptional counseling is essential before pregnancy is attempted. Acromegalic women have anovulation (69%) or may ovulate (31%), with the latter having better fertility outcomes. Common causes of anovulation include hyperprolactinemia, mass effect, and increased GH/idiopathic guttate hypomelanosis (IGH) levels. Most women ovulate after correcting underlying pathology. 174 pregnant patients with acromegaly have been documented in the literature, with 33 patients being included in the literature review. Most women have had no complications in their pregnancy.[8]

The best screening test is a serum IGF1 with age, gender, and Tanner stage corrections. Suppression tests are done to prognosticate therapy response. Diagnosis is confirmed by high GH levels (>10 ng/mL) after an oral glucose test or elevated IGF1 levels in patients suspected to have acromegaly.

Additionally, MRI with gadolinium contrast will be able to detect adenomas of the pituitary, and computed tomography (CT) scan of the abdomen will detect tumors of the ovary, pancreas, or adrenal glands, which may secrete GH.

Somatostatin analogs such as depot octreotide or lanreotide, dopamine agonists, or GH receptor antagonists may be used in newly identified pregnant patients and is the first line of management. Transsphenoidal surgery is recommended in patients with pituitary tumors prior to pregnancy and is preferred in older women.

THYROID AND REPRODUCTION

The thyroid gland consists of numerous follicles made of a simple secretory epithelium around a gelatinous lumen containing thyroglobulin and thyroxine (T4). Functions of the thyroid are enumerated in **Box 2**.

Iodide is taken up from the blood, converted to iodine, and the resulting monoiodo or diiodotyrosine is incorporated into the thyroglobulin. Organification occurs with the coupling of two diiodotyrosine to form T4 or one mono and one diiodotyrosine to form triiodothyronine (T3). Both iodination and organification are done by the enzyme thyroid peroxidase (TPO) **(Fig. 1)**. Autoantibodies to this enzyme are common and result in various pathologies of the thyroid gland.

The majority of the T4 in the circulation is bound to plasma proteins [70% to thyroxine-binding globulin (TBG), 20% to transthyretin, and 10% to albumin], and changes in the protein concentration have a profound impact on the free T4 concentration.

Prevalence

Thyroid disorders are more prevalent in women than men and most of them unsurprisingly have an autoimmune etiology.[9] Most common causes of hypothyroidism (Hashimoto's thyroiditis) and hyperthyroidism (Graves' disease) have associated antithyroid antibodies.

About 2.3% of subfertile women and 1.5% of women in the general population are found to have hyperthyroidism. About 3.1% of reproductive-age women are hypothyroid, with most of them having menstrual symptoms and anovulation. *Subclinical hypothyroidism*, which presents

BOX 2: Functions of the thyroid.[3]

- The thyroid controls the basal metabolic rate through triiodothyronine and thyroxine
- The thyroid is essential for the growth and development of the central nervous system, especially the brain
- Both hypothyroidism and hyperthyroidism are known to affect reproduction
- Patients with antithyroid antibodies are known to have adverse pregnancy outcomes despite being euthyroid

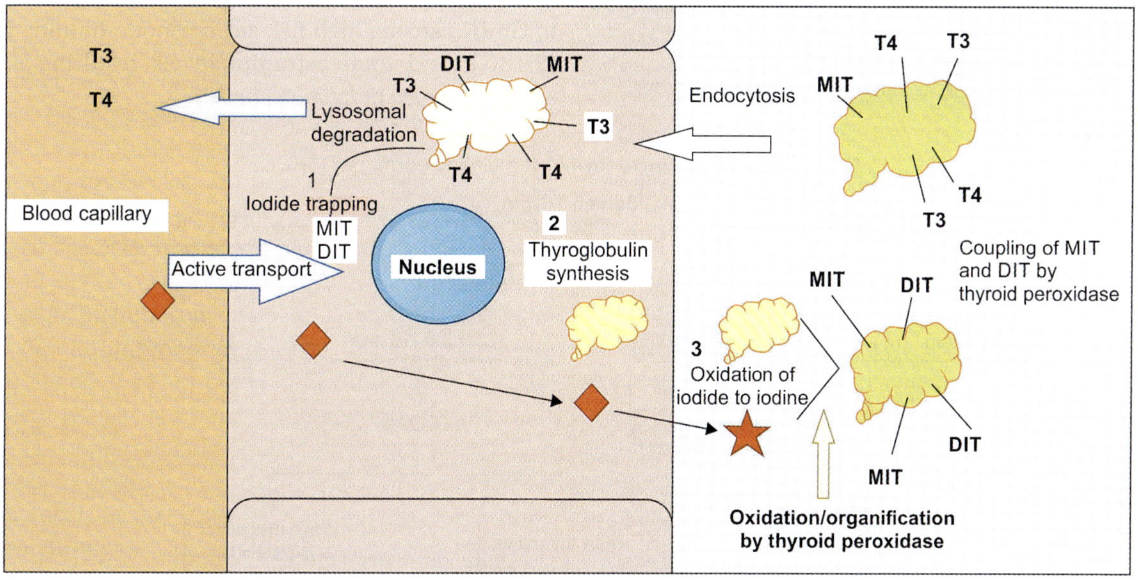

Fig. 1: Synthesis of triiodothyronine (T3) and thyroxine (T4) hormones.
(DIT: diiodotyrosine; MIT: monoiodotyrosine; ◊: iodide; *: iodine; : thyroglobulin)

with normal T4 levels (9–25 pmol/L) but raised thyroid-stimulating hormone (TSH) (>4.5 µM/mL), affects 2–4% of reproductive-age women.

All women who are infertile or in the initial stages of their pregnancy are evaluated to find the risk of thyroid disease according to **Box 3**. India is a high prevalence country where universal screening of all infertile and pregnant women may be recommended **(Flowchart 1)**.

Hypothyroidism[10]

- Hypothyroidism inhibits the pulsatile release of gonadotropin-releasing hormone (GnRH), preventing cyclical follicle-stimulating hormone (FSH) and luteinizing hormone (LH) release, causing anovulation.
- Children or adolescents with hypothyroidism present with delayed sexual development.
- Adults may manifest with menstrual irregularities such as oligomenorrhea, menorrhagia or amenorrhea, and hyperprolactinemia. Weight gain, intolerance to cold, sleepiness, dry skin, and hair loss may be other manifestations.
- Hypothyroidism is common in infertile women and controlled ovarian stimulation causes high estradiol levels, resulting in higher binding of T4 to TBG, temporarily making euthyroid women hypothyroid.

BOX 3: Screening for thyroid disorders.[3]

- History of hyper/hypothyroidism or recent thyroid disorders
- Goiter present or presence of thyroid antibodies
- History of thyroid surgery or neck irradiation
- More than 30 years of age
- Autoimmune diseases including type I diabetes
- Morbid obesity >40 kg/m^2
- Resides in area of high iodine deficiency
- History of previous pregnancy loss, infertility, or preterm birth
- Multipara >2 pregnancies
- Intake of lithium, amiodarone, or radioiodine contrast
- Family history of thyroiditis or autoimmune thyroid disorder

- Correcting both subclinical and overt hypothyroidism has been shown to improve implantation, pregnancy, and live birth rates in assisted reproductive technology (ART) pregnancies. It has been therefore recommended to maintain TSH levels of <4 mU/L in the preconceptional period as well as in the first trimester of pregnancy.[11]

Investigations[12]

The American Thyroid Association recommends screening from 35 years, once every 5 years. High-risk patients such as pregnant women, women >60 years, those with autoimmune disease, or with a history of irradiation to the neck require more monitoring.

Serum TSH and T4 are checked to detect overt hypothyroidism or subclinical hypothyroidism. If TSH is >2.5 mU/L, TPO antibody levels should be measured.

Treatment[12]

- Levothyroxine (LT4) replacement is the sole therapy with titration required for the dose.
- Young adults will usually require 50–75 µg and can be started with the full replacement dose.
- Older patients and those with cardiac disease may need to be started with a smaller dose and increased gradually to a higher dosage.
- Improvement of symptoms is seen within about 3–5 days, and dose adjustments are done every 6–8 weeks.[11]

Hyperthyroidism

Patients having hyperthyroidism typically present with palpitations, anxiety, involuntary weight loss, increased sweating, intolerance to heat, and excessive bowel movements.

Women with hyperthyroidism have a higher sensitivity to GnRH causing high LH, sex hormone-binding globulin (SHBG), and total estradiol levels resulting in either *oligomenorrhea* or *hypomenorrhea*.

Flowchart 1: Screening of thyroid-stimulating hormone (TSH).

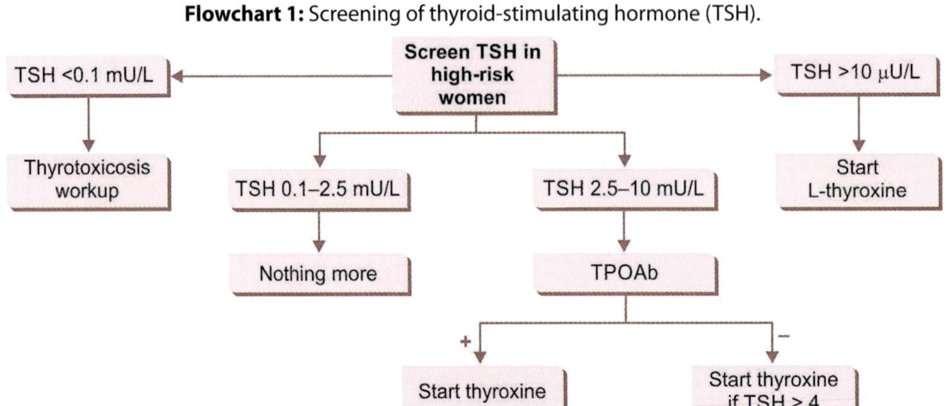

(TPOAb: thyroid peroxidase antibody)

Source: Vanderpump MP. The epidemiology of thyroid disease. Br Med Bull. 2011;99(1):39-51.

Most women with hyperthyroidism are *ovulatory* despite having these menstrual irregularities, and therefore treating hyperthyroidism generally does not increase the ovulation rate but does improve the quality of life in affected women. Pregnant women with thyrotoxicosis must be differentiated from those with hyperemesis gravidarum, molar pregnancies, and women having physiological changes in pregnancies.

Graves' disease, the most common cause of hyperthyroidism, occurs due to anti-TSH receptor antibodies (TRAb), causing unregulated stimulation of thyroid hormone production. On examination, affected patients have a classical protuberant gaze with exophthalmos due to the paralysis of extraocular muscles with periorbital infiltration and ophthalmopathy, resting tachycardia, tremors, and proximal muscle weakness. Pregnant women affected by Graves' disease have an increased risk of fetal or neonatal thyrotoxicosis due to the transplacental transport of the antibodies.

Men with Graves' disease present with hypogonadism, with low free testosterone levels despite high SHBG and high total testosterone. Low sperm counts unresponsive to human chorionic gonadotropin (hCG) and gynecomastia may also be present.

Inflammation of the thyroid gland causes thyroiditis, with subsequent release of the stored thyroid hormone into the circulation causing thyrotoxicosis. There is immediate hyperthyroidism, which may last up to 8 weeks followed by transient hypothyroidism and subsequent euthyroid state in most patients. Typically, both serum thyroglobulin and erythrocyte sedimentation rate are elevated in subacute thyroiditis.

Subacute thyroiditis (de Quervain's disease) may present with the classical symptoms of neck pain, fever, and tender thyroid gland following a viral infection in the recent past.

Other causes of hyperthyroidism include toxic adenoma, where a germline mutation results in a solitary tumor autonomously producing T3 and T4 or toxic multinodular goiter producing.

Diagnosis of Hyperthyroidism

Triiodothyronine, T4, and TSH are essential to make a diagnosis of hyperthyroidism in symptomatic patients.

Low TSH levels (<0.5 μIU/mL) with high free T4 and total T3 levels are seen in thyrotoxicosis. Subclinical hyperthyroidism presents with normal FT4/T3 and low TSH levels.

Antibodies[13]

Autoantibodies are an important cause of hyperthyroidism. Anti-TPO antibodies are specific for autoimmune thyroiditis and are significantly elevated in Graves' disease. Other causes of hyperthyroidism such as toxic multinodular goiter and toxic adenoma have a normal or slight increase in anti-TPO antibodies. About 8–10% of the population has a slight increase in anti-TPO antibodies, and hence a universal screening is not recommended.

Radioactive iodine (RAI) uptake by the thyroid gland can also be used to differentiate the etiology of hyperthyroidism, with a diffuse uptake seen in Graves' disease and focal areas of uptake seen in toxic adenoma and multinodular goiter. Both iodine-123 (^{123}I) and technetium-99m (^{99m}Tc) have been used for scintigraphy of the thyroid.

Treatment[12]

Management of Graves' disease involves a multidisciplinary approach with interventions for the ophthalmopathy, dermopathy, and β-blockers for the cardiac and neurological signs.

Antithyroid medications such as methimazole and propylthiouracil are the mainstay of treatment in children, pregnant women, and adults awaiting radioiodine therapy. They inhibit the synthesis of thyroid hormones and act over 2–8 weeks. Titration of drug dosage is done by measuring hormones every 4–6 weeks until the euthyroid state is obtained.

Methimazole is a more potent antithyroid drug with ease of once-a-day dosage due to its longer action as compared to propylthiouracil which is given in two to three doses. Propylthiouracil is safer in the first trimester of pregnancy, in patients intolerant to methimazole. In patients with thyroid storm, propylthiouracil inhibits the peripheral conversion of T4 to T3. Hepatotoxicity is a known adverse effect of the medication, and it is recommended to do liver function tests within 6 months of therapy, with discontinuation if results are abnormal.

About 1–5% of patients may have an intolerance to antithyroid medications and manifest as fever, arthralgia, and rash. This must be differentiated from the more serious aplastic anemia, agranulocytosis, hepatitis, or vasculitis, which are also known to occur.

Radioactive iodine is preferred in all other patients as it is given as a single oral capsule, is more effective, with lesser adverse effects. The gland undergoes fibrosis over a while, with patients becoming hypothyroid. It is avoided in pregnant, lactating women and young children.

Surgery is preferred in pregnant women with noncompliance or intolerance to antithyroid drugs, patients with large goiters, and those who reject radiotherapy or need a rapid correction to the euthyroid state.

THYROID AND SUBFERTILITY[12]

- Evidence suggests routine screening for thyroid disorders by a TSH and thyroid peroxidase antibody (TPOAb) is beneficial in infertile women. If TSH is <2.5, no further tests are needed. However, a TSH of >2.5 needs to be repeated along with antithyroid antibodies [TPOAb and thyroglobulin antibody (TgAb)]. LT4 supplementation with repeat TSH measurements done 6 weeks thereafter, until TSH is <2.5, is recommended. Women with overt thyroid disorders should be promptly treated.

- Routine screening of thyroid disorders in male partners is not recommended. Men with abnormal semen parameters, erectile, or ejaculatory disorders may benefit from the evaluation of thyroid function. Unless semen parameters are grossly affected, ART treatment may proceed despite thyroid abnormalities in males. If RAI is done, it is recommended to wait for 120 days before attempting conception/ART procedures. Sperm banking, family planning, and fertility should be discussed before offering RAI. RAI for thyroid cancers must not be delayed for fertility reasons.[14]
- Thyroid function tests are to be done either before or about 2 weeks after controlled ovarian stimulation. If TSH >4 mIU/L, with or without thyroid autoimmunity (TAI), LT4 needs to be started to keep TSH <2.5 mIU/L.
- Autoimmune disorders such as antiphospholipid antibodies (APLA), type I diabetes, systemic lupus erythematosus (SLE), and premature ovarian failure (POF) are common in infertile patients, and the significance of antithyroid antibodies has long been debated. Common thyroid disorders such as Hashimoto's thyroid disease, postpartum thyroiditis, and Graves' disease have autoantibodies as the etiology. Elevated levels of antithyroid antibodies are also seen in PCOS and endometriosis.[15]
- Infertile euthyroid women with antithyroid antibodies have a poorer pregnancy outcome with lower fertilization, bad embryos, and reduced pregnancy rates when compared to infertile women without autoantibodies. Intracytoplasmic sperm injection (ICSI) is to be offered for fertilization in cases of thyroid antibodies in females.[11] Higher levels of antibodies are also seen in ovarian follicular fluid with higher natural killer (NK) cell activity in the uterus. Limited evidence suggests an improvement in pregnancy outcomes with the treatment of thyroid antibodies.

THYROID AND PREGNANCY[11]

- The WHO recommends all pregnant women ingest 250 μg of iodine per day.
- Universal salt iodination is the most cost-effective method for increasing iodine intake, and it is to be supplemented 3 months before planning a pregnancy.
- Low iodine causes high TSH leading to compensatory goiter in both mother and fetus. This also causes long-term effects such as cognitive dysfunction and cretinism in the infant.
- All pregnant women should be asked about their history of thyroid disorders and intake of medications for the same. About 50–80% of hypothyroid women will need a change in dosage of LT4 in pregnancy and TSH must be kept <2.5 mU/L.
- All thyroid nodules can undergo fine-needle aspiration cytology (FNAC) during pregnancy. Radioiodine uptake studies are avoided in pregnancy.
- Surveillance of fetuses is done in all women with severe hyperthyroidism or with high TRAb (more than three times normal).
- Postpartum thyroiditis affects about 5% of women and is usually asymptomatic. If women are identified in the thyrotoxicosis phase, β-blockers are the first line of management. TSH should be measured about 4–8 weeks later to look for hypothyroidism.
- Antithyroid medications methimazole (up to 20 mg/day) and propylthiouracil (up to 450 mg/day) are found to be safe during pregnancy and lactation, although the lowest possible dose is to be recommended. Propylthiouracil is preferred in the first 16 weeks of pregnancy.
- ^{131}I is contraindicated during lactation, and if at all used, breast milk should be discarded for the next 3–4 days.
- Women with newly detected hypothyroidism in pregnancy on <50 μg of LT4 per day may discontinue it in the postpartum period and reassess thyroid function 6 weeks postpartum.

ADRENAL DISORDERS

The adrenal gland, embryologically and anatomically, is divided into the cortex and medulla, with the latter being a part of the sympathetic nervous system, producing epinephrine. The more important adrenal cortex has the aldosterone-secreting zona glomerulosa controlled by the renin–angiotensin–aldosterone system (RAAS), the cortisol-secreting zona fasciculata and the dehydroepiandrosterone (DHEAS)-secreting zona reticularis, both of which are regulated by the adrenocorticotropic hormone (ACTH). Adrenal glands are the major source of testosterone in women and their disorders are known to have reproductive implications, the most important of which is subfertility due to hyperandrogenemia.[16]

Cushing Syndrome

Cushing syndrome occurs due to prolonged exposure to glucocorticoids and may be classified into iatrogenic or endogenous, depending on the source of the steroids. Cushing syndrome of endogenous origin is further categorized as being ACTH-dependent or -independent.

Adrenocorticotropic hormone-producing pituitary tumors are the most common cause of Cushing syndrome and indeed are labeled as Cushing disease. Other sources of ACTH causing the syndrome are carcinomas, bronchial carcinoids, and neuroendocrine tumors. Cushing disease commonly affects women of reproductive age who present with infertility due to high DHEAS.[16]

The disease in its initial stages is most amenable to treatment but is difficult to diagnose. Cortisol causes a redistribution of fat and change in the body habitus causing central obesity with the classical dorsocervical deposition of fat (buffalo hump), supraclavicular fat pads, and hirsutism, along with facial and upper chest plethora.

Pathognomonic features of Cushing syndrome include proximal muscle weakness and extreme thinning of skin along with easy bruisability or striae. Affected individuals typically have difficulty in getting up from a chair, combing hair, climbing stairs, or changing light bulbs.

Young women with PCOS (oligomenorrhea, polycystic ovarian morphology, and hirsutism) should be evaluated for Cushing syndrome if they have dermatological manifestations of Cushing disease.

Diagnosis[17]

In affected individuals, an excessive amount of cortisol production occurs with a loss of the normal diurnal variation. A 24-hour free cortisol measurement in the urine and serum or salivary cortisol level both will reflect the excess steroid production. The dexamethasone suppression test also fails to reduce cortisol levels in the blood.

Adrenocorticotropic hormone measurements are done to detect ACTH-dependent or independent causes of the Cushing syndrome, and a CT scan of the adrenal gland is done if ACTH levels are low to seek out local causes. Conversely, an MRI with gadolinium contrast of the pituitary is done to look for adenomas in cases of high ACTH.

Adrenocorticotropic hormone levels in the blood of both petrosal sinuses after a bovine corticotropin-releasing hormone (CRH) challenge (100 μg bolus) are measured and compared to that in peripheral blood to help in reliably detecting the pituitary origin of ACTH.

Treatment

Surgery is the modality of choice in patients with Cushing syndrome. Transsphenoidal pituitary adenectomy is done in those with Cushing disease and, if unsuccessful, may require radiotherapy or bilateral adrenalectomy.

Medical management including ketoconazole, mifepristone, and cabergoline has been tried. Mifepristone has been shown to improve metabolic features, although largely ineffective for the associated hypertension. Cabergoline may be effective if pituitary adenoma contains dopamine type 2 receptors. Pasireotide has also been found to be effective in a few patients.

Bilateral or unilateral adrenalectomy is done in cases of non-ACTH-dependent Cushing syndrome and treatment-resistant Cushing disease.

Congenital Adrenal Hyperplasia

Congenital adrenal hyperplasia (CAH) is a group of autosomal recessive metabolic disorders characterized by abnormalities in the cholesterol pathway, leading to low levels of cortisol. It affects 1 in 10,000–20,000 people with a higher incidence seen in inbreeding populations such as the Ashkenazi Jews. More than 90% of affected individuals are known to have 21-hydroxylase deficiency, with mutations occurring in the *CYP21A2* gene on chromosome 6.

Depending on the severity of enzyme deficiency and age at presentation, the disease is categorized into classical virilizing CAH, simple virilizing CAH, and nonclassical CAH.

Classical CAH presents with typical ambiguous genitalia in newborn girls and is associated with salt-wasting, failure to thrive, and death due to electrolyte imbalance in affected male and female neonates. It is highly advisable to ask for newborn screening for CAH as a routine by Guthrie cards, as early diagnosis and treatment have been seen to reduce morbidity and mortality.

Simple virilizing CAH patients present with precocious puberty or clitoromegaly, virilization, and early skeletal maturity.

Late-onset CAH or nonclassical CAH presents in peripubertal girls who come with complaints of primary amenorrhea or oligomenorrhea, hirsutism, clitoromegaly, or acne. Ultrasound of the pelvis will show a polycystic ovarian morphology picture, and such patients are often labeled as having PCOS.

Serum cortisol level of <50 ng/mL with 17-hydroxy-progesterone (17-OHP) of >10,000 with high 24-hour urinary 17-ketosteroid is definitive of a diagnosis. In cases of nonclassical CAH, a Synacthen test will have to be done.

Synacthen Test

Synacthen (synthetic ACTH) testing is done to detect cases of CAH. A fasting early morning 17-OHP, cortisol, and ACTH are done, followed by an injection of Synacthen 250 mg intravenously. Repeat measurement of 17-OHP and cortisol is done after 30 minutes. Heterozygotes and homozygotes for 21-hydroxylase deficiency will have 17-OHP of 35 and >60 nmol/L.

Management[18]

All newborns with ambiguous genitalia must undergo a karyotype, abdominal scan to look for the uterus and ovaries, and a screen for CAH.

Extensive psychological support is required for all individuals suffering from CAH in all its spectrums, as issues of gender identity and infertility are common.

Glucocorticoids supplementation is the mainstay of treatment in late-onset CAH in symptomatic individuals. Counseling is also needed about the possibilities of the conception of a child with classical CAH.

ENDOCRINE-DISRUPTING COMPOUNDS

Manmade synthetic chemicals in pesticides, heavy metals, additives, and contaminants in food and personal products have been known to alter reproductive functions in both males and females. They have been thought to be responsible for the increased incidence of breast cancers, alteration in growth patterns, preterm labor, decreasing age at puberty, abnormal semen parameters, immune abnormalities, and neurodevelopmental delay in children.

Endocrine-disrupting compounds (EDC) are defined as exogenous synthetic chemicals or a mixture of chemicals that interfere with any aspect of hormone action.[19]

They can be inhaled in the air, ingested by food, water, absorbed through the skin, transferred across the placenta, or secreted in the breast milk. These chemicals have been identified by the WHO as an important cause of morbidity and mortality, with pregnant women and children being most vulnerable to their exposure.

The United Nations Environment Programme and WHO have released a joint statement on EDC and its effect on various aspects of fertility and the endocrine system. Policies must be made to reduce exposure and thereby reduce morbidity due to EDC.

CONCLUSION

Endocrine disorders affecting reproduction can have multiple etiology. This is especially pertinent when evaluating the infertile patient. Attention must be given to the common organs affecting reproduction—hypothalamus, pituitary, thyroid, adrenal gland, and ovaries. Each of these may individually or in synchrony affect reproduction. It is essential to individualize treatment based on a careful evaluation of the same.

REFERENCES

1. Goodman NF, Cobin RH, Futterweit W, Glueck JS, Legro RS, Carmina E, et al. American Association of Clinical Endocrinologists, American College of Endocrinology, and Androgen Excess and PCOS Society Disease State clinical review: guide to the best practices in the evaluation and treatment of polycystic ovary syndrome—part 2. Endocr Pract. 2015;21(12):1415-26.
2. Perez-Castro C, Renner U, Haedo MR, Stalla GK, Arzt E. Cellular and molecular specificity of pituitary gland physiology. Physiol Rev. 2012;92(1):1-38.
3. Chang AY, Auchus RJ. Endocrine disturbances affecting reproduction. In: Barbieri RL, Strauss JF (Eds). Yen & Jaffe's Reproductive Endocrinology, 7th edition. Philadelphia: WB Saunders; 2014. pp. 551-64.
4. Serri O, Chik CL, Ur E, Ezzat S. Diagnosis and management of hyperprolactinemia. CMAJ. 2003;169(6):575-81.
5. Melmed S, Casanueva FF, Hoffman AR, Kleinberg DL, Montori VM, Schlechte JA, et al. Diagnosis and treatment of hyperprolactinemia: an Endocrine Society clinical practice guideline. J Clin Endocrinol Metab. 2011;96(2):273-88.
6. La Torre D, Falorni A. Pharmacological causes of hyperprolactinemia. Ther Clin Risk Manag. 2007;3(5):929-51.
7. Katznelson L, Laws Jr ER, Melmed S, Molitch ME, Murad MH, Utz A, et al. Acromegaly: an endocrine society clinical practice guideline. J Clin Endocrinol Metab. 2014;99(11):3933-51.
8. Assal A, Malcolm J, Lochnan H, Keely E. Preconception counselling for women with acromegaly: more questions than answers. Obstet Med. 2016;9(1):9-14.
9. Vanderpump MP. The epidemiology of thyroid disease. Br Med Bull. 2011;99(1):39-51.
10. Boelaert K, Franklyn JA. Thyroid hormone in health and disease. J Endocrinol. 2005;187(1):1-15.
11. Alexander EK, Pearce EN, Brent GA, Brown RS, Chen H, Dosiou C, et al. 2017 guidelines of the American Thyroid Association for the diagnosis and management of thyroid disease during pregnancy and the postpartum. Thyroid. 2017;27(3):315-89.
12. Poppe K, Bisschop P, Fugazzola L, Minziori G, Unuane D, Weghofer A. 2021 European Thyroid Association guideline on thyroid disorders prior to and during assisted reproduction. Eur Thyroid J. 2021;9:281-95.
13. Ross DS, Burch HB, Cooper DS, Greenlee MC, Laurberg P, Maia AL, et al. 2016 American Thyroid Association guidelines for diagnosis and management of hyperthyroidism and other causes of thyrotoxicosis. Thyroid. 2016;26(10):1343-421.
14. Negro R, Formoso G, Coppola L, Presicce G, Mangieri T, Pezzarossa A, et al. Euthyroid women with autoimmune disease undergoing assisted reproduction technologies: the role of autoimmunity and thyroid function. J Endocrinol Invest. 2007;30(1):3-8.
15. Fröhlich E, Wahl R. Thyroid autoimmunity: role of anti-thyroid antibodies in thyroid and extra-thyroidal diseases. Front Immunol. 2017;8:521.
16. Raff H, Sharma ST, Nieman LK. Physiological basis for the etiology, diagnosis, and treatment of adrenal disorders: Cushing's syndrome, adrenal insufficiency, and congenital adrenal hyperplasia. Compr Physiol. 2014;4(2):739-69.
17. Sharma ST, Nieman LK, Feelders RA. Cushing's syndrome: epidemiology and developments in disease management. Clin Epidemiol. 2015;7:281-93.
18. Auchus RJ, Arlt W. Approach to the patient: the adult with congenital adrenal hyperplasia. J Clin Endocrinol Metab. 2013;98(7):2645-55.
19. Bergman Å, Heindel JJ, Jobling S, Kidd KA, Zoeller RT. State of the Science of Endocrine Disrupting Chemicals 2012: Summary for Decision-Makers. United Nations Environment Programme. World Health Organization; 2013.

CHAPTER 12

Hirsutism

Anjali Sharma

INTRODUCTION

Hirsutism is defined as the presence of terminal coarse hairs in a female in the androgen-dependent areas in a male-like pattern.[1] The prevalence of hirsutism is around 5–10%, and many women present in the dermatology department for cosmetic reasons.[2] Hirsutism is usually seen in patients with hormonal imbalance although very rarely may be associated with androgen-producing tumors. It is very important to identify the exact cause and offer appropriate treatment accordingly. Due to a generous contribution from adrenals and ovaries, these women are characterized by increased levels of androgens in their blood.[3] Sometimes, hirsutism can be idiopathic, where androgen levels are normal.

NORMAL DEVELOPMENT AND REGULATION OF GROWTH

Out of 50 million hair follicles distributed over the entire body, 100,000–150,000 are present on the scalp. Lips, palms of hands, and soles of the feet are the hairless areas of the body.

Hairs are classified into three categories based on their structure **(Fig. 1)**:

1. Lanugo is a soft hair that covers the skin of a neonate and gets shed off between the first and the fourth month of the postnatal phase of life.
2. Vellus hairs are longer than lanugo hairs but are similar in their texture. Vellus hairs cover the allegedly hairless areas of the body and are generally nonpigmented with a length of <2 mm.
3. Terminal hairs are longer, pigmented, and coarse in texture. The body and facial hair of men along with the eyelashes, eyebrows, scalp, axillary, and pubic hair in both sexes are terminal in nature.[4] Terminal hairs are often illustrated as being "medullated." The "medulla" is the innermost area of a terminal hair follicle and is made-up of a "collapsed protein", although the exact composition of this portion is still unknown. The lanugo and vellus hairs are nonmedullated.

There are three phases of hair growth shown in **Figure 2**.

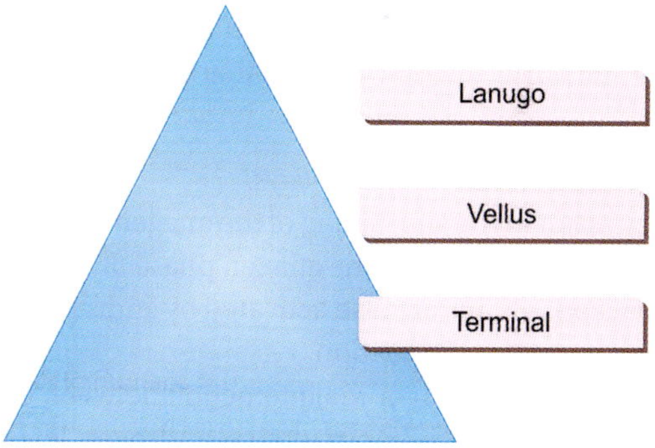

Fig. 1: Classification of hairs based on their structure.

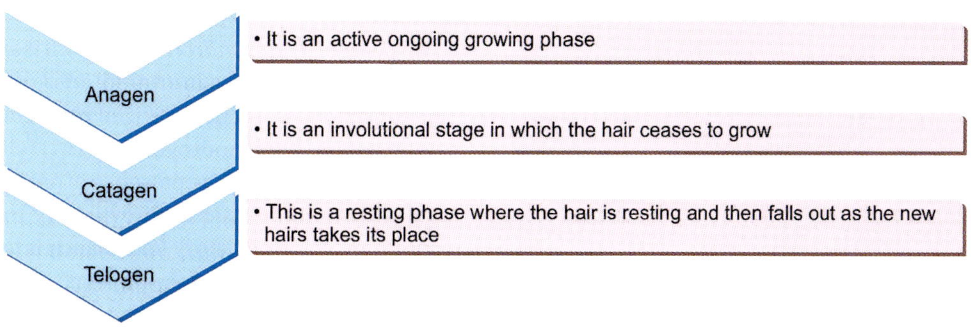

Fig. 2: Three phases of hair growth.

The hairs seem to be growing continuously due to the asynchrony in the growth phase of different hair follicles; some hairs are in the active phase while others are in the resting phase and vice versa, giving the illusion of continuous growth.

Regulatory Factors in Hair Growth

- *Local and systemic factors:* Various growth factors and cytokines have been observed to affect the hair growth.[5] These factors act by increasing the synthesis of stromelysin, which is a matrix metalloproteinase that acts on the dermal papilla to boost the growth of the hair follicle.

  Other hormones such as thyroid and growth hormone can also affect the hair growth. The anagen–telogen ratio in the scalp gets changed due to the deficiency of these hormones.[6,7] So, when patients with hypothyroidism and growth hormone deficiency are treated, regrowth of scalp hairs is seen within approximately 8 weeks, which is not associated with an increase in circulating androgens in the dermal papilla.[8]
- *Sex steroids:* The type and distribution of hairs are determined by the androgen levels in the body. The main androgens in the serum of a woman with a normal menstrual cycle in decreasing order of serum levels are dehydroepiandrosterone sulfate (DHEA-S), DHEA, androstenedione, testosterone, and dihydrotestosterone (DHT) **(Fig. 3)**.

  Testosterone and DHT activate androgen receptors, which result in gene transcription. DHEA, DHEA-S, and androstenedione are considered to be prohormones as they do not bind to the androgen receptors. Androgens can transform the hair follicles that produce vellus-type hairs into terminal hairs.

Androgens act in the following ways:
- They result in the shortening of the anagen phase of scalp hairs while prolonging the anagen phase of body hairs.[9]
- Sebaceous glands are also activated by androgens, which result in sebum production.

Hirsutism is a result of the interaction between the local androgen concentration, circulating androgen levels, and the sensitivity of the hair follicles to androgens. Yet, it has been seen that the severity of hirsutism is not associated with high androgen levels. There is an interindividual variation in the response of hair follicles to the circulating androgen levels explaining the varied response. However, some women with raised androgen levels are asymptomatic, and others may have seborrhea, acne, or alopecia even with normal androgen levels.

Hypertrichosis is a clinical entity that needs to be differentiated from hirsutism, where excessive growth of vellus hair is seen, which can be due to the intake of certain medications, such as glucocorticoids, phenytoin, minoxidil, and cyclosporine, or can be hereditary in nature. The hairs are distributed in a generalized nonsexual pattern.

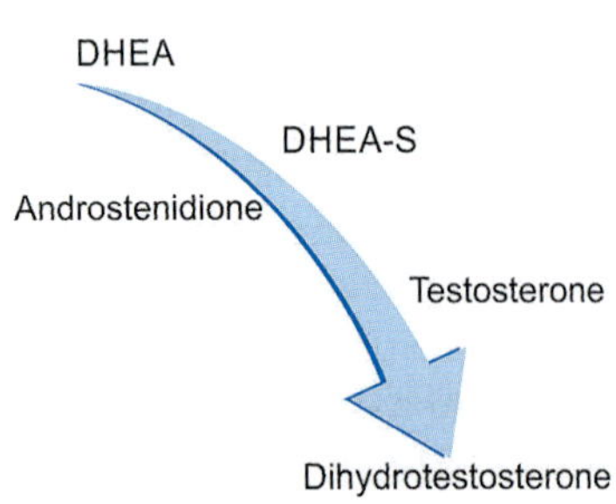

Fig. 3: Main androgens in the serum of a woman with a normal menstrual cycle in decreasing order of serum levels. (DHEA-S: dehydroepiandrosterone sulfate)

DIAGNOSIS OF HIRSUTISM

Several hirsutism scoring systems are available, of which the modified Ferriman–Gallwey score **(Fig. 4)** has now become the gold standard for the evaluation of hirsutism.[10]

This method scores 9 out of the 11 body areas (upper lip, chin, chest, upper and lower back, upper and lower abdomen, arm, forearm, thigh, and lower leg).

- *Score 0:* If terminal hair growth is not seen in the above areas
- *Score 1:* Minimally visible terminal hair growth is present
- *Score 2:* If hair growth is more than minimal, but not equivalent to that of an adult male.
- *Score 3:* If hair growth is that of a not very hairy male
- *Score 4:* Observed in well-virilized healthy adult males

  Total scores range from 0 to 36.

Hirsutism has been graded as:
- *Mild:* Up to a score of 15
- *Moderate:* For a score of 16–25
- *Severe:* Above the score of 25.

ETIOLOGY OF HIRSUTISM

Figure 5 shows the etiology of hirsutism.
- *Idiopathic hirsutism:* This term is used when a hirsute patient has normal ovulatory cycles and normal androgen levels. The pathophysiology is presumed to be the increased activity of 5α-reductase enzyme or an alteration in the androgen receptor function. It is seen in 4–7% of the patients.
- *Ovarian causes:*
  - *Polycystic ovarian syndrome (PCOS):* It is an endocrine disorder, which is seen in around 70%[11] of women with hirsutism. PCOS is characterized by oligoovulation or anovulation, hyperandrogenism (HA) (either clinical or biochemical), and the presence of polycystic ovaries on ultrasound. Classical anovulatory form is most common, while ovulatory form which is less common is seen in around 20% of the patients.
  - *Ovarian neoplasm:* Very rarely, women with ovarian malignancies, which include arrhenoblastoma,

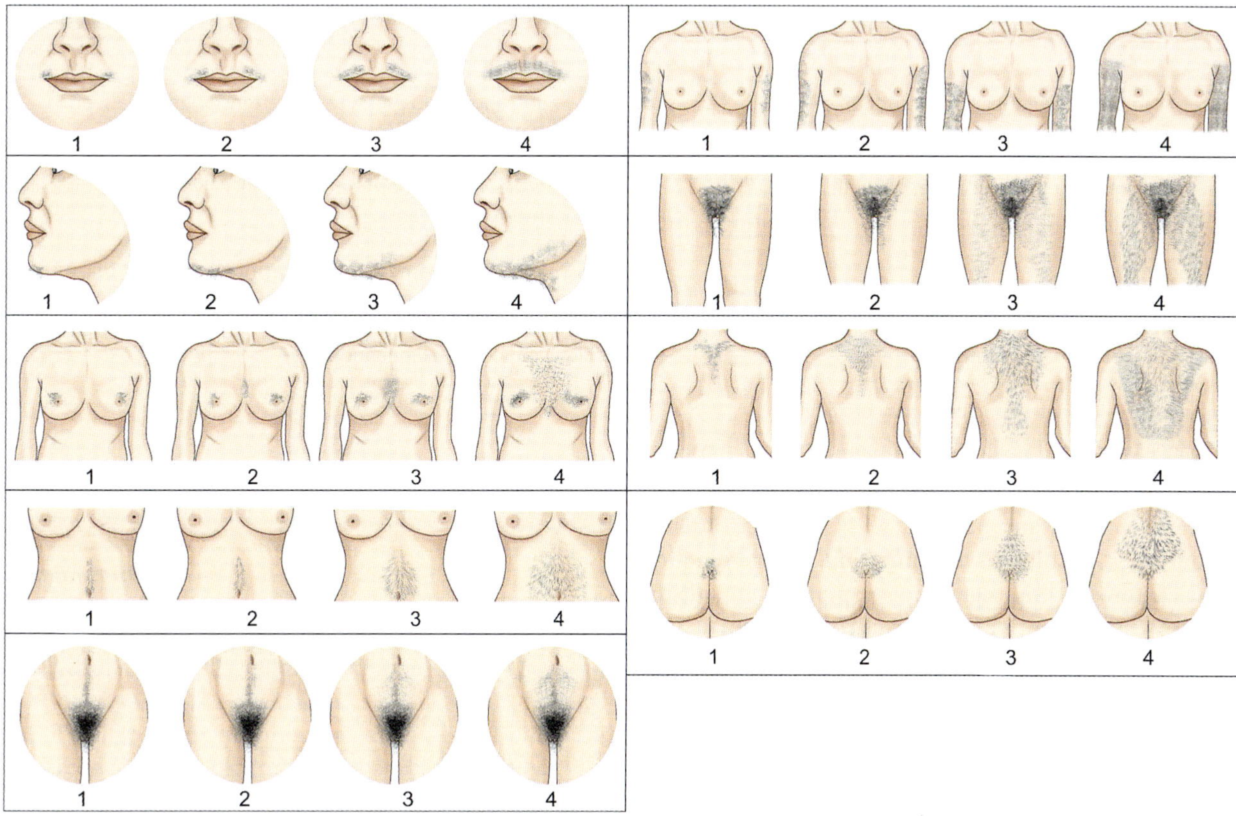

Fig. 4: Modified Ferriman–Gallwey (F–G) hirsutism scoring system. Each of the nine body areas is rated from 0 (absence of terminal hairs) to 4 (extensive terminal hair growth), and the numbers in each area are added for a total score. A modified F–G score ≥6 generally defines hirsutism.

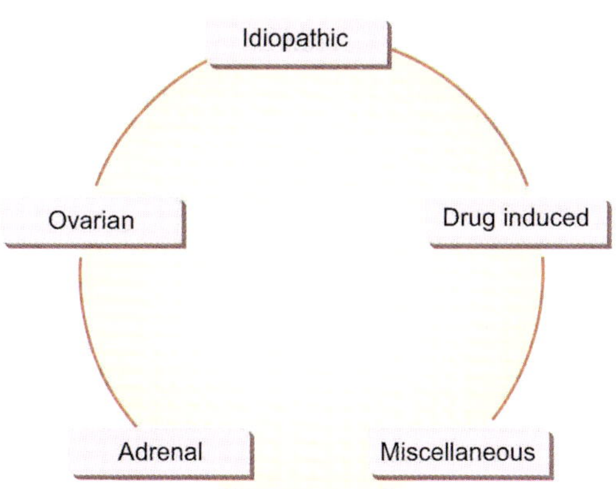

Fig. 5: Etiology of hirsutism.

Leydig cell tumor, and hilus cell tumor, can also present with hirsutism.

- *Adrenal causes:*
  - *Enzymatic deficiencies:*
    - 21-Hydroxylase deficiency (P-450c21)
    - 11β-Hydroxylase deficiency (P-450c11)
    - 3β-Hydroxysteroid dehydrogenase deficiency.

Adrenal hyperplasia is seen in around 5% of the patients with hirsutism, where due to a defect in adrenal cortisol synthesis, the precursors are redirected into the androgen synthesis pathway. Cases of classic adrenal hyperplasia are diagnosed at birth by ambiguous genitalia, while nonclassical congenital adrenal hyperplasia (NCCAH) can remain undiagnosed till puberty, when women develop menstrual irregularity along with anovulatory cycles and hirsutism.

  - *Neoplasms:*
    - Virilizing adrenal adenoma
    - Virilizing adrenal carcinoma.

These are very rare causes that are present in <0.2% of cases of hirsutism.

- *Drug induced:* Various medications that have been implicated as a cause of hirsutism are listed here:
  - Carbamazepine
  - Clonazepam
  - Corticosteroids
  - Cyclosporine
  - Diazoxide
  - Donepezil
  - Estrogens
  - Fluoxetine
  - Interferon alfa
  - Isotretinoin
  - Lamotrigine
  - Olanzapine

TABLE 1: History and the physical examination of hirsutism.

History	*Physical examination*
• Onset of symptoms whether slow or sudden with the extent of hair growth • Menstrual and reproductive history (PCOS patients may present with menstrual irregularities with infertility) • Weight gain • Breast discharge • Medication history • Skin changes (acne, striae) • Symptoms of virilization (changes in voice, atrophy of breast and muscle mass, amenorrhea, etc.) • Use of hair removal methods • Family history (idiopathic hirsutism may be familial)	• Height, weight, and blood pressure (hypertension may be seen in patients with nonclassical CAH) • Documentation of hair amount distribution • Skin changes (i.e., acne, seborrhea, thick dark velvety skin at the back (seen in acanthosis nigricans) • Galactorrhea • Signs of Cushing's syndrome (central obesity, abdominal stria, muscle weakness, and moon-like faces) • Signs of virilization • Abdominal and pelvic examination

(CAH: congenital adrenal hyperplasia; PCOS: polycystic ovarian syndrome)

- *Miscellaneous:* Many patients with hypothyroidism, acromegaly, Cushing's syndrome, and hyperprolactinemia can present with signs and symptoms of hirsutism. HAIR-AN syndrome[2] is another cause of hirsutism, which is defined as a constellation of HA, insulin resistance (IR), and acanthosis nigricans (AN).

INVESTIGATIONS AND MANAGEMENT

History and Examination

A complete and precise clinical history along with the physical examination, including the Ferriman-Gallwey scoring system, remains instrumental for the diagnosis of hirsutism. Idiopathic hirsutism shows an onset at the time of puberty with a slow progression over the years **(Table 1)**.[12]

Hormonal Evaluation (Table 2)

Free testosterone level measurement is of utmost importance as compared to the total testosterone level for the diagnosis of hyperandrogenic disorders. The significance of measuring serum androstenedione and DHEA-S levels in patients with hirsutism is questionable.[13]

Other hormonal evaluation may include:

- *Tests to rule out NCCAH:*
  - Cosyntropin stimulation test
  - 17α-Hydroxyprogesterone level >1,000 ng/dL is taken as cut-off for the diagnosis.
- Serum prolactin levels—if the patient presents with irregular menstruation and galactorrhea

TABLE 2: Hormonal evaluation.

Androgen	*Normal value in females*
Total testosterone	20–80 ng/dL
Free testosterone	0.3–1.9 ng/dL
Bioavailable testosterone	0.8–10 ng/dL
Free androgen index (T/SHBG × 100)	0.7–1
Androgen-producing tumors	>200 ng/dL

(SHBG: sex hormone-binding globulin; T: testosterone)

Metabolic Profile

For a patient presenting with obesity and PCOS, the recommended tests, including metabolic screening should be:

- Measurement of blood pressure, waist circumference, and body mass index (BMI)
- Complete lipid profile, including total cholesterol, low-density lipoprotein cholesterol, nonhigh-density lipoprotein (HDL) cholesterol, HDL cholesterol, and triglycerides
- *A 2-hour post 75 -g oral glucose tolerance test:* In patients with a family history of type 2 diabetes, personal history of gestational diabetes, or advanced age (>40 years), this test is recommended.

Ultrasound Evaluation

In addition to clinical findings and hormonal assays, ultrasound evaluation is also helpful in the evaluation of any patient with hirsutism. Ultrasound is helpful in the detection of polycystic ovarian morphology; it is also helpful in the detection of other rare disorders, such as NCCAH or androgen-secreting tumors.

TREATMENT AND MANAGEMENT

Treatment of hirsutism depends on various factors such as the severity of the condition and the amount of distress it is causing to the patient. A decision regarding the mode of treatment depends on the reproductive status of the patient; also, we need to take into consideration the potential side effects. The women should be well educated about the principles of management that the treatment will never be curative and it may take several months before the effects of treatment to become evident and the need for monitoring by an expert **(Fig. 6)**.

Lifestyle Modifications

Obesity is associated with increased serum androgen levels, and it has been seen that weight reduction improves the efficacy of other medical treatments. It has been noted that weight reduction results in a decrease in total and free testosterone and an increase in sex hormone-binding globulin (SHBG) levels; however, there is no convincing evidence to support the reduction in hirsutism following such measures.[14]

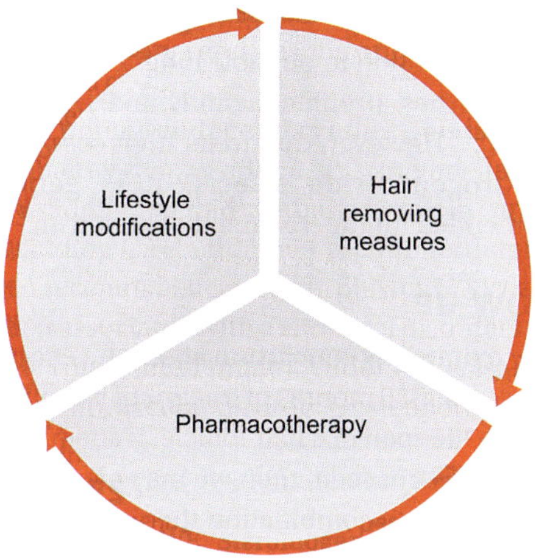

Fig. 6: Treatment and management of hirsutism.

Hair-Removing Measures

Various methods of hair removal are available, which may be used as a temporary measures or permanent measures **(Table 3)**.

Pharmacological Measures

Drug therapy is advocated for those patients who do not have any fertility issues. However, the efficacy of these drugs varies from person to person. Various pharmacological agents that can be used have been listed here.

Oral Contraceptive Pills

Combined oral contraceptives (OC) act by reducing the free androgen levels by increasing SHBG and inhibiting ovarian androgen production. The Endocrine Society recommends OC as the first-line medication for those women where infertility is not an issue.[1] Third-generation oral contraceptive pills (OCPs) are better in terms of efficacy; however, second-generation OCPs are better in terms of safety profile.

Antiandrogens

Table 4 shows list of drugs, their dose, and side effects.

While prescribing an antiandrogen, the following things should be taken into consideration:

TABLE 3: Temporary and permanent measures of hair removal.

Temporary methods	*Permanent methods*
Shaving: It is a simple, easy, and effective method, but has to be done at regular intervals. Also, the regrowth of hairs is coarser in nature because of the tip, which is blunt rather than tapered	*Electrolysis:* It is not a very popular method due to the pain. Also, it is a time-taking procedure because every follicle needs to be removed individually. It is of two types: Galvanic and thermal
Chemical depilation: It acts by dissolving the hairs, but may result in inflammation and dermatitis	*Laser therapy:* It is a more accepted form of treatment as it is less agonizing and faster than electrolysis, but it is relatively an expensive form of therapy. A recent Cochrane review of hair removal methods has found it to be less effective.[15] Diode and Alexandrite lasers are commonly used, and they reduced hair by almost 50%. Laser therapy works best in light-skinned women. Hyperpigmentation is a common adverse effect
Epilation methods: These include waxing or plucking, which removes the hairs from the roots, but comes with the side effects of folliculitis, hyperpigmentation, and sometimes scarring	

TABLE 4: List of drugs, their dose, and side effects.

Type of drug	*Drug*	*Dose*	*Side effects*	*Comments*
Androgen receptor blocker	Spironolactone	100–200 mg/day	Hyperkalemia, mild diuretic effect, postural hypotension, and irregular menses	Because of the dangers of antiandrogenic effects on fetal genital development, it is recommended that spironolactone should be given along with an oral contraceptive agent
	Cyproterone acetate	2 mg along with 35 μg of ethinylestradiol as a contraceptive pill	Nausea, fatigue, mastalgia, loss of libido, and weight gain	Should be given with ethinyl estradiol to prevent menstrual irregularities and ovulation
	Flutamide	250–750 mg/day	Liver toxicity	It is not approved for the treatment of hirsutism by the Endocrine Society because of the risk of liver failure
5α-Reductase inhibitor	Finasteride	5–7.5 mg/day	Gastrointestinal disturbances, headache, dry skin, and decreased libido	

- It can be combined with OCPs in women who do not reach a satisfactory result using OCPs alone after 1 year of treatment.
- It can be used as a single agent where OCPs are contraindicated, provided that the patient is using a reliable contraceptive method.

Topical Eflornithine

Eflornithine (13.9%) is a topical agent that reduces hair growth by inhibiting the enzyme ornithine decarboxylase, which catalyzes the conversion of ornithine to putrescine, a polyamine that is required to regulate the cell growth and differentiation within the hair follicle.[16] The effect is seen after 8 weeks of the therapy. It can be used alone or in conjunction with other therapies. However, it has been observed that the hair growth restarts after the discontinuation of the therapy. Eflornithine is currently approved for the treatment of unwanted facial hairs only.

Insulin Sensitizers

Insulin sensitizers improve IR and menstrual dysfunction and may decrease serum androgen concentrations.[17] According to a recent Cochrane review, in adult women with PCOS and hirsutism, either metformin alone or the OCP alone may be less effective in improving hirsutism as compared to metformin combined with the OCP.[18]

Miscellaneous Agents (Fig. 7)

- *Glucocorticoids:* The role of glucocorticoids in the treatment of hirsutism is controversial. They may be used in patients with NCCAH along with antiandrogens for better remission.[19] The drug used is prednisolone with a dosage of 5–10 mg daily. Currently, available studies suggest that they are less effective as compared with OCPs and antiandrogens.[20]
- *Ketoconazole:* It is an adrenal enzyme inhibitor that is used at a dosage of 400 mg/day. However, due to its side effects such as hepatotoxicity, its use is limited to the subjects of Cushing's syndrome, while waiting for definite treatment.

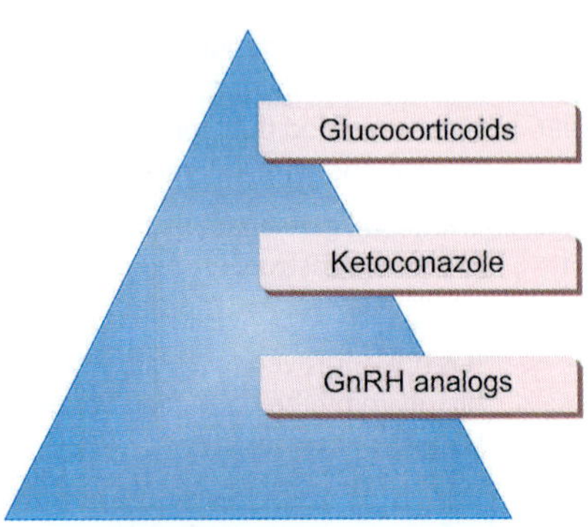

Fig. 7: Miscellaneous agents.
(GnRH: gonadotropin-releasing hormone agonist)

- *Gonadotropin-releasing hormone agonist (GnRH) analogs:* Long-acting GnRH agonists (e.g., leuprolide depot, 3.75 mg/month) have been found to be useful and may be required to suppress the hypothalamic–pituitary–ovarian axis in severely androgenized or hyperinsulinemic patients. Two to three months of treatment may be required for the full suppressive effect of the agonist to occur. GnRH analogs should be reserved for use in women who do not respond to combination hormonal therapy or those who cannot tolerate OCs. GnRH analogs should be used cautiously with particular attention to possible long-term consequences (e.g., hot flushes, atrophic vaginitis, and demineralization of bones).[21] However, due to its high cost and adverse hypoestrogenic side effects, it is generally not recommended for the treatment of hirsutism.

FOLLOW-UP

To be able to draw any conclusion about the effectiveness of any therapy, at least 6 months of treatment is required, which is the average life span of a hair follicle. If adequate response after 6 months is not seen, then we may consider switching the agents or using a combination therapy. The rationale of measuring serum androgen levels is not convincing, but if a decrease in serum androgen levels is documented during the treatment, then it may increase the patient's confidence in the therapy, especially while waiting for the clinical response to be evident.

KEY POINTS

- Hirsutism needs to be evaluated, especially if rapidly progressing, although may be idiopathic at times.
- A thorough history-taking, including history of medications and complete physical examination, needs to be done in all cases of hirsutism.
- The investigations that need to be done depend on the finding in history and examination to make a final diagnosis.
- Management again depends on the severity of symptoms and definitive diagnosis and includes both nonpharmacological and pharmacological measures.
- Any pharmacotherapy needs to be given for at least 6 months to draw any conclusion about its effectiveness.

REFERENCES

1. Martin KA, Chang RJ, Ehrmann DA, Ibanez L, Lobo RA, Rosenfield RL, et al. Evaluation and treatment of hirsutism in premenopausal women: an Endocrine Society clinical practice guideline. J Clin Endocrinol Metab. 2008;93(4):1105-20.
2. Azziz R, Woods KS, Reyna R, Key TJ, Knochenhauer ES, Yildiz BO. The prevalence and features of the polycystic ovary syndrome in an unselected population. J Clin Endocrinol Metab. 2004;89(6):2745-9.

3. Rosenfield RL. Clinical practice. Hirsutism. N Engl J Med. 2005;353:2578-88.
4. Uno H. Biology of hair growth. Semin Reprod Endocrinol. 1986;4:131-41.
5. Jankovic SM, Jankovic SV. The control of hair growth. Dermatol Online J. 1998;4:2.
6. Comaisch JS. The thyroid and hair growth. Semin Dermatol. 1985;4:4-8.
7. Blok GJ, de Boer H, Gooren LJ, van der Veen EA. Growth hormone substitution in adult growth hormone-deficient men augments androgen effects on the skin. Clin Endocrinol (Oxf). 1997;47:29-36.
8. Lobie PE, Breipohl W, Lincoln DT, García-Aragón J, Waters MJ. Localization of the growth hormone receptor/binding protein in skin. J Endocrinol. 1990;126:467-71.
9. Randall VA. Androgens and human hair growth. Clin Endocrinol (Oxf). 1994;40:439-57.
10. Yildiz BO, Bolour S, Woods K, Moore A, Azziz R. Visually scoring hirsutism. Hum Reprod Update. 2010;16:51-64.
11. Escobar-Morreale HF, Sanchón R, San Millán JL. A prospective study of the prevalence of nonclassical congenital adrenal hyperplasia among women presenting with hyperandrogenic symptoms and signs. J Clin Endocrinol Metab. 2008;93:527-33.
12. Hunter MH, Carek PJ. Evaluation and treatment of women with hirsutism. Am Fam Physician. 2003;67(12):2565-72.
13. Azziz R, Carmina E, Dewailly D, Diamanti-Kandarakis E, Escobar-Morreale HF, Futterweit W, et al. The androgen excess and PCOS society criteria for the polycystic ovary syndrome: the complete task force report. Fertil Steril. 2009;91:456-88.
14. Moran LJ, Hutchison SK, Norman RJ, Teede HJ. Lifestyle changes in women with polycystic ovary syndrome. Cochrane Database Syst Rev. 2011;(2):CD007506.
15. Haedersdal M, Gøtzsche PC. Laser and photoepilation for unwanted hair growth. Cochrane Database Syst Rev. 2006;(4):CD004684.
16. Balfour JAB, McClellan K. Topical eflornithine. Am J Clin Dermatol. 2001;2:197-201.
17. Lord JM, Flight IHK, Norman RJ. Insulin-sensitising drugs (metformin, troglitazone, rosiglitazone, pioglitazone, D-chiro-inositol) for polycystic ovary syndrome. Cochrane Database Syst Rev. 2003;(3):CD003053.
18. Fraison E, Kostova E, Moran LJ, Bilal S, Ee CC, Venetis C, et al. Metformin versus the combined oral contraceptive pill for hirsutism, acne, and menstrual pattern in polycystic ovary syndrome. Cochrane Database Syst Rev. 2020;8(8):CD005552.
19. Carmina E, Lobo RA. The addition of dexamethasone to antiandrogen therapy for hirsutism prolongs the duration of remission. Fertil Steril. 1998;69:1075-9.
20. Devoto E, Aravena L, Rios R. Treatment of hirsutism with spironolactone and with spironolactone plus dexamethasone. Rev Med Chil. 2000;128:868-75.
21. Pazos F, Escobar-Morreale HF, Balsa J, Sancho JM, Varela C. Prospective randomized study comparing the long-acting gonadotropin-releasing hormone agonist triptorelin, flutamide, and cyproterone acetate, used in combination with an oral contraceptive, in the treatment of hirsutism. Fertil Steril. 1999;71:122-8.

CHAPTER 13

Luteal Phase Defect

Deepti Sharma

INTRODUCTION

- Luteal phase of menstrual cycle starts after ovulation and leads to formation of corpus luteum (CL), which produces progesterone as a major hormone.[1]
- If pregnancy is not achieved, there is a drop in progesterone levels after failure of CL, leading to onset of menses.[2]
- However, whenever there is establishment of pregnancy, CL is rescued by luteotropic effect of human chorionic gonadotropin (hCG) produced by implanting embryo. hCG supports production of progesterone from CL by upregulating steroidogenic acute regulatory (StAR) protein and vascular endothelial growth factor (VEGF) gene expression.
- The progesterone produced from CL is essential for maintenance of early pregnancy until placental function is established.
- The concept of luteal phase defect (LPD), also known as luteal phase deficiency, was first described by Georgeanna Seegar Jones in 1949 as decreased production of progesterone during the luteal phase.[3]
- The potential causes of LPD include inadequate progesterone levels, inadequate progesterone duration, or resistance of endometrium to progesterone.[4]
- Luteal phase defect leads to dysfunctional endometrial development during the interval when embryo is present in uterine cavity, which in turn leads to impairment of implantation or maintenance of pregnancy.[5,6]
- LPD has been a controversial topic with doubts regarding its clinical relevance, due to a lack of reliable diagnostic criteria and treatment options.[7]
- As of now, LPD has not been proven as an independent cause of infertility or recurrent pregnancy loss.[4]

DEFINITION

- Luteal phase defect or luteal phase deficiency is a condition in which endogenous hormone production from ovaries is not of enough quantity or for enough duration so as to maintain the secretory endometrium for embryo implantation and growth.[4]
- *Clinical LPD* is defined as a luteal phase length of ≤10 days.[8]

INCIDENCE AND PREVALENCE

- The incidence of LPD is between 6.6 and 51%, estimated by endometrial biopsy in normally fertile women.[9] Endometrial biopsy timed during luteal phase and analyzed according to Noyes criteria remains the gold standard for many years.[10]
- Its prevalence is 8.1% in normo-ovulatory primary or secondary infertile patients.[11]
- In women with recurrent miscarriages, it is about 32.5%.[12]

PHYSIOLOGY OF LUTEAL PHASE

Corpus Luteum Formation

- Luteinizing hormone (LH) surge leads to resumption of meiosis in primary oocyte in dominant follicle and release of the first polar body and secondary oocyte, and the follicle remnant forms the CL.
- Corpus luteum contains steroidogenic cells along with immune cells and endothelial cells.[13] Steroidogenic cells are derived from granulosa and theca cells of follicle.[14]
- Formation of CL is characterized by neovascularization of granulosa cells. After ovulation, tissue remodeling takes place, and blood vessels from thecal vasculature invade granulosa cells.[15] This leads to formation of CL, which is the most vascular organ with blood flow of 6–10 mL/g/min, which is highest in the body.[16]

Progesterone Production

- Following LH surge, during luteinization, granulosa cells start expressing set of genes necessary to encode for progesterone production, which includes those required for side-chain cleavage for cholesterol esters (P450scc) and 3β-hydroxysteroid dehydrogenase (3β-HSD).[17]

- Steroidogenic acute regulatory protein is required for transfer of cholesterol from outer to inner mitochondrial membrane.[18] *StAR* gene is expressed in granulosa cells only after LH surge, thus enabling them to synthesize progesterone.[19]
- For progesterone biosynthesis, CL uptakes low-density lipoprotein (LDL) and high-density lipoprotein (HDL) from blood while cholesterol esters from intracellular stores. All these are then transported inside mitochondria with the help of StAR protein, where they are converted to pregnenolone with action of enzyme P450cc, which enters cytoplasm and gets converted to progesterone by 3β-HSD.[13]
- Daily production rate of progesterone during midluteal phase is 25 mg/day[20] and is under the control of LH pulse frequency (177/min) and amplitude (0.26 mIU/mL/min).[21]
- Progesterone acts on estrogen-primed endometrium to induce secretory changes, which are necessary for implantation of embryo. During these changes, glands become tortuous and secretory, and there is increased stromal vascularity.[22]

Estrogen Production

- During luteal phase, LH acts on small luteal cells for androgen production, which is then converted to estrogen in large luteal cells with the help of enzyme P450 aromatase expressed by follicle-stimulating hormone (FSH).[23]
- In luteal cells, steroidogenic action of FSH is augmented by LH and insulin-like growth factors.[24]
- The exact role of luteal estrogen is unknown; however, in primates, it appears to play a role in luteolysis.[25] But in humans, due to the presence of both types of estrogen receptors, estrogen is supposed to have local action also in luteal function.[26]
- Daily estradiol production is 0.25 mg/day during the midluteal phase.[20]

Luteolysis

- Corpus luteum undergoes a process of regression known as luteolysis in nonfertile cycles **(Fig. 1)**. It includes loss of functional as well as structural integrity of the gland.[27]
- Functional luteal regression consists of reduced production of progesterone levels, which in turn is due to decreased expression of *StAR* gene. Other molecules, including prostaglandin F2α, tumor necrosis factor-α, interleukin-1β, endothelin, monocyte chemoattractant-1, estrogens, and reactive oxygen species, have been implicated in the luteolytic process.[28]
- For structural regression, apoptosis is one of the mechanisms along with autophagy and necrosis.[29,30] So unscheduled activation of luteolysis can lead to LPD.

Corpus Luteum Rescue

- In a fertile cycle after implantation of blastocyst, CL is rescued structurally and functionally with the help of hCG secreted by the trophoblastic cells.
- It has been shown in vitro in CL that there is increased expression of *StAR* gene expression when hCG is administered in mid- and late luteal phase, not in early luteal phase.[31] In clinical terms, it means that for luteal phase support (LPS), hCG should be given from midluteal phase.[32]
- In addition, hCG rescues CL by stimulating angiogenesis so that the second wave of vascular development takes place.[33]
- The molecular mechanism by which hCG rescues CL is not completely understood. It has been postulated that it prevents apoptosis by interfering at various stages of apoptotic process, which includes inhibition of *Fas* and *Bax* gene expression and stimulating that of B-cell lymphoma-2 (Bcl-2) and increasing survivin, a molecule that inhibits action of caspases-3.[34]

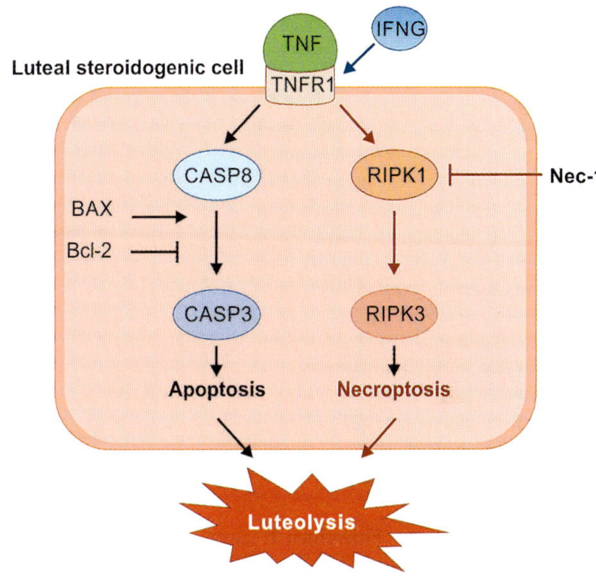

Fig. 1: Schematic representation of possible mechanisms to induce cell death in the bovine LSCs. Proinflammatory cytokines, tumor necrosis factor (TNF) and interferon-gamma (IFNG), can induce at least two cell death pathways, i.e., caspase (CASPs)-dependent apoptotic pathway and receptor-interacting serine/threonine protein kinase (RIPKs)-dependent necroptotic pathway, in the bovine luteal steroidogenic cells (LSCs). Apoptotic pathway is mediated by CASP8 and CASP3; Bcl2-associated X protein (BAX) and B-cell lymphoma-2 (Bcl-2) can play as inducer and inhibitor of apoptotic pathway, respectively. In necroptotic pathway, RIPK1 and RIPK3 play a central role to induce cell death. RIPK1 inhibitor, Nec-1, can inhibit necroptotic pathway. (BAX: Bcl2-associated X protein; Bcl-2: B-cell lymphoma-2; CASP: caspase; IFNG: interferon gamma; RIPK1: receptor-interacting serine/threonine protein kinase 1; TNF: tumor necrosis factor; TNFR1: tumor necrosis factor receptor 1.
Source: Principles and Practices of Assisted Reproductive Technology; second edition;166.

PATHOPHYSIOLOGY OF LUTEAL PHASE DEFECT IN NATURAL CYCLES

Several different mechanisms may be involved.

- *Abnormal follicular phase* leading to lower levels of luteal phase estrogen and progesterone: A follicular phase with low levels of FSH and estrogen, altered FSH/LH ratio and abnormal FSH and LH pulsatility was found to be associated with short luteal phase[8] and also with low levels of estrogen and progesterone in luteal phase.[35]
- *Endometrial resistance to progesterone:* The endometrium of patients with underlying diseases, e.g., polycystic ovarian syndrome (PCOS) and endometriosis, has been found to have altered the response to progesterone, which may lead to infertility.[36,37]
- *Abnormal luteal phase:* Various physiologic and pathologic conditions (as mentioned in **Box 1**) that lead to altered gonadotropin-releasing hormone (GnRH) and LH pulsatility can lead to abnormal luteal phase and hence to LPD.

BOX 1: Factors associated with luteal phase defect in natural cycles.[6,38-51]

- Short menstrual cycles
- Unexplained infertility
- Endometriosis
- First-trimester pregnancy loss
- Premenstrual spotting
- Excessive exercise
- Stress
- Starvation
- Eating disorders
- Extremes of reproductive ages
- Postpartum and lactation
- Renal transplant
- Thyroid and prolactin disorders
- Increased β-endorphin levels
- Obesity
- Hyperandrogenism
- 21-Hydroxylase deficiency

- *Idiopathic LPD or true isolated LPD:* It is the pathologic condition of luteal phase when no underlying disease process could be identified that is responsible for negatively affecting the normal LH support of CL.[4] However, it has not been found that idiopathic LPD can lead to infertility.[39]

PATHOPHYSIOLOGY OF LUTEAL PHASE DEFECT IN CONTROLLED OVARIAN STIMULATION CYCLES

Following the advent of controlled ovarian stimulation (COS) cycles, it was soon recognized that luteal phase was defective in COS cycles **(Flowchart 1, Fig. 2)**. Both gonadotropin-releasing hormone agonist (GnRH-a) and GnRH antagonist cycles are associated with LPD **(Box 2)**. An LPS is a must in all COS cycles to optimize the outcome.

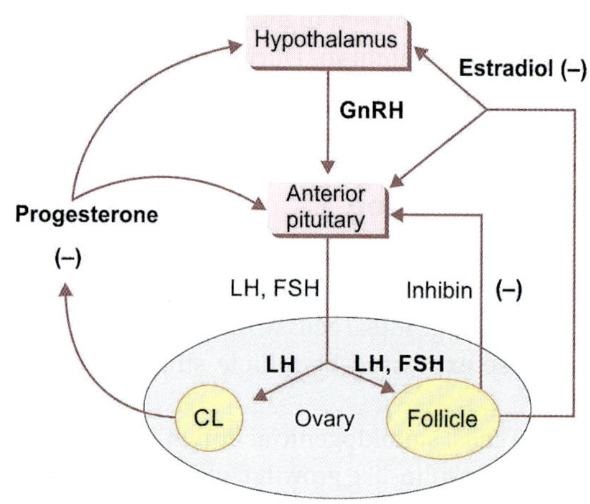

Fig. 2: Luteal phase defect due to supraphysiological steroid levels in controlled ovarian stimulation cycles. (CL: corpus luteum; FSH: follicle-stimulating hormone; GnRH: gonadotropin-releasing hormone; LH: luteinizing hormone)

Source: Adapted from Blockeel C. The Luteal Phase in a Natural and Stimulated Cycle. Brussel: Universitair Ziekenhuis; 2010.

Flowchart 1: Luteal phase defect (LPD) in controlled ovarian stimulation cycles (COS).[59,60]

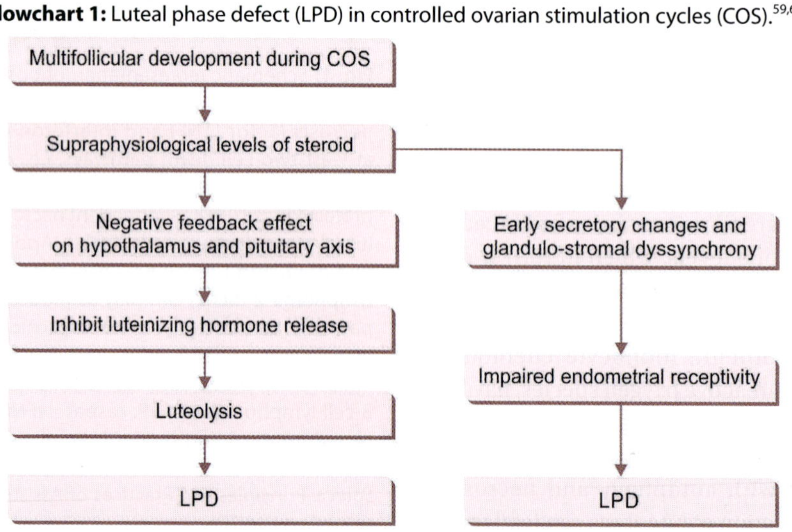

BOX 2: Theories regarding luteal phase defect (LPD) in controlled ovarian stimulation (COS) cycles.

- Destruction of granulosa cells during follicular aspiration, which was destined to form CL[52]
- In GnRH-a cycles, LPD is supposed to be due to prolonged suppression of pituitary LH secretion; usually for up to 3 weeks after downregulation has been achieved[53]
- In GnRH antagonist cycles, it has been found to have low levels of LH in early and midluteal phases irrespective of agent used for final oocyte maturation[54]
- Further adding GnRH-a as a trigger in antagonist cycles leads to short LH surge, which is not sufficient enough to support CL, thus leading to early luteolysis, and diminished estrogen and progesterone levels, and thereby LPD[55,56]
- Multifollicular development in COS leading to supraphysiological steroid levels leads to suppression of LH secretion from the pituitary; hence, a sufficient amount of LH is not available to support CL, thus leading to LPD[57,58]
- Various studies comparing the endometrium in COS cycles with natural cycles have demonstrated early secretory changes and glandular-stromal dyssynchrony in COS cycles leading to impaired endometrial receptivity[57]

(CL: corpus luteum; GnRH: gonadotropin-releasing hormone; LH: luteinizing hormone)

DIAGNOSIS OF LUTEAL PHASE DEFECT

According to the American Society for Reproductive Medicine (ASRM) 2021 guidelines, LPD is a clinical diagnosis.[4] Various diagnostic tests have been described to diagnose, ranging from clinical to biochemical to histological.

- *Length of luteal phase of menstrual cycle*
    - Luteal phase length can be assessed by monitoring basal body temperature (BBT) or by urinary LH surge detection as they substantiate ovulation.
    - BBT method is based upon the rise in body temperature following ovulation[61] and because of its inaccuracy and inconvenience, it is no longer practiced, and the recent studies have used LH surge detection kits to detect the time of ovulation.
    - Length of luteal phase ranges from 11 to 17 days, with an average duration of 14 days.[62] A duration of <9–11 days from the day of LH peak to the onset of menses has been described as "short luteal phase" in various studies.[4,8,42]
    - In one of the recent studies, luteal phase of <10 days was found in 13% of ovulatory menstrual cycles.[8]
    - In another prospective time to pregnancy cohort study, a short luteal phase of ≤11 days was found in 18% of menstrual cycles.[63]
    - Further in this study, it was noted that women with a short luteal phase have low chances of pregnancy in their immediate next menstrual cycles, but their cumulative fecundity for over 12 months was not lower.[63]
    - Given the various durations of short luteal phase described in literature, ASRM 2021 has considered LPD as clinical when the luteal phase duration is <10 days.[4]
- *Serum progesterone levels*
    - Measurement of serum progesterone levels in response to LH during the luteal phase is one of the proposed diagnostic methods for LPD.
    - Progesterone secretion occurs in pulses in normal ovulatory cycles, and its level may fluctuate up to eight times in 90 minutes;[64] therefore, single random serum progesterone value is not of any significance.
    - In one of the recent studies, it was shown that even in ovulatory cycles 8.4% times luteal progesterone is <5 ng/mL, which is called "biochemical LPD" and 31.3% times it is <10 ng/mL.[8]
    - Although it was suggested that the sum of three midluteal levels taken between 5 and 9 days post ovulation when >30 ng/mL has 100% sensitivity and 80% specificity,[65] this has neither been clinically validated nor is clinically practical.
    - Furthermore, the function of CL varies from cycle to cycle in fertile women, so progesterone levels cannot be taken as a diagnostic tool for LPD.[4]
- *Menstrual cycle length and luteal serum progesterone levels combined together*
    - In BioCycle study, it has been proposed to diagnose LPD by combining clinical LPD (luteal phase length <10 days) and biochemical LPD (midluteal serum progesterone <5 ng/mL), which had an 8.2% prevalence in the study.[8]
    - This study has paved the path for future clinical research in the direction of this diagnostic tool for LPD.
- *Endometrial biopsy and other endometrial markers*
    - Histological analysis of endometrial biopsy tissue is considered a means to determine the presence of adequate progesterone production during the luteal phase.
    - Any abnormality in this has been considered as a gold standard for LPD diagnosis in previous studies.[66]
    - With time, as the research has advanced, it has been shown that for implantation, it is not only the microscopic endometrial appearance that is important it also involves various other factors, e.g., cytokines, pinopodes, growth factors.[67,68]
    - Further, endometrium maturation may vary from one endometrial region to other; hence, the clinical criteria that define luteal phase endometrial development accurately are still evolving and under research.[4]
    - A randomized controlled study (RCT), which has included regularly cycling fertile females, concluded

that histological endometrial dating has considerable intrasubject, intersubject, and interobserver variabilities. It does not have accuracy to provide as a method to diagnose luteal phase insufficiency or to guide in the management of females with reproductive failures.[69]

- Another multicentric RCT that included 847 women with regular menstrual cycles to assess the ability of histological dating to discriminate between the women of fertile and infertile couples has shown that out-of-phase biopsy results poorly discriminate between women in fertile and infertile couples in either midluteal or late luteal phase.[70]
- Hence, these studies have confirmed that histological endometrial dating via endometrial biopsy is neither a valid diagnostic tool for identification of infertile population nor suitable for diagnosis of LPD.
- As far as markers for endometrial receptivity are concerned, there has been no RCT that is validated to differentiate fertile and infertile women. It is still experimental and not a valid tool to diagnose LPD.[4]

Hence,

- According to ASRM practice committee guidelines 2021, at present, there is no reproducible and clinically practical and gold standard method to diagnose LPD and to differentiate infertile and fertile women.[4]
- It does not recommend the luteal phase progesterone, endometrial biopsy, or other tests to diagnose LPD.[4]

COLOR DOPPLER IN LUTEAL PHASE DEFECT

- During normal menstrual cycles, resistance index (RI) of preovulatory follicle (0.4–0.48)[71] decreases following ovulation (RI 0.35–0.50),[72] and it further decreases till late luteal phase, when it again increases in nonconception cycles.
- RI of CL is suggested to correlate with plasma progesterone levels as an index of luteal function.[73]
- In LPD, RI of CL is increased (RI: 0.52–0.60) and maintained throughout the luteal phase.[74]
- In LPD, endometrium appears thin and nonechogenic with increased resistance in spiral arteries (RI 0.66–0.72). This may be an underlying mechanism in unexplained infertility.[75]

TREATMENT OF LUTEAL PHASE DEFECT

- The first and foremost thing to consider in the treatment of LPD is to identify any underlying cause for it (e.g., thyroid dysfunction, hyperprolactinemia) and to treat accordingly. If, however, no underlying cause is found (i.e., idiopathic or true isolated LPD), the treatment becomes empirical and has very minimal reliable data available.
- Empirical treatment consists of treatment to promote endometrial maturation, enhance endometrial receptivity, support implantation and development of early pregnancy.
- It includes:
    - Supplementation in the form of luteal phase progesterone, estrogen, hCG, and GnRH-a

      or
    - Ovulation induction: It has been postulated that there is a continuity between follicular and luteal phases, and improved preovulatory follicular development leads to improved CL function.

Clomiphene Citrate

- Luteal phase LH levels were found to be higher in clomiphene citrate (CC) cycles as compared to that with gonadotropins.[76] When CC is administered, it causes occupancy and depletion of estrogen receptors in the hypothalamus. This leads to increase in endogenous FSH and LH secretion resulting in higher estrogen (E) and progesterone (P4) levels in the luteal phase. The ability of CC to augment CL function has led to its potential use as a treatment modality for patients with inadequate luteal phase endogenous P4 secretion.[12,77]
- In a systematic review and meta-analysis by Hill et al., it has been concluded that there is no role of luteal phase progesterone supplementation in patients undergoing ovulation induction with CC.[78]
- However, in a study by Cook et al., it has been concluded that CC use may be associated with a high risk of LPD induction as diagnosed by endometrial biopsy, except in women with PCOS.[79]
- However, ovulation induction has not been found to be a treatment modality for LPD.[80,81]

Progesterone

- Besides inducing secretory changes in endometrium, progesterone also:
    - Improves endometrial receptivity in estrogenized endometrium[82]
    - Stabilizes lysosomal membrane, which leads to quiescent uterus[82]
    - Leads to uterine relaxation by blocking chemokines which cause inhibition of prostaglandin synthesis, reduce calcium intracellularly, and help in nitric oxide synthesis[82]
    - Has immunomodulatory effect, and it prevents the conceptus from rejection along with hCG and cortisol[82]
    - Regulates natural killer cells, HOX10, and human leukocyte antigen (HLA) genes, thus, positively shifting to TH2 cell type[83]

- It is thus considered the mainstay of treatment for LPD.
- Cochrane systematic review 2015 has established the beneficial effect of progesterone on live birth and ongoing pregnancy rates in in vitro fertilization (IVF) cycles, irrespective of its route of administration.[84]
- European Society of Human Reproduction and Embryology (ESHRE) Ovarian Stimulation for IVF/intracytoplasmic sperm injection (ICSI) 2019 guidelines has recommended progesterone for LPS in IVF/ICSI cycles.[85]
- Also, Cochrane Database of Systematic Reviews 2019 has shown that progesterone supplementation therapy in women with unexplained recurrent miscarriages may reduce the risk of miscarriage in subsequent pregnancies.[86]
- However, in a multicentric, double-blind, placebo-controlled, and randomized trial, progesterone use in first trimester has not been shown beneficial in terms of live births in women with unexplained recurrent miscarriage.[87]
- Progesterone can be given orally, intramuscularly, vaginally, subcutaneously, and rectally.
- As of now, the only well-documented evidence of intramuscular or vaginal progesterone in luteal phase is in assisted reproductive technology (ART), GnRH-a, and antagonist cycles.[88,89]
- There is no evidence that progesterone use is beneficial in unstimulated cycles.
- Intramuscular or vaginal route of natural progesterone administration yields better results than oral micronized form of natural progesterone due to less bioavailability of oral progesterone.[90]
- ESHRE ovarian stimulation for IVF/ICSI 2019 guidelines recommends the use of any of the above-mentioned routes except the oral, for natural progesterone as LPS.[85]
- Oral synthetic form of progesterone is now emerging as an option for LPS.
- A recent meta-analysis including eight randomized controlled trials (RCTs) with 3,386 women has reported similar reproductive outcomes of oral dydrogesterone as compared to vaginal progesterone in terms of live birth/ongoing pregnancy rate.[91]
- Lotus I trial, a multicentric RCT, has shown noninferiority of oral synthetic progesterone in a dose of 10 mg TDS as compared to micronized vaginal progesterone (MVP) (200 mg thrice daily) in terms of clinical pregnancy and live birth rates.[92]
- Lotus II trial, a randomized multicentric trial conducted in 10 countries, has also demonstrated the noninferiority of 30 mg daily of dydrogesterone to 8% MVP gel (90 mg daily) for the presence of fetal heartbeat at 12 weeks of gestation in fresh IVF cycles.[93]
- ESHRE guideline has recommended the probable use of dydrogesterone as LPS.[85]
- Progesterone supplementation is to be started in the window from the evening of the day of oocyte retrieval till day 3 after it[85,94] and is usually administered until the first positive β-hCG test.[85,95]

Human Chorionic Gonadotropin

- Due to structural similarity of hCG with LH, supplementation with hCG in luteal phase stimulates corpora lutea to secrete endogenous estrogen and progesterone in ART cycles.
- It has been documented that delivery rates are more and miscarriage rates are less in ART cycles supplemented with hCG as compared with those without hCG.[88,89]
- However, hCG supplementation is associated with the risk of ovarian hyperstimulation syndrome (OHSS). Cochrane 2015 has shown that the risk of OHSS is less with progesterone as compared to hCG.[84]
- ESHRE 2019 guidelines do not recommend hCG as LPS in hCG-triggered ovarian stimulation cycles.[85]

Estrogen

- As after luteolysis, there is deficiency of estrogen also; it has been postulated that estrogen along with progesterone is required in IVF cycles.
- A recent meta-analysis has shown the beneficial effect of progesterone plus estradiol on clinical pregnancy rates [odds ratio (OR) 1.617; confidence interval (CI): 1.059–2.471; $p = 0.026$] as compared to progesterone alone.[96]
- In an RCT by Turgut et al., it has been concluded that in ART cycles with GnRH-a protocol, addition of 4 mg of estrogen along with progesterone in luteal phase leads to significantly increased pregnancy and implantation rates and decreased miscarriage rates as compared to progesterone alone.[97]
- However, Cochrane Systematic Analysis 2015 has shown no significant benefit of adding estrogen in terms of ongoing pregnancy rate and live birth rates.[84]
- ESHRE 2019 guidelines do not recommend the addition of estradiol to progesterone as LPS.[85]

Gonadotropin-releasing Hormone Agonist

- Various hypotheses of beneficial effect of GnRH-a in ART cycles are:
    - Direct support of CL by secretion of LH from pituitary or by acting at GnRH receptors on endometrium[98]
    - Direct effect of GnRH on embryo has also been postulated as there is evidence of increased hCG secretion[99]
- In a study by Bar-Hava et al., intranasal GnRH-a (nafarelin 400 μg/day) was found to be an effective LPS in itself without progesterone; in GnRH-a triggered fresh embryo transfer cycles in high responders and it also helps in avoiding OHSS.[100]

- In an RCT, it was found that administration of 0.1 mg Decapeptyl bolus on day 6 after oocyte retrieval, in addition to routine LPS, can lead to improved implantation and pregnancy rates in women with previous IVF failures.[101]
- A recent meta-analysis by Song et al. including eight RCTs has shown that administration of a single dose of GnRH-a on day 5/6 after oocyte retrieval along with regular LPS led to higher clinical, ongoing, and even multiple pregnancy rates per transfer in GnRH antagonist downregulated IVF cycles but not in long-acting GnRH-a cycles.[102]
- Another evidence is from Cochrane Systematic Review 2015, including seven RCTs and 1,708 women, which has shown that the live birth and ongoing pregnancy rates were lower in the progesterone-only group than the progesterone plus GnRH-a group (OR 0.62, 95%; CI 0.48–0.81).[84]
- ESHRE 2019 guidelines recommend the use of GnRH-a as LPS in hCG-triggered IVF/ICSI cycles only in clinical trials.[85]

IN NATURAL CYCLES

- According to ASRM practice committee guidelines of 2021, there is no treatment of LPD to improve pregnancy rates in natural and unstimulated cycles.[4]
- There is no evidence that progesterone use is beneficial in fertility treatment in natural cycles and in the LPD treatment.[4]
- As of now, there is no evidence to support routine use of progesterone to prevent miscarriage in early and mid-pregnancy, although some benefit is found in unexplained recurrent miscarriage patients.[86]

IN INTRAUTERINE INSEMINATION CYCLES

- Systematic review and meta-analysis by Katherine et al., including 11 RCTs, have demonstrated benefit of supplementing progesterone in intrauterine insemination (IUI) cycles in terms of clinical pregnancy rate and live birth rate.[103]
- Furthermore, benefit of progesterone in luteal phase has been found only in IUI cycles where ovulation induction was achieved with exogenous gonadotropins and not with CC or both gonadotropins and CC.
- This can be explained by the effect of exogenous gonadotropins on ovaries leading to increased serum estradiol levels, which will exert negative feedback effect on the hypothalamus–pituitary axis leading to abnormal LH secretion and thereby reduced progesterone secretion from CL.[59]
- While in CC cycles, due to antiestrogenic effect of CC on hypothalamus, there is increased LH secretion from pituitary.[104]

IN CONTROLLED OVARIAN STIMULATION CYCLES

- For LPS in IVF cycles, vaginal progesterone is the mainstay of treatment because of the ease of administration and efficacy equivalent to intramuscular form.[105]
- It is directly absorbed avoiding first-pass metabolism and having higher progesterone concentration in the endometrium as compared to serum.[106]
- However, vaginal progesterone use may lead to vaginal irritation, discharge, and bleeding[84] and hence there is emerging research to use oral synthetic progesterone.
- In Lotus I and II trials, oral synthetic progesterone has been proven noninferior to vaginal progesterone in fresh embryo transfer IVF cycles and is probably recommended for LPS in IVF/ICSI cycles.[85,92,93]
- Progesterone can be started from the day of oocyte retrieval to 2 or 3 days thereafter without affecting the ongoing pregnancy rates,[107] and usually continued till 8 weeks of pregnancy or longer; most studies have shown no benefit of progesterone support after positive hCG.[85,95]
- Although hCG can be used, it is better avoided in patients having a higher risk of OHSS.[89]

IN FROZEN EMBRYO TRANSFER CYCLES AND DONOR–RECIPIENT CYCLES

- There are various protocols for frozen embryo transfer (FET) cycles depending upon the method of endometrial preparation used.
- Natural cycle FET does not involve exogenous hormone use for endometrial preparation.
- Whereas in artificial FET cycles and in donor–recipient cycles, exogenous estrogen is given for endometrial proliferation, and exogenous progesterone is given to induce secretory changes.
- In these artificial and donor–recipient cycles as there is no CL, there is no source of progesterone to support pregnancy.
- After embryo transfer, progesterone and estrogen supplementation is given.
- As evidenced by a randomized trial, there is no difference in ongoing pregnancy rate while comparing intramuscular to vaginal progesterone in donor–recipient cycles.[108]
- However, in a recent meta-analysis, it has been shown that the use of vaginal progesterone in natural FET cycles does not improve clinical pregnancy rates.[109]

CONLUSION

- Although LPD has been proposed as a clinical entity 70 years back that may lead to infertility and early pregnancy loss, there is still a controversy regarding its definition, diagnosis, and clinical relevance apart from known pathological conditions suppressing LH pulses.

- Until further research is done, at present true isolated LPD is not considered as a clinical entity that causes infertility or early pregnancy loss.
- At present, testing and treatment of LPD is not recommended in non-IVF cycles.

REFERENCES

1. Mesen TB, Young SL. Progesterone and the luteal phase: a requisite to reproduction. Obstet Gynecol Clin North Am. 2015;42(1):135-51.
2. Harlow SD, Ephross SA. Epidemiology of menstruation and its relevance to women's health. Epidemiol Rev. 1995;17(2):265-86.
3. Jones GS. The luteal phase defect. Fertil Steril. 1976;27:351-6.
4. Practice Committees of the American Society for Reproductive Medicine and the Society for Reproductive Endocrinology and Infertility. Diagnosis and treatment of luteal phase deficiency: a committee opinion. Fertil Steril. 2021;115:1416-23.
5. Sonntag B, Ludwig M. An integrated view on the luteal phase: diagnosis and treatment in subfertility. Clin Endocrinol (Oxf). 2012;77(4):500-7.
6. Muechler EK, Huang KE, Zongrone J. Superovulation of habitual aborters with subtle luteal phase deficiency. Int J Fertil. 1987;32(5):359-65.
7. Practice Committee of the American Society for Reproductive Medicine. Current clinical irrelevance of luteal phase deficiency: a committee opinion. Fertil Steril. 2015;103(4):e27-32.
8. Schliep KC, Mumford SL, Hammoud AO, Stanford JB, Kissell KA, Sjaarda LA, et al. Luteal phase deficiency in regularly menstruating women: prevalence and overlap in identification based on clinical and biochemical diagnostic criteria. J Clin Endocrinol Metab. 2014;99:E1007-14.
9. Davis OK, Berkeley AS, Naus GJ, Cholst IN, Freedman KS. The incidence of luteal phase defect in normal, fertile women, determined by serial endometrial biopsies. Fertil Steril. 1989;51(4):582-6.
10. Noyes RW, Hertig AT, Rock J. Dating the endometrial biopsy. Fertil Steril. 1950;1:3-25.
11. Rosenberg SM, Luciano AA, Riddick DH. The luteal phase defect: the relative frequency of, and encouraging response to, treatment with vaginal progesterone. Fertil Steril. 1980;34(1):17-20.
12. Balasch J, Vanrell JA. Luteal phase deficiency: an inadequate endometrial response to normal hormone stimulation. Int J Fertil. 1986;31(5):368-71.
13. Messinis IE, Messini CI, Dafopoulos K. Luteal-phase endocrinology. Reprod Biomed Online. 2009;19:4314.
14. Retamales I, Carrasco I, Troncoso JL, Las Heras J, Devoto L, Vega M. Morpho-functional study of human luteal cell subpopulations. Hum Reprod. 1994;9(4):591-6.
15. Fraser HM, Wulff C. Angiogenesis in the corpus luteum. Reprod Biol Endocrinol. 2003;1:88.
16. Niswender GD, Juengel JL, Silva PJ, Rollyson MK, McIntush EW. Mechanisms controlling the function and life span of the corpus luteum. Physiol Rev. 2000;80(1):1-29.
17. McNatty KP, Makris A, DeGrazia C, Osathanondh R, Ryan KJ. The production of progesterone, androgens, and estrogens by granulosa cells, thecal tissue, and stromal tissue from human ovaries in vitro. J Clin Endocrinol Metab. 1979;49(5):687-99.
18. Miller WL. Mechanism of StAR's regulation of mitochondrial cholesterol import. Mol Cell Endocrinol. 2007;265-266:46-50.
19. Kiriakidou M, McAllister JM, Sugawara T, Strauss 3rd JF. Expression of steroidogenic acute regulatory protein (StAR) in the human ovary. J Clin Endocrinol Metab. 1996;81(11):4122-8.
20. Baird DT, Fraser IS. Blood production and ovarian secretion rates of estradiol-17β and estrone in women throughout the menstrual cycle. J Clin Endocrinol Metab. 1974;38:l009-17.
21. Sollenberger MJ, Carlsen EC, Johnson ML, Veldhuis JD, Evans WS. Specific physiological regulation of luteinizing hormone secretory events throughout the human menstrual cycle: new insights into the pulsatile mode of gonadotropin release. J Neuroendocrinol. 1990;2(6):845-52.
22. Ghanem ME, Al-Boghdady LA. Luteal phase support in ART: an update. In: Darwish AMM (Ed). Enhancing Success of Assisted Reproduction. UK: InTech Publishers; 2012.
23. Sanders SL, Stouffer RL. Localization of steroidogenic enzymes in macaque luteal tissue during the menstrual cycle and simulated early pregnancy: immunohistochemical evidence supporting the two-cell model for estrogen production in the primate corpus luteum. Biol Reprod. 1997;56(5):1077-87.
24. Devoto L, Kohen P, Vega M, Castro O, González RR, Retamales I, et al. Control of human luteal steroidogenesis. Mol Cell Endocrinol. 2002;186(2):137-41.
25. le Nestour E, Marraoui J, Lahlou N, Roger M, de Ziegler D, Bouchard P. Role of estradiol in the rise in follicle-stimulating hormone levels during the luteal-follicular transition. J Clin Endocrinol Metab. 1993;77:439-42.
26. Hosokawa K, Ottander U, Wahlberg P, Ny T, Cajander S, Olofsson IJ. Dominant expression and distribution of oestrogen receptor β over oestrogen receptor α in the human corpus luteum. Mol Hum Reprod. 2001;7(2):137-45.
27. Stocco C, Telleria C, Gibori G. The molecular control of corpus luteum formation, function, and regression. Endocr Rev. 2007;28(1):117-49.
28. Devoto L, Vega M, Kohen P, Castro O, Carvallo P, Palomino A. Molecular regulation of progesterone secretion by the human corpus luteum throughout the menstrual cycle. J Reprod Immunol. 2002;55(1-2):11-20.
29. Vega M, Urrutia L, Iñiguez G, Gabler F, Devoto L, Johnson MC. Nitric oxide induces apoptosis in the human corpus luteum in vitro. Mol Hum Reprod. 2000;6(8):681-7.
30. Fraser HM, Lunn SF, Harrison DJ, Kerr JB. Luteal regression in the primate: different forms of cell death during natural and gonadotropin-releasing hormone antagonist or prostaglandin analogue-induced luteolysis. Biol Reprod. 1999;61(6):1468-79.
31. Kohen P, Castro O, Palomino A, Muñoz A, Christenson LK, Sierralta W, et al. The steroidogenic response and corpus luteum expression of the steroidogenic acute regulatory protein after human chorionic gonadotropin administration at different times in the human luteal phase. J Clin Endocrinol Metab. 2003;88(7):3421-30.
32. Tay PY, Lenton EA. The optimum time for exogenous human chorionic gonadotropin to rescue the corpus luteum. J Assist Reprod Genet. 1999;16(9):495-9.

33. Wulff C, Dickson SE, Duncan WC, Fraser HM. Angiogenesis in the human corpus luteum: simulated early pregnancy by HCG treatment is associated with both angiogenesis and vessel stabilization. Hum Reprod. 2001;16(12):2515-24.
34. Sugino N, Okuda K. Species-related differences in the mechanism of apoptosis during structural luteolysis. J Reprod Dev. 2007;53(5):977-86.
35. Schweiger U, Laessle RG, Tuschl RJ, Broocks A, Krusche T, Pirke KM. Decreased follicular phase gonadotropin secretion is associated with impaired estradiol and progesterone secretion during the follicular and luteal phases in normally menstruating women. J Clin Endocrinol Metab. 1989;68: 888-92.
36. Savaris RF, Groll JM, Young SL, deMayo F, Jeong JW, Hamilton A, et al. Progesterone resistance in PCOS endometrium: a microarray analysis in clomiphene citrate-treated and artificial menstrual cycles. J Clin Endocrinol Metab. 2011;96:1737-46.
37. Patel BG, Rudnicki M, Yu J, Shu Y, Taylor RN. Progesterone resistance in endometriosis: origins, consequences and interventions. Acta Obstet Gynecol Scand. 2017;96:623-32.
38. Moszkowski E, Woodruff JD, Jones GE. The inadequate luteal phase. Am J Obstet Gynecol. 1962;83(3):363-72.
39. Blacker CM, Ginsburg KA, Leach RE, Randolph J, Moghissi KS. Unexplained infertility: evaluation of the luteal phase; results of the National Center for Infertility Research at Michigan. Fertil Steril. 1997;67(3):437-42.
40. Jones GS, Madrigal-Castro V. Hormonal findings in association with abnormal corpus luteum function in the human: the luteal phase defect. Fertil Steril. 1970;21:1-13.
41. Jones GS. Luteal phase defect: a review of pathophysiology. Curr Opin Obstet Gynecol. 1991;3:641-8.
42. Strott CA, Cargille CM, Ross GT, Lipsett MB. The short luteal phase. J Clin Endocrinol Metab. 1970;30(2):246-51.
43. Suh BY, Betz G. Altered luteinizing hormone pulse frequency in early follicular phase of the menstrual cycle with luteal phase defect patients in women. Fertil Steril. 1993;60(5):800-5.
44. Swyer GI, Daley D. Progesterone implantation in habitual abortion. BMJ. 1953;1:1073-7.
45. Fatemi HM, Popovic-Todorovic B, Papanikolaou E, Donoso P, Devroey P. An update of luteal phase support in stimulated IVF cycles. Hum Reprod Update. 2007;13(6):581-90.
46. De Souza MJ, Van Heest J, Demers LM, Lasley BL. Luteal phase deficiency in recreational runners: evidence for a hypometabolic state. J Clin Endocrinol Metab. 2003;88(1): 337-46.
47. De Souza MJ, Leidy HJ, O'Donnell E, Lasley B, Williams NI. Fasting ghrelin levels in physically active women: relationship with menstrual disturbances and metabolic hormones. J Clin Endocrinol Metab. 2004;89(7):3536-42.
48. Milenković L, D'Angelo G, Kelly PA, Weiner RI. Inhibition of gonadotropin hormone-releasing hormone release by prolactin from GT1 neuronal cell lines through prolactin receptors. Proc Natl Acad Sci U S A. 1994;91(4):1244-7.
49. Yildirim Y, Tinar S, Yildirim YK, Inal M. Comparison of pituitary-ovarian function in patients who have undergone successful renal transplantation and healthy women. Fertil Steril. 2005;83(5):1553-6.
50. Shaarawy M, Shaaban HA, Eid MM, Abdel-Aziz O. Plasma β-endorphin level in cases of luteal phase defect. Fertil Steril. 1991;56(2):248-53.
51. Díaz S, Cárdenas H, Brandeis A, Miranda P, Salvatierra AM, Croxatto HB. Relative contributions of anovulation and luteal phase defect to the reduced pregnancy rate of breastfeeding women. Fertil Steril. 1992;58(3):498-503.
52. Kerin JF, Broom TJ, Ralph MM, Edmonds DK, Warnes GM, Jeffrey R, et al. Human luteal phase function following oocyte aspiration from the immediately preovular graafian follicle of spontaneous ovular cycles. Br J Obstet Gynaecol. 1981;88(10):1021-8.
53. Smitz J, Erard P, Camus M, Devroey P, Tournaye H, Wisanto A, et al. Pituitary gonadotrophin secretory capacity during the luteal phase in superovulation using GnRH-agonists and hMG in a desensitization or flare-up protocol. Hum Reprod. 1992;7(9):1225-9.
54. Beckers NG, Macklon NS, Eijkemans MJ, Ludwig M, Felberbaum RE, Diedrich K, et al. Nonsupplemented luteal phase characteristics after the administration of recombinant human chorionic gonadotropin, recombinant luteinizing hormone, or gonadotropin-releasing hormone (GnRH) agonist to induce final oocyte maturation in in vitro fertilization patients after ovarian stimulation with recombinant follicle-stimulating hormone and GnRH antagonist cotreatment. J Clin Endocrinol Metab. 2003;88:4186-92.
55. Duffy DA, Manzi D, Benadiva C, Maier D, Saunders M, Nulsen J. Impact of leuprolide acetate on luteal phase function in women undergoing controlled ovarian hyperstimulation and intrauterine insemination. Fertil Steril. 2006;85:407-11.
56. Bachus KE, Hughes Jr CL, Haney AF, Dodson WC. The luteal phase in polycystic ovary syndrome during ovulation induction with human menopausal gonadotropin with and without leuprolide acetate. Fertil Steril. 1990;54(1):27-31.
57. Tavaniotou A, Albano C, Smitz J, Devroey P. Impact of ovarian stimulation on corpus luteum function and embryonic implantation. J Reprod Immunol. 2002;55:123-30.
58. Albano C, Grimbizis G, Smitz J, Riethmüller-Winzen H, Reissmann T, Van Steirteghem A, et al. The luteal phase of nonsupplemented cycles after ovarian superovulation with human menopausal gonadotropin and the gonadotropin-releasing hormone antagonist cetrorelix. Fertil Steril. 1998;70(2):357-9.
59. Bourgain C, Devroey P. The endometrium in stimulated cycles for IVF. Hum Reprod Update. 2003;9(6):515-22.
60. Fatemi HM. The luteal phase after 3 decades of IVF: what do we know? Reprod Biomed Online. 2009;19(Suppl. 4):4331.
61. Ayers-de-Campos D, Silva-Carvalho JL, Oliveria C, Martins-da-Silva I, Silva-Carvalho J, Pereira-Leite L. Inter-observer agreement in analysis of basal body temperature graphs from infertile women. Hum Reprod. 1995;10(8):2010-6.
62. Lenton EA, Landgren BM, Sexton L. Normal variation in the length of the luteal phase of the menstrual cycle: identification of the short luteal phase. Br J Obstet Gynaecol. 1984;91:685-9.
63. Crawford NM, Pritchard DA, Herring AH, Steiner AZ. Prospective evaluation of luteal phase length and natural fertility. Fertil Steril. 2017;107:749-55.
64. Filicori M, Butler JP, Crowley Jr WF. Neuroendocrine regulation of the corpus luteum in the human. Evidence for pulsatile progesterone secretion. J Clin Invest. 1984;73:1638-47.
65. Jordan J, Craig K, Clifton D, Soules MR. Luteal phase defect: the sensitivity and specificity of diagnostic methods in common clinical use. Fertil Steril. 1994;62(1):54-62.

66. Noyes RW, Hertig AT, Rock J. Dating the endometrial biopsy. Am J Obstet Gynecol. 1975;122:262-3.
67. Vlahos NF, Lipari CW, Bankowski BJ, Lai TH, King JA, Shih IM, et al. Effect of luteal-phase support on endometrial L-selectin ligand expression after recombinant follicle-stimulating hormone and ganirelix acetate for in vitro fertilization. J Clin Endocrinol Metab. 2006;91:4043-9.
68. Lédée-Bataille N, Bonnet-Chea K, Hosny G, Dubanchet S, Frydman R, Chaouat G. Role of the endometrial tripod interleukin-18, -15, and -12 in inadequate uterine receptivity in patients with a history of repeated in vitro fertilization–embryo transfer failure. Fertil Steril. 2005;83:598-605.
69. Murray MJ, Meyer WR, Zaino RJ, Lessey BA, Novotny DB, Ireland K, et al. A critical analysis of the accuracy, reproducibility, and clinical utility of histologic endometrial dating in fertile women. Fertil Steril. 2004;81(5):1333-43.
70. Coutifaris C, Myers ER, Guzick DS, Diamond MP, Carson SA, Legro RS, et al. Histological dating of timed endometrial biopsy tissue is not related to fertility status. Fertil Steril. 2004;82(5):1264-72.
71. Kurkak A, Kupesic-Urek S. Infertilty. In: Kurjak A (Ed). Transvaginal Color Doppler. Carnforth, UK: Parthenon Publishing; 1991. pp. 33-8.
72. Kupesic S, Kurjak A. The assessment of normal and abnormal luteal function by transvaginal color Doppler sonography. Eur J Obstet Gynecol Reprod Biol. 1997;72(1):83-7.
73. Glock JL, Brumsted JR. Color flow pulsed Doppler ultrasound in diagnosing luteal phase defect. Fertil Steril. 1995;64(3):500-4.
74. Tamura H, Takasaki A, Taniguchi K, Matsuoka A, Shimamura K, Sugino N. Changes in blood-flow impedance of the human corpus luteum throughout the luteal phase and during early pregnancy. Fertil Steril. 2008;90(6):2334-9.
75. Kupesic S, Bekavac I, Bjelos D, Kurjak A. Assessment of endometrial receptivity by transvaginal color Doppler and three-dimensional power Doppler ultrasonography in patients undergoing in vitro fertilization procedures. J Ultrasound Med. 2001;20(2):125-34.
76. Tavaniotou A, Albano C, Smitz J, Devroey P. Effect of clomiphene citrate on follicular and luteal phase luteinizing hormone concentrations in in vitro fertilization cycles stimulated with gonadotropins and gonadotropin-releasing hormone antagonist. Fertil Steril. 2002;77(4):733-7.
77. Engman L, Luciano AA. Luteal phase deficiency: what we now know. OBG Manag. 2003;15(8):41-61.
78. Hill MJ, Whitcomb BW, Lewis TD, Wu M, Terry N, DeCherney AH, et al. Progesterone luteal support after ovulation induction and intrauterine insemination: a systematic review and meta-analysis. Fertil Steril. 2013;100:1373-80.
79. Cook CL, Schroeder JA, Yussman MA, Sanfilippo JS. Induction of luteal phase defect with clomiphene citrate. Am J Obstet Gynecol. 1984;149(6):613-6.
80. Bukulmez O, Arici A. Luteal phase defect: myth or reality. Obstet Gynecol Clin North Am. 2004;31:727-44.
81. Kusuhara K. Clinical importance of endometrial histology and progesterone level assessment in luteal-phase defect. Horm Res. 1992;37:53-8.
82. Nigam A. Luteal phase support: why, when and how. Pan Asian J Obs Gyn. 2018;1(2):6-10.
83. Szekeres-Bartho J, Balasch J. Progestagen therapy for recurrent miscarriage. Hum Reprod Update. 2008;14(1):27-35.
84. Van der Linden, Buckingham K, Farquhar C, Kremer JA, Metwally M. Luteal phase support for assisted reproduction cycles. Cochrane Database Syst Rev. 2015;2015:CD009154.
85. Guideline of the European Society of Human Reproduction and Embryology. Ovarian stimulation for IVF/ICSI. ESHRE Reproductive Endocrinology Guideline Group. 2019. pp. 106-12.
86. Haas DM, Hathaway TJ, Ramsey PS. Progestogen for preventing miscarriage in women with recurrent miscarriage of unclear etiology. Cochrane Database Syst Rev. 2018;10:CD003511.
87. Coomarasamy A, Williams H, Truchanowicz E, Seed PT, Small R, Quenby S, et al. A randomized trial of progesterone in women with recurrent miscarriages. N Engl J Med. 2015;373:2141-8.
88. Pritts EA, Atwood AK. Luteal phase support in infertility treatment: a meta-analysis of the randomized trials. Hum Reprod. 2002;17(9):2287-99.
89. Daya S, Gunby J. Luteal phase support in assisted reproduction cycles. Cochrane Database Syst Rev. 2004;(3):CD004830.
90. Licciardi FL, Kwiatkowski A, Noyes NL, Berkeley AS, Krey LL, Grifo JA. Oral versus intramuscular progesterone for in vitro fertilization: a prospective randomized study. Fertil Steril. 1999;71(4):614-8.
91. Barbosa MWP, Valadares NPB, Barbosa ACP, Amaral AS, Iglesias JR, Nastri CO, et al. Oral dydrogesterone vs. vaginal progesterone capsules for luteal-phase support in women undergoing embryo transfer: a systematic review and meta-analysis. JBRA Assist Reprod. 2018;22(2):148-56.
92. Tournaye H, Sukhikh GT, Kahler E, Griesinger G. A phase III randomized controlled trial comparing the efficacy, safety and tolerability of oral dydrogesterone versus micronized vaginal progesterone for luteal support in in vitro fertilization. Hum Reprod. 2017;32(5):1019-27.
93. Griesinger G, Blockeel C, Sukhikh TG, Patki A, Dhorepatil B, Yang DZ, et al. Oral dydrogesterone versus intravaginal micronized progesterone gel for luteal phase support in IVF: a randomized clinical trial. Hum Reprod. 2018;33(12):2212-21.
94. Connell MT, Szatkowski JM, Terry N, DeCherney AH, Propst AM, Hill MJ. Timing luteal support in assisted reproductive technology: a systematic review. Fertil Steril. 2015;103(4):939-46.e3.
95. Liu XR, Mu HQ, Shi Q, Xiao XQ, Qi HB. The optimal duration of progesterone supplementation in pregnant women after IVF/ICSI: a meta-analysis. Reprod Biol Endocrinol. 2012;10(1):107.
96. Zhang XM, Lv F, Wang P, Huang XM, Liu KF, Pan Y, et al. Estrogen supplementation to progesterone as luteal phase support in patients undergoing in vitro fertilization: systematic review and meta-analysis. Medicine (Baltimore). 2015;94(8):e459.
97. Var T, Tonguc EA, Doğanay M, Gulerman C, Gungor T, Mollamahmutoglu L. A comparison of the effects of three different luteal phase support protocols on in vitro fertilization outcomes: a randomized clinical trial. Fertil Steril. 2011;95(3):985-9.
98. Pirard C, Donnez J, Loumaye E. GnRH agonist as luteal phase support in assisted reproduction technique cycles: results of a pilot study. Hum Reprod. 2006;21(7):1894-900.

99. Tesarik J, Hazout A, Mendoza C. Enhancement of embryo developmental potential by a single administration of GnRH agonist at the time of implantation. Hum Reprod. 2004;19(5):1176-80.
100. Bar-Hava I, Mizrachi Y, Karfunkel-Doron D, Omer Y, Sheena L, Carmon N, et al. Intranasal gonadotropin-releasing hormone agonist (GnRHa) for luteal-phase support following GnRHa triggering, a novel approach to avoid ovarian hyperstimulation syndrome in high responders. Fertil Steril. 2016;106:330-3.
101. Zafardoust S, Jeddi-Tehrani M, Akhondi MM, Sadeghi MR, Kamali K, Mokhtar S, et al. Effect of administration of single dose GnRH agonist in luteal phase on outcome of ICSI-ET cycles in women with previous history of IVF/ICSI failure: a randomized controlled trial. J Reprod Infertil. 2015;16(2):96-101.
102. Song M, Liu C, Hu R, Wang F, Huo Z. Administration effects of single-dose GnRH agonist for luteal support in females undertaking IVF/ICSI cycles: a meta-analysis of randomized controlled trials. Exp Ther Med. 2020;19:786-96.
103. Green KA, Zolton JR, Schermerhorn SM, Lewis TD, Healy MW, Terry N, et al. Progesterone luteal support after ovulation induction and intrauterine insemination: an updated systematic review and meta-analysis. Fertil Steril. 2017;107(4):924-33.e5.
104. Rossmanith WG, Laughlin GA, Mortola JF, Johnson ML, Veldhuis JD, Yen SS. Pulsatile cosecretion of estradiol and progesterone by the midluteal phase corpus luteum: temporal link to luteinizing hormone pulses. J Clin Endocrinol Metab. 1990;70(4):990-5.
105. Zarutskie PW, Phillips JA. A meta-analysis of the route of administration of luteal phase support in assisted reproductive technology: vaginal versus intramuscular progesterone. Fertil Steril. 2009;92(1):163-9.
106. Miles RA, Paulson RJ, Lobo RA, Press MF, Dahmoush L, Sauer MV. Pharmacokinetics and endometrial tissue levels of progesterone after administration by intramuscular and vaginal routes: a comparative study. Fertil Steril. 1994;62(3):485-90.
107. Mochtar MH, Van Wely M, Van der Veen F. Timing luteal phase support in GnRH agonist down-regulated IVF/embryo transfer cycles. Hum Reprod. 2006;21(4):905-8.
108. Gibbons WE, Toner JP, Hamacher P, Kolm P. Experience with a novel vaginal progesterone preparation in a donor oocyte program. Fertil Steril. 1998;69(1):96-101.
109. Seol A, Shim JY, Kim WS, Kim SK, Lee JR, Jee BC, et al. Effect of luteal phase support with vaginal progesterone on pregnancy outcomes in natural frozen embryo transfer cycles: a meta-analysis. Clin Exp Reprod Med. 2020;47(2):147-52.

CHAPTER 14

Anovulation

Ashwini Sidhmalswamy G

INTRODUCTION

"The key to growth is the introduction of higher dimensions of consciousness into our awareness"

—Lao Tzu

Anovulation is one large spectrum in reproductive endocrinology. To know everything of a big spectrum is so much more of a challenge. Anovulation presents itself with various clinical manifestations that include amenorrhea, infertility, hirsutism, and menstrual irregularities.

Anovulation accounts for infertility in 15–20% of infertile women.[1] Infertility caused by anovulation can be classified according to the deficiency of the hypothalamic–pituitary–ovarian (HPO) axis at different levels **(Box 1)**. Anovulation is defined as a state where there is no release of oocyte due to failure of rupture of a mature follicle.[2] This is the working definition of anovulation accepted at present. Ovum release involves many steps and any blockage during one of these stages could lead to anovulation.

CLASSIFICATION

The World Health Organization (WHO) classification[3] offers a useful frame for diagnosis and treatment of anovulation. **Box 1** shows the WHO classification of anovulation.

BOX 1: World Health Organization (WHO) classification of anovulation.

WHO class I: Hypogonadotropic hypogonadal anovulation (hypothalamic amenorrhea)

These women have low or low-serum follicle-stimulating hormone (FSH) concentrations and low-serum estradiol concentrations due to decreased hypothalamic secretion of gonadotropin-releasing hormone (GnRH) or pituitary unresponsiveness to GnRH

WHO class II: Normogonadotropic normoestrogenic anovulation

These women may secrete normal amounts of gonadotropins and estrogens. However, FSH secretion during the follicular phase of the cycle is subnormal. This group includes women with polycystic ovary syndrome (PCOS). Some ovulate occasionally, especially those with oligomenorrhea

WHO class III: Hypergonadotropic hypoestrogenic anovulation

The primary causes are premature ovarian failure (absence of ovarian follicles due to early menopause) and ovarian resistance (follicular form)

Hyperprolactinemic anovulation

These women are anovulatory because hyperprolactinemia inhibits gonadotropin and therefore estrogen secretion; they may have regular anovulatory cycles, but most have oligomenorrhea or amenorrhea. Their serum gonadotropin concentrations are usually normal

ETIOPATHOGENESIS

The complex interaction of neuroendocrine and intra-ovarian mechanism that regulates the normal ovulatory cycle is controlled by the HPO axis **(Fig. 1)**. Disruption at any level of this axis causes anovulation.

Anovulation can be one of the earliest symptoms of functional or organic hypothalamic diseases, pituitary disease or inappropriate feedback by the peripheral hormones, and primary ovarian insufficiency. Ovarian dysfunction in relation to anti-Müllerian hormone (AMH), inhibin B, and follicle-stimulating hormone (FSH) is depicted in **Figure 2**.

In women of reproductive age group, there are multiple causes of anovulation; these are shown in **Box 2**. Anovulation is managed according to the causes as discussed later.

Hypogonadotropic Hypogonadism Causes (WHO Group I)

The main feature of hypogonadotropic hypogonadism is that there is no luteinizing hormone (LH) and FSH release as there is no production of these hormones by pituitary. There is physiological decrease in the production of gonadotropin-releasing hormone (GnRH) from hypothalamus, which causes amenorrhea.

The most common cause is overexercising usually seen in athletes and the other common cause is being underweight with low body mass index (BMI).

Sheehan's syndrome (panhypopituitarism), usually occurring after severe postpartum hemorrhage or trauma, causing infarction of the anterior pituitary venous complex causes hypogonadotropic hypogonadism. Kallmann syndrome, wherein amenorrhea is present along with anosmia, is caused by congenital absence of production of GnRH by hypothalamus. Cerebral irradiation, which affects hypothalamus or the pituitary, in children treated for a craniopharyngioma or leukemia can cause secondary hypogonadotropic hypogonadism.

Normogonadotropic Normogonadism (WHO Group II)

Ovarian causes are included in this group. The most common is the polycystic ovary syndrome (PCOS).

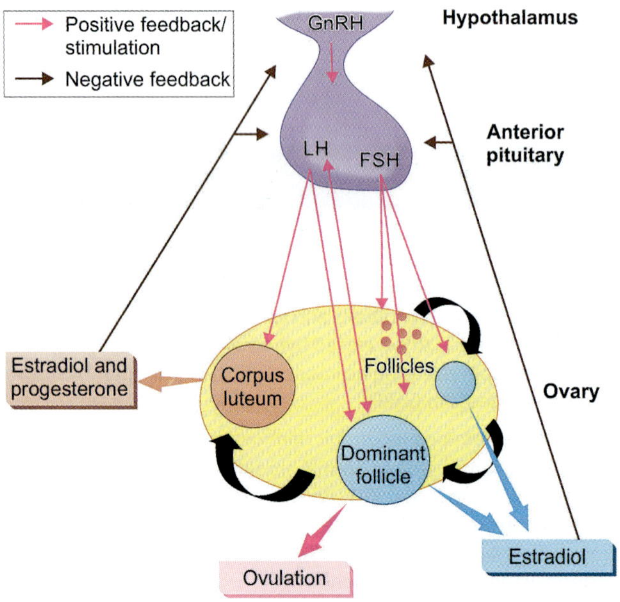

Fig. 1: Hypothalamic–pituitary–ovarian axis.
(FSH: follicle-stimulating hormone; GnRH: gonadotropin-releasing hormone; LH: luteinizing hormone)
Source: Fairley DH, Taylor A. Anovulation. BMJ. 2003;327(7414):546-9.

BOX 2: Causes of anovulation according to the World Health Organization (WHO) classification.

Hypogonadotropic hypogonadism (WHO group I)
- Functional hypothalamic dysfunction (e.g., excessive exercise, over stress, weight loss such as in anorexia nervosa, drug intake, iatrogenic)
- Pan-pituitary infarct as in Sheehan's syndrome, pituitary tumor
  - Kallmann syndrome where there is isolated gonadotropin deficiency along with anosmia
  - Idiopathic hypogonadotropic hypogonadism

Normogonadotropic normogonadism (WHO group II): Polycystic ovary syndrome (PCOS)

Hypergonadotropic hypogonadism (WHO group III)
- Iatrogenic as in postradiotherapy, surgical menopause, or chemotherapy
- Genetic disorders such as Turner syndrome
- Infectious cause such as mumps oophoritis
- Autoimmune causes
- Idiopathic

Other various endocrinopathies: Such as thyroid disorders, including hyperprolactinemia, congenital adrenal hyperplasia, ovarian and adrenal tumors, which are secreting androgens, are to be considered cause of anovulation

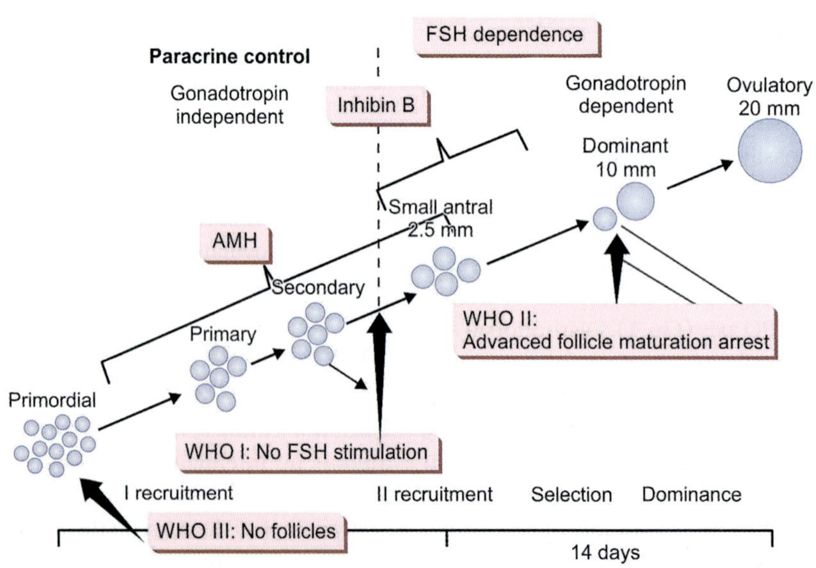

Fig. 2: Ovarian dysfunction in relation to anti-Müllerian hormone (AMH), inhibin B, and follicle-stimulating hormone (FSH). (WHO: World Health Organization)

Polycystic Ovary Syndrome

Polycystic ovary syndrome accounts for 70% of infertility occurring due to anovulation.[4] In PCOS, the excess production of androgens within the ovary results in recruitment of increased numbers of preovulatory follicles. No dominant follicle is produced. Insulin resistance is the main pathophysiological abnormality and is seen in only 10–15% of PCOS women who are slim and 20–40% of PCOS women who are obese.[5]

The prevalence of polycystic ovary syndrome depends on the criteria used to diagnose PCOS and it also depends on what population the study is conducted. Previously, the National Institutes for Health consensus[6] definition was used and prevalence was about 7%.[7] When Rotterdam consensus[8] was used for diagnosis of PCOS, the prevalence rate was around 20–25%. According to Rotterdam 2003 criteria, PCOS is defined as presence of (1) oligo- or anovulation, (2) clinical and/or biochemical signs of hyperandrogenism, or (3) polycystic ovaries (PCO) after excluding related disorders such as thyroid disorders, hyperprolactinemia, and congenital adrenal hyperplasia. If any two of the above features are present, then the woman is diagnosed to have PCOS.

Serum FSH concentration can be normal, but majority of times FSH is reduced in women with PCO when compared to women whose ovaries are normal.[9] FSH action in women with PCOS is inhibited. It is shown that AMH counteract the actions of FSH;[10,11] it is also in a way involved in causing anovulation in these women. the severity of the ovulatory dysfunction is greater when there is increased concentration of AMH.[9,12] Another contributory factor of AMH to anovulation is its direct relation with LH concentrations.[9,13] PCOS is separately dealt with in a separate chapter.

Obesity and Anovulation

In obese women, peripheral conversion of androgens to estrogens increases, causing imbalance in the secretion of gonadotropins. There is also decrease in the sex hormone-binding globulin in the blood, along with decrease in growth hormone secretion, and also decrease in insulin-like growth factor binding proteins and increase in leptin levels, causing alteration in the HPO axis. This causes ovulatory dysfunction.

Increased BMI is associated with infertility,[14-16] which causes ovulatory disorders in obese women. Obesity plays an adverse role in causing anovulation in PCOS.[17] However, not every woman who is obese suffers from PCOS, and not every woman diagnosed with PCOS is obese.[18,19] So, obesity may present with anovulation regardless of PCOS. This shows that there might be other factors causing an anovulatory disorder.[20,21]

Hypergonadotropic Hypogonadism (Ovarian Failure) (WHO Group III)

Premature Ovarian Failure

This condition cannot be reversed. This can only be treated by in vitro fertilization (IVF) with donor oocytes. Hormone replacement therapy is given for menopause symptoms and to prevent loss of bone density.

Genetic Abnormalities

One of the most common genetic abnormalities is Turner syndrome (45,X), in which the ovaries are underdeveloped (streak) and so there is primary ovarian failure. In this case, hormone replacement is done for the uterus to be adequate for implantation, so that the woman can conceive with IVF by using donated eggs. Some X chromosome translocations and deletions can also cause ovarian failure.

Androgen insensitivity syndrome, also called testicular feminization, can cause primary amenorrhea. These women have testes, but they are phenotypically female. The karyotype is 46,XY with intra-abdominal gonads. The androgen receptors are either absent or nonfunctioning. Pregnancy is impossible as there is absence of uterus and the vagina ends blindly.

Other Endocrinopathies

Hyperprolactinemia

The WHO classification did not include hyperprolactinemia in any of the category. *The cause of this condition* is usually pituitary microadenoma. In hyperprolactinemia, the pulsatile secretion of GnRH is hindered and this in turn impairs normal ovarian function. This leads to a decrease in pituitary LH production and also decrease in FSH. Secondary amenorrhea is usually the presenting symptom; some women may have galactorrhea. AMH levels to some extent can be used further to categorize women as the AMH levels are low in typical class I and class III WHO classification and the levels are high in class II.

DIAGNOSIS

Anovulatory infertility is a condition with several underlying causes. This can be systematically evaluated by proper history, physical examination, and basic investigations along with hormonal status. **Flowchart 1** shows schematic representation of hormonal status in relation to classification of anovulation.

History and Physical Examination

Women with ovulatory disorder present with history of infertility. Apart from this, anovulatory women present with scanty menses or oligomenorrhea, they can also present with amenorrhea, and few of the women can have regular menstrual cycles as well. So, menstrual history has to be taken properly. Hyperprolactinemia symptoms such as galactorrhea, headache, and visual disturbance have to be looked for. Symptoms of thyroid dysfunction are asked for. History of any drug intake or any other relevant medical history pertaining to menstrual cycle disturbance is to be noted. Hyperandrogenic symptoms such as hirsutism, acne, and male-pattern baldness are looked for in PCOS women.

Physical examination has to be done to note development of secondary sexual characteristics, and calculation of BMI is done. Abnormal genital development is also noted if any.

Apart from routine blood investigation that includes thyroid-stimulating hormone (TSH), free T4, and serum prolactin, further specific investigations are done to diagnose a particular type of anovulation. They are as follows:

- *Hypogonadotropic hypogonadism (WHO group I):* In these conditions, serum estradiol value is <40 pg/mL,[3] there is no withdrawal bleeding after progesterone challenge, and the endometrium is thin and atrophic, which measures <5 mm on ultrasound.[22]
- *Normogonadotropic anovulation (WHO group II):* These patients are more likely to have PCO. In these women, serum values of FSH may be normal and LH values are either raised or are within normal limits. Sometimes, there is some disturbance in the secretion pattern of GnRH.[23] They will have withdrawal bleeding in response to progesterone challenge.
- *Hypergonadotropic hypogonadism (WHO group III):* In these conditions, the plasma level of FSH is usually >20 mIU/mL on repeated measurements.[24] The women are hypoestrogenic and do not respond to the progesterone challenge; the most important test is karyotyping. If there is presence of Y chromosome, removal of the gonad through surgery is suggested as there is a risk of malignant transformation.[25]

Flowchart 1: Schematic representation of hormonal status in relation to classification of anovulation.

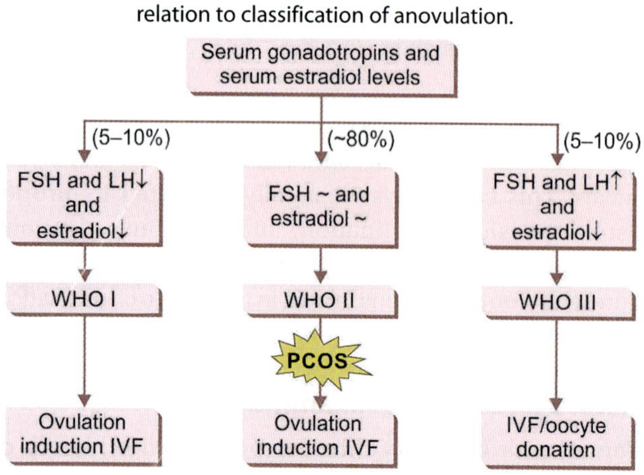

(FSH: follicle-stimulating hormone; IVF: in vitro fertilization; LH: luteinizing hormone; PCOS: polycystic ovary syndrome; WHO: World Health Organization)

Further Evaluation to Exclude Other Disorders

- *Autoimmune evaluation:* This should be done in young women with premature ovarian insufficiency, who are also usually at a high risk of developing autoimmune hypothyroidism. So, apart from regular thyroid testing with TSH, the levels of thyroid-peroxidase autoantibodies should also be checked. Other disorders associated with autoimmune polyglandular syndrome should be kept in mind and evaluated accordingly depending on the symptoms of the woman.
- *Karyotype:* This is done to evaluate chromosomal abnormalities specifically in women with premature ovarian insufficiency. Secondary infertility cases who have delivered one normal child may also develop premature ovarian insufficiency. This happens in women with X chromosome abnormalities, so it becomes necessary to evaluate the women with a karyotype. Any chromosomal abnormality on karyotyping mandates change in the treatment. Presence of Y chromosome material mandates oophorectomy as there is a high risk of gonadal malignancy.

TREATMENT

Treatment of anovulation is done according to the cause. **Box 3** shows the types of anovulation that are treatable and **Box 4** shows conditions that are not amicable to the treatment.

Flowchart 2 shows the treatment in relation to causative factors of anovulation.

Lifestyle Changes and Weight Management

Numerous studies have shown improvement in the hormonal levels and reproduction with weight loss in obese women. Losing weight improves insulin sensitivity, up to 5–10% of

BOX 3: Causes of anovulation treatable with ovulation induction.

Hypogonadotropic hypogonadism causes (WHO group I)
- *Hypothalamic*
  - Low concentration of gonadotropin-releasing hormone (hypogonadotropic hypogonadism)
  - Weight or exercise-related amenorrhea
  - Kallmann syndrome
  - Stress
  - Idiopathic
- *Pituitary*
  - Pituitary failure (hypogonadotropic hypogonadism)
  - Sheehan's syndrome
  - Craniopharyngioma or hypophysectomy
  - Cerebral radiotherapy

Normogonadotropic anovulation (WHO group II)
- *Ovarian*
  - Polycystic ovaries
- *Other endocrinopathies*
  - Hypothyroidism
  - Hyperprolactinemia
  - Congenital adrenal hyperplasia

(WHO: World Health Organization)

loss in total body weight can decrease up to 30% of central fat, and there can be ovulation.[26,27] Lifestyle modification is a key component in overweight anovulatory women.

Hyperprolactinemia

There are three ways to increase fertility in women with anovulatory hyperprolactinemia—surgery, treating with dopamine agonists, and release of ovum by ovarian stimulation. For idiopathic disease and prolactinoma, the treatment of choice is dopaminergic agents. Bromocriptine is the most common drug used. It is given as 2.5–20 mg in two or three divided doses per day.[28] This brings back the serum prolactin level to normal in about 80% of patients with microprolactinoma, leading to normalization of ovarian function in about 85% of women. In about 65% of patients with macroprolactinoma, the prolactin level becomes normal, with normalization of gonadal function in over 50%. The effective dopaminergic agent is cabergoline.[29] This is given in the dose of 0.5–1.0 mg/week. In women who do not ovulate with prolactin concentration being normal, bromocriptine can be given along with antiestrogens.[30]

BOX 4: Causes of anovulation not treatable with ovulation induction.

Ovarian failure
- Idiopathic
- Radiotherapy or chemotherapy
- Surgical removal
- Genetic
- Autoimmune

Chromosomal
- Turner syndrome (45,X)
- Androgen insensitivity syndrome (46,XY)

Hypogonadotropic Anovulation (WHO Group I)

Acute or chronic emotional stress is associated with acquired forms of hypogonadotropic amenorrhea. A proportion of fat tissue is needed to initiate menarche and maintain ovulation in women, which is about 27% of body weight. Thorough counseling is required when anovulation is associated with behavioral conditions and with weight issues such as underweight or overexercise.

Surgery is recommended for space-occupying tumors in the central nervous system (CNS). Proper counseling and reassurance are the initial steps of the treatment. GnRH given in pulsatile fashion induces ovulation in women with anovulation due to overweight. Other alternatives are menotropins. The advantages of pulsatile GnRH over menotropins are that the risk of hyperstimulation is minimal and the need for monitoring is also lessened.[31] In case anovulation is caused due to pituitary failure, ovulation is induced with gonadotropins. Human menopausal gonadotropin (hMG) is used as LH activity is required to stimulate proper estrogen production.[32] Serial ultrasonography is necessary to monitor the follicular growth.

Flowchart 2: Treatment in relation to causative factors of anovulation.

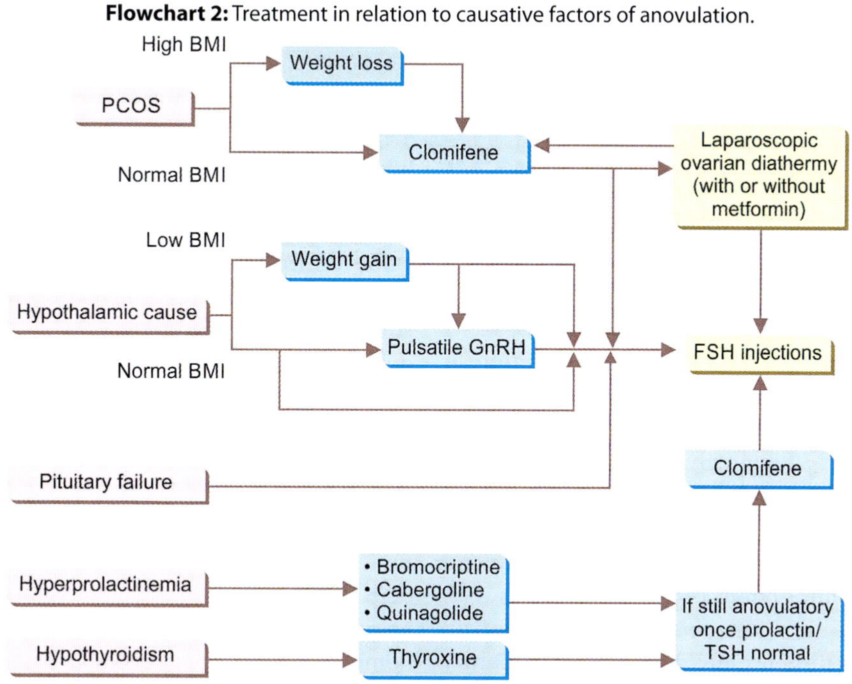

(BMI: body mass index; FSH: follicle-stimulating hormone; GnRH: gonadotropin-releasing hormone; PCOS: polycystic ovary syndrome; TSH: thyroid-stimulating hormone)

Source: Fairley DH, Taylor A. Anovulation. BMJ. 2003;327(7414):546-9.

Normogonadotropic Anovulation (WHO Group II)

Women in this group, when stimulated, have a greater risk of ovarian hyperstimulation and sometimes there also can be a decreased response. Treatment with antiestrogen is most effective; the drugs usually used are clomiphene citrate or tamoxifen. Clomiphene citrate is started in the dose of 50 mg/day for 5 days, starting from the second day of menses for 5 days, after induced or spontaneous bleeding. If no dominant follicle is developed, the dose can be increased by 50 mg each cycle. The treatment is monitored by serial ultrasound. Ultrasound monitoring is necessary as there can be development of more than one follicle leading to twins and triplets due to uncontrolled ovarian stimulation with clomiphene. If adrenal androgens are high [dehydroepiandrosterone sulfate (DHEAS) >30 ng/L], the addition of dexamethasone to clomiphene may be helpful.[33] The pregnancy rate is increased by 5.5-fold with clomiphene.[34]

The second line of treatment with normogonadotropic anovulation is ovarian stimulation with hMG preparations. The risk of ovarian hyperstimulation and multiple pregnancies is high. Low-dose regimen that is modification to the traditional regimen of gonadotropin treatment has been suggested for these patients.[35-37] With these regimens, the FSH threshold exceeds marginally, recruiting and selecting only few follicles leading to one or rarely two follicles to attain dominance. Multiple pregnancies are lower and even the abortion rate is minimal.

If the medical line of treatment fails, then ovarian drilling[38] is the next line of management. The sensitivity of the ovary to the gonadotropins is increased post this procedure, increasing the ovarian response to stimulatory drugs.

Medical Options for Ovulation Induction

Antiestrogens

Clomiphene citrate: This is the treatment of choice for WHO group II anovulation. Through its antiestrogenic effect, it displaces endogenous estrogen from estrogen receptors in the hypothalamic-pituitary axis; this in turn reduces its negative feedback and hence increases the secretion of endogenous GnRH and gonadotropins, which therefore induces ovulation.[39]

The starting dose is 50 mg daily for 5 days and can go up to 150 mg/day. The treatment is started on the second day of menses after a spontaneous or withdrawal bleeding. Follicular monitoring and endometrial response are studied by transvaginal pelvic ultrasound. The ovulation rate is 73%, and pregnancy and live birth rates are 36 and 29% per woman, respectively. Treatment is usually done for six ovulatory cycles.[40] The adverse effects may occur with clomiphene. Rarely these require discontinuation of treatment in some patients.

Tamoxifen: This mimics clomiphene citrate structurally; it is a triphenylethylene derivative. It is used in the dose of 20–40 mg/day for 5 days after a spontaneous period or withdrawal bleeding. According to a meta-analysis,[31] both tamoxifen and clomiphene citrate have similar ovulatory and pregnancy rates per cycle.

Insulin-Sensitizing Agents

In women with PCOS, there is insulin resistance. Insulin-sensitizing agents are used in these cases to increase the insulin responsiveness in tissues, which reduces the hyperinsulinemic condition. This improves ovulatory function. Metformin, a biguanide, is the common insulin sensitizer used; the dose is 850 mg twice daily with meals. According to a Cochrane review,[41] metformin used alone improves the ovulation rate and clinical pregnancy rate when compared with placebo or no treatment, but there was no significant change in live birth rate. When compared with clomiphene citrate, metformin has a lower ovulation rate, and there was no significant change in live birth rate.

Aromatase Inhibitors

Aromatase inhibitors block the production of estrogen by hindering the conversion of androstenedione to estrone and testosterone to estradiol, and the negative feedback to the hypothalamic–pituitary axis is decreased, causing increase in endogenous FSH secretion. It is used for ovulation induction in women with PCOS.

Letrozole, a third-generation aromatase inhibitor, is used for ovulation induction. It has a shorter half-life, so the endometrium suppression is minimal. It is used in the dose of 2.5–5 mg/day for 5 days starting on the second day of spontaneous or induced bleeding,[42] or as a single dose of 20 mg on day 3 of the period.[43] Serial ultrasound is done to monitor follicular growth. Letrozole is usually used in women who are resistant to clomiphene citrate. With this regimen, 70–84% women achieved ovulation and the pregnancy rate achieved was about 20–27% per cycle. Letrozole showed teratogenicity that has been described only in animal studies. On a larger sample size, a retrospective study was done, which found no difference in the rates of major and minor congenital malfo`rmations in newborns of mothers who took letrozole or clomiphene citrate treatments.[44]

Gonadotropin-Releasing Hormone

In hypogonadotropic anovulation caused by hypothalamic dysfunction, GnRH is given for the treatment, but this is of no help in the pituitary problem; it is given in a pulsatile fashion using a battery-operated pump, which causes growth of a dominant follicle. It is given subcutaneously or intravenously. An 80% cumulative pregnancy rate is noted after six cycles and 93% has been noted after 12 cycles of treatment.[44] The risk of multiple pregnancy is between 3.8 and 13.5%.

Gonadotropin

A combined preparation containing both FSH and LH gives a better outcome than only FSH in women with hypogonadotropic hypogonadism because LH activity is required for steroidogenesis in ovary to achieve optimal proliferation of endometrium. Exogenous gonadotropins are used to overcome the FSH threshold required for follicular development.

Chronic Low-Dose Step-Up Protocol

Chronic low-dose step-up protocol is the recommended protocol. The principle is to avoid excessive stimulation and aim at monofollicular development by determining the FSH threshold gradually. Follicle stimulation is started with a low dose (37.5–75 IU/day) of gonadotropins for at least 10–14 days,[26] and if there is no response, the dose is stepped up by 37.5 IU at weekly intervals, up to a maximum of 225 IU/day. Once follicular growth is observed, which is monitored by serial ultrasound scans, the same dose is maintained. Human chorionic gonadotropin (hCG) is given to trigger ovulation when one or two follicles are 18–20 mm in size. Once the maximum dose for follicular response is known, in subsequent cycle, the stimulation can be directly started with the maximum dose. **Figure 3** shows the low-dose step-up protocol.

Step-Down Protocol

The step-down protocol is more physiological. Gonadotropin is started from day 2 or 3 of the menstrual cycle at a dose of 150 IU/day, and the ovarian response is monitored by serial ultrasound every 2–3 days until one of the follicle size is 10 mm, and follicular growth is monitored by ultrasound every 2–3 days. Once there is response, the dose is reduced to 112.5 IU/day for 3 days and it is then further reduced to 75 IU/day until the follicle attains the size of 18–20 mm, and then ovulation trigger is done by hCG. The duration of stimulation in this protocol is shorter than the step-up protocol, but ovarian hyperstimulation syndrome risk is increased, and also there is a lower ovulation rate. There is no significant change in the pregnancy rate between the two regimens.[45]

With low-dose gonadotropin regimens, there is development of monofollicle and the ovulation rate is about 70% and the pregnancy rate is about 20% with a cumulative pregnancy rate of 55–70%. Multiple pregnancy rates are about 6% and ovarian hyperstimulation syndrome accounts to 1%. This is better than the conventional regimens of gonadotropin, in which there is a significant higher risk of multiple pregnancy and severe ovarian hyperstimulation syndrome.[26]

It is important to do strict ultrasound monitoring with titration of the gonadotropin dosage. When there is development of more than two dominant follicles, the cycle should be abandoned and the starting dose for stimulation in subsequent cycles should be reduced. **Figure 4** shows the step-down protocol.

A recent randomized-controlled trial[46] suggested that with low-dose FSH as the first-line treatment in women with PCOS, the outcome in terms of live birth rate for first cycle, time to pregnancy, and cumulative live birth rate over three cycles was significantly better than with clomiphene citrate. Further studies are required to know the cost effectiveness of such treatment and to choose between the two treatment modalities.

Laparoscopic Ovarian Drilling Surgery

Another way to induce ovulation in anovulatory women, especially with PCOS, is ovarian drilling by diathermy or laser through laparoscopy. A Cochrane review found that the cumulative ongoing pregnancy rate of 6–12 months post laparoscopic drilling is similar to ovulation induction with gonadotropins for three to six cycles.[47] However, the rate of multiple pregnancies is low in women who conceived with ovarian drilling.

As in all cases surgical methods carry more risk than the medical management, so they are reserved and used only when medical treatment fails or in selective women, where other fertility factors are properly assessed and where it mandates the use of laparoscopic ovarian drilling.

Hypergonadotropic Anovulation (WHO Group III)

There is no treatment available for women with hypergonadotropic anovulation. Fertility in these patients can be obtained by IVF with egg donation program.

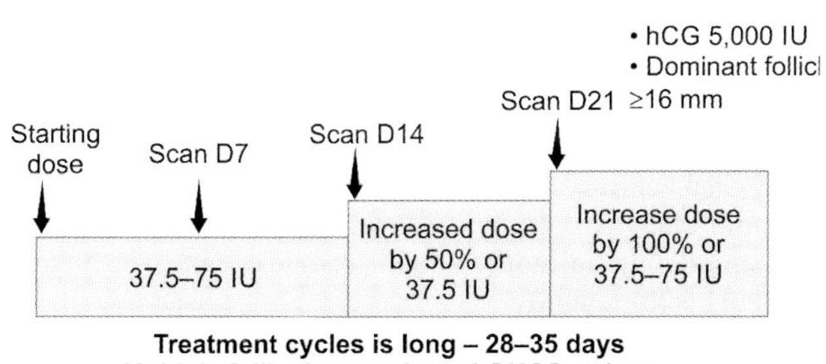

Fig. 3: Representation of low-dose step-up protocol.
(hCG: human chorionic gonadotropin; OHSS: ovarian hyperstimulation syndrome)

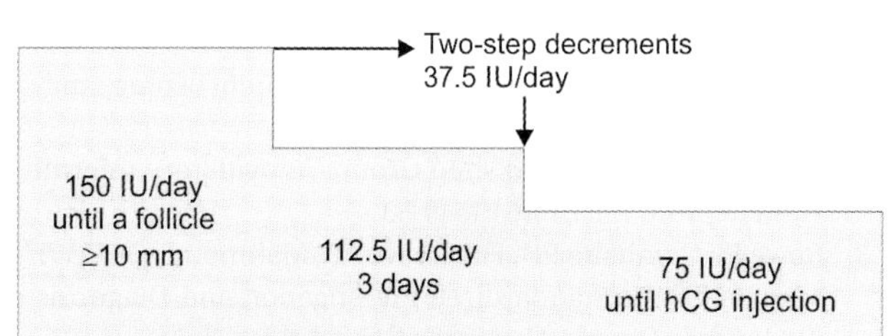

Fig. 4: Step-down protocol representation.
(hCG: human chorionic gonadotropin)

Flowchart 3: Diagnosis and treatment of anovulation.

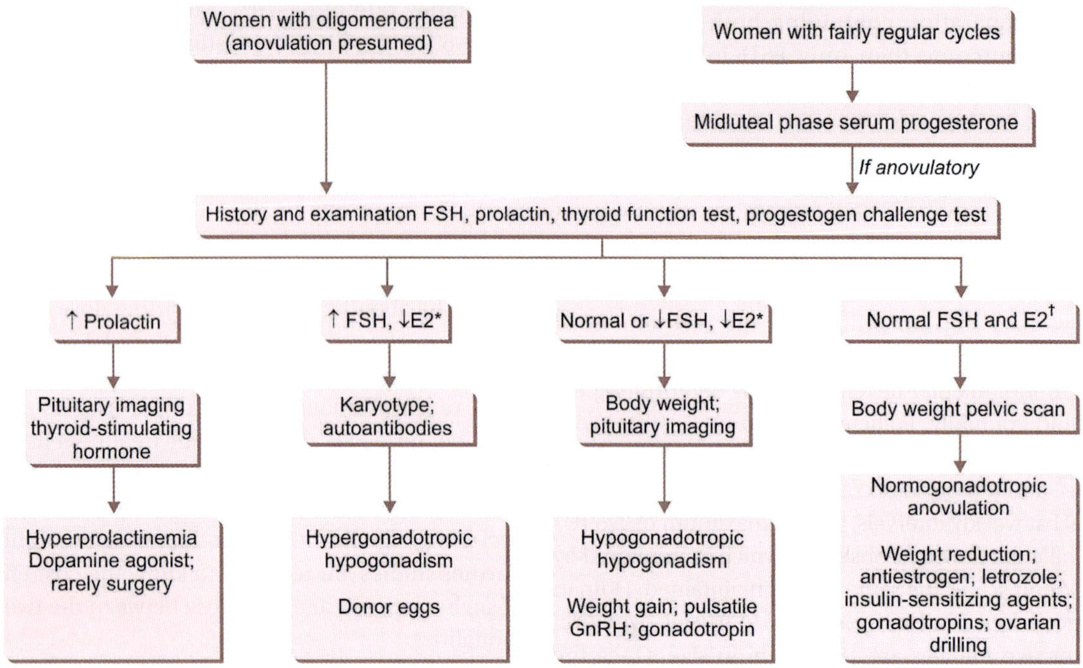

(E2: estradiol; FSH: follicle-stimulating hormone; GnRH: gonadotropin-releasing hormone)
*Absence of withdrawal bleeding after progestogen challenge in typical cases.
†Presence of withdrawal bleeding after progestogen challenge.

Flowchart 3 summarizes the treatment options for fertility in patients with chronic anovulation.

KEY POINTS

- Most of anovulatory patients can be successfully treated after proper diagnostic procedures.
- There are effective treatments available.
- A few women respond poorly to specific stimulation; in such a case, simpler and milder forms of individualized ovarian stimulation programs are being developed.
- The positive and added effect resulting from normalization of body weight in obese and underweight patients is very encouraging.
- Better ovarian stimulation depends on carefully choosing the available drugs to improve ovarian response in women who are poor responders and also to avoid multiple pregnancies.

REFERENCES

1. Templeton A. Infertility and the establishment of pregnancy—overview. Br Med Bull. 2000;56(3):577-87.
2. The ESHRE Capri Workshop Group. Anovulatory infertility. Hum Reprod. 1995;10(6):1549-53.
3. Rowe PJ, Comhaire FH, Hargreave TB, Mahmoud AMA. WHO Manual for the Standardized Investigation and Diagnosis of the Infertile Couple. Cambridge: Cambridge University Press; 1993.
4. Balen A, Michelmore K. What is polycystic ovary syndrome? Are national views important? Hum Reprod. 2002;17(9):2219-27.
5. Legro RS, Castracane VD, Kauffman RP. Detecting insulin resistance in polycystic ovary syndrome: purposes and pitfalls. Obstet Gynecol Surv. 2004;59(2):141-54.
6. Zawadzki JK, Dunaif A. Diagnostic criteria for polycystic ovary syndrome: towards a rational approach. In: Dunaif A, Givens JR, Haseltine FP, Merriam GR (Eds). Polycystic Ovary Syndrome. Boston: Blackwell Scientific; 1992. pp. 377-84.
7. Azziz R, Woods KS, Reyna R, Key TJ, Knochenhauer ES, Yildiz BO. The prevalence and features of the polycystic ovary syndrome in an unselected population. J Clin Endocrinol Metab. 2004;89(6):2745-9.
8. Rotterdam ESHRE/ASRM-Sponsored PCOS Consensus Workshop Group. Revised 2003 consensus on diagnostic criteria and long-term health risks related to polycystic ovary syndrome (PCOS). Hum Reprod. 2004;19(1):41-7.
9. Laven JS, Mulders AG, Visser JA, Themmen AP, De Jong FH, Fauser BC. Anti-Müllerian hormone serum concentrations in normoovulatory and anovulatory women of reproductive age. J Clin Endocrinol Metab. 2004;89(1):318-23.
10. Pellatt L, Rice S, Mason HD. Anti-Müllerian hormone and polycystic ovary syndrome: a mountain too high? Reproduction. 2010;139(5):825-33.
11. Pellatt L, Rice S, Dilaver N, Heshri A, Galea R, Brincat M, et al. Anti-Müllerian hormone reduces follicle sensitivity to follicle-stimulating hormone human granulosa cells. Fertil Steril. 2011;96(5):1246-51.
12. Pigny P, Merlen E, Robert Y, Cortet-Rudelli C, Decanter C, Jonard S, et al. Elevated serum level of anti-Müllerian hormone in patients with polycystic ovary syndrome: relationship to the ovarian follicle excess and to the follicular arrest. J Clin Endocrinol Metab. 2003;88(12):5957-62.

13. Piouka A, Famakiotis D, Katsikis I, Macut D, Gerou S, Panidis D, et al. Anti-Müllerian hormone levels reflect severity of PCOS but are negatively influenced by obesity: relationship with increased luteinizing hormone levels. Am J Physiol Endocrinol Metab. 2009;296(2):E238-43.
14. Castillo-Martínez L, López-Alvarenga JC, Villa AR, González-Barranco J. Menstrual cycle length disorders in 18- to 40-y-old obese women. Nutrition. 2003;19(4):317-20.
15. Parihar M. Obesity and infertility. Rev Gynaecol Pract. 2003; 3:120-6.
16. Bhattacharya S, Porter M, Amalraj E, Templeton A, Hamilton M, Lee AJ, et al. The epidemiology of infertility in the north east of Scotland. Hum Reprod. 2009;24:3096-107.
17. Ben-Shlomo I, Grinbaum E, Levinger U. Obesity-associated infertility—the earliest known description. Reprod Biomed. 2008;17:5-6.
18. Practice Committee of American Society for Reproductive Medicine. Obesity and reproduction: an educational bulletin. Fertil Steril. 2008;90(5 Suppl.):S21-9.
19. Metwally M, Li TC, Ledger WL. The impact of obesity on female reproductive function. Obes Rev. 2007;8(6):515-23.
20. Loret de Mola JR. Obesity and its relationship to infertility in men and women. Obstet Gynecol Clin North Am. 2009;36(2):333-46.
21. Jungheim ES, Travieso JL, Carson KR, Moley KH. Obesity and reproductive function. Obstet Gynecol Clin North Am. 2012;39(4):479-93.
22. Steinkampf MP. Ultrasonography in infertility management. In: Behrman SJ, Patton Jr. GW, Holz G (Eds). Progress in Infertility. Boston: Little Brown and Co.; 1990. pp. 339-69.
23. Moult PJA, Rees H, Besser GM. Pulsatile gonadotrophin secretion in hyperprolactinaemic amenorrhoea and the response to bromocriptine therapy. Clin Endocrinol (Oxf). 1982;16(2):153-62.
24. Baird DT. Amenorrhoea, anovulation and dysfunctional uterine bleeding. In: DeGroot LJ (Ed). Endocrinology. London: W.B. Saunders; 1995. pp. 2059-79.
25. Layman LC, Reindollar RH. The genetics of hypogonadism. Infertil Reprod Med Clin North Am. 1994;1:53-68.
26. Thessaloniki ESHRE/ASRM-Sponsored PCOS Consensus Workshop Group. Consensus on infertility treatment related to polycystic ovary syndrome. Hum Reprod. 2008;23(3):462-77.
27. Moran LJ, Pasquali R, Teede HJ, Hoeger KM, Norman RJ. Treatment of obesity in polycystic ovary syndrome: a position statement of the Androgen Excess and Polycystic Ovary Syndrome Society. Fertil Steril. 2009;92(6):1966-82.
28. Crosignani PG, Ferrari C, Liuzzi A, Benco R, Mattei A, Rampini P, et al. Treatment of hyperprolactinemic states with different drugs: a study with bromocriptine, metergoline and lisuride. Fertil Steril. 1982;37(1):61-7.
29. Webster J, Piscitelli G, Polli A, Ferrari CI, Ismail I, Scanlon MF, et al. A comparison of cabergoline and bromocriptine in the treatment of hyperprolactinemic amenorrhea. Cabergoline Comparative Study Group. N Engl J Med. 1994;331(14):904-9.
30. Diamant YZ, Yarkoni S, Evron S. Combined clomiphene-bromocriptine treatment in anovulatory, oligomenorrheic and hyperprolactinemic women resistant to separate clomiphene or bromocriptine regimens. Infertility. 1980;3:11-21.
31. Filicori M, Flamigni C, Meriggiola MC, Cognigni G, Valdiserri A, Ferrari P, et al. Ovulation induction with pulsatile gonadotrophin-releasing hormone: technical modalities and clinical perspectives. Fertil Steril. 1991;56(1):1-13.
32. Couzinet B, Lestrat N, Brailly S, Forest M, Schaison G. Stimulation of ovarian follicular maturation with pure follicle-stimulating hormone in women with gonadotrophin deficiency. J Clin Endocrinol Metab. 1988;66(3):552-6.
33. Daly DC, Walters CA, Soto-Albors CE, Tohan N, Riddick DH. A randomized study of dexamethasone in ovulation induction with clomiphene citrate. Fertil Steril. 1984;41(6):844-8.
34. Connaughton JF, Garcia CR, Wallach EE. Induction of ovulation with cisclomiphene and a placebo. Obstet Gynecol. 1974;43(5):697-701.
35. Hamilton-Fairley D, Kiddy D, Watson H, Paterson C, Franks S. Association of moderate obesity with a poor pregnancy outcome in women with polycystic ovary syndrome treated with low dose gonadotrophin. Br J Obstet Gynaecol. 1992;99(2): 128-31.
36. Fauser BC, Donderwinkel P, Schoot DC. The step-down principle in gonadotrophin treatment and the role of GnRH analogues. Baillieres Clin Obstet Gynaecol. 1993;7(2):309-30.
37. Schoemaker J, van Weissenbruch MM, Scheele F, van der Meer M. The FSH threshold concept in clinical ovulation induction. Baillieres Clin Obstet Gynaecol. 1993;7(2):297-308.
38. Li TC, Saravelos H, Chow MS, Chisabingo R, Cooke ID. Factors affecting the outcome of laparoscopic ovarian drilling for polycystic ovarian syndrome in women with anovulatory infertility. BJOG. 1998;105(3):338-44.
39. Wu CH, Winkel CA. The effect of therapy initiation day on clomiphene citrate therapy. Fertil Steril. 1989;52(4):564-8.
40. Homburg R. Clomiphene citrate—end of an era? A mini-review. Hum Reprod. 2005;20(8):2043-51.
41. Tang T, Lord JM, Norman RJ, Yasmin E, Balen AH. Insulin-sensitising drugs (metformin, rosiglitazone, pioglitazone, D-chiro-inositol) for women with polycystic ovary syndrome, oligo amenorrhoea and subfertility. Cochrane Database Syst Rev. 2012;(5):CD003053.
42. Badawy A, Abdel Aal I, Abulatta M. Clomiphene citrate or letrozole for ovulation induction in women with polycystic ovarian syndrome: a prospective randomized trial. Fertil Steril. 2009;92(3):849-52.
43. Mitwally MF, Biljan MM, Casper RF. Pregnancy outcome after the use of an aromatase inhibitor for ovarian stimulation. Am J Obstet Gynecol. 2005;192(2):381-6.
44. Tulandi T, Martin J, Al-Fadhli R, Kabli N, Forman R, Hitkari J, et al. Congenital malformations among 911 newborns conceived after infertility treatment with letrozole or clomiphene citrate. Fertil Steril. 2006;85(6):1761-5.
45. Christin-Maitre S, Hugues JN, Recombinant FSH Study Group. A comparative randomized multicentric study comparing the step-up versus step-down protocol in polycystic ovary syndrome. Hum Reprod. 2003;18(8):1626-31.
46. Amer SA, Li TC, Cooke ID. Laparoscopic ovarian diathermy in women with polycystic ovarian syndrome: a retrospective study on the influence of the amount of energy used on the outcome. Hum Reprod. 2002;17(4):1046-51.
47. Farquhar C, Vandekerckhove P, Lilford R. Laparoscopic "drilling" by diathermy or laser for ovulation induction in anovulatory polycystic ovary syndrome. Cochrane Database Syst Rev. 2001;(4):CD001122.

CHAPTER 15

Declining Fertility

Mahesh Koregol, Soumya Mahesh Koregol, Navya N

INTRODUCTION

Over the past 70 years, fertility rates have decreased worldwide, with nearly a 50% decline overall. Increased life expectancy, along with lower fertility rates, is creating an aging population which in turn puts pressure on healthcare systems globally. The total fertility rate (TFR) is the total number of offspring that would be born to each woman if she were to live to the end of her fertile age. In the last 50 years, there has been a consistent fall in the global TFR markedly in the more developed nations of the world.

TOTAL FERTILITY RATE TRENDS

Until 1870, the global TFR had been relatively static at around 5.7 children per woman. After 1870, there was a gradual decline that was made up for by the relative prosperity following World War II. The fertility rates gained momentum during the 1950s and peaked around the 1960s. Thereafter, there has been an astounding downward trend in global TFR.

Replacement level fertility is the level of fertility at which a population exactly replaces itself from one generation to the next. In simple words, it is the minimum fertility needed to keep the population unchanged from one generation to the next. The TFR should be at least 2 to ensure replacement for the parents. An additional 0.1 has been included to account for the infant mortality rate. Shockingly in 2017, TFR was only just above replacement levels.[1,2]

THE INDIAN SCENARIO

The Indian numbers are not very different from those of the more developed countries. There has been a striking decline in TFR from 2.2 (reported in 2015–2016) to 2.0 at the all-India level. This is as per the latest National Family Health Survey of India-5 (NFHS-5) (phase 2) released by the Union Health Ministry.[3] TFR is currently 1.6 in urban areas, 2.1 in rural areas, and an average of 2.0 all over India. The NFHS-5 for 2019–2021 was conducted in about 6.1 lakh sample households from 707 districts of India. This covered 724,115 women and 101,839 men to provide the estimates up to district level.

MAJOR CAUSES OF FERTILITY DECLINE: SHORT TERM AND LONG TERM

There are two major factors responsible for the fall in TFR. The "*short-term*" decline in human TFR is mainly a result of social, economic, and educational factors. This may be addressed by changes in policy, support to pregnant working women, and attitude of people in general. In parallel, there are more challenging "*long-term*" changes occurring, driven by a combination of drastic environmental, lifestyle, and genetic factors. These have the potential to result in permanent damage to the fertility of the human species and are less malleable to human interventions.

EDUCATION—"THE MOST EFFECTIVE CONTRACEPTION"

One of the biggest causes of large families is illiteracy, or more specifically, the lack of awareness and knowledge. The World Bank has found a negative correlation between women's education and fertility. It has been observed across countries and time. Literacy has been proven to be one of the most effective ways to achieve gender parity at a global level. There is a clear association between female education and reduced fertility.[4] The reasons behind this strong link are complex. Reduced fertility means that there are fewer children and all, including the daughters, get the advantage of gaining better education. This somewhat reduces the gender disparity level as there are increased job opportunities and independence for women.[5] Higher education comes with increased economic autonomy. These empowered women are more likely to make major decisions concerning fertility and family.[6] On the flip side, a relatively negative consequence of female education and career development is that women contemplate having a family at a later age at which fertility declines naturally.

The average age of women attending in vitro fertilization (IVF) clinics is around 36 years, when fertility is beginning its irrevocable age-dependent decline via mechanisms that assisted reproductive technology (ART) cannot reverse.[7]

WORKING WOMEN AND THE MYTH OF "HAVING IT ALL"

The present generation of men, women, and families has high aspirations for life. Having children will lead to a conflict with these aspirations. In fact, professional women find it challenging even to be married—for most cultures, a prerequisite for having children. Postponement of childbearing is a new behavioral change seen in many countries. A wide range of complex personal, psychological, and social factors affect the decision to have children. There is a lack of social and structural support for women to have their children at a time in their lives when their fertility is likely to be more viable. This will in turn mean women will have to compromise their education, career, and economic goals, which is also likely to peak in the same time period of their lives. Mostly a pause in career to have and raise children will result in an invariable struggle to reengage in the professional world.[8]

ECONOMY—"MONEY MAKES MANY THINGS"—DOES IT HOLD TRUE FOR HAVING CHILDREN

As nations become more prosperous, healthcare facilities and life expectancy improve. This increases the confidence of couples to have a smaller family as the risk of unexpected infant and childhood mortality rate decreases. This results in a decline in TFR which is temporarily unchanged by a parallel rise in life expectancy. As a result of this trend, we are seeing "super-old" populations like in Japan, Finland, Italy, or Germany. In these countries, over 20% of the society is over the age of 65 years.[9] As a consequence of these changes, these affluent nations are seeing their population pyramid turn on its head. In the long term, this is likely to build huge economic stress on these countries.

CHANGING RELATIONSHIP DYNAMICS—IT IS SIMPLY COMPLICATED

Marriage is a social institution that has been around for thousands of years. It ensures a stable relationship which is a prerequisite for expanding the family. We would assume that this social ritual is unlikely to change over time. However, developments since the middle of the 20th century show that this assumption is wrong. Marriage is no longer considered as a priority or even relevant to today's society. All over the world, fewer couples are becoming married. For example, plots of marriage rate against TFR for the Netherlands have revealed a drastic decline in the incidence of marriage as the TFR falls to a sub-replacement level.[10] The decrease in marriage rates have been accompanied by an increase in the age at which people are getting married in several countries. So, marriages are becoming less common, people are marrying much later, and unmarried couples are increasingly choosing to live together. There is also a shocking phenomenon in several countries where we are seeing a "decoupling" of parenthood and marriage. This will definitely cause a fall in fertility rates at present;[10] however, in future, it seems likely that more and more children will be born out of wedlock. This might become common and might not affect couples' decisions to bear children.

IS ASSISTED REPRODUCTIVE TECHNOLOGY GENETICALLY AFFECTING HUMAN FECUNDITY? LESSONS FROM THE CATTLE INDUSTRY

The mechanism of evolution heavily relies on the principle of "natural selection." Organisms that are more adapted to their environmental challenges are most likely to survive and pass on the genes that aided their survival. This process causes species to evolve and diverge over time toward better sustenance. In the early stages of human evolution and propagation on this planet, high rates of mortality essentially meant that natural selection involved choosing individuals with higher fertility genes. One had to be fertile enough to bear several offspring as high mortality would mean that only the best one or two would survive to pass their genetic material to the next generation.

Over the past few decades, the use of ART has increased rapidly, and the reasons for treatment are gradually broadening as more same-sex couples, single women, and surrogates are making use of advanced fertility treatments. While this is indeed a boon to many infertile couples, there is a long-term interference in nature's rule of selecting the best possible genotypes for the propagation of the human species. The spread of low fertility genotypes will be subsequently encouraged by the IVF industry itself, thereby setting off a vicious cycle of fertility problems. This might sound very theoretical, but the experience in the dairy industry has already proven this to be a real problem. There is a conscious effort to choose the most fertile domestic animals for breeding; otherwise, there is a subsequent decrease in the fertility of the next generation of the breed. A similar phenomenon may be expected in humans that will not be noticed for a few decades, but if we do not actively select for fertility, we will ultimately lose it in decades to come.[11] The fertility rates may remain unaffected by this in the immediate future as ART is responsible for <0.5% of births worldwide. However, it has been already noticed in most developed countries that one of the inadvertent consequences of ART is that, when conducted at a large scale, ART will help poor fertility genes be retained within the population and will get passed on to the next generation.

A shocking instance of ART facilitating the propagation of low fertility genotypes is seen in the management of severely oligozoospermic men with azoospermia factor c (AZFc) deletions on their Y-chromosome. These individuals need intracytoplasmic sperm injection (ICSI) to conceive, and the sons inherit the same male factor infertility. So, they will also require the same intervention once they wish to have a family.[12] There is already enough evidence to suggest that male offspring conceived by ICSI have lower sperm counts than their naturally conceived children of the same generation.[13] Of course, these data will need lot of substantiation, but they are quite consistent with the ability of ART to promote the transmission of poor fertility genotypes in humans. This situation is complex as any mutations that compromise fertility by acting on the quality of gametes or fertilization and early embryogenesis will potentially persist within the human population by the upsurge in the practice of ART, particularly ICSI.[14-16] The offspring born out of ART are more likely to carry aneuploidies[17] and abnormal DNA methylation profiles[18] as well as genetic mutations,[19] which are very much likely to be passed on to the upcoming generations.

The ART industry is indeed putting conscious efforts to avoid such problems through the development of high-end embryo selection processes and increasing use of genetic screening protocols.[20] The increased application of ART may also discourage research into the effect of environmental and lifestyle factors on human fertility by treating and achieving pregnancy in subfertile individuals. This will obscure the serious problem of falling human fecundity and fail to create political pressure to address these larger issues.

DECLINE IN MALE FERTILITY

There are several lifestyle and environmental factors acting to suppress human fecundity; the impact is likely to be more permanent. This is most evident in the rising incidence of male infertility. Human semen quality is consistently degrading all over the world.[21] The sperm counts have almost decreased by 50% over the last 50 years in both the West and the East.[22] This rapid and widespread change cannot be attributed to genetic causes alone. There must be a more generalized environmental cause.

The mechanism by which the environmental factors are affecting male fertility is being studied and there are few interesting observations. One such finding is simultaneous decline in serum testosterone levels. The fall in circulating testosterone levels might, in turn, be caused by increased exposure to estrogenic compounds from various sources.[23] Obesity is a pandemic known to be associated with low testosterone and high estrogen levels. This is due to a rise in aromatase activity, particularly in people with long tetranucleotide TTTA repeat polymorphisms in their aromatase gene.[24] Dairy products, such as milk and cheese, are known to contain significant quantities of natural estrogens. The increased intake of dairy along with phytoestrogens via the diet has been shown to lower serum testosterone levels in some studies.[25] Also, the exposure to synthetic estrogens in our environment, such as ethinyl estradiol or xenoestrogens, including bisphenol A or phthalate esters, is known to have a dual effect of suppressing gonadotropin production and reducing testosterone levels in humans.[26]

A reduction in sperm counts may not necessarily be associated with a simultaneous decrease in fecundity. Nevertheless, if the current trends continue, then, as Shanna Swan has pointed out, human fertility will become compromised due to poor sperm numbers.[22] The seriousness of the condition is emphasized by the rising incidence of testicular cancer which, according to the testicular dysgenesis syndrome hypothesis, has a similar origin to the global decline in sperm counts. Both share the common etiology of environmental endocrine disruptors with estrogen-like activity.[27]

ROLE OF FERTILITY SPECIALISTS: INCREASE AWARENESS AND OPTIMIZE NATURAL FERTILITY

As clinicians, we frequently encounter nonpregnant women, men, and couples in their reproductive age, which is an opportunity for us to create awareness in them about wellness and healthy habits to optimize their reproductive outcomes. The fact that the likelihood of conception is generally highest in the first few months of unprotected intercourse and declines gradually thereafter is unknown to many.[28] They are under the wrong assumption that pregnancy can be planned any time and fail to understand that modern ART techniques will not be able to overcome the effect of age on fertility. Fertility varies among populations, may be related to other health-based and environmental factors, and declines irreversibly with age in both sexes, the effects of age being much more pronounced in women.[29,30] There is a well-recognized age-related decline in the chances of pregnancy and live birth in older women. Also, there is a higher risk of aneuploidies, miscarriage, and medical complications of pregnancy with maternal aging, which further lowers fecundity.[31]

Apart from increasing awareness regarding the declining fertility, we should also inculcate a healthy "reproductive routine." Intercourse every day or alternate days during the fertile window should help maximize fecundability. Recreational drugs and smoking should be discouraged in couples attempting pregnancy. Caffeine and alcohol use should be limited to a minimum to moderate use while trying to conceive. There is no substitute for a healthy lifestyle and diet for couples attempting to achieve pregnancy and also for their general well-being. They should be encouraged, to the extent possible, to limit their exposure to endocrine-disrupting chemicals in food, air, water, and personal care products and exposure to air pollution. The limitations in the available options of ART should be frankly discussed.

KEY POINTS

- Over the past 70 years, fertility rates have declined worldwide.
- TFR is defined as the total number of children that would be born to each woman if she were to live to the end of her reproductive years.
- A TFR of 2.1 ensures the replacement for the couple giving birth to her offspring.
- The *short-term* decrease in human TFR is mainly a result of socioeconomic and educational factors that are relatively easier to tackle with change in attitude of the society.
- The *long-term* changes are driven by a combination of drastic environmental, lifestyle, and genetic factors, which could potentially result in permanent damage to the fertility of the human species.
- With large-scale ART practice, we may encourage the persistence of poor fertility genotypes within the population.
- As clinicians, we frequently encounter nonpregnant women, men, and couples in their reproductive age, which is an opportunity for us to create awareness in them about wellness and healthy habits to optimize their reproductive outcomes.

REFERENCES

1. Craig J. Replacement level fertility and future population growth. Popul Trends. 1994;78:20-2.
2. Vollset SE, Goren E, Yuan C-W, Cao J, Smith AE, Hsiao T, et al. Fertility, mortality, migration, and population scenarios for 195 countries and territories from 2017 to 2100: a forecasting analysis for the Global Burden of Disease Study. Lancet. 2020;396:1285-306.
3. International Institute for Population Sciences (IIPS) and ICF. National Family Health Survey (NFHS-5), 2019-21: India. Mumbai: IIPS; 2021.
4. Liu DH, Raftery AE. How do education and family planning accelerate fertility decline? Popul Dev Rev. 2020;46:409-41.
5. Wu X, Ye H, He GG. Fertility decline and women's status improvement in China. Chin Soc Rev. 2014;46(3):3-25.
6. Nomura K, Karita K, Araki A, Nishioka E, Muto G, Iwai-Shimada M, et al. For making a declaration of countermeasures against the falling birth rate from the Japanese Society for Hygiene: summary of discussion in the working group on academic research strategy against an aging society with low birth rate. Environ Health Prev Med. 2019;24:14.
7. Human Fertilization and Embryology Authority. (2021). Fertility treatment 2019: trends and figures. (online) Available from: https://www.hfea.gov.uk/about-us/publications/research-and-data/fertility-treatment-2019-trends-and-figures/. [Last accessed September, 2021].
8. Leridon H, Slama R. The impact of a decline in fecundity and of pregnancy postponement on final number of children and demand for assisted reproduction technology. Hum Reprod. 2008;23(6):1312-9.
9. Nakatani H. Population aging in Japan: policy transformation, sustainable development goals, universal health coverage, and social determinates of health. Glob Health Med. 2019;1:3-10.
10. Jones GW. Delayed marriage and very low fertility in Pacific Asia. Popul Dev Rev. 2007;33:453-8.
11. Whitfield L. Milk production, fertility and the modern dairy cow. Livestock. 2020;25:72-5.
12. Golin AP, Yuen W, Flannigan R. The effects of Y chromosome microdeletions on in vitro fertilization outcomes, health abnormalities in offspring and recurrent pregnancy loss. Transl Androl Urol. 2021;10:1457-66.
13. Belva F, Bonduelle M, Roelants M, Michielsen D, Van Steirteghem A, Verheyen G, et al. Semen quality of young adult ICSI offspring: the first results. Hum Reprod. 2016;31:2811-20.
14. Chen D, Liang Y, Li J, Zhang X, Zheng R, Wang X, et al. A novel CCDC39 mutation causes multiple morphological abnormalities of the flagella in a primary ciliary dyskinesia patient. Reprod Biomed Online. 2021;43:920-30.
15. Ferreux L, Bourdon M, Chargui A, Schmitt A, Stouvenel L, Lorès P, et al. Genetic diagnosis, sperm phenotype and ICSI outcome in case of severe asthenozoospermia with multiple morphological abnormalities of the flagellum. Hum Reprod. 2021;36:2848-60.
16. Mazaheri Moghaddam M, Mazaheri Moghaddam M, Hamzeiy H, Baghbanzadeh A, Pashazadeh F, Sakhinia E. Genetic basis of acephalic spermatozoa syndrome, and intracytoplasmic sperm injection outcomes in infertile men: a systematic scoping review. J Assist Reprod Genet. 2021;38:573-86.
17. Belva F, Bonduelle M, Buysse A, Van den Bogaert A, Hes F, Roelants M, et al. Chromosomal abnormalities after ICSI in relation to semen parameters: results in 1114 fetuses and 1391 neonates from a single center. Hum Reprod. 2020;35:2149-62.
18. Caramaschi D, Jungius J, Page CM, Novakovic B, Saffery R, Halliday J, et al. Association of medically assisted reproduction with offspring cord blood DNA methylation across cohorts. Hum Reprod. 2021;36:2403-13.
19. Aitken RJ. The male is significantly implicated as the cause of unexplained infertility. Semin Reprod Med. 2020;38:3-20.
20. Sang Q, Zhou Z, Mu J, Wang L. Genetic factors as potential molecular markers of human oocyte and embryo quality. J Assist Reprod Genet. 2021;38:993-1002.
21. Agarwal A, Mulgund A, Hamada A, Chyatte MR. A unique view on male infertility around the globe. Reprod Biol Endocrinol. 2015;13:37.
22. Swan SH, Colino S. Countdown: How Our Modern World is Threatening Sperm Counts, Altering Male and Female Reproductive Development, and Imperiling the Future of the Human Race. New York: Scribner; 2021.
23. Skakkebaek NE. Sperm counts, testicular cancers, and the environment. BMJ. 2017;359:j4517.
24. Mazur A, Westerman R, Mueller U. Is rising obesity causing a secular (age-independent) decline in testosterone among American men? PLoS One. 2013;8:e76178.
25. Reed KE, Camargo J, Hamilton-Reeves J, Kurzer M, Messina M. Neither soy nor isoflavone intake affects male reproductive

hormones: an expanded and updated meta-analysis of clinical studies. Reprod Toxicol. 2021;100:60-7.
26. Cariati F, D'Uonno N, Borrillo F, Iervolino S, Galdiero G, Tomaiuolo R. Bisphenol A: an emerging threat to male fertility. Reprod Biol Endocrinol. 2019;17:6.
27. Fénichel P, Chevalier N. Is testicular germ cell cancer estrogen dependent? The role of endocrine disrupting chemicals. Endocrinology. 2019;160:2981-9.
28. Gnoth C, Godehardt D, Godehardt E, Frank-Herrmann P, Freundl G. Time to pregnancy: results of the German prospective study and impact on the management of infertility. Hum Reprod. 2003;18:1959-66.
29. Howe G, Westhoff C, Vessey M, Yeates D. Effects of age, cigarette smoking, and other factors on fertility: findings in a large prospective study. Br Med J. 1985;290:1697-700.
30. Menken J, Trussell J, Larsen U. Age and infertility. Science. 1986;233:1389-94.
31. Practice Committee of the American Society for Reproductive Medicine. Fertility evaluation of infertile women: a committee opinion. Fertil Steril. 2021;116:1255-65.

SECTION

3 Combined Topics

CHAPTER 16

Evaluation of Infertility

Dipti Das, Kamini A Rao

INTRODUCTION

Since ancient times, humankind has been obsessed with fertility. With both biological and social imperatives driving us to have children, it is no surprise that, even today, the lack of fertility is perceived by many, especially the infertile, as a curse. In India, this has resulted in many social evils such as stigmatization and isolation and, in turn, has caused much trauma in the affected individuals. Further compounded by ignorance, this situation has engendered much quackery. Thus, the proper diagnosis of infertility is of paramount importance not only to the physical well-being of an affected couple but also to their mental and social well-being.

DIAGNOSIS OF INFERTILITY (MALE)

Definition

Infertility is the inability of a sexually active, noncontracepting couple to achieve spontaneous pregnancy in 1 year.[1]

About 8–12% of couples in the reproductive age group do not achieve pregnancy within 1 year and seek medical treatment for infertility. Eventually, <5% remain unwillingly childless.[2] The age-standardized prevalence of infertility has increased annually by 0.370% in women and by 0.291% in men.[3]

Male Infertility

- Male factor infertility may be explained by:
  - Abnormal semen analysis
  - Sperm function defects
  - Functional male defects.

A male factor is solely responsible in about 20–30% of infertile couples and contributes in another 20% of couples.[4]

Goals of Evaluation

There are various conditions causing male infertility, of which, many—but not all—can be identified and treated. Further, in cases of males who were previously fertile, the current condition of infertility implies that a newly acquired secondary factor of male infertility may be present, thus necessitating identical sequences of evaluation for either type of infertility—primary (having never caused a pregnancy) or secondary (having previously caused a pregnancy).[5]

The aims of evaluation, as per the American Urological Association (AUA) guidelines, are to correctly identify the following:[6]

- Potentially reversible conditions contributing to male infertility due to either obstruction within the reproductive tract or treatment of endocrinopathies
- Irreversible conditions amenable to assisted reproductive techniques using the sperm of the male partner
- Irreversible conditions that are not open to the above, and for which donor insemination or adoption is a possible option
- Life- or health-threatening conditions that may underlie the infertility and require medical attention
- Genetic abnormalities that may affect the health of offspring if assisted reproductive techniques are to be employed.

History

The reproductive history should cover the following:

- Sexual history, including:
  - Timing of puberty
  - Frequency and timing of coitus
  - Type of lubricants used
  - Libido, erectile, and ejaculatory dysfunction
  - Duration of infertility and previous fertility
  - Sexually transmitted infections
- Medical history, including:
  - Medical illnesses
    - Neurological conditions (spinal cord injury and multiple sclerosis), diabetes mellitus
    - Infections (urinary infections, epididymitis or prostatitis, tuberculosis, and mumps orchitis)

- Cryptorchidism and anosmia
- History of testicular torsion
- History of testicular trauma
- Previous surgery
  - Orchidopexy, herniorrhaphy, vasectomy, and prostatic surgery
  - Medications and allergies
  - Childhood illnesses and developmental history
  - Exposures to gonadotoxins (including environmental and chemical toxins and heat)
  - Malignancy
- Social history or lifestyle, including:
  - Current and/or past use of anabolic steroids, recreational drugs, tobacco, and alcohol
- Family history:
  - Infertility
  - Cystic fibrosis (CF)
  - Androgen receptor deficiency.

Physical Examination

Obviously, a general physical examination is a basic part and a starting point of the evaluation of infertile men. This should include the following:

- Calculating the body mass index (BMI)
- Examining the penis and noting the location of the urethral meatus
- Palpating and measuring the testes (normal volume 12–30 mL)
- Noting the presence and consistency of the epididymis and both vasa
- Noting the presence or absence of a varicocele
- Noting secondary sex characteristics, including physique (including arm span, muscle development), voice, hair distribution, and/or breast development
- Digitally examining the rectum for cysts, seminal vesicles, and prostate
- Diagnosing for the congenital bilateral absence of the vas deferens (CBAVD).

Varicocele

Varicoceles, defined as abnormally dilated scrotal veins, are present in almost 15% of the normal male population and in approximately 40% of infertile men. Primarily diagnosed by palpating the scrotum of the patient in both upright and recumbent positions, a palpable varicocele feels like a "bag of worms," which disappears or is significantly reduced when the patient is recumbent. Since only clinically palpable varicoceles have been clearly associated with infertility, in cases where physical examination has been inconclusive, scrotal ultrasonography is sufficient to confirm the presence of a varicocele.[7] Classification of varicoceles is shown in **Table 1**.[7]

TABLE 1: Classification of varicoceles by Dubin and Amelar.[7]

Grades of varicoceles	
Grade	***Characteristics***
1	Palpable only with Valsalva maneuver
2	Palpable without Valsalva maneuver
3	Detectable by visual inspection

Timing of Evaluation

Once the couple meets the definition for infertility, they should be referred for further investigations. The American Society for Reproductive Medicine (ASRM)[6] and the European Association of Urology (EAU)[8] both recommend an initial evaluation consisting of a reproductive history and at least two semen analyses.

However, there are certain circumstances where earlier evaluation may be required:

- Female partner is >35 years
- Predisposing factors for infertility
- Imminent treatment is planned for malignancy that may result in infertility (chemotherapy/radiotherapy).

Semen Analysis

The lynchpin of the diagnosis of infertility in men, semen analysis forms the basis of an evaluation of the male partner in subfertile couples and allows planning of further investigation and management **(Flowchart 1)**. The body stores sperm in the pair of epididymides as a concentrated suspension, which is mixed only during ejaculation with fluids from the other accessory sex glands—the prostate gland, the seminal vesicles, and the bulbourethral glands. The fluids amount to around 90% of the total semen volume, much of it from the prostate gland and the seminal vesicles with the remaining from the bulbourethral glands.

The analysis is done on the semen ejaculated, which is collected as a result of either:

- Masturbation into a sterile wide-necked container (at home or in a room close to the laboratory) or
- Intercourse using a special nonspermicidal condom (at home)

The quality of the ejaculated sample and, thus, the interpretation of the analysis vary as per:

- *Method of producing ejaculate:* The ejaculate produced by masturbation tends to be of lower quality than that produced by intercourse, perhaps due to a difference in the arousal level.
- *Completeness of the sample:* Ejaculation is done in a series of spurts, the first of which contains most of the sperm, while the subsequent ones contain very little.
- *Period of sexual abstinence:* The body stores the sperm in the epididymides which, when filled, allow the sperm to overflow into the urethra, to be passed out with urine.

Flowchart 1: Diagnosis algorithm of male partner in an infertile couple.

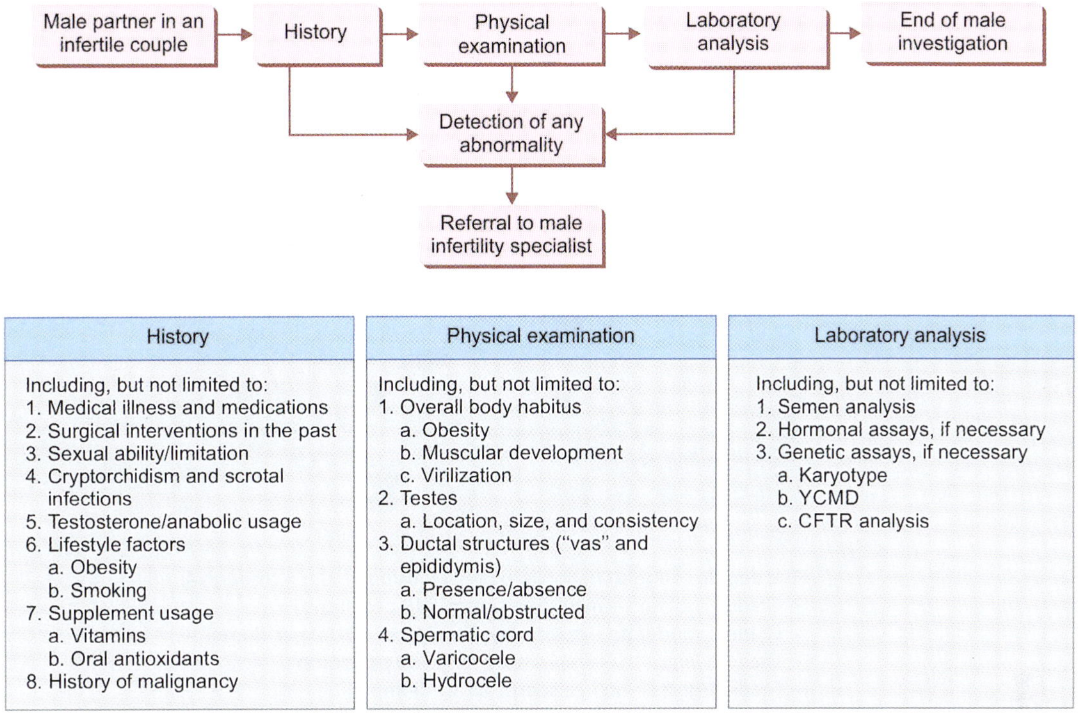

(CFTR: cystic fibrosis transmembrane conductance regulator; YCMD: Y chromosome microdeletions)

TABLE 2: Macroscopic examination of semen.

Liquefaction	The complete semen sample usually liquefies within 15 minutes and sometimes, up to 60 minutes
Viscosity	Viscosity is estimated after liquefaction; the sample should be aspirated into a pipette of around 1.5 mm diameter and then allowed to drop due to gravity while watching for threads. Normal semen usually forms small individual drops; the presence of threads longer than 2 cm indicates abnormal viscosity
Semen volume	Volume is best measured by collecting directly in a graduated measuring container. Decanting from the collection container into the measuring container or even aspirating into a pipette or syringe would cause a loss in volume
Semen pH	The seminal vesicle secretions are alkaline, while the prostatic secretions are acidic; thus, the pH value demonstrates the equilibrium between the secretions of the accessory sex glands. A sample of low volume combined with azoospermia and a pH below 7 strongly indicates the congenital bilateral absence of the vas deferens (CBAVD) or other ejaculatory duct obstruction(s). Semen pH increases with time, reducing the clinical usefulness of the value

- *Size of the testes:* The size of the testes affects both the total number of sperm per ejaculate and the morphology of the sperm.
- *Age of the male patient:* The total number of sperm and the total volume of semen ejaculated tend to reduce as age increases.
- For optimum results, physicians should give their patients a standardized set of instructions for semen collection, advising sexual abstinence—for 2 days at a minimum and 5 days at a maximum—prior to semen collection, and careful collection of the whole ejaculate.

The primary characteristics of semen are the total sperm number and the total semen volume. The total sperm number is a function of the sperm-production capacity of the testes. The total semen volume is a function of secretion capacity of the accessory sex glands. Both these characteristics are also a function of the degree of openness of the respective ducts of the reproductive tract.

Routine Tests

Macroscopic Examination

Table 2 shows the macroscopic examination of semen.

Microscopic Examination

Table 3 shows the microscopic examination of semen.

Many textbooks go into detail about available methods of semen analysis, but the gold standard is the World Health Organization (WHO) Laboratory Manual for the Examination and Processing of Human Semen.

TABLE 3: Microscopic examination of semen.

Agglutination	Though sperm move vigorously, they sometimes clump together. 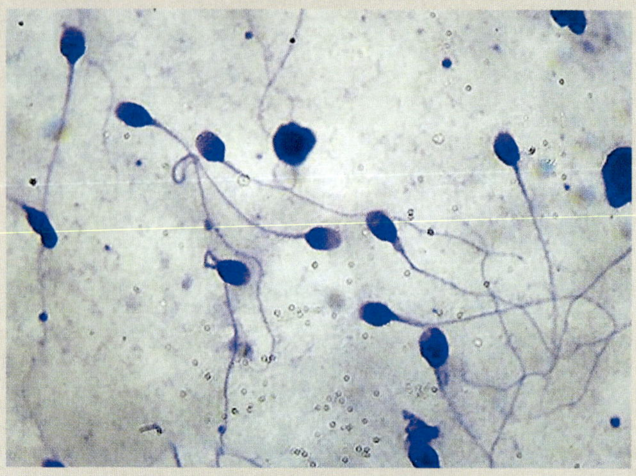 (*Courtesy:* Dr. Sarita Suresh, Aaradhya Fertility Center) The degree of agglutination is expressed using grades 1 through 4: • Grade 1, isolated—many free sperm; <10 per clump • Grade 2, moderate—quite a few free sperm; 10–50 per clump • Grade 3, large—a few sperm are free; >50 per clump • Grade 4, gross—no free sperm; all are clumped The site of attachment should be recorded, whether they are head-to-head, tail-to-tail, tail-tip-to-tail-tip, mixed, or tangled
Motility	Progressive sperm motility is linked to pregnancy rates. To reduce errors due to deterioration of the sample with time, motility should be determined soon after liquefaction, within 30 minutes or at most within 60 minutes. Motility is graded as: • Progressive motility (PR): Active movement, linear, or circular • Nonprogressive motility (NP): Any other pattern of movement • Immotility (IM): No movement Fast progressive (1), slow progressive (2), nonprogressive (3), and immotile (4)
Vitality	Sperm vitality is an estimate based on the percentage of sperm cells with an intact plasma membrane. Vitality is particularly important in the cases of samples with less than about 40% progressively motile sperm,[9] because the percentage of dead sperm should not be greater than the percentage of immotile sperm. Either of two methods is usually used: • *Dye exclusion—eosin-nigrosin one-step technique:* The plasma membrane of live sperm cells does not allow dyes such as eosin (yellow in color) to permeate into the cell. However, the membrane of a dead sperm cell is damaged and allows the eosin dye to stain the cell. Nigrosin (black in color) increases the contrast between the background and the sperm heads, making it easier to discern the dead sperm cells. Slides can be stored, allowing for reevaluation and quality control • *Hypoosmotic swelling (HOS):* On the other hand, the HOS test is used to discern live sperm cells because, in a hypotonic solution, only the cells with their plasma membranes intact would swell. This is an advantageous alternative because spermatozoa staining must be avoided in some cases, such as choosing spermatozoa for intracytoplasmic sperm injection (ICSI)
Sperm concentration Sperm number	Sperm are counted per slide, then concentration and number are calculated for the sample
Round cells number	Calculation of round cells is done relative to the number of sperm
Morphology	Like the "strict criteria" detailed by Dr. Thinus F. Kruger (Tygerberg Hospital, South Africa), the World Health Organization (WHO) criteria classify rather few sperm as having normal morphology, even in semen collected from fertile men. Morphological anomalies can be found—in more than one part—in the head, neck, mid-piece, and tail. Defective spermatogenesis and epididymal pathologies may increase the percentage of abnormal sperm morphology. Sperm with abnormal morphology generally have a lower ability to cause fertilization

Contd...

Contd…

Abnormal sperm

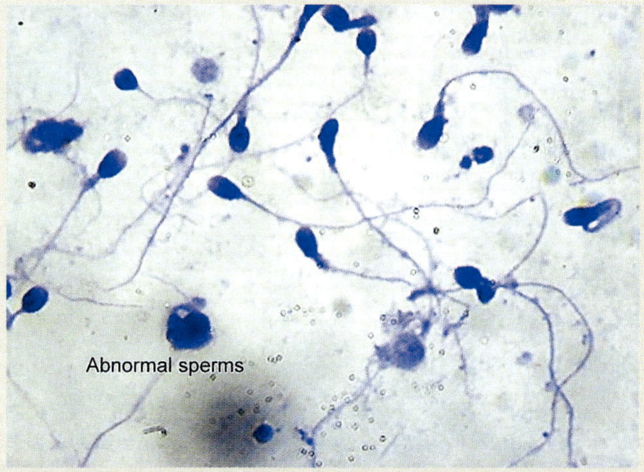

(*Courtesy:* Dr. Sarita Suresh, Aaradhya Fertility Center)

Bent neck sperm

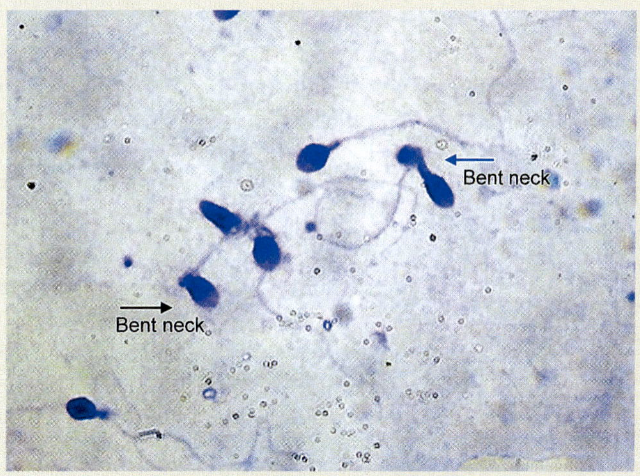

(*Courtesy:* Dr. Sarita Suresh, Aaradhya Fertility Center)

Double tail sperm

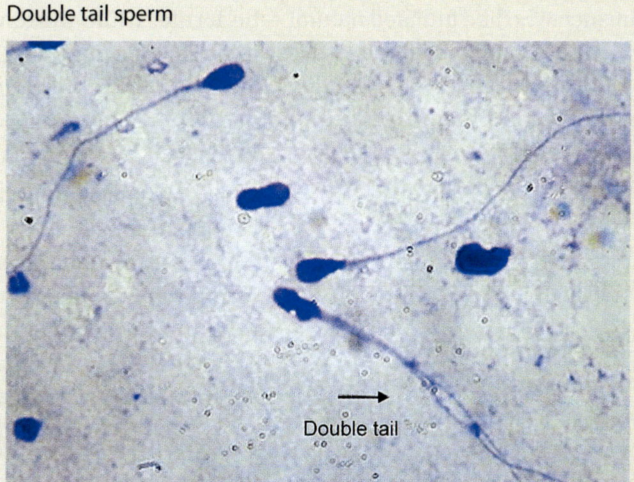

(*Courtesy:* Dr. Sarita Suresh, Aaradhya Fertility Center)

TABLE 4: Lower reference limits (fifth centiles and their 95% confidence interval) for some semen characteristics.

Parameter	*WHO 5th edition*[9]	*WHO 6th edition*[1]
Semen volume (mL)	1.5 (1.4–1.7)	1.4 (1.3–1.5)
Total sperm number (10^6/ejaculate)	39 (33–46)	39 (35–40)
Sperm concentration (10^6/mL)	15 (12–16)	16
Total motility (PR + NP, %)	40 (38–42)	42 (40–43)
Progressive motility (PR, %)	32 (31–34)	30 (29–31)
Nonprogressive (NPR, %)	1	1 (1–1)
Immotile	22	20 (19–20)
Vitality (live spermatozoa, %)	58 (55–63)	54 (50–56)
Sperm morphology (normal forms, %)	4 (3.0–4.0)	4 (3.9–4)

(WHO: World Health Organization)

TABLE 5: Consensus threshold values for other semen characteristics.[1]

Parameter	*Threshold value*
pH	7.2
Peroxidase-positive leukocytes (10^6/mL)	≥1.0
Mixed antiglobulin reaction (MAR) test (% motile spermatozoa with bound particles)	<50
Immunobead test (% motile spermatozoa with bound beads)	<50
Seminal zinc (μmol/ejaculate)	≥2.4
Seminal fructose (μmol/ejaculate)	≥13
Viscosity	≤2 cm thread after liquefaction
Sperm agglutination	Absent

TABLE 6: Basal hormone levels in various clinical states.[11]

Clinical condition	*FSH*	*LH*	*T*	*PRL*
Normal spermatogenesis	Normal	Normal	Normal	Normal
Hypogonadotropic hypogonadism	Low	Low	Low	Normal
Abnormal spermatogenesis	High/normal	Normal	Normal	Normal
Complete testicular failure or hypergonadotropic hypergonadism	High	High	Normal/low	Normal
PRL-secreting pituitary tumor	Normal/low	Normal/low	Low	High
Androgen excess	Normal/low	Normal	High	Normal
Hypothyroidism	Low	Low	High	
Hyperthyroidism	High	High	Low	
Insulin disorders	Decreased spermatogenesis, reduced vacuolization in the Sertoli cells, decreased fertility, decreased semen parameters, decreased Leydig cells count, decreased testosterone			

(FSH: follicle-stimulating hormone; LH: luteinizing hormone; PRL: prolactinomas; T: testosterone)

Note that the reference limits provided in **Tables 4 and 5** are from semen samples from men who had initiated natural conceptions; so, they represent the semen characteristics those are associated with the couples in the WHO study who achieved pregnancy during a 12-month period of unprotected sexual intercourse. Thus, these limits can only be used as guidelines and should not be used to distinguish between fertile and infertile men. Further, though these limits could indicate that a man needs treatment for infertility, they should not be used to ascertain the nature of the treatment.

Although each of the sperm parameters in **Tables 4 and 5** could be used to predict fertility and subfertility, the terms "normozoospermia," "asthenozoospermia," "necrozoospermia," and "teratozoospermia" are voluntarily removed in the WHO 6th manual as no single one is a powerful discriminator. Most importantly, these so-called normal values do not actually correspond to normal sperm concentrations in the general population, and, as such, the values cannot be considered as the minimum sufficient for conception. Men with out-of-range semen values could be fertile, while those with values within range could be infertile.[3] The male partner should be counseled for a repeat analysis if the result of the first is abnormal.

HORMONAL EVALUATION

One to two percent of male infertility is occasionally related to endocrinopathies.[10]

The international societies have evaluation limited to men with a sperm concentration below 10 × 10^6/mL or impaired sexual function, or if endocrinopathy is suspected.[6,8] However, a customized approach of the case would enable timely treatment and restoration of infertility.

Inhibin B: This is produced in males exclusively by Sertoli cells in the testis. It leads to negative feedback for follicle-stimulating hormone (FSH) secretion. Inhibin B, FSH, and testicular volume are important markers of the competence of Sertoli cells and spermatogenesis in a man. There is a positive correlation between sperm count and serum level of inhibin B and testicular volume. The adult reference level of 170 pg/mL is standard. Inhibin B can be used as a discriminatory biomarker to differentiate nonobstructive azoospermia (NOA) patients from obstructive azoospermia patients.[12,13]

EXTENDED SEMEN ANALYSIS

Sperm function tests analyze the functional aspects of spermatozoa and therefore augment semen analysis **(Box 1)**.[14]

The clinical application of these tests:[15]

- Clinical varicocele
- Unexplained infertility or intrauterine insemination (IUI) failure or recurrent pregnancy loss
- In vitro fertilization (IVF) failure, or intracytoplasmic sperm injection (ICSI) failure, or both
- Borderline abnormal (or normal) semen parameters with risk factor.

However, with the development of ICSI, hemizona or acrosome function assays have lost their significance because the penetrating capability of sperm is bypassed by ICSI.

The most commonly applied deoxyribonucleic acid (DNA) integrity tests, none indicate the specific DNA sequences that might be affected; rather, each provides a semiquantitative estimate of the general state of the DNA being studied.

- *Sperm chromatin structure assay (SCSA):*[16] It utilizes flow cytometry of fluorescently labeled sperm to determine the proportion of sperm susceptible to DNA damage (red fluorescence) compared with normal sperm (green fluorescence). Sperm samples diluted with a 1× TNE buffer are exposed for 30 seconds to a 1.2 pH acid detergent solution. Acridine orange (AO), a DNA-binding fluorescent dye, is then added. Normal range is 25–27%.
- *Terminal deoxynucleotidyl transferase-mediated dUTP nick end labeling (TUNEL) assay*: This utilizes flow cytometry of sperm fluorescently labeled at DNA strand breaks to determine the degree of DNA damage; the fluorescence intensity is proportional to the number of strand breaks. Normal is <36%.

BOX 1: Sperm function tests.

- Sperm zona pellucida binding—hemizona assay
- Sperm DNA fragmentation—SCD, TUNEL, SCSA, comet assay
- Acrosome reaction–acrosome reaction
- Reactive oxygen species—chemiluminescence (luminometer) ORP (MiOXSYS)
- Mitochondrial function—mitochondrial membrane potential

(DNA: deoxyribonucleic acid; MiOXSYS: Male Infertility Oxidative System; ORP: oxidation–reduction potential; SCD: sperm chromatin dispersion; SCSA: sperm chromatin structure assay; TUNEL: terminal deoxynucleotidyl transferase-mediated dUTP nick end labeling)

- *Single-cell gel electrophoresis assay (SCGE, also known as comet assay):* Fluorescently labeled sperm cells are embedded in an agarose gel, lysed to relax the DNA, and electrophoresed. The electrophoresis causes structures resembling comets, hence the name. DNA damage is proportional to the displacement between the nuclear material and the tail material.
- *Sperm chromatin dispersion (SCD) test:* This utilizes fluorescence microscopy to discriminate between cells with intact DNA (large halo) and sperm cells with damaged DNA (small or absent halo).
- *Oxidation-reduction potential (ORP) assay:* ORP levels can lend support to routine semen analysis. In patients with idiopathic male infertility, abnormal ORP levels are particularly useful in pinpointing altered sperm function, thereby improving the accuracy of therapy management.[17]

Chemiluminescent or fluorescent techniques can have prognostic value in the evaluation of oxidation-reduction potential with a cutoff value of <102.2 RLU/s/10^6 sperm/mL to distinguish between men who are fertile and men with infertility.[18,19]

Genetic Screening

Fifteen percent of men with infertility can be attributed to genetic mutations in embryos leading to repeated ICSI failure, recurrent miscarriage, or vertical transmission of paternal genetic defects.[20]

International societies agree on recommending karyotype analysis for men with azoospermia or severe oligozoospermia (sperm count $<5 \times 10^6$/mL).[21] EAU recommends the use of genetic screening also if there is a family history of recurrent spontaneous abortions, malformations, or intellectual disability,[22] regardless of the sperm concentration.

The most common genetic abnormalities associated with male factor infertility are:

- *Chromosomal abnormalities:* The most common chromosomal abnormalities in azoospermic men are abnormalities involving the sex chromosomes, which are found in approximately 4% of these men. Due to these abnormalities, proper chromosome pairing during meiosis is impaired, giving rise to spermatogenic disruption and the infertility phenotype. The most frequent abnormality is called Klinefelter syndrome, in which patients show a 47,XXY karyotype.
- *Karyotypic chromosomal abnormalities:* The incidence of chromosomal abnormalities is higher in infertile men and is inversely proportional to their sperm count; the incidence is 10–15% in azoospermic men, 5% in men with severe oligozoospermia (<5 million/mL), and <1% in men with normal sperm concentrations.[5]

For infertile men with such abnormalities, karyotype analysis is strongly recommended—either before using ejaculated sperm in performing ICSI or before testicular sperm extraction/aspiration (TESE/TESA). Prior knowledge of a chromosomal translocation would beneficially alter therapeutic planning to include the use of preimplantation genetic screening in discarding chromosomally unbalanced embryos, thus allowing the transfer of balanced or normal embryos.

- *Y chromosome microdeletions (YCMD):* Over 40 years ago, in 1976, Tiepolo and Zuffardi first suspected Y chromosome involvement in male infertility when they detected obvious terminal deletions. At that time, they postulated that infertility resulted from defects in the gene controlling spermatogenesis; it was called the azoospermia factor (*AZF*) gene. In 1996, Vogt et al. discovered three separate deletion intervals named AZFa, AZFb, and AZFc. A meta-analysis by Kohn et al. showed that the majority of YCMD occur in men with sperm counts of $<1 \times 10^6$/mL.[23]

  The latest EAU guidelines recommend Y chromosome microdeletion testing if sperm concentrations are $<5 \times 10^6$/mL and make such testing mandatory for sperm concentrations of $<1 \times 10^6$/mL.[8]

  Y chromosome microdeletions transmitted from fathers to sons by ICSI may maintain the same characteristics and size; though, without single-cell amplification, the stability of the boundary of the deletion cannot be determined with certainty. Such men had higher incidence of abnormal sperm karyotypes, and spermatozoa of men with AZFc or partial AZFb deletions will successfully fertilize and generate offspring at the same rate as nondeleted infertile men. Though deletions in the AZF regions apparently do not adversely affect the psychological and physical development of the children, men with such microdeletions must be informed of the risk of transmission of genetic defects as well as their infertile testis phenotype.[24]

  Although standard Y-deletion screening can detect deletions of AZFa, AZFb, and/or AZFc, there might be other, as yet undetected, deletions on the Y chromosome. The availability of the complete Y sequence will facilitate more precise research on Y chromosome integrity. Further research into the other numerous testis-specific genes, which are not part of the Y chromosome, would definitely help to illuminate the complex spermatogenesis process while also enabling screening for genetic aberrations in male partners of couples planning for ICSI.

  All infertile males should be provided genetic counseling, irrespective of whether an abnormality is detected or whether Y-deletion testing has even been done. The frequency of detection of genetic aberrations in infertile males using karyotyping and standard Y-deletion screening is <15%. Even so, some deletions might remain undetected because standard screening needs much improvement. Also, some suspected deletions may turn out to be polymorphisms, thus having no clinical significance. Finally, despite the apparent lack of cytogenetic or Y chromosomal abnormality in an infertile male patient, a genetic cause for his azoospermia or severe oligozoospermia may well be present.[25]
- *Cystic fibrosis:* The cystic fibrosis transmembrane conductance regulator (*CFTR*) gene is responsible for the production of a protein called the cystic fibrosis (CF) transmembrane conductance regulator protein. This protein acts as a channel to allow ions such as those of chloride and sodium to cross the membranes of cells. The movement of chloride ions controls the movement of water in and out of tissues and thus is critical in the production of mucus. For men with structural abnormalities of the vas deferens, it is recommended that both partners be tested for *CFTR* mutations containing a minimal panel of common point mutations and the 5T allele.[8]

Antisperm Antibodies

An uncommon cause of male infertility, antisperm antibodies (ASAs) may be detected in the serum, in the seminal plasma or directly bound to sperm. Consequent to a rupture in the blood–testis barrier, ASAs can form if the immune system is exposed to large quantities of sperm antigens. Risk factors for ASA formation include trauma, torsion, biopsy, orchitis, testicular cancer, and vasectomy.

Testing for ASAs is usually done when the semen analysis shows sperm agglutination or isolated asthenospermia (while sperm concentration is normal). ASAs in the serum or seminal plasma are detected using indirect antibody agglutination assays, while ASAs (immunoglobulin G and A) bound to the sperm head or tail are detected using a direct immunobead test. Sperm-bound ASAs could be important in clinical practice because of their cascade of effects—decreased motility, reducing the penetration of the cervical mucus, in turn reducing fertilization, and thus, greatly decreasing the likelihood of conception.

Antisperm antibodies are usually managed using ICSI. Therefore, if ICSI has been planned, testing for ASAs is unnecessary since its helpfulness in practice is unclear.[26] ASA testing should not be a part of routine male infertility evaluation. ASAs do not hamper the pregnancy rates of IVF or ICSI, which, therefore, become treatment options.[27]

Microbiological Assessment

Conditions indicating microbiological assessment include abnormal urine samples, urinary tract infections, male accessory gland infections (MAGIs), and sexually transmitted diseases. The combination of low ejaculate volume and the presence of white blood cells in the semen could mean ejaculatory duct obstruction, perhaps partial, resulting from an infection of the prostate or seminal vesicles. Genital tract obstruction can also result from *Neisseria gonorrhoeae* and *Chlamydia trachomatis* infections. Further, genital infections could provoke the production of spermatotoxic oxygen radicals. Antibiotic procedures for MAGI might improve sperm quality but not the probability of conception.

Viral Screening

Screening for human immunodeficiency virus (HIV), hepatitis B surface antigen, and hepatitis C virus should be offered to couples undergoing IVF or opting for semen freezing.

Ultrasonography

Almost the entire male genital tract can be easily and accurately imaged using ultrasonography; therefore, it is used to detect abnormalities that adversely affect fertility. However, it is required only in a minority of cases.

Transrectal Ultrasonography

Usually, seminal vesicles are <1.5 cm in the anteroposterior diameter. Thus, when dilated seminal vesicles or ejaculatory ducts and/or midline cystic prostatic structures are seen in transrectal ultrasonography (TRUS), this suggests—without establishing by itself—partial or complete ejaculatory duct obstruction. Typically, the ejaculate is low-volume and acidic, containing neither sperm nor fructose. Similar findings are seen for men with CBAVD because they often have absent or atrophic seminal vesicles. Unsurprisingly, partial ejaculatory duct obstruction often manifests low-volume ejaculate, oligoasthenospermia, and poor progressive motility. Outside of consensus, a few experts advocate routine TRUS for men with normal testicular size and normal serum T but with oligospermia, low-volume ejaculate, and palpable vasa.

Scrotal Ultrasonography

Most scrotal pathology, such as varicoceles, spermatoceles, absent vasa, epididymal induration, and testicular masses, can be identified via careful physical examination. Though scrotal ultrasonography can be used to identify varicoceles that are not palpable, they have no clinical significance because only palpable varicoceles have been linked with infertility. However, scrotal ultrasonography is more useful in clarifying vague or ambiguous physical examination findings or abnormalities such as apparent masses. It is also useful in cases with testes located in the upper scrotum, a small scrotal sac, or anatomy hindering examination. Further, scrotal ultrasonography is recommended for men with infertility and risk factors for testicular cancer, such as cryptorchidism or a previous testicular neoplasm, but not as a routine screening procedure.

Conclusion

Knowing the prevalence of a disease is central in the endeavor to manage patients, provide resources, estimate impact, present rational research questions, and effectively make arguments on the health economy. However, on a global level and across all health economies, there is a severe lack of clinical data on the extent of reproductive health problems and infertility in men.

The best estimates on infertility are based on demographic health studies which depend on heterosexual women to self-report a problem with becoming pregnant, and which further assume female infertility (due to minimal reporting of clinical diagnosis), or possibly, an infertile relationship. This, coupled with an even more severe lack of male diagnosis and management of infertility in low- and middle-income countries, renders any male infertility prevalence values which are based upon demographic health reports or reports from small private clinics to be, at best, greatly extrapolated and highly inaccurate. Consequently, and unsurprisingly, there is inadequate information on basic but crucial indicators such as the socioeconomic impact of infertility and other diseases or disorders on the individual as well as the society as a whole.

Improving the care of couples and expanding the collective knowledge of the scale of the problem depend on highlighting the criticality of male partner engagement in the assessment of the infertile couple and public awareness and education about male infertility. Equally crucial is the need to ascertain the potential consequences of male infertility; this is an extensive investigation which goes beyond the confines of the couple and their immediate relationships, to find out, for example, the relationship of infertility with other diseases and the associated impact.

RECOMMENDATIONS

- *Assess several ejaculate parameters:* For a more accurate prediction of fertility success
- *A single ejaculate is sufficient:* To determine the most appropriate investigation and treatment pathway (can repeat semen analysis if abnormalities are found)
- *Perform karyotype and YCMD testing:* On all males with severe oligozoospermia ($<5 \times 10^6$/mL) or NOA prior to any therapeutic procedure
- *Offer CFTR mutation analysis:* To all males with CBAVD or CF.[10]

DIAGNOSIS OF INFERTILITY (FEMALE)

Female Infertility

Failing to achieve pregnancy after 12 months or more of regular and unprotected sexual intercourse is an indication for couples to undergo diagnostic evaluation for infertility. As roughly 85% of couples usually achieve an unassisted natural pregnancy in 12–18 months, around 15% of couples would require evaluation for infertility. A couple in which the woman is over 35 years of age, after 6 months of attempting to conceive naturally, should soon undergo evaluation. This may also be necessary in cases with:

- History of oligo- or amenorrhea
- Known or suspected uterine/tubal/peritoneal disease or stage III–IV endometriosis
- Known or suspected male subfertility.

When appropriate for the couple, both partners should undergo evaluation at the same time. Women who intend to attempt pregnancy by donor insemination would benefit by undergoing evaluation before starting treatment.[28,29]

History and Physical Examination

Preferably, this should be done during the first consultation, allowing enough time for gathering a complete history (medical, reproductive, family, and social/lifestyle), carrying out a detailed physical examination, and counseling the patient about preconception care and about screening for any pertinent pathological and/or genetic conditions.

History

A comprehensive history should cover and document the following:

- *Sexual history, including:*
  - Frequency and timing of coitus
  - Sexual dysfunction
  - Previous methods of contraception
  - Duration of infertility and previous fertility
  - Previous evaluation and treatment
  - Menstruation (menarche, cycle, molimina, and dysmenorrhea)
  - Pregnancy (gravidity, parity, outcome, and complications).
- *Medical history, including:*
  - Surgery (procedures, indications, and outcomes), hospitalizations, serious illnesses or injuries, pelvic inflammatory disease, or sexually transmitted infections
  - Thyroid disease, galactorrhea, hirsutism, pelvic or abdominal pain, and dyspareunia
  - Previous abnormal Pap smears and any subsequent treatment
  - Current medications and allergies
  - Family history of birth defects, mental retardation, early menopause, or reproductive failure or compromise.
- *Social/lifestyle history, including:*
  - Occupation
  - Exposures to gonadotoxins (including environmental and chemical toxins and heat)
  - Use of tobacco, alcohol, and recreational drugs.

Physical Examination

A thorough physical examination should cover and document the following:

- Weight, BMI, blood pressure, and pulse
- Thyroid enlargement and presence of any nodules or tenderness
- Breast secretions and their character
- Signs of androgen excess
- Vaginal or cervical abnormality, secretions, or discharge
- Pelvic or abdominal tenderness, organ enlargement, or masses
- Uterine size, shape, position, and mobility
- Adnexal masses or tenderness
- Cul-de-sac masses, tenderness, or nodularity.

Diagnostic Evaluation

Evaluation should progress according to the couple's preferences, partner ages, duration of infertility, and significant features of their medical history and physical examination.

Ovulatory Function

Between 15 and 45% of cases of infertility in women arise from ovulatory dysfunction. Common causes of anovulation include polycystic ovary syndrome (PCOS), excess weight gain, thyroid disorders, and strenuous exercise. Though the detection of ovulation is of use, it is eminently more useful for the practice of assisted reproduction to identify the fertility window, which starts, due to sperm lifespan, about 3–5 days before ovulation, and ends, due to oocyte lifespan, about 1–2 days after ovulation.

Methods of evaluating ovulatory function are discussed below.

Menstrual History

A regular 25–35-day cycle indicates normal ovulation. Amenorrhea and oligomenorrhea indicate anovulation.

Basal Body Temperature

Ovulatory cycles typically exhibit a biphasic pattern of temperature change of dip followed by a rise, whereas anovulatory cycles show a single pattern. However, predicting ovulation using basal body temperature (BBT) is not reliable.

Serum Progesterone

Traditionally, the serum progesterone test has been considered to reliably predict ovulation. The adrenal glands produce progesterone and, prior to ovulation, provide a steady baseline serum progesterone value between 1.5 and 3 ng/mL. After ovulation, a corpus luteum forms and starts producing progesterone, raising the value over 3 ng/mL to a peak between 10 and 20 ng/mL on day 21 of a regular 28-day cycle (or, for longer cycles, 7 days before the start of the next cycle). Serum progesterone >3 ng/mL indicates ovulation, whereas serum progesterone >10 ng/mL indicates the quality of luteal function. However, since the corpus luteum secretes progesterone in pulses, the figures may vary depending on the time of day when the blood is drawn.[30,31]

Luteinizing Hormone Detection Kits

The dominant follicle produces the serum estradiol (E2), which, after reaching a threshold concentration level of over 200 pg/mL and being maintained for about 50 hours, causes the pituitary gland to abruptly release luteinizing hormone (LH) into the bloodstream, this is called the LH surge, and it is followed by ovulation in a day or two. A study of 35 women over 155 cycles found that, in the majority (85%), the LH surge begins between midnight and 8 am. Detecting the LH surge, whether in urine or in serum, can sensitively and reliably indicate ovulation.

Obviously, the detection of urinary LH is noninvasive and preferable to multiple drawings of blood. Urinary LH concentrations during the surge vary from 20 to 100 mIU/mL. Highly sensitive over-the-counter kits, detecting as little as 22 mIU/mL, make it extremely convenient for women to inexpensively test themselves in the privacy and comfort of their homes. For a reliable prediction of the ovulation day, women should test themselves over several menstrual cycles—starting on the 10th or 11th day of each cycle, once or twice a day for 5 days.[32]

In a study of 951 cycles of IUI, urine samples taken at four different times of the day were tested for LH. The distribution of the first positive test is shown in **Table 7.**[33]

Endometrial Biopsy

Lacking precision, endometrial biopsy is not an acceptable test of ovulation; thus, it is no longer recommended.

Transvaginal Sonography

Transvaginal sonography (TVS) is considered the standard reference examination for determining the time of ovulation, using signs such as:
- Collapse of follicle or abrupt decrease in size
- Increase in echogenicity of both follicle and endometrium
- Free fluid in the pelvis.

TABLE 7: Distribution of the first positive test.

Early morning 04:00–10:00	*Lunch time 11:00–15:00*	*Tea time 16:00–20:00*	*Bed time 21:00–00:00*
27%	44.5%	15.7%	12.8%

Further, it allows the identification of the number and size of growing follicles as well as the identification of any uterine and/or adnexal pathologies. However, TVS is expensive because it must be performed by an experienced professional (radiologist or gynecologist) and requires the patient to come to the clinic for a series of examinations. As such, it is slightly invasive, somewhat uncomfortable, and quite inconvenient.

Other tests include thyroid stimulating hormone (TSH) and prolactin.

Ovarian Reserve

Ovarian reserve is generally explained as the number of oocytes in a female at any given time. Formally, it is the concept that reproductive potential is a result of the number and quality of extant oocytes in a female.[34] In practice, ovarian reserve is assessed on the consideration that the number and quality of antral and mature follicles that form in response to endogenous or exogenous ovarian stimulation are proportional to the available reserve of oocytes in the ovaries of a woman.[35] Thus, when regularly menstruating women of reproductive age are found to have a poor response (less than three to four dominant follicles with a diameter >12 mm) to ovarian stimulation (using a minimum of 150 IU of FSH) than other women of comparable age, they are classified as having "poor ovarian reserve/diminished ovarian reserve (POR/DOR)."[36]

Established ovarian reserve tests (ORTs) include day 3 measurements of serum FSH, E2, and inhibin B; clomiphene citrate challenge test (CCCT); and the two most sensitive—antral follicle count (AFC) and serum anti-Müllerian hormone (AMH)—levels.

The tests may have predictive value for women at increased risk of DOR, such as those:
- Over 35 years of age
- With unexplained infertility
- Whose family has a history of early menopause
- Demonstrating poor response to gonadotropin stimulation
- Planning treatment with assisted reproductive technology (ART)
- With a single ovary or a history of previous ovarian surgery, chemotherapy, or pelvic radiation therapy.

It is important to remember that, rather than substantiating a diagnosis of DOR, ORTs help predict ovarian response to exogenous gonadotropin stimulation and, to a smaller degree, the prospect of pregnancy using ART. Equally importantly, poor test results are not an indication of an inability to conceive. Although ORTs are widely applied, there is an ongoing debate over their ability to predict three outcomes, which are linked but quite separate—quality of oocytes, quantity of oocytes, and fecundity. Ovarian reserve testing aims to provide additional prognostic information useful in counseling and planning, thus helping couples choose among treatment options.

Follicle-stimulating Hormone

Follicle-stimulating hormone is the first hormone to be linked with declining ovarian function. It is secreted by the anterior pituitary gland and stimulates the growth of antral follicles into dominant follicles. As the age of a woman increases, so do the concentrations of her basal serum FSH of the second, third, or fourth day of the menstrual cycle.[37]

However, though many studies have found that, independent of age, women with high FSH concentrations respond poorly to ovarian stimulation and thus have lower pregnancy rates, a lack of consensus in defining "high FSH concentration" has caused difficulties in test interpretation.[38] Further, considerable inter- and intra-cycle variability in the assays for FSH limits their reliability. Thus, high values are linked to but cannot be used to predict poor ovarian response and lack of conception.[37]

For clinicians trying, in their practice, to apply FSH cutoff points in medical literature, additional confusion arises due to a change in standard, from International Reference Preparation (IRP)-human menopausal gonadotropin (hMG) to the World Health Organization (WHO) Second International Standard (IRP 78/549). Cutoff point values of the two standards are compared in **Table 8**.

Assays which have been standardized against the WHO second International Standard exhibit high specificity (83–100%) in prediction of poor ovarian response to stimulation (<2–3 follicles or ≤4 retrieved oocytes) using several cutoff points over 10 IU/L (10–20 IU/L). Nevertheless, for the purpose of identifying poor responders, FSH assay sensitivity varies too widely (10–80%), decreasing with increasing FSH cutoff points.[37]

A study of 293 patients found that over 90% of those achieving a live birth lacked a high FSH.[38] Many studies have concluded that the utility of basal FSH is, at best, limited to that of a screening test.[37,38]

Estradiol

Like FSH, basal E2 of the second, third, or fourth day of the menstrual cycle has poor reliability as an ORT because it has diurnal, inter-, and intra-cycle variation. Additionally, test results can be misinterpreted because reproductive aging typically features increased serum E2 concentrations which may produce feedback suppression of FSH, lowering the level into the normal range. The presence of seemingly "normal" basal FSH concentration but too low or too high (<20 or >60–80 pg/mL) E2 level early in the follicular phase has been linked with the poor ovarian response, though *not* with lower pregnancy rates. Further, with a substantial majority of studies finding no difference in basal E2 values between normal women and women with DOR, the test has no predictive value and, thus, is not recommended for routine clinical practice.[34,37,39]

TABLE 8: Comparison of cutoff point values of the International Reference Preparation-human menopausal gonadotropin (IRP-hMG) to the World Health Organization (WHO) second International Standard (IRP 78/549).

Reference standard	Cutoff point		
	High	Moderately high	Normal
IRP-hMG	25	17	<15
IRP 78/549	16.7	11.4	<10

Inhibin B

Inhibin B, a heterodimeric glycoprotein secreted by the granulosa cells of growing follicles, downregulates pituitary FSH. Upon gonadotropin-releasing hormone (GnRH) or FSH stimulation (the basis of dynamic tests of ovarian reserve) during the luteal-follicular transition, inhibin B serum levels rise, peaking halfway through the follicular phase, while also varying significantly between menstrual cycles, thereby exhibiting high intra- and inter-cycle variability. Further, though, with age, the inhibin B levels taper off and perhaps cause the subsequent rise in FSH levels. It is a late marker of ovarian reserve decline. The cutoff point for low inhibin B as a marker of poor response varies widely among studies (40–141 pg/mL).[37,40]

With most studies proving that inhibin B, by itself, is of little value in predicting ovarian reserve and response, it is not recommended for routine use. Due to the low accuracy, attempting to use the levels as a diagnostic or screening test for ART programs will lead to needless rejection of patients. At best, the information can be used for counseling.[37,39-41]

Clomiphene Citrate Challenge Test

Clomiphene citrate, a synthetic compound, is an ovulation-inducing fertility drug that, taken orally, binds to estrogen receptors in the brain, thereby binding the hypothalamus–pituitary axis to the circulating endogenous estrogen, consequently stimulating the pituitary gland to release FSH and attempting to normalize the luteal phase.[42] Therefore, the CCCT is both a treatment and a test. It involves measuring serum FSH on cycle day 3, dosing the patient daily with 100 mg of clomiphene citrate on cycle days 5–9, and measuring serum FSH again on cycle day 10.[41]

While the group of growing follicles produces increasing inhibin B and E2 levels, which suppress FSH in women with responsive ovaries, the smaller follicles that respond in women with DOR generate less inhibin B and E2, reducing negative feedback inhibition of FSH secretion and, consequently, increasing stimulated serum FSH levels. Thus, a high serum FSH level after clomiphene stimulation suggests DOR.[37,41]

However, systematic reviews of the CCCT found that, though the test has higher sensitivity than basal FSH in predicting poor ovarian response, it has lower specificity and significant inter-cycle variability, leading them to conclude that the test does not improve prediction accuracy.[37,40] Additionally, clomiphene citrate has a list of side effects:

- Formation of cysts
- Development of multiple follicles (superovulation), thereby increasing the risk of multiple pregnancies (when fertilized in vivo)
- An adverse peripheral antiestrogenic action on the cervical mucus and endometrium (reduction in thickness), significantly reducing pregnancy rates
- Development of resistance to it (25% incidence), forcing poor responders to use another drug for fertility treatment.[42]

Further, although the drug itself is cheap, the CCCT is expensive and time-consuming to conduct. Thus, it has relatively little value in clinical practice.[39,42]

Anti-Müllerian Hormone

Performing a fundamental role in sex differentiation, the AMH is a glycoprotein and, such as inhibins and activins, is a member of the transforming growth factor-β (TGF-β) superfamily of tissue growth and differentiation factors.[43]

In women, ovarian AMH production starts around birth; however, it is barely detectable in the serum.[44] The levels rise during puberty, peak between 20 and 25 years, then taper off with age, becoming undetectable by menopause.[45] Many studies have confirmed age-related AMH serum level decline.[46]

Since AMH is produced mainly by the granulosa cells of preantral and antral follicles, serum levels are a significant marker of ovarian reserve.[47] A study involving 42 women undergoing oophorectomy found a high correlation of both AMH and AFC with the number of primordial follicles in their ovaries. Further, during normal menstrual cycles, follicular phases do not affect AMH serum levels. Whereas, inhibin B, E2, and FSH are not only menstrual-cycle-dependent, but also comparatively late in marking primordial follicle pool depletion. Thus, AMH is easier to use clinically.[46]

In the context of ART, AMH testing can be used to predict an individual woman's response to controlled ovarian hyperstimulation (COH). The accumulating evidence suggests that, of the available ORTs, the AMH test is the most sensitive and specific.[28,29] Analysis of results of the first IVF treatment cycle of 4,700 women proved the accuracy of a single AMH test for individual women.[36]

When attempting to predict follicular status and responsiveness to COH, there are two noteworthy points regarding AFC: (1) Ultrasound technology cannot differentiate between atretic and healthy follicles and (2) common clinical practice counts follicles as small as 2 mm and as large as 12 mm.[41,48] Atretic follicles neither respond to FSH stimulation nor produce AMH. Thus, the AMH test is a better predictor of responsive follicles. In the ovary, AMH exerts an inhibiting role on many follicular functions, including granulosa cell sensitivity to FSH. Supporting this, antral follicle responsiveness to exogenous gonadotropins, clinically assessed by the Follicular Output RaTe (FORT), is inversely correlated with serum AMH.[49]

Antral Follicle Count

Antral follicle count is done by counting the antral follicles observed early in the follicular phase using transvaginal ultrasonography. AFC has good inter-cycle reliability and, with experienced radiologists and doctors, interobserver reliability as well. Studies vary in defining the size of the antral follicles: 2–6 mm, 3–8 mm, 7–10 mm, 2–10 mm, and 2–12 mm.[37,41,48]

A study of 474 subfertile, ovulatory patients found that the number of smaller follicles (2–6 mm) reduced with age, whereas the number of larger follicles (7–10 mm) remained constant. The study had also conducted other ORTs—basal FSH, basal inhibin B, clomiphene citrate challenge, and, after dosing with clomiphene citrate, inhibin B. The study found that the number of larger follicles correlated only with basal inhibin B, while the number of smaller follicles, independent of age, correlated highly with all the other ORTs used. The study concluded that the smaller follicles (2–6 mm, the ones mainly producing AMH) better represent the ovarian reserve.[48]

The consensus cutoff counts for ovarian stimulation are 3 AFC as poor response, 8–10 as normal, while 14 and over is hyperresponse. Other than AMH, AFC is viewed as the best discriminator for poor ovarian response. However, AFC has not proved reliable in predicting failure to conceive. Thus, AFC should not be the sole measure used in ART practice.[37]

Ovarian Volume

Measuring the three perpendicular dimensions (D1, D2, and D3) of an ovary and using the formula for the volume of an ellipsoid ($D1 \times D2 \times D3 \times \pi/6$) yields the ovarian volume. Total basal ovarian volume (BOV) is the sum of the volumes of both ovaries. Mean ovarian volume is, obviously, BOV/2. Ovarian volume is not a reliable test of ovarian reserve. Average ovarian volume does decline a little with age but only in the perimenopausal period (over 40 years), and thereby, it is a late marker of ovarian reserve, adding no predictive value to other ORTs.[37,39]

Ovarian Response

The ORTs reviewed above facilitate assessment of the ovarian reserve at a particular time in a woman's life, whereas the ovarian response is dynamic and depicts the performance of a woman's ovaries following endogenous or exogenous stimulation. A poor ovarian response is defined as a reduced follicular response to maximal stimulation, with a subsequent reduction in the number of oocytes retrievable for use in IVF. At their Bologna convention, the working group of the European Society for Human Reproduction and Embryology (ESHRE) standardized the definition by proposing that the presence of any two of the criteria below is required to classify a specific low response to stimulation as poor ovarian response:

- Advanced maternal age or other poor ovarian response risk factor
- A previous poor ovarian response
- An abnormal ORT[37]

According to a retrospective study of 1,190 patients <40 years old, definitions of poor response should include the degree of ovarian stimulation used. The study found that if <3,000 IU FSH/cycle was sufficient to cause the ovaries to produce oocytes 18 mm in diameter, pregnancy (detected fetal heartbeat) rates were an encouraging 29% even if <4 oocytes were retrieved, and 33% when >4 were retrieved. On the other hand, when >3,000 IU FSH/cycle was required, pregnancy rates were 25% only if >4 oocytes were retrieved, compared to a mere 7% when <4 were retrieved.[50]

Combined Ovarian Reserve Testing

Since any ORT lacks 100% sensitivity and specificity in identifying women with DOR, some investigators have attempted to improve test characteristics by combining biochemical and imaging assays.[37,51]

Using a mean of two cycles of day 3 FSH and one of day 10 inhibin B, one study achieved a sensitivity of 71%, a specificity of 98%, and a receiver operator characteristic (ROC) curve of 0.92. Similarly, another study, using a combination of day 3 FSH, basal inhibin B, and AFC, achieved 75% sensitivity, 95% specificity, and 0.92 ROC. Though these were better characteristics than those of any single ORT, the results did not explain the prevalence of DOR in women of different ages.[51]

Standardizing ORT combinations is difficult because of variations in assay selection and cutoff points across studies, affecting their validity and reliability for use in clinical practice. In one review,[52] it can be seen that, while some combinations improved sensitivity, they decreased specificity, and other combinations did the reverse. Further, it can be observed that, for the same combination of ORTs, there is wide variation between studies. Thus, using >1 ORT does not consistently improve the prediction of ovarian reserve.

Tubal Evaluation of Infertility

Tubal disease accounts for 25–35% of female factor infertility with more than half of cases due to salpingitis. Proximal tubal disease accounts for 10–25% of tubal obstruction, and distal tubal obstruction accounts to 75–90% of cases.

Hysterosalpingography

The traditional and standard method for evaluating tubal patency, hysterosalpingography (HSG) is an invasive radiological procedure done by injecting a water-soluble contrast media (WSCM) or a lipid-soluble one (an iodine-based dye)[53] into the uterine cavity (delivered by a catheter pushed through the vaginal canal and past the cervix) and using either X-ray film or a fluoroscopy to visualize the travel of the contrast material through the fallopian tubes, Which if open, allows the contrast medium to spill into the peritoneal cavity. The medium sometimes flushes out blockages in the tubes and contributes to a higher pregnancy rate. According to a review of 13 trials that analyzed 2,494 women, those who underwent HSG with oil-soluble contrast media (OSCM) had a higher rate of live birth (odds ratio 3.09) and ongoing pregnancy (odds ratio 3.59) compared to women who did not undergo HSG. The review found no evidence that WSCM had a similar effect.[54]

Hysterosalpingography can prove salpingitis isthmica nodosa and can help reveal tubal architectural detail of potential prognostic value, such as proximal and distal tubal occlusion. Also, HSG may suggest the presence of fimbrial phimosis or peritubular adhesions when escape of contrast is delayed or becomes loculated, respectively. Findings suggesting proximal tubal obstruction (PTO) require further evaluation to exclude artifacts resulting from transient tubal/myometrial contractions or relating to catheter position.

Hysterosalpingography had a high specificity for proximal obstruction, but a low sensitivity. Distal obstruction, absence of hydrosalpinx, and adhesions had a poor accuracy. The likelihood ratio for the presence of hydrosalpinx was high. In conclusion, PTO detected on HSG changes the pretest probability of PTO from 16 to 50%. Proximal tubal patency detected on HSG changes the pretest probability of proximal tubal patency from 16 to 9%.

In conclusion, we can say that HSG has limited use in detecting tubal patency, defined as the absence of PTO and distal tubal obstruction. However, it is able to detect proximal tubal occlusion. The lack of sensitivity is not caused by a lack of reproducibility. The usefulness of HSG for detecting distal tubal obstruction is also limited. HSG is a good test to detect hydrosalpinx, but not very useful in ruling out this condition.

Saline Infusion Sonography

Saline infusion sonography (SIS) enhances visualization of the endometrial lining. It can also be used as a test to determine tubal patency using fluid and ultrasound, though of limited utility because the normal fallopian tube lacking the defined interfaces that produce clear organ outlines relative to catheter position is a poor reflector of ultrasound. Although tubal patency can be observed by the appearance of fluid in the cul-de-sac with the saline infusion, the test does not differentiate between unilateral and bilateral patency.

Laparoscopy

Laparoscopy with chromopertubation is widely accepted as the "gold standard" method for evaluating tubal patency. At present, it is considered the most accurate diagnostic test available for evaluating tubal-related subfertility. Its advantages include an ability to simultaneously evaluate the abdominal cavity and other pelvic structures for an enhanced diagnostic evaluation of other etiologies of subfertility. The National Institute for Health and Care Excellence (NICE) recommends that women who are thought to have comorbidities should be offered laparoscopy and dye so that tubal and other pelvic pathology (such as pelvic inflammatory disease, previous ectopic pregnancy, or endometriosis) can be assessed at the same time.[55] According to a meta-analysis by Jacobson et al. (2004b), the ablation of endometriotic lesions with adhesiolysis to improve fertility in minimal and mild endometriosis is effective compared to diagnostic laparoscopic surgery (DLS) alone.

Unilateral and bilateral tubal occlusion, as per HSG and laparoscopy, are linked to treatment-independent pregnancy. HSG-visible one-sided tubal occlusion had an adjusted fecundity rate ratio (FRR) of 0.80, whereas two-sided tubal occlusion had an FRR of 0.49. With laparoscopy, one-sided and two-sided tubal occlusion had FRRs of 0.51 and 0.15, respectively. In 5% of the patients, a laparoscopy showing two-sided occlusion after a normal or one-sided occluded HSG was found; the treatment-independent conception rate was practically zero. In 42% of patients, a normal laparoscopic examination after two-sided occluded HSG was found; in these cases, fertility prospects were only slightly impaired with a 3-year cumulative ongoing intrauterine pregnancy rate of 9%.

Hysterosalpingo-contrast Sonography

Hysterosalpingo-contrast sonography (HyCoSy) is an ultrasound contrast technique that uses the instillation of an echogenic contrast medium into the uterine cavity through a catheter inserted through the cervical os. Saline mixed with air, which produces a contrast fluid due to the presence of air bubbles, is a cost effective option or ex-foam (created by diluting gel containing glycerol and hydroxyethyl cellulose) can be used. HyCoSy is usually done in the mid-proliferative phase (days 6–10 of a 28-day cycle) of the menstrual cycle.

The NICE recommends where appropriate expertise is available, screening for tubal occlusion using hysterosalpingo-contrast-ultrasonography should be considered because it is an effective alternative to HSG for women who are not known to have comorbidities.[55]

Hysteroscopy

Hysteroscopic tubal catheterization in patients with PTO can be used both as a diagnostic method and, considerably effectively, as a therapeutic one. First, efforts using hysteroscopic proximal tube catheterization and balloon dilatation for recanalization were intraoperatively successful in >80% of the cases. With laparoscopy, the hysteroscopic approach enables tubal cannulation and evaluation of the entire pelvis.

Falloposcope

Falloposcope has been successfully used without complications to characterize normal and abnormal epithelial changes, document endo tubal lesions ranging from accumulated debris, nonobstructive intraluminal adhesions, stenosis, polyps, to total fibrotic obstruction, as well as the identification of the segmental location of tubal pathology. Falloposcopic cannulation has been performed hysteroscopically under laparoscopic guidance by dilation and coaxial catheters, and nonhysteroscopically with the linear eversion cannula (LEC). Higher recanalization success rates have been reported with falloposcopic cannulation using the LEC compared with those achieved with coaxial cannulation.

Peritoneal Factors

Endometriosis, pelvic or adnexal adhesions, and other such peritoneal factors may play a role or may result in infertility. History and/or physical examination findings could evoke suspicion, but are hardly ever sufficient for diagnosis. Peritoneal factors may be causative in women with otherwise unexplained infertility. Transvaginal ultrasonography could uncover an endometrioma and other such previously unidentified pelvic pathology with reproductive implications.

Thus, it is evident that laparoscopy is necessary for women who have no other clear indications for ART (e.g., severe male factor infertility) but have symptoms, risk factors, or an abnormal HSG or ultrasonography; it has low utility for asymptomatic women with normal imaging. Diagnostic laparoscopy may benefit certain individuals, such as young women who have been infertile for longer than 3 years, but without recognized abnormalities.

Cervical Factors

Abnormalities of cervical mucus regarding production or its interaction with sperm are seldom the only cause of infertility. Nevertheless, examination of cervical mucus could provide confirmation of chronic cervicitis requiring treatment.

The traditional method for diagnosing cervical factor infertility has been the postcoital test (PCT). As the name suggests, within hours after intercourse just prior to expected ovulation, a cervical mucus specimen is extracted and then examined under a microscope for the presence of motile sperm.

However, the PCT is not recommended anymore as an evaluation of infertility for three reasons. Firstly, the test is inconvenient to the patient; secondly, since it is subjective and has poor reproducibility, it is unable to predict the inability to conceive; finally, it seldom influences clinical management.

Chlamydial Antibody Testing

Chlamydial antibody testing (CAT) helps in avoiding unnecessary and invasive diagnostic testing and long-term expectative management, because in CAT-positive women, further testing can be performed early.[56] A conventional meta-analysis reported that accurate estimates of CAT for individual studies ranged between 21 and 90% for sensitivity and between 29 and 100% for specificity, with a summary ROC estimating the accuracy of CAT to be moderate and comparable to that of HSG.[57] Tubal pathology is linked to chlamydia antibody presence; although a positive test requires follow-up evaluation if the test is negative, tubal pathology at laparoscopy is unlikely (7–12%).

Conclusion

Female factors are a common cause of subfertility, which are often multifactorial and may be lifestyle related. Delay in childbirth that has a strong impact on the outcome of fertility treatment. Ovarian reserve testing may inform patients regarding their reproductive lifespan and also aid in counseling and treatment strategy. Though controversies persist regarding the diagnostic modalities and management of female infertility, the advances in the field of ART has given hope to women with the rising success rates.

KEY POINTS

- Both partners of a couple should be involved in counseling, and they must be investigated together.
- Investigations can identify the cause(s) of infertility and guide them about necessary treatment.
- The investigations and treatment cause a lot of stress in a couple, and therefore, they require a lot of support and care.
- Evaluation of ovulatory function should be an initial diagnostic step in the evaluation of all infertile women.
- If the menstrual history is obviously abnormal, further evaluation is *not* required to diagnose anovulation. If not, an objective measure of the ovulatory function is necessary. Properly timed, a serum progesterone concentration above 3 ng/mL provides reliable objective evidence for recent ovulation.
- In anovulatory infertile women, failure to achieve pregnancy after three to six cycles of successful ovulation induction should be viewed as an indication to perform the additional diagnostic evaluation or, if the evaluation is complete, to consider alternative treatments.
- Ovarian reserve should be assessed in select women at increased risk of DOR. Options include cycle day 3 FSH and E2, CCCT, ultrasound to assess AFC, or serum AMH.
- Histologic endometrial dating is not a valid method for the evaluation of luteal function.
- Examination of the uterine cavity is an important part of the evaluation of infertile women and can be accomplished using HSG, sonohysterography, or hysteroscopy.
- Evaluation of tubal patency is a key component of the diagnostic evaluation of infertile women. All methods for the evaluation of tubal patency have technical limitations that must be considered when interpreting test results. A second and different test should be considered when the diagnosis remains in doubt.
- Laparoscopy may be indicated when there is evidence or strong suspicion of advanced stages of endometriosis, tubal occlusive disease, or significant adnexal adhesions.
- Overall, FSH is the most commonly used screening test for DOR, but AFC and AMH exhibit less variability and therefore are promising predictors. A single FSH value has very limited reliability because of inter- and intra-cycle variability.
- Emerging evidence suggests that a low AMH level (e.g., undetectable AMH) has high specificity as a screen for poor ovarian response, but insufficient evidence to suggest its use to screen for failure to conceive.
- There is fair evidence to support that a low AFC (<6) has moderate-to-high specificity as a screening test for poor ovarian response and insufficient evidence to support the use of AFC as a screening test for failure to conceive.
- There is fair evidence against the use of basal inhibin B as a screening test for DOR.
- There is fair evidence against the use of ovarian volume as a screening test for ovarian reserve.
- There is fair evidence against the use of basal E2 concentration as a single screening test for DOR, but there is fair evidence that the basal E2 concentration helps in the accurate interpretation of basal FSH concentrations used to screen for DOR.

REFERENCES

1. World Health Organization, Department of Reproductive Health and Research. WHO Laboratory Manual for the Examination and Processing of Human Semen, 6th edition. Geneva: World Health Organization; 2021.
2. Vander Borght M, Wyns C. Fertility and infertility: definition and epidemiology. Clin Biochem. 2018;62:2-10.
3. Sun H, Gong TT, Jiang YT, Zhang S, Zhao YH, Wu QJ. Global, regional, and national prevalence and disability-adjusted life-years for infertility in 195 countries and territories, 1990–2017: results from a Global Burden of Disease Study, 2017. Aging (Albany NY). 2019;11:10952-91.
4. Anderson JE, Farr SL, Jamieson DJ, Warner L, Macaluso M. Infertility services reported by men in the United States: national survey data. Fertil Steril. 2009;91:2466-70.
5. Practice Committee of the American Society for Reproductive Medicine. Diagnostic evaluation of the infertile male: a committee opinion. Fertil Steril. 2015;103(3):e18-25.
6. Schlegel PN, Sigman M, Collura B, De Jonge CJ, Eisenberg ML, Lamb DJ, et al. Diagnosis and treatment of infertility in men: AUA/ASRM guideline part 1. Fertil Steril. 2021;115:54-61.
7. Dubin L, Amelar R. Varicocele size and results of varicocelectomy in selected subfertile men with varicocele. Fertil Steril. 1970;21(8):606-9.
8. Salonia A, Bettocchi C, Carvalho J, Corona G, Jones TH, Kadioglu A, et al. EAU guidelines on sexual and reproductive health. Eur Urol. 2020.
9. World Health Organization. (2010). WHO Laboratory Manual for the Examination and Processing of Human Semen, 5th edition. Geneva, Switzerland: WHO Press. [online] Available from: https://apps.who.int/iris/handle/10665/44261 [Last accessed October, 2022].
10. Kim HH, Schlegel PN. Endocrine manipulation in male infertility. Urol Clin North Am. 2008;35:303-18.
11. Sengupta P, Dutta S, Karkada IR, Chinni SV. Endocrinopathies and male infertility. Life (Basel). 2021;12:10.
12. Jankowska K, Suszczewicz N, Rabijewski M, Dudek P, Zgliczyński W, Maksym RB. Inhibin-B and FSH are good indicators of spermatogenesis but not the best indicators of fertility. Life (Basel). 2022;12:511.
13. Kong X, Ye Z, Chen Y, Zhao H, Tu J, Meng T, et al. Clinical application value of inhibin B alone or in combination with other hormone indicators in subfertile men with different spermatogenesis status: a study of 324 Chinese men. J Clin Lab Anal. 2021;35(8):e23882.
14. Agarwal A, Baskaran S, Parekh N, Cho CL, Henkel R, Vij S, et al. Male infertility. Lancet. 2021;397(10271):319-33.
15. Agarwal A, Cho CL, Majzoub A, Esteves SC. The Society for Translational Medicine: clinical practice guidelines for sperm DNA fragmentation testing in male infertility. Transl Androl Urol. 2017;6(Suppl. 4):S720-33.
16. Evenson D, Wixon R. Meta-analysis of sperm DNA fragmentation using the sperm chromatin structure assay. Reprod Biomed Online. 2006;12(4):466-72.
17. Agarwal A, Chandrakumar R, Arafa MM, Elbardisi H, Okada H, Suzuki K, et al. Multi-center evaluation of oxidation reduction potential assay in the infertile male. Fertil Steril. 2017;108(3):e317.
18. Venkatesh S, Shamsi MB, Dudeja S, Kumar R, Dada R. Reactive oxygen species measurement in neat and washed semen: comparative analysis and its significance in male infertility assessment. Arch Gynecol Obstet. 2011;283:121-6.
19. Agarwal A, Ahmad G, Sharma R. Reference values of reactive oxygen species in seminal ejaculates using chemiluminescence assay. J Assist Reprod Genet. 2015;32:1721-9.
20. Cariati F, D'Argenio V, Tomaiuolo R. The evolving role of genetic tests in reproductive medicine. J Transl Med. 2019;17:267.
21. Practice Committee of the American Society for Reproductive Medicine. Management of nonobstructive azoospermia: a committee opinion. Fertil Steril. 2018;110:1239-45.
22. Ventimiglia E, Capogrosso P, Boeri L, Pederzoli F, Cazzaniga W, Scano R, et al. When to perform karyotype analysis in infertile men? Validation of the European Association of Urology guidelines with the proposal of a new predictive model. Eur Urol. 2016;70:920-3.
23. Kohn TP, Kohn JR, Owen RC, Coward RM. The prevalence of Y-chromosome microdeletions in oligozoospermic men: a systematic review and meta-analysis of European and North American studies. Eur Urol. 2019;76:626-36.
24. Katagiri Y, Neri QV, Takeuchi T, Schlegel PN, Megid WA, Kent-First M, et al. Y chromosome assessment and its implications for the development of ICSI children. Reprod Biomed Online. 2004;8(3):307-18.
25. Silber SJ, Repping S. Transmission of male infertility to future generations: lessons from the Y chromosome. Hum Reprod Update. 2002;8(3):217-29.
26. Check ML, Check JH, Katsoff D, Summers-Chase D. ICSI as an effective therapy for male factor with antisperm antibodies. Arch Androl. 2000;45(3):125-30.
27. Zini A, Fahmy N, Belzile E, Ciampi A, Al-Hathal N, Kotb A. Antisperm antibodies are not associated with pregnancy rates after IVF and ICSI: systematic review and meta-analysis. Hum Reprod. 2011;26(6):1288-95.
28. Practice Committee of the American Society for Reproductive Medicine. Testing and interpreting measures of ovarian reserve: a committee opinion. Fertil Steril. 2012;98(6):1407-15.
29. Practice Committee of the American Society for Reproductive Medicine. Diagnostic evaluation of the infertile female: a committee opinion. Fertil Steril. 2012;98(2):302-7.
30. Filicori M, Butler JP, Crowley Jr WF. Neuroendocrine regulation of the corpus luteum in the human. Evidence for pulsatile progesterone secretion. J Clin Invest. 1984;73(6):1638-47.
31. Practice Committee of the American Society for Reproductive Medicine. Diagnosis and treatment of luteal phase deficiency :a committee opinion. Fertil Steril. 2021;115(6):1416-23.
32. Su HW, Yi YC, Wei TY, Chang TC, Cheng CM. Detection of ovulation, a review of currently available methods. Bioeng Transl Med. 2017;2(3):238-46.
33. Khattab AF, Mustafa FA, Taylor PJ. The use of urine LH detection kits to time intrauterine insemination with donor sperm. Hum Reprod. 2005;20(9):2542-5.
34. Jirge PR. Poor ovarian reserve. J Hum Reprod Sci. 2016;9(2):63-9.
35. Kwee J, Elting ME, Schats R, McDonnell J, Lambalk CB. Ovarian volume and antral follicle count for the prediction of

low and hyper responders with in vitro fertilization. Reprod Biol Endocrinol. 2007;5:9.
36. Broer SL, Dólleman M, van Disseldorp J, Broeze KA, Opmeer BC, Bossuyt PM, et al. Prediction of an excessive response in in vitro fertilization from patient characteristics and ovarian reserve tests and comparison in subgroups: an individual patient data meta-analysis. Fertil Steril. 2013;100(2):420-9.e7.
37. Practice Committee of the American Society for Reproductive Medicine. Testing and interpreting measures of ovarian reserve: a committee opinion. Fertil Steril. 2015;103(3):e9-17.
38. Esposito MA, Coutifaris C, Barnhart KT. A moderately elevated day 3 FSH concentration has limited predictive value, especially in younger women. Hum Reprod. 2002;17(1):118-23.
39. Jirge PR. Ovarian reserve tests. J Hum Reprod Sci. 2011; 4(3):108-13.
40. Broekmans FJ, Kwee J, Hendriks DJ, Mol BW, Lambalk CB. A systematic review of tests predicting ovarian reserve and IVF outcome. Hum Reprod Update. 2006;12(6):685-718.
41. Bukman A, Heineman MJ. Ovarian reserve testing and the use of prognostic models in patients with subfertility. Hum Reprod Update. 2001;7(6):581-90.
42. Kamath MS, George K. Letrozole or clomiphene citrate as first line for anovulatory infertility: a debate. Reprod Biol Endocrinol. 2011;9:86.
43. La Marca A, Sighinolfi G, Radi D, Argento C, Baraldi E, Artenisio AC, et al. Anti-Müllerian hormone (AMH) as a predictive marker in assisted reproductive technology (ART). Hum Reprod Update. 2010;16(2):113-30.
44. Rajpert-De Meyts E, Jørgensen N, Graem N, Müller J, Cate RL, Skakkebaek NE. Expression of anti-Müllerian hormone during normal and pathological gonadal development: association with differentiation of Sertoli and granulosa cells. J Clin Endocrinol Metab. 1999;84:3836-44.
45. Hudson PL, Douglas I, Donahoe PK, Cate RL, Epstein J, Pepinsky RB, et al. An immunoassay to detect human müllerian inhibiting substance in males and females during normal development. J Clin Endocrinol Metab. 1990;70(1): 16-22.
46. Broer SL, Broekmans FJ, Laven JS, Fauser BC. Anti-Müllerian hormone: ovarian reserve testing and its potential clinical implications. Hum Reprod Update. 2014;20(5):688-701.
47. Fanchin R, Schonäuer LM, Righini C, Guibourdenche J, Frydman R, Taieb J. Serum anti-Müllerian hormone is more strongly related to ovarian follicular status than serum inhibin B, estradiol, FSH and LH on day 3. Hum Reprod. 2003; 18(2):323-7.
48. Haadsma ML, Bukman A, Groen H, Roeloffzen EM, Groenewoud ER, Heineman MJ, et al. The number of small antral follicles (2-6 mm) determines the outcome of endocrine ovarian reserve tests in a subfertile population. Hum Reprod. 2007;22(7):1925-31.
49. Dewailly D, Andersen CY, Balen A, Broekmans F, Dilaver N, Fanchin R, et al. The physiology and clinical utility of anti-Müllerian hormone in women. Hum Reprod Update. 2014;20(3):370-85.
50. Kailasam C, Keay SD, Wilson P, Ford WC, Jenkins JM. Defining poor ovarian response during IVF cycles, in women aged <40 years, and its relationship with treatment outcome. Hum Reprod. 2004;19(7):1544-7.
51. Sun W, Stegmann BJ, Henne M, Catherino WH, Segars JH. A new approach to ovarian reserve testing. Fertil Steril. 2008;90(6):2196-202.
52. Verhagen TE, Hendriks DJ, Bancsi LF, Mol BW, Broekmans FJ. The accuracy of multivariate models predicting ovarian reserve and pregnancy after in vitro fertilization: a meta-analysis. Hum Reprod Update. 2008;14(2):95-100.
53. Lim CP, Hasafa Z, Bhattacharya S, Maheshwari A. Should a hysterosalpingogram be a first-line investigation to diagnose female tubal subfertility in the modern subfertility workup? Hum Reprod. 2011;26(5):967-71.
54. Mohiyiddeen L, Hardiman A, Fitzgerald C, Hughes E, Mol BW, Johnson N, et al. Tubal flushing for subfertility. Cochrane Database Syst Rev. 2015;2015(5):CD003718.
55. National Institute for Health and Care Excellence. Fertility: Assessment and treatment for people with fertility problems. NICE Clinical Guideline CG156. February 2013.
56. den Hartog JE, Lardenoije CM, Severens JL, Land JA, Evers JL, Kessels AG. Screening strategies for tubal factor subfertility. Hum Reprod. 2008;23:1840-8.
57. Mol BW, Dijkman B, Wertheim P, Lijmer J, van der Veen F, Bossuyt PM. The accuracy of serum chlamydial antibodies in the diagnosis of tubal pathology: a meta-analysis. Fertil Steril. 1997;67:1031-7.

CHAPTER 17

Immunology and Infertility

Tity Chacko, Anupama Patil

INTRODUCTION

The immunology of pregnancy is complex and must allow the mother to not only remain immunocompetent to fight infections but also become tolerant to a semi-allograft fetus. Knowledge of the immunology of pregnancy helps us to understand this paradox. Maternal and fetal immune cells must actively participate for implantation, placental growth, and fetal development. During pregnancy, maternal and fetal cells come close to each other. Fetal cells have the potential to trigger an immune response in the mother.

IMMUNE SYSTEM

Our immune system consists of innate and adaptive immunity.

Innate Immunity

Natural Killer Cells

The natural killer (NK) is the most common leukocyte in the uterus during pregnancy. The decidual NK (dNK) cells are different from those present in peripheral blood. Most NK cells in blood (90%) have low CD56 and high CD16 expression ($CD56^{dim}/CD16^{bright}$); in the uterine decidua, dNK cells have high CD56 expression ($CD56^{bright}$). $CD56^{bright}$ cells produce cytokines, while $CD56^{dim}$ cells found in peripheral blood are cytolytic. Gravid uterus has high levels of $CD56^{bright}$ NK cells. NK cells also help in remodeling of spiral arteries and thus have a role in normal placentation.

Adaptive Immunity

Adaptive immunity consists of B and T cells (lymphocytes). Fetal cells express paternal genes, which are foreign to the mother's immune system.

Humoral Immune Response

B cells protect the body by secreting immunoglobulins. A unique population of B cells, called regulatory B (Breg) cells, produces interleukin (IL)-10, which is a powerful anti-inflammatory cytokine. Breg cells also inhibit production of the proinflammatory cytokine tumor necrosis factor alpha (TNF-α); hence, they help in preventing rejection of fetal allograft.

Helper T-cell Subsets

There are two types of T helper (Th) cells—Th1 and Th2 subsets. Regulatory T (Treg) cells play an important role in the maternal immune tolerance. Th1 cells threaten maternal tolerance of the fetus. In contrast, Th2 cells suppress Th1 cell differentiation. Maternal dendritic cells present antigens derived from fetal trophoblast apoptotic debris to the T cells in the maternal lymph nodes and the spleen. A mother's immune cells recognize "fetal" alloantigens of paternal origin before pregnancy in the lymph nodes draining the uterus after intercourse with genital tract exposure to the male partner's seminal fluid.

Progesterone

Progesterone, the important hormone of pregnancy, is initially produced by the corpus luteum. Subsequently, the placenta is responsible for almost all progesterone synthesis. Progesterone alters the ratio of Th1 to Th2 cells and inhibits the production of TNF-α. Treg cells, which are critical mediators of tolerance, become more numerous in pregnancy and produce IL-10, which appears to play a role in maintaining pregnancy. Human chorionic gonadotropin (hCG) in early pregnancy stimulates proliferation of Breg cells, whose action is similar to Treg cells. The implications of some of the immunomodulatory features of progesterone remain to be proven in the clinical setting; it is likely that dydrogesterone mimics the effects of progesterone through binding to progesterone receptors.

EXPLORING TREATMENT OPTIONS FOR TACKLING FETAL REJECTION

Adjuvant immunotherapies have been tried to improve the implantation rates in patients with recurrent implantation failures. Immunotherapies may improve the immunological imbalance.

Aspirin

Aspirin causes vasodilation and tries to increase the blood flow to the uterus and hence increase the endometrial thickness and receptivity.[1,2] While four randomized controlled trials (RCTs) failed to show any benefit of aspirin on the implantation rate,[3-6] one trial showed an improvement which was statistically significant.[7] Recipients of oocyte donation, who had thin endometrium and so received Aspirin, had improved implantation rates but not the both rates.[8]

Summary Statement[9]

Routine use of low-dose aspirin in assisted reproductive technology (ART) cycles in the general population is not recommended.

Corticosteroids

Corticosteroids are produced in the adrenal cortex in response to adrenocorticotropic hormone from the anterior pituitary.[10,11] They decrease elevated androgen levels, which are detrimental to normal folliculogenesis and thus improve ovulation rates.[12,13] 290 patients were randomized to 1 mg dexamethasone or placebo in a double-blinded RCT. Although there was reduction in the rate of cancellation of cycle for poor response (2.8% vs. controls 12.4%, $p < 0.02$), there were no significant differences in fertilization, implantation, or clinical pregnancy rate per cycle start.

Peri-implantation Corticosteroids

Overactivity of NK cells has been hypothesized as one of the causes of implantation failure and early pregnancy loss.[14-17] Corticosteroids around the time of implantation have been tried to normalize NK cell activity and thereby increase endometrial receptivity.[14,18,19] Patients with anti-thyroglobulin and thyroid peroxidase antibodies ($n = 60$; age 38 years) were randomized to receive either 5 mg prednisolone daily from day of oocyte retrieval to pregnancy test or no treatment.[20] The treatment group had higher clinical pregnancy and live birth rates compared with the control group (clinical pregnancy: 46.6 vs. 16.6%, $p = 0.03$; live birth: 46.6 vs. 20%, $p = 0.055$).[21] Men with antisperm antibodies were randomized to receive 20 mg of prednisolone daily for 2 weeks before in vitro fertilization (IVF) and found that there was no improvement in the ART outcome.[22]

Summary Statements[9]

Routine use of corticosteroids during stimulation is not recommended in ART cycles in the general population. The routine use of corticosteroids during the implantation window to improve the outcome of live birth in ART cycles in the general population is not recommended. Subgroups that may benefit from peri-implantation corticosteroids need to be identified by additional studies.

Granulocyte Colony-stimulating Factor

Granulocyte colony-stimulating factor (G-CSF) and their receptors have been found in the reproductive system.[20] One level 1 study found no benefit of administering G-CSF during ovarian stimulation on the euploidy rate.[23] Another level 1 study found an increase in the endometrial thickness in women with a thin endometrium.[24] Another RCT of granulocyte-macrophage colony-stimulating factor (GM-CSF) treatment found an improvement in the implantation rate and live birth rate in women with recurrent miscarriage, and this was statistically significant.[25]

Summary Statement[9]

There is insufficient evidence to recommend for or against G-CSF or GM-CSF administered locally or systemically to improve IVF outcomes.

Intravenous Fat Emulsions

296 women with unexplained secondary infertility, recurrent spontaneous abortion, and elevated NK cell activity (>12%) were randomized to receive intravenous fat emulsions.[26] There was a statistically significant increase in the ongoing pregnancy rate and live birth rate. Another prospective cohort study on the effectiveness of intravenous fat emulsions on outcomes of women aged 40–42 years undergoing IVF-embryo transfer (ET) was terminated early because preliminary data showed no live births in the intravenous fat emulsion group and a 30% live birth rate in the untreated controls.[27]

Summary Statement[9]

There is no sufficient evidence to recommend routine intravenous fat emulsions for infertile women pursuing IVF.

Intravenous Immunoglobulin

Intravenous immunoglobulin (IVIG) has anti-inflammatory activity. IVIG was associated with improved implantation rate [treatment group 8/45 (17.7%) vs. placebo 4/61 (6.5%), $p < 0.05$] but not live birth rate [treatment group 6/18 (33.3%) vs. placebo 4/21 (19.1%)].[28-30] Two cohort studies employed analysis of Th1:Th2 ratio in the peripheral blood for immune stratification of treatment and response.[31,32] One of these studies was observational, retrospective, and with an unusually high live birth rate. While the other study, also retrospective, demonstrated an improvement in implantation rate, specifically in patients with an elevated Th1:Th2 ratio (45% IVIG vs. 22% control).[32]

Summary Statements[9]

There is no sufficient evidence to recommend IVIG administration to improve IVF outcomes.

Subpopulations that benefit from treatment may exist, but additional RCTs are needed to define indications and to explore risks and benefits.

Adalimumab

Disease-modifying agents such as adalimumab (TNF-α blocking antibody) have been used to treat autoimmune diseases. It was investigated if patients with abnormally high TNF secretion may benefit from treatment in conjunction with IVF by a single collaborative group of investigators[33-36] on a heterogenous population. Adalimumab should only be used in the context trials.

Long-term use (>12 weeks) has been associated with an increased risk of serious infection and malignancy.[37]

Summary Statement[9]

There is insufficient evidence to recommend adalimumab treatment toimprove IVF outcomes.

Peripheral Blood Mononuclear Cells

The rationale of peripheral blood mononuclear cells (PBMCs) intrauterine infusion in patients with recurrent implantation failure was that maternal immune cells are necessary to achieve immune tolerance to embryo. One RCT investigated the efficacy of PBMCs[38] and they compared a group with recurrent implantation failure who received autologous PBMCs instilled into the endometrial cavity prior to transfer or to standard ET without pretreatment.[38] The treatment group experienced a significantly increased clinical pregnancy rate ($p < 0.05$) and reduced, but not significant, early pregnancy loss rate.

Summary Statement[9]

Sufficient evidence is not available to recommend intrauterine infusion of autologous peripheral mononuclear cells prior to ET.

Seminal Plasma

Instillation of seminal plasma into the uterus and/or cervix at the time of oocyte pickup for IVF has been investigated as a strategy to improve pregnancy rates in fresh ET cycles. A meta-analysis of seven RCTs showed a statistically significant improvement in clinical pregnancy rate but no significant improvement in ongoing pregnancy or live birth rate with seminal plasma insemination.[39]

Tacrolimus

Recurrent implantation failure is associated with a high peripheral blood Th1/Th2 ratio. A Th1 immune response is associated with allograft, as well as embryo, rejection.[40,41] A prospective study[42] evaluated the success rates of 1–3 mg of tacrolimus for 2 days prior to ET. Patients with recurrent implantation failure had elevated peripheral blood Th1/Th2 ratios. The treated cohort had significantly higher clinical pregnancy (per ET, treated 64% vs. untreated 0%, $p < 0.0001$) and live birth rates (treated 60% vs. untreated 0%, $p < 0.0001$).[42] But the study was subject to selection bias due to lack of randomization and a small sample size.

Summary Statement[9]

There is insufficient evidence to recommend tacrolimus to improve IVF-ET outcomes.

HARMS AND BENEFITS OF IMMUNOTHERAPY

Immunotherapies have their own adverse effects. For example, IVIG use has been associated with fever, hypotension, tachycardia, thromboembolic complications, and anaphylactic reactions.[43] As a pooled blood product, IVIG use is also associated with an inherent risk of infectious disease. While intravenous fat emulsion infusions are generally well tolerated, jaundice and hyperthermia have been reported.[44] Cytokines such as G-CSF are used in healthy donors in the setting of blood and marrow transplantation. In this setting, common side effects associated with systemic administration include bone pain and myalgias. Tacrolimus is most commonly used as an immunosuppressant to prevent whole-organ rejection. In this setting, known side effects include nephrotoxicity, neurotoxicity, hypertension, and diabetogenic effects. Medications such as aspirin and corticosteroids are inexpensive, while others such as IVIG and adalimumab are costly. Most of these therapies should only be used under Institutional Review Boards (IRB)-approved protocols.

REFERENCES

1. Haapsamo M, Martikainen H, Räsänen J. Low-dose aspirin and uterine haemodynamics on the day of embryo transfer in women undergoing IVF/ICSI: a randomized, placebo-controlled, double-blind study. Hum Reprod. 2009;24(4):861-6. doi: 10.1093/humrep/den489. Epub 2009 Jan 18. PMID: 19153091.
2. Steer CV, Campbell S, Tan SL, Crayford T, Mills C, Mason BA, et al. The use of transvaginal color flow imaging after in vitro fertilization to identify optimum uterine conditions before embryo transfer. Fertil Steril. 1992;57:372-6.
3. Duvan CI, Ozmen B, Satiroglu H, Atabekoglu CS, Berker B. Does addition of low-dose aspirin and/or steroid as a standard treatment in nonselected intracytoplasmic sperm injection cycles improve in vitro fertilization success? A randomized, prospective, placebo-controlled study. J Assist Reprod Genet. 2006;23:15-21.
4. Lambers MJ, Hoozemans DA, Schats R, Homburg R, Lambalk CB, Hompes PG. Low-dose aspirin in non-tubal IVF patients

with previous failed conception: a prospective randomized double-blind placebo-controlled trial. Fertil Steril. 2009;92: 923-9.

5. Moini A, Zafarani F, Haddadian S, Ahmadi J, Honar H, Riazi K. Effect of low dose aspirin therapy on implantation rate in women undergoing in-vitro fertilization cycles. Saudi Med J. 2007;28:732-6.
6. Urman B, Mercan R, Alatas C, Balaban B, Isiklar A, Nuhoglu A. Low-dose aspirin does not increase implantation rates in patients undergoing intracytoplasmic sperm injection: a prospective randomized study. J Assist Reprod Genet. 2000;17:586-90.
7. Rubinstein M, Marazzi A, Polak de Fried E. Low-dose aspirin treatment improves ovarian responsiveness, uterine and ovarian blood flow velocity, implantation, and pregnancy rates in patients undergoing in vitro fertilization: a prospective, randomized, double-blind placebo-controlled assay. Fertil Steril. 1999;71:825-9.
8. Weckstein LN, Jacobson A, Galen D, Hampton K, Hammel J. Low-dose aspirin for oocyte donation recipients with a thin endometrium: prospective, randomized study. Fertil Steril. 1997;68:927-30.
9. Achilli C, Duran-Retamal M, Saab W, Serhal P, Seshadri S. The role of immunotherapy in in vitro fertilization and recurrent pregnancy loss: a systematic review and meta-analysis. Fertil Steril. 2018;110(6):1089-100.
10. Keay SD, Lenton EA, Cooke ID, Hull MG, Jenkins JM. Low-dose dexamethasone augments the ovarian response to exogenous gonadotrophins leading to a reduction in cycle cancellation rate in a standard IVF programme. Hum Reprod. 2001;16:1861-5.
11. Best R, Nelson SM, Walker BR. Dexamethasone and 11-dehydrodexamethasone as tools to investigate the isozymes of 11 beta-hydroxysteroid dehydrogenase in vitro and in vivo. J Endocrinol. 1997;153:41-8.
12. Kalampokas T, Pandian Z, Keay SD, Bhattacharya S. Glucocorticoid supplementation during ovarian stimulation for IVF or ICSI. Cochrane Database Syst Rev. 2017;3:CD004752.
13. Harlow CR, Jenkins JM, Winston RM. Increased follicular fluid total and free cortisol levels during the luteinizing hormone surge. Fertil Steril. 1997;68:48-53.
14. Boomsma CM, Kamath MS, Keay SD, Macklon NS. Peri-implantation glucocorticoid administration for assisted reproductive technology cycles. Cochrane Database Syst Rev. 2012;30:CD005996.
15. Ledee-Bataille N, Dubanchet S, Coulomb-L'hermine A, Durand-Gasselin I, Frydman R, Chaouat G. A new role for natural killer cells, interleukin (IL)-12, and IL-18 in repeated implantation failure after in vitro fertilization. Fertil Steril. 2004;81:59-65.
16. Ledee-Bataille N, Bonnet-Chea K, Hosny G, Dubanchet S, Frydman R, Chaouat G. Role of the endometrial tripod interleukin-18, -15, and -12 in inadequate uterine receptivity in patients with a history of repeated in vitro fertilization-embryo transfer failure. Fertil Steril. 2005;83:598-605.
17. Quenby S, Kalumbi C, Bates M, Farquharson R, Vince G. Prednisolone reduces preconceptual endometrial natural killer cells in women with recurrent miscarriage. Fertil Steril. 2005;84:980-4.
18. Hill JA. Immunological mechanisms of pregnancy maintenance and failure: a critique of theories and therapy. Am J Reprod Immunol. 1990;22:33-41.
19. Pountain GD, Keogan MT, Hazleman BL, Brown DL. Effects of single dose compared with three days' prednisolone treatment of healthy volunteers: contrasting effects on circulating lymphocyte subsets. J Clin Pathol. 1993;46:1089-92.
20. Robertson SA. GM-CSF regulation of embryo development and pregnancy. Cytokine Growth Factor Rev. 2007;18:287-98.
21. Litwicka K, Arrivi C, Varricchio MT, Mencacci C, Greco E. In women with thyroid autoimmunity, does low-dose prednisolone administration, compared with no adjuvant therapy, improve in vitro fertilization clinical results? J Obstet Gynaecol Res. 2015;41:722-8.
22. Lahteenmaki A, Rasanen M, Hovatta O. Low-dose prednisolone does not improve the outcome of in vitro fertilization in male immunological infertility. Hum Reprod. 1995;10:3124-9.
23. Agerholm I, Loft A, Hald F, Lemmen JG, Munding B, Sorensen PD, et al. Culture of human oocytes with granulocyte-macrophage colony-stimulating factor has no effect on embryonic chromosomal constitution. Reprod Biomed Online. 2010;20:477-84.
24. Sarvi F, Arabahmadi M, Alleyassin A, Aghahosseini M, Ghasemi M. Effect of increased endometrial thickness and implantation rate by granulocyte colony-stimulating factor on unresponsive thin endometrium in fresh in vitro fertilization cycles: a randomized clinical trial. Obstet Gynecol Int. 2017;2017:3596079.
25. Ziebe S, Loft A, Povlsen BB, Erb K, Agerholm I, Aasted M, et al. A randomized clinical trial to evaluate the effect of granulocyte-macrophage colony stimulating factor (GM-CSF) in embryo culture medium for in vitro fertilization. Fertil Steril. 2013;99:1600-9.
26. Dakhly DM, Bayoumi YA, Sharkawy M, Gad Allah SH, Hassan MA, Gouda HM, et al. Intralipid supplementation in women with recurrent spontaneous abortion and elevated levels of natural killer cells. Int J Gynaecol Obstet. 2016;135:324-7.
27. Check JH, Check DL. Intravenous intralipid therapy is not beneficial in having a live delivery in women aged 40-42 years with a previous history of miscarriage or failure to conceive despite embryo transfer undergoing in vitro fertilization-embryo transfer. Clin Exp Obstet Gynecol. 2016;43:14-5.
28. Chernyshov VP, Dons'koi BV, Sudoma IO, Goncharova YO. Multiple immune deviations predictive for IVF failure as possible markers for IVIG therapy. Immunol Lett. 2016;176: 44-50.
29. Coulam CB, Krysa LW, Bustillo M. Intravenous immunoglobulin for in-vitro fertilization failure. Hum Reprod. 1994; 9:2265-9.
30. Moraru M, Carbone J, Alecsandru D, Castillo-Rama M, Garcia-Segovia A, Gil J, et al. Intravenous immunoglobulin treatment increased live birth rate in a Spanish cohort of women with recurrent reproductive failure and expanded CD56(+) cells. Am J Reprod Immunol. 2012;68:75-84.
31. Ramos-Medina R, Garcia-Segovia A, Gil J, Carbone J, Aguaron de la Cruz A, Seyfferth A, et al. Experience in IVIg therapy for selected women with recurrent reproductive failure and NK cell expansion. Am J Reprod Immunol. 2014;71:458-66.

32. Winger EE, Reed JL, Ashoush S, El-Toukhy T, Ahuja S, Taranissi M. Elevated preconception CD56+ 16+ and/or Th1:Th2 levels predict benefit from IVIG therapy in subfertile women undergoing IVF. Am J Reprod Immunol. 2011;66:394-403.
33. Winger EE, Reed JL, Ashoush S, Ahuja S, El-Toukhy T, Taranissi M. Treatment with adalimumab (Humira) and intravenous immunoglobulin improves pregnancy rates in women undergoing IVF. Am J Reprod Immunol. 2009;61:113-20.
34. Winger EE, Reed JL, Ashoush S, El-Toukhy T, Ahuja S, Taranissi M. Birth defect rates in women using adalimumab (Humira®) to treat immunologic-based infertility in IVF patients. Am J Reprod Immunol. 2011;66:237-41.
35. Winger EE, Reed JL, Ashoush S, El-Toukhy T, Ahuja S, Taranissi M. Degree of TNF-alpha/IL-10 cytokine elevation correlates with IVF success rates in women undergoing treatment with adalimumab (Humira) and IVIG. Am J Reprod Immunol. 2011;65:610-8.
36. Winger EE, Reed JL, Ashoush S, El-Toukhy T, Taranissi M. Die-off ratio correlates with increased TNF-α:IL-10 ratio and decreased IVF success rates correctable with Humira. Am J Reprod Immunol. 2012;68:428-37.
37. Bongartz T, Sutton AJ, Sweeting MJ, Buchan I, Matteson EL, Montori V. Anti-TNF antibody therapy in rheumatoid arthritis and the risk of serious infections and malignancies: systematic review and meta-analysis of rare harmful effects in randomized controlled trials. JAMA. 2006;295:2275-85.
38. Madkour A, Bouamoud N, Louanjli N, Kaarouch I, Copin H, Benkhalifa M, et al. Intrauterine insemination of cultured peripheral blood mononuclear cells prior to embryo transfer improves clinical outcome for patients with repeated implantation failures. Zygote. 2016;24:58-69.
39. Crawford G, Ray A, Gudi A, Shah A, Homburg R. The role of seminal plasma for improved outcomes during in vitro fertilization treatment: review of the literature and meta-analysis. Hum Reprod Update. 2015;21:275-84.
40. Kwak-Kim JY, Chung-Bang HS, Ng SC, Ntrivalas EI, Mangubat CP, Beaman KD, et al. Increased T helper 1 cytokine responses by circulating T cells are present in women with recurrent pregnancy losses and in infertile women with multiple implantation failures after IVF. Hum Reprod. 2003;18:767-73.
41. Ng SC, Gilman-Sachs A, Thaker P, Beaman KD, Beer AE, Kwak-Kim J. Expression of intracellular Th1 and Th2 cytokines in women with recurrent spontaneous abortion, implantation failures after IVF-ET or normal pregnancy. Am J Reprod Immunol. 2002;48:77-86.
42. Nakagawa K, Kwak-Kim J, Ota K, Kuroda K, Hisano M, Sugiyama R, et al. Immunosuppression with tacrolimus improved reproductive outcome of women with repeated implantation failure and elevated peripheral blood TH1/TH2 cell ratios. Am J Reprod Immunol. 2015;73:353-61.
43. Katz U, Achiron A, Sherer Y, Shoenfeld Y. Safety of intravenous immunoglobulin (IVIG) therapy. Autoimmun Rev. 2007; 6:257-9.
44. Hansen LM, Hardie BS, Hidalgo J. Fat emulsion for intravenous administration: clinical experience with intralipid 10%. Ann Surg. 1976;184:80-8.

CHAPTER 18

Cytogenetics and Subfertility

CV Kannaki Uthraraj, KS Mangayarkarasi

INTRODUCTION

Genetics plays an important and ever-expanding role in basic reproductive biological processes from gonadal sex determination, reproductive organ development, gametogenesis, fertilization, implantation, and early embryonic development. Various disruptions in the genetic profile resulting from chromosomal aberrations including microdeletions and microduplications, single-gene disorders, polygenic influences, or epigenetic mechanisms can in turn affect the reproductive functions. This chapter presents an overview of basic cytogenetics, its role in subfertility, and its application in the management of a subfertile couple.

ROLE OF GENETICS IN INFERTILITY

Subfertility affects about 1 in 10 couples in the reproductive age group and has a multifactorial basis. In nearly half of these, an underlying genetic cause is implicated. However, in the majority of cases, the etiology for subfertility remains unclear and linking basic research to clinical practice is the path that will offer solutions to the affected couples. An in-depth understanding and application of cytogenetics, molecular tools, and epidemiological studies are therefore essential in the management and treatment of an infertile couple.

BASICS OF CYTOGENETICS

Cytogenetics is the study of chromosomes and combines cytology and genetics.

Chromosomes

Chromosomes are thread-like structures that represent the genetic material contained in the nucleus of a cell. In humans, nearly all nucleated body cells contain a diploid set consisting of 23 pairs of chromosomes ($2n$) **(Fig. 1)**.

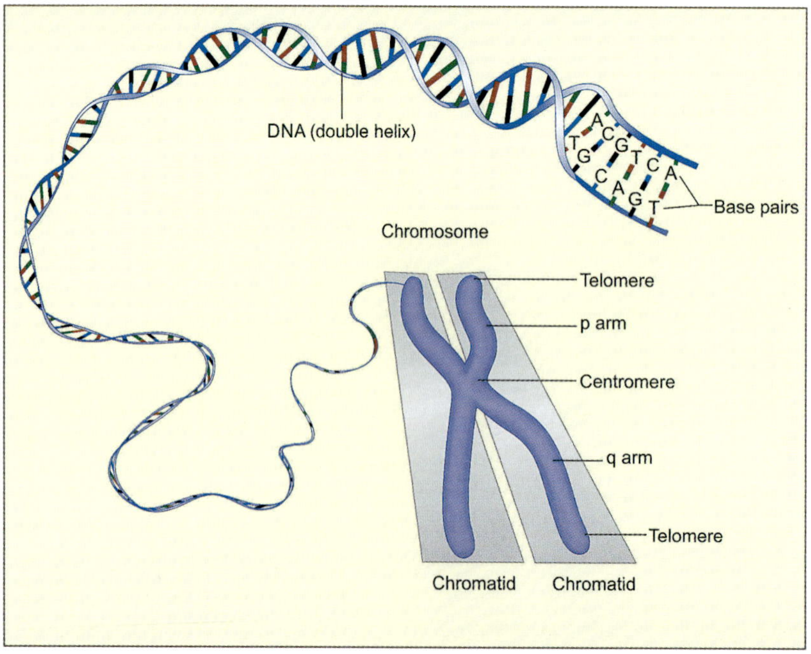

Fig. 1: Basic structure and subunits of a chromosome. (DNA: deoxyribonucleic acid).

In exception, the mature male and female gametes contain a haploid set containing half the number ($n = 23$) of chromosomes. The chromosomes 1–22 are the autosomes and the 23rd pair is the sex chromosomes, which is an X and X in females and an X and a Y in males. Chromosomes contain regions called genes. Genes code for proteins and are made up of deoxyribonucleic acid (DNA).

Cell Cycle

The genetic information present in each cell is transmitted in both mitosis and meiosis during cell division. The reason for the existence of two types of cell division is that somatic cells need a full diploid complement of chromosomes, whereas the gametes need only half the complement (haploid), as they will ultimately fuse with the other gamete during fertilization to become diploid in the zygote.

The transition from interphase to cell division (mitosis) and back to interphase is called cell cycle. The time when the cell is not dividing is called the interphase and this is the time when the nucleus is most metabolically active. Knowledge of the various phases of the cell cycle are important to understand the dynamics of cell division, segregation of chromosomes to daughter cells, and the processes of mitosis and meiosis in gametogenesis.

There are four distinct stages in the *interphase state* of the cell cycle **(Fig. 2 and Table 1)**:

1. G1 phase—9 hours
2. S phase (synthesis)—5 hours
3. G2 phase (interphase)—3 hours
4. M phase (mitosis)—1 hour.

M phase is itself composed of two tightly coupled processes:

1. *Karyokinesis:* Cell's chromosomes are divided.

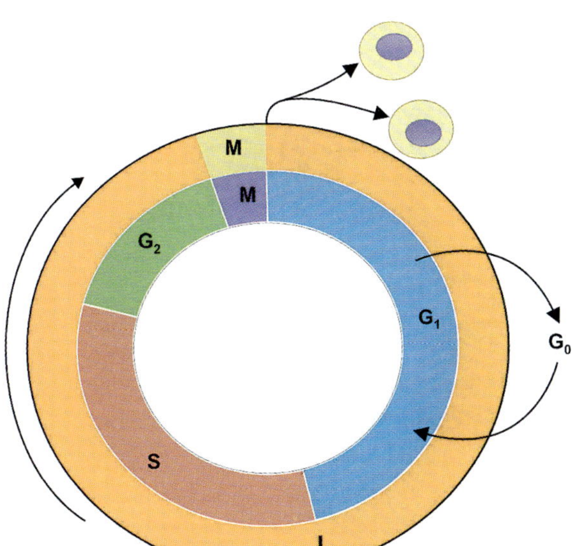

Fig. 2: Schematic of the cell cycle. Outer ring: I = interphase, M = mitosis; inner ring: M = mitosis, G_1 = gap 1, G_2 = gap 2, S = synthesis.

2. *Cytokinesis:* Cell's cytoplasm divides into two daughter cells. Each phase for its activation depends on the proper development and completion of the previous one. Cells that have temporarily or irreversibly stopped dividing are said to have entered a state of quiescence called G phase (G_0).

Cell Division—Mitosis and Meiosis

Meiosis, often called the reduction division, transforms primary spermatocytes and primary oocytes in the male and female into haploid spermatids and ova, respectively. Meiosis has two nuclear divisions, *meiosis I* and *meiosis II*.

In meiosis I, the homologous chromosomes separate, and in meiosis II, the chromatids separate. This results in four cells with a haploid set of chromosomes. In the female, only one of this becomes a viable ovum and the rest become polar bodies. In the male, all four spermatids mature into spermatozoa.

Compared with mitosis, meiosis is a lengthy and complicated process. Each stage of meiosis contains prophase, metaphase, anaphase, and telophase as in mitosis. Prophase I **(Figs. 3A and B)** is further divided into five consecutive substages: Leptotene, zygotene, pachytene, diplotene, and diakinesis.

There is no true prophase II in human meiosis; the cells pass directly into the second meiotic metaphase **(Fig. 2)**. The 23 chromosomes, each composed of two chromatids, move to the equatorial plate (metaphase II). Although only a haploid set of chromosomes is present, in one of each homolog, there is still a diploid amount of DNA since the replicated strands have not separated. In anaphase and telophase, the two chromatids have separated and go to two daughter cells, so that the end product of meiosis is four haploid cells, each with one complete but different set of genetic material. In females, the spindle is off-center, thus giving rise to a huge cell called the ovum and a second polar body. The first polar body also undergoes meiosis creating two additional polar bodies, but of the resulting four haploid cells only the ovum is theoretically viable gamete.

Chromosomal Variations

Chromosomal variations are commonly classified as follows:

- Numerical
- Structural[1,2]

Numerical Abnormalities

Numerical abnormalities, also known as *aneuploidies*, are the most commonly encountered.[3] Aneuploidies are alterations in chromosome numbers, and the presence/absence of chromosomes in haploid or diploid is termed monosomy or trisomy. Aneuploidy is more prevalent in spontaneous abortions and developmental errors in

TABLE 1: Phases of cell cycle.

State	*Phase*	*Abbreviation*	*Description*
Resting	Gap 0	G_0	A phase where the cell has left the cycle and has stopped dividing
Interphase	Gap 1	G_1	Cells increase in size in gap 1. The *G checkpoint* control 1 mechanism ensures that everything is ready for deoxyribonucleic acid (DNA) synthesis
	Synthesis	S	DNA replication occurs during this phase
	Gap 2	G_2	During the gap between DNA synthesis and mitosis, the cell will continue to grow. The *G checkpoint* control mechanism ensures that everything is ready to enter the M (mitosis) phase and divide
Cell division	Mitosis	M	Cell growth stops at this stage and cellular energy is focused on the orderly division into two daughter cells. A checkpoint in the middle of mitosis (*metaphase checkpoint*) ensures that the cell is ready to complete cell division

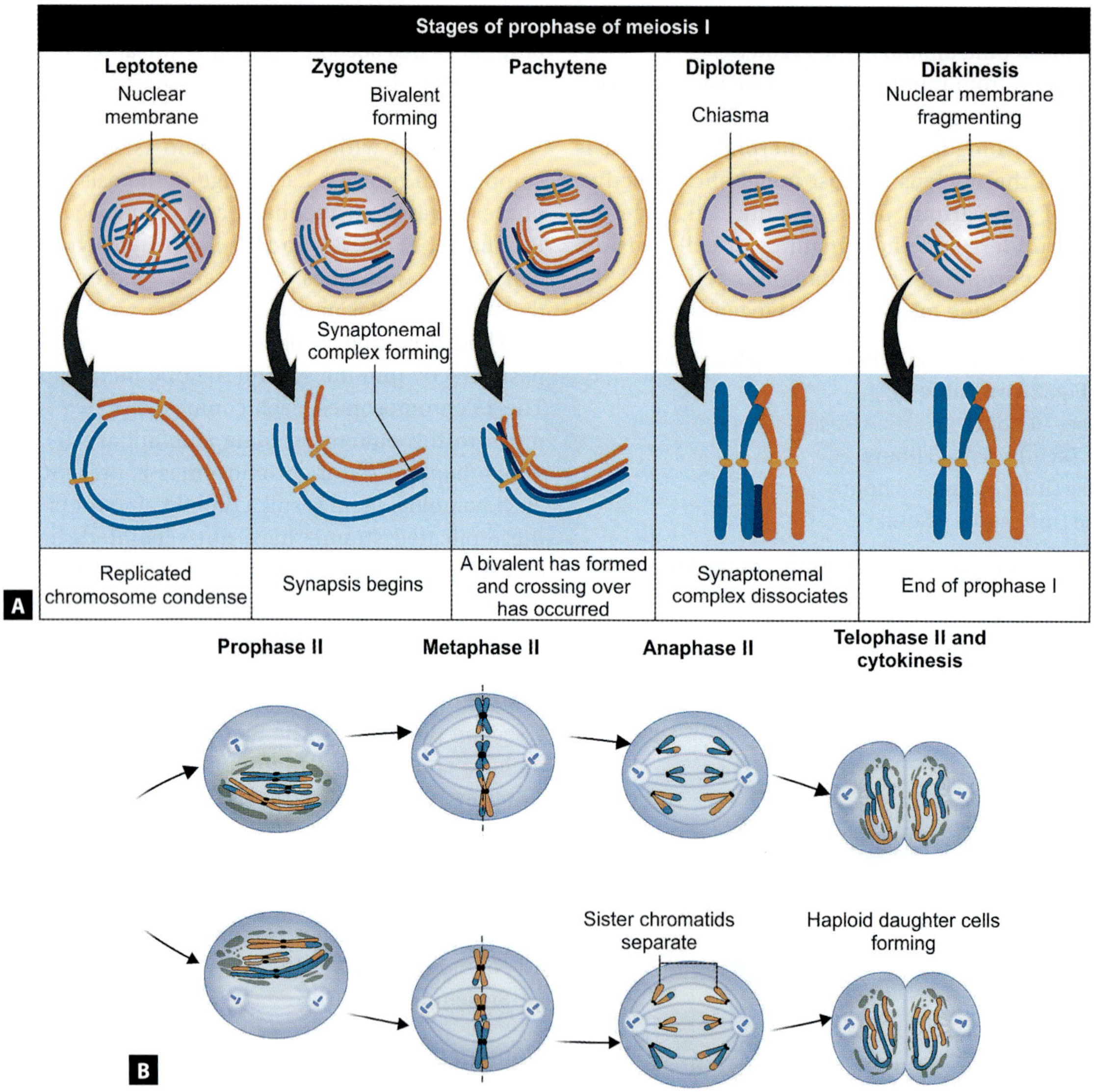

Figs. 3A and B: Meiosis I and II.

humans.[4] Of the aneuploidies, *trisomy is more common than monosomy*.[1] In some cases, the chromosomal variations may be present in only a few populations of cells due to postzygotic occurrence, and the individual then has two populations of cells and is, therefore, *mosaic* for the normal complement and the variation.

Structural Abnormalities

Structural variations include several types of rearrangements:

- Translocations—balanced and unbalanced **(Fig. 4)**
- Inversion **(Fig. 5)**
- Insertion **(Fig. 6)**
- Deletion and duplication **(Figs. 7 and 8)**
- Ring chromosomes **(Fig. 9)**
- Microdeletions.

Cytogenetics includes the study of chromosomes under the microscope.

The various cytogenetic techniques are described below:

- *Karyotyping:* It is the gold standard in the basic workup of any genetic testing in spite of advanced technology. The karyotype of an individual is the microscopic description of their chromosome complement. Here, the chromosomes are visualized as colored bodies with a specific structure containing a central constriction called centromere to which are attached two linear arms, the shorter "p" arm and the longer "q" arm. The appearance of the chromosomes varies in the different phases of the cell cycle. In karyotype, the metaphase spread is analyzed. The metaphase spread is the collection of

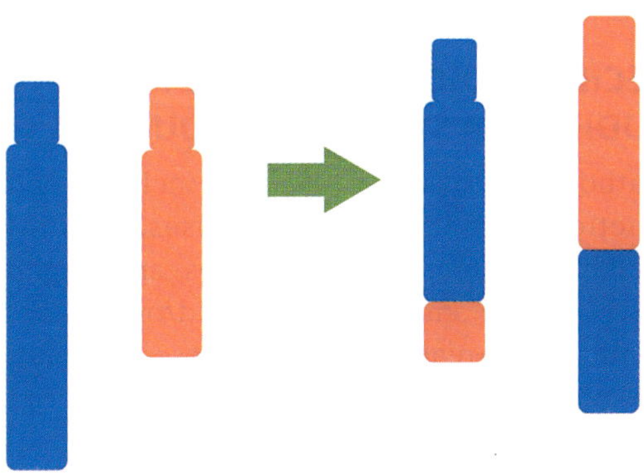

Fig. 4: Translocation of chromosomes.

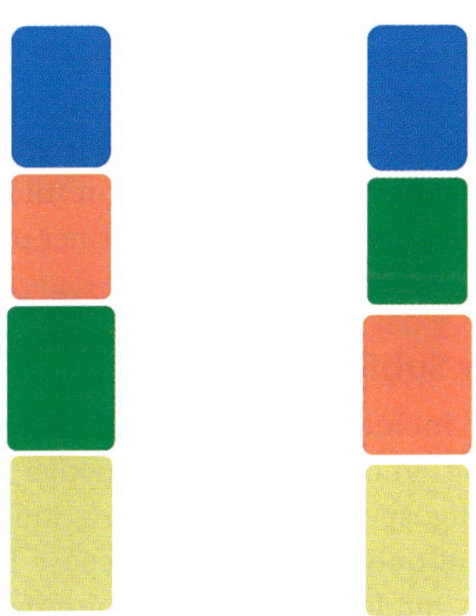

Fig. 5: Inversion of chromosomes.

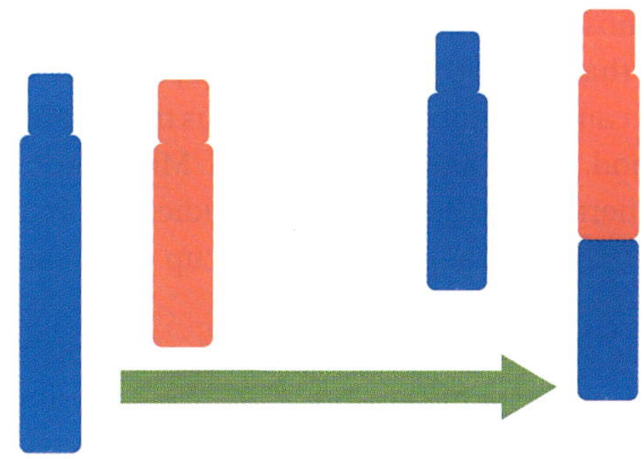

Fig. 6: Insertion of chromosomes.

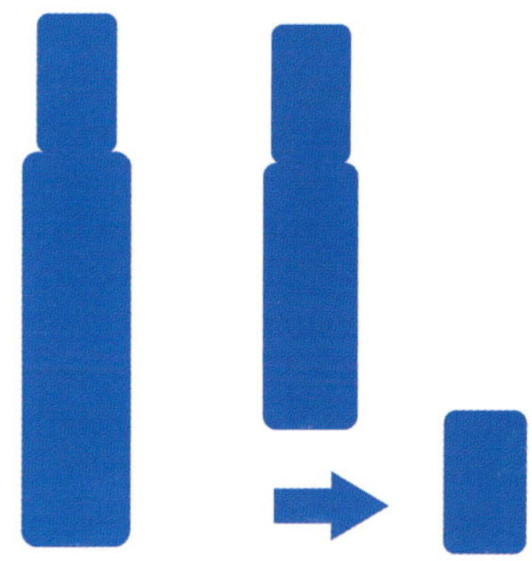

Fig. 7: Deletion of chromosomes.

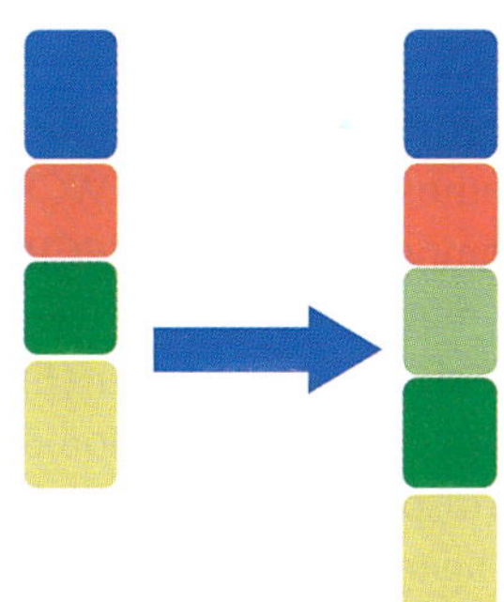

Fig. 8: Duplication of chromosomes.

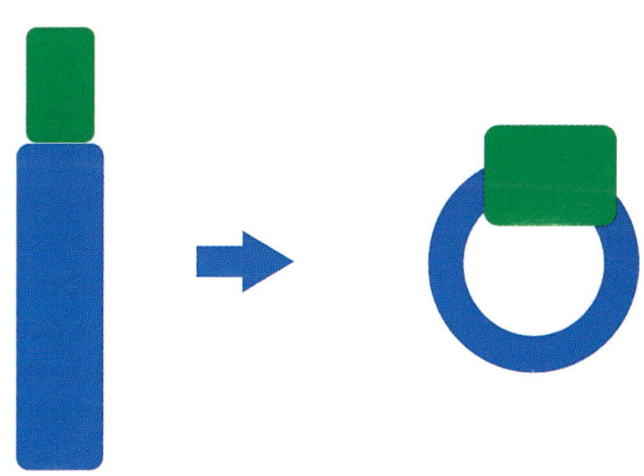

Fig. 9: Ring chromosomes.

chromosomes from one cell, visible in the condensed form that is assumed during metaphase. A karyotype study can be performed from various tissue samples such as blood, saliva, and skin fibroblast. Most commonly, the peripheral blood leukocytes are studied. A karyotype can detect chromosomal imbalances up to a resolution of approximately 5 megabases (Mb).

The peripheral blood sample is taken in a blood container containing sodium heparin, ensuring that the blood is mixed well soon after collection to prevent clots. Common causes for failed culture are lack of leukocytes, clotted blood, and inadequate sample, and therefore this may require a repeat sample.

This process involves cell culture, harvesting, slide preparation, staining, and analysis. Though manual processing is still necessary, much of the analysis has been automated with technological advances. Banding patterns are used to elucidate the breakpoints and chromosome constituents involved in chromosome translocations, deletions, and inversions within an individual chromosome can be identified and described using standard banding patterns. G-banding that utilizes trypsin and Giemsa allows visualization of banding patterns under bright field microscopy. Diagrams identifying the chromosomes based on banding patterns are called "idiograms."

- *Fluorescent in situ hybridization:* Fluorescent probes are for specific chromosomes in interphase. The following are modifications of the probes according to the indication:
  - Locus-specific probes
  - Repetitive sequence-specific probes
  - Whole chromosome painting (WCP) probes
  - Partial chromosome painting (PCP) probes.

  The above-mentioned probes use at least two-color fluorescent in situ hybridization (FISH) experiment, one probe as specific for the region of interest and the other as control probe. Multicolor FISH uses at least three different ligands and fluorochromes for the specific labeling of DNA, enabling staining of each of the 24 human chromosomes.

  Fluorescent in situ hybridization is done on metaphase spreads or interphase spreads, and at least 10–15 metaphases should be analyzed per probe. In case of suspected mosaicism, about 50–100 spreads are to be analyzed.

  The most commonly used FISH application in infertility is in preimplantation genetic testing and SRY locus detection in 46,XX males. Other applications include study of sperm nuclei to ascertain the aneuploidy rate, assessing the cytogenetic quality in post-chemotherapy scenarios, or to determine the percentage of unbalanced gametes in male balanced translocation carriers.

  Fluorescent in situ hybridization is a powerful tool due to its reliability and quickness; however, it should be offered only together with banding cytogenetics.
- *Single nucleotide polymorphism and comparative genomic hybridization:* Comparative genomic hybridization (CGH) is a molecular cytogenetic tool used to detect submicroscopic copy number changes. In this technique, the test and the control DNA are differentially labeled with fluorescent dyes and hybridized simultaneously in situ to normal metaphase spreads. Various array designs have been designed and used for diagnostic purposes and they include bacterial artificial chromosome (BAC)/P1-derived artificial chromosome (PAC) array, targeted array, and single nucleotide polymorphism (SNP) array.

  Array-CGH (a-CGH) is used to identify incidence of *mosaicism*, where routine chromosome analysis identifies as little as 3% of the cells on the basis of mitogen-induced metaphase counts. It finds applications in recognizing known and unknown chromosome syndrome by giving a detailed and comprehensive rearrangement pattern. a-CGH also helps in characterization of small supernumerary marker chromosomes (sSMC) that cannot be unambiguously recognized by conventional cytogenetics.

SPECIFIC INDICATIONS FOR CYTOGENETIC STUDIES IN A SUBFERTILE COUPLE

The pathological basis of infertility includes endocrine dysfunction, inflammatory diseases, genital tract abnormalities, gametogenesis failures, and implantation failures.[5] Lifestyle, environmental, and/or genetic factors are some of the reasons behind these pathologies. As 15–30% of the male infertility has a genetic origin, it is important to understand their genetic background. It may be chromosomal or single-gene anomalies[5] and around 2–14% of male infertility[4] and as much as 10% of female infertility[6] have a chromosomal origin.

In managing a couple with fertility issues, a karyotype may be needed in certain specific cases. This could be for either the partner or the couple or at times the product of conception depending on the clinical indication.

The following are the common indications for determining the karyotype in either partner presenting with infertility.

Male Factor Subfertility

Broadly this includes males with hypergonadotropic hypogonadism, idiopathic nonobstructive azoospermia, and severe oligospermia. Ascertaining the karyotype in these cases not only establishes the cause for the semen abnormalities, but it also helps in appropriate counseling and management.

For example, in case of males with Klinefelter syndrome (KS) (47,XXY), the chance of having male babies with an extra X chromosome exists and this needs to be explained.

Female Factor Subfertility

The most common indication for performing karyotype in a female partner is to investigate the cause for hypergonadotropic hypogonadism presenting as primary amenorrhea or premature ovarian failure (POF).

Couple Karyotype

Recurrent Pregnancy Loss

Screening for genetic causes in recurrent pregnancy losses (RPL) in the products of conception may reveal numerical or structural chromosomal abnormalities. The aim of investigating the chromosomes in a couple with RPL by karyotyping is to detect causative balanced structural chromosomal rearrangements in either of them that may have contributed to chromosomal imbalances in the conceptus. The incidence of balanced chromosomal translocations in couples with RPL is 2–5%, which is much higher compared to 0.2% incidence in the general population.

Generally, these are considered to have no phenotypic consequences in the individual carrying them as the exchange involves no loss or gain of genetic material. However, in some cases depending on the chromosomal breakpoints involved, there may be some clinical implications. For example, males with X autosome translocations are known to have low sperm counts.

There are, however, reproductive implications for carriers of balanced chromosomal translocations. In gametogenesis during meiosis, it is possible to have daughter cells with either a normal chromosome complement, or a balanced derivative chromosome number or unbalanced gametes with partial monosomy or trisomy in varying proportions. The latter two outcomes may result in abnormal embryos, which may subsequently result in miscarriage or an anomalous fetus.

Genetic counseling is recommended in such couples prior to testing and post-testing to discuss the recurrence risk, preconceptional and prenatal preventive options, and implications for the extended family. In each of their future pregnancy, prenatal testing by chorionic villi sampling or amniocentesis is recommended. Preimplantation genetic testing for aneuploidy (PGT-A) can be offered. The options of donor gamete may be considered by some couples.

Chromosomal Disorders in Male Infertility

Azoospermic men with severe oligospermia have a one in five chances of harboring a chromosomal aberration as a cause for their subfertility.[4,7] In males, autosomal ring chromosomes often cause oligospermia and azoospermia, probably due to gamete instability at meiosis.[8] Both numerical and structural variations are known.

Men with nonobstructive azoospermia have a greater incidence of aneuploidy in their chromosomes, particularly in their sex chromosomes with occasional fertilization and transmission of the defect to the progeny, e.g., KS 47,XXY karyotype or its variants.

NUMERICAL ABNORMALITIES/ ANEUPLOIDIES

Klinefelter Syndrome (47,XXY)

Klinefelter syndrome is the most common gonosomal (sex chromosomal) abnormality detected in 0.1–0.2% of newborns and 19% of men with severe oligospermia and in as high as 67% of azoospermic men.[9,10] Nondisjunction in male or female meiosis results in the extra X chromosome resulting in azoospermia in 74% of these men[11] **(Fig. 10)**. There are two variants of the syndromes:[12]

- Nonmosaic Klinefelter 47,XXY: 90% of KS falls into this category[13] and some can have sperms in the ejaculate.
- Mosaic Klinefelter 47,XXY/46,XY: 10% of the KS patients are mosaic and can have residual spermatogenesis.

In rare cases, more than two copies of X chromosome are found, for example, 48,XXXY and 49,XXXXY[13] resulting in severe conditions.

Clinically, features of androgen deficiency proven by a decline in serum testosterone levels and elevated follicle-stimulating hormone (FSH) and luteinizing hormone (LH) levels are noted along with germ cell degeneration in testicular biopsies.[11,12,14] As to their fertility potential, though the sperm of Klinefelter men have 23X or 23Y haploid genome, their offspring are reported to have an increased number of autosomal and sex chromosome aneuploidies.[15] The risk of transferring the abnormality by intracytoplasmic sperm injection (ICSI) with their sperms is present[16] though some studies have produced successful results with ICSI. Appropriate counseling should be offered for couples seeking treatment in such situations. Preimplantation

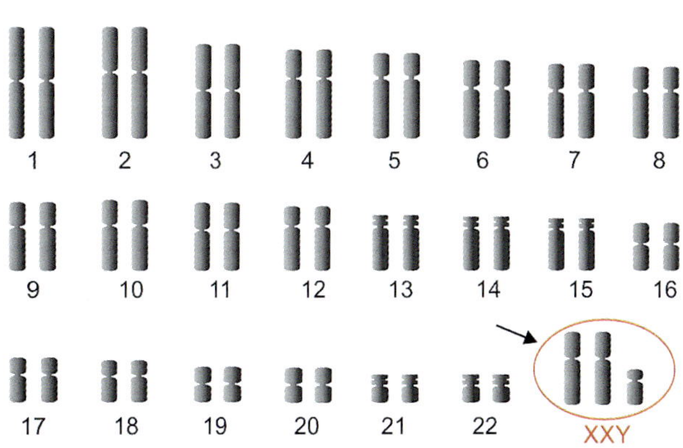

Fig. 10: Karyotype of a male with Klinefelter syndrome.

genetic diagnosis is indicated in such cases to ensure euploidy in the offspring.

47,XYY Syndrome/Jacob Syndrome

Jacob syndrome (JS) is the second most common gonosomal abnormality[17] occurring in 1:1,000 newborns. Most cases of JS are not inherited, but parental nondisjunction at meiosis II before conception leads to an additional Y chromosome 47,XYY in the affected offspring.[18,19] Extra Y chromosome in 47,XYY leads to infertility in adulthood, behavioral and cognitive disorders, facial dysmorphism, curved penis with nonpalpable testes, and decreased testosterone,[19] which eventually leads to sperm apoptosis and subsequent oligozoospermia and azoospermia[4,12,20] **(Fig. 11)**.

Some men expressing JS are fertile; here, additional Y chromosome is lost before meiosis, thereby preventing infertility.[18]

Translocations

Autosomal translocations are 4–10 times more in infertile men when compared to normal men, the most common being the Robertsonian translocation (RT) (0.8% prevalence in infertile men, 9 times higher than in general population).[21] RT results in a derivative chromosome (der) composed of two long arms from two acrocentric chromosomes.[22,23] Infertility, abortions, and aberrations in the child are the risks in RT carriers though they are healthy by themselves. The most frequent RTs are der (13;14) and der (14;21), with incidences of 1:1,000 and 1:5,000, respectively.[4,12,20,24,25] Nearly 20% of male carriers of der (13;14) are infertile.[24] Most mature spermatozoa with RT are normal or balanced (75–90%) as a result of alternate segregation. However, these translocations are associated with disrupted pairing in crossing over leading to trivalent formation and subsequent meiotic arrest, and result in oligozoospermia or azoospermia.[24,25] Male carriers of RTs involving chromosome 21 are more likely to have the disomic gametes that are likely to produce embryos with trisomy 21. Male RT carriers are often subfertile,[4] thereby reducing the chance of producing embryos. Loss of genetic material at breakpoints of genes can also occur due to translocations.

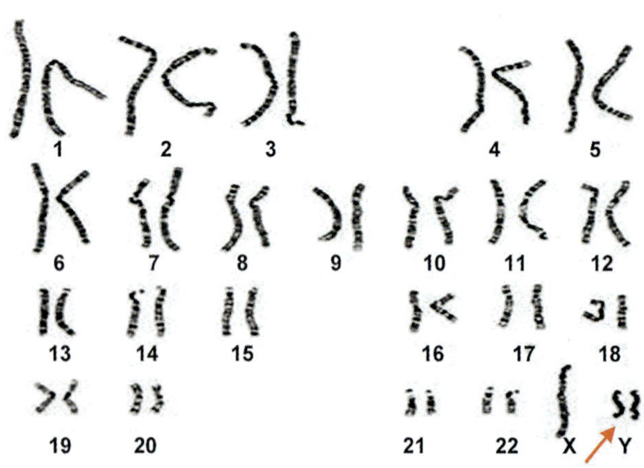

Fig. 11: Karyotype from a male with 47,XYY Jacob syndrome.

Y Chromosome Microdeletions (Table 2)

The critical genes that direct development of gonads and spermatogenesis are located on the Y chromosome, which is male-specific. This is the smallest of the human chromosomes and has a short arm (Yp) and a long arm (Yq) with a 60 Mb size and has the least number of genes.[14,23,26] Y chromosome microdeletions (YCMD) occur in 15% of azoospermic and 5% of oligozoospermic males **(Table 2)**. The genes identified are 27 in number, of which 9 are located in the Yp arm and 18 are located in the Yq arm. The male-specific region of the Y (MSY) is a complete sequence of the euchromatin segment. PAR represents the pseudoautosomal region and NRY, the region outside the PAR, represents the nonrecombining region.[27] The euchromatin lies in the Yp and the proximal part of Yq and the distal part of Yq is the heterochromatin segment. The mapping of the Y chromosome by molecular methods has shown deletion intervals and subintervals.[28] Tiepolo and Zuffardi[29] were the first to postulate the link between YCMD and infertility. It was proposed that at least one genetic Y factor required for male germ cell development is located on the distal Yq11.[30] It is defined as Y-borne fertile gene or azoospermia factor (AZF).

TABLE 2: Y chromosome microdeletions.[29,30]

Gene	*Location*	*Function*	*Deletion/shortening*
USP9Y	AZFa	Efficiency of spermatogenesis	Azoo/oligo/ oligoasthenospermia
DBY	AZFa	Premeiotic germ cell development	
RBMY	AZFb	RNA-binding protein/ testis splicing factor	Reduced expression in azoospermia
PRY	AZFb	Apoptosis regulation	
DAZ	AZFc	Regulation of translation, meiosis, and germ cell population; codes for RNA-binding proteins	Reduced expression in azoospermic men. Partial deletions related to oligospermia
sY153	AZFd	Spermatogenesis	Mild oligospermia/ normal semen parameters
CDY	Yq	Involved in histone replacement	
TSPY	Yp	Regulates timing of spermatogenesis	Greater copy number in infertile patients

(AZF: azoospermia factor; RNA: ribonucleic acid)

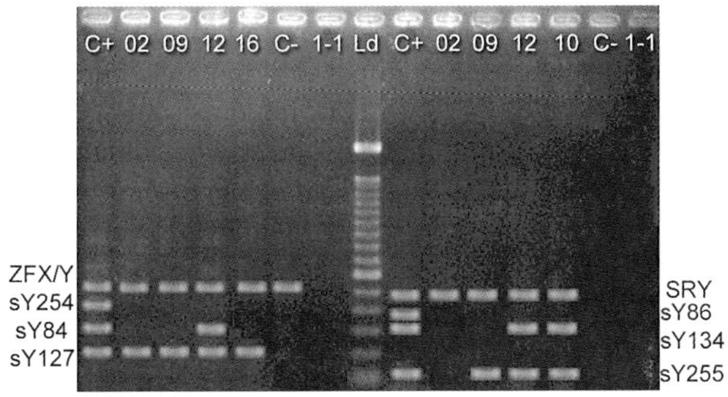

Fig. 12: Electrophoresis on a 1.5% agarose gel showing deletion in the azoospermia factor (AZF) region of the Y chromosome. Ld, molecular weight 100 bp (invitrogen); ZFX/Y, 495 bp; SRY, 472 bp; sY255, 126 bp; sY254, 400 bp; sY134, 301 bp; sY127, 274 bp; sY86, 320 bp; sY84, 326 bp. Lanes 02 and 09, azoospermic patients. Lanes 12 and 16, severe oligozoospermic patients.

Thus, deletions of genes of this region had a spectrum of impacts on spermatogenesis.[26] The deletion affects has three distinct regions—AZFa, AZFb, and AZFc.[30,31] AZFa is a nearly 0.8 Mb region that maps to proximal region Yq11.21. AZFb and AZFc map to regions Yq11.22 and Yq11.23, respectively **(Fig. 12)**.

AZFa region: The two main genes in AZFa are USP9Y and DBY (DDX3Y). When both are deleted, the result is Sertoli cell-only syndrome.[32] The *DBY* gene expresses in the testis and is involved in the development of the premeiotic germ cells.[33-35] The deletion or shortening of the *USP9Y* gene causes oligoasthenospermia, azoospermia, or oligospermia.[36-39] However, this gene is involved only in the efficacy of spermatogenesis because it can be carried to the offspring. Thus, the *DBY* gene plays a more important role in the spermatogenesis.

AZFb region: RBMY is the main gene of this region that codes for a ribonucleic acid (RNA)-binding protein,[15] a testis-specific splicing factor, conveyed in the nuclei of spermatogonia. A family of *PRY* genes in the AZFb region in regulation of apoptosis is for the regulation of abnormal sperms. However, if both are removed, arrest of spermatogenesis results indicating that both are vital for spermatogenesis.

AZFc region: The AZFc deletions cause approximately 12% of nonobstructive azoospermia and 6% of severe oligospermia.[31] The AZFa and AZFb regions are required to start spermatogenesis, but the process will not be completely normal without AZFc.[40] The AZFc deletion can be a result of a previous deletion or a de novo one, which when total may lead to a Y chromosome loss resulting in sexual reversal. Also, several studies have found this to be a permutation for 45,XO and for mosaic 45,X/46,XY.[15,20] Partial deletions may produce a wide variety of phenotypes from azoospermia to normospermia influenced by the background genetic makeup and the environment as exemplified by the ethnic variations.[41]

The three most frequent subdeletions are gr/gr, b1/b3, and g1/g3.[30,42] The deletions and their effects on spermatogenesis and fertility have not been uniform across ethnic groups and geographical regions illustrating the impact of environment on fertility genes.[43]

DAZ gene: Deleted in azoospermia (*DAZ*) genes having four copies are considered to play various roles in spermatogenesis because they are expressed in all stages of germ cell development.[44-46] They control code for germ cell-specific RNA-binding proteins, translation, and are involved in the control of maintenance of primordial germ cell population and meiosis. Thus, their deletion can cause a range of phenotypes such as oligospermia and azoospermia.[42]

Other genes on the Y chromosome: The CDY gene located on Yq is expressed exclusively in the testis and facilitates histone replacement spermatogenesis. It also grants the proteins that regulate transcription access to the postmeiotic sperm DNA. It is interesting to note that this gene has divulged from its homolog on chromosome 6 and subsequently migrated to the Y chromosome during evolution, reflecting the consolidation of the genes involved in spermatogenesis on the Y chromosome.[47] The *TSPY* gene, which is located on the short arm of the Y chromosome Yp, and has copies on the long arm, is expressed in the testis and its protein is identified in the spermatogonia. It may regulate timing of spermatogenesis and signaling of spermatogonia to enter spermatogenesis. More studies are needed on this gene as more copies of it were found in the infertile patients.

AZFd region: This is the region between AZFb and AZFc. No candidate gene has been identified till now, though sY153 has been implicated and patients with microdeletions in this region may present with mild oligospermia or even normal spermatogenesis.[48,49]

Recent genome-wide copy number variation (CNV) array studies using modern versions of the CGH technique began to uncover additional CNV linked to male infertility. Interestingly, a generally increased CNV burden seems to be associated with male infertility.[50-53] Several such aberrations including mutations within *TEX11* gene have been mapped to the X chromosome, which houses many germs cell-specific genes, and in analogy to the Y contains palindromic regions that facilitate rearrangements.[50]

Autosomal Genetic Aberrations

A number of candidate genes have been investigated for their role in male infertility. In patients with congenital bilateral absence of the vas deferens (CBAVD), *the cystic fibrosis transmembrane conductance regulator* (*CFTR*) gene on chromosome 7 is mutated in 60–90% of patients.[54,55] The F508del-CFTR is seen in 60–70% of patients with CBAVD, the male presenting with obstructive azoospermia. When shortening is seen on *SHBG* gene on chromosome 17, the spermatogenesis was increased and showed higher sperm concentrations.

Gene Polymorphisms

ESR1 and 2 on chromosome 6 has many polymorphisms and the promoter region of *ESR1* has a variable number of tandem repeats TA *n*. The high number of repeats of TA *n* polymorphism is correlated with[33] lower levels of spermatogenesis. Further studies are needed. *FSHR* located on chromosome 2 may undergo changes due to SNPs and may have effects on spermatogenesis. The polymorphism *677C/T* interferes with the activity of methylenetetrahydrofolate reductase (*MTHFR*) gene located on the short arm of chromosome 1 affecting coding for folate synthesis, which in turn can affect the methylation of the genomic DNA important for spermatogenesis.

Mutations on the *INSL3* gene on chromosome 19 and its receptor *LGR8* on chromosome 13 have been linked to cryptorchidism seen in 5% of such patients.[56] The *INSLR 3* gene may also have a role in testicular dysgenesis syndrome (TDS) consisting of a variety of disorders such as cryptorchidism, hypospadias, testicular cancer, and infertility. TDS is thought to result from the combination of genetic environmental and lifestyle factors.[57]

X-linked Genes

Spermatogenesis is considered to be linked to many X-linked genes expressed in the testis. The *AR* gene, located on the long arm of X chromosome, has an important role to play in the conversion of spermatocytes to round spermatids. Mutations of *AR* gene can result in a spectrum of disorders ranging from oligoasthenospermia to androgen insensitivity syndrome and Kennedy syndrome (a neurogenetic disorder with abnormal spermatogenesis).[46] A synergistic effect of *SHBG* gene and *AR* gene can influence sperm motility. Variations in the *UPPS26* gene on the long arm of the X chromosome may influence spermatogenesis, resulting in azoospermia. The *TAF7L* gene expressed in the testis is related to the autosomal TAF gene and its role as a transcription factor in spermatogenesis is important for regulation. Thus, the SNP at exon 13 is a risk for an infertile phenotype combined with other polymorphisms.[58,59]

The idiopathic hypogonadotropic hypogonadism with anosmia—Kallmann syndrome is yet another condition which has X-linked and autosomal inheritance. Stunted sexual development, anosmia, cognitive impairments, ocular abnormalities, midfacial cleft, and renal agenesis constitute this syndrome. Two genetic deletions found in these patients are in KAL1 (KS1 sequence) located on the short arm of the X chromosome and directing gonadotropin-releasing hormone neuronal migration as well as coding for the anosmin. This mutation is responsible for 30–70% of Kallmann syndrome in patients.

The fibroblast GF receptor (FGFR1) on chromosome 8 can cause anosmic or hyposmic Kallmann syndrome.[40,60] Patients with Kallmann syndrome need to be counseled regarding transmission to the offspring.

Mitochondrial Deoxyribonucleic Acid Deletions

The mitochondrial DNA deletions can affect spermatogenesis and impair motility.

Monogenic Disorders

More than 50 disorders by Mendelian inheritance are associated with the male infertility.

Epigenetic Disorders

Spermatogenesis is a several-step process where a single error or an accumulation of errors can lead to the SNP at exon 13, which is a risk for an infertile phenotype if combined with other polymorphisms. Severe disorders in spermatogenesis result. Epigenetics refers to alteration of the genetic code changing the[61] transcription and gene expression without affecting the basic DNA sequence.

Sperms harvested from the testis before maturation may not have a fully functional *centrosome. If* the *protamines P1 and P2 are* translated too early, spermatogenesis is arrested at the spermatid stage and the nucleus condenses prematurely. Also, an unequal P1:P2 ratio has been observed in the infertile men.

An SNP of the gene *G197T*, which codes for P1 may be the reason for sperm DNA fragmentation and teratozoospermia. *Histones* are important players in the transmission of epigenetic information. Their role in male fertility is under investigation.

Imprinting Disorders

Imprinting is the methylation of DNA during the last phase of spermatogenesis and determines which genes from the paternal genomes are to be expressed in the embryo. New imprints in the germ cells are made possible by reset of parental imprints in every cycle and are achieved by the different processes. In the normal men, paternally differentially methylated regions (DMR) of the DNA should be methylated and the maternal DMRs should be unmethylated.[63]

A study by Kobayashi et al. showed that 14% of infertile patients had abnormalities in the DMR of the paternal imprint and 21% of the infertile patients had abnormalities in the maternal imprint. Most patients with abnormalities in both imprints were oligospermic. These men had low success rates with assisted reproductive technology (ART). It was also found that these men have a higher risk of transmitting the imprinting errors to their children.[64]

The use of immature sperms in ART, when the epigenetic code is not well established, may result in an offspring with an imprinting disorder. The abnormalities in the centrosome, and sperm nuclear protein may not permit activation of the oocyte by the immature sperm. Thus, control of methylation may be the key point in regulation of the first few steps of fertilization in ART.[65] However, many studies have shown conflicting results of the occurrence of imprinting disorders such as Angelman and Beckwith-Wiedemann syndrome in infertile men.[66]

Defects in messenger RNA transcripts (mRNA), telomere length, mitochondrial DNA degradation in infertile men, and their impact on fertility and transmission to offspring are under evaluation by the use of novel technologies of genomics, proteomics, metabolomics, and microarray techniques.[67]

The exact transmission of genetic and epigenetic information is essential for fertility. The consolidation of new molecular techniques when processed for clinical application will enable the clinician to make the right decisions in ART.

Genetics of Female Infertility

The genetic control of reproduction in the female is complex as the genital tract development, gametogenesis, and the endocrine control of reproduction all come under the genes. However, complete knowledge in this area is still under research. During sexual development, in utero genetic misdirections can lead to congenital malformations of the reproductive tract that manifest as anatomical abnormalities of the Müllerian ducts, uterus, endometrium, fallopian tubes, and ovaries resulting in subfertility. Another facet of the genetics includes a wide spectrum such as POF, polycystic ovary syndrome (PCOS), endometriosis, and leiomyoma. As in male subfertility, genetic syndromes that manifest in female infertility are fragile X syndrome, myotonic dystrophy, Noonan's syndrome, Fanconi anemia, sickle cell anemia, β-thalassemia, etc.[68]

Chromosomal Disorders in Female Infertility

Sex Chromosomal Aneuploidies

47,XXX syndrome: The *47,XXX syndrome*, also known as trisomy X, is one of the most common causes of premature ovarian insufficiency (POI); the incidence is 1:1,000 female births. The extra X chromosome is due to maternal nondisjunction at meiosis I and there is an association with increased maternal age. As the extra X chromosomes are inactivated only after embryonic development, abnormalities occur. A few women with trisomy X may have primary ovarian insufficiency or genitourinary tract malformations, but majority are normal.[69]

Clinical features include:
- Small for gestational age at birth
- Ovarian dysfunction—rare
- Fertility may not be affected
- Risk of transmission to offspring is increased
- Mild-to-moderate problems in central nervous system (CNS) function as in motor, speech, language, and learning.

The treatment is directed holistically to speech and occupational therapy if needed.

The *48,XXXX syndrome* presents with mild-to-moderate mental retardation, facial, skeletal dysplasia, impaired secondary sexual characteristics, and fertility impairment due to POF in most cases. However, chromosomally normal offspring can be born.

The *49,XXXXX syndrome* presents with more severe mental retardation and microcephaly, congenital heart, and renal anomalies. Pregnancies have been reported.

Turner syndrome: Turner syndrome, also known as monosomy X or 45,XO chromosome disorder in females, has an incidence of 1:2,000 births **(Figs. 13 and 14)**. During meiosis, chromosomal nondisjunction results in the loss of chromosome X. No parental age effect has been reported.[70]

Clinical features include:
- Spontaneous abortions
- Newborns show decreased birth weight, neck webbing, posteriorly rotated ears, and lymphedema of the hands
- Older children and adults have facial, skeletal, renal, and congenital heart defects and primary amenorrhea with lack of secondary streak gonads
- The short stature homeobox gene (*SHOX*) the located is on the Xp escapes inactivation and single functional copy for SHOX causes short stature and skeletal features.

Ovarian function also declines rapidly in milder phenotypes of Turner mosaic as in 45,X/47,XXX.

45,X0/46,XY mosaicism: Mixed gonadal dysgenesis (45,X/46,XY mosaicism) is a rare sex chromosome

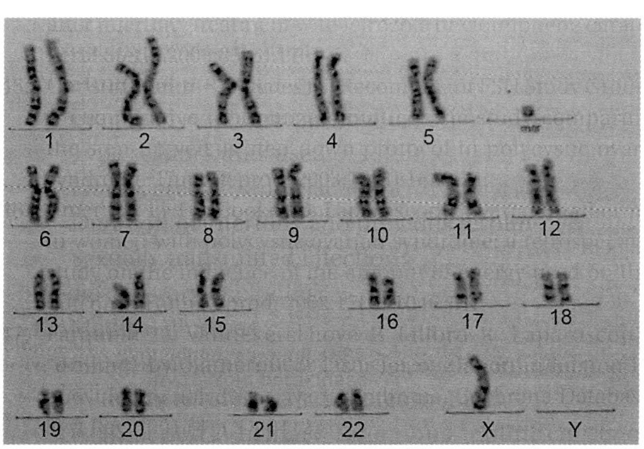

Fig. 13: Karyotype in Turner syndrome—the missing X.

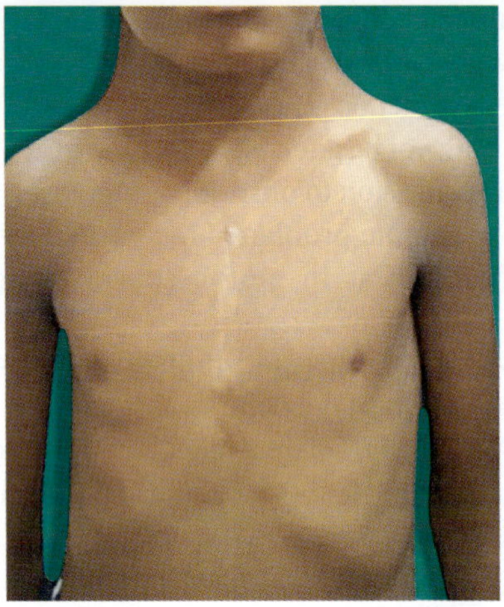

Fig. 14: Clinical picture in Turner syndrome.

aneuploidy with a prevalence of approximately 1 in 15,000 newborns.[71] Here, two cell lines exist, of which one has 45,X karyotype (X monosomy) and the other has a normal male karyotype (46,XY). The two cell lines are differently distributed in individuals and is responsible for the varied phenotypes expressed by the affected individuals.[72] 45,X/46,XY mosaicism is most often caused by the loss of the Y chromosome through nondisjunction in some somatic cells after normal fertilization.[72,73] Both the 46,XY and 45,X cell lines divide nonstop, resulting in a baby with 45,X/46,XY. The 45,X/46,XY karyotype is also formed by the deletions, or translocations of Y chromosome segments.[72] This abnormality can repress the *SRY* genes, resulting in abnormal genitals (incomplete sexual differentiation) and testosterone levels.[71]

STRUCTURAL ANOMALIES OF CHROMOSOMES

The chromosomes can have structural rearrangements, either inherited or occurring de novo.

Balanced Translocations

Balanced translocations between X chromosome and autosomes mutate the genes, which when expressed results in variable phenotypes. A process of inactivation spreads from the translocated X segment to autosomal material and inactivates the genes causing mutations.

The features expressed may range from primary or secondary ovarian failure with often normal phenotypes. Learning problems and developmental delays can be seen. A phenotypically normal mother with an X autosome translocation can have a daughter with phenotypic abnormalities and mental retardation. De novo translocations are associated with significantly higher abnormal outcome. In a female with a balanced X autosome translocation, a 20–40% risk of a live-born child with a structural and/or functional aneuploidy is expected. Counseling X autosomal translocations becomes extremely difficult due to the variable phenotypes.[74]

Unbalanced translocation between the X chromosome and the autosome expresses a range of phenotypical abnormalities from mental retardation and multiple congenital anomalies to mild behavioral problems. This again makes counseling extremely difficult in a patient with prenatal detection of an unbalanced translocation.[74]

Deletions

Xp and Xq deletion in a female is associated with short stature and POF of varying degrees. Xp deletions often mimic Turner syndrome.

Duplications

Xp and Xq duplications have a spectrum of phenotypes ranging from normal to Turner syndrome features. Xq duplications can manifest as short stature, microcephaly, and gonadal dysgenesis.

Inversions

The X chromosome inversions can present in highly varied phenotypes ranging from normal intelligence quotient (IQ) to mental retardation and gonadal dysgenesis to mild menstrual irregularities. The phenotype depends on the site of inversion.

Ring Chromosome

A ring chromosome is a chromosome abnormality, where two ends of the chromosome break and the broken ends fuse to form a ring.[75] It often occurs spontaneously and is rarely inherited due to instability of ring chromosomes during cell division and so may be lost.[76] If transmitted, they form new rings and are transmitted to the offspring and coexist with normal karyotype and cause a mosaic karyotype in the maternal and fetal karyotypes. Ring chromosomes rarely impair female fertility. However, low ovarian reserve has been reported in women expressing ring chromosomes.[77]

Genomic Aberrations, Copy Number Variants

Newer techniques such as microarray have enabled studies of relationship of complex female subfertility factors such as endometriosis and primary ovarian failure to genomic loci paving the pathway for the whole genome analysis and findings of new genes related to the disease process. Multiple genes such as *PLCB1*, *RB1CC1*, *MAP4K4*, *RBBP8*, *IMMP2L*, *FER1L6*, and *MEIG1* are involved in meiosis. DNA repair or folliculogenesis was identified as possible candidate genes for POF and ovarian dysfunction. Following CGH studies identified new infertility-associated candidate genes and unveiled new details of the pathophysiology of female subfertility.[78]

Single-gene Disorders

Fragile X Syndrome

Fragile X syndrome is a disorder characterized mainly by mental retardation, long face, large ears, and prominent jaws. The syndrome was first reported in 1969 with constriction of the long arm on the X chromosome.[79] It has an incidence of 1:5.[80] The critical gene for fragile X is fragile X mental retardation gene (*FMR1*), located at Xq27.3. The pathology is caused by the expansion of the CGG repeat in the gene's 50 untranslated region to a premutation state of between 56 repeats and 199 repeats (a complete mutation has over 200 repeats). Generally, *FMR1* premutations are found in 16% of POF females with about 2% of the cases being sporadic and 14–21% familial.[81,82] Carrier screening of *FMR1* premutation is recommended for women of advanced maternal age or with a family history of fragile X.

Primary Ovarian Failure

Primary ovarian failure is defined as either complete or incomplete failure of the ovaries (also known as primary ovarian insufficiency). Recently, several genes have been discovered that show incomplete loss of function of the ovary, leading to the term "primary ovarian insufficiency." A number of genes have been associated with POF or POI. X-linked genes include *FMR1* and bone morphogenetic protein 15 (BMP15) located in the Xp11.2 region. Many autosomal mutations are often found in women with POF or POI such as *AR*, *CDKN1B*, *CYP19A1*, *GDF9*, *FIGLA*, *FOXL2*, *FOXO1a*, *FOXO3a*, *INHA*, *LHX8*, *NOBOX*, and *NANOS3*, located at the Xp11.2 region.[83]

Polygenic Complex Female Infertility

Endometriosis

Endometriosis is a complex disease characterized by the inflammation and colonization of functional endometrium in extra endometrial sites with multiple pathological effects. In the case of endometriosis, the five to eight times higher prevalence rate has a genetic basis authenticated by the identification of candidate genes, SNPs and CNVs. Follow-up studies are needed, however, to close down on critical regions. A significant linkage to *10q26* gene was identified although more clarity was needed to point to a single gene.[84] Among two genome-wide association studies (GWAS) conducted in 2010 and 2011,[85,86] only one common locust was found in the 1p36 region, which contains *WNT4*, a gene responsible for cell proliferation, which plays a key role in embryogenesis. Earlier studies have noted association of this gene locus in endometriosis.

Polycystic ovarian syndrome has a dominant inheritance; however, no specific gene has been identified. The gene for insulin resistance *INSR* has a direct correlation as shown by the GWAS study. Three additional loci (2p16.3, 2p21, 9q33.3) were also identified.[87] Some studies have identified the gene of interest *DENND1A*, a guanine nucleotide exchange factor. As yet, the cause of PCOS is unknown; both genetic and environmental factors must be taken into consideration.

Leiomyoma

Leiomyoma is commonly known as fibroids and interfere with female fertility depending on the size and location. Mutations in mediator complex subunit 12 (MED 12), cytogenetic anomalies, and aberrant DNA methylation or demethylation have been observed. A direct cause of genetics in genesis of fibroids has been observed. Mutations in fumarate hydrates (*FH*) gene can cause renal cell carcinoma and hereditary leiomyomatosis.[88,89]

Mutations in *HMG1C* and *HMG1Y* have been implicated in origin of leiomyomas.[90]

Müllerian Anomalies

Some of the uterine malformations may result from spontaneous mutations, while majority are due to environmental factors. The *EMX2* gene mutation has been implicated as the cause of uterus didelphys in some females.[91]

Gene Polymorphisms

Follicle-stimulating hormone receptor polymorphisms coded in chromosome 2 can present as a range of symptoms ranging from POF to varied response to FSH administration to ovarian hyperstimulation syndrome. Polymorphisms of the genes for FSH and LH are now being studied for use in clinical medicine for identifying poor response to controlled ovarian stimulation in ART. In a recent study, the link between LHCGR N312S polymorphism and the difference in dosage requirement in women homozygous and heterozygous for serine was noted. Subsequently, alteration in recombinant human luteinizing hormone (r-hLH) dose according to the polymorphism resulted in a significant increase in pregnancy rates.[92] Thus, algorithms for controlled ovarian stimulation based on genomic profiles could improve results in ART.

CONCLUSION

The genetics and the molecular basis of male and female infertility are the forefront of research in reproductive medicine where the future holds specific targeted treatments, which will yield better clinical outcome. On the other hand, the increased risk of transmission of the genome necessitates the importance of accurate diagnosis and appropriate counseling, especially in assisted reproduction. Cytogenetic screening is indicated in suspected situations and counseling is mandatory prior to ART. The role of cytogenetics in reproductive medicine is not only in the diagnosis of the cause, but also in enhancing fertility rates, prevention of transmission of genetic aberrations, and future prenatal diagnosis. With the advances in infertility treatments, cytogenetics has parallelly developed into a highly sophisticated field with karyotyping, array technology, and preimplantation genetic testing.

KEY POINTS

- Newer applications of cytogenetics and molecular techniques have enabled diagnosis of genetic basis of many factors causing infertility.
- Subtle disturbances in mitosis and meiosis during gametogenesis and embryogenesis,can amplify these aberrations and cause infertility.
- Diagnosis of certain chromosomal and genomic factors are possible now and can guide the clinician in treatment and counselling in infertility.
- Knowledge and application of cytogenetics in infertility is also crucial to ascertain the risk of transmission of the abnormal factors across generation and hence is of epidemiological importance.

REFERENCES

1. Genetic Alliance, The New York-Mid-Atlantic Consortium for Genetic and Newborn Screening Services. Understanding Genetics: A New York, Mid-Atlantic Guide for Patients and Health Professionals. Washington, DC: Genetic Alliance; 2009. [online] Available from: https://pubmed.ncbi.nlm.nih.gov/23304754/. [Last accessed November, 2022].
2. National Human Genome Research Institute (NHGRI). (2020). Chromosome Abnormalities Fact Sheet. [online] Available from: https://www.genome.gov/about-genomics/fact-sheets/Chromosome-Abnormalities-Fact-Sheet. [Last accessed November, 2022].
3. Gersen LG, Keagel MB. The Principles of Clinical Cytogenetics. New Jersey: Humana Press; 2005. p. 596.
4. Harton GL, Tempest HG. Chromosomal disorders and male infertility. Asian J Androl. 2012;14(1):32-3.
5. Okutman O, Rhouma MB, Benkhalifa M, Muller J, Viville S. Genetic evaluation of patients with non-syndromic male infertility. J Assist Reprod Genet. 2018;35(11):1939-51.
6. Vicdan A, Vicdan K, Günalp S, Kence A, Akarsu C, Işik AZ, et al. Genetic aspects of human male infertility: the frequency of chromosomal abnormalities and Y chromosome microdeletions in severe male factor infertility. Eur J Obstet Gynecol Reprod Biol. 2004;117(1):49-54.
7. Chandley AC, Edmond P, Christie S, Gowans L, Fletcher J, Frackiewicz A, et al. Cytogenetics and infertility in man. I. Karyotype and seminal analysis: results of a five-year survey of men attending a subfertility clinic. Ann Hum Gen. 1975;39(2):231-54.
8. Rajesh H, Freckmann M-L, Chapman M. Azoospermia and paternal autosomal ring chromosomes: case report and literature review. Reprod Biomed Online. 2011;23: 466-70.
9. Huynh T, Mollard R, Trounson A. Selected genetic factors associated with male infertility. Hum Reprod Update. 2002;8: 183-98.
10. Mau-Holzmann UA. Somatic chromosomal abnormalities in infertile men and women. Cytogenet Genome Res. 2005; 111:317-36.
11. Oates RD. The natural history of endocrine function and spermatogenesis in Klinefelter syndrome: what the data show. Fertil Steril. 2012;98(2):266-73.
12. Walsh TJ, Pera RR, Turek PJ. The genetics of male infertility. Semin Reprod Med. 2009;27(2):124-36.
13. Bonomi M, Rochira V, Pasquali D, Balercia G, Jannini EA, Ferlin A. Klinefelter syndrome (KS): genetics, clinical phenotype and hypogonadism. J Endocrinol Invest. 2017;40(2):123-34.
14. O'Flynn O'Brien KL, Varghese AC, Agarwal A. The genetic causes of male factor infertility: a review. Fertil Steril. 2010; 93(1):1-12.
15. Hennebicq S, Pelletier R, Bergues U, Rousseaux S. Risk of trisomy 21 in offspring of patients with Klinefelter's syndrome. Lancet. 2001;357(9274):2104-5.
16. Jaruzelska J, Korcz A, Wojda A, Jedrzejczak P, Bierla J, Surmacz T, et al. Mosaicism for 45, X cell line may accentuate the severity of spermatogenic defects in men with AZFc deletion. J Med Genet. 2001;38:798-802.
17. Chantot-Bastaraud S, Ravel C, Siffroi JP. Genetic and epigenetic aspects of assisted reproduction: underlying karyotype abnormalities in IVF/ICSI patients. Reprod Biomed Online. 2008;16(4):514-22.
18. Kim IW, Khadilkar AC, Ko EY, Sabanegh ES. 47, XYY syndrome and male infertility. Rev Urol. 2013;15(4):188-96.
19. Latrech H, Skikar I, Gharbi ME, Chraïbi A, Gaouzi A. Disorder of sexual development and congenital heart defect in 47XYY: clinical disorder or coincidence? Case Rep Endocrinol. 2015;2015:802162.
20. Martin RH. Cytogenetic determinants of male fertility. Hum Reprod Update. 2008;14(4):379-90.
21. De Braekleer M. Cytogenetic studies in male infertility. Hum Reprod. 1991;2:245-50.
22. Marchetti F, Wyrobek AJ. Mechanisms and consequences of paternally-transmitted chromosomal abnormalities. Birth Defects Res C Embryo Today. 2005;75(2):112-29.
23. Reijo R, Lee TY, Salo P, Alagappan R, Brown LG, Rosenberg M, et al. Diverse spermatogenic defects in humans caused by Y chromosome deletions encompassing a novel RNA-binding protein gene. Nat Genet. 1995;10(4):383-93.
24. Roux C, Tripogney C, Morel F, Joanne C, Fellmann F, Clavequin MC, et al. Segregation of chromosomes in sperm of Robertsonian translocation carriers. Cytogenet Genome Res. 2005;111(3-4):291-6.
25. Engels H, Eggermann T, Caliebe A, Jelska A, Schubert R, Schüler HM, et al. Genetic counselling in Robertsonian translocations der(13;14): frequencies of reproductive outcomes and infertility in 101 pedigrees. Am J Med Genet A. 2008;146A(20):2611-6.
26. Reijo R, Alagappan RK, Patrizio P, Page DC. Severe oligozoospermia resulting from deletions of azoospermia factor gene on Y chromosome. Lancet. 1996;347(9011):1290-3.
27. Jorgez CJ, Weedin JW, Sahin A, Tannour-Louet M, Han S, Bournat JC, et al. Aberrations in pseudoautosomal regions (PARs) found in infertile men with Y-chromosome microdeletions. J Clin Endocrinol Metab. 2011;96(4):E674-9.
28. Volrath D. The human Y chromosome a 43 interval map based on natural deletions. Science. 1992;258(5079):52-9.

29. Tiepolo L, Zuffardi O. Localization of factors controlling spermatogenesis in the nonfluorescent portion of the human Y chromosome long arm. Hum Genet. 1976;34(2):119-24.
30. Vogt PH, Edelmann A, Kirsch S, Henegariu O, Hirschmann P, Kiesewetter F, et al. Human Y chromosome azoospermia factors (AZF) mapped to different subregions in Yq11. Hum Mol Genet. 1996;5(7):933-43.
31. Kuroda-Kawaguchi T, Skaletsky H, Brown LG, Minx PJ, Cordum HS, Waterston RH, et al. The AZFc region of the Y chromosome features massive palindromes and uniform recurrent deletions in infertile men. Nat Genet. 2001;29(3):279-86.
32. Tuttelmann F, Simoni M, Kliesch S, Ledig S, Dworniczak B, Wieacker P, et al. Copy number variants in patients with severe oligozoospermia and Sertoli cell-only syndrome. PLoS One. 2011;6(4):e19426.
33. Nuti F, Krausz C. Gene polymorphisms/mutations relevant to abnormal spermatogenesis. Reprod Biomed Online. 2008;16:504-13.
34. Lardone MC, Parodi DA, Valdevenito R, Ebensperger M, Piottante A, Madariaga M, et al. Quantification of DDX3Y, RBMY1, DAZ and TSPY mRNAs in testes of patients with severe impairment of spermatogenesis. Mol Hum Reprod. 2007;13:705-12.
35. Tyler-Smith C. An evolutionary perspective on Y-chromosomal variation and male infertility. Int J Androl. 2008;31:376-82.
36. Galan JJ, Guarducci E, Nuti F, Gonzalez A, Ruiz M, Ruiz A, et al. Molecular analysis of estrogen receptor alpha gene AGATA haplotype and SNP12 in European populations: potential protective effect for cryptorchidism and lack of association with male infertility. Hum Reprod. 2007;22:444-9.
37. Brown GM, Furlong RA, Sargent CA, Erickson RP, Longepied G, Mitchell M, et al. Characterisation of the coding sequence and fine mapping of human DFFRY gene and comparative expression analysis and mapping to the Sxrb interval of the mouse Y chromosome of the Dffry gene. Hum Mol Genet. 1998;7:97-107.
38. Elliott DJ. The role of potential splicing factors including RBMY, RBMX, hnRNPG-T and STAR proteins in spermatogenesis. Int J Androl. 2004;27:328-34.
39. Krausz C, Degl'Innocenti S, Nuti F, Morelli A, Felici F, Sansone M, et al. Natural transmission of USP9Y gene mutations: a new perspective on the role of AZFa genes in male fertility. Hum Mol Genet. 2006;15:2673-81.
40. Vogt PH. Azoospermia factor (AZF) in Yq11: towards a molecular understanding of its function for human male fertility and spermatogenesis. Reprod Biomed Online. 2005;10:81-93.
41. Lardone MC, Parodi DA, Ebensperger M, Penaloza P, Cornejo V, Valdevenito R, et al. AZFc partial deletions in Chilean men with severe spermatogenic failure. Fertil Steril. 2007;88:1318-26.
42. Elliot DJ, Cooke HJ. The molecular genetics of male infertility. Bioessays. 1997;19(9):801-9.
43. Rozen SG, Marszalek JD, Irenze K, Skaletsky H, Brown LG, Oates RD, et al. AZFc deletions and spermatogenic failure: a population-based survey of 20,000 Y chromosomes. Am J Hum Genet. 2012;91(5):890-6.
44. Reynolds N, Cooke HJ. Role of the DAZ genes in male fertility. Reprod Biomed Online. 2005;10:72-80.
45. Teng YN, Lin YM, Sun HF, Hsu PY, Chung CL, Kuo PL. Association of DAZL haplotypes with spermatogenic failure in infertile men. Fertil Steril. 2006;86(1):129-35.
46. Lavery R, Glennon M, Houghton J, Nolan A, Egan D, Maher M. Investigation of DAZ and RBMY1 gene expression in human testis by quantitative real-time PCR. Arch Androl. 2007;53:71-3.
47. Lahn B, Page DC. Retroposition of autosomal mRNA yielded testis-specific gene family on human Y chromosome. Nat Genet. 1999;21:429-33.
48. Kent-First MG, Muallem A, Shultz J, Pryor J, Roberts K, Nolten W, et al. Defining regions of the Y chromosome responsible for male infertility and identification of a fourth AZF region (AZFd) by Y chromosome microdeletion detection. Mol Reprod Dev. 1999;53:27-41.
49. Sao Pedro SL, Fraisetta R, Spaine D, Porto CS, Srougi M, Cedenho AP, et al. Prevalence of Y chromosome deletions in a Brazilian population of non-obstructive azoospermic and severely oligozoospermic men. Braz J Med Biol Res. 2003;36:787-93.
50. Krausz C, Giachini C, Lo Giacco D, Daguin F, Chianese C, Ars E, et al. High resolution X chromosome-specific array-CGH detects new CNVs in infertile males. PLoS One. 2012;7(10):e44887.
51. Lopes AM, Aston KI, Thompson E, Carvalho F, Gonçalves J, Huang N, et al. Human spermatogenic failure purges deleterious mutation load from the autosomes and both sex chromosomes, including the gene DMRT1. PLoS Genet. 2013;9(3):e1003349.
52. Aston KI, Krausz C, Laface I, Ruiz-Castané E, Carrell DT. Evaluation of 172 candidate polymorphisms for association with oligozoospermia or azoospermia in a large cohort of men of European descent. Hum Reprod. 2010;25(6):1383-97.
53. Aston KI, Carrell DT. Genome-wide study of single- nucleotide polymorphisms associated with azoospermia and severe oligozoospermia. J Androl. 2009;30(6):711-25.
54. Costes B, Girodon E, Ghanem N, Flori E, Jardin A, Soufir JC, et al. Frequent occurrence of the CFTR intron 8 (TG)n 5T allele in men with congenital bilateral absence of the vas deferens. Eur J Hum Genet. 1995;3(5):285-93.
55. Riordan JR, Rommens JM, Kerem B, Alon N, Rozmahel R, Grzelczak Z, et al. Identification of the cystic fibrosis gene: cloning and characterization of complementary DNA. Science. 1989;245(4922):1066-73.
56. Ferlin A, Foresta C. The INSL3-LGR8 hormonal system in humans: testicular descent, cryptorchidism and testicular functions. Curr Med Chem. 2005;5:421-30.
57. Olesen IA, Sonne SB, Hoei-Hansen CE, Rajpert-De Meyts E, Skakkebaek NE. Environment, testicular dysgenesis and carcinoma in situ testis. Best Pract Res Clin Endocrinol Metab. 2007;21:462-78.
58. Akinloye O, Gromoll J, Callies C, Nieschlag E, Simoni M. Mutation analysis of the X-chromosome linked, testis-specific TAF7L gene in spermatogenic failure. Andrologia. 2007;39:190-5.
59. Stouffs K, Willems A, Lissens W, Tournaye H, Van Steirteghem A, Liebaers I. The role of the testis-specific gene hTAF7L in the aetiology of male infertility. Mol Hum Reprod. 2006;12:263-7.
60. Bhagavath B, Layman LC. The genetics of hypogonadotropic hypogonadism. Semin Reprod Med. 2007;25:272-86.

61. Downer, J. 2002. Epigenetics and imprinted genes. http://www.hopkinsmedicine.org/press/2002/November/epigenetics.htm.
62. Rawe VY, Terada Y, Nakamura S, Chillik CF, Brugo Olmedo S, Chemes HE. A pathology of the sperm centriole responsible for defective sperm aster formation, syngamy and cleavage. Hum Reprod. 2002;17:2344-9.
63. Lawrence LT, Moley KH. Epigenetics and assisted reproductive technologies: human imprinting syndromes. Semin Reprod Med. 2008;26:143-52.
64. Kobayashi H, Sato A, Otsu E, Hiura H, Tomatsu C, Utsunomiya T, et al. Aberrant DNA methylation of imprinted loci in sperm from oligospermic patients. Hum Mol Genet. 2007;16:2542-51.
65. Kimura Y, Yanagimachi R. Mouse oocytes injected with testicular spermatozoa or round spermatids can develop into normal offspring. Development. 1995;121:2397-405.
66. Maher ER, Brueton LA, Bowdin SC, Luharia A, Cooper W, Cole TR, et al. Beckwith–Wiedemann syndrome and assisted reproduction technology (ART). J Med Genet. 2003;40:62-4.
67. Practice Committee of American Society for Reproductive Medicine. The clinical utility of sperm DNA integrity testing. Fertil Steril. 2008;90:S178-80.
68. Matzuk MM, Lamb DJ. The biology of infertility: research advances and clinical challenges. Nat Med. 2008;14(11):1197-213.
69. Tartaglia NR, Howell S, Sutherland A, Wilson R, Wilson L. A review of trisomy X (47, XXX). Orphanet J Rare Dis. 2010;5:8.
70. Simpson JL, Rajkovic A. Ovarian differentiation and gonadal failure. Am J Med Genet. 1999;89(4):186-200.
71. Johansen ML, Hagen CP, Meyts ER, Kjærgaard S, Petersen BL, Skakkebæk NE, et al. 45,X/46,XY mosaicism: phenotypic characteristics, growth, and reproductive function—a retrospective longitudinal study. J Clin Endocrinol Metab. 2012;97(8):E1540-9.
72. Rosa RF, D'Ecclesiis WF, Dibbi RP, Rosa RC, Trevisan P, Graziadio C, et al. 45,X/46,XY mosaicism: report on 14 patients from a Brazilian hospital. A retrospective study. Sao Paulo Med J. 2014;132(6):332-8.
73. Telvi L, Lebbar A, Del Pino O, Barbet JP, Chaussain JL. 45,X/46,XY mosaicism: report of 27 cases. Pediatrics. 1999;104(2):304-8.
74. Talwar P. Manual of Cytogenetics in Reproductive Biology. New Delhi: Jaypee Brothers Medical Publishers (P) Ltd.; 2014.
75. Shchelochkov OA, Cooper ML, Ou Z, Peacock S, Yatsenko SA, Brown CW, et al. Mosaicism for r(X) and der(X) del(X)(p11.23) dup(X)(p11.21p11.22) provides insight into the possible mechanism of rearrangement. Mol Cytogenet. 2008;1:16.
76. Yip MY. Autosomal ring chromosomes in human genetic disorders. Transl Pediatr. 2015;4(2):164-74.
77. Lazer T, Friedler S. Gene deletions due to ring chromosome 16 are associated with low reproductive potential, a novel observation. Ann Gynecol Obstet. 2019;3(1):39-42.
78. Ledig S, Ropke A, Wieacker P. Copy number variants in premature ovarian failure and ovarian dysgenesis. Sex Dev. 2010;4(4-5):225-32.
79. Lubs HA. A marker X chromosome. Am J Hum Genet. 1969;21(3):231-44.
80. Coffee B, Keith K, Albizua I, Malone T, Mowrey J, Sherman SL, et al. Incidence of fragile X syndrome by newborn screening for methylated FMR1 DNA. Am J Hum Genet. 2009;85(4):503-14.
81. Sherman S, Pletcher BA, Driscoll DA. Fragile X syndrome: diagnostic and carrier testing. Genet Med. 2005;7(8):584-7.
82. Fridovich-Keil JL, Gubbels CS, Spencer JB, Sanders RD, Land JA, Rubio-Gozalbo E. Ovarian function in girls and women with GALT-deficiency galactosemia. N Engl J Med. 1981;304(17):994-8.
83. Cordts EB, Christofolini DM, Dos Santos AA, Bianco B, Barbosa CP. Genetic aspects of premature ovarian failure: a literature review. Arch Gynecol Obstet. 2011;283(3):635-43.
84. Treloar SA, Wicks J, Nyholt DR, Montgomery GW, Bahlo M, Smith V, et al. Genome wide linkage study in 1,176 affected sister pair families identifies a significant susceptibility locus for endometriosis on chromosome 10q26. Am J Hum Genet. 2005;77(3):365-76.
85. Uno S, Zembutsu H, Hirasawa A, Takahashi A, Kubo M, Akahane T, et al. A genome-wide association study identifies genetic variants in the CDKN2BAS locus associated with endometriosis in Japanese. Nat Genet. 2010;42(8):707-10.
86. Painter JN, Anderson CA, Nyholt DR, Macgregor S, Lin J, Lee SH, et al. Genome-wide association study identifies a locus at 7p15.2 associated with endometriosis. Nat Genet. 2011:43(1):51-4.
87. Chen ZJ, Zhao H, He L, Shi Y, Qin Y, Shi Y, et al. Genome-wide association study identifies susceptibility loci for polycystic ovary syndrome on chromosome 2p16.3, 2p21 1nd 9q33.3. Nat Genet. 2011;43(1):55-9.
88. Stewart EA, Morton CC. The genetics of uterine leiomyomata: what clinicians need to know. Obstet Gynecol. 2006;107(4):917-21.
89. Pedeutour F, Ligon AH, Morton CC. Génétiques des léiomyomes utérines [Genetics of uterine leiomyomata]. Bull Cancer. 1999;86(11):920-8. French. PMID: 10586108.
90. Styer AK, Rueda BR. The epidemiology and genetics of uterine leiomyoma. Best Pract Res Clin Obstet Gynaecol. 2016;34:3-12.
91. Taylor HS. The role of EMX 2 in uterine development. Fertil Steril. 2016;103(3):633-4.
92. Ramaraju GA, Cheemakurthi R, Prathigudupu K, Balabomma KL, Kalagara M, Thota S, et al. Role of LH polymorphisms and r-hLH supplementation in GnRH agonist treated cycles: a cross sectional study. Eur J Obstet Gynecol Reprod Biol. 2018;222:119-25.

CHAPTER

19 Obesity and Infertility

Nupur Garg

"Take care of your body it is the only place that you have to live."

—**Jim Rohn**

INTRODUCTION

There has been a rising trend in obesity and overweight population in the past few years which has become an epidemic worldwide. According to the recent World Health Organization (WHO) global estimates, the worldwide prevalence of obesity has nearly tripled between 1975 and 2016.[1] In 2016, more than 1.9 billion adults aged 18 years and older were overweight. Of these, over 650 million adults were obese. Almost half of the children under 5 years of age who were overweight or obese in 2019 lived in Asia. Obesity has become a pandemic because of the changes in lifestyle resulting in a more obesogenic environment (inexpensive calorie-dense food, reduced physical activity, and inexpensive nonphysical entertainment). Genetics has also been implicated as a possible cofactor.[2,3] Women are affected most due to their small size and extra weight which is gained with each pregnancy.

Obesity has adverse effects on all systems, including reproductive health. It leads to increased health risks such as diabetes mellitus, hypertension, coronary heart disease, and osteoarthritis and is associated with various malignancies, particularly endometrium, breast, and colon cancers. Obesity also plays a significant role in reproductive disorders, particularly in women. It is associated with anovulation, menstrual disorders, infertility, difficulties in assisted reproduction, miscarriage, and adverse pregnancy outcomes.

OBESITY AND IMPAIRED REPRODUCTIVE POTENTIAL

Hippocrates recognized the adverse effect obesity has on fertility and wrote that "*People* of *such constitution cannot* be *prolific* ... *fatness* and *flabbiness* are to *blame*. The *womb* is *unable* to *receive* the *semen* and *they menstruate infrequently* and *little*."[4]

Several studies have shown a lower fertility in overweight and obese women. A Dutch study prospectively evaluated the effect obesity has on fecundity and found that an increase in waist-hip ratio (WHR) by 0.1 unit led to a decrease in the probability of conception by 30% per cycle.[5] Similarly, a health study in nurses comparing 2,527 married nulliparous women with anovulatory subfertility with 46,718 married multiparous women determined the relative risk of infertility for each body mass index (BMI) category found that above a BMI of 23.9, there is a significantly high risk of subfertility.[6]

Obese women suffer from menstrual cycle disturbances and anovulation more often than nonobese women. Menstrual cycle disturbance was found to be 3.1 times more common in obese than in normal-weight women.[7] Negative effect of excess fat was reinforced by the fact that weight-loss programs led to the resumption of normal menstrual cyclicity, normal ovulation, and natural pregnancies.[8]

Obese women are also found to have increased chances of miscarriages following natural conception, ovulation induction, and assisted conception. A recent meta-analysis found an increased risk of miscarriage among women (BMI 30 kg/m^2) undergoing assisted conception [in vitro fertilization (IVF)/intracytoplasmic sperm injection (ICSI)].[9] A further meta-analysis also found that patients with a BMI of 25 kg/m^2 were found to have a significantly elevated odds of miscarriage regardless of the mode of conception.[10]

FERTILITY RISKS IN OBESITY

Obesity is associated with greater risks for adverse health outcomes across the reproductive spectrum:[11-19]

- Higher rates of infertility[12]
- Subfertility (increased time to pregnancy)[13]

- Early pregnancy loss[10,14,15]
- Fetal deaths, stillbirths, and neonatal deaths[15]
- Congenital anomalies[16]
- Pregnancy complication[17]
- Greater risk of cesarean delivery and poor wound healing[18]
- Increased difficulty and shorter duration of breastfeeding.[19]

DIAGNOSIS AND CLASSIFICATION OF OBESITY

Obesity is defined as the condition of excess body fat that negatively impacts the health. As excess fat is the main variable that defines obesity, diagnosis of obesity requires measurement of body fat. There are several methods available to assess body fat.

Methods of Assessment of Body Fat

Body Mass Index

- The most widely accepted measure of obesity is the BMI [weight (kg)/height (m^2)] with cutoff points of 25 kg/m^2 (overweight) and 30 kg/m^2 (obese), as recommended by the National Heart, Lung, and Blood Institute's North American Association for the Study of Obesity expert committee.[20]
- BMI cutoff points are generated to predict health risks associated with increasing BMI.
- BMI is useful but a crude indicator of obesity. It does not distinguish dangerous adiposity (such as waistline intra-abdominal fat) from potentially less harmful fat in other areas of the body or healthy "nonfat" body mass such as muscle.
- In South Asians, body fat is more centralized with mean WHR being higher for a given level of BMI compared to Europeans.[21] Among Asians, morbidity and mortality were found to be occurring at lower BMI compared to Europeans[22,23] and hence BMI cutoffs have been redefined in Asian population with cutoff for overweight >23 kg/m^2 and obesity >25 kg/m^2 **(Table 1)**.

Distribution of Fat

- Fat deposition in abdominal or visceral region is important clinically as it plays the most significant role in the pathogenesis of metabolic syndrome.
- Visceral adipose tissue can be measured with the help of magnetic resonance imaging (MRI), computed tomography (CT) scan, and dual-energy X-ray absorptiometry (DEXA) performed at the level of L3/L4 and visceral fat area is calculated **(Fig. 1)**. An area >130 cm^2 has been associated with increased risk, whereas an area <110 cm^2 has been associated with low risk.

Waist Circumference Measurement

- Simple clinical measurement of visceral fat is waist circumference. WHO recommendations for the measurement of waist circumference involve the subject standing with feet 25–30 cm apart, weight evenly

TABLE 1: Comparison of body mass index (BMI) among European and Asian populations with respect to cardiovascular risk [World Health Organization (WHO), 2000].

Classification	*WHO BMI (kg/m²)*	*Asian BMI (kg/m²)*	*Cardiovascular risk*
Underweight	<18.5	<18.5	Low
Normal range	18.5–24.9	18.5–22.9	Average
Overweight	25–29.9	23–24.9	Increased
Obese I	30–34.9	25–29.9	Moderate
Obese II	35–39.9	= 30	Severe
Obese III	= 40		Very severe

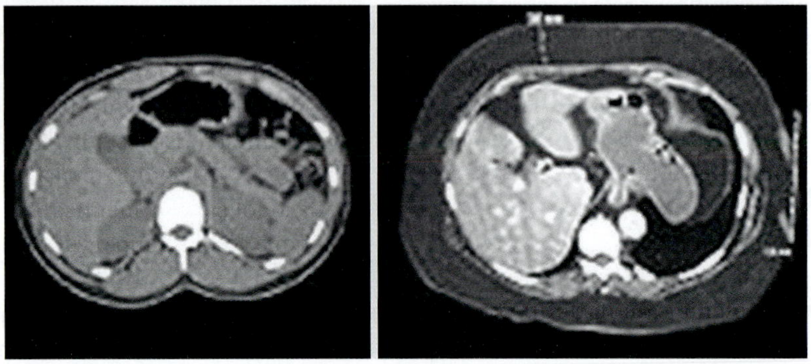

Fig. 1: Cross-sections of lumbar region of a normal-weight (left) and an obese person (right), taken by computed tomography (CT) scan. Note the increased thickness of subcutaneous fat of the obese person.

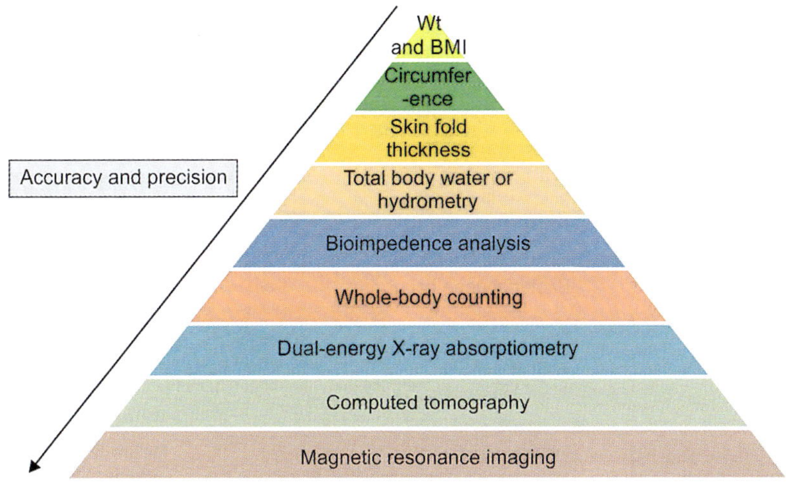

Fig. 2: Techniques in body composition.
(BMI: body mass index; Wt: weight)

distributed, and measurement taken midway between the inferior margin of the last rib and the crest of ilium in a horizontal plane. For hip circumference, measurement is taken around the pelvis at the level of maximum protrusion of the buttocks.[24]

- Waist circumference cutoff for increased risk of metabolic disease in Americans has been found to be ≥102 cm in men and ≥88 cm in women. The cutoff for waist circumference in Asians is ≥90 cm in men and ≥80 cm in women.[25]

Waist–hip Ratio

Waist–hip ratio is also used to measure abdominal obesity. In Caucasians, a WHR >1 for men and WHR >0.85 for women are used as a measurement of visceral adiposity.[26] However, waist circumference is preferred over WHR for measuring abdominal obesity.[27]

CONCEPT OF NORMAL-WEIGHT OBESITY

Excessive body fat despite normal body weight has been described as normal-weight obesity (NWO) syndrome.[28] NWO is a condition in which a person has an adequate BMI but an increased body fat percentage and a greater risk of developing noncommunicable chronic diseases. It is important to accurately diagnose individuals with excess body fat using more precise parameters other than BMI **(Fig. 2)**.

PATHOPHYSIOLOGY OF OBESITY

In Utero Programing

Barker's Hypothesis: Fetal Origin of Adult-onset Diseases

- Undernutrition and unfavorable intrauterine environment during early life can cause irreversible changes (in both structure and function) in developing systems of the fetus (i.e., programing).

Flowchart 1: Fetal origin of obesity.

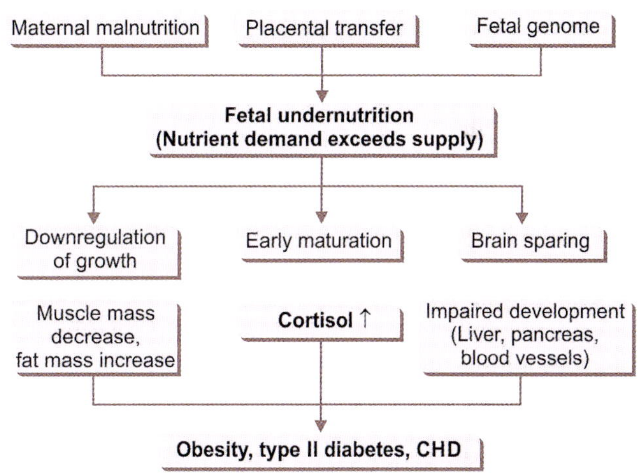

(CHD: congenital heart disease)

- This may present as a disease over a period of time due to "dysadaptation" with changed environmental circumstances **(Flowchart 1)**.[29]
- Research has found that children born small for gestation tend to develop adiposity and hyperinsulinemia.[30] Precocious puberty (appearance of pubic hair before 8 years of age) has also been demonstrated as a part of this sequence, as well as anovulatory and hyperinsulinemic hyperandrogenism in late adolescence and adulthood.[31]

ROLE OF GUT MICROBIOME IN ORIGIN OF OBESITY

The gut microbiome is now recognized as a separate endocrine system and is involved in the body's homeostatic process. A diet loaded with excess fat increases gut permeability, resulting in increased levels of lipopolysaccharides

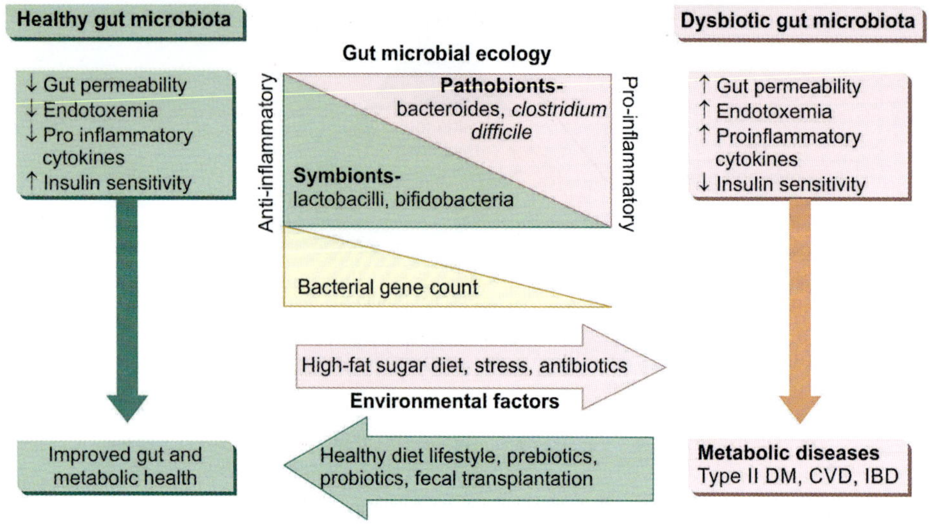

Fig. 3: Effects of a healthy gut microbiota and dysbiosis on the gut and metabolic health of the host. (CVD: cardiovascular diseases; DM: diabetes mellitus; IBD: inflammatory bowel disease)

in the body's systemic circulation. Lipopolysaccharides are endotoxins that are linked to inflammation-related processes such as obesity and insulin resistance.[32] Altered gut microbiome influences gut epithelium and motility, leading to the extraction of more calories from food, increased calorie absorption, and fat storage. Gut microbiota also affects many other regulatory processes in the body, such as mitochondrial fatty acid oxidation, ketogenesis, glucose uptake/insulin sensitivity, insulin secretion, increased lipogenesis, and cholesterol and triglyceride synthesis.[32] These processes all contribute to metabolic disease and obesity **(Fig. 3)**.

ENDOCRINE FUNCTION OF ADIPOSE TISSUE—THE ROLE OF ADIPOKINES

- Adipose tissue is a highly developed, endocrine and paracrine organ, which produces a variety of adipokines such as leptin, adiponectin, resistin, visfatin, omentin, ghrelin, and inflammatory cytokines such as tumor necrosis factor alpha (TNF-α), interleukin 6 (IL-6), and monocyte chemoattractant protein 1 (MCP-1). Adipokines are cytokines mainly secreted by adipocytes.
- Adipokines function as signaling molecules (hormones), and any abnormality in adipokines can cause inflammation and abnormal cell signaling which in turn can negatively affect cell metabolism and function **(Fig. 4)**.[33]
- The changes in body mass affect the levels of these adipokines. The direct effect of these adipokines on reproductive function during obesity has not been proven definitely, although they act indirectly by disturbing other regulatory systems. It has been seen that an excess or deficiency of adipose tissue results in sexual maturation disorders, pubertal disorders, and fertility disorder.[34]

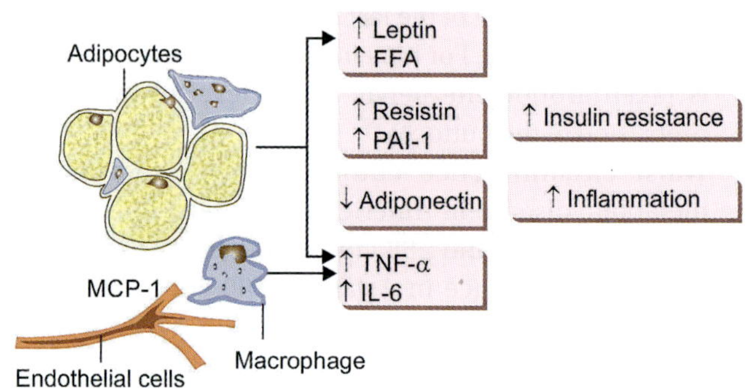

Fig. 4: In obesity, adipocytes release MCP-1, which attracts macrophages into the adipose tissue, which further increases the production of proinflammatory adipokine (TNF-α) and decreases adiponectin production, resulting in insulin resistance and inflammation.[35] (FFA: free fatty acid; IL-6: interleukin 6; MCP-1: monocyte chemoattractant protein 1; PAI-1: plasminogen activator inhibitor 1; TNF-α: tumor necrosis factor alpha)

Physiological Role of Adipokines

Leptin

- Adipokine that has been most studied and identified in more than 30 biochemical products secreted by adipocytes is leptin. Leptin is a peptide hormone with 167 amino acids and a molecular weight of 16 kDa and is synthesized from the "*ob*" gene in adipocytes. Its secretion is pulsatile, which increases with food intake and decreases during starvation. It thus reduces food intake and maintains energy homeostasis.
- It is a key signaling protein, relays the magnitude of the peripheral energy stores to the brain (hypothalamus), and also has metabolic and reproductive functions. Leptin has varied effects on reproduction and the target organs include hypothalamus, ovary, and endometrium.
- In the hypothalamic-pituitary axis, leptin has a stimulatory effect.[36] It has been hypothesized that an

elevated leptin level beyond a certain threshold is required for the activation of the hypothalamic–pituitary axis and the onset of puberty. The nutritional level of a person influences this central effect, with fasting causing a decrease in leptin levels resulting in the inactivation of gonadotropin-releasing hormone (GnRH) pulsatility. On the contrary, in well-fed state or energy-positive state also, no effect on GnRH secretion is seen due to the development of central leptin resistance leading to dysregulatory state in obesity.

- Leptin also influences steroidogenesis and folliculogenesis in ovarian cells. It modulates the stimulatory actions of gonadotropins and regulates perifollicular blood flow by promoting endothelial cell proliferation and angiogenesis.[37] Leptin also regulates the levels of reproductive hormones such as progesterone during the menstrual cycle and estradiol and human chorionic gonadotropin (hCG) during pregnancy.[38]
- Studies have shown that leptin may also affect oocyte maturation and early embryo development.[39] The endometrium and developing placenta express both leptin and its receptor[40] suggesting a possible role in the implantation of embryo and fetal growth.
- Leptin is produced in increased amounts with increasing adipose tissue. With high leptin levels as seen in obesity, a dysfunctional energetic state occurs suggesting a possible development of leptin resistance and altered leptin receptor sensitivity. This adversely affects leptin-mediated actions in the reproductive system and fertility.

Different adipokines and their effects on obesity are summarized in **Table 2**.

TABLE 2: Effects of the adipokines on reproduction.

Adipokines	*Serum levels in obesity*	*Effect in obesity*
Leptin[41]	Increase	• Dysregulation of GnRH secretion • Altered ovarian steroidogenesis • Dysregulation of folliculogenesis and perifollicular blood flow
Adiponectin[42]	Decrease	• Increased insulin resistance • Interference with folliculogenesis • Modulation of sex steroid secretion
IL-6[43]	Increase	• Increased insulin resistance • Impaired LH secretion • Impaired response to LH • Impaired estrogen secretion
PAI-1[44]	Increase	• Increased PAI-1 directly correlate with the development of metabolic syndrome • Increased miscarriage risk
TNF-α[45]	Increase	• Reduced insulin sensitivity • Inhibition of gonadotropin secretion • Impaired steroidogenesis • Induces corpus luteum regression • Impaired endometrial development

(GnRH: gonadotropin-releasing hormone; IL-6: interleukin 6; LH: luteinizing hormone; PAI-1: plasminogen activator inhibitor 1; TNF: tumor necrosis factor)

Pathophysiology of obesity and female fertility may be considered at the following levels:

- Central effects on the hypothalamus and pituitary
- Peripheral effects on the ovary and oocyte
- Direct effects on the embryo
- Effects on the endometrium
- Effects on pregnancy.

Effect of Obesity on Hypothalamus and Pituitary

- Obese women have higher circulating levels of free fatty acids, which stimulate increased insulin release and also lead to insulin resistance which together combined lead to hyperinsulinemia.[46]
- The ovary is a target organ for insulin action via both insulin receptor and insulin-like growth factor 1 (IGF-1) receptor. Hyperinsulinemia, as seen in obesity, stimulates androgen production from the ovary directly by activating ovarian theca cells or indirectly by suppressing the synthesis of sex hormone-binding globulin (SHBG) from liver which in turn leads to increased free androgen levels. It also decreases the synthesis of IGF-binding proteins 1 and 2 in liver leading to high free IGF-1 levels which in turn stimulates androgen synthesis from adrenals and ovarian theca cells.[47]
- Raised androgen is aromatized to estrogen at increasing rates in the periphery owing to excess adipose tissue. This leads to negative feedback on the hypothalamic–pituitary–ovarian (HPO) axis and affects gonadotropin production[48] **(Flowchart 2)**. This manifests as *menstrual abnormalities* and *ovulatory dysfunction*.

Furthermore, in obesity, there is altered hypothalamic leptin receptor expression.[49] An increased neuropeptide-Y level is seen in the hypothalamus, leading to reduced central leptin sensitivity and decreased GnRH pulsatility.

Effect of Obesity on Ovary and Oocyte Quality

Ovarian responsiveness to gonadotropins is impaired in obese women. Possible reasons suggested are as follows:

- Altered follicular environment with high levels of triglycerides, insulin, and inflammatory markers such as C-reactive protein (CRP)[50]
- Elevated follicular leptin levels have an inhibitory effect on follicle-stimulating hormone (FSH).[51]
- Insulin resistance has been associated with a relative gonadotropin resistance.[52]
- Altered pharmacodynamics of gonadotropins though suggested has not been found to be responsible for increased dose requirement in obese women.[53]

Flowchart 2: Obesity leading to dysregulation of hypothalamic–pituitary–ovarian axis.

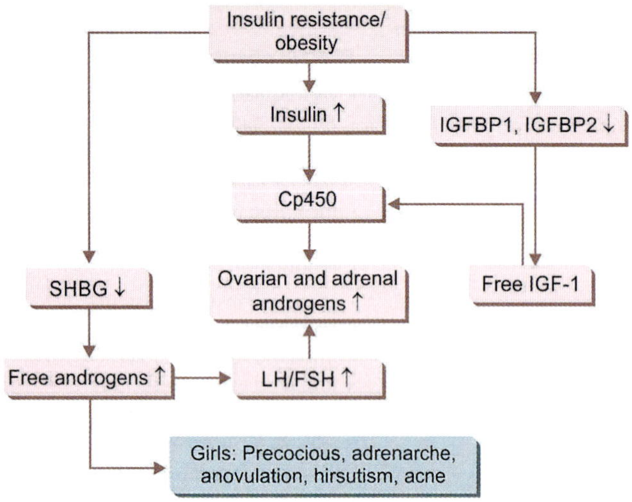

(FSH: follicle-stimulating hormone; IGF: insulin-like growth factor; IGFBP1: insulin-like growth factor-binding protein 1; LH: luteinizing hormone; SHBG: sex hormone-binding globulin)

- Animal studies have shown that obesity affects oocyte quality resulting in more number of aneuploid oocytes, apoptotic follicles, and intracellular organelle damage.[54] The mechanism suggested has been lipotoxicity, which generates reactive oxygen species leading to disarrayed meiotic spindles, mitochondrial and endoplasmic reticulum stress, and apoptosis.[55,56]

Effect on Embryo

- Embryos may also be susceptible to lipotoxicity as previously discussed regarding the oocyte.
- There occurs an imbalance between omega 3 and omega 6 fatty acids required for the normal development of embryo resulting in poor blastocyst rates with fewer cells in the trophectoderm with poor glucose uptake and high levels of triglycerides resulting in poor pregnancy rate.[57,58]
- The metabolomic profile of spent culture media of day 3 embryos from obese women has shown significant reductions in the concentration of saturated fatty acids compared to normal-weight women.[59]
- In addition, hyperleptinemia exerts a direct negative effect on the developing embryo.[60]

Effect on Endometrium

The histopathological and molecular effect of obesity on the endometrium remains to be fully elucidated. Studies have shown poor implantation rates in obese women.

Possible mechanisms suggested for compromised endometrial receptivity and poor implantation rates are as follows:

- Low leukemia inhibitory factor (LIF) levels in endometrium[61]
- Relative hyperestrogenemia is found to be detrimental to endometrial receptivity.[62]
- Elevated insulin levels have been associated with a reduced glycodelin and insulin-like growth factor-binding protein 1 (IGFBP1).[63]
- Elevated levels of acute-phase proteins and proinflammatory cytokines [including IL-6, plasminogen activator inhibitor 1 (PAI-1) and TNF-α]; these inflammatory markers are thought to exert a negative effect upon implantation and early embryonic development.[63]
- Altered endometrial gene expression.[64]

Animal studies have shown:

- Poor endometrial decidualization in obese mice[65]
- Decreased implantation sites[65]
- Decreased response to hormonal stimulation in the endometrial stromal cells[65]
- Poor embryo-endometrial crosstalk, as embryo quality also suffers in obesity
- Dysregulation of leptin expression in endometrium.[66]

Pathophysiology of obesity and its effect on fertility has been summarized in **Flowchart 3**.

Effect on Pregnancy

Decidualization and implantation defects may negatively affect the placentation process. Many of the pregnancy complications seen in obese women are linked to placental dysfunction, including stillbirth and pregnancy-induced hypertension. All the causes listed above may result in poor implantation, placentation, and adverse pregnancy outcomes **(Flowchart 4)**. A recent meta-analysis has confirmed increased odds of maternal, fetal, and neonatal complications in pregnant obese mothers compared with standard BMI mothers.[67]

OBESITY AND POLYCYSTIC OVARY SYNDROME

Obese women with polycystic ovary syndrome (PCOS) have a more severe phenotype and had a higher prevalence (78%) of:

- Disturbed menstrual cyclicity[68]
- Increased insulin resistance[69]
- Impaired response to gonadotropin during superovulation[70]
- Increased chance of cycle cancellation
- Reduced ovulation rates
- Reduced chance of treatment success following assisted reproductive technology (ART)[71]
- Increased risk of miscarriage.[71]

OBESITY AND ASSISTED CONCEPTION

The majority of the studies suggest that obesity has a deleterious effect on ART. Obesity has been reported to affect ovarian stimulation in women undergoing treatment.

Flowchart 3: Pathophysiology of obesity and its effect on fertility.

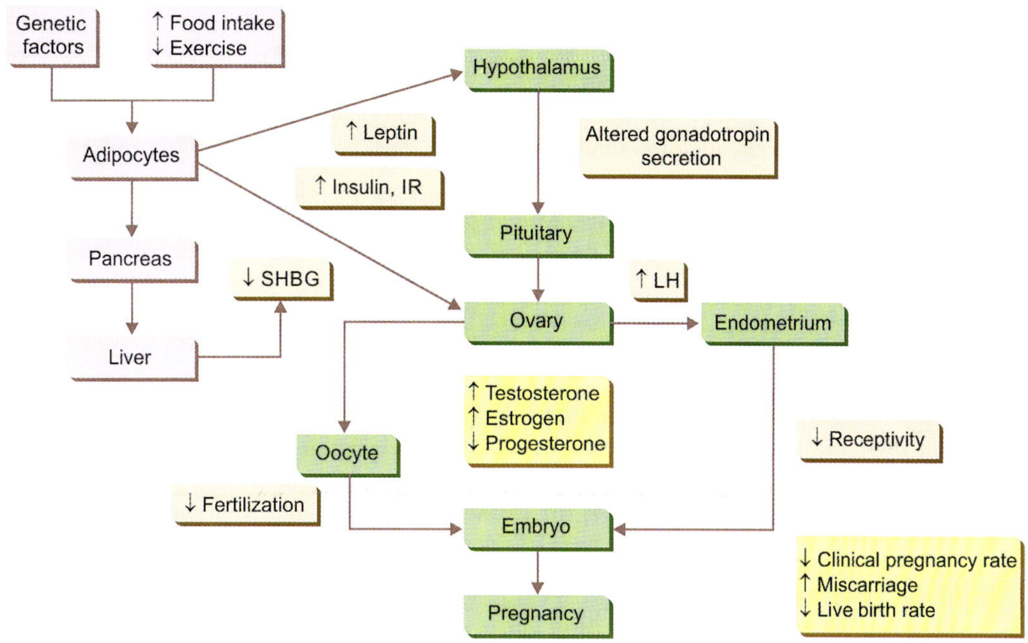

(IR: insulin resistance; LH: luteinizing hormone; SHBG: sex hormone-binding globulin)

Flowchart 4: Possible causes of miscarriages in obese women.

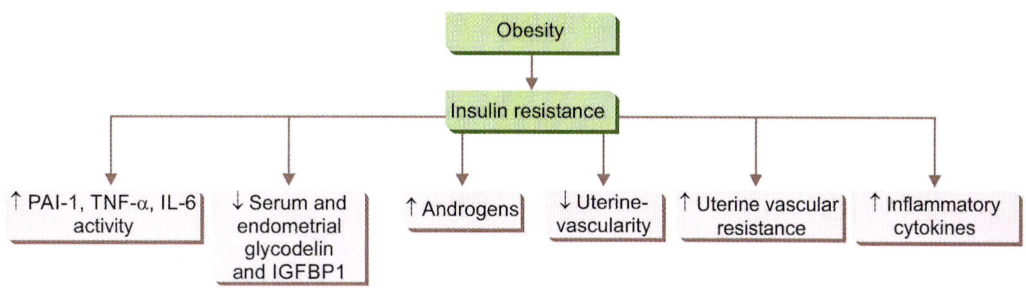

(IGFBP1: insulin-like growth factor-binding protein 1; IL-6: interleukin 6; PAI-1: plasminogen activator inhibitor 1; TNF-α: tumor necrosis factor alpha)

RESPONSE TO GONADOTROPIN STIMULATION AND CYCLE CANCELLATION

- Obesity impairs ovarian responsiveness to gonadotropin stimulation, requiring higher dosages and longer stimulation, and fewer mature follicles are obtained.[72-74] Several studies have documented a higher risk of cycle cancellation with increasing maternal BMI, with adjusted odds ratios (ORs) for women with BMI > 40 kg/m^2 compared with normal-weight women ranging from 2.73 [95% confidence interval (CI) 1.49–5.00] to 3.46 (95% CI 1.85–6.49).[71]
- In a cohort study of women with PCOS undergoing ovulation induction with either clomiphene or gonadotropins, it was observed that elevated BMI negatively affected ovulation rates. In this study,[75] obese patients had significantly lower ovulation rates at 6 months of treatment: 79% in women with a BMI of 18–24 kg/m^2 compared with 15.3% with a BMI of 30–34 kg/m^2 and 12% if BMI is 35 kg/m^2. Some authors, however, have been unable to demonstrate any difference in ovarian response to stimulation in obese women.[76,77]

Fertilization Rates

Obesity alters oocyte morphology,[78] reduces fertilization in some[79] but not all[78,80] studies, and impairs embryo quality in women less than 35 years of age.[80]

Implantation and Pregnancy Rates (Embryo vs. Endometrium)

- A national study of ART in the United States reported reduced clinical pregnancy rates with increasing BMIs with the use of autologous but not donor oocytes and reduced live birth rates with increasing BMIs regardless of oocyte source and embryo status.[81] Even studies limited to obese women using donor oocytes and eliminating the potential effect of older maternal age and lower quality of the embryos have reported significantly reduced implantation and pregnancy rates and higher abortion rates.[82] This suggests that oocyte quality is a primary, but not the only factor impairing IVF outcomes in obese women using autologous oocytes.

- Obesity also appears to alter endometrial receptivity during IVF since third-party surrogate women with a BMI >35 kg/m^2 have a lower live birth rate (25%) compared with those with a BMI <35 kg/m^2.[83]

Miscarriage Rate

- Obesity has been linked with increased pregnancy loss in many[84,85] except few studies.[86] A meta-analysis in 2008 of both spontaneous and assisted reproductive conception showed that women with a BMI >25 kg/m^2 had a significantly higher risk of miscarriage at <20 weeks of gestation, with an OR of 1.67.[87]
- A meta-analysis of 33 IVF studies including 47,967 cycles concluded that overweight or obese women have a higher rate of miscarriage compared with normal-weight women (BMI <25 kg/m^2).[84]
- In women with a history of recurrent pregnancy loss (RPL), obesity is a known risk factor for miscarriage in a subsequent pregnancy.[88]
- A chromosomal analysis of 117 miscarriage specimens from patients with RPL demonstrated that obese women had a much higher rate of euploid miscarriage, again suggesting a potential independent effect of obesity on the endometrium.[89]

Live Birth Rate

Obese women undergoing IVF/ICSI have lower live birth rates. It is thought that this is the cumulative effect of lower implantation and pregnancy rates, higher miscarriage rates, and increased obstetric complications.[90] Some authors have reported lower pregnancy and live birth rates in obese women undergoing assisted conception treatments.[91-93]

Others have been unable to demonstrate a reduction in success rates in obese women.[77,94]

Technical Difficulties During In Vitro Fertilization

Obese women are significantly more likely to encounter difficulty in observing the air bubble during ultrasound-guided embryo transfer and are more likely to have blood on or in the catheter after embryo transfer.[77] The effect of obesity in ART has been summarized in **Box 1**.

BOX 1: Summary of effects of obesity on assisted reproductive technology.

Effect of obesity on ART
- Impaired USS image quality due to adipose tissue[77]
- Increased duration of stimulation
- Increased total gonadotropin dose required[70]
- Increased follicular asynchrony[70]
- Increased cycle cancellation[70]
- Poor response to superovulation[75]
- Reduced follicular hCG concentration on the day of ovum pickup[95]
- Relative reduction in the number of cumulus–oocyte complex recovered at ovum pickup[9]
- Relative reduction in metaphase II oocytes recovered at ovum pickup[9]
- Relative number of surplus good quality embryos available for cryopreservation[80]
- Reduced pregnancy rates[9]
- Increased miscarriage rates[90]

(ART: assisted reproductive technology; hCG: human chorionic gonadotropin; USS: ultrasound scan)

OBESITY AND MALE INFERTILITY

- Obesity has a negative effect on male fertility. In 2006, Sallmen et al. illustrated a dose–response relationship between BMI and male infertility, with worsening male fertility for every three-point increase in BMI >25 kg/m^2, with an OR[96] of 1.12. These results were later confirmed in several other studies.[97,98]
- The mechanism suggested for the effect of obesity on male fertility includes thermal effects, hyperestrogenism, hypogonadotropic hypogonadism, diabetes mellitus, sexual dysfunction, and sperm epigenetic perturbations.

Sperm Parameters

The impact of obesity on sperm parameters is complex and likely multifactorial. Obese men are at a higher risk of:

- Oligozoospermia[99,100]
- Decreased total progressive motility[100]
- Raised deoxyribonucleic acid (DNA) fragmentation index.[101]

The mechanisms suggested are as follows **(Flowchart 5)**:

- Obesity is associated with the risk of diabetes and insulin resistance. Hyperinsulinemia leads to a reduction of sex hormone-binding globulin levels. This allows greater free testosterone levels, which aromatizes to estrogen in the periphery.[102] This hyperestrogenemic state has a detrimental effect on the androgen axis affecting semen quality.
- Hyperestrogenemia downregulates the release of kisspeptin from kisspeptin neurons and decreases the activity of hypothalamic–pituitary–gonadal (HPG) axis by negative feedback and thus of FSH and luteinizing hormone (LH).[103]
- Leptin resistance seen in obese men with hyperleptinemia results in the failure of leptin to stimulate HPG axis.[104]
- Sleep apnea is commonly found in obese men. Nocturnal sleep disturbances affect nocturnal LH pulsatility

Flowchart 5: Hormonal pathway responsible for male infertility.

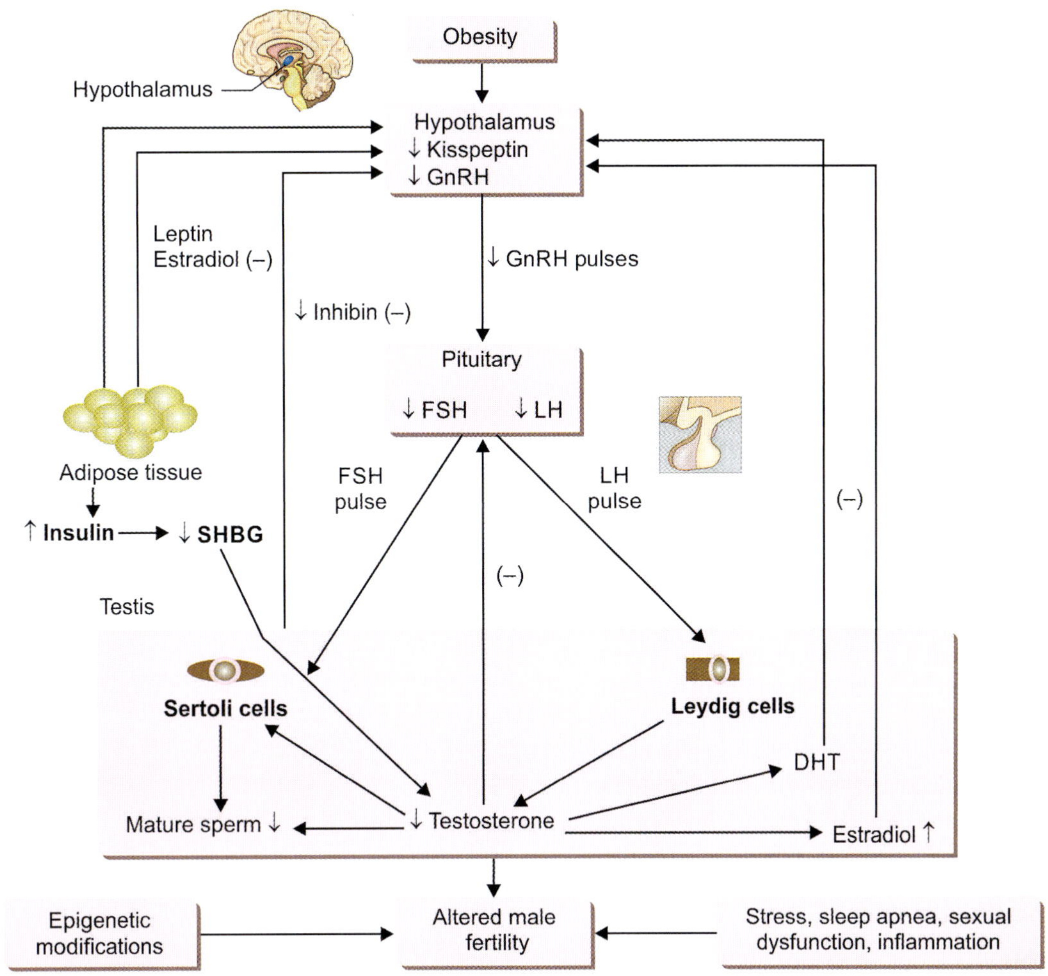

(DHT: dihydrotestosterone; FSH: follicle-stimulating hormone; GnRH: gonadotropin-releasing hormone; LH: luteinizing hormone; SHBG: sex hormone-binding globulin)

reducing testosterone levels. Intermittent hypoxia associated with sleep apnea can affect gene expression, sperm motility, and fertility.[105]

- Many environmental toxins are fat-soluble favoring adipose tissue for their accumulation making obese men susceptible to perturbation of the male endocrine axis and spermatogenesis.[106]
- Increased lower abdominal and thigh fat leads to increased testicular temperature. This negatively impacts both testosterone synthesis and spermatogenesis.[107]
- Obese men often suffer from sexual dysfunction resulting from decreased testosterone levels and vascular endothelial dysfunction secondary to inflammation.[108]
- Obesity alters fertility by affecting the epigenetic patterns of sperm, that is, sperm micro-RNA content and DNA methylation variations. These important markers in sperm, when altered, are thought to be implicated in abnormal phenotypes in the offspring and perturbations in embryogenesis.[109]

Male Obesity and Advanced Reproductive Technology Outcome

- The impact of male obesity on ART outcome is conflicting. Some studies suggest that obese men undergoing ART have a statistically significant decrease in live birth rate compared with normal-weight men.[110] Another study has reported a lower pregnancy rate in males undergoing IVF, but no significant difference if ICSI was used for ART therapy. In contrast, Thomsen et al. have reported no decrease in semen quality or IVF outcome in obese men undergoing ART.[111] Further research is required to assess the exact impact of male obesity on ART outcome.
- Despite the associations between obesity and semen parameters, it is clear that men with high levels of body fat are, in general, still capable of siring offspring, which may be accounted by the fact that in some cases lower maternal age results in improved oocyte quality, which may independently improve outcomes but may also

provide an improved opportunity for correction of some defects, such as sperm epigenetic abnormalities, after fertilization.[112]

Management

Lifestyle Modification

Weight management can be achieved through a lifestyle modification program that combines dietary modification, physical activity, and behavioral interventions, including psychological, behavioral, and stress management strategies.[113] Current recommendations for lifestyle modification for obesity include a weight loss of 7% of body weight and increased physical activity to at least 150 minutes weekly of moderate activity such as walking.[114]

Diet and Weight Loss

Calorie restriction is the mainstay of successful weight loss.[115] Calorie restriction of up to 500–1,000 kcal/day from daily dietary intake leads to a weight loss of 0.5–1 kg weight loss per week. Dietary composition plays a less important role in weight loss. Though few authors have published about "fertility diets," characterized by low content of trans fats and animal protein and more of low-glycemic carbohydrates, high-fat dairy, and multivitamins.[116-119] Similarly few observational studies have suggested the potential benefits of the Mediterranean diet, and found a lower risk of infertility and increased chances of pregnancy on adhering to the diet.[120]

Exercise and Weight Loss

Physical activity alone is less effective in producing weight loss. The addition of physical activity on top of a diet modification enhances weight loss.[121]

Studies examining the effect of physical activity on obese infertile population independent of weight loss have shown improved fertility. A recent study reported more than threefold higher pregnancy and live birth rates in obese women who exercised regularly compared with obese women who were not physically active.[122] Because exercise reduces the oxidative stress characteristic of overweight and obesity, it may represent the best therapy currently available.

Exercise Programs

At present, there are no evidence-based guidelines on exercise training programs to improve fertility. The following is the recommended framework for prescribing aerobic exercises to people who are overweight and obese[123] **(Table 3)**.

Patients starting a program of moderate exercise (e.g., walking) do not require prescreening, whereas those starting vigorous-intensity programs should be screened for cardiovascular and respiratory adequacy.

Drugs for Weight Loss

Few medicines are available for the treatment of obesity. Examples of the Food and Drug Administration (FDA)-approved drugs that may be considered for the long-term treatment of obesity include orlistat, lorcaserin, the combinations of phentermine and extended-release topiramate, and the fixed-dose combination of bupropion and naltrexone **(Table 4)**. According to Endocrine Society Guidelines, pharmacotherapy for weight loss is indicated in patients with a BMI ≥30 kg/m^2 or ≥ 27 kg/m^2 along with associated comorbidities (e.g., diabetes, hypertension).[124] Drugs for weight loss are indicated in addition to caloric restriction and increased physical activity. The patient should be reassessed by week 12. If a patient fails to lose at least 5% of baseline body weight, drugs should be discontinued, as it is unlikely that the patient will achieve and sustain clinically meaningful weight loss with continued treatment.

Weight-loss medications target important neurotransmitters involved in feeding behavior.[125]

Neurotransmitters govern the body's response to starvation and dietary intake.

- *Norepinephrine and dopamine:* Released by sympathetic nervous system in response to food intake. Fasting and starvation lead to decreased levels of these neurotransmitters.

TABLE 3: Recommended exercise program for weight loss in obese.

	Recommendations
Frequency	≥5 days per week
Intensity	• Moderate to vigorous intensity • If body mass index (BMI) >35 kg/m^2, vigorous intensity is not appropriate • Gradual shift to vigorous intensity after an initial 4–12-week period of moderate-intensity activity
Time	The ultimate minimum goal should be to achieve 30–60 minutes of continuous aerobic exercise 5–7 times per week
Type	• *Aerobic isotonic exercise* is of the greatest value for persons who are obese • *Brisk walking*: Ideal for obese, sedentary individuals constitute moderate-intensity physical activity • *Cycling, swimming, water aerobics*: Ideal for BMI >35 kg/m^2 and joint problems constitute moderate-intensity physical activity • *Anaerobic isotonic exercises*, e.g., weight lifting and resistance training can be cautiously added as an adjunct after the aerobic goal described above is achieved • Not indicated for patients with hypertension and heart diseases

TABLE 4: Mechanism of action of Food and Drug Administration (FDA)-approved drugs for weight loss.[126]

Drug	*Mechanism of action*	*Dosage*	*Side effects*	*Comments*
Orlistat	Pancreatic lipase inhibitor	120 mg b.d.	Flatulence, fecal urgency, fecal incontinence, steatorrhea	• Reduce absorption of fat-soluble vitamins • Recommended for patients with cardiovascular disease
Bupropion–naltrexone	Dopamine-NE reuptake inhibitor/ opioid receptor antagonist	360 mg/32 mg	Constipation, headache, nausea, insomnia, tremors	Weight loss: 1-year: 5%
Lorcaserin	Selective serotonin 2c receptor agonist	10 mg b.d.	Dry mouth, constipation, headache, dizziness, nausea, fatigue	Weight loss: 1-year: 5–6%
Phentermine–topiramate	Norepinephrine-releasing/Na^+ GABA modulating agent	18.5–37.5 mg/96–192 mg	• Hypertension, palpitations, tachyarrhythmia • Insomnia, dry mouth, constipation, depression, anxiety	• CI: Hypertension, glaucoma • Hyperthyroid • Weight loss: 1-year: 5–11%
Liraglutide	GLP-1 receptor agonist	3 mg s.c. daily	Nausea, vomiting, risk of pancreatitis	Recommended for patients with cardiovascular disease

(CI: contraindicated; GABA: γ-aminobutyric acid; GLP-1: glucagon-like peptide 1; NE: norepinephrine)

- *Serotonin:* Low serotonin levels and high neuropeptide Y levels are associated with a craving for carbohydrate food.
- *Proopiomelanocortin* (POMC): Integrates multiple energy signals. Increased firing leads to the release of norepinephrine and dopamine and weight loss.
- β*-Endorphins:* Endogenous opioid peptide inhibits POMC firing, thus increasing appetite and cravings. Cravings for fatty and sugary foods among obese and bulimic patients involve the endorphin system.
- *Glucagon-like peptide 1* (GLP-1): It is a gut peptide. It amplifies glucose-dependent insulin release, inhibits glucagon release, suppresses appetite, and slows gastric emptying.

Metformin has been proposed as a weight-loss medication. It is a biguanide that inhibits hepatic glucose production and increases peripheral tissue sensitivity to insulin, resulting in reduced circulating insulin and androgen levels accompanied by decreased body weight and visceral fat.[127] Metformin alone is not associated with weight loss; however, when metformin is combined with a low-calorie diet, weight loss has been demonstrated. Drugs such as fenfluramine, dexfenfluramine, sibutramine, and rimonabant are no longer used due to adverse effects associated with them.

ROLE OF PRE- AND PROBIOTICS

A promising new treatment/preventive intervention for obesity has been proposed based on the principle of modulation of the intestinal microbial community in the form of probiotics and prebiotics in order to reduce the susceptibility to obesity.[128] Probiotics are defined as "live microorganisms, which exert health benefits to host by supplying a healthier and more diverse population of microorganisms." Animal studies on probiotic-fed animals have shown less weight gain, fat accumulation, and white adipose tissue compared to placebo-treated animals. Specific strains belonging to *Lactobacillus* (*L. casei*, *L. gasseri*, *L. rhamnosus*, and *L. plantarum*) and *Bifidobacterium* species have been widely used as probiotic treatment.

Prebiotics are "nondigestible food ingredients and supplements that enhance the effect of probiotics by selectively stimulating the growth and/or activity of one or a limited number of bacterial species already established in the colon, e.g., galacto-oligosaccharides (GOSs), fructo-oligosaccharides (FOSs), soybean oligosaccharides, inulin, gluco-oligosaccharides, xylo-oligosaccharides, lactulose, and lactosucrose." Pre- and probiotics exert their beneficial effect by changes in gut microbiota, correction of intestinal pH, lower inflammation, lower insulin resistance, and greater satiety.[128]

MATCHING WEIGHT-LOSS MEDICATION TO A PATIENT'S PROFILE[124]

- Nonsympathomimetic agents such as lorcaserin or orlistat should be considered for patients with a history of cardiovascular disease (CVD) or uncontrolled hypertension.
- GLP-1 agonist liraglutide should be considered as the first line in patients with diabetes; patients with both diabetes and CVD might also do well.
- For individuals with obesity and depression who are taking a selective serotonin reuptake inhibitor (SSRI) or serotonin and norepinephrine reuptake inhibitor (SNRI),

lorcaserin is not recommended due to the potential for serotonin syndrome. Phentermine/topiramate or phentermine alone should be considered.
- Orlistat is safe for all individuals.

BARIATRIC SURGERY

Bariatric surgery is generally considered for patients with BMI >40 kg/m^2 or patients with BMI >35 kg/m^2 and associated comorbidities or failure of other treatments for weight control.[129,130] It is associated with significant and rapid weight loss. But, it is an expensive procedure.

Salient features of bariatric surgery:
- Weight loss at 12 months, with gastric bypass averages close to 40% of the initial body weight
- Complete resolution or improvement of hyperlipidemia, hypertension, type II diabetes mellitus, and obstructive sleep apnea in >60% of patients
- Restores menstrual regularity, more ovulations owing to shorter follicular phase, reduces serum testosterone
- Improves sexual function in both males and females and increased chances of pregnancy
- Benefits maintained up to 10 years after surgery.

Bariatric surgery may not be so beneficial for male fertility. There are some case reports of worsening of semen parameters following bariatric surgery, perhaps from postoperative nutritional deficiencies, causing secondary infertility from spermatogenic arrest[131,132] and impaired IVF pregnancy outcome. In another case series, however, semen parameters of three obese men remained stable up to 1 year following bariatric surgery.[133] Without larger studies to confirm the impact of bariatric surgery on sperm quality, individualized management with cryopreservation of semen samples should be considered in selected circumstances.

Bariatric procedures are of three types **(Figs. 5A to C)**:
1. Restrictive
   a. Sleeve gastrectomy (SG)
   b. Laparoscopic adjustable gastric band (LAGB).

Restrictive procedures create a small gastric pouch with staples or a band that fills rapidly to induce early satiety.

2. Malabsorptive
   a. Biliopancreatic diversion.

Reduces absorption by anatomical modification

3. Combined restrictive and malabsorptive
   a. Roux-en-Y gastric bypass (RYGB).

The RYGB creates a small stomach pouch and attaches it to a loop of jejunum to shorten the length of the intestinal tract, restricting food intake and causing malabsorption.

In Vitro Fertilization and Pregnancy after Bariatric Surgery

There are limited studies on the effect of bariatric surgery on reproductive outcome. Available evidence suggests that IVF after bariatric surgery is safe. Surgically induced weight loss

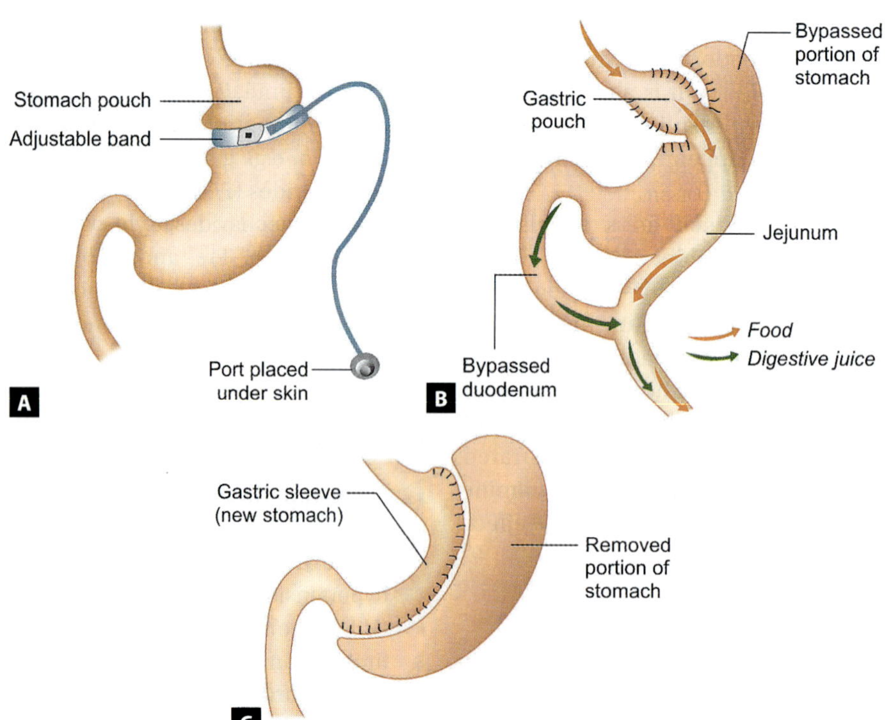

Figs. 5A to C: Types of bariatric procedures. (A) Adjustable gastric band (Lap band); (B) roux-en-Y gastric bypass (RYGB); (C) vertical sleeve gastrectomy.

reduces pregnancy complications associated with obesity such as gestational diabetes, preeclampsia, hypertensive disorders, and macrosomia. Surgical complications such as bowel obstructions, internal hernia, gastric ulcer, band events, and staple-line stricture can occur in pregnancy, but are rare.[134,135] Some reports also suggest increased chances of preterm births and small-for-gestation age births in women undergoing bariatric surgery. Postsurgical nutritional deficiencies owing to rapid weight loss have been suggested as the possible cause and are most commonly seen in malabsorptive rather than restrictive procedures.

Therefore, it is recommended that pregnancy should be delayed for a period of 1–2 years after the surgery and patient be supplemented with essential micronutrients. Sexually active women should be prescribed nonoral hormonal contraceptives as oral contraceptives may exhibit decreased efficacy due to malabsorption.

Preconceptional Weight Loss: Is it Worth the Wait?

The benefits of postponing pregnancy in women to achieve preconceptional weight loss must be balanced against the risk of declining fertility with advancing age, although optimizing weight gain during pregnancy can lower the incidence of gestational diabetes.[136]

Benefits are as follows:

- Spontaneous ovulation. Improved chance of unassisted conception[9,136]
- Improved sperm count and morphology and increased testosterone levels[137]
- Higher percentage and number of metaphase II oocytes in IVF[138]
- Decreased anesthesia-related morbidity associated with oocyte retrieval[139]
- Decreased pregnancy complications related to obesity.[140]

Weight Loss and In Vitro Fertilization Outcome

The research on weight loss and IVF outcomes has shown mixed results. There is insufficient evidence to suggest that preconception weight loss improves clinical pregnancy rates and live birth rates in IVF.[141] In fact, the use of very-low-calorie diets has been shown to have a negative effect on IVF outcomes.[142] There are some studies that have shown improved conception rates and improved live birth rates following weight loss.[143,144] Though outcomes after weight loss have been conflicting, we should keep in mind the possible benefits of decreased pregnancy risks and complications associated with obesity.

OBESITY AND ETHICAL DILEMMAS

Many International Programs and National Health System recommend a BMI threshold for access to IVF to women with obesity above which fertility treatment is denied until the patient loses weight.[145] Assuming weight loss as an achievable goal, increased anesthetic, surgical, and obstetric risks with obesity and fertility treatment are the most common cited reasons. There are several oppositions to this thought as denying a patient solely on the basis of arbitrary BMI cutoff violates the ethical principles of patient autonomy, beneficence/nonmaleficence, and justice. Regarding safety concerns, a recent evidence suggests that retrievals can be performed safely in women with class 3 and above obesity managed in the appropriate clinical setting.[146] Individualized approach based on BMI should be practiced, patients with comorbidities should be evaluated before the day of surgery, and the anesthesia team should be consulted.

TRANSGENERATIONAL EFFECTS

Evidence suggests that maternal obesity may confer a risk of metabolic dysfunction through multiple generations. Children born to obese mothers are more likely to develop obesity, type II diabetes, and cardiovascular disease as adults.[147] This may be due to epigenetic modifications in utero. Some studies have suggested that metabolic syndrome may be passed down generations through aberrant oocytes with defective mitochondria.[148]

NUTRIGENOMICS

Nutrigenomics is a newer field of genomic science. It is the study of the effects of nutrients on the gene expression. Nutrigenomics aims to study the influence of one's genetic constitution on nutrient's metabolism with respect to its absorption, elimination, or biological effects using the technology of microarray and single nucleotide polymorphism (SNP). Due to genetic variability, every individual responds differently to a certain diet. Nutrigenomics aims to devise the means to optimize or personalize nutrition according to the patient's genotype and thus prevent obesity.[149] Still in the research process, nutrigenomics will revolutionize the treatment of obesity and other nutrition-based diseases by identifying the ideal diet or nutrition based on one's genetic composition which will prevent lifestyle diseases and ensure proper function of all pathways involved in the maintenance of genome.

CONCLUSION

Obesity is the gravest health problem that we face today. It has now become a global epidemic. It has vast effects on all the systems of the body including the reproductive system in both males and females. High BMI has a strong association with adverse fertility outcomes. Weight loss through diet and multidisciplinary approaches such as exercise and behavioral modification has been found to benefit greatly in terms of improved fertility, fecundity, and decreased risks associated with pregnancy. Preconceptional counseling in an obese women should address the reproductive and maternal–fetal consequences of obesity and preconception weight loss should be encouraged. At the same time, pregnancy should not be delayed for weight loss due to declining ovarian reserve with increasing age. Obese women undergoing IVF should be carefully evaluated with a multidisciplinary team to determine the safety of oocyte retrieval under anesthesia. There is no available evidence to deny women IVF treatment based solely on BMI threshold. The obesity-associated reproductive morbidity is directly proportional to the duration of obesity. This makes obese children and young population, especially vulnerable in terms of their future reproductive potential. This population of obese adolescents should be the target of primary prevention such as lifestyle modification.

KEY POINTS

- Obesity is associated with decreased fertility and poor pregnancy outcomes.
- MRI is the most accurate and precise method for assessment of body fat.
- In utero programming and Gut microbiome may play an important role in onset of obesity.
- Preconception counseling and lifestyle modification are most important to improve the outcome in such patients.
- Pre-Pro Biotics and GLP-1 agonists are the promising new treatment in management of obesity.
- Obesity has deleterious effect on ART outcome.
- Although weight loss has not been shown to improve the IVF outcome it does decreases the pregnancy risks and complications associated with obesity.
- It is not recommended to delay IVF treatment to achieve ideal body weight, though lifestyle modification should continue.
- Multidisciplinary approach is recommended in obese women with multiple morbidities undergoing IVF.
- Nutrigenomics is the breakthrough science to deal with personalized nutrition based on ones genes.

REFERENCES

1. World Health Organization. (2021). Obesity and Overweight Newsroom. [Online] Available from: https://www.who.int/news-room/fact-sheets/detail/obesity-and-overweight [Last accessed December, 2022].
2. Speliotes EK, Willer CJ, Berndt SI, Monda KL, Thorleifsson G, Jackson AU, et al. Association analyses of 249,796 individuals reveal 18 new loci associated with body mass index. Nat Genet. 2010;42(11):937-48.
3. Hindorff LA, Sethupathy P, Junkins HA, Ramos EM, Mehta JP, Collins FS, et al. Potential etiologic and functional implications of genome-wide association loci for human diseases and traits. Proc Natl Acad Sci U S A. 2009;106(23):9362-7.
4. Hippocrates. In: Lloyd GER (Ed.) Hippocratic writings. London: Penguin Books; 1978.
5. Zaadstra BM, Seidell JC, Van Noord PA, te Velde ER, Habbema JD, Vrieswijk B, et al. Fat and female fecundity: prospective study of effect of body fat distribution on conception rates. BMJ. 1993;306(6876):484-7.
6. Rich-Edwards JW, Goldman MB, Willett WC, Hunter DJ, Stampfer MJ, Colditz GA, et al. Adolescent body mass index and infertility caused by ovulatory disorder. Am J Obstet Gynecol. 1994;171(1):171-7.
7. Grodstein F, Goldman MB, Cramer DW. Body mass index and ovulatory infertility. Epidemiology. 1994;5(2):247-50.
8. Clark AM, Ledger W, Galletly C, Tomlinson L, Blaney F, Wang X, et al. Weight loss results in significant improvement in pregnancy and ovulation rates in anovulatory obese women. Hum Reprod. 1995;10(10):2705-12.
9. Maheshwari A, Stofberg L, Bhattacharya S. Effect of overweight and obesity on assisted reproductive technology—a systematic review. Hum Reprod Update. 2007;13(5):433-44.
10. Metwally M, Ong KJ, Ledger WL, Li TC. Does high body mass index increase the risk of miscarriage after spontaneous and assisted conception? A meta-analysis of the evidence. Fertil Steril. 2008;90(3):714-26.
11. Yogev Y, Catalano PM. Pregnancy and obesity. Obstet Gynecol Clin North Am. 2009;36(2):285-300,viii.
12. van der Steeg JW, Steures P, Eijkemans MJ, Habbema JD, Hompes PG, Burggraaff JM, et al. Obesity affects spontaneous pregnancy chances in subfertile, ovulatory women. Hum Reprod. 2008;23(2):324-8.
13. Wise LA, Rothman KJ, Mikkelsen EM, Sørensen HT, Riis A, Hatch EE. An internet-based prospective study of body size and time-to-pregnancy. Hum Reprod. 2010;25(1):253-64.
14. Bellver J, Melo MA, Bosch E, Serra V, Remohí J, Pellicer A. Obesity and poor reproductive outcome: the potential role of the endometrium. Fertil Steril. 2007;88(2):446-51.
15. Veleva Z, Tiitinen A, Vilska S, Hyd_en-Granskog C, Tom_as C, Martikainen H, et al. High and low BMI increase the risk of miscarriage after IVF/ICSI and FET. Hum Reprod. 2008;23(4):878-84.
16. Stothard KJ, Tennant PW, Bell R, Rankin J. Maternal overweight and obesity and the risk of congenital anomalies: a systematic review and meta-analysis. JAMA. 2009;301(6):636-50.
17. Dokras A, Baredziak L, Blaine J, Syrop C, VanVoorhis BJ, Sparks A. Obstetric outcomes after in vitro fertilization in obese and morbidly obese women. Obstet Gynecol. 2006;108(1):61-9.
18. Sarsam SE, Elliott JP, Lam GK. Management of wound complications from cesarean delivery. Obstet Gynecol Surv. 2005;60:462-73.
19. Kitsantas P, Gallo S, Palla H, Nguyen V, Gaffney K. Nature and nurture in the development of childhood obesity: early infant feeding practices of overweight/obese mothers differ compared to mothers of normal body mass index. J Matern Fetal Neonatal Med. 2016;29(2):290-3.
20. North American Association for the Study of Obesity, National Heart, Lung, and Blood Institute, National Institutes of Health. The practical guide: identification, evaluation, and treatment of overweight and obesity in adults. Rockville, MD: National Institutes of Health; 2000.
21. McKeigue PM, Shah B, Marmot MG. Relation of central obesity and insulin resistance with high diabetes prevalence and cardiovascular risk in South Asians. Lancet. 1991;337(8738):382-6.

22. Deurenberg-Yap M, Yian TB, Kai CS, Deurenberg P, VAN Staveren WA. Manifestation of cardiovascular risk factors at low levels of body mass index and waist-to-hip ratio in Singaporean Chinese. Asia Pacific J Clin Nutr. 1999;8(3): 177-83.
23. Ko GT, Chan JC, Cockram CS, Woo J. Prediction of hypertension, diabetes, dyslipidaemia or albuminuria using simple anthropometric indexes in Hong Kong Chinese. Int J Obes. 1999;23(11):1136-42.
24. WHO/IOTF/IASO. The Asia-Pacific Perspective: Redefining Obesity and its treatment. Geneva: World Health Organization; 2000.
25. Han TS, van Leer EM, Seidell JC, Lean ME. Waist circumference action levels in the identification of cardiovascular risk factors: prevalence study in a random sample. Br Med J. 1995;311(7017):1401-5.
26. James WPT. The epidemiology of obesity. In: Chadwick DJ, Cardew G (Eds). Ciba Foundation Symposium 201 - The Origins and Consequences of Obesity: The Origins and Consequences of Obesity: Ciba Foundation Symposium 201. Switzerland: Novartis Foundation Symposia; 1996. pp. 1-16.
27. World Health Organization. (2000). Obesity: Preventing and Managing the Global Epidemic: report of a WHO consultation. [Online] Available from: https://apps.who.int/iris/handle/10665/42330 [Last accessed December, 2022].
28. Franco LP, Morais CC, Cominetti C. Normal-weight obesity syndrome: diagnosis, prevalence, and clinical implications. Nutr Rev. 2016;74(9):558-70.
29. Hales CN, Barker DJP. Type 2 (non-insulin-dependent) diabetes mellitus: the thrifty phenotype hypothesis. Diabetologica. 1992;35(7):595-601.
30. Ibáñez L, Suárez L, Lopez-Bermejo A, Díaz M, Valls C, de Zegher F. Early development of visceral fat excess after spontaneous catch-up growth in children with low birth weight. J Clin Endocrinol Metab. 2008;93(3):925-8.
31. Ibáñez L, Potau N, Zampolli M, Street ME, Carrascosa A. Girls diagnosed with premature pubarche show an exaggerated ovarian androgen synthesis from the early stages of puberty: Evidence from gonadotropin-releasing hormone agonist testing. Fertil Steril. 1997;67(5):849-55.
32. Boulange CL, Neves AL, Chilloux J, Nicholson JK, Dumas ME. Impact of the gut microbiota on inflammation, obesity, and metabolic disease. Genome Med. 2016;8(1):42.
33. Jungheim ES, Travieso JL, Carson KR, Moley KH. Obesity and reproductive functions. Obstet Gynecol Clin North Am. 2012;39(4):479-93.
34. Mircea CN, Lujan ME, Pierson RA. Metabolic fuel and clinical implications for female reproduction. J Obstet Gynaecol Can. 2007;29(11):887-902.
35. van Kruijsdijk RC, van der Wall E, Visseren F L. Obesity and cancer: the role of dysfunctional adipose tissue. Cancer Epidemiol Biomarkers Prev. 2009;18(10):2569-78.
36. Kennedy GC. The role of depot fat in the hypothalamic control of food intake in the rat. Proc R Soc Lond B Biol Sci. 1953;140(901):578-96.
37. Brannian JD, Hansen KA. Leptin and ovarian folliculogenesis: implications for ovulation induction and ART outcomes. Semin Reprod Med. 2002;20(2):103-12.
38. Henson MC, Castracane VD. Leptin in pregnancy. Biol Reprod. 2000;63(5):1219-28.
39. Craig J, Zhu H, Dyce PW, Petrik J, Li J. Leptin enhances oocyte nuclear and cytoplasmic maturation via the mitogen-activated protein kinase pathway. Endocrinology. 2004;145(11):5355-63.
40. Masuzaki H, Ogawa Y, Sagawa N, Hosoda K, Matsumoto T, Mise H, et al. Nonadipose tissue production of leptin: leptin as a novel placenta-derived hormone in humans. Nat Med. 1997;3(9):1029-33.
41. Mantzoros CS. Role of leptin in reproduction. Ann N Y Acad Sci. 2000;900:174-83.
42. Carmina E, Bucchieri S, Mansueto P, Rini G, Ferin M, Lobo RA. Circulating levels of adipose products and differences in fat distribution in the ovulatory and anovulatory phenotypes of polycystic ovary syndrome. Fertil Steril. 91(4 Suppl):1332-5.
43. Deura I, Harada T, Taniguchi F, Iwabe T, Izawa M, Terakawa N. Reduction of estrogen production by interleukin-6 in a human granulose tumor cell line may have implications for endometriosis-associated infertility. Fertil Steril. 2005;83(Suppl 1):1086-92.
44. Glueck CJ, Wang P, Bornovali S, Goldenberg N, Sieve L. Polycystic ovary syndrome, the G1691A factor V Leiden mutation, and plasminogen activator inhibitor activity: associations with recurrent pregnancy loss. Metabolism. 2003;52(12):1627-32.
45. Bruun JM, Verdich C, Toubro S, Astrup A, Richelsen B. Association between measures of insulin sensitivity and circulating levels of interleukin-8, interleukin-6 and tumor necrosis factor-alpha. Effect of weight loss in obese men. Eur J Endocrinol. 2003;148(5):535-42.
46. Matthaei S, Stumvoll M, Kellerer M, Haring HU. Pathophysiology and pharmacological treatment of insulin resistance. Endocr Rev. 2000;21(6):585-618.
47. Pasquali R, Gambineri A. Metabolic effects of obesity on reproduction. Reprod Biomed Online. 2016;12(5):542-51.
48. Poretsky L, Cataldo NA, Rosenwaks Z, Giudice LC. The insulin-related ovarian regulatory system in health and disease. Endocr Rev. 1999;20(4):535-82.
49. El-Haschimi K, Pierroz DD, Hileman SM, Bjorbaek C, Flier JS. Two defects contribute to hypothalamic leptin resistance in mice with diet-induced obesity. J Clin Invest. 2000;105(12):1827-32.
50. Robker RL, Akison LK, Bennett BD, Thrupp PN, Chura LR, Russell DL, et al. Obese women exhibit differences in ovarian metabolites, hormones, and gene expression compared with moderate-weight women. J Clin Endocrinol Metab. 2009;94(5):1533-40.
51. Zachow RJ, Magoffin DA. Direct intraovarian effects of leptin: impairment of the synergistic action of insulin-like growth factor-I on follicle-stimulating hormone-dependent estradiol-17 beta production by rat ovarian granulosa cells. Endocrinology. 1997;138(2):847-50.
52. Homburg R, Orvieto R, Bar-Hava I, Ben-Rafael Z. Serum levels of insulin-like growth factor-1, IGF binding protein-1 and insulin and the response to human menopausal gonadotrophins in women with polycystic ovary syndrome. Human Reprod. 1996;11(4):716-9.
53. Steinkampf MP, Hammond KR, Nichols JE, Slayden SH. Effect of obesity on recombinant follicle-stimulating hormone absorption: subcutaneous versus intramuscular administration. Fertil Steril. 2003;80(1):99-102.

54. Luzzo KM, Wang Q, Purcell SH, ChiM, Jimenez PT, Grindler N, et al. High fat diet induced developmental defects in the mouse: oocyte meiotic aneuploidy and fetal growth retardation/brain defects. PLoS One. 2012;7(11):e49217.
55. Sorensen TI, Virtue S, Vidal-Puig A. Obesity as a clinical and public health problem: is there a need for a new definition based on lipotoxicity effects? Biochim Biophys Acta. 2010; 1801(3):400-4.
56. Igosheva N, Abramov AY, Poston L, Eckert JJ, Fleming TP, Duchen MR, et al. Maternal diet-induced obesity alters mitochondrial activity and redox status in mouse oocytes and zygotes. PLoS One. 2010;5(4):e10074.
57. Jungheim ES, Macones GA, Odem RR, Patterson BW, Moley KH. Elevated serum alpha-linolenic acid levels are associated with decreased chance of pregnancy after in vitro fertilization. Fertil Steril. 2011;96(4):880-3.
58. Leary C, Leese HJ, Sturmey RG. Human embryos from overweight and obese women display phenotypic and metabolic abnormalities. Hum Reprod. 2015;30(1):122-32.
59. Bellver J, de los Santos MJ, Alama P, Castello D, Privitera L, Galliano D, et al. Day-3 embryo metabolomics in the spent culture media is altered in obese women undergoing in vitro fertilization. Fertil Steril. 2015;103(6):1407-15.
60. Magarinos MP, Sanchez-Margalet V, Kotler M, Calvo JC, Varone CL. Leptin promotes cell proliferation and survival of trophoblastic cells. Biol Reprod. 2007;76(2):203-10.
61. Metwally M, Tuckerman EM, Laird SM, Ledger WL, Li TC. Impact of high body mass index on endometrial morphology and function in the peri-implantation period in women with recurrent miscarriage. Reprod Biomed Online. 2007;14(3): 328-334.
62. Tamer Erel C, Senturk LM. The impact of body mass index on assisted reproduction. Curr Opin Obstet Gynecol. 2009;21(3): 228-35.
63. Levens ED, Skarulis MC. Assessing the role of endometrial alteration among obese patients undergoing assisted reproduction. Fertil Steril. 2008;89(6):1606-8.
64. Bellver J, Martínez-Conejero JA, Labarta E, Alama P, Melo MA, Remohí J, et al. Endometrial gene expression in the window of implantation is altered in obese women especially in association with polycystic ovary syndrome. Fertil Steril. 2011;95(7):2335-41,e1-8.
65. Rhee JS, Saben JL, Mayer AL, Schulte MB, Asghar Z, Stephens C, et al. Dietinduced obesity impairs endometrial stromal cell decidualization: a potential role for impaired autophagy. Hum Reprod. 2016;31:1315-26.
66. Tanaka T, Umesaki N. Leptin regulates the proliferation and apoptosis of human endometrial epithelial cells. Int J Mol Med. 2008;22(5):683-9.
67. Harsh Vats, Saxena R, Sachdeva MP, Walia GK, Gupta V. Impact of maternal pre-pregnancy body mass index on maternal, fetal and neonatal adverse outcomes in the worldwide populations: A systematic review and meta-analysis. Obes Res Clin Pract. 2021;15(6):536-45.
68. Kiddy DS, Hamilton-Fairley D, Bush A, Short F, Anyaoku V, Reed MJ, et al. Improvement in endocrine and ovarian function during dietary treatment of obese women with polycystic ovary syndrome. Clinl Endocrinol. 1992;36(1):105-11.
69. Dunaif A. Insulin resistance and the polycystic ovary syndrome: mechanism and implications for pathogenesis. Endocr Rev. 1997;18(6):774-800.
70. Mulders AG, Laven JS, Eijkemans MJ, Hughes EG, Fauser BC. Patient predictors for outcome of gonadotrophin ovulation induction in women with normogonadotrophic anovulatory infertility: a meta-analysis. Hum Reprod Update. 2003;9(5):429-49.
71. Hamilton-Fairley D, Kiddy D, Watson H, Paterson C, Franks S. Association of moderate obesity with a poor pregnancy outcome in women with polycystic ovary syndrome treated with low dose gonadotrophin. Br J Obstet Gynaecol. 1992; 99(2):128-31.
72. Shah DK, Missmer SA, Berry KF, Racowsky C, Ginsburg ES. Effect of obesity on oocyte and embryo quality in women undergoing in vitro fertilization. Obstet Gynecol. 2011; 118(1):63-70.
73. Luke B, Brown MB, Missmer SA, Bukulmez O, Leach R, Stern JE. The effect of increasing obesity on the response to and outcome of assisted reproductive technology: a national study. Fertil Steril. 2011;96(4):820-5.
74. Pinborg A, Gaarslev C, Hougaard CO, Nyboe Andersen A, Andersen PK, Boivin J, et al. Influence of female bodyweight on IVF outcome: a longitudinal multicentre cohort study of 487 infertile couples. Reprod Biomed Online 2011;23(4):490-9.
75. Al-Azemi M, Omu FE, Omu AE. The effect of obesity on the outcome of infertility management in women with polycystic ovary syndrome. Arch Gynecol Obstet. 2004;270(4):205-10.
76. Lashen H, LedgerW, Bernal AL, Barlow D. Extremes of body mass do not adversely affect the outcome of superovulation and in-vitro fertilization. Hum Reprod. 1999;14(3):712-5.
77. Martinuzzi K, Ryan S, Luna M, Copperman AB. Elevated body mass index (BMI) does not adversely affect in vitro fertilization outcome in young women. J Assist Reprod Genet. 2008;25(5):169-75.
78. Depalo R, Garruti G, Totaro I, Panzarino M, Vacca MP, Giorgino F, et al. Oocyte morphological abnormalities in overweight women undergoing in vitro fertilization cycles. Gynecol Endocrinol. 2011;27(11):880-4.
79. Zhang D, Zhu Y, Gao H, Zhou B, Zhang R, Wang T, et al. Overweight and obesity negatively affect the outcomes of ovarian stimulation and in vitro fertilisation: a cohort study of 2628 Chinese women. Gynecol Endocrinol. 2010;26(5):325-32.
80. Metwally M, Cutting R, Tipton A, Skull J, Ledger WL, Li TC. Effect of increased body mass index on oocyte and embryo quality in IVF patients. Reprod Biomed Online. 2007;15(5):532-8.
81. Jungheim ES, Schon SB, Schulte MB, DeUgarte DA, Fowler SA, Tuuli MG. IVF outcomes in obese donor oocyte recipients: a systematic review and meta-analysis. Hum Reprod. 2013;28(10):2710-7.
82. Sarais V, Pagliardini L, Rebonato G, Papaleo E, Candiani M, Vigano P. A comprehensive analysis of body mass index effect on in vitro fertilization outcomes. Nutrients. 2016;8(3):109.
83. Deugarte D, Deugarte C, Sahakian V. Surrogate obesity negatively impacts pregnancy rates in third-party reproduction. Fertil Steril. 2010;93(3):1008-10.
84. Wang JX, Davies MJ, Norman RJ. Obesity increases the risk of spontaneous abortion during infertility treatment. Obes Res. 2002;10(6):551-4.
85. Rittenberg V, Sobaleva S, Ahmad A, Oteng-Ntim E, Bolton V, Khalaf Y, et al. Influence of BMI on risk of miscarriage after single blastocyst transfer. Hum Reprod. 2011;26(10):2642-50.

86. Souter I, Baltagi LM, Kuleta D, Meeker JD, Petrozza JC. Women, weight, and fertility: the effect of body mass index on the outcome of superovulation/intrauterine insemination cycles. Fertil Steril. 2011;95(3):1042-7.
87. Nohr EA, Bech BH, Davies MJ, Frydenberg M, Henriksen TB, Olsen J. Prepregnancy obesity and fetal death: a study within the Danish National Birth Cohort. Obstet Gynecol. 2005;106(2):250-9.
88. Metwally M, Saravelos SH, Ledger WL, Li TC. Body mass index and risk of miscarriage in women with recurrent miscarriage. Fertil Steril. 2010;94(1):290-5.
89. Boots CE, Bernardi LA, Stephenson MD. Frequency of euploid miscarriage is increased in obese women with recurrent early pregnancy loss. Fertil Steril. 2014;102(2):455-9.
90. Bellver J, Busso C, Pellicer A, Remohi J, Simon C. Obesity and assisted reproductive technology outcomes. Reprod Biomed Online. 2006;12(5):562-8.
91. Petersen GL, Schmidt L, Pinborg A, Kamper-Jørgensen M. The influence of female and male body mass index on live births after assisted reproductive technology treatment: a nationwide register-based cohort study. Fertil Steril. 2013;99(6):1654-62.
92. Koning AM, Mutsaerts MA, Kuchenbecker WK, Broekmans FJ, Land JA, Mol BW, et al. Complications and outcome of assisted reproduction technologies in overweight and obese women. Hum Reprod. 2012;27(2):457-67.
93. Rittenberg V, Seshadri S, Sunkara SK, Sobaleva S, Oteng-Ntim E, El-Toukhy T. Effect of body mass index on IVF treatment outcome: an updated systematic review and meta-analysis. Reprod Biomed Online. 2011;23(4):421-39.
94. Dechaud H, Anahory T, Reyftmann L, Loup V, Hamamah S, Hedon B. Obesity does not adversely affect results in patients who are undergoing in vitro fertilization and embryo transfer. Eur J Obstet Gynecol Reprod Biol. 2006;127(1):88-93.
95. Carrell DT, Jones KP, Peterson CM, Aoki V, Emery BR, Campbell BR. Body mass index is inversely related to intrafollicular HCG concentrations, embryo quality and IVF outcome. Reproductive Biomedicine Online. 2001;3(2):109-11.
96. Sallmen M, Sandler DP, Hoppin JA, Blair A, Baird DD. Reduced fertility among overweight and obese men. Epidemiology. 2006;17(5):520-3.
97. Ramlau-Hansen CH, Thulstrup AM, Nohr EA, Bonde JP, Sorensen TI, Olsen J. Subfecundity in overweight and obese couples. Hum Reprod. 2007;22(6):1634-7.
98. Nguyen RH, Wilcox AJ, Skjaerven R, Baird DD. Men's body mass index and infertility. Hum Reprod. 2007;22(9):2488-93.
99. Jensen TK, Andersson AM, Jorgensen N, Andersen AG, Carlsen E, Petersen JH, et al. Body mass index in relation to semen quality and reproductive hormones among 1,558 Danish men. Fertil Steril. 2004;82(4):863-70.
100. Hammoud AO, Wilde N, Gibson M, Parks A, Carrell DT, Meikle AW. Male obesity and alteration in sperm parameters. Fertil Steril. 2008;90(6):2222-5.
101. Dupont C, Faure C, Sermondade N, Boubaya M, Eustache F, Clement P, et al. Obesity leads to higher risk of sperm DNA damage in infertile patients. Asian J Androl. 2013;15(5): 622-5.
102. Kley HK, Deselaers T, Peerenboom H, Kruskemper HL. Enhanced conversion of androstenedione to estrogens in obese males. J Clin Endocrinol Metab. 1980;51(5):1128-32.
103. George JT, Millar RP, Anderson RA. Hypothesis: kisspeptin mediates male hypogonadism in obesity and type 2 diabetes. Neuroendocrinology. 2010;91:302-7.
104. Brennan AM, Mantzoros CS. Drug insight: the role of leptin in human physiology and pathophysiology—emerging clinical applications. Nat Clin Pract Endocrinol Metab. 2006;2(6):318-27.
105. Torres M, Laguna-Barraza R, Dalmases M, Calle A, Pericuesta E, Montserrat JM, et al. Male fertility is reduced by chronic intermittent hypoxia mimicking sleep apnea in mice. Sleep. 2014;37(11):1757-65.
106. Magnusdottir EV, Thorsteinsson T, Thorsteinsdottir S, Heimisdottir M, Olafsdottir K. Persistent organochlorines, sedentary occupation, obesity and human male subfertility. Hum Reprod. 2005;20(1):208-15.
107. Shafik A, Olfat S. Lipectomy in the treatment of scrotal lipomatosis. Br JnUrol. 1981;53(1):55-61.
108. Burnett AL, Strong TD, Trock BJ, Jin L, Bivalacqua TJ, Musicki B. Serum biomarker measurements of endothelial function and oxidative stress after daily dosing of sildenafil in type 2 diabetic men with erectile dysfunction. J Urol. 2009;181(1):245-51.
109. Soubry A, Guo L, Huang Z, Hoyo C, Romanus S, Price T, et al. Obesity-related DNA methylation at imprinted genes in human sperm: results from the TIEGER study. Clin Epigenetics. 2016;8:51.
110. Campbell JM, Lane M, Owens JA, Bakos HW. Paternal obesity negatively affects male fertility and assisted reproduction outcomes: a systematic review and meta-analysis. Reprod Biomed Online. 2015;31(5):593-604.
111. Thomsen L, Humaidan P, Bungum L, Bungum M. The impact of male overweight on semen quality and outcome of assisted reproduction. Asian J Androl. 2014;16(5):749-54.
112. Jenkins TG, Carrell DT. The sperm epigenome and potential implications for the developing embryo. Reproduction. 2012;143(6):727-34.
113. Wadden TA, Webb VL, Moran CH, Bailer BA. Lifestyle modification for Obesity: new developments in diet, physical activity, and behavior therapy. Circulation. 2012;125(9):1157-70.
114. Wyatt HR. Update on treatment strategies for obesity. J Clin Endocrinol Metab. 2013;98(4):1299-306.
115. Sacks FM, Bray GA, Carey VJ, Smith SR, Ryan DH, Anton SD, et al. Comparison of weight-loss diets with different compositions of fat, protein, and carbohydrates. N Engl J Med. 2009;360(9):859-73.
116. Chavarro JE, Rich-Edwards JW, Rosner BA, Willett WC. Dietary fatty acid intakes and the risk of ovulatory infertility. Am J Clin Nutr. 2007;85(1):231-7.
117. Chavarro JE, Rich-Edwards JW, Rosner BA, Willett WC. Protein intake and ovulatory infertility. Am J Obstet Gynecol. 2008;198(2):210.e1-7.
118. Chavarro JE, Rich-Edwards JW, Rosner BA, Willett WC. Use of multivitamins, intake of B vitamins, and risk of ovulatory infertility. Fertil Steril. 2008;89(3):668-76.
119. Chavarro JE, Rich-Edwards JW, Rosner B, Willett WC. A prospective study of dairy foods intake and anovulatory infertility. Hum Reprod. 2007;22(5):1340-7.
120. Vujkovic M, de Vries JH, Lindemans J, Macklon NS, van der Spek PJ, Steegers EA, et al. The preconception

Mediterranean dietary pattern in couples undergoing in vitro fertilization/intracytoplasmic sperm injection treatment increases the chance of pregnancy. Fertil Steril. 2010;94(6): 2096-101.
121. NHS Education for Scotland. Management of obesity. A national clinical guideline. Edinburgh (Scotland): Scottish Intercollegiate Guidelines Network (SIGN); 2010.
122. Palomba S, Falbo A, Valli B, Morini D, Villani MT, Nicoli A, et al. Physical activity before IVF and ICSI cycles in infertile obese women: An observational cohort study. Reprod Biomed Online. 2014;29(1):72-9.
123. American College of Sports Medicine. Exercise Prescription for Other Clinical Populations. In: Thompson WR, Gordon NF, Pescatello LS (Eds). ACSM's guidelines for exercise testing and prescription, 8th edition. Philadelphia: Lippincott Williams & Wilkins; 2010. p. 254.
124. Apovian CM, Aronne LJ, Bessesen DH, McDonnell ME, Murad MH, Pagotto U, et al. Pharmacological management of obesity: an endocrine society clinical practice guideline. J Clin Endocrinol Metab. 2015;100(2):342-62.
125 Ulrich-Lai YM, Ryan KK. Neuroendocrine circuits governing energy balance and stress regulation: functional overlap and therapeutic implications. Cell Metab. 2014;19(6): 910-25.
126. GW Kim, JE Lin, ES Blomain, SA Waldman. Antiobesity Pharmacotherapy: New Drugs and Emerging Targets. Clin Pharmacol Ther. 2014;95(1):53-66.
127. Pasquali R, Gambineri A, Biscotti D, Vicennati V, Gagliardi L, Colitta D, et al. Effect of long-term treatment with metformin added to hypocaloric diet on body composition, fat distribution, and androgen and insulin levels in abdominally obese women with and without the polycystic ovary syndrome. J Clin Endocrinol Metab. 2000;85(8):2767-74.
128. Tomás Cerdó, García-Santos JA, G Bermúdez M, Campoy C. The role of probiotics and prebiotics in the prevention and treatment of obesity. Nutrients. 2019;11(3):635.
129. NIH Conference. Gastrointestinal surgery for severe obesity. Consensus Development Conference Panel. Ann Intern Med. 1991;115(12):956-61.
130. Guelinckx I, Devlieger R, Vansant G. Reproductive outcome after bariatric surgery: a critical review. Hum Reprod Update. 2009;15(2):189-201.
131. Sermondade N, Massin N, Boitrelle F, Pfeffer J, Eustache F, Sifer C, et al. Sperm parameters and male fertility after bariatric surgery: three case series. Reprod Biomed Online. 2012;24(2):206-10.
132. di Frega AS, Dale B, Di Matteo L, Wilding M. Secondary male factor infertility after Roux-en-Y gastric bypass for morbid obesity: case report. Hum Reprod. 2005;20(4):997-8.
133. Legro RS, Kunselman AR, Meadows JW, Kesner JS, Krieg EF, Rogers AM, et al. Time-related increase in urinary testosterone levels and stable semen analysis parameters after bariatric surgery in men. Reprod Biomed Online. 2015;30(2): 150-6.
134. Moore KA, Ouyang DW, Whang EE. Maternal and fetal deaths after gastric bypass surgery for morbid obesity. N Engl J Med. 2004;351(7):721-2.
135. Hezelgrave NL, Oteng-Ntim E. Pregnancy after bariatric surgery: a review. J Obes. 2011;2011:501939.
136. Clark AM, Thornley B, Tomlinson L, Galletley C, Norman RJ. Weight loss in obese infertile women results in improvement in reproductive outcome for all forms of fertility treatment. Hum Reprod. 1998;13(6):1502-5.
137. Hakonsen LB, Thulstrup AM, Aggerholm AS, Olsen J, Bonde JP, Andersen CY, et al. Does weight loss improve semen quality and reproductive hormones? Results from a cohort of severely obese men. Reprod Health. 2011;8:24.
138. Chavarro JE, Ehrlich S, Colaci DS, Wright DL, Toth TL, Petrozza JC, et al. Body mass index and short-term weight change in relation to treatment outcomes in women undergoing assisted reproduction. Fertil Steril. 2012;98(1):109-16.
139. Sankar A, Johnson SR, Beattie WS, Tait G, Wijeysundera DN. Reliability of the American Society of Anesthesiologists physical status scale in clinical practice. Br J Anaesth. 2014; 113(3):424-32.
140. American College of Obstetricians and Gynecologists. Practice bulletin no 156: Obesity in pregnancy. Obstet Gynecol. 2015;126(6):e112-26.
141. Sim KA, Partridge SR, Sainsbury A. Does weight loss in overweight or obese women improve fertility treatment outcomes? A systematic review. Obes Rev. 2014;15(10):839-50.
142. Tsagareli V, Noakes M, Norman RJ. Effect of a very-low-calorie diet on in vitro fertilization outcomes. Fertil Steril. 2006;86(1):227-9.
143. Kort JD, Winget C, Kim SH, Lathi RB. A retrospective cohort study to evaluate the impact of meaningful weight loss on fertility outcomes in an overweight population with infertility. Fertil Steril. 2014;101(5):1400-3.
144. Sim KA, Dezarnaulds GM, Denyer GS, Skilton MR, Caterson ID. Weight loss improves reproductive outcomes in obese women undergoing fertility treatment: a randomized controlled trial. Clin Obes. 2014;4(2):61-8.
145. Kaye L, Sueldo C, Engmann L, Nulsen J, Benadiva C. Survey assessing obesity policies for assisted reproductive technology in the United States. Fertil Steril. 2016;105(3):703-6.e2.
146. Romanski PA, Farland LV, Tsen LC, Ginsburg ES, Lewis EI. Effect of class III and class IV obesity on oocyte retrieval complications and outcomes. Fertil Steril. 2019;111(2):294-301.e1.
147. van Dijk SJ, Molloy PL, Varinli H, Morrison JL, Muhlhausler BS; Members of Epi S. Epigenetics and human obesity. Int J Obes (Lond). 2015;39(1):85-97.
148 Saben JL, Boudoures AL, Asghar Z, Thompson A, Drury A, Zhang W, et al. Maternal metabolic syndrome programs mitochondrial dysfunction via germline changes across three generations. Cell Rep. 2016;16(1):1-8.
149. Doo M, Kim Y. Obesity: interactions of genome and nutrients intake. Prev Nutr Food Sci. 2015;20(1):1-7.

CHAPTER 20

Unexplained Infertility

Abha Bhat

INTRODUCTION

Conception is by far one of the most elaborate and magnificent choreographies of nature, with each component working in complete harmony and synchrony with the other. The challenges in investigating and evaluating conception are twofold. Many steps in this complex set of events, though reasonably well understood, are not all easy to evaluate with currently available technologies with any degree of accuracy and ease, for example, the process of sperm capacitation and the ability of spermatozoa to bind to and penetrate zona pellucida (ZP), the quality of eggs, bidirectional tubal motility, etc. Certain steps have as yet eluded complete comprehension and understanding such as implantation and its determinants and are therefore impossible to diagnose. The unexplained therefore ranges from the not-so-easily diagnosed to the not-so-well understood. This chapter is an attempt to understand the "diagnosis" of unexplained infertility (UI) in current practice and the management thereof.

Average natural fecundity of human beings is only about 20% per month, and approximately 90% of couples achieve conception within a year of unprotected intercourse.[1,2] Those who are unable to conceive within this time frame are said to be subfertile and should be evaluated. Of these, 15–30% of couples will have no abnormality when subjected to standard fertility investigations, namely semen analysis, tubal patency tests, and ovulation studies. This group is classified as having UI. The fecundity rate in this group has been reported as 2–4% per menstrual cycle.[3] 50% of these couples will conceive in the subsequent year and another 12% in the year after.[4] It is in this group that management should be individualized based on patient characteristics as well as patient choice as many of the pregnancies that occur in this group following treatment may have occurred naturally without intervention. Several prediction models have been proposed to help clinicians in counseling patients.[5]

INCIDENCE

There is no universal consensus on the standard tests to be done for fertility evaluation. As such, the incidence of UI varies with the diagnostic criteria used. Many of the steps leading to conception cannot be routinely evaluated; hence, many reproductive disorders may not be amenable to detection. It may be speculated that the incidence of UI will decrease with advances in diagnostic modalities.[6,7]

CAUSES

The contributory causes may be in the male and/or the female partner.

UNEXPLAINED MALE INFERTILITY

Male partners who have a normal medical history, normal physical examination, a semen analysis reported as normal and, in whose partner, no female factors have been identified are classified as having unexplained male infertility (UMI). The average incidence of UMI is 15% (range: 6–37%). Possible factors leading to UMI may be the presence of antisperm antibodies (ASAs), sperm deoxyribonucleic acid (DNA) damage, elevated levels of reactive oxygen species (ROS), genetic defects, and sperm dysfunction. Coital factors (inappropriate timing of intercourse, erectile dysfunction, or anejaculation) may also contribute. A thorough initial assessment is therefore imperative in all couples and should include detailed sexual history and appropriate investigations **(Box 1)**.[8]

Sperm Deoxyribonucleic Acid Damage

Deoxyribonucleic acid damage may be present in the form of single or double DNA strand breaks, base deletion or modification, interstrand or intrastrand cross-linkage, or DNA-protein cross-linkage. The most common cause of DNA fragmentation is oxidative stress (OS). It may be associated with advanced paternal age, inadequate diet, drug abuse, tobacco use, environmental factors such as pesticide

BOX 1: Unexplained male infertility.

- Sperm DNA damage
- Immune infertility
- Oxidative stress
- Genetic defects
- Fertilization defects
- Coital factors:
  - Inappropriate timing of intercourse
  - Erectile dysfunction
  - Anejaculation

(DNA: deoxyribonucleic acid)

exposure or air pollution, varicocele, systemic diseases, and genital inflammation. DNA damage has been reported in 5–8% of normozoospermic men.[9] In a small controlled study on 28 normozoospermic individuals, sperm integrity defect as measured by sperm chromatin structure assay (SCSA) was reported to be 89.2%.[10]

Immune Infertility

Binding of autoantibodies to the antigens present in the male or female gametes may lead to immune infertility. Formation of ASA results from exposure of immune system to sperm antigens following a breach in blood–testis barrier. The breach may occur as a result of trauma, infection, or obstruction.[11]

There is evidence of ASA-induced functional deficit in the sperms. In the presence of ≤80% of sperms with sperm-bound ASA, a fertilization rate of 72% was seen, and if ≥80% of sperms contained sperm-bound ASA, the fertilization rate was 27%. There was no clear correlation between localization and fertilization capacity of spermatozoa. Complement in the female cervical mucus can bind to antibodies and cause lysis of sperm cell, reduce motility, and inhibit the ability of sperms to penetrate cervical mucus. ASA can also interfere with spontaneous and induced acrosome reaction (AR), spontaneous capacitation reaction, and recognition of sperm-binding sites on ZP. DNA fragmentation too has been found to be more frequent than fertile controls and ASA-negative patients.[8,11]

Presence of ASA correlates well with sperm agglutination, but this rarely affects a significant proportion of motile sperms even if all ejaculated sperms are coated with antibodies. Furthermore, several substances are present in semen that inhibit the seminal complement system activation.[8] This may be the reason for finding normal semen parameters in many men with immune fertility and the inconsistent correlation of ASA with infertility.

Oxidative Stress

Reactive oxygen species represent a broad category of molecules that are byproducts of oxidative metabolism. These may be either in the form of oxygen-free radicals (hydroxyl and superoxide ions), nonradical species (hydrogen peroxide and lipid peroxide), or reactive nitrogen species (nitrous oxide, nitroxyl ion, and peroxynitrite).[8] ROS in small amounts play a physiological role in capacitation, hyperactivation (HA), motility, AR, and fertilization.[12,13] ROS may also have a role in the regulation of nuclear maturation in spermatozoa.[14] The level of ROS is restricted by seminal antioxidants such as β-mercaptoethanol, protein, vitamin E, vitamin C, cysteamine, cysteine, taurine, and hypotaurine. However, elevated levels of ROS can overwhelm the body's natural antioxidant defense mechanisms and lead to damage of lipids, proteins, and DNA of spermatozoa, a condition called oxidative stress. Critical phases of spermiogenesis as well as sperms are vulnerable to ROS-induced damage. Sperm chromatin condensation is very vulnerable to damage by ROS as sperms do not have DNA repair mechanisms. The plasma membrane of sperm has high levels of polyunsaturated fatty acids and is especially susceptible to oxidative damage by ROS.[8] The antioxidant enzymes that are naturally present in the sperm cannot prevent tail and acrosome membranes from lipid peroxidation leading to reduced sperm motility and impaired sperm–oocyte interactions. Clinically, OS can be the underlying cause of reduced fertilization rates, failure of implantation, impaired embryonic development, recurrent pregnancy loss, and poor assisted reproductive technology (ART) outcomes.

Peroxides-positive leukocytes and morphologically abnormal spermatozoa (especially those with residual cytoplasm or cytoplasmic droplet) are the main sources of ROS. In spermatozoa, mitochondria and plasma membrane are the two major sites of ROS generation. Activated leukocytes in response to infection and inflammation can produce up to 100-fold higher levels of ROS compared to nonactivated leukocytes.[15] As such, even low-level leukocytospermia [$<1 \times 10^6$ white blood cells (WBCs)/mL of semen] has been associated with OS, and antibiotic therapy results in improvement in pregnancy rates.[16] Alcohol consumption, cigarette smoking, presence of varicocele, obesity, diabetes, too much physical exercise, psychological stress aging, environmental factors [such as nitric oxide (NO), lead, and electromagnetic waves from cell phones], and infections have also been etiologically associated with an induction of OS.[15]

Genetic Defects

Gene mutations and polymorphisms have been recognized in infertile men with normal spermiogram. Examples are *CatSper* gene 1 mutation and cytosine-adenine-guanine (CAG) repeat polymorphism in the gene coding for polymerase gamma, and sperm from these men have reduced oocyte penetration ability and fertilization rates.[17]

Fertilization Defects

The intricate and complex process of fertilization commences with capacitation which occurs in vivo during the travel of sperm through the female reproductive tract. In vitro, it can be induced by removal of seminal plasma and addition of culture media. This prepares the sperm cell to undergo HA and AR. "Hyperactivation motility" is characterized by lateral head displacement, high curvilinear velocity, and large amplitudinal flagellar waves and is essential for fertilization. The physiological mechanism is an increased intracellular calcium entry through sperm calcium channels called *CatSper1–4*.[8,18] Individuals with mutated *CatSper1* gene are infertile with poor HA response despite normal count, motility, and morphology.

Sperm binding to ZP is a crucial step in fertilization and a precursor to AR. Defects in ZP binding have been observed in 15% of infertile men with normal semen. Sperm-ZP binding triggers the release of hydrolyzing enzymes known as AR. AR is critical to enable sperm cell to penetrate the ZP and exposes the site of sperm that fuses with the plasma membrane of the oocyte. The processes should also occur in tandem for optimal fertilization potential. If AR occurs in a sperm before ZP binding, it would be unable to bind or penetrate the ZP.[8]

FEMALE INFERTILITY

Diagnosis of UI in the female partner is as ambiguous as in the male partner. Often the diagnosis of endometriosis, tubal infertility, premature ovarian aging, and immune infertility are missed **(Box 2)**.

Endometriosis

Endometriosis has been reported to be associated with infertility even in its mildest forms.[19,20] Severe endometriosis can be diagnosed on ultrasound. However, minimal to mild disease is not so easily picked up and has been reported as a dominant finding in women with UI.[21] The mechanism by which mild disease impacts infertility is less well understood. Peritubal adhesions that lead to altered tubal motility and function, toxic effect of peritoneal inflammation on the oocyte and sperms, and reduced endometrial receptivity may be the underlying factors contributing to infertility.

BOX 2: Causes of female unexplained infertility.

- Endometriosis
- Undiagnosed tubal factor
- Premature ovarian aging
- Immune infertility
- Poor oocyte quality
- Uterine cavity abnormalities:
  - Endometrial synechiae
  - Endometrial polyps
  - Chronic endometritis

Undiagnosed Tubal Factor

Fallopian tubes are crucial for sperm movement, oocyte capture and transport, and early embryo development. Through variations in tubal peristalsis or ciliary activity which may impact one or both fallopian tubes, subtle tubal abnormalities may cause defective transport of oocyte and impaired fertilization. Tubal diverticulitis, paratubal cysts, accessory fallopian tube, accessory ostium of fallopian tube, phimosis, agglutination, and sacculation have all been linked to infertility.[22]

Ovarian Aging

Ovarian reserve, generally defined as the number of oocytes remaining in the ovaries, may also influence the chances of conception. Being closely linked to age, the ovarian reserve decreases with age. Though this may impact the chances of conception, women with a low reserve continue to have regular ovulatory cycles.[23] Ovarian aging, which leads to poor ovarian response and poor follicular growth, may also contribute to unexplained female subfertility if found in chronologically young women well within the reproductive age bracket.[24]

Immune Infertility

In addition to the "self-tolerance," which is determined by the absence of autoantibodies, there exists a "natural tolerance" in the context of reproductive health. This tolerance extends to seminal fluid and its components (including sperm) as well as the semi-allogeneic embryo. The decidual cellular immune system comprises T helper cells, T follicular helper (Tfh) cells, and regulatory T cells. The humoral system consists of autoantibodies and pro- and anti-inflammatory cytokines. Alterations in any of the compartments of the immune system may interfere with the immune tolerance and lead to UI.

There may be an overall activation of the immune system or a production of autoantibodies specifically directed toward ovarian antigens. Majority of the antiovarian autoantibodies are directed against the β-subunit of follicle stimulating hormone (anti-FSH). Autoantibodies have been implicated in the causation of premature ovarian failure (POF), polycystic ovary syndrome, tubal infertility, endometriosis, and UI. Failure in differentiation of T cells into T-regulatory cells has been suggested as a mechanism of UI. Since the prevalence of antiovarian antibodies (AOAs) was similar in POF and UI, the latter may represent an early stage of autoimmune POF.[25]

The T helper 1 (Th1) cells inhibit while the T helper 2 (Th2) cells promote the trophoblastic invasion. The Th1/Th2 ratio has a crucial role in allowing the fetus to implant. For a successful pregnancy, the balance should therefore shift toward a Th2 response. The T helper 17 (Th17) cells play a fundamental role in the acceptance or rejection of the fetus and some studies have suggested that high numbers of cells of Th17 subset may lead to UI and unexplained recurrent spontaneous miscarriages. Serum IL-17 has been shown to be an indicator of increased Th17 cells in the peripheral circulation. The different types of Tfh cells formed from the interaction of $CD4^+$ T cells and B cells may lead to the production of potential autoantibodies that trigger an inflammatory process during pregnancy and lead to infertility. $CD8^+$ $CD28^-$ Tregs, a subset of regulatory T cells (formerly called T suppressor cells) have a modulatory effect on the immune response that leads to the tolerance of the semi-allogeneic fetus, and a decreased number may therefore lead to infertility.[26]

Our understanding of the physiology, however, is insufficient and more studies are required to understand how autoimmunity can lead to infertility before manipulation of immunological milieu can be recommended to improve implantation or to cure infertility.[26]

Oocyte Quality

Good quality and maturity of oocytes are essential for fertilization and formation of good-quality embryos which progress to become blastocysts and then hatch before successful implantation. Quality of the oocytes may be affected by ovarian aging, endometriosis, and OS.[24,27,28] No biomarkers have been identified to date to evaluate the quality of the female gamete. Oocyte morphology can only be evaluated in the event of in vitro fertilization (IVF) process; hence, it can only be diagnosed retrospectively. Natural aging, which is strongly linked to decreased mitochondrial efficiency as well as increased OS, is the most common and obvious cause of decline in oocyte quality. In younger women, the quality may be compromised due to accelerated aging or due to genetic mutations that impact oocyte and embryo development. Since the quality of oocytes cannot be evaluated, many women may be wrongly classified as UI.[29]

Uterine Cavity Abnormalities

Congenital uterine anomalies are found in approximately 4.3% of fertile women, 3.5% of infertile women, and as many as 13% of women with recurrent miscarriages.[30] The most common anomaly is septate uterus accounting for approximately 35% of women followed by bicornuate uterus (25%) and arcuate uterus (20%). The general consensus is that malformations do not cause infertility but may be associated with reproductive loss, preterm delivery, malpresentations, and perinatal mortality. It is therefore prudent to offer hysteroscopic corrective surgery not only to symptomatic patients but also as a prophylactic procedure in asymptomatic patients.[31,32]

Acquired anomalies such as fibroids, synechiae, and polyps may be diagnosed on hysteroscopy. Fibroids may vary in size and may distort the uterine cavity. The evidence linking fibroids to infertility is not conclusive. The current evidence supports surgical correction of cavity-distorting myomas since it is correlated with improved pregnancy rates and lower risk of early pregnancy loss. The impact on live-birth rate (LBR) is however insufficient.[33] Non-cavity-distorting fibroids are unlikely to impact conception and LBR in women with UI.[34]

Uterine synechiae are commonly missed as the symptoms do not necessarily correlate with severity of adhesions, and mild cases of adhesions may be missed on the transvaginal ultrasound scan. They have been reported to be present in 1.5% of women undergoing hysterosalpingography (HSG)[35] and in 5–39% of women with recurrent miscarriages.[36] Patients with history of uterine instrumentation, miscarriage, endometritis, and tuberculosis should be evaluated and any suspicion should be confirmed by hysteroscopy.

Endometrial polyps have been reported in up to 24% of symptomatic patients and in >11% of subfertile women.[37,38] Hysteroscopic polypectomy should be offered to subfertile women as pregnancy rate as well as at term delivery rate increases, especially since it is a safe procedure with a low recurrence rate.[39] Interestingly, Stamatellos et al. reported no difference in the fertility rates and the total spontaneous abortion rate between patients who had a polyp ≤1 cm and those with polyp >1 cm or with multiple polyps.[40]

Chronic endometritis (CE) may exert a negative impact on the implantation potential of endometrium due to impaired decidual transformation. There is growing evidence of an association of CE with recurrent implantation failure (RIF) but a causal relationship with UI has not yet been established. In a study of 910 women, Cicinelli et al. found fluid hysteroscopy to be very reliable in the diagnosis of CE. The combination of focal or diffuse hyperemia, stromal edema, and polypoidal endometrium had a diagnostic accuracy of 93.4%. The incidence of CE in women with UI in this study was 40.7%.[41] In a further study by the same group, women with UI referred for hysteroscopy over the period of 1 year underwent endometrial sampling for histology and culture. The prevalence of CE in this group was 56.8%.

Women diagnosed with CE who have a successful resolution of inflammation following antibiotics have a higher rate of spontaneous pregnancy as well as live birth.[42,43] However, evaluation of infertile couples for CE cannot be recommended routinely, at least till a consensus is reached on the diagnostic criteria and specific treatment of this condition.[44]

Evaluation of Unexplained Infertility

At present, there is no consensus on the standard set of investigations to be done for a couple presenting with delay in conception. Significant differences exist in the tests that are carried out with respect to criteria for normality and for their prognostic utility. The general agreement is that abnormal tests should only be correlated with infertility if the treatment of cause improves fecundity when compared to no treatment. It may therefore be better to perform a limited number of specific tests instead of a broad range of tests of dubious value.

INVESTIGATIONS OF THE MALE PARTNER

Semen Analysis

Semen analysis reports from different andrology laboratories suffer from a lack of uniformity. The highest variability is found for morphology, followed by count and motility.[39] The significant overlap in semen parameters between fertile and subfertile men makes semen analysis a suboptimal tool for assessment of male fertility potential.

The World Health Organization (WHO) guideline published in 2010 has revised the lower reference values of count to 15×10^6/mL, progressive motility to 32%, vitality to 58%, and normal morphology to 4%. With the change in the reference values, the previous estimation of prevalence of UI is likely to increase. Lack of standardization and training of staff in the andrology laboratories as well as wide biological variation in the semen parameters in ejaculates (of different men as well as in different ejaculates of the same man) limit the prognostic usefulness of semen analysis test.[45] A single analysis will falsely identify 10% of men as abnormal. Repeating the test when the first test is abnormal reduces the false-positive rate to 2%.[46] The lower limit of the reference range is taken as the 5th centile. The assessment of the fertilization potential may be more thorough if the 50th centile is also taken into account as this may give a more realistic understanding of the patient's seminal profile.[8] Computer-assisted semen analysis varies in its ability to predict fertilization and, therefore, is of limited use in practice.[46] In the absence of robust and cost-effective sperm function tests that reliably assess fertilization potential, it is not possible to diagnose or rule out male factor infertility, and men with suboptimal spermatozoa may be classified as normal and vice versa.

Antisperm Antibodies

Antisperm antibodies have been reported in 42% of men with IU, 10.7% of men undergoing fertility evaluation, and 10% of couples undergoing IVF treatment but only 2% of fertile men.[8] The role of ASA in causing male infertility, however, remains ambiguous at best.

Tests for Reactive Oxygen Species

Tests to assess OS are expensive, complex, and require extensive technical training and can quantify either the ROS or the antioxidants. Currently, available tests include chemiluminescence for ROS, total antioxidant capacity (TAC) for antioxidants, and malondialdehyde (MDA) assay for post-hoc damage from lipid peroxidation.[47] Recently, Agarwal et al. have suggested the use of MiOXSYS system to detect OS by measuring oxidation-reduction potential (ORP). This enables a direct evaluation of the redox balance between the ROS and the antioxidants. The authors claim that this simplified laboratory test can be a valuable tool in the male infertility workup and guide treatment of OS-induced male infertility.[47]

Sperm Deoxyribonucleic Acid Damage Assays

Sperm DNA integrity may be accepted as a specific marker of male infertility, but its utility is undermined by the lack of general consensus on a standardized objective assessment of DNA damage. Tests described for sperm DNA fragmentation are single cell gel electrophoresis (COMET) assay, SCSA, acridine orange test (AOT), terminal deoxynucleotidyl transferase (TdT)-mediated deoxyuridine triphosphate (dUTP) nick-end labeling (TUNEL) assay, and sperm chromatin dispersion (SCD) test.

Need for Better Tests for Male

Newer technologies need to be developed to fix the shortcomings of routine semen analysis. This may be through cost-effective and reliable techniques to assess OS, DNA fragmentation, and other subcellular defects that seem to be clinically relevant. The techniques of genomics, transcriptomics, proteomics, and metabolomics, which are presently very expensive and relatively inaccessible, may enable precise and comprehensive investigation of male UI in future.[8] Defects in sperm-oocyte interaction and fertilization may be diagnosed during an IVF cycle for the very first time, thereby placing the couple erroneously in the "unexplained" cases. With tests that can test the functions of spermatozoa, it may be possible to diagnose these defects earlier, thus enabling an optimal management plan with a shorter time to pregnancy.

INVESTIGATIONS OF THE FEMALE PARTNER

Hormonal Assays

Hormonal assays are routinely done assessment of ovarian reserve during the early follicular phase. This includes basal FSH, luteinizing hormone, and anti-Müllerian hormone (AMH). These tests are useful in predicting the outcomes of IVF including the number of oocytes, number of embryos, and number of clinical pregnancy. Use of age in conjunction with AMH, antral follicle count (AFC), and basal FSH also helps in prediction of poor ovarian response in an IVF cycle.[48,49] In addition, prolactin and thyroid hormones are also routinely assessed as these have an impact on the ovarian function directly and indirectly.

Ovulation Studies

Serum progesterone measurement that is timed approximately 1 week before the expected onset of menses is a cost-effective method of confirmation of ovulation, although this may need to be repeated weekly in women with irregular cycles.[50] There is however no consensus on reference values of serum progesterone for the purpose of confirmation of an ovulatory cycle. Values >18 nmol/L are considered by WHO as indicative of ovulation, while Hull et al. suggested a level >30 nmol/L.[51] The secretion of progesterone by the corpus luteum is pulsatile and fluctuates widely in the mid and late luteal phase raising the question of reliability of a single progesterone test for the assessment of ovulation and adequacy of luteal phase.[52] Ovulation studies, however, do not provide any information on the quality of oocyte released and hence have limited value in the diagnosis of UI.

Tubal Patency and Peritoneal Factors

Available tests to assess fallopian tubes are all directed to testing the structural patency of the tubes. However, it is known that tubal peristalsis and the internal milieu of the fallopian tubes are critical for fertilization of oocyte and normal implantation of the embryo. Presently, there are no tests that can assess the functional integrity of fallopian tubes.

Hysterosalpingogram is a less invasive, less expensive, and well-tolerated outpatient procedure and is generally the first-line investigation for evaluating tubal patency. Hysterosalpingo-contrast sonography is an alternative test with comparable accuracy.[53,54] HSG, however, may fail to detect tubal abnormalities, at least some of which are secondary to undiagnosed endometriosis.[55]

Laparoscopy is considered a gold standard in the diagnosis of endometriosis and should be offered to couples with UI prior to embarking on assisted reproductive techniques. Women diagnosed with mild endometriosis may be offered surgical removal of the endometriosis and this approach has been reported to improve postoperative pregnancies.[56] Women with hitherto undiagnosed endometriosis having severe tubal disease will benefit from assisted reproductive techniques without a period of expectant management.

De Cicco et al. compared 170 women with UI who underwent combined hysteroscopy and laparoscopy surgery with 100 women who refused surgery and ART treatment. 49.4% of patients who underwent combined surgery had pelvic pathologies. Of the 86 women who had no abnormalities, 28 achieved a spontaneous pregnancy and 23 conceived after ART. The authors concluded that combined laparoscopy and hysteroscopy should be done in women with UI as this may reveal the underlying pathology and indicate patients who would benefit from ART. They also concluded that those without an abnormal surgical finding would be unlikely to benefit from ART.[57]

In a large case-control study, Mahran et al. studied 600 infertile women who were subjected to laparoscopy or combined laparoscopy and hysteroscopy over a 3-year period. Of these, 38.2% of women had UI. Following surgery, women were treated with different options—expectant management (15.3%), ovulation induction with antiestrogens or gonadotropins (62%), intrauterine insemination (IUI) (10.7%), and IVF/intracytoplasmic sperm injection (ICSI) in (10.7%). 180 patients (30%) achieved pregnancy within a year of laparoscopy. The most favorable outcome was in women with UI (36.7%) while the worst was in women with endometriosis.[58] It may be inferred that women with UI may be offered laparoscopy to complete the evaluation. Following surgery, those with an underlying pathology may be offered ART while those without a pathology may be given the option of expectant management.

Laparoscopy is, however, not recommended by all. In a large prospective randomized clinical trial, Badawy et al. evaluated the role of laparoscopy in 512 patients with UI. The 255 women in the study group had laparoscopy followed by ovarian stimulation and timed intercourse for six cycles, while the 257 women in the control group had six cycles of ovarian stimulation with timed intercourse. The clinical pregnancy rates (CPRs) as well as miscarriage rates were not statistically significant in the two groups. The authors concluded that in patients with UI, laparoscopy may be done after ovarian stimulation with timed intercourse was found to be unsuccessful.[59]

Evaluation of Uterine Cavity

Transvaginal ultrasound is the preferred and almost universally used screening tool for the assessment of uterine cavity. Saline hysterosonography can be performed to enhance the diagnostic ability of ultrasonogram (USG) in select cases. Alternatively, 3D ultrasound can be done to evaluate both uterine structural anomalies and fibroids and intracavitary abnormalities.

Hysteroscopy is another tool available to diagnose uterine cavity abnormalities. It is both more expensive and invasive. Office hysteroscopy has made this test a lot less invasive than in the past; however, more randomized controlled trials are required before routine use of hysteroscopy in subfertile women can be recommended.

The alterations of endometrial microenvironment observed in CE may hamper endometrial receptivity, potentially causing female infertility.[4,5] Nevertheless, different studies have previously showed that CE is highly prevalent in patients affected by infertility, especially in case of repeated IVF failures,[10,11] with a prevalence of up to 57.55%.[12] Intriguingly, different studies demonstrated that antibiotic therapy is able to restore normal endometrial histology as well as to improve the implantation rate in such patients,[10-12] suggesting a causal relationship between CE and defective endometrial receptivity. Although the correlations between CE and RIF have been largely evaluated, no study has still investigated the impact of CE on "unexplained infertility." UI is diagnosed in about 15% of couples seeking medical advice when standard investigations fail to identify any abnormality.[13] Due to a poor spontaneous pregnancy rate (between 2 and 4% per menstrual cycle)[14-16] and the lack of clear targets for therapy, such patients are often submitted to ARTs with limited results.[17]

"Diagnosis" of female UI is thus a diagnosis of exclusion. Many investigations available may shed light on the probable cause, but it is the clinician's responsibility to do investigations not to satisfy curiosity but to enable a prognostic evaluation and plan management. It may not be wise to do investigations that are not cost-effective and do not help in tailoring the treatment strategy. Laparoscopy may be advised to diagnose and treat endometriosis and to evaluate tubal patency. However, there is a knowledge gap regarding evaluation of oocyte quality, immune infertility, and implantation failure. Research in these areas may help decipher the enigma of "unexplained infertility" better.

MANAGEMENT

The couples diagnosed to have UI by definition have no underlying reason for infertility. This is thus a heterogeneous group with undiagnosed but varied subtle or molecular defects. The prognosis, where the duration of infertility is 3 years or more, is worse.[60] Age-related infertility is associated with poor oocyte quality that is independent of a lower ovarian reserve.[61] Counseling the patient on the reason for infertility and on prognosis is therefore difficult.

Many patients with UI conceive while awaiting treatment. It has not been possible so far to identify patients who would benefit from an expectant management in order to prevent unnecessary medical interventions. The latest Cochrane systematic review of the interventions for UI showed insufficient evidence of difference between expectant management and the four interventions—ovarian stimulation, IUI, ovarian stimulation with intrauterine insemination (OS-IUI), and IVF/ICSI. The odds of multiple pregnancy rate (MPR) may be expected to increase in OS and OS-IUI but not with IVF/ICSI when compared with expectant management.[62]

Fertility treatments have cost implications, at the same time, the "cost" of waiting, of the stress of undergoing repeated cycles of treatment in any form, of the disappointment with every failure, and cost of managing complications arising from multiple pregnancies cannot be minimized. Individualized management must therefore be planned for each patient taking into account their clinical circumstances, beliefs, and expectations of time to pregnancy.

Expectant Management

Management of patients with UI is at best empiric. Many studies have observed high spontaneous pregnancy rates in couples with UI. The cumulative pregnancy rates at the end of 12 months have been reported to vary from 14.3 to 27.4%.[63] Guzick et al. published a retrospective review of 45 studies in which average fecundity was 1.3–4.1% in the untreated group; this was lower than most other treatment groups.[64]

A large observational study was conducted in the Netherlands of 5,962 patients (of which 1,236 patients were diagnosed with UI) who were on the national waiting list for IVF or ICSI. Of these, 80 patients conceived spontaneously. The cumulative ongoing pregnancy rate was calculated to be approximately 13%. Patients of this group had 2 years or more duration of infertility and may have had a poorer prognosis.[65]

Younger women <30 years of age with shorter durations of infertility are more likely to conceive and a period of 6–12 months may be offered expectant management. This option has the lowest cost. It may be offered where limited resources are a concern, especially when the female partner is young and ovarian reserve is ample. This approach does not seem to compromise ongoing birth rates and is as effective as offering assisted reproduction immediately.

The National Institute for Health and Care Excellence (NICE) guidelines and the Royal College of Obstetricians and Gynaecologists (RCOG) guidelines advise a period of 2 years expectant management prior to offering IVF.[66] The American College of Obstetricians and Gynecologists (ACOG) guidelines advise a period of up to 6 months for a woman with UI who is 35–40 years old. However, this approach is likely to increase the time to pregnancy and may not be acceptable to patient.[67]

Superovulation and/or Intrauterine Insemination

Women who fail to conceive after a period of expectant treatment may be offered superovulation either alone or in conjunction with IUI. The thought behind this strategy is a combination of multiple ovulations and a higher density of motile sperm in the vicinity of the oocytes, which would positively impact the likelihood of fertilization and conception. This would also benefit women with cervical factors and subtle ovulation disorders. The understandable repercussion of this would be the risk of multiple pregnancies resulting from multiple ovulations. Unlike in the anovulatory patient where monofollicular ovulation is the desired goal, multiple ovulations are desirable in patients with UI. Multiple ovulations may be achieved with clomiphene citrate (CC), letrozole, or gonadotropins.

Clomiphene citrate is a commonly used ovulation induction agent that has been used in the treatment of UI. Studies comparing CC with placebo or no treatment have failed to show a clear benefit. The Cochrane collaborative systematic review compared CC with no treatment in 1,159 patients with UI (data obtained from seven trials). There was no evidence of superiority of CC over expectant management (either with or without IUI) in achieving a clinical pregnancy.[68] These studies employed a standard protocol of treatment employing fixed doses of drugs without reporting multiple follicular developments or escalating the dose of drugs if the monofollicular response was seen. The objective of multiple ovulations was not always achieved and the confounding role of endometrial quality (which can be expected in CC therapy) was also not studied. This may be the reason for the lack of benefit seen with CC therapy.

Aromatase inhibitor induces ovulation without the disadvantage of antiestrogenic effect of CC. In a study of 214 patients, Fouda et al. demonstrated an improved ongoing pregnancy rate with letrozole plus IUI (33%) when compared with CC plus IUI (19%). On the other hand, DIAMOND trial studied 900 patients randomized to three arms: Letrozole (5 mg on cycle days 3–7), CC (100 mg on cycle days 3–7), and FSH (150 UI from cycle day 3 onwards). LBR was 23.3% in the CC group, 18.7% in the letrozole group, and 32.2% in the FSH group. While the difference in LBR in CC in comparison to the letrozole group was not significant, the LBR was significantly higher in the FSH group.[63]

Gonadotropins can also be used to achieve multiple ovulations. A review of a Cochrane database published in 2009 found insufficient evidence of a difference in LBR between oral and injectable ovulation-inducing agents. When data from three studies that had CPR as the outcome was combined, a significantly higher CPR was seen in the group treated with human menopausal gonadotropins.[68] The cost of treatment and patient's convenience should be taken into account before choosing the method of treatment. Patients should also be counseled regarding the risk of multiple gestations and ovarian hyperstimulation syndrome (OHSS).

In Vitro Fertilization

In vitro fertilization has been recommended by NICE for all patients who fail to conceive after expectant treatment for a period of 2 years. It is considered to be the most effective method of treatment as it helps with ovarian dysfunction, cervical factors, abnormal sperm-oocyte interaction, and tubal dysfunction. It is also expensive and invasive and has the additional risk of high multiple pregnancy and OHSS. Cochrane review on the role of IVF in UI showed higher CPR and LBR than expectant management.[68] Goverde et al. examined the efficacy of gonadotropins with IUI against IVF. No statistically significant difference was found. They also found IUI cycles more cost-effective than IVF.[63] On comparing IVF and natural cycle IUI, they found no significant difference in LBR (39% vs. 24%). ICSI was not found to be superior to IVF in terms of fertilization rate, CPR, and LBR.[63]

The FASTT (Fast Track and Standard Treatment) trial studied two arms with time to pregnancy as an endpoint. Reindollar et al. randomized patients to one of two arms: (1) A conventional arm with three cycles of CC (100 mg on days 3–7) and IUI followed by three cycles of gonadotropins (at a starting dose of 150 IU) and IUI and then up to six cycles of IVF or (2) an accelerated arm with three cycles of CC with IUI followed by up to six cycles of IVF. This study also reviewed per-cycle pregnancy rates and found no benefit to gonadotropin treatment after failed oral superovulation. The accelerated arm had a shorter time to pregnancy.[63]

To conclude, IVF may be offered to those couples who fail to conceive after 2 years of expectant management.[66] However, ovulation induction with oral or injectable agents may be offered in conjunction with IUI in an attempt to limit over-medicalization. IVF is probably the most effective management strategy once the 3–6 cycles of Ovulation Induction + IUI fail. It also provides an opportunity to rule out poor oocyte quality and abnormal sperm-oocyte interaction which would otherwise remain undiagnosed with currently available tests.

CONCLUSION

Unexplained infertility continues to confound and challenge fertility specialists the world over. Clinical experience and research have over the years implicated many factors as the possible cause of subfertility in these cases; however, most have not shown any direct correlation with fecundity. The causality remains ambivalent and tentative at best. This makes the management of UI much more difficult. The prognosis swings widely between those who conceive spontaneously or with treatment, who fortunately form the bigger group to those who are refractory to all treatments. It is this group of recalcitrant that are difficult to explain and understand and they continue to remain unexplained until age or a decreasing reserve becomes a definite factor needing correction. The way forward continues to remain an individualized tailor-made approach for each patient depending upon their clinical features, age and other logistical considerations, and the clinician's experience and judgment. More will hopefully be known to us in the future and the management will subsequently be a lot more assured and unequivocal.

KEY POINTS

- Causes of UI range from not so easily diagnosed to not so well understood.
- There is no standard prescribed list of investigations for evaluation. Most clinicians rely on their own experience as well as availability and cost of tests to guide them.
- The significant overlap in semen parameters between fertile and subfertile men makes semen analysis a suboptimal tool for assessment of male fertility.

- The correlation of ASA is inconsistent with infertility. Many men with immune infertility may have normal semen parameters.
- OS may affect fertility potential in both men and women, but it is difficult to diagnose.
- Sperm DNA integrity may be accepted as a specific marker of male infertility, but its utility is undermined by the lack of general consensus on a standardized objective assessment of DNA damage.
- Tubal peristalsis and the internal milieu of the fallopian tubes are critical for fertilization of oocyte and normal implantation of the embryo. Presently, there are no tests for the functional integrity of the tubes.
- It is known that the immune system has an important role in implantation, but our understanding of the physiology is insufficient to recommend manipulation of the immunological milieu to improve implantation.
- Hysteroscopy and laparoscopy may assist in the diagnosis and management of patients with endometriosis and uterine cavity abnormalities.
- The prognosis where the duration of infertility is 3 years or more is worse.
- Age-related infertility is associated with poor oocyte quality that is independent of a lower ovarian reserve.
- Management of patients with UI is at best empiric.
- High spontaneous pregnancy rates have been observed in couples with UI with expectant management.
- Cost of fertility treatments should also take into account the "cost" of waiting, of the stress of undergoing repeated cycles of treatment in any form, of the disappointment with every failure, and the cost of managing complications arising from multiple pregnancies cannot be minimized.
- Individualized management must therefore be planned for each patient taking into account their clinical circumstances, beliefs, and expectations of time to pregnancy.

REFERENCES

1. Wang X, Chen C, Wang L, Chen D, Guang W, French J. Conception, early pregnancy loss, and time to clinical pregnancy: a population-based prospective study. Fertil Steril. 2003;79:577-84.
2. Weinberg CR, Gladen BC. The beta-geometric distribution applied to comparative fecundability studies. Biometrics. 1986;42:547-60.
3. Polyzos NP, Tzioras S, Mauri D, Tsappi M, Cortinovis I, Tsali L, et al. Treatment of unexplained infertility with aromatase inhibitors or clomiphene citrate: a systematic review and meta-analysis. Obstet Gynecol Surv. 2008;63:472-9.
4. te Velde ER, Eijkemans R, Habbema HD. Variation in couple fecundity and time to pregnancy, an essential concept in human reproduction. Lancet. 2000;355:1928-9.
5. van Eekelen R, Scholten I, Tjon-Kon-Fat RI, van der Steeg JW, Steures P, Hompes P, et al. Natural conception: repeated predictions over time. Hum Reprod. 2017;32:346-53.
6. ESHRE Capri Workshop Group. Diagnosis and management of the infertile couple: missing information. Hum Reprod Update. 2004;10:295-307.
7. Gleicher N, Barad D. Unexplained infertility: does it really exist? Hum Reprod. 2006;21:1951-5.
8. Hamada A, Esteves SC, Nizza M, Agarwal A. Unexplained male infertility: diagnosis and management. Int Braz J Urol. 2012;38:576-94.
9. Shefi S, Turek PJ. Definition and current evaluation of subfertile men. Int Braz J Urol. 2006;32:385-97.
10. Venkatesh S, Shamsi MB, Deka D, Saxena V, Kumar R, Dada R. Clinical implications of oxidative stress and sperm DNA damage in normozoospermic infertile men. Indian J Med Res. 2011;134:396-8.
11. Bozhedomov VA, Nikolaeva MA, Ushakova IV, Lipatova NA, Bozhedomova GE, Sukhikh GT. Functional deficit of sperm and fertility impairment in men with antisperm antibodies. J Reprod Immunol. 2015;112:95-101.
12. de Lamirande E, Gagnon C. A positive role for the superoxide anion in triggering hyperactivation and capacitation of human spermatozoa. Int J Androl. 1993;16:21-5.
13. Olugbenga OM, Olukole SG, Adeoye AT, Adejoke AD. Semen characteristics and sperm morphological studies of the West African Dwarf Buck treated with Aloe vera gel extract. Iran J Reprod Med. 2011;9:83-8.
14. Aitken R. Possible redox regulation of sperm motility activation. J Androl. 2000;21:491-6.
15. Sabeti P, Pourmasumi S, Rahiminia T, Akyash F, Talebi AR. Etiologies of sperm oxidative stress. Int J Reprod Bio Med. 2016;14:231-40.
16. Agarwal A, Makker K, Sharma R. Clinical relevance of oxidative stress in male factor infertility: an update. Am J Reprod Immunol. 2008;59:2-11.
17. Garrido N, Martínez-Conejero JA, Jauregui J, Horcajadas JA, Simón C, Remohí J, et al. Microarray analysis in sperm from fertile and infertile men without basic sperm analysis abnormalities reveals a significantly different transcriptome. Fertil Steril. 2009;91(Suppl. 4):1307-10.
18. Lishko PV, Kirichok Y. The role of Hv1 and CatSper channels in sperm activation. J Physiol. 2010;588:4667-72.
19. Holoch KJ, Lessey BA. Endometriosis and infertility. Clin Obstet Gynecol. 2010;53(2):429-38.
20. Bancroft K, Vaughan Williams CA, Elstein M. Minimal/mild endometriosis and infertility. A review. Br J Obstet Gynaecol. 1989;96:454-60.
21. Meuleman C, Vandenabeele B, Fieuws S, Spiessens C, Timmerman D, D'Hooghe T. High prevalence of endometriosis in infertile women with normal ovulation and normospermic partners. Fertil Steril. 2009;92:68-74.
22. Guan J, Watrelot A. Fallopian tube subtle pathology. Best Pract Res Clin Obstet Gynaecol. 2019;59:25-40.
23. Goverde AJ, McDonnell J, Schats R, Vermeiden JP, Homburg R, Lambalk CB. Ovarian response to standard gonadotrophin stimulation for IVF is decreased not only in older but also in younger women in couples with idiopathic and male subfertility. Hum Reprod. 2005;20(6):1573-7.
24. May-Panloup P, Boucret L, Chao de la Barca JM, Desquiret-Dumas V, Ferré-L'Hotellier V, Morinière C, et al. Ovarian ageing: the role of mitochondria in oocytes and follicles. Hum Reprod Update. 2016;22(6):725-43.

25. Haller-Kikkatalo K, Salumets A, Uibo R. Review on autoimmune reactions in female infertility: antibodies to follicle stimulating hormone. Clin Dev Immunol. 2012;2012: 762541.
26. Ehsani M, Mohammadnia-Afrouzi M, Mirzakhani M, Esmaeilzadeh S, Shahbazi M. Female unexplained infertility: a disease with imbalanced adaptive immunity. J Hum Reprod Sci. 2019;12(4):274-82.
27. Sanchez AM, Vanni VS, Bartiromo L, Papaleo E, Zilberberg E, Candiani M, et al. Is the oocyte quality affected by endometriosis? A review of the literature. J Ovarian Res. 2017; 10(1):43.
28. Mihalas BP, Redgrove KA, McLaughlin EA, Nixon B. Molecular mechanisms responsible for increased vulnerability of the ageing oocyte to oxidative damage. Oxid Med Cell Longev. 2017;2017:4015874.
29. Homer HA. The role of oocyte quality in explaining "unexplained" infertility. Semin Reprod Med. 2020;38(1):21-8.
30. Grimbizis GF, Camus M, Tarlatzis BC, Bontis JN, Devroey P. Clinical implications of uterine malformations and hysteroscopic treatment results. Hum Reprod Update. 2001;7(2): 161-74.
31. Pundir J, El Toukhy T. Uterine cavity assessment prior to IVF. Womens Health (Lond). 2010;6(6):841-7.
32. Practice Committee of the American Society for Reproductive Medicine. Removal of myomas in asymptomatic patients to improve fertility and/or reduce miscarriage rate: a guideline. Fertil Steril. 2017;108(3):416-25.
33. Styer AK, Jin S, Liu D, Wang B, Polotsky AJ, Christianson MS, et al. Association of uterine fibroids and pregnancy outcomes after ovarian stimulation-intrauterine insemination for unexplained infertility. Fertil Steril. 2017;107(3):756-62.e3.
34. Dmowski WP, Greenblatt RB. Asherman's syndrome and risk of placenta accreta. Obstet Gynecol. 1969;34:288-99.
35. Ventolini G, Zhang M, Gruber J. Hysteroscopy in the evaluation of patients with recurrent pregnancy loss: a cohort study in a primary care population. Surg Endosc. 2004;18:1782-4.
36. Gelbaya TA, Potdar N, Jeve YB, Nardo LG. Definition and epidemiology of unexplained infertility. Obstet Gynecol Surv. 2014;69(2):109-15.
37. van Bogaert LJ. Clinicopathologic findings in endometrial polyps. Obstet Gynecol. 1988;71:771-3.
38. Silló-Seidl G. The analysis of the endometrium of 1,000 sterile women. Hormones. 1971;2:70-5.
39. Filimberti E, Degl'Innocenti S, Borsotti M, Quercioli M, Piomboni P, Natali I, et al. High variability in results of semen analysis in andrology laboratories in Tuscany (Italy): the experience of an external quality control (EQC) programme. Andrology. 2013;1:401-7.
40. Stamatellos I, Apostolides A, Stamatopoulos P, Bontis J. Pregnancy rates after hysteroscopic polypectomy depending on the size or number of the polyps. Arch Gynecol Obstet. 2008;277:395-9.
41. Cicinelli E, Resta L, Nicoletti R, Tartagni M, Marinaccio M, Bulletti C, et al. Detection of chronic endometritis at fluid hysteroscopy. J Minim Invasive Gynecol. 2005;12:514-8.
42. Cicinelli E, Matteo M, Trojano G, Mitola PC, Tinelli R, Vitagliano A, et al. Chronic endometritis in patients with unexplained infertility: prevalence and effects of antibiotic treatment on spontaneous conception. Am J Reprod Immunol. 2018;79(1).
43. Kuroda K, Horikawa T, Moriyama A, Nakao K, Juen H, Takamizawa S, et al. Impact of chronic endometritis on endometrial receptivity analysis results and pregnancy outcomes. Immun Inflamm Dis. 2020;8(4):650-8.
44. Espinós JJ, Fabregues F, Fontes J, García-Velasco JA, Llácer J, Requena A, et al. Impact of chronic endometritis in infertility: a SWOT analysis. Reprod Biomed Online. 2021;42(5):939-51.
45. Björndahl L. What is normal semen quality? On the use and abuse of reference limits for the interpretation of semen analysis results. Hum Fertil (Camb). 2011;14:179-86.
46. Opsahl MS, Dixon NG, Robins ER, Cunningham DS. Single vs. multiple semen specimens in screening for male infertility factors. A comparison. J Reprod Med. 1996;41(5):313-5.
47. Agarwal A, Bui AD. Oxidation-reduction potential as a new marker for oxidative stress: correlation to male infertility. Investig Clin Urol. 2017;58(6):385-99.
48. Wang X, Jin L, Mao YD, Shi JZ, Huang R, Jiang YN, et al. Evaluation of ovarian reserve tests and age in the prediction of poor ovarian response to controlled ovarian stimulation—a real-world data analysis of 89,002 patients. Front Endocrinol (Lausanne). 2021;12:702061.
49. Tehraninezhad ES, Mehrabi F, Taati R, Kalantar V, Aziminekoo E, Tarafdari A. Analysis of ovarian reserve markers (AMH, FSH, AFC) in different age strata in IVF/ICSI patients. Int J Reprod BioMed. 2016;14(8):501-6.
50. Crosignani PG, Collins J, Cooke ID, Diczfalusy E, Rubin B. Recommendations of the ESHRE workshop on 'unexplained infertility'. Anacapri, August 28-9, 1992. Hum Reprod. 1993;8:977-80.
51. Hull MG, McLeod FN, Joyce DN, Ray BD, Mcdermott A. Human in-vitro fertilisation, in-vivo sperm penetration of cervical mucus, and unexplained infertility. Lancet. 1984;324: 245-6.
52. Filicori M, Butler JP, Crowley Jr WF. Neuroendocrine regulation of the corpus luteum in the human. Evidence for pulsatile progesterone secretion. J Clin Invest. 1984;73(6):1638-47.
53. Maheux-Lacroix S, Boutin A, Moore L, Bergeron ME, Bujold E, Laberge P, et al. Hysterosalpingosonography for diagnosing tubal occlusion in subfertile women: a systematic review with meta-analysis. Hum Reprod. 2014;29(5):953-63.
54. Mandia L, Personeni C, Antonazzo P, Angileri SA, Pinto A, Savasi V. Ultrasound in infertility setting: optimal strategy to evaluate the assessment of tubal patency. Biomed Res Int. 2017;2017:3205895.
55. Karande VC, Pratt DE, Rabin DS, Gleicher N. The limited value of hysterosalpingography in assessing tubal status and fertility potential. Fertil Steril. 1995;63(6):1167-71.
56. De Cicco S, Tagliaferri V, Selvaggi L, Romualdi D, Di Florio C, Immediata V, et al. Expectant management may reduce overtreatment in women affected by unexplained infertility confirmed by diagnostic laparoscopy. Arch Gynecol Obstet. 2017;295(2):427-33.
57. Miller PB, Savaris RF, Forstein DA, Likes CE, Nichols C, Cooper LJ, et al. Laparoscopic surgery improves pregnancy outcomes in women with suspected endometriosis with or without pathological confirmation. Clin Exp Obstet Gynecol. 2016;43(1):31-6.
58. Mahran A, Abdelraheim AR, Eissa A, Gadelrab M. Does laparoscopy still has a role in modern fertility practice? Int J Reprod Biomed. 2017;15(12):787-94.

59. Badawy A, Khiary M, Ragab A, Hassan M, Sherif L. Laparoscopy—or not—for management of unexplained infertility. J Obstet Gynaecol. 2010;30:712-5.
60. Hansen KR, He AL, Styer AK, Wild RA, Butts S, Engmann L, et al. Predictors of pregnancy and live-birth in couples with unexplained infertility after ovarian stimulation-intrauterine insemination. Fertil Steril. 2016;105(6):1575-83.e2.
61. ESHRE Capri Workshop Group. A prognosis-based approach to infertility: understanding the role of time. Hum Reprod. 2017;32(8):1556-9.
62. Wang R, Danhof NA, Tjon-Kon-Fat RI, Eijkemans MJ, Bossuyt PM, Mochtar MH, et al. Interventions for unexplained infertility: a systematic review and network meta-analysis. Cochrane Database Syst Rev. 2019;9(9):CD012692.
63. Gunn DD, Bates GW. Evidence-based approach to unexplained infertility: a systematic review. Fertil Steril. 2016; 105(6):1566-74.e1.
64. Guzick DS, Sullivan MW, Adamson GD, Cedars MI, Falk RJ, Peterson EP, et al. Efficacy of treatment for unexplained infertility. Fertil Steril. 1998;70(2):207-13.
65. Eijkemans MJC, Lintsen AME, Hunault CC, Bouwmans CA, Hakkaart L, Braat DD, et al. Pregnancy chances on an IVF/ICSI waiting list: a national prospective cohort study. Hum Reprod. 2008;23(7):1627-32.
66. National Collaborating Centre for Women's and Children's Health (UK). NICE Clinical Guidelines, No. 156. London: Royal College of Obstetricians & Gynaecologists; 2013.
67. American College of Obstetricians and Gynecologists Committee on Gynecologic Practice and Practice Committee. Female age-related fertility decline. Committee Opinion No. 589. Fertil Steril. 2014;101(3):633-4.
68. Ray A, Shah A, Gudi A, Homburg R. Unexplained infertility: an update and review of practice. Reprod Biomed Online. 2012;24(6):591-602.

CHAPTER 21

Fertility Preservation

Sonia Malik, Aneesha Grover

INTRODUCTION

Fertility preservation can be defined as a means for preserving an individual's ability to reproduce at will or at a chosen time.[1] Fertility preservation has given a new dimension to assisted reproductive technology (ART) services. With a post-thaw embryo/gamete survival rate of around 90% and around 50% implantation rate, the infertility specialists confidently offer cryopreservation to all who want to delay childbearing or whose fertility is at risk.[2] Both men and women have been benefited by it.

Concomitantly, there is a marked increase in the incidence of cancer worldwide in all age groups.[3] Childhood cancers are increasing and so are the young cancer survivors.[4] Moreover, with men and women delaying childbearing, there is a growing pool of cancer patients who require to save their fertility.

There are other noncancer patients as well whose fertility is at risk and will be benefited by this, for example, autoimmune disorders, and delayed marriages.

Many options are available to these patients; some are well established while some are emerging. Embryo/oocyte and semen cryopreservation are well-accepted methods of fertility preservation in postpubertal patients.[5-7] New techniques for mitigating the negative effect of cancer treatments, protecting ovarian function and preserving fertility are constantly being developed. Both existing and emerging techniques in fertility preservation will be dealt with in detail in this chapter.

INDICATIONS OF FERTILITY PRESERVATION

Both oncologic and nononcologic diseases can affect the fertility potential of an individual, either directly by the disease process itself or due to their fertility-threatening therapy. The main objective of fertility preservation intervention is to minimize or eliminate the disease burden and also preserve the individual's chance of achieving pregnancy.

Fertility preservation may be sought by both men and women for either cancer or noncancer indications.

FERTILITY PRESERVATION IN WOMEN

The European Society of Human Reproduction and Embryology (ESHRE) guidelines on fertility preservation, 2020, divided the subpopulation of women requiring fertility preservation into four subgroups,[8] namely:

1. Postpubertal women diagnosed with cancer undergoing gonadotoxic treatments
2. Postpubertal women with benign diseases undergoing gonadotoxic treatments or with genetic conditions predisposing to premature ovarian insufficiency (POI), for example, Turner syndrome
3. Transgender men (assigned female at birth)
4. Women considering oocyte cryopreservation for age-related fertility loss.

Cancer therapy in the form of chemotherapy or radiotherapy leads to POI. The degree of ovarian damage is related to the type and dose of chemotherapy and the dose and field of radiation.[9] The age of the patient and the ovarian reserve at the time of initiation of therapy are other prognostic factors for fertility decline after therapy. Decanter et al. found that the anti-Müllerian hormone (AMH) levels declined substantially after the initiation of chemotherapy.[10] Among the chemotherapeutic agents, it is the alkylating agents such as cyclophosphamide, chlorambucil, busulfan, and mechlorethamine, which have the maximum negative impact on the fertility potential of the woman. These agents cause single- and double-strand deoxyribonucleic acid (DNA) breaks in ovarian cells. They are also seen to cause cortical fibrosis and blood vessel damage in the ovarian tissue. These agents are thus associated with acute ovarian insufficiency, premature menopause, and poor reproductive outcomes.[9]

Figures 1A and B describe the follicle development in the ovary and the mechanism of chemotherapeutic damage of the ovary.[11]

Radiotherapy not only damages the ovaries but also reduces uterine vascularity and causes myometrial fibrosis, endometrial damage, and reduction in uterine volume.[9] It

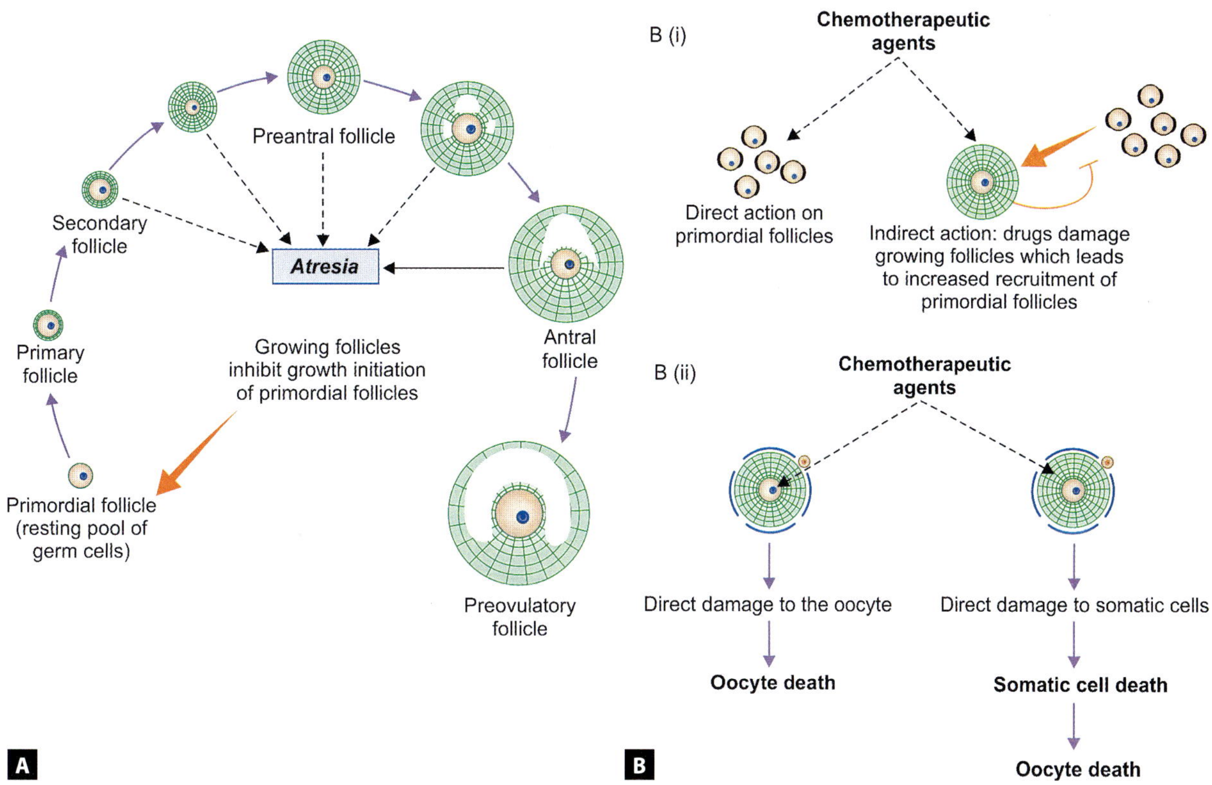

Figs. 1A and B: Mechanism of cellular damage in ovary after cytotoxic therapy.
Source: Adapted from Morgan et al. 2012;18(5):525-35.

had been seen that an irradiation dose of as less as 2 Gy can destroy 50% of the primordial follicles in the ovary. It has also been seen that an abdominal irradiation dose of 20–30 Gy in childhood resulted in 97% of women to suffer from ovarian failure and 67% of women who received irradiation in prepuberty to suffer from ovarian failure.[9] Also, cancer debulking surgeries involving removal or damage to the reproductive organs can also result in loss of fertility.

Chemotherapy and radiotherapy may be advised before hematopoietic stem cell transplantation or bone marrow transplantation for nononcologic conditions such as thalassemia major, aplastic anemia, sickle cell anemia, and other myeloproliferative and myelodysplastic diseases. Alkylating agents may also be used in the treatment of autoimmune diseases such as systemic lupus erythematosus (SLE), Behçet's syndrome, Sjögren's syndrome, steroid-resistant glomerulonephritis, inflammatory bowel disease, and scleroderma, thereby putting the fertility potential of these individuals at risk.[9]

Some genetic disorders such as Turner syndrome, fragile X syndrome, and galactosemia (autosomal recessive disorder of galactose metabolism) predispose an individual to POI.

Some gynecologic diseases such as endometriosis are associated with declining fertility, not only due to the disease process but also because of the corrective surgeries done as treatment. The local inflammation caused by the endometrioma increases the follicular burnout and the cystectomy surgery for removal of the endometrioma has a negative impact on the ovarian reserve due to loss of germinal vesicles (GV) attached to the cyst. Fertility preservation should be offered in endometriosis if:[9]

- There is quantitative alteration in ovarian reserve due to repetitive surgeries
- Recurrent endometriosis
- Bilateral endometrioma
- A large (>5 cm) unilateral endometrioma.

Female fertility starts declining after the age of 32 years and this decline accelerates after the age of 37 years. Women who delay childbearing should therefore consider oocyte freezing in order to preserve their fertility.[12]

Sex affirmation procedures in transgender men who have been assigned female at birth involve surgical removal of ovaries and cross-sex hormone therapy. This has a deleterious effect on the fertility of these individuals. Therefore, fertility preservation may be offered to them before they undergo any of the sex-changing treatments.

FERTILITY PRESERVATION IN MALES

Men requiring fertility preservation can be subgrouped as per their indications:[13]

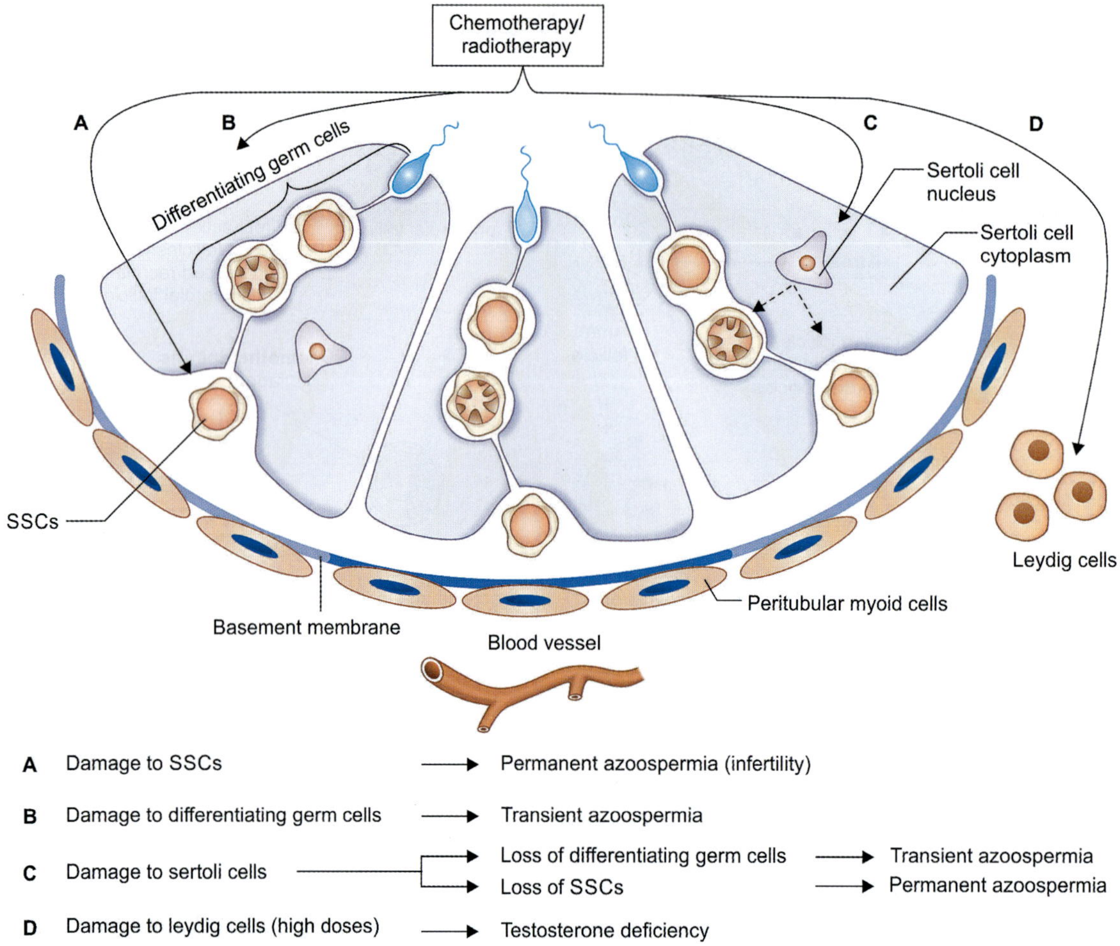

Fig. 2: Mechanism of cellular damage in testis after cytotoxic therapy.
(SSC: spermatogonial stem cell)
Source: Adapted from Anderson et al. 2015.

- *For medical indications*
  - Oncologic treatment: Adults/adolescents/prepubertal boys planned for gonadotoxic treatment in view of cancer
  - Human immunodeficiency virus (HIV) infection
  - Prevasectomy
  - Posthumous sperm retrieval
  - Men undergoing gender reassignment
- *Nonmedical conditions*
  - Social.

Cancer is one of the primary indications for fertility preservation in men. Radiotherapy and chemotherapeutic drugs, especially alkylating agents, adversely affect the spermatogonial stem cells and result in fertility problems.

Figure 2 describes the mechanism of cellular damage in the testis after cytotoxic therapy.[14]

It has been seen that the sperm quality is impaired even when the initial diagnosis of cancer is made, even before the initiation of any form of treatment.[9] Also if there is an adequate number of spermatogonial stem cells at the time of initiation of the cancer treatment, it has been observed that adverse effect of the treatment on fertility may be reversible.[15]

Surgical interventions can affect spermatogenesis both directly and indirectly. Direct damage to spermatogenesis occurs in procedures such as orchidectomy, while indirect impairment can occur due to damage to the sympathetic and parasympathetic nervous systems resulting in ejaculatory and erectile dysfunction.[16]

There are some nononcologic medical conditions which result in impaired fertility, either due to the disease process itself or due to the gonadotoxic nature of its treatment. Autoimmune diseases such as SLE, multiple sclerosis, and Crohn's disease are associated with abnormal sperm parameters and erectile and ejaculatory dysfunction.[17] Hematopoietic stem cell transplantation may be required in the treatment of these diseases. This in turn requires chemotherapy and radiotherapy to damage the diseased blood-forming cells and marrow, which also damage the spermatogonia.[18] The other nononcologic conditions associated with infertility include spinal cord injuries and nerve injuries during abdominopelvic surgeries resulting in ejaculatory and erectile dysfunction.

Human immunodeficiency virus infection has a direct impact on fertility. It is associated with reduced seminal fluid volume, sperm concentration, vitality, motility, morphology, and fertilizing capacity of the sperms. The degree of impact is related to the duration of infection, age of the patient, and the presence of concomitant sexually transmitted disease (STD) infection. A low $CD4^+$ count has been directly correlated with reduced semen quality.[19,20]

Vasectomy is a permanent method for contraception. Only those men who are certain that they do not want to biologically father children in the future are offered this procedure. However, it has been observed that up to 6% of men who have undergone vasectomy request a reversal of the procedure due to a change in their life circumstances.[21] Hence, the option of fertility preservation before vasectomy may be discussed.

Posthumous sperm retrieval raises many ethical, moral, and legal issues for the patients, their families, and the clinicians. This is dealt with in greater detail later in the chapter. Perimortem sperm retrieval can be done either with the help of electroejaculation or through surgical sperm retrieval techniques. Postmortem sperm retrieval is done surgically through partial/complete orchiectomy, epididymectomy, or testicular aspiration and should be done within 36 hours of death in order to obtain viable spermatozoa.[9]

Gender reassignment procedure involves hormonal and surgical interventions. Hormone therapy causes decreased spermatogenesis and surgical intervention involves orchiectomy. Thus, cryopreservation of the spermatozoa should be contemplated if the patient wishes to father a genetic offspring in the future with the help of ART.[9]

One of the most upcoming indications for fertility preservation is for social reasons. There is now increasing evidence that advancing age of males is associated with increased risk of heritable disease-causing mutations in the offspring. Paternal age of >40 years is associated with declining sperm quality, increased risk of pregnancy complications, birth defects, childhood cancers, autism, and some psychiatric disorders.[9]

Table 1 describes the risk of developing infertility after anticancer treatment.[5]

TABLE 1: Risk of developing infertility after anticancer treatment.

Degree of risk	*Type of anticancer treatment in women*	*Type of anticancer treatment in men*
High risk (>80% risk of permanent amenorrhea in women; prolonged azoospermia in men)	• HSC transplantation with cyclophosphamide/TBI or cyclophosphamide/busulfan • External beam radiation to a field that includes the ovaries • CMF, CEF, CAF, TAC × 6 cycles in women ≥40 years	• Radiation >2.5 Gy to testis • Chlorambucil (1.4 g/m^2) • Cyclophosphamide (19 g/m^2) • Procarbazine (4 g/m^2) • Melphalan (140 mg/m^2) • Cisplatin (500 mg/m^2) • BCNU (1 g/m^2) and CCNU (500 mg/m^2)
Intermediate risk (40–60% risk of permanent amenorrhea in women; likelihood of azoospermia in men, especially when given with other sterilizing agents)	• BEACOPP • CMF, CEF, CAF, TAC × 6 cycles in women aged 30–39 years • AC × 4 cycles in women ≥40 years • AC or EC × 4 → taxanes	• Busulfan (600 mg/kg) • Ifosfamide (42 g/m^2) • BCNU (300 mg/m^2) • Nitrogen mustard • Actinomycin D
Low risk (<20% risk of permanent amenorrhea in women; only temporary reductions in sperm counts in men, especially when not given with other sterilizing agents)	• ABVD in women ≥32 years • CHOP × 4–6 cycles • CVP • AML therapy (anthracycline/cytarabine) • ALL therapy (multi-agent) • CMF, CEF, CAF, TAC × 6 cycles in women ≤30 years • AC × 4 cycles in women ≤40 years	• Carboplatin (2 g/m^2) • Doxorubicin (770 mg/m^2) • Thiotepa (400 mg/m^2) • Cytosine arabinoside (1 g/m^2) • Vinblastine (50 g/m^2) • Vincristine (8 g/m^2)
Unknown risk (risk of permanent amenorrhea in women; effect on sperm production in men)	• Monoclonal antibodies (trastuzumab, bevacizumab, cetuximab) • Tyrosine kinase inhibitors (erlotinib, imatinib)	• Oxaliplatin • Irinotecan • Monoclonal antibodies (trastuzumab, bevacizumab, cetuximab) • Tyrosine kinase inhibitors (erlotinib, imatinib) • Taxanes

(ABVD: adriamycin, bleomycin sulfate, vinblastine sulfate, and dacarbazine; AC: doxorubicin, cyclophosphamide; ALL: acute lymphocytic leukemia; AML: acute myeloid leukemia; BCNU: carmustine; BEACOPP: bleomycin, etoposide, doxorubicin, cyclophosphamide, vincristine, procarbazine, and prednisone; CAF: cyclophosphamide, adriamycin, fluorouracil; CCNU: lomustine; CEF: cyclophosphamide, epirubicin, fluorouracil; CHOP: cyclophosphamide, hydroxydaunorubicin, oncovin, prednisone; CMF: cyclophosphamide, methotrexate, fluorouracil; CVP: cyclophosphamide, vincristine, prednisone; EC: epirubicin, cyclophosphamide; HSC: hematopoietic stem cell; TAC: taxotere, adriamycin, and cyclophosphamide; TBI: total body irradiation)

Flowchart 1: Model of care for patients seeking fertility preservation.

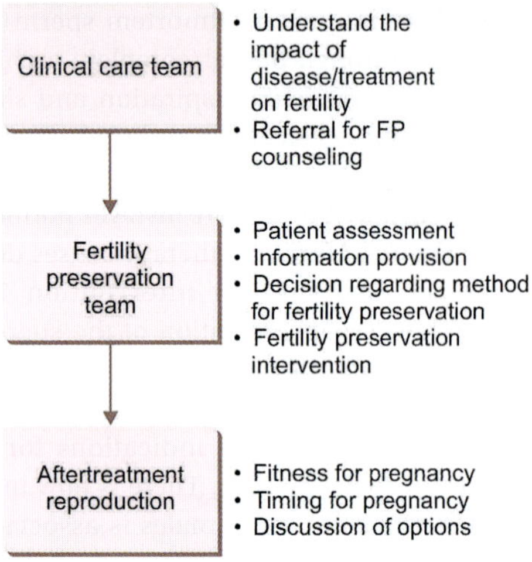

(FP: family planning)

MODEL OF CARE FOR PATIENTS SEEKING FERTILITY PRESERVATION[8]

The model of care for patients seeking fertility preservation is shown in **Flowchart 1**.

CRITERIA FOR SELECTION OF PATIENTS WHO CAN BE OFFERED FERTILITY PRESERVATION

Fertility preservation should be offered only after careful individual assessment in terms of indication and risk assessment. A checklist for patient assessment and selection for fertility preservation is given below:[8,22]

- *Intrinsic factors:*
  - Assessment of health status of the patient
    - Surgical/anesthetic risk including thrombosis and infection
    - Malignant contamination of the gonad
  - The need to obtain fully informed consent (patient/parent)
  - Age of the patient (upper and lower limits for safety and efficacy)
  - Assessment of ovarian reserve in girls/young women
  - Assessment of pubertal stage in boys/young men (including testicular volume)
- *Extrinsic factors:*
  - Nature of predicted treatment (high/medium/low/uncertain risk)
  - Time available
  - Expertise available.

At the time of counseling, it is important to discuss with the patient about her risk of developing ovarian insufficiency after the oncologic treatment and also decide the method of fertility preservation that can be offered to her. Also, it is imperative to know the baseline ovarian reserve before any treatment modality can be offered. The parameters used to determine this are the age of the patient, the AMH levels, and the antral follicle count (AFC) in the ovaries.

The American Society of Clinical Oncology (ASCO) in 2006 proposed to stratify the patients into three categories (low, intermediate, and high) based on their risk of developing ovarian insufficiency.[23]

It is not recommended to offer fertility preservation to women with overt POI.[8]

INTERVENTIONS FOR FERTILITY PRESERVATION

All patients who are at substantial risk of posttreatment fertility loss should receive information about the fertility preservation options in a timely manner.[6,7] Because of the ever-expanding number of options for treating cancer and preserving fertility, there is now an opportunity to take a precision medicine approach by informing patients about the fertility risks associated with their cancer treatment and the options of fertility preservation available to them. It is then entirely their prerogative whether they wish to opt for it or not. Currently, sperm, egg, and embryo cryopreservation are standards of care for preserving fertility in reproductive-age cancer patients; ovarian tissue cryopreservation (OTC) is still considered experimental.[23] Adoption and surrogacy may also need to be considered in a few cases.

Flowchart 2 and Figures 3 and 4 graphically represent the fertility-preserving interventions available at present.[14]

Techniques of Fertility Preservation in Males

Sperm cryopreservation is a standard and well-accepted method of fertility preservation in postpubertal men. It should be offered prior to the start of cancer therapy as per the American Society for Reproductive Medicine (ASRM) and ASCO recommendations. There is not much to offer in fertility preservation for prepubertal boys as testicular tissue cryopreservation is still in the experimental stage and the utility of fertiprotectant agents such as gonadotropin-releasing hormone (GnRH) analogs is still not proven.

Sperm Cryopreservation

Sperm cryopreservation is the most common technique utilized for fertility preservation in pubertal and postpubertal males. Sperm banking may provide both a sense of security and reassurance of the future as both young cancer patients and their parents wish to be offered fertility preservation options.[24-26] Most often, sperm samples are collected by masturbation and cryopreserved after a period of abstinence of 2–3 days. Ideally, samples should be collected prior to initiation of cancer treatment to ensure sperm quality. Sperm collection can be challenging in adolescents and in those with ejaculatory dysfunctions. In case of azoospermia,

Flowchart 2: Summary of the available fertility preservation interventions.

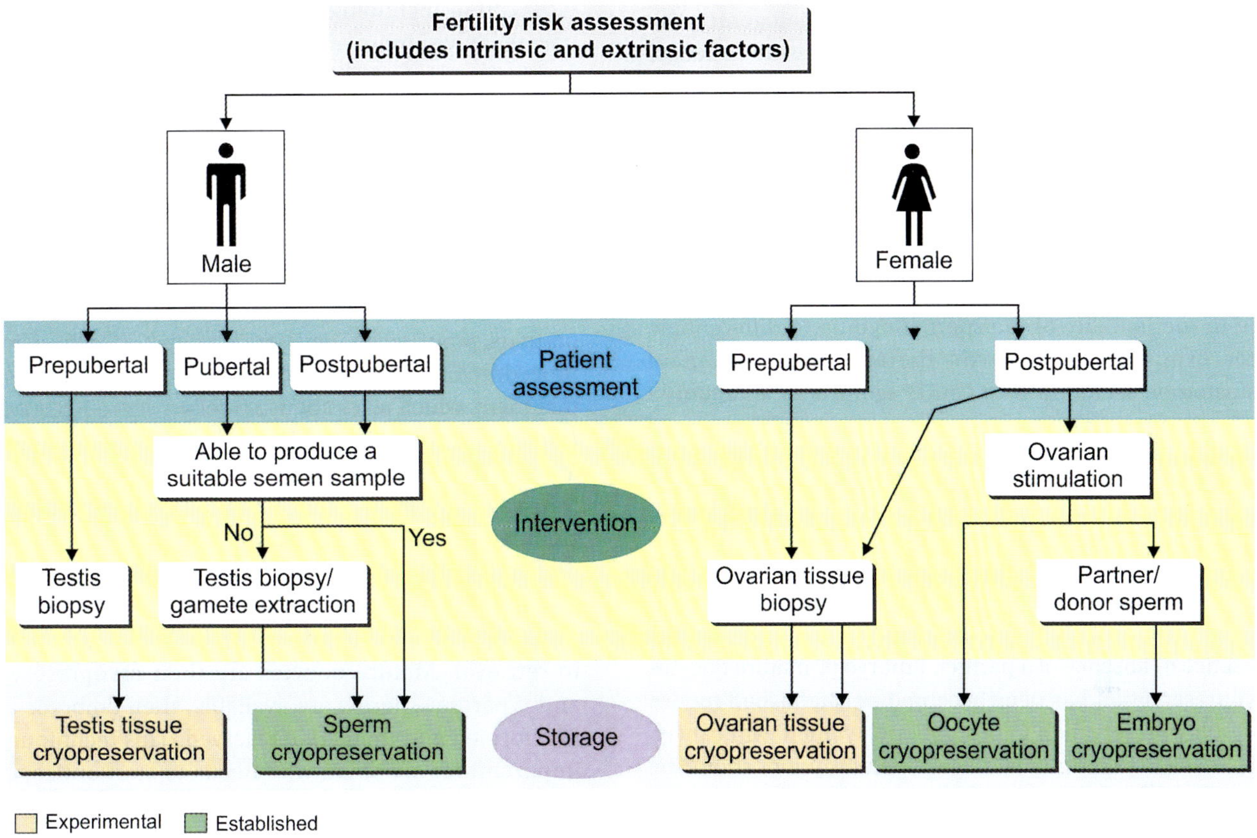

Source: Adapted from Anderson et al. 2015.

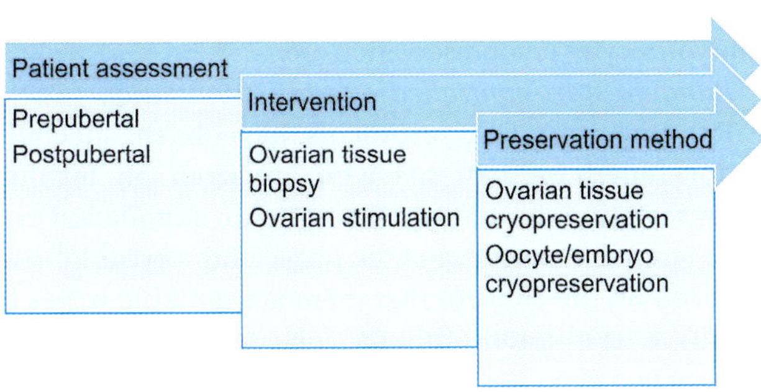

Fig. 3: Fertility preservation interventions in females.
Source: Adapted from Anderson et al. 2015.

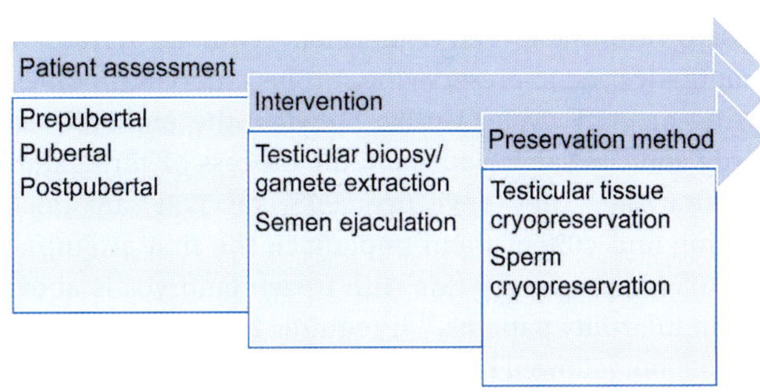

Fig. 4: Fertility preservation interventions in males.
Source: Adapted from Anderson et al. 2015.

sperm can be obtained by testicular sperm aspiration (TESA) or microdissection testicular sperm extraction (micro-TESE) in special cases. These sperms are cryopreserved for future use. Pregnancy rate of 33–56% has been reported in these patients. Although the exact length of time that cryopreserved sperm remains viable is unknown, successful paternity has been demonstrated with sperm stored up to 28 years.[27-29]

Testicular Tissue Cryopreservation

It is an option for prepubertal patients who have not initiated spermatogenesis, though it is still in experimental stage. Testicular tissue cell suspensions or direct testicular tissue preservation are achieved through mechanical and/or enzymatic digestion of testicular tissue followed by preservation in media, including agents such as ethylene glycerol, dimethyl sulfoxide (DMSO), and propanediol.[30-34] Again, tissue processing and cryopreservation result in decreased cell survival, with a post-thaw viability of 60%.[35,36] Till date, no study has demonstrated a technique to transform the immature, cryopreserved testicular tissue into functional gametes either in vivo or in vitro. Further, there is always a concern regarding the potential for reseeding the cancer when the cryopreserved tissue is reintroduced into the native host.[37]

Gonadal Shielding

Radiation treatment can damage the spermatogenic stem cells in the testes and cause infertility. This is unavoidable if both testes need to be radiated directly. However, when the radiation is directed at other structures in the pelvis, the testicular injury can be prevented by covering the testicles with a lead shield.

Gonadal Suppression

Infertility after exposure to radio- or chemotherapy results due to the inability of the spermatogonia to differentiate after exposure to the toxic therapy. Suppression of testosterone secretion with GnRH agonists or antagonists before or after the cytotoxic insult may help in recovery of spermatogenesis.[38]

Techniques of Fertility Preservation in Females

The choice of the optimal method for fertility preservation depends on the time available to start cancer treatment, cancer type and its treatment, age of the patient, and presence or absence of a partner. Embryo or mature oocytes cryopreservation has been accepted as established modes of fertility preservation in postpubertal women with cancer. OTC is still in experimental stage.[7,39] These options should be discussed as early as possible with the patient, ideally before starting treatment (ASRM and ASCO guidelines).[6,7]

Embryo Cryopreservation

Embryo vitrification is an established technique in ART.[6,7] It is routinely used to preserve the surplus embryos produced during an ART cycle. Unlike oocytes, the embryos are sturdy and can safely withstand the process of vitrification and thawing. They have over 90% survival rate post-thawing and 40% of them implant in the first attempt.[40] Cumulative pregnancy rate with frozen embryos is above 65% in infertility patients.[41] It requires 2 weeks for ovarian stimulation, followed by egg retrieval and cryopreservation. This can be a limitation for women with highly malignant tumors requiring immediate initiation of treatment and in prepubertal girls.

Oocytes Cryopreservation

Since 2013, oocyte cryopreservation is no longer considered an experimental procedure.[42-44] It is an ideal method for women without partners. Limitations of oocyte cryopreservation are similar to embryo cryopreservation. Additionally, being single-celled, they are more likely to be damaged during the process of vitrification and thawing. Mature [metaphase II (MII)] oocytes cryopreservation is preferred; however, even immature ones [GV/metaphase I (MI)] can be grown in lab through the process of in vitro maturation (IVM) and then frozen the next day.

- *Mature oocyte cryopreservation:* With advanced vitrification technology, pregnancy rates with mature oocytes have improved dramatically. A post-thawing survival rate of >90% and pregnancy rate of 45–50% have been reported with mature cryopreserved oocytes. Frozen oocytes yield similar pregnancy rates compared to fresh oocytes without increasing the risk of chromosomal abnormalities. So far, more than 900 children are born out of frozen oocytes with no apparent increase in congenital abnormalities.[38,45,46] It is the preferred method in postpubertal girls and in women without partners, provided enough time is available for the whole procedure of oocytes collection prior to starting cancer treatment, which takes about 2 weeks.
- *Immature oocyte cryopreservation and IVM:* IVM is a technique where immature oocytes are retrieved transvaginally from either unstimulated or minimally stimulated ovary. It takes 24–48 hours for the immature oocytes to mature in vitro once kept in a specially formulated medium.[47] Results are better if priming with human chorionic gonadotropin (hCG) is done prior to retrieval. Mature oocytes are then cryopreserved and if partner sperms are available, then embryos are first formed and then cryopreserved. This technique is important for a woman who needs to start anticancer treatment immediately or who has a hormone-sensitive tumor. So far, over 2,000 healthy infants have been born with this technique.[6,48,49]

The ovarian stimulation protocols which can be used for embryo/oocytes cryopreservation are:

- *Random-start controlled ovarian stimulation (COS)*: Random-start COS protocols have been specially developed for patients who are keen on fertility preservation. In this protocol, ovarian stimulation can be started irrespective of the phase of the cycle.[50-53] It is based on the concept that there are multiple waves of follicle recruitment within a single menstrual cycle.[54,55] Also, one need not bother about the synchronization of ovarian stimulation with endometrial development as no transfer will take place.
- *Role of tamoxifen aromatase inhibitors in patients with hormone-sensitive cancer/nonmalignant disease:* COS involves use of drugs which increase the serum estrogen levels. There is thus an apprehension that these drugs may activate hormone-sensitive diseases. It is thus suggested to use aromatase inhibitors such as letrozole, which causes multiple egg formation without much increase in serum estradiol (E2) levels.[56] For women who have hormone-sensitive cancers such as breast cancer, 5 mg of letrozole has been suggested from the second to third day of the cycle, followed by initiation of gonadotropins.[57] To start ovarian stimulation, initially GnRH antagonist is started at any point in the cycle

and once plasma E2 is below 50 pg/mL, oral letrozole administration at a dose of 5 mg/day is started from the second or third day of the cycle and then continued until the day of hCG administration. After 2 days of letrozole administration, 150 U of gonadotropins are added. A GnRH antagonist is administered when a follicle reaches 14–15 mm or the E2 level exceeds 250 pg/mL and hCG trigger is given when the lead follicles are 20 mm. Letrozole administration is however continued until the appearance of menses. Various studies have suggested no increase in risk of birth defects in babies post-letrozole intake in mothers.[58] Also, prospective data regarding the risk of breast cancer recurrence in patients undergoing COS with the letrozole protocol are reassuring when compared to the risk of recurrence in women with breast cancer who did not undergo COS.[59]

Figures 5A to E diagrammatically describe the stimulation protocols which can be used in women undergoing ovarian stimulation for fertility preservation.[60]

Ovarian Tissue Cryopreservation

It is a suggested method for patients where ovarian stimulation cannot be performed, mostly in prepubertal girls and in cases where anticancer treatment cannot be delayed. However, this procedure is invasive and requires general anesthesia and surgical removal of ovarian tissue. In addition, it needs medical expertise, which may not be available easily. As ovarian reserve declines with age, it should not be offered to women above 39 years of age (Oncofertility Consortium).[61,62] As per the ESHRE Guidelines on Female Fertility Preservation (2020), OTC can be offered under the following conditions:[8]

- In patients undergoing gonadotoxic treatment where oocyte/embryo cryopreservation is not feasible or if the patient so prefers.
- In patients with POI-associated genetic and chromosomal disorders

Ovarian tissue cryopreservation may also be considered in prepubertal girls.

However, OTC should not be offered to patients with low ovarian reserve (AMH <0.5 ng/mL and AFC <5) or advanced age (>36 years).[8]

Ovary can be cryopreserved as a whole or just the cortical tissue which contains follicles. The method of choice for OTC is slow freezing and not vitrification. Cryopreserved ovarian tissue can be used in two ways: (1) Thawed ovarian tissue can be transplanted back into the cancer survivor or (2) IVM can be performed on the follicles obtained from thawed ovarian tissue.

The replacement of the cryopreserved ovarian tissue is called ovarian tissue transplantation (OTT), which can be either at orthotopic (site of ovarian fossa) or at heterotopic (site other than ovarian fossa). Of the two, OTT at the orthotopic site is recommended to restore fertility.

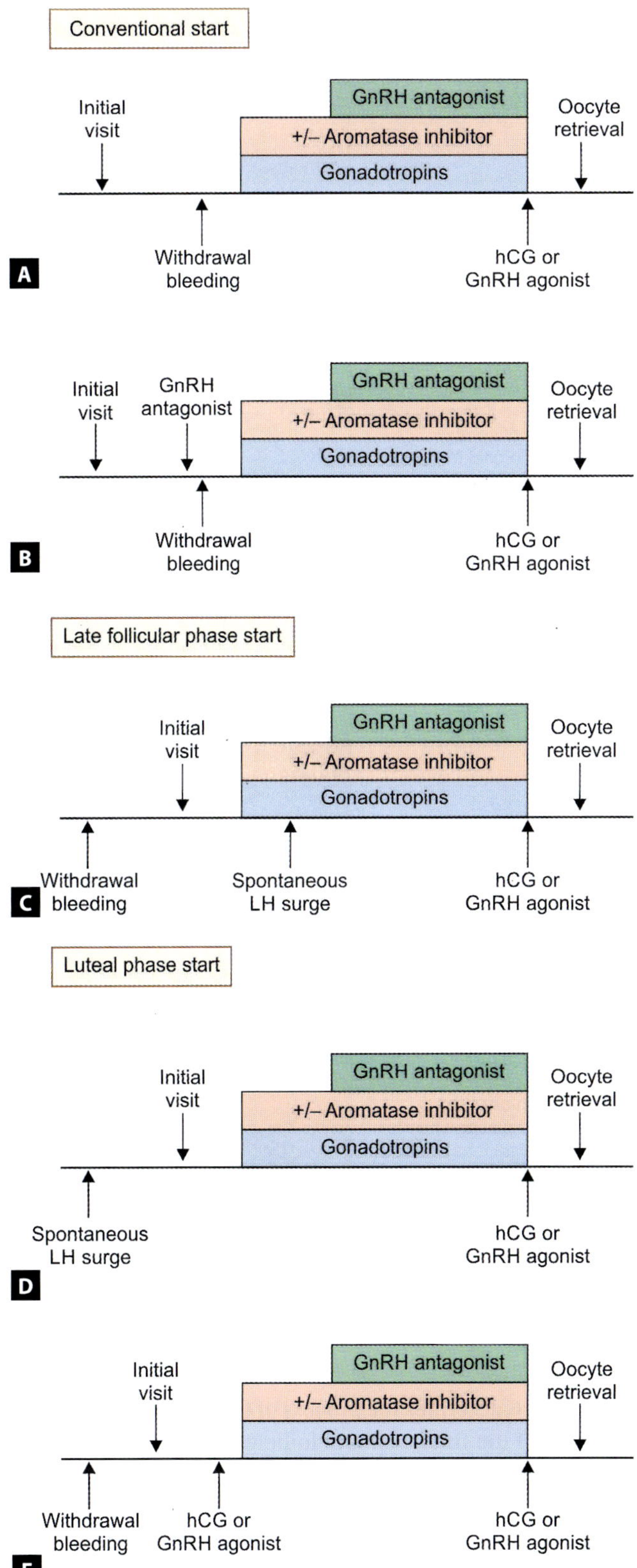

Figs. 5A to E: Controlled ovarian stimulation (COS) protocols for women undergoing fertility preservation.[9] (GnRH: gonadotropin-releasing hormone; hCG: human chorionic gonadotropin; LH: luteinizing hormone)

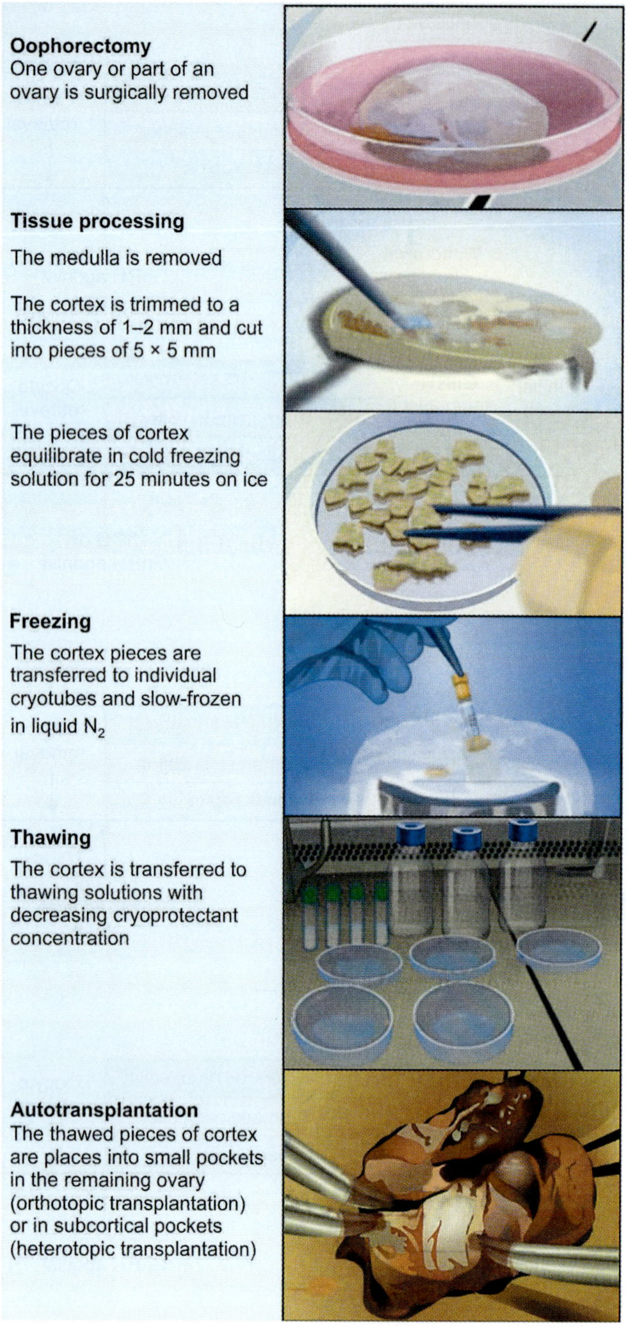

Fig. 6: Process of ovarian tissue cryopreservation.

Figure 6 describes the process of OTC.[63]

Most of the time, >50% of follicles are lost due to cryo-induced injury and ischemic damage.[64] Till date, 60 live births have been reported from either natural conception or with in vitro fertilization (IVF) after reimplantation of cryopreserved ovarian tissue.[65] It takes 4–6 months for this tissue to become functional.[66] Following transplantation, ovarian function continues for approximately 5 years.[65,67] It is imperative that before cryopreservation and transplantation of ovarian tissue, it should be checked for malignancy. Whole ovary cryopreservation with its blood vessels and stromal structure is still in experimental stage and needs further studies before it is applied in clinical practice.

Hormonal Suppression

Anticancer treatment kills fast dividing cells of the body, including germ cells. Based on this concept, GnRH agonists have been used during chemotherapy as a way to reduce the toxic effects of cancer treatment on growing ovarian follicles and their enclosed oocytes. It reduces ovarian activity by blocking the hypothalamic–pituitary–gonadal axis. It takes at least 10 days for its effect to come and should be continued 2 weeks post-chemotherapy.[68] Nevertheless, recent studies have demonstrated protective effects of GnRH agonists with a highly significant reduction in amenorrhea and ovarian insufficiency.[69,70]

This can be offered to premenopausal women with breast cancer who are receiving chemotherapy. However, there is not much evidence available regarding its protective effect on the ovarian reserve.[8]

It may also be offered in premenopausal women with autoimmune diseases receiving cyclophosphamide. However, limited evidence is available regarding usefulness of this approach.[8]

Transposition of Ovaries

In this technique, ovaries are moved out of the field of pelvic irradiation, also known as oophoropexy.[71] However, although the ovaries are out of direct irradiation field, the scatter dose may cause significant ovarian damage.[72] Ovarian transposition may be offered to women who are going to undergo radiotherapy without chemotherapy. However, it should not be offered to women who are at risk of having ovarian metastasis or have a low ovarian reserve.[8]

Flowchart 3 summarizes the various options available for fertility preservation in women.[63]

EMERGING TECHNOLOGIES

Ovarian Follicle Culture In Vitro

In patients with highly malignant cancer such as acute lymphoblastic leukemia or acute myeloblastic leukemia (AML), where treatment cannot be delayed, in them, OTC appears to be the only option for fertility preservation. However, this ovarian tissue might contain malignant tumor cells,[73] which could be reintroduced into patients when the tissue is transplanted.[74,75] Cancer recurrence after transplantation of cryopreserved ovarian tissue has been reported in some studies.[76] To mitigate the risks of reintroducing cancer cells with transplanted ovarian tissue, methods to isolate and culture individual follicles from banked tissue are practical approaches. The aim of this method is to develop oocytes from in vitro culture of follicles and later produce viable embryos for transfer to the uterus.

Flowchart 3: Options for fertility preservation in women.

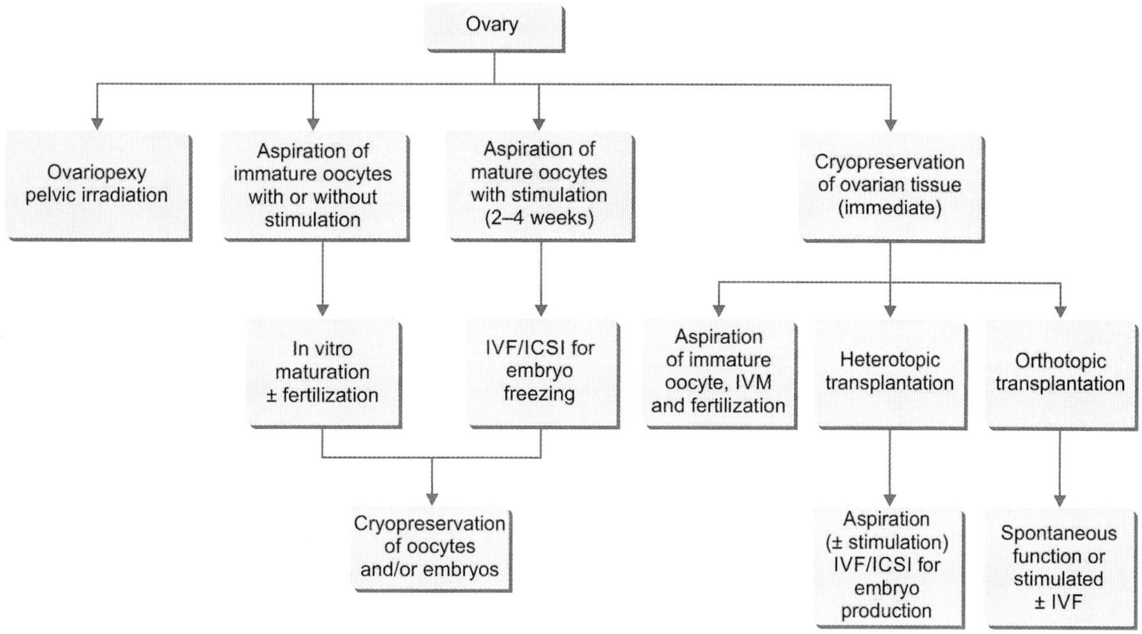

(ICSI: intracytoplasmic sperm injection; IVF: in vitro fertilization; IVM: in vitro maturation)

A lot of work has been going on in animals on this technology; however, it still remains experimental in humans.[77,78]

Ovarian Follicle Transplantation (Artificial Ovary)

Researchers have been working hard to develop an artificial ovary comprising cryopreserved ovarian tissue along with other ovarian cells, which are assembled on a 3D matrix scaffold. The artificial ovary comprises a biodegradable scaffold made of substances such as alginate hydrogel, which maintains the interaction between the oocyte and the granulosa cells during the time revascularization occurs at the transplanted site. This helps in creating an optimal microenvironment for the growth and survival of follicles and ovarian cells and also reduces the risk of transmission of malignant cells.

The artificial ovary would potentially restore both fertility and endocrine function once transplanted into the patient.[79-82] Animal studies have shown production of ovarian follicle, sex hormones (estrogen and progesterone),[83] and development of vascularization in these ovarian grafts. However, further robust trials are needed before it comes into clinical practice.

Oogonial Stem Cells

Oogonial stem cells (OSCs) are an option for cancer patients when no healthy follicles are retrieved from the ovarian tissue. Then, other sources of cells carrying the patient's genetic material are considered, including OSCs, embryonic stem (ES) cells, or induced pluripotent stem (iPS) cells.[84] Recently, a study reported successful production of oocytes from ES cells, also in mice.[85] These findings provide proof-of-concept support for future methods that may be able to produce new oocytes for cancer patients who have lost all of their oocytes as a result of chemo- or radiation therapy. These methods might also have applications in the treatment of premature ovarian failure (POF).

In Vitro Activation of Ovarian Follicles

Ovarian tissues collected from prepubertal cancer patients contain immature primordial follicles that must be activated in order to enter the growing pool and produce mature oocytes that can be fertilized. The same is true for ovarian tissues from patients with primary ovarian insufficiency who have a reduced ovarian reserve.[86] Researchers have been successful in inducing primordial follicle activation using ovarian fragmentation, drilling, and laser techniques.[87] These approaches disrupt the ovarian Hippo signaling pathway and promote actin polymerization in somatic and granulosa cells, which activates the growth of primordial follicles in the ovarian reserve.[88] This work supports the hypothesis that primordial ovarian follicles are held by surrounding cells in a state of restricted growth and that local Hippo signaling regulates the location of growing follicles and interfollicle communication.[82] Once activated, the follicles are treated with Akt stimulators, PI3K activators, and PTEN inhibitors before being used in autotransplantation.[89,90] This approach has resulted in a successful live birth.

Figure 7 summarizes the potential applications of the whole ovary and cortex fragments cryopreserved for fertility preservation in women.[91]

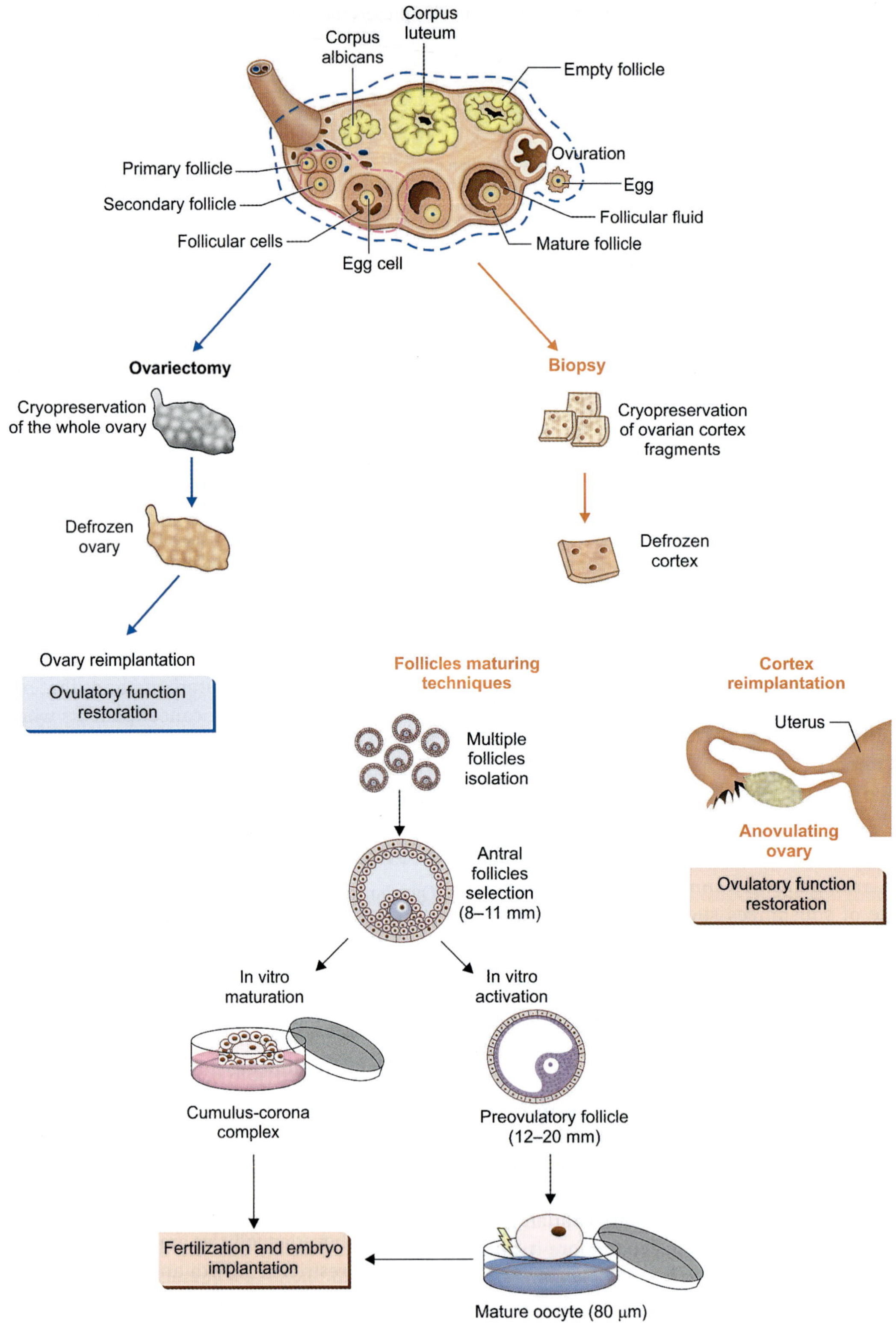

Fig. 7: Potential techniques for fertility preservation in women.[91]

Administration of Drugs for Specific Target Tissues

Use of Nanoparticles

A chemotherapeutic agent encapsulated inside nanoparticles has the specialty to reach target cancer cells without causing any systemic side effects. A lot of research is going on in animals to confirm its efficacy.[92,93]

Use of Fertiprotective Reagents

Fertiprotective reagents are drugs which not only kill cancer cells but also at the same time protect oocytes against

TABLE 2: Comparison of various fertility preservation methods in women.

FP method	Ideal patient	Success rate	Advantages	Disadvantages
Oocyte cryopreservation	Postpubertal women without a male partner or who do not wish to use donor sperm	Pregnancy rate per cycle of 50.2% or per embryo transfer 55.4%	• Well-established method • Can be offered to single women also • No risk of reimplanting malignant cells	• Time is required for ovarian stimulation • Can be done in postpubertal women only
Embryo cryopreservation	• Has a male partner or is willing to use a donor • Has time for ovarian stimulation before start of treatment	Cumulative pregnancy rate of 66% among women with cancer	• Well-established method • No risk of reimplanting malignant cells	• Can be offered to postpubertal women who have a male partner • Time is required for ovarian stimulation
Ovarian tissue cryopreservation	Prepubertal girls or young women who do not have time for ovarian stimulation to retrieve eggs	Pregnancy rate of 25% among women with cancer	• Can be offered to prepubertal girls also • Can be done at any time and thus does not delay start of oncologic treatment	• Age limitation can be done only at the age of <35 years • Involves laparoscopic surgery for procurement and transplantation of ovarian tissue • Risk of retransmission of malignancy
Fertility sparing surgery	Women with certain early-stage gynecological malignancies	• Cumulative conception rate after trachelectomy 53% • Pregnancy rate after progestin therapy for endometrial cancer 34.8%	Ovaries and/or uterus are preserved	
Hormone suppression			• May have some medical benefits not invasive • Does not need delaying in oncologic therapy • Can be used in association with cryopreservation techniques • Reduce the risk of hypermenorrhea associated with hematologic malignancies or myelosuppressive treatments • Low cost	• Uncertain efficacy for fertility preservation • Symptoms of estrogenic deprivation • Transient alterations of bone metabolism not significant for therapy duration <6 months • Limited clinical evidences in patients with disease other than breast cancer

(FP: family planning)

chemoradiation. Tamoxifen, granulocyte colony-stimulating factor (G-CSF), imatinib, AS101, sphingosine-1-phosphate, and triiodothyronine (T3) are various fertiprotective reagents which are under research. They all protect oocytes by blocking/altering apoptotic pathways involved in follicular growth.[94-97]

Wallace et al., Angarita et al., and Brancati et al. in their articles discussed about the various methods available for fertility preservation and their pros and cons. These are summarized in **Table 2.**[22,98,99]

POSTHUMOUS REPRODUCTION

What is Posthumous Reproduction?

Posthumous reproduction refers to the retrieval of gametes and reproductive tissue after a person's death or after they have become incapacitated and their death is imminent. It also deals with the storage and the use of these gametes and reproductive tissue after the person's death. It refers to a situation where the person will be deceased at the time their gametes are used and any resulting child is born.

The Opinion of the Ethics Committee of the American Society for Reproductive Medicine on the posthumous retrieval and use of embryos (2018):[100]

- Posthumous retrieval and use of gametes or embryos for reproductive purposes is ethically justifiable if written documentation from the deceased authorizing the procedure is available.
- In the absence of written documentation, centers may consider requests for posthumous reproduction only if such requests are initiated by the surviving partner.

- Adequate time for grieving and counseling is imperative before initiating the process of posthumous reproduction.

The psychological, ethical, and legal considerations in posthumous reproduction:

- The deceased will not be present to rear the child born through posthumous reproduction. The well-being of any children resulting from posthumous reproduction needs to be considered.
- To consider the choice or interests of the surviving partner regarding the use of the deceased's gametes/embryos or the choices of others who cared about the deceased such as surviving partner. However, their interests need to be weighed against the interests of the deceased.
- Can tissue be taken from a person who has not consented to its retrieval?
- If tissue is retrieved, who holds responsibility for its storage and use?
- If a child is conceived with a deceased person's gamete, what are that child's inheritance rights?
- The impact of posthumous reproduction on the deceased's wider family, including any existing children/ siblings.

The only guideline available in India regarding posthumous reproduction is "The Assisted Reproductive Technologies (Regulation) Rules - 2010" drafted by the Indian Council of Medical Research (ICMR), New Delhi. Section 3.16.5 of "Guidelines for ART Clinics in India" allows insemination of the women with husband's semen after death of the husband. However, it states that sperm must have been collected while the husband was alive and who may or may not be under imminent death but was in sound mind. Consent is therefore taken at the time of cryopreservation from the male/female partner in case of sperm or oocyte freezing and from both partners in case of a couple regarding the fate of the cryopreserved gametes/embryos in case of their death. However, there are no guidelines for postmortem retrieval of sperm from the deceased husband.[101]

As per the ART Regulation Bill 2020, "prior consent" of the commissioning couple is needed before posthumous collection of gametes can take place. However, in situations of sudden death where no prior gamete retrieval has been performed by clinics or banks and there is no written consent for posthumous reproduction, inferred consent may be ascertained from the surviving partner of the deceased to determine if the deceased had discussed a wish for posthumous gamete retrieval and would have approved of such a procedure. While a child born to a woman artificially inseminated with the stored sperm of her dead husband is considered as the legitimate child of the couple, the legal status of the child born through the process of postmortem sperm retrieval (PMSR) still needs to be defined.

The New York hospital guidelines, also known as the Cornell guidelines, are the only wholesome guidelines available related to PMSR and may be referred to in the Indian scenario. Some important considerations addressed in these guidelines are as follows:[94]

- In the absence of the deceased's consent, only the consent of the wife matters as the next of kin because she is the woman with whom the deceased had intended to have children.
- Sperm retrieval and its cryopreservation should be done within 24 hours.
- There should be a gap of at least 1 year before the use of retrieved sperm by the wife. This time period will help the wife to go through the period of bereavement and not take any emotional decisions.
- Psychological counseling of the wife must be done so that she can understand the procedure, success rate, potential benefits, limitations, and risks of such procedures. She should also be counseled about rearing a child single-handedly and about the legal status of the child.

Posthumous reproduction is banned in Canada, France, Germany, and Sweden.[102-104] The ethical committee of ASRM suggests that posthumous use of stored sample is justifiable provided written consent from the deceased authorizing the procedure is available.[105] In the absence of written documentation, such requests should only be entertained if it comes from the surviving spouse. It is very important to allow adequate time for grieving and counseling prior to the posthumous use of gametes or embryos for reproduction. The ESHRE Task Force on ethics and law on posthumous reproduction recommends a waiting period of 1 year before any such procedure is initiated.[97]

Social Egg Freezing

In 2013, the ASRM declared that oocyte cryopreservation was no longer an experimental procedure and could be used as an option for fertility preservation.[106]

Argyle et al. in 2016 conducted a study to compare the results from fresh versus frozen oocytes. They found that IVF pregnancy rates with frozen oocytes are similar to those with fresh oocytes.[107]

The term "social freezing" is used when eggs are frozen for nonmedical causes and used later in life. It is also referred to as "anticipated gamete exhaustion (AGE) banking" (oocyte banking for AGE) as it involves cryopreservation of oocytes to protect the woman against age-related fertility decline and ineffective fertility treatments at older ages.[108] It also enhances a woman's reproductive autonomy and allows them to feel more socially, psychologically, and financially stable before motherhood. Oocyte cryopreservation allows a woman to conceive with children who are biologically related to her at a later age.

The most common reasons for opting for egg freezing include:

- Delay in marriage due to absence of a partner suitable for creating a family
- Professional reasons where the woman feels that delay in childbearing is required in order to complete her education, for her career advancement, or due to inflexibility at her workplace.

The Australasian Certificate of Reproductive Endocrinology and Infertility (CREI) constituted an expert panel to evaluate the best practices for oocyte cryopreservation to guide clinicians who are working with women who are considering oocyte cryopreservation for fertility preservation.[109]

Their recommendations are referred to as the ACCEPT (Australasian Certification in Reproductive Endocrinology and Infertility Consensus Expert Panel on Trial evidence) consensus and are summarized in **Table 3**.

Varlas et al. in 2021 published a review article on social egg freezing.[108] The main findings of their review are highlighted below:

- Oocyte cryopreservation is an elective method for fertility preservation for age-related infertility and involves ovarian hormonal stimulation, oocyte retrieval, freezing, and oocyte storage.
- Ovarian stimulation protocols can be initiated at any moment in the menstrual cycle and the protocols which can be used are random start or DuoStim.
- Ovarian stimulation does not raise the embryo aneuploidy rate.
- Vitrification is the technique of choice for oocyte cryopreservation. It is associated with a 90–97% survival rate, 71–79% fertilization rate, 17–41% implantation rate, and 4.5–12% clinical pregnancy rate per vitrified oocyte.
- Women's age at the time of storage and the number of mature oocytes retrieved are predictors for future live births. The optimal timing for a woman to freeze her eggs is under 35 years. Mesen et al. found maximum benefits when cryopreservation is performed between 32 and 37 years, with little benefit at ages of 25–30 years.[110]
- The number of oocytes retrieved depends upon the patient's age, clinical profile, and the ovarian reserve. A woman can attempt a maximum of four oocyte retrieval cycles. A total of 15–20 oocytes retrieved will ensure a balance between the procedure's safety and efficacy with individualized stimulation protocols. Goldman et al. proposed a mathematical model to predict the probability of live birth rate based on the number of cryopreserved oocytes and the woman's age at the moment of cryostorage and said that 10, 20, and 61 eggs are required to obtain a 75% cumulative live birth rate (CLBR), for women at ages 34 years, 37 years or 42 years respectively.[111]
- Artificial intelligence (AI) has been introduced recently to assess the quality of embryos and oocytes in order to

TABLE 3: ANZSREI ACCEPT consensus statement on elective oocyte cryopreservation.

Recommendation	*Level of evidence*
Vitrification is currently the most effective method for mature (MII) oocyte cryopreservation	Level 1A
Women should be made aware that not all oocytes will survive warming	Level 1A
To minimize the risk of OHSS, the recommended stimulation strategy is an FSH/GnRH antagonist regimen with planned GnRH agonist trigger	Level 4
Ovarian reserve testing should be offered to women prior to oocyte cryopreservation and counseling provided regarding expected oocyte yield per stimulated cycle	Level 4
Women should be informed that microinjection of sperm is required to fertilize warmed oocytes	Level 4
Women should be aware that warmed oocytes may create fewer blastocysts compared with fresh oocytes	Level 1B
The best age to freeze oocytes is before the age of 35 years. Women over 35 years achieve poorer pregnancy outcomes from vitrified oocytes related to oocyte quality deterioration with advancing maternal age	Level 4
Women should be informed that there is a chance that they may not need to use their frozen oocytes and oocyte cryopreservation does not guarantee future live birth	Level 3
Safety outcomes for births from vitrified oocytes are to date reassuring with no evidence of increased risk compared with IVF births. Safety data remain preliminary. Long-term follow-up studies for all cryopreservation techniques remain essential	Level 3
Women should be counseled at the time of cryopreservation of oocytes that if they achieve pregnancy at an advanced maternal age, they will be at increased risk of perinatal and obstetric complications	Level 3
The probability of live birth is mainly dependent on the number of mature oocytes and the age of the woman at the time of storage	Level 2A

(ACCEPT: Australasian Certification in Reproductive Endocrinology and Infertility Consensus Expert Panel on Trial evidence; ANZSREI: Australian and New Zealand Society for Reproductive Endocrinology and Infertility; FSH: follicle-stimulating hormone; GnRH: gonadotropin-releasing hormone; IVF: in vitro fertilization; MII: metaphase II; OHSS: ovarian hyperstimulation syndrome) create a highly predictable model for ART. Cavalera et al. used AI to differentiate between competent and incompetent oocytes with an accuracy of 91.03%.[112] Yanez et al. reported that a lack of embryonic viability is associated with certain gene expression transcriptomes of oocyte maturation.[113]

- Neonatal outcomes and risk of genetic diseases and congenital anomalies are the same when using vitrified oocytes as compared to natural conception or following IVF treatment with fresh oocytes. Also, prolonged cryopreservation in liquid nitrogen does not affect the euploidy rate or IVF success.

Counseling, both at the beginning and at the end of the cycle, has to be done to ensure that the women who have undergone oocyte cryopreservation for fertility preservation should not have a false sense of security regarding their fertility potential later in life. It is also important to spread awareness regarding the availability of this fertility-preserving technique. It is also important for women to understand that the success of oocyte cryopreservation resulting in live birth is strongly dependent on the age of the woman at the time of egg freezing. In a survey conducted by Anderson et al., it was observed that most women opted for oocyte freezing at age above 35 years, where the success rates are limited.[106]

RECOMMENDATIONS FOR FERTILITY PRESERVATION

Although continuous work has been going on in the field of fertility preservation, there are still several controversial issues which need to be addressed. As recommended by the ASCO and the European Society for Medical Oncology (ESMO), sperm cryopreservation and embryo/oocyte cryopreservation are standard strategies for fertility preservation in male and female patients, respectively. Other strategies (e.g., pharmacological protection of the gonads and gonadal tissue cryopreservation) are still generally considered experimental techniques. However, still there are several unanswered controversial questions regarding safety and efficacy of fertility preservation in cancer survivors.

International recommendations for fertility preservation according to the ASCO and ESMO Clinical Practice Guidelines for Fertility Preservation in cancer patients are as follows:[5,7,16,114]

- Ovarian stimulating drugs with standard treatment protocols may be administered in subfertile/infertile women without increasing the risk of developing breast cancer (III, B). The long-term use of clomiphene outside the current limited indications [i.e., first-line therapy of World Health Organization (WHO) group II anovulatory infertility] should be discouraged because of a possible increase in breast cancer risk (III, B).
- Pregnancy in cancer survivors, after adequate treatment and follow-up, should not be discouraged, including among patients with endocrine-sensitive breast cancer (III, A).
- All patients with potential interest in keeping their fertility should be referred to a fertility unit for adequate determination of risk of infertility, chances of future conception, and how to proactively preserve it (V, A). However, some cancer patients will not require the help of a fertility clinic after cancer treatment (V, B). Since several patient- and treatment-related factors are associated with the risk of developing infertility, the oncofertility counseling should be tailored to the individual patient (V, A).
- In men, sperm cryopreservation is an easily accessible and widely available option in >95% of patients and should be encouraged for those who want to preserve fertility (III, A). On the contrary, from 2 to 65% of women undergo one of the available cryopreservation options: Oncologists should discuss with them the fertility issues and secure proper counseling in appropriate centers prior to cancer treatment (IV, A).
- Paucity of data is available on fatherhood after cancer. Although most of the published data are reassuring, some recent conflicting results suggest a potential increased risk of birth defects, particularly among the children born closer to a paternal cancer diagnosis, and caution should be taken in counseling these patients (V, B for discussion with patients); data on children conceived after ART are too scarce to draw any conclusion although in the general population, available evidence for the outcomes of progeny after ART suggests safety of the techniques themselves (V, B for discussion with patients).
- The current limited data suggest the safety of a COS in cancer patients (III, B). "Random start protocols" can be employed to avoid delays in anticancer treatment initiation (III, B). GnRH agonist ovulation triggering should be adopted in patients at moderate-high risk for ovarian hyperstimulation syndrome (OHSS) (I, A). Letrozole (or tamoxifen) should be incorporated in the protocol for COS in cancer patients with hormone-responsive tumors (III, B).
- Embryo and oocyte cryopreservation are standard options for fertility preservation (III, B). Vitrification showed a better performance than slow freezing (II, B). During oncofertility counseling, patients should be aware that data on the success of these strategies derive from infertile women in general and that a different ovarian response to stimulation might be expected in cancer patients (IV, B).
- The best candidates for OTC are prepubertal girls (III, A). The technique may also be proposed to patients scheduled for treatments with a high risk of POI who cannot delay anticancer treatments or who have already received chemotherapy or with contraindications to

COS (III, B). Patients with cancer with a high risk of malignant contamination to the ovaries (e.g., aggressive hematologic malignancies) should not be considered eligible for ovarian tissue autotransplantation (V, B).

- In order to optimize the procedure in terms of both patient management and cost-effectiveness, the harvesting of the tissue can be performed locally but subsequent sample freezing and storage should be centralized (III, B). A well-organized network between fertility units is required (III, B).
- Ovarian suppression with the use of GnRH agonist during chemotherapy should be considered a reliable strategy to preserve ovarian function and fertility, at least in breast cancer patients, given the availability of new data suggesting that both the safety and the efficacy of the procedure have become available (I, A).

The recommendations for fertility preservation as given by the Fertility Preservation Society (India) are given below:[115]

- *Recommendations for family planning (FP) in prepubertal children:*
  - Parents of children and adolescents should be informed about the risk to fertility with cancer treatment. Adolescents need to be counseled individually and with parents (II, A).
  - For prepubertal children, the only fertility-preservation options are ovarian and testicular cryopreservation. Testicular tissue freezing is still investigational, but OTC is no longer experimental (III, B).
  - In postpubertal children, established methods of fertility preservation such as semen or oocyte cryopreservation should be offered (III, B).
- *Should ovarian reserve testing be done routinely prior to initiation of computed tomography (CT)?*
  - Ovarian reserve should be assessed before cancer therapy by estimating AMH and AFC (III, A).
  - AMH levels should be done before and 1 year after gonadotoxic therapy as they predict recovery of ovarian function (III, A).
  - Pretreatment AMH levels should not be used as an indicator of posttreatment fertility (IV, D).
  - When estimating the risk of posttreatment ovarian insufficiency, age, proposed gonadotoxic treatment type and dose, and pretreatment AMH levels should be taken into consideration (IV, B)
- *Fertility preservation in the male:*
  - Sperm cryopreservation is effective and sperm banking should be advised to postpubertal males receiving cancer treatment (II, A).
  - Testicular tissue cryopreservation and reimplantation is still experimental but is the only option in prepubertal boys for fertility preservation and should be considered as a part of clinical trials.
  - Hormonal therapy in men is not successful in preserving fertility. It is not recommended (I, C).
  - All male patients should be informed about the potentially higher risk of genetic damage in sperm collected after initiation of chemotherapy (II, B).
- *What is the role of fertility-sparing surgeries in the men?*
  - Partial orchiectomy should be done in selected patients when the testicular mass is small.
  - Sperm banking prior to surgery, even in patients undergoing partial orchiectomy, is advisable (III B).
  - In men with azoospermia undergoing orchidectomy, sperms can be extracted from the epididymis and vas deferens of the orchiectomy specimen or contralateral noncancerous testis.
- *Fertility preservation in the females:*
  - Embryo and oocyte vitrification are established methods of cryopreservation (II, A).
  - OTC in prepubertal, postpubertal girls, and women. OTC is considered as an established technique now (II, B).
  - Patients with high risk of secondaries in ovaries should not be considered eligible for ovarian tissue autotransplantation (IV, B).
- *Effect of COS on cancer prognosis:*
  - For ovarian stimulation in women seeking fertility preservation for medical reasons, the GnRH antagonist protocol is recommended for its feasibility in urgent situations, short time, and safety reasons (IV, A).
  - Random-start protocols can be employed to avoid delays in anticancer treatment initiation (II, C).
  - Double stimulation can be considered if time is available so that more number of oocytes/embryos can be cryopreserved (II, D).
  - GnRH agonist ovulation triggering should be adopted in patients to prevent OHSS (I, A).
  - Letrozole or tamoxifen should be incorporated in the protocol for COS in cancer patients with hormone-responsive tumors.
  - Where pelvic radiotherapy is planned, women may be offered ovarian transposition with the aim to protect the ovaries from radiation to prevent POI (IV, C).
  - Women with decreased ovarian reserve and women at risk of having ovarian metastases should not be offered ovarian transposition.
- *After treatment and pregnancy in cancer patients:*
  - Before the use of stored material, fitness for pregnancy should be evaluated, taking into consideration the late effects of treatment, age of the patient, and the interval since the last gonadotoxic treatment (IV, B).
  - Preconception counseling and appropriate obstetric monitoring in consultation with oncologist and physician are recommended in women intending

    to become pregnant after gonadotoxic treatments (II, A).
  - A minimum interval of at least 1 year is suggested before attempting pregnancy following chemotherapy completion in order to reduce the risk of pregnancy complications (IV, A).
- *Fatherhood after cancer:*
  - Fatherhood after cancer treatment is safe (IV, B).

CONCLUSION

Fertility preservation is gaining importance as to complete management of cancer in young survivors. It requires a multidisciplinary approach involving oncologists, oncosurgeons, infertility specialists, and embryologists. Infertility specialists/oncologists must discuss regarding potential gonadotoxicity caused by cancer treatment and options available to preserve the same. Ideally, fertility preservation should be done prior to initiating cancer treatment. Sperm cryopreservation in men and embryo/oocyte cryopreservation in women are the established methods of fertility preservation. In prepubertal girls, OTC can be offered. In prepubertal boys, testicular tissue can be cryopreserved, but strategies for transplantation need to be established. Instructions should be specified about the disposition of stored gametes, embryos, or gonadal tissue in the event of the patient's death, unavailability, or any other contingency.

REFERENCES

1. Noyes N, Melzer K, Druckenmiller S, Fino ME, Smith M, Knopman JM. Experiences in fertility preservation: lessons learned to ensure that fertility and reproductive autonomy remain options for cancer survivors. J Assist Reprod Genet. 2013;30:1263-70.
2. De Vos M, Smitz J, Woodruff TK. Fertility preservation in women with cancer. Lancet. 2014;384:1302-10.
3. Dursun P, Doğan NU, Ayhan A. Oncofertility for gynecologic and non-gynecologic cancers: fertility sparing in young women of reproductive age. Crit Rev Oncol Hematol. 2014;92:258-67.
4. Mahajan N. Fertility preservation in female cancer patients: an overview. J Human Reprod Sci. 2015;8(1):3-13.
5. Lambertini M, Del Mastro L, Pescio M, Andersen CY, Azim Jr HA, Peccatori FA, et al. Cancer and fertility preservation: international recommendations from an expert meeting. BMC Med. 2016;14:1.
6. Ethics Committee of American Society for Reproductive Medicine. Fertility preservation and reproduction in patients facing gonadotoxic therapies: a committee opinion. Fertil Steril. 2013;100(5):1224-31.
7. Loren AW, Mangu PB, Beck LN, Brennan L, Magdalinski AJ, Partridge AH, et al. Fertility preservation for patients with cancer: American Society of Clinical Oncology clinical practice guideline update. J Clin Oncol. 2013:31:2500-10.
8. The ESHRE Guideline Group on Female Fertility Preservation, Anderson RA, Amant F, Braat D, D'Angelo A, de Sousa Lopes SMC, et al. ESHRE guidelines: female fertility preservation. Hum Reprod Open. 2020;2020(4):hoaa052.
9. Hussein RS, Khan Z, Zhao Y. Fertility preservation in women: indications and options for therapy. Mayo Clin Proc. 2020; 95(4):770-83.
10. Decanter C, Morschhauser F, Pigny P, Lefebvre C, Gallo C, Dewailly D. Anti-Müllerian hormone follow-up in young women treated by chemotherapy for lymphoma: preliminary results. Reprod Biomed Online. 2010;20(2):280-5.
11. Morgan S, Anderson RA, Gourley C, Wallace WH, Spears N. How do chemotherapeutic agents damage the ovary? Hum Reprod Update. 2012;18(5):525-35.
12. Stoop D, van der Veen F, Deneyer M, Nekkebroeck J, Tournaye H. Oocyte banking for anticipated gamete exhaustion (AGE) is a preventive intervention, neither social nor nonmedical. Reprod Biomed Online. 2014;28(5):548-51.
13. Grin L, Girsh E, Harlev A. Male fertility preservation—methods, indications and challenges. Andrologia. 2020;53:e13635.
14. Anderson RA, Mitchell RT, Kelsey TW, Spears N, Telfer EE, Wallace WHB. Cancer treatment and gonadal function: experimental and established strategies for fertility preservation in children and young adults. Lancet Diabetes Endocrinol. 2015;3:556-67.
15. Rodriguez-Wallberg KA, Oktay K. Fertility preservation during cancer treatment: clinical guidelines. Cancer Manag Res. 2014;6:105-17.
16. Foster RS, McNulty A, Rubin LR, Bennett R, Rowland RG, Sledge GW, et al. Fertility considerations in nerve-sparing retroperitoneal lymph-node dissection. World J Urol. 1994;12(3):136-8.
17. Fode M, Krogh-Jespersen S, Brackett NL, Ohl DA, Lynne CM, Sønksen J. Male sexual dysfunction and infertility associated with neurological disorders. Asian J Androl. 2012;14(1):61-8.
18. Snowden JA, Badoglio M, Labopin M, Giebel S, McGrath E, Marjanovic Z, et al. Evolution, trends, outcomes, and economics of hematopoietic stem cell transplantation in severe autoimmune diseases. Blood Adv. 2017;1(27):2742-55.
19. Nicopoullos JD, Almeida P, Vourliotis M, Gilling-Smith C. A decade of the sperm-washing programme: correlation between markers of HIV and seminal parameters. HIV Med. 2011;12(4):195-201.
20. Wang D, Li L, Xie Q, Hou Z, Yu X, Ma M, et al. Factors affecting sperm fertilizing capacity in men infected with HIV. J Med Virol. 2014;86(9):1467-72.
21. Sandlow JI, Nagler HM. Vasectomy and vasectomy reversal: important issues. Preface. Urol Clin North Am. 2009: 36(3):xiii-xiv.
22. Wallace WH, Critchley HO, Anderson RA. Optimizing reproductive outcome in children and young people with cancer. J Clin Oncol. 2012;30:3-5.
23. Pinelli S, Basile S. Fertility preservation: current and future perspectives for oncologic patients at risk for iatrogenic premature ovarian insufficiency. Biomed Res Int. 2018; 2018:6465903.
24. Nieman CL, Kinahan KE, Yount SE, Rosenbloom SK, Yost KJ, Hahn EA, et al. Fertility preservation and adolescent cancer patients: lessons from adult survivors of childhood cancer and their parents. Cancer Treat Res. 2007;138:201-17.
25. Schover LR. Psychosocial aspects of infertility and decisions about reproduction in young cancer survivors: a review. Med Pediatr Oncol. 1999;33:53-9.

26. Ginsberg JP, Ogle SK, Tuchman LK, Carlson CA, Reilly MM, Hobbie WL, et al. Sperm banking for adolescent and young adult cancer patients: sperm quality, patient, and parent perspectives. Pediatr Blood Cancer. 2008;50:594-8.
27. Feldschuh J, Brassel J, Durso N, Levine A. Successful sperm storage for 28 years. Fertil Steril. 2005;84:1017.
28. Horne G, Atkinson AD, Pease EH, Logue JP, Brison DR, Lieberman BA. Live birth with sperm cryopreserved for 21 years prior to cancer treatment: case report. Hum Reprod. 2004;19:1448-9.
29. Sanger WG, Olson JH, Sherman JK. Semen cryobanking for men with cancer—criteria change. Fertil Steril. 1992;58: 1024-7.
30. Kvist K, Thorup J, Byskov AG, Høyer PE, Møllgård K, Yding Andersen C. Cryopreservation of intact testicular tissue from boys with cryptorchidism. Hum Reprod. 2006;21:484-91.
31. Keros V, Hultenby K, Borgström B, Fridström M, Jahnukainen K, Hovatta O. Methods of cryopreservation of testicular tissue with viable spermatogonia in pre-pubertal boys undergoing gonadotoxic cancer treatment. Hum Reprod. 2007;22:1384-95.
32. Keros V, Rosenlund B, Hultenby K, Aghajanova L, Levkov L, Hovatta O. Optimizing cryopreservation of human testicular tissue: comparison of protocols with glycerol, propanediol and dimethylsulphoxide as cryoprotectants. Hum Reprod. 2005;20:1676-87.
33. Goossens E, Frederickx V, Geens M, De Block G, Tournaye H. Cryosurvival and spermatogenesis after allografting prepubertal mouse tissue: comparison of two cryopreservation protocols. Fertil Steril. 2008;89:725-7.
34. Wyns C, Curaba M, Vanabelle B, Van Langendonckt A, Donnez J. Options for fertility preservation in prepubertal boys. Hum Reprod Update. 2010;16:312-28.
35. Brook PF, Radford JA, Shalet SM, Joyce AD, Gosden RG. Isolation of germ cells from human testicular tissue for low temperature storage and autotransplantation. Fertil Steril. 2001;75:269-74.
36. Hovatta O. Cryopreservation of testicular tissue in young cancer patients. Hum Reprod Update. 2001;7:378-83.
37. Franck P, Duffner U, Schulze-Seemann W, Riede U, Dördelmann M, Niemeyer CM. Testicular relapse after 13 years of complete remission of acute lymphoblastic leukemia. Urol Int. 1998;60:239-41.
38. Shetty G, Meistrich ML. Hormonal approaches to preservation and restoration of male fertility after cancer treatment. JNCI Monographs. 2005;2005(34):36-39. https://doi.org/10.1093/jncimonographs/lgi002
39. Babayev SN, Arslan E, Kogan S, Moy F, Oktay K. Evaluation of ovarian and testicular tissue cryopreservation in children undergoing gonadotoxic therapies. J Assist Reprod Genet. 2013;30(1):3-9.
40. Mandelbaum J, Belaisch-Allart J, Junca AM, Antoine JM, Plachot M, Alvarez S, et al. Cryopreservation in human assisted reproduction is now routine for embryos but remains a research procedure for oocytes. Hum Reprod. 1998;13 Suppl. 3:161-74.
41. Senn A, Vozzi C, Chanson A, De Grandi P, Germond M. Prospective randomized study of two cryopreservation policies avoiding embryo selection: the pronucleate stage leads to a higher cumulative delivery rate than the early cleavage stage. Fertil Steril. 2000;74:946-52.
42. Practice Committees of the American Society for Reproductive Medicine, Society for Assisted Reproductive Technology. Mature oocyte cryopreservation: a guideline. Fertil Steril. 2013;99:37-43.
43. Borini A, Bianchi V. Cryopreservation of mature and immature oocytes. Clin Obstet Gynecol. 2019;53:763-74.
44. Huang JY, Chian RC, Gilbert L, Fleiszer D, Holzer H, Dermitas E, et al. Retrieval of immature oocytes from unstimulated ovaries followed by in vitro maturation and vitrification: a novel strategy of fertility preservation for breast cancer patients. Am J Surg. 2010;200:177-83.
45. Forman EJ, Li X, Ferry KM, Scott K, Treff NR, Scott Jr RT. Oocyte vitrification does not increase the risk of embryonic aneuploidy or diminish the implantation potential of blastocysts created after intracytoplasmic sperm injection: a novel, paired randomized controlled trial using DNA fingerprinting. Fertil Steril. 2012;98:644-9.
46. Goldman KN, Kramer Y, Hodes-Wertz B, Noyes N, McCaffrey C, Grifo JA. Long-term cryopreservation of human oocytes does not increase embryonic aneuploidy. Fertil Steril. 2015;103:662-8.
47. Chian RC. In-vitro maturation of immature oocytes for infertile women with PCOS. Reprod Biomed Online. 2004;8:547-52.
48. Chen H, Lv JQ, Ge HS, Wu XM, Xi HT, Chi HH, et al. Live birth following vitrification of in vitro matured oocytes derived from sibling smaller follicles at follicle selection phase in the context of in vitro fertilization. Gynecol Endocrinol. 2014;30:624-6.
49. Oktay K, Buyuk E, Rodriguez-Wallberg KA, Sahin G. In vitro maturation improves oocyte or embryo cryopreservation outcome in breast cancer patients undergoing ovarian stimulation for fertility preservation. Reprod Biomed Online. 2010;20:634-8.
50. Bedoschi GM, de Albuquerque FO, Ferriani RA, Navarro PA. Ovarian stimulation during the luteal phase for fertility preservation of cancer patients: case reports and review of the literature. J Assist Reprod Genet. 2010;27:491-4.
51. Nayak SR, Wakim AN. Random-start gonadotropin-releasing hormone (GnRH) antagonist-treated cycles with GnRH agonist trigger for fertility preservation. Fertil Steril. 2011;96:e51-4.
52. Sonmezer M, Türkçüoğlul, Coşkun U, Oktay K. Random-start controlled ovarian hyperstimulation for emergency fertility preservation in letrozole cycles. Fertil Steril. 2011;95:2125. e9-11.
53. de Mello Bianchi PH, Serafini P, da Rocha AM, Hassun PA, Alves da Motta ELA, Baruselli PS, et al. Review: follicular waves in the human ovary: a new physiological paradigm for novel ovarian stimulation protocols. Reprod Sci. 2010;17:1067-76.
54. Cakmak H, Katz A, Cedars MI, Rosen MP. Effective method for emergency fertility preservation: random-start controlled ovarian stimulation. Fertil Steril. 2013;100:1673-80.
55. Kim JH, Kim SK, Lee HJ, Lee JR, Jee BC, Suh CS, et al. Efficacy of random-start controlled ovarian stimulation in cancer patients. J Korean Med Sci. 2015;30:290-5.
56. Garcia-Velasco JA, Moreno L, Pacheco A, Guillén A, Duque L, Requena A, et al. The aromatase inhibitor letrozole increases the concentration of intraovarian androgens and improves in vitro fertilization outcome in low responder patients: a pilot study. Fertil Steril. 2005;84:82-7.

57. Oktay K, Hourvitz A, Sahin G, Oktem O, Safro B, Cil A, et al. Letrozole reduces estrogen and gonadotropin exposure in women with breast cancer undergoing ovarian stimulation before chemotherapy. J Clin Endocrinol Metab. 2006;91:3885-90.
58. Tulandi T, Martin J, Al-Fadhli R, Kabli N, Forman R, Hitkari J, et al. Congenital malformations among 911 newborns conceived after infertility treatment with letrozole or clomiphene citrate. Fertil Steril. 2006;85:1761-5.
59. Azim AA, Costantini-Ferrando M, Oktay K. Safety of fertility preservation by ovarian stimulation with letrozole and gonadotropins in patients with breast cancer: a prospective controlled study. J Clin Oncol. 2008;26:2630-5.
60. Cakmak H, Mitchell PR. Ovarian stimulation in cancer patients. Fertil Steril. 2013;99(6):1476-84.
61. Donnez J, Dolmans MM. Fertility preservation in women. Nat Rev Endocrinol. 2013;9:735-49.
62. Waimey KE, Duncan FE, Su HI, Smith K, Wallach H, Jona K, et al. Future directions in oncofertility and fertility preservation: a report from the 2011 oncofertility consortium conference. J Adolesc Young Adult Oncol. 2013;2:25-30.
63. Andersen CY, Kristensen SG, Greve T, Schmidt KT. Cryopreservation of ovarian tissue for fertility preservation in young female oncological patients. Future Oncol. 2012;8(5):595-608.
64. Donnez J, Dolmans MM, Demylle D, Jadoul P, Pirard C, Squifflet J, et al. Livebirth after orthotopic transplantation of cryopreserved ovarian tissue. Lancet. 2004;364:1405-10.
65. Donnez J, Dolmans MM. Ovarian cortex transplantation: 60 reported live births brings the success and worldwide expansion of the technique towards routine clinical practice. J Assist Reprod Genet. 2015;32:1167-70.
66. Donnez J, Jadoul P, Squifflet J, Van Langendonckt A, Donnez O, Van Eyck AS, et al. Ovarian tissue cryopreservation and transplantation in cancer patients. Best Pract Res Clin Obstet Gynaecol. 2010;24:87-100.
67. Donnez J, Dolmans MM, Pellicer A, Diaz-Garcia C, Sanchez Serrano M, Schmidt KT, et al. Restoration of ovarian activity and pregnancy after transplantation of cryopreserved ovarian tissue: a review of 60 cases of reimplantation. Fertil Steril. 2013;99:1503-13.
68. Xu M, Pavone ME, Woodruff T. Fruitful progress to fertility: preserving oocytes from chemodestruction. Nat Med. 2011;17:1562-3.
69. Moore HC, Unger JM, Phillips KA, Boyle F, Hitre E, Porter D, et al. Goserelin for ovarian protection during breast-cancer adjuvant chemotherapy. N Engl J Med. 2015;372:923-32.
70. Del Mastro L, Ceppi M, Poggio F, Bighin C, Peccatori F, Demeestere I, et al. Gonadotropin-releasing hormone analogues for the prevention of chemotherapy-induced premature ovarian failure in cancer women: systematic review and meta-analysis of randomized trials. Cancer Treat Rev. 2014;40:675-83.
71. Arian SE, Goodman L, Flyckt RL, Falcone T. Ovarian transposition: a surgical option for fertility preservation. Fertil Steril. 2017;107(4):e15.
72. Farber LA, Ames JW, Rush S, Gal D. Laparoscopic ovarian transposition to preserve ovarian function before pelvic radiation and chemotherapy in a young patient with rectal cancer. MedGenMed. 2005;7(1):66.
73. Meirow D, Hardan I, Dor J, Fridman E, Elizur S, Ra'anani H, et al. Searching for evidence of disease and malignant cell contamination in ovarian tissue stored from hematologic cancer patients. Hum Reprod. 2008;23:1007-13.
74. Dolmans MM, Jadoul P, Gilliaux S, Amorim CA, Luyckx V, Squifflet J, et al. A review of 15 years of ovarian tissue bank activities. J Assist Reprod Genet. 2013;30:305-14.
75. Rosendahl M, Greve T, Andersen CY. The safety of transplanting cryopreserved ovarian tissue in cancer patients: a review of the literature. J Assist Reprod Genet. 2013;30:11-24.
76. Ernst EH, Offersen BV, Andersen CY, Ernst E. Legal termination of a pregnancy resulting from transplanted cryopreserved ovarian tissue due to cancer recurrence. J Assist Reprod Genet. 2013;30:975-8.
77. Skory RM, Xu Y, Shea LD, Woodruff TK. Engineering the ovarian cycle using in vitro follicle culture. Hum Reprod. 2015;30:1386-95.
78. Xu M, Barrett SL, West-Farrell E, Kondapalli LA, Kiesewetter SE, Shea LD, et al. In vitro grown human ovarian follicles from cancer patients support oocyte growth. Hum Reprod. 2009;24:2531-40.
79. Soares M, Sahrari K, Chiti MC, Amorim CA, Ambroise J, Donnez J, et al. The best source of isolated stromal cells for the artificial ovary: medulla or cortex, cryopreserved or fresh? Hum Reprod. 2015;30:1589-98.
80. Vanacker J, Luyckx V, Dolmans MM, Des Rieux A, Jaeger J, Van Langendonckt A, et al. Transplantation of an alginate-matrigel matrix containing isolated ovarian cells: first step in developing a biodegradable scaffold to transplant isolated preantral follicles and ovarian cells. Biomaterials. 2012;33:6079-85.
81. Luyckx V, Dolmans MM, Vanacker J, Scalercio SR, Donnez J, Amorim CA. First step in developing a 3D biodegradable fibrin scaffold for an artificial ovary. J Ovarian Res. 2013;6:83.
82. Luyckx V, Dolmans MM, Vanacker J, Legat C, Fortuno Moya C, Donnez J, et al. A new step toward the artificial ovary: survival and proliferation of isolated murine follicles after autologous transplantation in a fibrin scaffold. Fertil Steril. 2014;101:1149-56.
83. Sittadjody S, Saul JM, Joo S, Yoo JJ, Atala A, Opara EC. Engineered multilayer ovarian tissue that secretes sex steroids and peptide hormones in response to gonadotropins. Biomaterials. 2013;34:2412-20.
84. White YA, Woods DC, Takai Y, Ishihara O, Seki H, Tilly JL. Oocyte formation by mitotically active germ cells purified from ovaries of reproductive-age women. Nat Med. 2012;18:413-21.
85. Hayashi K, Ogushi S, Kurimoto K, Shimamoto S, Ohta H, Saitou M. Offspring from oocytes derived from in vitro primordial germ cell-like cells in mice. Science. 2012;338:971-5.
86. Farquhar C, Brown J, Marjoribanks J. Laparoscopic drilling by diathermy or laser for ovulation induction in anovulatory polycystic ovary syndrome. Cochrane Database Syst Rev. 2012;6:CD001122.
87. Hsueh AJ, Kawamura K, Cheng Y, Fauser BC. Intraovarian control of early folliculogenesis. Endocr Rev. 2015;36:1-24.
88. Baker SJ, Spears N. The role of intra-ovarian interactions in the regulation of follicle dominance. Hum Reprod Update. 1999;5:153-65.

89. Suzuki N, Yoshioka N, Takae S, Sugishita Y, Tamura M, Hashimoto S, et al. Successful fertility preservation following ovarian tissue vitrification in patients with primary ovarian insufficiency. Hum Reprod. 2015;30:608-15.
90. Cheng Y, Kim J, Li XX, Hsueh AJ. Promotion of ovarian follicle growth following mTOR activation: synergistic effects of AKT stimulators. PLoS One. 2015;10:e0117769.
91. Silvestris E, De Palma G, Canosa S, Palini S, Dellino M, Revelli A, Paradiso AV. Human ovarian cortex biobanking: a fascinating resource for fertility preservation in cancer. Int J Mol Sci. 2020;21:3245.
92. Ahn RW, Chen F, Chen H, Stern ST, Clogston JD, Patri AK, et al. A novel nanoparticulate formulation of arsenic trioxide with enhanced therapeutic efficacy in a murine model of breast cancer. Clin Cancer Res. 2010;16:3607-17.
93. Ahn RW, Barrett SL, Raja MR, Jozefik JK, Spaho L, Chen H, et al. Nano-encapsulation of arsenic trioxide enhances efficacy against murine lymphoma model while minimizing its impact on ovarian reserve in vitro and in vivo. PLoS One. 2013;8:e5849.
94. Li F, Turan V, Lierman S, Cuvelier C, De Sutter P, Oktay K. Sphingosine-1-phosphate prevents chemotherapy-induced human primordial follicle death. Hum Reprod. 2014; 29:107-13.
95. Skaznik-Wikiel ME, McGuire MM, Sukhwani M, Donohue J, Chu T, Krivak TC, et al. Granulocyte colony-stimulating factor with or without stem cell factor extends time to premature ovarian insufficiency in female mice treated with alkylating chemotherapy. Fertil Steril. 2013;99:2045-54.e3.
96. Ting AY, Petroff BK. Tamoxifen decreases ovarian follicular loss from experimental toxicant DMBA and chemotherapy agents cyclophosphamide and doxorubicin in the rat. J Assist Reprod Genet. 2010;27:591-7.
97. Mahran YF, El-Demerdash E, Nada AS, Ali AA, Abdel-Naim AB. Insights into the protective mechanisms of tamoxifen in radiotherapy-induced ovarian follicular loss: impact on insulin-like growth factor 1. Endocrinology. 2013;154:3888-99.
98. Angarita AM, Johnson CA, Fader AN, Christianson MS. Fertility preservation: a key survivorship issue for young women with cancer. Front Oncol. 2016;6:102.
99. Brancati S, Gozzo L, Longo L, Vitale DC, Russo G, Drago F. Fertility preservation in female pediatric patients with cancer: a clinical and regulatory issue. Front Oncol. 2021;11: 641450.
100. Ethics Committee of the American Society for Reproductive Medicine. Posthumous retrieval and use of gametes or embryos: an Ethics Committee opinion. Fertil Steril. 2018; 110(1):45-9.
101. Sikary AK, Murty OP, Bardale RV. Postmortem sperm retrieval in context of developing countries of Indian subcontinent. J Hum Reprod Sci. 2016;9(2):82-5.
102. Ethics Committee of the American Society for Reproductive Medicine. Posthumous collection and use of reproductive tissue: a committee opinion. Fertil Steril. 2013;99:1842-5.
103. Lansac J. French law concerning medically-assisted reproduction. Hum Reprod. 1996;11:1843-7.
104. Smith GP. Australia's frozen 'orphan' embryos: a medical, legal and ethical dilemma. J Fam Law. 1985;24:27-41.
105. Pennings G, de Wert G, Shenfield F, Cohen J, Devroey P, Tarlatzis B. ESHRE Task Force on Ethics and Law 11: posthumous assisted reproduction. Hum Reprod. 2006;21(12):3050-53.
106. Anderson RA, Davies MC, Lavery SA. Elective egg freezing for non-medical reasons: Scientific Impact Paper No. 63. BJOG. 2020;127:e113-21.
107. Argyle CE, Harper JC, Davies MC. Oocyte cryopreservation: where are we now? Hum Reprod Update. 2016;22:440-9.
108. Varlas VN, Bors RG, Albu D, Penes ON, Nasui BA, Mehedintu C, et al. Social freezing: pressing pause on fertility. Int J Environ Res Public Health. 2021;18:8088.
109. Lew R, Foo J, Kroon B, Boothroyd C, Chapman M, Australasian CREI Consensus Expert Panel on Trial evidence (ACCEPT) Group. ANZSREI consensus statement on elective oocyte cryopreservation. Aust N Z J Obstet Gynaecol. 2019;59:616-26.
110. Mesen TB, Mersereau JE, Kane JB, Steiner AZ. Optimal timing for elective egg freezing. Fertil Steril. 2015;103:1551-6.
111. Goldman RH, Racowsky C, Farland LV, Munné S, Ribustello L, Fox JH. Predicting the likelihood of live birth for elective oocyte cryopreservation: a counseling tool for physicians and patients. Hum Reprod. 2017;32:853-9.
112. Cavalera F, Zanoni M, Merico V, Bui TTH, Belli M, Fassina L, et al. A neural network-based identification of developmentally competent or incompetent mouse fully-grown oocytes. J Vis Exp. 2018;56668.
113. Yanez LZ, Han J, Behr BB, Pera RAR, Camarillo DB. Human oocyte developmental potential is predicted by mechanical properties within hours after fertilization. Nat Commun. 2016;7:10809.
114. Peccatori FA, Azim Jr HA, Orecchia R, Hoekstra HJ, Pavlidis N, Kesic V, et al. Cancer, pregnancy and fertility: ESMO clinical practice guidelines for diagnosis, treatment and follow-up. Ann Oncol. 2013;24 Suppl 6:vi160-70.
115. Mahajan NK, Patil M, Jirge PR. Fertility preservation for patients on gonadotoxic treatment: recommendations for clinical practice by Fertility Preservation Society (India). Onco Fertil J. 2020;3:48-107.

CHAPTER

22 Counseling in Infertility

Prathap Tharyan, Sudeepa Chaparala

INFERTILITY IS A GLOBAL PROBLEM

Infertility is a common problem worldwide. Precise epidemiological estimates of its reported prevalence vary considerably, depending on the variations in different aspects of the definition of infertility.[1] These include the source of the sample (population vs. clinic); the time period used to define infertility (1 year, 2 years, or more); whether primary or secondary infertility is estimated; the role of current contraception versus the continuous use of contraception; the intent or desire to conceive; whether single, regularly cohabiting, or married; and the outcome measure used (pregnancy or live births).[1,2] Shorter exposure times such as 1–2 years are important from a clinical perspective to initiate treatment, but from an epidemiological and population perspective, these tend to misclassify women as infertile, since some women could give birth without any intervention if longer exposure times such as 5 years are used. Applying a standard definition of infertility that estimated live births in sexually active women over a 5-year period to data from 53 selected demographic and health surveys done in 26 countries in Africa, Asia, the Middle East, Eastern Europe, and South America from 1990 to 2008, age-standardized estimates for primary infertility were 0.6–3.4% and 8.7–32.6% for secondary infertility.[2]

Based on these estimates, it can therefore be assumed that roughly a tenth to a third of the population of women in the reproductive age group across the world do not have children in spite of attempts to have one. There are also indications that infertility is more common, and the childless state also more perceived as undesirable in less developed countries than in more developed countries.[3,4]

INFERTILITY, AND ITS TREATMENT, IS ASSOCIATED WITH CONSIDERABLE DISTRESS

Infertility can be due to factors in the male, the female, both, or due to unknown causes. Parenthood is generally considered by couples and society as a desired social role and the desire to have a child can be considered, with some exceptions, a universal phenomenon. The nature and extent of distress caused by childlessness varies between men and women, and though men also experience pressures and distress related to infertility, affected women worldwide tend to show more distress. This is, in part, related to the greater importance that women attach to having a child; with childlessness perceived more as a direct blow to their identity as women, while for men, the effects are largely mediated by the effects of childlessness on their wives, and due to a sense of responsibility for this distress.[4] However, women's reactions to childlessness are also largely influenced by gender-specific cultural expectations and societal reactions. In many traditional societies in low- and middle-income countries, particularly in South Asia, women are considered responsible for childlessness, even when the cause of infertility is due to the male partner, as the female is blamed for this state by their in-laws, often their male partners, and by society; and infertile women are often stigmatized, and subjected to various forms of emotional, verbal, and physical abuse, discrimination, separation, and social ostracism.[4-10]

The psychological reactions seen in infertile couples include depression and anxiety, grief, guilt, shame, suicidal attempts, feelings of inadequacy, low self-esteem, social isolation, dissatisfaction with marital and sexual functioning, and impaired quality of life.[4,11-13] Socioeconomic status, societal and personal expectations, religious beliefs, and attitudes influence the distress associated with childlessness. Individual copying styles and previous psychological status; the quality of marital functioning; the duration of infertility; the availability of social networks and support structures; and whether professional services are available or used, and the quality of these services are also important mediators of the distress associated with infertility.

Infertile couples are increasingly seeking assistance to have children, and advances in medical technology such as in vitro fertilization (IVF) and microinjection [intracytoplasmic sperm injection (ICSI)] have helped millions of infertile couples worldwide. The numerous claims of success of assisted reproductive technologies (ARTs) also contribute to expectations of success in childless couples, and to distress and disappointment at failures. Estimates of successful pregnancies and live births vary. The best estimates are that around 50% of those seeking treatment will have a child, but in many surveys, the rates of success with ART are considerably lower.[14,15] Many couples also drop out of treatment after their first experience of failure. Although, infertility is considered a crisis (often ranked in impact similar to having a life-threatening illness or having lost a loved one),[16] and reactions to crises typically resolve with time; resolution of the crisis caused by childlessness may not be possible for many, and unresolved grief and depression continue to be experienced by women and men, after unsuccessful ART, many years after discontinuing treatment.[17]

Couples seeking ART may also experience considerable distress, inconveniences, and costs associated with the treatment. Couples often have to not only understand complex biological processes and treatment procedures, or face delays and failures, and the emotional effects of intensive, protracted, and invasive medical treatments; they also have to face complex decisions associated with choice of techniques, disposal of embryos, the possibility of complications associated with treatments (often related to the causes of infertility) that may result in pregnancy or birth complications, more frequent need for assisted deliveries, low birth-weight or premature babies, and babies with congenital abnormalities, leading to poorer neonatal outcomes.[18] There is also the possibility of multiple pregnancies and choices may have to be made related to fetal reduction. Many couples may have ethical and religious issues associated with donated sperm and embryos, and surrogacy. Those in contact with ART services as donors or surrogates also face considerable stresses that may require formal supportive services.[12] Some of these techniques also have legal implications that vary in different parts of the world.

Thus, people with infertility seeking ART as patients, donors, or surrogates, face complex issues, which span biological, psychological, social, legal, spiritual, and ethical domains and the attention paid to the medical and technical aspects of ART should not overshadow these needs or neglect these domains.

COUNSELING IN INFERTILITY AND ASSISTED REPRODUCTIVE TECHNOLOGY

Counseling refers to a confidential interaction between a health professional and a client aimed at enabling the client to cope with stressful situations and take personal decisions related to problem areas. Counseling aims to enable people to arrive at realistic solutions to their situations, and improve their ability to cope with stresses and thereby develop a sense of control, and reduce distress associated with their situation.

The aims of counseling in the context of infertility are to help couples to explore, understand, and resolve issues arising from infertility and infertility treatment, and to help them identify ways of dealing with these more effectively. The counseling process should consider the needs of the patient as well as any other person who might be affected by the treatment process (not ignoring the rights of the unborn child), and the decisions that have to be made. Considering the range of complex issues faced by couples with infertility, counseling in infertility often involves discussions of matters far beyond the medical or biological aspects of infertility; though these are also integral to the content of counseling.

The Need for Counseling in People with Infertility

While studies have documented higher levels of distress and psychological indices of ill-health in infertile couples compared to control populations, not all couples or individuals surveyed have been found to express such levels of distress after the initial reaction to the diagnosis; and studies have also documented that many couples who were offered counseling support do not take up this offer. On average, only around 20–30% avail counseling services, even when they are available.[19] The remaining 70–80% of people who do not take up counseling services are presumed to have coping mechanisms that are adequate to meet the demands imposed by their childless state.[20] However, this premise has not been systematically studied in less developed countries, where infertile women face more stigma and rejection within families and in their social circles.

In recent times, the concept of resilience has emerged as a possible protective factor against distress caused by life's vicissitudes, and resilient individuals develop coping skills and a problem-solving approach to improve their self-esteem, their social relationships, and their quality of life in spite of adversity.[21] Systematic enquiry in infertile couples has documented that resilience can be considered as a nonspecific protective factor against infertility-specific distress and poor quality of life, and this suggests that improving the resilience of distressed infertile couples who seek help should be considered a goal of counseling, irrespective of the outcomes of ART.[22]

Specific Indications for Counseling in Infertility

While not everyone requires counseling (though ideally every couple seeking ART should be offered psychosocial help and counseling), counseling is specially indicated under certain circumstances. These include people experiencing high distress, those undergoing social pressures, marital problems, unrealistic expectations, and prior failures;

people who need donated gametes, surrogacy, adoption, or fetal reduction; those with past histories of psychiatric or psychological problems; and those who require genetic counseling. In addition, counseling may be required at treatment-related time points, for mood fluctuations, failures, commencements, and delays associated with treatment.

Legal Mandate for Counseling

The nature, scope, and timing of counseling in infertility; who delivers counseling and their qualifications; and the specific aspects of ART services where counseling is considered mandatory are often decided by legal requirements in force in Australia, Canada, and some countries in Europe, UK, USA, and New Zealand. In many of these jurisdictions, counseling can only be provided by a trained and certified mental health professional, often requiring additional special training in the setting of infertility services, and requiring demonstration of involvement in continuous professional education.[23] In resource-constrained countries, such mandated requirements are impractical, considering the scarcity of trained mental health professionals to meet the demands of standard mental health needs. Numerous professional bodies also endorse the provision of psychological care and support to people seeking ART, and the guidelines of these bodies delineate the specific counseling requirements for different aspects of ART.[23] The endorsement for the need for psychological support is also echoed in surveys of people seeking help with assisted reproduction, who often report dissatisfaction with the lack of sensitivity provided for their emotional and psychological needs; however, integrated care within the context of the multidisciplinary team where their psychosocial needs were also attended was valued more frequently than specialized psychological referral and treatment, except in those with high infertility-related distress or with interpersonal problems or due to the social consequences of infertility.[24]

Outcomes with Counseling for Infertility

Whether psychological stress is a causative factor for infertility is an area surrounded by controversy, with no reliable evidence to support a causative role for stress in the majority of people with infertility. Some studies have suggested that pretreatment anxiety and depression affect outcomes with ART.[25] Based on this notion, psychosocial treatments have been devised to improve pregnancy outcomes with ART.[26] However, a systematic review of psychosocial interventions concluded that current evidence, from the eight studies identified of which three suggested benefit, was not robust enough to support this view, or to recommend psychosocial interventions as a primary method of improving pregnancy outcomes with ART.[27]

However, this systematic review did find that certain form of psychosocial interventions showed evidence of positive effects in reducing distress and improving mood in people presenting with infertility-related distress, though not changing preexisting maladaptive patterns of behavior, or dysfunctional relationships.[27] The beneficial psychosocial interventions were those that provided education specific to people's problems with infertility and that improved coping skills and problem-solving abilities; while interventions aimed only at providing support and an opportunity to ventilate their distress, or at exploring the meaning of childlessness were associated with less wide-ranging benefits.[27] The results of this systematic review are concordant with the literature on the potential benefits of increasing resilience in general as a useful goal for counseling and psychosocial care in infertile couples, irrespective of whatever specific theoretical models of psychological support are used.[22]

Psychiatric Interventions in Infertility

Not all people with infertility-related distress require psychiatric assessment or treatment, as psychological methods are usually what is required. However, people with preexisting psychiatric disorders or those who develop psychiatric problems, such as major depression, severe anxiety, or obsessive symptoms, are best dealt with in liaison with a psychiatrist, preferably one who has had some experience with the biological and psychosocial issues related to infertility. People with depression undergoing ART and treated with a combination of antidepressants and psychological support have better mental health and pregnancy-related outcomes than those not undergoing this treatment.[28]

The couples undergoing the infertility treatment have stress and anxiety. Couples should be given proper time to discuss the issues, and patient hearing and interactive discussion help decrease anxiety. Counseling regarding the need of stress management and impact of stress and anxiety on the treatment outcome have to be discussed. Stress and anxiety levels are elevated in most patients. Studies show that women with lower stress and anxiety levels on the day prior to oocyte retrieval had a higher pregnancy rate.[29]

Types of Counseling, Psychosocial Support, and Care in Infertility and with Assisted Reproductive Technology

Evaluation and Screening

Traditionally, the role of a mental health professional in infertility treatment clinics had been to screen aspiring couples and individuals for their vulnerabilities, expectations, social supports, coping skills, and financial solvency, in order to identify those couples who would be most suitable for ART. Often, in the absence of trained counselors or mental health professionals, this eligibility screening was done by a doctor or a nurse with a special interest and some experience of counseling. In some countries, this screening or evaluation of couples seeking ART now also requires assessment of their suitability to be parents, keeping the welfare of the child as a priority. This may require background checks for criminal records, or records of sexual assault or had a child in there care removed away by a child protection order. Such eligibility assessments are often more stringent in the case of embryo donors or those wishing to be surrogates.[23] Current roles of counseling in ART clinics go far beyond screening couples for suitability, though this continues to be an expectation of the role of mental health professionals in ART services.

Various tools have been developed to help identify couples likely to be distressed with IVF procedures, though they are less widely used in developing countries. SCREEN IVF is a pretreatment screening tool that helps medical staff to identify patients with positive scores that predict high levels of distress with treatment, and who need referral to psychological support services.[30] An internationally validated tool exists that can help assess the quality of life of people with infertility. The Fertility Quality of Life Tool (FertiQoL) is a sensitive, reliable, and valid measure of quality of life for men and women experiencing fertility problems, and the 36-item self-rated questionnaire assesses the subjective rating of the excellence of the infertile patient's life within their cultural, emotional, social, and environmental context. FertiQoL assesses the influences of fertility problems in multiple domains of the infertile person, such as self-esteem, emotions, general health, partnership, family and social relationships, work life, and future life plans.[31] An optional FertiQoL treatment module assesses the potential burden and tolerability of fertility treatment, and can aid assessment of risk factors for poor adjustment to infertility treatment. FertiQoL is available for free download from //psych.cf.ac.uk/fertiqol/download/index.html, and the scoring key is also available from //psych.cf.ac.uk/fertiqol/scoring/index.html.

The Continuum of Patient-Centered Care, Counseling, and Psychotherapy

A distinction is also made between those aspects of care that are considered part of good clinical practice, such as providing information, discussing options, and assessing implications, versus the more specialized psychological techniques for helping distressed people.[32] These often form a continuum with some degree of overlap in the middle of the continuum that are often provided both by medical personal and nurses in the infertility clinic as well as by mental health professionals, while the ends of this continuum are best dealt with by the respective specialists. The domains of this continuum are described in **Table 1**[32] and the contents and focus are elaborated subsequently.

Information Gathering and Assessment

Assessing people presenting with infertility is the primary responsibility of the medical and nursing staff of the infertility clinic. Presenting people with information about infertility, the common emotional and other problems associated with infertility and its treatment, and the specific issues related to ART can be done using written material, videos, and even by telephone to supplement face-to-face discussions with clinic staff, and through self-help groups of patients that can empower them, aid information sharing, as well as normalize the experience of infertility.[33] However, these issues often come up in counseling sessions, and

TABLE 1: The continuum of patient-centered care, counseling, and psychotherapy in relation to infertility and assisted reproductive technology (ART).[32]

Domain in the continuum	*Type of counseling*	*Focus*	*Delivered by*
Patient-centered care	• Information gathering and assessment • Implication and decision making	• Evaluation of medical and biological factors associated with infertility and eligibility for ART • Discussing the implications of infertility and options for treatment and helping people make decisions regarding treatment	Medical and nursing staff of fertility clinic
Infertility counseling	• Supportive counseling • Crisis counseling	• Providing emotional support to patients in distress • Short-term support in crises (e.g., acute grief) • Long-term support for people with multiple or longer term problems	Trained clinic counselor (medical or nursing staff or mental health professional such as a counselor, psychologist, psychiatric social worker)
Psychotherapy	Therapeutic counseling	Specific psychotherapeutic techniques such as problem-solving, interpersonal therapy, cognitive behavior therapy for long-standing problems	Qualified mental health professional (counselor, psychologist, psychotherapist, psychiatrist)

infertility counselors need to be conversant with these issues as well.

Implications and Decision-making Counseling

Patients need to be helped to understand the implications of infertility on their lives and their emotional reactions; the implications of the different forms of ART offered or chosen; the implications of dealing with failures; and also the implications of success and their roles as parents of a child born through ART. The primary role of medical personnel in this is to provide accurate information, provide opportunities for patients to clarify their doubts, express their concerns, and to work with them to understand the implications of their choices and make necessary practical arrangements. Counselors may also be required to help patients make sense of these decisions and fully understand the implications and the changes required in their lifestyles to ensure better outcomes. Implication counseling is specially important in the context of sperm and egg donation and surrogacy, and is also important when discussing issues such as adoption, termination of treatment, disclosure to future children of the circumstances associated with their conception, and the impact of their changed status as parents as well. This discussion may also help them identify patients at potentially high risk of distress and to arrange for more formal support, if needed.

Supportive Counseling

Supportive counseling aims to support patients experiencing distress arising from the psychosocial problems related to infertility, the desire to have a child, the financial pressures, and practical difficulties associated with ART, and the limitations of these technologies in guaranteeing success. Concerned family members may also need support. Supportive counseling may be needed at specific periods associated with treatments such as for men facing the pressure to perform, the waiting period or during delays in treatment, during phases of intensive assessment, and with failure to achieve pregnancy, and when there are conflicts between partners related to treatment options, or with clinical staff in relation to treatment options or termination of treatment. Clinic-based counselors may sometimes need to refer some patients to mental health services outside the clinic if these latter conflicts impede the counseling and therapeutic relationship.

The principles of supportive counseling include the facilitation of the expression of concerns and the distress experienced, the validation of these concerns and distress, the normalization of such experiences, provision of information, and correction of misconceptions or unwarranted misgivings, strengthening coping mechanisms (encouraging resilience), and mobilizing social and family support. A problem-solving approach and specific techniques to aid relaxation are also useful in some patients experiencing high levels of distress.

Crisis Counseling

Patients with infertility often face acute emotional crises related to their infertile state as well as to specific issues of ART treatment that for some are more distressing than for others. Failure of an IVF cycle, miscarriages, and abortions, or exacerbations of marital conflicts or interpersonal problems are often traumatic. Acute grief reactions can follow losses and can be devastating for some patients. In such situations, patients need immediate help and assessment of their coping and support. Working with grieving patients requires knowledge of the stages of normal grief: From numbness and disbelief, through anger and protest, to despair and depression, till eventual resolution as they make new plans, and reinvest in life. Normalizing these experiences while using the principles of supportive counseling, supplemented by specific techniques related to grief work, help many patients come to terms with their losses. These crises are best averted by supportive counseling that aims to provide patients with opportunities to anticipate potential losses, and to learn and practice new adaptive behaviors that could enhance their ability to cope with infertility and the associated medical procedures, and failures. The emphasis should be on providing both positive and negative information, identifying coping strategies and strengthening resilience, and helping them redefine their future, if treatment fail's; and helping to strengthen their relationships.

Psychotherapy

Psychotherapy may be required for people going through specific issues arising out of infertility or of failed treatment, or the consequences of treatment. Mental health professionals often use specific psychological techniques, such as psychodynamically oriented psychotherapy; cognitive behavior therapy aimed at identifying dysfunctional attitudes and beliefs and cognitive distortions that influence emotional responses, and providing alternate rational explanations; interpersonal therapy aimed at dealing with distressing relationships; and problem-solving approaches.

However, the features common to all forms of psychotherapy and supportive counseling that are likely to benefit patients in distress, irrespective of the theoretical models employed,[34] are:

- Having an unconditional positive regard for the patient
- Providing the opportunity for a confiding relationship with a helping person, often with the participation of a group or others to help.
- Facilitating the expression of distress and of emotional arousal; this is often a prerequisite to attitudinal and behavioral changes.

- Providing a rational explanation of the cause of the patient's distress and a method for relieving it.
- Provision of new information concerning the nature and sources of the patient's problems and possible alternative ways of dealing with them.
- Strengthening the patient's expectations of help through the personal qualities of the therapist that emphasize compassionate professionalism; this is often enhanced by the status (or reputation) of the therapist in society and the setting in which he or she works.
- Providing patients with hope and the experience of success, in coping with their problems through simple practical measures, which can further heighten the patient's hopes and also enhance their sense of mastery, interpersonal competence, or capability.

Specific Issues in Counseling for Infertility

Gender, Sexuality, and Sexual Functioning

Gender differences in the reactions of infertility in couples who seek help relate to the greater distress and the need to express distress, and the need for emotional support in women; while men tend to use problem-solving approaches more. Male partners of infertile women often tend to be seen as emotionally unsupportive due to these differences in dealing with emotional distress, and couples need to be helped to understand these differences and to support each other. Women also tend to avoid reminders of their childlessness due to the distress it arouses, and helping them confront, rather than avoid, these issues and enhance resilience and coping mechanisms, using practical suggestions is important. Infertile couples also have many problems with their sexual lives, and the pressure of timed intercourse with IVF treatments is one of the causes of this dissatisfaction that will need to be dealt with by enhancing the pleasurable aspects of their sexual relationship, rather than focusing on pregnancy outcomes. Couples need to be approached with the view that, irrespective of pregnancy outcomes, the principal focus of counseling is on strengthening their marital relationship and their quality of life, while helping them cope with the pressures of treatment.

Dealing with Multiple Gestations

Since the possibility exists for multiple gestations, information sharing and implication counseling is an opportunity to broach this possibility and encourage reflections on the implications of dealing with multiple pregnancies. This is in keeping with the expectations of counselors to always keep the welfare of the unborn child or children as part of the focus of counseling. Early discussion of potentially distressing issues such as fetal reduction, if required, is also important to prevent subsequent distress, if multiple gestations occur.

Counseling in Serodiscordant Couples

The discordant couples either of who is human immunodeficiency virus (HIV) positive should be counseled regarding how to prevent transmission to their partner and child, and advantages of ART procedures in decreasing the risk of HIV sexual transmission.

- *HIV-positive men:* Sperms are not infected by HIV virus. Most recent studies show that sperms lack the CD4 and CCR5 receptors on the surface, which allow viruses to bind and enter the cell. HIV is probably found in higher concentration in the white cells in the semen. To prevent transmission to HIV-negative wife, options can be given to couple regarding:
  - Intrauterine insemination (IUI) with washed semen sample
  - IVF
  - ART with donor semen.
- *HIV-positive women:* They should be counseled regarding the ART options available and advantages, the retroviral treatment and blood tests, and frequent visits needed. Counseling is done regarding the risk of transmission to child, importance of delivery in multidisciplinary setting involving relevant health professionals, and measures to be taken to decrease the risk of spread to child.

Donor Insemination, Egg Sharing, Oocyte Donations, and Other Third-Party Treatments

There are many aspects of ART that require the involvement of a third party, other than the couple, that may need to be dealt with in counseling. Some of these include: semen donation, oocyte donation, embryo donation, surrogates, gestational surrogacy, lesbian couples, single women without a partner, disclosure of information to donor-conceived children or adults, concluding treatment without achieving pregnancy, adoption, and fertility preservation for medical or social reasons.[23]

Some issues to focus on in counseling are as follows:

- Helping couples understand the implications of third-party treatments on their relationships, particularly the implications for the genetically unrelated partner.
- The emotional reactions and motivations of the third-party donor who will not conceive and the future boundaries and expectations of the third-party donor.
- The legal, moral, spiritual, and emotional issues raised by third-party treatments.
- Issues related to confidentiality, the nature and timing of disclosure to future offspring, family, and others of third-party treatments.[34]
- Counseling and assuring of the patient regarding the prior screening of donors with communicable diseases that endangers the recipient health.

Counseling in situations of third-party treatments is particularly difficult and limited evidence indicates that considerable distress exists long after the treatments in people who were involved in such treatments, often related to the lack of counseling, but sometimes perceived to be due to the mandated provision of counseling that left them feeling stigmatized.

There is insufficient qualitative or quantitative research from developing countries on the distress associated with third-party treatments and the provision of counseling services to those involved.

NEGATIVE COUNSELING

The need of negative counseling is more in the patients where the IVF success rate is low due to low ovarian reserve, advanced maternal age, highly compromised semen parameters, recurrent pregnancy loss, etc., as there is high risk of aneuploidies, and increase in financial burden. But the routine negative counseling of patients may increase the stress and anxiety, which may impact the outcome.

KEY POINTS

- Infertility is a common problem and affects between a third and a tenth of women worldwide.
- Infertility is associated with considerable distress that is influenced by personal expectations and coping styles, and interpersonal relations, but influenced considerably by gender-specific special pressures and attributions.
- Women all over the world experience more distress due to infertility than men, but in parts of the developing world, also face considerable stigma, discrimination, abuse, and neglect.
- ARTs have brought hope to millions of infertile couples, but couples entering treatment with these technologies are not guaranteed success; the treatment is complex and protracted; and associated with psychological, social, financial, legal, religious or spiritual, and medical challenges and dilemmas that require the offer and provision of psychosocial support and care.
- Counseling in infertility includes evaluation, patient-centered care, infertility counseling, and psychotherapy that overlap to form a continuum of care.
- This continuum hopes to provide suitable patients and couples information and help with understanding their condition, treatment options, and their implications, in order to reduce the distress associated with their chosen treatments and the outcomes.
- Some couples will also require supportive and crisis counseling, and fewer still will require psychotherapeutic help from trained mental health professionals.
- Legal provisions exist in some countries as to what aspects of this continuum are mandatory and who is qualified to provide such services.
- In developing countries, all members of the treating team need to have knowledge and some expertise in the provision of patient-centered care and infertility counseling, though therapeutic counseling is best done by trained mental health professionals.
- The forms of psychosocial treatments that have shown the best outcomes in infertile couples are those that improve their sense of mastery and control, and problem-solving techniques that enhance reliance, rather than only providing the opportunity for emotional expression and introspection.
- Counseling for infertility and with ART is a developing field that needs more trained professionals and further research to better delineate who needs to be counseled, the components of counseling that are effective, and the perceptions of those being counseled, particularly from the developing world.
- Finally, reversing the state of childlessness is the focus of treatment of the medical team, while strengthening the relationship of the couple and improving their quality of life, irrespective of pregnancy outcomes, should be the focus of infertility counseling.

CONCLUSION

Counseling should be given by trained and certified professional, who makes couple understand, explore and to resolve issues arising from infertility and infertility treatment. Psychological impact on infertility is no longer considered a negligible area as studies show evidence of positive effects on improving ART outcome after treating the stress.

In patients with psychosocial disturbances counseling should not be a single step procedure, counselors should help couple make sense of the decisions and fully understand the implications, lifestyle changes required. Support patients experiencing the distress arising from psychological problems and to deal with emotional crisis (like miscarriage, abortions etc.,) psychotherapy may be required for people going through special issues arising out of infertility or failed treatment or consequence of treatment.

REFERENCES

1. Gurunath S, Pandian Z, Anderson RA, Bhattacharya S. Defining infertility—a systematic review of prevalence studies. Hum Reprod Update. 2011;17:575-88.
2. Mascarenhas MN, Cheung H, Mathers CD, Stevens GA. Measuring infertility in populations: constructing a standard definition for use with demographic and reproductive health surveys. Popul Health Metr. 2012;10:17.
3. Boivin J, Bunting L, Collins JA, Nygren KG. International estimates of infertility prevalence and treatment-seeking: potential need and demand for infertility medical care. Hum Reprod. 2007;22:1506-12.
4. Greil A, Slauson-Blevins K, McQuillan J. The experience of infertility: a review of recent literature. Social Health Illn. 2010;32(1):140-62.

5. Leung TW, Ng EHY, Leung WC, Ho PC. Intimate partner violence among infertile women. Int J Gynaecol Obstet. 2003;83:323-4.
6. Sami N, Ali TS. Domestic violence against infertile women in Karachi, Pakistan. Asian Rev Soc Sci. 2012;1:15-20.
7. Moghadam ZB, Ardabily HE, Salsali M, Ramezanzadeh F, Nedjat S. Physical and psychological violence against infertile women. J Fam Reprod Health. 2010;4:65-7.
8. Yilidizhan R, Adali E, Kolusari A, Kurdoglu M, Yildizhan B, Sahin G. Domestic violence against infertile women in a Turkish setting. Int J Gynaecol Obstet. 2009;104:110-2.
9. Mumtaz Z, Shahid U, Levay A. Understanding the impact of gendered roles on the experiences of infertility amongst men and women in Punjab. Reprod Health. 2013;10:3.
10. Dyer SJ, Abrahams N, Mokoena NE, Lombard CJ, van der Spuy ZM. Psychological distress among women suffering from couple infertility in South Africa: a quantitative assessment. Hum Reprod. 2005;20(7):1938-43.
11. Noorbala AA, Ramezanzadeh F, Abedinia N, Yazdi SAB, Jafarabadi M. Study of psychiatric disorders among fertile and infertile women and some predisposing factors. J Fam Reprod Health. 2007;1(1):6-11.
12. Cousineau TM, Domar AD. Psychological impact of infertility. Best Pract Res Clin Obstet Gynaecol. 2007;21:293-308.
13. Valsangkar S, Bodhare T, Bele S, Sai S. An evaluation of the effects of infertility on marital and sexual satisfaction indices and health-related quality of life in women. J Hum Reprod Sci. 2011;4(2):80-5.
14. Jose-Miller AB, Boyden JW, Frey KA. Infertility. Am Fam Physician. 2007;75:849-56.
15. Pinborg A, Hougaard CO, Andersen AN, Molbo D, Schmidt L. Prospective longitudinal cohort study on cumulative 5-year delivery and adoption rates among 1338 couples initiating infertility treatment. Hum Reprod. 2009;24:991-9.
16. Domar AD, Zuttermeister P, Friedman R. The psychological impact of infertility: a comparison with patients with other medical conditions. J Psychosom Obstet Gynaecol. 1993;14(Suppl):45-52.
17. Volgsten H, Avanberg AS, Olsson P. Unresolved grief in women and men in Sweden three years after undergoing unsuccessful in vitro fertilization treatment. Acta Obstet Gynecol Scand. 2010;89:1290-7.
18. Barnes M, Roiko A, Reed R, Williams C, Willcocks K. Outcomes for women and children following assisted conception. Implications for perinatal education, care, and support. J Perinat Educ. 2012;21(1):18-23.
19. Verhaak CM, Smeenk JM, Evers AW, Kremer JA, Kraaimaat FW, Braat DD. Women's emotional adjustment to IVF: a systematic review of 25 years of research. Hum Reprod Update. 2007;13(1):27-36.
20. Boivin J, Scanlan LC, Walker SM. Why are infertile patients not using psychosocial counseling? Hum Reprod. 1999;5:1384-91.
21. Ridenour AF, Yorgason JB, Peterson B. The infertility resilience model: assessing individual, couple, and external predictive factors. Contemp Fam Ther. 2009;31:34-51.
22. Herrmann D, Scherg H, Verres R, von Hagens C, Strowitzki T, Wischmann T. Resilience in infertile couples acts as a protective factor against infertility-specific distress and impaired quality of life. J Assist Reprod Genet. 2011;28:1111-7.
23. Blyth E. Guidelines for infertility counseling in different countries: is there an emerging trend? Hum Reprod. 2012;27(7):2046-57.
24. Schmidt L, Holstein BE, Boivin J, Sångren H, Tjørnhøj-Thomsen T, Blaabjerg J, et al. Patients' attitudes to medical and psychosocial aspects of care in fertility clinics: findings from the Copenhagen Multi-Centre Psychosocial Infertility (COMPI) Research Programme. Hum Reprod. 2003;18(3):628-37.
25. Smeenk JM, Verhaak CM, Eugster A, van Minnen A, Zielhuis GA, Braat DD. The effect of anxiety and depression on the outcome of in-vitro fertilization. Hum Reprod. 2001;16:1420-3.
26. Domar AD, Seibel M, Benson H. The mind/body program for infertility: a new behavioral treatment approach for women with infertility. Fertil Steril. 1990;53:246-9.
27. Boivin J. A review of psychosocial interventions in infertility. Soc Sci Med. 2003;57:2325-41.
28. Ramezanzadeh F, Noorbala AA, Abedinia N, Forooshani AR, Naghizadeh MM. Psychiatric intervention improved pregnancy rates in infertile couples. Malays J Med Sci. 2011;18(1):16-24.
29. Turner K, Reynolds-May MF, Zitek EM, Tisdale RL, Carlisle AB, Westphal LM. Stress and anxiety scores in first and repeat IVF cycles: a pilot study. PLoS One. 2013;8(5):e63743.
30. Verhaak CM, Lintsen AM, Evers AW, Braat DD. Who is at risk of emotional problems and how do you know? Screening of women going for IVF treatment. Hum Reprod. 2010;25:1234-40.
31. Boivin J, Takefman J, Braverman A. The fertility quality of life (FertiQoL) tool: development and general psychometric properties. Hum Reprod. 2011;26(8):2084-91.
32. Peterson B, Boivin J, Norré J, Smith C, Thorn P, Wischmann T. An introduction to infertility counseling: a guide for mental health and medical professionals. J Assist Reprod Genet. 2012;29:243-8.
33. Frank JD. Common features of psychotherapy. Aust N Z J Psychiatry. 1972;6:34-40.
34. Boivin J, Appleton TC, Baetens P, Baron J, Bitzer J, Corrigan E, et al. Guidelines for counseling in infertility: outline version. Hum Reprod. 2001;16(6):1301-4.

CHAPTER 23

Assisted Reproductive Technology in Patients with Chronic Medical Disorders

Anuradha Kumari, Devi R

INTRODUCTION

The majority of women undergoing assisted reproduction are healthy and relatively young. However, the tendency to postpone the marriage and childbearing to later on in life is leading to the concurrent conditions that may have implications for in vitro fertilization (IVF), pregnancy, and its outcome. Assisted reproductive technology (ART) treatments in women with underlying chronic diseases have become increasingly frequent. Some of the most prevalent chronic diseases in women during their reproductive years are ulcerative colitis, Crohn's disease, rheumatoid arthritis, multiple sclerosis, epilepsy, hypertension, and diabetes mellitus (DM). Patients at risk for thrombosis could pose tremendous challenges during assisted reproduction treatment and subsequent pregnancy. The research area on the efficacy of ART in women with different chronic diseases is still new, and the amount of literature is limited.

PRECONCEPTION COUNSELING

Despite tremendous advances in prenatal care, certain adverse pregnancy outcomes such as preterm delivery and birth defects have not changed. The principal goal of preconception counseling is to maximize the quality of fetal, maternal, and newborn life through primary prevention. The four main components of preconception care are—(1) risk assessment, (2) health promotion, (3) interventions to eliminate risk factors, and (4) adequate counseling.

ASSISTED REPRODUCTION IN PATIENTS AT RISK OF THROMBOSIS

The clinical association between VTE and IVF is primarily due to ovarian hyperstimulation syndrome (OHSS) in which thromboembolic complications may have fatal consequences. Sometimes patients presenting for IVF might have a previous history of VTE or may be at increased risk of developing thromboembolic complication while undergoing IVF treatment due to a pre-existing condition which increases the risk for the same. The prevalence of venous thromboembolism (VTE) in patients undergoing assisted reproduction (0.1–0.2%) is 10x higher than the general population (2.2/10,000).[1,2] This risk is increased to 100-fold in patients who develop ovarian hyperstimulation (1.7%).[1] Although the absolute numbers of VTE events in assisted reproduction are low, it can be potentially fatal with serious morbidity or mortality. With increasing use of assisted reproductive techniques (ARTs), especially in women with advanced age, obesity, and smoking, it is extremely important as clinicians to identify women who are at increased risk, provides appropriate counseling, and risk-reduction strategies to make treatment safer.

Mechanism of Thrombosis in Assisted Reproductive Technology

The pathogenesis of venous thrombosis is complex. The hyperestrogenism resulting from ovarian hyperstimulation is a known thrombotic agent. It causes increase in procoagulant factors (fibrinogen, von Willebrand factor, factors VIII and V, and increased activated protein C resistance), enhanced activation of coagulation (D-dimer), reduced fibrinolysis (reduced tissue plasminogen activator and plasminogen activator inhibitor type I), and reduced natural anticoagulants (antithrombin III and protein S).[3,4] Changes in Von Willebrand factor and Von Willebrand factor-cleaving protease have also been reported. Tissue factor pathway inhibitor values progressively and significantly decreased throughout the ovarian stimulation and negatively correlated with estradiol.[5] Indeed, during IVF treatment, the action of coagulation factors seems to be associated less with the level of serum estradiol concentrations (which may reach levels 10x higher than in physiological cycles but remain below those occurring in pregnancy) than with the biochemical changes that occur after the triggering of final oocyte maturation with human chorionic gonadotropin (hCG). The predominant contribution of hCG rather than estradiol to the etiology of

VTE after ovarian stimulation is supported by the clinical observation that frozen thaw cycles (when estrogens but not hCG are administered) are not associated with an increased risk compared to natural conceptions. It has been seen that activation of the coagulation cascade system (fibrinogen and factors II, V, VII, VIII, and IX) was elevated within 2 days after hCG, reaching a maximum approximately 8 days after hCG administration.[6] Although hemostatic risk is more during the stimulation phase, the final event is often attributable to exogenous hCG. In severe OHSS excessive vasoactive substances produced by the ovaries causes increased permeability of blood vessels leading to escape of fluid from the vascular compartment to the third space (ascites, hydrothorax, and hydropericardium) and contribute to hemoconcentration, hypovolemia, and thromboembolism. Careful monitoring and preventive measures to avoid OHSS are important in patients at risk of thrombosis.

Risk Assessment and Screening

All patients proceeding to IVF treatment should be individually assessed for their risk of thrombotic complications. Women who should be considered at increased risk include those with congenital or acquired thrombophilias, hyperhomocysteinemia, previous history of OHSS, advanced age, smoking, and obesity.[1] Women with a previous episode of VTE are at increased risk for recurrence, particularly when exposed to high-risk conditions.[7] Universal screening for thrombophilia in pregnancy or prior to IVF is not recommended routinely for the prevention of VTE. However, screening for thrombophilia should be considered in women with a history of recurrent miscarriage or personal or family history of VTE. Screening should include plasma antithrombin III, activated proteins S and C resistance, antiphospholipid antibodies, and testing for factor V Leiden mutation and MTHFR 677T.[8]

In Vitro Fertilization Management

- Risk assessment for thrombosis before starting the treatment.
- Couples should be counseled in detail about risk of thromboembolism during IVF stimulation[9] and pregnancy and genetic counseling should be provided in indicated cases.
- Modifiable risk factors, e.g., medical conditions and obesity, should be optimized prior to starting treatment.
- IVF stimulation and embryo transfer protocol should be modified to prevent thrombosis as stimulation with higher dose of gonadotropins elevated estradiol levels hCG trigger, OHSS, multiple pregnancy and use of exogenous estrogen for frozen-thawed embryo transfer (FET) increase the risk of developing thromboemolism.
- Mild stimulation, antagonist protocol for ovarian stimulation with use of GnRH agonist trigger.
- Coadministration of letrozole with gonadotropin during ovarian stimulation. Letrozole is an aromatase inhibitor, lowers the level of estrogen by preventing conversion of androgen to estrogen and decreased estrogen concentrations in serum possibly reduces the risk of OHSS and thromboembolic events.[10] Letrozole can be used in a dose of 5 mg/day in two divided doses from day 1 of controlled ovarian hyperstimulation till the day of trigger.
- Preventing OHSS.
- Frozen embryo transfer (FET), in natural cycle, avoiding hCG exposure.
- Single embryo transfer and avoiding multiple pregnancies.
- Use of prophylactic or therapeutic anticoagulation if indicated.
- If the patient develops OHSS and is pregnant, thromboprophylaxis should continue till 12 + 6 weeks. If not pregnant, it should be continued for 4 weeks after resolution of OHSS.[11]

Thromboprophylaxis

All women should be assessed for risk of VTE as per the Royal College of Obstetricians and Gynaecologists[12] or ACOG guidelines before starting stimulation.

Indications of thromboprophylaxis are enumerated in **Box 1**.[11]

Thromboprophylaxis should be initiated at the start of stimulation. Women who have suffered previous episodes of VTE having an underlying cause, already under long-term anticoagulant therapy with warfarin presenting for IVF, should be switched to low-molecular-weight heparins (LMWH) prior to starting ovarian stimulation and should be stopped 24 hours prior to the procedure, restarting in the evening or next day after oocyte retrieval. Advised doses of LMWH in this case are enoxaparin 0.5–1 mg/kg 12 hourly or dalteparin 5,100 IU/kg 12 hourly, with an aim of achieving anti-Xa levels of 0.7–1.0.[9]

If therapeutic doses of LMWH are required, enoxaparin 1 mg/kg 12 hourly or dalteparin 90 IU/kg 12 hourly are advised. Specialist advice will be required to determine the

BOX 1: Indications of thromboprophylaxis.[13]

- Previous history of deep venous thrombosis (DVT)
- Severe ovarian hyperstimulation syndrome (OHSS) and moderate OHSS requiring hospital admission
- Antithrombin deficiency
- Acquired or hereditary thrombophilias in combination with other risk factors such as age over 40 years and/or smoking
- When multiple risk factors such as high BMI, poor mobility, and smoking are identified
- Women with mechanical heart valves, VTE with APAS, recurrent VTE, or antithrombin deficiency

(APAs: antiphospholipid antibodies; BMI: body mass index; VTE: venous thromboembolism)

TABLE 1: Management strategies for various clinical conditions before and after ovarian stimulation.[9]

Clinical situations	*Management*
• Single previous VTE (not pregnancy- or "pill"-related) associated with a transient risk factor and no additional current risk factors such as obesity	Surveillance or prophylactic doses of LMWH +/compression stockings.
• Single previous idiopathic VTE or single previous VTE with underlying thrombophilia and not on long-term anticoagulant therapy, or single previous VTE and additional current risk factor(s) (e.g., obesity)	Prophylactic doses of LMWH from starting of ovarian stimulation +/ compression stockings.
• More than one previous episode of VTE, with no thrombophilia and not on long-term anticoagulant therapy	Prophylactic doses of LMWH with graduated elastic compression stockings at time of starting controlled ovarian stimulation and continued throughout pregnancy
• Previous episode(s) of VTE in women receiving long-term anticoagulants (e.g., with underlying thrombophilia)	Switch from oral anticoagulants to LMWH therapy prior to controlled ovarian stimulation and continue throughout pregnancy +compression stockings
• Thrombophilia (confirmed laboratory abnormality) but no prior VTE	Surveillance or prophylactic LMWH +/compression stockings. The indication for LMWH prophylaxis in the antenatal period is stronger in antithrombin deficiency women than the other thrombophilias, in symptomatic family members compared to asymptomatic relatives and also where additional risk factors are present
• Risk factors for VTE present prior to controlled ovarian stimulation but no previous VTE or thrombophilia	Risk assessment for VTE. If multiple risk factors present or if single major risk factor present, consider LMWH thromboprophylaxis +/ compression stockings
• Develops VTE	Therapeutic doses of LMWH with specialist advice for duration of therapy, but usually for at least 6 months with therapeutic or prophylactic treatment continued until at least 6 weeks postpartum

(LMWH: low molecular weight heparins; VTE: venous thromboembolism)

TABLE 2: Prophylactic and therapeutic dose of LMWH (RCOG recommendations).[12]

	Enoxaparin	*Dalteparin*	*Tinzaparin*
Prophylactic dose:			
<50 kg	20 mg/day	2,500 units/day	3,500 units/day
50–90 kg	40 mg/day	5,000 units/day	4,500 units/day
>90–130 kg	60 mg/day	7,500 units/day	7,000 units/day
131–170 kg	40 mg/12 hourly	10,000 units/day	9,000 units/day
>170 kg	0.6 mg/kg/day	75 U/kg/day	75 U/kg/day
Therapeutic dose	1 mg/kg 12 hourly	90 U/kg 12 hourly	90 U/kg 12 hourly

(LMWH: low-molecular-weight heparins; RCOG: Royal College of Obstetricians and Gynaecologists)

duration of therapy, but normally a minimum of 6 months of therapeutic dose is advised, followed by prophylactic doses continuing until 6 weeks postpartum.[9,11]

Management strategies for various clinical conditions before and after ovarian stimulation are enumerated in **Table 1**.[9]

Prophylactic and therapeutic dose of LMWH are enumerated in **Table 2.**[12]

SUMMARY

- Occurrence of thrombosis after ovarian stimulation is usually very uncommon.
- Ovarian hyperstimulation must be prevented by use of antagonist cycle, cotreatment with letrozole during stimulation, mild stimulation and use of gonadotropin-releasing hormone (GnRH) agonist trigger.
- Thromboprophylaxis with LMWH is started along with the stimulation in high risk cases.
- On the day of oocyte retrieval, the dose should be omitted and to be restarted the following day or in the evening after oocyte retrieval. Prophylactic or therapeutic dose is decided based on the risk factors and in association with hematologist advice.
- Cryopreservation of all embryos and natural cycle FET avoids the use of hCG completely.
- Single embryo transfer is preferable to avoid the risk of multiple pregnancies.

AUTOIMMUNITY AND IN VITRO FERTILIZATION

INTRODUCTION

Systemic autoimmune diseases (SADs) comprise a heterogeneous group of chronic immune-mediated disorders including systemic lupus erythematosus (SLE), antiphospholipid antibody syndrome (APS), rheumatoid arthritis (RA), systemic sclerosis (SSc), Sjogren's syndrome (SS), mixed connective tissue disease (MCTD), idiopathic inflammatory myopathies (IIM), and vasculitis. SADs often occur in women of childbearing age and can affect fertility.

SYSTEMIC LUPUS ERYTHEMATOSUS

It is a chronic multisystem autoimmune disease with a heterogeneous pattern of clinical and serological manifestations with unpredictable course, alternating between periods of flares with remissions. Disease etiology is not fully known, but a strong genetic component has been shown to play a key role in the predisposition of this disease. Genes of the major histocompatibility complex (MHC), particularly *HLA-A1*, *B8*, and *DR3*, have been linked to SLE, as well as certain single-nucleotide polymorphisms (SNPs) that are associated with its clinical manifestation.[14]

Pathogenesis of this disease involves a complex interaction between gene susceptibility, hormonal influences, and certain environmental triggers which induce autoantibody production, formation of immune complexes, activation of T-lymphocytes, dysregulation of apoptosis, and production of proinflammatory cytokines.[15] The prevalence ranges from 20 to 150 cases per 100,000 persons and appears to be increasing due to better diagnosis and survival.[16] It occurs nine times more often in women than in men, especially in women of childbearing age, and tends to be more severe among the black population.[17] The predilection for women, particularly of childbearing age, combined with improved survival has led to increasing numbers of women with lupus considering pregnancy.

The reproductive system may be affected in women and men, as a result of disease activity and through iatrogenic cytotoxic treatments. Autoantibody positivity does not appear to impact fertility but it has been found to be associated with a decreased rate of embryo implantation and clinical pregnancy.[18]

Classification criteria for SLE are enumerated in **Table 3**.[19]

TABLE 3: Classification criteria for SLE (American College of Rheumatology).[19]

Clinical criteria	*Laboratory criteria*
• Malar rash • Discoid rash • Photosensitivity • Oral ulcers • Nonerosive arthritis • Pleuritis/pericarditis • Renal disorder(Persistent proteinuria or cellular casts) • Neurological disorder(seizure or psychosis)	• Hematological disorder (hemolytic anemia with reticulocytosis or leukopenia or lymphopenia or thrombocytopenia • Immunological disorder (anti-dsDNA or anti-Sm or antiphospholipid antibodies) • Antinuclear antibodies
Four out of the 11 clinical or laboratory criteria to be met for diagnosis of SLE (95% specificity and 85% sensitivity).	

(anti-dsDNA: anti-double stranded DNA; anti-SmAb: anti-Smith antibody)

ANTIPHOSPHOLIPID ANTIBODY SYNDROME

Antiphospholipid syndrome (APS) is an acquired thrombophilic disorder in which autoantibodies are produced to a variety of phospholipids and phospholipid-binding proteins.[20] Secondary APS occurs in 30% of SLE patients and is well recognized to cause spontaneous abortions, stillbirths and premature births as well as venous and arterial thrombotic events. A more direct link, however, between aPL and infertility remains controversial and assessment for aPL is not routinely indicated in women undergoing IVF.

Revised Sapporo criteria for diagnosis of APS are mentioned in **Table 4**.[21]

Causes of Infertility in Patient with Systemic Lupus Erythematosus and Antiphospholipid Syndrome

According to recent evidence autoimmunity per se is not a likely cause of infertility. Nonrheumatic autoimmune disease of thyroid, ovary, and adrenal failure may cause infertility by interfering with endocrine function. Therefore, in the absence of severe disease and with a normal ovarian function, fertility in women with lupus is similar to that of the general population.

- *Age:* Onset of SLE is often during the early reproductive years and patients are counseled to avoid pregnancy while disease is active and advised to wait for a period of disease remission and drug washout before conception. These patients get older when they try to conceive and may encounter age-related difficulties and reduced fertility.[22]
- *Menstrual disturbances:* Amenorrhea may occur, not only as a result of cyclophosphamide (CYC) treatment causing ovarian failure, but also as a result of the disease itself. Episodes of amenorrhea has been found to be associated with anticorpus luteum antibodies and with raised follicle-stimulating hormone (FSH) levels, suggestive of an autoimmune, SLE-related menstrual dysfunction. Menstrual irregularities have also been attributed to high-dose corticosteroids administration.

TABLE 4: Revised Sapporo criteria (Miyakis et al.) for diagnosis of APS.[21]

Clinical criteria	*Laboratory criteria*
• Vascular thrombosis in any tissue or organ • Pregnancy morbidity • ≥3 unexplained consecutive spontaneous abortions (<10 weeks of gestation) • ≥1 unexplained fetal death (>10 weeks gestation) of morphologically normal fetus • ≥1 premature delivery (<34 weeks gestation) of morphologically normal fetus due to eclampsia, severe preeclampsia or placental insufficiency	• Positive LAC (on two occasions at least 12 weeks apart) • Positive medium or high titers of IgG OR IgM anticardiolipin antibodies (>40 GPL or MPL, or >99th centile) on two occasions at least 12 weeks apart • Positive titers of IgG or IgM anti-β2-glycoprotein-1 antibodies (>99th centile) on 2 occasions at least 12 weeks apart
One clinical plus one laboratory criteria to be met for diagnosis of APS	

(APS: antiphospholipid syndrome; GPL: immunoglobulin G phospholipids units; IgG: immunoglobulin G; IgM: immunoglobulin M; LAC: lupus anticoagulant; MPL: immunoglobulin M phospholipids units)

- *Hypothalamic-pituitary-ovarian (HPO) axis dysfunction due to renal failure:* Patients with chronic renal failure secondary to lupus nephritis may develop infertility through hypothalamic-pituitary dysfunction due to raised prolactin that reduces the production of gonadotropin-releasing hormone from the hypothalamus, which manifests as a menstrual irregularity and anovulatory cycles.[23]
- *Premature ovarian failure (POF):* Cyclophosphamide (CYC) is a known gonadotoxic agent that can cause POF by depleting the healthy oocytes. Its toxicity is associated with the cumulative dose of CYC and the age at which the drug is administered.[24] It is recommended to delay the conception, until at least 3 months after the last dose, to avoid the risk of teratogenicity.
- *Luteinized unruptured follicle (LUF):* The use of nonsteroidal anti-inflammatory drugs NSAIDs in women with lupus might increase the risk of infertility due to persistent luteinized unruptured follicles. Women having problems in conceiving should be advised to stop NSAIDs, but not all women on NSAIDs who wish to become pregnant have to stop them on the basis of present evidence.[25]
- *Psychosocial aspects influencing fertility:* SLE is associated with fatigue and depression and subsequent loss of libido/sexual function in women as well as men. Therefore, an apparent reduction in fertility may actually reflect reduced frequency of sexual intercourse. Moreover, drugs used in the treatment of SLE may diminish libido further.[26]

Systemic Lupus Erythematosus in Male

- *Testicular damage:* A study by Kenney et al., showed a significant reduction in testicular volume in men with SLE as determined by ultrasound imaging, which correlated with the degree of sperm abnormalities.[27] It was suggested that this reduction was most likely due to damage by SLE to the seminiferous tubules.
- *Impaired spermatogenesis:* Cyclophosphamide (CYC) destroys dividing cells, thereby impairing the spermatogenesis during treatment.[27] Methotrexate (MTX) and sulfasalazine (SSZ) used in the treatment of SLE, can also reduce sperm count leading to infertility.

TREATMENT STRATEGIES TO PRESERVE FERTILITY

General Principle

When CYC is prescribed for patients with severe lupus activity, it should be at the lowest effective dose and for the shortest duration. When it is necessary to give CYC to prevent renal failure, gonadal protection should be considered in those patients due to increased risk of premature ovarian failure.

Patients should be counseled properly for disease recurrence during pregnancy and must be assessed for disease remission, disease burden, presence of organ involvement such as lupus nephritis, the presence of aPL and anti-Ro antibodies, medication regime prior to conception, to ensure avoidance of any drugs that are not safe in pregnancy.

Gonadotropin-releasing Hormone Agonist (Leuprolide)

Treatment with gonadotropin releasing hormone (GnRH) agonists during CYC therapy is used to minimize ovarian toxicity, although the degree of benefit is still debatable. Mechanisms by which GnRH agonist reduces chemotherapy induced gonadotoxicity are—(i) simulating prepubertal hypogonadotropic effect, (ii) decreased ovarian perfusion due to hypoestrogenism, (iii) direct ovarian effect, (iv) upregulating sphingosine-1-phosphate (an ovarian protecting molecule), and (v) germ-line stem cell preservation.[28]

A study conducted by Brunner et al., suggested that GnRH-a should be administered 22 days before CYC is started. It is nevertheless recommended to start the GnRH-a prior or concomitantly to initiation of CYC.[29] GnRH agonist therapy should not be started during the follicular phase, as it can stimulate the ovaries and worsen ovarian damage.

Oocyte and Embryo Cryopreservation

Cryopreservation of either oocyte or embryo may be considered as a fertility preservation option for stable inactive SLE patients.

Ovarian Tissue Cryopreservation

This domain is primarily a research procedure at this time but improved techniques in the future could make this an ideal method for fertility preservation in prepubertal SLE patients requiring CYC therapy.

IMPACT OF ASSISTED REPRODUCTION TECHNIQUE ON SYSTEMIC LUPUS ERYTHEMATOSUS AND ANTIPHOSPHOLIPID SYNDROME

Women with SLE and APS undergoing controlled ovarian hyperstimulation (COH) and IVF are at increased risk of hormone-associated flare and venous and arterial thromboembolism due to the hypercoagulable state induced by high serum estradiol (E2) concentrations, as well as enhanced risk of maternal and fetal complications.[30,31] A planned individualized ovarian stimulation with administration of prophylactic corticosteroids and anticoagulants, in the stable phase of the disease, is safe and reduces the risk of complications.

EFFECT OF SYSTEMIC LUPUS ERYTHEMATOSUS AND ANTIPHOSPHOLIPID SYNDROME ON PREGNANCY

Pregnancy in women with SLE/APS is associated with the increased risk of fetal complications due to placental insufficiency, including miscarriage, intrauterine death, hypertension, preeclampsia, FGR, low birth weight, and preterm delivery. There is increased risk of fetal heart block and cutaneous neonatal lupus in women with positive anti-Ro or anti-La antibodies and may lead to fetal demise.[32]

There is an increased risk of maternal death due to pulmonary hypertension and is reported in 14% of patients with lupus.[33]

PRECONCEPTION COUNSELING

Couples should be counseled about the risk of disease flares, thromboembolism, maternal and fetal complications, and risk of neonatal lupus syndromes in pregnancy. They must be educated about the need for optimal disease control with pregnancy safe medications before conception.

MANAGEMENT DURING IN VITRO FERTILIZATION

Assisted reproductive technology are generally safe, if the patient has quiescent disease and is on appropriate prophylactic therapy with antithrombotic or immunosuppressants if aPL positive. Efficacy of IVF in terms of pregnancy rate is comparable with that in the general population (up to 30%).[31]

For IVF cycle programming, combined OC pills may be given, using the lowest possible dose of ethinylestradiol (30–35 mg), if disease is in remission phase, without high titers of antiphospholipid antibodies, negative lupus anticoagulant, no previous clinical history of thrombosis, and no previous exacerbation of the lupus activity with administration of estradiol.[34,35] In ovulation induction, antiestrogen is the first line of treatment, with clomiphene citrate being the drug of choice.[36] Letrozole would also be an alternative option. At present, no particular type of gonadotropin offers any advantage over others in terms of reducing the risk of thrombosis.[37]

Contraindications of ovarian stimulation/pregnancy in women with SLE are enumerated in **Box 2.**[31]

It is recommended to use friendly ovarian stimulation to avoid high serum estrogen and OHSS using antagonist protocol, mild stimulation protocols, GnRH agonists trigger, embryo freezing and single-embryo transfer to reduce complications related to multiple pregnancies.[31] To minimize the risk of OHSS and thrombosis due to very high estrogen levels, aromatase inhibitors (letrozole) can be used in these patients during ovarian stimulation to lower the levels of serum estrogen.[38] Risk of both lupus flare and thrombosis is greater if the diagnosis of SLE is not known at the start of the cycle.[31]

Coadjuvant therapy (anticoagulation, corticosteroids, and immunosuppressants) should be advised during and after ovarian stimulation for the prevention of thrombosis or lupus flares.[39] The natural cycle should be considered as the first option in case of FET. When estrogens are used for endometrial preparation, less procoagulant natural estrogens should be used and transdermal route should be preferred over oral. Similarly, natural progesterone through

BOX 2: Contraindications of ovarian stimulation/pregnancy in women with systemic lupus erythematosus (SLE).[31]

- Acute flare (and the following 6–12 months)
- Pulmonary hypertension
- Uncontrolled arterial hypertension
- Severe renal impairment
- Severe restrictive lung disease
- Valvulopathy or heart disease
- High titer of antiphospholipid antibodies and anti-Ro/anti-La antibodies

Flowchart 1: Systemic lupus erythematosus and antiphospholipid antibody syndrome.

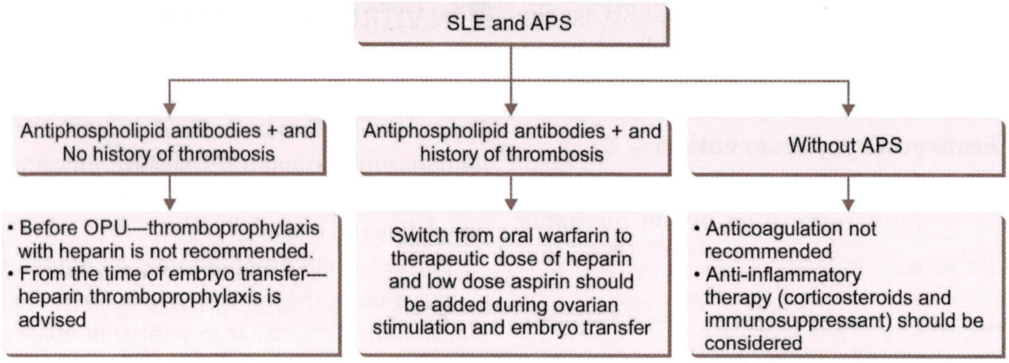

(APS: antiphospholipid antibodies syndrome; SLE: systemic lupus erythematosus)

vaginal administration is preferable compared to synthetic progesterone because it avoids the first-passage effect in the liver.[31]

Sometimes, patients with severe lupus damage such as significant renal insufficiency, may be suitable for IVF stimulation but not for pregnancy, as they might tolerate ovarian hyperstimulation but not the hemodynamic stress of pregnancy. So, IVF followed by embryo transfer to a gestational surrogate would be an option for such patients.

With respect to anticoagulation in women with SLE and APS the most appropriate approach seems to be the following **(Flowchart 1)**.[40]

KEY POINTS

- Preconception counseling and planning pregnancy in remission phase.
- Friendly ovarian stimulation
- GnRH agonist trigger
- Avoid OHSS
- Single embryo transfer
- *Coadjuvant therapy*: Anticoagulation, corticosteroids, and immunomodulators
- *Frozen embryo transfer*: Natural cycle, natural estradiol, transdermal route to be preferred.
- *Luteal phase support*: Natural progesterone and vaginal route.

FERTILITY AND ASSISTED REPRODUCTIVE TECHNOLOGY IN WOMEN WITH CHRONIC KIDNEY DISEASE AND RENAL TRANSPLANT RECIPIENTS

INTRODUCTION

Chronic kidney disease (CKD) is associated with reduced fertility and decreased pregnancy rates compared to the general population[41] and are estimated to affect 3% of women of reproductive age.[42] Women with end-stage renal disease can manifest with sexual dysfunction and infertility resulting from endocrine disturbance, vasomotor dysfunction leading to reduced libido, medications and psychological factors.[43] Overall, it can be estimated that pregnancy rates in the kidney transplant population is approximately 10% of the pregnancy rates of the general population, and pregnancy rates in the dialysis population are approximately 1% of the general population.[41]

FACTORS AFFECTING FERTILITY IN WOMEN WITH CHRONIC KIDNEY DISEASE

Endocrine Disturbances

The kidney plays an important role in the regulation of female sex hormones. In patients with CKD there is loss of GnRH pulsatility, which results in impaired luteinizing hormone (LH) and FSH cyclicity leading to hypoestrogenemia. The lack of cyclicity of gonadotropins and ovarian hormones, as well as persistent hypoestrogenemia and elevated LH and FSH results in anovulation.[44] Serum FSH concentration is normal or just slightly elevated due to loss of pulsatile GnRH release.

Graphic representation of the normal menstrual cycle and the menstrual cycle in chronic kidney disease is depicted in **Figures 1A and B.**[41]

Prolactin levels are also increased in 30–65% women with CKD, which may contribute to an anovulatory state. In women with CKD, reduction in renal clearance leads to increased serum prolactin, as well as decreased sensitivity to dopaminergic inhibition of prolactin synthesis causes upregulation of its production.[45] An increased serum prolactin concentration also contributes to HPO axis dysfunction. High prolactin inhibits gonadotropin secretion, leading to hypogonadotropic hypogonadism.

Mechanism of hypothalamic-pituitary-ovarian dysfunction in women with CKD is depicted in **Figure 2.**[41]

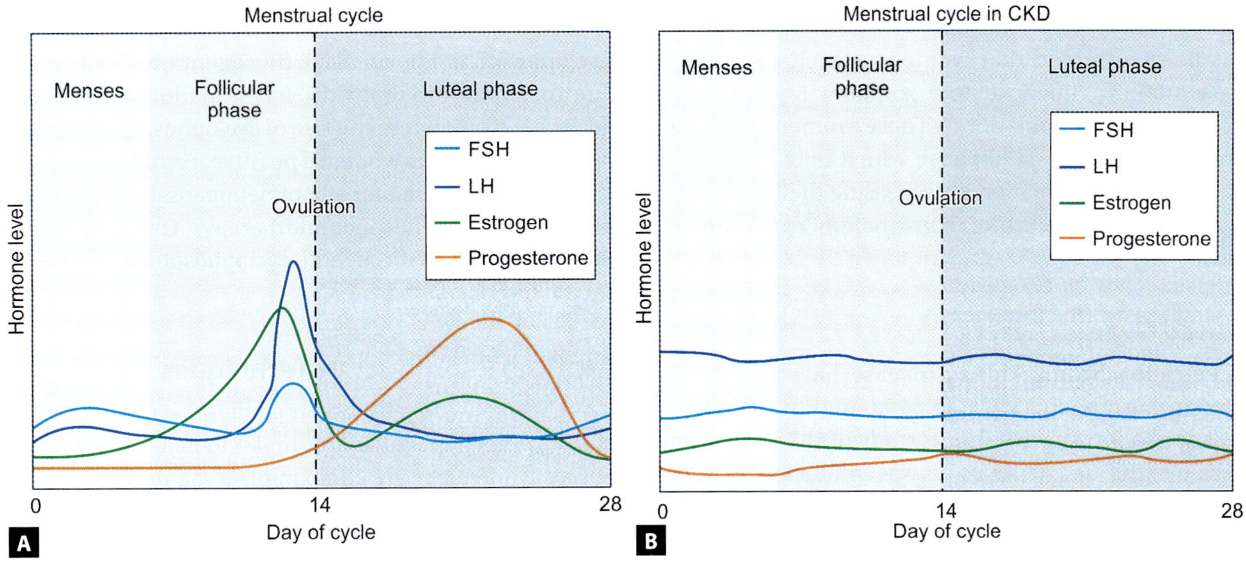

Figs. 1A and B: Graphic representation of the normal menstrual cycle and the menstrual cycle in chronic kidney disease.
(FSH: follicle-stimulating hormone; LH: luteinizing hormone)
Courtesy: Adapted from Wiles et al.[41]

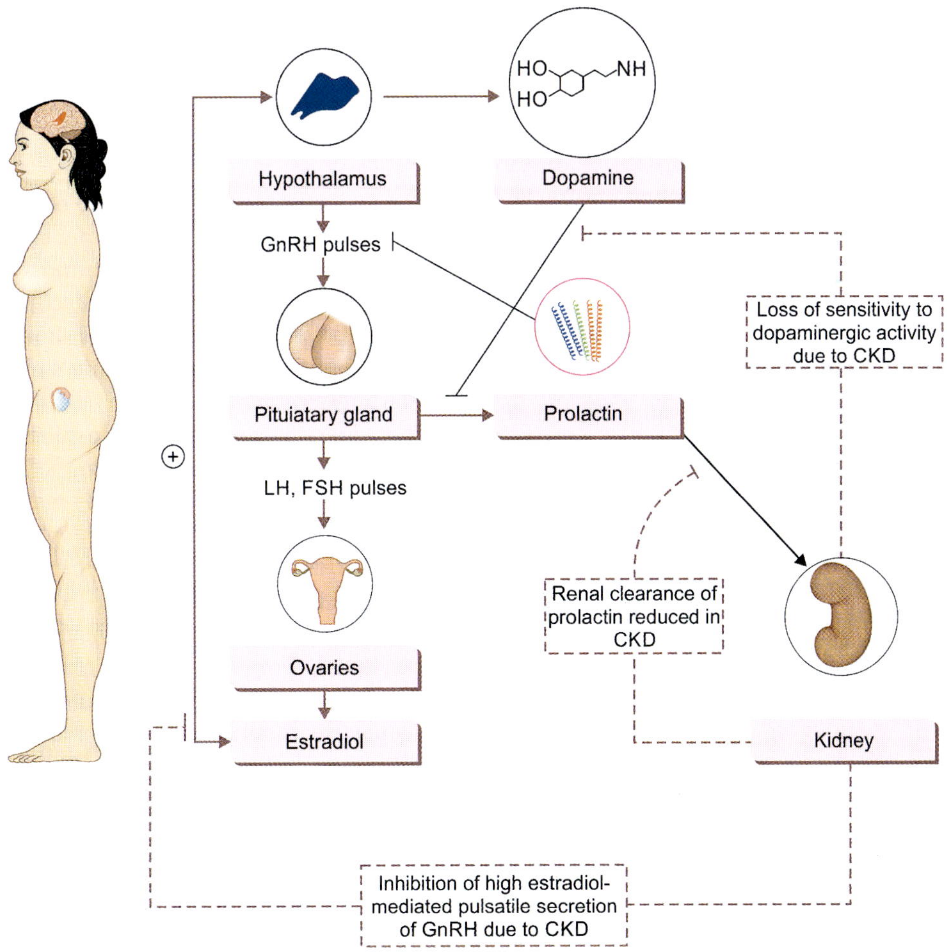

Fig. 2: Mechanism of hypothalamic-pituitary-ovarian dysfunction in women with CKD.
(CKD: chronic kidney disease; FSH: follicle-stimulating hormone; GnRH: Gonadotropin-releasing hormone; LH: luteinizing hormone)
Courtesy: Adapted from Wiles et al.[41]

Menstrual Disorders and Functional Menopause

It has been observed that women with chronic kidney disease attain menopause approximately 5 years earlier than the general population.[46] These women often have a functional state of menopause which may be reversed after kidney transplantation or increasing the frequency of hemodialysis, with return of menstruation, ovulation, and fertility.[47]

Reduced Ovarian Reserve

Women with chronic kidney disease have lower anti-Mullerian hormone (AMH), as compared to the general population. A prospective cohort study of 163 women with CKD vs. healthy matched controls was conducted by Wiles K et al., and serum AMH levels were compared among these two groups and it was observed that AMH levels were significantly lower in women with CKD (stage 1–5).[48] It has been postulated that the interaction of uremic toxins and the ovary may play a role in decreased AMH secretion. Furthermore, CKD is a chronic inflammatory state, the inflammatory changes related to kidney dysfunction may be, in part, responsible for the reduction in ovarian reserve.[49]

Reduced Libido and Sexual Dysfunction

Sexual dysfunction among women with CKD is due to psychological and/or organic factors. Among chronically hemodialyzed women, 60–70% suffers from sexual dysfunction.[50]

MANAGEMENT OF INFERTILITY IN WOMEN WITH CHRONIC KIDNEY DISEASE

These approaches include intensive hemodialysis, kidney transplantation, and ART.

Intensive Hemodialysis

The effect of dialysis modality on fertility in women with end stage kidney disease (ESKD) is poorly understood. Various studies reveal that the pregnancy rates for women on hemodialysis are approximately twice the pregnancy rates for women on peritoneal dialysis.[51] The reason for the same is unclear.

Kidney Transplantation

Hypothalamic-pituitary-ovarian axis improvement after successful kidney transplantation in women with end stage renal disease, leads to return of menses and ovulation resulting in ten-fold increase of pregnancy rate as compared to women on hemodialysis. However, despite this improvement the pregnancy rate in kidney-transplanted women remains 10% of the general population.[47]

Fertility Preservation

Cyclophosphamide, an alkylating agent used to treat CKD due to glomerulonephritis, has gonadotoxic effect and decreases ovarian reserve. Use of cyclophosphamide should be avoided in young women if possible. Fertility preservation should be considered for all premenopausal women prior to initiation of cyclophosphamide therapy.[27] Ovarian protection with GnRH agonist throughout cyclophosphamide treatment should be considered.

Artificial Reproductive Techniques

It has been observed in various studies that the success rates of IVF in this population are similar to healthy controls and obstetric outcomes are comparable to natural pregnancy in stable kidney transplant recipients.[52]

IVF MANAGEMENT

- Women with renal transplantation should be counseled to plan pregnancy after 1 year of receiving renal transplant as the risk of rejection is highest in the first year.[53]
- Couples should be informed about risks involved with IVF treatment as well as the maternal and fetal risks during pregnancy including risk of OHSS, graft rejection, hypertension, and risk of prematurity and inherited renal disease.
- The patient should be advised to consult a nephrologist before planning fertility treatments to optimize renal function and shifting to immunosuppressant drugs that are safe in pregnancy. Mycophenolate mofetil should be stopped and patients should be switched to using tacrolimus or azathioprine 3 months prior to the infertility treatment.[54]
- The American Society of Transplantation Consensus Opinion recommends optimizing renal function before planning the pregnancy (serum creatinine <1.5 mg/dL, with <500 mg/24 h protein excretion).[55]
- If a patient is taking antihypertensive drugs like angiotensin-converting enzyme (ACE) inhibitors, then it should be replaced with pregnancy safe antihypertensives (i.e., labetalol or methyldopa) before pregnancy.[53,55]
- There should be no concurrent infections, no rejection in the past year and maintenance immunosuppression at stable dose before starting treatment.[55]
- Ovarian stimulation should be done with GnRH antagonist protocol using low dose gonadotropin and GnRH agonist trigger for final oocyte maturation to reduce the risk of OHSS and should be monitored closely. As renal transplant recipients are at higher risk for OHSS compared to the general population due to reduced renal clearance of gonadotropins that may lead to enhanced effect as approximately 10% of

gonadotropin is excreted through the kidneys.[56] OHSS can result in increased risk of thromboembolism and acute kidney injury resulting from ischemia or obstructive nephropathy.[57]

- The position of the transplanted kidney should be known before starting IVF treatment, because if the allograft kidney is situated in the pelvis that might lead to difficulty in accessing the ovaries during ovum pick up.
- A senior IVF consultant should be involved throughout the IVF treatment and oocyte retrieval.
- Single embryo transfer should be done due to increased risks of preeclampsia, diabetes, prematurity, and low birth weight babies in multiple pregnancies.
- For conditions such as Alport's syndrome, polycystic kidney disease, and preimplantation genetic testing (PGT) should be considered with appropriate genetic counseling.[54]
- Lastly, in patients with proteinuria and/or antiphospholipid antibodies, low molecular weight heparin prophylaxis and aspirin should be considered during the IVF process to decrease the risk of thrombosis.[58]
- Recent data demonstrated a live birth rate of around 75% in women who conceived a pregnancy after renal transplantation,[46,51] miscarriage and ectopic pregnancy rates were similar to the general population[47]

MATERNAL AND FETAL RISKS IN PREGNANCY[54,56]

- Hypertension in pregnancy is reported in 52–69% renal transplant recipients. Preeclampsia or eclampsia is also common and has been seen in 27% of them.
- There is a slightly increased risk of graft loss in pregnancy. Risk factors for graft loss include; prepregnancy hypertension, elevated prepregnancy creatinine, and proteinuria.[55]
- Risks in pregnancy such as miscarriage, preeclampsia, thrombosis, fetal growth restriction (FGR), preterm delivery, and stillbirth are increased.[41]
- Slightly increased risk of urinary tract infection and risk of other infections such as *Cytomegalovirus*, toxoplasmosis, varicella, human immunodeficiency virus (HIV), herpes and hepatitis B or C virus due to immunosuppressive therapy.[41]
- Increased risk of anemia in pregnancy that can be treated with iron (oral/intravenous if necessary) and erythropoietin.[52]

INFLAMMATORY BOWEL DISEASE AND ASSISTED REPRODUCTIVE TECHNOLOGIES

BACKGROUND

Inflammatory bowel diseases (IBDs) include Crohn's Disease (CD) and ulcerative colitis (UC). Women with inflammatory bowel disease (IBD) are often young and of childbearing age. The disease per se along with the medications used for its treatment may reduce fertility.

IMPACT OF INFLAMMATORY BOWEL DISEASE ON FERTILITY

Ulcerative colitis without previous pelvic surgery and inactive Crohn's disease do not impair fertility and have similar infertility rates as the general population.[59] However, active disease can impair fertility via various mechanisms including pelvic inflammation of the fallopian tubes and ovaries, reduced ovarian reserve, dyspareunia secondary to perianal disease, and adhesion or scarring from previous surgeries. Voluntary nulliparity due to fear of intimacy and disease transmission to offspring, poor body image (colostomy, perianal disease) and depression also play a role in fertility reduction.[60] Ileal pouch anal anastomosis (IPAA) in patient with ulcerative colitis leads to tubal dysfunction due to postoperative adhesion and scarring resulting in reduced fertility.[61] Delaying abdominal surgeries that spare the pelvis, such as colectomy with ileorectal anastomosis/subtotal colectomy, rectal stump creation and ileostomy, until childbearing is complete; they are all temporary measures that may preserve female fertility. Inflammatory bowel disease may reduce the ovarian reserve due to chronic inflammation, altered immune response, and the indirect influence due to use of anti-IBD medicines.[62,63] Therefore, patients with IBD should be referred to ART earlier than the general population, even as early as 6–12 months of attempts.[59]

EFFECT OF IBD ON ART AND PREGNANCY

A nationwide large data based Danish study concluded that the chance of a live birth following an IVF treatment was reduced in women with ulcerative colitis and Crohn's disease, compared to normal women and live birth was significantly reduced further in women with history of prior surgery.[64] However, recent studies have reported that the pregnancy and live births rates after IVF in patients with ulcerative colitis and Crohn's disease are comparable to that of the general population.[65,66]

Women with IBD are more likely to have pregnancy complications compared to age-matched controls. These include spontaneous abortion, small for gestational age (SGA), preterm birth and labor, and delivery complications. They are correlated with disease activity. The risk of congenital abnormalities in offspring from women with inflammatory bowel disease does not seem to be increased.[67]

IMPACT OF PREGNANCY ON INFLAMMATORY BOWEL DISEASE

During implantation and pregnancy, many physiological changes occur leading to fluctuation of immunological states. During implantation phase, proinflammatory Th1 state is prevalent while later Th2 response predominates till just before delivery.[68] So, these two diseases behave differently in pregnancy because Crohn's disease is known to be a Th1/Th17 disease, whereas UC is more Th2/Th17 driven.[69] Women with IBD who conceive during the remission phase, approximately 80% of them remain in remission throughout the pregnancy and in the postpartum period.[70] A recent study by Nielson et al., also demonstrated that the relapse rates of IBD in pregnant women were similar to that in nonpregnant women.[71]

MANAGEMENT DURING IN VITRO FERTILIZATION

- Preconception counseling, reviewing and optimizing medications, confirming disease remission (fecal calprotectin/colonoscopy) and ensuring optimal levels of vitamin D and hemoglobin levels are important measures before planning pregnancy in these women.
- Patients should be advised to start supplemental folic acid preconceptionally. Higher doses of folic acid supplementation should be prescribed [4–5 mg/day] for women taking sulphasalazine[59]
- Women should be in remission for at least 3–6 months before conception.[59]
- Methotrexate should be discontinued at least 6 months prior to conception because it may persist in tissues for long periods.[72] Thalidomide should be discontinued at least 1 month before planning for pregnancy.[73]
- If a patient with IBD is not able to conceive 6 months after surgery, they should be counseled for ART.
- Couples should be informed about the risk of IBD in offspring. The risk is greater for Crohn's disease and is much greater when both parents are affected.[58] A population-based study have shown that the risk of CD in first degree relatives of a CD case is almost 8-fold increased, whereas the risk of ulcerative colitis (UC) in first degree relatives of a UC case is 4-fold increased When both parents have IBD, the risk of developing IBD in the offspring was approximately 30% in a population-based study.[74] In Crohn's disease, transmission is more common from mother to child than from father to child, and female offspring are at higher risk than male offspring **(Table 5)**.[75]

TABLE 5: Safety of inflammatory bowel diseases (IBD) drugs in pregnancy.[25]

Risk in pregnancy	*Drugs*
Low risk	Sulfasalazine, mesalazine, thiopurines, corticosteroids, and antitumor necrosis factor (TNF) agents
Contraindication Methotrexate and thalidomide	
Avoid in first trimester	Metronidazole and ciprofloxacin

- Couples should be counseled regarding higher risk of small for gestational age, low birth weight, stillbirth, preterm prelabor rupture of membranes, and preterm delivery.[58]
- IVF stimulation protocols or anti-inflammatory/immunosuppressive agents do not significantly reduce the chance of a live-born child and women should continue on their current IBD regimen to maintain disease remission.

A Cochrane review on use of preimplantation steroid use concluded that there is no evidence that steroids helped to improve live birth rates in ART, but the use of glucocorticoids in a subgroup of women undergoing IVF was associated with an improvement in the pregnancy rates of borderline statistical significance.[76] The use of prophylactic antibiotics should be at the discretion of the gynecologist, but most gastroenterologists would suggest that unless absolutely necessary, avoid the use of antibiotics as some can cause a flare of disease.[58]

SUMMARY

- It is very important to maintain disease remission preconception at least 3–6 months before and throughout pregnancy.
- Pelvic dissection surgery as is done with creation of an ileal pouch anal anastomosis markedly affects fecundity.
- Active disease at time of conception and during gestation has been shown to lead to worse pregnancy outcomes.
- Rates for IBD flares are comparable in pregnant women and nonpregnant controls in women with clinical remission.
- All IBD medications except for thalidomide and methotrexate can be continued in patients who are planning on conceiving and in pregnant patients.
- A patient, who had IBD surgery and not conceived after 6 months, should be counseled for ART.
- Pregnancy and IBD increase the risk of VTE events. VTE risk assessment should be performed before conception and during pregnancy, especially in patients with active disease.

ART IN PATIENT WITH EPILEPSY

INTRODUCTION

Epilepsy is a major public health problem in all countries including India. Women of childbearing age account for 25% of people with epilepsy, and 3–4 pregnancies in every thousand occur in women with epilepsy.[77] Women with epilepsy are high-risk, all pregnancies in women with epilepsy should be planned, with optimization of medication regimens and seizure control occurring preconceptually to improve the outcome.[78]

PATHOPHYSIOLOGY OF REPRODUCTIVE AND ENDOCRINE DYSFUNCTION IN EPILEPSY

Reproductive endocrine disorders are common among men and women with epilepsy, resulting in lower rates of childbearing and reduced fertility.[79,80] The reasons for the changes in reproductive endocrine function are multifactorial and include psychosocial factors, comorbidity, the use of antiepileptic drugs and the epilepsy itself. The possible explanations for reproductive endocrine disorders related to epilepsy or antiepileptic drugs are as follows:[81,82]

- Direct influence of the epileptogenic lesion, epilepsy, or antiepileptic drugs on the hypothalamic-pituitary axis.
- Effects of antiepileptic drugs on peripheral endocrine glands and the metabolism of hormones and binding proteins.
- Secondary endocrine dysfunction of antiepileptic drugs related to weight changes or changes of insulin sensitivity.

Epileptic seizures and interictal epileptiform discharges, particularly with temporal lobe involvement, may disrupt the hypothalamic-pituitary axis by interfering with gonadotropin-releasing hormone (GnRH) pulsatility.[83] Sexual dysfunction, hormonal and neuroendocrine abnormalities, hypothalamic amenorrhea, premature menopause, polycystic ovary syndrome (PCOS), and anovulatory cycles are more common in women with epilepsy compared to the general population.[84,85]

Antiepileptic drugs (AEDs) may also have an effect on fertility, which induce the cytochrome P450 system (carbamazepine, phenobarbital, phenytoin, oxcarbazepine, primidone, and eslicarbazepine acetate) and leads to abnormal sex hormone levels.[86] Among the antiepileptic drugs, valproate (VPA) is more commonly associated with reproductive endocrine disorders such as hyperandrogenism, polycystic ovaries, menstrual disorders, anovulatory cycles, and PCOS. It has been suggested that valproate inhibits the conversion of testosterone to estrogen and also directly induces androgen synthesis in ovarian theca cells.[87]

Studies of reproductive function and fertility in men with epilepsy are fewer, but altered testosterone metabolism, hyposexuality, reduced testicular volume, reduced sperm concentration and motility as well as increased incidence of morphologically abnormal sperm has all been reported in association with epilepsy or AEDs.[88]

EFFECT OF HORMONES ON EPILEPSY

Female sex hormones affect neuronal excitability, with estrogens being mainly proconvulsant and progesterone and its metabolites being anticonvulsant.[82]

Excitatory effect of estrogen is primarily by influencing N-methyl-D-aspartate (NMDA), but also non-NMDA types of glutamate receptors are involved. Neural tissue and pituitary contain the enzyme 5 alpha reductase, which is able to convert progesterone to 3α,5α-THP within the brain. Production of this very effective anticonvulsant neurosteroid and intracellular progesterone receptors are responsible for the anticonvulsant effect of progesterone and its metabolites.

EFFECT OF EPILEPSY AND ANTIEPILEPTIC DRUGS ON IN VITRO FERTILIZATION

Recent studies suggest that the chance of live birth per embryo transfer is similar after IVF in women with and without epilepsy.[89] Regarding antiepileptic drugs, data are reassuring that these medications do not reduce the chance of live birth rate.

IMPACT OF EPILEPSY AND ANTIEPILEPTIC DRUGS ON PREGNANCY

Obstetric Complications

Most women (around 93–95%) with epilepsy have uncomplicated pregnancies and normal deliveries.[90] However, pregnancies of women with epilepsy pose a greater risk of complications particularly premature contractions, premature labor, delivery, stillbirths and neonatal deaths.[90,91] The risks of trauma, status epilepticus, or even death due to seizures and the psychosocial consequences need to be considered in all these women.[92] Tonic-clonic seizures have the highest risk for sudden unexpected death in epilepsy (SUDEP) and seizure related injuries.[93]

Fetal Complications

Impact of Antiepileptic Drugs

Automated external defibrillators have an effect on fetal and embryonic development and lead to an increased risk for major congenital malformations, neurodevelopmental delay and maladaptive behaviors, minor congenital anomalies such as facial dysmorphism and intrauterine growth retardation.

The risk of congenital malformations in children of women with epilepsy not using AEDs is found in the range of 1.1–3.3% and is similar to the risk of malformations in the general population (2.1–2.9%).[94] The risk of congenital defects in children of women with epilepsy and using AEDs is 4–9% and further increases with valproate and polytherapy.[95-97]

Monotherapy with newer antiepileptic drugs such as levetiracetam, lamotrigine, and oxcarbazepine is relatively safe in pregnancy.[98-100] The incidence of defects in children of mothers treated with AEDs depends not only on the type of AED but also on its dose. The risk of a defect increases with higher doses of a drug.[99] If women with epilepsy are required to continue AEDs during pregnancy then it is safer to use single AED with low teratogenicity and at the lowest effective doses possible.

Impact of IVF and Pregnancy on Epilepsy

Majority of women with epilepsy (55–80%) do not have seizures during pregnancy, whereas a third of them may experience an increase in the number of epileptic seizures. The data from the Epilepsy Pregnancy Registry report that seizures are observed in 14–32% of pregnant women.[101] Literature suggests that lamotrigine performs worse in seizure control while levetiracetam is one of the best drugs among newer antiepileptic groups in controlling maternal seizures during pregnancy.[102] The number of epileptic seizures occurring before pregnancy may predict seizure control during pregnancy. The occurrence of seizures one month before pregnancy increases the risk of seizures during pregnancy by 15-fold.[103]

An increase in the frequency of epileptic seizures may be due to decrease of plasma antiepileptic drugs level that may be because of increase in the volume of distribution, reduced plasma protein concentrations, increased renal clearance, and enhanced metabolism.[104]

In addition to pharmacokinetic factors, physiological factors (e.g., sleep deprivation, nausea, and vomiting), metabolic factors (increased sodium and water retention), hormonal factors (changes in estrogen and progesterone levels), and psychological factors (stress, anxiety, and noncompliance) also contribute to the increased frequency of epileptic seizures in pregnant women.[105,106]

PRECONCEPTION COUNSELING

Preconception counseling is very important for women with epilepsy and is a time to inform these patients about optimal care before, during, and after pregnancy. Ideally a joint obstetrician and neurologist counseling service should be available.

- Women with epilepsy should be informed to control the seizure at least 9–12 months prior to conception, as the best predictor of seizure control during pregnancy is the seizure control prior to pregnancy.[101]
- Couples should be informed in detail about the course of epilepsy during pregnancy.
- Re-evaluation of the diagnosis and need for continuation of antiepileptic medications should be decided prior to planning conception and strict compliance to antiepileptic medications should be encouraged and ensured during IVF and pregnancy.[107]
- Women should be reassured that risk of congenital malformations is low if they are not exposed to antiepileptics in the periconceptional period.[94]
- Risks of teratogenicity and possible adverse effect on long-term cognitive and neuro-developmental delay of the newborn following in utero exposure to antiepileptics should be informed. Based on limited evidence, in utero exposure to carbamazepine and lamotrigine does not appear to adversely affect neurodevelopment of the offspring.[98,99]
- Risk of congenital abnormalities in the fetus is dependent on the type, number and dose of antiepileptics.[99]
- If treatment with AEDs is necessary, monotherapy, and controlled release drugs should be used if possible to avoid the increased risk of congenital malformations associated with polytherapy regimens.[96]
- Appropriate medicine at the lowest effective dose with the least teratogenic risk should be offered to control the severity and frequency of seizures. Lamotrigine and levetiracetam that are not associated with significant increased risks of congenital malformations.[95] Lamotrigine blocks voltage-gated sodium channels and stabilizes their inactive state and levetiracetam inhibits the release of the excitatory neurotransmitter by binding to synaptic vesicle protein synaptic vesicle glycoprotein 2A (SV2A).
- If a change of antiepileptic drug is necessary, it should be done before pregnancy. The risks and benefits of reducing or changing medication should be fully discussed with the patients.
- It is recommended that all women with epilepsy planning conception should take folic acid (5 mg/day) before and during the early stages of pregnancy, primarily to reduce the risk of major congenital malformations and in particular neural tube defects.[78] Prepregnancy folic acid may be helpful in reducing the risk of AED-related cognitive deficits.
- Genetic counseling should be done, especially in case of maternal/paternal idiopathic epilepsy and a positive family history. The risk of a child developing epilepsy is dependent on the type of seizure disorder and the number of affected relatives. The risk of passing epilepsy to the child is very low; however, in specific cases, there is a risk of ~5–20% if one affected first-degree relatives and 25% if two first-degree relatives are affected.[108]

The risk of inheritance is lower if only the father has epilepsy compared with if only the mother has epilepsy.

The overall risk of a mother passing on idiopathic generalized epilepsy is 9–12%.[109] Most of the inheritable syndromes which include epilepsy in their phenotype are autosomal recessive, and there is therefore a low risk of children developing the condition.

MANAGEMENT DURING ASSISTED REPRODUCTIVE TECHNOLOGY

Assisted reproductive technology treatment for women should be started once antiepileptic drug dose and seizure control are optimized. Neurologist consultation is a must for fitness for general anesthesia and also carrying the pregnancy. Women undertaking IVF treatment should be made aware of the potential influence of ovarian stimulation, effect of estrogen and the stress of IVF on seizure frequency. Strict compliance to medications must be ensured before and during the treatment. Standard protocol for ovarian stimulation can be used and OHSS should be avoided.

MANAGEMENT IN EARLY PREGNANCY

Ideally pregnant women with epilepsy are considered high risk and careful management by both neurological and obstetric teams is essential. Women should be encouraged to continue to take high-dose folic acid throughout pregnancy. Ultrasonography (USG) should be done at 11–13 weeks to identify the neural tube defects and maternal serum α-fetoprotein to be measured at 14–16 weeks. The fetal anomaly scan at 18 + 0 – 20 + 6 weeks of gestation can identify major cardiac defects in addition to neural tube defects.[104] Serial growth scans are required for detection of small-for-gestational-age babies and to plan further management in women taking antiepileptic drugs. Based on current evidence, routine monitoring of serum AED levels in pregnancy is not recommended routinely, however it may be considered if suspicion of nonadherence, toxicity and intractable seizures is present.[110]

ART IN WOMEN WITH HYPERTENSION

INTRODUCTION

Chronic hypertension currently affects 1–3% of women of childbearing age, and is continuing an upward trend due to increasing maternal age and rising obesity rates.[110]

IMPACT OF HYPERTENSION ON IN VITRO FERTILIZATION OUTCOMES

Risks of hypertension in IVF patients are mainly related to its association with an increased incidence of hypertensive disorders in pregnancy.[111] There is no evidence that hypertension directly affects the success rate of IVF in terms of ongoing pregnancy rates or incidence of first-trimester pregnancy loss.[112] However, patients who undergo IVF are generally older and primiparous, which can affect the prevalence of chronic hypertension, as well as the risk of obstetric complications. Women with pre-existing hypertension are at risk of abnormal placental development predisposing to preeclampsia, FGR, and small for gestational age, gestational diabetes mellitus (GDM), placental abruption, preterm delivery, and stillbirth.[113] However, in patients with hypertension secondary to renal disease, pregnancy may cause renal dysfunction with potential irreversible loss of kidney function.

IMPACT OF IN VITRO FERTILIZATION ON HYPERTENSION

Women who conceive through ART are at increased risk of hypertensive disorders in pregnancy, including preeclampsia,[114] although the risk is variable and depends on the presence of pre-existing conditions (including chronic hypertension, obesity and PCOS) and the multiple gestations. Recent evidence has shown that FET is associated with higher risk of preeclampsia compared to fresh embryo transfer.[115,116] Although the mechanism by which IVF/ICSI increases the risk is unknown, the possible cause is attributed to a larger proportion of multiple births and to a higher prevalence of preeclampsia risk factors among women who conceive through ART, such as advanced maternal age, obesity, and medical comorbidities compared to women who conceive spontaneously.[117] However, the altered hormonal profile due to ovarian stimulation or the technology in itself, may play a role. Supraphysiologic concentrations of estrogen due to ovarian stimulation and its effect on increment of angiotensinogen and insulin-like growth factor I production by liver, increased sympathetic activity and increased expression of angiotensin-1 (AT1) receptor in the kidneys may increase the risk of hypertension and preeclampsia.[118,119]

The possible mechanism for the increased risk of hypertensive disorders of pregnancy in autologous frozen and donor oocyte fresh and frozen transfer is absence of the corpus luteum. Recent data suggests that the absence of the corpus luteum is associated with deficient maternal circulatory adaptations during early gestation[120] and increases the incidence of preeclampsia.[121,122] With oocyte donation cycles, it is possible that autoimmune factors associated with the use of donor gametes[123] as well as increased maternal age may also contribute to increased risk for hypertensive disorders.

There is no evidence to suggest that IVF treatment per se worsens pre-existing chronic hypertension in the long term.

However, in patients with hypertension secondary to renal disease, pregnancy may aggravate renal dysfunction with potential irreversible loss of kidney function.

PRE IVF AND PRECONCEPTION WORKUP AND ADVICE

- A detailed history, examination, and relevant investigations should be done to identify the cause of hypertension, especially to exclude any secondary causes. The most common secondary causes of hypertension in patients of childbearing age are renal and cardiac diseases.
- Women with newly diagnosed hypertension, onset before 30 years of age and without any positive family history, who are not evaluated previously should be evaluated thoroughly before any fertility treatment.
- Women with hypertension considering pregnancy should undergo investigations including a complete blood count, blood urea, serum creatinine level, liver function test, and a 24-hour urine collection to test protein and creatinine clearance[124,125]
- Additional testing includes evaluation of target organ damage, i.e., electrocardiogram (ECG) to detect left ventricular hypertrophy. If hypertrophy is detected, obtaining an echocardiogram should be considered. Ophthalmological examination to rule out hypertensive retinopathy and renal ultrasound examination to exclude renal scarring and hydronephrosis, polycystic kidney disease (especially in those patients with a positive family history that suggests an autosomal dominant inheritance pattern) should be performed if indicated prior to planning conception.
- Couples should be counseled regarding the risk of adverse pregnancy outcomes, lifestyle modification (weight management, exercise, healthy diet, and lowering the amount of salt in diet), strict adherence to antihypertensive medications and need of close monitoring in pregnancy.
- Genetic counseling and prenatal screening may be required in case of hypertension secondary to a hereditary condition (e.g., polycystic kidney disease).
- Women with hypertension should be advised to meet a general physician/cardiologist for optimization of blood pressure preconception.
- Couples should be informed about the risk of congenital malformations, if patient is on angiotensin converting enzyme (ACE) inhibitors or angiotensin receptor blockers (ARBs) drugs and should be advised to stop these drugs and switch to pregnancy safe antihypertensives.[126,127]
- Women with chronic hypertension not on treatment and planning to conceive should be offered antihypertensive if they have sustained systolic blood pressure of 140 mm Hg or higher or sustained diastolic blood pressure of 90 mm Hg or higher.[124]
- Home blood pressure monitoring should be explained and target blood pressure (BP) should be 135/85 mm Hg.[125]

ANTIHYPERTENSIVE MEDICATIONS

Patients should be advised to continue antihypertensive medications if they are safe in pregnancy, if not, then change to safer ones. First-line antihypertensive drugs are labetalol (combined α and β-adrenergic blocking agents) and methyldopa (α-adrenergic agonist).[110] Long-acting formulations of nifedipine (a calcium channel blocker) can be used as an additional second-line agent if blood pressure is not adequately controlled by labetalol or methyldopa.[110,128]

Propranolol has been associated with premature labor, and atenolol has been associated with intrauterine growth restriction; thus, these drugs are best avoided.[129] Angiotensin-converting enzyme (ACE) inhibitors should be avoided, as they have been shown to cause fetal anomalies such as renal dysgenesis and malformations of the cardiovascular and central nervous systems.[126,127] Diuretics are also contraindicated because of their presumed effect on placental blood flow, although accurate studies are lacking.[130]

Notably, antihypertensive treatment in pregnancy does not reduce the incidence of preeclampsia, rather provides protection against adverse outcomes due to severe or malignant hypertension **(Table 6)**.

IN VITRO FERTILIZATION MANAGEMENT

Patients with chronic hypertension should have blood pressure monitoring before, during and after IVF treatment, and secondary causes of hypertension and relevant comorbidities (e.g., diabetes mellitus and obesity) should be treated and monitored accordingly. Some studies have reported a higher incidence of pregnancy-induced hypertension after OHSS[131] but this was not found by others.[132]

TABLE 6: Recommendation for anti-hypertensive drugs.[111,129]

Drugs	*Indication*	*FDA category*	*Initial dose*	*Maximum dose*	*Potential side effects*
Methyldopa	First line	B	125–250 mg BD	500 mg QID	Lethargy psychosis
Labetalol	First line	C	100 mg BD	400 mg QID	Asthma exacerbation
Nifedipine	Second line	C	10–20 mg BD	40 mg BD	Synergistic action with magnesium sulfate for neuromuscular depression

Aspirin supplementation has been shown to reduce the risk of preeclampsia in high risk patients (e.g., a previous episode of severe preeclampsia, chronic hypertension, chronic kidney disease, and autoimmune disease). Low dose aspirin (75–150 mg/day) should be started from 12 weeks of pregnancy and continued until delivery to prevent preeclampsia.[124] Based on a recent meta-analysis, routine use of aspirin in IVF patients did not reduce the risk of hypertensive complications of pregnancy or preterm delivery.[133] Routine use of aspirin in all patients undergoing IVF should not be recommended.

There is no conclusive data on prescription of calcium supplements prior to IVF treatment, making its safety, and efficacy in IVF patients questionable.[134] Antioxidants (including vitamin C and E supplementation) do not reduce hypertensive complications of pregnancy.[135]

In patients with chronic hypertension, natural cycle FET protocol is preferred to avoid exogenous estrogen and single-embryo transfer is recommended to reduce the risk of blood pressure related adverse pregnancy outcomes in multiple gestation.

ART IN WOMEN WITH DIABETES MELLITUS

INTRODUCTION

Diabetes mellitus is a major public health problem worldwide.[136] Although the incidence of type 1 diabetes is growing slowly, there has been a very steep rise in the number of young adults diagnosed with type 2 diabetes.[137,138]

Reproductive dysfunction is seen in 20–40% of women with type 1 diabetes, manifesting as delayed puberty, primary amenorrhea, menstrual cycle disturbance, subfertility, pregnancy complications, and early menopause.[139-141] Type 2 diabetes in young women, particularly in the second and third decades of life, is associated with potential fertility and pregnancy implications.[138] The mechanisms of reproductive dysfunction in type 2 diabetes could be largely attributable to concomitant obesity, PCOS, and endogenous and exogenous hyperinsulinemia.

DIABETES AND FERTILITY

In type 1 diabetes, hyperglycemia due to insulin deficiency and hyperinsulinemia due to exogenous insulin leads to hypogonadism, polycystic ovarian morphology, and hyperandrogenism, resulting in reduced fertility.[139] Hypogonadotropic hypogonadism is seen in patients with type 1 DM having absolute insulin deficiency, as insulin is an important regulator of the hypothalamic-pituitary-gonadal axis[142,143] and another postulated mechanism being inhibitory effect of hyperglycemia on the hypothalamic secretion of GnRH.[144]

Insulin, insulin resistance, and hyperglycemia contribute to ovarian dysfunction in both type 1 and type 2 diabetes.[145] Exogenous or endogenous hyperinsulinemia in diabetes leads to stimulation of ovarian granulosa cells, increasing follicular recruitment and prevents the recruitment and growth of dominant follicles, leading to anovulation, polycystic ovarian morphology, and subfertility **(Fig. 3)**.[146,147]

IMPACT OF DIABETES ON ASSISTED REPRODUCTIVE TECHNOLOGY OUTCOMES

Evidence on the efficacy of ART in women with type 1 and type 2 diabetes is sparse. A nationwide Danish cohort study was conducted by Larsen et al., and it was concluded that biochemical pregnancy and live birth rate per embryo transfer was significantly lower in women with type 2 diabetes as compared to women without diabetes and

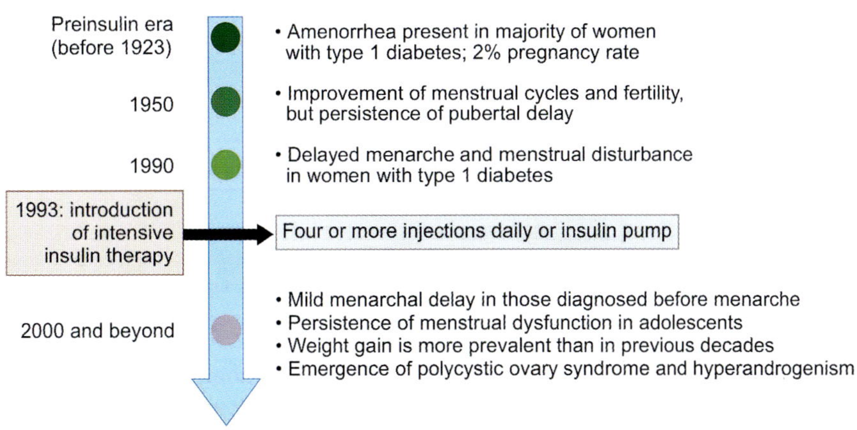

Fig. 3: Evolution of menstrual disorder in women with type 1 diabetes mellitus.
Source: Adapted from Thong et al.[148]

Flowchart 2: Mechanisms of interaction between type 1 diabetes and reproductive function.

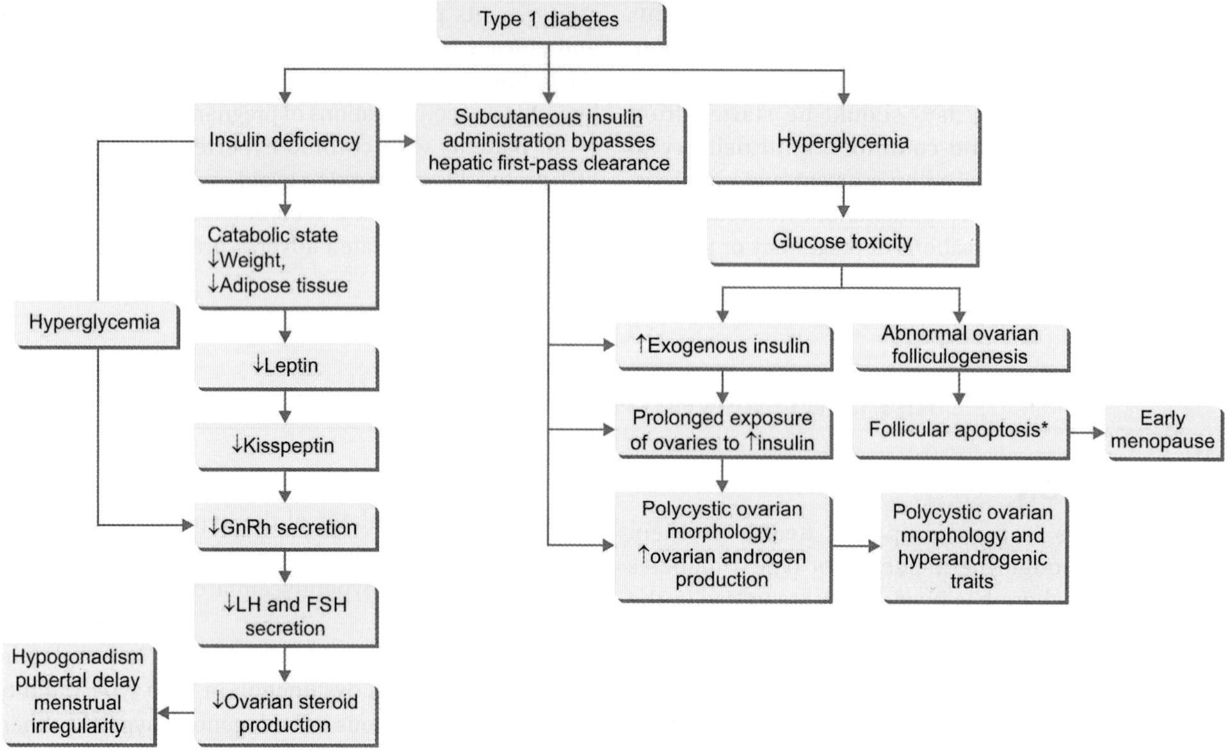

(FSH: follicle-stimulating hormone; GnRH: gonadotropin-releasing hormone; LH: luteinizing hormone)
Source: Codner et al.[139]

Flowchart 3: Mechanisms of interaction between type 2 diabetes and reproductive function.

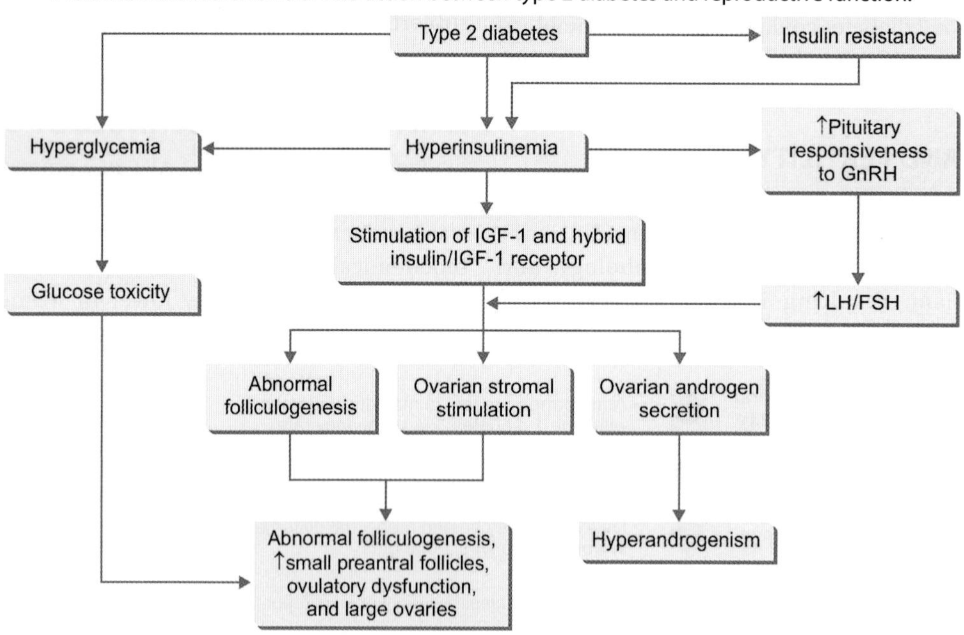

(FSH: follicle-stimulating hormone; IGF-1: Insulin-like growth factor 1; LH: luteinizing hormone)
Source: Adapted from Thong et al.[148]

similar results were observed in both normal weight and obese women.[148] While, women with type 1 diabetes had biochemical pregnancy, clinical pregnancy and live birth rate similar to women without diabetes **(Flowcharts 2 and 3)**.[149-151]

Maternal diabetes may impair oocyte quality and its developmental competence by disturbing the metabolism in granulosa cells and their communications with the oocyte.[152,153]

Risks due to DM in pregnancy for both mothers and children are well established, and could be influenced by the type and duration of diabetes, glycemic control, and diabetes related complications. Fetal risks include miscarriage, preterm delivery, stillbirth, perinatal mortality, congenital anomalies, small/large for gestational age (SGA/LGA), shoulder dystocia and birth injury, neonatal hypoglycemia, polycythemia, hypocalcaemia, and respiratory distress syndrome.[154]

EFFECT OF IVF AND PREGNANCY ON DIABETES

In vitro fertilization stimulation per se does not affect the blood sugar level. Various studies suggest that pregnancy resulting from ART treatment, particularly blastocyst transfer as compared to cleavage stage embryo, is associated with slightly increased risk of GDM, therefore proper monitoring is needed during pregnancy.[155] The higher rate of GDM in these patients, independent of age and parity, may be due to cause of infertility, types of drugs used, changes in the hormonal environment due to increased hormone levels during ovarian stimulation and early pregnancy and presence of underlying metabolic and vascular factors[156] However, recent studies has observed that ART was not associated with increased risk of GDM when adjusted for age, parity, and body mass index (BMI).[157] Women with diabetes may have progression of their disease during pregnancy, and careful management of diabetes is necessary before and during pregnancy. Maternal complications for women with preexisting diabetes include worsening of preexisting retinopathy and nephropathy, as well as increased risk for hypertension, preeclampsia and operative delivery.[158]

PRECONCEPTION CARE AND IN VITRO FERTILIZATION MANAGEMENT

- Prepregnancy planning and counseling in women with type 1 and type 2 DM has beneficial effects in terms of reducing congenital malformation by 50%, perinatal mortality by 80% and preterm delivery by 50%.[159]
- Couples should be counseled to achieve optimal diabetes control before planning the pregnancy, as glycemic control can avoid risk of malformations and reduce the risk of miscarriage, stillbirth, and neonatal death. The American Diabetes Association (ADA) 2016 guideline defines an optimal preconceptional control as preprandial glucose <100 mg/dL, postprandial <140 mg/dL and glycated hemoglobin (HbA1c) of <7%.[160]
- Couples should be informed and educated about the association between HbA1C levels >7.0% at the time of conception and increased risk for major congenital malformations.[160] Mechanism of congenital malformation is not clear, although animal studies have revealed that pregestational diabetes mellitus induces oxidative stress that activates cellular stress signaling leading to dysregulation of gene expression and excessive apoptosis in target organs, including neural tube and embryonic heart.[161]
- Patients should be counseled for behavioral modification (diet and exercise) and weight reduction before conception. American college of obstetricians and gynecologists (ACOG) 2018 guidelines on pregnancy and obesity recommends a 5–7% weight loss before conception.[162]
- Periconceptional folic acid 5 mg is recommended as diabetes increases the risk of neural tube defects by 3 fold.[160]
- Detailed history and evaluation should be done, all medications should be reviewed and drugs with teratogenic risks should be replaced with pregnancy safe medications. Glyburide and metformin are classified as Food and Drug Administration (FDA) category B drugs and can be continued in pregnancy if sugar level is well controlled on these two drugs.
- Couples should be counseled about maternal and fetal risks during pregnancy.
- Ophthalmological, renal and cardiac evaluation should be done before starting fertility treatment. Multidisciplinary team approach including obstetrician, fertility specialist, ophthalmologist, nephrologist, and cardiologist is advisable.
- Thyroid function tests should be done in women with type 1 diabetes, as 10–20% of these women have autoimmune thyroid disease.[159]
- Relative contraindications to pregnancy include retinopathy requiring light amplification by stimulated emission of radiation (LASER) treatment until treatment is undertaken or eye status is stabilized, nephropathy with serum creatinine >200 μmol/L or HbA1c level >10%.[159]
- IVF and embryo transfer should be planned only after adequate blood glucose control.
- Single embryo transfer is recommended to avoid complications due to multiple gestations.

CONCLUSION

Assisted reproductive technology treatments in women with underlying chronic medical conditions have become increasingly frequent and nowadays the average women's age at marriage and child bearing is increasing which further increases the risk of medical illnesses. These patients may pose a significant risk during ovarian stimulation, embryo transfer or during pregnancy as their medical problems may get aggravated or may cause life-threatening risk during pregnancy or teratogenic effects on the fetus or obstetric complications. Therefore, it is important for clinicians to identify women who are at increased risk, to provide appropriate and detailed counseling, and follow risk-reduction strategies. Prior identification and preparation of the patient at increased risk of complications will enable the clinician to avoid problems in advance, anticipate the necessary management and optimize the outcomes. A multidisciplinary team approach is necessary for management of these patients. All pregnancies in such women should be planned with optimization of the clinical conditions while in the remission phase of the disease to improve the maternal and fetal outcome. Presentation for fertility treatment offers an excellent opportunity for clinicians to improve the preconception health and maximize obstetric outcome in these patients. The literature on the efficacy of ART in women with different chronic diseases is still limited and further research is needed in future.

REFERENCES

1. Rova K, Passmark H, Lindqvist PG. Venous thromboembolism in relation to in vitro fertilization: an approach to determining the incidence and increase in risk in successful cycles. Fertil Steril. 2012;97(1):95-100.
2. Bates SM, Middeldorp S, Rodger M, James AH, Greer I. Guidance for the treatment and prevention of obstetric-associated venous thromboembolism. j Thromb Thrombolysis. 2016;41(1):92-128.
3. Curvers J, Nienhuis SJ, Nap AW, Hamulyak K, Evers JL, Rosing J. Activated protein C resistance during in vitro fertilization treatment. Eur J Obstet Gynecol Reprod Biol. 2001;95(2):222-4.
4. Chan WS. The "ART" of thrombosis: a review of arterial and venous thrombosis in assisted reproductive technology. Curr Opin Obstet Gynecol. 2009;21(3):207-18.
5. Romagnuolo I, Sticchi E, Fedi S, Cellai AP, Lami D, Liotta AA, et al. Is tissue factor pathway inhibitor a marker of procoagulable status in healthy infertile women undergoing ovarian stimulation for assisted reproduction? Blood Coagul Fibrinolysis. 2014;25(3):254-8.
6. Nelson SM. Venous thrombosis during assisted reproduction: novel risk reduction strategies. Thromb Res. 2013;131 (Suppl 1):S1-3.
7. Yinon Y, Pauzner R, Dulitzky M, Elizur SE, Dor J, Shulman A. Safety of IVF under anticoagulant therapy in patients at risk for thrombo-embolic events. Reprod Biomed Online. 2006;12(3):354-8.
8. Fábregues F, Tàssies D, Reverter JC, Carmona F, Ordinas A, Balasch J. Prevalence of thrombophilia in women with severe ovarian hyperstimulation syndrome and cost-effectiveness of screening. Fertil Steril. 2004;81(4):989-95.
9. Nelson SM. Prophylaxis of VTE in women-during assisted reproductive techniques. Thrombosis Research. 2009;123(Suppl 3):S8-15.
10. Eftekhar M, Saeed L. Effect of adding letrozole to gonadotropin on in vitro fertilization outcomes: An RCT. Int J Reprod Biomed. 2020;18(4):287-94.
11. Jacobsen AF, Sandset PM. Prior thromboembolic disease and assisted reproductive therapy. Seminars in reproductive medicine. 2021;39(5-06):180-5.
12. Royal College of Obstetricians & Gynaecologists. (2015). Reducing the risk of venous thromboembolism during pregnancy and the puerperium. [Online] Available from: https://www.rcog.org.uk/media/qejfhcaj/gtg-37a.pdf [Last accessed December, 2022].
13. Nordic Federation of Societies of Obstetrics and Gynecology. Guidelines. Clinical Guidelines and Nordic Collaboration presented by NFOG. [Online] Available from: http://www.nfog.org/files/guidelines/NFOG_Guideline_SWE_160116%20Thromboprophylaxis%20in%20IVF.pdf [Last accessed December, 2022].
14. Tsokos GC. Systemic lupus erythematosus. N Engl J Med. 2011;365(22):2110-21.
15. Pan Q, Chen J, Guo L, Lu X, Liao S, Zhao C, et al. Mechanistic insights into environmental and genetic risk factors for systemic lupus erythematosus. Am J Transl Res. 2019; 11(3):1241-54.
16. Rees F, Doherty M, Grainge MJ, Lanyon P, Zhang W. The worldwide incidence and prevalence of systemic lupus erythematosus: a systematic review of epidemiological studies. Rheumatology. 2017;56(11):1945-61.
17. Weckerle CE, Niewold TB. The unexplained female predominance of systemic lupus erythematosus: clues from genetic and cytokine studies. Clin Rev Allergy Immunol. 2011;40(1):42-9.
18. Practice Committee of the American Society for Reproductive Medicine. Anti-phospholipid antibodies do not affect IVF success. Fertil Steril. 2008;90(5 Suppl):S172-3.
19. Guidelines for referral and management of systemic lupus erythematosus in adults. American College of Rheumatology Ad Hoc Committee on Systemic Lupus Erythematosus Guidelines. Arthritis Rheum. 1999;42(9):1785-96.
20. Baker Jr WF, Bick RL. The clinical spectrum of antiphospholipid syndrome. Hematol Oncol Clin North Am. 2008;22(1):33-52.
21. Miyakis S, Lockshin MD, Atsumi T, Branch DW, Brey RL, Cervera RH, et al. International consensus statement on an update of the classification criteria for definite antiphospholipid syndrome (APS). J Thromb Haemost. 2006;4(2):295-306.
22. Jones A, Giles IP. Fertility and pregnancy in systemic lupus erythematosus. Indian J Rheumatol. 2016;11(6):128-34.
23. Gómez F, De La Cueva R, Wauters JP, Lemarchand-Béraud T. Endocrine abnormalities in patients undergoing long-term hemodialysis. The role of prolactin. Am J Med. 1980;68(4):522-30.
24. Boumpas DT, Austin HA, Vaughan EM, Yarboro CH, Klippel JH, Balow JE. Risk for sustained amenorrhea in patients with systemic lupus erythematosus receiving intermittent pulse cyclophosphamide therapy. Ann Intern Med. 1993;119(5):366-9.
25. Østensen M, Khamashta M, Lockshin M, Parke A, Brucato A, Carp H, et al. Anti-inflammatory and immunosuppressive drugs and reproduction. Arthritis research & therapy. 2006;8(3):209.
26. Kenney LB, Laufer MR, Grant FD, Grier H, Diller L. High risk of infertility and long term gonadal damage in males treated with high dose cyclophosphamide for sarcoma during childhood. Cancer. 2001;91(3):613-21.
27. Mersereau J, Dooley MA. Gonadal failure with cyclophosphamide therapy for lupus nephritis: advances in

fertility preservation. Rheum Dis Clin North Am. 2010;36(1): 99-108.
28. Brunner III, Silva CA, Reiff A, Higgins GC, Imundo L, Williams CB, et al. Randomized, double-blind, dose-escalation trial of triptorelin for ovary protection in childhood-onset systemic lupus erythematosus. Arthritis Rheumatol. 2015;67(5):1377-85.
29. Chan WS, Dixon ME. The "ART" of thromboembolism: a review of assisted reproductive technology and thromboembolic complications. Thromb Res. 2008;121(6):713-26.
30. Bellver J, Pellicer A. Ovarian stimulation for ovulation induction and in vitro fertilization in patients with systemic lupus erythematosus and antiphospholipid syndrome. Fertil Steril. 2009;92(6):1803-10.
31. Clowse ME, Jamison M, Myers E, James AH. A national study of the complications of lupus in pregnancy. Am J Obstet Gynecol. 2008;199(2):127-e1.
32. Ritchie J, Smyth A, Tower C, Helbert M, Venning M, Garovic VD. Maternal deaths in women with lupus nephritis: a review of published evidence. Lupus. 2012;21(5):534-41.
33. Petri M, Kim MY, Kalunian KC, Grossman J, Hahn BH, Sammaritano LR, et al. Combined oral contraceptives in women with systemic lupus erythematosus. N Engl J Med. 2005;353(24):2550-8.
34. Askanase AD. Estrogen therapy in systemic lupus erythematosus. Treat Endocrinol. 2004;3(1):19-26.
35. Wechsler B, Vauthier-Brouzes D, Duhaut P, Costedoat N, Lefebvre G, Piette JC. Importance of planning ovulation induction therapy in systemic lupus erythematosus and antiphospholipid syndrome: a single center retrospective study of 21 cases and 114 cycles. Semin Arthritis Rheum. 2002;32(3):174-188.
36. Ricci G, Cerneca F, Simeone R, Pozzobon C, Guarnieri S, Sartore A, et al. Impact of highly purified urinary FSH and recombinant FSH on haemostasis: an open-label, randomized, controlled trial. Hum Reprod. 2004;19(4): 838-48.
37. Mai Q, Hu X, Yang G, Luo Y, Huang K, Yuan Y, et al. Effect of letrozole on moderate and severe early-onset ovarian hyperstimulation syndrome in high-risk women: a prospective randomized trial. Am J Obstet Gynecol. 2017;216(1):42.e1-42. e10.
38. Guballa N, Sammaritano L, Schwartzman S, Buyon J, Lockshin MD. Ovulation induction and in vitro fertilization in systemic lupus erythematosus and antiphospholipid syndrome. Arthritis Rheum. 2000;43(3):550-6.
39. Udoff LC, Branch DW. Management of patients with antiphospholipid antibodies undergoing in vitro fertilization. J Autoimmun. 2000;15(2):209-11.
40. Lateef A, Petri M. Managing lupus patients during pregnancy. Best Pract Res Clin Rheumatol. 2013;27(3):435-47.
41. Wiles KS, Nelson-Piercy C, Bramham K. Reproductive health and pregnancy in women with chronic kidney disease. Nat Rev Nephrol. 2018;14(3):165-84.
42. Zhang QL, Rothenbacher D. Prevalence of chronic kidney disease in population-based studies: systematic review. BMC Public Health. 2008;8(1):1-3.
43. Rathi M, Ramachandran R. Sexual and gonadal dysfunction in chronic kidney disease: Pathophysiology. Indian J Endocrinol Metab. 2012;16(2):214-9.
44. Holley JL. The hypothalamic-pituitary axis in men and women with chronic kidney disease. Adv Chronic Kidney Dis. 2004;11(4):337-41.
45. Sievertsen GD, Lim VS, Nakawatase C, Frohman LA. Metabolic clearance and secretion rates of human prolactin in normal subjects and in patients with chronic renal failure. J Clin Endocrinol Metab. 1980;50(5):846-52.
46. Harlow SD, Gass M, Hall JE, Lobo R, Maki P, Rebar RW, et al. Executive summary of the Stages of Reproductive Aging Workshop + 10: addressing the unfinished agenda of staging reproductive aging. Menopause. 19(4):387-95.
47. Pietrzak B, Wielgos M, Kaminski P, Jabiry-Zieniewicz Z, Bobrowska K. Menstrual cycle and sex hormone profile in kidney-transplanted women. Neuro Endocrinol Lett. 2006;27(1-2):198-202.
48. Wiles K, Anckaert E, Holden F, Grace J, Nelson-Piercy C, Lightstone L, et al. Anti-Müllerian hormone concentrations in women with chronic kidney disease. Clinical Kidney J. 2021;14(2):537-42.
49. Stoumpos S, Lees J, Welsh P, Hund M, Geddes CC, Nelson SM, Mark PB. The utility of anti-Müllerian hormone in women with chronic kidney disease, on haemodialysis and after kidney transplantation. Reprod Biomed Online. 2018;36(2): 219-26.
50. Wang CJ, Cukor D, Johansen KL. Sexual Dysfunction Among Patients With Chronic Kidney Disease. In: Seminars in Nephrology. 2021;41(6):534-49.
51. Hladunewich M, Schatell D. Intensive dialysis and pregnancy. Hemodialysis International. 2016;20(3):339-48.
52. Norman E, Bergh C, Wennerholm UB. Pregnancy outcome and long-term follow-up after in vitro fertilization in women with renal transplantation. Hum Reprod. 2015;30(1):205-13.
53. Kasiske BL, Zeier MG, Chapman JR, Craig JC, Ekberg H, Garvey CA, et al. KDIGO Clinical practice guideline for the care of kidney transplant recipients: a summary. Kidney Int. 2010;77(4):299-311.
54. Wiles K, Chappell L, Clark K, Elman L, Hall M, Lightstone L, et al. Clinical practice guideline on pregnancy and renal disease. BMC Nephrol. 2019;20(1):401.
55. McKay DB, Josephson MA, Armenti VT, August P, Coscia LA, Davis CL, et al. Reproduction and transplantation: report on the AST Consensus Conference on Reproductive Issues and Transplantation. Am J Transplant. 2005;5(7):1592-9.
56. Shah S, Verma P. Overview of pregnancy in renal transplant patients. Int J Nephrol. 2016;2016:4539342.
57. Wiles K, Lightstone L. Glomerular disease in women. Kidney Int Rep. 2018;3(2):258-70.
58. Expert EB. Group on Renal Transplantation. European best practice guidelines for renal transplantation. Section IV: long-term management of the transplant recipient. IV.10. Pregnancy in renal transplant recipients. Nephrol Dial Transplant. 2002; 17(Suppl 4):50-5.
59. Van der Woude CJ, Ardizzone S, Bengtson MB, Fiorino G, Fraser G, Katsanos K, et al. The second European evidenced-based consensus on reproduction and pregnancy in inflammatory bowel disease. J Crohns Colitis. 2015;9(2):107-24.
60. Leenhardt R, Rivière P, Papazian P, Nion-Larmurier I, Girard G, Laharie D, et al. Sexual health and fertility for individuals with inflammatory bowel disease. World J Gastroenterol. 2019;25(36):5423-33.

61. Waljee A, Waljee J, Morris AM, Higgins PD. Threefold increased risk of infertility: a meta-analysis of infertility after ileal pouch anal anastomosis in ulcerative colitis. Gut. 2006;55(11):1575-80.
62. Zhao Y, Chen B, He Y, Zhang S, Qiu Y, Feng R, et al. Risk factors associated with impaired ovarian reserve in young women of reproductive age with Crohn's disease. Intest Res. 2020;18(2):200-9.
63. Şenateş E, Çolak Y, Erdem ED, Yeşil A, Coşkunpınar E, Şahin Ö, et al. Serum anti-Müllerian hormone levels are lower in reproductive-age women with Crohn's disease compared to healthy control women. J Crohns Colitis. 2013;7(2):e29-34.
64. Pottegård A, Schmidt SA, Wallach-Kildemoes H, Sørensen HT, Hallas J, Schmidt M. Data resource profile: the Danish national prescription registry. Intl J Epidemiol. 2017;46(3):798-f.
65. Hernandez-Nieto C, Sekhon L, Lee J, Gounko D, Copperman A, Sandler B. Infertile patients with inflammatory bowel disease have comparable in vitro fertilization clinical outcomes to the general infertile population. Gynecol Endocrinol. 2020;36(6):554-7.
66. Lavie I, Lavie M, Doyev R, Fouks Y, Azem F, Yogev Y. Pregnancy outcomes in women with inflammatory bowel disease who successfully conceived via assisted reproduction technique. Arch Gynecol Obstet. 2020;302(3):611-8.
67. Norgard BM, Larsen PV, Fedder J, de Silva PS, Friedman S. Live birth and adverse birth outcomes in women with ulcerative colitis and Crohn's disease receiving assisted reproduction: a 20-year nationwide cohort study. Gut. 2016;65(5):767-76.
68. Mor G, Aldo P, Alvero AB. The unique immunological and microbial aspects of pregnancy. Nat Rev Immunol. 2017;17(8):469-82.
69. van der Giessen J, Binyamin D, Belogolovski A, Frishman S, Tenenbaum-Gavish K, Hadar E, et al. Modulation of cytokine patterns and microbiome during pregnancy in IBD. Gut. 2020;69(3):473-86.
70. Reddy D, Murphy SJ, Kane SV, Present DH, Kornbluth AA. Relapses of inflammatory bowel disease during pregnancy: in-hospital management and birth outcomes. Am J Gastroenterol. 2008;103(5):1203-9.
71. Nielsen OH, Gubatan JM, Juhl CB, Streett SE, Maxwell C. Biologics for inflammatory bowel disease and their safety in pregnancy: a systematic review and meta-analysis. Clin Gastroenterol Hepatol. 2022;20(1):74-87.e3.
72. Dubinsky M, Abraham B, Mahadevan U. Management of the pregnant IBD patient. Inflamm Bowel Dis. 2008;14(12):1736-50.
73. Eriksson T, Björkman S, Höglund P. Clinical pharmacology of thalidomide. Eur J Clin Pharmacol. 2001;57(5):365-76.
74. Bennett RA, Rubin PH, Present DH. Frequency of inflammatory bowel disease in offspring of couples both presenting with inflammatory bowel disease. Gastroenterology. 1991;100(6):1638-43.
75. Akolkar PN, Gulwani-Akolkar B, Heresbach D, Lin XY, Fisher S, Katz S, et al. Differences in risk of Crohn's disease in offspring of mothers and fathers with inflammatory bowel disease. Am J Gastroenterol. 1997;92(12):2241-4.
76. Boomsma CM, Kamath MS, Keay SD, Macklon NS. Peri-implantation glucocorticoid administration for assisted reproductive technology cycles. Cochrane Database of Syst Rev. 2012;6:CD005996.
77. Olafsson E, Hallgrimsson JT, Hauser WA et al. Pregnancies of women with epilepsy: A population-based study in Iceland. Epilepsia. 1998;39(8):887-92.
78. National Institute for Health and Care. (2012). National Institute for Health and Care Excellence Clinical Guideline 137: The epilepsies: The diagnosis and management of the epilepsies in adults and children in primary and secondary care. [Online] Available from: http://www.nice.org.uk/cg137 [Last accessed December, 2022].
79. Olafsson E, Hauser WA, Gudmundsson G. Fertility in patients with epilepsy: A population-based study. Neurology. 1998;51(1):71-3.
80. Herzog AG, Seibel MM, Schomer DL, Vaitukaitis JL, Geschwind N. Reproductive endocrine disorders in women with partial seizures of temporal lobe origin. Arch Neurol. 1986;43(4):341-6.
81. Herzog AG, Coleman AE, Jacobs AR, Klein P, Friedman MN, Drislane FW, et al. Interictal EEG discharges, reproductive hormones, and menstrual disorders in epilepsy. Ann Neurol. 2003;54(5):625-37.
82. Bilo L, Meo R, Valentino R, DiCarlo C, Striano S, Nappi C. Characterization of reproductive endocrine disorders in women with epilepsy. J Clin Endocrinol Metab. 2001;86(7):2950-6.
83. Isojärvi JI, Tauboll E, Herzog AG. Effect of antiepileptic drugs on reproductive endocrine function in individuals with epilepsy. CNS Drugs. 2005;19(3):207-23.
84. Morrell MJ, Hayes FJ, Sluss PM, Adams JM, Bhatt M, Ozkara C, et al. Hyperandrogenism, ovulatory dysfunction, and polycystic ovary syndrome with valproate versus lamotrigine. Ann Neurol. 2008;64(2):200-11.
85. Herzog AG, Drislane FW, Schomer DL, Pennell PB, Bromfield EB, Dworetzky BA et al. Differential effects of antiepileptic drugs on sexual function and hormones in men with epilepsy. Neurology. 2005;65(7):1016-20.
86. Larsen MD, Jølving LR, Fedder J, Nørgård BM. The efficacy of assisted reproductive treatment in women with epilepsy. Reprod Biomed Online. 2020;41(6):1015-22.
87. Borthen I, Eide MG, Veiby G, Daltveit AK, Gilhus NE. Complications during pregnancy in women with epilepsy: population-based cohort study. BJOG. 2009;116(13):1736-42.
88. Lawn ND, Bamlet WR, Radhakrishnan K, O"Brien PC, So EL. Injuries due to seizures in persons with epilepsy: a population-based study. Neurology. 2004;63(9):1565-70.
89. Sveberg L, Svalheim S, Tauboll E. The impact of seizures on pregnancy and delivery. Seizure. 2015;28:35-8.
90. Cantwell R, Clutton-Brock T, Cooper G, Dawson A, Drife J, Garrod D, et al. Saving mothers" lives: reviewing maternal deaths to make motherhood safer: 2006–2008. The eighth report of the Confidential Enquiries into Maternal Deaths in the United Kingdom. BJOG. 2011;118(Suppl 1):1-203.
91. Tomson T, Xue H, Battino D. Major congenital malformations in children of women with epilepsy. Seizure. 2015;28:46-50.
92. Veroniki AA, Cogo E, Rios P, Straus SE, Finkelstein Y, Kealey R, et al. Comparative safety of anti-epileptic drugs during pregnancy: A systematic review and network meta-analysis of congenital malformations and prenatal outcomes. BMC Med. 2017;15(1):95.
93. Tomson T, Battino D, Bonizzoni E, Craig J, Lindhout D, Sabers A, et al. Dose-dependent risk of malformations

with antiepileptic drugs: an analysis of data from the EURAP epilepsy and pregnancy registry. Lancet Neurol. 2011;10(7):609-17.
94. Tomson T, Battino D, Bonizzoni E, Craig J, Lindhout D, Perucca E, et al. Declining malformation rates with changed antiepileptic drug prescribing: An observational study. Neurology. 2019;93(9):e831-40.
95. Veroniki AA, Rios P, Cogo E, Straus SE, Finkelstein Y, Kealey R, et al. Comparative safety of antiepileptic drugs for neurological development in children exposed during pregnancy and breast feeding: A systematic review and network meta-analysis. BMJ Open. 2017;7(7):e017248.
96. Weston J, Bromley R, Jackson CF, Adab N, Clayton-Smith J, Greenhalgh J, et al. Monotherapy treatment of epilepsy in pregnancy: Congenital malformation outcomes in the child. Cochrane Database Syst. Rev. 2016;11(11):CD010224.
97. Beydoun A, DuPont S, Zhou D, Matta M, Nagire V, Lagae L. Current role of carbamazepine and oxcarbazepine in the management of epilepsy. Seizure. 2020;83:251-63.
98. Battino D, Tomson T, Bonizzoni E, Craig J, Lindhout D, Sabers A, Perucca E, Vajda F, et al. Seizure control and treatment changes in pregnancy: Observations from the EURAP epilepsy pregnancy registry. Epilepsia. 2013;54(9):1621-7.
99. Ferri MM, Mayor PP, López-Fraile IP, Siquier AE, Moro MM, Berdusan MF. Comparative study of antiepileptic drug use during pregnancy over a period of 12 years in Spain. Efficacy of the newer antiepileptic drugs lamotrigine, levetiracetam, and oxcarbazepine. Neurología (Engl Ed). 2018;33(2):78-84.
100. Vajda FJ, O"Brien TJ, Graham JE, Hitchcock AA, Lander CM, Eadie M. Predicting epileptic seizure control during pregnancy. Epilepsy Behav. 2018;78:91-5.
101. Reisinger TL, Newman M, Loring DW, Pennell PB, Meador KJ. Antiepileptic drug clearance and seizure frequency during pregnancy in women with epilepsy. Epilepsy Behav. 2013;29(1):13-8.
102. Brodtkorb E, Reimers A. Seizure control and pharmacokinetics of antiepileptic drugs in pregnant women with epilepsy. Seizure. 2008;17(2):160-5.
103. Borgelt LM, Hart FM, Bainbridge JL. Epilepsy during pregnancy: focus on management strategies. Int J Womens Health. 2016;8:505-17.
104. Crawford P. Best practice guidelines for the management of women with epilepsy. Epilepsia. 2005;46(Suppl 9): 117-24.
105. Beck-Mannagetta G, Janz D, Hoffmeister U, Behl I, Scholz G. Morbidity risk for seizures and epilepsy in offspring of patients with epilepsy. In: Genetics of the Epilepsies. Berlin, Heidelberg: Springer; 1989. pp. 119-26.
106. Dreier JW, Ellis CA, Berkovic SF, Cotsapas C, Ottman R, Christensen J. Epilepsy risk in offspring of affected parents; a cohort study of the "maternal effect" in epilepsy. Ann Clin Transl Neurol. 2021;8(1):153-62.
107. Narayan B, Nelson-Piercy C. Medical problems in pregnancy. Clin Med (Lond). 2017;17(3):251-7.
108. Harden CL, Pennell PB, Koppel BS, Hovinga CA, Gidal B, Meador KJ, et al. Practice parameter update: management issues for women with epilepsy--focus on pregnancy (an evidence-based review): vitamin K, folic acid, blood levels, and breastfeeding: report of the Quality Standards Subcommittee and Therapeutics and Technology Assessment Subcommittee of the American Academy of Neurology and American Epilepsy Society. Neurology. 2009;73(2):142-9.
109. Pirie DA, Al Wattar BH, Pirie AM, Houston V, Siddiqua A, Doug M, et al. Effects of monitoring strategies on seizures in pregnant women on lamotrigine: a meta-analysis. Eur J Obstet Gynecol Reprod Biol. 2014;172:26-31.
110. Bateman BT, Hernandez-Diaz S, Huybrechts KF, Palmsten K, Mogun H, Ecker JL, et al. Patterns of outpatient antihypertensive medication use during pregnancy in a Medicaid population. Hypertension. 2012;60(4):913-20.
111. Roberts CL, Ford JB, Henderson-Smart DJ, Algert CS, Morris JM. Hypertensive disorders in pregnancy: a population-based study. Med J Aust. 2005;182(7):332-5.
112. Kharazmi E, Dossus L, Rohrmann S, Kaaks R. Pregnancy loss and risk of cardiovascular disease: a prospective population-based cohort study (EPIC-Heidelberg). Heart. 2011;97(1):49-54.
113. Akbar MI, Adibrata MA, Aditiawarman, Aryananda RA, Angsar MD, Dekker G. Maternal and perinatal outcome related to severity of chronic hypertension in pregnancy. Pregnancy Hypertension. 2019;16:154-60.
114. Almasi-Hashiani A, Omani-Samani R, Mohammadi M, Amini P, Navid B, Alizadeh A, et al. Assisted reproductive technology and the risk of preeclampsia: an updated systematic review and meta-analysis. BMC Pregnancy Childbirth. 2019;19(1):149.
115. Roque M, Valle M, Sampaio M, Geber S. Obstetric outcomes after fresh versus frozen-thawed embryo transfers: a systematic review and meta-analysis. JBRA Assist Reprod. 2018;22(3):253-60.
116. Wong KM, van Wely M, Mol F, Repping S, Mastenbroek S. Fresh versus frozen embryo transfers in assisted reproduction. Cochrane Database Syst Rev. 2017;3(3):CD011184.
117. Tandberg A, Klungsøyr K, Romundstad LB, Skjaerven R. Preeclampsia and assisted reproductive technologies: consequences of advanced maternal age, interbirth intervals, new partner and smoking habits. BJOG. 2015;122(7):915-22.
118. Farhi J, Haroush AB, Andrawus N, Pinkas H, Sapir O, Fisch B, et al. High serum oestradiol concentrations in IVF cycles increase the risk of pregnancy complications related to abnormal placentation. Reprod Biomed Online. 2010;21(3):331-7.
119. Ashraf MS, Vongpatanasin W. Estrogen and hypertension. Curr Hypertens Rep. 2006;8(5):368-76.
120. Conrad KP. Emerging role of relaxin in the maternal adaptations to normal pregnancy: implications for preeclampsia. Semin Nephrol. 2011;31(1):15-32.
121. Von Versen-Höynck F, Schaub AM, Chi YY, Chiu KH, Liu J, Lingis M, et al. Increased preeclampsia risk and reduced aortic compliance with in vitro fertilization cycles in the absence of a corpus luteum. Hypertension. 2019;73(3):640-9.
122. Von Versen-Höynck F, Narasimhan P, Tierney ESS, Martinez N, Conrad KP, Baker VL, et al. Absent or excessive corpus luteum number is associated with altered maternal vascular health in early pregnancy. Hypertension. 2019;73(3):680-90.
123. Masoudian P, Nasr A, de Nanassy J, Fung-Kee-Fung K, Bainbridge SA, El Demellawy D. Oocyte donation pregnancies and the risk of preeclampsia or gestational hypertension: a systematic review and metaanalysis. Am J Obstet Gynecol. 2016;214(3):328-39.
124. National Institute for Health and Care Excellence. (2019). Hypertension in Pregnancy: Diagnosis and Management.

[Online] Available from: https://wwwniceorguk/guidance/ng133 [Last accessed December, 2022].
125. Webster K, Fishburn S, Maresh M, Findlay SC, Chappell LC; Guideline Committee. Diagnosis and management of hypertension in pregnancy: summary of updated NICE guidance. BMJ. 2019;366:l5119.
126. Bateman BT, Patorno E, Desai RJ, Seely EW, Mogun H, Dejene SZ, et al. Angiotensin-converting enzyme inhibitors and the risk of congenital malformations. Obstetrics and gynecology. 2017;129(1):174-84.
127. Ahmed B, Tran DT, Zoega H, Kennedy SE, Jorm LR, Havard A. Maternal and perinatal outcomes associated with the use of renin-angiotensin system (RAS) blockers for chronic hypertension in early pregnancy. Pregnancy Hypertension. 2018;14:156-61.
128. Abalos E, Duley L, Steyn DW, Gialdini C. Antihypertensive drug therapy for mild to moderate hypertension during pregnancy. Cochrane Database Syst Rev. 2018(10).
129. Easterling TR, Carr DB, Brateng D, Diederichs C, Schmucker B. Treatment of hypertension in pregnancy: effect of atenolol on maternal disease, preterm delivery, and fetal growth. Obstet Gynecol. 2001;98(3):427-33.
130. Churchill D, Beevers GD, Meher S, Rhodes C. Diuretics for preventing preeclampsia. Cochrane Database Syst Rev. 2007;2007(1)P:CD004451.
131. Abramov Y, Elchalal U, Schenker JG. Obstetric outcome of in vitro fertilized pregnancies complicated by severe ovarian hyperstimulation syndrome: a multicenter study. Fertil Steril. 1998;70(6):1070-6.
132. Wiser A, Levron J, Kreizer D, Achiron R, Shrim A, Schiff E, et al. Outcome of pregnancies complicated by severe ovarian hyperstimulation syndrome (OHSS): a follow-up beyond the second trimester. Hum Reprod. 2005;20(4):910-4.
133. Groeneveld E, Lambers MJ, Lambalk CB, Broeze KA, Haapsamo M, De Sutter P, et al. Preconceptional low-dose aspirin for the prevention of hypertensive pregnancy complications and preterm delivery after IVF: a meta-analysis with individual patient data. Hum Reprod. 2013;28(6):1480-8.
134. Hofmeyr GJ, Duley L, Atallah A. Dietary calcium supplementation for prevention of pre-eclampsia and related problems: a systematic review and commentary. BJOG. 2007;114(8):933-43.
135. Poston L, Briley AL, Seed PT, Kelly FJ, Shennan AH; Vitamins in Preeclampsia (VIP) Trial Consortium. Vitamins in Preeclampsia (VIP) Trial Consortium. Vitamin C and vitamin E in pregnant women at risk for preeclampsia (VIP trial): randomised placebo-controlled trial. Lancet. 2006;367(9517):1145-54.
136. Centers for Disease Control and Prevention. (2022). National Diabetes Statistics Report. [Online] Available from: https://www.cdc.gov/diabetes/data/statistics-report/index.html [Last accessed December, 2022].
137. Lascar N, Brown J, Pattison H, Barnett AH, Bailey CJ, Bellary S. Type 2 diabetes in adolescents and young adults. Lancet Diabetes Endocrinol. 2018;6(1):69-80.
138. Mayer-Davis EJ, Lawrence JM, Dabelea D, Divers J, Isom S, Dolan L, et al. Incidence trends of type 1 and type 2 diabetes among youths, 2002–2012. N Engl J Med. 2017;376(15):1419-29.
139. Codner E, Merino PM, Tena-Sempere M. Female reproduction and type 1 diabetes: from mechanisms to clinical findings. Hum Reprod Update. 2012;18(5):568-85.
140. Kjaer K, Hagen C, Sandø SH, Eshøj O. Epidemiology of menarche and menstrual disturbances in an unselected group of women with insulin-dependent diabetes mellitus compared to controls. J Clin Endocrinol Metab. 1992;75(2):524-9.
141. Dorman JS, Steenkiste AR, Foley TP, Strotmeyer ES, Burke JP, Kuller LH, et al. Menopause in type 1 diabetic women: is it premature? Diabetes. 2001;50(8):1857-62.
142. Arrais RF, Dib SA. The hypothalamus–pituitary–ovary axis and type 1 diabetes mellitus: a mini review. Hum Reprod. 2006;21(2):327-37.
143. Salvi R, Castillo E, Voirol MJ, Glauser M, Rey JP, Gaillard RC, et al. Gonadotropin-releasing hormone-expressing neurons immortalized conditionally are activated by insulin: implication of the mitogen-activated protein kinase pathway. Endocrinology. 2006;147(2):816-26.
144. Pal L, Chu HP, Shu J, Topalli I, Santoro N, Karkanias G. In vitro evidence of glucose-induced toxicity in GnRH secreting neurons: high glucose concentrations influence GnRH secretion, impair cell viability, and induce apoptosis in the GT1-1 neuronal cell line. Fertil Steril. 2007;88(4 Suppl):1143-9.
145. Nandi A, Poretsky L. Diabetes and the female reproductive system. Endocrinology and Metabolism Clinics. 2013;42(4):915-46.
146. Escobar-Morreale HF, Roldán B, Barrio R, Alonso M, Sancho J, de la Calle H, et al. High prevalence of the polycystic ovary syndrome and hirsutism in women with type 1 diabetes mellitus. J Clin Endocrinol Metab. 2000;85(11):4182-7.
147. Fulghesu AM, Villa P, Pavone V, Guido M, Apa R, Caruso A, et al. The impact of insulin secretion on the ovarian response to exogenous gonadotropins in polycystic ovary syndrome. J Clin Endocrinol Metab. 1997;82(2):644-8.
148. Thong EP, Codner E, Laven JS, Teede H. Diabetes: a metabolic and reproductive disorder in women. Lancet Diabetes Endocrinol. 2020;8(2):134-49.
149. Larsen MD, Jensen DM, Fedder J, Jølving LR, Nørgård BM. Live-born children after assisted reproduction in women with type 1 diabetes and type 2 diabetes: a nationwide cohort study. Diabetologia. 2020;63(9):1736-44.
150. Mattsson K, Nilsson-Condori E, Elmerstig E, Vassard D, Schmidt L, Ziebe S, et al. Fertility outcomes in women with pre-existing type 2 diabetes-a prospective cohort study. Fertil Steril. 2021;116(2):505-13.
151. Zymperdikas CF, Zymperdikas VF, Mastorakos G, Grimbizis G, Goulis DG. Assisted reproduction technology outcomes in women with infertility and preexisting diabetes mellitus: a systematic review. Hormones (Athens). 2022;21(1):23-31.
152. Wang Q, Moley KH. Maternal diabetes and oocyte quality. Mitochondrion. 2010;10(5):403-10.
153. Jungheim ES, Moley KH. The impact of type 1 and type 2 diabetes mellitus on the oocyte and the preimplantation embryo. Semin Reprod Med. 2008;26(2):186-195.
154. Bell R, Bailey K, Cresswell T, Hawthorne G, Critchley J, Lewis-Barned N, et al. Trends in prevalence and outcomes of pregnancy in women with pre-existing type I and type II diabetes. BJOG. 2008;115(4):445-52.
155. Chen H, Li J, Cai S, Tang S, Zeng S, Chu C, et al. Blastocyst Transfer: A Risk Factor for Gestational Diabetes Mellitus in

Women Undergoing In Vitro Fertilization. J Clin Endocrinol Metab. 2022;107(1):e143-52.
156. Bosdou JK, Anagnostis P, Goulis DG, Lainas GT, Tarlatzis BC, Grimbizis GF, et al. Risk of gestational diabetes mellitus in women achieving singleton pregnancy spontaneously or after ART: a systematic review and meta-analysis. Hum Reprod Update. 2020;26(4):514-44.
157. Sesmilo G, Prats P, Álvarez M, Romero I, Guerrero M, Rodríguez I, et al. Gestational diabetes prevalence and outcomes in women undergoing assisted reproductive techniques (ART). Endocrinología, Diabetes y Nutrición. 2022;69(10):837-43.
158. Buchanan TA, Xiang AH, Page KA. Gestational diabetes mellitus: risks and management during and after pregnancy. Nat Rev Endocrinol. 2012;8(11):639-49.
159. Mahmud M, Mazza D. Preconception care of women with diabetes: a review of current guideline recommendations. BMC Women's Health. 2010;10:5.
160. American Diabetes Association. 14. Management of diabetes in pregnancy: Standards of medical care in diabetes-2019. Diabetes Care. 2019;42(Suppl 1): S165-72.
161. Mills JL. Malformations in infants of diabetic mothers. Teratology 25:385-94. 1982. Birth Defects Res A Clin Mol Teratol. 2010;88(10):769-78.
162. American College of Obstetricians and Gynecologists" Committee on Practice Bulletins—Obstetrics. ACOG Practice bulletin No. 201: Pregestational diabetes mellitus. Obstet Gynecol. 132(6):e228-48.

SECTION

4

Male Infertility

CHAPTER 24

Etiopathogenesis of Male Infertility

Haritha Mannem, Sathya Balasubramanyam

INTRODUCTION

Infertility has become a public health problem affecting approximately 1 in 10 couples globally.[1] Male infertility alone contributes to nearly 60% of the problem and has turned out to be a key health concern; the incidence of male infertility ranges from 2.5 to 12% across different regions around the world **(Fig. 1)**.[2]

The impaired spermatogenesis and functions can be associated with factors which act at pretesticular level, at the level of testis, or at post-testicular level. Primary testicular failure is responsible for nearly 75% of all infertility due to male factor, while genetic factors can be acknowledged in around 15% of cases [congenital hypogonadotropic hypogonadism (cHH), primitive testicular failure, and congenital absence of vas deferens (CAVD)].

The factors implicated in male infertility can also be grouped as:

- *Congenital factors:*[3]
  - Anorchia
  - CAVD
  - Cryptorchidism
  - Genetic anomalies [karyotype anomalies such as Klinefelter syndrome (KS), microdeletions in the Y chromosome, Kallmann syndrome (KLS), partial or mild androgen insensitivity syndrome, and mutations in genes which are involved in hypothalamic–pituitary–gonadal axis].
- *Acquired factors:*[3]
  - Testicular torsion
  - Testicular trauma
  - Subobstruction or obstruction of proximal and/or distal part of urogenital tract

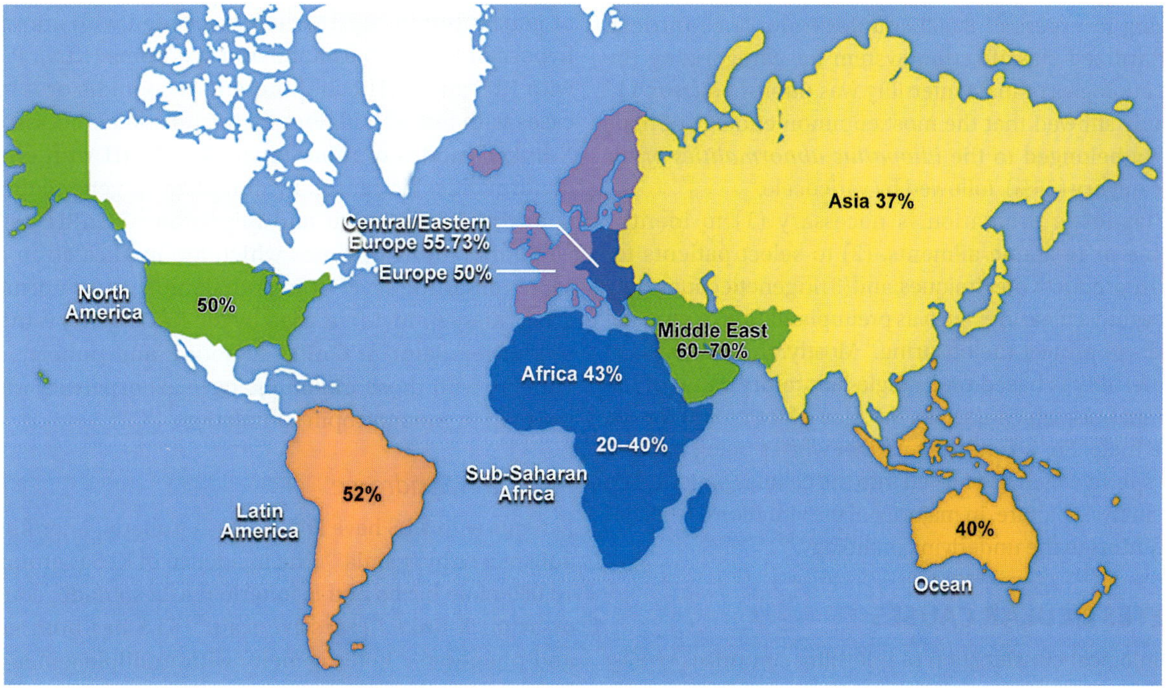

Fig. 1: World map containing percentages of infertility cases per region that are due to male factor.

BOX 1: Causes of male infertility [World Health Organization (WHO)].

- Idiopathic
- Isolated abnormalities of semen and sperm parameters
- Varicocele
- Immunological infertility
- Genital tract infection
- Primary testicular failure
- Kallmann syndrome
- Klinefelter syndrome
- Cryptorchidism
- Obstruction
- Ejaculatory dysfunction
- Erectile dysfunction
- Genetic causes: Y chromosome microdeletion

Note: The exact etiopathological mechanism through which varicocele and antisperm antibodies contribute to male infertility remains to be elucidated.

- Postinflammatory forms (orchitis, epididymitis)
- Recurrent urogenital infections, prostatitis, and prostatovesiculitis
- Systemic diseases such as cirrhosis of liver and renal failure
- Varicocele
- Exogenous factors such as medications, irradiation, cytotoxic drugs, and heat
- Surgeries which can cause damage to the testicular vascularization
- Erectile or ejaculatory dysfunction
- Acquired hypogonadotropic hypogonadism (AHH).

- Idiopathic forms:[3]
  - Unknown etiology (around 50%).

In a large World Health Organization (WHO) study (involving in excess of 8,500 couples from 25 countries), a standardized classification system for categorizing the several etiologies of male infertility was published **(Box 1)**.[4] This study showed that the most common etiology of male infertility belonged to the *idiopathic abnormalities of the semen* category (25%), followed by varicocele.[5]

A diagnostic evaluation is necessary (1) to identify reversible or treatable ailments, (2) to select patients for assisted reproductive techniques, and (3) in genetic counseling and preventive measures such as preimplantation or prenatal diagnosis to protect the offspring.[3] Mostly, the diagnosis of male infertility is based on a single laboratory value of the semen analysis, which decides the plan of treatment for the infertile male. So, it is not the patient who is being treated, but the sperm which has turned into the cellular patient. The semen analysis picture, in majority of the situations, does not give any hints to the underlying pathology.[6]

PRETESTICULAR CAUSES

This etiological classification of infertility comprises chiefly two types of pathological disorders, i.e., hypogonadotropic hypogonadism (HH) and coital disorders such as erectile dysfunction and ejaculatory disorders, i.e., ejaculatio precox and retrograde ejaculation.

Hypogonadotropic Hypogonadism

The deficit of follicle-stimulating hormone (FSH) and luteinizing hormone (LH) secretion can be congenital or acquired, i.e., associated with a primary lesion in the pituitary gland or secondary to inadequate hypothalamic gonadotropin-releasing hormone (GnRH) production.[7,8] Hypogonadotropic hypogonadism is of the following types:

- Congenital
- Secondary (hypogonadotropic) hypogonadism, i.e., secondary testicular failure
- Idiopathic HH
- Hyposmic or anosmic (KLS)
- Normosmic
- Acquired, i.e., tumors in:
  - Diencephalon such as craniopharyngioma or meningioma
  - Hypothalamus or pituitary
- Skull base fractures
- Empty sella syndrome
- Granulomatous illnesses
- Hyperprolactinemia
- Ischemia or hemorrhagic lesions in hypothalamus
- Radiotherapy
- Drugs or anabolic steroids.

Congenital Hypogonadotropic Hypogonadism

Patients with cHH have faulty or reduced secretion of GnRH, manifesting as pubertal delay and low levels of gonadotropins. cHH when associated with anosmia or hyposmia is known as Kallmann syndrome (KLS). Patients with KLS and cHH could present as sporadic or inherited cases with autosomal dominant, autosomal recessive, and X-linked modes of inheritance. KLS (cHH with olfactory abnormalities) is caused by mutations in genes concerned with the development and migration of GnRH neurons, while mutations in genes which are implicated in GnRH secretion at the level of hypothalamus cause normosmic cHH.[9] Kisspeptin-1 (encoded by the *KISS1* gene) is the most potent regulator of GnRH secretion and puberty onset. Patients with these mutations have azoospermia which is resistant to gonadotropin stimulation.[10,11]

Kallmann Syndrome

Patients with KLS have HH, delay in puberty, infertility, and anosmia or hyposmia.[12] The incidence of KLS is around 1 in 10,000 male births and is inherited as a sporadic condition or as an X-linked recessive trait.[13] KLS has both genetic and phenotypic heterogeneity with multiple genes.[14] KLS 1 (*KAL1*) and fibroblast growth factor receptor 1 (*FGFR1*) are the *KLS* genes which are most researched. As men with this syndrome have paucity of GnRH-releasing neurons, endocrine assessment shows untraceable levels of LH and FSH and very low testosterone. These males with failure to achieve puberty, barring a few cases of spontaneously reversible KLS,[15] have paucity of intratesticular testosterone, lack of FSH, and hence incomplete spermatogenesis. The defective development of the olfactory tract can be diagnosed by scanning with magnetic resonance imaging (MRI). In some cases, other defects such as cerebellar dysfunction, cleft palate, red–green color blindness, and congenital deafness are present.[16]

Diagnosis can be made by genetic testing guided by the pattern of inheritance and additional phenotypic features.[17,18] After diagnosing, hormonal treatment is planned to accomplish two key purposes: inducing virilization and normal development, thus improving fertility status. In patients with prepubertal hypogonadism, androgen replacement alone is sufficient to attain normal androgen levels and development of secondary sexual characteristics. On the other hand, stimulus for sperm production requires treatment with human chorionic gonadotropin (hCG), i.e., hCG in conjunction with human menopausal gonadotropins (hMGs) or recombinant FSH or urinary FSH, but if the origin of HH is hypothalamic, a substitute to hCG treatment is pulsatile GnRH.[19]

Acquired Hypogonadotropic Hypogonadism

Acquired hypogonadotropic hypogonadism, as opposed to cHH, is postnatal onset of disorders which damages or changes the functioning of pituitary gonadotroph cells and/or GnRH neurons. Though tumors of the pituitary gland (chiefly prolactinoma) are the major cause of AHH, other disorders such as tumors of the sella or hypothalamic or infundibular cyst, iron overload, infiltrative and vascular disorders, head trauma, pituitary surgery, and cranial or pituitary radiotherapy may also lead to AHH.[20,21] The clinical presentations of AHH are subject to age of onset, the rapidity of its onset, the amount of gonadotropin deficit, and the relationship to other pituitary deficiencies or excess. These men lack stamina, suffer from erectile dysfunction, and have decreased libido and overall poor quality of life with low self-esteem. If the hypogonadism is of acute onset, the general physical examination is typically normal. Decreased facial and body hair, reduced muscle mass, gynecomastia, facial wrinkles, and hypotrophic testes are seen in chronic and complete AHH.

Men with AHH having significant testosterone deficiency improve with testosterone replacement therapy, i.e., by using an injectable testosterone ester. Fertility can be restored rather fast as long as there is no primary testicular damage and the spouse is fertile.[22] Serious illness, acquired immunodeficiency syndrome (AIDS), stress, malnutrition, illicit drug intake, excessive alcohol consumption, exhausting exercise, systemic illnesses such as hemochromatosis, and sarcoidosis may also be linked with transient HH.[23]

Coital Disorders

This category includes disorders such as erectile dysfunction and ejaculatory disorders (ejaculatio precox and retrograde ejaculation). To make precise diagnosis, a systematic andrological workup is required so as to exclude organic causes of erectile dysfunction (i.e., neurogenic and vascular) and other coexisting morbidities. Retrograde ejaculation or anejaculation is seen in patients with diabetes mellitus, postretroperitoneal lymph node dissection, bladder neck surgery, multiple sclerosis, and in patients with spinal cord injury. Retrograde ejaculation is diagnosed on the basis of absence of spermatozoa in the semen but its presence in the urine postmasturbation, and in such circumstances in vitro fertilization with embryo transfer (IVF with ET) is the only dependable option. In patients with anejaculation caused by spinal cord injury, the effective methods for sperm retrieval are electroejaculation and vibrostimulation, while pregnancy can be achieved by intracytoplasmic sperm injection (ICSI). Medical treatment is an extensively available option for most patients with premature ejaculation and erectile dysfunction. Psychosexual therapy is an effective therapeutic choice for patients affected by psychogenic erectile dysfunction and premature ejaculation.[24,25]

TESTICULAR CAUSES

Primary Testicular Disease

Primary testicular disease is the most common type of decreased male fertility. Testicular deficiency is due to primary spermatogenic failure as a result of conditions barring hypothalamo-pituitary axis disorder and obstructed male genitourinary tract. Testicular deficiency has multiple etiologies, and it manifests as severe oligoasthenoteratozoospermia (OAT) or nonobstructive azoospermia (NOA).[26]

Etiologies of Testicular Deficiency

- Congenital, i.e., anorchia
- Genetic anomalies such as karyotypic aberrations and Y chromosome deletions
- Dysgenetic testes or cryptorchidism
- Acquired, i.e., trauma to the testis
- Torsion of the testis
- Testicular tumor
- Postinflammatory types, mainly mumps and orchitis
- Varicocele
- Systemic diseases such as cirrhosis of liver and renal failure
- Miscellaneous extrinsic factors such as anabolic or cytotoxic drugs, radiotherapy, and heat

- Surgical procedures which compromise testicular vascularization and cause testicular atrophy
- Unknown etiology: Idiopathic.

Testicular Dysgenesis Syndrome

Increasing trends have been observed in testicular malignancies and congenital abnormalities of the male reproductive tract with a drift toward poorer quality of semen. Additionally, many of these illnesses have similar risk factors. Skakkebæk et al. in the year 2001 recommended the term testicular dysgenesis syndrome (TDS) for this group of conditions that represent a syndrome of disorders caused by similar underlying entity, which leads to disturbance in the testicular development during fetal life.[27] TDS has an unclear etiology, but the rapid upsurge in male reproductive disorders in a few generations indicates environmental changes and changes in the lifestyle instead of genetic factors as the likely causes **(Flowchart 1)**.[28]

Testicular Dysfunction Syndrome

Basic etiological factors in TDS are genetically determined in utero and environmental factors such as endocrine disrupting compounds, toxins, and lifestyle factors like dietary habits, lack of exercise, and obesity act as contributing factors. The consequence is androgen insufficiency predisposing to testicular maldescent and Sertoli cell dysfunction leading to impaired spermatogenic function. Impaired germ cell (GC) differentiation can also lead to testicular carcinoma in situ.[27]

Cryptorchidism

Cryptorchidism is the most frequent congenital defect in male newborns. It can either occur as isolated defect or as syndromic cryptorchidism (i.e., in conjunction with other congenital anomalies).[28] Two key hormones and their receptor systems are involved in testicular descent, namely testosterone and its receptor, i.e., androgen receptor (AR) and insulin-like factor 3 (INSL3), and its G protein-coupled receptor, i.e., relaxin family peptide 2 (RXFP2).[29] The INSL3/RXFP2 system is vital for the first phase of descent of testis, while the inguinal phase requires the involvement of androgens. Syndromic cryptorchidism is predominately a result of mutations in the *AR* gene.[30] It is believed that increased temperature exposure to the intra-abdominal testicles leads to the damage of seminiferous tubules and GCs. Another contributing factor in partially maldescended testis positioned in the inguinal canal or at the root of the scrotal neck is much easily exposed to the risk of trauma. Possibility of torsion is also very high in a maldescended testis.[31,32]

GENETIC CAUSES

Chromosomal Abnormalities

Spermatogenesis needs the concerted action of more than 2,000 genes and mutation of any of these genes may be accountable for infertility. With progresses in genetics and diagnostic methods, a lot of the men previously labeled under "idiopathic" are reclassified as having genetic etiology of male infertility. The genetic factors can be transmitted as autosomal dominant, autosomal recessive, X-linked, and Y-linked traits.

There is a higher incidence of chromosomal aberrations among infertile men, mainly aneuploidy, and its incidence ranges from 2 to 15%, which depends on the severity of impairment of spermatogenesis.[33]

Autosomes can undergo recombination along their full length while pairing and recombination of X–Y sex chromosomes is limited to small homologous pseudoautosomal areas, and this is why sex chromosomal aneuploidies are the most common genetic anomalies in men.[34]

Flowchart 1: Schematic representation of pathogenetic links between the components of testicular dysgenesis syndrome.

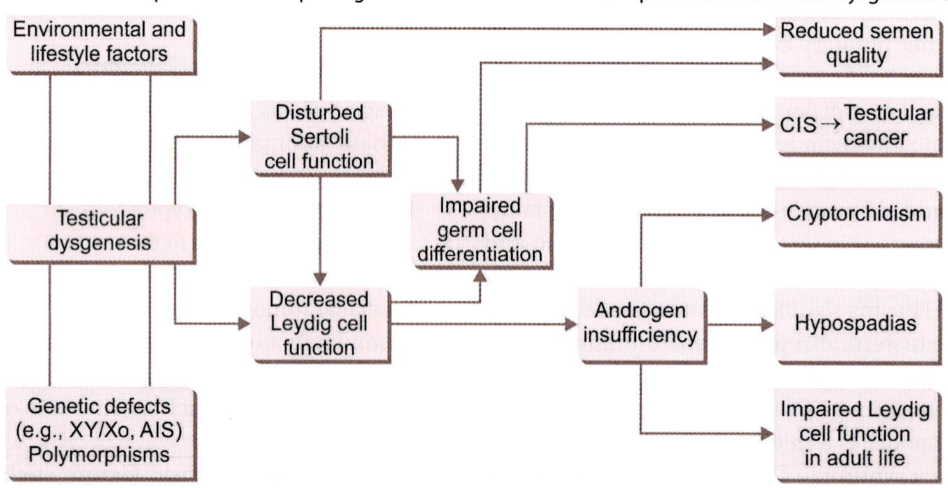

(AIS: androgen insensitivity syndrome; CIS: carcinoma in situ)

The majority of chromosome aberrations are caused during the meiotic phase.[35] Severely impaired production of sperm is often in association with a higher frequency of structural and numerical chromosomopathies.

Patients having less than 10 million sperms/mL have 10 times more incidence (i.e., around 4%) of autosomal structural defects in comparison to the common population. Men with severe oligozoospermia (i.e., less than 5 million sperms/mL) have an increased frequency (7–8%), while men with NOA have the highest frequencies (15–16%).[36]

Klinefelter Syndrome

Klinefelter syndrome (47,XXY) is the most common karyotyping aberration in males with severe infertility and azoospermia, followed by terminal deletions in the Y chromosome (Yq-) and structural autosomal aberrations. The incidence of KS is 1 in 500. Most patients with KS have 47,XXY karyotype while around 20% bear 47,XXY/46,XY mosaics or structurally abnormal X chromosome or higher grade sex chromosomal aneuploidy. The starting point of an extra X chromosome is nondisjunction in meiosis I. This extra X chromosome is derived paternally in around 60% of the patients with KS. Increased maternal age is associated with KS while increased paternal age is contentious.[37]

It manifests clinically as infertility, cognitive disorders, and hypergonadotropic hypogonadism. The spectrum of phenotype varies with the presence of mosaicism and the amount of genetic inactivation.[38,39] There is a progressive degeneration of Sertoli cells and GCs after puberty in patients with KS.[40] Microsurgical testicular sperm extraction (microTESE) (sperm recovery rate of 30–50%) with ICSI may allow patients with Klinefelter to have their own progenies.[41-45]

Fluorescence in situ hybridization (FISH) studies have questioned the genetic integrity of gametes and a research based on ICSI in combination with preimplantation genetic diagnosis (PGD) reported a substantial drop in the frequency of normal embryos in Klinefelter couples, i.e., 54% as compared to 77.2% in controls.[46]

Other Sex Chromosomal Abnormalities

The karyotype 47,XYY has an incidence of 1/1,000 live births and it is the second most common sex chromosomal aneuploidy.[47] Nondisjunction during meiosis II gives rise to the extra Y chromosome. These men may have a normal phenotype, but other characteristics such as infertility, clinodactyly, high stature, cognitive impairment, hypertelorism, and hostile behavior can be seen. Increased incidence of spermatozoa with chromosomal abnormality, especially sex chromosome disomies in the semen of men with this karyotype, is reported.[48,49]

A rare chromosomal anomaly is a 46,XX male which is seen in 0.9% of azoospermic males. Delay in puberty, infertility, and gynecomastia are the common manifestations, while genital ambiguity like cryptorchidism and hypospadias are a rarity. Two variations of this condition are known.

The first variant is the sex-determining region Y (SRY) + XX males, which accounts for majority (80–90%) of the cases and is due to the translocation of the *SRY* gene. Men with this variant usually have a normal male phenotype, but all are azoospermic.[50] The other variation is the SRY – XX males, in whom no copy of SRY is found. The male phenotype in these cases is either owing to mutations in X-linked genes or autosomal genes which are involved in the sex-determining cascade, such as *DAX1* and *SOX9* genes, that substitute the SRY. Patients with this variant are more probable to have incomplete masculinization.[51,52]

Autosomal Abnormalities

The commonly found abnormalities in men with oligozoospermia are Robertsonian translocations, paracentric inversions, reciprocal translocations, and marker chromosomes. The underlying relationship between chromosome abnormalities and impaired production of sperm is recommended to be a structural effect related to modifications in the chromosomal synapsis during meiosis.[53,54]

Robertsonian Translocations

Robertsonian translocations take place when there is a fusion of long arms of two acrocentric chromosomes (13, 14, 15, 21, and 22), resulting in genetic material loss on the short arms. These are the most common structural abnormalities, seen in 0.9% of infertile men and in 1/1,000 live births.[9] These men have a higher incidence of aneuploidy in the sperm with a likelihood of passing on the translocation to progeny.[55] Thus, chromosomal composition of their sperm should be analyzed; PGD should be done and genetic counseling for the couples should be offered.[56]

Autosomal Inversions

Autosomal inversions are structural chromosomal derangements, which do not cause loss of genetic material and are of utmost relevance for male infertility, seen in 3–5% of the men with infertility.[57,58] Carriers of inversions in chromosome 9 may show normozoospermia, oligospermia, azoospermia, or asthenozoospermia. These males have an increased incidence of sperm aneuploidy as well.[59]

Y Chromosome Microdeletions

It is the most common molecular genetic cause of severe spermatogenesis impairment, seen in around 10% of NOA and 3–5% of men with idiopathic oligozoospermia.[60] The euchromatin zone in the long arm of the Y

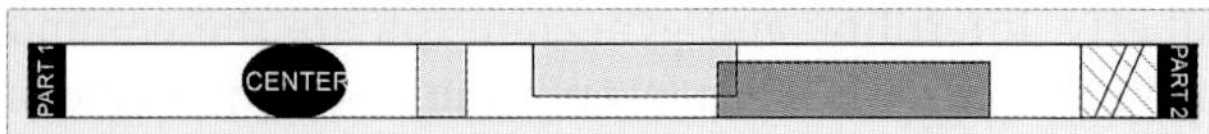

AZF regions	AZFa	AZFb	AZFc
Semen phenotype	Azoospermia		Azoospermia or severe OAT
Testis phenotype	SCOS pure	SGA pure	Hypospermatogenesis SCOS (mixed or pure)
Predicted TESE success	Virtually zero		Average 50%
Frequency of deletion type*	5%	10%	75%

Fig. 2: Classification of azoospermia factor (AZF) region. (OAT: oligoasthenoteratozoospermia; SCOS: Sertoli cell-only syndrome; SGA: spermatogenic arrest; TESE: testicular sperm extraction)

*Rest 10% of deletions are due to deletion of more than one AZF region.

chromosome (Yq11) contains the azoospermia factor (AZF) region, which has genes important for spermatogenesis. Based on their location, these genes are grouped into three groups, namely—AZFa, AZFb, and AZFc (**Fig. 2**).[61]

- The group AZFc is positioned in the distal part of Yq11 which accounts for 60% of all Y chromosome microdeletions.[62,63] AZFc group has numerous genes, and the DAZ (deleted in azoospermia), a group of four genes which are involved in spermatogenesis, has been the most researched.[64] Men who have AZFc deletions frequently present with severe azoospermia. By using microTESE, viable sperm can be collected in around 50–60% of the men with azoospermia.[65] Yq microdeletions have to be identified for diagnosing and in prognosticating prior to testicular biopsy (TESE).[66,67] Biopsy of the testis is not recommended when there are complete AZFa and AZFb deletions of the Y chromosome as the probability of finding spermatozoa is essentially zero. Y deletions which are compatible with the sperms being there in the ejaculate or in the testis are transmitted to the male progeny; thus, the role of genetic counseling is vital.

Mutations and Polymorphisms Affecting the Androgen Receptor

The *AR* gene is positioned in the long arm of the X chromosome (Xq11-12). *AR* gene mutations are infrequent, seen in 1/20,000–1/64,000 males. Around 300 mutations have been reported in the *AR* gene. These mutations lead to a variable phenotype from a phenotypic female in case of complete androgen insensitivity syndrome to an underandrogenized male having ambiguous genitalia in case of partial androgen insensitivity syndrome.[68-71]

Syndromic Monogenic Defects

Bardet–Biedl Syndrome

This group of disorders is characterized by mental retardation, obesity, hypogonadism, polydactyly, renal anomalies, and retinal pigmentary dystrophy.[72,73] Other additional characteristics are small stature, dental anomalies, diabetes mellitus, and deafness. Male hypogonadism includes micropenis, cryptorchidism, and hypospadias. It is a rare syndrome with incidence <1 in 100,000 newborns. Bardet–Biedl syndrome is mainly inherited as an autosomal recessive disorder, but other complex types of inheritance patterns exist.[74,75]

Prader–Willi Syndrome

Prader–Willi syndrome is a neurobehavioral group of disorders which affects both females and males and it manifests clinically as infantile hypotonia, mental retardation, delay in achieving developmental milestones, obesity, and hypogonadism. The prevalence of Prader–Willi syndrome ranges from 1/10,000 to 1/15,000.[76]

Primary Ciliary Dyskinesia

Primary ciliary dyskinesia is also called immotile cilia syndrome. It constitutes a group of disorders which are genetically heterogeneous, caused due to poor motility or complete immotility of the cilia leading to the lack of mucociliary clearance of the airways and other ciliated organs.[77] Most males suffering from primary ciliary dyskinesia are infertile due to functional and structural abnormalities in the central portion of the sperm flagella leading to immotile spermatozoa. About 50% of these patients also show situs inversus and then this condition is known as Kartagener syndrome. The mode of inheritance is autosomal recessive in the majority of cases.

Noonan Syndrome

Noonan syndrome is characterized by short stature, facial dysmorphism with posteriorly rotated ears, and congestive cardiac failure (mainly hypertrophic cardiomyopathy or pulmonary stenosis). 50% of the patients with this syndrome have oligozoospermia or azoospermia because of bilateral cryptorchidism. The mode of inheritance of Noonan syndrome is autosomal dominant with incidence around 1/1,000–1/5,000 newborns.[78]

Monogenic Defects in Post-testicular and Primary Testicular Forms of Male Infertility

Post-testicular Form: Congenital Absence of the Vas Deferens

The congenital unilateral absence of the vas deferens (CUAVD) is associated with oligozoospermia. Congenital bilateral absence of the vas deferens (CBAVD) is a post-testicular disease which is characterized by the absence of the vas deferens bilaterally, leading to blockade in transport of the spermatozoa from the testis or epididymis to the distal genitourinary tract. CBAVD is also seen in the majority of male patients with cystic fibrosis (CF), the most common autosomal recessive disease in Caucasians. CF has an incidence of 1 in 2,500 newborns.[79] It is caused by mutations in CF-transmembrane conductance regulator (*CFTR*) gene, present on chromosome no. 7 that encodes CFTR protein (anion channel) which is involved in chloride conduction across epithelial cell membranes like in the lung and pancreas.[80-82] In 80% of males with CBAVD, mutations in the *CFTR* gene are seen. In excess of 1,950 CFTR mutations have been recognized.[83] Patients with severe mutations progress to developing CF, the most common lethal genetic disease in Caucasians, whereas men with mild mutations may present only with CBAVD which is seen in about 1% of infertile men, and in up to 25% of men with obstructive azoospermia (OA). The ejaculatory ducts and seminal vesicles may also be absent in these patients.[84] A meta-analysis showed that 78% of men with CBAVD have a minimum of one CFTR mutation, and 46% with two mutations. Men with CBAVD are candidates for sperm retrieval from testis or epididymis coupled with ICSI.[85,86] Genetic testing for *CFTR* mutation is obligatory, not only for patients with CBAVD but also for their spouses, as 1 out of 25 individuals are asymptomatic carriers of a mutation.[79]

Association of CBAVD with OA and chronic sinopulmonary disease is known as Young syndrome, which was thought to be associated with CF. However, no increased frequency of *CFTR* mutations is found in these patients, suggestive of the fact that Young syndrome is a CF-independent disorder and probably owing to mercury poisoning in childhood.[87]

Epigenetics

Epigenetics is the study of various processes [such as deoxyribonucleic acid (DNA) methylation, chromatin remodeling, post-translational histone modifications, and regulation of microribonucleic acids (miRNAs)] which change the expression of genes without altering the DNA sequence. Changes in these epigenetic factors are involved in the pathophysiology of numerous male infertility conditions and are possibly accountable for various cases of idiopathic male infertility.[88] Additionally, these epigenetic processes may well be the mechanism by which various conditions such as obesity and environmental exposure affect spermatogenesis and thus affect the progeny.[89-91]

Deoxyribonucleic Acid Damage

Deoxyribonucleic acid damage is caused due to breaks in the single strand and double strand which are not repaired. These breaks in the strands are created during meiosis I, to let recombination happen, as well as during spermiogenesis, to avoid supercoiling and to allow unwinding of the nucleosomal structure.[92] These breaks may perhaps also be made due to the release of reactive oxygen species (ROS) because of various causes, such as prolonged epididymal transit, incomplete apoptosis, varicocele, environmental chemical exposures, and diabetes mellitus.[93-95] During spermatogenesis, GCs with more amount of irreparable DNA fragmentation may be directed toward apoptosis,[96] but some escape it and become defective sperm. Both these mechanisms lead to male infertility, and increased DNA fragmentation has been linked with decreased rates of pregnancy.[97-99]

Acquired Testicular Causes

Varicocele

Varicocele is defined clinically as a palpable, elongated, tortuous, and dilated testicular pampiniform plexus of veins in the spermatic cord. It is the most common treatable cause of infertility due to male factor. Its prevalence in men with primary infertility is around 35%,[100,101] whereas approximately 70–85% of men with secondary infertility present with varicocele.[102] As per a study involving 9,034 men, varicocele affected 11.7% of the total male population. This estimate has risen to 25.4% among infertile males with abnormal semen parameters. Likewise, decline in the motility and concentration of sperm has been seen in men with varicocele.[103,104]

Torsion Testis

Testicular torsion is a surgical emergency which is due to twisting of the spermatic cord and its contents. Its annual incidence is 3.8 per 100,000 males (<18 years).[105] Torsion testis is a diagnosis which is made clinically, with manifestations such as severe acute pain in the unilateral scrotum, nausea, and vomiting.[106-108] The degree of damage caused by torsion directly depends on time duration between the onset of torsion and intervention. Sometimes, this is misdiagnosed as epididymo-orchitis and the patient is put on conservative management for many days and ends up with complete loss of testicular function.

The various mechanisms which cause testicular deterioration in cases of torsion are:

- Cellular hypoxia or ischemia
- Ischemia or reperfusion injury
- Microcirculation changes
- Leukocyte or endothelin interaction
- Reactive nitrogen species and ROS
- GC apoptosis or caspase pathway
- Postinflammatory obstruction
- Proteolytic enzymes.[109]

Subfertility is seen in 36–39% of the patients following torsion. In long-term follow-up of these cases, only 5–50% may have normal semen analysis. Detorsion with early surgical intervention (with mean torsion time <13 hours) preserves fertility. Fertility is jeopardized with prolonged periods of torsion (mean torsion time ~70 hours) and following orchiectomy.[110]

Trauma

Trauma to the testis is fairly uncommon regardless of the vulnerable location of the testis. The likely reason attributed to low incidence of severe injuries is the mobility of scrotum. Injuries to the testis deserve a cautious approach as it is important to preserve fertility. On the basis of mechanism of injury, there are three types of testicular injuries: (1) Blunt trauma, (2) penetrating trauma, and (3) degloving trauma. These kinds of traumatic injuries are usually seen in the 15–40 years age group.[111]

There are two factors that provide protection to the testes from minor trauma:

1. Physiologic hydrocele: Small amount of serous fluid which separates the tunica albuginea from the tunica vaginalis so that the testis can slide freely within the scrotal sac.
2. The testes are allowed to move freely within the genital area because they are suspended by spermatic cord within the scrotum.

Secondary to trauma, intratesticular hematoma and edema develop which exert pressure on the vascular architecture of testis compromising the arterial supply which in turn leads to ischemic injury.[112]

Infections (Orchitis)

This is another common cause of acute scrotum, which usually coexists with epididymitis. The causative agents may be subdivided into viral and bacterial. Viral orchitis is most common because of the hematogenous spread, and the causative organisms may be paramyxovirus (the virus that results in mumps), coxsackie, varicella, lymphocytic choriomeningitis, and Marburg virus.[113,114] Mumps orchitis is rare in prepubertal boys but may occur in 15–30% of pubertal or postpubertal men. Mumps orchitis may be associated with infertility in 25% of bilateral cases and testicular atrophy is a sequelae in 30–50% of affected testicles. Bacterial orchitis may be caused by the spread of bacteria from the epididymis. Common pathogens include gonorrhea, chlamydia, gram-negative bacilli (*Escherichia coli, Klebsiella pneumoniae, Pseudomonas*), and gram-positive cocci. Orchitis may present with testicular swelling, pain, fever, and acute hydrocele. Acute infections may be associated with a transient reduction in semen parameters, which often recover after resolution of the infection. In addition, orchitis may affect fertility by the direct effect of the organism as well as pressure-induced necrosis of the seminiferous tubules due to parenchymal edema within the testicle.[115-117]

Tumors (Testicular Cancer)

It is one of the most common cancers among young men. Its etiology is unclear; however, it has been proposed that testicular cancer in situ (CIS), which is a precancerous condition of testicular GC tumor, starts during the fetal life, and thus the disease originates prenatally.[118,119] Testicular cancer leads to impaired quality of semen and infertility even before the cancer develops.[120,121] Its incidence has risen over the past 40–50 years in most of the developed countries.[122,123]

Gonadotoxic Drugs and Radiation

Ionizing radiation poses risk of damage in all living creatures, but the testes in mammals are far more susceptible to damage by ionizing radiation as they lie outside the body.[124] The level of damage is proportional to the dose of radiation and exposure time to radiation. It has been reported that there is reduction in sperm count after treatment with low-dose irradiation to testis while moderate- to high-dose irradiation can result in severe reduction in sperm count or even azoospermia. On an average, a person is exposed to 2.1 mSv natural radiation annually.[125] Sources of artificial radiations include radionuclides present in eating and drinking materials, X-rays used in medical diagnostic procedures, and gamma rays produced as by-products in the nuclear industry and products formed during atmospheric nuclear testing.

A multicenter prospective study conducted at Center for the Study and Conservation of Eggs and Human Sperm (CECOS) network of France has published interesting data on radiotherapy and sperm parameters. The results showed significant reduction in sperm count and sperm motility at 3 months postirradiation, which remained significantly low until 12 months. The sperm count and motility reached control values only after 24 months postirradiation.[126,127] Spermatozoa cryopreservation must be advised to all patients before treatment. It may be advisable to go for GC preservation in patients who have not achieved puberty and in whom spermatogenesis has not yet begun.

A large number of patients need medications for a long duration of time starting at an early age. These medications can affect male reproduction through direct gonadotoxic effects, central hormonal effects, effects on sperm function, etc., but these effects are often inadequately considered and studied **(Table 1)**.[128]

Immunological

Antisperm antibodies (ASA) are present in 3–12% of men being evaluated for infertility. Their production may arise from:

TABLE 1: Medications negatively affecting male fertility.

Drug class	Specific medications
Antibiotics	Erythromycin, gentamicin, neomycin, nitrofurantoin (high dose), tetracycline
Antihypertensives	Alpha-blockers, beta-blockers, CCBs, spironolactone, thiazide diuretics
Chemotherapeutic agents	Busulfan, carmustine, chlorambucil, cisplatin cyclophosphamide, cytarabine, lomustine, melphalan, mustine, nitrogen mustard, procarbazine, vinblastine
Hormones	Anabolic steroid, antiandrogens, estrogens, progesterone derivatives, testosterone
Miscellaneous agents	Allopurinol, cimetidine, colchicine, cyclosporine, sulfasalazine
Psychotherapeutic agents	Lithium, MAOIs, phenothiazines, SSRIs, TCAs

(CCB: calcium channel blocker; MAOIs: monoamine oxidase inhibitors; SSRIs: selective serotonin reuptake inhibitors; TCAs: tricyclic antidepressants)

- Breakdown of blood-testis barrier (BTB)
- Inoculation of host with sperm antigens
- Failure of immunosuppression.

Infection of the genitourinary tract is a potential risk factor for developing ASA. It has been postulated that ASA affects fertility by the agglutination of sperm, prevention of cervical mucous penetration, and the inhibition of the oocyte-sperm fusion.[113]

Lifestyle Factors

Reports of decreasing semen quality have prompted interest in the potential impact of environment and lifestyle on male reproductive potential. For the last 40 years, there has been a dramatic turnaround in the factors which can cause changes in semen parameters. These factors include the excessive use of cell phones, sudden upsurge in usage of marijuana,[129] opioids, and growth in the population of cigarette smokers.[130] Moreover, obesity rates have rapidly increased,[131] and physical activity rates and levels of environmental pollution have decreased. Meanwhile, global surface temperatures have increased substantially. It is important for providers and patients to recognize and manage modifiable risk factors that can improve fertility potential for men.[132]

Post-testicular Causes

Post-testicular causes constitute around 15% of all infertility in the male. This category includes the subobstructive or obstructive lesions of the seminal tract (proximal or distal), inflammations and infectious illnesses of accessory glands, and autoimmune infertility. In bilateral obstructive lesions, there is azoospermia, i.e., no spermatozoa in the ejaculate. Disorders which affect the accessory glands characteristically have low volume of ejaculate since around 90% of the ejaculate finds its origin from the seminal vesicles and prostate. However, in other post-testicular conditions, a different grade of impairment in the sperm parameters (i.e., sperm count, motility, and morphology) is seen.[133] The presence of leukocytes in excess of 1 million/mL is suggestive of inflammation of accessory glands. In cases labeled as having autoimmune infertility (seen in <5% of infertile males), there is an autoimmune reaction against the spermatozoa. The ASA are the result of past inflammations and infectious diseases of the testis or epididymis, which led to the disruption of the hematotesticular barrier. If >80% of motile spermatozoa are coated by ASA, it is suggestive of a pure immunological factor as the likely cause and the lone therapeutic option available in such a scenario is IVF.[134,135]

Obstructive Lesions

Obstructive lesions that affect the male genital tract can be congenital or acquired. Intratesticular obstruction is infrequent and can involve seminiferous tubules or the rete testis. Intratesticular obstruction is seen in 15% of males with OA.[136] Acquired forms (i.e., postinflammatory or post-traumatic) are more common compared to the congenital forms. The network channels which form the rete in the mediastinum of the testis are obliterated by fibrous tissue. There is no reduction in testicular size as sperm production is normal.

- *Epididymal obstruction:* This is the most common cause of OA, which affects 30–67% of men with azoospermia. Congenital obstruction of the epididymis frequently manifests as CBAVD and is often in association with at least single mutation of the *CF* gene in approximately 82% of the cases.[137] Congenital epididymal obstruction comprises Young syndrome, i.e., chronic sinopulmonary infections. On the other hand, acquired forms which are secondary to subclinical (e.g., chlamydial) and acute (e.g., gonococcal) epididymitis are the most common. Trauma or surgical interventions may be the other causes.[136,138]
- *Vas deferens obstruction:* This is the most common cause of acquired obstruction after vasectomy; therefore, around 2–6% of these patients undergo vasectomy reversal.[139-142] Vas deferens obstruction may also happen following repair of hernia. CBAVD is the most common congenital cause of vas deferens obstruction, which is frequently accompanied by CF. Unilateral agenesis is associated with contralateral seminal duct anomalies in 80% of the cases, while it is associated with renal agenesis in 26% of the cases.[143,144]
- *Ejaculatory duct obstruction:* This is seen in around 1–3% of cases of OA[145] and has two main types: cystic or postinflammatory. Postinflammatory obstructions commonly occur due to urethroprostatitis,[146,147] while

cystic obstructions are mostly congenital (i.e., Müllerian duct cyst or ejaculatory duct cysts or urogenital sinus) and are classically located in the midline. Complete obstructions are usually associated with low semen volume, acidic pH, and decreased or nil seminal fructose. There is typical dilatation of seminal vesicles (anterior-posterior diameter >15 mm).[137,148,149]

- *Functional obstruction of the distal seminal ducts:* This abnormality might be accredited to local neuropathy, which is frequently in association with urodynamic dysfunction. There is impairment in transport of sperm which may be idiopathic or due to selective serotonin reuptake inhibitor (SSRI) medication.[150,151]

INFLAMMATION

The effect of any inflammation or infection of the male reproductive tract on fertility relies on many factors, including the chronic versus acute nature of the disease and the type of invading pathogen **(Flowchart 2)**. Nonetheless, noninfectious inflammatory reactions may also affect the male reproductive tract. The key mediators of the inflammatory response in the male reproductive tract are the proinflammatory cytokines, interleukin (IL)-1a, IL-1b, and tumor necrosis factor-alpha (TNF-α).[152,153]

Inflammation of the testicles may cause spermatogenic arrest and a decline in serum levels of testosterone and LH, thus affecting the dual functions of spermatogenesis and steroidogenesis.[154,155]

The secretion of both TNF-α and IL-1a during the inflammatory response causes an inhibition of steroidogenesis by Leydig cells.[156,157] In inflammatory states of the male reproductive tract, oxidative stress is generated primarily by the infiltrating leukocytes and the proinflammatory cytokines. Phagocytosis by infiltrating phagocytes causes enhanced oxygen consumption and generation of large amounts of ROS.[158,159]

Inflammatory and infectious conditions of the male reproductive tract may also cause infertility owing to damage of the reproductive tract organs affecting their function (changing the production or release of the secretions required to support sperm function) and due to scarring of the delicate ductal systems and following anatomic obstruction. Nonregenerative epithelial cells lining the epididymis and testis are mainly vulnerable to scarring.[160] The result of such scarring is stricture formation, which may occur in the ejaculatory ducts, thus leading to a reduced ejaculatory volume and impaired fertility.[161]

INFECTIONS—EFFECT ON THE MALE REPRODUCTIVE TRACT

Male genitourinary tract infections are possibly correctable etiologies of male infertility. According to the WHO, urethritis, orchitis, epididymitis, and prostatitis are considered to be male accessory gland infections (MAGIs).[25] Infectious organisms could have a direct negative influence on sperm by directly interacting with sperm cells or potentially have a negative influence on fertility by a secondary effect either through the inflammatory process inherent in the infection or due to the release of toxins. Any infection of the male genital tract causes an inflammatory response whereby the body's immune system tries to fight off this infection. Gram-negative bacteria are one of the main causative infectious agents implicated in the male reproductive tract, which induce an inflammatory response due in part to the release of the endotoxin lipopolysaccharide which is present in the cell wall **(Fig. 3)**.

Flowchart 2: Possible mechanisms of impaired male fertility due to reproductive tract inflammation.

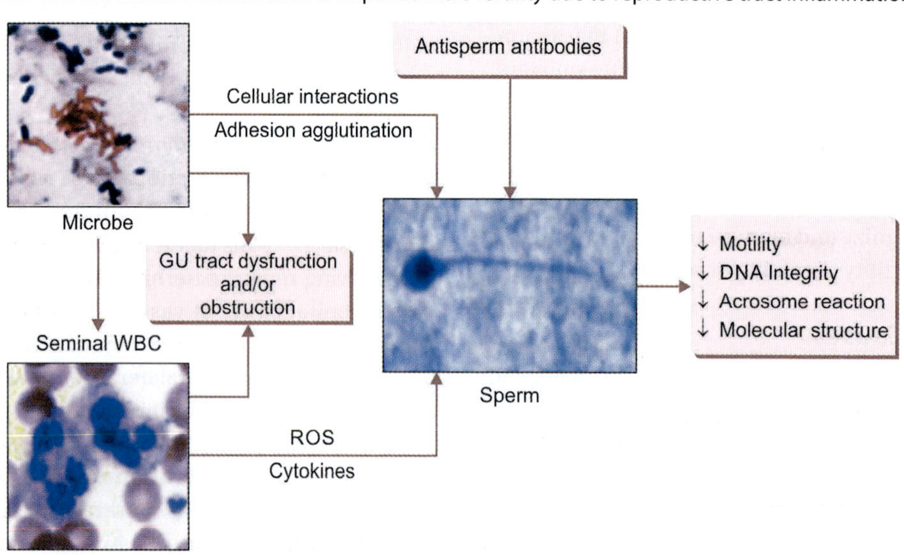

(DNA: deoxyribonucleic acid; GU: genitourinary; ROS: reactive oxygen species; WBC: white blood cells)

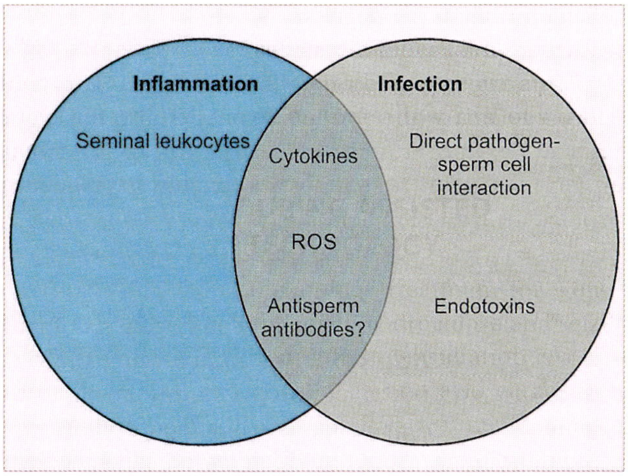

Fig. 3: Synergistic effect of inflammation and infection leading to male reproductive tract dysfunction and/or obstruction. (ROS: reactive oxygen species)

Infections may also impair fertility due to the direct effect of the pathogen on the sperm cell. Several bacterial and viral pathogens are also known to interact with and cause damage to spermatozoa, including *Chlamydia trachomatis, Ureaplasma urealyticum, E. coli*, and hepatitis B virus (HBV).[162,163] *E. coli* is known to adhere to spermatozoa and can lead to sperm agglutination, while *U. urealyticum* impairs sperm nuclear chromatin integrity. HBV reduces sperm motility by triggering a loss of mitochondrial membrane potential.[164]

The post-testicular type is diagnosed on the basis of physical examination (testicular volume is classically normal, signs of vas deferens or epididymal agenesis or cyst or obstruction), normal FSH values, and sonography of the scrotum with or without transrectal ultrasound (to pinpoint the level of obstruction and better visualize the accessory glands). Additionally, microbiological tests should be done in suspected cases of prostatitis or prostatovesiculitis or epididymitis and in patients with history of recurrent urogenital tract infections (in the patient or in his partner). The pathogens such as Chlamydia and Ureaplasma should be searched for using a urethral swab, while other pathogens can be analyzed in the urine and seminal fluid. Screening for *CFTR* gene mutations in case of CAVD (without kidney malformations) and congenital epididymal malformations is required both in the patient and in his partner.

REACTIVE OXYGEN SPECIES

Presently, almost 50% of men suffering from infertility cannot be diagnosed with a definite cause for their problem. This condition in men is labeled as unexplained infertility and is defined as couples in whom routine semen examination is normal, and the factors accounting for female infertility have been extensively ruled out.[165] There are substantial amounts of data that associate oxidative stress with the etiology of male infertility.[166] ROS production is linked to sperm physiology owing to its role in various sperm processes, including maturation, capacitation, hyperactivation, acrosome reaction, and sperm–oocyte interaction.[167] Pathological ROS levels are similarly implicated in causing significant damage to proteins, lipids, and nucleic acids (both nuclear and mitochondrial genomes) in human spermatozoa.[168]

The key sources of ROS production in seminal fluid include activated leukocytes, mainly neutrophils and macrophages in the seminal plasma. Semen leukocytes produce 1,000 times more ROS than spermatozoa. Immature and morphologically abnormal spermatozoa are other key sources of ROS in semen. However, the main cause of ROS production in human spermatozoa is oxidative phosphorylation reaction in sperm mitochondria.[169] Intrinsic origins of ROS can be attributed to deficient or damaged sperm and several other etiologies, such as infection or inflammation, varicocele, cryptorchidism, testicular torsion, and aging.

A major difference in DNA fragmentation between fertile and general population men could be explained by an environmental attack on the latter. Spermatozoa have limited defense mechanisms against oxidative attack on their DNA, mainly due to the tight packaging of sperm DNA and the absence of a precise DNA repair system. In such cases, the ROS metabolites attack DNA bases (guanine in particular) and phosphodiester bonds, destabilizing these molecules and thus creating the conditions which eventually lead to DNA fragmentation. The essential requirement for accurate transmission of genetic material and the birth of healthy progeny is sperm DNA integrity. It has also been recognized that the male factor is accountable not only for fertilization, but also for correct embryo development.[170,171]

EFFECTS OF CORONAVIRUS DISEASE 2019 ON MALE FERTILITY

The world has faced a major pandemic threat through the outbreak of novel coronavirus disease 2019 (COVID-19). The various studies conducted during this period have concluded that COVID-19 not only affects lungs but also causes functional and histopathological changes in various other organs including male genital tract.

The severe acute respiratory syndrome coronavirus 2 (SARS-CoV-2) enters host cells through a complex process, which starts with the interaction of its spike protein with angiotensin-converting enzyme 2 (ACE2) (receptor) on host cells.[172]

As testis is protected by a BTB, it is partially immune to many microorganisms; however, some viruses, such as the mumps virus, were shown to cross the BTB and cause localized testis inflammation in the form of orchitis.[173,174] It has been shown that ACE2 is strongly expressed at the protein levels in the testicular cells. This high expression suggests that testes in the COVID-19 infected males may have a significant role in the viral persistence and replication.[175] More specifically, ACE2 is expressed in seminiferous tubules cells along with Leydig and Sertoli cells in testes.[176] It was also observed that ACE2 expression in testes is age-dependent. According to this, the highest and lowest expressions of ACE2 occurs in patients aged 30 and 60, respectively.[177] It was observed that cells which express TMPRSS2 for S protein (which can initiate the viral internalization process) on their surface have enhanced SARS-CoV-2 isolation in them.[178]

The TMPRSS2 expression is prominently found in the epithelial cells of the human prostate gland more specifically in the apical surface of the luminal cells. This high TMPRSS2 expression in the prostate can also be related to COVID infection and can be another point of weakness of the male reproductive system.[179] The SARS-CoV-2 can also have a role in affecting the production of LH, FSH, and testosterone as well.[180] In a study conducted, SARS-CoV-2 was isolated in semen in 26.70% of COVID-19 patients in the acute phase and 8.70% of the patients in the recovery phase.[181] COVID infection also causes inflammatory response in the body, which leads to leukocyte infiltration even in testis. This can interfere with the Leydig cells' normal function and testosterone production and also cause BTB damage and seminiferous epithelium destruction. Additionally, leukocytes can lead to autoantibody development and autoimmune responses in seminiferous tubules via inflammatory cytokines.[182] An increase in levels of serum IgG was reported in both SARS and COVID-19 patients. Therefore, SARS-CoV-2 might trigger secondary autoimmune responses in testis and result in autoimmune orchitis.[183] Most of the viral infections including COVID-19 result in redox homeostasis abnormalities in the body leading to ROS overproduction and developing an ideal situation for replication of the virus further.[184]

The negative effects noticed in the male semen characteristics can also be due to unexpected side effects of unindicated and overuse of COVID-19 medications such as steroids.

Still, at this point of research, the clinical and epidemiological evidence regarding the effects of COVID-19 on reproductive health and future infertility of male patients is scarce to conclude. As COVID-19 is a newly emerged disease with recurring waves, further follow-up studies on reproductive effects and outcomes of affected and recovered patients as well (especially those who are of the reproductive age group) are required.

FACTORS THAT HELP IN PROGNOSTICATING MALE INFERTILITY

Factors that help in prognosticating male infertility are:

- Infertility duration
- Types of infertility—primary or secondary
- Semen analysis parameters
- Partner's age and fertility status.

In infertile couples on follow-up for 2 years with oligozoospermia as the chief cause of infertility, the overall pregnancy rate is around 27%.[185] The age of the female partner is the single most important variable that influences the outcome in assisted reproduction.[186]

KEY POINTS

- Understanding the etiology and pathogenesis of male infertility will help clinicians in achieving the right diagnosis and offering appropriate counseling to the patient about the pathology and treatment options.
- Multidisciplinary input between reproductive medicine specialists, endocrinologists, and surgeons may be required in some cases to optimize treatment.
- As our understanding about etiology and pathogenesis improves, novel treatment options are bound to come, and many conditions might be tackled by medical and lifestyle management rather than opting for assisted reproduction technology (ART).

REFERENCES

1. Boivin J, Bunting L, Collins JA, Nygren KG. International estimates of infertility prevalence and treatment-seeking: potential need and demand for infertility medical care. Hum Reprod. 2007;22(6):1506-12.
2. Agarwal A, Mulgund A, Hamada A, Chyatte MR. A unique view on male infertility around the globe. Reprod Biol Endocrinol. 2015;13(1):37.
3. Csilla K. Male infertility: pathogenesis and clinical diagnosis. Best Pract Res Clin Endocrinol Metab. 2011;25:271-85.
4. World Health Organization. Who Laboratory Manual for the Examination and Processing of Human Semen, 5th edition. Geneva: World Health Organization; 2010.
5. Comhaire F. Towards more objectivity in the management of male infertility. The need for a standardized approach. Int J Androl. 1987;7:1-53.
6. Cummins JM, Jequier AM. Treating male infertility needs more clinical andrology, not less. Hum Reprod. 1994;9(7):1214-9.
7. Huhtaniemi I, Alevizaki M. Mutations along the hypothalamic-pituitary-gonadal axis affecting male reproduction. Reprod Biomed Online. 2007;15:622-32.
8. Bianco SD, Kaiser UB. The genetic and molecular basis of idiopathic hypogonadotropic hypogonadism. Nat Rev Endocrinol. 2009;5:569-76.
9. Mau-Holzmann UA. Somatic chromosomal abnormalities in infertile men and women. Cytogenet Genome Res. 2005;111:317.
10. Franco B, Guioli FB, Pragliola AS, Incerti B, Bardoni B, Tonlorenzi R, et al. A gene deleted in Kallmann's syndrome shares homology with neural cell adhesion and axonal path-finding molecules. Nature. 1991;353:529-36.
11. Silveira LG, Noel SD, Silveira-Neto AP, Abreu AP, Brito VN, Santos MG, et al. Mutations of the KISS1 gene in disorders of puberty. J Clin Endocrinol Metab. 2010;95:2276-80.

12. Della Valle E, Vezzani S, Rochira V, Granata AR, Madeo B, Genovese E, et al. Prevalence of olfactory and other developmental anomalies in patients with central hypogonadotropic hypogonadism. Front Endocrinol. 2013;4:70.
13. Hardelin JP, Petit C. A molecular approach to the pathophysiology of the X chromosome-linked Kallmann's syndrome. Baillieres Clin Endocrinol Metab. 1995;9: 489-507.
14. Mitchell AL, Dwyer A, Pitteloud N, Quinton R. Genetic basis and variable phenotypic expression of Kallmann syndrome: towards a unifying theory. Trends Endocrinol Metab. 2011;22:249-58.
15. Zhang S, Wang T, Yang J, Liu Z, Wang S, Liu J. A fertile male patient with Kallmann syndrome and two missense mutations in the KAL1 gene. Fertil Steril. 2011;95:1789.e3-6.
16. Santen RJ, Paulsen CA. Hypogonadotropic eunuchoidism. I. Clinical study of the mode of inheritance. J Clin Endocrinol Metab.1973;36:47-54.
17. Boehm U, Bouloux PM, Dattani MT, de Roux N, Dodé C, Dunkel L, et al. Expert consensus document: European consensus statement on congenital hypogonadotropic hypogonadism—pathogenesis, diagnosis and treatment. Nat Rev Endocrinol. 2015;11:547-64.
18. Layman LC. Clinical genetic testing for Kallmann syndrome. J Clin Endocrinol Metab. 2013;98:1860-2.
19. Schopohl J, Mehltretter G, von Zumbusch R, Eversmann T, von Werder K. Comparison of gonadotropin-releasing hormone and gonadotropin therapy in male patients with idiopathic hypothalamic hypogonadism. Fertil Steril. 1991;56(6):1143-50.
20. Darby E, Anawalt BD. Male hypogonadism: an update on diagnosis and treatment. Treat Endocrinol. 2005;4(5):293-309.
21. Hayes FJ, Seminara SB, Crowley Jr WF. Hypogonadotropic hypogonadism. Endocrinol Metab Clin North Am. 1998;27(4):739-63.
22. Salenave S, Trabado S, Maione L, Brailly-Tabard S, Young J. Male acquired hypogonadotropic hypogonadism: diagnosis and treatment. Ann Endocrinol (Paris). 2012;73(2):141-6.
23. Dobs AS, Dempsey MA, Landenson PW, Polk BF. Endocrine disorders in men infected with human immunodeficiency virus. Am J Med. 1988;84:611-6.
24. Brackett NL, Lynne CM, Ibrahim E, Ohl DA, Sønksen J. Treatment of infertility in men with spinal cord injury. Nat Rev Urol. 2010;7:162-72.
25. Colpi G, Weidner W, Jungwirth A, Pomerol J, Papp G, Hargreave T, et al. EAU guidelines on ejaculatory dysfunction. Eur Urol. 2004;46:555-8.
26. World Health Organization. WHO Manual for the Standardized Investigation, Diagnosis and Management of the Infertile Male. Cambridge, UK: Cambridge University Press; 2000.
27. Skakkebæk NE, Rajpert-De Meyts E, Main KM. Testicular dysgenesis syndrome: an increasingly common developmental disorder with environmental aspects. Hum Reprod. 2001;16(5):972-8.
28. Main KM, Skakkebaek NE, Virtanen HE, Toppari J. Genital anomalies in boys and the environment. Best Pract Res Clin Endocrinol Metab. 2010;24:279-89.
29. Virtanen HE, Toppari J. Epidemiology and pathogenesis of cryptorchidism. Hum Reprod Update. 2008;14:49-58.
30. Gottlieb B, Beitel LK, Wu JH, Trifiro M. The androgen receptor gene mutations database (ARDB): 2004 update. Hum Mutat. 2004;23:527-33.
31. Toppari J, Kaleva M. Maldescendus testis. Horm Res. 1999;51:261-9.
32. Wilson JD, George FW, Renfree MB. The endocrine role in mammalian sexual differentiation. Recent Prog Horm Res.1995;50:349-64.
33. Ferlin A, Raicu F, Gatta V, Zuccarello D, Palka G, Foresta C. Male infertility: role of genetic background. Reprod Biomed Online. 2007;14:734-45.
34. Hinch AG, Altemose N, Noor N, Donnelly P, Myers SR. Recombination in the human pseudoautosomal region PARl. PLoS Genet. 2014;10:e1004503.
35. Martin RH. Meiotic errors in human oogenesis and spermatogenesis. Reprod Biomed Online. 2008;16:523-31.
36. Vincent MC, Daudin M, De MP, Massat G, Mieusset R, Pontonnier F, et al. Cytogenetic investigations of infertile men with low sperm counts: a 25-year experience. J Androl. 2002;23:18-22.
37. Iitsuka Y, Bock A, Nguyen DD, Samango-Sprouse CA, Simpson JL, Bischoff FZ. Evidence of skewed X-chromosome inactivation in 47,XXY and 48,XXYY Klinefelter patients. Am J Med Genet. 2001;98:25-31.
38. Groth KA, Skakkebæk A, Høst C, Gravholt CH, Bojesen A. Clinical review: Klinefelter syndrome—a clinical update. J Clin Endocrinol Metab. 2013;98:20-30.
39. Samplaski MK, Lo KC, Grober ED, Millar A, Dimitromanolakis A, Jarvi KA. Phenotypic differences in mosaic Klinefelter patients as compared with non-mosaic Klinefelter patients. Fertil Steril. 2014;101:950-5.
40. Wosnitzer MS, Paduch DA. Endocrinological issues and hormonal manipulation in children and men with Klinefelter syndrome. Am J Med Genet C Semin Med Genet. 2013;163C:16-26.
41. Kamischke A, Baumgardt A, Horst J, Nieschlag E. Clinical and diagnostic features of patients with suspected Klinefelter syndrome. J Androl. 2003;24:41-8.
42. Tournaye H, Staessen C, Liebaers I, Van Assche E, Devroey P, Bonduelle M, et al. Testicular sperm recovery in nine 47,XXY Klinefelter patients. Hum Reprod. 1996;11:1644-9.
43. Westlander G, Ekerhovd E, Granberg S, Hanson L, Hanson C, Bergh C. Testicular ultrasonography and extended chromosome analysis in men with nonmosaic Klinefelter syndrome: a prospective study of possible predictive factors for successful sperm recovery. Fertil Steril. 2001;75:1102-5.
44. Rucker GB, Mielnik A, King P, Goldstein M, Schlegel PN. Preoperative screening for genetic abnormalities in men with nonobstructive azoospermia before testicular sperm extraction. J Urol. 1998;160:2068-71.
45. Fullerton G, Hamilton M, Maheshwari A. Should non-mosaic Klinefelter syndrome men be labelled as infertile in 2009? Hum Reprod. 2010;25:588-97.
46. Staessen C, Tournaye H, Van Assche E, Michiels A, Van Landuyt L, Devroey P, et al. PGD in 47,XXY Klinefelter's syndrome patients. Hum Reprod Update. 2003;9:319-30.
47. Abramsky L, Chapple J. 47,XXY (Klinefelter syndrome) and 47,XYY: estimated rates of and indication for postnatal diagnosis with implications for prenatal counselling. Prenat Diagn. 1997;17:363-8.

48. Gonzalez-Merino E, Hans C, Abramowicz M, Englert Y, Emiliani S. Aneuploidy study in sperm and preimplantation embryos from nonmosaic 47,XYY men. Fertil Steril. 2007;88:600-6.
49. Wu C, Wang L, Iqbal F, Jiang X, Bukhari I, Guo T, et al. Preferential Y-Y pairing and synapsis and abnormal meiotic recombination in a 47,XYY man with non obstructive azoospermia. Mol Cytogenet. 2016;9:9.
50. Anik A, Çatli G, Abaci A, Böber E. 46,XX male disorder of sexual development: a case report. J Clin Res Pediatr Endocrinol. 2013;5:258-60.
51. Li TF, Wu QY, Zhang C, Li WW, Zhou Q, Jiang WJ, et al. 46,XX testicular disorder of sexual development with SRY-negative caused by some unidentified mechanisms: a case report and review of the literature. BMC Urol. 2014;14:104.
52. Hyon C, Chantot-Bastaraud S, Harbuz R, Bhouri R, Perrot N, Peycelon M, et al. Refining the regulatory region upstream of SOX9 associated with 46,XX testicular disorders of sex development (DSD). Am J Med Genet A. 2015;167A:1851-8.
53. Johannisson R, Schwinger E, Wolff HH, vom Ende V, Löhrs U. The effect of 13;14 Robertsonian translocations on germ-cell differentiation in infertile males. Cytogenet Cell Genet. 1993;63:151-5.
54. Odorisio T, Rodriguez TA, Evans EP, Clarke AR, Burgoyne PS. The meiotic checkpoint monitoring synapsis eliminates spermatocytes via p53-independent apoptosis. Nat Genet. 1998;18:257-61.
55. Keymolen K, Van Berkel K, Vorsselmans A, Staessen C, Liebaers I. Pregnancy outcome in carriers of Robertsonian translocations. Am J Med Genet A. 2011;155A:2381-5.
56. Godo A, Blanco J, Vidal F, Sandalinas M, Garcia-Guixé E, Anton E. Altered segregation pattern and numerical chromosome abnormalities interrelate in spermatozoa from Robertsonian translocation carriers. Reprod Biomed Online. 2015;31:79-88.
57. Dana M, Stoian V. Association of pericentric inversion of chromosome 9 and infertility in Romanian population. Maedica (Bucur). 2012;7:25-9.
58. Mozdarani H, Meybodi AM, Karimi H. Impact of pericentric inversion of chromosome 9 [INV (9) (p11q12)] on infertility. Indian J Hum Genet. 2007;13:26-9.
59. Collodel G, Moretti E, Capitani S, Piomboni P, Anichini C, Estenoz M, et al. TEM, FISH and molecular studies in infertile men with pericentric inversion of chromosome 9. Andrologia. 2006;38:122-7.
60. Krausz C, Degl'Innocenti S. Y chromosome and male infertility: update, 2006. Front Biosci. 2006;11:3049-61.
61. Vogt PH, Edelmann A, Kirsch S, Henegariu O, Hirschmann P, Kiesewetter F, et al. Human Y chromosome azoospermia factors (AZF) mapped to different subregions in Yq11. Hum Mol Genet. 1996;5:933-43.
62. Hopps CV, Mielnik A, Goldstein M, Palermo GD, Rosenwaks Z, Schlegel PN. Detection of sperm in men with Y chromosome microdeletions of the AZFA, AZFB and AZFC regions. Hum Reprod. 2003;18:1660-5.
63. Asero P, Calogero AE, Condorelli RA, Mongioi' L, Vicari E, Lanzafame F, et al. Relevance of genetic investigation in male infertility. J Endocrinol Invest. 2014;37:415-27.
64. Saxena R, de Vries JW, Repping S, Alagappan RK, Skaletsky H, Brown LG, et al. Four *DAZ* genes in two clusters found in the *AZFc* region of the human Y chromosome. Genomics. 2000;67:256-67.
65. Stahl PJ, Masson P, Mielnik A, Marean MB, Schlegel PN, Paduch DA. A decade of experience emphasizes that testing for Y microdeletions is essential in American men with azoospermia and severe oligozoospermia. Fertil Steril. 2010;94:1753-6.
66. Brandell RA, Mielnik A, Liotta D, Ye Z, Veeck LL, Palermo GD, et al. AZFb deletions predict the absence of spermatozoa with testicular sperm extraction: preliminary report of a prognostic genetic test. Hum Reprod. 1998;13:2812-5.
67. Krausz C, Quintana-Murci L, McElreavey K. Prognostic value of Y deletion analysis: what is the clinical prognostic value of Y chromosome microdeletion analysis? Hum Reprod. 2000;15:1431-4.
68. Giwercman YL, Nikoshkov A, Byström B, Pousette A, Arver S, Wedell A. A novel mutation (N233K) in the transactivating domain and the N756S mutation in the ligand binding domain of the androgen receptor gene are associated with male infertility. Clin Endocrinol (Oxf). 2001;54:827-34.
69. Hiort O, Holterhus PM, Horter T, Schulze W, Kremke B, Bals-Pratsch M, et al. Significance of mutations in the androgen receptor gene in males with idiopathic infertility. J Clin Endocrinol Metabol. 2000;85:2810-5.
70. Wang Q, Ghadessy FJ, Yong EL. Analysis of the transactivation domain of the androgen receptor in patients with male infertility. Clin Genet. 1998;54:185-92.
71. Yong EL, Loy CJ, Sim KS. Androgen receptor gene and male infertility. Hum Reprod Update. 2003;9:1-7.
72. Beales PL, Elcioglu N, Woolf AS, Parker D, Flinter FA. New criteria for improved diagnosis of Bardet-Biedl syndrome: results of a population survey. J Med Genet. 1999;36:437-46.
73. Green JS, Parfrey PS, Harnett JD, Farid NR, Cramer BC, Johnson G, et al. The cardinal manifestations of Bardet-Biedl syndrome, a form of Laurence-Moon-Biedl syndrome. N Engl J Med. 1989;321:1002-9.
74. Katsanis N, Ansley SJ, Badano JL, Eichers ER, Lewis RA, Hoskins BE, et al. Triallelic inheritance in Bardet-Biedl syndrome, a Mendelian recessive disorder. Science. 2001;293:2256-9.
75. Mykytyn K, Nishimura DY, Searby CC, Beck G, Bugge K, Haines HL, et al. Evaluation of complex inheritance involving the most common Bardet-Biedl syndrome locus (BBS1). Am J Hum Genet. 2003;72:429-37.
76. Vogels A, Fryns JP. The Prader-Willi syndrome and the Angelman syndrome. Genet Couns. 2002;13:385-96.
77. Cardenas-Rodriguez M, Badano JL. Ciliary biology: understanding the cellular and genetic basis of human ciliopathies. Am J Med Genet C Semin Med Genet. 2009;151C:263-80.
78. Elsawi MM, Pryor JP, Klufio G, Barnes C, Patton MA. Genital tract function in men with Noonan syndrome. J Med Genet. 1994;31:468-70.
79. Castellani C, Picci L, Tamanini A, Girardi P, Rizzotti P, Assael BM. Association between carrier screening and incidence of cystic fibrosis. JAMA. 2009;302:2573-9.
80. Dubin L, Amelar RD. Etiologic factors in 1294 consecutive cases of male infertility. Fertil Steril. 1971;22:469-74.
81. Kerem B, Rommens JM, Buchanan JA, Markiewicz D, Cox TK, Chakravarti A, et al. Identification of the cystic fibrosis gene: genetic analysis. Science. 1989;245:1073-80.
82. Rommens JM, Iannuzzi MC, Kerem B, Drumm ML, Melmer G, Dean M, et al. Identification of the cystic

fibrosis gene: chromosome walking and jumping. Science. 1989;245:1059-65.

83. Sharma H, Mavuduru RS, Singh SK, Prasad R. Increased frequency of CFTR gene mutations identified in Indian infertile men with non-CBAVD obstructive azoospermia and spermatogenic failure. Gene. 2014;548:43-7.
84. Goldstein M, Schlossberg S. Men with congenital absence of the vas deferens often have seminal vesicles. J Urol. 1988;140:85-6.
85. Elhanbly S, El-Saied MA, Fawzy M, El-Refaeey A, Mostafa T. Relationship of paternal age with outcome of percutaneous epididymal sperm aspiration-intracytoplasmic sperm injection, in cases of congenital bilateral absence of the vas deferens. Fertil Steril. 2015;104:602-6.
86. Llabador MA, Pagin A, Lefebvre-Maunoury C, Marcelli F, Leroy-Martin B, Rigot JM, et al. Congenital bilateral absence of the vas deferens: the impact of spermatogenesis quality on intracytoplasmic sperm injection outcomes in 108 men. Andrology. 2015;3:473-80.
87. Hendry WF, A'Hern RP, Cole PJ. Was Young's syndrome caused by exposure to mercury in childhood? BMJ. 1993;307:1579-82.
88. Dada R, Kumar M, Jesudasan R, Fernández JL, Gosálvez J, Agarwal A. Epigenetics and its role in male infertility. J Assist Reprod Genet. 2012;29:213-23.
89. Anway MD, Cupp AS, Uzumcu M, Skinner MK. Epigenetic transgenerational actions of endocrine disruptors and male fertility. Science. 2005;308:1466-9.
90. Donkin I, Versteyhe S, Ingerslev LR, Qian K, Mechta M, Nordkap L, et al. Obesity and bariatric surgery drive epigenetic variation of spermatozoa in humans. Cell Metab. 2016;23:369-78.
91. Stuppia L, Franzago M, Ballerini P, Gatta V, Antonucci I. Epigenetics and male reproduction: the consequences of paternal lifestyle on fertility, embryo development, and children lifetime health. Clin Epigenetics. 2015;7:120.
92. González-Marin C, Gosálvez J, Roy R. Types, causes, detection and repair of DNA fragmentation in animal and human sperm cells. Int J Mol Sci. 2012;13:14026-52.
93. Aitken RJ, De Iuliis GN. On the possible origins of DNA damage in human spermatozoa. Mol Hum Reprod. 2010;16:3-13.
94. Greco E, Scarselli F, Iacobelli M, Rienzi L, Ubaldi F, Ferrero S, et al. Efficient treatment of infertility due to sperm DNA damage by ICSI with testicular spermatozoa. Hum Reprod. 2005;20:226-30.
95. Neto FT, Bach PV, Najari BB, Li PS, Goldstein M. Spermatogenesis in humans and its affecting factors. Semin Cell Dev Biol. 2016;59:10.
96. Aitken RJ, Koppers AJ. Apoptosis and DNA damage in human spermatozoa. Asian J Androl. 2011;13:36-42.
97. Spanò M, Bonde JP, Hjøllund HI, Kolstad HA, Cordelli E, Leter G. Sperm chromatin damage impairs human fertility. The Danish First Pregnancy Planner Study Team. Fertil Steril. 2000;73:43-50.
98. Zidi-Jrah I, Hajlaoui A, Mougou-Zerelli S, Kammoun M, Meniaoui I, Sallem A, et al. Relationship between sperm aneuploidy, sperm DNA integrity, chromatin packaging, traditional semen parameters, and recurrent pregnancy loss. Fertil Steril. 2016;105:58-64.
99. Osman A, Alsomait H, Seshadri S, El-Toukhy T, Khalaf Y. The effect of sperm DNA fragmentation on live birth rate after IVF or ICSI: a systematic review and meta-analysis. Reprod Biomed Online. 2015;30:120-7.
100. Jarow JP, Coburn M, Sigman M. Incidence of varicoceles in men with primary and secondary infertility. Urology. 1996;47(1):73-6.
101. Sayfan J, Soffer Y, Orda R. Varicocele treatment: prospective randomized trial of 3 methods. J Urol. 1992;148(5):1447-9.
102. Gorelick JI, Goldstein M. Loss of fertility in men with varicocele. Fertil Steril. 1993;59(3):613-6.
103. Trum JW, Gubler FM, Laan R, van der Veen F. The value of palpation, varicoscreen contact thermography and colour Doppler ultrasound in the diagnosis of varicocele. Hum Reprod. 1996;11(6):1232-5.
104. World Health Organization. The influence of varicocele on parameters of fertility in a large group of men presenting to infertility clinics. Fertil Steril. 1992;57(6):1289-93.
105. Zhao LC, Lautz TB, Meeks JJ, Maizels M. Pediatric testicular torsion epidemiology using a national database: incidence, risk of orchiectomy and possible measures toward improving the quality of care. J Urol. 2011;186(5):2009-13.
106. Davis JE, Silverman M. Scrotal emergencies. Emerg Med Clin North Am. 2011;29(3):469-84.
107. Molokwu CN, Somani BK, Goodman CM. Outcomes of scrotal exploration for acute scrotal pain suspicious of testicular torsion: a consecutive case series of 173 patients. BJU Int. 2011;107(6):990-3.
108. Srinivasan A, Cinman N, Feber KM, Gitlin J, Palmer LS. History and physical examination findings predictive of testicular torsion: an attempt to promote clinical diagnosis by house staff. J Pediatr Urol. 2011;7(4):470-4.
109. Hadziselimovic F, Geneto R, Emmons LR. Increased apoptosis in the contralateral testes of patients with testicular torsion as a factor for infertility. J Urol. 1998;160:1158-60.
110. EAU Guidelines; 2010. https://uroweb.org/guidelines
111. Chandra RV, Dowling RJ, Ulubasoglu M, Haxhimolla H, Costello AJ. Rational approach to diagnosis and management of blunt scrotal trauma. Urology. 2007;70(2):230-4.
112. Beni-Israel T, Goldman M, Bar Chaim S, Kozer E. Clinical predictors for testicular torsion as seen in pediatric ED. Am J Emerg Med. 2010;28(7):786-9.
113. Lipshultz L, Howards S, Niederberger C. Infertility in the Male, 4th edition. Cambridge, UK: Cambridge University Press; 2009.
114. Nieschlag E, Behre HM, Nieschlag S. Andrology: Male Reproductive Health and Dysfunction, 3rd edition. Heidelberg, Germany: Springer; 2009.
115. Cunningham KA, Beagley KW. Male genital tract chlamydial infection: implications for pathology and infertility. Biol Reprod. 2008;79:180-9.
116. Raheem AA, Ralph D, Minhas S. Male infertility. BJMSU. 2012;5:254-68.
117. Davis NF, McGuire BB, Mahon JA, Smyth AE, O'Malley KJ, Fitzpatrick JM. The increasing incidence of mumps orchitis: a comprehensive review. BJU Int. 2010;105(8):1060-5.
118. Skakkebæk NE, Berthelsen JG, Giwercman A, Müller J. Carcinoma-in-situ of the testis: possible origin from gonocytes and precursor of all types of germ cell tumours except spermatocytoma. Intl J Androl. 1987:10(1):19-28.
119. Rajpert-De Meyts E. Developmental model for the pathogenesis of testicular carcinoma in situ: genetic and environmental aspects. Human Reprod Update. 2006;12(3): 303-23.

120. Jacobsen R, Bostofte E, Engholm G, Hansen J, Olsen JH, Skakkebaek NE, et al. Risk of testicular cancer in men with abnormal semen characteristics: cohort study. BMJ. 2000;321(7264):789-92.
121. Møller H, Skakkebaek NE. Risk of testicular cancer in subfertile men: case-control study. BJM. 1999;318(7183):559-62.
122. Huyghe E, Matsuda T, Thonneau P. Increasing incidence of testicular cancer worldwide: a review. J Urol. 2003;170(1):5-11.
123. Huyghe E, Plante P, Thonneau PF. Testicular cancer variations in time and space in Europe. Eur Urol. 2007;51(3):621-8.
124. Abuelhija M, Weng CC, Shetty G, Meistrich ML. Rat models of post-irradiation recovery of spermatogenesis: interstrain differences. Andrology. 2013;1:206-15.
125. Du Plessis SS, Agarwal A, Sabanegh Jr ES. Male Infertility: A Complete Guide to Lifestyle and Environmental Factors. New York: Springer; 2014.
126. Bujan L, Walschaerts M, Moinard N, Hennebicq S, Saias J, Brugnon F, et al. Impact of chemotherapy and radiotherapy for testicular germ cell tumors on spermatogenesis and sperm DNA: a multicenter prospective study from the CECOS network. Fertil Steril. 2013;100:673-80.
127. Di Bisceglie C, Bertagna A, Composto ER, Lanfranco F, Baldi M, Motta G, et al. Effects of oncological treatments on semen quality in patients with testicular neoplasia or lymphoproliferative disorders. Asian J Androl. 2013;15:425-9.
128. Samplaski MK, Nangia AK. Adverse effects of common medications on male fertility. Nat Rev Urol. 2015;12(7):401-13.
129. Fronczak CM, Kim ED, Barqawi AB. The insults of illicit drug use on male fertility. J Androl. 2012;33(4):515-28.
130. Meri ZB, Irshid IB, Migdadi M, Irshid AB, Mhanna SA. Does cigarette smoking affect seminal fluid parameters? A comparative study. Oman Med J. 2013;28(1):12-5.
131. Palmer NO, Bakos HW, Fullston T, Lane M. Impact of obesity on male fertility, sperm function and molecular composition. Spermatogenesis. 2012;2(4):253-63.
132. Hansen J, Sato M, Ruedy R. Perception of climate change. Proc Natl Acad Sci U S A. 2012;109(37):E2415-23.
133. Weidner W, Anderson RU. Evaluation of acute and chronic bacterial prostatitis and diagnostic management of chronic prostatitis/chronic pelvic pain syndrome with special reference to infection/inflammation. Int J Antimicrob Agents. 2008;31(Suppl. 1):S91-5.
134. Schneider H, Ludwig M, Hossain HM, Diemer T, Weidner W. The 2001 Giessen cohort study on patients with prostatitis syndrome—an evaluation of inflammatory status and search for microorganisms 10 years after a first analysis. Andrologia. 2003;35:258-62.
135. Krausz C, Mills C, Rogers S, Tan SL, Aitken RJ. Stimulation of oxidant generation by human sperm suspensions using phorbol esters and formyl peptides: relationships with motility and fertilization in vitro. Fertil Steril. 1994;62:599-605.
136. Jequier AM. Obstructive azoospermia: a study of 102 patients. Clin Reprod Fertil. 1985:3:21-36.
137. Hendry W. Azoospermia and surgery for testicular obstruction. In: Hargreave TB (Ed). Male Infertility. Berlin: Springer Verlag; 1997.
138. Hendry WF, Parslow JM, Stedronska J. Exploratory scrototomy in 168 azoospermic males. Br J Urol. 1983;55(6):785-91.
139. Pierik FH, Vreeburg JT, Stijnen T, De Jong FH, Weber RF. Serum inhibin B as a marker of spermatogenesis. J Clin Endocrinol Metab. 1998;83(9):3110-4.
140. Oates RD, Amos JA. The genetic basis of congenital bilateral absence of the vas deferens and cystic fibrosis. J Androl. 1994;15(1):1-8.
141. Handelsman DJ, Conway AJ, Boylan LM, Turtle JR. Young's syndrome. Obstructive azoospermia and chronic sinopulmonary infections. N Engl J Med. 1984;310(1):3-9.
142. Schoysman R. Vaso-epididymostomy—a survey of techniques and results with considerations of delay of appearance of spermatozoa after surgery. Acta Eur Fertil. 1990;21(5):239-45.
143. Silber SJ, Grotjan HE. Microscopic vasectomy reversal 30 years later: a summary of 4010 cases by the same surgeon. J Androl. 2004;25(6):845-59.
144. Jarvi K, Zini A, Buckspan MB, Asch M, Ginzburg B, Margolis M. Adverse effects on vasoepididymostomy outcomes for men with concomitant abnormalities in the prostate and seminal vesicle. J Urol. 1998;160(4):1410-2.
145. Matthews GJ, Schlegel PN, Goldstein M. Patency following microsurgical vasoepididymostomy and vasovasostomy: temporal considerations. J Urol. 1995;154(6):2070-3.
146. Borovikov A. Treatment of large vasal defects. In: Goldstein M (Ed). Surgery of Male Infertility. Philadelphia: WB Saunders; 1995. pp. 77-95.
147. Shin D, Lipshultz LI, Goldstein M, Barmé GA, Fuchs EF, Nagler HM, et al. Herniorrhaphy with polypropylene mesh causing inguinal vasal obstruction: a preventable cause of obstructive azoospermia. Ann Surg. 2005;241(4):553-8.
148. Schlegel PN, Shin D, Goldstein M. Urogenital anomalies in men with congenital absence of the vas deferens. J Urol. 1996:155(5):1644-8.
149. Schroeder-Printzen I, Ludwig M, Köhn F, Weidner W. Surgical therapy in infertile men with ejaculatory duct obstruction: technique and outcome of a standardized surgical approach. Hum Reprod. 2000;15(6):1364-8.
150. Kuligowska E, Baker CE, Oates RD. Male infertility: role of transrectal US in diagnosis and management. Radiology. 1992;185(2):353-60.
151. Colpi GM, Casella F, Zanollo A, Ballerini G, Balerna M, Campana A, et al. Functional voiding disturbances of the ampullo-vesicular seminal tract: a cause of male infertility. Acta Eur Fertil. 1987;18(3):165-79.
152. Chan PTK, Schlegel PN. Inflammatory conditions of the male excurrent ductal system. Part I. J Androl. 2002;23(4):453-60.
153. Bols B, Jensen L, Jensen A, Braendstrup O. Immunopathology of in situ seminoma. Int J Exp Pathol. 2000;81(3):211-7.
154. Sarkar O, Bahrainwala J, Chandrasekaran S, Kothari S, Mathur PP, Agarwal A. Impact of inflammation on male fertility. Front Biosci. 2011;3:89-95.
155. Liew SH, Meachem SJ, Hedger MP. A stereological analysis of the response of spermatogenesis to an acute inflammatory episode in adult rats. J Androl. 2007;28(1):176-85
156. Hong CY, Park JH, Ahn RS, Im SY, Choi HS, Soh J, et al. Molecular mechanism of suppression of testicular steroidogenesis by proinflammatory cytokine tumor necrosis factor alpha. Mol Cell Biol. 2004;24(7):2593-604.
157. Calkins JH, Guo H, Sigel MM, Lin T. Tumor necrosis factor-alpha enhances inhibitory effects of interleukin-1 beta on Leydig cell steroidogenesis. Biochem Biophys Res Commun. 1990;166(3):1313-8.
158. Fraczek M, Kurpisz M. Inflammatory mediators exert toxic effects of oxidative stress on human spermatozoa. J Androl. 2007;28(2):325-33.

159. Whittington K, Ford WC. Relative contribution of leukocytes and of spermatozoa to reactive oxygen species production in human sperm suspensions. Int J Androl. 1999;22(4):229-35.
160. Hedger MP. Immunophysiology and pathology of inflammation in the testis and epididymis. J Androl. 2011;32(6):625-40.
161. Weidner W, Krause W, Ludwig M. Relevance of male accessory gland infection for subsequent fertility with special focus on prostatitis. Hum Reprod Update. 1999;5(5):421-32.
162. Diemer T, Huwe P, Michelmann HW, Mayer F, Schiefer HG, Weidner W. Escherichia coli-induced alterations of human spermatozoa. An electron microscopy analysis. Int J Androl. 2000;23(3):178-86.
163. Kang X, Xie Q, Zhou X, Li F, Huang J, Liu D, et al. Effects of hepatitis B virus S protein exposure on sperm membrane integrity and functions. PLoS One. 2012;7(3):e33471.
164. Reichart M, Kahane I, Bartoov B. In vivo and in vitro impairment of human and ram sperm nuclear chromatin integrity by sexually transmitted Ureaplasma urealyticum infection. Biol Reprod. 2000;63(4):1041-8.
165. Hamada A, Esteves SC, Nizza M, Agarwal A. Unexplained male infertility: diagnosis and management. Int Braz J Urol. 2012;38(5):576-94.
166. Agarwal A, Prabakaran S, Allamaneni SS. Relationship between oxidative stress, varicocele and infertility: a meta-analysis. Reprod Biomed Online. 2006;12(5):630-3.
167. Du Plessis SS, Agarwal A, Halabi J, Tvrda E. Contemporary evidence on the physiological role of reactive oxygen species in human sperm function. J Assist Reprod Genet. 2015;32(4):509-20.
168. Kothari S, Thompson A, Agarwal A, du Plessis SS. Free radicals: their beneficial and detrimental effects on sperm function. Indian J Exp Biol. 2010;48(5):425-35.
169. Koppers AJ, De Iuliis GN, Finnie JM, McLaughlin EA, Aitken RJ. Significance of mitochondrial reactive oxygen species in the generation of oxidative stress in spermatozoa. J Clin Endocrinol Metab. 2008;93(8):3199-207.
170. Aitken RJ, Smith TB, Jobling MS, Baker MA, De Iuliis GN. Oxidative stress and male reproductive health. Asian J Androl. 2014;16(1):31-8.
171. Gil-Villa AM, Cardona-Maya W, Agarwal A, Sharma R, Cadavid A. Role of male factor in early recurrent embryo loss: do antioxidants have any effect? Fertil Steril. 2009;92(2):565-71.
172. Zhou P, Yang XL, Wang XG, Hu B, Zhang L, Zhang W, et al. A pneumonia outbreak associated with a new coronavirus of probable bat origin. Nature. 2020;579(7798):270-3.
173. Cheng CY, Mruk DD. The blood-testis barrier and its implications for male contraception. Pharmacol Rev. 2012;64(1):16-64.
174. Chen Y, Guo Y, Pan Y, Zhao ZJ. Structure analysis of the receptor binding of 2019-nCoV. Biochem Biophys Res Commun. 2020;525(1):135-40.
175. Holshue ML, DeBolt C, Lindquist S, Lofy KH, Wiesman J, Bruce H, et al. First case of 2019 novel coronavirus in the United States. New Engl J Med. 2020;382(10):929-36.
176. Wang Z, Xu X. scRNA-seq profiling of human testes reveals the presence of the ACE2 receptor, a target for SARS-CoV-2 infection in spermatogonia, Leydig and Sertoli cells. Cells. 2020;9(4):920.
177. Shen Q, Xiao X, Aierken A, Yue W, Wu X, Liao M, et al. The ACE2 expression in Sertoli cells and germ cells may cause male reproductive disorder after SARS-CoV-2 infection. J Cell Mol Med. 2020;24(16):9472-7.
178. Hoffmann M, Kleine-Weber H, Schroeder S, Krüger N, Herrler T, Erichsen S, et al. SARS-CoV-2 cell entry depends on ACE2 and TMPRSS2 and is blocked by a clinically proven protease inhibitor. Cell. 2020;181(2):271-80.
179. Chen Y-W, Lee M-S, Lucht A, Chou F-P, Huang W, Havighurst TC, et al. TMPRSS2, a serine protease expressed in the prostate on the apical surface of luminal epithelial cells and released into semen in prostasomes, is misregulated in prostate cancer cells. Am J Pathol. 2010;176(6):2986-96.
180. Ma L, Xie W, Li D, Shi L, Mao Y, Xiong Y, et al. Effect of SARS-CoV-2 infection upon male gonadal function: a single center-based study. MedRxiv. 2020.
181. Li D, Jin M, Bao P, Zhao W, Zhang S. Clinical characteristics and results of semen tests among men with coronavirus disease 2019. JAMA Netw Open. 2020;3(5):e208292.
182. Xu J, Qi L, Chi X, Yang J, Wei X, Gong E, et al. Orchitis: a complication of severe acute respiratory syndrome (SARS). Biol Reprod. 2006;74(2):410-6.
183. Ma H, Zeng W, He H, Zhao D, Jiang D, Zhou P, et al. Serum IgA, IgM, and IgG responses in COVID-19. Cell Mol Immunol. 2020;17(7):773-5.
184. Checconi P, De Angelis M, Marcocci ME, Fraternale A, Magnani M, Palamara AT, et al. Redox-modulating agents in the treatment of viral infections. Int J Mol Sci. 2020;21(11):4084.
185. Snick HK, Snick TS, Evers JL, Collins JA. The spontaneous pregnancy prognosis in untreated subfertile couples: the Walcheren primary care study. Hum Reprod. 1997;12(7):1582-8.
186. Rowe T. Fertility and a woman's age. J Reprod Med. 2006;51(3):157-63.

CHAPTER 25

Clinical and Endocrinological Evaluation of Infertile Male

Radha Pandiyan, S Sowbarnika, D Ramesh Raja, N Pandiyan

INTRODUCTION

Male infertility evades a precise definition. Semen analysis gives a descriptive picture about the spermatozoa and does not necessarily confirm whether the man is fertile or infertile except in extreme situations such as azoospermia, aspermia, total asthenozoospermia, total necrozoospermia, and total teratozoospermia.

World Health Organization (WHO) defines infertility as "A disease affecting the physical, mental, and psychological well-being of the individual." Recent statistics from WHO[1] quote that infertility affects 15% of couples worldwide, while male factor infertility has been acknowledged widely to contribute to 40–50% of the infertile couples.[2]

An unpublished observation for a duration of 2 years, in the Department of Andrology and Reproductive Medicine, Chettinad Academy of Research and Education, Chennai, India, states that the incidence of male factor infertility accounts for about 14% among the total infertile couples.

Sadly, the role of the male partner is diminished to that of a "spermiator" providing semen samples on demand in many infertility clinics. It was also wrongly believed that there is no role for the Andrologist in the present intracytoplasmic sperm injection (ICSI) era.

As the field of human reproduction is ever evolving to reach newer heights, male factor infertility too deserves equal focus, if not more than the female partner. Assisted reproduction is often performed today for male factor infertility. It is needless to say that there is a compelling need to train not only specialists in andrology but also provide working knowledge to the general practitioners in the field of andrology—to identify correctable problems and to refer them to the proper center as early as possible for the correct approach and management.

AIM OF EVALUATION OF THE INFERTILE MALE

This primarily targets the assessment of spermatogenic and endocrine function:

- To identify the probable cause and treat it for achieving spontaneous pregnancy, if possible
- To refer patients with irremediable causes for higher reproductive technologies
- To diagnose and offer concurrent genetic counseling in specific circumstances
- To diagnose testicular malignancies and pituitary lesions, which may be associated with infertility[3] as the leading complaint. This latter may become a cause for sexual dysfunction **(Table 1 and Box 1)**.

TABLE 1: Causes for male infertility.[3]

Causes	*Percentage*
Varicocele (?)	12
Primary idiopathic testicular failure	10
Male accessory gland infection	7
Abnormal sperm morphology	6
Sexual problems	2
Other seminal fluid abnormalities	4
Decreased sperm motility	4
Immunological causes	3
Azoospermia owing to obstruction	1
Endocrine and other causes	4
No demonstrable cause	47

BOX 1: Provocative causes for male infertility.

Provocative causes

Lifestyle factors:[4]
- Smoking
- Alcohol, drug usage
- Obesity

Environmental factors:
- Endocrine-disrupting chemicals[5] (plastics, perfumes, food additives, food storage materials, children's products)
- Environmental toxins[6] (fertilizers, industrial solvents, lubricants, pesticides)

Pharmaceutical drugs[7]

Radiation[8,9]
- Mobile phones, laptops, microwaves, Wi-Fi gadgets, wireless devices, X-rays, nuclear radiation

PRINCIPLES OF MANAGEMENT OF THE MALE PARTNER

Evaluation and management of a male partner should focus on the following:

- Initiating and maintaining spermatozoa production
- Testicular endocrine function
- Treatment of genital tract infections, if any
- Management of retrograde ejaculation
- Decreasing free radicals and enhancing spermatozoa motility
- Correcting sexual dysfunction, if present.

PART I: CLINICAL EVALUATION OF INFERTILE MALE

History

A detailed history brings the significant factors[10] affecting the fertility of the individuals to light and a simple correction of them would restore their fertility. Gametes being the single and specialized cells in the human body are very much liable to be influenced by any disturbances in the health status of the individual. The following sections will help in understanding various factors influencing fertility of the individual.

Prerequisites for History Taking

- The consultation room should offer total privacy, a calm atmosphere, and a comfortable setting for the couple.
- The female partner is encouraged to be present along with the male partner during history taking—at least initially; this is preferable, unless not desired by either or both of them.
- Patients should be allowed to present their history without interrupting their flow of thoughts, at the same time guiding them back to the point, if they go astray. A recent study found that patients are often interrupted within 40 seconds of their narration.[11]
- It is the clinician's duty to provide adequate time to the couple for discussion. Questions should be encouraged from both partners for free discussion and guidance.

Age of the Male Partner

Though the age of the female markedly influences the outcome of treatment to a greater extent, the age of the male partner, especially after 40 years,[12] has a significant impact too. Aneuploidies are more common in the embryos generated by older men leading to increased pregnancy losses.[13,14]

There is a natural decline in testosterone levels in aging men; they may also have other underlying systemic illnesses, both leading to sexual dysfunction as a result of the illnesses per se and/or as side effects of the medications used.[15]

Occupational and Environmental History

Specifically, occupations involving direct handling of chemicals, pesticides, and radiation[9] would certainly impact semen parameters and lead to infertility.[16,17] A pilot study by Benziger et al. clearly brought out the impact of mobile phone irradiation on the motility of semen samples.[8]

Kesari et al. also explain in their review paper that exposure to radiofrequency electromagnetic fields (RF-EMFs) inhibits the cellular metabolism which leads to oxidative stress, which in turn raises the reactive oxygen species (ROS), and is likely to lead to male infertility. They express concerns about "electrosmog" and emphasize the need to restrict the usage of wireless and electronic gadgets, especially by the younger generation, though there is no final word about the impact of their ill effects on health and reproduction.[9]

Similarly, any history of exposure to high heat, disturbed sleep, and nutrition and/or increased stress would also influence semen quality.[10]

Exposure to volatile compounds[18] can result in temporary suppression of gonadotropin secretion and increase in prolactin levels. They have a major impact on spermatozoa production and sexual function.

Substance Abuse: A Truly Reversible Cause

This history is often not considered or ignored by both the patients and physicians. Cigarette smoking, either active or passive, primary, secondary, or tertiary is a well-known cause of deranged seminal parameters—a truly reversible cause for male infertility.[19,20] Similarly, excessive alcohol intake is known to impair sexual function.[21] Hard drugs such as cannabis/marijuana and cocaine hamper the sexual desire and decrease the performance.[21]

Sexual History: The Basic Step in Reproduction

Though it is a very sensitive subject, a detailed sexual history (frequency/week, erection, intravaginal penetration and ejaculation) is mandatory to ensure proper coital practice, which is the basic step in natural reproduction. This can also reveal a correctable cause of infertility such as the use of lubricants during the act. Spermatozoa are known to survive only in the natural vaginal secretions and not in any other artificial solutions/liquid. Most of these lubricants are either spermiostatic or spermicidal. Pregnancies have happened by simply stopping the use of lubricants.[22] Nonconsummation of marriage, infrequent sexual intercourse, and improper techniques are potentially treatable causes for male infertility. Though there is no prescribed norm for sexual frequency, sexual intercourse on at least alternate days optimizes the chances of natural pregnancy.[23]

Fertility History

Duration of marriage; past conception if any, either with the present partner or previous partner, or other partners; and any previous treatment for infertility are all crucial to ascertain the current fertility potential of the male partner.

Sexual Dysfunction

Sexual dysfunction includes both erectile and ejaculatory dysfunction. Many men with normal sexual function start developing sexual dysfunction after the diagnosis of infertility. It could be due to the diagnosis per se or due to the rigmarole of semen collection on demand or performance anxiety (sex on demand).[24] Many a times, couples report to us for only infertility, masking their sexual dysfunction. There are also men who cannot masturbate and situational anejaculation is a common mini-emergency in the infertility clinics. Sexual dysfunction (erectile dysfunction) and infertility can also be due to hyperprolactinemia. This again is another medically treatable cause for male infertility.[25]

Some medical drugs administered for other diseases can also impair sexual dysfunction **(Table 2)**.[7] This is often unnoticed or not paid enough importance. Statins are the most widely used drug. They may cause sexual dysfunction.[26]

A detailed history and guidance by the andrologist would go a long way in alleviating this problem. Retrograde ejaculation should be suspected, if there is no history of antegrade ejaculate or history of passing cloudy urine postcoitally.

Medical History

Past/present medical illnesses such as diabetes mellitus, hypertension, liver and renal failure, urinary tract infections, sexually transmitted infections, and other infections such as chlamydia, gonococcus, and tuberculosis may impair a man's fertility either by the disease per se or due to the long-term use of medications affecting both spermatogenesis and sexual function[7,27] **(Table 3)**.

Gastroesophageal reflux disease (GERD) or acid peptic disease is a common condition often treated by H2-receptor antagonists. These drugs are known to impair sexual function.[28] Agents such as salazopyrin used for the treatment of ulcerative colitis cause changes in semen quality.[29]

Men with azoospermia visit chest clinic repeatedly due to bronchiectasis which could be because of Kartagener's syndrome (immotile cilia syndrome)[30] or cystic fibrosis associated with congenital bilateral absence of the vas deferens (CBAVD).[31]

History of chronic diseases such as bronchiectasis or sinusitis may suggest obstruction of excurrent ducts from testes due to inspissated testicular secretions, in a condition called Young's syndrome.

Another aspect of history is the treatment for malignancies with chemotherapy and/or radiations. If fertility preservation was not done prior to the therapy, it may lead to irremediable infertility.[7]

Surgical History

- Childhood history of inguinal surgeries such as orchidopexy, inguinal hernia repair, correction of hypospadias, and epispadias are to be enquired. Hernia repair surgery can lead to inadvertent damage to the vas deferens. Vas is extremely vulnerable in childhood operations such as herniotomy.
- In adulthood, history of vasectomy, varicocelectomy, hydrocelectomy, torsion correction, bladder neck surgeries, or urethral stricture corrections is to be enquired. Each of these surgical techniques has possible future implications on the fertility of the individual.
- Any history of surgery in para-aortic region including retroperitoneal node dissection and lumbar sympathectomy may lead to sexual dysfunction.

TABLE 2: Medical drugs impairing sexual dysfunction.[7]

Effect of treatment	*Drugs or group of drugs*
Loss of libido and erectile dysfunction due to increased prolactin concentration	*H2-receptor antagonists:* Cimetidine, ranitidine
Loss of libido and erectile dysfunction (due to increased prolactin concentration), ejaculatory dysfunction (retrograde ejaculation)	*Antipsychotic drugs:* Phenothiazine
Erectile dysfunction	*Antihypertensives:* Clonidine, guanethidine, hydralazine, methyldopa, prazosin, beta-blockers
Erectile dysfunction, ejaculatory dysfunction (retrograde ejaculation)	*Anticonvulsants:* Spironolactone, finasteride, ketoconazole
Anticholesterol medication	Statins[26]

TABLE 3: Medical drugs impairing spermatozoa parameters.[7]

Effect of treatment	*Drugs or group of drugs*
Suppression of spermatogenesis: Reversible	• *Antibiotics:* Gentamicin, neomycin, penicillin G, cephalothin, ampicillin, spiramycin • *Antibacterials:* Nitrofurantoin, sulfasalazine, cotrimoxazole • *Testosterone and its esters*: Injected testosterone
Arrest of spermatogenesis leading to azoospermia: Often irreversible	*Antimitotics/antimetabolites:* Cyclophosphamide, colchicine
Impairment of spermatozoa motility: Reversible	• *Antibiotics:* Tetracyclines, neomycin, erythromycin, lincomycin, tylosin, dicloxacillin • *Antibacterials:* Sulfasalazine, cotrimoxazole, quinolones • *Antiepileptics:* Phenytoin • *Antimalarial:* Quinine
Fertilization failure	*Calcium channel blockers and antihypertensive:* Nifedipine

Developmental/Childhood History

History of mumps, rubella, viral illness, testicular injury, and torsion,[32] any sexual developmental disturbances during puberty, sexual infantilism, and testicular maldescent are to be enquired. Local trauma causes testicular edema and varying degree of ischemia, leading to seminiferous tubular dysfunction.

Family History

It is crucial to ascertain any history of infertility in the family members, especially male siblings. Conditions such as CBAVD, cryptorchidism,[33] and metabolic/endocrine disorders can run in families.

PART II: CLINICAL EVALUATION OF INFERTILE MALE

Nutritional Status and Body Mass Index

- The global pandemic of obesity also has its toll on the fertility of the male as well.[34] Though obesity is more commonly observed in infertile females (many of them having polycystic ovarian syndrome), the males are not exempt from the repercussions of poor lifestyle and diet. Obesity in the reproductive age group men is more likely to impair spermatogenesis[34] sexual function and is often associated with metabolic disorders.[35]
- Associated medical illnesses such as diabetes mellitus, hypertension, and drugs used to treat[23] can also confound the infertility problem by causing sexual dysfunction.

Evidence of Androgenization

This directly reflects the role of testosterone and in turn, the endocrine axis. A hypoandrogenized male exhibits signs of reduced or absence of facial and body hair, female habitus, and gynecomastia. These indicate reduction in testosterone production or malfunctioning of Leydig cells. He needs evaluation for hypogonadotropic hypogonadism.[36] This, if identified, is a potentially curable cause of male infertility with successful medical management.

Eunuchoidal male with gynecomastia and soft small testis may prove to be a case of Klinefelter's syndrome.

Cardiovascular System and Lungs

Blood pressure and routine heart monitoring need to be done to identify any associated abnormal findings. Chest auscultation will pick up pulmonary problems (especially bronchiectasis and tuberculosis) which may be associated with azoospermia;[37] CBAVD in the former and obstructive azoospermia in the later. Chest auscultation will also pick up dextrocardia in situs inversus which is associated with bronchiectasis (immotile cilia syndrome).

Thyroid Disorder

Thyroid disorders are not common[38] in the infertile male unlike infertile women; hypothyroidism if present may be associated with hyperprolactinemia which in turn may result in erectile dysfunction and in turn infertility.

Breast Examination

Besides gynecomastia (as a part of hypogonadism, i.e., Klinefelter's syndrome), rarely one can demonstrate galactorrhea due to increased prolactin; any palpable tumor of the male breast may be revealed in the routine examination. This will lead to early diagnosis and treatment of the pathology detected.

Abdominal Examination

Liver enlargement may indicate chronic hepatitis or tumors. Men with cirrhosis may also present a hypoandrogenized picture. Any visible scar in the lower abdomen/inguinal region may be a telltale evidence of previous varicocelectomy, hernia surgery, or correction of undescended testes.

Genital Examination

This is best done both in the supine and standing position. Penile pathologies such as displaced urinary meatus, leading to hypospadias or epispadias, urethral or meatal strictures, and phimosis are indicative of faulty or no semen deposition into the female genital tract. Simple correction may ameliorate the sexual dysfunction and infertility.

Testes

Well-distended scrotum with rugae is indicative of descended testes into the normal position in the scrotal sac. Size of the testis is assessed by the Prader orchidometer. This can also be assessed by ultrasound, bedside examination, or with a vernier caliper **(Figs. 1 to 3)**.

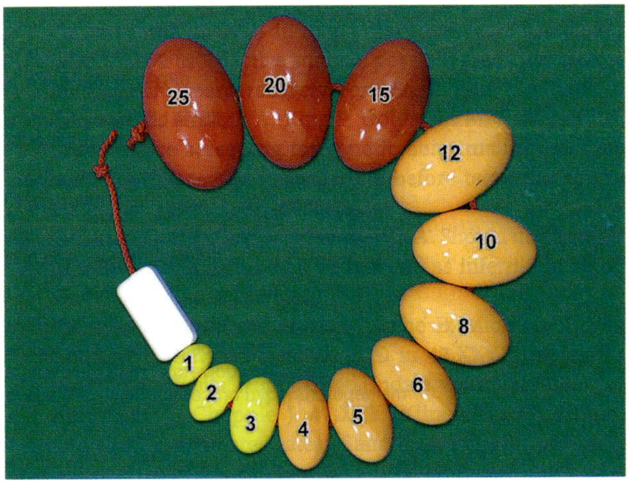

Fig. 1: Prader orchidometer.

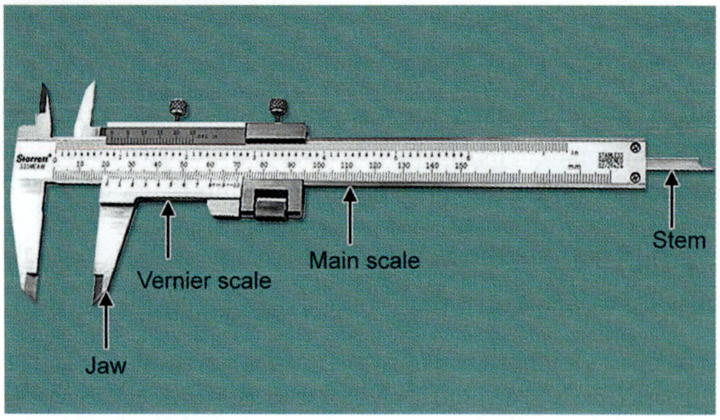

Fig. 2: Vernier caliper.
Idea courtesy: Dr Eswar.
Image courtesy: Dr Ramesh Raja.

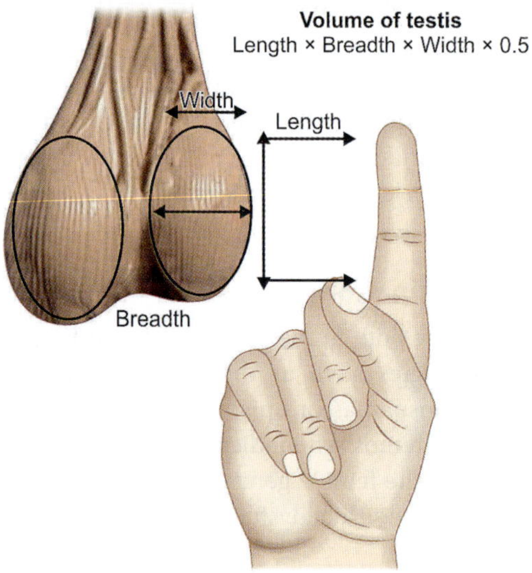

Fig. 3: Bedside clinical assessment of testicular volume.
Idea courtesy: Professor Dr N Pandiyan.
Image courtesy: Dr Ramesh Raja.

Volume of testis:

- Normal volumes (8–15 cm^3)—indicate the presence of a significant amount of the seminiferous tubules. Seminiferous tubules constitute 80% of testicular volume.
- Low volume (<8 cm^3)—soft, shrunken testis is suggestive of hypogonadotropic hypogonadism or seminiferous tubular failure.
- High volume (>20 cm^3)—hydrocele, hematocele (tenderness +), tumors, filariasis.

Testicular sensation:

- Mildly painful sensation to touch—normal male
- Exquisite tenderness—torsion, infection
- Absent or reduced sensation—seminoma testes, leprosy, seminiferous tubular dysfunction.

Epididymis

It is felt on the posterolateral aspects of testes—it is often distended and enlarged in cases of obstructive azoospermia where the obstruction is at the cauda of epididymis, vas, or ejaculatory duct.

Vas Deferens

It is felt as a cord-like structure in the spermatic cord at the root/neck of the scrotum, between thumb and index finger. It snaps when rolled between the fingers. It is absent in cases of CBAVD also called as vasal aplasia.

Varicocele

It is often best felt in the erect standing position; it feels like a bag of worms at the neck of the scrotum. Venous bruit and reversal of blood flow in pampiniform plexus during Valsalva maneuver is often detected with Doppler ultrasound. Cough impulse elicits an inguinal hernia, which may be missed in the lying position.

Rectal Examination

Absence of seminal vesicle by rectal examination adds to the suspicion of vasal aplasia.

INVESTIGATIONS FOR MALE INFERTILITY

Semen Analysis

It is the most important test available for assessing man's fertility, despite its limitations and fluctuations. Various artifacts exist in the assessment of semen analysis—collection artifacts, analysis artifacts, and interpretation artifacts. These have to be addressed/given cognizance while interpreting the seminogram. Spermatological diagnosis is arrived at the overall picture of ejaculate and not the individual parameters. The andrologist correlates the previous and present analyses in conjunction with the clinical and endocrine evaluation and can come to a diagnosis and decide on further management options for the couples.

Semen analysis is performed as per WHO 2021 manual[39] in current day practice **(Table 4)**.

Figure 4 shows the variability of semen picture in the same fertile male over 120 weeks. **Figure 5** depicts the varying spermatozoa concentration and motility from time to time in the same individual. This clearly brings to light the inherent variable nature of spermatogenesis.

Hence, the fertility potential of the individual cannot be assessed with a single semen analysis. Repeated semen tests at 2–3-month intervals are needed to confirm the seminal abnormalities, whereas a normal semen report can be taken as a reassuring step to proceed with further treatment of the couple. However, in most men, the exact cause of the semen abnormalities and infertility remains unknown and could be genetic **(Table 5)**.[40]

Endocrine Workup for Infertile Men

Figure 6 explains the neuroendocrinological control of testicular function. However, routine endocrine workup is not required in all men presenting with infertility. The common biochemical tests done are: serum follicle-stimulating hormone (S. FSH), luteinizing hormone (LH), total and free testosterone, and prolactin. They indicate seminiferous tubular function, Leydig cell function, and the role of anterior pituitary gland on gonadal function. Rarely seminal fructose estimation is needed as a qualitative test in men with azoospermia as a diagnostic aid to identify obstructive azoospermia due to vasal aplasia or ejaculatory duct obstruction.

TABLE 4: Distribution of semen examination results from men in couples starting a pregnancy within 1 year of unprotected sexual intercourse leading to a natural conception.

	Centiles	
	5th	***(95% CI)***
Semen volume (mL)	1.4	(1.3–1.5)
Sperm concentration (10^6/mL)	16	(15–18)
Total sperm number (10^6 per ejaculate)	39	(35–40)
Total motility (PR + NP, %)	42	(40–43)
Progressive motility (PR, %)	30	(29–31)
Nonprogressive motility (NP, %)	1	(1–1)
Immotile spermatozoa (IM, %)	20	(19–20)
Vitality (%)	54	(50–56)
Normal forms (%)	4	(3.9–4.0)

Source: Campbell et al. Fifth percentile given with variability (95% confidence interval).[39]

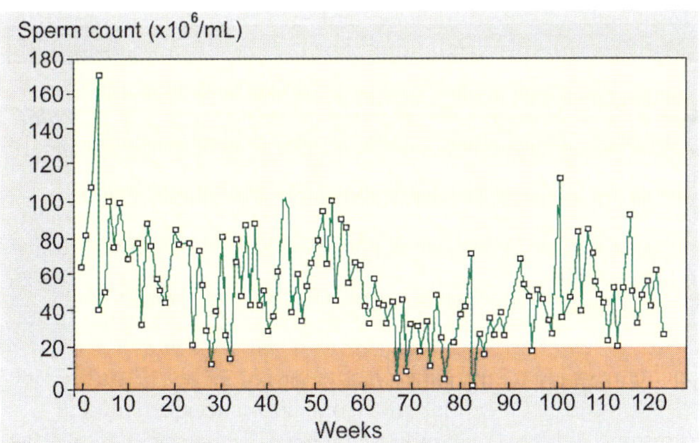

Fig. 4: Variability of spermatozoa concentration of a male over a period of time.[41]

Indications

- More often serum follicle-stimulating hormone (S. FSH) is the only hormonal test required when spermatozoa count is <10 million/mL, men with azoospermia, and in patients with persistent oligozoospermia **(Tables 6 and 7)**. These tables help in the differential diagnosis of azoospermia.

TABLE 5: Nomenclature for seminal abnormalities.

Aspermia	No ejaculate or retrograde ejaculation
Azoospermia	No spermatozoa in the neat sample and centrifuged pellet
Oligozoospermia	Total number (or concentration, depending on outcome reported) of spermatozoa below the lower reference limit[43]
Asthenozoospermia	Percentage of progressively motile (PR) spermatozoa below the lower reference limit[43]
Teratozoospermia	Percentage of morphologically normal spermatozoa below the lower reference limit[43]
Oligoasthenoteratozoospermia	Total number (or concentration, depending on outcome reported) of spermatozoa, and percentages of both PR and morphologically normal spermatozoa, below the lower reference limits[43]
Cryptozoospermia	Spermatozoa absent from fresh preparations but observed in a centrifuged pellet[43]
Normozoospermia	Total number (or concentration, depending on outcome reported) of spermatozoa, and percentages of PR and morphologically normal spermatozoa, equal to or above the lower reference limits[43]
Necrozoospermia	Dead spermatozoa in the ejaculate

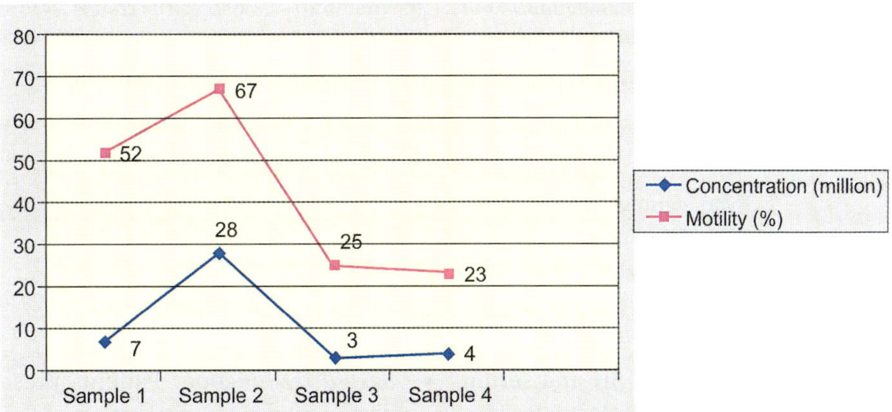

Fig. 5 : Variation in spermatozoa concentration and motility over time.[42]

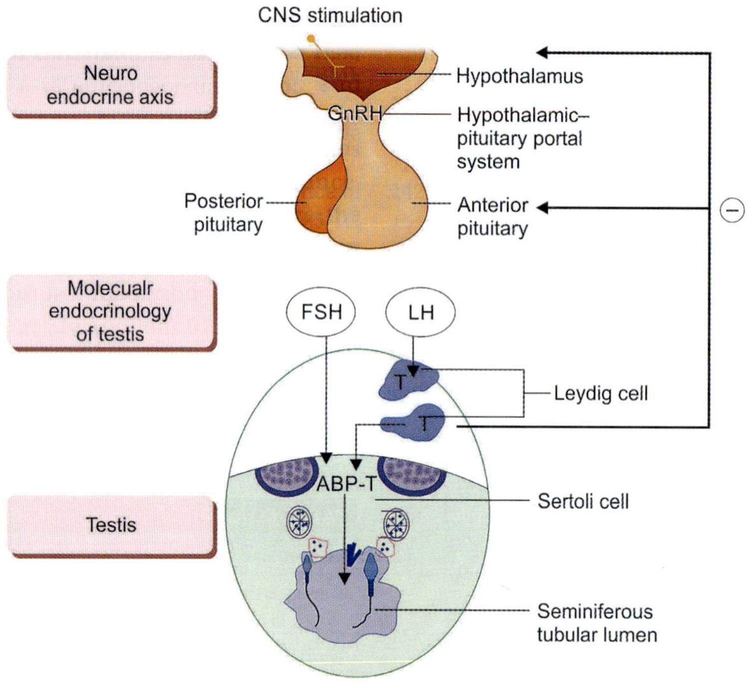

Fig. 6: Male endocrine axis.
(ABP: androgen-binding protein; CNS: central nervous system; FSH: follicle-stimulating hormone; GnRH: gonadotropin-releasing hormone; LH: luteinizing hormone)

TABLE 6: Diagnosis of types of obstructive azoospermia.

Condition	***Ejaculatory duct obstruction***	***Absence of vas deferens (CBAVD)***	***Obstruction of vas deferens as in vasectomy***	***Epididymal obstruction***	***Intra-testicular obstruction***
Serum follicle-stimulating hormone	Normal	Normal	Normal	Normal	Normal
Testicular size	Normal	Normal	Normal	Normal	Normal
Semen volume	Very low	Very low	Normal	Normal	Normal
Fructose	Absent	Absent	Present	Present	Present

(CBAVD: congenital bilateral absence of the vas deferens)
Source: Adapted from Pandiyan N. Male infertility and its management. Handbook of Andrology. T R Publications; 1999. pp. 21-46.

TABLE 7: Diagnosis of types of nonobstructive azoospermia.

Condition	***Hypogonadotropic hypogonadism***	***Seminiferous tubule failure***	***Borderline azoospermia***
Follicle-stimulating hormone (FSH)	Low or undetectable FSH, low LH, low testosterone, normal prolactin	Raised	Normal range or mild elevation
Testes size	Small	Small	Normal, small
Semen volume	Normal	Normal	Normal
Feature	Hypo/anosmia as in Kallmann's syndrome	–	HPE: Maturation arrest, hypospermatogenesis

(HPE: Histopathological examination; LH: luteinizing hormone)
Source: Adapted from Pandiyan N. Male infertility and its management. Handbook of Andrology. TR Publications; 1999. pp. 21-46.

- Hypogonadal (eunuchoidal) male: S. FSH and serum LH (S. LH), free and total testosterone, prolactin besides karyotyping
- *Sexual dysfunction:* Patients presenting with sexual dysfunction need evaluation of S. FSH, total and free testosterone, S. LH, and serum prolactin.

- *Rarely TSH estimation:* Along with prolactin in the case of sexual dysfunction
- *Anti-Müllerian Hormone (AMH) in male infertility:* Estimating AMH level in female gives an idea of ovarian reserve, whereas it is not of much clinical significance in men.[44]

GENETICS IN MALE INFERTILITY

Genetic analysis is recommended in men with severe oligo-, astheno-, teratozoospermia, and azoospermia. Genetic study requires not only karyotyping but also evaluation of Y-chromosome microdeletions. When diagnosed with Y-chromosome microdeletions, detailed counseling is to be done for the couple regarding possible transmission of deletion to the male offspring.[45] Genetic testing is also indicated when there is clinical suspicion of Klinefelter's or Kallmann's syndrome. Rarely autosomal abnormalities such as translocation[46] can also be the cause for seminal abnormalities.

Cystic fibrosis transmembrane conductance regulator (CFTR) gene mutation evaluation is advised in all cases of vasal aplasia, preferably for both the partners prior to surgical sperm retrieval for assisted reproductive techniques, as the presence of these mutations are indicative of the risk of pulmonary cystic fibrosis and consequent morbidity and mortality in the offspring.[47]

In selective cases of male infertility, genetic testing (especially for Y-chromosome microdeletions) and detailed counseling need to be done regarding possible genetic transmission to the male offspring.

Impact of Severe Acute Respiratory Syndrome Coronavirus 2 on Male Reproduction

COVID-19 is a novel coronavirus affecting humans in late 2019. It has resulted in a pandemic with reports of many systems and organs getting affected in the infected individuals. The reproductive system of the male has been found to have more susceptibility for the viral impact than women due to greater presence of angiotensin-converting enzyme (ACE) 1 and 2 receptors. ACE2 receptor is highly expressed by several cell types in the testes including Leydig cells, Sertoli cells, and the germ line.[48] They are required for viral attachment and propagation.[49]

Research of the impact of COVID-19 on human reproduction is in a very nascent stage. Conclusions are yet to be derived, but still concerns have been raised on COVID-19 virus affecting male fertility. In this continuing pandemic scenario, routine inclusion of reverse transcription-polymerase chain reaction (RT-PCR) test in the initial assessment of the couple and prior to the actual treatment is a good clinical practice.

COVID-19 Vaccination and Male Fertility

Concerns have been raised about the risks to male fertility due to COVID-19 vaccination. Though these fears appear unfounded as the vaccination does not contain the active virus and therefore unlikely to produce active disease or affect testes, yet these fears remained until a recent original article in *JAMA* quelled the fear with its observations of semen parameters before and after vaccination and found no deterioration in semen quality.[50]

CONCLUSION

Diagnosis of Male infertility is devastating to the individuals concerned, their partners and even their families. It has profound emotional, marital, and social issues. It is vital that every practitioner involved in the care of infertile couples is well versed with evaluation of the male partners also. Detailed history remains the pivotal point of examination, strengthened by thorough physical examination and supported by properly done semen analysis and necessary biochemical, radiological, and genetic testing. A clear diagnosis goes a long way in treating the possible causes and directing the couples to undergo the recommended treatment in their journey towards parenthood.

KEY POINTS

- It is explicit from the above detailed narration that it is vital to elicit an exhaustive history, which may give us a clue to the possible cause of infertility and its remedy. This also brings the importance of systemic influence on gonadal functions to light and the need to look at the infertility issue from a holistic point of view.
- A thorough clinical examination is essential to identify features of androgenization and evaluation of genitalia for obvious causes for seminal abnormality.
- Routine endocrine evaluation is not required in all men with infertility. It is indicated in conditions such as severe oligozoospermia, azoospermia, hypogonadal state, and in sexual dysfunction.
- Though the contributions by the male for the couple's infertility problem have been widely acknowledged, sadly there has not been much awareness among public and medical professionals for the need to evaluate the male partner thoroughly.
- The right approach to evaluate male infertility should be a combination of dedicated and detailed history taking and thorough clinical examination with relevant investigations.
- This chapter has attempted to provide a basic understanding of the various clinical and endocrinological methods used to evaluate the issue of male factor infertility and to identify the possible cause and plan appropriate treatment.

REFERENCES

1. Agarwal A, Mulgund A, Hamada A, Chyatte MR. A unique view on male infertility around the globe. Reprod Biol Endocrinol. 2015;13:37.
2. Kumar N, Singh AK. Trends of male factor infertility, an important cause of infertility: a review of literature. J Hum Reprod Sci. 2015;8(4):191-6.
3. WHO Biennial Report. Research in Human Reproduction. Geneva: WHO; 1992.
4. Siddharth C, Ramesh Raja D, Prathima T. Lifestyle and environmental factors influencing male infertility. Chettinad Health City Med J. 2014;3(4):156-60.
5. Perheentupa A. Male infertility and environmental factors. Global Reprod Health. 2019;4(2):e28.
6. Selvaraju V, Baskaran S, Agarwal A, Henkel R. Environmental contaminants and male infertility: effects and mechanisms. Andrologia. 2021;53:e13646.
7. Pandiyan N. Medical management of male infertility. Reprod Biomed Online. 2000;1(1):13-6.
8. Benziger A, Ramesh Raja D, Pandiyan N. Impact of radiation emitted by mobile phone during call mode on the ejaculated semen. Chettinad Health City Med J. 2014;3(4):144-8.
9. Kesari KK, Agarwal A, Henkel R. Radiations and male fertility. Reprod Biol Endocrinol. 2018;16(1):118.
10. Jequier AM. The importance of diagnosis in the clinical management of infertility in the male. Reprod Biomed Online. 2006;13(3):331-5.
11. Ospina NS, Phillips KA, Rodriguez-Gutierrez R, Castaneda-Guarderas A, Gionfriddo MR, Branda ME, et al. Eliciting the patient's agenda: secondary analysis of recorded clinical encounters. J Gen Intern Med. 2019:34;36-40.
12. Khan SD. Aging and male reproduction. In: Pandiyan N, Khan SD (Eds). A Clinical Approach to Male Infertility. New Delhi: Springer; 2017. pp. 197-206.
13. Kovac JR, Addai J, Smith RP, Coward RM, Lamb DJ, Lipshultz L. The effects of advanced paternal age on fertility. Asian J Androl. 2013;15(6):723-2.
14. Sharma R, Agarwal A, Rohra VK, Assidi M, Abu-Elmagd M, Turki RF. Effects of increased paternal age on sperm quality, reproductive outcome and associated epigenetic risks to offspring. Reprod Biol Endocrinol. 2015;13:35.
15. Gökçe Mİ, Yaman Ö. Erectile dysfunction in the elderly male. Turk J Urol. 2017;43(3):247-51.
16. Jeng HA. Exposure to endocrine disrupting chemicals and male reproductive health. Front Public Health. 2014;2:55.
17. Bonde JP. Male reproductive organs are at risk from environmental hazards. Asian J Androl. 2010;12(2):152-6.
18. Sharpe RM. Environmental/lifestyle effects on spermatogenesis. Philos Trans R Soc Lond B Biol Sci. 2010;365(1546):1697-712.
19. Harlev A, Agarwal A, Gunes SO, Shetty A, du Plessis SS. Smoking and male infertility: an evidence-based review. World J Mens Health. 2015;33(3):143-60.
20. Sharma R, Harlev A, Agarwal A, Esteves SC. Cigarette smoking and semen quality: a new meta-analysis examining the effect of the 2010 World Health Organization laboratory methods for the examination of human semen. Eur Urol. 2016;70(4):635-45.
21. Kulkarni M, Hayden C, Kayes O. Recreational drugs and male fertility. Trends Urol Mens Health. 2014;5(5):19-23.
22. Johnson S, Marriott L, Reay M, Parsons P. Vaginal lubricant use among women trying to conceive: insights from a survey of over 1000 participants. Fertil Steril. 2016;106(3):287.
23. Practice Committee of the American Society for Reproductive Medicine in Collaboration with the Society for Reproductive Endocrinology and Infertility. Optimizing natural fertility: a committee opinion. Fertil Steril. 2013;100(3):631-7.
24. Lotti F, Corona G, Castellini G, Maseroli E, Fino MG, Cozzolino M, et al. Semen quality impairment is associated with sexual dysfunction according to its severity. Hum Reprod. 2016;31(12):2668-80.
25. Pandiyan N, Ramesh RD, Radha P. Treatment options arising from different semen analyses. In: Mehta Jayant G, Bryan W (Eds). Male Infertility: Sperm Diagnosis, Management and Delivery. New Delhi, India: Jaypee Digital Explore Health Science; 2014. pp. 65-70.
26. Corona G, Boddi V, Balercia G, Rastrelli G, De Vita G, Sforza A, et al. The effect of statin therapy on testosterone levels in subjects consulting for erectile dysfunction. J Sex Med. 2010;7:1547-56.
27. Pandiyan N. Medical drugs impairing fertility. In: Nicolopoulou-Stamati P, Hens L, Howard C (Eds). Reproductive Health and the Environment. Environmental Science and Technology Library. Dordrecht: Springer; 2007. pp. 187-205.
28. Mondillo C, Varela ML, Abiuso AMB, Vázquez R. Potential negative effects of anti-histamines on male reproductive function. Reproduction. 2018;155(5):221-7.
29. Semet M, Paci M, Saias-Magnan J, Metzler-Guillemain C, Boissier R, Lejeune H, et al. The impact of drugs on male fertility: a review. Andrology. 2017;5(4):640-63.
30. Pandit S, Choudhury S, Das A, Basuthakur S, Das SK. A rare case of Kartagener's syndrome. J Nat Sci Biol Med. 2014;5(1):175-7.
31. Ong T, Marshall SG, Karczeski BA, Sternen DL, Cheng E, Cutting GR. Cystic fibrosis and congenital absence of the vas deferens. In: Adam MP, Ardinger HH, Pagon RA, Wallace SE, Bean LJH, Mirzaa G, et al. (Eds). GeneReviews. Seattle (WA): University of Washington, Seattle; 2017.
32. Monga M, Hellstrom WJ. The Effects of Testicular Torsion on Fertility: Male Infertility and Sexual Dysfunction. New York: Springer; 1997. pp. 323-34.
33. Agoulnik AI, Feng S. The Genetics of Cryptorchidism. The Genetics of Male Infertility. Totowa, NJ: Humana Press; 2007. pp. 185-98.
34. Palmer NO, Bakos HW, Fullston T, Lane M. Impact of obesity on male fertility, sperm function and molecular composition. Spermatogenesis. 2012;2(4):253-63.
35. Craig JR, Jenkins TG, Carrell DT, Hotaling JM. Obesity, male infertility, and the sperm epigenome. Fertil Steril. 2017;107(4):848-59.
36. Sermondade N, Faure C, Fezeu L, Shayeb AG, Bonde JP, Jensen TK. BMI in relation to sperm count: an updated systematic review and collaborative meta-analysis. Hum Reprod Update. 2013;19(3):221-31.

37. Mishra M, Kumar N, Jaiswal A, Verma AK, Kant S. Kartagener's syndrome: a case series. Lung India. 2012;29(4):366-9.
38. Krassas GE, Poppe K, Glinoer D. Thyroid function and human reproductive health. Endocr Rev. 2010;31(5):702-55.
39. WHO Laboratory Manual for the Examination and Processing of Human Semen, 6th edition. Geneva: World Health Organization; 2021.
40. Esteves SC. A clinical appraisal of the genetic basis in unexplained male infertility. J Hum Reprod Sci. 2013;6(3): 176-82.
41. WHO Laboratory Manual for the Examination of Human Semen and Sperm-cervical Mucus Interaction, 4th edition. Cambridge University Press; 2000.
42. Pandiyan N. Semen analysis: a numbers game. Chettinad Health City Med J. 2012;1(1):2-3.
43. WHO Laboratory Manual for the Examination and Processing of Human Semen, 5th edition. Geneva: WHO Press; 2010.
44. La Marca A, Sighinolfi G, Radi D, Argento C, Baraldi E, Artenisio AC. Anti-Müllerian hormone (AMH) as a predictive marker in assisted reproductive technology (ART). Hum Reprod Update. 2010;16(2):113-30.
45. Colaco S, Modi D. Genetics of the human Y chromosome and its association with male infertility. Reprod Biol Endocrinol. 2018;14:16.
46. Pandiyan N, Jequier AM. Mitotic chromosomal anomalies among 1210 infertile men. Hum Reprod. 1996;11(12):2604-8.
47. Moskowitz SM, Chmiel JF, Sternen DL, Cheng E, Gibson RL, Marshall SG, et al. Clinical practice and genetic counseling for cystic fibrosis and CFTR-related disorders. Genet Med. 2008;10(12):851-68.
48. Aitken RJ. COVID-19 and human spermatozoa—potential risks for infertility and sexual transmission? Andrology. 2021; 9(1):48-52.
49. Khalili MA, Leisegang K, Majzoub A, Finelli R, Panner Selvam MK, Henkel R, et al. Male fertility and the COVID-19 pandemic: systematic review of the literature. World J Mens Health. 2020;38(4):506-20.
50. Gonzalez DC, Nassau DE, Khodamoradi K, Ibrahim E, Blachman-Braun R, Ory J, et al. Sperm parameters before and after COVID-19 mRNA vaccination. JAMA. 2021;326(3): 273-4.

CHAPTER

26 Sexual Dysfunction in Male Infertility

Vasan SS, Fahim L Rajwate, Ankur

INTRODUCTION

In recent years, infertility has become the subject of significant media attention and public discussion, particularly in light of new advances in the technology of assisted reproduction. Male factor infertility plays a role in approximately 50% of infertility cases with male factor as a sole cause in about 35%. It has been proposed that a man who fails at fertility is likely to evaluate himself as sexually inadequate and may experience temporary impotence and decreased libido. Constant worry about the problem may arouse inhibitory nerves and interfere with smooth muscle relaxation in the penis, thus causing partial or complete failure of erection.

In India, approximately 15% of couples are unable to initiate a pregnancy without some form of assistance or therapy. These patients are said to be "primarily infertile." In approximately 2% of these couples there are factors other than seminal abnormalities, which prevent conception. It is imperative that these groups of patients are properly diagnosed and treated to enable them to achieve conception.

Some of the uncommon problems seen in males leading to infertility are as follows:

- Nonconsummation of marriage
- Ejaculatory disturbances
- Erectile dysfunction.

Treatment of these problems entails proper understanding of the physiology of erection and ejaculation. The majority of contemporary knowledge on the physiology of erection has been assembled during the past thirty years. It consists of basic biological response and mechanics of pelvic floor muscles and sphincters, during erection, and ejaculation.

BIOLOGICAL BASIS OF MALE SEXUAL RESPONSE

Depending on the situation, a person can be sexually aroused by a variety of factors, both physical and mental. The welcome physical stimulation of an erogenous zone or acts of foreplay can result in arousal, especially if it is accompanied with the anticipation of imminent sexual activity. The potential stimuli for sexual arousal vary from person to person and from one time to another, as does the level of arousal.

Stimuli can be classified according to the sense involved—somatosensory (touch), visual, and olfactory (scent). Auditory stimuli are also possible, though they are generally considered secondary in role to the other three. Erotic stimuli that can result in sexual arousal can include conversation, reading, films, or images or a smell or setting, any of which can generate erotic thoughts and memories in a person.

Five brain areas were found to be more active during the sexual act, they are as follows:

1. The first was the inferior temporal cortex, a region also corresponding to the visual associative zone. The researchers inferred that the subject was assessing and analyzing the visual stimulus when this zone was activated, corresponding to the perceptive cognitive component of sexual arousal.
2. The second region was the right orbitofrontal cortex, which might be related to emotional and motivational phenomena.
3. The third area was the left anterior cingulate cortex, which appears to control primary physiological responses (endocrine and autonomic), but also affective responses, to sexual stimuli. In other words, it would govern physical and psychological preparation for sexual activity.
4. The fourth region was the right insula, which could be involved in subjective perception of physiological modifications associated with arousal (heart rate acceleration, penile erection, etc.).
5. Finally, the right caudate nucleus probably controls whether sexual arousal is followed by sexual activity.

The stimuli from a receptive female and/or sexual act itself leads to the release of dopamine (DA) in at least three integrative hubs.[1] The nigrostriatal system promotes somatomotor activity; the mesolimbic system subserves numerous types of motivation; and the medial preoptic area (MPOA) focuses the motivation onto specifically sexual targets, increases sexual rate and efficiency, and coordinates genital reflexes. The previous (but not necessarily concurrent) presence of testosterone is permissive for DA release in the MPOA, both during the basal conditions and in response to a female. One means by which testosterone may increase DA release is by upregulating nitric oxide synthase, which produces nitric oxide, which in turn increases DA release. Finally, while DA is facilitative to sexual activity, 5-hydroxy tryptamine (5HT) is generally inhibitory. 5HT is released in the lateral hypothalamic area (LHA), but not in the MPOA, at the time of ejaculation. Thus reciprocal changes in DA and 5HT release in different areas of the brain may promote sexual activity and sexual satiety, respectively. Other factors such as medication, alcohol, and other health problems can modify the biological impact of hormones on libido.

As to the mediators at the cavernosal level, acetylcholine and nitric oxide (NO) released from the endothelium are involved along with noradrenaline, vasoactive intestinal polypeptide (VIP), calcitonin gene related peptide (CGRP) and prostaglandins.[2] Nitric oxide and VIP play the most important roles in the phase of erection. Erection takes the following course (simplified) erotic stimuli—impulses from brain via hypothalamus—stimulation of parasympathetic (PNS) spinal erection center (T11-L2, S2, 3, 4)—release of acetylcholine, no at PNS nerve endings and at cavernous nerve - sinusoids smooth muscle relaxation and rapid filling with blood (tumescence stage)— veno-occlusive mechanism prevents blood egress—full erection phase—erotogenic stimuli lead to the stimulation of the parasympathetic nerve→vasodilating substances are released→the sinusoids are filled with blood (tumescence stage)→the veno-occlusive mechanism starts to work—thus complete erection occurs. Then the contractions of the musculature of the perineum compress the proximal portions of the corpora cavernosa—this leads to rigid erection. Detumescence (which occurs as a rule after ejaculation) is due to released noradrenaline (active stage) and the reduced tonus of the smooth muscles of the blood vessels (released endothelin and neuropeptide Y).

Pelvic Floor Muscles and Sphincters during Erection and Ejaculation

The pelvic floor muscles involved in maintaining an erection[3] consists of puborectalis (PR), levator ani (LA) and, external anal sphincters (EAS) and external urethral sphincters (EUS). The increased PR activity might express the prostatic secretions into the posterior urethra. Levator ani contraction seems to elevate the prostate and partially straightens the prostato membranous urethral kink that might occur during erection. The EAS and EUS contractions are believed to abort the urge to defecate or urinate and prevent leak of feces, flatus, or urine during coitus. The rhythmic EUS contraction at ejaculation might act as a "suction ejection pump," sucking the genital fluid into the posterior urethra while being relaxed, and ejecting it into the bulbous urethra upon contraction.

NONCONSUMMATION OF MARRIAGE

The main factor associated with an unconsummated marriage is the intense social pressure to accomplish hasty sexual activity[4] with an unfamiliar woman (some men having had no social contact with their new bride), and in the presence of relatives waiting nearby for evidence of the bride's virginity and confirmation of sexual act. This initial problem will then be further compounded with resultant erectile failure caused by anxiety about sexual performance. In addition to psychological causes and a lack of sexual education, the social circumstances in which partners are obliged to initiate and complete sexual act are important factors in the etiology of unconsummated marriage.

There may be many reasons for nonconsummation.

- *These may include:*
  - Lack of emotional involvement
  - Fear of sexual act
  - Inappropriate advice or information from friends and family before marriage about first night and sex
  - Vaginismus (terrible cramp at the entrance of the vagina, which makes penetration impossible)
  - Lack of arousal and less lubrication for the female
  - Dyspareunia (painful intercourse)
  - Thick hymen
  - Erection problems or an inability to copulate
  - Fear of pregnancy
  - Sexual abuse in childhood
- *Signs of nonconsummation:*
  - Lack of desire for sex
  - Irritating or painful experience while attempting intercourse
  - Difficulty in insertion of penis into vagina
  - Softening of penis while performing intercourse
  - Ejection of semen before penetration
  - Inability to consummate medically is caused by:
    - Premature ejaculation in 23%
    - Erectile dysfunction in 61%
    - Combination of factors in 16%.

Erectile dysfunction in some form or other may contribute to the problem. It is the clinician's obligation to establish the etiology of impotence, namely end organ vascular failure versus neurologic dysfunction versus psychosexual dysfunction, classify the severity of that dysfunction, and select a therapy that is not only acceptable to the patient but also addresses his pathology. The most commonly utilized diagnostic tests for erectile dysfunction are mentioned underneath.

Combined Injection and Stimulation Test or CIS Test

They consist of intracavernous injection and visual rating of the subsequent erection. It is simple, minimally invasive, and performed without monitoring equipment. Hemodynamic investigations suggest that a positive injection test is associated with normal veno-occlusion, but not necessarily with normal arterial function. When the penile response to pharmacotesting is suboptimal or equivocal, diagnostic testing with duplex Doppler assessment should be performed.

Nocturnal Penile Tumescence

Nocturnal penile tumescence (NPT) to measure man's nocturnal erections have been measured by each of the following methods—stamp test, snap gauges, strain gauges, NPTR (Rigiscan and Osborn Medical Systems), and sleep laboratory NPTR.[5] Normal nocturnal penile tumescence and rigidity (NPTR) depends on both the integrity of the corticospinal efferents to the penis and vascular responsiveness of the penile tissues to those nerve signals. When nocturnal erections are of appropriate duration and strength, the central and peripheral neuroeffectors and intracorporal regulators of penile hemodynamics are intact. Unfortunately, abnormal NPTR is of little value in determining the etiology or classifying the severity of vascular impotence, the most prevalent kind of end organ failure.

Blood Flow Studies

Insufficient penile blood flow and inefficient corporal veno-occlusion is implicated in up to 30% of patients, and in their evaluation numerous diagnostic tests have been employed to evaluate penile hemodynamics.[6] The more popular ones are color duplex Doppler ultrasound, selective internal pudendal pharmacoangiography and dynamic infusion cavernosometry/cavernosography (DICC). Duplex ultrasound, which measures penile blood flow, provides an objective, minimally invasive evaluation of arterial pattern in a suboptimal/equivocal erectile response.

The diagnosis and demonstration of venous leakage requires complete smooth muscle relaxation. Veno-occlusive dysfunction is associated with poorly sustained erections; this pathology has traditionally been evaluated with dynamic infusion cavernosometry and cavernosography. Dynamic infusion cavernosometry/cavernosography is an invasive test, and is now primarily reserved for patients considering the option of vascular reconstructive procedure.

Neurological Assessment

The sacral reflex arc of erection consists of somatosensory afferents via the dorsal and pudendal nerves and autonomic efferents via the pelvic and cavernous nerves. These afferents have been measured indirectly by somatosensory evoked potentials (SSEP) and bulbocavernosus reflex latency (BCR). These at present are used in research situations, as it does not principally aid in the patient management.

Penile EMGs (CCEMG) have been used to measure corpora cavernosal smooth muscle electrical activity and is far from standardized.[5] Computer-assisted interpretations of penile electrical potentials may eventually differentiate afferent nerve pathologies so long inferred in diabetes, spinal cord injury and following radical pelvic surgery.

Erectile dysfunction evaluation is based on the clinical judgment and not all these tests may be necessary for evaluation. Proper evaluation of nonconsummation will aid in treatment planning. Various options in management are psychotherapy, sexual education, oral medications (sildenafil citrate, tadalafil, vardenafil, udenafil, and uprima), intracavernosal injection and specific treatment directed for organic cause. Most cases respond to medications and counseling with surgical options being reserved for resistant organic causes.

EJACULATORY DISTURBANCES

Diagnosis of Infertility: Psychological Aspects-infertility Investigation

The semen needed for a spermiogram should be collected by masturbation, which can be disturbing to infertility patients. Men may have an erection failure at this time. Masturbation is still often a taboo and the setting is not erotic. Men may fear the judgment of the biologist regarding their semen and this may lead to impotence. Guilt over their felt inadequacy can make impotence persist. In this context, some men suffer scrotal pain, asthenia and depression. They often describe the impression of having a "cold penis."

The use of standard techniques for evaluating medical problems in general such as complete history, physical examination, and laboratory tests which are beyond the scope of this chapter, are essential for this purpose.

A secondary goal of the infertility evaluation is to identify any underlying health conditions that may be contributing to difficulties with conception. This could include any conditions that would contribute to problems with ejaculation such as undiagnosed diabetes, or problems with erection, such as might be caused by a significant smoking history, severe hypercholesterolemia, or hypogonadism. A full discussion of the diagnosis and treatment of erectile dysfunction (ED) is beyond the scope of this article; however, it is not uncommon for men to report some stress-related ED during the course of the infertility evaluation and treatment.

These patients may benefit from a prescription for a phosphodiesterase-5 (PDE5) inhibitor or a dopaminergic drug, apomorphine for enhancing sexual response cycle. Alprostadil (Muse) is not recommended since its potential effect on the ejaculate is not known.

Patients who complain of the difficulty with ejaculation and climax need to be checked for psychotherapeutic agents usage that block dopamine production and consequently blunt the hypothalamic pituitary axis and possibly decrease libido. Other psychotherapeutic agents can decrease vasodilatation and decrease the quality of erections. Tricyclic antidepressants, selective-serotonin reuptake inhibitors, and monoamine oxidase inhibitors can lead to ED, an ejaculation and decreased libido. These patients can have their regimen changed, or may be offered other means of medically managing their complaints, such as a PDE5 inhibitor.

The most widely accepted theory to explain ejaculation consists of two phases:[7]

1. A phase of accumulation of the various constituents of semen inside the prostatic urethra.
2. A phase of expulsion with opening of the striated sphincter, while the smooth sphincter of the bladder neck remains closed.

These events are mediated by the sympathetic nervous system via T10 to L3 level preganglionic fibers. Ejaculation is the forceful antegrade expulsion of semen from the posterior urethra through the urethral meatus. This event is secondary to the rhythmic contraction of periurethral and pelvic floor smooth muscle, mediated by parasympathetic outflow (S2, 3, and 4) and somatic efferents, and occurs in conjunction with closure of the bladder neck, which is sympathetically stimulated.

Ejaculatory Disorders

- Premature ejaculation
- Retrograde ejaculation
- Anejaculation
- Deficient or retarded ejaculation.

On the basis of the history and simple investigations, the various disorders are relatively easy to differentiate. History taking should include information about the ability to ejaculate, including nocturnal emission and the ability to experience an orgasm.

Premature Ejaculation

All men know what it feels like to sometimes want sexual intercourse to last longer. But premature ejaculation (PE; also called early ejaculation, rapid ejaculation or ejaculation praecox or inability to control ejaculation) is much more than just feeling like you want to last longer from time to time. It is a very real condition with real impact on people's life and it is measured by the average intravaginal ejaculation latency time (IELT).

Deficiency in ejaculation appears to be caused by sympathetic, motor pudendal or suprasacral lesion. An altered perception of genital sensations due to a lesion in the afferent pudendal pathway appears to be present in premature ejaculation.[8]

The exact reason why some people have a faster sexual response is not yet fully clear. In the past, PE was thought to be a purely a psychological condition, but Janssen et al.,[9] in their study of IELT in Dutch men with life-long premature ejaculation found serotonin transporter promoter region (*5-HTTLPR*) polymorphism which might explain a genetic basis in some men.

It is proposed that there are two broad causes of premature ejaculation:

1. Biogenic and
2. Psychogenic

There are two different types of premature ejaculation:

1. Primary (lifelong)
2. Secondary (acquired).

The traditional assumption among sex therapists is that premature ejaculation is almost universally caused by psychological features and is easily treated with sex therapy and behavioral techniques. This is questionable, as results from systematic investigations have shown that behavioral treatments for premature ejaculation remain beneficial to only a minority of men three years after treatment ends, suggesting that this male dysfunction is difficult to treat effectively with behavioral techniques.

With proper assessment and identification a specific diagnosis of premature ejaculation can be made and accurate treatment designed to address the particular type of disorder, with long-term benefits, can be achieved.

The commonly used medications in this disorder are fluoxetine, paroxetine, and clomipramine either singly or in combination. Recently, there has been emphasis on pelvic floor rehabilitation as a form of treatment for this disorder.

Retrograde Ejaculation

Retrograde ejaculation is an uncommon cause of male infertility. Antegrade ejaculation requires intact anatomy and innervation of the bladder neck. Retrograde ejaculation can be defined as the escape of seminal fluid from the posterior urethra into the bladder.[10] The etiology may be anatomic, neurogenic, pharmacologic, or idiopathic. *Anatomic causes* include prostatectomy (open or transurethral) or bladder neck surgeries (YV plasty, transurethral incision of the bladder neck). *Neurogenic causes* include spinal cord injury, retroperitoneal surgery, and diabetes mellitus. *Pharmacologic agents* implicated in causing retrograde ejaculation include neuroleptics, tricyclic antidepressants, α-blockers used in the treatment of prostatism and certain antihypertensives. Also congenital and idiopathic causes have been described.[11]

It should be suspected in any case of persistent low volume ejaculate (<1.5 mL), absent ejaculate or rarely azoospermia. It can easily be differentiated from partial ejaculatory obstruction by transrectal ultrasound. The diagnosis of ejaculatory duct obstruction is suggested by the presence of a cyst posterior to the prostatic urethra, with or without dilatation of the seminal vesicles. The differential diagnosis for a prostatic cyst includes Müllerian duct cysts, utricle cysts, prostatic retention cysts, seminal vesicle cysts, and ejaculatory duct cysts. Such cysts can be classified according to their location and the presence or absence of sperm in the fluid aspirated from them.

Investigations which Aid in the diagnosis

- Demonstration of sperm in the postmasturbation urine.
- Analysis of the ejaculate.
- Determination of the secretion markers of the adnexa.
- Ultrasonographic (abdominal and transrectal) examination of the genital organs.

The patient is instructed to void immediately following ejaculation and the diagnosis of retrograde ejaculation can be confirmed by examination of postejaculate urine (PEU). A sample of the specimen is evaluated microscopically for sperm density and motility. Alternatively, the specimen may be centrifuged and the pellet resuspended in a medium such as human tubular fluid, and then analyzed for sperm density and motility. Presence of >15 sperms/high-pass filter (HPF) is confirmatory of retrograde ejaculation.

Principles of management of retrograde ejaculation (Glander 1998)

- Conversion of retrograde into antegrade ejaculation by drug therapy.
- Harvesting of sperm from postejaculatory urine.

In the treatment of retrograde ejaculation, an initial trial of medical therapy is warranted. Medical management aims to increase the tone of the bladder neck, preventing retrograde flow of semen into the bladder. This can be achieved either by stimulating sympathetic activity (closure of the bladder neck is under sympathetic control) or by blocking parasympathetic input.

The agents commonly utilized are α-adrenergic agonists such as ephedrine, pseudoephedrine, tricyclic antidepressants–imipramine, and antihistamines brompheniramine, and phenylpropanolamine. When pharmacological attempts to restore antegrade ejaculation fail, the spermatozoa should be recovered from postejaculation urine, to be applied in one of the modern techniques of assisted reproduction. The successful recovery of viable spermatozoa from the urine is dependent upon careful regulation of pH and osmolarity of the urine at the time of ejaculation. Careful handling of the retrieved spermatozoa enables isolation of sperm cells with good quality for insemination of ovulated oocytes (in vivo) or retrieved oocytes (in vitro), and is timed to coincide with the wife's ovulation. There are several protocols for urinary alkalinization, however, the protocol outlined below yields the best sperm retrieval rates.

Protocol for urinary alkalinization: Patient is instructed to use sodium bicarbonate tablets 2 g TID and Sudafed 60 mg TID for 3 days prior to anticipated day of ovulation and to monitor his urinary pH with pH strips to assess the efficacy of alkalization.

On the day of sample collection, pH and osmolarity of spontaneous urine is measured. The aim is that the pH should reach 7.3 and the osmolarity should be 280 mOsmol. If not, dissolve 2.0 g sodium bicarbonate in 200 mL of distilled water and administer to the patient. After 30 minutes repeat the measurement and if the desired value has not been attained repeat the procedure by reducing the amount of sodium bicarbonate and measure again in 30 minutes (this is the time the sodium bicarbonate needs to reach the bladder).

It should be remembered that the reducing bicarbonate is dependent on pH level and if the correct pH and osmolarity are reached, the patient is instructed to empty his bladder completely just prior to ejaculation (the closer the better). Then catheterize the bladder, drain it to completion, and administer a small volume of media. The patient then ejaculates and collects his antegrade sample. Then recatheterize, collect the bladder sample and if needed irrigate the bladder with media to collect the rest of the retrograde specimen prior to sending them all off to the laboratory for processing. It is necessary to use media at room temperature and minimal lubrication while catheterizing to enhance sperm recovery.

Most cases of retrograde ejaculation can be managed either by conversion to antegrade by pharmacological manipulation or sperm recovered from the bladder by urinary alkalinization, and surgical treatment is anecdotal in the era of assisted reproduction.

The goal of surgical intervention is restoration of bladder neck integrity. Limited data are available regarding the use of surgical intervention in the treatment of retrograde ejaculation. However, Reynolds, McCall, Kim, and Lipshultz (1998) successfully injected collagen into the bladder neck of a male with retrograde ejaculation, achieving antegrade ejaculation, two subsequent pregnancies, and one live birth. However, this approach is fraught with complications and is currently not recommended as a treatment option.

Anejaculation

Anejaculation and ejaculatory dysfunction are the terms used to describe the inability of a man to have an ejaculation.

The common types are:
- Orgasmic
- Nonorgasmic.

It is a relatively uncommon disorder that can occur as a result of spinal cord injury, retroperitoneal lymph node dissection, or other retroperitoneal surgery, diabetes mellitus, transverse myelitis, or multiple sclerosis.[12] In addition the etiology may be psychogenic or idiopathic. The nerves that are responsible for carrying the signal for ejaculation, exit the spinal cord and course along the aorta, in the posterior part of the abdomen. These nerves are most commonly injured after spinal trauma resulting in paraplegia or quadriplegia, major bowel or vascular surgery, or surgery for testicular cancer. In the past, men with ejaculatory dysfunction were considered infertile because they could not ejaculate but presently there are treatment options available.

Anejaculation, resulting from the damage to the afferent or efferent neural pathways (reflex arc) responsible for emission and/or ejaculation, can be treated with electroejaculation. In cases where the reflex arc is intact or is partially damaged, vibratory stimulation is useful. Some researchers have tried medical therapy in both these types and were generally unsuccessful.

VIBRATORY STIMULATION

Penile vibratory stimulation mimics rapid and repetitive manual/hand stimulation of the penis, which is a natural aspect of human sexual behavior. Vibratory stimulation (VS) employs a custom designed mechanical vibrator (store bought vibrators do not work for many patients) that is applied to the underside of the glans penis and set to vibrate at designated frequency and wave amplitude. This vibration travels along the sensory nerves to the spinal cord and may induce a reflex ejaculation. This technique only works in patients with an intact ejaculatory reflex arc. The results are dependent on the level of spinal cord injury and are most effective in patients with upper cord lesions. This is an office procedure that requires no anesthesia or sedation to perform. However, it is suggested that all the patients, irrespective of the level of injury in the spinal cord, have an initial trial with vibratory therapy, as many a times the lesion may be incomplete. When vibratory stimulation is unsuccessful, electroejaculation often works quite well. After standard bladder preparation (detailed below), a handheld, electrically driven vibrator is applied initially to the dorsum of the glans and then to the frenulum and penoscrotal area. The slow movement of the vibrator often identifies a "trigger" point, which is often reproducible from one cycle to another.[13] The selection of a frequency of 100 Hz and a peak-to-peak amplitude of 2.5 mm may be important for successful ejaculation. Patients who ejaculate using this form of stimulation need to be trained properly in its usage and ejaculatory interval may vary from 10 to 180 minutes depending on the pathology. People who are likely to respond to vibrators develop penile tumescence and pelvic floor contractions. In the absence of these signs electroejaculation is a better option. Most patients who respond to vibratory stimulation will exhibit antegrade ejaculation, but catheterization must be performed because these patients frequently have incomplete closure of the bladder neck, and may also have a significant retrograde component.

The presence of bulbocavernosus and hip flexion reflexes are useful in predicting response of penile vibratory stimulation. When both reflexes were present, 80% of the men ejaculated in response to stimulation, compared to only 8% of men in whom neither reflex was present. Poor prognostic indicators are spinal cord injury within the last 6 months, the absence of reflex hip flexion and lesion below T12 level.

The common types of vibrators available are as follows:
- Ferticare
- Viberect

Electroejaculation

Initially used in veterinary medicine and animal husbandry, electroejaculation produces seminal emission by sinusoidal electrical stimulation of sympathetic efferent fibers and smooth muscle. The best site for inducing seminal emission is in front of the bifurcation of the aorta, between the rectum and obturator nerves, where both preganglionic and postganglionic sympathetic fibers reside. Unfortunately, because electroejaculation does not stimulate the somatically mediated events of ejaculation or coordinate bladder neck closure essential to antegrade emission, pulsatile expulsion of seminal fluid does not occur. Rather, semen either dribbles from the meatus or is deposited retrograde into the bladder.[14,15]

A complete urologic evaluation is required prior to electroejaculation in order to detect and treat any urinary tract infections. Men with spinal cord injuries often have a problem of poor sperm production as well as ejaculatory difficulty. A diagnostic trial of electroejaculation is attempted to obtain and examine the quality of the semen specimen. Good quality samples are frozen for future use as a backup. A fresh specimen is obtained at the time of the women's ovulation. Unlike vibratory stimulation, electroejaculation is uniformly successful, irrespective of the duration and level of the spinal lesion.

Electroejaculation is performed with a device known as an electroejaculator. A specially designed electric probe is inserted into the rectum next to the prostate. A current generated by the machine is applied to stimulate the nerves and produce contraction of the pelvic muscles resulting in ejaculation.[16] The procedure begins by first catheterizing the patient in supine position and emptying the bladder completely. The use of betadine is to be avoided because of its spermicidal effect. Instead, the urethra is lubricated with glycerin for catheterization. The pH of urine should be assessed to ensure its alkalinity (pH >7.0). Oral sodium bicarbonate may be used if necessary. Because retrograde ejaculation occurs frequently in this procedure, an additional 10 cc of the medium is instilled into the bladder to help preserve any sperm inside the bladder. The catheter is then removed. Although it is possible to perform the procedure in lithotomy position, lateral decubitus position is preferred, as it allows easier access to both the penis and rectum.

Rhythmic delivery of current is performed by manually turning the dial to increase the voltage delivery progressively for a few seconds. After a few initial stimulations, the voltage is reduced to zero. Voltage is then gradually increased until erection/ejaculation has occurred. The voltage at which the first erection/ejaculation occurs is noted and it is then increased to a level 30–50% higher, depending on patient's tolerance and the rectal temperature, which is constantly monitored and displayed. Ejaculation may be entirely retrograde and in such cases, sweating, piloerection, goose bumps on the thighs, buttocks, and partial erection may be the only signs that the patient is adequately stimulated and ejaculated. The number of stimulations, the current, and the voltage necessary to produce a maximum erection are noted, as this information will be useful for subsequent procedure if needed. The ejaculate is collected directly into a cup containing a sperm friendly buffer.

The collected semen specimen is processed in the andrology laboratory and if the specimen is of very good quality,[17] then it can be used for intrauterine insemination (IUI). If there are few sperms, or the sperms have low motility, then the specimen can be used with in vitro fertilization/intracytoplasmic sperm injection (ICSI) to establish a pregnancy. Electroejaculation must be performed under general anesthesia in all patients who have abdominal and perirectal sensation. Anesthesia is not required for spinal cord injured men who have high level injuries and are without sensation. Anyone who has a history of autonomic dysreflexia must have blood pressure and heart rate monitored as electroejaculation may cause a significant increase in blood pressure.

Initial results in terms of the ability to obtain motile sperm were variable, but with refinements in the equipment and techniques, sperm can now be obtained in approximately 90% of anejaculatory patients. These patients have excellent sperm densities averaging 180–300 million/cc. Despite success in the induction of ejaculation, sperm motility has continued to be low, limiting fertility in these patients. Mean sperm motilities of 20% have been reported in several series.[18] This poor motility appears to be secondary to intrinsic factors such as elevated scrotal temperature and recurrent genitourinary tract infection rather than to the electroejaculation procedure. The use of assisted reproductive techniques, especially ICSI, has become increasingly important in this patient population.[19] Because these patients often have supranormal sperm densities with low motility, semen processing with Percoll gradients may be beneficial in removing non motile sperm, white blood cells, and debris before insemination.

Research on persistent low motility in these patients suggests that psychogenic anejaculation is associated with increased incidence of antisperm autoimmunity explaining poor motility.[20] The majority of antibodies were directed against the sperm heads. Surface antibodies were mainly IgA isotype whereas serum antibodies were IgG isotype. Further research on sperm motility and effects of electrical current on sperm behavior in vitro exhibited a significant two fold decrease in motility percentage and viability. Superoxide dismutase (SOD) activity decreased significantly in sperm subjected to direct electric current, in comparison to the control groups.[21] These studies indicate that in vitro and in vivo electrical stimulation generates reactive oxygen species, which affects superoxide dismutase (SOD) activity, which in part is responsible for decreased sperm motion and viability.

Electroejaculation and vibratory stimulation have enabled many men who suffer from ejaculatory failure to conceive children of their own but it is imperative to plan for multiple sittings to maximize benefit.

Patient Preparation

Pretreatment: 24–48 hours alkalinization with sodium bicarbonate, 2 g PO TID.

- Bladder wash + medium optional*
- *They may need*:
  - Prophylactic antibiotics, if there is a history of urinary tract infection
  - Alpha agonist (e.g., Sudafed) to prevent retrograde ejaculation
  - Nifedipine (sublingual), if there is autonomic dysreflexia
  - Several proprietary media are available for sperm preservation
  - Currently, employing this technique, semen can be obtained in >90% of neurologically impaired men. More than 40% of the couples achieve pregnancy with IUI or IVF. Pregnancy rates are slightly better among couples in whom the male partner had spinal cord injury (43%) or idiopathic anejaculation (33%) than in those who had undergone retroperitoneal lymph node dissection (20%) or had diabetes.

Types of electroejaculators:

- Saeger
- Brindley

Retarded Ejaculation

Retarded ejaculation is the persistent difficulty or inability to ejaculate despite the presence of adequate sexual desire, erection, and stimulation (Glander HJ, 1998). Ejaculatory episodes are either partial, without pleasure or with pain. The causes of this dysfunction may be organic, i.e. medical illness or drug induced (particularly medications with antiadrenergic effects), the result of surgical interventions, or secondary to inhibiting psychological factors. With regard to psychological determinants, fear, guilt, and resentment have all been implicated.

Medical therapy is helpful in patients with severe psychological factors, and behavioral therapy or vibratory therapy helps most patients.

Orgasmic Disturbances

- Primary
- Secondary.

Primary absolute anorgasmia is the inability to have an orgasm and ejaculation during any kind of sexual activity while awake, in men with normal erectile function and nocturnal emission.[22] Though some men are occasionally found to have a neurological basis for the problem (occult spinal dysraphism with tethered cord, MS, etc.), primarily it is psychogenic with very few cases reported in literature. Primary modality of treatment of this condition is by:

- Sexual behavioral therapy—where in majority are refractory to treatment.
- Electroejaculation—may require multiple sittings and is usually successful.
- Vasal aspiration and ICSI is used in resistant cases.

Secondary anorgasmia is mainly associated with psychotropic drugs such as sertraline and gabapentin. Clinicians are increasingly faced with the need to identify, treat, and counsel patients regarding psychotropic drug induced sexual dysfunction. Antipsychotic and antidepressant drugs have both rational mechanisms to explain their effects on sexual function and established literature documenting these effects. Sexual dysfunction secondary to the use of antidepressants, especially clomipramine or SSRI's is an adverse effect that is often underestimated. This can affect approximately 60% of the patients. These patients may present with decrease in libido, alterations in the ability to reach orgasm/ejaculation, erectile dysfunction and anorgasmia. These dysfunctions appear to be related to the increase in serotonin, which occurs with the stimulation of serotonin 5 HT receptors. Nefazodone, amantadine, cyproheptadine, sildenafil, and serotonin antagonist mianserin are some of the drugs used in secondary anorgasmia but are ineffective. Failing drug therapy, electroejaculation, or vibratory stimulation is generally successful.

ERECTILE DYSFUNCTION INTRODUCTION

Virtually every male can regain sexual function if he so chooses. The silent suffering experienced by over 50% of males can come to an end with a wide spectrum of treatment forms from well-known means Sildenafil to not so commonly known ones like penile implants.

Sexual dysfunction as a consequence of drug therapy has been reported with a range of drugs, notably antihypertensives, antipsychotics, and antidepressants. The overall incidence of drug-induced sexual dysfunction is difficult to quantify. Patients are often unwilling to raise the issue of sexual health with health professionals leading to under reporting of problems. In addition, many diseases can affect sexual function, making it difficult to establish causality with a drug rather than concurrent illness. Antihypertensive medications are associated with erectile dysfunction and are often prescribed for hypertension in patients with diabetes, which itself may cause impotence. Other factors that can influence sexual function in men and women are age, alcohol consumption, smoking, drugs of abuse, over the counter medicines, and exposure to environmental or occupational toxins. Most of the published literature relates to the adverse effects of drugs on male sexual function. It is more difficult to assess these effects in women and this aspect of drug safety has seldom been considered in clinical studies **(Table 1)**.

The era of safe and effective surgery for the management of erectile dysfunction. The penile implant came to represent the "energizer bunny" approach to male sexual dysfunction, emphasizing the importance of a durable on demand rigid erection. The evaluation and management of male sexual dysfunction switched from the psychiatrist's couch to the urologist office and the operating room. If the "phallocentric approach" was born out of surgical zeal to fix something that was broken, it was also nurtured by industry's correct perception of the financial health market. The chance discovery in 1982 that a vasodilator could produce a normal erection in the absence of sexual stimulation began *the age of physiology and pathophysiology* of erectile dysfunction. This was a decade of directed research that culminated in 1993 with the first National Institutes of Health (NIH) Consensus Conference on impotence where the various aspects of male sexual function (interest, performance, and satisfaction) were addressed and erectile dysfunction was specifically defined.[23-40]

The participants looked at multiple strategies for correctly identifying and evaluating ED; they were most impressed by the statistical associations with increasing age, and the concurrence of distinct medical illnesses—diabetes, atherosclerotic peripheral and coronary artery disease, hypertension, cigarette smoking, and chronic renal insufficiency. In the clinical arena the "goal-directed" was formulated to conserve health care dollars and minimize morbidity to patients from excessive testing. The goal

TABLE 1: The major risk factors for the development of erectile dysfunction (ED).	
Aging	Men who are aged 50–90 are 10 times more likely to develop erectile dysfunction than men younger than 50
Comorbidities	Certain medical conditions can increase the risk of erectile dysfunction, including diabetes and cardiovascular disease. Arteriosclerosis (hardening of arteries), chronic kidney disease, liver failure, Peyronie's disease (bending of the penis caused by scar tissue), endocrine disorders neurological disorders (such as multiple sclerosis, peripheral neuropathy, and stroke), hypertension (high blood pressure), psychiatric disorders (such as anxiety, depression, and schizophrenia)
Traumatic conditions	Vascular surgery, urologic surgery, pelvic surgeries (particularly for prostate cancer), and spinal cord injury
Lifestyle behavior	Certain behaviors increase the risk of erectile dysfunction, including—alcohol use, illegal drug, anabolic steroid use, heavy smoking, interpersonal conflicts with a sexual partner
Medications	Medications increasing the risk of erectile dysfunction, include antihypertensives, antihistamines, antidepressants, tranquilizers, and antipsychotics

directed approach was based on a very limited number of options for ED, and recognition that the main purpose of testing to establish a diagnosis should be to formulate a treatment plan. In an era when there were no cause-specific treatments a good sexual history with assessment of medical risks, permitted most patients to be safely directed to therapy based solely on preference. Without testing efficacy and satisfaction were matters of chance.

Among patients referred to urology clinics for ED, the subgroups having decreased libido, testicular damage/abnormality, arterial disease, insulin resistance, or diabetes were more likely to have hypogonadism. The evidence is less consistent concerning such factors as the severity of ED, duration of ED, or sexual disorders (e.g., premature ejaculation).

Laboratory Testing

Laboratory testing needs tailoring to the patient's complaints and risk factors. Patients may need a fasting blood glucose or HbA1c [preferred over fasting blood sugar (FBS) or random blood sugar (RBS)], and lipid profile, if these are not assessed recently. Hormonal tests include an early morning total testosterone. If indicated, the bio-available or calculated-free testosterone may be needed to corroborate total testosterone measurements. However, the threshold of testosterone required to maintain an erection is low, and ED is usually a symptom of more severe cases of hypogonadism. For levels >8 nmol/L relationship between circulating testosterone and sexual functioning is quite low. Additional laboratory tests may be considered in selected patients [e.g., prostate-specific antigen (PSA), prolactin, and luteinizing hormone]. Although physical examination and laboratory evaluation of most men with ED may not reveal the exact diagnosis, they present opportunities to identify critical comorbid conditions that should not be missed.

This new age of effective oral pharmacotherapy presents the possibility of cause specific therapy. Currently under clinical evaluation are multiple oral agents with distinct pharmacological mechanisms: central initiators of erection, central conditioners of sexual behavior and peripheral modulators of penile blood flow. Currently, we are compelled to categorize patients simplistically as oral agent responsive or oral agent resistant erectile dysfunction. When available treatments grow into a "laundry list of options" the role of impotence testing will assume a two-fold importance—establishing an etiology specific diagnosis and formulating an effective treatment plan. Patients seeking the expertise of urologists will want to know why a specific agent has failed. We will return to erectile testing to produce vascular profiles, to predict which oral drug or combination of drugs (oral, cutaneous, urethral, and intracavernosal) will effectively restore their erections, or to determine whether patients would best be served by the placement of a penile prosthesis.

How Has Oral Pharmacotherapy Changed ED Practice?

Evidence-based assessments of erectile dysfunction have taken a secondary role in the evaluation process; the introduction of effective oral pharmacotherapy for vascular impotence has dramatically altered my approach to ED testing much like injectable vasoactive agents almost two decades prior. It is clinically pragmatic to begin every evaluation of male sexual dysfunction with a good medical history to determine the patient's relative risks for vascular ED—hypertension, atherosclerotic coronary and peripheral vascular disease, diabetes mellitus, and smoking. Sex questionnaires are a good way of structuring the male sexual history for the novice, but it is unclear whether they accurately distinguish psychogenic from vasculogenic dysfunction or whether they can qualify the severity of erectile dysfunction, no matter what the etiology. It is pragmatic to use an oral agent in a diagnostic role and to characterize the patient as having "oral agent responsive" or "oral agent resistant ED."

Pharmacotherapy: Rationale

The physiology of the smooth muscle cell (SMC) in the trabeculae of the cavernosal sinusoids and in the walls of the cavernosal and helicine arteries is central to the unique erectile function of the penis. The functional state of the penis is a neurovascular event representing the balance between the degree of relaxation and that of contraction of the SMC.

Nitric oxide (NO), produced by the vascular endothelium and the nonadrenergic noncholinergic parasympathetic nerve endings under the influence of the various isoforms of NO synthase, is the principal chemomediator for SMC relaxation, thus penile erection, through the production of cyclic guanosine monophosphate (cGMP). While neuronal NO initiates erection, endothelial NO maintains the erectile response. Alongside this, through the cyclic adenosine monophosphate (cAMP) pathway, prostanoids and vasoactive intestinal polypeptide also contribute to SMC relaxation.

Smooth muscle cell contraction, on the other hand, is brought about principally by noradrenaline via the α1 sympathetic pathway, and is responsible for penile flaccidity and detumescence. Other chemotransmitters for SMC contraction include endothelin, neuropeptide Y and prostanoids. Currently available pharmacotherapeutic agents for ED act mainly by enhancing SMC relaxation through the selective and nonselective inhibition of the phosphodiesterases.[41,42]

Role of Testosterone in Erectile Dysfunction

Testosterone modulates the expression of NO synthase in the corpus cavernosum and the production of NO, and acts on the cavernosal arterioles enhancing penile rigidity. It influences genital sensitivity and pleasurable enhancement of erectile activity. Testosterone deficiency is an infrequent cause of ED. However, if it is the confirmed cause, treatment with testosterone supplementation is rewarding. Correction of androgen deficiency not only restores erectile function but also improves general well-being and libido. As it influences NO production through hits modulating effect on NO synthase, testosterone enhances the treatment outcome for ED with PDE5 inhibitors.[43-46]

There is no universally accepted method of identifying men with clinically relevant hypogonadism affecting erectile function. The implications of androgen status for erectile dysfunction and its treatments continue to remain controversial. Given the current gaps in knowledge, the most adequate and cost-effective laboratory test for hormonal evaluation is unclear. The two differing guideline statements available reflect this problem.[25]

The American Urological Association recommends testosterone testing based on initial clinical assessment results or failure of prior management with PDE5 inhibitors. However, the European Urological Association mandates testosterone measures (bioavailable or calculated-free testosterone begin preferred over total levels) for all men with ED. These two associations have similar guidelines, which suggest that further laboratory investigations including prolactin, luteinizing hormone (LH), and follicle stimulating hormone (FSH) testing are indicated when low testosterone levels are detected.

Recommendations

Testosterone therapy is not indicated for the treatment of erectile dysfunction in the patient with a normal serum testosterone level.

Combination Pharmacotherapy for the Hard-to-Treat Erectile Dysfunction

Although response to the currently available pharmacotherapy is mostly satisfactory, a significant number of patients with ED are unable to achieve an adequate response. There is, therefore, the need to explore if there may be beneficial outcomes from a rational combination of the therapeutic agents in current use, until newer agents become available. At least three plausible combinations would merit consideration:

- Combination of a centrally acting agent with a peripherally acting agent, e.g., sublingual apomorphine with oral PDE5 inhibitor.
- Combination of an agent acting via the cGMP pathway with one via the cAMP pathway, e.g., oral PDE5 inhibitor with intracavernosal alprostadil.
- Combination of an agent enhancing SMC relaxation with one decreasing SMC contraction, e.g., oral PDE5 inhibitor with α-1 adrenergic blocker.

Further research will be needed to confirm the usefulness of such combinations as intracavernosal alprostadil and oral PDE5 inhibitor and provide rational guidelines for this and other combinations of proven value to be part of the management strategy for ED. The risk of possible side effects may be minimized if the relevant exclusion criteria and prerequisites, based on a sound understanding of the pharmacological properties of the agents used, are strictly observed and treatment protocol meticulously followed.

How Much Testing is Needed in the Era of Effective Oral Pharmacotherapy?

The selection of a treatment for erectile dysfunction (ED) in the 1970s was relatively simple. Sex therapy was the treatment of choice for psychogenic ED, and penile prosthesis implantation was the only reasonable treatment option for organic ED. Today we have a variety of treatment options including: sex therapy, systemic therapy, vacuum erection devices, intraurethral pharmacotherapy, penile injection therapy, penile prosthesis implantation, vascular surgery and the most recent addition penile shock wave therapy. The introduction of the concept of intracavernous vaso active drug injection in 1983 significantly changed both the evaluation and the treatment of ED. Now the following tests based on vasoactive drug injection are available—test injection, cavernosometry, cavernosography, and duplex ultrasonography.

Which of These Tests, If Any, Should be Performed and How Valid are these Tests?

Vasoactive intracorporeal drug injection triggers two responses. The first is increased arterial inflow, which leads to tumescence. The second is corporeal smooth muscle relaxation which if complete leads to corporovenous occlusion and rigidity. Both of the responses can be blunted by anxiety, but this is much more likely to occur with the second response. Psychogenic ED has two subtypes. The man with high performance anxiety remains completely flaccid. The man with a lesser amount of anxiety develops tumescence but either does not obtain full rigidity or cannot maintain it. Responses to diagnostic testing involving vasoactive drug injection often parallel what occurs in men with psychogenic ED; thus these tests are not reliable for differentiating psychogenic from organic ED. Because vasoactive drug injection does not invariably produce complete smooth muscle relaxation, the validity of tests involving these injections comes under question.

In terms of a diagnostic test injection, if a man responds with a full, sustained erection, he may be normal, he may have neurogenic ED, or he may have mild vasculogenic ED. On the other hand, if he fails to respond to a test injection, nothing can be said about the etiology of his ED.

Duplex ultrasonography study of the penile arteries after vasoactive drug injection has two components. The assessment of peak systolic velocities in the cavernous arteries is probably reasonably accurate as this phase of the erection response to these drugs seems less influenced by anxiety than the corporovenous occlusive phase. However, since complete smooth muscle relaxation is quite subject to anxiety, one should be cautious about making the diagnosis of corporal venous occlusive disease/dysfunction (CVOD) if the end diastolic velocity does not return to zero.

There has been a disturbing trend in recent years toward over reliance on tests involving vasoactive drug injections. This is often associated with taking an incomplete sexual history. This is unfortunate because some important elements of the evaluation can only be ascertained by taking a good sexual history. For example, a man with premature ejaculation often presents with the complaint of problems with erections. An incomplete history fails to uncover the fact that his problem is in fact with ejaculatory control. The patient is then subjected to unnecessary testing which often leads to the false diagnosis of CVOD and unnecessary surgery. Another disturbing trend is the abandonment of NPT testing, a diagnostic technique which has been well validated by studies in normal subjects.

Diagnosis and treatment of erectile dysfunction is given in an Analytic framework depicted in the **Figure 1**.

In the Era of Goal Directed Therapy are Any Tests Necessary?

If a man and his partner select a nonsurgical treatment, then a thorough sexual and medical history, physical examination, and laboratory studies to rule out occult systemic disease and hypogonadism should suffice. If a man elects surgical treatment, then further testing is usually desirable.

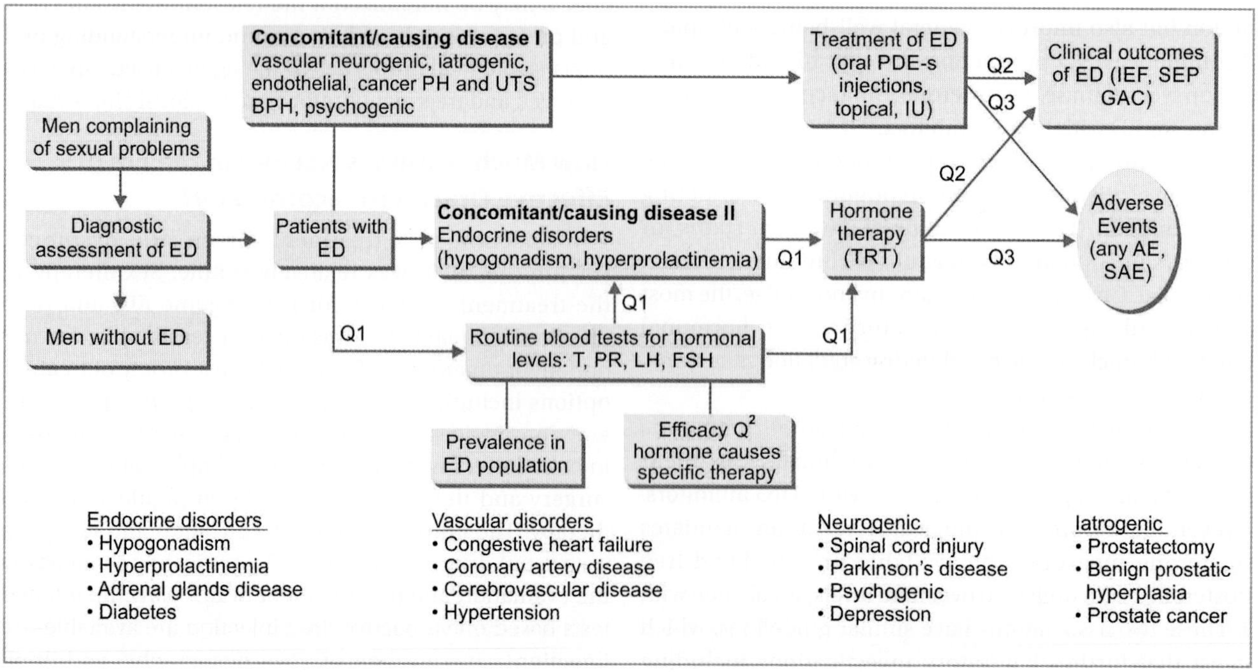

Fig. 1: Analytic framework for the diagnosis and treatment of erectile dysfunction.

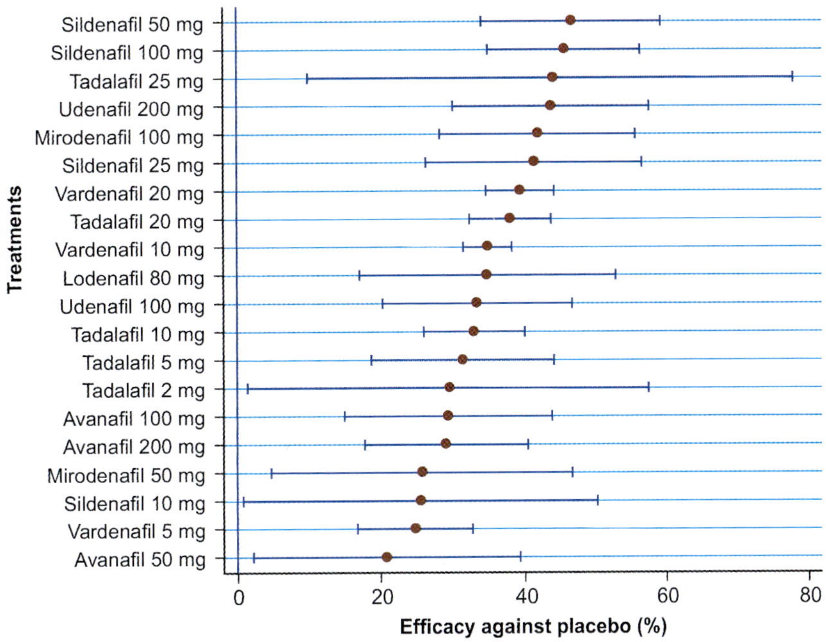

Fig. 2: Efficacy of phosphodiesterase type 5 inhibitor as per trade-off analysis. Sildenafil 50 mg had the greatest efficacy.
Source: Chen L, Staubli SE, Schneider MP, Kessels AG, Ivic S, Bachmann LM, et al. Phosphodiesterase 5 inhibitors for the treatment of erectile dysfunction: a trade-off network meta-analysis. Eur Urol. 2015;68(4):674-80.

Erectile Dysfunction Assessment and Treatment Protocol Evaluation-diagnostic Algorithm for ED (Fig. 1)

- Sexual history (validated questionnaire)
- Psychological profile
- Medical history

Physical Examination Assessment of Cardiac Risks

Investigations:

- Fasting blood sugar
- Lipid profile if indicated
- Serum testosterone if needed

Management/Treatment

- Educate patients regarding treatment options and associated risks and benefits.
- Manage risk factors for erectile dysfunction (e.g., lifestyle modifications to prevent or reverse erectile dysfunction).
- Consider comorbidities when managing patients with ED (e.g., provide appropriate management of patients with ED in the presence of cardiovascular disease).
- *Pharmacologic therapy*:
    - Phosphodiesterase type-5 (PDE5) inhibitors (sildenafil, tadalafil, and vardenafil) **(Figs. 2 and 3) (Table 2)**
    - Alprostadil intraurethral suppositories
    - Intracavernous injection with alprostadil, papaverine, or phentolamine or combinations.
- Vacuum constriction devices:
- *Surgery*:
    - Penile prosthesis implantation with preoperative administration of antibiotics
    - Vascular surgery (penile arterial reconstructive surgery).
- Periodic follow-up of efficacy, side effects, and change in health status.

Primary Interventions

- *Suspicion of predominantly psychogenic impotence*: Psychotherapy
- *Low testosterone and no contraindications*: Testosterone replacement
- *Performance anxiety + mild organic risk factors*: NO donors + mood elevators +/− *sildenafil/tadalafil/vardenafil moderate organic risk factors*: Sildenafil-tadalafil or vardenafil-titrate dosage

Option of intracavernous injection (I/C) therapy for failures or combination therapy of oral drug + I/C injection.

Third Line Therapy—Penile Prosthesis

In **Tables 2 and 3**, we see that penile prosthesis implantation is the only treatment option, which is applicable under all circumstances. VED's (vacuum devices) have the next broadest usage (however this is popular in US but not in India due to cultural reasons and feeling that it is too artificial) but they require reasonably intact corpora, MUSE or ICI require reasonably intact arterial inflow and corpora, and systemic therapy requires that some of all 3 determinants be present.

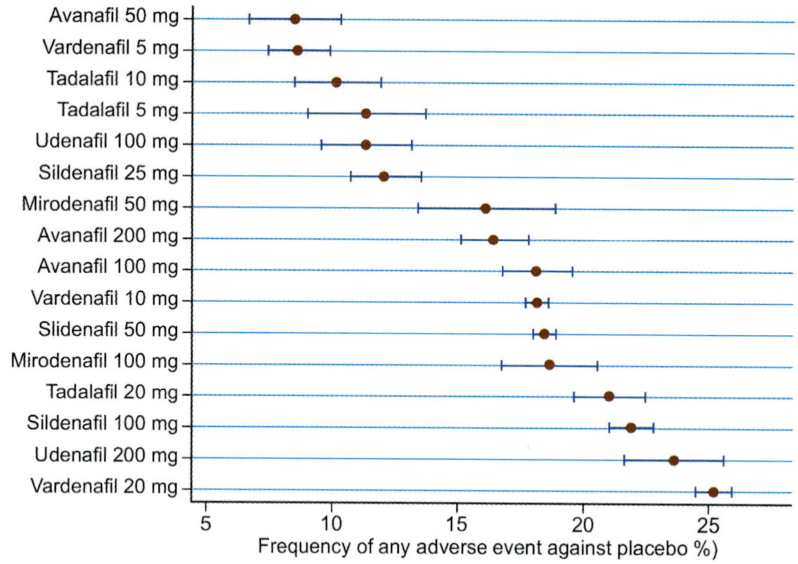

Fig. 3: Safety of phosphodiesterase type 5 inhibitor as per trade-off analysis. Tadalafil 10 mg had the lowest overall rate of all adverse events. *Source:* Chen L, Staubli SE, Schneider MP, Kessels AG, Ivic S, Bachmann LM, et al. Phosphodiesterase 5 inhibitors for the treatment of erectile dysfunction: a trade-off network meta-analysis. Eur Urol. 2015;68(4):674-80.

TABLE 2: Requirements for treatment success.

Rx modality	*Nerves*	*Arteries*	*Corpora*
Oral agents	+	+	+
MUSE/intracavernosal injection (ICI)	–	+	+
VED	–	–	+
Implant	–	–	–

When there are significant problems with the corpora in terms of abnormalities of the tunica albuginea and/or the cavernosal smooth muscle, penile prosthesis implantation may be the only reasonable treatment alternative. This includes men with corporeal fibrosis following removal of an infected penile prosthesis or following priapism and men with erectile deformity secondary to Peyronie's disease if they also have significant ED.

Future Therapies in Management of Erectile Dysfunction

Extracorporeal shock wave therapy (ESWT) is currently used in the treatment of urinary stones in orthopedics, cardiology, wound healing, plastic surgery and neurology. Shockwaves are being successfully used around the world since 2005 to treat reversible ischemic tissues in the heart, inducing neovascularization and developing new collaterals which improves the blood supply to tissues.[47] The same modality is used for treatment of vascular based (poor blood flow) erectile dysfunction problems. This therapy aims to provide improvement and possible cure for ED. It allows a man to return to a more normal erection.

With ESWT, it has been possible for the first time to establish a rapid, effective, and cost-effective outpatient therapy that can be used as often as required without any side effects. Short term results are extremely encouraging. Pharmacotherapeutic strategies for ED either promote proerectile mechanisms or suppress antierectile mechanisms, or do both. These objectives are based on the knowledge that the erectile state represents a finely controlled equilibrium between proerectile and antierectile mechanisms that influence corporal smooth muscle tone.

Promoting proerectile action can be achieved by either—(i) inducing smooth muscle relaxation through cell receptor agonists or direct activators of tissue relaxant pathways [e.g., stimulating second messenger cyclic nucleotide (cGMP or cAMP) synthesis] or (ii) inhibiting the deactivation of smooth muscle relaxation pathways. In the latter strategy, for example, inhibition of phosphodiesterases, enzymes that inactivate cAMP or cGMP, results in the accumulation of these nucleotides, which in turn diminishes contractility of smooth muscle tissue and thus maintains the muscle relaxation necessary for erection. Suppressing antierectile action can be achieved by decreasing smooth muscle contraction through receptor antagonists of tissue contractile pathways [e.g., alpha 2 adrenergic (nor epinephrine) inhibitors].

Indications for treatment for ED are enumerated in **Table 3**.

Treatment approaches may also be directed toward the central nervous system (i.e., brain or spinal cord. Similar to peripheral mechanisms, these either promote proerectile pathways (e.g., agonists of dopaminergic receptors in the medial hypothalamus or suppress antierectile pathways [e.g., antagonists of 5(HT.sub.lA/2) serotonergic receptors in the spinal cord] **(Table 4)**.

TABLE 3: Indications for treatment.

Rx modality	*Nerves*	*Arteries*	*Corpora*
Oral agents	+	+	+
MUSE/intracavernosal injection (ICI)	+/–	+	+
VED	+/-	+/–	+
Implant	+/–	+/–	+/–

TABLE 4: Phosphodiesterase-5 pharmacokinetic comparison.

Generic name	*Udenafil*	*Sildenafil*	*Tadalafil*	*Vardenafil*
Onset	30–40 minutes	30–60 minutes	45–120 minutes	30–60 minutes
Duration time	12–24 hours	4–8 hours	36 hours	6–8 hours
Half-life	11–13 hours	4 hours	17.5–20 hours	4 hours

Onset of action–sildenafil = udenafil < tadalafil
Duration of action–tadalafil > udenafil > sildenafil

SUMMARY

Infertility is an emotional crisis and a physical challenge because it interferes with one of the most fundamental human activities. From a list of 87 items of stressful life events, infertility has been ranked as one of the most negative stressful situations—akin to the death of a son or a spouse.

Fertility related concerns are significant for the spinal cord injured male because of his young age and loss of ejaculatory function. Fortunately, using electroejaculation and vibratory stimulation, the successful recovery of sperm has become routine. However, because of the poor quality of the sperm obtained, the assisted reproductive techniques of intrauterine insemination and in vitro fertilization have had only modest pregnancy results. The revolutionary technique of intracytoplasmic sperm injection (ICSI), which involves the injection of a single sperm into an oocyte, is particularly applicable for these patients and has been very successful in initiating pregnancies. The potential for improvement in semen recovery and processing is great and must be considered a challenge for the immediate future. Finally, fertility issues in men may be quite complex and clearly needs a multidisciplinary management approach.

KEY RECOMMENDATIONS

Common Sexual Problem in Clinical Practice and History

As per The Diagnostic and Statistical Manual of Mental Disorders, 2013, all these problems should be present for minimum 6 months and should be associated with personal distress to term as dysfunction. Sexual history taking is very

Flowchart 1: Pathogenesis—erectile dysfunction (ED) due to metabolic syndrome.

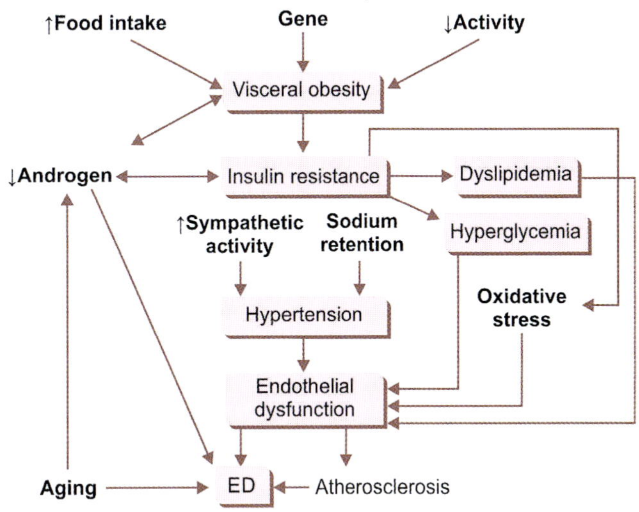

Source: Suetomi T, Kawai K, Hinotsu S, Joraku A, Oikawa T, Sekido N, et al. Negative impact of metabolic syndrome on the responsiveness to sildenafil in Japanese men. J Sex Med. 2008;5(6):1443-50.

Flowchart 2: Pathogenesis—erectile dysfunction is a vascular disease.

Pathophysiology of vascular disease

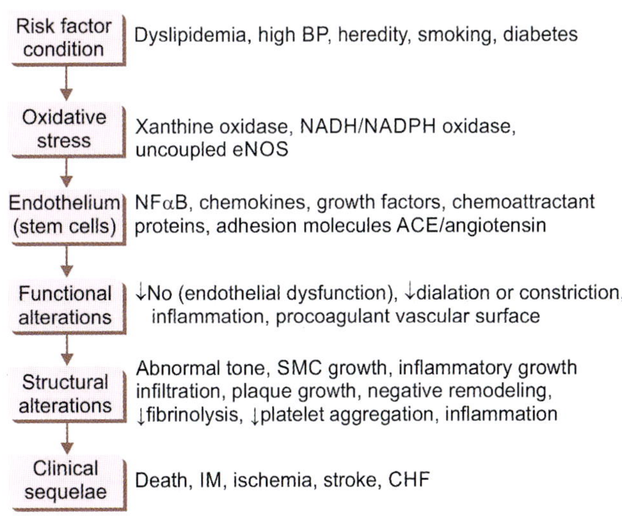

(ACE: angiotensin-converting enzyme; BP: blood pressure; CHF: congestive heart failure; eNOS: endothelial nitric oxide synthase; NADH: nicotinamide adenine dinucleotide; NADPH: nicotinamide adenine dinucleotide phosphate; NO: nitric oxide; SMC: smooth muscle cell)

Source: Pepine CJ. Why vascular biology matters. Am J Cardiol. 2001;88(8A):5K-9K.

important and crucial first step in arriving to the etiology of sexual dysfunction. Almost 70% cases of sexual problems can be diagnosed by meticulous history taking alone.

Sexual history can be taken by verbal or nonverbal methods including various questionnaires such as Arizona Sexual Experience Scale and The International Index of Erectile Function.

Brief screening questions like "many people have sexual concerns, I wonder what yours might be?" provide high yield of information related to sexual health when it is covered as part of routine history in patients with other health problems.

Almost 64% of men reported some concomitant illness associated with erectile dysfunction; 29% having one comorbidity; 20% having two comorbidities; 11% having three comorbidities, and 5% having four or more comorbid conditions. The common comorbid conditions associated with erectile dysfunction (ED) are angina, hypertension, depression, diabetes, hypercholesterolemia, etc.

Erectile dysfunction and cardiovascular disease have common risk factors, which are dependent on endothelial function all over the body. Smoking, blood pressure, diabetes, and cholesterol all are the common risk factors for both **(Flowcharts 1 and 2)**.

As the diameter of the penile artery is less compared to coronary artery, ED often occurs before other vascular diseases. Hence, it is important to evaluate cardiovascular status as well in young patients presented with ED.

Almost three out of four diabetic patients have reported erectile problems, and as the prevalence of diabetes increases, so the prevalence of ED. Hence, it is important to ask every patient of diabetes coming to the clinic regarding erectile function.

Endothelial dysfunction is a significant marker to predict hypertension and diabetes. As per one study in postmenopausal women, endothelial dysfunction leads to 5.8-fold increase in developing hypertension and sixfold increase in developing diabetes over a period of 3–5 years.

Diagnosis of endothelial dysfunction helps in early diagnosis of cardiovascular and metabolic events.

Flowchart 3: Canadian Urology Association—Erectile Dysfunction (ED) Management Guideline.

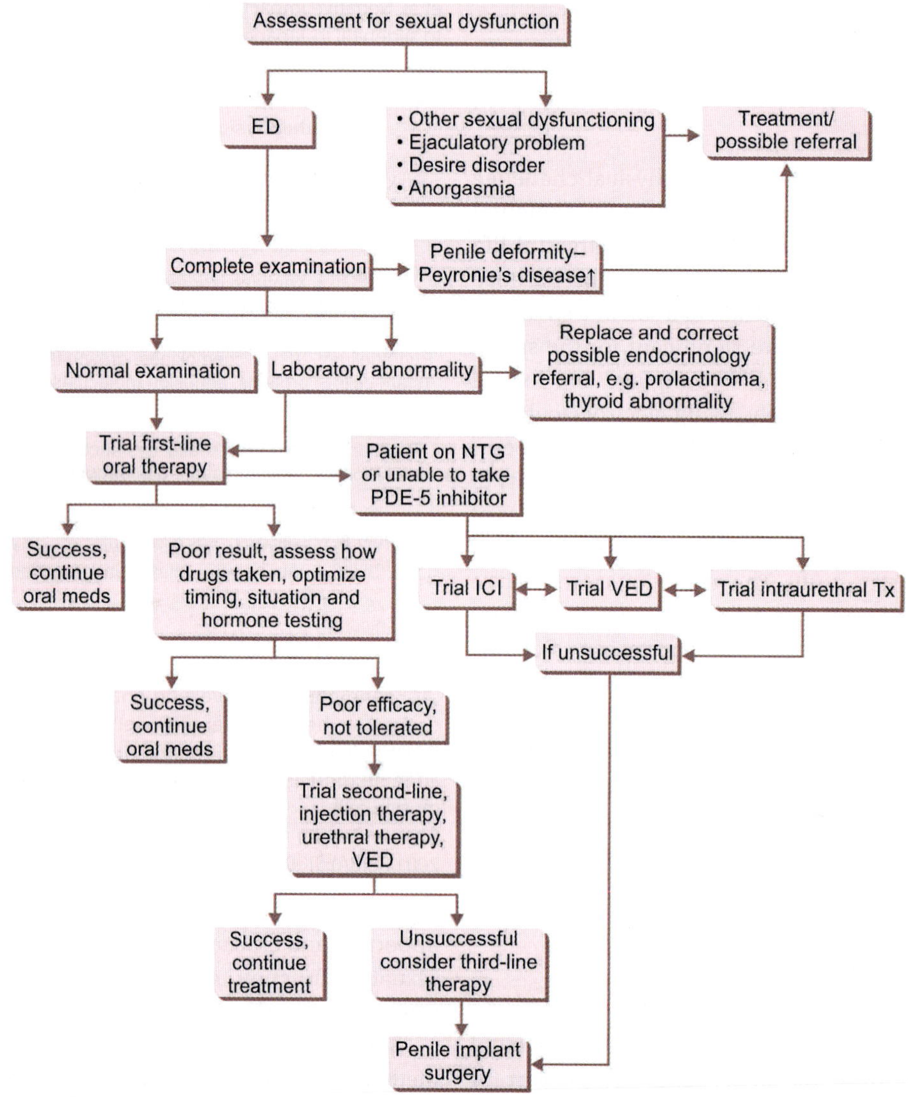

(ICI: intracavernosal injections; VED: vacuum erection device; NTG: nitrates/nitroglycerine)

Source: Bella AJ, Lee JC, Carrier S, Bénard F, Brock GB. 2015 CUA Practice guidelines for erectile dysfunction. Can Urol Assoc J. 2015;9(1-2):23-9.

Flowchart 4: Erectile dysfunction (ED) in hypertensive patients on medication—management algorithm.

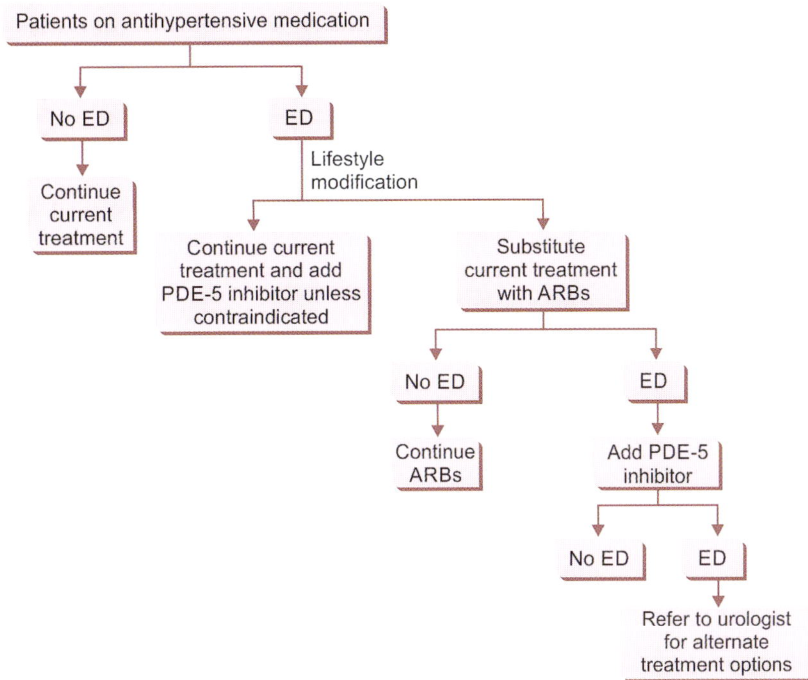

(PDE5: phosphodiesterase-5; ARBs: angiotensin receptor blockers)
Source: Doumas M, Douma S. The effect of antihypertensive drugs on erectile function: a proposed management algorithm. J Clin Hypertens (Greenwich). 2006;8(5):359-64.

Flowchart 5: Algorithm for erectile dysfunction (ED) medication prescription.

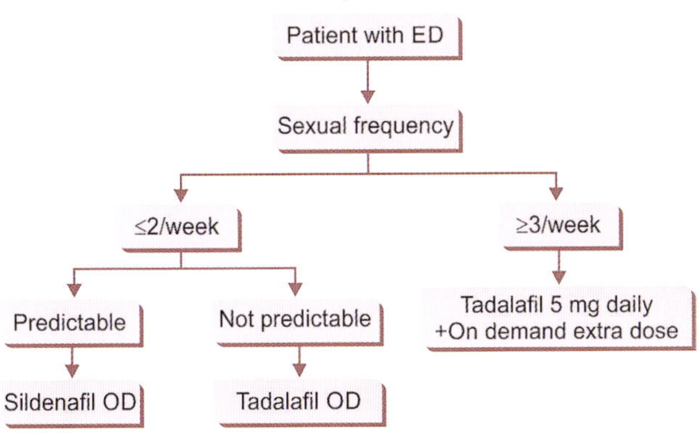

Start with max dose-reduce for side effects

The Erection Hardness Score is a simple measure to diagnose the hardness of penis, which is an old method of ED evaluation.

Assessment of penile endothelial function can help detect early systemic derangement and facilitate ED or vascular risk assessment (*see* **Flowcharts 3 to 5**). Brachial artery reactivity test is a standardized test to assess the terminal arteriolar health. A reactivity index obtained by this test could indicate penile arteriolar vascular health and endothelial derangement. Tissue perfusion of oxygen is an indirect measure of nitric oxide level, which can be measured by FDA, approved devices. Systemic involvement of endothelial dysfunction can be evaluated by assessment of medium size arteries with pulse wave velocity. Abnormal findings of these tests in ED evaluation suggest that such patients are at high risk of developing future cardiovascular events. Shock wave therapy is one of additional modality of management of arteriogenic ED.

It is hypothesized to increase the nitric oxide level and vascular reactivity as assessed in rat model and cardiac muscle. As per a global study, the effect usually lasts for about 12–14 months with peak effect reported till 6–8 months. Who will benefit? Only those who have the sexual health inventory for men score >8 and mainly arteriogenic ED.

CONCLUSION

In today's era, any patient of sexual dysfunction is treated according to identifying which part of sexual cycle is invovled and keeping his and his partner's goal. The idea is not to be judgmental of patient's preferences but appropriately counsel them about all options, to lead a satisfactory and fulfilling sexual life, which will ultimately enhance their quality of life, which is the main goal of medical practice in this century.

KEY POINTS

In today's era, we can ensure that every patient of ED is treated according to his and his partner's goal. The idea is not to be judgmental of patient's preferences but appropriately counsel them about all options, to lead a satisfactory and fulfilling sexual life, which will ultimately enhance their quality of life, which is the main goal of medical practice in this century.

REFERENCES

1. Hull EM, Lorrain DS, Du J, Matuszewich L, Lumley LA, Putnam SK, et al. Hormone-neurotransmitter interactions in the control of sexual behavior. Behav Brain Res. 1999; 105(l):105-16.
2. Hora M, Vozeh F. The physiology of erection Urologicka Klinika LF UK a FN, Plzen Cas Lek Cesk. 1997;136(12):363-6.
3. Shafik A. Pelvic floor muscles and sphincters during erection and ejaculation. Arch Androl. 1997;39(l):71-8.
4. Zaragooshi J. Unconsummated marriage: Clarification of aetiology; treatment with intracorporeal injection. BJU Int. 2000;86(l):75-9.
5. Broderick GA. Evidence based assessment of erectile dysfunction. Int J Impot Res. 1998;(Suppl 2):S64-73; discussion S77-9.
6. McMahon CG, Touma K. Predictive value of patient history and correlation of nocturnal penile tumescence, colour duplex Doppler ultrasonography and dynamic cavernosometry and cavernosography in the evaluation of erectile dysfunction. Int J Impot Res. 1999;11(1):47-51.
7. Hermabessiere J, Guy L, Boiteux JP. Human ejaculation: Physiology, surgical conservation of ejaculation. Prog Urol. 1999;9(2):305-9.
8. Metz ME, Pryor JL, Nesvacil LJ, et al. Premature ejaculation: a psychophysiological approach for assessment and management. J Sex Marital Ther. 2000;26(4):293-320.
9. Janssen PK, Waldinger MD. The mathematical formula of the intravaginal ejaculation latency time (IELT) distribution of lifelong premature ejaculation differs from the IELT distribution formula of men in the general male population. Investig Clin Urol 2016;57:119-26; discussion 126-8. 10.4111/icu.2016.57.2.119
10. Malossinni G, Ficarra V, Caleffi G. Retrograde ejaculation. Arch Ital Urol Androl. 1999;71(3):185-96
11. Glander HJ. Disorders of ejaculation. Fortschr Med. 1998; 116(26):26-8,30-l.
12. Witt MA, Grantmyre JE. Ejaculatory failure. World J Urol. 1993;11(2):89-95.
13. Sonksen J, Biering-Sørensen F, Kristensen JK. Ejaculation induced by penile vibratory stimulation in men with spinal cord injuries. The importance of the vibratory amplitude. Paraplegia. l994;32(10):651-60.
14. Ohl DA, Sonksen J, Menge AC, McCabe M, Keller LM. Electroejaculation versus vibratory stimulation in spinal cord injured men: Sperm quality and patient preference. J Urol. 1997;157(6):2147-9.
15. Ohl DA, Bennett CJ, McCabe M, Menge AC, McGuire EJ. Predictors of success in electroejaculation of spinal cord injured men. J Urol. 1989;142(6):1483-6.
16. Eid JF. Electroejaculation. AUA Update Series, Volume XI, Lesson. 1992;10:73-80.
17. Chung PH, Verkauf BS, Mola R, Skinner L, Eichberg RD, Maroulis GB. Correlation between semen parameters of electroejaculates and achieving pregnancy by intrauterine insemination. Fertil Steril. 1997;67(1):129-32.
18. Hirsch IH, Sedor J, Jeyendran RS, Stass WE. The relative distribution of viable sperm in the antegrade and retrograde portions of ejaculates obtained after electrostimulation. Fertil Steril. 1992;57(2):399-401.
19. Nehra A, Werner MA, Bastuba M, Title C, Oates RD. Vibratory stimulation and rectal probe electroejaculation as therapy for patients with spinal cord injury: Semen parameters and pregnancy rates. J Urol. 1996;155(2):554-59.
20. Bubanouic I, Najmah S, Kojic S. New immunomodulatory treatment for infertile men with antisperm antibodies. Fertil Steril. 2004;81(3):S7-31;p:20.
21. Rajasekaran M, Hellstrom WJ, Sparks RL, Sikka SC. Sperm-damaging effects of electric current: Possible role of free radicals. Reprod Toxicol. 1994;8(5):427-32.
22. Michetti PM, Rossi R, Travaglia S, Barrese F, Franco G, Leone P, et al. Primary absolute anorgasmy in the male. Report of three clinical cases. Minerva Urol Nefrol. 999;51(l):23-6.
23. Lizza EF, Rosen RC. Definition and classification of erectile dysfunction: Report of the Nomenclature Committee of the International Society of Impotence Research. Int J Impot Res. 1999;11(3):141-3.
24. Korenman SG. Epidemiology of erectile dysfunction. Endocrine. 2004;23(2-3):87-91.
25. Shabsigh R, Perelman MA, Lockhart DC, Lue TF, Broderick GA. Health issues of men: Prevalence and correlates of erectile dysfunction. J Urol. 2005;174(2):662-7.
26. Mallis D, Moisidis K, Kirana PS, Papaharitou S, Simos G, Hatzichristou D. Moderate and severe erectile dysfunction equally affects life satisfaction. J Sex Med. 2006;3(3):442-9.
27. Kupelian V1, Shabsigh R, Araujo AB, O'Donnell AB, McKinlay JB. Erectile dysfunction as a predictor of the metabolic syndrome in aging men: Results from the Massachusetts male aging study. J Urol. 2006;176(l):222-6.
28. Sun P, Cameron A, Seftel A, Shabsigh R, Niederberger C, Guay A. Erectile dysfunction--An observable marker of diabetes mellitus? A large national epidemiological study. J Urol. 2006;176(3):1081-5.
29. Shabsigh R, AG Anastasiadis. Erectile dysfunction. Annu Rev Med. 2003;54:153-68.
30. Watts GF, Chew KK, Stuckey BG. The erectile-endothelial dysfunction nexus: new opportunities for cardiovascular risk prevention. Nat Clin Pract Cardiovasc Med. 2007;4(5):263-73.
31. Eaton CB, Liu YL, Mittleman MA, Miner M, Glasser DB, Rimm EB. A retrospective study of the relationship between biomarkers of atherosclerosis and erectile dysfunction in 988 men. Int J Impot Res. 2007;19(2):218-25.
32. Muller A, Mulhall JP. Cardiovascular disease, metabolic syndrome and erectile dysfunction. Curr Opin Urol. 2006; 16(6):435-43.
33. Kirby M, Jackson G, Simonsen U. Endothelial dysfunction links erectile dysfunction to heart disease. Int J Clin Pract. 2005;59(2):225-9.
34. Thompson IM, Tangen CM, Goodman PJ, Probstfield JL, Moinpour CM, Coltman CA. Erectile dysfunction and subsequent cardiovascular disease. JAMA. 2005;294(23): 2996-3002.
35. Stuckey BG, Walsh JP, Ching HL, Stuckey AW, Palmer NR, Thompson PL, et al. Erectile dysfunction predicts generalised cardiovascular disease: Evidence from a case-control study. Atherosclerosis. 2007;194(2):458-64.
36. Burnett AL. Erectile dysfunction. J Urol. 2006;175(3 Pt 2): S25-31.

37. Feldman HA, Goldstein I, Hatzichristou DG, Krane RJ, McKinlay JB. Impotence and its medical and psychosocial correlates: results of the Massachusetts male aging study. J Urol. 1994;151(1):54-61.
38. Grover SA, Lowensteyn I, Kaouache M, et al. The prevalence of erectile dysfunction in the primary care setting: Importance of risk factors for diabetes and vascular disease. Arch Intern Med. 2006;166(2):213-9.
39. Nicollerat JA. Implications of the United Kingdom Prospective Diabetes Study (UKPDS) results on patient management. Diabetes Educ. 2000;(Suppl 26):8-10.
40. Kloner RA. NIH Consensus Conference. Impotence. NIH Consensus Development Panel on Impotence. JAMA. 1993; 270(1):83-90.
41. Hamed EA Meki AR, Gaafar AA, Hamed SA. Role of some vasoactive mediators in patients with erectile dysfunction: Their relationship with angiotensin-converting enzyme and growth hormone. Int J Impot Res. 2003;15(6):418-25.
42. El Melegy, Ali ME, Awad EM. Plasma levels of endothelin-1, angiotensin II, nitric oxide and prostaglandin E in the venous and cavernosal blood of patients with erectile dysfunction. BJU Int. 2005;96(7):1079-86.
43. Mikhail N. Does testosterone have a role in erectile function? Am J Med. 2006;119(5):373-82.
44. Greco EA, Spera G, Aversa A. Combining testosterone and PDE5 inhibitors in erectile dysfunction: Basic rationale and clinical evidences. Eur Urol. 2006;50(5): 940-7.
45. Martine-Jabaloyas JM, Queipo-Zaragoza A, Poster-Hernandez F, Gil-Salom M, Chuan-Nuez P. Testosterone levels in men with erectile dysfunction. BJU Int. 2006;97(6): 1278-83.
46. Vignozzi L, Corona G, Petrone L, Filippi S, Morelli AM, Forti G, et al. Testosterone and sexual activity. J Endocrinol Invest. 2005;28(3 Suppl):39-44.
47. Young SR, Dyson M: The effect of therapeutic ultrasound on angiogenesis. Ultrasound Med Biol. 990;16(3):261.

CHAPTER 27

Ultrasound in Male Infertility

Kuldeep Jain, Bharti Jain, Maansi Jain

INTRODUCTION

Infertility incidence is increasing and as per estimate, 15% population in the reproductive age group is affected from infertility[1] and a large number of infertile couples opt for treatment because of increasing awareness, availability of infertility-related services, and advancement in all fields of infertility management. Studies have shown that male and female factors coexist in approximately 30% of cases; 30% are because of female problems, while rest are due to male factor. Therefore, it is important to evaluate the male partner concurrently as it may be contributing in as high as 60% of cases.[2]

The primary screening investigation of male infertility is the semen analysis. Male factor can be safely excluded if the semen parameters are normal as per the World Health Organization (WHO) criteria. However, if abnormal, further investigations are required to exclude the causes of infertility and characterize them as testicular, pretesticular, and post-testicular.

ETIOLOGICAL DISTRIBUTION

Table 1 shows the etiological distribution as per a study of 7,057 men.[3]

TABLE 1: Etiological distribution as per a study of 7,057 men.

Factors	*Percentage*
Sexual factor	1.7
Urogenital infection	6.6
Congenital anomalies	2.1
Acquired factors	2.6
Varicocele	12.3
Endocrinal disturbances	0.6
Immunological factors	3.1
Other abnormalities	3.0
Idiopathic oligoasthenoteratozoospermia (OAT)	75.1

As it is evident from the table, >75% of cases do not have any demonstrable cause and usually no investigation is helpful in management.[3]

In the diagnostic protocol, ultrasound (US) has become an integral part of infertility management because it is noninvasive and the entire male genital tract can be imaged easily and accurately. However, ultrasonography (USG) is only indicated for a minority of infertile male patients,[4-7] and the use of USG in male infertility is surrounded by several controversies. This chapter aims to look into the technique of USG and delineate the clinical relevance in male infertility and to evaluate various controversies and recommendations.

Routine USG of male genitalia may not be helpful in diagnostic management of all cases of male infertility and so is not required in all cases. There are certain specific conditions where USG may be helpful in confirming pathology as well as in decision-making. Scrotal USG provides a panoramic view and is very helpful in confirming suspected abnormalities on physical examination, differentiating between testicular and paratesticular pathology, and transrectal ultrasonography (TRUS) is indicated to exclude obstructive azoospermia, mainly the congenital absence of vas deferens (CAVD), seen in 10–20% cases. The aim of the imaging modality is to identify a pathology which can correct a potentially correctable cause and select the best method for retrieving a sperm capable of fertilizing the ova-like sperm aspiration from epididymis and testicular seminiferous tubules which can be used later for intracytoplasmic sperm injection (ICSI).

INDICATIONS OF SCROTAL ULTRASOUND[4,8]

The indications of scrotal ultrasound are as follows:

- *Testicular abnormalities:*
    - Absent testes/cryptorchidism **(Fig. 1)**
    - Atropic/small testes **(Fig. 2)**
    - Ectopic location
    - Enlarged testes/hydrocele **(Figs. 3A and B)**
    - Testicular tumor/neoplasm
    - Abnormalities associated with obstruction
    - Mediastinal cyst

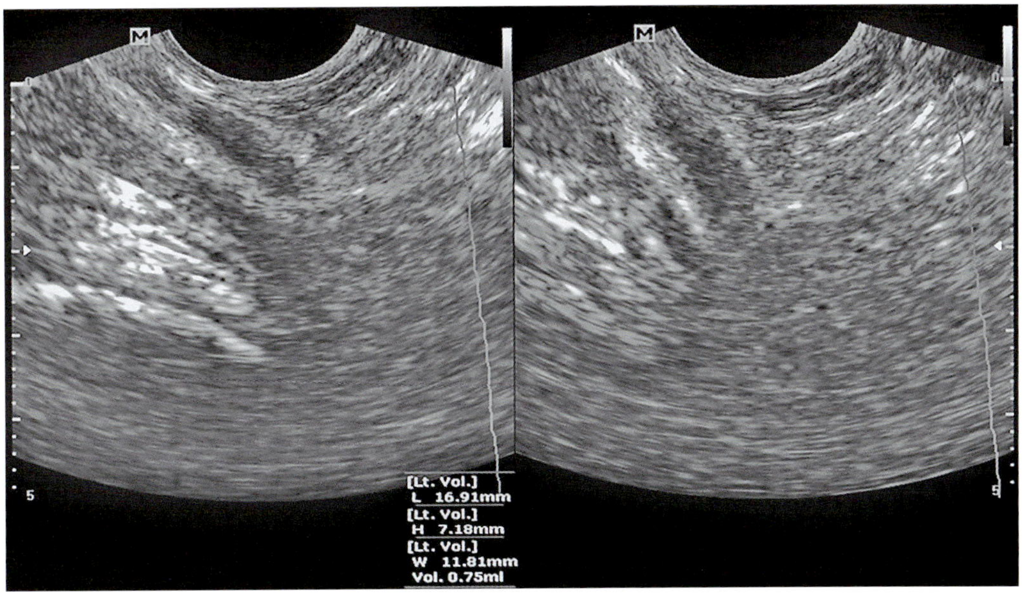

Fig. 1: Absent testis—undescended testis.

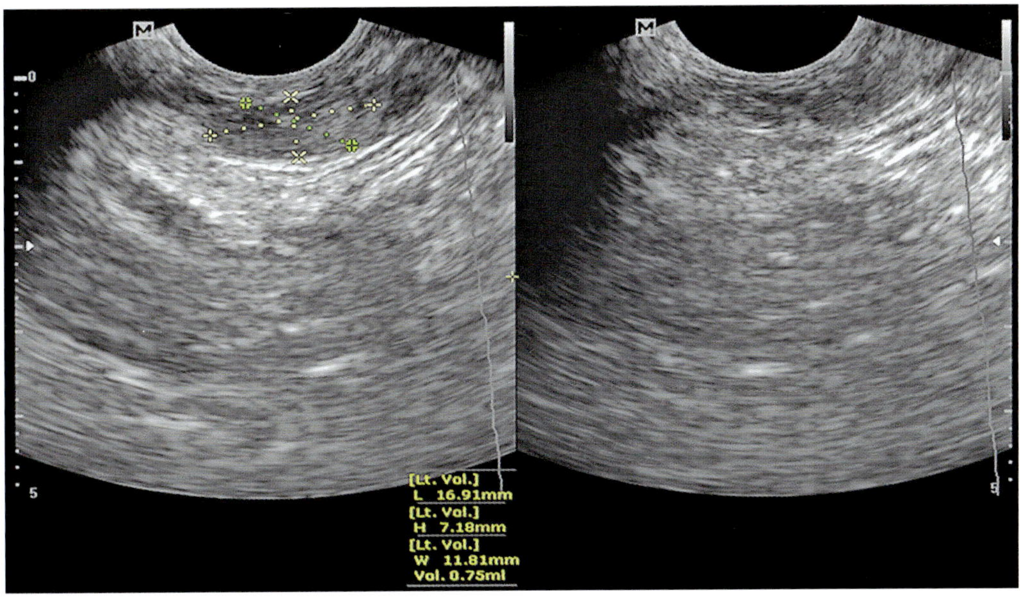

Fig. 2: Atropic testis.

- *Inflammatory disorders:* Acute and chronic orchitis/epididymo-orchitis **(Fig. 4)**
- *Epididymal abnormalities:*
    - Acute and chronic epididymitis
    - Epididymal cyst
    - Spermatocele
    - Tubular ectasia
- *Paratesticular abnormalities:* Varicocele—especially in inconclusive physical examination **(Fig. 5)**
- To differentiate between obstructive and nonobstructive azoospermia.

Technique of Scrotal Sonography

Scrotal US is done using a high-frequency (7–15 MHz) transducer. The patient lies supine with penis resting in the suprapubic region. Scanning is done in transverse, longitudinal, and oblique planes. The size, volume, and echotexture of testes are seen. Testes are ellipsoidal, measuring 3–5 cm (length), 2–4 cm (width), and 3 cm (anteroposterior). Testicular volume (TV) can be estimated by applying the following formula:

$$\text{Length} \times \text{width} \times \text{anteroposterior diameter} \times 5.2 = \text{Volume (cm}^3\text{)}.$$[9]

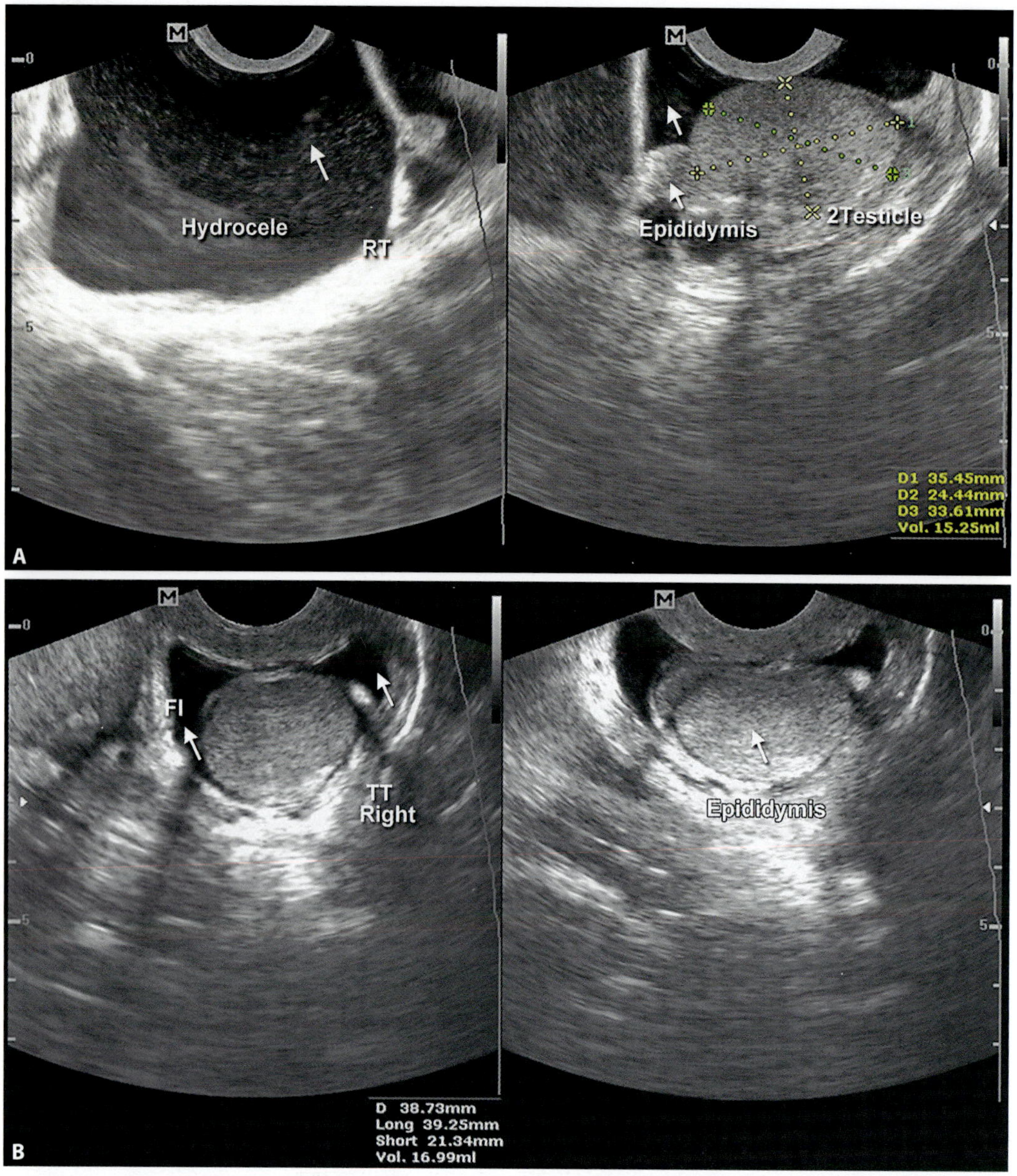

Figs. 3A and B: (A) Gross hydrocele—post-traumatic; (B) Hydrocele with thick wall. (FL: fluid; RT: right testis; TT: testicular tissue)

Nowadays, almost all machines are equipped with software which can calculate volume by different methods. Normal testicular volume is 15–20 Cu Cms. Normal testes have homogenous granular uniformly distributed echoes with an eccentric hyperechoic line (mediastinum testes).

Epididymis (head, body, and tail) and proximal vas deferens (VD) are evaluated in longitudinal and transverse axes. Epididymis is posterolateral to testes, with head in relation to the upper part and tail related to the lower part of the testes. Head measures 5–12 mm, body 2–4 mm, and tail 2–4 mm. Head is of a higher echotexture, and rest are slightly hypoechoic. In a scrotal scan, proximal VD is seen as a straight duct arising from the tail of epididymis. On TRUS, seminal vesicles look like bow-tie with the deferential ampullas medially placed in transverse scans.

CLINICAL APPLICATIONS

The role of scrotal US is to exclude testicular pathologies in *nonobstructive azoospermia* and indications are:

- Hypergonadotropic hypogonadism
- Cryptorchidism
- Testicular atrophy
- Torsion and infarction
- Mumps
- Neoplasm
- Hydrocele
- Varicocele evaluation.[10]

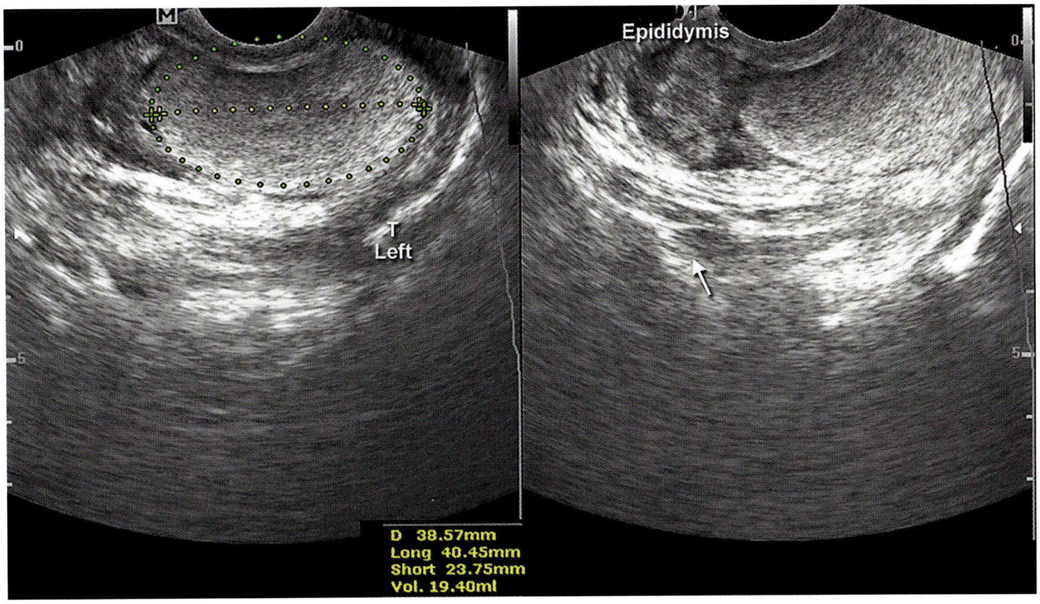

Fig. 4: Chronic epididymitis.

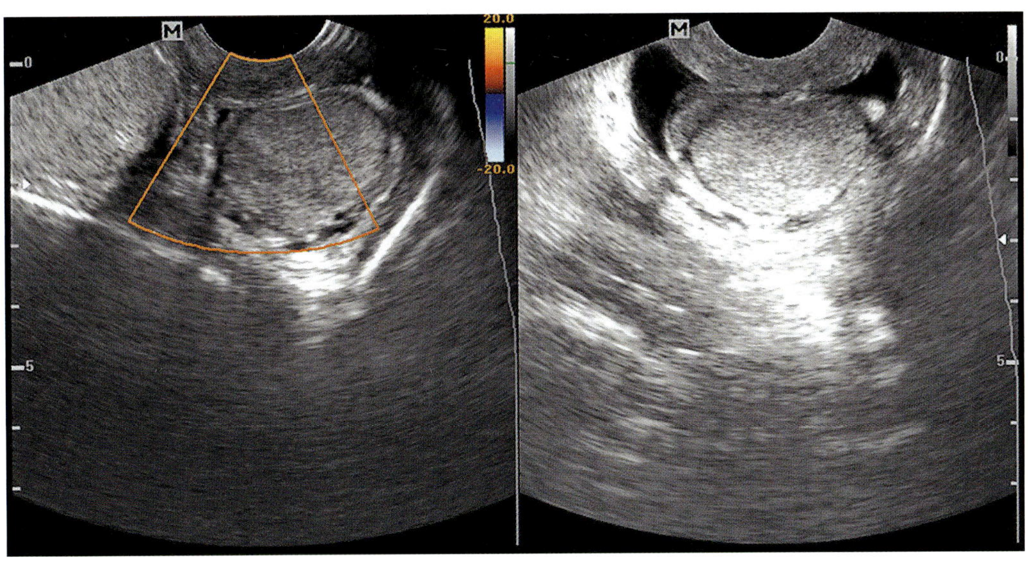

Fig. 5: Absent venous reflux on Valsalva.

Clinically, if testes are not palpable, either there is absence of testis or there are atrophic or undescended testes. US helps in confirming the diagnosis and planning further management. In undescended testes, even though physical examination suffices, USG helps in localizing the testis and seeing the echotexture. Most clinicians believe that there is a limited/doubtful role of USG prior to orchiopexy planning related to infertility management. However, it is useful for general health care follow-up of cryptorchid testis and to exclude risk of malignancy and evaluation contralateral testis.

Testicular volume is significantly higher in obstructive azoospermia (7.7–25.8 cm^3; median 11.6 cm^3) compared to nonobstructive azoospermia (1.2–16.4 cm^3; median 8.3 cm^3) **(Fig. 6)**. Prader orchidometer (PO)-derived TV very well correlates with USG-TV; US scores over PO even though the latter is reliable enough in clinical practice. However, USG is useful when PO has limitations, i.e., when there are testicular pathologies, such as inguinal testis, enlarged epididymis, and large hydrocele. There is a definite positive correlation of TV with the sperm availability and hormonal parameters. Hence, estimating TV should be a part of evaluating the male partner in compromised semen parameters. A volume <50% of the normal is related to suboptimal sperm and hormonal parameters [low testosterone, increased follicle-stimulating hormone (FSH) and luteinizing hormone (LH)]. These cases are less likely to yield sperm recovery

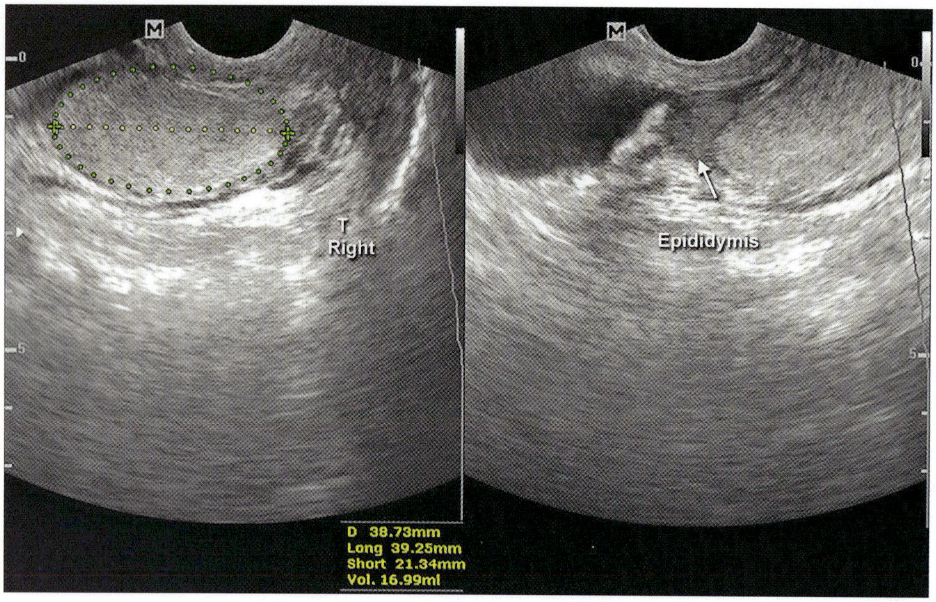

Fig. 6: Normal testis and epididymis.

during percutaneous epididymal sperm aspiration (PESA)/ testicular sperm aspiration (TESA). USG determination of TV is not mandatory in fertility as clinical assessment of TV suffices.

Echogenicity of the testis depends on germ cell representation and seminiferous tubules maturation. Echo-pattern abnormalities such as testicular inhomogeneity are associated with testicular function impairment (reduction of seminiferous tubules and interstitial proliferation).

When gross inhomogeneity or microcalcifications are found, malignancy should be excluded on follow-up scans, especially in the presence of other risk factors in interests of general health care. There is a debatable role of biopsy in the presence of microcalcifications. Doppler adds to the diagnostic confidence by seeing the testicular vascularization—reduced in torsion and infarction and increased in orchiepididymitis or some tumors. Few studies have shown positive correlation of testicular lesions, echotexture, and vascularization with sperm parameters and retrieval by TESE. But as of now, assessing these parameters on USG is not a part of any recommended/standardized protocol for male factor infertility assessment and assessment prior to TESE for probabilities of sperm retrieval.

EPIDIDYMAL DIAMETERS

- US is more accurate than physical examination in evaluating epididymal size. Enlarged epididymis, altered echotexture, and hyperemia may be due to past or present inflammation, which may be associated with oligoasthenospermia. In oligo/azoospermia, if epididymis is absent or dilated, distal obstruction should be excluded by USG evaluation of the prostate-vesicular region.
- Scrotal US is very useful in cases of PESA to identify the position of epididymis, which may yield maximum recovery of sperms as one-third cases of vassal agenesis are associated with hypoplasia of distal two-thirds of epididymis.

SCROTAL ULTRASOUND IN VARICOCELE

Surgical treatment of varicocele is controversial as only few randomized controlled trials (RCTs) evaluating the benefit of varicocelectomy on sperm parameters are available. On the contrary, there is sufficient evidence to suggest harmful effects of varicocele on testicular function and seminal parameters.[11-13] Detrimental effects are reduced TV, slightly increased FSH, LH, and prostatitis-related premature ejaculation due to intrapelvic venous congestion. The effect of varicocele on testosterone levels is debatable. A meta-analysis by Li et al. showed that there is an increase in testosterone after surgical treatment of varicocele. Controversially, it has been seen that 75% of patients with varicocele have normal semen parameters.[14,15]

The current recommendation for varicocele treatment is very clear, and one must take these recommendations into consideration when suggesting varicocelectomy to these infertile men.[16,17] The American Urological Association (AUA)/American Society for Reproductive Medicine (ASRM) recommends treatment for varicocele when in an infertile couple, the female partner is normal or has a potentially treatable cause of infertility, varicocele is palpable on clinical examination, and the semen parameters are deranged. Treatment of varicocele is not indicated in subclinical varicocele or in patients with normal semen parameters.[3] Color Doppler and US (CDUS) is an important and more sensitive modality for diagnosis of varicocele, especially in cases of clinical doubt such as tight scrotum and obese patients (sensitivity 97% and specificity 94%).[18] The diagnosis of varicocele on USG requires greater than three vessels of size >2–3 mm on Doppler. Varicoceles are seen superior and lateral to testes and extend posteriorly and inferiorly if severe. Varicocele evaluation includes extension, size, and number of vessels. Complete evaluation involves noting the presence of spontaneous flow in upright position and seeing the duration of retrograde flow during Valsalva. There should be a mention of the volume and echotexture of the affected testes and comparison with the contralateral testes.[19] The current recommendations by the ASRM, the AUA (practice committee of ASRM 2008), and the European Association of Urology (EAU) on male infertility suggest that varicocele should be evaluated clinically as only palpable varicoceles have been seen to be associated with infertility.[17] However, the EAU guidelines on male infertility recommend that the diagnosis should be confirmed on Doppler, especially when examination is inconclusive (EAU/ASRM, 2008), and that Doppler is the imaging modality of choice to detect and grade varicocele. Clinical examination has 70% sensitivity, and CDUS has 90% sensitivity in varicocele detection.

Caution: Practice of varicocelectomy only on US finding (subclinical varicocele) should be discouraged as there is no evidence to suggest that varicocele diagnosed on US only required correction.[15,18]

Indication of Ultrasound and Color Doppler for Varicocele Evaluation

- Suspected case of varicocele to confirm (grades II and III).
- Difficult physical evaluation as in cases of tight scrotum, hydrocele, thick skin, and obesity.
- Evaluation of contralateral testes for the presence of subclinical varicocele before varicocele correction.[15]

Scrotal US in obstructive azoospermia: Evaluation of epididymis and testes is important in distinguishing obstructive azoospermia from nonobstructive azoospermia in infertile men with a sensitivity, specificity, and accuracy of 82.1%, 100%, and 87.5%, respectively.[19]

Significant findings are dilatation of proximal seminal duct (mediastinum, testes, epididymis, and intrascrotal portion of VD). Epididymis abnormalities are a significant finding in obstructive azoospermia. Distal genital duct obstruction causes secondary changes—dilated proximal genital tract (terminal vas, ampulla of vas, seminal vesicle, and ejaculatory duct), formation of intratesticular cyst, and epididymal cyst in obstruction of the seminal tract. These obstructive pathologies may be managed by epididymovasostomy or by PESA/TESA and ICSI.[20]

Transrectal ultrasonography and male infertility: The role of TRUS is now firmly established in diagnosing post-testicular causes of infertility. It can clearly visualize the prostrate and distal genital tract (vas ampulla, seminal vesicle, and ejaculatory duct). Low ejaculate volume is one of the most important indications of TRUS. The modality provides complete visualization of the ductal system. TRUS is noninvasive, accepted by most of patients, and provides valuable information, especially in azoospermic patients. It identifies correctable defects and helps in counseling of patients in cases of noncorrectable etiologies for advanced assisted reproductive techniques.

Assessing prostrate volume by USG shows greater accuracy than physical examination. It is not very useful in the management of male infertility; reduced volume may suggest hypogonadism.

Echotexture and vascular abnormalities are suggestive of past or present inflammation and their effect on fertility is not proven. Median cyst of prostrate points toward obstructive azoospermia. Large cysts may cause ejaculatory duct obstruction and aspiration may lead to the improvement of semen parameters.

Seminal vesicles appear as paired saccular structures posterior–superior to prostrate, between the bladder and the rectum. They have bow-tie appearance on transverse scans and are club shaped in longitudinal scans. Seminal vesicles are said to be normal if >25 mm is length, are labeled hypoplastic if <25 mm and >16 mm, and atrophic if found <16 mm in length[21] **(Fig. 7)**. Abnormality of seminal vesicles is significantly higher in the azoospermic group than the nonazoospermic population. The incidence of seminal vesicles anomalies such as atrophy or hypoplasia or vassal agenesis is higher in azoospermic patients and may be found in >75% of patients, while there were no abnormalities in 60% of nonazoospermic patients.[22]

- Evaluation of the ejaculatory duct is useful in defining obstructive azoospermia causes. Ejaculatory duct cyst and seminal vesicle agenesis may indicate *CFTR* gene evaluation. Increased volume of seminal vesicles after ejaculation is suggestive of partial ejaculatory duct obstruction. Giant cyst may indicate genitourinary anomalies. Abnormalities of echotexture may indicate inflammation or stasis.

INDICATIONS OF TRANSRECTAL ULTRASOUND[4,8]

- Low seminal volume
- Suspected distal obstruction
- Seminal vesicle enlargement **(Fig. 8)**
- Midline prostatic obstruction
- Ejaculatory duct obstruction
- CAVD **(Fig. 9)**
- Absent seminal vesicles
- Severe oligospermia
- Anejaculation

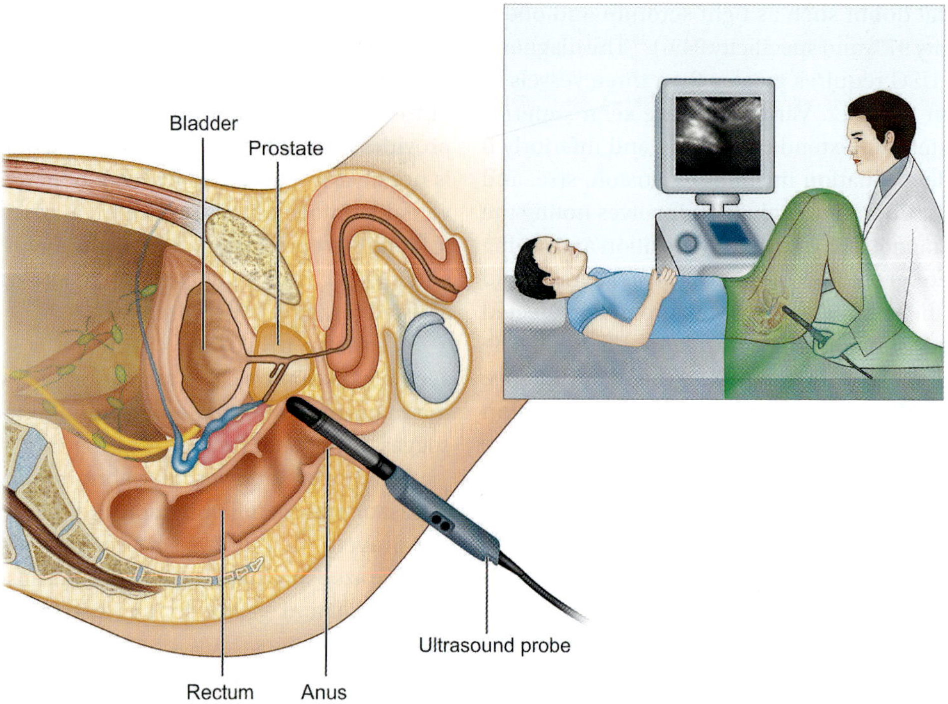

Fig. 7: Technique of transrectal ultrasonography (TRUS).

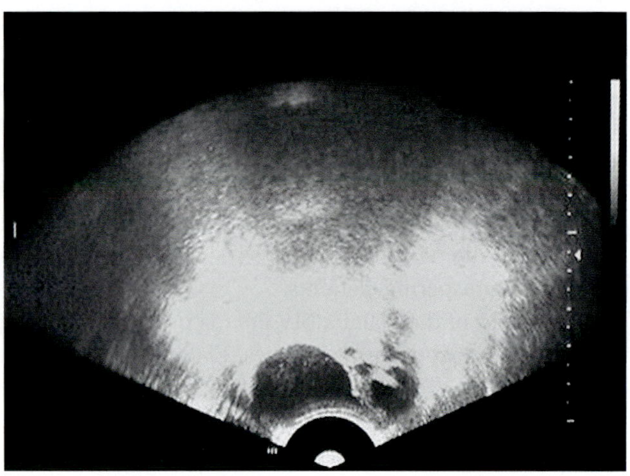

Fig. 8: Seminal vesical cyst—calcification.

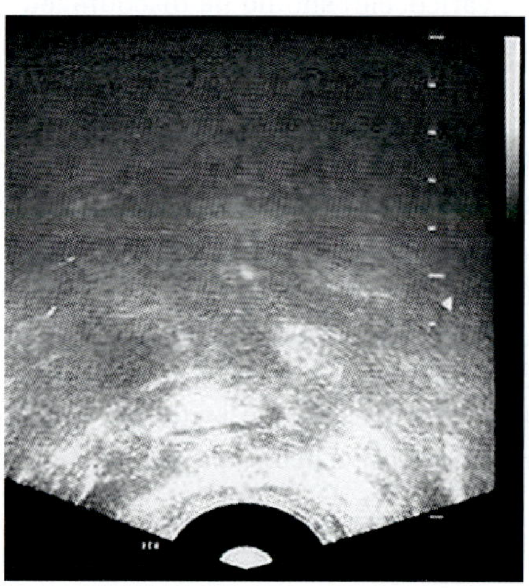

Fig. 9: Absent seminal vesicle/vas.

- Painful ejaculation
- Retrograde ejaculation
- Hematospermia.

Various abnormalities that are seen on TRUS are:

- Vasal agenesis—unilateral or bilateral, partial or complete
- Echogenic vas—calcification
- Cyst of VD or calculi
- Absent seminal vesicle
- Hypoplastic seminal vesicle
- Seminal vesicular cyst
- Ejaculatory duct cyst
- Ejaculatory duct calcification or dilatation **(Fig. 10)**.

Though TRUS is a noninvasive modality, however, it is not enough and reliable tool for diagnosis for ejaculatory duct obstruction and requires an invasive test such as vesiculography and seminal vesicle aspiration to confirm the diagnosis before planning for surgery.

In a study of 70 patients of suspected ejaculatory duct obstruction, 55 patients were diagnosed on TRUS of having ejaculatory duct obstruction; however, only 27 patients were confirmed with seminal vesicle aspiration[22,23] **(Fig. 11)**.

According to recent guidelines published by EAU, scrotal US performed by a high-resolution transducer may be helpful in finding the signs of obstruction, dilatation of rete testes, enlarged epididymis or absent VD, or signs of testicular

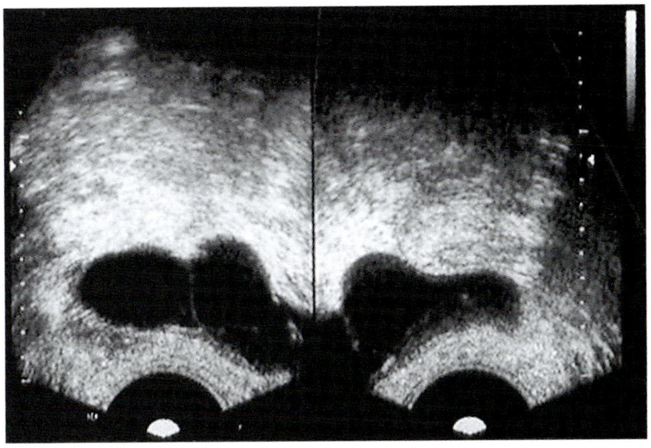

Fig. 10: Bilateral cystic dilatation/ejaculatory duct dilation.

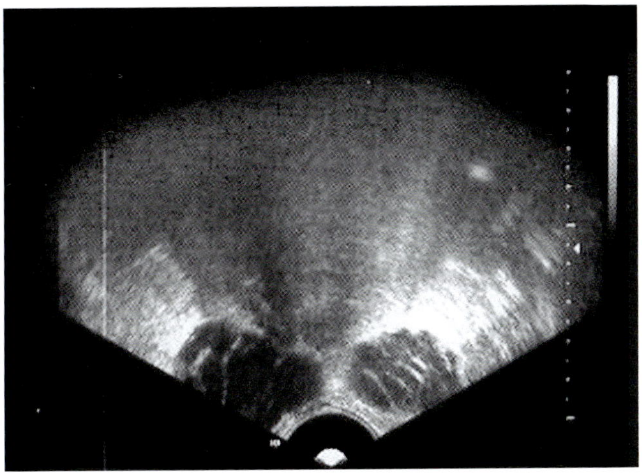

Fig. 11: Midline cyst in periurethral location.

dysgenesis (nonhomogeneous testicular architecture or microcalcification).

It is also indicated in assessment of blood reflex in men with varicocele.

Transrectal ultrasonography is indicated in low seminal volume and suspected ejaculatory duct obstruction. It can also detect testicular microlithiasis, which might indicate carcinoma in situ.

Recently, *TRUS-guided seminal vesiculography* is advocated in a patient with suspected ejaculatory duct obstruction. The seminal vesicles are aspirated using a long needle through a transrectal transducer. It is now preferred over surgical vasography.[24]

CONCLUSION

- Diagnostic and therapeutic measures in treating male infertility have limitations as there is paucity of evidence-based treatment.
- The prime screening modality is semen analysis; hormonal assessment is an adjunct. The role of USG lies in specific decision-making situations.
- Scrotal US is helpful in testicular evaluation and proximal obstruction (e.g., dilatation of rete testis, enlarged epididymis).
- TV can be adequately assessed by either PO or USG, scrotal US is more precise, but PO suffices in clinical practice except when physical examination is unreliable.
- Scrotal US is suggestive of testicular damage, dysgenesis, cryptorchidism, and malignancy in nonobstructive azoospermia, but fails to predict sperm retrieval in nonobstructive azoospermia.
- USG has limitations in surgical sperm extraction decision-making.
- Physical examination is sufficient for diagnosis and decision making in varicocele treatment (AUA/ASRM, 2008); even though EAU guidelines on male infertility require confirmation by Doppler.
- In obstructive azoospermia, USG helps in planning the management, such as TRUS-guided cyst aspiration (large prostatic cyst), surgical treatment (ejaculatory duct abnormalities), or surgical sperm extraction [congenital bilateral absence of the vas deferens (CBAVD)].
- The EAU guidelines on male infertility recommend TRUS to assess distal obstruction, especially when semen volume is <1.5 mL.
- TRUS and scrotal US are useful in diagnosing CBAVD or congenital unilateral absence of the vas deferens (CUAVD) (EAU guidelines on male infertility), followed by *CFTR* gene and urinary tract evaluation by US; surgical sperm extraction is recommended.

To conclude, sonographic imaging of the male genital tract lacks standardization. Multicenter RCTs aimed at defining the indications of USG—scrotal and TRUS—and defining the USG criteria of the pathological abnormalities for standardization of male infertility evaluation and treatment.

KEY POINTS

- Investigations in an infertile male are aimed to find out correctable cause, if any, and to counsel regarding the possibility of further treatment.
- US plays an important role in differentiating obstructive and nonobstructive azoospermia. TRUS further identifies the site of obstruction as well as the cause of obstruction.
- Use of color Doppler for varicocele is though controversial but used to quantify. However, it may not help in management as subclinical varicocele surgery is not recommended and it is clinical varicocele that only requires treatment.[5,25,26]
- Findings suggestive of obstructive azoospermia on scrotal US are to be followed by TRUS to delineate proximal from distal obstruction. This will help plan the management as vasoepididymal anastomosis (VEA) is useful in cases of proximal obstruction.
- In patients with distal obstruction, TRUS or magnetic resonance imaging (MRI) may diagnose the cause and exact site of distal obstruction.

- However, further management is usually based on more invasive tests to confirm or opt for surgical retrieval of sperm and assisted reproductive technique.

REFERENCES

1. Fisch H, Kang YM, Johnson CW, Goluboff ET. Ejaculatory duct obstruction. Curr Opin Urol. 2002;12:509-15.
2. Sigman M, Lipshultz LI, Howards SS. Evaluation of the subfertile male. In: Lipshults LI, Howard SS (Eds). Infertility in the Male, 3rd edition. St. Louis: Mosby; 1997. pp. 173-93.
3. Jungwirth A, Giwercman A, Tournaye H, Diemer T, Kopa Z, Dohle G, et al. European Association of Urology guidelines on Male Infertility: the 2012 update. Eur Assoc Urol. 2012;62(2):324-32.
4. Practice Committee of American Society for Reproductive Medicine. Diagnostic evaluation of the infertile male: a committee opinion. Fertil Steril. 2012;98:294-301.
5. Joshi M. Role of ultrasound in assessment of male infertility. Biomed Imaging Interv J. 2007;3:e12-47.
6. Mathers MJ, Sperling H, Rübben H, Roth S. The undescended testis: diagnosis treatment and long-term consequences. Dtsch Arztebl Int. 2009;106:527-32.
7. Schurich M, Aigner F, Frauscher F, Pallwein L. The role of ultrasound in assessment of male fertility. Eur J Obstet Gynecol Reprod Biol. 2009;144(Suppl. 1):S192-8.
8. Jungwirth A, Giwercman A, Tournaye H, Diemer T, Kopa Z, Dohle G, et al. European Association of Urology guidelines on male infertility: the 2012 update. Eur Urol. 2012;62(2): 324-32.
9. Osvaldopardon, Agarwal A. The use of diagnostic ultrasonography in evaluation of infertile males. In: Allahabadia G (Ed). Transvaginal Sonography in Infertility. Mumbai: Rotunda Medical Technologies; 1998. pp. 137-43 (Chapter 24).
10. Donkol RH. Imaging in male factor obstructive infertility. World J Radiol. 2010;2(5):172-9.
11. Zorba UO, Sanli OM, Tezer M, Erdemir F, Shavakhabov S, Kadioglu A. Effect of infertility: duration on postvaricocelectomy sperm count and pregnancy rates. Urology. 2009; 73:767-71.
12. Romeo C, Santoro G. Varicocele and infertility: why a prevention? J Endocrinol Invest. 2009;32:559-61.
13. Zheng YQ, Gao X, Li ZJ, Yu YL, Zhang ZG, Li W. Efficacy of bilateral and left varicocelectomy in infertile men with left clinical and right subclinical varicoceles: a comparative study. Urology. 2009;73:1236-40.
14. Li F, Yue H, Yamaguchi K, Okada K, Matsushita K, Ando M, et al. Effect of surgical repair on testosterone production in infertile men with varicocele: a meta-analysis. Int J Urol. 2012;19:149-54.
15. Zini A, Boman JM. Varicocele: red flag or red herring? Semin Reprod Med. 2009;27:171-8.
16. Practice Committee of American Society for Reproductive Medicine. Report on varicocele and infertility. Fertil Steril. 2008;90s:244-9.
17. Cocuzza M, Cocuzza MA, Bragais FMP, Agarwal A. The role of varicocele repair in the new era of assisted reproductive technology. Clinics. 2008;63:395-404.
18. Yamamoto M, Hibi H, Hirata Y, Miyake K, Ishigaki T. Effect of varicocelectomy on sperm parameters and pregnancy rates in patients with varicocele repair: a randomized prospective controlled study. J Urol. 1996;155:1636-8.
19. Chiou RK, Anderson JC, Wobig RK, Rosinsky DE, Matamoros Jr A, Chen WS, et al. Color Doppler ultrasound criteria to diagnose varicocele: correlation of new scoring system with physical examination. Urology. 1997;50:953-6.
20. Kantartzi PD, Goulis CD, Goulis GD, Papadimas I. Male infertility and varicocele: myths and reality. Hippokratia. 2007;11:99-104.
21. Moon MH, Kim SH, Cho JY, Seo JT, Chun YK. Scrotal US for evaluation of infertile men with azoospermia. Radiology. 2006;239:168-73.
22. Beedy P, Geoghegan T, Browne RF, Torreggiani WC. Testicular varicoceles. Clin Radiol. 2005;60:1248-55.
23. Purohit RS, Wu DS, Shinohara K, Turek PJ. A prospective comparison of 3 diagnostic methods to evaluate ejaculatory duct obstruction. J Urol. 2004;171:232-5.
24. Engin G, Kadioglu A, Orhan I, Akdol S, Rozanes I. Transrectal US and endorectal MR imaging in partial and complete obstruction of seminal duct system. A comparative study. Acta Radiol. 2000;41:288-95.
25. Jones TR, Zagoria RJ, Jarow JP. Transrectal US guided and seminal vesiculography. Radiology. 1997;205:276-8.
26. Ammar T, Sindhu PS, Wilkins CJ. Male infertility: the role of imaging in diagnosis and management. Br J Radiol. 2012; 85(Spec No. 1):S59-68.

CHAPTER 28

Medical Management of Male Infertility

Sonal Agarwal, Vinay Kumar

INTRODUCTION

Since the past two decades, there is an increase in the rate of infertility due to delayed childbearing, late marriages, acquiring sexually transmitted diseases, use of contraception, and higher medical care and assistance for infertility. Male factor is responsible in approximately 50% of infertile couples with 30% of cases having male factor as the sole reason for infertility.[1] Thus along with female partner treatment, male partner management of infertility is equally important. In the past, empirical treatment used to be done in infertile men when surgical treatment was either unavailable or had failed. Recent trend is to identify the cause and then provide a specific treatment for it. Cases where a specific cause **(Fig. 1)** cannot be identified are considered under idiopathic category and given empirical treatment.

This chapter provides an evidence-based overview for medical management of male infertility. Efforts have been done to make this chapter fascinating and interesting to read for reproductive endocrinologists, urologists, fertility specialists, gynecologists, and general practitioners.[2]

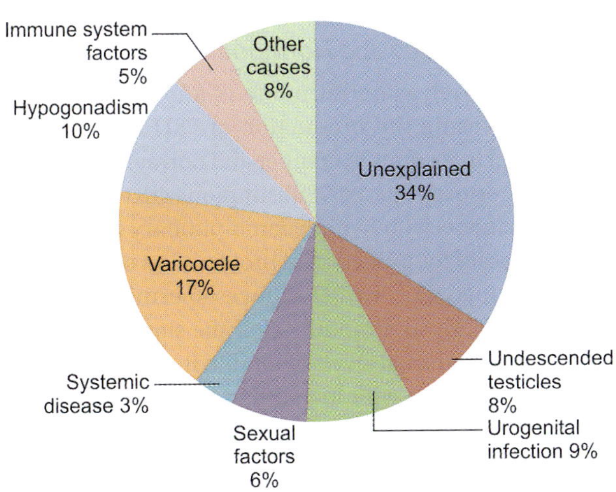

Fig. 1: Causes of male infertility.

MEDICAL THERAPY

Medical therapy is divided into two categories:

1. Specific therapy for endocrine disorders, male accessory gland infections (MAGI), and ejaculatory disorders. It is further divided into subcategories such as:
   a. To enhance sperm production and gonadal function
   b. To prevent and treat genital tract infection
   c. To correct sexual dysfunction [anejaculation, anorgasmic, ejaculatory, and erectile dysfunction (ED)]
   d. To look for free radicals so as to increase sperm motility
   e. To manage infertility related to obesity
2. Nonspecific therapy as empirical treatment for idiopathic causes in the form of antiestrogens, aromatase inhibitors, gonadotropins, and antioxidants.

SPECIFIC THERAPY

To Enhance Sperm Production and Gonadal Function

The classical treatment of infertility can be put under the following points:

- *Lifestyle modifications:* Professional exposure to thermal stress or toxic substances such as pesticides and hot baths should be avoided.[3] Cigarette and alcohol consumption also have a role in infertility.
- *Treatment of systemic illness:* Semen analysis should be done at least after 3 months of febrile illness. Zinc supplementation and improving nutritional status are necessary in renal diseases, cirrhosis, and sickle cell anemia.
- *Treatment of endocrinopathies:* Endocrinopathies dealt with in this chapter are listed in **Box 1**.

Hypogonadotropic Hypogonadism

About 2–5% of male infertility is due to hypothalamic and pituitary causes.[4] Follicle-stimulating hormone (FSH) is

BOX 1: List of endocrinopathies causing male infertility.

- Hemochromatosis
- Hypogonadotropic hypogonadism
- Kallmann syndrome
- Cushing's disease
- Gonadotropin secreting adenoma
- Diabetes mellitus
- Congenital adrenal hyperplasia
- Liver disease
- Thyroid disease
- Androgen resistance
- Acromegaly
- Hyperprolactinemia
- Anabolic steroid abuse

required to initiate spermatogenesis and testosterone, and luteinizing hormone (LH) is needed for processes of spermiogenesis and spermiation. Human chorionic gonadotropin (hCG) is longer acting and is used in place of LH as no commercial preparations of LH are available. Advantage of giving gonadotropins is that initiation of spermatogenesis and secondary sexual development occur simultaneously. Replacement with gonadotropin injections is accepted for effective management of associated infertility.[5]

Gonadotropin replacement therapy can be by any of the following methods:

- hCG
- Human menopausal gonadotropin (hMG) (mimics LH and FSH)
- Purified FSH
- Pulsatile GnRH in Kallmann syndrome.

Gonadotropin replacement for hypogonadotropic hypogonadism with only a few pubertal signs is as follows:

- Initially, hCG has to be given intramuscularly (IM) or subcutaneously (SC) 2,000 IU/thrice a week until adequate serum testosterone levels are detected in 6 weeks followed by addition of FSH 75 or 100 IU 3 times/week.[6]
- Human menopausal gonadotropin 75 or 150 IU 3 times/week restores serum testosterone levels and normal spermatogenesis after 6–9 months of treatment. If satisfactory, FSH can be suspended, and spermatogenesis may be maintained with hCG alone.[7] The dose has to be doubled if no response in fertility is seen in 3–6 months or no increase in gonadal size within 3 months of the start of treatment.[8] If spermatogenic cells are nonfunctioning even after 6 months of treatment, recombinant follicle-stimulating hormone (rFSH) injections have to be added.[9]

Treatment of prepubertal adult:

- hCG 2,000 IU thrice weekly IM for 6 weeks
- At the end of 6 weeks, 37.5 IU FSH thrice a week is added.[10]

Treatment with FSH can be started when adequate serum testosterone levels are detected with hCG. hCG combined with FSH has shown results in 94% of men.[11]

In resistant cases, therapy may be for a longer duration of 1–2 years. In cryptorchid patients, even after testicular descent, prognosis for fertility is poor.[12]

Treatment of a postpubertal adult: In patients with incomplete hypogonadism or adult with hypogonadotropic hypogonadism, only hCG is sufficient for both androgenization and fertility.[13]

Disadvantages of hCG injection:

- Cost
- Increasing resistance to hCG is because of frequent injections due to induced downregulation of receptors. With adequate spacing of injections, it can be prevented
- Antibody formation blocking action of hCG may also occur but it is rare.

In such men, once fertility is achieved, cryopreservation of sample should be done for future fertility issues. One study by Esteves et al.[14] worked on clinical efficacy and safety of recombinant hCG to restore spermatogenesis and androgen production of hypogonadotropic hypogonadal men and found that 10 out of 11 patients had restoration of spermatogenesis and improvement in virilization, libido, and erectile function.

Positive predictive factors of gonadotropin replacement response are:

- Larger volume of testis
- Prior intake of gonadotropin therapy
- Postpubertal status
- Absence of bilateral maldescended testes.

Negative prognostic factors for treatment with gonadotropins are:

- Extreme gonadotropin insufficiency
- Obesity
- Cryptorchidism
- Small testicles.

Gonadotropin-releasing Hormone Therapy

Gonadotropin-releasing hormone is a more physiologic drug in increasing the production of FSH and LH when administered in a pulsatile manner and normalizing the LH–Leydig cell–testosterone axis. Substitution with GnRH is most pivotal in patients with hypothalamo-pituitary insufficiency as it is necessary for induction of proliferation of Sertoli cells and spermatogonia.[15] GnRH induces spermatogenesis in up to 85% as early as 4 months after the start of treatment. Achievement of normal levels of inhibin B, testosterone, and gonadotropins along with increase in testicular volume are predictors of successful treatment with GnRH.[16]

Dosage: 100 or 500 mg of gonadorelin is given in a pulsatile form through the SC/intravenous (IV) route with the help of an electric-driven pump at a rate of 90 minutes apart with doses around 25 ng/kg body weight. It provides 1–2 mg/pulse. In cases of profound suppression of hypothalamus, doses can reach up to 300 ng/kg body weight. This should result in a rise in gonadotropin and testosterone levels after about 7 days of treatment.

Disadvantages:

- High cost
- Anaphylactic reaction
- Pump is visible through clothes
- Hindrance in swimming and other outdoor recreational activities.

Causes of failure of GnRH therapy:

- Patients who develop GnRH antibodies during the course of therapy resulting in deterioration of testosterone and gonadotropin levels
- Mutation of the GnRH receptor gene.

Androgen Therapy

Testosterone replacement therapy (TRT) (androgen therapy) causes pubertal development in the form of increased muscle mass, pubic hair, beard growth, penile growth, normal sexual behavior, and cognitive function in men.[17] Pituitary hormones may be needed to stimulate testicle growth. Starting with an initial low dose and then gradually increasing, it causes less adverse effects and mimics hormonal status during physiological puberty. It is a useful means to restore sexual functionality and in a person with hypogonadotropic hypogonadism who is not desirous of fertility at that point of time. It has the advantage of cost over gonadotropins and can be used for inducing puberty.[18] Natural testosterone can be taken orally and undergoes rapid degradation by hepatic metabolism. Chemical changes such as 17-alpha alkylation and modified ring are done to lessen enterohepatic circulation.[19]

Mechanisms of testosterone action: Testosterone in a way acts as three hormones due to different biologic effects. It directly binds to androgen receptors, can act via dihydrotestosterone (more avidity than testosterone) which acts after conversion by enzyme 5-alpha reductase, and acts as estrogen after conversion through the aromatase enzyme.

Routes of administration: The particular route of administration depends on preference, side effects, compliance, and cost of that method.

- *Injection:* Testosterone enanthate or testosterone propionate or decanoate 100–250 mg IM injection every 3–4 weeks. This will result in attaining steady levels of androgen in the majority of patients. In prepubertal patients, start with lesser doses and increase as pubertal maturation ensues. Testosterone undecanoate (Aveed) was recently approved by the Food and Drug Administration (FDA).
- *Crystalline pellet form (testosterone implant):* 100 and 200 mg doses. A special introducer helps in the insertion of pellet every 3–6 months. Though it is expensive, it will save patients from monthly injections.
- *Oral preparation of testosterone undecanoate (Andriol):* 120–160 mg/day
- *Modified androgen mesterolone (Proviron):* 50–75 mg daily doses
- *Transdermal preparation in patch or cream form:* Recently developed Androderm patch is applied each night to the back, abdomen, upper arm, or thigh. The site of application should be rotated in order to maintain at least a 7-day interval between the same site application so as to lessen skin reactions. Adverse effects of patch include pruritus, erythema, vesicle formation, induration, headache, depression, rash, and gastrointestinal bleeding.
- *Gel:* Different gel preparations are available. Gel is either rubbed into your skin on the upper arm or shoulder (AndroGel, Testim, Vogelxo) or applied in each armpit with an applicator (Axiron) or a pump on the front and inner thigh (Fortesta). No bath should be taken for 4–5 hours after application for complete absorption. Gel causes lesser skin reactions as compared to patches. Avoid skin-to-skin contact until it gets dried, otherwise the risk of transferring medication to another person is there. Nasal route gel is also available. It avoids the risk of transfer of medicine through skin contact. It should be applied twice in each nostril three times a day, but this method does not have better compliance due to inconvenience.
- *Gum and cheek testosterone replacement (Striant)* in the form of a putty-like substance delivers testosterone through the natural depression above your top teeth at the junction of the gum and upper lip. Quick absorption is there.

Long-term use of alkylated preparations can lead to liver damage and thus precautions should be kept in mind. All patients should be carefully monitored for changes in hematocrit, liver function, lipid parameters, and prostate-specific antigen (PSA). The dose should be increased gradually to full adult dosage over 18–24 months to prevent abrupt virilization and bone maturation. Maintain serum sex steroid concentration in mid-normal adult range. The Institute of Medicine recommends 1 g of calcium and 600 IU vitamin D per day for men aged between 19 and 70 years along with hormone therapy. In men of >70 years of age, 1200 mg of calcium and 800 IU of vitamin D are needed.

A multicenter trial has demonstrated restoration of serum testosterone levels and increased desire and libido, mood, and bone markers after testosterone administration. It showed that the earliest improvement in androgenic features is seen with TRT.[20]

Debate between urologists and infertility specialists: Urologists and general practitioners generally use TRT in patients with hypogonadism due to testicular failure with intentions of improving muscle strength and bone loss prevention.[21] Men receiving such replacement usually experience increase in energy, sex drive, erectile function, and a sense of well-being.

Fertility specialists believe that in pituitary causes, gonadotropin therapy should be given to stimulate sperm production. Testosterone therapy should be reserved for those whose concern is not fertility. Androgen in the form of exogenous testosterone is detrimental for spermatogenesis to occur and has a contraceptive effect due to negative feedback on the hypothalamus and pituitary.

Guidelines

Recent ED consensus guidelines have recommended evaluation of bioavailable testosterone and free testosterone in patients of suspected hypogonadism and sexual dysfunction. These guidelines have titled gonadotropin therapy as first line of management and TRT as second line of management.[22]

Thyroid Disease

Hypothyroidism: Prevalence of hypothyroidism is 0.6% in males. There is loss of libido and reduced potency. It is often associated with hyperprolactinemia but its contribution toward male infertility is unknown. Young males are at increased risk. Sperm quality is also severely affected.[23]

Treatment of hypothyroidism: Aim is to resolve hypothyroidism.

Hyperthyroidism: Prevalence of hyperthyroidism is 0.9% in males. It causes weight loss and varying degrees of hypogonadotropic hypogonadism. Excessive thyroxine production sensitizes pituitary gonadotrophs to GnRH, as such response is enhanced but despite it, gonadotropins and testosterone levels remain the same.

Treatment of hyperthyroidism: Hyperthyroidism can be managed by antithyroid medication and treatment of underlying cause.

Hyperprolactinemia

Presentation of hyperprolactinemia in men as compared to women is subtle and may take years to get diagnosed. Its prevalence in males is 11%. Tumors of pituitary tend to be large, often causing loss of peripheral vision and invading cavernous sinuses causing ophthalmoplegia. Excess prolactin secretion results in decrease in frequency of LH pulses. It causes overall reduction in testosterone secretion,[24] although more effect on sexual dysfunction such as loss of libido, retrograde ejaculation, and impotence is seen in such men.

Treatment of hyperprolactinemia: Medical treatment is appropriate. Dopamine agonist cabergoline (Dostinex) 0.5–2 mg/wk and bromocriptine are also used for this purpose. In large tumors, treatment may be needed lifelong. Gonadotropin therapy is also required in patients having hypospermatogenesis.

Cushing's Disease

Prevalence of Cushing's disease is between 1.2 and 2.4 cases per million. Usually, due to high adrenocorticotropic hormone (ACTH), adrenal gland produces high levels of cortisol; there is reduction in serum levels of LH and FSH, causing hypogonadism.[25] Prolactinemia may be associated with it. Loss of libido and reduced potency are there in more than half of the men.

Treatment of Cushing's disease: Surgery results in rise in LH and testosterone. Ablation of pituitary tumor can be done by irradiation therapy too. Normal adrenal function will soon ensue resulting in recovery in sexual function and semen quality. If no adenoma is present, ketoconazole medical therapy can be given to block steroid synthesis.

Gonadotropin-secreting Adenoma

Clinical presentation of gonadotropin-secreting tumors in males is rare because excess FSH secretion produces fewer symptoms, which remain undetectable for a longer time. Tumors take time to reach a considerable size. Serum FSH levels are elevated.[26]

Treatment of gonadotropin-secreting tumors: They can be removed by surgery or irradiation. Reduction in size can occur following bromocriptine therapy.

Diabetes Mellitus

Diabetes mellitus is one of the most common endocrine diseases. It interferes with normal sexual function. Both neurological and vascular factors cause erectile failure in diabetics and autonomic neuropathy causes ejaculatory disturbances in patients. Impotence is a very common complication of diabetes and occurs in almost 50% of all. Nocturnal penile tumescence is reduced because of an organic lesion. Retrograde ejaculation progresses to ejaculatory failure. Testicular biopsies from impotent diabetic patients show a huge range of changes varying from minimal reduction in spermatogenesis to completely hyalinized and nonfunctional seminiferous tubules.

Treatment of infertility due to diabetes mellitus: It depends on the severity of dysfunction and infertility. If testes are reduced in size with FSH raised, primary testicular disease is suspected and significant damage to sperm production will be there. Thus, diabetic patients are susceptible to developing sperm maturation disorders. If a patient is able to produce good fertile ejaculate, it is wise to cryopreserve semen for future insemination because primary testicular disease or ejaculatory failure may occur any time.

Congenital Adrenal Hyperplasia

Congenital adrenal hyperplasia is a genetically inherited autosomal recessive disease due to deficiency of enzymes needed for production of steroid precursors of cortisol.[27] This results in enhanced pituitary ACTH secretion. Only nonclassical nonsalt losing congenital adrenal hyperplasia (NCAH) is diagnosed in men late in life. It is not a very common disease with an incidence of 1 in 2,500 adults. The patient will present with a history of precocious puberty. Nonclassical CAH has normal androgenic features but testes are reduced in size. Semen analysis may show severe oligozoospermia or azoospermia. Testicular biopsy shows hyalinization in seminiferous tubules and spermatogenic arrest along with reduced number of Leydig cells.

Treatment: Dexamethasone may improve Leydig cell hypoplasia.

Liver Disease

In relation with alcoholic cirrhosis, liver disease may be seen associated with infertility. Hepatocellular damage affects gonadotropin secretion and spermatogenesis.

Treatment of liver disease: Liver disease can be treated by abstinence from alcohol and treatment of underlying pathology of liver.

Acromegaly

Occasionally, men suffer from infertility and sexual dysfunction due to it. There is acidophilic adenoma of pituitary causing overproduction of growth hormone. Rise in prolactin causes relative LH deficiency.

Treatment of acromegaly: Acromegaly can be treated by surgical removal of pituitary adenomas or radiotherapy. Treatment with bromocriptine can also result in shrinkage in size of tumor.

Androgen Resistance

Androgen resistance is also known as androgen insensitivity syndrome or testicular feminizing syndrome. It is genetically determined. Depending on severity, four types of phenotypic and endocrine abnormalities have been determined. Androgen receptor resistance is present. In typical syndrome, male pseudohermaphroditism is there. Patients are thus hypogonadal with LH and testosterone levels increased. Genital abnormalities such as hypospadias, cryptorchidism, and bifid scrotum are associated.

Excess androgens are converted to estrogens resulting in gynecomastia. Penile size is reduced and prostate is markedly reduced in size. Histology may reveal maturation arrest.

Treatment: Reduced chances of improving semen quality as this disease is genetically predetermined. Thus, some form of assisted reproduction is required in such cases.

Kallmann Syndrome

Kallmann syndrome is an X-linked disease with hypogonadotropic hypogonadism resulting in absent pubertal maturation and maldevelopment of midline structures such as hypothalamus. Anosmia is associated with aplasia of the olfactory tract. Severe hypogonadism is associated.

Treatment of Kallmann syndrome: Gonadotropin-replacement therapy can be used to treat Kallman syndrome.

Hemochromatosis

In anterior pituitary cells, there is deposition of iron causing decreased secretion of FSH and LH. Sexual dysfunction may be associated along with it. Males usually present with complaints of impotence, loss of libido, hypoandrogenization, and reduced testes size. Gonadotropin levels decrease causing reduced testosterone levels. Histological section of testis shows hypospermatogenesis and absent or reduced Leydig cells with no iron deposition.

Treatment: Depletion of iron from tissues is important for attaining normal testicular and sexual function. Phlebotomy can be done to achieve this. The main cause is pituitary insufficiency, so treatment with gonadotropin therapy is of utmost importance.

Anabolic Steroid Abuse

Anabolic steroid abuse is seen in sports persons, athletes, and weightlifters so as to increase their muscle mass. This in turn causes profound suppression of gonadotropins. Due to illegal transactions of such agents, patients hide this while history-taking. Such men present with impotence and azoospermia. At first, these patients may have few signs visible along with loss of libido. Serum hormones have negligible levels with hypospermatogenesis.[28]

Treatment: Gonadotropin therapy can be used to treat anabolic steroid abuse.

Treatment of Antisperm Antibodies and Infection

Incidence varies between 8 and 21% among infertile men.[29] Antisperm antibodies affect fertilization by inhibiting cervical mucus penetration and facilitate destruction of coated sperm by uterine leukocytes, inhibiting capacitation, binding to zona, and acrosome reaction. In cases of antisperm antibodies, treatment with prednisone at a dose of 40–60 mg/day for 10 days corresponding to the female partner's first 10 days of menstrual cycle has been tried. Ejaculation into Tyrode's buffer solution has been tried too, to dilute antibodies secreted by the prostate. Intrauterine insemination (IUI) and in vitro fertilization (IVF) can be tried but due to high rates of fertilization failure, intracytoplasmic sperm injection (ICSI) is more successful.

One of the potentially correctable causes of male infertility is symptomatic and asymptomatic infection of the male urogenital tract. Etiology is given in **Table 1**.

Infection causes male infertility in the following ways:[30]

- Affects normal functioning of the male reproductive system
- Disrupts blood–testis barrier
- Semen parameter changes occur
- Disrupts normal morphology, biochemistry, and sperm function
- Reactive oxygen species (ROS) production increases
- Impairs sperm–oocyte interaction
- Accessory glands' normal functioning is impaired
- Duct system is occluded.

Basic ejaculate analysis does not reveal a link between accessory gland infection and impaired sperm characteristics. Antibiotic treatment gives symptomatic relief, eradicates microorganisms, and no positive effect is there on inflammatory alterations. It cannot reverse functional deficits and anatomical dysfunctions and cannot always enhance the probability of conception.[31]

Comhaire et al.[32] suggested that the presence of any two of the following parameters indicates diagnosis of abnormal semen samples:

- History of genitourinary infection and/or abnormal rectal examination
- Abnormally expressed prostatic secretion and/or urinary sediment after prostatic massage
- $\geq 10^3$ bacteria/mL or $\geq 10^4$ nonpathogenic bacteria/mL in a dilution of 1:2 of seminal plasma
- $\geq 10^6$ leukocytes/mL of ejaculate.

TABLE 1: Etiology and distribution (%) of male infertility among 7,057 men.

Etiology	%
No demonstrable cause	48.5
Sexual factors	1.7
Urogenital infection	6.6
Congenital anomalies	2.1
Acquired factors	2.6
Varicocele	12.3
Endocrine disturbances	0.6
Immunological factors	3.1
Idiopathic abnormal semen (oligoasthenoteratozoospermia syndrome)	26.4
Other abnormalities	3.0

Source: Dohle GR, Colpi GM, Hargreave TB, Papp GK, Jungwirth A, Weidner W, et al. EAU guidelines on male infertility. Eur Urol. 2005;48(5):703-11.

Guidelines and Recommendations

The World Health Organization (WHO) guidelines (2010) for seminal tract infections:

- Significant bacteriospermia—$\geq 10^3$ bacteria/mL ejaculate
- Detection of *Neisseria gonorrhea* or *Chlamydia trachomatis* or *Ureaplasma urealyticum*
- Significant leukocytospermia—$\geq 10^6$ peroxidase-positive leukocytes/mL of ejaculate.

Treatment according to Centers for Disease Control and Prevention (CDC) guidelines for uncomplicated genital chlamydial infection is given in **Box 2**.

Partner management: Male accessory glands are reservoirs for organisms (*C. trachomatis* and *Mycoplasma genitalium*); hence, they increase transmission to the partners.[34] Sex partners of the infected person should be evaluated and tested. They have to be treated if sexual contact was done within 60 days preceding the onset of symptoms or diagnosed with *Chlamydia*. The most recent sexual partner has to be evaluated and treated even if the time of last sexual contact was >60 days from the time of the start of patient's symptoms and diagnosis.

For *M. genitalium*, azithromycin 1 g single dose has been considered superior to doxycycline 100 mg BD for 7 days. Moxifloxacin (400 mg daily × 7, 10, or 14 days) has been successfully used to treat *M. genitalium* in men and women with previous treatment failures or persistent nongonococcal urethritis (NGU) Centers for Disease Control and Prevention (CDC 2015). Unlike female sterility, the significance of genital infections for male infertility is still in debate. Leukocytospermia does not always indicate infection.[35] Instead of classical parameters, for example, the determination of microorganisms and/or counting leukocytes, functional parameters such as cytokines, ROS, or other indicators of inflammation should be estimated if available. Proper antibiotic treatment directed against the specific organism in symptomatic men and not empirical treatment is important

BOX 2: Treatment of uncomplicated genital chlamydial infections in adults.[33]

Recommended regimens:
- Azithromycin 1 g orally single dose or
- Doxycycline 100 mg orally twice a day for 7 days

Alternative regimens:
- Erythromycin base 500 mg orally four times a day for 7 days or
- Erythromycin ethylsuccinate 800 mg orally four times a day for 7 days or
- Ofloxacin 300 mg orally twice a day for 7 days or
- Levofloxacin 500 mg orally once a day for 7 days

for eradicating microorganism, improvement of symptom, prevention of transmission to others, and decrease of potential complications, for example, stricture, obstruction, or atrophy, and improvement of semen quality.

To Correct Sexual Dysfunction

The aim is to retrieve spermatozoa for use in assisted reproductive technology (ART).[36] Psychotherapy is of not much use. For anejaculation, vibratory or electroejaculation can be tried. Retrograde ejaculation can be either medically or surgically treated.

- *Medical treatment of retrograde ejaculation:*[37] It is directed to control the internal sphincter by use of sympathomimetics **(Table 2)**. Alkalization of urine has to be done before collection of urine post ejaculation to recover spermatozoa.
- *Surgical:* To restore bladder neck integrity. Recently, collagen injection in the bladder neck has been tried to allow antegrade ejaculation who has a history of previous V-Y plasty. This is for people in whom medical therapy and IUI have failed.

For detailed etiology, diagnosis, and management of sexual dysfunction.[38]

TABLE 2: Medication for retrograde ejaculation.

Medication	***Dose***
Pseudoephedrine (sympathomimetic)	60 mg orally four times per day
Imipramine (tricyclic antidepressants)	25 mg orally two times per day
Ephedrine (sympathomimetic)	25–50 mg orally four times per day
Phenylpropanolamine (sympathomimetic)	75 mg po bid
Brompheniramine maleate (antihistamine)	8 mg bid
Desipramine (tricyclic antidepressants)	50 mg every alternate day

To Decrease Free Radicals and Enhance Sperm Motility

Antioxidants

Reactive oxygen species such as hydroxyl radicals and superoxide anions are released out of leukocytes and abnormal immature forms. Seminal plasma has antioxidant activity. ROS is associated with dysfunction of sperm and deoxyribonucleic acid (DNA) damage resulting in impaired motility of sperm and sperm membrane damage and lipid peroxidation **(Flowchart 1)**.

Classification:

- *Enzymatic:* Superoxide dismutase, catalase, and glutathione peroxidase. These inactivate ROS. These are metal-containing enzymes, which catalyze superoxide in O_2 and H_2O_2 which are less toxic.
- *Nonenzymatic:* Ascorbic acid, alpha-tocopherol, and carnitine. These neutralize ROS.

Flowchart 1: Depiction of balance between oxidative stress and antioxidants.

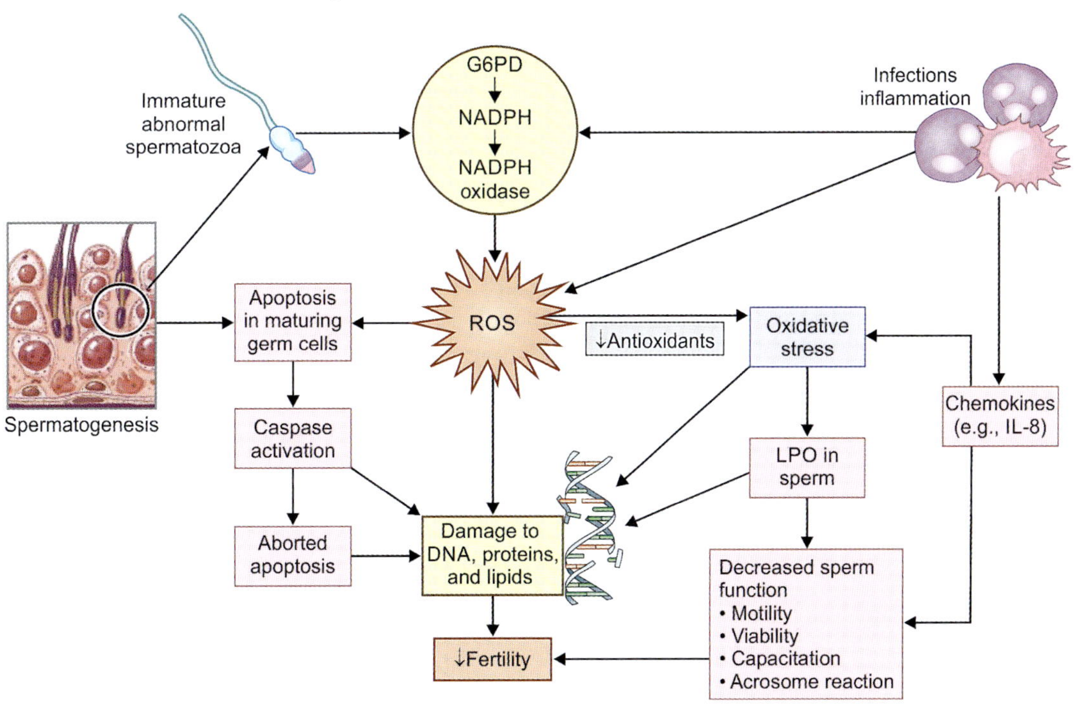

(DNA: deoxyribonucleic acid; G6PD: glucose-6-phosphate dehydrogenase; IL-8: Interleukin-8; LPO: lipid peroxidation; NADPH: nicotinamide adenine dinucleotide phosphate; ROS: reactive oxygen species)

About 30–80% of male infertility is due to the damaging and harmful effect of oxidative stress. Oral antioxidants may improve sperm quality by causing reduction in oxidative stress. Cochrane (2014) analysis concluded that antioxidants cause statistically significant increase in pregnancy and live birth rate.[39] There is no protocol as such to take over-the-counter antioxidant supplementation for improving semen parameters and pregnancy outcomes.[40] There are many confounding factors such as duration of treatment, control for dietary intake, and lack of standardized dose regimens.[41] No conclusive results have been obtained yet. A systemic analysis of 17 randomized studies evaluated the effect of antioxidants (carnitine, carotenoids, zinc, selenium, folate, vitamin C and E) on sperm parameters and pregnancy rates in 1,655 infertile men. 82% of trials showed either improved sperm quality or pregnancy rate after therapy.[42]

Overtreatment with antioxidants should not be done as it causes asynchronous chromosomal condensation and cytoplasmic fragments in embryo, resulting in decreasing pregnancy rates.[42] In a study, 47 normogonadotropic men with idiopathic asthenozoospermic were divided randomly and given 1,200 mg of pentoxifylline/day for 6 months. Sperm motility increased following pentoxifylline treatment after 3 and 6 months from 25.5 (21.0–30.0) to 35.5 (31.5–39.0) ($p < 0.00001$) and to 42.0 (38.0–46.0) ($p < 0.00001$), respectively.[43] **Table 3** depicts various antioxidants and their role with

TABLE 3: Various antioxidants and their role and rationale behind use.

Antioxidant	*Rationale*	*Parameter improved*	*Evidence*
N-Acetylcysteine	Lowers ROS and protects from xanthine oxidase-induced damage	Motility	Oeda et al.[44]
Vitamin E	Lowers LPO and protects sperm from loss of motility	Motility	Verma and Kanwar[45]
Dithiothreitol, catalase, SOD, and GSH		Motility	Griveau and Le Lannou[46]
Ferulic acid	Increases sperm cAMP and cGMP	Motility	Zheng and Zhang[47]
EDTA/Catalase	Reduces centrifugation-induced ROS and protects from xanthine/xanthine oxidase-induced loss of motility	Motility and DNA integrity	de Lamirande and Gagnon[48]
GSH/Hypotaurine	Protects from xanthine/xanthine oxidase-induced loss of motility	Lessen DNA damage	Lopes et al.[49]
Isoflavones (genistein, equol) or vitamin C/E	Protects from H_2O_2-induced DNA damage		Sierens et al.[50]
Vitamins C, E, zinc, and β-carotene	Vitamin C expresses genes involved in intracellular redox pathways. Its concentration in seminal plasma is 10 times more than in blood plasma *Dosage:* 1,000 µg *Dose <200 µg:* no benefit	DNA damage decreased from 22 to 9% after 2 months of vitamins C and E 1 g each Six out of nine couples got pregnant after 3 months of vitamins C and E, 1 g each	Greco et al.[51] and Gil-Villa et al.[52]
Vitamins C and E (400 mg), zinc, selenium, and β-carotene	Vitamin E protects integrity of phospholipid bilayer of cell membrane and mitochondrial sheath by preventing lipid peroxidation. Enhances production of antioxidant enzymes and decreases MDA concentrations (a marker for lipid peroxidation)	Rx (90 days): ↓ Sperm% DFI (32→26%: By 19%)	Menezo et al.[53]
Menevit (lycopene, vitamins C, E, zinc, selenium, folate, and garlic)	Decrease in ROS production and increased sperm protamination	Rx (3 months): 39% ICSI pregnancy rate, but no ↑ in embryo quality	Tremellen et al.[54]
		Rx (3 months): ↓ Differential diagnosis (22→18%)	Tunc et al.[55]
Vitamins C, E, β-glucan, papaya, and lactoferrin		Rx (90 days): ↑ motility and morphology	Piomboni et al.[56]
Vitamin C, E, and glutathione (400 mg)		Rx (2 months)	Kodama et al.[57]

Contd...

Contd...

Antioxidant	***Rationale***	***Parameter improved***	***Evidence***
Astaxanthin 16 mg for 3 months	Acts like vitamin E	Motility	Comhaire et al.[58]
Vitamin E 300 mg: 6 months		Asthenospermia	Suleiman et al.[59]
Glutathione 600 mg alternate days for 2 months	Glutathione protects plasma membrane from lipid peroxidation, scavenges superoxide, and prevents O_2 formation	Motility and morphology increased in men with varicocele and infection	Lenzi et al.[60]
Vitamin E + selenium		Motility	Keskes-Ammar et al.[61]
L-carnitine + L-acetyl carnitine	• Carnitine increases expression of antioxidant enzymes (heme oxygenase and endothelial nitric oxide synthetase) • Helps in membrane stability and in sperm development and maturation	6 months: Motility	Balercia et al.[62]
Selenium 100 mg or/with vitamin A 1 mg, vitamin C 10 mg, and vitamin E 15 mg	Selenium increases glutathione peroxidase expression, which destroys H_2O_2 molecules	3 months: Motility	Scott et al.[63]
LC ± LAC ± cinnoxicam		Improved concentration, motility, and morphology in men with varicocele except in high-grade varicocele men	Cavallini et al.[64]
NAC 600 mg for 3 months	NAC increases availability of glutathione Acts as ROS scavenger	Improved volume, motility, and viscosity	Ciftci et al.[65]
Folic acid 5 mg and zinc 66 mg	Folic acid reduces homocysteine levels	Improves concentration	Ebisch et al.[66]
LC 2 mg 6 months		Improves concentration and motility	Lenzi et al.[67]
Zinc 400 mg ± vitamin E 20 mg—3 months	• Zinc has membrane-stabilizing activity by inhibiting membrane-bound oxidative enzymes • Immunological function		Omu et al.[68]
β-Glucan 20 mg, papaya 50 mg, lactoferrin 97 mg, vitamin C 30 mg, and vitamin E 5 mg for 3 months		Motility and morphology	Piomboni et al.[56]
Selenium 200 mg ± NAC 600 mg 300 mg coenzyme Q10 for 26 weeks	Coenzyme Q10 inhibits lipid peroxidation	• Motility, morphology, and concentration • Acrosome reaction had increased from 14 ± 8% and 15 ± 8% to 31 ± 11% and 16 ± 10% in the coenzyme Q10 and placebo groups, respectively ($p = 0.01$)	Safarinejad and Safarinejad[69]
Folic acid 5 mg and zinc 66 mg		Concentration	Wong et al.[70]
NAC 600 mg + vitamins—minerals		Concentration	Paradiso et al.[71]
Pentoxifylline	Methylxanthine increases intracellular cAMP levels, which improves sperm motility hyperactivation and acrosome reaction	Curvilinear velocity, path velocity, straight-line velocity, lateral head displacement, beat cross frequency, and sperm hyperactivation	Tesariki et al.[72]

(cAMP: cyclic adenosine monophosphate; cGMP: cyclic guanosine monophosphate; DNA: deoxyribonucleic acid; DFI: DNA fragmentation index; EDTA: ethylenediaminetetraacetic acid; GSH: glutathione; ICSI: intracytoplasmic sperm injection; LC: L-carnitine; LAC: L-acetyl carnitine; LPO: lipid peroxidation; MDA: malondialdehyde; NAC: N-Acetylcysteine; ROS: reactive oxygen species; SOD: superoxide dismutase)

TABLE 4: Recommended daily allowance (RDA) of antioxidants.[76]

Vitamins/Minerals	*RDA*
A (carotenoids)	800 µg
E (tocopherols)	12 mg
C (ascorbic acid)	80 mg
B1 (thiamine)	1.1 mg
B2 (riboflavin)	1.4 mg
B3 (niacin)	16 mg
B5 (pantothenic acid)	6 mg
B6 (pyridoxine)	1.4 mg
B7 (biotin)	50 µg
B12 (cobalamin)	2.5 µg
Zinc	10 mg
Selenium	55 µg
Copper	1 mg
Chrome	40 µg
Magnesium	2 mg
Iron	14 mg

evidence supporting it. Candidates for oral antioxidant therapy are infertile men with ROS after indirect or direct assessment of it.

Indirect assessment methods are lipid peroxidation (malondialdehyde), protein oxidation products (8-OHdG), and sperm DNA integrity. Direct assessment methods are measuring total antioxidant capacity, seminal ROS levels, and detection of superoxide anion.[73] A quick way to detect sperm DNA fragmentation is sperm chromatin dispersion test in which sperms detected with absent halos are the ones with DNA strand breaks. It is a quantitative assay. Once the oxygen species is diagnosed, our focus should be on identifying the source and controlling it. Conditions such as genital infection, varicocele, smoking, medication, drug abuse, systemic diseases, pollution, and radiation are some of the attributable causes, which can be corrected. Differentiation between leukocytes and sperm should be done to know the source of ROS. Antioxidants should be selected according to their formulation and dosage. Recommendations for daily allowance of antioxidants are given in **Table 4**. Earlier, it was believed that antioxidant therapy should be given for 80 days at least[74] but now the latest concept of 60 days has come up depending on the time taken for sperm to undergo the process of differentiation and maturation.[75]

To Treat Obesity-related Infertility

Obesity is a risk factor for male infertility in various ways.[77] Effects of obesity on fertility are depicted in **Box 3**.

BOX 3: Effects of obesity.

Physical effects:
- Increased erectile dysfunction
- Increased scrotal temperature
- Increased sleep apnea

Seminal effects:
- Oligozoospermia[80]
- Increased DFI
- Decreased seminal volume

Hormonal:
- Increased estrogen, insulin, and leptin
- Decreased testosterone

Erectile dysfunction or disorders

(DFI: DNA fragmentation index)

Treatment Modalities

- *Lifestyle and nutritional changes:* Diet and exercise should be included. Patients should be counseled about negative effects of smoking cigarettes and marijuana and alcohol.[78]
  Exposure to harmful substances should be avoided. Psychological counseling and stress-relief therapy can be done.[79]
- *Pharmacological intervention:*
  - Appetite suppressants such as sibutramine
  - Weight loss drugs such as orlistat: It is the only FDA drug approved for this purpose.
  - Aromatase inhibitors such as anastrozole and letrozole.[80] Peripheral androgen aromatization is enhanced in men with increased body mass index (BMI). Obese men have increased plasma estradiol and low testosterone levels. Aromatase inhibitors lower estradiol levels and thus there is increase in LH and FSH, in turn increasing testosterone levels. This indirectly stimulates spermatogenesis.
- *Surgical:* Morbid obese men can go through bariatric surgery or scrotal lipectomy can also be tried.
- *ART:* It is the last modality if all fails.

NONSPECIFIC TREATMENT (EMPIRICAL THERAPY)

According to WHO 2010 analysis, oligospermia is defined as less than 15 million sperms/mL, asthenospermia as less than 40% motility, and teratospermia as less than 4% normal sperms (Tygerberg criteria). Such healthy men present with infertility but are eugonadotropic with normal androgenic features and virilization with subnormal seminal characteristics. No specific etiology is known for such people.

Nonspecific or Empirical Drug Treatment

Indications:
- Patient with oligospermia, asthenospermia, or teratospermia of unknown origin
- Other specific treatments have failed.

In such cases, empirical treatment can be tried to improve sperm count and motility only if FSH levels are normal. These are:

- Antiestrogens
- AIs
- Gonadotropins
- Adjuvants.

Antiestrogens

Antiestrogens such as clomiphene and tamoxifen act on estrogen receptors of hypothalamus to prevent negative feedback by estrogens.[81] It results in increased secretion of FSH and LH, which act on Leydig cells to secrete testosterone and possibly spermatogenesis. Clomiphene citrate is most commonly used in treating idiopathic oligospermia by binding to estrogen receptors. It decreases peripheral conversion of testosterone.[82] It is less likely to be efficacious in men with elevated levels of gonadotropins with markedly abnormal semen analysis or testicular biopsy.[83] Studies have shown conflicting results in sperm counts, morphology, motility, and pregnancy rates. A meta-analysis of 10 controlled studies involving 738 men when treated with clomiphene or tamoxifen for idiopathic oligo- or asthenospermia had positive hormonal effect, but no improvement in pregnancy rate was seen.[84] One randomized controlled trial (RCT) assessed the effect of treatment with clomiphene and vitamin E on the incidence of pregnancy and sperm variables in men with idiopathic oligoasthenozoospermia and infertility. Patients were randomly assigned in two groups with one group getting 25 mg/day of clomiphene and 400 mg/day of vitamin E and the other group placebo for 6 months. Significant higher pregnancy rates were found in the treatment group with increase in sperm count and progressive sperm motility. Nonsignificant changes in total sperm motility, percentage of abnormal forms, and volume were present.[85] A number of meta-analyses have shown a significant elevation in FSH, LH, and testosterone levels on treatment with selective estrogen receptor modulators (SERMs).[86]

Aromatase Inhibitors

Aromatase enzyme belongs to the cytochrome P450 group of enzymes, which is involved in synthesis of aldosterone, cortisol, and androgens.

Mechanism of action:

- Aromatase inhibitors block the conversion of androgens to estrogens and thus increase testosterone levels.
- Aromatase inhibitors block inhibitory feedback of testosterone on the hypothalamic–pituitary–gonadal (HPG) axis and convert into more potent estrogen without any increase in circulating estrogens and E2 receptor modulators.[87]

The most commonly used are letrozole and anastrozole. For AIs to work, the HPG axis should be functional. Altered estrogen-to-testosterone ratio impairs spermatogenesis. Aromatase inhibition is dose-dependent, thus as a result of which aromatase is less suppressed in testis than in adipose tissue and muscle tissue. This is beneficial as it prevents excess reduction of estradiol levels. Semen parameters and testosterone/estradiol ratios improved in a study of nonobstructive azoospermic and cryptozoospermic patients.[88] Treatment of infertile males with the aromatase inhibitors testolactone, anastrozole (1 mg/day), and letrozole (2.5 mg/day) have been associated with increased sperm production and return of sperm to the ejaculate in men with excess aromatase activity [abnormal testosterone/estradiol (T/E) ratios].[89]

Adverse effects: There may be detrimental effects on mineralization. Decrease in high-density lipoprotein (HDL) and increase in hemoglobin level may be present.

Contraindications:

- Elevated liver enzymes and liver diseases
- Estrogen deficiency—osteopenia or osteoporosis
- High blood pressure
- Alopecia, peripheral edema, rashes, and acne.

Gonadotropins

Follicle-stimulating hormone is beneficial in a subset group with normal levels of inhibin B and FSH with hypospermatogenesis but without maturation defects.[90] Four RCTs in a Cochrane analysis of 278 participants had better pregnancy rate per couple with idiopathic subfertility after completing 3 months of treatment [odds ratio (OR) 3.03, 95% confidence interval (CI) 1.30–7.09]. Pregnancy rate was 13.4% (19/142) in the gonadotropin group and 4.4% (6/136) in the control group.[91] The number of participants and trials was small and thus evidence is insufficient to decipher any conclusion. Large multicenter trials with more participants are needed.

Adjuvants

Products such as arginine, pentoxifylline, growth hormone, testolactone, GnRH, kallikrein, prostaglandin inhibitors, and antioxidants have not shown any beneficial effect in controlled studies in normogonadotropic patients. In one controlled study by indomethacin (50–75 mg/day for 60 days) was found to significantly improve both semen parameters and pregnancy rates compared with no improvement in the placebo group. More studies are needed to add this in daily practice.

EFFECT ON MALE INFERTILITY IN COVID-19 ERA

Angiotensin-converting enzyme 2 (ACE2) is expressed in spermatogonia, Sertoli, and Leydig cells of testes, which might lead to testicular dysfunction in patients infected with severe acute respiratory syndrome coronavirus 2 (SARS-CoV-2). This damage to testes may be allocated to inflammatory response and fever-associated inflammation. Testicular inflammation caused by viral infection causes increase in interleukins and tumor necrosis factor-α resulting in defective spermatogenesis. Testicular dysfunction may also be caused by disease-related medications, glucocorticoids, and disease-related stress.[92] This may affect semen parameters such as motility and concentration for 72–90 days post-COVID-19 infection. Changes in semen quality are either a direct impact on spermatogenesis caused by viruses or an indirect effect of cytokine excess due to disease and oxidative stress. Achua et al.[93] performed immunofluorescence analysis of testicular biopsy samples of six patients to exhibit association between spermatogenesis dysfunction and increased ACE2 levels, thus stipulating the mechanism of testicular infection by SARS-CoV-2.

Ma et al.[94] detected an increase in circulating LH levels and reduced testosterone: LH ratio in COVID-19 patients, suggesting a negative impact on Leydig cell function. Damage affects not only fertility but mental and psychological well-being also. These effects may subside with time, though further studies are required to validate the point.

Gonzalez et al.[95] studied semen parameters before and after two doses of COVID-19 messenger ribonucleic acid (mRNA) vaccine (Pfizer and Moderna) and found no significant decrease in semen parameters. This may be due to the fact that the vaccines contain mRNA and not the live virus and thus it is highly unlikely that the vaccine would affect sperm parameters. This cannot be predicted for the long-term future due to limitations of the study. Abdel-Moneim[96] has affirmed that precautions should be taken to minimize the risk of transmitting infection via sexual intercourse as also advised by American Society for Reproductive Medicine (ASRM). Miller et al.[97] have demonstrated the importance of telemedicine in the COVID-19 era. Agarwal et al.[98] have recently developed a novel test for oxidative stress measurement called MiOXSYS, which can be used in this COVID-19 era.

Follow-up studies are needed to identify the actual effect on reproductive functions of male patients before any definitive statement can be issued in public as limitations are present in all aforementioned studies.[99] Recently, a project PROTEGGIMI is developed for making an international collaborated registry to fill gaps within the association of SARS-CoV-2 and male fertility.[100]

KEY POINTS

- When a clinician faces male factor infertility, an affirmative and diligent search has to be done to reach up to proper and correct diagnosis. Early diagnosis and intervention along the correct line of management is the key to success.
- A fully functioning basic andrology laboratory along with embryology laboratory should be mandatory in a tertiary-level infertility clinic.
- Understanding of basic HPG axis with basics of endocrinology is of utmost importance.
- Majority of male infertility causes are idiopathic.
- Gonadotropin replacement therapy results in improving androgenic and seminal parameters.
- Primary focus is on optimizing testosterone production through Leydig cells and FSH production to stimulate Sertoli cells and spermatogenesis.
- Despite the fact that testosterone is necessary for virilization and spermatogenesis, exogenous androgens in the form of testosterone should be avoided as they have contraceptive effects by inhibiting LH stimulation on intratesticular testosterone and FSH stimulation of Sertoli cells.
- Aromatase inhibitors play a significant role in men with abnormal testosterone-to-estrogen ratio.

REFERENCES

1. Damani MN, Shaban SF. Medical treatment of male infertility. Glob Libr Women's Med; 2008.
2. World Health Organization. Task Force on the Diagnosis and Treatment of Infertility. Towards More Objectivity in Diagnosis and Management of Male Infertility. Int J Androl. 1987;7(Suppl.):1–53.
3. Kandeel FR, Swerdloff RS. Role of temperature in regulation of spermatogenesis and the use of heating as a method for contraception. Fertil Steril. 1988;49:1-23.
4. Kim HH, Schlegel PN. Endocrine manipulation in male infertility. Urol Clin North Am. 2008;35:303-18.
5. Anawalt BD. Approach to male infertility and induction of spermatogenesis. J Clin Endocrinol Metab. 2013;98:3532-42.
6. Burris AS, Rodbard HW, Winters SJ, Sherins RJ. Gonadotropin therapy in men with isolated hypogonadotropic hypogonadism: the response to human chorionic gonadotropin is predicted by initial testicular size. J Clin Endocrinol Metab. 1988;66(6):1144-51.
7. Zitzmann M, Nieschlag E. Hormone substitution in male hypogonadism. Mol Cell Endocrinol. 2000;161(1-2):73-88.
8. Madani AH, Falahatkar S, Heidarzadeh A, Roshan ZA, Sazgari E, Zareian M. Sensitivity and specificity of serum FSH and testis size in predicting the existence of spermatogenesis in azoospermic infertile men. Andrologia. 2012;44:205-9.
9. Darby E, Anawalt BD. Male hypogonadism: an update on diagnosis and treatment. Treat Endocrinol. 2005;4(5):293-309.
10. Raivio T, Wikstrom AM, Dunkel L. Treatment of gonadotropin-deficient boys with recombinant human FSH: long-term observation and outcome. Eur J Endocrinol. 2007;156(1):105-11.
11. Miyagawa Y, Tsujimura A, Matsumiya K, Takao T, Tohda A, Koga M, et al. Outcome of gonadotropin therapy for male hypogonadotropic hypogonadism at university affiliated male infertility centers: a 30-year retrospective study. J Urol. 2005;173:2072-5.

12. Viswanathan V, Eugster EA. Etiology and treatment of hypogonadism in adolescents. Pediatr Clin North Am. 2011;58(5):1181-200.
13. Bakircioglu ME, Erden HF, Ciray HN, Bayazit N, Bahçeci M. Gonadotropin therapy in combination with ICSI in men with hypogonadotropic hypogonadism. Reprod Biomed Online. 2007;15(2):156-60.
14. Esteves SC, Papanikolaou V. Clinical efficacy, safety and tolerability of recombinant human chorionic gonadotropin to restore spermatogenesis and androgen production of hypogonadotropic hypogonadal men. Fertil Steril. 2011;96(3):S230.
15. Jarow JP, Zirkin BR. The androgen microenvironment of the human testis and hormonal control of spermatogenesis. Ann N Y Acad Sci. 2005;1061:208-20.
16. Pitteloud N, Hayes FJ, Dwyer A, Boepple PA, Lee H, Crowley Jr WF. Predictors of outcome of long-term GnRH therapy in men with idiopathic hypogonadotropic hypogonadism. J Clin Endocrinol Metab. 2002;87:4128-36.
17. Bhasin S, Cunningham GR, Hayes FJ, Matsumoto AM, Snyder PJ, Swerdloff RS, et al. Testosterone therapy in men with androgen deficiency syndromes: an Endocrine Society clinical practice guideline. J Clin Endocrinol Metab. 2010;95:2536-59.
18. Byrne M, Nieschlag E. Testosterone replacement therapy in male hypogonadism. J Endocrinol Invest. 2003;26(5):481-9.
19. Finkelstein JS, Lee H, Burnett-Bowie SAM, Pallais JC, Yu EW, Borges LF, et al. Gonadal steroids and body composition, strength, and sexual function in men. N Engl J Med. 2013; 369:1011-22.
20. Seftel AD, Mack RJ, Secrest AR, Smith TH. Restorative increases in serum testosterone levels are significantly correlated to improvements in sexual functioning. J Androl. 2004;25:963-72.
21. Seal JL. Male hypogonadism and testosterone replacement therapy. Medicine. 2017;45(9):532-7.
22. Bella AJ, Lee JC, Carrier S, Bénard F, Brock GB. 2015 CUA practice guidelines for erectile dysfunction. Can Urol Assoc J. 2015;9(1-2):23-9.
23. Jaya Kumar B, Khurana ML, Ammini AC, Karmarkar MG, Ahuja MM. Reproductive endocrine functions in men with primary hypothyroidism: effect of thyroxine replacement. Horm Res. 1990;34:215-8.
24. Gillam MP, Molitch ME, Lombardi G, Colao A. Advances in the treatment of prolactinomas. Endocr Rev. 2006;27:485-534.
25. Pavlovich CP, King P, Goldstein M, Schlegel PN. Evidence of a treatable endocrinopathy in infertile men. J Urol. 2001; 165:837-41.
26. Layman LC. Hypogonadotropic hypogonadism. Endocrinol Metab Clin North Am. 2007;36(2):283-96.
27. Arlt W, Willis DS, Wild SH, Krone N, Doherty EJ, Hahner S, et al. Health status of adults with congenital adrenal hyperplasia: a cohort study of 203 patients. J Clin Endocrinol Metabol. 2010;95(11):5110-21.
28. Menon DK. Successful treatment of anabolic steroid-induced azoospermia with human chorionic gonadotropin and human menopausal gonadotropin. Fertil Steril. 2003;79(Suppl. 3):1659-61.
29. Schuppe HC, Pilatz A, Hossain H, Diemer T, Wagenlehner F, Weidner W. Urogenital infection as a risk factor for male infertility. Dtsch Arztebl Int. 2017;114:339-46.
30. Chan PT, Schlegel PN. Inflammatory conditions of the male excurrent ductal system. Part I. J Androl. 2002;23:453-60.
31. Wein AJ (Ed). Campbell-Walsh Urology, 9th edition. Philadelphia: Saunders/Elsevier; 2007.
32. Comhaire F, Verschraegen G, Vermeulen L. Diagnosis of accessory gland infection and its possible role in male infertility. Int J Androl. 1980;3:32-45.
33. Eley A, Pacey AA, Galdiero M, Galdiero M, Galdiero F. Can *Chlamydia trachomatis* directly damage your sperm? Lancet Infect Dis. 2005;5:53-7.
34. Hosseinzadeh S, Brewis IA, Pacey AA, Moore HD, Eley A. Coincubation of human spermatozoa with *Chlamydia trachomatis* in vitro causes increased tyrosine phosphorylation of sperm proteins. Infect Immun. 2000;68:4872-6.
35. Hamada A, Agarwal A, Sharma R, French DB, Ragheb A, Sabanegh Jr ES. Empirical treatment of low-level leukocytospermia with doxycycline in male infertility patients. Urology. 2011;78:1320-5.
36. Dunsmuir WD, Holmes SA. The aetiology and management of erectile, ejaculatory, and fertility problems in men with diabetes mellitus. Diabet Med. 1996;13:700-8.
37. Jefferys A, Siassakos D, Wardle P. The management of retrograde ejaculation: a systematic review and update. Fertil Steril. 2012;97:306-12.
38. Ohl DA, Quallich SA, Sonksen J, Brackett NL, Lynne CM. Anejaculation and retrograde ejaculation. Urol Clin North Am. 2008;35:211-20.
39. Showell MG, Brown J, Yazdani A, Stankiewicz MT, Hart RJ. Antioxidants for male subfertility. Cochrane Database Syst Rev. 2011;CD007411.
40. Ko EY, Sabanegh Jr ES. The role of over-the-counter supplements for the treatment of male infertility—fact or fiction? J Androl. 2012;33(3):292-308.
41. Gharagozloo P, Aitken RJ. The role of sperm oxidative stress in male infertility and the significance of oral antioxidant therapy. Hum Reprod. 2011;26(7):1628-40.
42. Ross C, Morriss A, Khairy M, Khalaf Y, Braude P, Coomarasamy A, et al. A systematic review of the effect of oral antioxidants on male infertility. Reprod Biomed Online. 2010;20(6):711-23.
43. Merino G, Martínez Chéquer JC, Barahona E, Bermúdez JA, Morán C, Carranza-Lira S. Effects of pentoxifylline on sperm motility in normogonadotropic asthenozoospermic men. Arch Androl. 1997;39(1):65-9.
44. Oeda T, Henkel R, Ohmori H, Schill WB. Scavenging effect of N-acetyl-L-cysteine against reactive oxygen species in human semen: a possible therapeutic modality for male factor infertility. Andrologia. 1997;29:125-31.
45. Verma A, Kanwar KC. Effect of vitamin E on human sperm motility and lipid peroxidation in vitro. Asian J Androl. 1999;1:151-4.
46. Griveau JF, Le Lannou D. Effects of antioxidants on human sperm preparation techniques. Int J Androl. 1994;17:225-31.
47. Zheng RL, Zhang H. Effects of ferulic acid on fertile and asthenozoospermic infertile human sperm motility, viability, lipid peroxidation, and cyclic nucleotides. Free Radic Biol Med. 1997;22:581-6.
48. de Lamirande E, Gagnon C. Reactive oxygen species and human spermatozoa. I. Effects on the motility of intact spermatozoa and on sperm axonemes. J Androl. 1992;13: 368-78.

49. Lopes S, Jurisicova A, Sun JG, Casper RF. Reactive oxygen species: potential cause for DNA fragmentation in human spermatozoa. Hum Reprod. 1998;13:896-900.
50. Sierens J, Hartley JA, Campbell MJ, Leathem AJC, Woodside JV. In vitro isoflavone supplementation reduces hydrogen peroxide-induced DNA damage in sperm. Teratog Carcinog Mutagen. 2002;22:227-34.
51. Greco E, Iacobelli M, Rienzi L, Ubaldi F, Ferrero S, Tesarik J, et al. Reduction of the incidence of sperm DNA fragmentation by oral antioxidant treatment. J Androl. 2005;26:349-53.
52. Gil-Villa AM, Cardona-Maya W, Agarwal A, Sharma R, Cadavid A. Role of male factor in early recurrent embryo loss: do antioxidants have any effect? Fertil Steril. 2009;92:565-71.
53. Menezo YJ, Hazout A, Panteix G, Robert F, Rollet J, Cohen-Bacrie P, et al. Antioxidants to reduce sperm DNA fragmentation: an unexpected adverse effect. Reprod Biomed Online. 2007;14:418-21.
54. Tremellen K, Miari G, Froiland D, Thompson J. A randomised control trial examining the effect of an antioxidant (Menevit) on pregnancy outcome during IVF-ICSI treatment. Aust N Z J Obstet Gynaecol. 2007;47:216-21.
55. Tunc O, Thompson J, Tremellen K. Improvement in sperm DNA quality using an oral antioxidant therapy. Reprod Biomed Online. 2009;18:761-8.
56. Piomboni P, Gambera L, Serafini F, Campanella G, Morgante G, De Leo V. Sperm quality improvement after natural antioxidant treatment of asthenoteratospermic men with leukocytospermia. Asian J Androl. 2008;10:201-6.
57. Kodama H, Yamaguchi R, Fukuda J, Kasai H, Tanaka T. Increased oxidative deoxyribonucleic acid damage in the spermatozoa of infertile male patients. Fertil Steril. 1997;68:519-24.
58. Comhaire FH, El Garem Y, Mahmoud A, Eertmans F, Schoonjans F. Combined conventional/antioxidant "Astaxanthin" treatment for male infertility: a double blind, randomized trial. Asian J Androl. 2005;7:257-62.
59. Suleiman SA, Ali ME, Zaki ZM, el-Malik EM, Nasr MA. Lipid peroxidation and human sperm motility: protective role of vitamin E. J Androl. 1996;17:530-7.
60. Lenzi A, Culasso F, Gandini L, Lombardo F, Dondero F. Placebo-controlled, double-blind, cross-over trial of glutathione therapy in male infertility. Hum Reprod. 1993;8:1657-62.
61. Keskes-Ammar L, Feki-Chakroun N, Rebai T, Sahnoun Z, Ghozzi H, Hammami S, et al. Sperm oxidative stress and the effect of an oral vitamin E and selenium supplement on semen quality in infertile men. Arch Androl. 2003;49:83-94.
62. Balercia G, Regoli F, Armeni T, Koverech A, Mantero F, Boscaro M. Placebo-controlled double-blind randomized trial on the use of L-carnitine, L-acetylcarnitine, or combined L-carnitine and L-acetylcarnitine in men with idiopathic asthenozoospermia. Fertil Steril. 2005;84:662-71.
63. Scott R, MacPherson A, Yates RW, Hussain B, Dixon J. The effect of oral selenium supplementation on human sperm motility. Br J Urol. 1998;82:76-80.
64. Cavallini G, Ferraretti AP, Gianaroli L, Biagiotti G, Vitali G. Cinnoxicam and L-carnitine/acetyl-L-carnitine treatment for idiopathic and varicocele-associated oligoasthenospermia. J Androl. 2004;25:761-70.
65. Ciftci H, Verit A, Savas M, Yeni E, Erel O. Effects of N-acetylcysteine on semen parameters and oxidative/antioxidant status. Urology. 2009;74:73-6.
66. Ebisch IM, Pierik FH, de Jong FH, Thomas CMG, Steegers-Theunissen RPM. Does folic acid and zinc sulphate intervention affect endocrine parameters and sperm characteristics in men? Int J Androl. 2006;29:339-45.
67. Lenzi A, Lombardo F, Sgro P, Salacone P, Caponecchia L, Dondero F, et al. Use of carnitine therapy in selected cases of male factor infertility: a double-blind crossover trial. Fertil Steril. 2003;79:292-300.
68. Omu AE, Al-Azemi MK, Kehinde EO, Anim JT, Oriowo MA, Mathew TC. Indications of the mechanisms involved in improved sperm parameters by zinc therapy. Med Princ Pract. 2008;17:108-16.
69. Safarinejad MR, Safarinejad S. Efficacy of selenium and/or N-acetyl-cysteine for improving semen parameters in infertile men: a double-blind, placebo controlled, randomized study. J Urol. 2009;181:741-51.
70. Wong WY, Merkus HM, Thomas CM, Menkveld R, Zielhuis GA, Steegers-Theunissen RP. Effects of folic acid and zinc sulfate on male factor subfertility: a double-blind, randomized, placebo-controlled trial. Fertil Steril. 2002;77:491-8.
71. Paradiso Galatioto G, Gravina GL, Angelozzi G, Sacchetti A, Innominato PF, Pace G, et al. May antioxidant therapy improve sperm parameters of men with persistent oligospermia after retrograde embolization for varicocele? World J Urol. 2008;26:97-102.
72. Tesariki J, Thébault A, Testart J. Effect of pentoxifylline on sperm movement characteristics in normozoospermic and asthenozoospermic specimens. Hum Reprod. 1992;7(9):1257-63.
73. Esteves SC, Hamada A, Kondray V, Pitchika A, Agarwal A. What every gynecologist should know about male infertility: an update. Arch Gynecol Obstet. 2012;286(1):217-29.
74. Misell LM, Holochwost D, Boban D, Santi N, Shefi S, Hellerstein MK, et al. A stable isotope-mass spectrometric method for measuring human spermatogenesis kinetics in vivo. J Urol. 2006;175:242-6.
75. Esteves SC, Agarwal A. Novel concepts in male infertility. Int Braz J Urol. 2011;37(1):5-15.
76. Walczak-Jedrzejowska R, Wolski JK, Slowikowska-Hilczer J. The role of oxidative stress and antioxidants in male fertility. Cent European J Urol. 2013;66(1):60-7.
77. Sallmén M, Sandler DP, Hoppin JA, Blair A, Baird DD. Reduced fertility among overweight and obese men. Epidemiology. 2006;17:520-3.
78. Magnusdottir EV, Thorsteinsson T, Thorsteinsdottir S, Heimisdottir M, Olafsdottir K. Persistent organochlorines, sedentary occupation, obesity and human male subfertility. Hum Reprod. 2005;20:208-15.
79. Stokes VJ, Anderson RA, George JT. How does obesity affect fertility in men - and what are the treatment options? Clin Endocrinol (Oxf). 2015;82:633-8.
80. Ribeiro MA, Gameiro LF, Scarano WR, Briton-Jones C, Kapoor A, Rosa MB, et al. Aromatase inhibitors in the treatment of oligozoospermic or azoospermic men: a systematic review of randomized controlled trials. JBRA Assist Reprod. 2016;20:82-8.
81. Tsourdi E, Kourtis A, Farmakiotis D, Katsikis I, Salmas M, Panidis D. The effect of selective estrogen receptor modulator administration on the hypothalamic-pituitary-testicular axis in men with idiopathic oligozoospermia. Fertil Steril. 2009;91(4 Suppl.):1427-30.

82. Komm BS, Mirkin S. An overview of current and emerging SERMs. J Steroid Biochem Mol Biol. 2014;143:207-22.
83. Mazzola CR, Katz DJ, Loghmanieh N, Nelson CJ, Mulhall JP. Predicting biochemical response to clomiphene citrate in men with hypogonadism. J Sex Med. 2014;11(9):2302-7.
84. Vandekerckhove P, Lilford R, Vail A, Hughes E. Clomiphene or tamoxifen for idiopathic oligo/asthenospermia. Cochrane Database Syst Rev. 2000;(2):CD000151.
85. Ghanem H, Shaeer O, El-Segini A. Combination clomiphene citrate and antioxidant therapy for idiopathic male infertility: a randomized controlled trial. Fertil Steril. 2010;93:2232-5.
86. Chua ME, Escusa KG, Luna S, Tapia LC, Dofitas B, Morales M. Revisiting oestrogen antagonists (clomiphene or tamoxifen) as medical empiric therapy for idiopathic male infertility: a meta-analysis. Andrology. 2013;1(5):749-57.
87. Yasser E, Ibrahim F. Aromatase inhibitors in the treatment of male infertility. Hum Androl. 2011;1:35-8.
88. Cavallini G, Biagiotti G, Bolzon E. Multivariate analysis to predict letrozole efficacy in improving sperm count of non-obstructive azoospermic and cryptozoospermic patients: a pilot study. Asian J Androl. 2013;15:806-11.
89. Schlegel PN. Aromatase inhibitors for male infertility. Fertil Steril. 2012;98:1359-62.
90. Foresta C, Bettella A, Garolla A, Ambrosini G, Ferlin A. Treatment of male idiopathic infertility with recombinant human follicle-stimulating hormone: a prospective, controlled, randomized clinical study. Fertil Steril. 2005;84:654-61.
91. Attia AM, Al-Inany HG, Farquhar C, Proctor M. Gonadotrophins for idiopathic male factor subfertility. Cochrane Database Syst Rev. 2007;CD005071.
92. Fainberg J, Kashanian JA. Recent advances in understanding and managing male infertility. F1000Res. 2019;8:670.
93. Achua JK, Chu KY, Ibrahim E, Khodamoradi K, Delma KS, Iakymenko OA, et al. Histopathology and ultrastructural findings of fatal COVID-19 infections on testis. World J Mens Health. 2021;39:65-74.
94. Ma L, Xie W, Li D, Shi L, Ye G, Mao Y, et al. Evaluation of sex-related hormones and semen characteristics in reproductive-aged male COVID-19 patients. J Med Virol. 2021;93(1):456-62.
95. Gonzalez DC, Nassau DE, Khodamoradi K, Ibrahim E, Blachman-Braun R, Ory J, et al. Sperm parameters before and after COVID-19 mRNA vaccination. JAMA. 2021;326(3):273-4.
96. Abdel-Moneim A. COVID-19 pandemic and male fertility: clinical manifestations and pathogenic mechanisms. Biochemistry (Mosc). 2021;86(4):389-96.
97. Miller D, Vukina J. Recent advances in clinical diagnosis and treatment of male factor infertility. Postgrad Med. 2020;132(sup4):28-34.
98. Agarwal A, Sharma R, Roychoudhury S, Du Plessis S, Sabanegh E. MiOXSYS: a novel method of measuring oxidation reduction potential in semen and seminal plasma. Fertil Steril. 2016;106(3):566-73.e10.
99. Illiano E, Trama F, Costantini E. Could COVID-19 have an impact on male fertility? Andrologia. 2020;52(6):e13654.
100. Dutta S, Sengupta P. SARS-CoV-2 and male infertility: possible multifaceted pathology. Reprod Sci. 2021;28(1):23-6.

CHAPTER 29

Azoospermia: Evaluation and Management

Ameya Rangnath Sangle, Tarun Dilip Javali

INTRODUCTION

Infertility affects nearly 10–15% of couples who are unable to conceive after 1 year of unprotected intercourse. Male factor infertility accounts for nearly 20–50% of these couples.[1] Of these men, azoospermia is diagnosed in nearly 10–15%.[2] Aspermia is distinct pathology where no ejaculate is produced.

TERMINOLOGY

As per the 2010 World Health Organization (WHO) standards (5th edition) for the evaluation of human semen,[3] the terminologies that are most used in andrology practice are given in **Table 1**.

DEFINITION

The diagnosis of azoospermia requires the absence of sperm from at least two separate centrifuged semen samples. The WHO Laboratory Manual for the Examination of Human Semen and Semen-Cervical Mucus Interaction recommends that the seminal fluid be centrifuged for 15 minutes at a centrifugation speed of, preferably, 3,000 × *g* or greater.[4]

CLASSIFICATION OF AZOOSPERMIA

The classification of azoospermia has been shown in **Flowchart 1**.

CLINICAL CLASSIFICATION OF AZOOSPERMIA

The clinical classification of azoospermia has been shown in **Flowchart 2**.

TABLE 1: Terminology.

Aspermia	No ejaculate (0 mL)
Asthenospermia	<40% total motility
Azoospermia	0 sperm on two centrifuged specimens
Normospermia	>39 million sperm/ejaculate
Oligospermia	<39 million sperm/ejaculate
Teratospermia	<4% normal morphology

EVALUATION OF A MALE PATIENT WITH AZOOSPERMIA

The initial evaluation of the azoospermic male should begin with a standard reproductive history and physical examination.

History should include:[5]

- *Fertility history:*
  - Duration of infertility
  - Whether the infertility is primary or secondary
  - Any treatments to date
  - Libido
  - Sexual function
  - Sexual activity.
- *General health:*
  - *Diabetes:* Long-standing diabetes may lead to ejaculatory dysfunction and erectile dysfunction.

Flowchart 1: Classification of azoospermia.

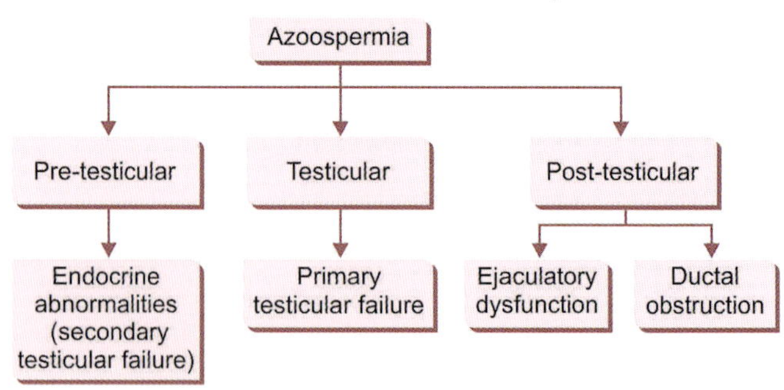

Flowchart 2: Clinical classification of azoospermia.

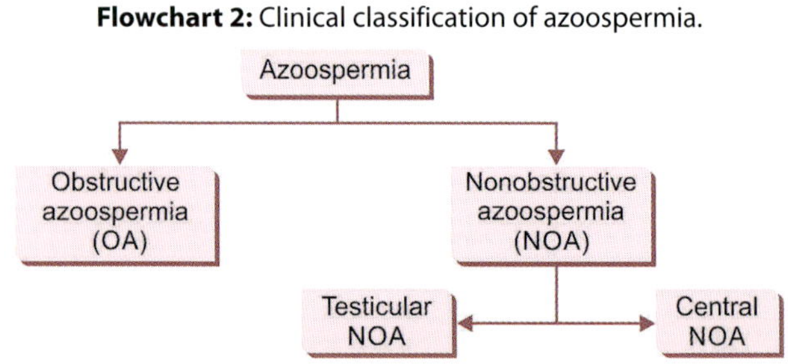

- *Respiratory illness:* Recurrent respiratory tract infections may be due to cystic fibrosis, Young's syndrome, and Prune belly syndrome.
- *Recent illness:* Acute viral fever may cause temporary suppression of testicular function but is usually reversible within 3 months.
- *Smoking:* It causes oxidative stress and deoxyribonucleic acid (DNA) damage of spermatozoa.

- *Genitourinary infections:*
  - Mumps-orchitis
  - Epididymo-orchitis
  - Sexually transmitted infections.
- *Prior surgeries:*
  - Testis cancer
  - Undescended testis
  - Hydrocelectomies
  - Spermatocelectomies
  - Varicocelectomies
  - Vasectomies
  - Testicular torsion.
- *Medication history:*
  - *Hormone or steroid therapy:* Anabolic steroids have a negative impact on the hypothalamic–pituitary–gonadal axis.
  - *Antibiotics:* High dose of nitrofurantoin may affect sperm maturation. Erythromycin and tetracycline may impair sperm motility. Sulfasalazine decreases sperm density, motility, and morphology.
  - *α-blockers:* They cause retrograde ejaculation.
  - 5-α-reductase inhibitors
  - *Chemotherapeutic agents and radiation:* Almost all chemotherapeutic agents are gonadotoxic. Chances of recovery are poor with agents such as bleomycin, etoposide, cisplatin, procarbazine, and vincristine. Cryopreservation should be considered in young patients prior to initiation of chemotherapy.
  - Narcotics
  - Recreational drugs and alcohol.
- History of genetic abnormalities in the family or patient himself
- *Environmental/occupational hazards:*
  - Pesticides
  - Excessive heat on testicles
  - *Occupation:* Welders/coal miners, etc.

Physical examination should focus on evaluating:

- *State of virilization:* Development of secondary sexual characters
  - *Facial, truncal, axillary, and pubic hair:* Sparse in primary and secondary hypogonadism
  - *Voice:* High pitched in hypogonadism
  - Presence of gynecomastia.
- *Scrotal examination:*
  - Presence of testis in scrotum
  - Size of the testis
  - Consistency of the testis
  - Presence and grade of varicocele
  - Palpation of vas deferens
  - Presence of testicular mass.
- *Abdominal examination:*
  - Presence of abdominal mass
  - Presence of scars over abdomen indicative of previous surgeries.

Laboratory Investigations

- *Semen analysis:* Azoospermia in men, by definition, is the absence of sperms in the ejaculate. For further evaluation, the following semen parameters are of importance:
  - *Volume:* Threshold volume is 1.5 mL.
  - *Liquefaction:* Semen is aspirated into a pipette and length of the drop which forms is measured. Length should be no longer than 2 cm.
  - *Semen pH:* Semen pH is generally alkaline. Acidic pH may indicate obstruction or infection.
  - *Fructose:* Patients with obstructive azoospermia tend to have absent fructose whereas those with nonobstructive azoospermia generally have fructose-positive semen.
- *Endocrine evaluation:* Hormonal abnormalities of the hypothalamic–pituitary–testicular axis are well-recognized, though not common causes of male infertility; they form an important component in the evaluation of an azoospermic male **(Tables 2 and 3)**. An endocrine evaluation should include:
  - Serum follicle-stimulating hormone (FSH)
  - Total testosterone
  - Luteinizing hormone (LH)
  - Estradiol
  - Prolactin
  - Free testosterone levels
  - Inhibin B.
- *Urine analysis:* In males with low ejaculate volume (<1.5 mL) and normal hormone levels, postejaculate urine analysis is an important initial test to evaluate for retrograde ejaculation.

TABLE 2: Endocrine parameters in various types of azoospermia.

	FSH	*LH*	*Testosterone*	*Inhibin B*
Obstructive azoospermia	Normal	Normal	Normal	Normal
Hypogonadotropic hypogonadism	Low	Low	Low	Low
Hypergonadotropic hypogonadism	High	High	Low	Low

(FSH: follicle-stimulating hormone; LH: luteinizing hormone)

TABLE 3: Endocrine and semen parameters in azoospermia based on etiology.

Etiology		Semen volume	Total testosterone	Serum FSH
Pre-testicular	Hypogonadotropic hypogonadism	Normal	Low	Low
	Exogenous androgens	Normal	Elevated/normal/low	Low
Testicular	Primary testicular failure	Normal	Low	Elevated
Post-testicular	Epididymal obstruction, vasectomy	Normal	Normal	Normal
	Ejaculatory duct obstruction	Low	Normal	Normal/elevated

(FSH: follicle-stimulating hormone)

Radiological Evaluation

Imaging in a case of infertility is not indicated for routine evaluation or as a part of initial workup. However, it plays an important role in aiding the diagnosis and imaging modalities should be chosen as per clinical indication.

- *Scrotal ultrasound:*
  - To assess testicular size and volume
  - Color Doppler can be used to assess varicocele.
- *Transrectal ultrasound (TRUS):*
  - TRUS is recommended when semen analysis is suggestive of obstructive azoospermia (i.e., acidic, fructose negative, azoospermic, semen volume <1.5 mL, with normal serum testosterone, palpable vas deferens). TRUS evidence of ejaculatory duct obstruction includes:[6]
    - Seminal vesicle anteroposterior (AP) diameter >1.5 cm
    - Seminal vesicle cyst may or may not be present.
  - TRUS can also be used for chromotubation, wherein seminal vesicles can be aspirated to check for sperms and a dilute dye (methylene blue or indigo carmine) can be injected, and cystoscopy can be done to see if the dye flows from the ductal orifice.[7]
- *Vasography:* It is currently rarely performed. It is usually done at the time of vasal reconstructive procedures, wherein contrast is injected in the vasal lumen toward the abdominal end to assess the site of obstruction. Indications for vasography:
  - Hernia or pelvic surgery
  - Semen volume <1 mL
  - Fructose-negative azoospermia with palpable vas.

Testicular Biopsy

The current role of testicular biopsy in patients with male factor infertility is:

- To differentiate between obstructive and nonobstructive azoospermia in case of uncertainty in diagnosis
- To assess the presence or absence of focal spermatogenesis in nonobstructive azoospermia **(Fig. 1)**. The biopsy or aspirate is performed with the additional ability to examine the tissue for sperm and to cryopreserve it, potentially avoiding the need for a second procedure.

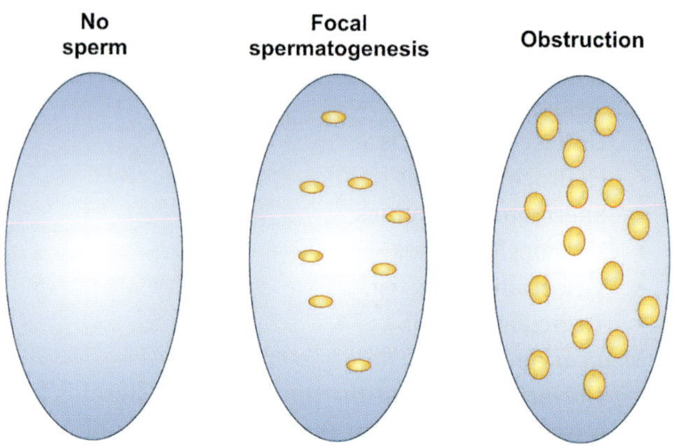

Fig. 1: New interpretation of testicular biopsy.

ETIOLOGY OF AZOOSPERMIA

The etiology of azoospermia is given in **Table 4**.

Obstructive Azoospermia

Congenital Bilateral Absence of the Vas Deferens

The most common cause of congenital bilateral absence of the vas deferens (CBAVD) is the cystic fibrosis transmembrane conductance regulator (*CFTR*) gene mutation. Diagnosis can be easily made by physical examination. Imaging studies and surgical exploration are generally not necessary to confirm the diagnosis but may be useful for diagnosing abnormalities associated with vasal agenesis such as seminal vesicle aplasia. The American Urological Association (AUA) recommends genetic counseling and testing for *CFTR* mutation for both partners. However, failure to identify a CFTR abnormality in a man with CBAVD does not rule out the presence of a mutation as many are undetectable by routine testing methods. In patients with unilateral absence of vas, contralateral segmental atresia of the vas deferens or seminal vesicle and ipsilateral renal anomalies may be present.[8] Treatment options include:

- Intrauterine insemination using epididymal sperm (3–5% pregnancy rate)
- Percutaneous epididymal sperm aspiration (PESA)-intracytoplasmic sperm injection (ICSI) (30–40% pregnancy rate).

TABLE 4: Etiology of azoospermia.

	Nonobstructive		
	Testicular failure	***Hypogonadotropic hypogonadism (HH)***	***Obstructive***
Most common etiology	• Y chromosome microdeletions • Klinefelter syndrome • Cryptorchidism • Postinfectious (mumps) • Radiotherapy • Chemotherapy • Testicular trauma/torsion • Idiopathic	• Congenital [e.g., Kallmann syndrome, normosmic HH), Prader–Willi] • Acquired (e.g., pituitary tumor, steroid abuse)	• Postsurgical (e.g., vasectomy, epididymal cysts removal, hernia repair, scrotal surgery, prostatectomy) • CBAVD • Postinfectious • Ejaculatory duct obstruction • Idiopathic
Physical examination	• Either small-sized (long axis <6.6 cm) or normal testis • Normal epididymis • Palpable vas	• Small-sized testes (volume <15 mL and long axis <4.6 cm) • Small epididymis • Palpable vas	• Either normal or enlarged epididymis • Palpable or nonpalpable vasa (e.g., CBAVD) • Normal-sized testes (volume ≥15 mL and long axis >4.6 cm)
Semen analysis	• Normal (>1.5 mL) ejaculate volume • pH (>7.2) • Hypospermia (<1.5 mL) may be found with hypogonadism	Low ejaculate volume (<1.5 mL) and normal pH	Either normal or low pH and ejaculate volume (e.g., CBAVD and EDO)
Endocrine profile	• Either elevated (>7.6 mIU/mL) or normal FSH levels • Either elevated or normal LH levels • Either low (<300 ng/dL) or normal testosterone	• Low FSH and LH levels (<1.2 mIU/mL) • Low testosterone (<300 ng/dL)	• Normal FSH (300 ng/dL) • Normal LH • Normal testosterone
Genetic testing	• Nonmosaic (47,XXY) and mosaic (46,XY/47,XXY) Klinefelter syndrome • AZF Yq microdeletions seen in about 15% of cases	*KAL1, FGFR1, PROK2, PROKR2, CHD7,* and *FGF8* gene mutations can be found in congenital HH	Cystic fibrosis transmembrane conductance regulator gene mutations usually found in males with CBAVD
Testicular biopsy	• Hypospermatogenesis • Maturation arrest • Sertoli cell-only • Tubular atrophy • Mixed pattern	Not applicable	Normal spermatogenesis

(AZF: azoospermia factor; CBAVD: congenital bilateral absence of the vas deferens; EDO: ejaculatory duct obstruction; FSH: follicle-stimulating hormone; LH: luteinizing hormone)

Treatment of Obstructive Azoospermia

Treatment options for men with obstructive azoospermia include **(Flowchart 3)**:

- Surgical correction of the obstruction which obviates the need for assisted reproductive technology (ART)
- Retrieval of sperm from the male reproductive system for in vitro fertilization or ICSI.

Surgical treatment: Surgical options include microsurgical reconstruction of vas and/or epididymis, and transurethral resection of ejaculatory duct (TURED) in case of ejaculatory duct obstruction. The AUA recommends evaluation of female factor infertility prior to microsurgical reconstruction of vas and/or epididymis.

Ejaculatory duct obstruction: Ejaculatory duct may be obstructed in patients with previous genital infection, calcification, stones in ampulla, tuberculosis, Müllerian or Wolffian duct abnormality, and previous surgical trauma. Ejaculatory duct obstruction may be of two types: (1) Fibrous (associated with normal TRUS) and (2) cystic (associated with dilated seminal vesicles). Patients usually present with infertility, anejaculation or scanty ejaculate, hematospermia, pyospermia, and pain or dysuria. Diagnosis can be confirmed with TRUS, which shows dilated ejaculatory duct, seminal vesicles, calcification, and/or stones in ejaculatory duct. Treatment is by TURED at the point where the duct enters the distal prostatic urethra near the verumontanum. TURED results in the appearance of sperm in the ejaculate in about 50–75% of cases. A 25% pregnancy rate can be expected following TURED (AUA Guidelines).

Microsurgical reconstruction: Microsurgical reconstruction, introduced by Silber and Owen, is considered the gold standard for reconstructive surgery for treatment of men with obstructive azoospermia. Vasovasostomy or vasovasal

Flowchart 3: Management of obstructive azoospermia.

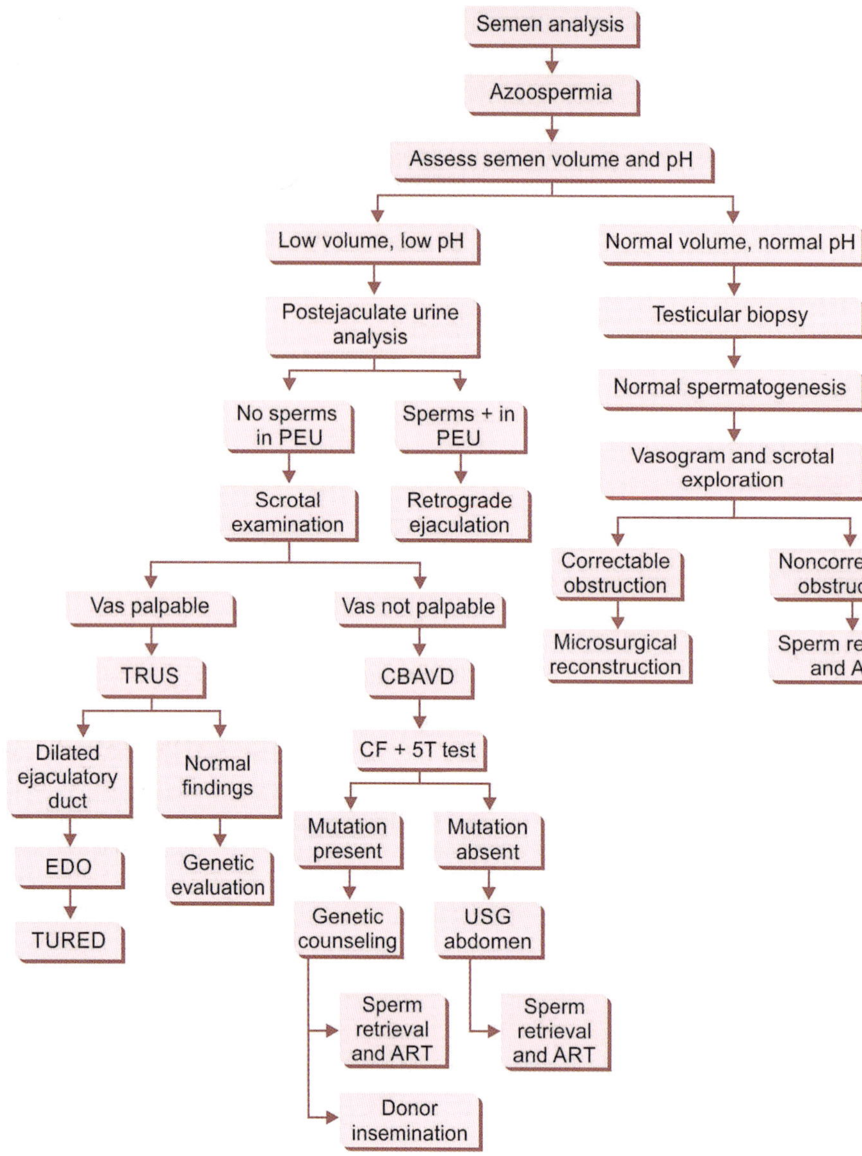

(ART: assisted reproductive techniques; CBAVD: congenital bilateral absence of the vas deferens; CF: cystic fibrosis; EDO: ejaculatory duct obstruction; PEU: postejaculate urinalysis; TRUS: transrectal ultrasound; TURED: transurethral resection of ejaculatory duct; USG: ultrasonography)

anastomosis (VVA) and vasoepididymostomy (VEA) are the microsurgeries commonly performed. Microsurgical reconstruction is preferred in younger couples, and the advantage is that it is less expensive and conception can be achieved by natural means. However, the disadvantage is the high failure rate and the need for special expertise.

Vasovasal anastomosis is usually performed following vasectomy (2–6%) or following injury to the vas during hernia surgery (6%). VVA is usually performed under general anesthesia or spinal anesthesia with an epidural using a high scrotal approach for vasectomy reversal or an inguinal approach in case of vasal injuries following hernia surgeries. Initial vasography is performed to assess the length and site of obstruction. Fluid from the proximal end of vas is analyzed prior to VVA **(Table 5)**. Testicular vasal fluid may be watery and copious or thick and creamy in consistency and have one of the following microscopic characteristics:

TABLE 5: Fluid analysis prior to vasovasal anastomosis (VVA).

Clear fluid, sperm +ve	VVA
Thick copious fluid, no sperm	Barbotage with 0.1 mL saline and reanalyze; sperm present: VVA; sperm absent: VEA (secondary epididymal obstruction)
Vas dry, no sperm	Vasoepididymostomy

(VEA: vasoepididymostomy)

- *Grade 1:* Mainly normal motile sperm
- *Grade 2:* Mainly normal nonmotile sperm
- *Grade 3:* Mainly sperm heads
- *Grade 4:* Only sperm heads
- *Grade 5:* No sperm.

Vasovasostomy should be performed for grades 1–4. For grade 5 vasal fluid, vasovasostomy should be performed if the fluid is watery and copious. Vasoepididymostomy should be performed in other cases.[9,10]

Vasovasal anastomosis is performed by multilayer microdot technique with 10-0 monofilament nylon suture in a mucosa-to-mucosa, watertight, tension-free interrupted fashion followed by a seromuscular and adventitial suture. Following VVA, the return of sperm to the ejaculate occurs in 70–95% of the patients and spontaneous pregnancy in 10–75% of the couples. The Canadian Urological Association (CUA) recommends that all men be offered the option to cryobank sperm retrieved during the course of the operation in case the surgery is not successful (level of evidence: 3; grade of recommendation: C) **(Fig. 2)**.[5]

Vasoepididymostomy: This is indicated in patients with secondary epididymal obstruction, wherein no sperm is aspirated from the vasal lumen with normal spermatogenesis on testicular biopsy. Conventional VEA is an approximation rather than an anastomosis, wherein the adjoining vas is anastomosed to the epididymal tunica with the hope that a fistula would form. This technique was associated with poor results. Newer techniques of VEA include:

- Vasoepididymal ductal end-to-side anastomosis (VEDSA) **(Fig. 3A)**
- Triangulation technique **(Fig. 3B)**
- Longitudinal intussusception vasoepididymostomy (LIVE) **(Fig. 3C)**.

Following VEA, sperm is present in ejaculate in 85% of the patients with spontaneous pregnancy seen in over 50% of the couples.[11]

Sperm retrieval techniques: Sperm retrieval may be used in patients with postvasectomy obstruction as a primary therapy for obstructive and nonobstructive azoospermia or as an adjunct to microsurgical reconstructive procedures in cases of obstructive azoospermia. It is indicated in patients with obstructive azoospermia with CBAVD, failed VEA, unreconstructable causes of OA, and older males. Types of sperm retrieval technique are given in **Table 6**.

Sperm Retrieval techniques ***(Flowchart 4)****:*

- *Microsurgical epididymal sperm aspiration (MESA):*[12,13] The epididymis is exposed through a scrotal incision. Under microscope magnification, the epididymal tunica is incised and an epididymal ductule is mobilized. The ductule is opened and spermatic fluid is aspirated. The aspirated fluid is evaluated for the presence of sperm. If an adequate sample is aspirated, the ductule is sutured. If no sperms are retrieved, another ductule is opened.
- *Open fine needle aspiration (OFNA):*[14] It is an open technique of sperm retrieval in which the epididymis is exposed and a ductule is directly punctured through the tunica without dissection. A 26G needle is used for aspiration of the epididymal fluid. The epididymal fluid continues to flow out after withdrawing the needle. This fluid, too, is aspirated from the epididymal surface.
- *PESA:*[15] The head of epididymis is stabilized between the thumb and index finger. A 26G needle is used to puncture the epididymis through the skin. Sperms are aspirated using a tuberculin syringe. The syringe is filled with 0.1 mL of sperm washing medium. A small amount of air is kept between the rubber and this

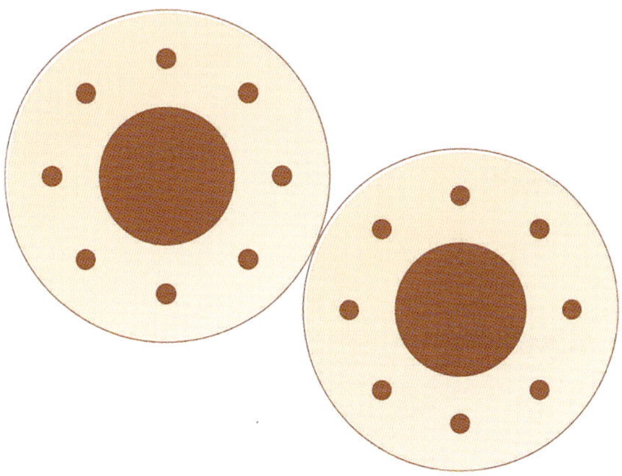

Fig. 2: Microdot technique.

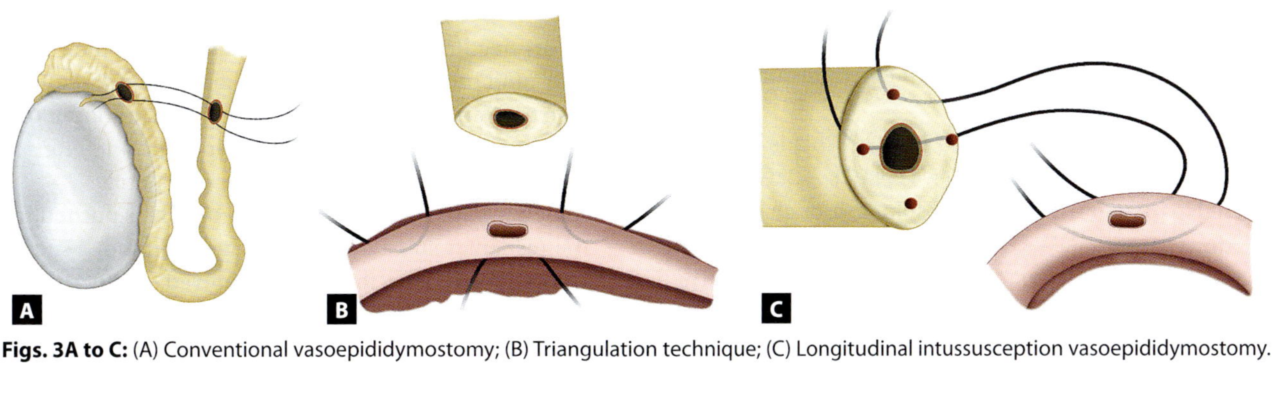

Figs. 3A to C: (A) Conventional vasoepididymostomy; (B) Triangulation technique; (C) Longitudinal intussusception vasoepididymostomy.

TABLE 6: Types of sperm retrieval technique.

	Advantages	*Disadvantages*
Microsurgical epididymal sperm aspiration (MESA)	• Large quantities of sperm obtained suitable for several in vitro fertilization/intracytoplasmic sperm injection cycles in one procedure • Individual epididymal tubes identified and aspirated under microscopic vision • Best pregnancy rates • Minimum complications	• Requires microsurgical skills • Incision with postoperative discomfort • Higher cost compared to percutaneous procedures • Requires anesthesia (GA/sedation)
Percutaneous epididymal sperm aspiration (PESA)	• No microsurgical skills required • Fast and repeatable • Minimum postoperative discomfort • OPD procedure • Done under LA • Can be repeated if needed	• Fewer sperm retrieved • Risk of epididymal damage • Risk of hematoma
Testicular sperm extraction (TESE) and micro-TESE	No microsurgical skills required except when micro-TESE performed	• Risk of testicular damage with multiple biopsies • Incision with postoperative discomfort • Higher cost compared to percutaneous procedures
Percutaneous testicular sperm aspiration (TESA)	• No microsurgical skills required • Fast and easy • Minimum postoperative discomfort • Minimally invasive	Fewer sperm retrieved
Open testicular biopsy	• No microsurgical skills required • Done under LA • Sperm yield comparable to MESA • Tissue diagnosis to determine cause of infertility is possible	• Possible testicular damage • Lower live birth rates as compared to MESA
Percutaneous testicular biopsy (PercBiopsy)	• No microsurgical skills required • Done under LA • Tissue diagnosis to determine cause of infertility is possible • Multiple pass can be performed • Minimum postprocedure discomfort	• Same as open biopsy • Sperm yield is lower

(GA: general anesthesia; LA: local anesthesia; OPD: outpatient department)

Flowchart 4: Sperm retrieval techniques.

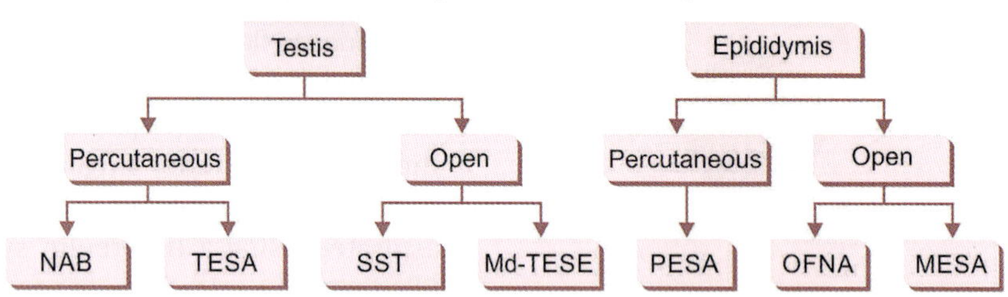

(MESA: micro epididymal sperm aspiration; Md-TESE: micro dissection testicular sperm aspiration; NAB: needle aspiration biopsy; OFNA: open fine needle aspiration; PESA: percutaneous epididymal sperm aspiration; SST: single seminiferous tubule biopsy; TESA: testicular sperm aspiration)

medium. The needle is manipulated within the epididymis in different directions while maintaining continuous suction.

- *Testicular sperm aspiration (TESA):*[16] This is similar to fine needle aspiration cytology (FNAC). A 22G needle is used to puncture testicular substance through the scrotal skin. A continuous suction is applied using a 20cc syringe, and the aspirate is examined for the presence of sperm.
- *Single seminiferous tubule (SST) biopsy:*[14,17] Scrotum is incised and testis is exposed. Testis is punctured with a 26G needle through an avascular area in the tunica. The puncture is dilated with microscopic forceps till a seminiferous tubule is exposed. The tubule is then examined under an operating microscope and biopsy is done and evaluated for the presence of sperm.
- *Needle aspiration biopsy:*[14] An 18G needle is pushed into the testicular substance and under continuous suction with a 10cc syringe, the needle is moved to and fro in the testicular parenchyma till aspirate is noted. The needle is then withdrawn from the testis. Along with the needle,

a loop of seminiferous tubule is pulled out and biopsy is done. The aspirate and the tissue are examined for sperms. The procedure is repeated until an adequate sample is obtained.
- *Microdissection testicular sperm extraction (Md-TESE):*[18] Testis is incised to expose the parenchyma. The seminiferous tubules are separated gently and examined under an operating microscope. Healthy tubules are biopsied and examined for sperms. Dissection and biopsy are done till an adequate sample is obtained.

Microsurgical testicular sperm extraction is the preferred sperm retrieval technique in patients with nonobstructive azoospermia and failed MESA (AUA recommendation). In obstructive azoospermia, MESA or PESA is the preferred technique. AUA recommends that the timing of sperm retrieval in relation to oocyte retrieval should be based upon local preference and expertise because there is no evidence that either fertilization or pregnancy rates are different using either fresh or thawed cryopreserved sperm from patients with either obstructive or nonobstructive azoospermia.[19,20]

Some of the recent advances in sperm retrieval techniques are as follows:
- *Multiphoton microscopy (MPM):* It is a technique which helps to identify the presence of sperm within the tubules without the need for extraction of testicular tissue. MPM uses a low-energy infrared femtosecond pulse laser which excites photons and produces autofluorescence which in turn can be translated to produce detailed images of underlying tissue.[21] The MPM technique has shown promising results that can enhance the ability of the surgeon to improve sperm retrieval by correctly identifying seminiferous tubules and also decrease operative time.[22]
- *Full-field optical coherence tomography (FFOCT):* It uses the principle of white light interference microscopy to produce high-resolution images of unstained tissue.[23] The high-resolution images obtained demarcate the seminiferous tubules, the layers of germ cells that line the tubule, and the distinct tubule lumen with intraluminal sperm. This technique is helpful in reducing the number of biopsies and the operating time. The one disadvantage of FFOCT is its inability to identify cellular and nuclear details.[22]
- *Raman spectroscopy:* It utilizes laser-based optics to determine the biochemical structures of living tissue. The advantage of this technique is that it is nondestructive, and the sperms extracted can be used for ICSI.
- *Sperm antibody detection:* This technique utilizes fluorescent microscopy to identify antibody-labeled sperm in seminiferous tubules during micro-TESE. Sperm-specific monoclonal antibodies are injected into the rete testis prior to surgery and thus help the surgeon in identifying sperms during extraction.

BOX 1: Etiology of primary testicular failure.

Genetic abnormalities
- Klinefelter syndrome
- Y chromosome microdeletion

Acquired
- Torsion testis/trauma
- Postinflammatory (mumps)
- Exogenous factors (Chemo-/radiotherapy)
- Testicular cancer
- Systemic diseases (CKD/CLD)
- Varicocele

Idiopathic

(CKD: chronic kidney disease; CLD: chronic liver disease)

Nonobstructive Azoospermia

Primary Testicular Failure

Etiology of primary testicular failure (PTF) is discussed in **Box 1**.

Genetic Abnormalities

Klinefelter syndrome: The most common identified genetic cause of male infertility is the presence of a supernumerary X chromosome yielding 47,XXY or Klinefelter syndrome.[24] This syndrome affects 1 in 500–1,000 live births, and over 95% of the affected adults have azoospermia.[24] Body morphology features such as increased height and sparse secondary sexual characters are seen in 30% of the affected patients.[24] A nonmosaic 47,XXY karyotype is seen in 80–90% of men with Klinefelter syndrome.[25]

Only about 8% of the patients with Klinefelter syndrome have sperm in ejaculate, while the remainders are azoospermic. Many of these patients are prescribed exogenous testosterone, which suppresses native spermatogenesis if present. Patients with Klinefelter syndrome are managed by surgical extraction of sperm at early or mid-puberty before initiation of testosterone therapy or donor insemination.[26]

Structural chromosomal anomalies: Y chromosome microdeletions are associated with azoospermia or oligospermia. Investigators researched three regions of the Y chromosome which may be responsible and designated them as:
1. Azoospermia factor a (AZFa)
2. Azoospermia factor b (AZFb)
3. Azoospermia factor c (AZFc).

Microdeletions of AZFa and AZFb are almost always associated with the absence of retrievable sperm from the testis. Deletion of the entire AZFa region is associated with the severe testicular phenotype, Sertoli cell-only syndrome. Complete removal of the AZFb region is associated with spermatogenic arrest at meiosis.[25] AZFc is the most frequent deletion of the Y chromosome and is associated with a wide range of phenotypes, including complete absence

Flowchart 5: Evaluation of nonobstructive azoospermia.

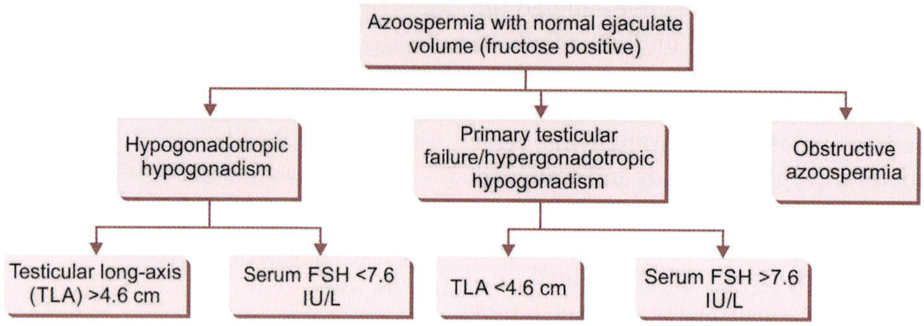

(FSH: follicle-stimulating hormone)

of germ cells in the testes, reduction in germ cells—hypospermatogenesis, and maturation arrest.[27] Patients with AZFc microdeletions have nearly 70% sperm retrieval rate.

Acquired Causes: The various acquired causes of testicular failure include torsion testis, trauma, mumps, testicular neoplasm, chemotherapy and radiotherapy, and varicocele. The first step in the management of these patients is to rule out reversible causes of testicular failures such as varicocele. Approximately 20% of men with nonobstructive azoospermia and large varicocele will show appearance of sperm after varicocele ligation. However, sperm counts may still remain low and most patients may still require ICSI.[5]

Management of Patients with Primary Testicular Failure: Patients with a clinical diagnosis of PTF typically have azoospermia, small testis, raised FSH and LH, and low testosterone. Reversible causes such as large varicocele have to be diagnosed and treated. Patients with irreversible PTF should undergo genetic testing to rule out Klinefelter syndrome and Y chromosome microdeletion. Patients with AZFa and AZFb are best treated with donor insemination or adoption. Patients who are eligible for sperm retrieval can undergo mapping microsurgical testicular biopsies to assess the presence or absence of focal spermatogenesis. Patients with focal spermatogenesis can undergo micro-TESE-ICSI. Sperm retrieval rates in patients with nonobstructive azoospermia are around 40%, and live birth rates after micro-TESE-ICSI are around 20% and 40% with donor sperm-ICSI **(Flowchart 5)**.[28]

BOX 2: Etiology of hypogonadotropic hypogonadism.

Congenital
- Kallmann syndrome
- Prader–Willi syndrome

Acquired
- Pituitary tumor
- Steroid abuse
- Testosterone replacement therapy

Flowchart 6: Management of primary testicular failure (PTF).

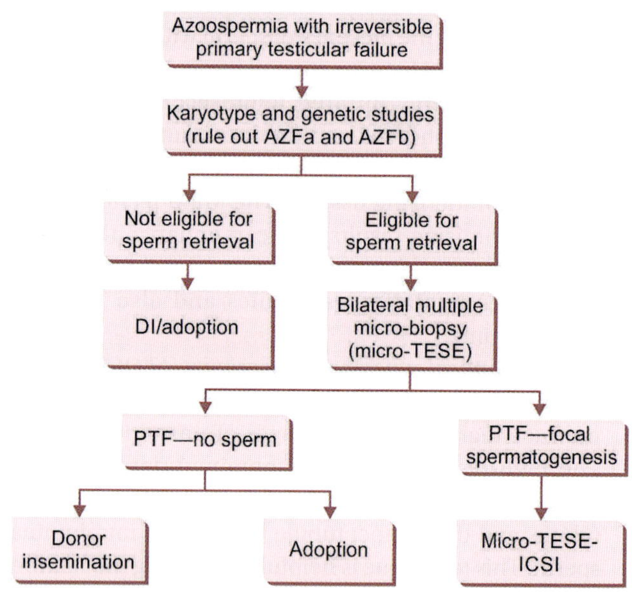

(AZFa: azoospermia factor a; DI: donor insemination; ICSI: intracytoplasmic sperm injection; Micro-TESE: microsurgical testicular sperm extraction)

Nonobstructive Azoospermia Due to Hypogonadotropic Hypogonadism

Patients with hypogonadotropic hypogonadism typically have azoospermia, small testis, and low FSH, LH, and testosterone. Both congenital and acquired causes are described in **Box 2**.

Congenital Causes

Kallmann syndrome: It is a syndrome associated with pituitary dysfunction and anosmia. Various genes have been found to be responsible, including *KAL1* which codes for anosmin-1 and is responsible for neurotropic growth factors during embryogenesis, genes coding for gonadotropin releasing hormone (GnRH) receptor, *PIT1*, Kisspeptin receptor, and homeobox genes. Treatment includes replacement of LH with human chorionic gonadotropin (hCG) and replacement of FSH with recombinant FSH (rFSH) or human menopausal gonadotropin. Treatment with hCG alone may initiate spermatogenesis. A typical dose of hCG is 1,500–5,000 IU two/three times per week **(Flowchart 6)**.

Prader–Willi syndrome: It is a syndrome characterized by failure to thrive in infancy associated with poor suck reflex followed by loss of satiety which may lead to early onset obesity. Other features include hypogonadism, small testis, growth hormone deficiency, and dysmorphic facies. The precise pathophysiology of this syndrome is still uncertain, but it is believed to be due to hypothalamic dysfunction with growth hormone deficiency and hypogonadism. Genetic malformation in Prader–Willi syndrome is loss of expression of genes located on chromosome 15q11-q13. In Prader–Willi syndrome, genes located on maternal chromosome 15q11-q13 are active, and those on the paternal ones are inactive, whereas in healthy individuals, the paternal genes are active.

Acquired Causes

Pituitary tumors and diseases: Space-occupying lesions in sella turcica and such as micro- and macroadenomas and craniopharyngiomas may compress pituitary resulting in FSH and LH suppression. Most pituitary tumors secrete prolactin and are associated with erectile dysfunction. Patients with raised prolactin of >50 μg/L should undergo a cranial magnetic resonance imaging (MRI). Functioning microadenomas may be treated with dopamine agonists such as bromocriptine and cabergoline whereas macroadenomas are treated with surgery.

CONCLUSION

- Azoospermia is a encountered in 10–15% of males during evaluation of infertility.
- Algorithmic approach to azoospermia is essential for proper management of infertility.
- Multiple options are available for treatment of obstructive azoospermia with high success rates.
- Micro TESE is the method of choice for surgical sperm retrieval in nonobstructive azoospermia.

KEY POINTS

- Management of azoospermia has evolved with advances in ART and microsurgical techniques.
- Management of azoospermia today is complex, challenging, but rewarding.

REFERENCES

1. Thonneau P, Marchand S, Tallec A, Ferial ML, Ducot B, Lansac J, et al. Incidence and main causes of infertility in a resident population (1,850,000) of three French regions (1988-1989). Hum Reprod. 1991;6(6):811-6.
2. Jarow JP, Espeland MA, Lipshultz LI. Evaluation of the azoospermic patient. J Urol. 1989;142(1):62-5.
3. Morshedi M. New 2010 WHO standards (5th edition) for the evaluation of human semen. [online] Available from: https://www.aab.org/images/aab/pdf/2014/CRBPPT14/NotesMM%20WHO.pdf. [Last accessed February, 2018].
4. World Health Organization. (2010). WHO laboratory manual for the examination and processing of human semen, 5th edition. [online] Available from: http://apps.who.int/iris/bitstream/10665/44261/1/9789241547789_eng.pdf. [Last accessed February, 2018].
5. Jarvi K, Lo K, Grober E, Mac V, Fischer A, Grantmyre J, et al. CUA guideline: the workup and management of azoospermic males. Can Urol Assoc J. 2015;9(7-8):229-35.
6. Schlegel PN, Sigman M, Collura B, De Jonge CJ, Eisenberg ML, Lamb DJ, et al. Diagnosis and treatment of infertility in men: AUA/ASRM guideline part I. Fertil Steril. 2021;115(1):54-61.
7. Purohit RS, Wu DS, Shinohara K, Turek PJ. A prospective comparison of 3 diagnostic methods to evaluate ejaculatory duct obstruction. J Urol. 2004;171(1):232-5.
8. Hall S, Oates RD. Unilateral absence of the scrotal vas deferens associated with contralateral mesonephric duct anomalies resulting in infertility: laboratory, physical and radiographic findings, and therapeutic alternatives. J Urol. 1993;150(4):1161-4.
9. Belker AM, Thomas Jr AJ, Fuchs EF, Konnak JW, Sharlip ID. Results of 1,469 microsurgical vasectomy reversals by the Vasovasostomy Study Group. J Urol. 1991;145:505-11.
10. Sigman M. The relationship between intravasal sperm quality and patency rates after vasovasostomy. J Urol. 2004;171:307-9.
11. Chawla A, O'Brien J, Lisi M, Zini A, Jarvi K. Should all urologists performing vasectomy reversals be able to perform vasoepididymostomies if required? J Urol. 2004;172(3):1048-50.
12. Silber SJ, Nagy ZP, Liu J, Godoy H, Devroey P, Van Steirteghem AC. Conventional in-vitro fertilization versus intracytoplasmic sperm injection for patients requiring microsurgical sperm aspiration. Hum Reprod. 1994;9:1705-9.
13. Girardi SK, Schlegel PN. Microsurgical epididymal sperm aspiration: review of techniques, preoperative considerations, and results. J Androl. 1996;17:5-9.
14. Shah RS. Surgical and non-surgical methods of sperm retrieval. In: Hansotia M, Desai S, Parihar M (Eds). Advanced Infertility Management. New Delhi: Jaypee Brothers; 2002. pp. 253-8.
15. Shrivastav P, Nadkarni P, Wensvoort S, Craft I. Percutaneous epididymal sperm aspiration for obstructive azoospermia. Hum Reprod. 1994;9:2058-61.
16. Craft I, Tsirigotis M. Simplified recovery, preparation and cryopreservation of testicular spermatozoa. Hum Reprod. 1995;10:1623-6.
17. Shah RS. Operative sperm retrieval for ART. In: Goenka ML, Goenka D, (Eds). Recent Advances in Infertility Management. Guwahati: Goenka; 2001. pp. 179-83.
18. Schlegel PN. Nonobstructive azoospermia: a revolutionary surgical approach and results. Semin Reprod Med. 2009;27:165-70.
19. Verheyen G, Vernaeve V, Van Landuyt L, Tournaye H, Devroey P, Van Steirteghem A. Should diagnostic testicular sperm retrieval followed by cryopreservation for later ICSI be the procedure of choice for all patients with non-obstructive azoospermia? Hum Reprod. 2004;19(12):2822-30.

20. Practice Committee of the American Society for Reproductive Medicine. New techniques for sperm acquisition in obstructive azoospermia. Fertil Steril. 2004;82:S186-93.
21. Najari BB, Ramasamy R, Sterling J, Aggarwal A, Sheth S, Li PS, et al. Pilot study of the correlation of multiphoton tomography of ex vivo human testis with histology. J Urol. 2012;188(2):538-43.
22. Ran R, Kohn TP, Ramasamy R. Innovations in surgical management of nonobstructive azoospermia. Indian J Urol. 2016;32(1):15-20.
23. Jain M, Shukla N, Manzoor M, Nadolny S, Mukherjee S. Modified full-field optical coherence tomography: a novel tool for rapid histology of tissues. J Pathol Inform. 2011;2(1):28.
24. Groth KA, Skakkebæk A, Høst C, Gravholt CH, Bojesen A. Klinefelter syndrome—a clinical update. J Clin Endocrinol Metab. 2013;98(1):20-30.
25. Maiburg M, Repping S, Giltay J. The genetic origin of Klinefelter syndrome and its effect on spermatogenesis. Fertil Steril. 2012;98(2):253-60.
26. Mehta A, Paduch DA. Klinefelter syndrome: an argument for early aggressive hormonal and fertility management. Fertil Steril. 2012;98(2):274-83.
27. Li Q, Song NH, Cao WZ, Shao Q, Xie JJ, Liu C, et al. Relationship between AZFc deletions and testicular histology in infertile South Chinese men with azoospermia and severe oligospermia. Springerplus. 2016;5(1):1805.
28. Esteves SC, Prudencio C, Seol B, Verza S, Knoedler C, Agarwal A. Comparison of sperm retrieval and reproductive outcome in azoospermic men with testicular failure and obstructive azoospermia treated for infertility. Asian J Androl. 2014;16(4):602-6.

CHAPTER 30

Varicocele and Infertility

Ameya Rangnath Sangle, Varun Huilgol, Tarun Dilip Javali

INTRODUCTION

Varicocele is a vascular abnormality due to the enlargement and elongation of the veins of the pampiniform plexus within the spermatic cord. It is considered as the most common cause of male infertility. The overall prevalence of varicocele in different studies ranges from 4.4 to 22.6% in general population.[1,2] Left-sided varicoceles are more frequent than right ones due to venous reflux because the perpendicular termination compromises flow from the left spermatic vein in the presence of elevated left renal venous pressure. With a bilateral incidence of 10% of patients and an isolated right varicocele in <1%, the left side is more prevalent than the right.[3] Varicoceles, in majority, are clinically insignificant. A small number of varicoceles can cause pain, infertility, and/or impairment in testicular growth.[4] The temperature in the testis is usually 2–4° lower than the core body temperature for the sperm to mature and function. The pampiniform plexus causes this by acting as a heat exchanger with a countercurrent flow, thereby reducing the temperature of the blood in the testicular artery before it enters the testicles.[5] Increased temperature due to varicocele causes impairment in the function of testis further leading to infertility.[6] There have been theories that hypoxia, oxidative stress (OS), and food deprivation are a combination of genetic and other molecular variables that together induce varicocele-mediated infertility (VMI) rather than being the sole cause.[7] However, even after receiving surgery, antioxidant therapy, or other treatments, some patients never restore their fertility. It was reported that this condition affects between 15 and 20% of adult males. Further, almost 40% of men who are being tested for infertility have varicocele.[3]

ETIOLOGY OF VARICOCELE

In majority, the left internal spermatic vein drains into the left renal vein lateral to the vertebral column.[8] The right internal spermatic vein usually drains into the inferior vena cava (IVC) just below the right renal vein. Variations in these findings are found quite frequently in studies examining cadaver specimens.[9] Most commonly, this classic anatomic configuration is seen on the right in 78% and on the left in 79% of patients. Anomalous drainage patterns described on the right include termination of the testicular vein in the renal vein in 8% and multiple veins terminating in the IVC and the renal vein in 16%. Anomalous drainage patterns described on the left include multiple veins terminating in the renal vein in 20%. Infrequently, one of the multiple branches may terminate in the infrarenal IVC.[8,10] The exact etiology of varicocele is not fully explained; however, multiple factors have been postulated for the origin of varicocele, one of the factors being hydrostatic pressure. Due to the anatomical structure of the veins, there is higher hydrostatic pressure in the left spermatic vein in comparison with the right side, which is said to predispose the left side to varicocele formation.[11] Another factor for varicocele formation is said to be incompetent or absent valves in the spermatic veins that predispose to varicose information. Based on these, two types of varicocele have been described: Stop type and shunt type.[12] However, this concept is controversial as the absence of valves has been noted in men without varicoceles on autopsy. Ahlberg et al.[13] identified absent valves in approximately 40% of left spermatic veins and 23% of right spermatic veins. The third mechanism that may result in varicocele formation is the nutcracker effect. It is also known as the left renal vein entrapment syndrome. Compression of the left renal vein by the abdominal aorta and the superior mesenteric artery or common iliac artery causes pressure elevation in the renal vein, which is transferred to the left internal spermatic vein and pampiniform plexus.[14] Nevertheless, the adverse effects of varicocele on spermatogenesis are multifactorial.

PATHOGENESIS

The presence of a varicocele has a detrimental effect on the processes of spermatogenesis, testicular volume, standard semen parameters, sperm function, fertilization, implantation, and the outcomes of embryos. The effects of varicocele on the male reproductive system are potentially mediated through elevated scrotal temperature, reflux of toxic metabolites into the internal spermatic vein, hypoxia, antisperm antibodies, hormonal dysfunction, and OS. However, despite the clear evidence of the adverse effects, the underlying pathophysiological mechanisms have not yet been completely elucidated.[15,16]

OXIDATIVE STRESS

In mitochondrial respiration, highly reactive oxygen-containing species are released as unavoidable by-products.[17] The primary sources of seminal reactive oxygen species (ROS) are believed to be immature sperm cells and leukocytes.[18] ROS are vital products for optimal sperm function by regulating capacitation processes—hyperactivation and acrosomal reaction—and, consequently, fertilization. Despite such important physiologic effects, excessive amounts of ROS can be harmful as they can exacerbate sperm deoxyribonucleic acid (DNA) damage, lipid peroxidation, and abortive apoptosis.[19] Patients with varicocele are associated to have higher OS in their semen leading to infertility. There is evidence that says varicocelectomy is associated with decreased sperm DNA fragmentation and increase in fertility.[20,21]

IMPAIRMENT OF SPERMATOGENESIS BY SCROTAL HYPERTHERMIA

The ideal temperature range for spermatogenesis, which is temperature-sensitive and operates best between 35 and 36°C, is maintained. Varicoceles cause the temperature of the scrotum to increase by 2.6°C, which leads to impaired spermatogenesis.[22] A rise in scrotal and intratesticular temperature in males with varicoceles can be produced by retrograde blood flow into the pampiniform plexus, which abnormally encourages spermatozoa and leukocytes to generate more ROS.[23] A decrease in the quantities of antioxidants as well as a downregulation in the expression of antioxidant enzymes can both be caused by heat stress. In cryptorchidism in which chronic elevation in testicular temperature is a primary factor for the impairment of testicular function, a similar increase in ROS has been seen. This is because cryptorchidism affects the testicles. In addition, some animal models have shown that scrotal hyperthermia can inhibit the production of androgen, increase the rate of death in germ cells, and decrease the expression of heat shock proteins.[24,25]

Molecular mechanisms of heat stress causing impaired spermatogenesis are decreased production of proteins and key enzymes such as topoisomerase 1, DNA polymerase, and heat shock proteins.[26-28]

Impairment of Blood Flow in Testis

Venous blood flow is decreased in varicocele and may result in localized testicular hypoxia. Research suggests that there is increase in the expression of hypoxia-inducible factor-1 (HIF-1) in the testicular tissues of rats with varicoceles. HIF-1 regulates numerous genes' transcription and translation in hypoxia to improve cellular survival rates. HIF-1 may, paradoxically, restrict stem cell proliferation in the presence of decompensated or persistent hypoxia.[29] Numerous authors have proposed that elevated HIF-1 expression causes elevated p53 expression, which in turn speeds up the apoptotic process in testicular tissue.[17] Recent proteomic studies have revealed that HIF-1 is responsible for the lower expression of heat shock proteins in individuals who have unilateral varicocele. This study also revealed an increase in reduced nicotinamide adenine dinucleotide (NADH) and a decrease in the expression of oxidative phosphorylation proteins, which shows that the spermatozoa from affected men had inefficient mitochondria and low redox capabilities.[30] To better understand the significance of these measures and assess how well they might predict the degree of hypoxia, more research is needed.

DEOXYRIBONUCLEIC ACID DAMAGE AND APOPTOSIS

Varicocele-induced OS may cause sperm pathology. Varicocelectomy improves spermatogenesis and DNA integrity as well as spontaneous and assisted reproductive technique (ART) pregnancy rates. A morphologically normal spermatozoon may also have inadequate chromatin compaction. The effect of sperm DNA damage on pregnancy, embryonic development, and offspring health is a cause for concern. Sperm DNA compaction/fragmentation can be additional diagnostic and prognostic markers for subfertile men with varicocele. Standardization and clinical implementation of sperm DNA fragmentation tests are recommended.[31,32]

Apoptosis, or programmed cell death, is involved in varicocele pathogenesis. Developing germ cells, testicular tissues, and ejaculated spermatozoa show higher apoptosis in men with varicocele. ROS, cadmium, and genetics can induce apoptosis. Cadmium is a metal ion that promotes apoptosis. Left varicocele patients with bilaterally elevated testicular cadmium levels had higher apoptosis, inverse association to postoperative semen parameter improvement. Spermatozoa apoptosis was higher in men with varicocele.

Colloidal microbeads coupled with annexin V can be used to select spermatozoa for intracytoplasmic sperm injection (ICSI). Neuronal apoptosis inhibitory protein (NAIP) and survivin prevent apoptosis. In rats with varicocele, these proteins were drastically reduced, along with spermatogenesis. Polydeoxyribonucleotide (PDRN) administration before varicocele production in rats blocked these effects. PDRN may increase spermatogenesis following experimental varicocele.[33]

TABLE 1: Grading of varicocele.

Grade	Description
Grade 1	Palpable during Valsalva maneuver and in standing position
Grade 2	Palpable without performing Valsalva maneuver and in standing position
Grade 3	Visible through the scrotal skin and palpable in standing position

CLINICAL GRADING

A clinical varicocele is one that is only palpable during the Valsalva maneuver; a grade 2 varicocele is easily palpable with or without Valsalva but is not visible, and a large varicocele that is easily palpable and detected by visual inspection of the scrotum is classified as grade 3. Clinical varicoceles are detected and graded based on physical examination. **Table 1** describes the different grading of varicocele based on the criteria described by Dubin and Amelar.[34]

MANAGEMENT

Evaluation

Varicoceles are mainly diagnosed on clinical examination. Various imaging modalities are available to improve detection rates and provide further anatomic detail of varicoceles. However, the benefit of obtaining imaging studies in a subset of varicoceles that are only found on imaging and not appreciated on physical examination has been debated. The current guidelines from the American Urological Association/American Society for Reproductive Medicine (AUA/ASRM) recommend against the use of routine imaging studies for the detection and screening of subclinical varicocele.[35]

Ultrasonography

Ultrasonography is the primary imaging modality for diagnosing varicocele. The characteristic appearance of a varicocele is described as "multiple, anechoic, serpiginous, tubular structures" near the superior and lateral aspects of the testis.[36] Numerous classification systems have been described for grading of varicoceles based on ultrasound and Doppler findings. The most widely accepted systems are the Sarteschi and Chiou classifications mentioned in **Tables 2 and 3**, respectively.

Another classification used in ultrasound is the Chiou et al. scoring system **(Table 3)**.[38]

TABLE 2: Sarteschi classification for color Doppler ultrasound diagnosis of varicocele.[37]

Grade	Description
1	Venous reflux at the emergence of the scrotal vein only during the Valsalva maneuver; hypertrophy of the venous wall without stasis
2	Supratesticular reflux only during the Valsalva maneuver; venous stasis without varicosities
3	Peritesticular reflux during the Valsalva maneuver; overt varicocele with early stage varices of the cremasteric vein
4	Spontaneous basal reflux that increases during the Valsalva maneuver, possible testicular hypotrophy, overt varicocele, varicosities in the pampiniform plexus
5	Spontaneous basal reflux that does not increase during the Valsalva maneuver, testicular hypotrophy, overt varicocele, varicosities in the pampiniform

TABLE 3: Chiou et al. scoring system for color Doppler ultrasound diagnosis of varicocele.

	Score
Maximum vein diameter (mm)	
<2.5	0
2.5–2.9	1
3.0–3.9	2
≥4.0	3
Plexus/sum of diameter of veins	
No plexus identified	0
Plexus (+) with sum diameter <3 mm	1
Plexus (+) with sum diameter 3–5.9 mm	2
Plexus (+) with sum diameter ≥6 mm	3
Change of flow velocity on Valsalva maneuver	
<2 cm/s or duration <1 s	0
2–4.9	1
5–9.9	2
≥10	3
Total score	0–9

Note: Total score of >4 is defined as varicocele.

Computed Tomography

Computed tomography (CT) has gained popularity since its introduction in the 1970s and has become a mainstay in the evaluation of abdominal pathology. Small vessels, including the gonadal veins, are better evaluated by using submillimeter thickness slice and multiplanar image reconstruction.[39] However, the increased radiation exposure and ease of availability of ultrasound have reduced the desirability of this investigation. The role of CT in the evaluation of varicoceles has mainly been limited to investigating retroperitoneal pathology. CT is the study of choice when a retroperitoneal abnormality is suspected. Causes of varicocele formation that could be identified on CT imaging include renal tumors, retroperitoneal tumors causing compression, vena caval thrombi, and retroaortic renal veins.[40-43]

Magnetic Resonance Imaging

Early changes within the tissue parenchyma can be detected early by using diffusion-weighted imaging (DWI).[44] The effects of varicocele on fertility can be potentially quantified by using magnetic resonance imaging (MRI). Çekiç et al. showed that decreased apparent diffusion coefficient (ADC) values calculated from DWI in patients with varicoceles correlated with semen parameters.[45]

Venography

Percutaneous venography has now become obsolete and diagnostic modality of historical significance and research interest. In today's practice, venography is a useful adjunct to guide intraoperative decision-making. It has also been described for the planning of definitive treatment in cases where varicoceles recur.[46]

Thermography and Scintigraphy

Thermography evolved as a screening tool to identify areas of hyperthermia for subclinical varicocele. It measures the temperature and surface of scrotal skin and utilizes a film with heat-sensitive liquid crystals. The World Health Organization (WHO) Task Force on Diagnosis and Treatment of Infertility compared contact thermography with ultrasound to the gold standard of retrograde venography. In this multicenter series, ultrasound combined with contact thermography had the highest diagnostic accuracy with a 1% false-negative result and 44% false-positive results.[47]

Scintigraphy has now been rendered to be largely of historical and research interest due to the time required and impracticality compared to other modalities. The patient's red blood cells (RBCs) are labeled by intravenous administration of pyrophosphate 20 mCi prior to administration of ^{99m}Tc pertechnetate. The patient is then examined standing with the penis strapped in the midline to the abdomen. The scrotum is located in the lower third of the area of interest, while a gamma camera evaluates the accumulation of radioactive tracer-labeled RBCs.[48]

Varicocele Repair

Varicocele repair has been shown to improve both semen parameters and testosterone production in hypogonadal males with subfertility.[49,50] Varicocele repair in azoospermic and oligozoospermic patients improves pregnancy rates and live birth rates following the use of ART, even if azoospermia or oligozoospermia persists **(Table 4)**.[21]

Open Varicocele Repair

Open macroscopic, varicocele repair was the standard of care till the 1970s when microsurgery took over.[51] The traditional inguinal open varicocele repair (Ivanissevich technique) is done by making a skin crease incision in the inguinal region above and lateral to the ipsilateral pubic tubercle and extending laterally. External oblique aponeurosis is sharply incised along the length of the fibers to open the inguinal ring and expose the spermatic cord. External spermatic fascia is then incised to access the vascular structures within. Venous structures, including the internal spermatic vein, cremasteric veins, external spermatic veins, gubernacular veins, and periarterial veins, are identified and ligated.[52] Varicocele is also performed using the Palomo technique through either open or laparoscopic approach. The open retroperitoneal approach or open Palomo technique was first described by Palomo in 1949.[53] In Palomo's initial series, a 4 cm incision was made

TABLE 4: Comparison between different techniques of varicocele repair.

Procedure	*Advantages*	*Disadvantages*	*Recurrence*	*Complications*
Embolization	Minimal pain	Difficult canalization of the right spermatic vein	3.2–19.3%	• Extravasation NR • Thrombophlebitis NR
Laparoscopic	Simplified vascular anatomy, short operating time, can address bilateral varices simultaneously	• Difficulty visualizing lymphatics • Artery usually not spared	4.3%	Hydrocele 2.8–20%
Microscopic subinguinal	Adequate anatomic visualization, possibly less pain	Complex vascular anatomy	1.05%	Hydrocele 0–0.4%
Microscopic inguinal	Simplified vascular anatomy, adequate visualization	Pain at incision site	2.1%	Hydrocele 0.7%
Loupe-assisted high ligation	Simplified vascular anatomy	Incisional pain, poor visualization of structures	14.9%	Hydrocele 8.2–13%

(NR: not reported)

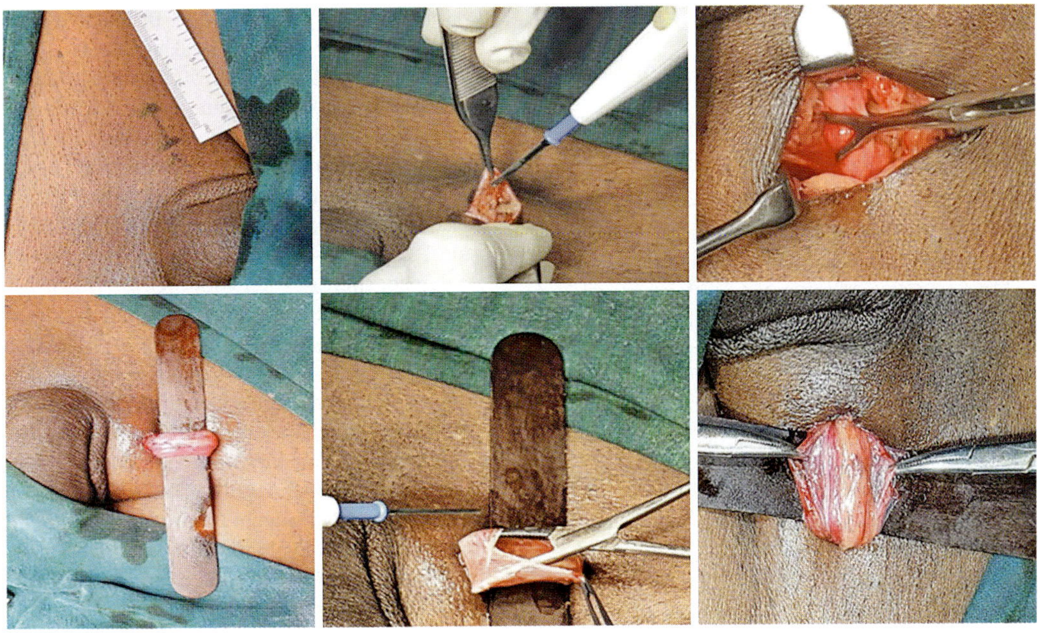

Fig. 1: Subinguinal microscopic varicocelectomy.

3 cm above the internal inguinal ring, and the large spermatic veins and testicular artery were ligated together at this location. Currently, an open Palomo technique uses Gibson incision and ligates the internal spermatic vein between the anterior superior iliac spine and renal vein.

Laparoscopic Varicocele Repair

Palomo technique can be performed laparoscopically and is the preferred technique in adolescent patients. Three transperitoneal ports are placed with a camera port at the umbilicus, one working port at midline between umbilicus and pubic symphysis and a third port lateral to ipsilateral inferior epigastric vessels. The peritoneum is opened 3 cm proximal to the deep inguinal ring. Spermatic vessels are dissected from surrounding tissues. Veins are then ligated with clips and divided. The testicular artery may or may not be spared.[54]

Microscopic Varicocele Repair

Microscopic varicocele repair is currently considered as the gold standard for varicocele repair.[55] It can be done by inguinal and subinguinal approaches. The subinguinal approach provides the highest success with least complications. For the subinguinal approach, a 2 cm incision is made along Langer lines located above the superficial inguinal ring. The incision is then deepened to open the wound in layers. Blunt dissection is carried out till spermatic cord identification. The cord is then delivered atraumatically using a Babcock clamp. The cord is placed over a 1" Penrose drain or a sterile scale to provide for stability and to allow for the use of countertraction for dissection. Under the magnification of an operating microscope, the external spermatic fascia is split, and the vascular structures within the cord are accessed. Once the vas deferens is identified, it is isolated. Veins are identified and ligated with sutures (usually 4-0 silk) or dissected using a bipolar cautery. Micro-Doppler is used for the effective identification of testicular artery and avoidance of inadvertent arterial injury. After all veins have been ligated, the cord can be repositioned back. The external spermatic fascia may or may not be closed. Care should be taken to preserve at least two to three lymphatic vessels to prevent hydrocele formation. Finally, the incision is closed in layers using absorbable sutures **(Fig. 1)**.

Embolotherapy

The main indications for interventional treatment are pain, infertility, and recurrence after surgical ligation. This recurrence is usually attributed to collateral circulation that was missed during surgery.[56]

The most frequently used agents for embolization are sodium tetradecyl sulfate (STS), endovascular coils, vascular plugs, glue, and absolute ethanol. Complications to varicocele embolization include groin pain, hematoma formation, contrast agent reactions, fever, nausea, and thrombophlebitis. The risk of hydrocele formation is said to be the least in this technique.[57]

CONCLUSION

- Varicocele is one of the important causes of male infertility
- Prompt diagnosis and correction of the condition leads to improved fertility results.
- Microscopic varicocelectomy is the gold standard in varicocele repair.

KEY POINTS

- Varicocele
- Male infertility
- Microscopic varicocelectomy.

REFERENCES

1. Jarow JP, Coburn M, Sigman M. Incidence of varicoceles in men with primary and secondary infertility. Urology. 1996;47(1):73-6.
2. Will MA, Swain J, Fode M, Sonksen J, Christman GM, Ohl D. The great debate: varicocele treatment and impact on fertility. Fertil Steril. 2011;95(3):841-52.
3. Leslie SW, Sajjad H, Siref LE. Varicocele. StatPearls [Internet]. Treasure Island (FL): StatPearls Publishing; 2022. Available from: http://www.ncbi.nlm.nih.gov/books/NBK448113/. [Last accessed September 2022].
4. Paick S, Choi WS. Varicocele and testicular pain: a review. World J Mens Health. 2019;37(1):4-11.
5. Ismail E, Orlando G, Pompa P, Gabrielli D, Di Donato L, Cardone D,et al. Time-domain analysis of scrotal thermoregulatory impairment in varicocele. Front Physiol. 2014; 5:342.
6. Ioannidou PG, Papanikolaou DA, Bosdou JK, Goulis DG, Lambropoulos AF, Grimbizis GF, et al. Improvement in sperm quality by oral antioxidant supplementation in infertile men with varicocele who have not undergone surgical repair: systematic review and meta-analysis. Andrologia. 2022;54:e14533.
7. Eisenberg M, Lipshultz L. Varicocele-induced infertility: newer insights into its pathophysiology. Indian J Urol. 2011; 27(1):58.
8. Lechter A, Lopez G, Martinez C, Camacho J. Anatomy of the gonadal veins: a reappraisal. Surgery. 1991;109(6):735-9.
9. Favorito LA, Costa WS, Sampaio FJ. Applied anatomic study of testicular veins in adult cadavers and in human fetuses. Int Braz J Urol. 2007;33(2):176-80.
10. Valji K. Endocrine, exocrine and reproductive system. In: Valji K (Ed). The Practice of Interventional Radiology, with Online Cases and Video, 1st edition. Philadelphia: Elsevier Saunders; 2012. p. 424.
11. Kass EJ. Adolescent varicocele. Pediatr Clin N Am. 2001; 48:1559.
12. Mohseni MJ, Nazari H, Amini E, Javan-Farazmand N, Baghayee A, Farzi H, et al. Shunt-type and stop-type varicocele in adolescents: prognostic value of these two different hemodynamic patterns. Fertil Steril. 2011;96(5):1091-6.
13. Ahlberg NE, Bartley O, Chidekel N. Right and left gonadal veins: an anatomical and statistical study. Acta Radiol Diagn (Stockh). 1966;4:593-601.
14. Gat Y, Gornish M, Chakraborty J, Perlow A, Levinger U, Pasqualotto F. Azoospermia and maturation arrest: malfunction of valves in erect poster of humans leads to hypoxia in sperm production site. Andrologia. 2010;42(6):389-94.
15. Liang M, Wen J, Dong Q, Zhao LG, Shi BK. Testicular hypofunction caused by activating p53 expression induced by reactive oxygen species in varicocele rats. Andrologia. 2015;47(10):1175-82.
16. Kimura M, Nagao K. Role of varicocele repair for male infertility in the era of assisted reproductive technologies. Reprod Med Biol. 2014;13(4):185-92.
17. Sharma RK, Agarwal A. Role of reactive oxygen species in male infertility. Urology. 1996;48:835-50.
18. Kessopoulou E, Tomlinson MJ, Barratt CL, Bolton AE, Cooke ID. Origin of reactive oxygen species in human semen: spermatozoa or leucocytes? J Reprod Fertil. 1992;94:463-70.
19. Burton GJ, Jauniaux E. Oxidative stress. Best Pract Res Clin Obstet Gynaecol. 2011;25:287-99.
20. Esteves SC, Sánchez-Martín F, Sánchez-Martín P, Schneider DT, Gosálvez J. Comparison of reproductive outcome in oligozoospermic men with high sperm DNA fragmentation undergoing intracytoplasmic sperm injection with ejaculated and testicular sperm. Fertil Steril. 2015;104:1398-405.
21. Kirby EW, Wiener LE, Rajanahally S, Crowell K, Coward RM. Undergoing varicocele repair before assisted reproduction improves pregnancy rate and live birth rate in azoospermic and oligospermic men with a varicocele: a systematic review and meta-analysis. Fertil Steril. 2016;106:1338-43.
22. Erfani Majd N, Sadeghi N, Tavalaee M, Tabandeh MR, Nasr-Esfahani MH. Evaluation of oxidative stress in testis and sperm of rat following induced varicocele. Urol J. 2019;16:300.
23. Ko EY, Sabanegh Jr ES, Agarwal A. Male infertility testing: reactive oxygen species and antioxidant capacity. Fertil Steril. 2014;102(6):1518-27.
24. Garolla A, Torino M, Miola P, Caretta N, Pizzol D, Menegazzo M, et al. Twenty-four-hour monitoring of scrotal temperature in obese men and men with a varicocele as a mirror of spermatogenic function. Hum Reprod. 2015;30(5):1006-13.
25. Hosseinifar H, Gourabi H, Salekdeh GH, Alikhani M, Mirshahvaladi S, Sabbaghian M, et al. Study of sperm protein profile in men with and without varicocele using two-dimensional gel electrophoresis. Urology. 2013;81:293-300.
26. Fujisawa M, Yoshida S, Kojima K, Kamidono S. Biochemical changes in testicular varicocele. Arch Androl. 1989;22:149-59.
27. Shiraishi K, Takihara H, Matsuyama H. Elevated scrotal temperature, but not varicocele grade, reflects testicular oxidative stress-mediated apoptosis. World J Urol. 2010; 28(3):359-64.
28. Tawadrous GA, Aziz AA, Mostafa T. Seminal soluble fas relationship with oxidative stress in infertile men with varicocele. Urology. 2013;82(4):820-3.
29. Wang YJ, Zhang RQ, Lin YJ, Zhang RG, Zhang WL. Relationship between varicocele and sperm DNA damage and the effect of varicocele repair: a meta-analysis. Reprod Biomed Online. 2012;25(3):307-14.
30. Swain N, Samanta L, Agarwal A, Kumar S, Dixit A, Gopalan B, et al. Aberrant upregulation of compensatory redox molecular machines may contribute to sperm dysfunction in infertile men with unilateral varicocele: a proteomic insight. Antioxid Redox Signal. 2020;32(8):504-21.
31. Almeida C, Correia S, Rocha E, Alves A, Ferraz L, Silva J, et al. Caspase signalling pathways in human spermatogenesis. J Assist Reprod Genet. 2013;30(4):487-95.
32. Coughlan C, Clarke H, Cutting R, Saxton J, Waite S, Ledger W, et al. Sperm DNA fragmentation, recurrent implantation failure and recurrent miscarriage. Asian J Androl. 2015;17(4):681.
33. Minutoli L, Arena S, Antonuccio P, Romeo C, Bitto A, Magno C, et al. Role of inhibitors of apoptosis proteins in testicular function and male fertility: effects of polydeoxyribonucleotide administration in experimental varicocele. BioMed Res Int. 2015;2015:1-9.

34. Dubin L, Amelar RD. Varicocele size and results of varicocelectomy in selected subfertile men with varicocele. Fertil Steril. 1970;21(8):606-9.
35. Schlegel PN, Sigman M, Collura B, De Jonge CJ, Eisenberg ML, Lamb DJ, et al. Diagnosis and treatment of infertility in men: AUA/ASRM guideline part I. J Urol. 2021;205(1):36-43.
36. Sommers D, Winter T. Ultrasonography evaluation of scrotal masses. Radiol Clin N Am. 2014;52(6):1265-81.
37. Sarteschi M. Lo studio del varicocele con eco-color-Doppler. G Ital Ultrasonologia. 1993;4:43-9.
38. Chiou RK, Anderson JC, Wobig RK, Rosinsky DE, Matamoros Jr A, Chen WS, et al. Color Doppler ultrasound criteria to diagnose varicoceles: correlation of a new scoring system with physical examination. Urology. 1997;50(6):953-6.
39. Karcaaltincaba M. Demonstration of normal and dilated testicular veins by multidetector computed tomography. Jpn J Radiol. 2011;29(3):161-5.
40. Hanna GB, Byrne D, Townell N. Right-sided varicocele as a presentation of right renal tumours. Br J Urol. 1995;75(6): 798-9.
41. Thompson JN, Abraham TK, Jantet GH. Metastasis to pampiniform plexus from left renal adenocarcinoma presenting with acute varicocele. Urology. 1984;24(6):621-2.
42. Roy 2nd CR, Wilson T, Raife M, Horne D. Varicocele as the presenting sign of an abdominal mass. J Urol. 1989; 141(3):597-9.
43. Arslan H, Etlik O, Ceylan K, Temizoz O, Harman M, Kavan M. Incidence of retro-aortic left renal vein and its relationship with varicocele. Eur Radiol. 2005;15(8):1717-20.
44. Koh DM, Collins DJ. Diffusion-weighted MRI in the body: applications and challenges in oncology. AJR Am J Roentgenol. 2007;188(6):1622-35.
45. Çekiç B, Kiliç KK, Toslak IE, Şükun A, Sağlik S, Savaş M, et al. Correlation between semen analysis parameters and diffusion-weighted magnetic resonance imaging of the testicles in patients with varicocele: a pilot study. J Comput Assist Tomogr. 2018;42(3):423-8.
46. Morag B, Rubinstein ZJ, Madgar I, Lunnenfeld B. The role of spermatic venography after surgical high ligation of the left spermatic veins: diagnosis and percutaneous occlusion. Urol Radiol. 1985;7(1):32-4.
47. World Health Organization. Comparison among different methods for the diagnosis of varicocele. Fertil Steril. 1985; 43(4):575-82.
48. Vanlangenhove P, Dhondt E, Everaert K, Defreyne L. Pathophysiology, diagnosis and treatment of varicoceles: a review. Minerva Urol Nefrol. 2014;66(4):257-82.
49. Abdel-Meguid TA, Al-Sayyad A, Tayib A, Farsi HM. Does varicocele repair improve male infertility? An evidence-based perspective from a randomized, controlled trial. Eur Urol. 2011;59:455-61.
50. Chen X, Yang D, Lin G, Bao J, Wang J, Tan W. Efficacy of varicocelectomy in the treatment of hypogonadism in subfertile males with clinical varicocele: a meta-analysis. Andrologia. 2017;49.
51. Marmar JL. The evolution and refinements of varicocele surgery. Asian J Androl. 2016;18:171-8.
52. Chan P. Management options of varicoceles. Indian J Urol. 2011;27:65-73.
53. Palomo A. Radical cure of varicocele by a new technique: preliminary report. J Urol. 1949;61:604-7.
54. Johnson D, Sandlow J. Treatment of varicoceles: techniques and outcomes. Fertil Steril. 2017;108:378-84.
55. Marmar J, Kim Y. Subinguinal microsurgical varicocelectomy: a technical critique and statistical analysis of semen and pregnancy data. J Urol. 1994;152(4):1127-32.
56. Puche-Sanz I, Flores-Martín JF, Vázquez-Alonso F, Pardo-Moreno PL, Cózar-Olmo JM. Primary treatment of painful varicocoele through percutaneous retrograde embolization with fibred coils. Andrology. 2014;2:716.
57. Storm DW, Hogan MJ, Jayanthi VR. Initial experience with percutaneous selective embolization: a truly minimally invasive treatment of the adolescent varicocele with no risk of hydrocele development. J Pediatr Urol. 2010;6(6):567-71.

CHAPTER 31

Spinal Cord Injuries and Male Infertility

Yalavarthi Pavan Ganesh, Tarun Dilip Javali, Mahendra V Javali

INTRODUCTION

Spinal cord injury (SCI) is a devastating neurological condition.[1] SCI is one of the most disabling events that involves the central nervous system. It causes temporary or permanent loss of muscle function, sensation, or autonomic function in the parts of the body served by the spinal cord below the level of the injury. SCI affects every aspect of the life of an injured person ranging from their normal day-to-day activities to their reproductive health including fertility. It is more commonly seen in young men.[1,2] The role of SCI in affecting female fertility is limited as compared to male infertility. In women, the challenges are usually restricted to self-care during pregnancy, labor, delivery, and for activities of daily functioning. Infertility following SCI in men occurs due to a combination of erectile dysfunction (ED), ejaculatory dysfunction, and semen abnormalities.[1,3] The treatment of ED in SCI can be done through similar therapies as used in the general population. Treatments that are effective in non-SCI male factor infertility are effective for management in couples with SCI male factor infertility. But the major difference in symptoms between SCI-related male factor infertility and non-SCI-related male factor infertility is higher occurrence of atypical profile of the semen and anejaculation in men with SCI. The role of health professionals is of paramount importance in identifying people with SCI-related male factor infertility and educating them and their family about the problem, ways to approach them, and types of support available for them to have children. A lot of advances have been made over the years in the field of medical sciences with regard to SCI-related infertility. This chapter will provide an overview of SCI-related male factor infertility and its management.

SPINAL CORD INJURY

Definition

The term "Spinal Cord Injury" can be defined as any damage to the spinal cord that results from trauma or due to a disease or due to degenerative conditions or disorders like cancer. Around 90% of the cases of SCI occur due to trauma.[2,3]

Epidemiology

Majority of SCIs occur in young men, who are at the peak of their reproductive health.[1] According to the reports of World Health Organization (WHO), globally around 2,50,000–5,00,000 people suffer from SCI.[2] The annual incidence of SCI is estimated globally to be around 40–80 cases per million population, according to WHO. There were 0.93 million new cases of SCI with 95% confidence interval (CI) of 0.78–1.16 million in 2016. The prevalence was 27.04 million with 95% CI of 24.98–30.15 million. SCI was responsible for 9.5 million years lost due to disability in 2016.[3] There are no reliable countrywide estimates of SCI in India **(Fig. 1)**.

Majority of them occur due to causes that are preventable such as road traffic crashes, violence, or falls. Falls and road injuries were the leading causes of new cases of SCI and traumatic brain injury (TBI) in most regions.[3]

Males are more commonly affected than females in the ratio of 1:1 to 8:1. Males are four times more likely to sustain an SCI in comparison with females.[4] SCI subjects are likely to die, two to five times more prematurely, on comparing them to those without SCI. The survival rates in subjects with SCI are low in countries belonging to low- and middle-income groups. SCI is associated with substantial individual and

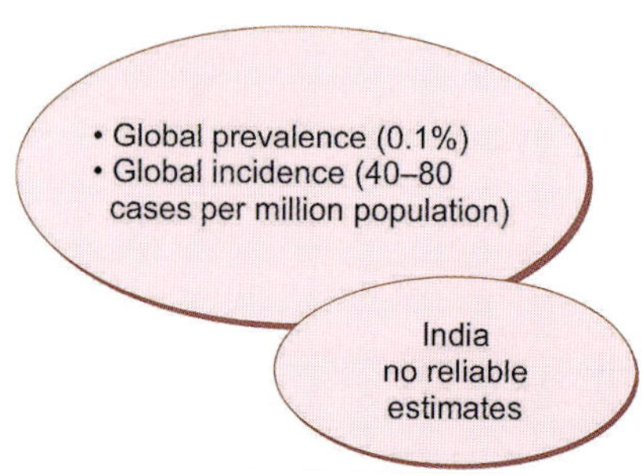

Fig. 1: Estimates of global prevalence and incidence of spinal cord injury (SCI) in relation with India.

societal costs, besides lower rates of school enrolment and economic participation. Approximately 78% of new cases of SCI occur in men in the United States of America.[5] According to SCI data in United States, the average age at injury has increased in the recent decades from 29 (1970s) to 43 years.[5]

A report of the WHO shows that 15% of the world's population is affected by disability, 0.1% by SCI.[6] The incidence of SCI varies substantially between countries. Only a very few countries have a countrywide SCI registry system. The incidence estimates are often extrapolated from data available from a region. Also, there is no central worldwide registry. Population-based surveys are also rare for estimating the SCI in the general population. It was reported in 2012 that nearly 20,000 cases of SCI are added every year in India and there are 1.5 million people with SCI in India.[7] There is a lack of population-based studies in India. Epidemiological data are available only from various hospital-based studies.[8-10]

Spinal cord injury can be primary, secondary, or immune response SCI. Primary injury is due to input from primary mechanical forces while secondary injury is due to a series of biological phenomena that occurs following the primary injury. The neuroinflammation can be beneficial or detrimental following an SCI.

Etiology

Based on etiology, SCI can be classified as:

- Traumatic SCI
- Nontraumatic SCI.

Majority (90%) of SCI occurs due to trauma.[2,3] The most common global causes for traumatic SCI are road traffic accidents followed by falls and violence.[11] Traumatic causes of SCI include:

- Falls from height
- Road traffic accidents
- Sports-related accidents
- Violence
- Other causes of injury.

Nontraumatic causes include diseases or degenerative conditions or disorder such as cancer. The etiology of nontraumatic SCI includes:

- Vertebral spondylosis
- Compression due to tumors
- Vascular ischemia
- Injuries due to congenital disease.

Nontraumatic SCI is commonly seen in older age groups on comparison with the predominance of traumatic SCI in younger age groups. With increase in lifespan in the recent decades, incidence of nontraumatic SCI can increase and can overtake that of traumatic SCI.[12] In nontraumatic SCI, the etiology varies according to the region like infectious diseases such as human immunodeficiency virus (HIV) and nutritional disorders.[13,14]

Clinical Presentation

A typical presentation of SCI includes a young male, with a history of trauma. Symptoms of SCI may range from partial or total loss of sensation to loss of movements of arms, legs, and the body. Bowel and bladder control, breathing, heart rate, and blood pressure are affected in most severe SCIs. The symptoms depend on the location of injury on the spinal cord and severity of injury. They may include:

- Partial or complete loss of sensory function and/or motor function
- Inability to move arms, legs, and/or body
- Loss of control of bladder and bowel
- Unnatural positioning of neck
- Chronic pain
- Unconsciousness
- Signs of sock.

Spinal cord injury can affect almost every aspect of the reproductive system in males like ED, sexual dysfunction, poor spermatogenesis, and ejaculation problems.[15,16] Complete loss of sensory function or motor function bilaterally below a certain level indicates a complete SCI.[17] Respiratory function may be impaired due to loss of central ventilatory drive, loss of ventilatory muscle function, chest wall injury, lung injury like hemothorax and pneumothorax. Vital capacity is severely affected in high lesions at C1 to C2 while respiratory dysfunction is minimal for injuries at T11.[18] In case of a complete injury above T11, the ability to achieve psychogenic erection is lost. Sacral nerve root injuries impact the reflex or tactile erections.[19] In SCIs of T11 to L2, the ability to achieve erection by one or both pathways is variable[20] **(Fig. 2)**.

Natural Progression

Spinal cord injury is a devastating condition that can lead to death. In SCI due to traumatic injuries, the course is more or less well defined, depending on the level of injury.[21] Depending on the severity of the lesion and level of the lesion, death can occur within a few days to months. Pneumonia can occur in lesions of the high cervical cord due to respiratory function impairment. Lack of therapeutic measures can lead to death in the long run. Depending on the lesion level, pressure sores, urinary tract infections can also occur. With establishment of dedicated rehabilitative therapies, the life expectancy and the quality of life have increased in SCI. The disease course now mainly depends on the functional recovery.[22]

The life expectancy in subjects with SCI has increased over the last few decades but it still remains lower in comparison with age-matched able-bodied individuals.

The American Spinal Injury Association Impairment Scale (AIS) standardizes a careful, detailed documentation of the injury.[23] It has tremendous prognostic value as it guides further assessment radiographically and management.

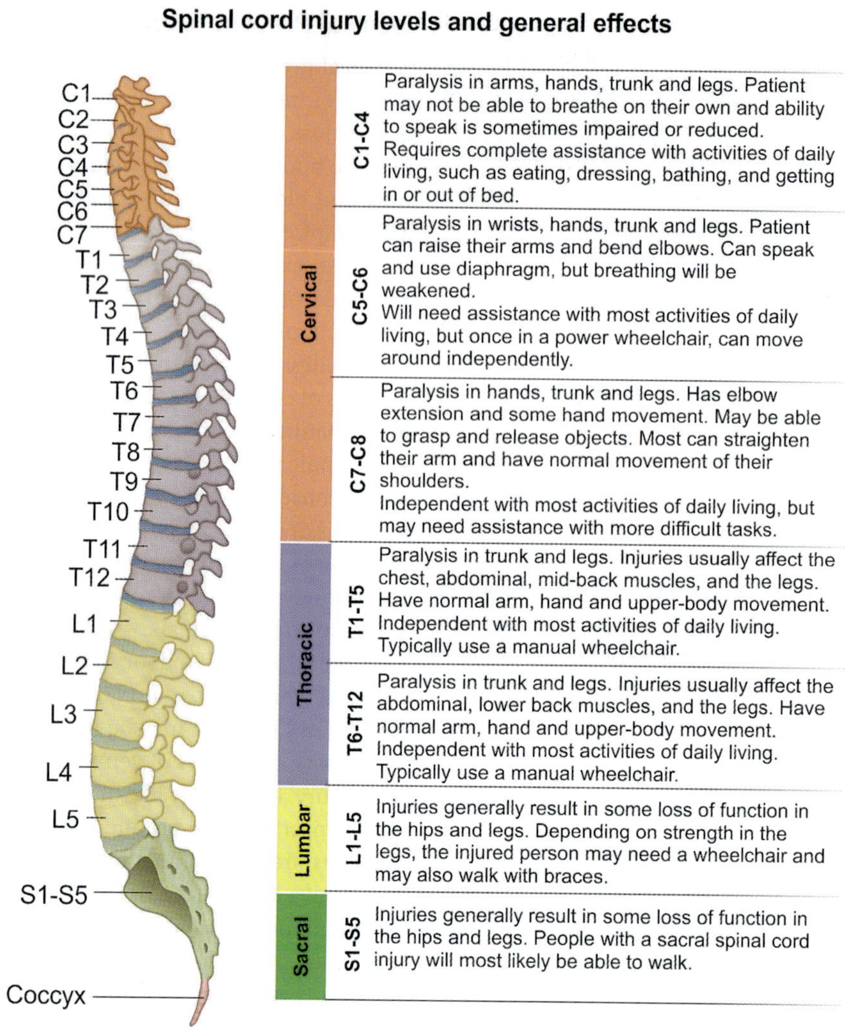

Fig. 2: Levels of spinal cord injury and corresponding clinical presentation.
Source: BY MATT LALANDE in Spinal Cord Injuries on May 01, 2021, (https://injured.ca/what-is-a-cervical-spinal-cord-injury/)

It determines the injury as complete or incomplete. AIS also allows for better counseling of the patient regarding expectation of recovery.[23]

MALE INFERTILITY DUE TO SPINAL CORD INJURIES

The natural fertility rate in men after a complete SCI lesion is estimated to be around 5–10%.[24,25] They may be unable to achieve either erection or ejaculation or both.

Male infertility is the condition where in the female partner has reduced the chances of getting pregnant in spite of being normal.

Spinal cord injury occurs commonly in young men, who are most probably at the peak of their reproductive health. It leads to infertility in them. Three major complications that are responsible for infertility in men with SCI are:[16]

- ED
- Ejaculatory dysfunction
- Abnormal quality of the semen.

Sexuality and Fertility in Men with SCI

In males, SCI can affect almost every aspect of the reproductive system. ED, sexual dysfunction, endocrine dysfunction, poor spermatogenesis, and problems in ejaculation and semen emission may occur.[15,16] After SCI, majority of the men may experience severely impaired fertility. The sexual dysfunction arising in neurological disorders has several causes. A model proposed for multiple sclerosis consisting of primary, secondary, and tertiary sexual dysfunction is considered valid for all neurological problems causing sexual dysfunction **(Figs. 3A and B and 4A to D)**.[26-28]

Primary sexual dysfunction is due to neurological lesions that affect the pathways responsible for sexual function. Lesions affecting the nervous system from the cerebrum to the peripheral nerves including the autonomic nervous system (ANS) can cause sexual dysfunction. It may manifest in the form of decreased libido or loss in libido, altered orgasmic response, and painful genital sensation like burning. There is also difficulty in erection, its maintenance, and ejaculation.

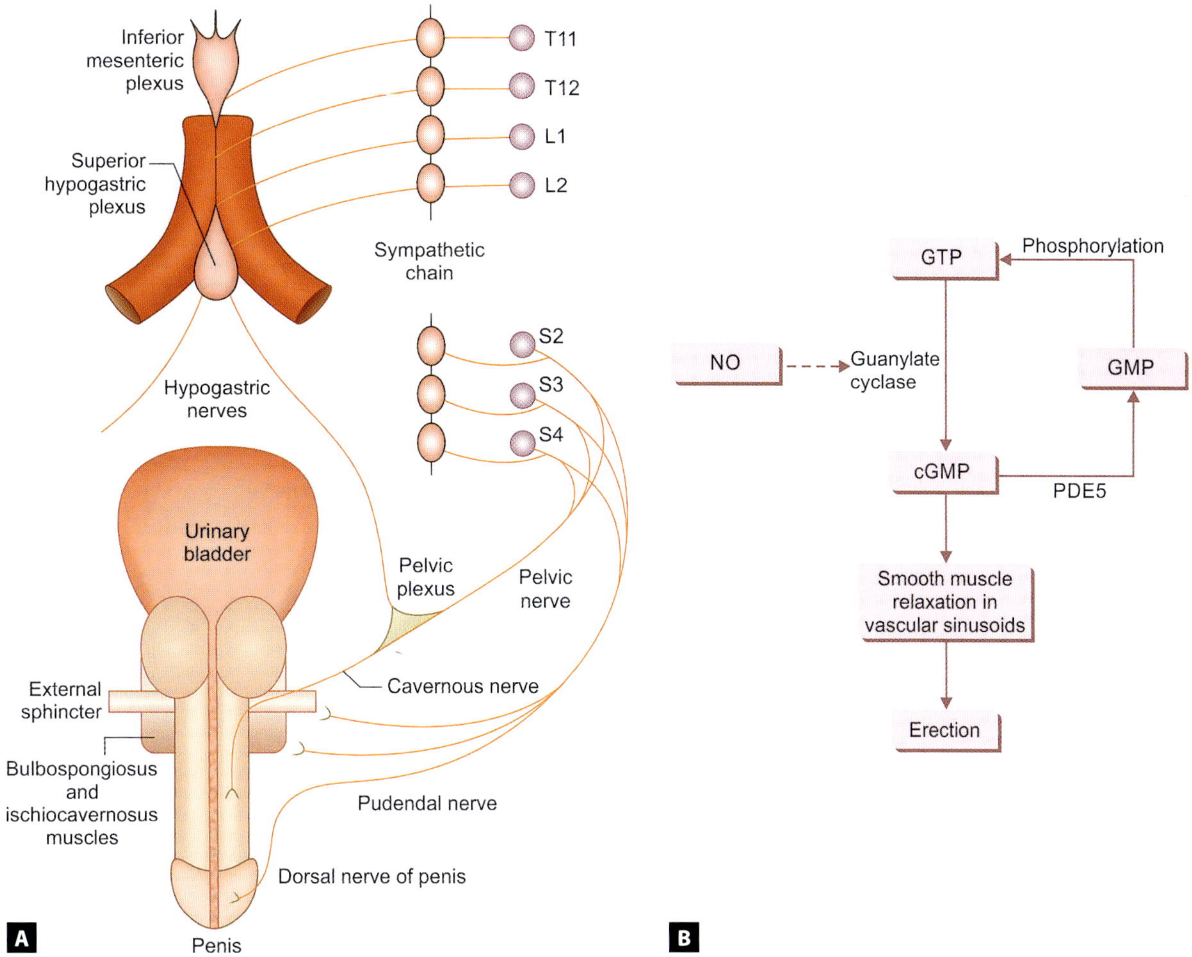

Figs. 3A and B: Neurophysiology of normal penile erection. (A) Sympathetic and parasympathetic penile innervation, pudendal nerve innervation. (B) Cyclic guanosine monophosphate (cGMP) pathway responsible for ejection. (GTP: guanosine triphosphate; NO: nitric oxide; PDE5: phosphodiesterase-5)

Source: Brackett NL et al. (2010b) 24 and Ibrahim E et al. (2016).[29]

Secondary sexual dysfunction can be due to fatigue, weakness of muscles, cognitive impairment, poor bladder control, and medications. It can also arise due to non-neurological comorbidities, such as depression, hypertension, diabetes mellitus, and obesity.

Tertiary sexual dysfunction is associated with psychological, psychosocial, and cultural issues affecting sexual response.

Loss of muscle movement, loss of touch sensation, and loss of sexual reflexes can occur commonly after SCI. The effect on one's sexuality such as arousal, orgasm, and their fertility is dependent on the level of injury and the type of injury as complete or incomplete injury.

Erection, Emission, and Ejaculation in SCI

The process of erection can be classically divided into:

- Reflex
- Tactile or psychogenic.

They are dependent on intact lower motor sacral nerves and spinal cord, respectively.[30] A complete injury above T11 may lead to loss of psychogenic erection. Injuries at the level of sacral nerve root impact the reflex or tactile erections.[19] In SCIs of T11 to L2, the ability to achieve erection by one or both pathways is variable.[20]

Emission involves the process by which semen is deposited in the urethra. It involves afferent signals from penile nerves and sympathetic input from T11 to L2 sympathetic nerve roots. It induces rhythmic contraction of vas deferens, seminal vesicles, and ejaculatory ducts.[20]

Ejaculation involves adequate deposit of semen in an antegrade fashion. It needs a closed bladder neck besides the somatically controlled rhythmic contraction of bulbocavernosus and ischiocavernosus muscles with concomitant relaxation of the external sphincter.[31]

The process of erection, emission, and ejaculation is a highly coordinated one. In a male with SCI, this process can break down and can result in infertility without medication or assisted reproductive technology. The completeness and level of injury determine the ability to ejaculate naturally in an antegrade fashion.

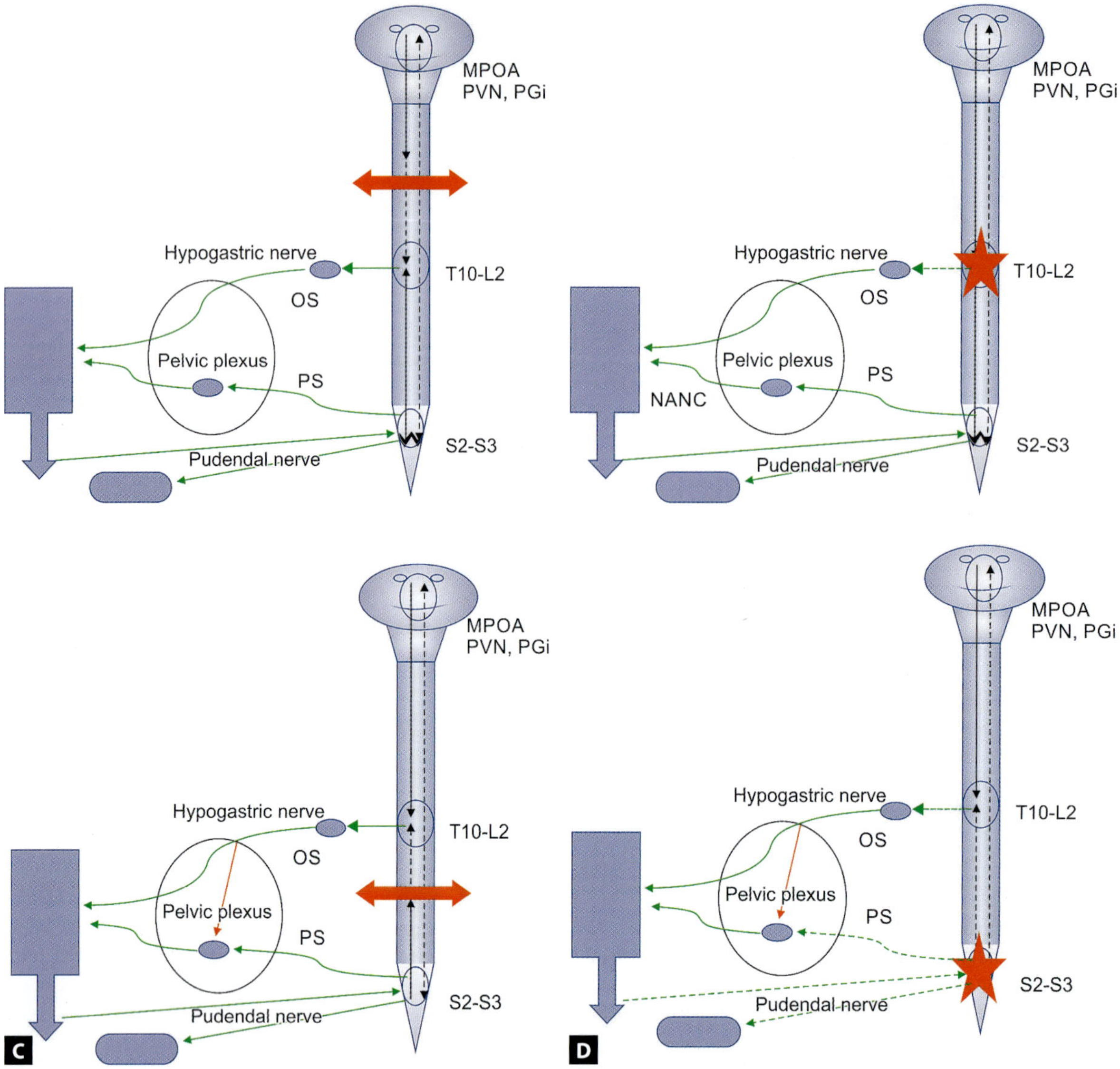

Figs. 4A to D: Neuroanatomy and neurophysiology related to sexual dysfunction due to lesions of spinal cord.
(OS: orthosympathetic, PS: parasympathetic, PGi: nucleus paragigantocellularis)
Source: Everaert K, de Waard W, Van Hoof, T. et al. Neuroanatomy and neurophysiology related to sexual dysfunction in male neurogenic patients with lesions to the spinal cord or peripheral nerves. Spinal Cord. 2010;48:182-191. https://doi.org/10.1038/sc.2009.172

It has also been reported that only 18% retain the ability to ejaculate after lower motor neuron injury. In case of complete upper motor neuron injury, only around 11% can ejaculate.[32,33]

Erectile Dysfunction, Neurophysiology and Evaluation of Erectile Dysfunction in SCI Patients

Neurogenic ED encompasses the disorders, which impair erections because of neurologic compromise or dysfunction. The disorders can be central, peripheral, or both. Neurogenic ED accounts for about 10–19% of all ED causes.[28,34] Several components of the normal pathway can be affected in SCI, leading to ED. Much emphasis has been placed on penile smooth muscle function and cavernosal hemodynamics with regards to penile erection. Although the neuroanatomy and neurophysiology of erection has been extensively characterized, there is still some poor understanding of the full extent of the process.[28]

The penile innervation is derived from both:
- ANS (sympathetic and parasympathetic) and
- Somatic innervation supplying sensory and motor inputs **(Fig. 5)**.[30,31]

The sympathetic preganglionic neurons rise from T11 to L2 while parasympathetic preganglionic neurons come from S2 to S4. Somatic innervation comes from the Onuf's nucleus in the lumbosacral region.

Reflexogenic erection needs intact S2 to S4 nerve roots. It happens by direct stimulation of genital region by involving

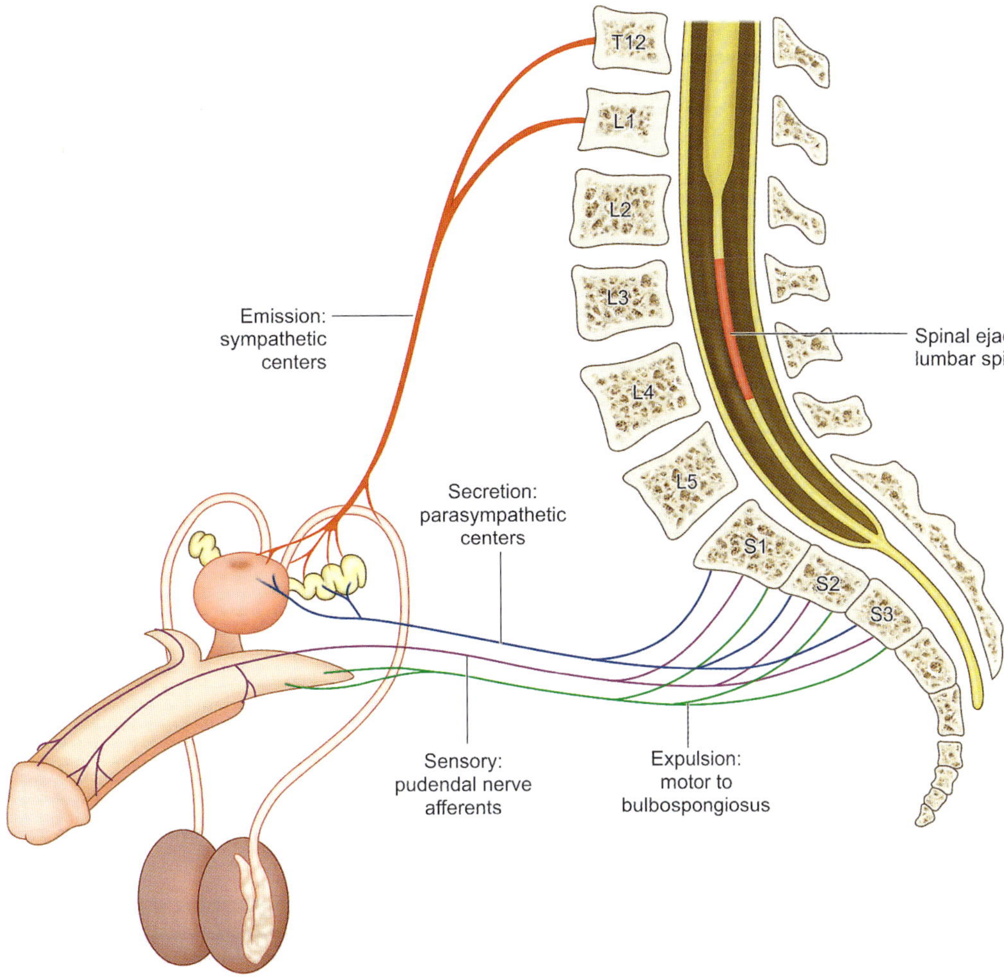

Fig. 5: Neuroanatomy and neurophysiology of erection, emission, and ejaculation.
Source: Celigoj FA, Coward RM, Matthew D, Timberlake, Smith RP. Management of Sexual Dysfunction in Men and Women: An Interdisciplinary Approach 1st ed. Anatomy and Physiology of Erection, Ejaculation, and Orgasm.

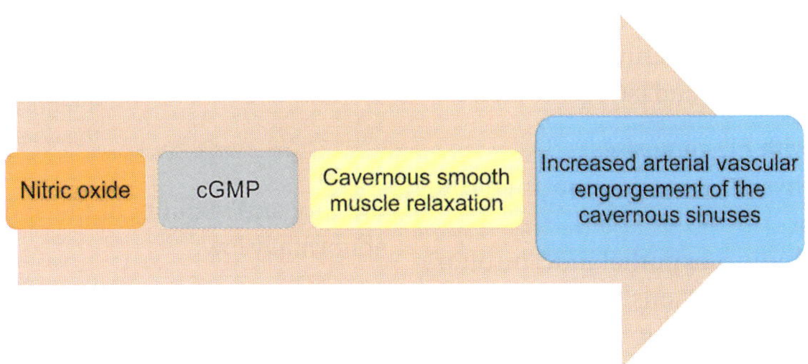

Fig. 6: Vascular process for erection.
(cGMP: cyclic guanosine monophosphate)

the dorsal nerve of the penis, which is a sensory branch of the pudendal nerve.

Independent of this direct genital stimulation, psychotic stimulation can happen with erotic stimuli and thoughts. It needs an intact thoracolumbar nerve root. In injuries of the thoracic and cervical spinal cord, it is often lost. The maintenance of erection during sexual intercourse is mainly due to psychogenic erection. Balance between the relaxing and contracting factors controlling corpora cavernosa is essential for initiating and maintaining penile erection. The NO (nitric oxide)-guanylate cyclase-cGMP (cyclic guanosine monophosphate) pathway is the relaxing factor which allows for rapid engorgement of venous sinuses of corpus cavernosum **(Fig. 6)**. Inhibition of erection is due

Flowchart 1: Management of erectile dysfunction (ED).

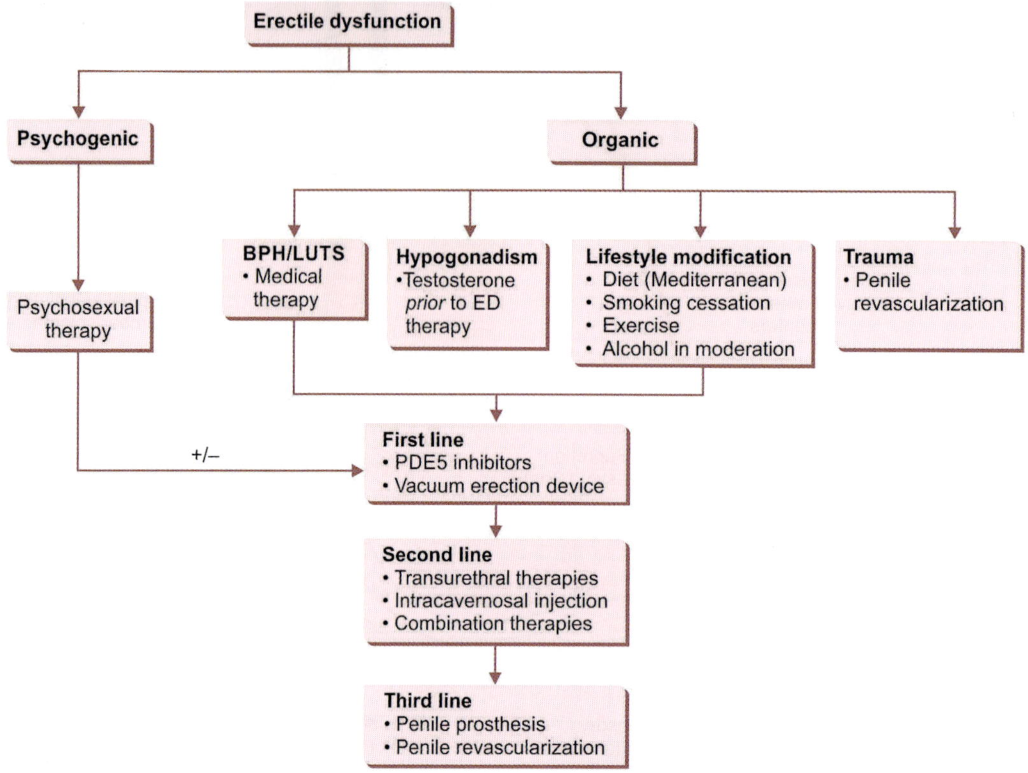

(BPH: benign prostatic hyperplasia; LUTS: lower urinary tract symptoms; PDE5: phosphodiesterase-5)

to phosphodiesterase-5 (PDE5) activity. PDE5 inhibits the engorgement of the cavernosal sinuses by causing persistent cyclic nucleotide signaling, resulting in penile detumescence.

Erectile dysfunction in SCI is mainly neurogenic **(Flowchart 1)**. But other causes of ED should also be evaluated such as psychogenic, penile factors, organic, vasculogenic, medical disorders, endocrine disorders, urological disorders, and drug-induced and iatrogenic factors.[35]

The evaluation of the men with ED comprises:

- Clinical history and physical examination including psychosocial assessment
- Laboratory testing including hypothalamic pituitary gonadal axis and metabolic conditions
- Imaging and other adjunct modalities.

Sequelae of SCI that Affect Male Fertility

The integrity of both the sympathetic and parasympathetic branches of the ANS is responsible for the complex process of erection through ejaculation. The control of ANS is most often affected in SCI, leading to unmodulated reflexes **(Box 1)**.

BOX 1: Sympathetic and parasympathetic outflow necessary for erection, emission, and ejaculation.[27]

Sympathetic outflow from T11 to L2	• Psychogenic erections • Seminal emission • Closure of the bladder neck during ejaculation
Parasympathetic outflow from S2 to S4	• Initiation of reflexogenic erections • Pulsatile expulsion of the semen during ejaculation • Integrity of the pudendal nerve and the dorsal nerve of the penis

The vascular process seems to be intact in SCI in absence of any other injuries/comorbidities.

In SCI, spermatogenesis seems to be little affected as seen by the normal numbers in several ejaculates. But the motility and viability of the sperm in most of the men are abnormally low.[36-38]

Ejaculatory Dysfunction

Majority of the men cannot ejaculate after SCI, without medical assistance. It is dependent on spinal cord coordination and supraspinal input from the brain. Supraspinal stimulation with erotic thoughts can cause ejaculation without any peripheral stimulation, and also the vice versa. Anejaculation after SCI is the absence of seminal emission in the posterior urethra. It mainly results from neuromuscular dysfunction and involvement of ANS. Ejaculation is often possible in SCI, which are incomplete with techniques such as masturbation and/or non-vibrostimulatory methods **(Table 1)**.

TABLE 1: Level of injury in SCI and chances of ejaculation.

Damage to T12 to L2 region[39]	*Testicular atrophy, poor ability to ejaculate*
Complete upper motor neuron lesions above T11[40]	5–10% chances of ejaculation during sex or masturbation
Complete lower motor neuron lesions below L2[40]	18% chance of emission
If upper limit of spinal cord injury (SCI) is below T12	Psychogenic emission with motile spermatozoa can occur

In SCI patients, those with a level of injury which is at or rostral to T10 have increased chances of response to penile vibratory stimulation (PVS) in comparison with level of injury at T11 or caudal. This is because of the integrity of sympathetic and parasympathetic components of the ejaculatory reflex, and the dorsal nerve of the penis in lesions, that are at T10 or rostral to it. In many of the SCI cases, S2–S4 segments are intact, allowing the reflex action to occur. In 95% of males with upper motor neuron lesions, reflex action is preserved. Similarly in 25% of those with lower motor neuron lesions, reflex action is preserved.[41] These reflex erections are often inconvenient and do not last long.

Semen Abnormalities in Men with SCI

In men with SCI, sperm production is usually normal. But there could be deterioration of sperm quality leading to infertility.[1,16,42] Although they may not be able to achieve erection or ejaculation, semen could be collected from them using medical methods. After SCI, there is sufficient evidence to suggest the disturbance of sperm production, the maturation of the sperm, storage and transport because of the altered neuroendocrine milieu.[42]

The quality of semen in men with SCI is poor. The changes in the quality of semen are seen as early as 2 weeks after the time of injury.

- Abnormal sperm motility and
- Viability.

These are the distinguishing characteristics of poor quality of semen seen in men with SCI. The sperm count is not abnormal in the majority of the subjects with SCI. The total sperm count was commonly reported to be high (>100 million/mL) in men with SCI, but the motility of the sperm was poor (asthenozoospermia, that is usually <10%) with poor viability.[38,43,44] Although, it was previously thought there could be progressive decline in the spermatozoa number over the years, the spermatozoa number appears to be normal in spinal cord injured patients with regular urological follow up. Brackett et al. reported that there was no difference in the motility, total number, and concentration of spermatozoa in the ejaculate on consideration with time lapsed from the injury.[44] There was no relationship between decline in semen parameters and time post injury.[44] Momen et al. in their study reported that in SCI men, the seminogram is characterized by normal volume (2.3 ± 1.9 mL), normal sperm count ($85 \times 10^6 \pm 83.8 \times 10^6$/mL), decreased motility (11.6% ± 0.1%), decreased vitality (18.5% ± 5.2%), and normal forms (17.5% ± 3.4%) besides increased number of pus cells ($6 \times 10^6 \pm 8.2 \times 10^6$/mL).[38] They also observed that total motility and progressive motility were higher significantly in subjects having lower scrotal temperatures.[38]

Utida et al. observed that sperm motility is abnormal in SCI patients despite the normal spermatozoa number.[45] They reported that these changes are not related to changes in thermal regulation of scrotum, ejaculation frequency, or duration of spinal cord damage but are due to the factors related to seminal plasma. In spite of poor seminal quality, using techniques from simple homologous insemination to sophisticated assisted reproduction techniques, many SCI men have become fathers.[45] Kathiresan et al. observed that motility of the sperm was comparatively higher in men with SCI, who could ejaculate by masturbation compared to those who could not ejaculate by masturbation. This difference could be attributed to the level of completeness of injury.[43] In a follow-up study, it was observed that there was a decline in semen quality starting 16 days after SCI and it was also recommended to store semen within the first 2 weeks after injury for future use.[46]

Semen Quality and Factors Contributing to Poor Semen Quality in SCI

The quality of semen is reported to be normal for 6–10 days after injury. But after a period of 2 weeks from injury, it is reduced to levels as commonly seen in those chronic SCI, typically with reduced viability and abnormal sperm motility.[38,43,44] It was reported that men with SCI capable of ejaculation by masturbation had significantly higher sperm motility on comparison to those with SCI not capable of ejaculation by masturbation.[43] It was also reported that quality of semen collected by masturbation in SCI subjects had significantly lower sperm motility on comparison with normal control subjects without SCI.

The difference in the degrees of dysinnervation to seminal vesicles and prostate glands can result in abnormal constituents to the seminal plasma that are toxic to sperm.[43] The motility of the sperm tends to be higher in cases of incomplete SCI and lesions that are situated above the spinal ejaculation centers.[43]

Poor semen quality in men with SCI seems to be primarily due to post-spermatogenic causes, such as ANS dysfunction, impaired ejaculatory function, abnormal constituents of seminal plasma, dysfunction of the sperm, and type of bladder management.[42]

It has also been reported that around 51% of men with SCI have at least one hormonal abnormality and also

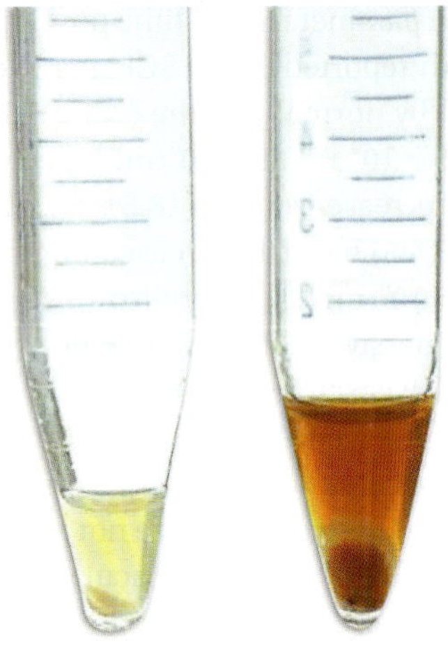

Fig. 7: Semen in spinal cord injury. Left tube shows prostatic fluid, right tube shows brown-colored semen.
Source: Image adapted from Wieder et al. (1999).[47]

that 86% of men with SCI have some abnormality of the hypothalamic-pituitary-testicular axis.[48]

There are multiple theories for the abnormal semen motility in subjects with SCI such as increased scrotal temperature, antisperm antibodies, leukospermia, and seminal plasma proteins and cytokines. The color of the ejaculate also appears to be brown or dark after SCI **(Fig. 7)**.[47] Many factors affecting the quality of semen in SCI are interconnected.

Seminal plasma was observed to be affecting the motility in SCI.[49] Seminal plasma in SCI men is characterized by high number of leukocytes, especially activated T-cells. They can secrete cytotoxic substances and cytokines. It has been reported that spermatogenesis may improve after an initial period of impairment.[50] The evidence is inconsistent regarding short- and long-term hormonal changes seen following SCI in men, which could affect the semen quality.[16] SCI affects multiple organs including testis. Testicular hypofunction and prostate gland dysfunction may also play a role.[51] SCI is a highly inflammatory process. The semen of SCI men was reported to have elevated cytokines and caspases. The factors affecting the semen quality are shown in **Figure 8**.

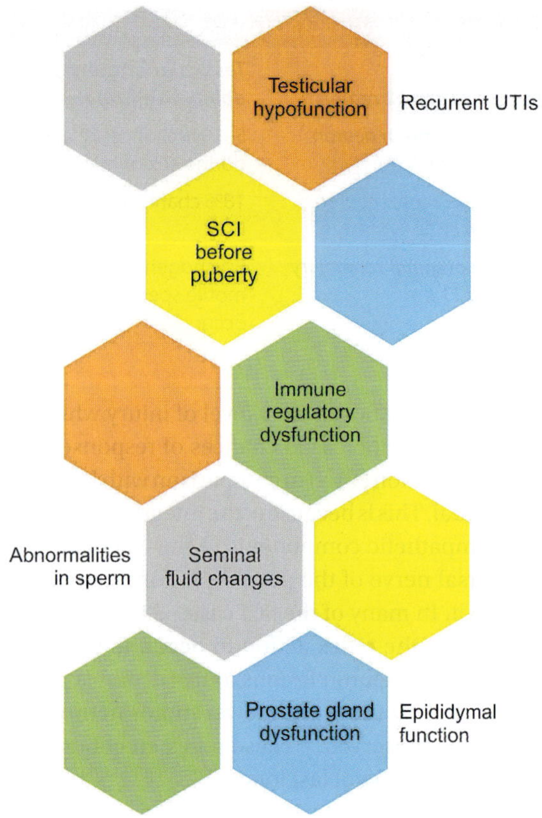

Fig. 8: Factors affecting semen quality in spinal cord injury (SCI). (UTIs: urinary tract infections)

MANAGEMENT OF COUPLES WITH SCI-RELATED MALE FACTOR INFERTILITY

Most men with SCI are infertile. ED, ejaculatory dysfunction, and semen abnormalities contribute to the problem. Treatments for ED include PDE5 inhibitors, intracavernous injections of alprostadil, intraurethral injections, penile prosthesis, and vacuum constriction devices besides psychosocial counseling.[1] In anejaculatory patients who wish to father children, semen retrieval is necessary. PVS is recommended as the first line of treatment. Patients who fail PVS can be referred for electroejaculation (EEJ). If this approach is not possible, prostate massage is an alternative. Surgical sperm retrieval should be considered as a last resort when other methods fail. Despite abnormalities, sperm from men with SCI can successfully induce pregnancy. In selected couples, the simple method of intravaginal insemination is a viable option. Another option is intrauterine insemination (IUI). The efficacy of IUI increases as the total motile sperm count inseminated increases. In vitro fertilization (IVF) and intracytoplasmic sperm injection (ICSI) are options in cases of extremely low total motile sperm count. Reproductive outcomes for SCI male factor infertility are similar to outcomes for general male factor infertility.

Administration of the PDE-5 inhibitors can be used for treating ED, as the vascular mechanism is intact and they help in maintaining erection during sexual activity. In case of inability to obtain a reflexogenic erection or failure of PDE-5 inhibitors to induce sustained erection, more invasive methods may be needed like intracavernous injection of prostaglandins. A combination of prostaglandins, phentolamine, and papaverine can also be tried on them.[52,53] The counseling of patients is essential with regard to side effects. There has been varied patient satisfaction rates and success rates in methods such as intraurethral application of alprostadil and vacuum constriction devices.[54,55] Penile prosthesis can also be surgically implanted as a last resort. Inflatable devices are usually preferred in men with SCI.[56]

Management of Anejaculation in Men with Spinal Cord Injury

Anejaculation occurs due to interference in the afferent or efferent innervation of the seminal vesicles, bladder neck, posterior urethra, or vas deferens after SCI. Treatment to improve dysfunction in the general population can be used to improve ejaculatory dysfunction in men with SCI. There can be disruption of the nerve pathways in SCI for ejaculation. Hence, medical assistance is required to procure sperm for insemination like:

- PVS
- EEJ
- Prostate massage
- Sperm retrieval surgically.

Although SCI patients with injury level above T9 experience frequently some degree of erectile impairment, the most important barrier to fertility in these subjects is complete absence of ejaculatory reflex.[57]

Penile vibratory stimulation is recommended as the first line of treatment for anejaculation in men with SCI.[58] PVS involves placing a vibrator on the dorsum or frenulum of the glans penis.[59] Ejaculation is induced by the ejaculatory reflex and hence it is more effective in men with intact ejaculatory reflex, that is, men with a level of injury T10 or higher. An intact dorsal penile nerve, which terminates in sacral spinal cord segments between S2 and S4, is required for a successful ejaculatory reflex.[60] On comparison with other methods, PVS is safe, cost-effective, and reliable method.[61] The success rate was reported to be 86% in subjects with neurological injury level at T10 or rostral. But one dangerous problem in PVS is the potential for occurrence of autonomic dysreflexia.

Patients who fail this therapy should be referred for EEJ.[24,32] It has a high success rate of 95%. In this procedure, ejaculation is induced by placing the patient in lateral decubitus position, inserting the probe with electrodes into rectum with electrodes facing prostate gland and seminal vesicles.[62,63] Then, electric current is delivered in a pattern of 5 seconds of stimulation followed by rest periods of approximately 20 seconds, during which ejaculation can occur. By this procedure, ejaculation occurs in a dribbling, nonprojectile manner. To retrieve as much semen as possible, the urethra should be milked. The delivery of current is increased in 2-volt increments if there is no ejaculation.[64] Majority of SCI men can undergo EEJ without anesthesia. But it can cause significant discomfort in men with preserved sensation, for whom sedation or general anesthesia may be required. Similar to PVS, it can also cause autonomic dysreflexia.

In *prostate massage*, the seminal vesicles and also the prostate are emptied by a physician by pressing on these structures using a finger inserted into the patient's rectum. It is based on the concept that sperm are stored in the ampulla of the vas deferens and in SCI, they are sequestered also in the seminal vesicles.[65] Hence, it is mechanically pushed out through the ejaculatory ductal system. The yield of sperm is low in prostate massage in comparison with EEJ or PVS. Hence, it is used in countries without access to EEJ, after PVS fails.[66]

Surgical semen retrieval (SSR): This involves retrieval of sperm from reproductive tissue, by aspiration or through surgical exploration. It is done through a variety of techniques such as testicular sperm aspiration, testicular sperm extraction, microepididymal sperm aspiration, percutaneous epididymal sperm aspiration, and aspiration of sperm from the vas deferens.[1,67,68] SSR was developed as a technique for retrieval of sperm from azoospermic men without SCI. But PVS and EEJ were developed to manage and treat anejaculation. SSR should be performed only when PVS or EEJ fail or are not feasible. Because they are less invasive and expensive in comparison with SSR. Also, there is a need for more expensive assisted reproductive techniques such as ICSI, with the use of SSR, as the yield often has low motile sperm count. Use of SSR as the first line of treatment for anejaculation in men with SCI is controversial, when other methods are available. The complications include hematoma, pain, and other risks associated with ICSI through IVF.

Reproductive Options and Outcomes

The options for fertility in male SCI-related infertility include:

- Intravaginal insemination
- IUI
- IVF (in vitro fertilization) or ICSI (intra cytoplasmic sperm injection).

"*In-home insemination*" is the least invasive and least expensive of the assisted reproductive options. It is also called *intravaginal insemination*. The couples should be evaluated at a clinic for determining the optimal method for ejaculation at home, which is effective and safe. The optimal method will be evaluated, and guidelines will be set regarding the number of intravaginal insemination cycles for choosing more advanced methods of assisted conception. Any tubal or uterine pathology should be evaluated for the female partner. She is counseled about timing of insemination and methods to detect ovulation. If semen cannot be ejaculated during intercourse, PVS can be used to collect it and can be deposited into the vagina with the help of a syringe. The success rate has been good at 43% pregnancy rate from a multicentric study.[69]

"*Intrauterine insemination*" involves collecting semen from male partner affected with SCI usually by PVS or EEJ. It is processed to separate sperm from the semen and for isolating motile from the nonmotile sperm. The processed sperm is then placed inside the uterus of the woman. In a study on 121 consecutive couples including 87 couples with SCI male partners, a pregnancy rate of 8.6% per cycle and 32.2% per couple was reported. EEJ was done in combination with assisted reproductive technology (gamete intrafallopian transfer or IVF) in these couples for treatment of anejaculatory infertility.[66] They also suggested that in couples with total motile sperm count of <4 million, high-level assisted reproductive technologies should be done directly as the pregnancy rates to 1.1% per cycle. They also suggested that around 3–6 cycles of IUI should be attempted before proceeding to IVF. It was also reported that with inseminated total motile sperm counts of >40 million, the pregnancy rate was 17.6% per cycle. IUI warrants consideration before taking up IVF.

Advanced assisted reproductive technology techniques like in vitro fertilization or ICSI are indicated in case of fertilization not being possible or not indicated by IUI. IVF involves placing the sperm retrieved from a man in a laboratory dish with ova retrieved from the woman. This mixture is then incubated for up to 5 days to allow for fertilization of ova. Then high quality embryos reaching blastocyst stage are placed into the uterine cavity.[70] When the number of motile sperm is too low for conventional IVF, the method of ICSI is often used to achieve fertilization. ICSI is a procedure in which a single sperm is injected directly into the egg. IVF and ICSI have been used to achieve pregnancy in couples with male partners with SCI.[71,72]

Semen Retrieval Methods

In men failing pharmacological conversion or who are contradicted to pharmacological conversion, assisted ejaculation may be used to harvest sperm. For men with SCI, who do not respond to medical management of

Flowchart 2: Semen retrieval methods.

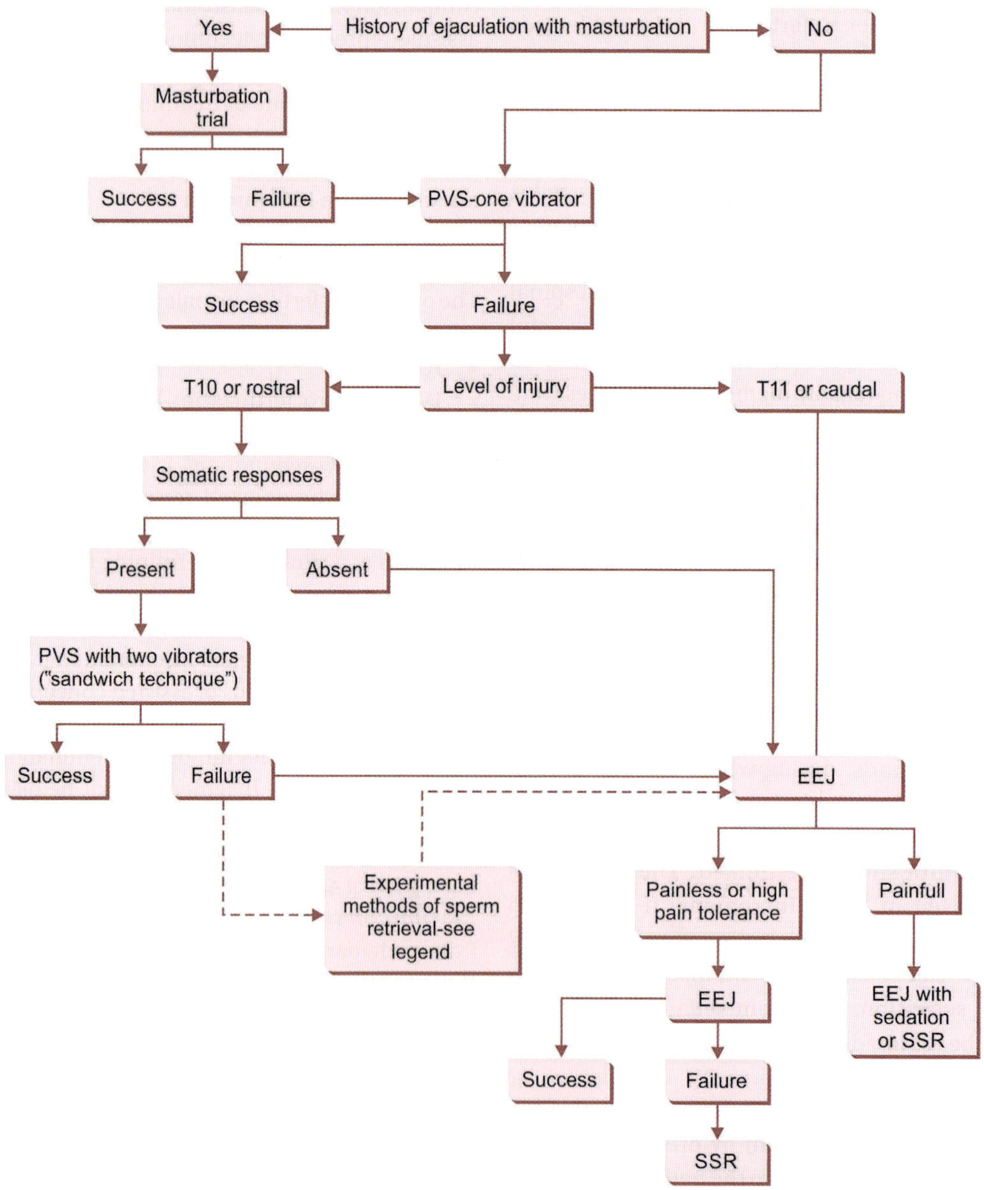

(EEJ: electroejaculation; PVS: penile vibratory stimulation; SSR: surgical semen retrieval)

anejaculation, sperm retrieval can be attempted using either PVS or EEJ. If no viable sperm can be retrieved with these methods, surgical sperm retrieval may be performed using microsurgical epididymal sperm aspiration, percutaneous epididymal sperm aspiration, testicular sperm aspiration, or testicular sperm extraction. Postejaculatory harvesting of sperm in the bladder can be done. Urinary sperm retrieval is achieved by alkalinization of urine using oral sodium bicarbonate. It is then catheterized to obtain a postejaculatory urine specimen and then centrifuged. The urine specimen is then resuspended in medium before using it for vaginal or IUI **(Flowchart 2)**.

The effects of sperm freezing were similar in both healthy patients and those with SCT. After thawing the decrease in motility was around 60–80%. Because of inferior seminal quality in SCI patients, there is no clear advantage with routine seminal cryopreservation. But it can be indicated in conditions such as personal wish of the patient, difficulty in transportation of ejaculate, or time constraints for transportation.[73]

Current Issues in Managing Couples with SCI-related Infertility in Men

Assisted conception is possible in couples with SCI in men, whose semen quality is impaired. The infertility treatment methods that are used for the general population can be used on them. But instead, these couples are preempted to surgical sperm retrieval and IVF/ICSI. Main problems faced by the couples are cost and lack of accessible procedures and equipment. In methods like PVS or EEJ, the main obstacles were a lack of equipment and lack of training.[63] IVF/ICSI is more invasive and expensive. In contrast, the ejaculate of men with SCI often has a sufficient number of motile sperm for considering IUI or intravaginal insemination.[63]

CONCLUSION

The majority of individuals with SCI are young men. ED, ejaculatory dysfunction, and semen abnormalities are the major obstacles for fertility in SCI. The treatment of these conditions and assisted reproductive techniques have the same use in SCI-related male infertility in comparison to those men who have infertility without SCI. Atypical semen profile and anejaculation are the main culprits in SCI for infertility. It is typically characterized by normal sperm concentration with low sperm motility and viability besides other factors affecting semen quality like altered seminal plasma. There is not much of a difference in pregnancy outcomes with sperm from SCI men in comparison with non-SCI men.

Penile vibratory stimulation is a safe, cost-effective, and reliable method and should be the first line of treatment for men with SCI. SSR should be performed only when PVS or EEJ fail or are not feasible because they are less invasive and expensive in comparison with SSR. Future research should focus on improving the semen quality in men with SCI and promoting natural ejaculation.

KEY POINTS

- Infertility following SCI in men occurs due to a combination of erectile dysfunction, ejaculatory dysfunction, and semen abnormalities.
- A lot of advances have been made over the years in the field of medical sciences with regard to SCI-related infertility.
- Treatments that are effective in non-SCI male factor infertility are effective for management in couples with SCI male factor infertility.
- Atypical semen profile and anejaculation are the main culprits in SCI for infertility.
- Penile vibratory stimulation is a safe, cost-effective, and reliable method and should be the first line of treatment for men with SCI.
- SSR should be performed only when PVS or EEJ fail or are not feasible.

REFERENCES

1. Brackett NL. Infertility in men with spinal cord injury: research and treatment. Scientifica (Cairo). 2012;2012:578257.
2. World Health Organization. (2013). Spinal cord injury. [online] Available from: https://www.who.int/news-room/fact-sheets/detail/spinal-cord-injury [Last accessed October, 2022].
3. GBD (2016). Traumatic Brain Injury and Spinal Cord Injury Collaborators. Global, regional, and national burden of traumatic brain injury and spinal cord injury, 1990-2016: a systematic analysis for the Global Burden of Disease Study 2016. Lancet Neurol. 2019;18(1):56-87.
4. Chamberlain JD, Deriaz O, Hund-Georgiadis M, Meier S, Scheel-Sailer A, Schubert M, et al. Epidemiology and contemporary risk profile of traumatic spinal cord injury in Switzerland. Inj Epidemiol. 2015;2(1):28.
5. National Spinal Cord Injury Statistical Center. (2019). Spinal cord injury facts and figures at a glance. [online] Available from: https://www.nscisc.uab.edu/Public/Facts%20and%20Figures%202019%20-%20Final.pdf [Last accessed November, 2022].
6. World Health Organization. (2013). International perspectives on spinal cord injury. [online] Available from: http://apps.who.int/iris/bitstream/10665/94190/1/9789241564663_eng.pdf [Last accessed November, 2022].
7. Singh R. Epidemiology of spinal cord injuries: Indian perspective. Epidemiol Spinal Cord Inj. 2012;157-68.
8. Mathur N, Jain S, Kumar N, Srivastava A, Purohit N, Patni A. Spinal cord injury: Scenario in an Indian state. Spinal cord. 2015;53(5):349-52.
9. Birua GJS, Munda VS, Murmu NN. Epidemiology of spinal injury in North East India: A Retrospective Study. Asian J Neurosurg. 2018;13(4):1084-6.
10. Manjeet S, Siddhartha S, Iftikhar W, Agnivesh T, Farid M, Nirdosh M, et al. Spine injuries in a tertiary health care

hospital in Jammu: A clinico-epidemiological study. Internet J Neurosurg. 2009;5:2.

11. Kang Y, Ding H, Zhou HX, Wei ZJ, Liu L, Pan DY, et al. Epidemiology of worldwide spinal cord injury: a literature review. Journal of Neurorestoratology. 2018;6:1-9.
12. New PW, Farry A, Baxter D, Noonan VK. Prevalence of non-traumatic spinal cord injury in Victoria, Australia. Spinal Cord. 2013;51(2):99-102.
13. Román GC. Tropical myelopathies. Handb Clin Neurol. 2014; 121:1521-48.
14. Modi G, Ranchhod J, Hari K, Mochan A, Modi M. Non-traumatic myelopathy at the Chris Hani Baragwanath Hospital, South Africa—the influence of HIV. QJM. 2011; 104(8):697-703.
15. Anderson R, Moses R, Lenherr S, Hotaling JM, Myers J. Spinal cord injury and male infertility-a review of current literature, knowledge gaps, and future research. Transl Androl Urol. 2018;7(Suppl 3):S373-S382.
16. Ibrahim E, Lynne CM, Brackett NL. Male fertility following spinal cord injury: an update. Andrology. 2016;4(1):13-26.
17. Bennett J, Das JM, Emmady PD. Spinal Cord Injuries. In: StatPearls [Internet]. Treasure Island (FL): StatPearls Publishing; 2022.
18. Alizadeh A, Dyck SM, Karimi-Abdolrezaee S. Traumatic spinal cord injury: an overview of pathophysiology, models and acute injury mechanisms. Front Neurol. 2019;10:282.
19. Courtois FJ, Goulet MC, Charvier KF, Leriche A. Posttraumatic erectile potential of spinal cord injured men: how physiologic recordings supplement subjective reports. Arch Phys Med Rehabil. 1999;80(10):1268-72.
20. Dean RC, Lue TF. Physiology of penile erection and pathophysiology of erectile dysfunction. Urol Clin North Am. 2005;32(4):379-95, v.
21. Schubert M. Natural Course of Disease of Spinal Cord Injury. In: Weidner N, Rupp R, Tansey KE (Eds). Neurological Aspects of Spinal Cord Injury. Cham: Springer International Publishing; 2017. pp. 77-105.
22. El Tecle NE, Dahdaleh NS, Bydon M, Ray WZ, Torner JC, Hitchon PW. The natural history of complete spinal cord injury: a pooled analysis of 1162 patients and a meta-analysis of modern data. J Neurosurg Spine. 2018;28(4):436-43.
23. Roberts TT, Leonard GR, Cepela DJ. Classifications In Brief: American Spinal Injury Association (ASIA) Impairment Scale. Clin Orthop Relat Res. 2017;475(5):1499-504.
24. Brackett NL, Lynne CM, Ibrahim E, Ohl DA, Sønksen J. Treatment of infertility in men with spinal cord injury. Nat Rev Urol. 2010;7(3):162-72.
25. State Spinal Cord Injury Service, NSW Agency for Clinical Innovation. (2020). Fertility following spinal cord injury. Sydney: ACI. Available from: https://aci.health.nsw.gov.au/__data/assets/pdf_file/0006/600855/ACI-SCI-Fertility-following-spinal-injury.pdf [Last accessed November, 2022].
26. Pöttgen J, Rose A, van de Vis W, Engelbrecht J, Pirard M, Lau S, et al. Sexual dysfunctions in MS in relation to neuropsychiatric aspects and its psychological treatment: a scoping review. PLoS One. 2018;13(2):e0193381.
27. Krassioukov A, Elliott S. Neural Control and Physiology of Sexual Function: Effect of Spinal Cord Injury. Top Spinal Cord Inj Rehabil. 2017;23(1):1-10.
28. Shridharani AN, Brant WO. The treatment of erectile dysfunction in patients with neurogenic disease. Transl Androl Urol. 2016;5(1):88-101.
29. Ibrahim E, Brackett NL, Lynne CM. Advances in the management of infertility in men with spinal cord injury. Asian J Androl. 2016;18(3):382-90.
30. Giuliano F, Clement P. Neuroanatomy and physiology of ejaculation. Annu Rev Sex Res. 2005;16:190-216.
31. Clement P, Giuliano F. Physiology and Pharmacology of Ejaculation. Basic Clin Pharmacol Toxicol. 2016;119 (Suppl 3): 18-25.
32. Brackett NL, Ibrahim E, Iremashvili V, Aballa TC, Lynne CM. Treatment for ejaculatory dysfunction in men with spinal cord injury: an 18-year single center experience. J Urol. 2010;183(6):2304-8.
33. Ohl DA, Bennett CJ, McCabe M, Menge AC, McGuire EJ. Predictors of success in electroejaculation of spinal cord injured men. J Urol. 1989;142(6):1483-6.
34. Aboseif S, Shinohara K, Borirakchanyavat S, Deirmenjian J, Carroll PR. The effect of cryosurgical ablation of the prostate on erectile function. Br J Urol. 1997;80(6):918-22.
35. Pastuszak AW. Current Diagnosis and Management of Erectile Dysfunction. Curr Sex Health Rep. 2014;6(3):164-76.
36. Chalas C, Jilet L, Wolf JP, Drouineaud V, Abdoul H, Patrat C, et al. Prospective analysis over time of semen parameters in spinal cord-injured patients: results of a pilot study. Andrology. 2022;10(1):120-7.
37. Celigoj FA, Ibrahim E, Aballa TC, Lynne CM, Brackett NL. Semen quality in men who sustained a spinal cord injury during the prepubertal period. J Urol. 2012;188(2): 521-5.
38. Momen MN, Fahmy I, Amer M, Arafa M, Zohdy W, Naser TA. Semen parameters in men with spinal cord injury: changes and aetiology. Asian J Androl. 2007;9(5):684-9.
39. Chapelle PA, Roby-Brami A, Yakovleff A, Bussel B. Neurological correlations of ejaculation and testicular size in men with a complete spinal cord section. J Neurol Neurosurg Psychiatry. 1988;51(2):197-202.
40. Sønksen J, Biering-Sørensen F. Fertility in men with spinal cord or cauda equina lesions. Semin Neurol. 1992;12(2):106-14.
41. Courtois FJ, Charvier KF, Leriche A, Raymond DP. Sexual function in spinal cord injury men. I. Assessing sexual capability. Paraplegia. 1993;31(12):771-84.
42. Patki P, Woodhouse J, Hamid R, Craggs M, Shah J. Effects of spinal cord injury on semen parameters. J Spinal Cord Med. 2008;31(1):27-32.
43. Kathiresan AS, Ibrahim E, Modh R, Aballa TC, Lynne CM, Brackett NL. Semen quality in ejaculates produced by masturbation in men with spinal cord injury. Spinal Cord. 2012;50(12):891-4.
44. Brackett NL, Ferrell SM, Aballa TC, Amador MJ, Lynne CM. Semen quality in spinal cord injured men: does it progressively decline postinjury? Arch Phys Med Rehabil. 1998;79(6): 625-8.
45. Utida C, Truzzi JC, Bruschini H, Simonetti R, Cedenho AP, Srougi M, et al. Male infertility in spinal cord trauma. Int Braz J Urol. 2005;31(4):375-83.
46. Mallidis C, Lim TC, Hill ST, Skinner DJ, Brown DJ, Johnston WI, et al. Collection of semen from men in acute phase of spinal cord injury. Lancet. 1994;343(8905):1072-3.

47. Wieder JA, Lynne CM, Ferrell SM, Aballa TC, Brackett NL. Brown-colored semen in men with spinal cord injury. J Androl. 1999;20(5):594-600.
48. Huang TS, Wang YH, Lee SH, Lai JS. Impaired hypothalamus-pituitary-adrenal axis in men with spinal cord injuries. Am J Phys Med Rehabil. 1998;77(2):108-12.
49. Brackett NL, Davi RC, Padron OF, Lynne CM. Seminal plasma of spinal cord injured men inhibits sperm motility of normal men. J Urol. 1996;155(5):1632-5.
50. Sánchez-Ramos A, Vargas-Baquero E, Martin-de Francisco FJ, Godino-Durán JA, Rodriguez-Carrión I, Ortega-Ortega M, et al. Early spermatogenesis changes in traumatic complete spinal cord-injured adult patients. Spinal Cord. 2017;55(6): 570-4.
51. Ibrahim E, Castle SM, Aballa TC, Keane RW, de Rivero Vaccari JP, Lynne CM, et al. Neutralization of ASC improves sperm motility in men with spinal cord injury. Hum Reprod. 2014;29(11):2368-73.
52. Conejero Sugrañes J, Muñoz Villellas A, Sarrias Lorenz F, Ramírez Garceran L. [Prostaglandin treatment in neurological patients with erectile dysfunction]. Arch Esp Urol. 2002;55(1):63-8.
53. Lebib Ben Achour S, Laffont I, Boyer F, Boiteau F, Dizien O. [Intracavernous injections in the treatment of erectile dysfunction in spinal cord injured patients: experience with 36 patients]. Ann Readapt Med Phys. 2001;44(1):35-40.
54. Bodner DR, Haas CA, Krueger B, Seftel AD. Intraurethral alprostadil for treatment of erectile dysfunction in patients with spinal cord injury. Urology. 1999;53(1):199-202.
55. Denil J, Ohl DA, Smythe C. Vacuum erection device in spinal cord injured men: patient and partner satisfaction. Arch Phys Med Rehabil. 1996;77(8):750-3.
56. Kim YD, Yang SO, Lee JK, Jung TY, Shim HB. Usefulness of a malleable penile prosthesis in patients with a spinal cord injury. Int J Urol. 2008;15(10):919-23.
57. Biering-Sørensen F, Sønksen J. Sexual function in spinal cord lesioned men. Spinal Cord. 2001;39(9):455-70.
58. Sønksen J, Ohl DA. Penile vibratory stimulation and electroejaculation in the treatment of ejaculatory dysfunction. Int J Androl. 2002;25(6):324-32.
59. Brackett NL. Semen retrieval by penile vibratory stimulation in men with spinal cord injury. Hum Reprod Update. 1999; 5(3):216-22.
60. Wieder JA, Brackett NL, Lynne CM, Green JT, Aballa TC. Anesthetic block of the dorsal penile nerve inhibits vibratory-induced ejaculation in men with spinal cord injuries. Urology. 2000;55(6):915-7.
61. Brackett NL, Padron OF, Lynne CM. Semen quality of spinal cord injured men is better when obtained by vibratory stimulation versus electroejaculation. J Urol. 1997;157(1):151-7.
62. Ohl DA, Sønksen J, Brackett NL, Lynne CM. Electroejaculation. Current Sexual Health Reports. 2008;5(1):3-5.
63. Kafetsoulis A, Brackett NL, Ibrahim E, Attia GR, Lynne CM. Current trends in the treatment of infertility in men with spinal cord injury. Fertil Steril. 2006;86(4):781-9.
64. Brackett NL, Ead DN, Aballa TC, Ferrell SM, Lynne CM. Semen retrieval in men with spinal cord injury is improved by interrupting current delivery during electroejaculation. J Urol. 2002;167(1):201-3.
65. Ohl DA, Menge AC, Jarow JP. Seminal vesicle aspiration in spinal cord injured men: insight into poor sperm quality. J Urol. 1999;162(6):2048-51.
66. Ohl DA, Wolf LJ, Menge AC, Christman GM, Hurd WW, Ansbacher R, et al. Electroejaculation and assisted reproductive technologies in the treatment of anejaculatory infertility. Fertil Steril. 2001;76(6):1249-55.
67. Craft I, Tsirigotis M, Courtauld E, Farrer-Brown G. Testicular needle aspiration as an alternative to biopsy for the assessment of spermatogenesis. Hum Reprod. 1997;12(7):1483-7.
68. Engin-Uml Stün Y, Korkmaz C, Duru NK, Başer I. Comparison of three sperm retrieval techniques in spinal cord-injured men: pregnancy outcome. Gynecol Endocrinol. 2006;22(5): 252-5.
69. Sønksen J, Fode M, Löchner-Ernst D, Ohl DA. Vibratory ejaculation in 140 spinal cord injured men and home insemination of their partners. Spinal Cord. 2012;50(1):63-6.
70. Balaban B, Urman B, Sertac A, Alatas C, Aksoy S, Mercan R. Blastocyst quality affects the success of blastocyst-stage embryo transfer. Fertil Steril. 2000;74(2):282-7
71. Sønksen J, Sommer P, Biering-Sørensen F, Ziebe S, Lindhard A, Loft A, et al. Pregnancy after assisted ejaculation procedures in men with spinal cord injury. Arch Phys Med Rehab. 1997; 78(10):1059-61.
72. Taylor Z, Molloy D, Hill V, Harrison K. Contribution of the assisted reproductive technologies to fertility in males suffering spinal cord injury. Aust N Z J Obstet Gynaecol. 1999;39(1):84-7.
73. Padron OF, Brackett NL, Weizman MS, Lynne CM. Semen of spinal cord injured men freezes reliably. J Androl. 1994;15(3):266-9.

CHAPTER

32 Algorithms for Genetic Evaluation of Infertile Males

Stacy Colaco, Deepak Modi

INTRODUCTION

Male infertility is most commonly caused by problems in the ejection of semen, absence of sperm or low sperm count, or abnormal shape (morphology) and movement (motility) of the sperm. The causes of male infertility include endocrine defects leading to hypogonadism, primary testicular defects, and post-testicular defects such as the absence of vas deferens. Genetic defects are reported in all forms of male fertility, and more than 200 genetic conditions are associated with male infertility. The genetic defects seen in infertile males are karyotype abnormalities, Y chromosome microdeletions, gene copy number variations, gene duplications, mutations, and polymorphisms. These genetic defects interfere with the development of the male gonads and the urogenital tract, cause degeneration of the germ cells, lead to arrest in spermatogenesis due to faulty meiosis or lead to the production of nonfunctional spermatozoa including defects in the flagella.

Irrespective of their clinical history, infertile men need to undergo genetic testing. Men with nonobstructive azoospermia (NOA) or oligozoospermia will require to undergo karyotyping and Y chromosome microdeletion testing, while for those with obstructive azoospermia cystic fibrosis transmembrane conductance regulator (*CFTR*) gene testing is recommended. Beyond abnormal sperm count, motility, and sperm head morphology defects, a condition termed multiple morphological abnormalities of the sperm flagella (MMAF) has been characterized. Men with MMAF have morphological abnormalities of the flagellum such as coiled, bent, irregular, short, or/and absent flagella. In MMAF, mutations in a set of autosomal genes are reported. Along with mutations in several autosomal genes, gene copy numbers, variations, deletions, and mutations in different autosomal genes and mitochondrial deoxyribonucleic acid (mtDNA) are reported in men with an abnormal seminogram.[1] However, most of these tests are in the research phase, and their applications in a clinical setup are restricted. **Table 1** provides the genetic tests to be offered to infertile males based on semen parameters.

TABLE 1: Genetic tests to be offered to infertile males.

Diagnosis	*Genetic testing to be done*
Nonobstructive azoospermia	Karyotyping and Y chromosome microdeletions
Obstructive azoospermia	CFTR gene mutation
Oligozoospermia	Karyotyping and Y chromosome microdeletions
Azoospermia and oligozoospermia with normal karyotype and no Y chromosome microdeletions	Exome analysis
Multiple morphological abnormalities of the sperm flagella (MMAF)	Panel for DNAH1, CFAP43, CFAP44, and CFAP69 genes or exome analysis
Asthenozoospermia	Exome analysis

(CFTR: cystic fibrosis transmembrane conductance regulator)

PRACTICAL APPROACH FOR GENETIC TESTING FOR INFERTILE MALES AND ITS APPLICATIONS IN CLINICAL PRACTICE

As per the clinical history and semen parameters, appropriate tests should be offered to infertile men **(Table 1)**. Clinical decisions can be made based on the results of these tests and as per the algorithms described below.

Nonobstructive Azoospermia and Oligozoospermia

Patients with azoospermia (absent or very few sperm in semen) must be thoroughly examined to be classified as obstructive or nonobstructive type. A differential diagnosis of these two conditions requires a thorough clinical examination of the presence or absence of vas deferens (see below). Along with clinical examination, serum follicle-stimulating hormone (FSH) is elevated in a subset of men with

Flowchart 1: Algorithm for genetic testing in men with nonobstructive azoospermia, oligozoopsermia, multiple morphological abnormalities of sperm flagella (MMAF).

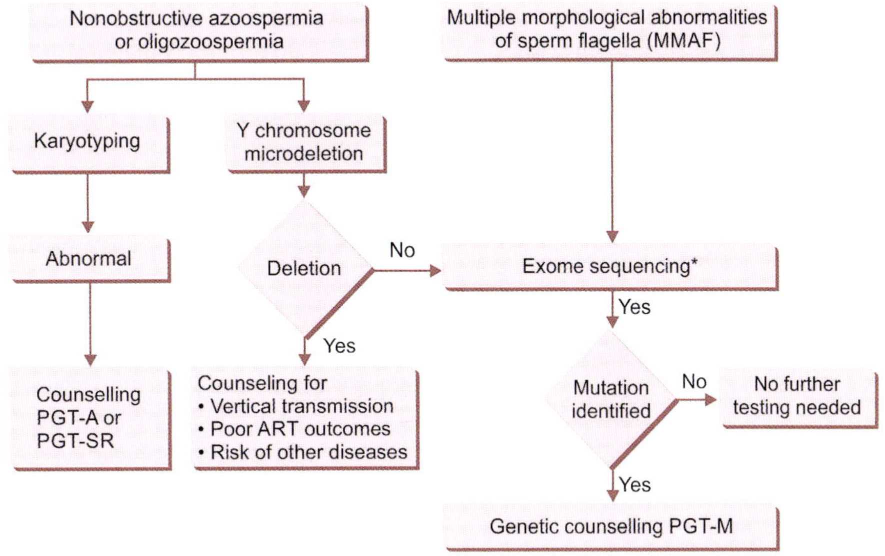

Mutations, *Still in research phase

(PGT-M: preimplantation genetic testing for mutations; PGT-A: preimplantation genetic testing for aneuploidies; PGT-SR: preimplantation genetic testing for structural rearrangements; ART: assisted reproductive technologies)

NOA and can be used as a guiding tool. However, not all men with NOA will have elevated FSH, and clinical examination is the only reliable method of diagnosis. Once the diagnosis of NOA or oligozoospermia is established, karyotyping and Y chromosome microdeletion testing are recommended. The algorithm for the same is given in **Flowchart 1**.

About 10–15% of men with NOA or oligozoospermia will have karyotype abnormalities. These will include mosaic or nonmosaic 47,XXY karyotype (Klinefelter syndrome), 45,X/46,XY mosaic, and 46,XX syndrome (de la Chapelle syndrome). Structural abnormalities include Robertsonian translocations, inversions, ring Y, truncated Y, or isodicentric Y. It must be remembered that polymorphic variants of certain chromosomes (commonly chromosomes 1, 9, 16, or Y) are often reported in karyotyping; these should be considered as normal variations and should not be considered as a genetic cause. A geneticist must be consulted to understand the prognosis and decide the course of action. Except in the case of 46,XX phenotypic males, there is a good possibility of obtaining sperm after testicular sperm aspiration (TESA). These sperm can be used in intracytoplasmic sperm injection (ICSI); however, the success rates of ICSI are quite low. TESA need not be performed in XX males as there is no chance of even focal spermatogenesis due to the absence of any of the genes required for spermatogenesis.

In couples where karyotype abnormalities are detected, a proportion of embryos are aneuploid and will result in implantation failure or miscarriage. In such couples, preimplantation genetic testing (PGT) for aneuploidy (PGT-A) or PGT for structural rearrangements (PGT-SR) is recommended to identify euploid embryos **(Flowchart 1)**. This should increase the chance of a successful pregnancy.

The European Academy of Andrology (EAA), American Society for Reproductive Medicine (ASRM), and Indian Council of Medical Research (ICMR) recommend testing for the Y chromosome microdeletions in all men with NOA and oligozoospermia. The Y chromosome microdeletions cannot be identified by standard karyotyping methods and need polymerase chain reaction (PCR) techniques. These microdeletions cause the removal of one or more azoospermia factor (AZF) loci on the long arm of the Y chromosome. There are three AZF loci on the Y chromosome, namely AZFa, AZFb, and AZFc. These loci are rich in genes required for spermatogenesis, and deletions in these regions cause azoospermia or oligozoospermia.[2] Another type of microdeletion called the AZFc sub-deletions, i.e., gr/gr, b1/b3, and b2/b3, are also associated with infertility. In the Indian population, the gr/gr deletions are found at a higher frequency in infertile males,[2,3] and hence, testing for gr/gr deletion as a part of Y chromosome microdeletions testing is imperative.

Y chromosome microdeletion testing is done by PCR and it requires a panel of sequence-tagged site (STS) markers to be used for accurate diagnosis. However, different laboratories use different numbers and types of STS markers. It must be borne in mind that the STS markers recommended by the EAA are not sufficient in all populations and there are reports of misdiagnosis.[4] Hence, clinicians must insist on Y chromosome microdeletion testing using the appropriate markers for their population.

The results of the Y chromosome microdeletion testing should aid clinicians in deciding management modalities, deciding to offer assisted reproduction, appropriate counseling, and predicting future risks of other diseases.[2,5]

Deciding Management Modalities

Various treatment modalities such as hormonal therapies and/or antioxidant supplementation, lifestyle changes, or surgery to treat varicocele are offered to men with low sperm count and motility in order to improve the seminogram. Although some men (mainly with oligozoospermia) show a marked improvement in semen quality, men with Y chromosome microdeletions will not respond to such treatment. Therefore, men with Y chromosome microdeletions should not be subjected to medical treatments to improve sperm count and motility.

Decision to Offer Assisted Reproduction

In general, men with AZFa and AZFb deletions will rarely have sperm in their testis, while AZFc-deleted men would have hypospermatogenesis.[4] Thus, TESA may be avoided in men with AZFa or AZFb microdeletions. In men with AZFc deletions, there is a good chance of focal spermatogenesis, and hence TESA can be considered for biological parenthood.

However, irrespective of the type of microdeletions, the embryos derived from sperm of men with Y chromosome microdeletions are poor in quality and have impaired blastocyst rate and result in lower overall success of assisted reproductive technology (ART).[2,3] Thus, patients with Y chromosome microdeletions must be appropriately counseled about the low success rates.

Counseling for Vertical Transmission of the Genetic Defects in the Family and Perpetuating Infertility

While men with Y chromosome microdeletions (especially AZFc deletion) can father a child via ICSI, all male offspring will inherit the paternal deletion and, in turn, will also be infertile. Thus, in men with Y chromosome microdeletion, the couple and the clinician must make an informed choice of having biological parenthood at the risk of perpetuating infertility in the family.

Risk of Other Diseases

With increased biomedical research, the role of the Y chromosome beyond the regulation of fertility is emerging. Studies show that the presence of Y chromosome microdeletions predisposes men to the development of testicular germ cell tumors.[2] Other studies have described instances where men with Y chromosome microdeletions have mild to severe neuropsychiatric disorders with increasing age.[5] The loss of the Y chromosome is associated with a spectrum of disorders such as the increased risk of heart failure, age-related macular degeneration,[6] and colorectal/prostate cancer.[6-8] Although these reports are preliminary, genetic counseling may be offered and regular checkups can be recommended for timely diagnosis of these life-threatening conditions.

Beyond karyotype and Y chromosome microdeletions, men with azoospermia and oligozoospermia have mutations in other autosomal genes, X chromosome genes, and in the mitochondrial genome.[1,9] Testing for these requires specific technologies such as exome sequencing or mtDNA sequencing to identify defects. While data from studies exploring these conditions look promising, the involvement is at best associative and the cause–effect relation is yet not conclusively established in most cases. Hence, these tests are not recommended to be offered routinely in a clinical setup but may be considered in research/academic applications.

Obstructive Azoospermia

Men with obstructive azoospermia have blocked flow in the male ductal system due to absence of vas deferens but have normal spermatogenesis. There are five phenotypes associated with obstructive azoospermia. These include (1) congenital bilateral absence of the vas deferens (CBAVD) with normal kidneys, (2) CBAVD with unilateral renal anomalies (CBAVD-URA), (3) congenital unilateral absence of the vas deferens (CUAVD), (4) CUAVD-URA, and (5) CBAVD/CUAVD with ejaculatory duct obstruction.[1] For differential diagnosis of obstructive and NOA, the presence of the vas deferens and the characteristics of the epididymis should always be determined. Patients with NOA typically have palpable vasa deferentia and flat and firm epididymis, whereas in obstructive azoospermia, the vasa is non-palpable and the epididymis is soft. As CBAVD may occur concurrent to unilateral renal agenesis, these men should undergo an ultrasound scan to uncover this potentially health-threatening condition. In contrast, most patients (~60%) with CUAVD are nonazoospermic. The algorithm to be followed for men with obstructive azoospermia is shown in **Flowchart 2**.

CFTR gene mutations are observed in 60–70% of men with CBAVD.[10] These are also detected in patients with cystic fibrosis; however, 30–40% of cases may have a genetic etiology other than *CFTR*. Two types of *CFTR* mutations are reported in men with CBAVD: the severe mutations that result in absence/inadequate amount or poorly functional *CFTR* protein and the mild mutations where a CFTR protein with sufficient residual *CFTR* activity is produced. If a patient has two severe mutations, he will have cystic fibrosis. Almost 90% of men with CBAVD have one mild and one severe *CFTR* mutation, while two mild *CFTR* mutations are reported in 10% of cases with CBAVD. F508del *CFTR* gene mutation is the most commonly reported defect in Caucasian men with CBAVD, while IVS-9 c.1210-12 is a commonly reported

Flowchart 2: Algorithm for genetic testing in men with obstructive azoospermia.

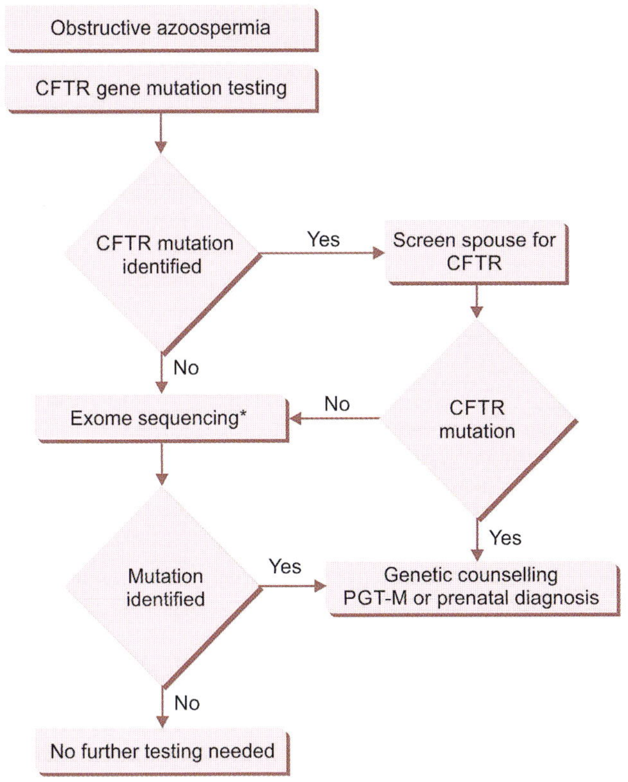

*Still in research phase

(PGT-M: preimplantation genetic testing for mutations; CFTR: cystic fibrosis transmembrane conductance regulator)

CFTR variant in non-Caucasian men with CBAVD.[10] Several other mutations are also observed in the *CFTR* gene, and there is a need for sequencing the entire gene and not just screening for the frequently reported mutations. In CBAVD men without *CFTR* gene mutations, pathogenic variants in the *ADGRG2*, *PANK2*, *SCNN1B*, and *CA12* genes are reported.[11] The functional significance of these mutations or how these genes cause CBAVD is yet not understood, and hence testing for these mutations is not applied in routine clinical use.

In men with *CFTR* gene mutation, there is active spermatogenesis and good-quality sperm can be retrieved. Thus, TESA–ICSI can be offered for biological parenthood in men with CBAVD. While having the mutation in the male partner alone will have no consequence, if the female partner is also a carrier for *CFTR* gene mutations (females are usually phenotypically silent), there is a high-risk cystic fibrosis in the offspring. Thus, it is mandatory that testing for the *CFTR* gene be performed on the female partner as well in such couples. If the female partner is a carrier for *CFTR* gene mutation, the couple should be counseled for the possible occurrence of CBAVD and cystic fibrosis in the offspring.

In the event of both partners having *CFTR* gene mutations, prenatal diagnosis or preimplantation genetic testing for monogenic disease (PGT-M) should be offered to prevent the birth of a child with cystic fibrosis. However, if the female partner has a normal *CFTR* gene, embryonic/prenatal testing is not mandatory. In the event of *CFTR* gene mutations not being identified, the couple may be tested via exome sequencing to identify rare mutations and appropriate genetic counseling followed by PGT-M may be offered in such cases **(Flowchart 2)**. Exome analysis in men with obstructive azoospermia is still in the research phase and must be applied with caution.

MULTIPLE MORPHOLOGICAL ABNORMALITIES OF THE SPERM FLAGELLA

Multiple morphological abnormalities of the sperm flagella are diagnosed in a semen sample as total asthenozoospermia with different sperm flagellar anomalies. These anomalies may be absent, short, irregular shaped, and/or angulated flagella. The current World Health Organization manual does not provide any classification for MMAF based on semen analyses, and hence MMAF will not be obtained in a diagnostic report. However, such patients are very likely to have genetic defects. The algorithm to be followed in men with MMAF is shown in **Flowchart 1**.

With the advent of the whole exome and genome analysis, mutations in many genes associated with flagella development or functions have been identified. In men with MMAF, mutations in the *DNAH1*, *CFAP43*, *CFAP44*, and *CFAP69* genes have been reported.[12] Presently, the detection of these mutations requires whole-exome sequencing and this is not feasible in a clinical laboratory. A network of molecular genetic laboratories and counselors will be required to offer genetic screening for MMAF in infertile males. However, it must be remembered that these genes account for only 30% of patients with MMAF and the cause in others is still unknown.

As men with MMAF have impaired sperm motility, medicinal therapies will not improve semen parameters making ICSI the only treatment option. There are limited reports on ICSI outcomes of men with MMAF. In general, in men with MMAF, rather than using immotile ejaculated sperm, testicular sperm is recommended for ICSI. The outcomes of ICSI suggest that the fertilization rates are relatively low (40–75%) and clinical pregnancy rates are almost 50%.[13] Thus, males with MMAF resulting from genetic defects are likely to experience disappointing outcomes in assisted reproduction.

In men with MMAF, mutations occur in the autosomal genes that are also functional in other tissues where ciliary/flagellar activity is required (like lungs and brain); there is a risk of the development of other defects apart from the sperm morphological defects. To date, there is no information on the health outcomes of offspring of men with MMAF due to genetic defects. Therefore, genetic counseling and PGT-M are a must for MMAF patients when ICSI is utilized **(Flowchart 1)**. However, the utility of gene mutation testing in MMAF is in its infancy, and extensive research in different populations is required to decide on its routine clinical use.

CONCLUSION

With a clear-cut cause–effect relationship between impaired spermatogenesis and abnormal karyotype or Y chromosome microdeletions, their testing is mandatory in clinical practice. The detection of *CFTR* mutations is recommended in men with obstructive azoospermia. These tests will not only allow the determination of the exact cause of male infertility but also aid in predicting the success rates of ART and offering PGT. Further, the infertile couples need to be aware that they will transmit their genetic defect to their future generations and may additionally also perpetuate other diseases along with infertility. With the proper implementation of androgenetic, the clinician and the patients will be able to decide on the appropriate and timely management of infertility.

ACKNOWLEDGMENTS

Stacy Colaco is thankful to the Department of Health Research for the Young Scientist Fellowship and the DM lab is supported by grants from ICMR. The manuscript bears the NIRRH ID: OTH/1291/08-2022.

REFERENCES

1. Sudhakar DVS, Shah R, Gajbhiye RK. Genetics of male infertility—present and future: a narrative review. J Hum Reprod Sci. 2021;14(3):217-27.
2. Colaco S, Modi D. Genetics of the human Y chromosome and its association with male infertility. Reprod Biol Endocrinol. 2018;16(1):14.
3. Sen S, Ambulkar P, Hinduja I, Zaveri K, Gokral J, Pal A, et al. Susceptibility of gr/gr rearrangements to azoospermia or oligozoospermia is dependent on DAZ and CDY1 gene copy deletions. J Assist Reprod Genet. 2015;32(9):1333-41.
4. Sen S, Pasi AR, Dada R, Shamsi MB, Modi D. Y chromosome microdeletions in infertile men: prevalence, phenotypes and screening markers for the Indian population. J Assist Reprod Genet. 2013;30(3):413-22.
5. Colaco S, Modi D. Consequences of Y chromosome microdeletions beyond male infertility. J Assist Reprod Genet. 2019;36(7):1329-37.
6. Duan Q, Gao Y, Cao X, Wang S, Xu M, Jones OD, et al. Mosaic loss of chromosome Y in peripheral blood cells is associated with age-related macular degeneration in men. Cell Biosci. 2022;12(1):73.
7. Sano S, Horitani K, Ogawa H, Halvardson J, Chavkin NW, Wang Y, et al. Hematopoietic loss of Y chromosome leads to cardiac fibrosis and heart failure mortality. Science. 2022;377(6603):292-7.
8. Fukami M, Miyado M. Mosaic loss of the Y chromosome and men's health. Reprod Med Biol. 2022;21(1):e12445.
9. Amor H, Hammadeh ME. A systematic review of the impact of mitochondrial variations on male infertility. Genes (Basel). 2022;13(7):1182.
10. Gaikwad A, Khan S, Kadam S, Shah R, Kulkarni V, Kumaraswamy R, et al. Cystic fibrosis transmembrane conductance regulator-related male infertility: relevance of genetic testing & counselling in Indian population. Indian J Med Res. 2020;152(6):575-83.
11. Cai Z, Li H. Congenital bilateral absence of the vas deferens. Front Genet. 2022;13:775123.
12. Wang WL, Tu CF, Tan YQ. Insight on multiple morphological abnormalities of sperm flagella in male infertility: what is new? Asian J Androl. 2020;22(3):236-45.
13. Sha YW, Xu X, Mei LB, Li P, Su ZY, He XQ, et al. A homozygous CEP135 mutation is associated with multiple morphological abnormalities of the sperm flagella (MMAF). Gene. 2017;633:48-53.

SECTION

5 Female Factor Infertility

CHAPTER 33

Uterine Factors in Infertility

Mala Arora, Mahesh Koregol, Soumya Mahesh Koregol, Navya N

INTRODUCTION

Around 1 in 500 reproductive age women is affected by uterine factor infertility (UFI).[1,2] Success in assisted reproductive techniques (ART) cycle involves transferring a good quality embryo atraumatically at the right time into a receptive endometrium for implantation. A healthy uterus is crucial in allowing a woman to achieve pregnancy and carry it to term successfully. Any structural and functional abnormalities of the uterus will affect success rates of both spontaneous and ART conception. When a patient first presents for evaluation of infertility, the uterine factors have to be assessed. Uterine factors encountered can be congenital or acquired. In this chapter we shall elaborate on the following conditions of the uterus:

- Congenital uterine anomalies (CUAs)/Müllerian anomalies
- Myomas
- Adenomyosis
- Intrauterine adhesions or polyps or foreign bodies
- Chronic endometritis (CE).

CONGENITAL UTERINE ANOMALIES

Congenital anomalies of the female reproductive tract may involve uterus, cervix, fallopian tubes, or vagina.[3] Cruveilhier and von Rokitansky first described uterine anomalies in the 1800s.[4] The prevalence of CUAs in general population is around 4.3–6.7% while the prevalence in the infertile population is around 3–13%. In patients with recurrent miscarriages, the CUAs are as high as 12.6–18.2%.[5] As reproductive medicine specialists, we are more likely to encounter not only infertile population but also those with recurrent first and second trimester losses. Therefore, we should have a high suspicion when assessing our cohort of patients right from the initial evaluation. It is prudent to make an accurate diagnosis as each anomaly has differing reproductive outcomes and treatment approaches.[5] Karyotypes are normal (46XX) in majority (92%) of women with Müllerian anomalies and abnormal in 7.7% of these women.[6,7]

Embryology of the Female Reproductive Tract and Etiology of Müllerian Anomalies

The development of the female gonads and the Müllerian system are separate processes. Women with Müllerian developmental anomalies will often have normal functioning ovaries and female hormones. The uterus and the fallopian tubes are developmentally derived from the paramesonephric (Müllerian) ducts, which arise lateral to the mesonephric (Wolffian) ducts from the coelomic epithelium of the urogenital ridge **(Fig. 1)**. This begins at around seventh week of intrauterine development. The paramesonephric ducts grow downward across the mesonephric duct to fuse in the midline to form the uterovaginal canal. The lower end of the uterovaginal canal connects with the urogenital sinus. Finally, the fused Müllerian ducts are canalized internally forming two channels separated by a septum. This septum is resorbed around 20 weeks in a caudal toward the cephalad direction. The uterus and the upper vagina are derived from the caudal portion of the Müllerian ducts. The upper portion becomes the fallopian tubes. The lower vagina is derived from the urogenital sinus and the sinovaginal bulb.[3]

Normal development of the Müllerian ducts depends on the completion of three phases:

- Organogenesis
- Fusion
- Septal resorption

Organogenesis leads to the formation of both Müllerian ducts. Failure of this results in uterine agenesis or hypoplasia

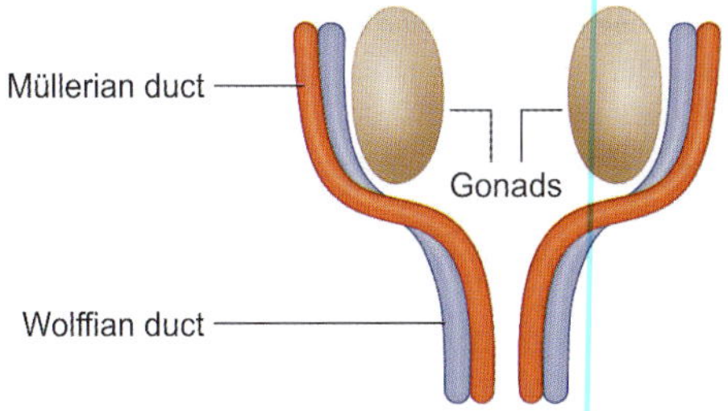

Fig. 1: Embryology of the female reproductive duct.

or a unicornuate uterus. Fusion of the ducts leads to formation of the normal uterus. Failure of this results in a bicornuate or didelphic uterus. Septal resorption defects result in a septate or arcuate uterus.[8] The etiology behind this failure is unknown and there have been no genetic linkages identified.[9]

Classification of Congenital Uterine Anomalies

Classification plays an important role in communicating diagnoses between clinicians (gynecologists, radiologists, etc.) and their patients. The very recent American Society of Reproductive Medicine (ASRM) 2021 and the European Society of Human Reproduction and Endocrinology/European Society of Gynecological Endoscopy (ESHRE/ESGE) consensus[9] (CONUTA—CONgenital UTerine Anomalies) classification 2013 (reaffirmed in 2016) are the two most important classifications currently.

American Society of Reproductive Medicine Müllerian Anomalies Classification 2021 (also referred to as MAC 2021)—What is New in This Classification?[10]

The old American Fertility Society (AFS) classification was only for the uterine anomalies, but this new one added the cervical and vaginal anomalies. The old AFS classification was no definite criteria whereas this new one has added clear measurements for each subtype type. The old one is not suitable for complex anomalies but the new one is suitable. Unlike the AFS classification, anomaly categories are no longer numbered but instead are identified by descriptive terminology **(Box 1 and Fig. 2)**.

ESHRE/ESGE Classification System (2013, 2016)

European Society of Human Reproduction and Endocrinology/European Society of Gynecological Endoscopy classifies female genital tract anomalies into the main classification for the uterine body (U) and supplemental classification for the cervix (C) and vagina (V).

The schematic and the diagrammatic representations of the classifications have been discussed in **Figures 3 to 5**.

So there are several thoughts from the various international societies regarding the classification of Müllerian anomalies. However, which of these methods is better is a moot point. Ludwin et al.[11] were of the opinion that application of the CONUTA classification leads to unnecessary overdiagnosis of septate uterus which will be elaborated later in the chapter.

BOX 1: American Society of Reproductive Medicine (ASRM) classification of mullerian anomalies 2021.

- Müllerian agenesis
- Cervical agenesis
- Unicornuate uterus
- Uterus didelphys
- Bicornuate uterus
- Septate uterus
- Longitudinal vaginal septum
- Transverse vaginal septum
- Complex anomalies

Clinical Presentation and Diagnostic Modalities

Most women are asymptomatic. Women may present with cyclic or noncyclic pelvic pain and dysmenorrhea suggestive of an obstructive anomaly, retrograde menstruation, and endometriosis.[9] Patients may present with primary amenorrhea as in the case of Müllerian agenesis or Mayer–Rokitansky–Küster–Hauser (MRKH) syndrome which involves congenital absence of the uterus and vagina (ASRM-Müllerian agenesis, CONUTA-U5b). Patients with septate uterus and uterus didelphys may present with abnormal uterine bleeding (AUB) because of the increased surface area of the endometrium and also in a longitudinal vaginal septum when only one tampon is used while two are required because of the two separate tracks. Endometriosis are more common in patients with congenital anomalies probably due to obstruction and retrograde menstruation which may also lead to infertility.[12]

Hysterosalpingography (HSG) helps in the assessment of uterine cavities and tubes, but it is limited by the nonvisualization of the external contour of the uterus.[13] The gold standard diagnostic modality for CUA is magnetic resonance imaging (MRI). 3D ultrasonography (USG), being noninvasive and better than 2D USG, has the potential to surpass MRI.[14,15]

Reproductive Outcomes

In an elaborate systematic review and meta-analysis, Venetis et al.[6] concluded that the presence of CUA is associated with a decreased, albeit not significantly so, probability of pregnancy achievement both in natural and ART cycles.

Women with a septated or bicornuate uterus had a higher probability of spontaneous miscarriage even in the first trimester, whereas in women with arcuate, didelphys, and unicornuate uterus the effect on reproduction is small and not statistically significant. Women with CUA are at increased risk of preterm birth and second trimester losses, which are the hallmark of all types of CUA. The implantation failure, spontaneous abortion, and impaired obstetrical outcome could be due to impaired vascularization of the endometrium, abnormal uterine contractility, and decreased uterine volume.[6]

Management

Management of the CUA depends on the type of the abnormality present and the obstetric goals of a patient. **Table 1** summarizes the treatment approach.[5]

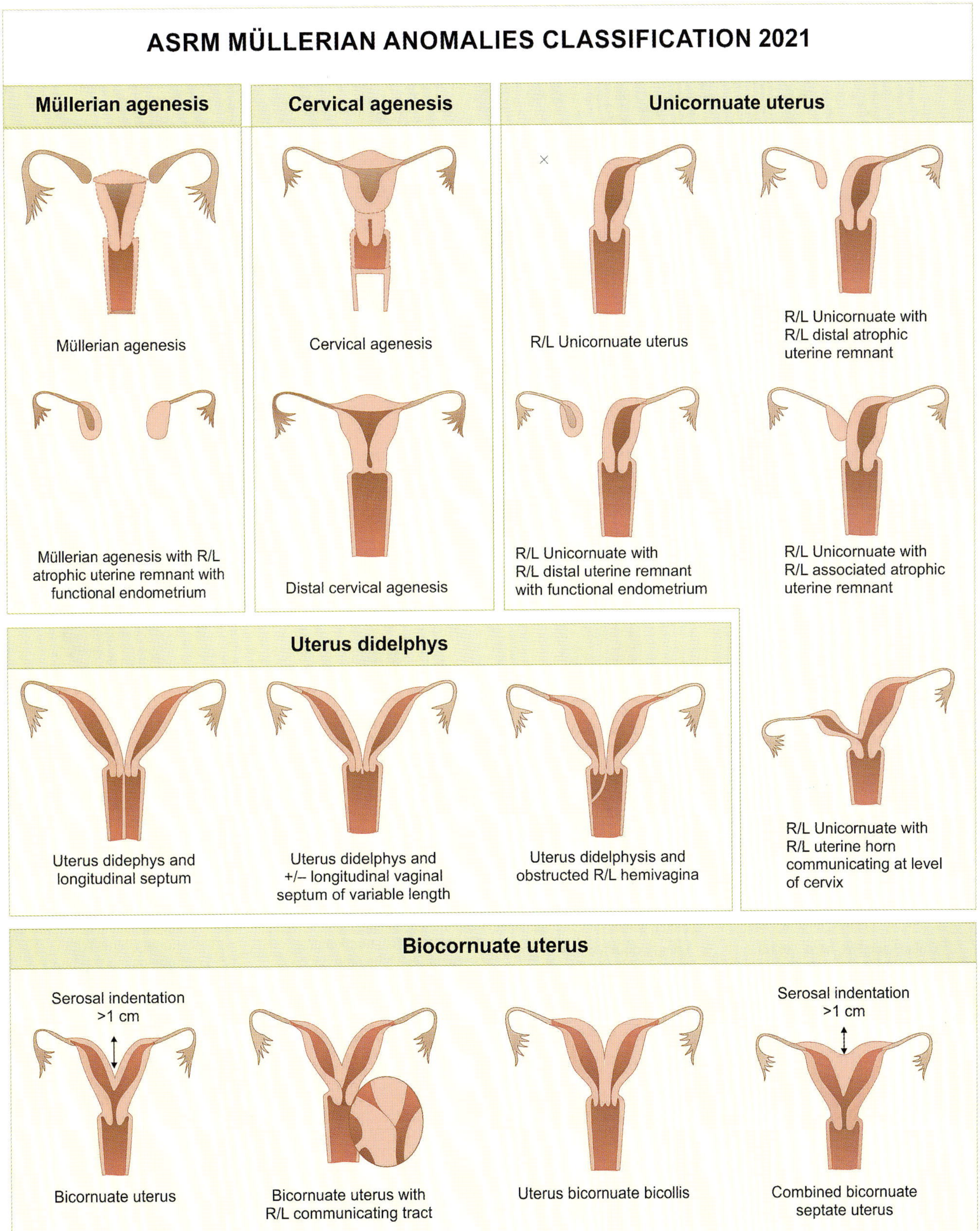
ASRM MÜLLERIAN ANOMALIES CLASSIFICATION 2021
Müllerian agenesis
Müllerian agenesis
Müllerian agenesis with R/L atrophic uterine remnant with functional endometrium
Cervical agenesis
Cervical agenesis
Distal cervical agenesis
Unicornuate uterus
R/L Unicornuate uterus
R/L Unicornuate with R/L distal atrophic uterine remnant
R/L Unicornuate with R/L distal uterine remnant with functional endometrium
R/L Unicornuate with R/L associated atrophic uterine remnant
R/L Unicornuate with R/L uterine horn communicating at level of cervix
Uterus didelphys
Uterus didephys and longitudinal septum
Uterus didelphys and +/– longitudinal vaginal septum of variable length
Uterus didelphysis and obstructed R/L hemivagina
Biocornuate uterus
Serosal indentation >1 cm
Bicornuate uterus
Bicornuate uterus with R/L communicating tract
Uterus bicornuate bicollis
Serosal indentation >1 cm
Combined bicornuate septate uterus

Contd...

Contd...

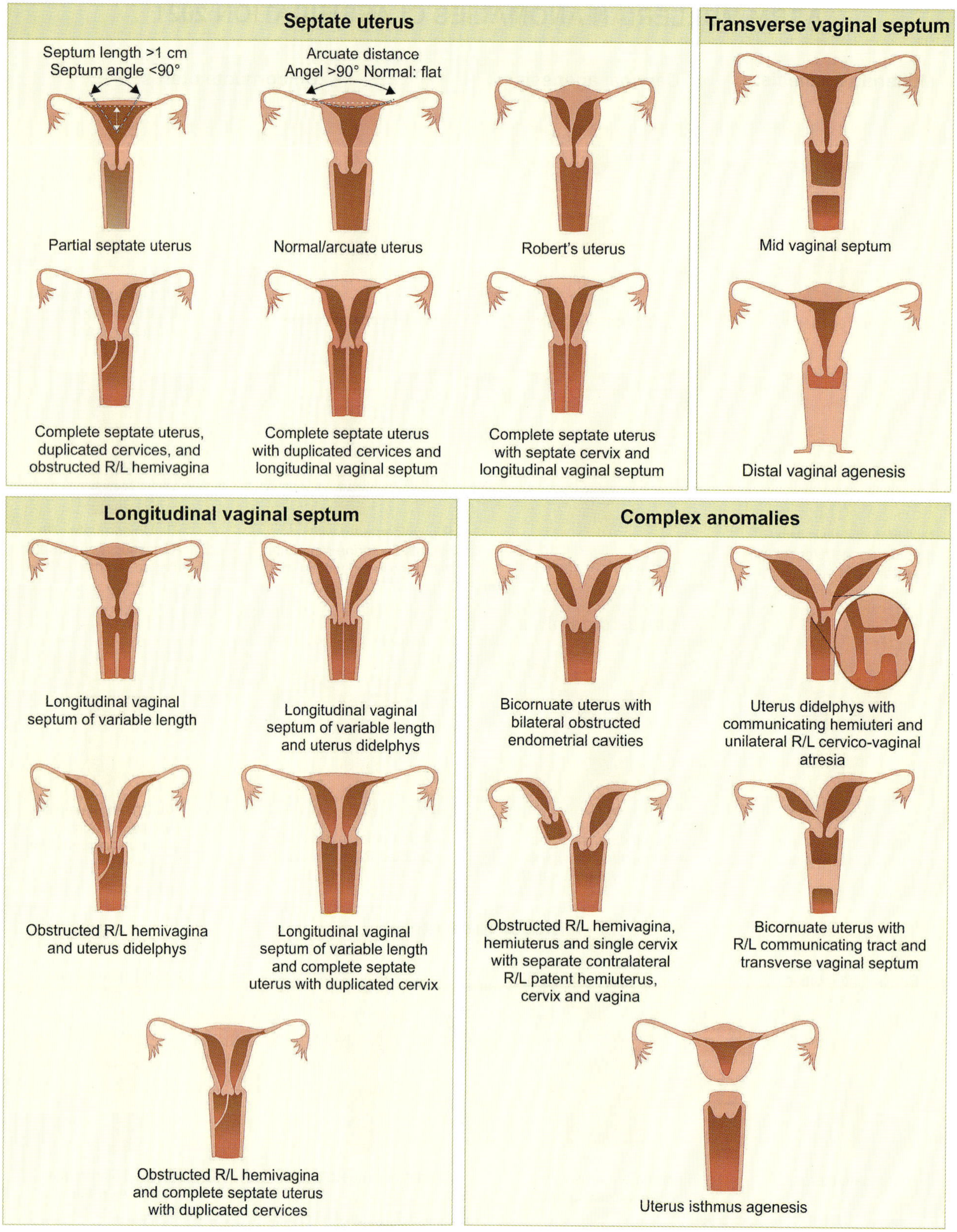

Fig. 2: ASRM classification of Müllerian anomalies.

ESHRE/ESGE classification
Female genital tract anomalies

Name .... **Birth Date:** ....

Diagnostic Method:

	Uterine anomaly		Cervical/vaginal anomaly	
	Main class	*Sub-class*	*Co-existent class*	
U0	Normal uterus		*C0*	*Normal cervix*
U1	Dysmorphic uterus	**a.** T-shaped **b.** Infantilis **c.** Others	*C1*	*Septate cervix*
			C2	*Double 'normal' cervix*
U2	Septate uterus	**a.** Partial **b.** Complete	*C3*	*Unilateral cervical aplasia*
			C4	*Cervical aplasia*
U3	Bicorporeal uterus	**a.** Partial **b.** Complete **c.** Bicorporeal septate	*V0*	*Normal vagina*
U4	Hemi-uterus	**a.** With rudimentary cavity (communicating or not horn) **b.** Without rudimentary cavity (horn without cavity/no horn)	*V1*	*Longitudinal non-obstructing vaginal septum*
			V2	*Longitudinal obstructing vaginal septum*
U5	Aplastic	**a.** With rudimentary cavity (bi- or unilateral horn) **b.** Without rudimentary cavity (bi- or unilateral uterine remnants/aplasia)	*V3*	*Transverse vaginal septum and/or imperforate hymen*
			V4	*Vaginal aplasia*
U6	Unclassified malformations			
U			*C*	*V*

Associated anomalies of non-Müllerian origin:

Fig. 3: Classification of female genital tract anomalies.

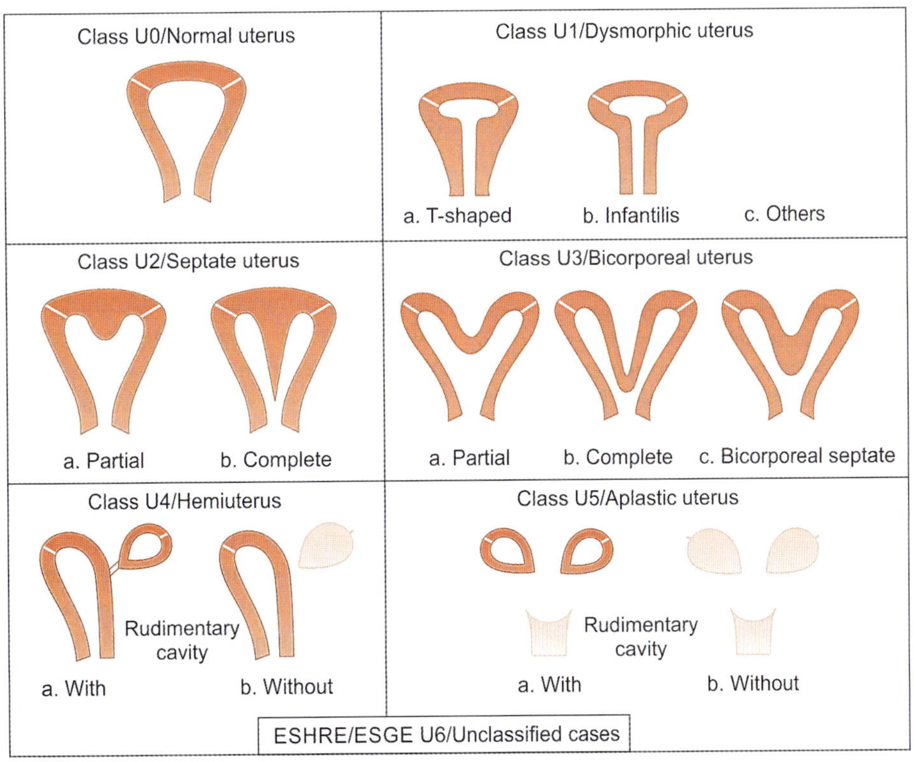

Fig. 4: European Society of Human Reproduction and Endocrinology/European Society of Gynecological Endoscopy (ESHRE/ESGE) classes of female genital tract anomalies.

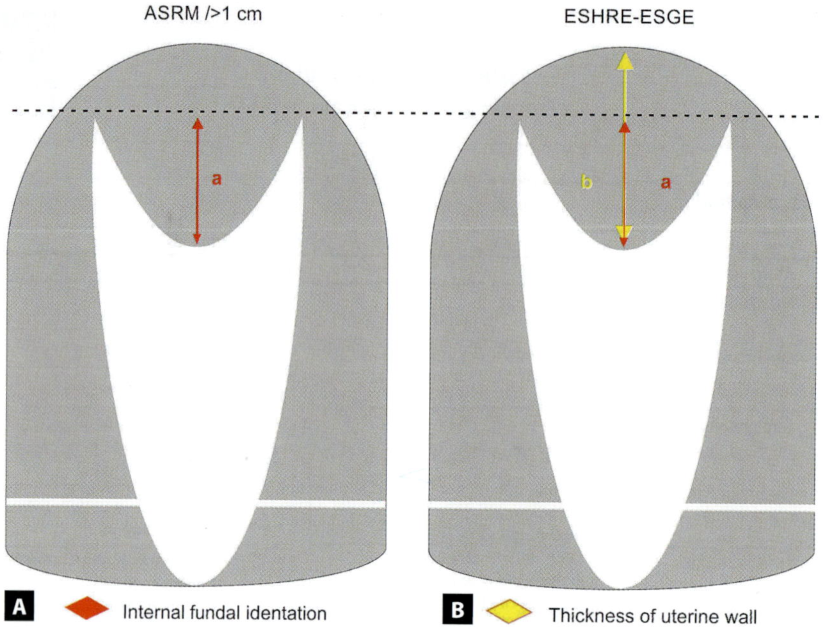

Figs. 5A and B: (A) American Society for Reproductive Medicine (ASRM) recommended considering a uterus as septate when there is both an indentation depth >10 mm and an indentation angle <90°, while a normal/arcuate uterus should have both an indentation depth <10 mm and an indentation angle >90°, and a uterus that does not fit these criteria would be left in an unclassifiable 'gray-zone'; (B) European Society for Gynecological Endoscopy (ESGE) recommended using an indentation-to-wall-thickness (I:WT) ratio >50% to diagnose septate uterus. Over diagnosis of uterine septum (50% of the septum is 4–5 mm if the myometrial wall thickness for example is 8 mm so if you measure the internal fundal indentaion more than 4 mm it will be considered as septum by the ESHRE/ESGE classfication.
(ASRM: American Society of Reproductive Medicine; ESHRE-ESGE: European Society of Human Reproduction and Endocrinology-European Society of Gynecological Endoscopy)

TABLE 1: Management of congenital uterine anomalies.

	Management
Müllerian agenesis	In vitro fertilization (IVF) of harvested ova and surrogacy
Unicornuate uterus: • Noncommunicating, cavitary horn • Noncommunicating, noncavitary horn • Communicating, cavitary horn • No horn	1. Always surgically resected, as it is associated with dysmenorrhea, hematometra, endometriosis, and ectopic pregnancy. 2. Surgery not currently recommended. No complications of endometriosis, etc., as there is no endometrium. 3. Also, surgically removed because pregnancy that implants in the rudimentary horn rarely is viable. 4. No treatment. Reproductive potential is possible.
Uterus didelphys	May consider metroplasty; however not usually advised, full term pregnancies have occurred
Bicornuate	Surgical intervention rarely needed; may consider metroplasty

In case of MRKH syndrome, apart from the fertility management, one has to consider the restoration of the vaginal anatomy and sexual function on priority. Emphasis should be placed here about the need for psycho-socio-sexual counseling, especially in cases of complete Müllerian agenesis.[16]

Mayer–Rokitansky–Küster–Hauser Syndrome

Serial Frank's dilators can be used for the creation of the neovagina without any surgery. The self-dilation to create a neovagina involves patients manually placing successive dilators on the vaginal dimple for 30 minutes to 2 hours per day. Alternatively, a bicycle seat stool can provide perineal pressure while allowing the patient to participate in other activities. A number of surgical techniques can be used to create a neovagina. The modified Abbè-McIndoe operation is the most common surgical procedure used to create a neovagina. This procedure involves the dissection of a space between the rectum and bladder, placement of a mold covered with a split-thickness skin graft into the space, and the diligent use of vaginal dilation postoperatively.[16] The laparoscopic Vecchietti procedure is a modification of the open technique where a neovagina is created using continuous dilation with an external traction device that is temporarily affixed to the abdominal wall.[17,18]

Use of a syringe mold with a split skin graft over the mold ensures patency of the passage.[18] Laparoscopic creation of a neovagina using an ileal loop has the advantage of providing adequate lubrication which is absent with the skin graft.[19]

Around 75–90% cases of a *bicornuate uterus* with rudimentary horn are noncommunicating. Literature suggests the need to remove the rudimentary horn through a laparoscopic approach.[20,21]

Bicornuate Uterus

When both the horns are equal in size and well developed, no further treatment is required. Most often one horn may be rudimentary and underdeveloped and the other of normal size. In such a scenario, conception is encouraged in the larger horn both at the time of ovarian stimulation and intrauterine insemination as well as embryo transfers. Another option is to place an intrauterine contraceptive device (IUCD) in the rudimentary horn to discourage implantation and subsequent pregnancy loss.[22]

In the event of a noncommunicating horn presenting as hematometra or pregnancy, evacuation of the horn should be followed by unification procedure or excision of that horn, whichever is feasible. Laparoscopic metroplasty is performed for recurrent poor reproductive outcomes.[23]

Septate Uterus

Diagnosis: The diagnosis depends on visualization of the external and internal contour of the uterus. The best diagnostic tool should be noninvasive, accurate, and inexpensive, and can evaluate the external and internal contour at the same time. HSG and hysteroscopy for example can evaluate the internal contour only. Laparoscopy can evaluate the external contour only. Combined laparoscopy and hysteroscopy can evaluate the external and internal contour but it is invasive and expensive.

Evaluation by 2D transvaginal ultrasound specially in the transverse plane with movement up and down from the fundus to the cervix can be used as a screening tool but not a diagnostic tool. Both MRI and 3DUS are adequate modalities for diagnosing women with Müllerian duct anomalies (MDAs) in trained hands. However, 3DUS is more sensitive and specific than MRI in categorizing some specific types of MDAs. The high sensitivity, specificity, and convenience of 3DUS makes it an ideal tool for identifying women with uterine anomalies. Hence, three-dimensional sonography has become the gold standard tool for the diagnosis of CUAs.

Uterine Septum

The ASRM 2021 criteria for diagnosis of the septum:[10] This new classification has changed the criteria for diagnosis of uterine septum from 1.5 cm in the ASRM guideline 2016 into more than 1 cm in the new 2021 classification **(Figs. 5A and B)**. ESGE recommended using an indentation-to-wall-thickness (I:WT) ratio >50% to diagnose septate uterus.[11] This may result in over diagnosis of uterine septum (50% of the septum is 4–5 mm if the myometrial wall thickness for example is 8 mm). So if you measure the internal fundal indentation >4 mm it will be considered as septum by the ESHRE/ESGE classification **(Figs. 5A and B)**. This is considered a limitation of the ESHRE/ESGE classification of uterine septum.[24]

Congenital Uterine Malformation by Experts (CUME) **(Figs. 6A to C)***:* For compiling a better criterion for distinguishing between normal/arcuate and septate uterus the following has been proposed:

- Indentation depth ≥10 mm
- Indentation angle <140°
- I:WT ratio >110%

They suggest using internal indentation depth ≥10 mm to distinguish between a normal/arcuate and a septate uterus, because it is the simplest and most reliable measurement of these three.[24]

Management: Incidentally diagnosed: treatment for incidentally diagnosed septum in infertile women is debatable and unproven [Royal College of Obstetricians and Gynaecologists (RCOG) Scientific Impact Paper November, 2019].

Uterine septum and miscarriage: This is what is mentioned in the ASRM 2016, ESHRE 2017, and RCOG 2019.

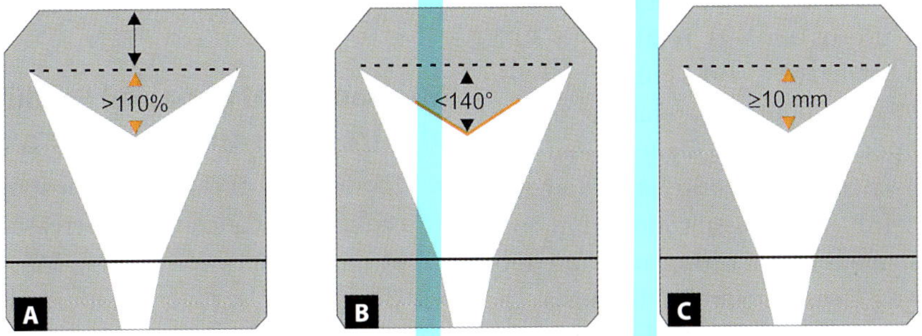

Figs. 6A to C: Congenital Uterine Malformation by Experts (CUME): Better criteria for distinguishing between normal/arcuateand septate uterus? The criteria are: (A) I:WT ratio >110%; (B) indentation angle <140°; (C) indentation depth ≥10 mm. They suggest using internal indentation depth ≥10 mm to distinguish between a normal/arcuate and a septate uterus, because it is the simplest and most reliable measurement of these three.

A meta-analysis evaluated the effect of CUAs on reproductive outcomes and found that septate uterus was noted to have a higher rate of first-trimester miscarriage when compared with controls [relative risk (RR): 2.65, 95% confidence interval (CI): 1.39–5.06]. ASRM guideline 2016 stated that there is fair evidence that a uterine septum contributes to miscarriage and preterm birth. Some limited studies indicate that hysteroscopic septum incision is associated with a reduction in subsequent miscarriage rates and improvement in live birth rates in patients with a history of recurrent pregnancy loss (RPL).[25]

A Cochrane review septate uterus could have no randomized controlled trials (RCTs) evaluating hysteroscopic metroplasty with expectant management in women with RPL.[26] Another meta-analysis which was not specific for RPL reported a significantly decreased risk of pregnancy loss in women who underwent hysteroscopic septotomy as compared to women who differed undergoing treatment (RR: 0.37; 95% CI: 0.25–0.55; $I^2 = 0\%$; five studies).[26]

European Society of Human Reproduction and Endocrinology guideline 2017 recommended that whether hysteroscopic septum resection has beneficial effects in improving live birth rates, and decreasing miscarriage rates, without doing harm needs further evaluation in the context of surgical trials in women with RPL and septate uterus.[27]

Royal College of Obstetricians and Gynaecologists Scientific Impact Paper 2019 has mentioned that high-quality evidence on the efficacy and safety of surgical treatment to improve reproductive in septate uterus outcomes is lacking. However, controlled studies have indicated that hysteroscopic septal division reduces miscarriage rates, resulting in improved live birth rates.[28] On this basis hysteroscopic resection of a uterine septum can be offered on an individualized basis for women with recurrent miscarriage by specialists after appropriate counseling.

Historically T-shaped uterus was secondary to diethylstilbestrol (DES) exposure in utero. This is managed by hysteroscopic metroplasty, which involves incision on lateral uterine walls to expand the uterine cavity.[29] It is important to diagnose a T-shaped uterus because many studies were recently published about the reproductive outcome of T-shaped uterus and its relation to RPL, infertility, and in vitro fertilization (IVF) failure and also many studies were published about the lateral metroplasty as a treatment of T-shaped uterus. The main limitation of these studies is the absence of clear criteria to diagnose T-shaped uterus. The ESHRE/ESGE classification mentioned dysmorphic uterus (T-shaped) with narrow cavity and thick lateral wall but there is no measurement for diagnosis. The ASRM 2021 classification did not mention the criteria for diagnosis of T-shaped uterus. The CUME has tried to solve this problem.[30] The diagnosis of T-shaped uterus is not simple and the agreement among top experts is only moderate. A single expert judgment is commonly insufficient for accurate diagnosis. The group of experts described,[30] what they considered reliable and accurate, a measurable criteria for the classification of T-shaped uterus.

1. Lateral indentation depth ≥7 mm
2. Lateral indentation angle ≤130°
3. T-angle ≤40°

If the three criteria are present, the case is T-shaped uterus. If two criteria are met, the case is borderline T-shaped uterus. In case one or no criteria is met, then it is a normal uterus. This classification should be applied only when there is no internal fundal indentation ≥10 mm (according to CUME). It is also mentioned that the clinical relevance of the non-DES-related T-shaped uterus is unknown. Moreover, the results may help in understanding and validating the quality of evidence on T-shaped uterus, and may help to improve the quality of studies and our understanding of this morphology. It may well be that non-DES-related T-shaped uterus is not a congenital anomaly and need not be treated as such. Further efforts should be aimed at determining whether a T-shaped uterus is a true uterine anomaly with clinical consequences.[30]

MYOMAS

Leiomyomas that distort the uterine cavity (submucosal or intramural with an intracavitary component) cause difficulty in conception and an increased risk of miscarriage.[31,32] Myomectomy is the preferred treatment modality for symptomatic women who desire future fertility in comparison to uterine artery embolization (UAE), high-intensity focused ultrasound (HIFU), and magnetic resonance-guided HIFU (MRgHIFU).

Impact of uterine myomas on fertility:

- Greater distance for sperm travel
- Encroachment on tubal ostium
- Distortion of uterine cavity
- Vascular changes
- Interfere normal rhythmic uterine contractions
- Impaired implantation
- Abnormal endometrial maturation
- Alteration on oxytocinase activity.

Mechanism of Impaired Fertility in Case of Intramural-submucosal Myoma

- The number of caveolae in host myometrium and fibromyomata is conceivably decreased compared to normal myometrium.
- This specific structural abnormality may affect calcium metabolism by causing a decrease in defect in calcium extrusion and thus raising the intracellular calcium.
- Increased intracellular calcium produces myometrial irritability and hyperactivity.

- Resulting in disruption of the rhythmical contraction process of the junctional zone (JZ).

Subendometrial tumors:

- Causing endometrial erosion with subsequent inflammation altering the nature of the intrauterine fluid, results in a hostile environment
- Disrupt the endometrial blood supply, affecting nidation and sustenance of early embryo.

Effect on fertility of noncavitary uterine myoma is still controversial. In patients with infertility or history of pregnancy loss, other causes should also be thoroughly looked at and involvement of uterine cavity is checked.[31] Buttram and Reiter reviewed 1,699 cases of myomectomy and determined that 27% of these women also had infertility.[33] When all other causes were ruled out, myomas were found to play a role in only 2.4% of the cases.[32] Hence, it was concluded that although myomas may be coincidentally present in 25% of the cases of infertility, myomectomy would directly benefit only 2.4% of these women, where all other infertility factors have been ruled out. The rest will conceive following treatment of an identifiable cause without resorting to myomectomy. The above concept is important to understand. Most gynecologists feel that operating on myomas would enhance fertility in all patients with myomas. On the contrary, myomectomy leads to peritubal adhesions and distortion of the tubo-ovarian relationship as well as the uterine cavity in a large number of patients that will actually reduce further fertility potential leaving IVF as the only treatment option post myomectomy.

Hence, the decision to perform myomectomy or not in an infertile patient with intramural myomas is a crucial one.[32] It must be taken only after all other identifiable factors have been treated, and pregnancy has not ensued. Indications are:

- Failure of three cycles of controlled ovarian stimulation and intrauterine insemination after optimizing all other factors
- Recurrent implantation failure (RIF)
- Intramural myoma >5 cm in size
- Intramural myomas with submucous extension.

Yet myomectomy will benefit some patients with infertility. A recent meta-analysis concluded that the presence of leiomyoma without cavity involvement reduces the success rate of ART cycles.[34,35]

Classification of Leiomyomas

The International Federation of Gynecology and Obstetrics (FIGO) proposed the leiomyoma classification system. It is based on the relationship between the leiomyoma and the endometrial and serosal surfaces of the uterus[36] **(Table 2)**.

TABLE 2: International Federation of Gynecology and Obstetrics classification of leiomyoma.

Submucous	0	Pedunculated intracavitary
	1	<50% intramural
	2	>50% intramural
Others	3	Contacts endometrium, 100% intramural
	4	Intramural
	5	Subserous ≥50% intramural
	6	Subserous <50% intramural
	7	Subserous pedunculated
	8	Others (specify, e.g., cervical and parasitic)

Submucous Myomas

For women desiring future fertility, or who are currently infertile, hysteroscopic myomectomy is required for all submucous myomas.

An abdominal approach to multiple submucous myomas should be considered in following situations:[37]

- Three or more submucous myomas
- When hysteroscopic myomectomy might be anticipated to damage a large portion of the endometrial surface
- When submucous myoma extends to the uterine serosa (e.g., type 2–5 or 2–6 lesions).

Concomitant laparoscopy or ultrasound in cases of hysteroscopic myomectomy of deep type 2 submucous myoma can be considered. Abdominal approach is also necessary to remove intramural (types 3 and 4) or large subserosal myomas (types 5, 6, or 7).

Among various techniques available for abdominal myomectomy in infertile women, preferably minimally invasive approaches like laparoscopic myomectomy should be selected. Robotic assisted laparoscopic myomectomy (RALM) is also an option but cost remains a limiting factor. Whichever approach is selected, surgeon should not only be skilled in proper enucleation of myoma but also in adequate suturing of the myoma bed in two layers with minimal possible blood loss.[32]

Preoperative Evaluation

Thorough medical history followed by abdominal pelvic examination is a must. On bimanual examination, the size, contour, and mobility of the uterus should be noted, along with any other pelvic pathology. Baseline complete blood count, blood grouping, and routine blood investigations are ordered. USG, saline infusion sonography, MRI, or hysteroscopy are important in evaluating an infertile female with submucous myoma. Abdominal and transvaginal USG is carried out for location, number, and size of myoma along with the measurement of the distance between endometrium and myoma or serosa and myoma, which should be documented prior to surgery.[35,36] Though ultrasound is highly sensitive for preoperative mapping of myomas, due to limited tactile sensation in laparoscopic and robotic myomectomy, MRI is preferred in cases of difficult USG.[37,38]

Preoperative Preparation

Preoperative informed consent with proper explanation of the available alternatives to the procedure and potential complications of the procedure must be discussed and documented. In patients seeking pregnancy, need of cesarean delivery in future should be explained.[34] Other steps include:

- Correction of anemia with preoperative iron supplements.
- Gonadotropin-releasing hormone agonists (GnRH-a) should be considered in large myomas.
- Blood should be crossmatched, especially in cases where excessive blood loss is anticipated. In suitable cases, autologous blood transfusion may be arranged.
- Bowel preparation in case of myomectomy through abdominal route is mandatory.
- Cervical ripening with laminaria tents or misoprostol prior to hysteroscopic myomectomy prevents traumatic complications related to cervical dilatation.[32]

Preoperative and Intraoperative Measures to Achieve Hemostasis

Hemorrhage is probably the most frequent complication of myomectomy. Various surgeons all over the world have tried following interventions to reduce the bleeding during myomectomy.[39]

- Interventions on uterine arteries:
  - Laparoscopic uterine artery dissection and temporary clipping of the uterine artery
  - UAE
  - Pericervical mechanical tourniquet
  - Vasopressin injection around the myoma, or a vasoconstrictive solution of bupivacaine plus epinephrine.
- Uterotonics such as ergometrine, oxytocin, and misoprostol.
- Atraumatic myoma dissection techniques, these include:
  - Hydrodissection
  - Myoma enucleation by morcellation
  - Use of laser dissectors or, use of electrocautery or harmonics
  - Pharmacologic manipulation of the coagulation cascade with antifibrinolytic agents such as tranexamic acid and gelatin-thrombin hemostatic sealant.

Recently, a Cochrane review[39] was done to assess the effectiveness, safety, tolerability, and costs of these interventions to reduce blood loss during myomectomy. The review highlighted the paucity of randomized data on the use of such techniques.[40] It found significant reductions in blood loss with misoprostol mean difference (MD): –149.00 mL, 95% CI: –229.24 to –68.76), vasopressin (MD: –298.72 mL, 95% CI: –593.10 to –4.34), bupivacaine plus epinephrine (MD: –68.60 mL, 95% CI: –93.69 to –43.51), tranexamic acid (MD: –243 mL, 95% CI: –46.0 to –25.98), pericervical tourniquet (MD: –289.44, 95% CI: –406.55 to –172.32), and gelatin-thrombin matrix (MD: –545.00 mL, 95% CI: –593.26 to –496.74). There was no evidence of an effect on blood loss with oxytocin or morcellation. The best option appeared to be vasopressin injection **(Fig. 7)**. None of the interventions significantly increased myomectomy-related complications.

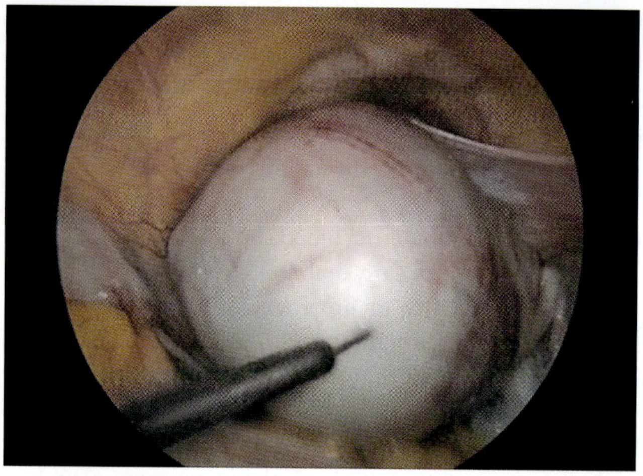

Fig. 7: Blanching of uterus due to vasopressin injection.
Courtesy: Dr Kamini Rao Hospital.

Role of Pretreatment with GnRH Analogs

Pretreatment with GnRH analogs before myomectomy is controversial. GnRH-a cause myoma shrinkage by reducing the circulating estrogen levels.[41] Drawbacks of preoperative GnRH therapy are that it increases the difficulty in identifying and dissecting the cleavage plane during myoma enucleation[39] and also increases the chance of myoma recurrence, as small myomas may be totally missed. Additionally, GnRH therapy is expensive and commonly associated with menopause-like side effects.[41] The role for GnRH administered for the purpose of reducing operating time, the amount of systemic absorption of distension media, and the risk of incomplete resection of submucous myomas has not been established. It can be considered a useful tool to correct anemia prior to surgery[37] or to obtain the shrinkage with consequent optimal mobilization of a single and very large myoma.[42]

Various Surgical Techniques for Myomectomy

Open Myomectomy

Abdominal myomectomy is performed through a laparotomy by taking transverse incision (Pfannenstiel) or in very large myomas a vertical incision. Size, number, location, and type of myoma are noted to accomplish the surgery. After taking measures to reduce blood loss, vertical, oblique or transverse uterine incision is taken, which is then extended down through myometrium and pseudocapsule to reach the myoma. Myoma is grasped by instruments such as tenaculum, allis, towel clip, or myoma screw and is further enucleated by blunt and sharp dissection.[43] In case of multiple myomas, removal of myoma by *tunneling* the same incision is preferred. Multiple incisions are taken when tunneling is not possible. Uterine defect is closed in a single or double layer with absorbable sutures. When the endometrial cavity is breached, it should be repaired with 5.0 Vicryl everting the endometrial edges toward the cavity. Inclusion of endometrial edges in the myometrium may cause foci of adenomyosis. Adequate tissue reapproximation and hemostasis is a must. The microsurgical principles inherent to all reproductive pelvic surgeries must be applied, namely atraumatic tissue handling, strict attention to hemostasis, continuous moistening of the pelvic tissues, and meticulous approximation of dissected tissue planes.[43-45]

Routine postoperative care includes monitoring of a patient's hemodynamic and fluid status, pain control, and reintroducing normal diet and activity. Early ambulation is preferred. Bleeding, fever, infection, visceral damage, ileus, bowel obstruction, pelvic abscess, and thromboembolism are reported as short-term complications of open myomectomy.[46] Long-term complications of abdominal myomectomy include pelvic adhesions, recurrent fibroids, and the risk of uterine rupture in subsequent pregnancies.[47,48]

Laparoscopic Myomectomy

The first laparoscopic myomectomy was performed by Dr Kurt Semm in 1979.[47] Laparoscopic myomectomy is an option in women with a uterus of less than 18 weeks' size, with ≤3 cm intramural or subserosal leiomyomas of ≤ 5 cm in diameter.[48] But with better instrumentation in laparoscopy and advanced surgical skills, laparoscopic myomectomy can be performed by experienced surgeons regardless of the size, number, or location of the myomas.[47]

The technique of laparoscopic myomectomy involves four steps:

- *Incision:* The incision on the uterus overlying the fibroid is created using a monopolar hook, monopolar needle electrode, harmonic scalpel, or sharp scissors. The direction of incision depends upon number, site and size of myoma, and surgeon preference. Horizontal incision minimizes blood loss as vessels run transversely along the uterine wall **(Fig. 8)**. Additionally, laparoscopic suturing is easier with horizontal and oblique incisions than with vertical incisions. Care must be taken to avoid extension and injury to fallopian tubes and ascending uterine vessels.[49]

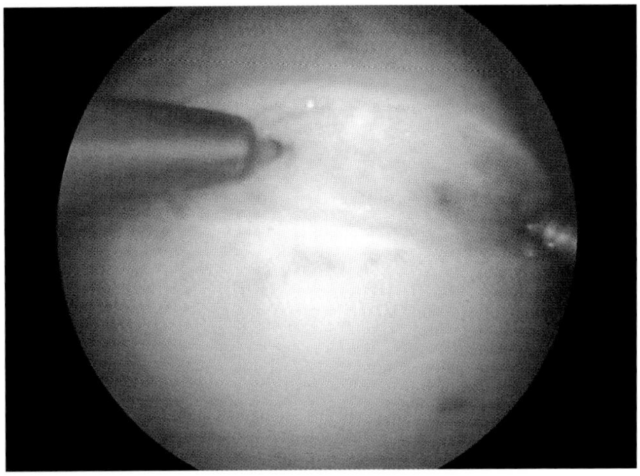

Fig. 8: Uterine incision by monopolar hook.
Courtesy: Dr Kamini Rao Hospital.

- *Enucleation:* Cleavage plane between myoma and pseudocapsule is created by blunt and sharp dissection. Traction is applied by myoma screw or tenaculum and myoma is then enucleated by gentle dissection and counter traction **(Fig. 9)**. Alternatively, hydrodissection with a suction irrigation cannula is convenient and atraumatic. Recognition of a proper cleavage plane between myoma and pseudocapsule is important to minimize bleeding and adequate enucleation. Bipolar coagulation of the vascular pedicle at the base of the myoma, prior to complete enucleation (after enucleation these vessels usually retract in the myometrium) will minimize blood loss.
- *Suturing:* Suturing is the key in laparoscopic myomectomy to avoid a number of complications ranging from postoperative bleeding to uterine rupture in subsequent pregnancy.[50] Depending upon the depth of defect, single or multilayer suturing is required **(Fig. 10)**. Delayed absorbable sutures such as polydioxanone, polyglactin, or a new kind of suture, bidirectional barbed thread is used. Barbed sutures consist of standard suture material with tiny barbs cut into the length of the filament facing in opposite directions from the midpoint with a needle on each end. It does not require knots, so decreases the mean suturing time and blood loss.[51,52] Excessive use of electrocautery during enucleation and for achieving hemostasis should be avoided as it causes necrosis of myometrium.
- *Myoma extraction*: Small myomas are removed by 10 mm primary port while large myoma requires electromechanical morcellation. Most surgeons perform morcellation after completion of myomectomy **(Fig. 11)**; however, morcellation of partially attached myoma can also be performed in case of large myoma. It should be performed with blade tips always under

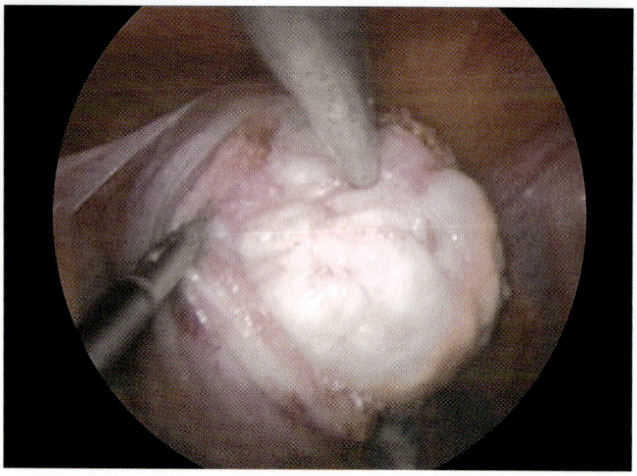

Fig. 9: Enucleation of myoma.
Courtesy: Dr Kamini Rao Hospital.

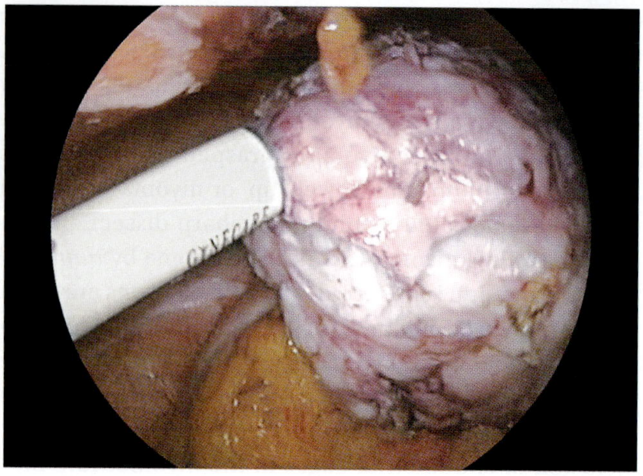

Fig. 11: Myoma retrieval by electromechanical morcillator.
Courtesy: Dr Kamini Rao Hospital.

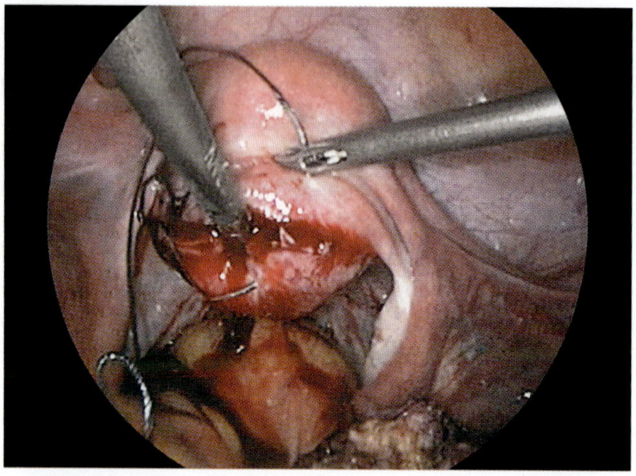

Fig. 10: Uterine reconstruction by intracorporeal suturing.
Courtesy: Dr Kamini Rao Hospital.

direct vision to prevent injury to bowel and adjacent structures. Special care must be taken to remove all myoma fragments to avoid iatrogenic parasitic myomas as complications. In order to prevent inadvertent peritoneal dissemination of leiomyosarcoma during morcellation, the Food and Drug Administration (FDA) issued a directive to perform morcellation in a bag in order to minimize the spill of cellular debris all over the peritoneum.[53] This also ensures complete removal of fragments and minimizes the chances of injury to the surrounding bowel.

Figures 8 to 11 show various steps of laparoscopic myomectomy.

Prevention of Postoperative Adhesions

Adhesions are of concern whether the abdominal or laparoscopic route is used. Besides good hemostasis, the use of barrier methods has been shown to be of some use. Removal of more than five myomas leads to significantly lower pregnancy rates due to subsequent formation of adhesions. Tulandi[54] performed a second look laparoscopy after initial myomectomy and observed a greater degree of adhesion formation after posterior wall myomectomy (93.7%) than with anterior wall myomectomy (55.5%). These adhesions may be prevented by the use of *Interceed*[55] (Johnson and Johnson, New Brunswick, New Jersey, USA) or *Gore Tex* (WL Gore and Associates Inc., Flagstaff, AZ, USA).[56]

Hysteroscopic Management of Submucous Myomas

In women with intracavitary filling defects due to submucous myomas, causing AUB, infertility, or RPL, hysteroscopic resection is preferred. This results in less blood loss and postoperative pain, reduced hospitalization, and recovery time and lower risk of postoperative pelvic adhesions. The Wamsteker[57] classification system, used by the ESGE, is based upon the degree of myoma within the uterine cavity.

- Type 0, the submucosal fibroid is entirely within the endometrial cavity
- Type 1 represents myoma which is more than 50% in the cavity
- Type 2 represents myoma which is less than 50% in the endometrial cavity.

Lasmer[58] and colleagues introduced the STEP-W (size, topography, extension, penetration, wall) classification system for submucous myoma in 2005 **(Table 3)** and recently demonstrated significant improvement in its prognostic capabilities as compared to the ESGE classification system.[59]

Techniques for Hysteroscopic Management of Myoma

Traditional Monopolar Resectoscope Technique

Neuwirth and Amin[60] reported the first case of using the urologist resectoscope for the treatment of submucosal

TABLE 3: STEP-W (size, topography, extension, penetration, wall) classification system for submucous myoma.

	Size (cm)	*Topography*	*Extension of the base*	*Penetration*	*Lateral wall*	*Total*
0	>2–5	Low	≤1/3	0	+1	
1	>2–5	Middle	>1/3–>2/3	≤50%		
2	>2	Upper	>2/3	>50%		
Score	+	+	+	+	+	
Score	**Group**	**Complexity and therapeutic options**				
0–4	I	Low complexity hysteroscopic myomectomy				
5–6	II	High complexity hysteroscopic myomectomy; consider use of GnRH preoperatively; consider two step hysteroscopic myomectomy				
7–9	III	Consider alternatives to hysteroscopic techniques				

(GnRH: gonadotropin-releasing hormone)

myoma in 1976. Resection of myoma is performed using a telescope from 0° to 30° and standard resectoscope between 24F and 28F and loop electrode with monopolar current and hypotonic distension media (glycine or sorbitol-mannitol).[61]

After cervical dilatation, a resectoscope fitted with a cutting loop is introduced and myoma is systematically resected under direct vision using cutting current of 60–120 watts **(Fig. 12)**. During resection:

- Resectoscope loop alone is moved toward the surgeon using the spring mechanism of the loop alone (short chip technique) or
- Moving the entire resectoscope toward the surgeon (long chip technique).

Care should be taken to minimize endometrial and myometrial damage. Myoma chips are removed at the end of the procedure unless it is a big myoma or the view is obstructed. Facilitation of uterine contractions by deflation, bimanual massage, or use of prostaglandins has been advocated as this squeezes the myoma into the uterine cavity. Cavity is then inspected to ensure hemostasis and completion of the procedure.

Bipolar Resectoscopic Technique

This is a safer technique of myoma resection. It requires isotonic distension media like normal saline so the risk of electrolyte imbalance related to fluid overload is less.[62]

Use of Vaporizing Electrodes

Bulk electrosurgical vaporization is performed with a large surface area electrode activated with low-voltage current to vaporize relatively large volumes of tissue.[63] As the electrode is moved through the myoma, it completely vaporizes the tissue so that there is no vision obstruction by myoma pieces. The drawback is that there is no tissue available for histopathological examination (HPE).[64]

Hysteroscopic Morcellation of Myoma

In order to minimize the complications of fluid overload and electrosurgical injuries related to traditional monopolar resection of myoma, hysteroscopic morcellators are also used.[65] These morcellators have a hollow cylindrical blade with a side aperture that is used to morcellate the myoma sequentially. It has an integrated suction removal system to remove tissue fragments from the uterine cavity for histopathology. Simultaneous removal of tissue fragments from uterine cavity makes this procedure quick and reduces the risks of perforation by maintaining visibility.[66] Mechanical morcellators allow resection of type 0 and type 1 myomas using normal saline as distension media without the use of electric current.[67] This minimizes damage to the endometrium which may give us better implantation rates.

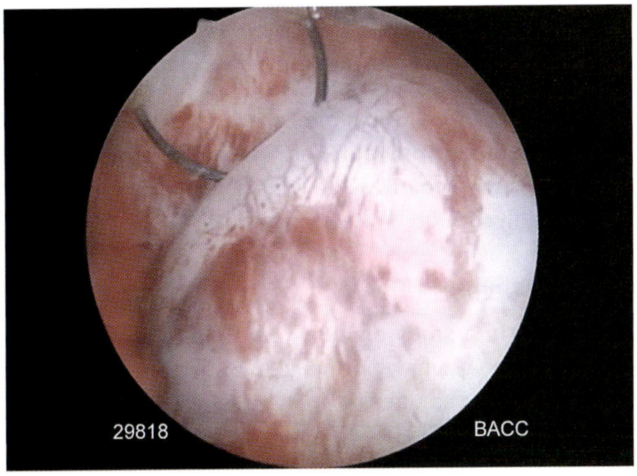

Fig. 12: Submucous myoma with loop electrode.

Complications Associated with Hysteroscopic Myomectomy

Following are the American Association of Gynecologic Laparoscopists (AAGL) recommendations to prevent complications:[37]

- Postoperative bleeding can be managed either with intracervical prostaglandin F2α (carboprost) or with tamponade by use of an inflated balloon catheter.
- Distension media complications can be minimized with strict monitoring of fluid deficit, preferably with weighted

monitoring systems and the adherence to institutionally predetermined fluid loss guidelines. The surgery should be abruptly terminated if the fluid deficit approaches 1,500 mL or the serum sodium level nears 125 mmol/L.
- *Thermal injury:* The risk of monopolar current diversion resulting in lower genital tract burns may be reduced by:
  - Maintaining contact of the external sheath with the cervix
  - Avoiding activation of the electrosurgical unit when the electrode is not in contact with tissue
  - Ensuring the sustained integrity of the electrode insulation
  - Minimizing the use of high-voltage ("coagulation") current when performing hysteroscopic submucous myomectomy.
- Post myomectomy intrauterine synechiae can be minimized if opposing tissue is not resected during a single surgery. These are more common after multiple submucous myomectomies. Moreover, when fertility is an issue, second-look hysteroscopy and appropriate adhesiolysis should be considered.[67,68]

Fertility Outcome after Hysteroscopic Myomectomy

Vercellini[68] in a study of 108 women that used the ESGE classification system reported 49%, 36%, and 33% fertility rates over a 3-year period in type 0, 1, and 2 myomas, respectively. Emanuel et al. reported 46% conception rate and 80.4% delivery rate after hysteroscopic resection of myoma.[69] In a systematic review of leiomyomas and fertility, Pritts et al. concluded that submucous myomas lower fertility rates and their removal enhances the rates of conception and live births.[70]

After hysteroscopic myomectomy, patients should wait for 2–3 months for endometrial healing prior to conception. As there are no reported cases of uterine rupture, patients may attempt vaginal delivery after hysteroscopic myomectomy.[71]

Vaginal myomectomy of intramural lower segment myomas is an alternative to laparoscopy or laparotomy. However, the chances of conversion are high as are the chances of pelvic infection. There are no good studies for comparative analysis.[72]

Cervical myomas account for about 5% of all myomas. They require excision if they restrict entry into the uterine cavity for ART procedures. Due to its close vicinity to bladder, rectum, ureter, and uterine vessels, the approach needs to be modified with relation to these surrounding vital structures. During laparoscopic myomectomy for cervical myoma, temporary blocking of uterine artery blood flow and the use of vasopressin are essential to decrease excessive bleeding.[73] Minimizing the risk of damage to surrounding organs by positioning the incision in the myometrium somewhat lateral to the uterine corpus and appropriate suturing to avoid leaving dead space are important. Hysteroscopic resection and vaginal myomectomy may be considered where appropriate. Embolization of the cervical branch of the uterine artery can be considered when removal is challenging.

Medical Management

Medical management with oral progesterone, progesterone intrauterine system (IUS), and oral contraceptive pills is seldom indicated in the infertile patient. However, in patients with multiple small myomas where surgery would be more traumatizing to the uterus, treatment with ulipristal acetate (UPA) may be indicated prior to ART cycles. UPA is a selective progesterone receptor modulator (SPRM) with antiproliferative effects on myoma cells.[74,75] UPA 5–10 mg daily helps in reducing myoma size and uterine volume; it also decreases pelvic pain and excessive bleeding, thereby normalizing anemia and restoring quality of life.[74-76] In women with large myomas, two courses of 3 months of UPA 5 mg daily can be given. Depending upon regression of myoma and restoration of uterine cavity, the patient may attempt a pregnancy after the second bleed following cessation of therapy.[77]

ADENOMYOSIS

Adenomyosis is a benign condition of the uterus, defined by the presence of endometrial glands and stroma within the myometrium.[78] Prevalence of adenomyosis is variable around 20% and increases with age reaching to about 32% in women aged 40–49 years.[78,79]

Adenomyosis may present with symptoms like:
- Infertility
- Dysmenorrhea
- Menorrhagia
- Pelvic pain

Variable symptomatology with difficult diagnosis of adenomyotic lesions at imaging makes this a challenging entity in gynecological practice.

Pathogenesis

A major pathogenetic mechanism suggests adenomyosis as a sex hormone-related disorder, in fact the most commonly used drugs are targeted or modulating estrogen/progesterone receptors (ER/PR). Studies have shown that polymorphisms in the ER-α gene are associated with a risk of adenomyosis.[80] Adenomyotic tissue is known to contain steroid receptors, apart from having increased activity of aromatase and sulfatase enzymes. These ER receptors under the influence of circulating and locally produced estrogens stimulate the growth of adenomyotic tissue.[81] Local hyperestrogenism is due to the action of aromatase and sulfatase enzymes converting estrone-3-sulfate to estrone. This explains the increased levels of estradiol (E2) in menstrual blood, but not in peripheral blood of women with adenomyosis. The reduction of PR expression can be related to the development and progression of adenomyosis and may explain the mechanism of action of progestin agents on adenomyosis.[82]

Investigations

Transvaginal USG and MRI are reliable tools for a noninvasive diagnosis of adenomyosis.[83,84] MRI is more accurate as it helps to assess JZ thickening and extent of myometrial involvement. It will also differentiate adenomyosis from myoma and identify associated endometriotic lesions. HPE of biopsy or hysterectomy specimens provides the most definitive diagnosis.

Impact on In Vitro Fertilization

Women with adenomyosis are commonly known to suffer from infertility. These women encounter low success rates even while undergoing ART cycles. There is significant:

- Reduction in ovarian response to stimulation.
- Reduced implantation of good quality embryos.
- Low clinical pregnancy rates.
- Increased risk of early pregnancy loss.
- Lower live birth rates in women with adenomyosis undergoing IVF.[85-88]

Medical Management

The management of patients with adenomyosis is difficult and conservative treatment is required for those who require preservation of fertility and improvement of quality of life. The objective of medical treatment is pain reduction, control excessive bleeding in AUB, and restore fertility. The present medical treatments for adenomyosis follow the principles of the management of endometriosis, which are usually aimed at reducing the production of endogenous estrogen or inducing endometrial differentiation with progestins.[89]

Nonhormonal medications, such as procoagulating agents, iron supplementation and nonsteroidal anti-inflammatory drugs (NSAIDs), are also aimed at controlling symptoms of AUB and pain in adenomyosis. Hormonal medications commonly used in the treatment of adenomyosis is similar to those for endometriosis. These include GnRH-a, progestins [danazol, levonorgestrel-intrauterine device (IUD), dienogest], and combined oral contraceptives (COC).

Progestins

Progestins act via decidualization and subsequent atrophy of endometrial tissue apart from modulation of mitotic activity, local growth factors, and their receptor. There are other paracrine mechanisms and anti-inflammatory mechanisms as well. [90,91,92]

Norethindrone Acetate

The use of norethindrone acetate (NETA) in adenomyosis is associated with a marked degree of pain relief and symptomatic relief. The onset of action seems to be slow but with longer duration of use the efficacy improves.[93] The role of NETA in the management of adenomyosis has been well demonstrated in women presenting moderate or severe pelvic pain and bleeding. There is a significant improvement of both dysmenorrhea and bleeding after treatment (dose 5 mg/day).[94] The progestin treatment started at the beginning of the menstrual cycle, and was taken orally as a three-weeks-on and one-week-off regime. Since maximum response was obtained at 3 months, NETA may be considered an effective, well-tolerated and inexpensive medical treatment for adenomyosis, with fewer and milder side effects.[94] A drawback of NETA therapy is the reduction of libido in around one-fifth of women.

Danazol

The mechanism of action of danazol is complex. It acts by lowering the mid-cycle luteinizing hormone (LH) surge, and increasing serum-free testosterone levels. It also acts directly on adenomyotic tissue in vitro to inhibit DNA synthesis and induce apoptosis. Its use results in an androgenic and hypoestrogenic environment.[93] The use of danazol is associated with relieved pain and clinical improvement in 55–93% of adenomyosis patients treated for a duration of 6 months.[95] However, danazol is not suitable for prolonged use because of its adverse side effects. A low-dose of danazol (200 mg/day) is daily administered by vaginal route for 6 months in young women with adenomyosis. The severity of blood loss and uterine volume are significantly reduced.[96]

Levonorgestrel-releasing Intrauterine System

Several mechanisms may explain the role of the levonorgestrel-releasing intrauterine system (LNG-IUS) in the treatment of adenomyosis.[97] After insertion of the system there is a decidualization of the endometrium, followed by atrophic changes, which produces a marked reduction in menstrual blood loss. Direct action is thought to occur due to direct absorption into the myometrium and action on adenomyotic foci. Additionally, downregulation of ER, in both glandular and stromal endometrial layers, occurs shortly after placement of the device and persists for at least the first year of use. The LNG-IUS is highly efficient in decreasing AUB and uterine volume at 12 months and in resolving pain associated with adenomyosis (moderate or severe dysmenorrhea and dyspareunia).[98] The main side effects include irregular bleeding and amenorrhea during the first few months.

Dienogest

Dienogest has been reported to show high selectivity for binding to progesterone receptors[99,100] and has inhibitory effects on the secretion of cytokines in endometriotic stromal cells.[101] It also directly inhibits cellular proliferation and also induces apoptosis in adenomyotic stromal cells. In a pilot study, dienogest was effective in relieving the pain symptoms associated with adenomyosis and uterine fibroids. The regimen used was adenomyosis oral dienogest on days 2–5 of menstruation and followed up every 8 weeks after beginning treatment.[102]

GnRH Agonist

Gonadotropin-releasing hormone agonists act by binding to their receptors inducing a state of reversible iatrogenic menopause. With the fall in estrogen levels there is atrophy of the adenomyotic lesions, which in turn results in a reduction in the uterine size. There is a decrease in expression of aromatase cytochrome P450 in eutopic endometrium, mainly by promoting a hypoestrogenic state.[103] In assisted reproductive technologies, long agonist stimulation protocols along with pretreatment with GnRH-a for differed embryo transfer improve pregnancy rates.[95] The main adverse effect is due to the hypoestrogenic state. These include vasomotor syndrome, reduced bone mineral density, genital atrophy, and mood instability. When used with adequate precautions, add-back therapy with various kinds of hormone preparations has been successfully used to reduce the GnRH-a-included adverse effects which enables an indefinite extension of the treatment period.

Combined Oral Contraceptives

Mechanism of action: Combined oral contraceptives are useful in the management of adenomyosis-related pain and AUB. They decrease menstrual flow, cause decidualization and subsequent atrophy of the endometrium. Aromatase expression in the eutopic endometrium and adenomyotic foci is also suppressed by COCs.[104]

Future Medical Treatments

Several new drugs have been introduced in the treatment of adenomyosis. Selective estrogen receptor modulators (SERMs), SPRMs, and aromatase inhibitors (AIs) are the main drugs under investigation.

Aromatase Inhibitors

Mechanism of action: Aromatase cytochrome P450 (CYP19A1) is a key enzyme in the synthesis of estrogen from androgens. It is involved in the conversion of androstenedione and testosterone to estrone and E2, respectively.[105] CYP19A1 has been identified immunohistochemically in the cytoplasm of glandular cells of adenomyotic tissues and of eutopic endometrium from patients with this adenomyosis.[106] It is therefore an ideal target for inhibition of the E2 synthesis because it is the final step in steroid biosynthesis. Thereby no important downstream enzymes to be affected.[105] A single clinical trial employing AIs in the management of adenomyosis has been done.[107] In a prospective randomized controlled study which compared the efficacy of letrozole versus GnRH-a for 12 weeks in treating premenopausal women with uterine adenomyosis, there was no significant difference in total uterine size based on post-treatment uterine volumes in the two groups. AIs demonstrated the same efficacy as GnRH-a in reducing adenomyoma volume and improving symptoms.[107] The adverse effects most commonly associated with AI include headaches, hot flashes, mood changes, muscle aches, and breakthrough bleeding. E2 levels are significantly suppressed with this treatment, without the vasomotor symptoms and agonist flare-up effects of GnRH-a.[107] Their use would also be interesting in obese patients due to antiestrogenic action on both ovarian and adipose tissues. Hence, AIs appear to have a promising future for adenomyosis in cases of resistance to other treatments though additional studies are needed.

Selective Estrogen Receptor Modulators

Mechanism of action: The ideal SERM for management of adenomyosis needs to have an antagonistic activity in the endometrium (adenomyotic lesion) and agonistic activity for bone and lipids. Basic clinical studies indicate major roles for estrogen and progesterone in the pathology of adenomyosis. There is a need to conduct RCTs on the pharmacological treatment of adenomyosis with SERMs.[108,109]

Selective Progesterone Receptor Modulators

Selective progesterone receptor modulators are a new class of progesterone receptor ligands, which exhibit both progesterone agonist and antagonist activities in the endometrium. They reduce pain, bleeding, cell proliferation, and inhibit inflammation.[110] Thus they are beneficial in the treatment of myomas or endometriosis.[109,111] Mifepristone influences the caspase 3 expression in adenomyotic tissue. The role of SPRMs requires investigations and well-designed RCTs to assess their long-term action and their clinical use in patients with adenomyosis.[111-113]

Conclusions

The medical treatment of adenomyosis is an open field with a great possibility of new advancement. No double-blind placebo-controlled study was ever conducted on the management of adenomyosis and only observational studies are reported in literature.

Surgery can be beneficial for women who have experienced previous IVF failures. It also increases spontaneous pregnancy rates.

- If the adenomyosis is localized, laparoscopic excision is advisable as it may improve implantation rates as well as symptom control. Women less than 39 years of age were shown to have benefit with uterus sparing adenomyomectomy. Both robotic-assisted adenomyomectomy and laparoscopic adenomyomectomy (LAM) have better results when compared to GnRH-a therapy in symptom control.[114,115]
- If the lesions are mainly subendometriotic, i.e., <2.5 cm deep, they may be dealt with by hysteroscopic resection with a resectoscope and commencing estrogen replacement therapy postoperatively.[116]
- However in diffuse adenomyosis, prolonged pretreatment with GnRH-a has been tried prior to ART cycles. However, pregnancy rates remain low.
- Harvesting the oocytes and pooling them prior to prolonged suppression and performing frozen embryo transfer (FET) is currently the best option.
- Medical management with UPA for one or two courses, of 3 months each, has also been tried prior to ART cycles. However, no studies are available on pregnancy rates following such treatment.
- Use of HIFU[116,117] and HIFU MRg;[118] a clinical trial is currently recruiting patients to see the efficacy of this modality.[119]
- In multiple failed IVF cycles, surrogacy offers the best chances for the couple.

ENDOMETRIAL FACTORS

Implantation of the embryo in the endometrium is the bottleneck for the success of ART. Today most ART laboratories achieve a fertilization rate of over 80% but a clinical pregnancy rate of 30–35%. The gap is due to defects in the embryo-like aneuploidy or subtle defects in the endometrial environment that lead to failure of the embryo to implant in the uterus. The endometrium undergoes cyclical changes to accommodate a window of implantation (WOI) each month that is short-lived. It is characterized by formation of pinopodes and microvilli to allow embryo adhesion as well as secretion of Th2 cytokines in preference to Th1 cytokines. Embryo transfer should be done during this WOI which can be assessed by performing endometrial receptivity analysis (ERA) test done at a precise time, i.e., natural cycle—LH surge or human chorionic gonadotropin (hCG) + 7 days and in hormone replacement cycle—progesterone + 5 days. A displaced WOI is seen in 20% of patients with RIF.[120]

In order to understand the diverse causes of failed implantation, let us understand the process of implantation. This can be divided into following phases:

- *Apposition*
- *Adhesion* of the embryo to the endometrium
- *Burrowing* of the embryo into the endometrium
- Escaping *immune rejection*
- Establishing a *vascular connection* to derive nutrition.

Apposition

The timing and technique of embryo transfer is very important to allow for apposition of the embryo and endometrium.

Embryo transfer should involve:

- Ultrasound visualization of embryo placement
- Placement of embryos in mid cavity
- Minimal volume of media
- Minimal transit time between incubator and uterus of less than 1 minute to maintain embryo viability
- Gentle release of embryos
- Maintaining steady pressure on the plunger to prevent backflow
- No blood in the cavity that can alter the pH of the endometrial secretions[120]
- Abolishing uterine contractions by:
  - Not stimulating the cervix
  - Giving prostaglandin inhibitors like indomethacin
  - Giving oxytocin receptor blockers like atosiban during embryo transfer in patients with increased endometrial contractions visible on transvaginal scan (TVS).

The pattern of uterine contractions is different in fresh and FET thereby the difference in clinical outcome.[122]

Adhesion

It is believed that the sulfhydryl groups of the endometrium are chemotactic for the embryo. The embryo initially derives nutrition from the secretions of endometrial glands. Hence, it will implant on one of the glandular openings. Thin endometrium with poor secretory change will not support the nutrition of the implanting embryo. With this premise, estradiol valerate is used to cause glandular proliferation in the follicular phase and induce progesterone receptors, followed by the use of micronized progesterone in the luteal phase to enhance endometrial secretions.

Pinopod formation in the endometrium lasts for only 24 hours, and puts forth an increased surface area of the endometrium in the form of microvilli for the adhesion of the embryo. Missing the WOI may prevent adhesion of the embryo to the endometrium.

Adhesion can only occur if the embryo has successfully hatched out of the zona pellucida. In cases of zona hardening and improper hatching, the embryo will be unable to adhere to the endometrium. Hence, *assisted hatching* procedures are useful in a select group of patients that include:[119]

- Frozen thawed embryos as it hardens the zona
- Thickened zona pellucida of more than 15 microns
- Age more than 37 years
- Elevated basal follicle-stimulating hormone (FSH) level of more than 10
- Previous two cycles with failed implantation
- Embryos with increased fragmentation and delayed development

The use of hyaluronic acid (HA) as an adhesion molecule in the embryo transfer media has shown slightly improved implantation rates and also a higher incidence of multiple pregnancies.[123]

Blastocyst culture has taught us that the blastocyst is sticky and will readily adhere, a quality that makes it survive in the endometrium. However most aneuploid embryos will arrest at 4–16 cell stage and will not proceed to form a blastocyst. Hence, it is worthwhile replacing blastocysts in patients with implantation failures.

Blastocysts can now be screened for aneuploidy by performing *preimplantation genetic screening (PGS)* by complete genomic hybridization (CGH) or fluorescent in situ hybridization (FISH) on trophectoderm cells. Women with RIF will benefit from PGS and those with recurrent 100% aneuploid embryos will benefit with oocyte or embryo donation.

Blastocyst culture fluid can now be analyzed for specific *implantation marker proteins* secreted by the blastocyst. Those with positive secretion of these markers can be preferably transferred in patients with RIF.

Adhesion is a dynamic process which involves secretion of factors both by the embryo and endometrium. Hence the use of *embryo glue* to promote adhesion met with limited success.

A number of *adhesion molecules* have also been identified in the endometrium. These are:

- *Integrins* are maximally expressed in the endometrium during the implantation window. AlphaV beta 3 ($\alpha V\beta 3$) integrin has been maximally studied as a potential marker for endometrial receptivity. It is secreted under the influence of progesterone. Low levels of this integrin were found in women with unexplained infertility[103,124]
- *Osteopontin* is a glycoprotein whose expression is increased in the endometrium during the implantation window, i.e., 7 days after the LH peak.[104,125]
- *Mucin 1 (MUC 1)* in the mouse model MUC 1 can prevent mouse embryo attachment to the polarized uterine endometrium. However in humans MUC 1 is maximally expressed during the implantation window. Expression of MUC 1 in the endometrium is regulated by estrogen and progesterone hormones, via the steroid receptors. It remains to be seen whether human MUC 1 is lost focally at the implantation site or undergoes a change in glycosylation to become an adhesive molecule.[126] Glandular MUC 1 levels were diminished in patients with recurrent miscarriages and implantation failures.

Burrowing

The burrowing of the embryo requires that the embryo should produce proteolytic enzymes like *matrix metalloproteinases* that will lyse the endometrium around it. This enzyme has to be produced in a controlled manner so that the path ahead is cleared without any buildup of free radicals, which means that its secretion needs to be regulated both spatially and quantitatively. Both over and under secretion of proteolytic enzymes will lead to failed implantation.

Failure to secrete these proteolytic enzymes will result in biochemical pregnancies without appearance of a gestational sac. On the other hand, buildup of free radicals in the endometrium will affect cell function and impair the secretion of growth-promoting cytokines. However, use of antioxidants and vitamin supplementation does not improve implantation rates in clinical studies.[127]

Chronic endometritis is identified in 15% of patients with infertility. It is generally asymptomatic and can be diagnosed on hysteroscopy and/or biopsy. The causative organisms are usually of low virulence, may be nonspecific but chlamydia and tuberculosis (TB) may also be responsible. A routine course of broad-spectrum antibiotics like doxycycline is often administered in the pre-IVF phase. CE will result in high levels of tumor necrosis factor alpha (TNF-α), free radicals or natural killer cells (NKC) that may hamper implantation. Hence, an endometrial biopsy is performed along with hysteroscopy to identify gross pathology in the endometrium like granulomas, leukocytic infiltration, or disordered proliferation. It is also postulated that hysteroscopy may help to remove bacterial biofilms and cure CE.[128]

In recent studies, *endometrial scratching* has shown to improve implantation rates by promoting secretion of growth factors and cytokines. However, it is still debatable whether maximum benefit comes from scratching the endometrium in the stimulated cycle or the cycle previous to ART.[129,130]

A multicenter randomized trial is recruiting patients for endometrial scratch in patients undergoing the first cycle of IVF.[131]

Immune Tolerance

The fetus is an allograft in the maternal body. Yet it is not rejected by the maternal immune system. The endometrium undergoes changes in its immune environment at the time of implantation so as to protect the developing embryo. The cytokine environment changes from a proinflammatory Th1 to an anti-inflammatory Th2 response.[132] There are reduced levels of proinflammatory cytokines like TNF-α. In cycles where there is an infective or autoimmune process activated in the endometrium the TNF-α levels are high that leads to implantation failure. In such cycles delaying embryo transfer to a cycle where these levels are downregulated will help embryo implantation.

Uterine natural killer cells (uNKC) are large granular lymphocytes. Unlike peripheral NKC they lack cell differentiation (CD) 16 and CD3 antigens. These cells are increased in number during the midluteal phase of the cycle. Their population may be controlled by progesterone. They express families of receptors that are capable of recognizing specific antigens on the surface of extravillous trophoblast. Furthermore, the extravillous trophoblast does not express the classical MHC type 2 HLA antigens but expresses HLA G, so as to prevent recognition by the maternal immune cells. Besides, uNKC possesses less cytotoxic activity than peripheral NKC and their cytotoxic activity is downregulated in the peri-implantation period. Hence, the fetus does not face rejection by the uNKC. However subclinical infections of the endometrium with chlamydia, TB, or Gram-negative bacteria will upregulate the population of uNKC that may mediate rejection of the implanting embryo, resulting in failed implantation or recurrent miscarriage.[133] Hence, treatment of these infections is advisable prior to ART cycles.

Immunocytochemical studies enable us to do uNKC count in a biopsy taken during the luteal phase of the cycle. A count of more than 300 uNK cells/mm^2 was seen in patients with unexplained recurrent miscarriages when endometrial biopsy was performed in the luteal phase.[134]

The endometrium can also be tested for presence of anti-implantation proteins like apolipoprotein A1. This is present in high concentrations in the ectopic endometrial implants seen in endometriosis.[135]

Genomic study has compiled a human gene expression endometrial database (HGEx-ERdb). It was showed that 179 genes could be defined as receptivity associated genes (RAG) which may prove useful in identifying endometrial receptivity.[136]

Therapeutic Options

- Downregulation of the NK cells with immune modulation has been tried with variable results. Currently, it is advisable to correct hypovitaminosis D prior to ART cycles. Vitamin D is known to have immunomodulatory properties.[137]
- Use of progesterone as an immune modulator in the luteal phase is a routine in all ART cycles. However, its role in enhancing immune modulation and preventing RIF is debatable. The PROMISE trial was a double-blind randomized trial controlled on patients with recurrent miscarriages and showed no benefit of supplementing progesterone to prevent miscarriages.[138] However, systematic reviews done earlier show a lower miscarriage rate with progesterone supplementation.[139]
- Using paternal lymphocytes or third-party cells carries the risk of disease transmission and has no beneficial effect.[140]
- A short course of *steroids* during the peri-implantation phase has been used in patients with autoimmune diseases to downregulate the uNKC activity and to enhance implantation rates and reduce the chances of immune rejection. Although current evidence does not support the use of steroids for implantation,[141] a RCT is currently on, for its use in patients with high NK cell count, and the results are awaited.[132]
- The use of *intravenous immunoglobulin* (IVIg) prior to embryo transfer has also been tried.[133] It is indicated in a small subset of women with IgG subclass deficiency.[134] However, it is not beneficial in all cases of implantation failure.
- *Intralipids* have been used by some for immune modulation prior to embryo transfer and repeated every 3 weeks thereafter.[135]
- *Granulocyte colony-stimulating factor* was proposed by Scarpellini to improve implantation rates.[136] It was concluded in an RCT that it increased the rate of biochemical pregnancies by facilitating implantation but whether that translates to a higher clinical pregnancy rate is still uncertain.[137]
    - Intrauterine installation of 300 μg on day of hCG in women with thin endometrium and/or
    - Subcutaneous administration of 1 μg/kg (50–60 μg) two or three times a week for 4 weeks.
- *Human chorionic gonadotropin* is administered to trigger ovulation and improve pregnancy rates in women with oligomenorrhea. It has been shown that it enhances secretion of pro-implantation cytokines and growth factors during the periovulatory period.[138]

However, we need randomized trials to prove the efficacy of these empirical therapies.

Vascular Connection

The expression of vascular endothelial growth factor (VEGF) is increased in the endometrium during the postimplantation phase.[139] This allows the maternal spiral arterioles to establish a rich vascular network in the subendometrial layer, which can be studied by power Doppler studies of the endometrium in the mid cycle. Cycles with poor subendometrial flow may be associated with poor pregnancy rates.[140] The administration of *vasodilators* like sildenafil is used to improve pregnancy rates but there are no randomized studies supporting its use.[141]

However, *Doppler studies of the uterine artery* are helpful in women with RIF to identify cycles with improved uterine artery blood flow indices that will enhance implantation rates. Also, presence of power Doppler flow signals in the basal layer of the endometrium ensures better implantation rates.[141]

Use of *low-molecular-weight heparin* enhances uterine artery blood flow indices in a select group of patients. It has been suggested as a potential therapy in ART cycles for implantation failure. However RCTs on the subject are still lacking.[142]

Identification of implantation markers by *proteomic analysis* of culture medium has met with limited success. Presence of proteins like *glycodelin A* and *uteroglobin* in uterine secretions during midcycle has met with limited success. *Leukemia inhibitory factor (LIF)*, which was an implantation marker in the mouse model, has not been of value in human endometrium.

Growth factors secreted by platelet-rich plasma (PRP) injected into the uterine cavity under ultrasound guidance or in the endometrium under hysteroscopic guidance have shown to improve the quality of endometrium.[143] However, the procedure is new and we need to await results in terms of pregnancy rates.

Use of hematopoietic stem cells (SCs) or in conjunction with PRP helps in regenerating damaged endometrium but its effect on enhancing pregnancy rates are still awaited.[144] Severely damaged uterine cavity, not amenable to corrective measures, is an indication for surrogacy. Uterine transplant has also reported a successful pregnancy but is a cumbersome surgical procedure with risk of immunosuppression and rejection. Currently, it requires a hysterectomy post child birth.[145]

ASHERMAN'S SYNDROME

The Asherman's syndrome (AS) is characterized by the presence of intrauterine adhesions or adhesions in the endocervix with consequent risk of hypomenorrhea/amenorrhea, reduced fertility, pregnancy loss, and abnormal placentation. It can develop secondary to pregnancy-related curettage, infection or surgery related to the uterus, and TB. The pathophysiology involves trauma to the basal layer of endometrium.

Diagnosis

Intrauterine adhesions can be visualized by HSG, USG including contrast sonohysterography (SHG), 3D USG, hysteroscopy, and MRI. Hysteroscopy is the gold standard.

Treatment

The treatment of AS is indicated in women with infertility and those with painful hypo-/amenorrhea. This involves the division of adhesions under hysteroscopic guidance beginning in the central and safe part of the uterus and moving laterally and toward the fundus.[146] Overall restoration of normal menstrual cycle is observed in 75–100%.[147,148] The pregnancy rate ranges between 25% and 76%.[149] To prevent recurrent adhesions, IUCD, intrauterine application of hyaluronic gel, and estrogen therapy can be used. Regeneration of endometrium through SC treatment has been evaluated both in animal models.[150,151] Future randomized trials are needed to prove if SC treatment will have a clinical role in AS.

GENITOURINARY TUBERCULOSIS

Genitourinary TB is a common form of extrapulmonary TB (EPTB) worldwide (27%) with genital TB alone accounting for 9% of all EPTB cases.[152] TB infects the genital tract by four routes: hematogenous route, descending direct spread, lymphatic spread, and rarely as primary infection of the genitalia through sexual transmission.[153] The genital organs affected by *Mycobacterium tuberculosis* are as follows: fallopian tubes (95–100%), uterine endometrium (50–60%), ovaries (20–30%), cervix (5–15%), uterine myometrium (2.5%), and vagina/vulva (1%).[154]

Diagnosis

Hysterosalpingography: The uterine changes due to TB may be seen as specific features such as "collar-stud abscess," "T-shaped" uterus, and "pseudo unicornuate" uterus or nonspecific features such as synechiae formation, uterine contour distortion, and obliteration of the uterine cavity. Chronic infection may lead to extensive destruction of the endometrium and myometrium resulting in complete narrowing of the uterine cavity resulting in what is known as the Netter syndrome.[155]

Treatment

The WHO treatment guidelines for TB[156] recommend that patients newly diagnosed with TB should receive a regimen containing rifampicin (R) for 6 months: intensive phase with isoniazid (H), R, ethambutol (E), and pyrazinamide (Z) for a duration of 2 months followed by continuation phase with HR for 4 months.

KEY POINTS

- Around 1 in 500 reproductive age women are affected by UFI, which can be congenital or acquired.
- *Prevalence of CUAs:* General population 4.3–6.7%, infertile population 3–13%, and in patients with recurrent miscarriages 12.6–18.2%. Normal karyotype is found in 92% of women with Müllerian anomalies.
- Women with Müllerian developmental anomalies often will have normal functioning ovaries and female hormones and hence good reproductive potential.
- ASRM 2021 and ESHRE/ESGE consensus[9] (CONUTA) classification 2013 (reaffirmed in 2016) are the two most important classifications currently.
- Gold standard diagnostic modality for CUA is MRI. 3D USG has the potential to surpass MRI.
- Significant effect on reproduction seen in septate or bicornuate uterus, whereas the effect is statistically insignificant in women with arcuate, didelphys, and unicornuate uterus.
- Fertility management, restoration of the vaginal anatomy, and sexual function with emphasis on psycho-socio-sexual counseling are needed in CUA.

- Leiomyomas that distort the uterine cavity cause difficulty in conception and an increased risk of miscarriage.
- For myomectomy in infertile women, preferably minimally invasive approaches like laparoscopic myomectomy should be selected.
- Adenomyosis may present with infertility, dysmenorrhea, menorrhagia, or pelvic pain.
- TVS and MRI are reliable tools for noninvasive diagnosis of adenomyosis, MRI being more accurate. HPE of biopsy or hysterectomy specimens provides the most definitive diagnosis.
- Women with adenomyosis commonly suffer from infertility, success rate being low even with ART.
- Medical treatment of adenomyosis is an open field with a great possibility of new advancement. Medication or surgery as pretreatment for adenomyosis does not significantly increase the pregnancy rates in infertile women with adenomyosis. Surgery can be beneficial in previous IVF failures.
- Due to implantation failure, in spite of a fertilization rate of over 80%, clinical pregnancy rate is 30–35%.
- Use of hematopoietic SCs or in conjunction with PRP helps in regenerating damaged endometrium but its effect on enhancing pregnancy rates are still awaited.

REFERENCES

1. Practice Committee of the American Society for Reproductive Medicine. Uterine septum: a guideline. Fertil Steril. 2016; 106(3):530-40.
2. Saravelos SH, Cocksedge KA, Li TC. Prevalence and diagnosis of congenital uterine anomalies in women with reproductive failure: a critical appraisal. Hum Reprod Update. 2008;14(5):415-29.
3. Rackow BW, Arici A. Reproductive performance of women with müllerian anomalies. Curr Opin Obstet Gynecol. 2007;19(3):229-37.
4. Doerr W. [Cruveilhier DWJ, Rokitansky CV, Virchow R. Fundamentals of pathology, thoughts on the 100th anniversary of Rokitansky's death]. Virchows Arch A Pathol Anat Histol. 1978;378(1):1-16.
5. Brucker SY, Rall K, Campo R, Oppelt P, Isaacson K. Treatment of congenital malformations. Semin Reprod Med. 2011;29(2):101-12.
6. Venetis CA, Papadopoulos SP, Campo R, Gordts S, Tarlatzis BC, Grimbizis GF. Clinical implications of congenital uterine anomalies: a meta-analysis of comparative studies. Reprod Biomed Online. 2014;29(6):665-83.
7. Harger JH, Archer DF, Marchese SG, Muracca-Clemens M, Garver KL. Etiology of recurrent pregnancy losses and outcome of subsequent pregnancies. Obstet Gynecol. 1983;62(5):574-81.
8. Chandler TM, Machan LS, Cooperberg PL, Harris AC, Chang SD. Mullerian duct anomalies: from diagnosis to intervention. Br J Radiol. 2009;82(984):1034-42.
9. Grimbizis GF, Gordts S, Di Spiezio Sardo A, Brucker S, De Angelis C, Gergolet M. The ESHRE/ESGE consensus on the classification of female genital tract congenital anomalies. Hum Reprod. 2013;28(8):2032-44.
10. Pfeifer SM, Attaran M, Goldstein J, Lindheim SR, Petrozza JC, Rackow BW, et al. ASRM müllerian anomalies classification 2021. Fertil Steril. 2021;116(5):1238-52.
11. Ludwin A, Ludwin I. Comparison of the ESHRE-ESGE and ASRM classifications of Müllerian duct anomalies in everyday practice. Hum Reprod. 2015;30(3):569-80.
12. Lin PC, Bhatnagar KP, Nettleton GS, Nakajima ST. Female genital anomalies affecting reproduction. Fertil Steril. 2002;78(5):899-915.
13. Grimbizis GF, Camus M, Tarlatzis BC, Bontis JN, Devroey P. Clinical implications of uterine malformations and hysteroscopic treatment results. Hum Reprod Update. 2001;7(2):161-74.
14. Fedele L, Bianchi S, Frontino G. Septums and synechiae: approaches to surgical correction. Clin Obstet Gynecol. 2006;49(4):767-88.
15. Deutch TD, Abuhamad AZ. The role of 3-dimensional ultrasonography and magnetic resonance imaging in the diagnosis of müllerian duct anomalies. J Ultrasound Med. 2008;27(3):413-23.
16. ACOG Committee Opinion. Müllerian Agenesis: Diagnosis, Management, And Treatment. Number 562. 2013 (replaces No. 355, December 2006).
17. Borruto F, Chasen ST, Chervenak FA, Fedele L. The Vecchietti procedure for surgical treatment of vaginal agenesis: comparison of laparoscopy and laparotomy. Int J Gynaecol Obstet. 1999;64(2):153-8.
18. Mishra B, Janavar G, Pradeep Y, Singh AK, Kumar V, Upadhyay DN, et al. Indigenous technique of fabricating vaginal mould for vaginal reconstruction and uterine drainage in McIndoe vaginoplasty using 10 ml syringe. Indian J Plast Surg. 2016;49(1):76-80.
19. Liguori G, Trombetta C, Bucci S, Salamè L, Bortul M, Siracusano S, et al. Laparoscopic mobilization of neovagina to assist secondary ileal vaginoplasty in male-to-female transsexuals. Urology. 2005;66(2):293-8.
20. Medeiros LR, Rosa DD, Silva FR, Silva BR, Ros MI. Laparoscopic approach of a unicornuate uterus with noncommunicating rudimentary horns. ISRN Obstet Gynecol. 2011;2011: 906138.
21. Whittaker MD, Garry R. Modern management of congenital abnormalities of the uterus. Curr Obstet Gynaecol. 1995;5(1):41-5.
22. Arora M, Kumar BH. No-surgical management of uterus didelphys. Saudi Med J. 1989;10(1):141-2.
23. Matsaseng T, Kruger TF. Laparoscopic Strassman's metroplasty for bicornuate uterus—is it relevant? S Afr J OG. 2012;18(3):85-7.
24. Ludwin A, Ludwin I, Coelho Neto MA, Nastri CO, Bhagavath B, Lindheim SR, et al. Septate uterus according to ESHRE/ESGE, ASRM and CUME definitions: association with infertility and miscarriage, cost and warnings for women and healthcare systems. Ultrasound Obstet Gynecol. 2019;54(6): 800-14.
25. Practice Committee of the American Society for Reproductive Medicine. Uterine septum: a guideline. Fertil Steril. 2016; 106(3):530-40.

26. Rikken JF, Kowalik CR, Emanuel MH, Mol BW, Van der Veen F, van Wely M, et al. Septum resection for women of reproductive age with a septate uterus. Cochrane Database Syst Rev. 2017;1(1):CD008576.
27. Bender Atik R, Christiansen OB, Elson J, Kolte AM, Lewis S, Middeldorp S, et al; ESHRE Guideline Group on RPL. ESHRE guideline: recurrent pregnancy loss. Hum Reprod Open. 2018;2018(2):hoy004.
28. Akhtar MA, Saravelos SH, Li TC, Jayaprakasan K; on behalf of the Royal College of Obstetricians and Gynaecologists. Reproductive Implications and Management of Congenital Uterine Anomalies: Scientific Impact Paper No. 62 November 2019. BJOG. 2020;127(5):e1-e13.
29. Garbin O, Ohl J, Bettahar-Lebugle K, Dellenbach P. Hysteroscopic metroplasty in diethylstilboestrol-exposed and hypoplastic uterus: a report on 24 cases. Hum Reprod. 1998;13(10):2751-5.
30. Ludwin A, Coelho Neto MA, Ludwin I, Nastri CO, Costa W, Acién M, et al. Congenital Uterine Malformation by Experts (CUME): diagnostic criteria for T-shaped uterus. Ultrasound Obstet Gynecol. 2020;55(6):815-29.
31. Klatsky PC, Tran ND, Caughey AB, Fujimoto VY. Fibroids and reproductive outcomes: a systematic literature review from conception to delivery. Am J Obstet Gynecol. 2008;198(4):357-66.
32. Falcone T, Parker WH. Surgical management of leiomyomas for fertility or uterine preservation. Obstet Gynecol. 2013;121(4):856-68.
33. Buttram VC Jr, Reiter RC. Uterine leiomyomata: etiology, symptomatology, and management. Fertil Steril. 1981;36(4):433-45.
34. Benecke C, Kruger TF, Siebert TI, Van der Merwe JP, Steyn DW. Effect of fibroids on fertility in patients undergoing assisted reproduction. A structured literature review. Gynecol Obstet Invest. 2005;59(4):225-30.
35. Sunkara SK, Khairy M, El-Toukhy T, Khalaf Y, Coomarasamy A. The effect of intramural fibroids without uterine cavity involvement on the outcome of IVF treatment: a systematic review and meta-analysis. Hum Reprod. 2010;25(2):418-29.
36. Munro MG, Critchley HO, Broder MS, Fraser IS; FIGO Working Group on Menstrual Disorders. FIGO classification system (PALM-COEIN) for causes of abnormal uterine bleeding in nongravid women of reproductive age. Int J Gynaecol Obstet. 2011;113(1):3-13.
37. American Association of Gynecologic Laparoscopists (AAGL): Advancing Minimally Invasive Gynecology Worldwide. AAGL practice report: practice guidelines for the diagnosis and management of submucous leiomyomas. J Minim Invasive Gynecol. 2012;19(2):152-71.
38. Dubuisson JB, Fauconnier A. Laparoscopic myomectomy. In: Donnez J (Ed). Atlas of Operative Laparoscopy and Hysteroscopy, 3rd edition. United Kingdom: Informa Healthcare; 2007. pp. 227-39.
39. Kongnyuy EJ, Wiysonge CS. Interventions to reduce haemorrhage during myomectomy for fibroids. Cochrane Database Syst Rev. 2011;(11):CD005355.
40. Friedman AJ, Harrison-Atlas D, Barbieri RL, Benacerraf B, Gleason R, Schiff I. A randomized, placebo-controlled, double-blind study evaluating the efficacy of leuprolide acetate depot in the treatment of uterine leiomyomata. Fertil Steril. 1989;51(2):251-6.
41. Campo S, Garcea N. Laparoscopic myomectomy in premenopausal women with and without preoperative treatment using gonadotropin-releasing hormone analogues. Hum Reprod. 1999;14(1):44-8.
42. Mattei A, Cioni R, Bargelli G, Scarselli G. Techniques of laparoscopic myomectomy. Reprod Biomed Online. 2011;23(1):34-9.
43. Munro MG. Uterine leiomyomas, current concepts: pathogenesis, impact on reproductive health, and medical, procedural, and surgical management. Obstet Gynecol Clin North Am. 2011;38(4):703-31.
44. Grande N, Catalano GF, Ferrari S, Marana R. Spontaneous uterine rupture at 27 weeks of pregnancy after laparoscopic myomectomy. J Minim Invasive Gynecol. 2005;12(4):301.
45. Nezhat C, Nezhat F, Nezhat C. Overview of complications. In: Nezhat C, Nezhat F, Nezhat C (Eds). Nezhat's Operative Gynecologic Laparoscopy and Hysteroscopy, 3rd edition. Cambridge: Cambridge University Press; 2008. pp. 582-600.
46. Dubuisson JB, Chavet X, Chapron C, Gregorakis SS, Morice P. Uterine rupture during pregnancy after laparoscopic myomectomy. Hum Reprod. 1995;10(6):1475-7.
47. Semm K. New methods of pelviscopy (gynecologic laparoscopy) for myomectomy, ovariectomy, tubectomy and adenectomy. Endoscopy. 1979;11(2):85-93.
48. Tulandi T. Reproductive issues in women with uterine leiomyomas. [online] Available from www.uptodate.com. [Last accessed September, 2009].
49. Sinha R, Hegde A, Mahajan C, Dubey N, Sundaram M. Laparoscopic myomectomy: do size, number, and location of the myomas form limiting factors for laparoscopic myomectomy? J Minim Invasive Gynecol. 2008;15(3):292-300.
50. Igarashi M. Value of myomectomy in the treatment of infertility. Fertil Steril. 1993;59(6):1331-2.
51. Angioli R, Plotti F, Montera R, Damiani P, Terranova C, Oronzi I, et al. A new type of absorbable barbed suture for use in laparoscopic myomectomy. Int J Gynaecol Obstet. 2012;117(3):220-3.
52. Einarsson JI, Vellinga TT, Twijnstra AR, Chavan NR, Suzuki Y, Greenberg JA. Bidirectional barbed suture: an evaluation of safety and clinical outcomes. JSLS. 2010;14(3):381-5.
53. Brölmann H, Tanos V, Grimbizis G, Ind T, Philips K, van den Bosch T. Options on fibroid morcellation: a literature review. Gynecol Surg. 2015;12(1):3-15.
54. Tulandi T, Murray C, Guralnick M. Adhesion formation and reproductive outcome after myomectomy and second-look laparoscopy. Obstet Gynecol. 1970;82(2):213-5.
55. The efficacy of Interceed (TC7)* for the prevention of reformation of postoperative adhesions on ovaries, fallopian tubes, and fimbriae in microsurgical operations for fertility: a multicenter study. Nordic Adhesion Prevention Study Group. Fertil Steril. 1995;63(4):709-14.
56. An expanded polytetrafluoroethylene barrier (Gore-Tex Surgical Membrane) reduces post-myomectomy adhesion formation. The Myomectomy Adhesion Multicenter Study Group. Fertil Steril. 1995;63(3):491-3.
57. Wamsteker K, Emanuel MH, de Kruif JH. Transcervical hysteroscopic resection of submucous fibroids for abnormal

uterine bleeding: results regarding the degree of intramural extension. Obstet Gynecol. 1993;82(5):736-40.
58. Lasmar RB, Lasmar BP, Celeste RK, da Rosa DB, Depes Dde B, Lopes RG. A new system to classify submucous myomas: a Brazilian multicenter study. J Minim Invasive Gynecol. 2012;19(5):575-80.
59. Lasmer RB, Xinmei Z, Indman PD, Celeste RK, Di Spiezio Sardo A. Feasibility of a new system of classification of submucus myomas: a multicenter study. Fertil Steril. 2011;95(6): 2073-7.
60. Neuwirth RS, Amin HK. Excision of submucous fibroids with hysteroscopic control. Am J Obstet Gynecol. 1976;126(1):95-9.
61. Charles J, Walsh A, Brodman M. Hysteroscopic myomectomy. In: Nezhat C, Nezhat F, Nezhat C (Eds). Nezhat's Operative Gynecologic Laparoscopy and Hysteroscopy, 3rd edition. Cambridge: Cambridge University Press; 2008. pp. 152-61.
62. Makris N, Vomvolaki E, Mantzaris G, Kalmantis K, Hatzipappas J, Antsaklis A. Role of a bipolar resectoscope in subfertile women with submucous myomas and menstrual disorders. J Obstet Gynaecol Res. 2007;33(6):849-54.
63. Clark TJ, Mahajan D, Sunder P, Gupta JK. Hysteroscopic treatment of symptomatic submucous fibroids using a bipolar intrauterine system: a feasibility study. Eur J Obstet Gynecol Reprod Biol. 2002;100(2):237-42.
64. Bettocchi S, Nappi L, Ceci O, Santoro A, Selvaggi L, Cormio G, et al. Treatment of submucosal and partially intramural myomas using the bipolar Versapoint system. J Am Assoc Gynecol Laparosc. 2004;11:S17-S18.
65. Emanuel MH, Wamsteker K. The Intra Uterine Morcellator: A new hysteroscopic operating technique to remove intrauterine polyps and myomas. J Minim Invasive Gynecol. 2005;12(1):62-6.
66. van Dongen H, Emanuel MH, Wolterbeek R, Trimbos JB, Jansen FW. Hysteroscopic morcellator for removal of intrauterine polyps and myomas: a randomized controlled pilot study among residents in training. J Minim Invasive Gynecol. 2008;15(4):466-71.
67. Indman PD. Hysteroscopic treatment of submucous myomas. Clin Obstet Gynecol. 2006;49(4):811-20.
68. Vercellini P, Zàina B, Yaylayan L, Pisacreta A, De Giorgi O, Crosignani PG. Hysteroscopic myomectomy: long-term effects on menstrual pattern and fertility. Obstet Gynecol. 1999;94(3):341-7.
69. Emanuel MH, Wamsteker K, Hart AA, Metz G, Lammes FB. Long-term results of hysteroscopic myomectomy for abnormal uterine bleeding. Obstet Gynecol. 1999;93(5 Pt 1): 743-8.
70. Pritts EA, Parker WH, Olive DL. Fibroids and infertility: an updated systematic review of the evidence. Fertil Steril. 2009;91(4):1215-23.
71. Guo XC, Segars JH. The impact and management of fibroids for fertility an evidence-based approach. Obstet Gynecol Clin North Am. 2012;39(4):521-33.
72. Faivre E, Surroca MM, Deffieux X, Pages F, Gervaise A, Fernandez H. Vaginal myomectomy: literature review. J Minim Invasive Gynecol. 2010;17(2):154-60.
73. Matsuoka S, Kikuchi I, Kitade M, Kumakiri J, Kuroda K, Tokita S. Strategy for laparoscopic cervical myomectomy. J Minim Invasive Gynecol. 2010;17(3):301-5.
74. Galliano D. Ulipristal acetate in uterine fibroids. Fertil Steril. 2015;103(2):359-60.
75. Donnez J, Donnez O, Matule D, Ahrendt HJ, Hudecek R, Zatik J. Long-term medical management of uterine fibroids with ulipristal acetate. Fertil Steril. 2016;105(1):165-73.e4.
76. Chabbert-Buffet N, Esber N, Bouchard P. Fibroid growth and medical options for treatment. Fertil Steril. 2014;102(3):630-9.
77. Liu J, Soper D, Lukes AS, Gee P, Kimble T, Kroll R. VENUS II: the second us-based phase 3 study of ulipristal acetate (UPA) for treatment of symptomatic uterine fibroids (UF). Fertil Steril. 2017;108(3):e27-e28.
78. Naftalin J, Hoo W, Pateman K, Mavrelos D, Holland T, Jurkovic D. How common is adenomyosis? A prospective study of prevalence using transvaginal ultrasound in a gynecology clinic. Hum Reprod. 2012;27(12):3432-9.
79. Naftalin J, Hoo W, Pateman K, Mavrelos D, Foo X, Jurkovic D. Is adenomyosis associated with menorrhagia? Hum Reprod. 2014;29(3):473-9.
80. Oehler MK, Greschik H, Fischer DC, Tong X, Schuele R, Kieback DG. Functional characterization of somatic point mutations of the human estrogen receptor alpha (hERalpha) in adenomyosis uteri. Mol Hum Reprod. 2004;10(12):853-60.
81. Kitawaki J. Adenomyosis: the pathophysiology of an oestrogen-dependent disease. Best Pract Res Clin Obstet Gynaecol. 2006;20(4):493-502.
82. Nie J, Liu X, Guo SW. Promoter hypermethylation of progesterone receptor isoform B (PR-B) in adenomyosis and its rectification by a histone deacetylase inhibitor and a demethylation agent. Reprod Sci. 2010;17(11):995-1005.
83. Bazot M, Darai E. Adenomyosis: "advances in diagnosis". Abstracts of the 24th Annual Meeting of ESHRE. Barcelona, Spain; 2008.
84. Sofic A, Husic-Selimovic A, Carovac A, Jahic E, Smailbegovic V, Kupusovic J. The Significance of MRI Evaluation of the Uterine Junctional Zone in the Early Diagnosis of Adenomyosis. Acta Inform Med. 2016;24(2):103-6.
85. Martínez-Conejero JA, Morgan M, Montesinos M, Fortuño S, Meseguer M, Simón C, et al. Adenomyosis does not affect implantation, but is associated with miscarriage in patients undergoing oocyte donation. Fertil Steril. 2011;96(4):943-50.
86. Fernandes HM, Healey MG, Vollenhoven BJ, Meagher SM. The association of sonographically diagnosed adenomyosis on ovarian response and the outcome of in vitro fertilization-embryo transfer. Fertil Steril. 2013;100(3):S79.
87. Younes G, Tulandi T. Effects of adenomyosis on in vitro fertilization treatment outcomes: a meta-analysis. Fertil Steril. 2017;108(3):483-90.e3.
88. Fernandes H, Higgins C, Vollenhoven BJ, da Silva Costa F, Healey M. The association between sonographically diagnosed adenomyosis and in vitro fertilization-embryo transfers. Fertil Steril. 2017;108(3):e260.
89. Kishi Y, Yabuta M, Taniguchi F. Who will benefit from uterus-sparing surgery in adenomyosis-associated subfertility? Fertil Steril. 2014;102(3):p802-7.e1.
90. Vercellini P, Viganò P, Somigliana E, Fedele L. Endometriosis: pathogenesis and treatment. Nat Rev Endocrinol. 2014; 10(5):261-75.
91. Schweppe KW. The place of dydrogesterone in the treatment of endometriosis and adenomyosis. Maturitas. 2009; 65(Suppl 1):S23-S7.
92. Lazzeri L, Luisi S, Petraglia F. Progestins for the Treatment of Endometriosis: An Update. J Endometr Pelvic Pain Disord. 2010;2(4):169-81.

93. Fedele L, Bianchi S, Frontino G. Hormonal treatments for adenomyosis. Best Pract Res Clin Obstet Gynaecol. 2008; 22(2):333-9.
94. Muneyyirci-Delale O, Chandrareddy A, Mankame S, Osei-Tutu N, von Gizycki H. Norethindrone acetate in the medical management of adenomyosis. Pharmaceuticals (Basel). 2012;5(10):1120-7.
95. Streuli I, Dubuisson J, Santulli P, de Ziegler D, Batteux F, Chapron C. An update on the pharmacological management of adenomyosis. Expert Opin Pharmacother. 2014;15(16): 2347-60.
96. Luisi S, Razzi S, Lazzeri L, Bocchi C, Severi FM, Petraglia F. Efficacy of vaginal danazol treatment in women with menorrhagia during fertile age. Fertil Steril. 2009;92(4): 1351-4.
97. Bahamondes L, Valeria Bahamondes M, Shulman LP. Non-contraceptive benefits of hormonal and intrauterine reversible contraceptive methods. Hum Reprod Update. 2015;21(5):640-51.
98. Matteson KA, Rahn DD, Wheeler TL 2nd, Casiano E, Siddiqui NY, Harvie HS, et al; Society of Gynecologic Surgeons Systematic Review Group. Nonsurgical management of heavy menstrual bleeding: a systematic review. Obstet Gynecol. 2013;121(3):632-43.
99. Oettel M, Breitbarth H, Elger W, Gräser T, Hübler D, Kaufmann G, et al. The pharmacological profile of dienogest. Eur J Contracept Reprod Health Care. 1999;4(Suppl):2-13.
100. Foster RH, Wilde MI. Dienogest. Drugs. 1998;56(5):825-33; discussion 834-5.
101. Horie S, Harada T, Mitsunari M, Taniguchi F, Iwabe T, Terakawa N. Progesterone and progestational compounds attenuate tumor necrosis factor alpha-induced interleukin-8 production via nuclear factor kappa B inactivation in endometriotic stromal cells. Fertil Steril. 2005;83(5):1530-5.
102. Hirata T, Izumi G, Takamura M, Saito A, Nakazawa A, Harada M, et al. Efficacy of dienogest in the treatment of symptomatic adenomyosis: A pilot study. Gynecol Endocrinol. 2014; 30(10):726-9.
103. Ishihara H, Kitawaki J, Kado N, Koshiba H, Fushiki S, Honjo H. Gonadotropin-releasing hormone agonist and danazol normalize aromatase cytochrome P450 expression in eutopic endometrium from women with endometriosis, adenomyosis, or leiomyomas. Fertil Steril. 2003;79(Suppl 1):735-42.
104. Niu Z, Chen Q, Sun Y, Feng Y. Long-term pituitary down-regulation before frozen embryo transfer could improve pregnancy outcomes in women with adenomyosis. Gynecol Endocrinol. 2013;29(12):1026-30.
105. Bulun SE, Sebastian S, Takayama K, Suzuki T, Sasano H, Shozu M. The human CYP19 (aromatase P450) gene: update on physiologic roles and genomic organization of promoters. J Steroid Biochem Mol Biol. 2003;86(3-5):219-24.
106. Kitawaki J, Noguchi T, Amatsu T, Maeda K, Tsukamoto K, Yamamoto T, et al. Expression of aromatase cytochrome P450 protein and messenger ribonucleic acid in human endometriotic and adenomyotic tissues but not in normal endometrium. Biol Reprod. 1997;57(3):514-9.
107. Badawy AM, Elnashar AM, Mosbah AA. Aromatase inhibitors or gonadotropin-releasing hormone agonists for the management of uterine adenomyosis: a randomized controlled trial. Acta Obstet Gynecol Scand. 2012;91(4):489-95.
108. Lee WL, Cheng MH, Chao HT, Wang PH. The role of selective estrogen receptor modulators on breast cancer: from tamoxifen to raloxifene. Taiwan J Obstet Gynecol. 2008;47(1):24-31.
109. Pinkerton JV, Thomas S. Use of SERMs for treatment in postmenopausal women. J Steroid Biochem Mol Biol. 2014;142:142-54.
110. Wagenfeld A, Saunders PT, Whitaker L, Critchley HO. Selective progesterone receptor modulators (SPRMs): progesterone receptor action, mode of action on the endometrium and treatment options in gynecological therapies. Expert Opin Ther Targets. 2016;20(9):1045-54.
111. Kashani BN, Centini G, Morelli SS, Weiss G, Petraglia F. Role of Medical Management for Uterine Leiomyomas. Best Pract Res Clin Obstet Gynaecol. 2015;34:85-103.
112. Angioni S, Cofelice V, Sedda F, Loi ES, Multinu F, Pontis A, et al. Progestins for symptomatic endometriosis: results of clinical studies. Current Drug Therapy. 2015;10(2):91-104.
113. Chong GO, Lee YH, Hong DG, Cho YL, Lee YS. Long-term efficacy of laparoscopic or robotic adenomyomectomy, with or without medical treatment, for severely symptomatic adenomyosis. Gynecol Obstet Invest. 2016;81(4):346-52.
114. Kim S, Kang SY, Min JY, Kwak S, Chung YJ, Kim JH. Conservative surgical treatment of focal adenomyosis by robot-assisted laparoscopic adenomyomectomy. Fertil Steril. 2013;100(3):S171.
115. McCausland V, McCausland A The response of adenomyosis to endometrial ablation/resection. Hum Reprod Update. 1998;4(4):350-9.
116. Zhang L, Zhang W, Orsi F, Chen W, Wang Z. Ultrasound-guided high intensity focused ultrasound for the treatment of gynecological diseases: A review of safety and efficacy. Int J Hyperthermia. 2015;31(3):280-4.
117. Chin W, Walbridge J, Quinn S. MR-guided focused ultrasound for the treatment of adenomyosis: current insights. Research and Reports in Focused Ultrasound. 2015;4:1-8.
118. ClinicalTrials.gov. (2019). Treatment of benign uterine disorders using high intensity focused ultrasound (MR-HIFU). Turku University hospital. [online] Available from https://clinicaltrials.gov/ct2/show/NCT02914704 [Last accessed November, 2022].
119. Hammadeh ME, Fischer-Hammadeh C, Ali KR. Assisted hatching in assisted reproduction: a state of the art. J Assist Reprod Genet. 2011;28(2):119-28.
120. Simon C, Vladimirov IK, Castillón G, Ortega I, Cabanillas S, Vidal C, et al. Prospective randomized study of the endometrial receptivity analysis (ERA) test in the infertility work up to guide personalized embryo transfer versus fresh transfer or deferred embryo transfer. Fertil Steril. 2016;106(3):e46-e47.
121. Derks RS, Farquhar C, Mol BW, Buckingham K, Heineman MJ. Techniques for preparation prior to embryo transfer. Cochrane Database Syst Rev. 2009;(4):CD007682.
122. Chung CH, Wong AW, Chan CP, Saravelos SH, Kong GW, Cheung LP, et al. The changing pattern of uterine contractions before and after fresh embryo transfer and its relation to clinical outcome. Reprod Biomed Online. 2017;34(3):240-7.
123. Bontekoe S, Heineman MJ, Johnson N, Blake D. Adherence compounds in embryo transfer media for assisted reproductive technologies. Cochrane Database Syst Rev. 2014; 2014(2):CD007421.

124. Kang YJ, Forbes K, Carver J, Aplin JD. The role of the osteopontin-integrin αvβ3 interaction at implantation: functional analysis using three different in vitro models. Hum Reprod. 2014;29(4):739-49.
125. Johnson GA, Burghardt RC, Bazer FW, Spencer TE. Osteopontin: roles in implantation and placentation. Biol Reprod. 2003;69(5):1458-71.
126. DeSouza MM, Surveyor GA, Zhou X, Julian J, Carson DD. Mucins provide a barrier to embryo implantation. In: Carsen DD (Ed). Embryo Implantation: Molecular, Cellular and Clinical Aspects. Germany: Springer; 1999. pp. 123-31.
127. Rumbold A, Middleton P, Pan N, Crowther CA. Vitamin supplementation for preventing miscarriage. Cochrane Database Syst Rev. 2011;(1):CD004073.
128. Park HJ, Kim YS, Yoon TK, Lee WS. Chronic endometritis and infertility. Clin Exp Reprod Med. 2016;43(4);185-92.
129. El Toukhy T, Khalaf Y, Sunkara S. Local endometrial injury and IVF outcome: a systematic review and meta-analysis. Reprod Biomed Online. 2012;25(4):345-54.
130. Karimzadeh MA, Ayazi Rozbahani M, Tabibnejad N. Endometrial local injury improves the pregnancy rate among recurrent implantation failure patients undergoing in vitro fertilisation/intra cytoplasmic sperm injection: a randomised clinical trial. Aust N Z J Obstet Gynaecol. 2009;49(6): 677-80.
131. Endometrial Scratch Trial. A multicentre randomised controlled trial of induced endometrial scratch in women undergoing first time in vitro fertilization (IVF). The University of Sheffield; 2017.
132. Raghupathy R. Cytokines and the success or failure of pregnancy. In: Arora M (Ed). Recurrent Pregnancy Loss. New Delhi: Jaypee Medical Publishers (P) Ltd; 2007.
133. Lissauer D, Goodyear O, Khanum R, Moss PA, Kilby MD. Profile of maternal CD4 T-cell effector function during normal pregnancy and in women with a history of recurrent miscarriage. Clin Sci (Lond). 2014;126(5):347-54.
134. Kuon RJ, Weber M, Heger J, Santillán I, Vomstein K, Bär C, et al. Uterine natural killer cells in patients with idiopathic recurrent miscarriage. Am J Reprod Immunol. 2017;78(4).
135. Brosens JJ, Hodgetts A, Feroze-Zaidi F, Sherwin JR, Fusi L, Salker MS. Proteomic analysis of endometrium from fertile and infertile patients suggests a role of apolipoprotein A-I in embryo implantation failure and endometriosis. Mol Hum Reprod. 2010;16(4):273-85.
136. Bhagwat SR, Chandrashekar DS, Kakar R, Davuluri S, Bajpai AK, Nayak S, et al. Endometrial receptivity: a visit to functional genomics studies on human endometrium and creation of HGEx-ERdb. PLoS One. 2013;8(3):e58419.
137. Preitl B, Treiber G, Peiber TR, Amrein K. Vitamin D and immune function. Nutrients. 2013;5(7):2502-21.
138. Coomarasamy A, Williams H, Truchanowicz E, Seed PT, Small R, Quenby S, et al. A Randomized Trial of Progesterone in Women with Recurrent Miscarriages. PROMISE trial. N Engl J Med. 2015;373(22):2141-8.
139. Haas DM, Ramsey PS. Progesterone for preventing miscarriage. Cochrane Database Syst Rev. 2013(10):CD003511.
140. Wong LF, Porter TF, Scott JR. Immunotherapy for recurrent miscarriage. Cochrane Database Syst Rev. 2014(10): CD000112.
141. Jeve YB, Davies W. Evidence-based management of recurrent miscarriages. J Hum Reprod Sci. 2014;7(3):159-69.
142. Allahbadia GN. Low-Molecular-Weight Heparin (LMWH) in Women with Repeated Implantation Failure. J Obstet Gynecol India. 2012;62(4):381-3.
143. Chang Y, Li J, Chen Y, Wei L, Yang X, Shi Y, et al. Autologous platelet rich plasma promotes endometrial growth and improves pregnancy outcome during in vitro fertilization. Int J Clin Exp Med. 2015;8(1):1286-90.
144. Mouhayar Y, Sharara FI. Modern management of thin lining. Middle East Fertil Soc J. 2017;22(1):1-12.
145. Bräannströom M, Johannesson L, Bokstrom H, Kvarnström N, Mölne J, Dahm-Kähler P, et al. Live birth after uterus transplantation. The Lancet. 2015;385(9968):607-16.
146. Sugimoto O. Diagnostic and therapeutic hysteroscopy for traumatic intrauterine adhesions. Am J Obstet Gynecol. 1978;131(5):539-47.
147. Pabuçcu R, Atay V, Orhon E, Urman B, Ergün A. Hysteroscopic treatment of intrauterine adhesions is safe and effective in the restoration of normal menstruation and fertility. Fertil Steril. 1997;68(6):1141-3.
148. Capella-Allouc S, Morsad F, Rongières-Bertrand C, Taylor S, Fernandez H. Hysteroscopic treatment of severe Asherman's syndrome and subsequent fertility. Hum Reprod. 1999;14(5):1230-3.
149. Yamamoto N, Takeuchi R, Izuchi D, Yuge N, Miyazaki M, Yasunaga M, et al. Hysteroscopic adhesiolysis for patients with Asherman's syndrome: menstrual and fertility outcomes. Reprod Med Biol. 2013;12(4):159-66.
150. Kilic S, Yuksel B, Pinarli F, Albayrak A, Boztok B, Delibasi T. Effect of stem cell application on Asherman syndrome, an experimental rat model. J Assist Reprod Genet. 2014; 31(8):975-82.
151. Domnina A, Novikova P, Obidina J, Fridlyanskaya I, Alekseenko L, Kozhukharova I, et al. Human mesenchymal stem cells in spheroids improve fertility in model animals with damaged endometrium. Stem Cell Res Ther. 2018;9(1):50.
152. Golden MP, Vikram HR. Extrapulmonary tuberculosis: an overview. Am Fam Physician. 2005;72(9):1761-8.
153. Sharma JB. Current Diagnosis and Management of Female Genital Tuberculosis. J Obstet Gynaecol India. 2015;65(6):362-71.
154. Das P, Ahuja A, Gupta SD. Incidence, etiopathogenesis and pathological aspects of genitourinary tuberculosis in India: A journey revisited. Indian J Urol. 2008;24(3):356-61.
155. Netter A, Musset R, Lambert A, Salomon Y, Montbazet G. Tuberculous endo-uterine symphysis; an anatomo-clinical and radiologically characteristic syndrome. Gynecol Obstet (Paris). 1955;54(1):19-36.
156. World Health Organization. (2010). Treatment of Tuberculosis: Guidelines, 4th edition. [online] Available from https://apps.who.int/iris/handle/10665/44165 [Last accessed November, 2022].

CHAPTER 34

Tubal Factors in Infertility

Pratap Kumar, Aswathy Kumaran

INTRODUCTION

The fallopian tubes named after Gabriele Falloppio (also spelled Falloppia), a 16th-century physician and surgeon, are appendages of the uterus located on either side at the superior portion of the uterine cavity. They are 10 cm long muscular tubes originating at the uterine cornua and opening distally into the peritoneal cavity. Each tube is divisible into four parts and runs laterally within the mesosalpinx. The proximal narrowest segment comprises the interstitium (1.25 cm long, 1 mm wide) and the isthmus (2.5 cm long, 2.5 cm wide). The ampulla, the middle segment (5 cm long, 2.5–5 mm wide), gradually widens and merges with the distal segment, the broad funnel-like infundibulum (1.25 cm long, 6 mm wide) of the tubes that lies in close proximity to the ipsilateral ovary. Infundibulum has fimbriae that help in capturing the cumulus oophorus complex at ovulation.

The uterine tubes form a conducting channel for gametes and embryos. The tubes assist and modulate sperm transport and regulate oocyte transport; the ampulla promotes fertilization, nurtures gametes and embryos, and ensures the timely passage of the embryo to the uterus.[1] The patent healthy functional tubes are hence important for fertility.

Tubal disease contributes to 25–35% of female factor infertility and 11–30% of infertility in general depending on the population characteristics.[2,3] The main cause for tubal infertility is salpingitis which accounts for >50% of the cases as well as tubal surgery.[2] Published literature reveals that 20–30% of women regret that they have had a tubal ligation.[4-6] Therefore prevention, diagnosis, and management of tubal factor-dependent subfertility are important in reproductive medicine.

CAUSES FOR TUBAL SUBFERTILITY

Congenital

Developmental or inherent anomalies of the fallopian tubes are rare and most do not require treatment. Absence of one or both tubes is almost always associated with absence of the uterus as well as other anomalies.[7] Rudimentary oviducts, infantile ones, duplication of ostia, and accessory tubes are some other uncommon developmental anomalies.

Acquired

Pelvic inflammatory disease (PID) is the most frequent cause for tubal disease of which the single largest cause is *Chlamydia trachomatis* infection. Bulk of tubal disease is acquired and may be categorized into—proximal, mid, and distal tubal disease.

Proximal and Mid-tubal Disease

Pathology and blockage of proximal tube account for 10–25% of tubal disease.[3] Proximal block may be due to pseudo-obstruction or true anatomic blockage of the fallopian tubes **(Table 1)**.[8,9]

Salpingitis isthmica nodosa (SIN) is thought to arise from tubal inflammation of unspecified origin and affects the proximal tube prominently. Involvement of the distal tube and adhesions in pelvis and perihepatic areas, similar to PID, are also noted. Laparoscopy shows fibrosed tubal segments. Myosalpingeal hypertrophy encasing endosalpingeal diverticula is noted on histopathological examination.[8,9]

Pelvic inflammatory disease and endometriosis can cause anatomic tubal occlusion by direct involvement or secondary to adhesions.

TABLE 1: Causes of proximal tubal disease.

Pseudo-obstruction	*True anatomic blockage*
Plugs of mucus and amorphous debris	Salpingitis isthmica nodosa
Mucosal agglutination and viscous secretions	Pelvic inflammatory disease
Cornual spasm	Endometriosis
	Cornual polyps
	Intrauterine synechiae

TABLE 2: Causes of distal tubal disease.

Pelvic inflammatory disease	85% sexually transmitted diseases • *Neisseria gonorrhoeae* • *Chlamydia trachomatis* • *Mycoplasma hominis* • 15% iatrogenic
Tuberculosis	
Peritonitis of any cause	
Tubal damage from previous surgery	
Endometriosis	

Mid-tubal disease is commonly caused by PID, endometriosis, or prior surgery-related inflammations and adhesions that cause steno-occlusions, bulbous termination, scarring, and fibrosis of tubes.

Distal Tubal Disease

Eighty-five percent of tubal infertility is due to distal tubal disease. Distal tubal disease includes hydrosalpinges and fimbrial phimosis. Hydrosalpinx is an end stage of distal tubal disease where the distal is completely occluded, whereas a stenosed fimbrial opening due to adhesions results in fimbrial phimosis.[8,9] Causes of distal tubal disease are enumerated in **Table 2.**

Iatrogenic

Tubal Sterilization

Tubal sterilization causes irreversible infertility unless tubal patency is restored. As many as 30% of women regret their decision for sterilization. Thus, tubal sterilization is an iatrogenic cause of tubal infertility that needs to be addressed.

Salpingectomy

Women who have had to have bilateral salpingectomy for ectopic gestations, tubal or tubo-ovarian pathology often needs assisted reproductive techniques (ARTs) to conceive.

EVALUATION FOR THE TUBAL FACTOR INFERTILITY—GUIDELINES AND RECOMMENDATIONS

When?

Evaluation of the fallopian tube function and patency is a component of the initial triad of diagnostic investigations for infertile couples and is the third in line after evaluation of semen and ovulation. Tests for tubal patency and function are recommended initially when the woman's history, examinations, and ultrasound evaluation are suggestive of a high risk for tubal disease. Tubal infertility should be suspected and ruled out in women with history of PID, endometriosis, prior pelvic surgery, or ectopic pregnancy. If she is considered unlikely to have tubal pathology, then evaluation of tubes is done only if she does not conceive for at least 3 months in spite of satisfactory ovulation and natural or artificial insemination around ovulation.[10] Invasive tubal patency testing should be offered depending on the treatment needs of the couple and is ideal in couples who need or opt for ovulation induction, natural conception, or intrauterine insemination (IUI).

Guidelines and Recommendations

Royal College of Obstetricians and Gynaecologists Guidelines for Investigation of Suspected Tubal and Uterine Abnormalities[11]

- Hysterosalpingography (HSG) should be offered to women with no suspicion of comorbidities (such as PID, previous ectopic pregnancy, or endometriosis) to screen for tubal occlusion.
- Where available, hysterosalpingo-contrast-ultrasonography (HyCoSy) screening for tubal patency should be considered because it is an effective alternative to HSG for women who are not known to have comorbidities.
- When comorbidities are suspected, laparoscopy and chromopertubation should be offered.
- Do not offer hysteroscopy as part of the initial investigation unless clinically indicated.

ESHRE Recommendations[12]

European Society of Human Reproduction and Embryology (ESHRE) Capri workshop in 2000 put forward three categories of tests that have established association with healthy pregnancy—semen analysis, tubal patency tests by HSG, or laparoscopy, and tests to detect ovulation.

The ESHRE 2008 guidelines recommend that semen analysis and ovulation assessment before a test of tubal patency is performed. Women suspected to have comorbidities should be offered laparoscopic assessment directly so that any treatable tubal or pelvic pathology can be evaluated and managed at the same time.

ASRM Recommendations[13]

American Society for Reproductive Medicine (ASRM) has suggested specific ruling out of tubal disease by tubal patency tests and chlamydia antibody testing.

Hysterosalpingography, saline infusion sonography (SIS), laparoscopy and chromotubation, and fluoroscopic or hysteroscopic selective tubal cannulation have all been put forward as complementary and not mutually exclusive methods for evaluating tubal patency.

More than one technique is often required for accurate diagnosis and effective treatment of tubal obstruction tests for tubal function.

ULTRASOUND EVALUATION OF FALLOPIAN TUBES

Transvaginal sonography (TVS) of the female pelvis provides valuable information with ease. In fertility evaluation, TVS is used universally almost like an extension to clinical examination. The clinical history and examination in conjunction with the TVS findings decide whether the patient has a high index of suspicion for tubal disease.

The healthy fallopian tubes are not seen on routine two-dimensional or three-dimensional (2D/3D) ultrasound imaging of the pelvis unless filled or surrounded by fluid.[14] The tubal wall is not sonologically discernible unless thickened or distended with fluid. The characteristic retort-shaped pseudoseptate appearance helps us diagnose hydrosalpinx.[15]

The diseased and distended fallopian tubes on the other hand can often be seen as adnexal masses.

The distended tubes on ultrasonography (USG) are:[15]

- Thin- or thick-walled (in chronic cases)
- Elongated or folded, tubular, and retort-shaped fluid distended structure
- Separate the uterus and ovary.

A "cogwheel" appearance from thickened longitudinal folds in a hydrosalpinx when imaged in cross section is pathognomonic of a hydrosalpinx. "Beads on a string" sign is noted when incomplete stations are present.[12]

Atypical hydrosalpinx appearance without any pseudo septation may lead it to be mistaken for an ovarian or paraovarian cyst. Densely adherent, thick, and multiloculated distended tubes may mimic a complex ovarian tumor.

TUBAL ASSESSMENT TESTS

Active pelvic infection is an absolute contraindication to performing tubal patency tests. Hence, the evaluation of fallopian tubes starts with ruling out of active pelvic infection. The testing may be performed after treatment and resolution of active pelvic infection. Thorough history taking and clinical examination play an invaluable role to assess whether a patient has a high index of suspicion for pelvic infection.

Evaluating for Pelvic Infections

Centers for Disease Control and Prevention Criteria to Diagnose and Manage PID

There is no single test or symptom that can diagnose salpingitis effectively. Even though laparoscopy was considered the gold standard to diagnose salpingitis, almost 20% of PID may show no evidence of salpingitis. The Centers for Disease Control and Prevention (CDC) criteria used to diagnose and manage PID is comprehensive and simple. PID may be treated following the parenteral or oral treatment regimens suggested by CDC as is described in the chapter on PID or may be managed in India following the syndromic management approach for sexually transmitted diseases (STDs).[16]

We should also realize that about 15% of PIDs are iatrogenic with endometrial curettage, biopsy, or HSG. Intrauterine contraceptive device insertion being the main causative procedure. Hence, maintaining meticulous asepsis during the above procedures and avoiding unwarranted investigations will help decrease tubal infertility from iatrogenic PID **(Table 3)**.

TABLE 3: Centers for Disease Control and Prevention (CDC) criteria to diagnose pelvic inflammatory disease (PID).

Minimum criteria	If one or more of following is present: • Cervical motion tenderness • Uterine tenderness • Adnexal tenderness
Additional criteria	• Oral temperature >101°F (>38.3°C) • Abnormal cervical discharge or cervical friability • Presence of lots of white blood cells on vaginal fluid microscopy • Elevated erythrocyte sedimentation rate • Elevated C-reactive protein • Laboratory confirmation of *Neisseria gonorrhoeae* or *Chlamydia trachomatis* infection
Most specific	• Endometrial biopsy showing endometritis • Transvaginal sonography or magnetic resonance imaging techniques showing thickened, fluid-filled tubes with or without free pelvic fluid or tubo-ovarian complex, or Doppler studies suggesting pelvic infection (e.g., tubal hyperemia) • Laparoscopic findings consistent with PID

Chlamydia Antibody Test[15,17]

Chlamydial infection is the most common infective cause of tubal disease. The detection of antibodies to *C. trachomatis* has been associated with tubal pathology. The meta-analysis by Broeze et al. (2011) evaluated the accuracy of different chlamydia antibody test (CAT) assays. They found that microimmunofluorescence (MIF) was significantly better than enzyme-linked immunosorbent assay (ELISA) or immunofluorescence (IF) assays.[15,17]

Chlamydia antibody test has sensitivity of only 40–50% and positive predictive value (PPV) of 60%, but high negative predictive value (NPV) of 80–90% for detection of distal tubal disease compared to laparoscopy.[15,18,19] ASRM suggests that the CAT has limited clinical utility. But in women with low index of suspicion for tubal disease based on history and clinical examination, a negative CAT test reliably rules out the chance of tubal obstruction. The infection can be treated by treating the couple with a 14–21 day course of doxycycline.

Testing for Tuberculosis (in Endemic Countries)

Female genital tuberculosis (FGTB) is an undisputed cause for subfertility in countries like India where tuberculosis (TB) is endemic (incidence up to 16% in subfertile women).[20] It causes extensive tubal and endometrial damage. The fallopian tubes are involved in 90–100% cases. Ruling out of TB and curative treatment when diagnosed should be done prior to tube testing, and is ideal in women with hypomenorrhea, thin endometrium, or features of chronic PID. FGTB often coexists with other causes of PID like chlamydia and gonorrhea.

Female genital TB diagnosis is challenging as isolation of *Mycobacterium tuberculosis* by culture which is considered the requisite for diagnosis is often unreliable. A high index of clinical suspicion and multimodality testing is recommended. Genital TB may be diagnosed when one or two of the tests turn positive for TB. Premenstrual endometrial aspiration or biopsy and nucleic acid amplification (NAA) [TB polymerase chain reaction (PCR)] allow for rapid diagnosis and help to detect mycobacterial DNA in 80.9% of genital TB-suspected patients.[21] However, the PCR cannot differentiate between active and latent infection and may be unreliable in identifying the cases that actually require treatment. Hence, endometrial sampling and TB stain, BACTEC culture, histopathological examination for tubercles, and diagnostic laparoscopy are used in conjunction with TB PCR to diagnose genital TB. The new self-contained cassette-based analysis (GeneXpert) is faster than PCR and helps to identify rifampicin-resistant TB also.[21] TB when diagnosed has to be treated with appropriate antitubercular agents for 9 months.

Tubal Patency Tests

The various tests used to assess tubal patency and functional integrity are enumerated in **Figure 1** in the order of their coming into vogue. HSG/HyCoSy are the screening tests that are to be considered for tubal patency evaluation in women with no history/examination suggestive of tubal disease. In women with or without suspicion of comorbidities that can cause tubal disease and in women with inconclusive or positive screening on HSG/HyCoSy laparoscopy accompanied by hysteroscopy is to be offered as the gold standard for testing tubal integrity.

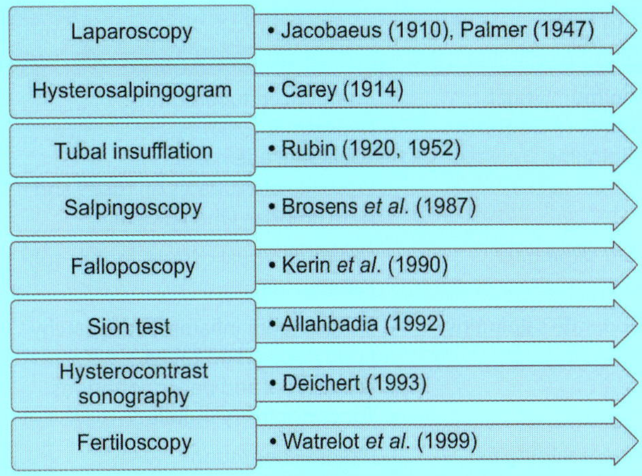

Fig. 1: Tests used to assess tubal patency and functional integrity.

Laparoscopy and Chromopertubation

Laparoscopy is the gold standard for diagnosing tubal patency and inflammation. It is a minimally invasive procedure which allows visualization of the pelvic anatomy and pathology, and spill of dye from the tube is seen. It allows diagnosis assessment and management of peritubal disease, adhesions, and endometriosis. Laparoscopy enables biopsy of suspicious lesions for further evaluation. Provided appropriate consent is taken, laparoscopy allows for surgical correction of pathology detected, where feasible.

Laparoscopy is a better predictor of fertility prognosis compared to other tubal tests like HSG and hence, the performances of other tests are compared to those of laparoscopy.[22] Although laparoscopy is considered the standard, it is not without error as around 3% of patients diagnosed with bilateral tubal block conceive spontaneously. Laparoscopy requires general anesthesia, creation of pneumoperitoneum as well as surgical skill and experience to perform. It is advocated in women suspected to have tubal infertility having comorbidities like PID, previous ectopic pregnancy, and endometriosis or history of appendicitis.

Laparoscopy has the distinct advantage that it can be complemented with hysteroscopy, falloposcopy, and salpingoscopy.

Falloposcopy introduced by Kerin is hysteroscopic proximal fallopian tube endoscopic examination using a flexible microendoscope (0.5 mm diameter, 1.73 mm length, 50× magnification), and guided catheterization.[23,24]

Salpingoscopy introduced by Brosens and Putemans (1987) is an endoscopic visualization of the distal tubal lumen via a laparoscopic approach. A 2.8-mm diameter telescope, within a 5 mm sheath that fits to the operating channel (5 cm longer than sheath), is used alongside a 10 mm operating laparoscope. A conical obturator helps the distal end of the sheath to enter the tubal ostium.

Laparoscopic Diagnosis and Grading of Salpingitis[25,26]

Laparoscopic diagnosis and grading of salpingitis are shown in **Table 4**.

TABLE 4: Jacobson and Weström laparoscopic criteria to diagnose and grade salpingitis.

Minimum visual criteria to diagnose salpingitis	• Pronounced tubal surface • Hyperemia • Tubal wall edema • Presence of exudates on tubes and from fimbriae when patent
Mild salpingitis	• Minimum visual criteria, mobile tubes • Patent ostia
Moderate salpingitis	• More evident inflammation, patchy fibrin deposits on tubes • Loose tubal and pelvic adhesions • Tubes not freely mobile
Severe salpingitis	• Intense congestion • Dense adhesions to pelvic structures • Pyosalpinx • Tubo-ovarian masses
Each adnexa should be graded separately	
The overall grade is that of the more severe pathology	

Hysterosalpingography

Hysterosalpingography is an inexpensive and widely available screening test to rule out unilateral or bilateral tubal block and provides a permanent visual record of the uterus and tubes.

It involves instillation of approximately 10 mL water-soluble radiocontrast transcervically and serial X-ray imaging of the pelvis to visualize the uterine cavity, delineate the tubes, and to assess peritoneal spill. Cornual tubal spasm is the main reason for lower accuracy of this diagnostic imaging technique. Gentle handling and administration of an antispasmodic tablet or injection prior to the procedure tackles this problem effectively. PID and pregnancy are the two contraindications for performing HSG. Therefore, it is ideally performed in the late follicular phase (day 7–12) following a normal menstrual cycle. Performing the HSG with an oil-based radiopaque dye has been associated with increased live birth rates. In spite of this, water-based dye is preferred due to better image quality and safety.[27] Oil-based dyes may cause oil embolization or granulomas. The conventional HSG is safe as radiation exposure is only 0.4–5.5 mGy, much below the 100 mGy safety threshold for teratogenicity.

Hysterosalpingography has a low sensitivity of 53–65% and a high specificity of 83–87%, PPV of 38%, and NPV of 94%, i.e., HSG is a reliable indicator of tubal patency if bilateral spill is noted on evaluation.[13,28]

An abnormal HSG helps predict proximal tubal blockage and hydrosalpinges with moderate accuracy while it is very inaccurate in diagnosing or ruling out distal tubal obstruction and peritubal adhesions. Although an HSG might look normal, hydrosalpinges remain undiagnosed.[24]

TABLE 5: Three hysterosalpingography (HSG)-based categories of tubal patency.[9]

Category 1 (normal)	***Category 2 (patent tube with tubal disease)***	***Category 3 (patent or blocked tubes, severe tubal disease)***
• Patency with free spill • Preserved distal tubal folds • Normal proximal, mid, distal tubal dimensions, and appearance • No fimbrial end clumping • No detected peritubal disease, normal tubal pressures with free flow • Lack of sharp pain on forceful flushing	• Patency with good spill • Almost fully preserved distal tubal folds, normal to slightly altered tubal dimensions • ±Fimbrial end clumping • ±Peritubal disease • Normal or elevated tubal pressures	• Patent/blocked tubes • Loss of distal tubal folds • Altered proximal, mid, distal tubal dimensions, and appearance with dilatation/narrowing/scarring/tubal rigidity • Fimbrial end dilatation/narrowing with clumping present peritubal disease may or may not be seen • Usually elevated tubal pressures but may be normal

Advanced HSG may be done with using fluoroscopic guidance, manipulation, tubal cannulation, and tubal pressure to yield more information and increase reliability of testing.[9] The information so gathered may be used to categorize tubal disease into three, based on which we can decide appropriate management.

- *Category 1:* Normal: Good chance for future fertility
  - Very low incidence of ectopic pregnancy
- *Category 2:* Patent tube with tubal disease:
  - 2a—mild tubal disease
  - 2b—moderate tubal disease
  - Moderate prognosis and outcome future fertility
  - Highest incidence of ectopic pregnancy
- *Category 3:* Patent or blocked tubes, severe tubal disease:
  - ART ideal
  - Very low incidence of ectopic pregnancy.

The HSG category allotment criteria are enumerated in **Table 5**.

Selective Salpingography and Tubal Catheterization/ Ultrasound or Hysteroscopy-guided Tubal Cannulation

Fluoroscopy-guided transcervical proximal tubal cannulation and selective salpingogram to identify and dislodge proximal tubal block were introduced by Corfmann and Taylor in 1966. Later, hysteroscopic and ultrasound-guided proximal tubal cannulation[29,30] became more commonly used modalities to identify and tackle proximal tubal obstruction due to spasm, plugs, and adhesions.

Sonohysterosalpingography

Sonohysterosalpingography is a test to determine tubal patency using transcervical fluid instillation, the filling and flow of which is monitored by transvaginal ultrasound monitoring. Although tubal patency can be observed by the appearance of fluid in the cul-de-sac with the saline infusion, the test does not differentiate between unilateral and bilateral patency.[13] The two common methods used are Sion's test or SIS and HyCoSy. Use of 3D ultrasound and color or power Doppler for sonographic visualization of insufflated tubes helps in identifying tubal and uterine pathology clearly.

The uterine cavity is insufflated slowly with about 300 mL plain saline (Sion's test), mixture of air and saline, or solution of galactose and 1% palmitic acid (Echovist, Levovist for HyCoSy), etc., after catheterizing the cervix with a narrow (no. 8 Foleys) catheter.

Where available, sonohysterosalpingography is a better alternative to HSG, as it has higher sensitivity and specificity of 76–96%, and 67–100%, respectively.[8,13]

Tubal Insufflation Test (Rubin's Test)

Rubin's insufflation test involves pushing air or carbon dioxide gas under pressure transcervically and noting whether it reaches the peritoneal cavity. Fall in pressure when the gas pressure rises above 120 mm Hg, hissing sound on auscultation at iliac fossa, and shoulder pain (due to gaseous irritation of diaphragm) were considered as signs of tubal patency. Tubal insufflation is now obsolete as patency testing is very subjective and unreliable and cannot identify the site or side of blockage.

Transvaginal Hydrolaparoscopy and Fertiloscopy

Transvaginal hydrolaparoscopy (THL) involves small diameter endoscopic visualization of the pelvis after instillation of 500 mL of a fluid medium through a needle inserted through posterior vaginal fornix. When hysteroscopy, falloposcopy, and distal tubal salpingoscopy are done along with THL, it is termed fertiloscopy.[31] Fertiloscopy provides a wealth of information, although consensus guidelines on how to interpret and put the findings into use has not yet been laid.

Fertiloscopy may be done in an outpatient procedure under local anesthesia. Minor adhesiolysis, endometriosis fulguration, etc. may be performed concurrently.[31]

The risk of bowel injury is much higher as compared to laparoscopy and THL is not useful in evaluating women with an obliterated pouch of Douglas.

Fertiloscopy findings are almost identical to laparoscopy findings and are reliable. The expensive instruments needed and lack of procedural experience may be the reason why THL is not commonly done.

The tubal assessment tests are summarized in **Table 6**.

MANAGEMENT OF TUBAL INFERTILITY

- Preventive approaches
- Identifying and treating pelvic infection/inflammation
- In established tubal disease, management depends on:
  - Site and extent of the tubal disease:
    - Unilateral or bilateral
    - Proximal or distal
    - Mild/moderate/severe tubal disease
  - Age of the patient
  - Duration of fertility
  - Ovarian reserve
  - Prior fertility
  - Presence of other infertility factors
  - Experience of the surgeon if tubal surgery is planned
  - Success rates of the in vitro fertilization (IVF) program or restorative surgery.

TABLE 6: Tubal assessment tests—summary.[8]

Test	*Sensitivity*	*Specificity*	*Limitations*	*Complications*
Laparoscopy—Gold standard	Unknown (no comparator)	Unknown	• Invasive • General anesthesia • Skill requirement expensive	Bowel/urological/vascular injury 0.13%
Hysterosalpingography	53–65%	83–87%	Failure to catheterize/cannulate, leak of dye around cervix, tubal spasm or debris causing false +ve report reporting errors	Anaphylaxis PID 3.1%—radiation exposure ~2 gray
HyCoSy	93.3%	89.7%		PID
SSTC	Unknown (lack of data)	Unknown	Unclear	Tubal perforation 2%
Fertiloscopy	86%	100%		Rectal injury 0.61%
Chlamydia antibody test	21–90%	29–100%		Unknown

(HyCoSY: hysterosalpingo contrast-ultrasonography; PID: pelvic inflammatory disease; SSTC: selective salpingography and tubal catheterization)

Prevention of Tubal Infertility

Prevention of tubal pathology from emerging is the best way to mitigate tubal causes of infertility.

Strategies include:

- General education and awareness to decrease the incidence of sexually transmitted infection (STI) and PID
- Proper precautions to reduce the incidence of iatrogenic PID/peritubal adhesions
- Early identification and treatment of STI and PID and treatment of the partners
- Identifying patients with unfavorable reproductive microbiome and optimizing their health to reduce the risk of infections.

Reproductive Tract Microbiome

Women undergoing IVF with tubal factor infertility (a pathology associated with infections) were found to be more likely to have a vaginal microbiota consistent with bacterial vaginosis (BV) by analysis of smears.[58] Studies have shown that presence of unfavorable non-lactobacillus dominant microbiomes are significantly more in infertile women.

Identification and Treatment of Sexually Transmitted Disease and Pelvic Inflammatory Disease

We should exert a high index of suspicion to diagnose and treat STI and PID in infertile couples as these are major culprits causing and worsening tubal infertility.

In Vitro Fertilization for Tubal Infertility

In vitro fertilization was originally developed to allow couples with untreatable tubal infertility to conceive and enjoy the joys of parenthood. Thus, IVF and embryo transfer (ET) remain ideal therapeutic options to achieve intrauterine pregnancy in women with absolute tubal infertility. Also, IVF is the treatment modality to be opted when there are other problems like male factor infertility, resistant anovulation, etc., contributing to infertility.

The ideal management of severe tubal disease, especially with hydrosalpinx and severe fimbrial phimosis is always IVF and ET after salpingectomy or occlusion of hydrosalpinges.[32]

However, IVF is an expensive treatment modality, and for some, unacceptable. IVF is also associated with complications like ovarian hyperstimulation syndrome (OHSS) and multiple pregnancies that cause significant morbidity and expenses. Women with mild or unilateral tubal disease may benefit from treatment approaches like IUI or tubal reconstructive surgery. Tuboplasty may be tried in women who cannot accept or afford IVF. The 2017 Cochrane review found that well-controlled randomized clinical trials (RCTs) or high-quality evidence comparing the post tuboplasty reproductive outcomes for diseased tubes with IVF are not available yet.[33]

Ovarian stimulation with IUI may be offered initially to patients with unilateral proximal tubal occlusion often obtaining satisfactory results. However in women with mid-distal or distal tubal occlusion on HSG, the IUI after ovarian stimulation is ineffective. They require laparoscopic evaluation and often IVF.[34]

On the other hand, tubal reanastomosis for infertility due to tubal sterilization offers a cumulative pregnancy rate that is comparable or even higher than IVF although the per cycle pregnancy rate is higher in IVF.[32] A cost-effectiveness analysis found that ongoing pregnancy rates were 75%, 66%, and 44% for maternal ages <35 years, 35–40 years, and >40 years in women undergoing tubal anastomosis while they were 46%, 35%, and 16% in women undergoing fresh IVF cycle for tubal infertility. They found that sterilization reversal was the most cost-effective approach for most women younger than 41 years, while IVF remained the best approach for women >41 years of age.[35]

Reconstructive Surgery for Tubal Infertility

Tubal surgery to overcome infertility is becoming an attractive option to many, as the benefits obtained from tubal surgery would potentially be sustained for many years and may allow conception through intercourse or IUI. However, tubal surgery requires specialized skill development.[33] Its efficacy has to be weighed against the cons of expenses, risk of tubal ectopic pregnancy (7–18%), reocclusion, and failure to conceive.[8]

Tubal restorative surgery is most effective in younger women with mild or moderate tubal disease. Integrity of the endosalpinx and mesosalpingeal thickening are the most important predictors of successful intrauterine conceptions following surgery. At least 50% of the endosalpinx should be healthy to ensure favorable outcomes. Tubal reconstructive surgeries include those for proximal tubal disease, distal tubal disease, and sterilization reversal **(Table 7)**.

Microsurgical Techniques[36]

Microsurgery was introduced into gynecology specifically to improve tubal reconstructive surgery outcomes. The microsurgical techniques should be applied universally for all tuboplasty irrespective of the approach (laparoscopy or laparotomy). The microsurgical principles include:

- Surgery under magnification—using a binocular microscope (20×) and/or loupe magnifier (6×)
- Gentle handling of tissues
- Use of lightweight microsurgical instruments (13–15 mm length)
- Use of fine sutures (7-0 to 10-0)
- Use of fine tapered needles (135° curvature, 50–150 μm diameter)

TABLE 7: Surgical management for hydrosalpinges.[32]

Method	*Advantages*	*Disadvantages*
Salpingectomy (laparoscopic)	• Total removal of chronically inflamed tissue • No further risk of abscess formation or torsion • Increased the accessibility of the ovary for oocyte pick up	• Invasive procedure, difficult if tube buried in adhesions • Interstitial/cornual pregnancy and rupture may rarely occur • May hamper with ovarian vascularity and function All chances of spontaneous conception lost
Tubal occlusion: • Electrocautery • Clips • Hysteroscopic-Essure microinsert	• Less invasive • Easier than salpingectomy when dense adhesions are present	Risk of abscess formation or torsion
Aspiration (Transvaginal/laparoscopic)	• Less invasive, easy • Tube retained	• May flare up infection • Recurrence of hydrosalpinx
Salpingostomy	Less invasive, easy	• Recurrence of hydrosalpinx • Increased risk of tubal ectopic pregnancy

- Meticulous hemostasis with electrocautery devices having microelectrodes, fingertip controls, and lowest current setting
- Copious irrigation
- Sharp precise dissection by an experienced surgeon who is ideally seated on the opposite site to the tube being operated on.

As laparoscopic visualization offers a significantly magnified view, the microsurgical approaches are applied more easily.

Surgery for Proximal Tubal Disease

Proximal tubal cannulation: Hysteroscopic proximal tubal cannulation or fluoroscopic selective salpingography and proximal tubal catheterization are effective modes to assess and treat proximal tubal obstruction due to tubal debris, sludge, and intraluminal adhesions. Proximal tubal cannulation may be done under sonological guidance too.[30] Ideally, proximal tubal cannulation is done after confirming that the distal tube is normal using prior laparoscopic evaluation. Gentle pressure and flushing by the cannula inserted through the cornual tubal ostia is enough to overcome mechanical obstruction of the proximal tube.[3,10] Tubal perforation may occur in 3–11% cases but does not cause any clinical consequences. Tubal cannulation relieves obstruction in approximately 85% and around half the patients conceive.[3,10] The meta-analysis by Holden et al. found that although fluoroscopic and hysteroscopic tubal canalization achieved similar patency rates, ongoing pregnancy rates were more following hysteroscopic tubal cannulation.

Tubal resection and reanastomosis: Proximal tube disease like SIN causes extensive intraluminal and mesenchymal damage of the proximal tube. IVF and ET are the best treatment options. Where IVF is not acceptable or possible, diseased proximal tubal resection and reanastomosis of tubes is the best option as it is associated with higher pregnancy rates compared to expectant management or proximal tubal cannulation.[37]

Surgery for Distal Tubal Disease

Surgical reconstruction for damaged distal tubes may be offered in mild to moderate disease where at least 50% of the endosalpinx and tubal wall is healthy.

Extent of tubal mucosal damage and increase in wall thickness are the most important determinants and are inversely related to successful tubal restorative surgery outcomes.[38]

The best prognosis is seen in patients with mildly dilated tubes (<3 cm) having thin and pliable walls, undamaged endosalpinx with intact mucosa, and only filmy adnexal adhesions.

Neosalpingostomy (opening up of a blocked distal tube) and *fimbrioplasty* (widening of stenosed distal tubal ostia) are commonly done to restore the fallopian tube patency. *Salpingo-ovariolysis* that involves the release of adhesions binding the tubes and ovaries restoring the normal tubo-ovarian relation is done alongside the above two options.[12,39]

American Society for Reproductive Medicine recommends that the reconstructive surgeries be done laparoscopically as they are less risky, less invasive, and associated with the same treatment outcomes as in laparotomy.[37]

Laparoscopic opening of mild or even moderately diseased tubes offers a satisfactory pregnancy outcome in comparison with IVF.[38]

Intrauterine and ectopic pregnancy rates after neosalpingostomy for mild hydrosalpinges range from 58% to 77% and from 2% to 8%, respectively. For severe disease, these values were 0–22% and 0–17%, respectively.[13,38,40]

Sterilization Reversal

Tubal sterilization reversal may be accomplished by opening the occluded ends of the proximal and distal segments and anastomosing them with fine nonreactive sutures using non-microsurgical or magnification and microsurgical techniques.[13] Microsurgical techniques require training and experience so that the gynecologist can operate using binocular or loupe magnification allowing precise placement of fine sutures (7-0 to 10-0) as well as undistorted and tension-free approximation of tissue edges. Tubal reanastomosis success depends on multiple factors including the woman's age, ovarian reserve, the sterilization procedure she underwent as well as the endoluminal and surface integrity of the tube left behind.

The age of the woman is the most important predeterminant for pregnancy rates following tubal reversal. The younger the woman, the better the pregnancy rates. Women <40 years have cumulative intrauterine pregnancy rates as high as 70% and 90%, respectively, following non-microsurgical and microsurgical reversal of tubal sterilization.[41] Another study noted that significantly higher cumulative pregnancy rates obtained and lesser cost per delivery incurred following tubal reanastomosis compared to IVF in women younger than 37 years.[42] The rate of ectopic pregnancy following tubal reanastomosis is 2–10%, compared to 2% for IVF.

Sterilization reversal success rate is inversely related to the extent of tubal damage that occurred during the sterilization procedure and directly related to the length of healthy tube retained. Understandably the reversal success rates are more when the tubes were either clipped or ringed, compared to sterilization by Pomeroy's method (as large lengths of tube may be removed) or by electrocautery where the cautery energy may cause irreversible functional damage to the tube. Some methods of sterilization like fimbriectomy are irreversible and IVF is the fertility option to be opted.

Isthmus to isthmus reanastomosis and longer final tubal lengths (>4 cm) are generally thought to yield higher success rates. Traditionally tubal reanastomosis is done via laparotomy as it is an easier approach to implement microsurgical tubal reanastomosis effectively. Laparoscopic microsurgical tubal reanastomosis requires good laparoscopic suturing skill and experience but have comparable outcomes to laparotomy sterilization reversal.[13] Recently, robotic laparoscopic tubal reconstruction is also being applied.

Destructive Tubal Surgery Followed by IVF—For Severe and Bipolar Tubal Disease and Hydrosalpinx

Tubal reconstruction is not beneficial for women with severe and/or bipolar (both proximal and distal) tubal disease. The presence of unresolving hydrosalpinx is pathognomonic of severe tubal disease and is associated with poor ART outcomes. In such cases salpingectomy, tubal occlusion or clipping followed by IVF is the preferred treatment to conceive. All sonologically detectable hydrosalpinges should be removed or occluded prior to applying ART.

In vitro fertilization was developed primarily to allow pregnancy in women with tubal infertility, but paradoxically it was noted that IVF outcomes were poorer in women with extensive tubal disease as in hydrosalpinges. Poor implantation rates and higher miscarriage rates were noted.[43-45] RCTs have reported that IVF and ET following salpingectomy restore the rates of pregnancy and live birth to levels similar to those of women without hydrosalpinx who were treated with IVF.[46,47]

It is believed that the hydrosalpinges adversely affect the various embryo-endometrial interactions involved in implantation. At the molecular level, hydrosalpinges have been associated with reduced $\alpha v\beta 3$ integrin and leukemia inhibitory factor (LIF) expressions as well as decreased *HOXA10* (homeobox gene) expression in the endometrium that hamper implantation.[48]

The hydrosalpingeal fluid is considered the main culprit for deleterious IVF outcomes though why it is so, is still unclear. It contains various cytokines and growth factors which may be toxic to gametes or embryos.[49] Bathing of the endometrial cavity in hydrosalpinx fluid may hinder embryo endometrium cross talk and cause potential embryo toxicity.[50,51] The mechanical effects exerted by hydrorrhea through the uterine cavity may cause changes in endometrial peristalsis that may washout or hinder implantation of the transferred embryo.[45] Furthermore, the hydrosalpinges provide unfavorable environment for early follicular recruitment.

The best method to detect hydrosalpinx is by routine 2D TVS (sensitivity: 84.6%; specificity: 99.7%). HyCoSy is ideal to assess the uterine cavity and tubes in women with two more unexplained implantation failures as sonography distending and visualizing the tubal and uterine lumen will reveal pathologies like intrauterine polyps or adhesions and hydrosalpinges that were not detected on routine evaluation.[8]

The less invasive laparoscopic salpingectomy is the preferred approach. The tube is delinked by coagulating and dividing the proximal tube close to the cornua. The mesosalpinx is then serially coagulated and cut, staying close to the tube to avoid compromising the ovarian blood supply.[13,37]

A Scandinavian RCT published in 1999 that included 141 women showed that salpingectomy prior to IVF in all transvaginal ultrasound detectable hydrosalpinges improved IVF outcomes in terms of increased pregnancy and delivery rates. This was especially proven in women with bilateral hydrosalpinges. The histopathological examination of the tubes showed that >90% of the tubes showed pathology that could not be corrected by restorative tubal surgery.[52] Thus hydrosalpinges that are detectable on ultrasound almost always represent dysfunctional and uncorrectable tubal pathology.

Strandell et al. in 2001 provided reassuring evidence that the salpingectomy prior to IVF does not compromise ovarian function.[53] Salpingectomy for hydrosalpinges also does not adversely influence the response to ovarian stimulation or alter IVF parameters.[53]

The 2010 Cochrane on surgical treatment of tubal disease for IVF reviewed five RCTs including 646 women. Outcomes following laparoscopic salpingectomy, laparoscopic tubal occlusion, and USG-guided aspiration were compared. They found that the ongoing pregnancy rates and clinical pregnancy rates were increased with laparoscopic salpingectomy prior to IVF, while laparoscopic tubal occlusion was associated with significant increase in clinical pregnancy. IVF outcomes following salpingectomy and tubal occlusion were similar. Ultrasound-guided aspiration of hydrosalpinx (covered with intravenous amoxicillin + clavulanic acid followed by oral azithromycin for 3 days) was found to be effective in one RCT although no significant improvement in pregnancy rates were noted.[54] The adverse effects following the different surgical techniques were not significantly different.[32]

They concluded that both laparoscopic salpingectomy and tubal occlusion (electrocautery delinking or proximal tubal clipping) prior to IVF improved pregnancy rates. Hence, the less invasive laparoscopic occlusion may be considered as an alternative to salpingectomy.[32]

Dreyer et al. (2016) noted that the ongoing pregnancy rates were significantly lower in ART cycles following hysteroscopic occlusion compared to laparoscopic salpingectomy.[55]

From the above discussion, it is clear that hydrosalpinges left unattended prior to IVF are associated with poorer pregnancy rates. So, all hydrosalpinges detected prior to IVF should ideally be occluded or removed. Concurrent transvaginal aspiration of hydrosalpinges noted during oocyte pick up reduces their presence at the time of ET but whether it improves clinical outcomes is still under debate.[32]

MANAGEMENT OF TUBAL ECTOPIC PREGNANCY

Management of ectopic pregnancy is being addressed here as ectopic pregnancy is often a consequence of tubal pathology which worsens the tubal integrity. When managing ectopic pregnancy, the aim is to restore the chance of natural fertility where feasible weighing is against the risks of life-threatening repeated occurrence of ectopic pregnancy. In women presenting with ectopic pregnancy who require surgical management, we need to provide the patient appropriate treatment, by educating her regarding the plausible intraoperative findings and factoring in her priorities and concerns before deciding the surgical treatment.

The UK guidelines state that in the event of an ectopic pregnancy requiring surgical management:

- A laparoscopic surgical approach is preferable to an open approach (unless the patient is decompensated, when laparotomy is the best strategy).
- In the presence of a healthy contralateral tube, salpingectomy is preferred to salpingotomy.
- In women with a history of fertility-reducing factors (previous ectopic pregnancy, contralateral tubal damage, previous abdominal surgery, previous PID), salpingotomy should be considered, after informing about the risk of persisting trophoblast and need for serial beta human chorionic gonadotropin (β-hCG) monitoring.

This rationale is based on reliable published evidence showing increased intrauterine pregnancy rates without resorting to assisted reproduction strategies, when salpingotomy was resorted to in women presenting with ectopic pregnancy, in whom the contralateral tube was likely to be diseased due to the presence of preexisting comorbidity or on appearance.[56-58]

KEY POINTS

- Pelvic inflammatory disease causing salpingitis and tubal infertility should be diagnosed early and treated following the CDC guidelines.
- HSG is the recommended first-line test to assess tubal patency, but where available sonohysterosalpingography using saline or contrast to visualize the uterine cavity and tubes is preferred.
- Laparoscopy and chromopertubation is the current gold standard to assess tubal patency and should be offered as a first-line test for women with a history of pelvic comorbidities like endometriosis and PID.
- IVF and ET is the best option to achieve intrauterine pregnancy in severe tubal disease.
- IVF is also the best option for tubal infertility when associated with other factors like abnormal semen parameters, anovulation, and rapidly declining ovarian reserve.
- Tubal cannulation is recommended for proximal tubal obstruction in young women with isolated tubal factors as it restores patency in most of the cases.
- Tubal reconstructive surgery—laparoscopic neosalpingostomy or fimbrioplasty improves fertility in young women with isolated tubal factor infertility due to mild distal tubal disease.
- Microsurgical tubal sterilization reversal is recommended in women younger than 40 years as the subsequent cumulative pregnancy rates are comparable if not higher than IVF pregnancy rates. It is also more cost-effective.

- Laparoscopic salpingectomy or proximal tubal occlusion is recommended prior to IVF in all cases of sonologically detected hydrosalpinges and severe tubal disease to improve IVF pregnancy rates.

REFERENCES

1. ESHRE Capri Workshop Group. Diagnosis and management of the infertile couple: missing information. Hum Reprod Update. 2004;10(4):295-307.
2. Evers JL. Female subfertility. Lancet. 2002;360(9327):151-9.
3. Honoré GM, Holden AE, Schenken RS. Pathophysiology and management of proximal tubal blockage. Fertil Steril. 1999;71(5):785-95.
4. Borrero SB, Reeves MF, Schwarz EB, Bost JE, Creinin MD, Ibrahim SA. Race, insurance status, and desire for tubal sterilization reversal. Fertil Steril. 2008;90(2):272-7.
5. Schmidt JE, Hillis SD, Marchbanks PA, Jeng G, Peterson HB. Requesting information about and obtaining reversal after tubal sterilization: findings from the U.S. Collaborative Review of Sterilization. Fertil Steril. 2000;74(5):892-8.
6. Chi IC, Jones DB. Incidence, risk factors, and prevention of poststerilization regret in women: an updated international review from an epidemiological perspective. Obstet Gynecol Surv. 1994;49(10):722-32.
7. Muckle C, Feinberg E. Developmental Abnormalities of the Female Reproductive Organs. Glob Libr Women's Med. 2008.
8. Suresh YN, Narvekar NN. The role of tubal patency tests and tubal surgery in the era of assisted reproductive techniques. Obstet Gynaecol. 2014;16:37-45.
9. Patil M. Assessing tubal damage. J Hum Reprod Sci. 2009;2(1):2-11.
10. Practice Committee of the American Society for Reproductive Medicine. Role of tubal surgery in the era of assisted reproductive technology: a committee opinion. Fertil Steril. 2021;115(5):1143-50.
11. NICE Clinical Guideline. Fertility: Assessment and Treatment for People with Fertility Problems. London: RCOG; 2013. pp. 1-555.
12. Practice Committee of the American Society for Reproductive Medicine. Optimal evaluation of the infertile female. Fertil Steril. 2006;86(5 Suppl 1):S264-7.
13. Committee on Gynecologic Practice for the American Society for Reproductive Medicine and the American College of Obstetricians and Gynecologists. Infertility Workup for the Women's Health Specialist: ACOG Committee Opinion, Number 781. Obstet Gynecol. 2019;133(6):e377-84.
14. Benjaminov O, Atri M. Sonography of the abnormal fallopian tube. Am J Roentgenol. 2004;183(3):737-42.
15. Mol BW, Dijkman B, Wertheim P, Lijmer J, van der Veen F, Bossuyt PM. The accuracy of serum chlamydial antibodies in the diagnosis of tubalpathology: a meta-analysis. Fertil Steril. 1997;67(6):1031-7.
16. Workowski KA. Centers for Disease Control and Prevention Sexually Transmitted Diseases Treatment Guidelines. Clin Infect Dis. 2015;61(Suppl 8):S759-62.
17. Broeze KA, Opmeer BC, Coppus SF, Van Geloven N, Alves MF, Anestad G, et al. Chlamydia antibody testing and diagnosing tubal pathology in subfertile women: an individual patient data meta-analysis. Hum Reprod Update. 2011;17(3):301-10.
18. den Hartog JE, Morré SA, Land JA. Chlamydia trachomatis-associated tubal factor subfertility: Immunogenetic aspects and serological screening. Hum Reprod Update. 2006;12(6):719-30.
19. Ubaldi F, Wisanto A, Camus M, Tournaye H, Clasen K, Devroey P, et al. The role of transvaginal ultrasonography in the detection of pelvic pathologies in the infertility workup. Hum Reprod. 1998;13(2):330-3.
20. Sharma JB. Current Diagnosis and Management of Female Genital Tuberculosis. J Obstet Gynaecol India. 2015;65(6):362-71.
21. Yadav S, Singh P, Hemal A, Kumar R. Genital tuberculosis: current status of diagnosis and management. Transl Androl Urol. 2017;6(2):222-33.
22. Papaioannou S, Bourdrez P, Varma R, Afnan M, Mol BW, Coomarasamy A. Tubal evaluation in the investigation of subfertility: a structured comparison of tests. BJOG. 2004;111(12):1313-21.
23. Kerin J, Daykhovsky L, Segalowitz J, Surrey E, Anderson R, Stein A, et al. Falloposcopy: a microendoscopic technique for visual exploration of the human fallopian tube from the uterotubal ostium to the fimbria using a transvaginal approach. Fertil Steril. 1990;54(3):390-400.
24. Dechaud H, Daures JP, Hedon B. Prospective evaluation of falloposcopy. Hum Reprod. 1998;13(7):1815-8.
25. Soper DE. Diagnosis and laparoscopic grading of acute salpingitis. Am J Obstet Gynecol. 1991;164(5 Pt 2):1370-6.
26. Westrom L, Mardh PA. Acute pelvic inflammatory disease (PID). In: Holmes KK, Mardh PA, Sparling PF, Lemon SM, Stamm WE, Piot P, Wasserheit JN (Eds). Sexually Transmitted Diseases, 2nd edition. New York: McGraw-Hill; 1990. pp. 593-613.
27. Luttjeboer F, Harada T, Hughes E, Johnson N, Lilford R, Mol BW. Tubal flushing for subfertility. Cochrane Database Syst Rev. 2007;18(3):CD003718.
28. Broeze KA, Opmeer BC, Van Geloven N, Coppus SF, Collins JA, Den Hartog JE, et al. Are patient characteristics associated with the accuracy of hysterosalpingography in diagnosing tubal pathology? An individual patient data meta-analysis. Hum Reprod Update. 2011;17(3):293-300.
29. Novy MJ. Transhysteroscopic techniques for tubal catheterization. Ref Gynecol Obstet. 1995;3:67-71.
30. Rahimunnisa S, Tanwar R, Prasad S. Ultrasound versus tactile cannulation in the treatment of proximal tubal obstruction. Int J Gynaecol Obstet. 2009;106(3):216-7.
31. Watrelot A, Nisolle M, Chelli H, Hocke C, Rongières C, Racinet C; International Group for Fertiloscopy Evaluation. Is laparoscopy still the gold standard in infertility assessment? A comparison of fertiloscopy versus laparoscopy in infertility. Results of an international multicentre prospective trial: the 'FLY' (Fertiloscopy–Laparoscopy) study. Hum Reprod. 2003;18(4):834-9.
32. Johnson N, van Voorst S, Sowter MC, Strandell A, Mol BW. Surgical treatment for tubal disease in women due to undergo in vitro fertilisation. Cochrane Database Syst Rev. 2010;2010(1):CD002125.
33. Chua S, Akande VA, Mol BJ. Surgery for tubal infertility. Cochrane Database Syst Rev. 2017;1(1):CD006415.
34. Farhi J, Haroush AB, Lande Y, Fisch B. Role of treatment with ovarian stimulation and intrauterine insemination

in women with unilateral tubal occlusion diagnosed by hysterosalpingography. Fertil Steril. 2007;88(2):396-400.
35. Messinger LB, Alford CE, Csokmay JM, Henne MB, Mumford SL, Segars JH, et al. Cost and efficacy comparison of in vitro fertilization and tubal anastomosis for women after tubal ligation. Fertil Steril. 2015;104(1):32-8.e4.
36. Siegler A. Microsurgical Tubal Reconstruction. Glob Libr Women's Med. 2008.
37. Gomel V, McComb PF. Microsurgery for tubal infertility. J Reprod Med. 2006;51(3):177-84.
38. Milingos SD, Kallipolitis GK, Loutradis DC, Liapi AG, Hassan EA, Mavrommatis CG, et al. Laparoscopic treatment of hydrosalpinx: factors affecting pregnancy rates. J Am Assoc Gynecol Laparosc. 2000;7(3):355-61.
39. Bontis JN, Theodoridis TD. Laparoscopic management of hydrosalpinx. Ann N Y Acad Sci. 2006;1092:199-210.
40. Nackley AC, Muasher SJ. The significance of hydrosalpinx in in vitro fertilization. Fertil Steril. 1998;69(3):373-84.
41. Kim JD, Kim KS, Doo JK, Rhyeu CH. A report on 387 cases of microsurgical tubal reversals. Fertil Steril. 1997;68(5):875-80.
42. Boeckxstaens A, Devroey P, Collins J, Tournaye H. Getting pregnant after tubal sterilization: surgical reversal or IVF? Hum Reprod. 2007;22(10):2660-4.
43. Steptoe PC, Edwards RG. Birth after the reimplantation of a human embryo. Lancet. 1978;2(8085):366.
44. Andersen AN, Yue Z, Meng FJ, Petersen K. Low implantation rate after in-vitro fertilisation in patients with hydrosalpinges diagnosed by ultrasonography. Hum Reprod. 1994; 9(10):1935-8.
45. Strandell A, Waldenström U, Nilsson L, Hamberger L. Hydrosalpinx reduces in-vitro fertilisation/embryo transfer pregnancy rates. Hum Reprod. 1994;9(5):861-3.
46. Déchaud H, Daurès JP, Arnal F, Humeau C, Hédon B. Does previous salpingectomy improve implantation and pregnancy rates in patients with severe tubal factor infertility who are undergoing in vitro fertilization? A pilot prospective randomized study. Fertil Steril. 1998;69(6):1020-5.
47. Kontoravdis A, Makrakis E, Pantos K, Botsis D, Deligeoroglou E, Creatsas G. Proximal tubal occlusion and salpingectomy result in similar improvement in in vitro fertilization outcome in patients with hydrosalpinx. Fertil Steril. 2006;86(6):1642-9.
48. Cakmak H, Taylor HS. Implantation failure: molecular mechanisms and clinical treatment. Hum Reprod Update. 2011;17(2):242-53.
49. Chen CD, Yang JH, Lin KC, Chao KH, Ho HN, Yang YS. The significance of cytokines, chemical composition, and murine embryo development in hydrosalpinx fluid for predicting the in-vitro fertilization outcome in women with hydrosalpinx. Hum Reprod. 2002;17(1):128-33.
50. Akman MA, Garcia JE, Damewood MD, Watts LD, Katz E. Hydrosalpinx affects the implantation of previously cryopreserved embryos. Hum Reprod. 1996;11(5):1013-4.
51. Mukhurjee T, Copperman AB, McCaffrey C Cook CA, Bustillo M, Obasaju MF. Hydrosalpinx fluid has embryotoxic effects on murine embryogenesis: a case for prophylactic salpingectomy. Fertil Steril. 1996;66(5):851-3.
52. Strandell A, Lindhard A, Waldenström U, Thorburn J, Janson PO, Hamberger L. Hydrosalpinx and IVF outcome: a prospective, randomized multicentre trial in Scandinavia on salpingectomy prior to IVF. Hum Reprod. 1999;14(11):2762-9.
53. Strandell A, Lindhard A, Waldenström U, Thorburn J. Prophylactic salpingectomy does not impair the ovarian response in IVF treatment. Hum Reprod. 2001;16(6):1135-9.
54. Hammadieh N, Coomarasamy A, Ola B, Papaioannou S, Afnan M, Sharif K. Ultrasound-guided hydrosalpinx aspiration during oocyte collection improves pregnancy outcome in IVF: a randomized controlled trial. Hum Reprod. 2008;23(5):1113-7.
55. Dreyer K, Lier MC, Emanuel MH, Twisk JW, Mol BW, Schats R, et al. Hysteroscopic proximal tubal occlusion versus laparoscopic salpingectomy as a treatment for hydrosalpinges prior to IVF or ICSI: an RCT. Hum Reprod. 2016;31(9):2005-16.
56. Elson CJ, Salim R, Potdar N, Chetty M, Ross JA, Kirk EJ. Diagnosis and management of ectopic pregnancy (Green-top Guideline No. 21). BJOG. 2016;123(13):e15-55.
57. Becker S, Solomayer E, Hornung R, Kurek R, Banys M, Aydeniz B, et al. Optimal treatment for patients with ectopic pregnancies and a history of fertility-reducing factors. Arch Gynecol Obstet. 2011;283(1):41-5.
58. Kroon SJ, Ravel J, Huston WM. Cervicovaginal microbiota, women's health, and reproductive outcomes. Fertil Steril. 2018;110(3):327-36.

CHAPTER 35

Infections and Infertility

Chandrika Kulkarni

INTRODUCTION

Infertility is a consequence of a number of factors. The causes could be hormonal, infectious, gonadal, or unexplained.[1] About one-third of women with fertility problems are, in fact, afflicted with tubal and peritoneal changes affecting the tubo-ovarian relationship. The specific and nonspecific bacterial infections of the genital tract majorly contribute to these alterations. The World Health Organization (WHO) estimated that nearly 1 million people become infected every day with any of the four curable sexually transmitted infections (STIs): Chlamydia, gonorrhea, syphilis, and trichomoniasis.[2] The complications of curable STIs include pelvic inflammatory disease (PID), ectopic pregnancy, infertility, chronic pelvic pain, seronegative arthropathy, and neurological and cardiovascular diseases.[3] Several STIs including *Chlamydia trachomatis* and *Neisseria gonorrhoeae* have been found to be important causal factors of infertility. However, there are no definitive evidence linking other organisms such as *Mycoplasma* and *Trichomonas vaginalis* (TV) to tubal damage and subsequent infertility.[4] Pelvic tuberculosis is an important cause of salpingitis and has been dealt with in detail in a different chapter.

Nontuberculous salpingitis can be divided into chlamydial, gonococcal, and nongonococcal-nonchlamydial disease based on the results of endocervical or peritoneal fluid cultures.[5]

CHLAMYDIA

Prevalence

Chlamydia remains the most commonly diagnosed bacterial STI in high-income countries despite widespread testing recommendations, sensitive and specific noninvasive testing techniques, and cheap effective therapy.[2] It is more common in sexually active young adults (15–24 years) and also in patients with secondary infertility.[6,7] Incidence varies widely, ranging between 2.2 and 10.7%.[8,9] Earlier studies had shown a higher prevalence of chlamydia to the tune of 20–28%.[6,8] Studies in developing countries such as India have shown a similar prevalence (19.9–23%).[10,11]

Microbiology

Chlamydiae are obligate intracellular bacteria. They are spherical or ovoid in shape. They have a peptidoglycan-free cell wall similar to that of gram-negative bacteria. Their intracellular nature differentiates them from other bacteria. Unlike viruses, chlamydia possesses both deoxyribonucleic acid (DNA) and ribonucleic acid (RNA). Chlamydia exists in two forms—the infective form, called the elementary body, is the extracellular form, and the intracellular form or the reticulate body is required for intracellular survival and multiplication.[12,13]

There are three types of chlamydial species which infect humans namely, *C. trachomatis, Chlamydia psittaci,* and *Chlamydia pneumoniae*. *C. trachomatis* is the species causing the STI.[14]

Pathophysiology

The main targets of chlamydia infection are the columnar epithelial cells.[15] The cells which are infected with chlamydia secrete chemokines which attract leukocytes and cytokines leading to inflammatory response.[16] The inflammatory response is also thought to be mediated through heat shock protein.[17] This inflammation leads to direct damage of the tissues and eventual fibrosis and scarring—the hallmark of chlamydia-induced oviduct disease.[18] *C. trachomatis* infection can lead to irrevocable damage in the fallopian tubes, including proximal and distal tubal occlusions. Multiple sequelae can result from *C. trachomatis* infection among women, the most serious of which include PID, ectopic pregnancy, and infertility.[7]

Infection of the endosalpinx can also produce peritonitis by contiguous spread, including perihepatitis (Fitz-Hugh-Curtis syndrome). Chlamydia also causes urethritis, cervicitis, epididymitis, proctitis, and reactive arthritis. PID is seen in 20% of the infected women and around 4% will have chronic pelvic pain. Infertility as a squeal is seen in 3% of women.[19]

Risk factors for chlamydial infection:

- Young age <25 years
- New sexual partner within the past year
- Use of nonbarrier contraception
- Poor socioeconomic status
- Other STIs.

Clinical Features

The incubation period for the onset of symptoms is longer in chlamydia when compared to other bacteria because of the longer half-life (24–48 hours). A large number of women (around 80%) are asymptomatic,[20] and some women may present with vaginal discharge, dysuria, intermenstrual bleeding, or postcoital bleeding. Untreated infection may lead to mucopurulent cervicitis, acute urethral syndrome, and PID.[21]

On examination, cervix may appear reddened and friable with contact bleeding. Patients with Fitz-Hugh–Curtis syndrome may present with right upper quadrant pain. Women with chlamydial infection may have gonorrhea and vice versa.[5]

Symptoms are more common in men with chlamydial infection when compared to women. The chief symptoms in men are dysuria and urethral discharge. They may also develop epididymo-orchitis with pain and swelling of testis or the epididymis.[20]

Diagnosis

Urogenital chlamydial infection can be diagnosed by testing the first-catch urine sample, swabs from endocervix or vagina, and swabs from urethra.[22] Culture confirms the presence of viable organisms. However, antigens, antibodies, and nucleic acid can be present even in the absence of viable organisms. Chlamydial antigens can be detected using commercially available enzyme immunoassays (EIAs).[20,23] The EIAs usually use monoclonal or polyclonal antibodies to detect the lipopolysaccharide (LPS). Nucleic acid amplification tests (NAATs) are more sensitive (90–95%) and specific (97–99%) than other tests such as culture, microscopy, and immunoassay and are therefore recommended.[19,22] The specimen of choice for detecting chlamydia in women is a vulvovaginal NAAT test, either self-collected or taken by the clinician. In men, a "first-catch urine sample" or urethral swab is the specimen of choice.

Management

Annual screening of all sexually active women aged <25 years is recommended, as is screening of older women at increased risk for infection (e.g., women aged ≥25 years who have a new sex partner, more than one sex partner, a sex partner with concurrent partners, or a sex partner who has an STI).[7,24] Contact tracing and treatment forms an important part of the treatment strategy. Infected patients should also be screened for other STIs such as human immunodeficiency virus (HIV), hepatitis B surface antigen (HBsAg), hepatitis C virus (HCV), and gonorrhea. Pregnant women with chlamydia should be treated to prevent transmission of infection to the neonate; however, doxycycline used in the regimen is contraindicated.[25]

To minimize disease transmission to sex partners, persons treated for chlamydia should be instructed to abstain from sexual intercourse for 7 days after single-dose therapy or until completion of a 7-day regimen and resolution of symptoms if present.[7]

Recommended antibiotic treatment according to Centres for Disease Control (CDC)[7] has been given in **Box 1**.

BOX 1: Recommended regimen for chlamydial infection among adolescents and adults.

- *Doxycycline* 100 mg orally 2 times/day for 7 days
  Alternative regimens:
- *Azithromycin* 1 g orally in a single dose
  or
- *Levofloxacin* 500 mg orally once daily for 7 days

GONORRHEA

Prevalence

Gonorrhea is still one of the important causes for infertility in developing Asian and African countries.[26] However, it is the second most common cause of bacterial STI in the United Kingdom and United States of America.[7] Gonococcal infection is most common in sexually active young people in the age group of 15–24 years. A study in Mumbai sexually transmitted disease (STD) clinic found a prevalence of 9.2%. It was found that the prevalence of gonococcal infection was more common than in those with HIV.[27]

Microbiology

Gonococcal infection is caused by *N. gonorrhoeae* which is found in the neutrophils of the infected host. In 1879, Albert Neisser isolated this gram-negative bacterium. *N. gonorrhoeae* is typically intracellular, aerobic, coffee bean shaped and appears in pairs (diplococci). *N. gonorrhoeae* and *N. meningitidis* are the only two pathogenic species of the total 11 species found in humans.[27,28] It can be cultured in Thayer-Martin media which is a chocolate-enriched agar in the presence of carbon dioxide.[27]

Pathophysiology

Traditionally, it was thought that *N. gonorrhoeae* gets attached to spermatozoan and ascends up the female genital tract. But this does not explain the transmission of the disease from female to male. Anderson et al.[29] suggest that rather than "surf" on wiggling sperm, the bacteria use pili which are hair-like structures to anchor to sperm surface proteins and move through semen.

Neisseria gonorrhoeae infects the mucous membranes of the urethra, endocervix, rectum, pharynx, and conjunctiva by direct inoculation of infected secretions. The most common site of *N. gonorrhoeae* infection is the urogenital tract. *N. gonorrhoeae* infects the nonciliated tubal cells, but the toxin produced also destroys the adjacent ciliated cells which play a major part in transport of fertilized eggs toward the uterus. The gonococcal LPS targets the ciliated cells by upregulating the tumor necrosis factor alpha.[30]

About 10–20% of infected women suffer from ascending infections resulting in PID. These PIDs can further lead to other complications such as salpingitis, endometritis, and tubo-ovarian abscess, which promote ectopic pregnancy, sterility, and chronic pelvic pain.[31]

Clinical Features

More than 50% of the women may be asymptomatic. Rest of those infected may present with nonspecific vaginal discharge, lower abdominal discomfort, and/or dysuria. The symptoms usually appear during or just after menses. On the other hand, most men are symptomatic with dysuria (>50%) and urethral discharge (>80%), both of which usually start within 2–5 days of exposure.[32] Subsequently, if the infection is left untreated, it may lead to urethral scarring. *N. gonorrhoeae* can also cause epididymo-orchitis and prostatitis.[28]

Diagnosis

There are two ways of detecting gonococcal infection. One is the culture method and the other is the nonculture techniques, which include Gram staining and NAAT. Culture is the method of choice which requires endocervical swabs in women and urethral swabs in men. Culture is more favored because it can also provide information about antimicrobial susceptibility. But, the NAAT as well as Gram staining have a very high sensitivity (96 and 95%) and specificity (both nearing 99%). Gram staining can only be used in symptomatic men, and it is not sufficiently sensitive to rule out infection in asymptomatic men. Culture is superior to nonculture techniques in case of treatment failure.[20,32]

Management

According to CDC 2015,[20] ceftriaxone 250 mg with azithromycin 1 g was considered as the treatment of choice. However, the first clinical failure with the above treatment was reported in 2016.[33] Therefore, a new treatment regime was formulated **(Boxes 2 and 3)**.[7]

In addition to antibiotic treatment, management also includes counseling, screening for other STIs, contact tracing/treatment, and advice on safe sex. Due to the emerging problem of antibiotic resistance, test of cure is recommended in all cases. In those with persistent symptoms, culture should be done 72 hours posttreatment, and in those who are asymptomatic, NAAT should be performed after 2 weeks.

BOX 2: Uncomplicated gonococcal infection of the cervix, urethra, or rectum.

- *Recommended regimen for uncomplicated gonococcal infection of the cervix, urethra, or rectum among adults and adolescents*
- *Ceftriaxone* 500 mg* intramuscular (IM) in a single dose for persons weighing <150 kg
- If chlamydial infection has not been excluded, treat for chlamydia with doxycycline 100 mg orally 2 times/day for 7 days

*For persons weighing ≥150 kg, 1 g ceftriaxone should be administered.

BOX 3: Alternative regimens if ceftriaxone is not available.

- *Gentamicin* 240 mg intramuscular (IM) in a single dose *plus*
- *Azithromycin* 2 g orally in a single dose
  or
- *Cefixime** 800 mg orally in a single dose

*If chlamydial infection has not been excluded, providers should treat for chlamydia with doxycycline 100 mg orally 2 times/day for 7 days.

NONGONOCOCCAL–NONCHLAMYDIAL INFECTIONS

Mycoplasma

Prevalence

In an analysis of 34 studies published from 1993 to 2011 involving men with nongonococcal urethritis, 13% of 7,123 tested positive for *M. genitalium*.[34]

Microbiology

Mycoplasmas are small membrane-bound (i.e., they lack a cell wall) free-living prokaryotes. They are the smallest organisms, capable of independent replication. Mycoplasma differs from viruses in that they can reproduce outside of living cells. They are unique among prokaryotes because they lack a cell wall. This absence of cell wall is responsible for their lack of a reaction to Gram stain and their lack of susceptibility to many commonly prescribed antimicrobial agents, including β-lactams.

Three types of mycoplasmas have been isolated from female genital mucosal surfaces:

1. *M. genitalium*
2. *M. hominis*
3. Ureaplasma urealyticum.

Pathophysiology

The exact role of mycoplasma in patients with infertility problems is not completely understood. Colonization with genital mycoplasmas happens mainly through sexual contact. Women are more commonly infected than men. The recently discovered *M. genitalium* may also have the ability to cause reproductive tract infections.[35] Whether this organism, alone or in combination with other microbes, contributes to fallopian tube occlusion is unclear.[5]

Clinical Features

Genital mycoplasmas may be associated with nonspecific urethritis, cervicitis, and vaginitis. They may also be responsible for some cases of acute salpingitis, fever after abortions, chorioamnionitis, and puerperal infections.[10] While evidence shows that *M. genitalium* is often present in or associated with PID cases,[34] more data is necessary to determine the role of this microorganism in the pathogenesis of PID and subsequent tubal factor infertility.[4] However, controlled studies have not demonstrated any significant difference in isolation of the organism in fertile and infertile couples.[36] Since its discovery, it has demonstrated that *M. genitalium* is strongly associated with male urethritis.[34]

Diagnosis and Management

Mycoplasma genitalium is diagnosed by NAAT testing of urine, urethral, vaginal, and cervical swabs and through endometrial biopsies.[5] There is little point in testing for mycoplasmas and ureaplasmas in culture due to the high level of colonization in the general population. In addition, these microorganisms are rarely isolated from pure cultures and may take a very long time to grow.[7,20]

Mycoplasma genitalium lacks a cell wall, and thus antibiotics targeting cell-wall biosynthesis (e.g., β-lactams including penicillins and cephalosporins) are ineffective against this organism. Because of the high rates of macrolide resistance with treatment failures[37] and efficient selection of additional resistance, a 1 g dose of azithromycin should not be used.

Two-stage therapy approaches, ideally using resistance-guided therapy, are recommended for treatment. Resistance-guided therapy has demonstrated cure rates of >90% and should be used whenever possible;[38,39] however, it requires access to macrolide-resistance testing. As part of this approach, doxycycline is provided as initial empiric therapy, which reduces the organism load and facilitates organism clearance, followed by macrolide-sensitive *M. genitalium* infections treated with high-dose azithromycin; macrolide-resistant infections are treated with moxifloxacin **(Box 4)**.[7,40,41]

BOX 4: Recommended regimens if *Mycoplasma genitalium* resistance testing is available.

- *If macrolide sensitive: Doxycycline* 100 mg orally 2 times/day for 7 days, followed by *azithromycin* 1 g orally initial dose, followed by 500 mg orally daily for 3 additional days (2.5 g total)
- *If macrolide resistant: Doxycycline* 100 mg orally 2 times/day for 7 days, followed by *moxifloxacin* 400 mg orally once daily for 7 days
- *Recommended regimen if M. genitalium resistance testing is not available*
- *If M. genitalium is detected by an FDA-cleared NAAT: Doxycycline* 100 mg orally 2 times/day for 7 days, followed by *moxifloxacin* 400 mg orally once daily for 7 days

(FDA: Food and Drug Administration; NAAT: nucleic acid amplification test)
Source: CDC (2021).[7]

Trichomonas

Prevalence

Trichomonas vaginalis is the most common nonviral STI.[42] More than 50% of the curable STIs can be attributed to TV.[43]

Microbiology

Trichomonas vaginalis is a flagellated protozoan. It is typically pyriform in shape and is an anaerobic obligate parasite.[44] TV is sometimes amoeboid in shape. TV possesses five flagella, out of which four arise from the anterior aspect of the organism. The fifth flagella are incorporated into the undulating membrane, giving it a characteristic motility.[45] TV generally reproduces by longitudinal binary fission.

Pathophysiology

The genital tract squamous epithelium is the main site of infection of TV. Humans are the only known hosts of TV. It is primarily transmitted via sexual intercourse.[42] The cell surface of the organism plays an important role in adhesion, host-parasite interaction, nutrition, and these functions may be mediated via the proteins and glycoproteins on the surface. There is alteration in the normal vaginal pH from 4.5 to >5.0.[35]

Clinical Features

Trichomoniasis in women may be classified as acute, chronic, or asymptomatic, depending on the severity. In acute infection, women have a copious vaginal discharge, which is typically copious, malodorous, frothy, yellow-green in color with or without vulval irritation.[7] The cervix and the vagina may appear speckled with small punctate hemorrhagic spots, referred to as a "strawberry appearance." However, this characteristic feature is seen only in 2% of the patients. In chronic infection, the symptoms are mild with pruritus and dyspareunia and the discharge is minimal.

Around 25–50% are asymptomatic carriers of TV. The long-term sequelae may include pyosalpinx, endometritis, and infertility. Trichomoniasis is also associated with increased HIV transmission.[46]

Male partners of women with trichomoniasis are likely to have infection. Trichomoniasis in men is largely asymptomatic, and these men are the carriers of TV. Occasionally it may produce symptoms in men with complaints of scanty, clear to mucopurulent discharge, dysuria, and mild pruritus or burning sensation immediately after sexual intercourse.[46] TV can also lead to epididymitis, prostatitis, and decreased sperm cell motility.

Diagnosis

Traditionally, direct observation of the organism on wet mount microscopy has been the method used. This must be performed within 10–20 minutes of collection of the sample, or the organisms will lose viability. But the test method has very poor sensitivity (51–65%);[46,47] therefore, NAAT which is highly sensitive has replaced the wet mount. Also, culture using specialized culture media is another method used and will be diagnostic in 95% of cases, but it may take as long as 2–7 days.[46,48]

Management

Metronidazole gives a cure rate of approximately 95%. During treatment and for at least 48 hours afterward, alcohol should not be taken because of the antabuse effect with metronidazole. Sexual partners should be treated, and abstinence is advised until treatment is completed. All patients should be screened for other STIs **(Box 5)**.[20]

Bacterial Vaginosis

Bacterial vaginosis (BV) is being included as an STI, despite it not being considered a traditional STI because an accumulating body of epidemiological and microbiological evidence suggests that sexual transmission is integral to its pathogenesis. It is the most prevalent urogenital disorder of women in reproductive age with reproductive and obstetric sequelae and is also highly resistant to treatment.[49,50] BV is a vaginal dysbiosis resulting from replacement of normal hydrogen peroxide and lactic acid-producing *Lactobacillus* species in the vagina with high concentrations of anaerobic bacteria, including *Gardnerella vaginalis*, *Prevotella* species, *Mobiluncus* species, *Atopobium vaginae*, and other BV-associated bacteria. BV is a highly prevalent condition and the most common cause of vaginal discharge worldwide.[7]

Although BV-associated bacteria can be identified on male genitalia, treatment of male sex partners has not been beneficial in preventing the recurrence of BV.[51]

Diagnostic Considerations

Bacterial vaginosis can be diagnosed by using clinical criteria (i.e., Amsel's diagnostic criteria)[52] or by determining the Nugent score from a vaginal Gram stain.[53]

A Nugent score of 0–3 is consistent with a *Lactobacillus*-predominant vaginal microbiota, 4–6 with intermediate microbiota (emergence of *G. vaginalis*), and 7–10 with BV.

Clinical diagnosis of BV by Amsel's criteria requires at least three of the following four symptoms or signs:

1. Homogeneous, thin discharge (milk-like consistency) that smoothly coats the vaginal walls.
2. Clue cells (e.g., vaginal epithelial cells studded with adherent bacteria) on microscopic examination.
3. pH of vaginal fluid >4.5.
4. A fishy odor of vaginal discharge before or after addition of 10% potassium hydroxide (KOH) (i.e., the whiff test).

Current treatments are associated with frequent recurrence. Recurrence after treatment might relate to evidence that suggests sexual transmission is integral to the pathogenesis of BV, which has substantial implications for the development of effective management approaches **(Boxes 6 and 7)**.[2]

BOX 5: Recommended regimen for trichomoniasis among women.

- *Metronidazole* 500 mg orally 2 times/day for 7 days
- *Recommended regimen for trichomoniasis among men*
- *Metronidazole* 2 g orally in a single dose
- *Alternative regimen for women and men*
- *Tinidazole* 2 g orally in a single dose

Source: CDC (2021).

BOX 6: Alternative regimens—clindamycin, secnidazole, and tinidazole.

Alternative regimens:
- *Clindamycin* 300 mg orally 2 times/day for 7 days
  or
- *Clindamycin ovules* 100 mg intravaginally once at bedtime for 3 days*
  or
- *Secnidazole* 2 g oral granules in a single dose†
  or
- *Tinidazole* 2 g orally once daily for 2 days
  or
- *Tinidazole* 1 g orally once daily for 5 days

*Clindamycin ovules use an oleaginous base that might weaken latex or rubber products (e.g., condoms and diaphragms). Use of such products within 72 hours after treatment with clindamycin ovules is not recommended.

†Oral granules should be sprinkled onto unsweetened applesauce, yogurt, or pudding before ingestion. A glass of water can be taken after administration to aid in swallowing.

BOX 7: Recommended regimens for bacterial vaginosis

- *Metronidazole* 500 mg orally 2 times/day for 7 days
  or
- *Metronidazole gel 0.75%* one full applicator (5 g) intravaginally, once daily for 5 days
  or
- *Clindamycin cream 2%* one full applicator (5 g) intravaginally at bedtime for 7 days

Pelvic Inflammatory Disease

Pelvic inflammatory disease comprises a spectrum of inflammatory disorders of the upper female genital tract, including any combination of endometritis, salpingitis, tubo-ovarian abscess, and pelvic peritonitis.[54,55]

Microbiology

Pelvic inflammatory disease is a polymicrobial infection of the upper genital tract (UGT). It is mainly caused by *N. gonorrhoeae* and *C. trachomatis* in many cases. However, of late, it has been found that the number of cases of PID attributable to the above organisms is decreasing; hardly around 50% of the cases test positive for these. PID can also be caused by a host of other organisms, including *G. vaginalis*, *Haemophilus influenzae*, enteric gram-negative rods, and *Streptococcus agalactiae*.[56]

Pathophysiology

Tubal damage is a very common sequela of PID, with the incidence of tubal occlusion being proportional to the number of episodes of PID. Tubal damage can ultimately lead to infertility and increased risk of ectopic pregnancy. Delay in treatment can also lead to chronic pelvic pain.

The likelihood of developing tubal-factor infertility after PID is related to the following:

- The number of episodes of PID
- Severity of the episodes
- Length of time before treatment
- The age of the woman.

Clinical Features and Diagnosis

No single historical, physical, or laboratory finding is both sensitive and specific for the diagnosis of acute PID. Women with lower abdominal or pelvic pain should be diagnosed with PID if at least one of the three minimum criteria are present. One or more of the additional criteria will enhance the specificity of the minimum clinical criteria and support a diagnosis of PID.[7,20]

Minimum criteria (any one) for the diagnosis of PID:

- Cervical motion tenderness
  or
- Uterine tenderness
  or
- Adnexal tenderness

Additional criteria:

- Oral temperature >101°F (>38.3°C)
- Abnormal cervical mucopurulent discharge or cervical friability
- Presence of abundant numbers of white blood count (WBC) on saline microscopy of vaginal fluid
- Elevated erythrocyte sedimentation rate
- Elevated C-reactive protein
- Laboratory documentation of cervical infection with *N. gonorrhoeae* or *C. trachomatis.*

Specific criteria:

- Endometrial biopsy with histopathologic evidence of endometritis
- Transvaginal sonography or magnetic resonance imaging techniques showing thickened, fluid-filled tubes with or without free pelvic fluid or tubo-ovarian complex, or Doppler studies suggesting pelvic infection (e.g., tubal hyperemia); or
- Laparoscopic findings consistent with PID.

BOX 8: Recommended intramuscular (IM) or oral regimens for pelvic inflammatory disease.

- *Ceftriaxone* 500 mg* IM in a single dose *plus*
- *Doxycycline* 100 mg orally 2 times/day for 14 days with *metronidazole* 500 mg orally 2 times/day for 14 days
  or
- *Cefoxitin* 2 g IM in a single dose and *probenecid* 1 g orally administered concurrently in a single dose *plus*
- *Doxycycline* 100 mg orally 2 times/day for 14 days with *metronidazole* 500 mg orally 2 times/day for 14 days
- *Other parenteral third-generation cephalosporin* (e.g., ceftizoxime or cefotaxime) *plus*
- *Doxycycline* 100 mg orally 2 times/day for 14 days with *metronidazole* 500 mg orally 2 times/day for 14 days

*For persons weighing >150 kg, 1 g of ceftriaxone should be administered.

Management

Treatment needs to be started no sooner than the presumptive diagnosis is made because prevention of long-term sequelae is related to the efficacious and urgent start of treatment.

Women with mild to moderately severe PID should be treated with oral regimen. In case of very severe infection or intolerance or no response, it is recommended to switch over to parenteral regimen **(Boxes 8 and 9)**.[7]

Hospitalization may be required in cases of:

- Pregnancy
- Tubo-ovarian abscess
- Inability to tolerate an outpatient oral regimen
- Absent response to oral therapy.

BOX 9: Recommended parenteral regimens for pelvic inflammatory disease.

- *Ceftriaxone* 1 g by every 24 hours *plus*
- *Doxycycline* 100 mg orally or intravenous (IV) every 12 hours *plus*
- *Metronidazole* 500 mg orally or IV every 12 hours

or

- *Cefotetan* 2 g IV every 12 hours *plus*
- *Doxycycline* 100 mg orally or IV every 12 hours

or

- *Cefoxitin* 2 g IV every 6 hours *plus*
- *Doxycycline* 100 mg orally or IV every 12 hours

Women should be instructed to avoid sexual intercourse until therapy is completed and symptoms have resolved. Sex partners should be appropriately treated.[7]

SEXUALLY TRANSMITTED VIRAL INFECTIONS

Around 4.2 million people of childbearing age in the United States of America are infected with HIV, HCV, hepatitis B virus (HBV), or a combination.[57]

Majority (around 75%) of the men and women infected with viral infections are in their reproductive age and many of these couples look for reducing the risk of transmission to their partners and child.[58] A few of them may require treatment for their fertility problems.

- Preconception counseling explaining the risks of transmission
- Treatment of infection when possible
- Usage of appropriate measures to prevent transmission.

Sperm-wash Methods

Sperm-wash procedures involving density-gradient centrifugation followed by a sperm swim-up step have been used to separate motile sperm from free HIV virus and HIV-infected somatic cells.[59-61] Quantitative assessment of HIV in semen before and after the sperm-wash procedure indicates that >99% of HIV is removed.[60] Virologic testing of the sperm fraction for the presence of residual detectable HIV before its use for insemination can provide an added measure of safety as up to 5–10% of samples may contain residual virus after this procedure.[61] Similar sperm preparation techniques have been used to separate HCV from sperm[62] and may be useful for other viral infections where the majority of virus is found in free form or associated with semen somatic cells (i.e., white blood cells, epithelial cells).

Management of Cryopreserved Tissue

Contamination with HIV, HBV, and HCV has been documented in assisted reproductive technology (ART) clinics[63] and blood banks.[64] Although there is no documentation of cross-contamination of cryopreserved stored human tissue, it is highly recommended that samples from viral carriers be processed in a separate laboratory or designated space within the main laboratory. HIV, HCV, HBV, and possibly other viruses can survive in liquid nitrogen, making it possible to cross-contaminate samples in liquid nitrogen storage tanks, although this risk is very low.

To protect cryopreserved specimens from the potential cross-contamination risk, it is advised that HIV, HBV, and HCV-infected specimens be stored in separate tanks.

The risks of cross contamination of samples in liquid nitrogen storage could be reduced by following the below-given measures:[58]

- Use of a closed-system vitrification device to avoid direct contact with liquid nitrogen
- Storage of samples in liquid nitrogen vapor instead of in the liquid phase of nitrogen itself
- Use of sperm-wash techniques to decrease the viral load before freezing semen samples.

Human Immunodeficiency Virus

Human immunodeficiency virus is a retrovirus because it uses enzyme reverse transcriptase to transcribe RNA to DNA. It binds to CD4+ T-lymphocytes and leads to their destruction. HIV leads to the development of acquired immunodeficiency syndrome (AIDS) once the CD4+ cell count drops below 200.[65]

Sexual transmission is the predominant mode of spread of HIV. The global prevalence of HIV is 0.7% (WHO–HIV 2020). It is highly prevalent in high-risk groups, including users of unscreened blood products, intravenous drug users, sex workers, and men who have sex with men (MSM). HIV is transmitted both sexually and vertically through blood, semen, vaginal secretions, and breast milk. The rate of HIV heterosexual transmission is relatively low (approximately 1/1,000 acts of unprotected intercourse). Risk factors for HIV transmission include genital-tract infections and ulceration, sexual practices that induce trauma or bleeding, and lack of male circumcision.[58]

Worldwide, approximately 73% of adults and children have access to highly active antiretroviral therapy (HAART), which is combined HAART where three or more antiretroviral drugs are used to control HIV infection [Joint United Nations Programme on HIV/AIDS (UNAIDS) factsheet 2021].[66]

HIV and Infertility

Semen parameters in HIV-positive men are impaired compared to WHO normal range. There is a decrease in sperm count, motility, and morphology.[67]

It has been found that these parameters are abnormal even though the patient is on HAART. HIV-positive women are prone to have reduced fertility with a decreased ovarian reserve when compared to HIV-negative individuals.

Patients on HAART have impaired oocyte quality because of the effect of the drugs on oocyte mitochondria.[68]

The American Society for Reproductive Medicine (ASRM) has stated that fertility services cannot be withheld ethically from individuals with chronic viral infections, including HIV, if a center has the resources to provide care.[58]

HIV-infected Individuals and Risk Reduction Strategies

In case of an uninfected partner of an HIV-positive individual, the rate of transmission is approximately 1 in 500–1,000 episodes of unprotected intercourse.[69]

The risk of transmission increases drastically if the viral load is high or if the HIV-negative partner has a concomitant genital infection, inflammation, or abrasions.[70]

Serodiscordant Couples with Near-normal Gamete Parameters

Earlier to 2008, there were controversies regarding the treatment of serodiscordant couples with European countries going in for sperm wash and intrauterine insemination (IUI).

In 2008, the Swiss Commission for HIV care[71,72] stated that an HIV-positive person (male or female) receiving HAART and with an undetectable viral load (<50 copies/mL) for 6 months and without genital infection does not transmit HIV by sex. Therefore, they can be allowed to conceive naturally. According to Cochrane review,[73] the risk of transmission of HIV to the uninfected partner in such cases is negligible. But despite this strong evidence, the United States of America still follows a conservative approach with sperm washing and intracytoplasmic sperm injection (ICSI) being the primary treatment modality in HIV-positive male with negative partner irrespective of the viral load.[57] Ongoing research now supports the CDC statement that people with HIV who take antiretroviral therapy as prescribed and achieve and maintain an undetectable viral load have effectively no risk of transmitting HIV through sex.[74]

Sperm washing may still be offered to couples (with male being HIV positive) if:

- Couple unwilling to conceive naturally despite counseling about negligible risk
- Inability to achieve low viral loads despite HAART
- Difficult to access HAART therapy as in underdeveloped countries.

In case of an HIV-infected woman with negative partner, ideally, HAART is advocated to reduce the risk of transmission to both the partner and the future child. However, if HAART is not fully effective, autoinsemination with the partner's sperm is a simple method to avoid the risk of transmission to the man.

Serodiscordant Couples with Abnormal Gamete Parameters

Men and women with conception problems can no longer be denied access to fertility treatment, citing HIV status. The modalities of treatment are the same as that of the noninfected patients. However, in view of the complexities involved in handling of the infected gametes, it is advisable according to the European Society of Human Reproduction and Embryology (ESHRE) 2015 and ASRM practice committee 2013 to assign a dedicated laboratory space and separate cryostorage facility for the purpose.[75,76]

Seroconcordant Couples for HIV

There is obviously no risk of infecting an uninfected partner in seroconcordant couple for HIV; however, there is a possibility of superinfection. There are increasing reports that one HIV-infected partner can transmit their unique strain of HIV to another infected partner.[77]

Therefore, it is worthwhile for both partners to have low viral loads before attempting conception. Also, in case of abnormal gamete parameters, fertility treatment must follow the accepted protocol.

Sperm-wash Techniques

Fiore et al.[78] in their unique experiment using semen samples preloaded with known concentration of HIV virus found that density gradient centrifugation is sufficient to clear the virus of samples containing 1 × 103–5 × 104 copies viral RNA/mL, density gradient followed by swim up is required for samples containing 1 × 105–5 × 105 copies viral RNA/mL. In semen samples containing 1–3 × 106 copies of viral RNA/mL, viral RNA was persistent in some even after the two standard washing procedures.

This study concludes that the effectiveness of the sperm-washing techniques is dependent on the viral load.[79]

Hepatitis B Virus

Hepatitis B virus is a DNA virus that attacks the liver and can cause both acute and chronic diseases. The virus is transmitted through contact with the blood or other body fluids of an infected person. It is a highly infectious virus which is 100 times more infective than HIV or HCV. It is also transmitted by sexual intercourse and is twice as infective as HIV by this modality. HBV vaccine was developed in 1982. The vaccine is 95% effective in preventing infection and the development of chronic disease and liver cancer due to hepatitis B. The vaccine also protects uninfected partner against sexual transmission.

Hepatitis B virus is one of the most common infectious diseases in the world; it has been estimated that 350 million people worldwide are HBV carrier. HBV can be transmitted parenterally, sexually, vertically, and via other routes of mucosal exposure. Approximately 25% of regular sexual contacts of HBV-infected persons will become seropositive for HBV, and HBV has been transmitted through artificial insemination.[58]

Hepatitis B virus is a disease that is transmitted through fluids; many studies also showed that HBV DNA can be detected in urine, saliva, and other tissues beyond the liver and blood. HBV is not only able to pass through the blood-testis barrier and enter the sperm cell but also integrate into their sperm chromosome.[80] When human sperm-mediated HBV genes were delivered into zona-free hamster oocytes via the in vitro fertilization (IVF) method, HBV genes were able to replicate and express in early embryonic cells.[81] Actually, the sperm-washing procedures could eliminate the presence of viruses, but the risk of HBV DNA integrated into sperm chromosome could not be eliminated.[82] These results suggest that sperm cells of HBV patients might act as vectors for transmitting the HBV genes during IVF and ICSI procedures.

All couples being evaluated for IVF should be screened for HBV via HBsAg. In couples who are discordant for HBV infection, the partner who is seronegative for HbsAg and has no evidence of immunity on additional serologic testing (i.e., is negative for HbsAb and core antibody) should be vaccinated against HBV. Fertility treatments may be initiated once the vaccinated partner's anti-HbsAb titer is positive. Modified sperm wash to reduce viral load is not required after the female partner is immunized against HBV.[58]

Hepatitis B virus-discordant couples can be allowed to conceive naturally once the negative individual is fully vaccinated. The effectiveness of HBV vaccination is measured by the presence of HBV surface antibody. 5% of the individuals are nonresponders, i.e., they do not produce HBV surface antibody. Such couples may be subjected to sperm wash and IUI.

All HBsAg-positive HBV-infected females should be offered referral to a hepatologist to determine if she is immune tolerant or has immune-active disease. Immune-tolerant individuals are a carrier of the virus with normal alanine transaminase and aspartate transaminase levels and do not have active hepatitis. Immune-active disease (previously termed chronic active hepatitis) occurs in those individuals who have elevated liver function tests associated with chronic hepatitis. For the immune-tolerant patient with HBV, the current recommendations would be to treat individuals with HBV DNA viral level >200,000 IU/mL with appropriate antiviral therapy.[58]

Vertical transmission accounts for over 40% of cases of chronic infection. In case of HBV-positive women, additionally, the newborn has to be given immunoprophylaxis (HBV vaccination and one dose of HBV immunoglobulins) immediately at birth (within 24 hours) and two more doses of vaccine at 1 and 6 months to minimize vertical transmission. In women with high viral load (>100,000 IU/mL) risk of transmission is much higher; therefore, antiviral therapy is advocated during pregnancy.[83]

Hepatitis B virus infection is associated with a reduced sperm motility and a higher proportion of apoptotic and necrotic sperm, resulting in lower fertility index.[84] HBV-positive men had decreased sperm motility and viability but normal morphology compared to the controls.[80]

Zhou et al.[85] reported ICSI could aggravate HBV transmission into the oocyte, and HBV-infected men had lower rates of 2 pro-nuclei (2PN) fertilization (70.9 vs. 74.0%), high-grade embryos acquisition (57.6 vs. 60.4%), implantation (18.3 vs. 24.2%), and clinical pregnancy (31.2 vs. 39.3%) in ICSI cycles. However, Lutgens et al.[82] thought sperm washing could effectively reduce the risk of vertical transmission and prevent introduction of HBV into the oocyte in the case of ICSI. As previous studies found that hepatotropism was a prominent feature of HBV infection, the HBV DNA level in semen was lower compared with that in serum.[86] In addition, these patients had been in a convalescent stage for >6 months, which exceed the spermatogenic cycle.

According to two similar studies, they found that the rates of HBV-positive embryos were only 16.6 and 21.3% in male HBsAg positive/female HBsAg-negative couples, respectively.[87,88] It can assume that HBV DNA integrate into human sperm chromosomes, causing adverse effects on human sperm function, but that those infected embryos could not be fully functional, and the HBV-positive males still have the opportunity to get uninfected sperm and embryos to fertilize and implant. These may explain why no adverse effect on outcomes of ICSI/IVF cycles was observed in the HBV-infected group. There is little information about HBV-positive males of IUI cycles. In our research, the significant difference in total motile sperm count before sperm preparation (50.0 ± 31.6 vs. 69.2 ± 47.1, $p < 0.01$) disappeared after preparation (23.5 ± 14.4 vs. 27.8 ± 17.4, $p > 0.05$). And the two groups showed similar clinical pregnancy rate and abortion rate. It showed that the use of semen processing was effective enough to improve the properties of the sperm, leading to a high chance of fertility. Therefore, IUI might be beneficial for improving HBV-infected males fertility outcomes. However, these findings are insufficient to make a definite conclusion on the subject.[80]

The presence of HBsAg and HBV–DNA has been detected in the ovary and the ovum of patients with chronic HBV infection.[89] There was no statistically significant association between HBV carrier status and clinical pregnancy, live birth, or miscarriage.[90]

Hepatitis C Virus

Hepatitis C virus is an RNA virus which affects the liver. It spreads primarily by parenteral route involving mainly blood. Occasionally, it may be transmitted sexually in MSM. Heterosexual transmission is not seen normally.[91] There is currently no vaccine available for HCV.

Natural conception is recommended for discordant couples; however, antiviral therapy is advocated for infected individuals before planning conception. In case of fertility problems, ART is indicated as per treatment protocol. Vertical transmission is seen in around 5–6% of HCV-positive women and is around 10–12% in women with concurrent HIV.[92] Cesarean delivery is not indicated, and breastfeeding is not contraindicated.

There is a small but measurable risk of HCV transmission via semen. All patients with hepatitis C should be counseled about the risks of transmission to their partner, which is rare through sexual transmission, and to their children through vertical transmission (occurring in 4–6%). They should be referred to a hepatitis specialist for discussion of potential treatment and cure. Current treatment of hepatitis C with direct-acting antiviral (DAA) therapy is 98% effective in achieving a sustained virologic response (SVR, i.e., a cure) within 8–12 weeks of treatment. An SVR is defined as a negative HCV RNA 12 weeks after treatment. With the ease, accessibility of insurance coverage, and short duration of therapy, it is recommended to treat all patients before IVF.[93]

CONCLUSION

The bacterial infections are associated with decreased fertility in view of alteration of the tubal factor and the semen parameters. Timely identification and treatment prevent occurrence of infertility. However, the viral infections and their treatment affect fertility. It is no longer ethically appropriate to deny treatment for any infertile couple based on their viral status. Necessary precautions need to be taken and required additional procedures offered in infected patients.

KEY POINTS

- Nontuberculous salpingitis can be divided into chlamydial, gonococcal and nongonococcal-nonchlamydial disease.
- Chlamydial infections are common in sexually active young adults.
- Culture is the method of diagnosis for *Neisseria gonorrhoeae*.
- Tubal damage is a very common sequela of PID (pelvic inflammatory disease).
- HIV, hepatitis B, hepatitis C are important sexually transmitted viral infections.

REFERENCES

1. Quaas A, Dokras A. Diagnosis and treatment of unexplained infertility. Rev Obstet Gynecol. 2008;1:69-76.
2. Unemo M, Bradshaw CS, Hocking JS, de Vries HJC, Francis SC, Mabey D, et al. Sexually transmitted infections: challenges ahead. Lancet Infect Dis. 2017;17:e235-79.
3. Holmes KK, Sparling PF, Stamm WE, Piot P, Wasserheit JN, Corey L, et al. Sexually Transmitted Diseases. New York: McGraw Hill Professional; 2008.
4. Tsevat DG, Wiesenfeld HC, Parks C, Peipert JF. Sexually transmitted diseases and infertility. Am J Obstet Gynecol. 2017;216:1-9.
5. Novy MJ, Eschenbach DA, Witkin SS. Infections as a cause of infertility. GLOWM. 2008.
6. Malik A, Jain S, Hakim S, Shukla I, Rizvi M. Chlamydia trachomatis infection & female infertility. Indian J Med Res. 2006;123:770-5.
7. Workowski KA, Bachmann LH, Chan PA, Johnston CM, Muzny CA, Park I, et al. Sexually transmitted infections treatment guidelines, 2021. MMWR Recomm Rep. 2021;70(4):1-187.
8. World Health Organization Task Force on the Prevention and Management of Infertility. Tubal infertility: serologic relationship to past chlamydial and gonococcal infection. Sex Transm Dis. 1995;22:71-7.
9. Rodríguez R, Hernández R, Fuster F, Torres A, Prieto P, Alberto J. Genital infection and infertility. Enferm Infecc Microbiol Clin. 2001;19(6):261-6.
10. Imudia AN, Detti L, Puscheck EE, Yelian FD, Diamond MP. The prevalence of Ureaplasma urealyticum, Mycoplasma hominis, Chlamydia trachomatis and Neisseria gonorrhoeae infections, and the Rubella status of patients undergoing an initial infertility evaluation. J Assist Reprod Genet. 2008;25(1):43-6.
11. Patel AL, Sachdev D, Nagpal P, Chaudhry U, Sonkar SC, Mendiratta SL, et al. Prevalence of chlamydia infection among women visiting a gynaecology outpatient department: evaluation of an in-house PCR assay for detection of Chlamydia trachomatis. Ann Clin Microbiol Antimicrob. 2010;9:24.
12. Malhotra M, Bala M, Muralidhar S, Khunger N, Puri P. Prevalence of sexually transmitted infections in patients attending a tertiary care hospital in North India—a retrospective study. Indian J Sex Transm Dis. 2008;29:82-5.
13. Malhotra M, Sood S, Mukherjee A, Muralidhar S, Bala M. Genital Chlamydia trachomatis: an update. Indian J Med Res. 2013;138(3):303-16.
14. Ward ME, Ridgway G. Chlamydia. In: Collier L, Balows A, Sussman A (Eds). Topley and Wilson's Microbiology and Microbial Infection, 9th edition. New York: Oxford University Press Inc; 1999. pp. 1331-6.
15. Kasper DL, Fauci AS, Hauser SL. Chlamydia trachomatis and Chlamydia psittaci. In: Kasper DL (Eds). Harrison's Manual of Medicine, 19th edition. New York: McGraw-Hill; 2016.
16. Darville T, Hiltke TJ. Pathogenesis of genital tract disease due to Chlamydia trachomatis. J Infect Dis. 2010;201(Suppl. 2):S114-25.
17. Rasmussen SJ, Eckmann L, Quayle AJ, Shen L, Zhang YX, Anderson DJ, et al. Secretion of proinflammatory cytokines by epithelial cells in response to chlamydia infection suggests a central role for epithelial cells in chlamydial pathogenesis. J Clin Invest. 1997;99(1):77-87.

18. Giakoumelou S, Wheelhouse N, Cuschieri K, Entrican G, Howie SE, Horne AW. The role of infection in miscarriage. Hum Reprod Update. 2016;22(1):116-33.
19. Dieterle S. Urogenital infections in reproductive medicine. Andrologia. 2008;40:117-9.
20. Workowski KA, Bolan GA. Sexually transmitted diseases treatment guidelines, 2015. MMWR Recomm Rep. 2015;64(3):1-137.
21. Rodriguez-Cerdeira C, Sanchez-Blanco E, Molares-Vila A, Alba A. Unveiling new molecular factors useful for detection of pelvic inflammatory disease due to Chlamydia trachomatis infection. ISRN Obstet Gynecol. 2012;2012:581725.
22. Chernesky MA, Mahony JB, Castriciano S, Mores M, Stewart IO, Landis SJ, et al. Detection of Chlamydia trachomatis antigens by enzyme immunoassay and immunofluorescence in genital specimens from symptomatic and asymptomatic men and women. J Infect Dis. 1986;154:141-8.
23. Chernesky MA. The laboratory diagnosis of *Chlamydia trachomatis* infections. Can J Infect Dis Med Microbiol. 2005;16(1):39-44.
24. LeFevre ML, U.S. Preventive Services Task Force. Screening for chlamydia and gonorrhea: US Preventive Services Task Force recommendation statement. Ann Intern Med. 2014;161:902-10.
25. Paavonen J. Immunopathogenesis of pelvic inflammatory disease and infertility—what do we know and what shall we do? J Br Fer Soc. 1996;1:42-5.
26. Divekar AA, Gogate AS, Shivkar LK, Gogate S, Badhwar VR. Disease prevalence in women attending the STD clinic in Mumbai (formerly Bombay), India. Int J STD AIDS. 2000;11(1):45-8.
27. O'Donnell JA, Gelone SP. Pelvic Inflammatory Disease. New York: Infobase Publishing; 2009.
28. Ryan KJ, Ray CG (Eds). Sherris Medical Microbiology, 4th edition. New York: McGraw Hill; 2004.
29. Anderson MT, Dewenter L, Maier B, Seifert HS. Seminal plasma initiates a Neisseria gonorrhoeae transmission state. mBio. 2014;5(2):e01004-13.
30. Apari P, de Sousa JD, Müller V. Why sexually transmitted infections tend to cause infertility: an evolutionary hypothesis. PLoS Pathog. 2014;10(8):e1004111.
31. Rosemond A, Lanotte P, Watt S, Sauget AS, Guerif F, Royère D, et al. Systematic screening tests for Chlamydia trachomatis, Mycoplasma hominis and Ureaplasma urealyticum in urogenital specimens of infertile couples. Pathol Biol (Paris). 2006;54:125-9.
32. Miller KE. Diagnosis and treatment of Neisseria gonorrhoeae infections. Am Fam Physician. 2006;73(10):1779-84.
33. Fifer H, Natarajan U, Jones L, Alexander S, Hughes G, Golparian D, et al. Failure of dual antimicrobial therapy in treatment of gonorrhea. N Engl J Med. 2016;374: 2504-6.
34. Lis R, Rowhani-Rahbar A, Manhart LE. Mycoplasma genitalium infection and female reproductive tract disease: a meta-analysis. Clin Infect Dis. 2015;61:418-26.
35. Taylor-Robinson D, McCormack WM. The genital mycoplasmas. N Engl J Med. 1980;302:1003-10.
36. Gump DW, Gibson M, Askikaga T. Lack of association between genital mycoplasmas and infertility. N Engl J Med. 1984;310:937-41.
37. Horner P, Donders G, Cusini M, Gomberg M, Jensen JS, Unemo M. Should we be testing for urogenital Mycoplasma hominis, Ureaplasma parvum and Ureaplasma urealyticum in men and women?—a position statement from the European STI Guidelines Editorial Board. J Eur Acad Dermatol Venereol. 2018;32:1845-51.
38. Read TRH, Fairley CK, Murray GL, Jensen JS, Danielewski J, Worthington K, et al. Outcomes of resistance-guided sequential treatment of Mycoplasma genitalium infections: a prospective evaluation. Clin Infect Dis. 2019;68:554-60.
39. Durukan D, Read TRH, Murray G, Doyle M, Chow EPF, Vodstrcil LA, et al. Resistance-guided antimicrobial therapy using doxycycline-moxifloxacin and doxycycline-2.5 g azithromycin for the treatment of Mycoplasma genitalium infection: efficacy and tolerability. Clin Infect Dis. 2020; 71:1461-8.
40. Li Y, Le WJ, Li S, Cao YP, Su XH. Meta-analysis of the efficacy of moxifloxacin in treating Mycoplasma genitalium infection. Int J STD AIDS. 2017;28:1106-14.
41. Mondeja BA, Couri J, Rodríguez NM, Blanco O, Fernández C, Jensen JS. Macrolide-resistant *Mycoplasma genitalium* infections in Cuban patients: an underestimated health problem. BMC Infect Dis. 2018;18:601.
42. Kissinger P. Trichomonas vaginalis: a review of epidemiologic, clinical and treatment issues. BMC Infect Dis. 2015;15: 307.
43. World Health Organization. (2012). Global incidence and prevalence of selected curable sexually transmitted infections; 2008. [online] Available from: https://apps.who.int/iris/bitstream/handle/10665/75181/9789241503839_eng.pdf [Last accessed December, 2022].
44. Harp DF, Chowdhury I. Trichomoniasis: evaluation to execution. Eur J Obstet Gynecol Reprod Biol. 2011;157(1):3-9.
45. Honigberg BM, King VM. Structure of Trichomonas vaginalis Donné. J Parasitol. 1964;50:345-64.
46. Petrin D, Delgaty K, Bhatt R, Garber G. Clinical and microbiological aspects of *Trichomonas vaginalis*. Clin Microbiol Rev. 1998;11(2):300-17.
47. Roth AM, Williams JA, Ly R, Curd K, Brooks D, Arno J, et al. Changing sexually transmitted infection screening protocol will result in improved case finding for Trichomonas vaginalis among high-risk female populations. Sex Transm Dis. 2011;38:398-400.
48. Peipert JF, Ness RB, Blume J, Soper DE, Holley R, Randall H, et al. Clinical predictors of endometritis in women with symptoms and signs of pelvic inflammatory disease. Am J Obstet Gynecol. 2001;184:856-63.
49. Fethers KA, Fairley CK, Hocking JS, Gurrin LC, Bradshaw CS. Sexual risk factors and bacterial vaginosis: a systematic review and meta-analysis. Clin Infect Dis. 2008;47:1426-35.
50. Liu CM, Hungate BA, Tobian AA, Ravel J, Prodger JL, Serwadda D, et al. Penile microbiota and female partner bacterial vaginosis in Rakai, Uganda. mBio. 2015;6:e00589.
51. Mehta SD. Systematic review of randomized trials of treatment of male sexual partners for improved bacteria vaginosis outcomes in women. Sex Transm Dis. 2012;39:822-30.
52. Amsel R, Totten PA, Spiegel CA, Chen KC, Eschenbach D, Holmes KK. Nonspecific vaginitis. Diagnostic criteria and microbial and epidemiologic associations. Am J Med. 1983;74:14-22.

53. Nugent RP, Krohn MA, Hillier SL. Reliability of diagnosing bacterial vaginosis is improved by a standardized method of gram stain interpretation. J Clin Microbiol. 1991;29: 297-301.
54. Wiesenfeld HC, Sweet RL, Ness RB, Krohn MA, Amortegui AJ, Hillier SL. Comparison of acute and subclinical pelvic inflammatory disease. Sex Transm Dis. 2005;32:400-5.
55. Burnett AM, Anderson CP, Zwank MD. Laboratory-confirmed gonorrhea and/or chlamydia rates in clinically diagnosed pelvic inflammatory disease and cervicitis. Am J Emerg Med. 2012;30:1114-7.
56. Ness RB, Kip KE, Hillier SL, Soper DE, Stamm CA, Sweet RL. A cluster analysis of bacterial vaginosis-associated microflora and pelvic inflammatory disease. Am J Epidemiol. 2005;162:585-90.
57. Jindal SK, Rawlins RG, Muller CH, Drobnis EZ. Guidelines for risk reduction when handling gametes from infectious patients seeking assisted reproductive technologies. Reprod Biomed Online. 2016;33:121-30.
58. Practice Committee of the American Society for Reproductive Medicine. Recommendations for reducing the risk of viral transmission during fertility treatment with the use of autologous gametes: a committee opinion. Fertil Steril. 2020;114(6):1158-64.
59. Semprini AE, Levi-Setti P, Bozzo M, Ravizza M, Taglioretti A, Sulpizio P, et al. Insemination of HIV-negative women with processed semen of HIV-positive partners. Lancet. 1992;340:1317-9.
60. Politch JA, Xu C, Tucker L, Anderson DJ. Separation of human immunodeficiency virus type 1 from motile sperm by the double tube gradient method versus other methods. Fertil Steril 2004;81:440-7.
61. Marina S, Marina F, Alcolea R, Expósito R, Huguet J, Nadal J, et al. Human immunodeficiency virus type 1—serodiscordant couples can bear healthy children after undergoing intrauterine insemination. Fertil Steril. 1998;70:35-9.
62. Pasquier C, Daudin M, Righi L, Berges L, Thauvin L, Berrebi A, et al. Sperm washing and virus nucleic acid detection to reduce HIV and hepatitis C virus transmission in serodiscordant couples wishing to have children. AIDS. 2000;14: 2093-9.
63. Lesourd F, Izopet J, Mervan C, Payen JL, Sandres K, Monrozies X, et al. Transmissions of hepatitis C virus during the ancillary procedures for assisted conception. Hum Reprod. 2000;15:1083-5.
64. Tedder RS, Zuckerman MA, Goldstone AH, Hawkins AE, Fielding A, Briggs EM, et al. Hepatitis B transmission from contaminated cryopreservation tank. Lancet. 1995;346: 137-40.
65. Doitsh G, Galloway NL, Geng X, Yang Z, Monroe KM, Zepeda O, et al. Cell death by pyroptosis drives CD4 T-cell depletion in HIV-1 infection. Nature. 2014;505:509-14.
66. UNAIDS. (2021). Global HIV and AIDS statistics—fact sheet. [online] Available from: https://www.unaids.org/en/resources/fact-sheet [Last accessed December, 2022].
67. Nicopoullos JD, Almeida P, Vourliotis M, Gilling-Smith C. A decade of the sperm-washing programme: correlation between markers of HIV and seminal parameters. HIV Med. 2011;12:195-201.
68. López S, Coll O, Durban M, Hernàndez S, Vidal R, Suy A, et al. Mitochondrial DNA depletion in oocytes of HIV-infected antiretroviral-treated infertile women. Antivir Ther. 2008;13:833-8.
69. Mandelbrot L, Heard I, Henrion-Géant E, Henrion R. Natural conception in HIV-negative women with HIV-infected partners. Lancet. 1997;349:850-1.
70. Le Tortorec A, Dejucq-Rainsford N. HIV infection of the male genital tract–consequences for sexual transmission and reproduction. Int J Androl. 2010;33:e98-108.
71. Vernazza P, Hirschel B, Bernasconi E, Flepp M. Les personnes séropositives ne souffrant d'aucune autre MST et suivant un traitement antirétroviral efficace ne transmettent pas le VIH par voie sexuelle. Bull Med Suisses. 2008;89:165-9.
72. Vernazza P, Bernard EJ. HIV is not transmitted under fully suppressive therapy: the Swiss Statement—eight years later. Swiss Med Wkly. 2016;146:w14246.
73. Anglemyer A, Rutherford GW, Baggaley RC, Egger M, Siegfried N. Antiretroviral therapy for prevention of HIV transmission in HIV-discordant couples. Cochrane Database Syst Rev. 2011;(8):CD009153.
74. Centers for Disease Control and Prevention. Effectiveness of prevention strategies to reduce the risk of acquiring or transmitting HIV. [online] Available from https://www.cdc.gov/hiv/risk/estimates/preventionstrategies.html. [Last accessed November, 2022].
75. ESHRE Guideline Group on Good Practice in IVF Labs; De los Santos MJ, Apter S, Coticchio G, Debrock S, Lundin K, Plancha CE, et al. Revised guidelines for good practice in IVF laboratories (2015). Hum Reprod. 2016;31(4):685-6.
76. Practice Committee of American Society for Reproductive Medicine. Recommendations for reducing the risk of viral transmission during fertility treatment with the use of autologous gametes: a committee opinion. Fertil Steril. 2013;99(2):340-6.
77. Redd AD, Quinn TC, Tobian AA. Frequency and implications of HIV superinfection. Lancet Infect Dis. 2013;13:622-8.
78. Fiore JR, Lorusso F, Vacca M, Ladisa N, Greco P, De Palo R. The efficiency of sperm washing in removing human immunodeficiency virus type 1 varies according to the seminal viral load. Fertil Steril. 2005;84:232-4.
79. Ethics Committee of American Society for Reproductive Medicine. Human immunodeficiency virus (HIV) and infertility treatment: a committee opinion. Fertil Steril. 2015;104:e1-8.
80. Wang Z, Liu W, Zhang M, Wang M, Wu H, Lu M. Effect of hepatitis B virus infection on sperm quality and outcomes of assisted reproductive techniques in infertile males. Front Med (Lausanne). 2021;8:744350
81. Ali BA, Huang TH, Salem HH, Xie QD. Expression of hepatitis B virus genes in early embryonic cells originated from hamster ova and human spermatozoa transfected with the complete viral genome. Asian J Androl. 2006;8:273-9.
82. Lutgens SP, Nelissen EC, van Loo IH, Koek GH, Derhaag JG, Dunselman GA. To do or not to do: IVF and ICSI in chronic hepatitis B virus carriers. Hum Reprod. 2009;24:2676-8.
83. Gilling-Smith C, Almeida P. HIV, hepatitis B and hepatitis C and infertility: reducing risk. Hum Fertil (Camb). 2003;6:106-12.
84. Moretti E, Federico MG, Giannerini V, Collodel G. Sperm ultrastructure and meiotic segregation in a group of patients

with chronic hepatitis B and C. Andrologia. 2008;40: 286-91.
85. Zhou XP, Hu XL, Zhu YM, Qu F, Sun SJ, Qian YL. Comparison of semen quality and outcome of assisted reproductive techniques in Chinese men with and without hepatitis B. Asian J Androl. 2011;13:465-9.
86. Qian WP, Tan YQ, Chen Y, Peng Y, Li Z, Lu GX, et al. Rapid quantification of semen hepatitis B virus DNA by real-time polymerase chain reaction. World J Gastroenterol. 2005;11:5385-9.
87. Nie R, Jin L, Zhang H, Xu B, Chen W, Zhu G. Presence of hepatitis B virus in oocytes and embryos: a risk of hepatitis B virus transmission during in vitro fertilization. Fertil Steril. 2011;95:1667-71.
88. Hu XL, Zhou XP, Qian YL, Wu GY, Ye YH, Zhu YM. The presence and expression of the hepatitis B virus in human oocytes and embryos. Hum Reprod. 2011;26:1860-7.
89. Ye F, Yue Y, Li S, Chen T, Bai G, Liu M, et al. Presence of HBsAg, HBcAg, and HBVDNA in ovary and ovum of the patients with chronic hepatitis B virus infection. Am J Obstet Gynecol. 2006;194:387-92.
90. Wang L, Li L, Huang C, Diao L, Lian R, Li Y, et al. Maternal chronic hepatitis B virus infection does not affect pregnancy outcomes in infertile patients receiving first in vitro fertilization treatment. Fertil Steril. 2019;112(2):250-7.e1.
91. Chan DP, Sun HY, Wong HT, Lee SS, Hung CC. Sexually acquired hepatitis C virus infection: a review. Int J Infect Dis. 2016;49:47-58.
92. Benova L, Mohamoud YA, Calvert C, Abu-Raddad LJ. Vertical transmission of hepatitis C virus: systematic review and meta-analysis. Clin Infect Dis. 2014;59:765-73.
93. AASLD-IDSA HCV Guidance Panel. Hepatitis C guidance 2018 update: AASLD-IDSA recommendations for testing, managing, and treating hepatitis C virus infection. Clin Infect Dis. 2018;67:1477-92.

CHAPTER 36

Tuberculosis and Infertility

JB Sharma, Sona Dharmendra, Gowri Rapaka

INTRODUCTION

Tuberculosis (TB) is caused by *Mycobacterium tuberculosis* complex (*M. tuberculosis, M. bovis, M. albicans* or atypical *Mycobacterium* species with human disease in immunocompetent persons mainly caused by *M. tuberculosis*[1,2]). It remains a major public health problem worldwide.[1-5] Most cases (95%) occur in developing countries with 3.2 million cases in women and 1.4 million deaths in the year 2019.[2] India has one of the highest incidences of TB in the world.[3] Coinfection with human immunodeficiency virus (HIV) and more liberal immigration has significantly increased the risk of developing TB all over the world.[3] Multidrug-resistant (MDR) and extreme drug-resistant TB, which are caused by poor case management, are causes of serious concern throughout the world.[1-5]

HISTORY

Morgagni in 1744 reported the first case of female genital tuberculosis (FGTB).[6]

Due to the high prevalence, mortality, and morbidity due to TB globally, World Health organization (WHO) promoted a new treatment strategy based on five essential elements named—directly observed treatment, short-course (DOTS) strategy.[2] India adopted DOTS, and achieved high cure rate, and has now planned to eliminate the disease from India by 2025.[3]

Extrapulmonary TB (EPTB) is gradually becoming more common.[1,3] FGTB, an important form of EPTB, develops secondary to TB elsewhere in the body.[4-7] It causes significant morbidity and short- and long-term sequelae like menstrual dysfunction and infertility for the affected women due to damage to endometrium and fallopian tubes.[4-9] Timely diagnosis and treatment may prevent permanent damage to genital organs.[4-9]

MICROBIOLOGY OF *MYCOBACTERIUM TUBERCULOSIS*

Staining

Acid-fast bacillus (AFB) microscopy is performed on endometrial sample by staining with Ziehl–Neelsen staining culture. Mycobacterial culture from endometrial aspirate can be done by Löwenstein–Jensen medium or Middlebrook 7H9 broth.[4-10] Their major disadvantage is that the results may take up to 6 weeks. Drug susceptibility tests take another 4 weeks (total 10 weeks).[4,10]

Modern Rapid Methods

These give reports faster and are reasonably sensitive and specific. They include BACTEC 460, MGIT 960 system, MB/Bact system, and liquid-based culture for TB using Versa TREK. They have better sensitivity (80–90%) with faster results (5–10 days). Molecular diagnostic tests like polymerase chain reaction, gene Xpert, and loop-mediated isothermal amplification (LAMP) are done with gene Xpert giving results in few hours and detect Rifampicin resistance also.

Serological tests have been banned by Government of India due to their low specificity.

EPIDEMIOLOGY OF FEMALE GENITAL TUBERCULOSIS

Female genital tuberculosis can manifest with infertility, abdominal or pelvic pain, and menstrual irregularities, in autopsy series, and recently in laparoscopy series of infertility cases and pelvic pain.[11,12] It can even coexist with other diseases like endometriosis.[13] Incidence of genital TB in infertility cases varies greatly depending upon the geographical location being 1% in infertility clinics of USA,[6] 1.4% in Sweden,[14] 3.5–20% in Pakistan,[15,16] 0.8% (2% in tubal factor) in Italy,[17] 4.2% in infertility patients in Saudi Arabia,[18] 16.7% in Nigeria,[19] 6.15–21.1% in South Africa,[20,21] and 1–19% in different areas of India.[8,9,22-24]

Incidence is more in tertiary centers like Delhi, where prevalence of FGTB in women of infertility was 26% and incidence of infertility in FGTB to be 42.5%, by referral cases from all over India, especially from states like Bihar, Jharkhand, and Uttar Pradesh with high prevalence of TB.[4,5]

Singh et al.[24] reported 48.5% prevalence in tubal factor sterility can produce many signs and findings.[25-32]

The prevalence of genital TB in infertility patients in various countries and different cultures in India is shown in **Table 1**. The incidence of infertility in genital TB patients is very high ranging from 44% to 90.6% with average being 70.6% as reported by Chaman Ara et al. **(Table 2)**.[33]

Female genital tuberculosis is encountered in younger women in developing countries with range being 20–40 years whereas in developed countries it is usually diagnosed in premenopausal women over the age of 40 years.[4,5,14] It could be due to younger age at marriage and childbearing in developing countries as compared to developed nations.[4,5]

TABLE 1: Prevalence of genital tuberculosis in infertile patients in different countries and different centers in India by different authors.

Study (Reference no.)	*Year*	*Country*	*Prevalence in infertile patients*
Malkani et al.[22]	1959	Delhi, India	10%
Schaefer et al.[6]	1976	USA	1%
Khan[15]	1985	Pakistan	23.08%
Chattopadhyay et al.[18]	1986	Saudi Arabia	4.2%
Oosthuizen et al.[21]	1990	South Africa	21%
Marana et al.[17]	1991	Italy	0.8% (2% in tubal factor)
Margolis et al.[20]	1992	South Africa	6.15%
Emembolu et al.[19]	1993	Nigeria	16.7%
Parikh et al.[8]	1997	Mumbai, India	39% (tubal factor)
Tripathy and Tripathy[23]	2002	Cuttack	3% (41% tubal factor)
Gupta et al.[9]	2007	Odisha	26%
Singh et al.[24]	2008	Delhi, India	48.6% in tubal factor
Shahzad[16]	2012	Pakistan	20%
Sharma et al.[32]	2020	India	18%

TABLE 2: Incidence of infertility in genital tuberculosis patients in different countries and different centers in India by different authors.

Study (Reference no.)	*Year*	*Country*	*Incidence in infertile patients*
Schaefer et al.[6]	1976	USA	55%
Sutherland et al.[7]	1980	UK	44%
Saracoglu et al.[25]	1992	Turkey	47.2%
Margolis et al.[20]	1992	South Africa	73.7%
Tripathy and Tripathy[23]	2002	Cuttack	53%
Zou SE et al.[28]	2014	Odisha	77.2%
Sharma et al.[31]	2008	Hyderabad, India	90.6%
Chaman Ara et al.[33]	2017	Iran	70.6%

PATHOGENESIS

The genital organs are secondarily infected from lungs through hematogenous route but can be affected through lymphatics or directly from gastrointestinal tract.[4-7] Rarely, the infection can be primary from infected semen of the male partner.[6]

Fallopian Tubes

They are infected in most (>90%) cases in genital TB and the involvement is usually bilateral. Various types of TB salpingitis can be TB endosalpingitis, exosalpingitis, interstitial TB salpingitis, and salpingitis isthmic nodosa.[4-7,14,26]

In TB endosalpingitis, the infection begins in endosalpinx, mostly hematogenously. The tube is swollen and edematous with hydrosalpinx and pyosalpinx with fibrosis and adhesions.[4-7,26]

Endosalpinx may be hyperplastic or edematous and may be totally destroyed with higher rate of sterility and ectopic gestation.[4-7,26]

In TB exosalpingitis, disease usually spreads from intestines and starts in the muscularis mucosa of the tubes with their hyperemia and tubercles on ovaries and peritoneum of the pouch of Douglas with flimsy adhesions, pyosalpinx, and pelvic adhesions.[4-7,11,26] Various grades of adhesions are formed between tubes and adjacent pelvic organs. In more severe cases, there may be multiple adhesions in peritoneal cavity with obliterated pouch of Douglas (frozen pelvis).[4-7,11,26] There may occur perihepatic adhesions (Fitz-Hugh-Curtis syndrome) in FGTB and abdominopelvic TB.[27]

Using laparoscopy and laparotomy, hydrosalpinx and tubal condition can be graded by taking into consideration the type of adhesions (peritubal, partial ovarian, extensive ovarian), patency (patent, partially patent, or blocked), morphology (soft or hydrosalpinx), morphology (soft, partially narrow in shift or hydrosalpinx, and fimbrial structure (complete, partially destroyed, and totally destroyed) which has prognostic significance.[28]

Uterus

The endometrium is involved in about 50–60% cases of FGTB.[4-7] The spread of infection from the fallopian tubes to uterus is usually hematogenous but can rarely be lymphatic or contagious.

Initially, there is no macroscopic disease but caseation and ulceration occurs and in advanced stages, distortion of the cavity occurs with adhesion formation and Asherman's syndrome causing amenorrhea and sterility.[4-7,31]

Microscopically, TB granulomas with or without caseation, granulomatous endometritis or focal collection of lymphocytes in endometrium may occur.[4-7,26]

Ovaries

Ovarian involvement occurs in 20–30% cases.[4-7] Ovarian function and reserve may also be affected in FGTB and abdominal pelvic TB.[34]

Peritoneum

Pelvic and abdominal peritoneum may be involved in widespread TB simulating ovarian neoplasm.[30]Ascitic fluid sampling for biochemical analysis and peritoneal biopsy may confirm the diagnosis of TB and thus avoiding a needless laparotomy.[4,5]

Quinsville grading of abdominal TB includes tubercular lymphadenopathy, peritoneal TB, which can be acute, chronic, visceral, and gastrointestinal TB.[35]

Cervix

The cervix may be involved in 5% cases of genital TB, usually as a downward extension of endometrial TB, but may rarely be a primary disease. It may present as polypoidal growth or ulceration and may resemble cervical cancer necessitating biopsy for confirmation of diagnosis.[6,7,26] Histopathological examination demonstrates granulomatous inflammation in cervical TB.[6,7,26]

Vagina and Vulva

They are rarely involved (1–2%) and are usually secondary to the downward extension but occasionally be primary infection from male partner.[6,7] There may be a hypertrophic lesion or a nonhealing ulcer on the vulva or vagina resembling malignancy necessitating biopsy and histopathological examination to confirm the diagnosis and to rule out malignancy and other differential diagnosis like syphilis, lymphogranuloma venereum, etc.[6,7]

PATHOGENESIS OF INFERTILITY IN GENITAL TUBERCULOSIS

Infertility is quite common in FGTB (40–80%). Pathogenesis of infertility in FGTB may be due to following factors:

- *Tubal factors causing infertility in FGTB:*
  - Blockage of one or both fallopian tubes due to their involvement in FGTB.[4,5,11]
  - Loss of tubal function due to ciliary damage in FGTB causing infertility and ectopic pregnancy.
  - Perisalpingitis causing adhesions and tubo-ovarian mass formation.
  - Unilateral or bilateral hydrosalpinx with or without obstruction occurs in 46% cases of FGTB, which adversely affects fertilization and embryonic implantation.[36] In in vitro fertilization (IVF) treatment, women with tubercular hydrosalpinx have very low pregnancy rate, which is worse with bilateral (12%) as compared to unilateral hydrosalpinx (24%). Clinical pregnancy rates can be increased with salpingectomy.[37] However, routine pre-IVF salpingectomy is not recommended with ultrasonologically visible hydrosalpinx but is performed if aspirated hydrosalpingeal fluid can be tested for toxin by Mouse Embryo Assay.[35,36]
- *Ovarian function causing infertility in FGTB:* Decreased ovarian function occurs in FGTB due to the tubo-ovarian mass formation, adhesions, anovulation, and poor ovarian reserve causing infertility by following mechanisms:[4,5,26]
  - Endocrine dysfunction can occur in FGTB.
  - Through chronic anovulation.
  - *M. tuberculosis* has antigonadotropic effect necessitating more ampoules of gonadotropins in IVF cycle.
  - Women with genital TB require higher number of gonadotropin ampoules than controls.[36]
  - Mycobacteria cause luteal phase defect, implantation failure, lower pregnancy rates, and higher abortion rates.[36]
  - In genital TB, quality of embryo tends to be poor due to "intrinsic oocyte factor" defect.[37] The harmful interleukins (ILs) induced by immune modulation or by the direct effect of toxins of mycobacteria adversely affect the oocyte development within the follicle.[37]
- *Uterine (endometrial) factors causing infertility:* Endometrial damage occurs in TB as follows—
  - Effect of genital TB on endometrial receptivity:
    - Female genital TB adversely impacts the endometrial markers which are essential to make the endometrium receptive for embryonic implantation.[31,38,39]
    - There is poor vascularization of endometrium in FGTB.
  - Through immunomodulation with production of enzyme procoagulase causing vascular thrombus formation.
  - Endometrial atrophy and synechiae formation: Involvement of endometrium by caseous or fibrocaseous lesions of FGTB causes Asherman's syndrome (uterine synechiae) which is common in endometrial TB.[31,38,39] We observed various grades of intrauterine adhesions in FGTB on hysteroscopy as—Grade-I 20.8%, Grade-II 28.5%, Grade-III 28.5%, and Grade-IV 17.5% with other findings of TB like tubercles and shaggy cavity with caseation on hysteroscopy.[39] We also observed increased difficulties and complications in hysteroscopy in women with genital TB.[40] Hysterosalpingographic findings in our study were irregular filling defect in 18.5%, and synechiae in 17.1% of women.[41]

- *Defective or failed implantation in FGTB:* It occurs by the following mechanism:[38]
  - There is release of harmful cytokines and growth factors (IL-2, IL-8, TNF-α) in the endometrium.
  - There is formation of symmetric antibodies.
  - There is production of natural killer (NK) cells.
  - There is production of lymphocyte activated killer (LAK) cells.
  - There is T helper 1 cell (Th1) response causing implantation failure as compared to Th2 response required for fertilized ovum implantation.
  - Hence, FGTB shifts Th2 response to ThI response in endometrium leading to implantation failure. In fact, Dam et al.[42] from Kolkata observed latent FGTB causing repeat IVF failure in their setting.

DIAGNOSIS

Clinical presentation of FGTB is shown in **Box 1**.[4-7,14,26] Prompt diagnosis by good history taking, thorough clinical examination, judicious testing, and timely treatment can prevent permanent damage.

BOX 1: Symptoms and signs in female genital TB.[4-7,14,26]

Symptoms:
- Asymptomatic (up to 12%)
- General symptoms:
  - Raised temperature
  - Loss of weight and anorexia
  - Poor or debilitated general condition
- Menstrual symptoms:
  - Menorrhagia (in early stages due to ulcerative lesions)
  - Dysmenorrhea
  - Oligomenorrhea (in late stage)
  - Hypomenorrhea (in late stage)
  - Amenorrhea (primary and secondary) (up to 10% cases) (in late stage due to endometrial atrophy and synechiae)
  - Opsomenorrhea
- Infertility (primary and secondary)
- Abdominal lump
- Dyspareunia
- Abdominal pain
- Chronic pelvic pain
- Acute abdomen
- Abnormal vaginal discharge

Signs:
- No physical sign
- Systemic examination:
  - Raised temperature
  - Enlarged lymph nodes (in TB lymphadenitis)
  - Rales on chest examination
  - Systemic signs as per site of extrapulmonary TB
- Abdominal examination:
  - Mass abdomen (vague or definite)
  - Doughy feel of abdomen
  - Ascites
- Vaginal examination:
  - Large uterus
  - Adnexal tenderness and fullness

INVESTIGATIONS

The investigations done in FGTB are demonstrated in **Box 2.**[4,5,10,43-47]

BOX 2: Investigations in genital tuberculosis.[4,5,10,43-47]

Blood investigations:
- Low Hb, leukocytosis, elevated lymphocytes, and ESR
- Moderate (up to 200 IU/mL) elevation of CA-125 in genital TB

Mantoux (Tuberculin) test and interferon gamma release assays; more than 10 mm

Skiagram chest:
- For pulmonary TB

Radiological methods:
- Ultrasound
- Computerized axial tomography **(Fig. 1)**.
- *Magnetic resonance imaging:*[43] Useful for tubo-ovarain masses **(Fig. 2)**.
- *Positron emission tomography (PET scan):*[44] Tubercular tubo-ovarian masses with increased FDG uptake **(Fig. 3)**.
- *Hysterosalpingography (HSG):*[41] Shrunken cavity, filling defects and lymphatic intravasation and blocked fallopian tubes **(Figs. 4 and 5)**.

Endometrial biopsy, curettage, or aspirate:
- *Histopathology:* Observation of epithelioid granuloma.
- *Mycobacterial smear and culture:* Using Löwenstein–Jensen (LJ) medium or BACTEC 460 or Mycobacteria growth inhibitor tube (MGIT)[4,5,45]
- *Polymerase chain reaction:* Rapid (1–2 days), sensitive, but less specific method for diagnosis of FGTB.[46] DNA PCR has also been used with higher specificity but is expensive and is not routinely available in most centers. Hence, ATT not be started only on PCR test.
- Gene Xpert if positive on endometrial biopsy is a reliable test for FGTB and treatment can be started on its basis.[32] It can also detect resistance to rifampicin. It has 33–50% sensitivity and 100% specificity for detection of genital TB.[32]

Endoscopy:
- *Hysteroscopy:* The endometrium is pale in color, may show tubercles or caseous nodules. The cavity is partially or completely obliterated by adhesions of varying grade (grade 1 to grade 4) often involving ostia **(Fig. 6)**. There may be a small shrunken cavity.[31,39]
- *Laparoscopy:* Useful modality for diagnosis of FGTB by direct visualization of disease like tubercles, adnexal masses **(Fig. 7)**, caseous nodules **(Fig. 8)**, fluid collect, pelvic adhesions, hydrosalpinx **(Fig. 9)**, pyosalpinx, beading of tubes, and inability to see tubes due to adhesions.[11,12] However, laparoscopy should be done by experts in FGTB as increased complications and difficulties have been observed on laparoscopy in FGTB patients.[45] Adhesions: Different adhesions are formed in FGTB causing hanging, gallbladder, and ascending colonic adhesions.[48] Being thick and vascular, adhesiolysis can cause bleeding and flare-up of the disease. There is very high prevalence (48%) of perihepatic adhesions on laparoscopy in FGTB cases.[27]

Combination of tests (algorithm): Can be useful in diagnosis[5,49] **(Flowchart 1)**.

(ATT: antitubercular treatment; DNA: deoxyribonucleic acid; ESR: erythrocyte sedimentation rate; FDG: fluorodeoxyglucose; FGTB: female genital tuberculosis; Hb: hemoglobin; PCR: polymerase chain reaction)

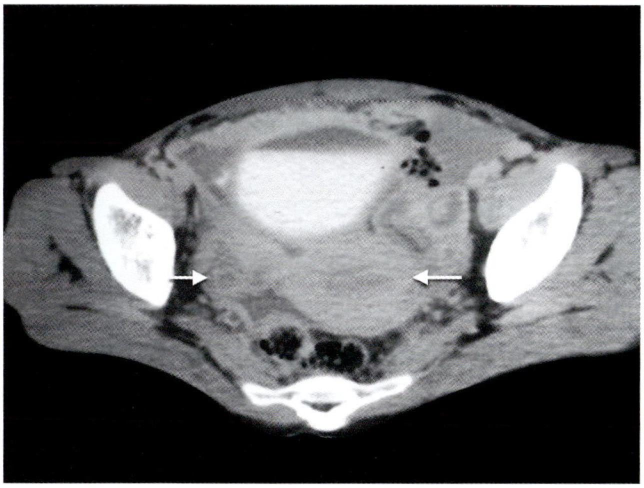

Fig. 1: CT scan findings in patient with female genital tuberculosis bilateral tubo-ovarian mass.

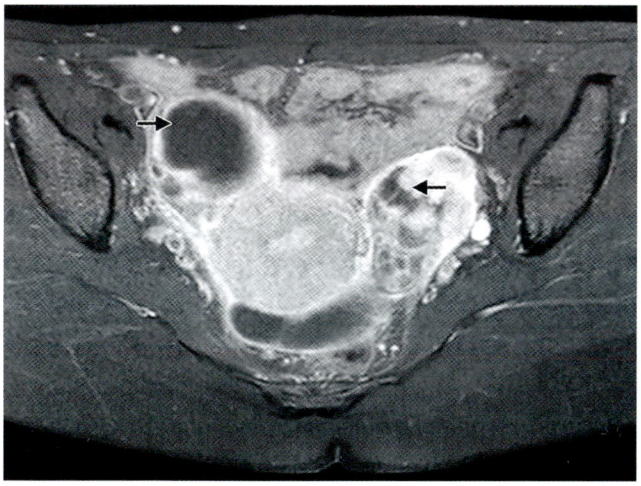

Fig. 2: MRI depicting adnexal masses (arrows) on both sides with enlarged lymph nodes.

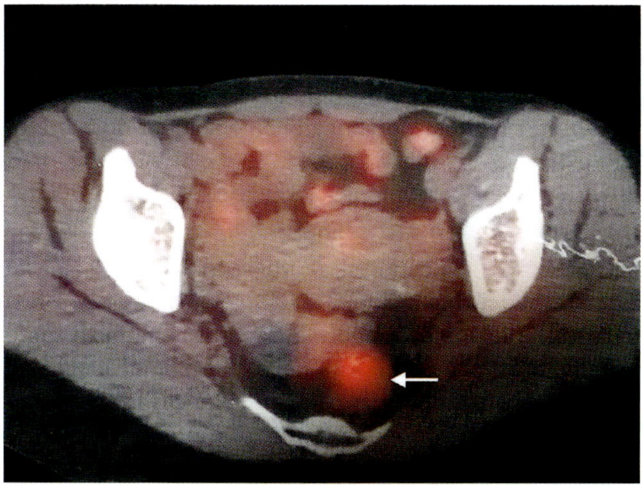

Fig. 3: Positron emission tomography CT scan showing tubercular adnexal mass (arrow) with enhanced fluorodeoxyglucose uptake.

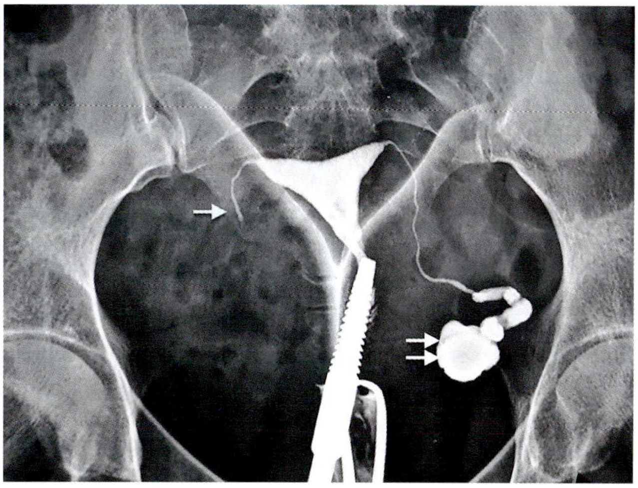

Fig. 4: Hysterosalpingography showing mid-tubal block (single arrow) on right side and fimbrial block with hydrosalpinx showing tobacco pouch appearance (double arrows) in left side in female genital tuberculosis (FGTB).

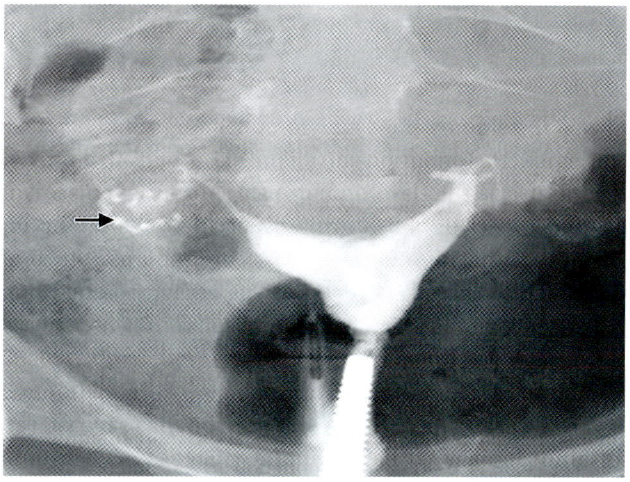

Fig. 5: Hysterosalpingograhpy depicting with "beaded" tube (arrow) on right side and left mild isthmic block in female genital tuberculosis (FGTB).

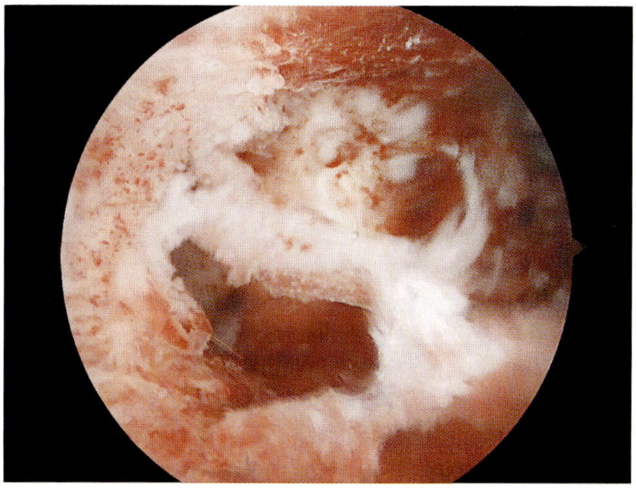

Fig. 6: Hysteroscopic picture showing Grade III adhesions in a case of female genital tuberculosis (FGTB).

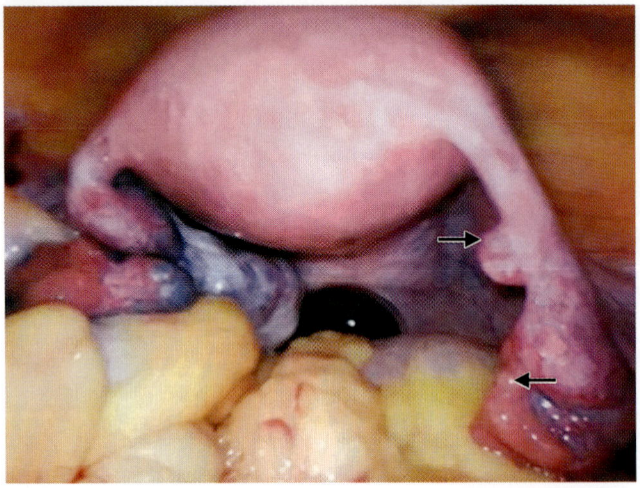

Fig. 7: Laparoscopy demonstrates congested, dilated, and inflamed fallopian tubes with tubercles (arrows) in female genital tuberculosis (FGTB).

Female genital TB is associated with increased complications in laparoscopy, hysteroscopy, and other techniques.[40,48]

Index-TB guidelines for EPTB including FGTB have been developed by Ministry of Health and Family Welfare and All India Institute of Medical Sciences in 2016 for guidance and management of FGTB.[49]

TREATMENT

Medical Treatment

Treatment of latent genital TB with positive PCR is controversial due to high false positivity. Many infertility experts routinely treat positive PCR women with higher pregnancy outcome, especially often in those women treated with antitubercular treatment (ATT) than without treatment. The logic of treating latent TB is that in early stage, it can be treated without causing permanent damage to endometrium and other genital organs with much better outcome.

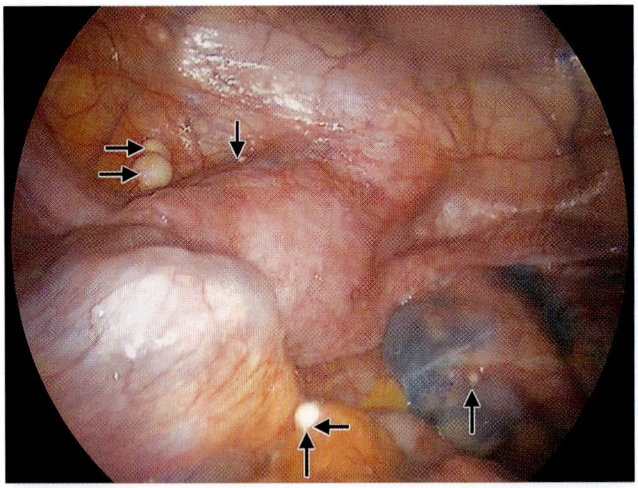

Fig. 8: Laparoscopy demonstrating caseous nodules on peritoneum fallopian tubes, and pouch of Douglas in female genital tuberculosis (FGTB).

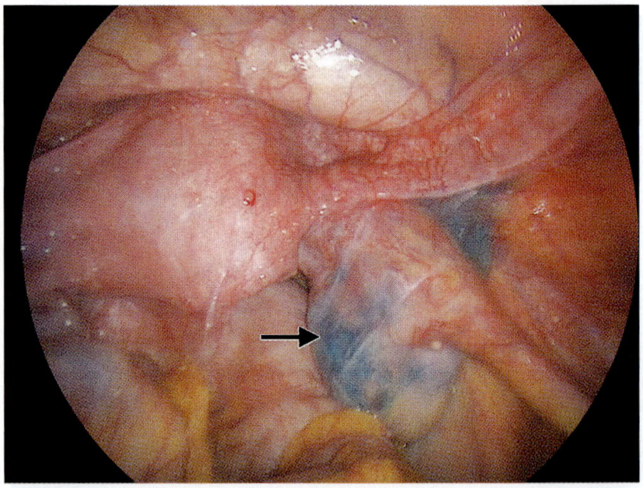

Fig. 9: Laparoscopy depicting hydrosalpinx (arrow) in female genital tuberculosis (FGTB).

Flowchart 1: Algorithm for diagnosis of female genital tuberculosis (FGTB).

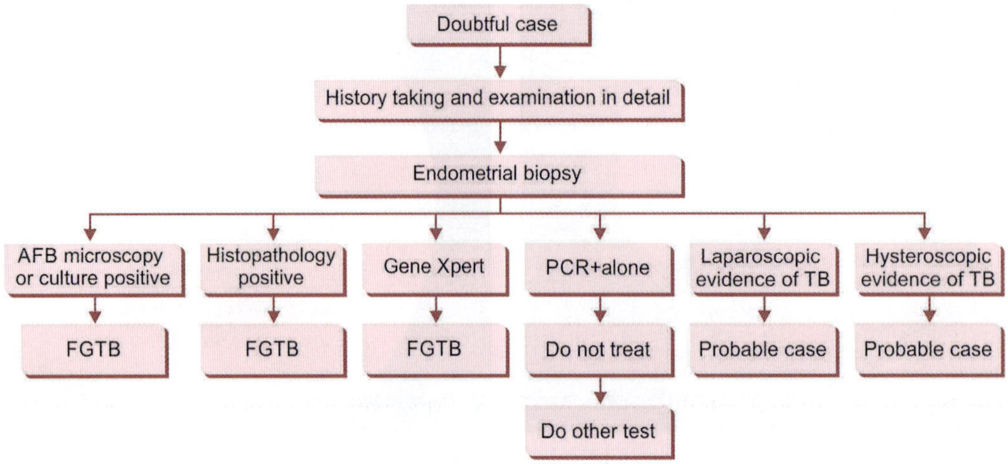

(AFB: acid-fast bacillus; PCR: polymerase chain reaction; TB: tuberculosis)

Jindal et al.[50] observed 30.8% conception rate in latent TB with ATT while Kulshrestha et al.[51] also obtained 31% pregnancy rate on ATT in TB PCR positive women. Latent genital TB has been found to be associated with recurrent IVF failure.[42] Even on migration to western countries, Indian women have poor prognosis with IVF as compared to Caucasian women despite similar embryo quality which could be due to latent FGTB in Indian women.[52] However, treating women with positive PCR is associated with risk of over treatment as many women without FGTB are then treated. ATT for 6 months is adequate effective for medical treatment of FGTB as seen in randomized controlled trial (RCT).[5,53]

DOTS Strategy Treatment

Directly observed treatment, short-course (DOTS) is favored by WHO and National Tuberculosis Elimination Program (NTEP) of India to prevent MDR and for better results. There have been recent changes in medical treatment of all types of TB including FGTB. Categories are not used anymore. All drug sensitive TB cases (both pulmonary and FGTB) including defaulters are given 2 months of 4 drugs orally daily (rifampicin [R], isoniazid [H], pyrizinamide [Z] and ethambutol [E]-intensive phase) followed by three drugs (RHE) orally daily for next 4 months (continuation phase).

DRUG TREATMENT OF DRUG SENSITIVE FGTB

Daily oral rifampicin (R), isoniazid (H), pyrazinamide (Z), and ethambutol (E) for 2 months. Then oral RHE for next 4 months orally daily as per DOTS. On an averege a 50 kg woman will require 450 mg rifampicin, 600 mg isoniazid, 1,500 mg pyrazinamid, and 1,200 mg ethambutol.

Treatment of Chronic Cases, Drug-resistant, and Multidrug-resistant FGTB

Although rare MDR FGTB is being observed in clinical practice. It is usually secondary to MDR TB in lungs or elsewhere but can be primary also if the initial infection occurs with MDR stains.[54] Treatment is same as for pulmonary MDR with second-line drugs in consultation with TB experts. Patients with HIV and TB should be treated with both ART and ATT in consultation with experts in the area. The MDR treatment is given either longer oral regimen for 18–24 months or shorter regimen for 9–12 months in consultation with experts. TB notification should be done to Government of India through Nikshay (TB notification portal).

Monitoring

Patients are regularly followed and monitored for compliance and side effects of drugs.

Surgical Treatment

Surgery is usually avoided in FGTB as modern short-course treatment is very effective. However, abscess should be drained surgically. Besides, there are difficulties increased chances of complications in various surgeries like hysteroscopy, laparoscopy, and laparotomy in women with genital TB with risk of injury to bowel necessitating a very difficult laparotomy and resection of injured bowel.[48,55] It is better to just take biopsies and avoid difficult surgery done for suspected pelvic tumors but found to be tubercular at laparotomy followed by full medical treatment. Laparoscopy and hysteroscopy can be done after ATT.

It is also useful to prognosticate and plan for further treatment. Outcome for fertility in FGTB is only good when ATT is started in early disease. However, cases of advanced TB with extensive adhesions in pelvis and uterus are usually not amenable to treatment with poor prognosis for fertility. Tuboplasty is avoided much as it runs the risk of flare-up of the disease and ectopic gestation.[56,57]

IN VITRO FERTILIZATION AND EMBRYO TRANSFER IN FGTB[23,58]

Most women with genital TB present with infertility and have poor prognosis for fertility in spite of ATT. The conception rate is low (19.2%) with live birth rate being still low (7%).[23] IVF with embryo transfer (ET) appears to be the only hope for some of these women whose endometrium is not damaged with pregnancy rate of 16.6% per transfer.[58-66] Jindal et al.[50] observed favorable infertility outcomes following ATT prescribed on sole basis of positive PCR test for endometrial TB. Singh et al.[67] observed poor endometrial blood flow in women with FGTB undergoing IVF–ET. We also observed decreased blood flow to endometrium and ovaries in FGTB patients which got improved on repeat examination after ATT.[34,68]

Malhotra et al.[69] studied perifollicular Doppler blood flow before oocyte recovery in patients with or without genital TB. They observed a trend of poor ovarian blood flow in FGTB women undergoing IVF or intracytoplasmic sperm injection (ICSI) in their center. IVF–ET has 17.3% conception rate in contrast to only 4.3% with tubal surgery in FGTB.[60] The pregnancy rate and take-home baby rate could be improved by early detection and timely treatment. The result of IVF and ET are poorer in FGTB than in other indications. The results of IVF–ET in FGTB by various authors are shown in **Table 3** and pregnancy rate vary from 9.1% to 38.3% with increased chances of miscarriage and ectopic gestation. Studies have shown poor result with IVF in FGTB due to following reasons:

- Most patients are poor responders.
- They require higher quantity of drugs.

TABLE 3: Fertility outcome in FGTB with IVF and ET by various authors.

Author (Reference) (Year)	*Frydman et al.*[66]	*Parikh et al.*[8]	*Marcus et al.*[61]	*Soussis et al.*[62]	*Gurgan et al.*[58]	*Bapna et al.*[65]	*Malik et al.*[60]	*Dai et al.*[63]
No. of patients	20	30	10	13	24	49	120	155
Pregnancy rate; No (%)	8 (25%)	5 (16%)	6 (60%)	6 (28.6%)	4 (9.1%)	17 (19.1%)	46 (38.3%)	94 (60.6%)
Implantation rate					5.8%			
Delivered No (%)	NA	16.2%	22.2%	37.5%	1 (25%)	–	45%	40.2%
Abortion No (%)	6 (30%)	5 (16%)	4 (40%)	4 (31%)	3 (75%)	37 (30.3%) 11/94 (11.7%)	37 (30.3%)	(24.5%)
Ectopic pregnancy; No (%)	1 (5%) (5%)	– 1 (3%)	1 (10%) 1 (10%)	2 (15%) –	5 (10.2%) 2 (1.6%)	9 (7.5%)	3/94 (3.2%)	

(ET: embryo transfer; FGTB: female genital tuberculosis; IVF: in vitro fertilization)

- Endometrium is invariably poorly developed.
- Quality of egg and fertilized ovum is suboptimal and pregnancy rate is poor.

Malik[60] observed a conception rate of 38.2% in FGTB patients with IVF–ET. ATT was given to the patients till the endometrial biopsy was negative and this varied from 6 to 18 months. IVF was done only after the biopsy was negative. No difference in pregnancy rate was noticed when patients were kept on or were taken off the ATT during the IVF cycle.

Hence, IVF–ET is an optimum treatment for tubal blockage but receptive endometrium in FGTB.

Gestational Surrogacy in Genital TB

It is recommended for blocked tube and Asherman's syndrome.

In gestational surrogacy another woman's uterus is used for implantation while ovum belongs to this woman and sperm belongs to her husband. She is thus the genetic mother of the fetus.

Samantha et al. recommended surrogacy for following case:

- Asherman's syndrome not amenable to hysteroscopic adhesiolysis
- Atrophic endometrium not responding to hormonal therapy
- Grossly reduced endometrial thickness (<7 mm) in spite of estrogen supplementation with high resistance subendometrial blood flow in the proliferative phase in repeated cycles
- Dense pelvic adhesions causing repeated IVF failure
- Unexplained repeated IVF failure with endometrium showing persistence of TB granuloma or PCR positivity despite adequate antitubercular chemotherapy
- MDR genital TB.

Surrogate host can be a family member or stranger but a forced friendship, must be established between host and the commissioning couple in surrogacy.

Samantha et al.[70] could achieve a viable delivery rate of 50% by surrogacy in FGTB patients with uterine synechiae, poor endometrial development, or repeated IVF failure.

Adoption: It is indicated for blocked tube, defective endometrium, and failed ovaries.

NEW TUBERCULOSIS RESEARCH

More research is being done in FGTB including immune markers, molecular tests, newer vaccines, newer and shorter drug regimen, and stem cell therapy. IVF–ET if performed on time has good success rate. There is need to improve pregnancy outcome by IVF–ET in FGTB. Gestational surrogacy has a role in some women. More research is needed on changing trends in prevalence and on better methods of diagnosis of FGTB as genital TB impacts both male and female infertility.[71-74]

CONCLUSION

Female genital tuberculosis is a common cause of sterility in India and requires early diagnosis and timely treatment with 6 months ATT followed by IVF–ET for most patients and surrogacy and adoption for some patients.

KEY POINTS

- Female genital tuberculosis is a common cause of sterility through tubal, endometrial, and ovarian factors.
- Early diagnosis by detailed history examination and selected tests including endoscopy is needed.
- Surrogacy and adoption may be needed in some women.
- Stem cell regeneration may be helpful in Asherman's syndrome.

REFERENCES

1. World Health Organization. (2019). Global Tuberculosis Report-2019. [online] Available from https://apps.who.int/iris/bitstream/handle/10665/329368/9789241565714-eng.pdf? [Last accessed October, 2022].

2. World Health Organization. (2020). Global tuberculosis report 2020: executive summary. [online] Available from https://apps.who.int/iris/bitstream/handle/10665/337538/9789240016095-eng.pdf [Last accessed October, 2022].
3. Central TB Division of Ministry of Health and Family Welfare under Government of India. National Strategic Plan for Tuberculosis: 2017-25 Elimination by 2025. [online] Available from https://tbcindia.gov.in/WriteReadData/National%20Strategic%20Plan%202017-25.pdf. [Last accessed October, 2022].
4. Sharma JB, Sharma E, Sharma S, Dharmendra S. Female genital tuberculosis: Revisited. The Ind J Med Res. 2018;148(Suppl 1):S71-S83.
5. Sharma JB. Tuberculosis and gynecological practice. In: Studd J, Tan SL, Chervenak FA. (Eds). Current Progress in Obstetric and Gynecology, 1st edition. Mumbai: Tree Life India; 2012. pp. 304-27.
6. Schaefer G. Female genital tuberculosis. Clin Obstet Gynecol. 1976;19(1):223-39.
7. Sutherland AM. Genital tuberculosis. Tubercle. 1980;79:66.
8. Parikh FR, Nadkarni SG, Kamat SA, Naik N, Soonawala SB, Parikh RM. Genital tuberculosis–a major pelvic factor causing infertility in Indian women. Fertil Steril. 1997;67(3):497-500.
9. Gupta N, Sharma JB, Mittal S, Singh N, Misra R, Kukreja M. Genital tuberculosis in Indian infertility patients. Int J Gynaecol Obstet. 2007;97(2):135-8.
10. Munne KR, Tandon D, Chauhan SL, Patil AD. Female genital tuberculosis in light of newer laboratory tests: a narrative review. Indian J Tuberc. 2020;67(1):112-20.
11. Sharma JB, Sneha J, Singh UB, Kumar S, Roy KK, Singh N, et al. Comparative study of laparoscopic abdominopelvic and fallopian tube findings before and after antitubercular therapy in female genital tuberculosis with infertility. J Minim Invasive Gynecol. 2016;23(2):215-22.
12. Malhotra N, Singh UB, Iyer V, Gupta P, Chandhiok N. Role of laparoscopy in the diagnosis of genital TB in infertile females in the era of molecular tests. J Minim Invasive Gynecol. 2020;27(7):1538-44.
13. Sharma JB, Goyal M, Kumar S, Roy KK, Sharma E, Arora R. Concomitant female genital tuberculosis and endometriosis. Indian J Tuberculosis. 2017;64(3):173-7.
14. Neonakis IK, Spandidos DA, Petinaki E. Female genital tuberculosis: a review. Scand J Infect Dis. 2011;43(8):564-72.
15. Khan SM. Incidence of genital tuberculosis in infertile women. J Pak Med Assoc. 1985;35(9):280-1.
16. Shahzad S. Investigation of the prevalence of female genital tract tuberculosis and its relation to female infertility: an observational analytical study. Iran J Reprod Med. 2012; 10(6):581-8.
17. Marana R, Muzil L, Lucisano A, Ardito F, Muscatello P, Bilancioni B, et al. Incidence of genital tuberculosis in infertile patients submitted to diagnostic laparoscopy: recent experience in an Italian University Hospital. Int J Fertil. 1991;36(2):104-7.
18. Chattopadhyay SK, Sengupta BS, Edrees YB, Al-Meshari AA. The pattern of female genital tuberculosis in Riyadh, Saudi Arabia. Br J Obstet Gynaecol. 1986;93(4):367-71.
19. Emembolu JO, Anyanwu DO, Ewa B. Genital tuberculosis in infertile women in northern Nigeria. West Afr J Med. 1993;12(4):211-2.
20. Margolis K, Wranz PA, Kruger TF, Joubert JJ, Odendaal HJ. Genital tuberculosis at Tygerberg Hospital-prevalence, clinical presentation and diagnosis. S Afr Med J. 1992;81(1): 12-5.
21. Oosthuizen AP, Wessels PH, Hefer JN. Tuberculosis of the female genital tract in patients attending an infertility clinic. S Afr Med J. 1990;77(11):562-4.
22. Malkani PK, Rajani CK. Pelvic tuberculosis. Obstet Gynecol. 1959;14:600-11.
23. Tripathy SN, Tripathy SN. Infertility and pregnancy outcome in female genital tuberculosis. Int J Gynaecol Obstet. 2002;76(2):159-63.
24. Singh N, Sumana G, Mittal S. Genital tuberculosis: a leading cause for infertility in women seeking assisted conception in North India. Arch Gynecol Obstet. 2008;278(4):325-7.
25. Saracoglu OF, Mungan T, Tanzer F. Pelvic tuberculosis. Int J Gynaecol Obstet. 1992;37:115-20.
26. Kumar S, Sharma JB. Female genital tuberculosis. In: Sharma SK, Mohan A (Eds). Tuberculosis, 3rd edition. New Delhi: Jaypee Brothers Medical Publishers (P) Ltd; 2016. pp. 311-24.
27. Sharma JB, Roy KK, Gupta N, Jain SK, Malhotra N, Mittal S. High prevalence of Fitz-Hugh-Curtis syndrome in genital tuberculosis. Int J Gynaecol Obstet. 2007;99(1):62-3.
28. Zou SE, Jin Y, Ko YL, Zhu J. A new classification system for pregnancy prognosis of tubal factor infertility. Int J Clin Exp Med. 2014;7(5):1410-6.
29. Sharma JB. Sharma's ascending colonic adhesion: a new sign in abdominopelvic tuberculosis with infertility. J IVF Lite. 2016;3:18-22.
30. Sharma JB, Jain SK, Pushparaj M, Roy KK, Malhotra N, Zutshi V, et al. Abdomino-peritoneal tuberculosis masquerading as ovarian cancer: a retrospective study of 26 cases. Arch Gynecol Obstet. 2010;282(6):643-8.
31. Sharma JB, Roy KK, Pushparaj M, Gupta N, Jain SK, Malhotra N, et al. Genital tuberculosis: an important cause of Asherman's syndrome in India. Arch Gynecol Obstet. 2008;277(1):37-41.
32. Sharma JB, Dharmendra S, Jain S, Sharma SK, Singh UB, Soneja M, et al. Evaluation of Gene Xpert as compared to conventional methods in diagnosis of Female Genital Tuberculosis. European Journal of Obstetrics & Gynecology and Reproductive Biology. 2020;255:247-52.
33. Chaman-Ara K, Bahrami MA, Bahrami E, Bahrami S, Bahrami MN, Moosazadeh M, et al. Prevalence of genital tuberculosis among infertile women: a systematic review and meta-analysis. International Journal of Medical Research & Health Sciences. 2016;5(4):208-15.
34. Sharma JB, Sneha J, Singh UB, Kumar S, Roy KK, Singh N, et al. Effect of antitubercular treatment on ovarian function in female genital tuberculosis with infertility. J Hum Reprod Sci. 2016;9(3):145-50.
35. Debi U, Ravishankar V, Prasad KK, Sinha SK, Sharma AK. Abdominal tuberculosis of the gastrointestinal tract: World J Gastroenterol. 2014;20(40):14831-40.
36. Chen CD, Yang JH, Lin KC, Chao KH, Ho HN, Yang YS. The significance of cytokines, chemical composition, and murine embryo development in hydrosalpinx fluid for predicting the IVF outcome in women with hydrosalpinx. Hum Reprod. 2002;17(1):128-33.
37. Caliskan E, Cakiroglu Y, Sofuoglu K, Doger E, Akar ME, Ozkan SO. Effects of salpingectomy and antituberculosis

treatments on fertility results in patients with genital tuberculosis. J Obstet Gynaecol Res. 2014;40(10):2104-9.
38. Chakravarty BN. Genital tuberculosis-ovarian function and endometrial receptivity. In: Mukherjee GG, Tripathy SN, Tripathy SN (Eds). Genital Tuberculosis, 1st edition. New Delhi: Jaypee Brothers Medical Publishers (P) Ltd; 2010. pp. 27-42.
39. Sharma JB, Roy KK, Pushparaj M, Kumar S. Hysteroscopic findings in women with primary and secondary infertility due to genital tuberculosis. Int J Gynecol Obstet. 2009;104(1): 49-52.
40. Sharma JB, Roy KK, Pushparaj M, Karmakar D, Kumar S, Singh N. Increased difficulties and complications encountered during hysteroscopy in women with genital tuberculosis. J Minim Invasive Gynecol. 2011;18(5):660-5.
41. Sharma JB, Pushparaj M, Roy KK, Neyaz Z, Gupta N, Jain SK, et al. Hysterosalpingographic findings in infertile women with genital tuberculosis. Int J Gynecol Obstet. 2008;101(2): 150-5.
42. Dam P, Shirazee HH, Goswami SK, Ghosh S, Ganesh A, Chaudhary k. Role of latent genital tuberculosis in repeated IVF failure in Indian clinical settings. Gynecol Obstet Invest. 2006;61(4):223-7.
43. Sharma JB, Karmakar D, Hari S, Singh N, Singh SP, Kumar S, et al. Magnetic resonance imaging findings among women with tubercular tubo-ovarian masses. Int J Gynecol Obstet. 2011;113(1):76-80.
44. Sharma JB, Kumar R, Singh U, Kumari A, Dharmendra S, Sachani H. Pre treatment and post treatment positron emission tomography-computed tomography (PET-CT) to evaluate treatment response in tuberculous Tubo-Ovarian masses. Eur J Obstet Gynecol Reprod Biol. 2021;264:128-34.
45. Neonakis IK, Gitti Z, Krambovitis E, Spandidos DA. Molecular diagnostic tools in mycobacteriology. J Microbiol Methods. 2008;75(1):1-11.
46. Bhanu NV, Singh UB, Chakraborty M, Suresh N, Arora J, Rana T, et al. Improved diagnostic value of PCR in diagnosis of female genital tuberculosis leading to infertility. J Med Microbiol. 2005;54(10):927-31.
47. Sharma JB, Roy KK, Pushparaj M, Kumar S, Malhotra N, Mittal S. Laparoscopic finding in female genital tuberculosis. Arch Gynecol Obstet. 2008;278(4):359-64.
48. Sharma JB, Mohanraj P, Roy KK, Jain SK. Increased complication rates associated with laparoscopic surgery among patients with genital tuberculosis. Int J Gynecol Obstet. 2010;109(3):242-4.
49. Ministry of Health and Family Welfare. Government of India and World Health Organization. (2016). Index-TB Guidelines for diagnosis and management of extra pulmonary tuberculosis (EPTB) in India. [online] Available from https://tbcindia.gov.in/WriteReadData/l892s/5585665076Index-TB%20 Guidelines.pdf. [Last accessed October, 2022].
50. Jindal UN, Verma S, Bala Y. Favorable infertility outcomes following anti-tubercular treatment prescribed on the sole basis of a positive polymerase chain reaction test for endometrial tuberculosis. Hum Reprod. 2012;27(5): 1368-74.
51. Kulshrestha V, Kriplani A, Agarwal N, Singh UB, Rana T. Genital tuberculosis among infertile women and fertility outcome after antitubercular therapy. Int J Gynaecol Obstet. 2011;113(3):229-34.
52. Shahine LK, Lamb JD, Lathi RB, Milki AA, Langen E, Westphal LM. Poor prognosis with in vitro fertilization in Indian women compared to Caucasian women despite similar embryo quality. PLOS One. 2009;4(10):e7599.
53. Sharma JB, Singh N, Dharmendra S, Singh UB, Kumar S, Roy KK, et al. Six months versus nine months anti-tuberculous therapy for female genital tuberculosis: a randomized controlled trial. Eur J Obstet Gynecol Reprod Biol. 2016;203:264-73.
54. Sharma JB, Kriplani A, Sharma E, Sharma S, Dharmendra S, Kumar S, et al. Multi drug resistant female genital tuberculosis: a preliminary report. Eur J Obstet Gynecol Reprod Biol. 2017;210:108-15.
55. Sharma JB, Mohanraj P, Jain SK, Roy KK. Surgical complications during laparotomy in patients with abdominopelvic tuberculosis. Int J Gynaecol Obstet. 2010;110(2):157-8.
56. Sharma JB, Naha M, Kumar S, Roy KK, Singh N, Arora R. Genital tuberculosis: an important cause of ectopic pregnancy in India. The Indian journal of tuberculosis. 2014 Oct 1;61(4): 312-7.
57. Singh N, Sharma AK, Dadhwal V, Gupta N, Mittal S. Postoperative flare-up of genital tuberculosis: a clinical reality. Int J Tuberc Lung Dis. 2008;12(8):981-3.
58. Gurgan T, Urman B, Yarali H. Results of in vitro fertilization and embryo transfer in women with infertility due to genital tuberculosis. Fertil Steril. 1996;65(2):367-70.
59. Chakravarty B, Shirazee HH, Vijay PK, Goswami SK. The place for IVF in genital tuberculosis. Hum Reprod. 2003;18(suppl.1):XVIII 126.
60. Malik S. IVF and tuberculosis. In: Mukherjee GG, Tripathy SN, Tripathy SN (Eds). Genital Tuberculosis, 1st edition. New Delhi: Jaypee Brothers Medical Publishers (P) Ltd.; 2010. pp.135-40.
61. Marcus SF, Rizle B, Fountain S, Brinsden P. Tuberculosis infertility and in vitro Fertilization. Am J Obstet Gynecol 1994;171(6):1593-96.
62. Soussis I, Trew G, Matalliotakis I, Margara R, Winston RM. In vitro fertilization treatment in genital tuberculosis. J Assist Reprod Genet. 1998;15(6):378-80.
63. Dai W, Ma L, Cao Y, Wu D, Yu T, Zhai J. In vitro fertilization outcome in women with endometrial tuberculosis and tubal tuberculosis. Gynecological Endocrinology. 2020; 36(9):819-23.
64. Tripathy SN, Tripathy SN. Tuberculosis. Manual of Obstetrics and Gynecologists, 1st edition. New Delhi: Jaypee Brothers Medical Publishers (P) Ltd;2015.
65. Bapna N, Swarnkar M, Kotia N. Genital tuberculosis and its consequences on subsequent fertility. J Obstet Gynaecol Ind. 2005;55;534-7.
66. Frydman R, Eibschitz I, Belaisch-Allart J G. In vitro fertilization in tuberculous infertility. J In Vitro Fert Embryo Transfer. 1985;4:184.
67. Singh N, Bahadur A, Mittal S, Malhotra N, Bhatt A. Comparative analysis of endometrial blood flow on the day of hCG by 2D Doppler in two groups of women with or without genital tuberculosis undergoing IVF-ET in a developing country. Arch Gynecol Obstet. 2011;283(1):115-20.

68. Sharma JB, Sneha J, Singh UB, Kumar S, Rpoy KK, Singh N, et al. Effect of antitubercular therapy on endometrial function in infertile women with female genital tuberculosis. Infect Disord Drug Targets. 2016;16(2):101-8.
69. Malhotra N, Bahadur A, Singh N, Kalaivani, Mittal S. Role of perifollicular Doppler blood flow in predicting cycle response in infertile women with genital tuberculosis undergoing in vitro fertilization/intracytoplasmic sperm injection. J Hum Reprod Sci. 2014;7(1):19-24.
70. Samantha J, Goswami SK, Mukherjee GG, et al. Gestational surrogacy in genital tuberculosis. In: Mukherjee GG, Tripathy SN, Tripathy SN (Eds). Gential Tuberculosis, 1st edition. New Delhi: Jaypee Brothers Medical Publishers (P) Ltd.; 2010. pp. 141-54.
71. Bhanothu V, Venkatesan V. Conventional polymerase chain reaction and amplification refractory mutation system-multi-gene/multi-primer PCR in the diagnosis of female genital tuberculosis. Archives of microbiology. 2019;201(3):267-81.
72. Scriba TJ, Netea MG, Ginsberg AM. Key recent advances in TB vaccine development and understanding of protective immune responses against Mycobacterium tuberculosis. Semin Immunol. 2020;50:101431.
73. Wang Y, Shao R, He C, Chen L. Emerging progress on diagnosis and treatment of female genital tuberculosis. Journal of International Medical Research. 2021;49(5):03000605211014999.
74. Chavan D. Fighting TB requires empowered patients. BMJ. 2017;356:i6344.

CHAPTER 37

Sonoendocrinology and Cycle Monitoring-Assisted Reproduction Technology

Sonal Panchal, Chaitanya Nagori

INTRODUCTION

Human reproductive system is a finely balanced highly dynamic orchestra involving several hormones. The hormones as they change their concentration and their role at different phases of the cycle lead to changes in ovarian and uterine morphology and vascularity that can be effectively studied by B-mode ultrasound, Doppler, and to some extent by three-dimensional (3D) ultrasound, and 3D power Doppler also. These morphological and vascular changes can be best studied by transvaginal ultrasound and Doppler. Correlating the morphological and vascular changes with their physiological and hormonal basis can interpret the hormonal changes occurring during the menstrual cycle whether natural or stimulated. These changes can be monitored by different imaging modalities.

IMAGING MODALITIES FOR ASSESSMENT OF REPRODUCTIVE SYSTEM

Transabdominal ultrasound was the approach used earlier but this approach has certain inherent disadvantages. It uses a low-frequency probe that has a low resolution. Moreover, the probe is placed far from the pelvic organs, and further reduces the precision of information available on scan. Apart from this, the patient requires to tolerate the discomfort of full bladder.

With the development of endocavity probes, transvaginal route became very popular for scanning the pelvic organs, uterus, ovaries, and fallopian tubes. It uses a high-frequency probe and the probe is placed very close to the uterus and ovaries—both help to achieve high-resolution images of uterus and ovaries. The resolution was further improved in high-end scanners by advanced features that are used to improve the B-mode image. These are harmonics, speckle reduction imaging (SRI), and compound resolution imaging (CRI). All these together made it possible to assess morphology of uterus and ovaries more precisely. Improvement in the Doppler sensitivity with advancing technology has made it possible to assess the blood flow changes in small blood vessels of ovarian stroma, follicle, and endometrium. Volume ultrasound further leads to assessment of global vascularity of ovary, follicle, and endometrium. Moreover, these volume studies are also used to assess the volumes of the organs or structures instead of just diameters. We shall now discuss the role of ultrasound for understanding the physiology in assessment and monitoring of natural and stimulated menstrual cycles, respectively, and correlate the hormonal changes with the ultrasound findings of ovaries and uterus in different phases of menstrual cycle. The discussion here is divided into three phases of the menstrual cycle—the baseline scan (day 2–3 scan), preovulatory scan, and luteal phase scan.

The hormones of major interest on the baseline scan are:

- Androgen
- Anti-Müllerian hormone (AMH)
- Follicle-stimulating hormone (FSH)
- Luteinizing hormone (LH)
- Estrogen
- Progesterone.

Of course other hormones like thyroid and prolactin also have an impact on fertility and it is insulin resistance (IR) that may also be of concern.

Androgen

The menstrual cycle starts on first day of the menstruation. But, actually, the recruitment of the follicles from preantral to primary antral and then secondary antral follicles start in the luteal phase of the previous cycle. The antral follicles are 2–9 mm in size and are then recognizable by ultrasound. Recruitment of these follicles is a function of androgen, and antral follicle count (AFC) represents the functional ovarian reserve. Higher androgen level would lead to more follicles being converted from preantral to antral and so higher AFC.[1] It is for this reason that patients with polycystic ovarian syndrome (PCOS), who have hyperandrogenemia, show higher AFC as compared to controls **(Figs. 1A to C)**.

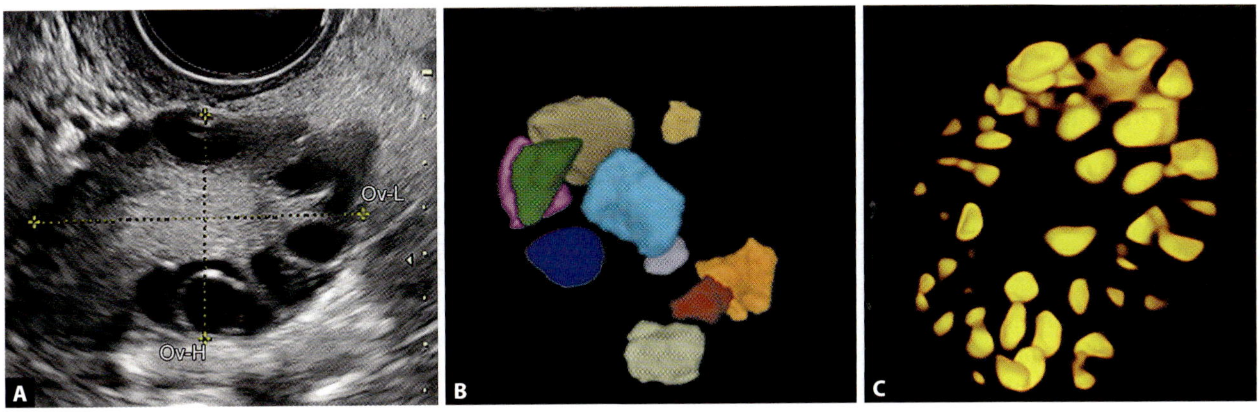

Figs. 1A to C: (A) Antral follicles seen in the ovary on B-mode; (B) Low-antral follicle count on sonography-based automated volume count (Sono-AVC); (C) High-antral follicle count (on inversion mode 3D-rendered image).

What Happens in PCOS Patients?

High-basal androgen levels in the PCOS patients lead to recruitment of more antral follicles. But androgen also leads to sensitizing of the follicles to FSH. As follicles get sensitized to FSH, these cannot grow further beyond a certain size (6–7 mm) without FSH. But due to increasing estrogen levels as a result of multiple follicular recruitment and conversion of the excess androgen to estrogen in PCOS patients, the FSH rise is dampened or may also be stopped in cases. This prevents follicular growth but also stimulates LH secretion, which leads to follicular atresia, increase in the theca cell population, and thus increased stroma. Thus, more androgen levels in PCOS patients are indicated by more antral follicles. Obesity and IR may enhance follicular excess by dysregulation of AMH through pathway of hyperandrogenemia.[2] AFC and ovarian volume showed significant correlation with AMH, total testosterone, and free androgen index.[2] The ovarian stroma/total ovarian volume ratio was the most accurate predictor of both hyperandrogenemia (area under the curve, 0.915; $P < 0.0001$) and hirsutism (area under the curve, 0.891; $P < 0.0001$).[3]

Moreover, androgen is responsible for smooth muscle tone. Uterine arteries have thick muscularis layer to allow the flexibility and dynamicity in its caliber during different phases of menstruation and also during pregnancy and labor. This layer consists of smooth muscle fibers and therefore androgen leads to increased tone in these muscles and therefore high-resistance flow in uterine arteries in PCOS patients during the whole cycle **(Fig. 2)**.[4]

High androgen is reflected as:

- More antral follicles
- Increased uterine artery resistance
- Stromal predominance.

Anti-Müllerian Hormone

Biochemically ovarian reserve can be assessed by AMH, FSH, and inhibin B.

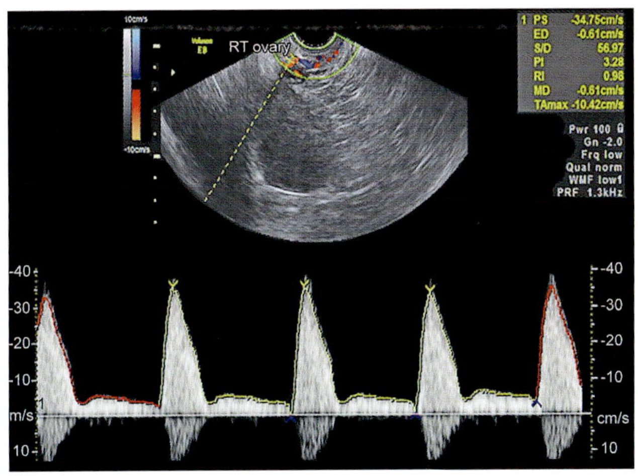

Fig. 2: High-uterine artery resistance.

The AMH is produced by granulosa cells of preantral and small antral follicles of between 2 and 6 mm, before they become sensitive to FSH. It is a regulator of recruitment of follicles. AMH has an advantage that it can be tested in any phase of cycle, though threshold in late luteal phase may be different.

Antral follicle count can be correlated to AMH. AFC and ovarian volume showed significant correlation with AMH. The number of small antral follicles (2–6 mm) is significantly related to age and also, independent of age, to all endocrine ovarian reserve tests, and suggesting that the number of small antral follicles represents the functional ovarian reserve.[5]

Serum AMH levels have been shown to strongly correlate with the number of antral follicles[6,7] and have appeared to be cycle independent.[8,9] AFC and ovarian volume provide direct measurements of ovarian reserve, while AMH, inhibin B, and estradiol are released from growing follicles and so their levels reflect the size of developing follicle cohort.[10]

The receiver operating characteristic (ROC) curves do not suggest a clearly better predictive ability for AMH than for AFC, and the difference was not statistically significant (P¼.73). This implies that the best poor response predictor to date, AFC,[11] has obtained company from a test that may have some crucial advantages.

Sensitivity and specificity for AMH were 82% and 76%, respectively, and 82% and 80%, respectively, for AFC. Comparison of the summary estimates and ROC curves for AMH and AFC showed no statistical difference in this study, which shows that both AMH and AFC are accurate predictors of excessive response to ovarian hyperstimulation. Moreover, both tests appear to have clinical value.[12] Small AFC and AMH have similar predictive accuracy for high-ovarian response with area under curve of 0.961 and 0.922, respectively. The sensitivity and specificity for prediction of high-ovarian response were 89% and 92% for small AFC and 93% and 78% for AMH at the cutoff values of ≥16 and ≥34.5 pmol/L, respectively.[13] In our study, we compared the efficacy of AFC and AMH in PCO and non-PCO group. The results show that correlation of AFC and follicles >12 mm on day of human chorionic gonadotropin (hCG) in PCO group is 0.56 and non-PCO group is 0.63; and for AMH and follicles >12 mm on day of hCG in PCO group is 0.42 and non-PCO group is 0.47. A correlation of AFC was found with number ova retrieved on oocyte pick-up (OPU) in PCO group is 0.44 and for non-PCO group is 0.50. The value for AMH is 0.39 in PCO and 0.43 for non-PCO group (significance of correlation at 0.01 level is required to be higher than 0.283).[14] In a meta-analysis by Broer et al., it has been shown that AMH has at least the same level of accuracy and clinical value for the prediction of poor response and nonpregnancy as AFC.[15]

The AMH can be closely correlated with AFC **(Fig. 3)** and can also be used as a test of ovarian reserve instead of AMH without compromising the accuracy and efficacy. It will be worth mentioning here that androgen is the cause and AMH is the effect of recruited antral follicles.

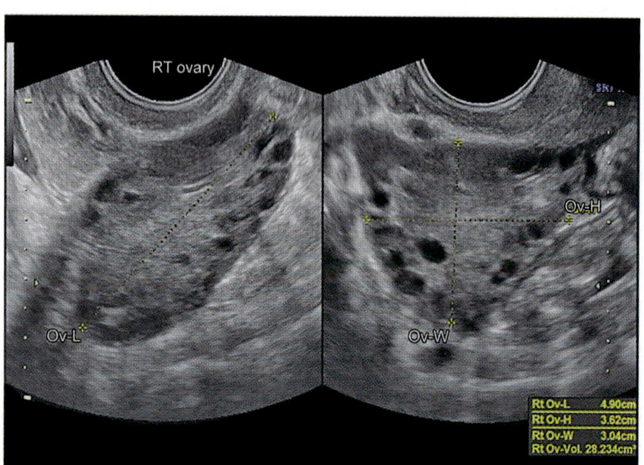

Fig. 3: Small antral follicles.

Correlation of AFC with Hyperinsulinemia and AMH in PCOS Patients

Hyperinsulinemic PCOS patients had an increased vascularity of the ovarian stroma.[16] Increased ovarian stromal blood flow in PCOS may be because of overexpression of vascular endothelial growth factor (VEGF), which modulates the permeability of theca cells and increases insulin-like growth factor 1 (IGF-1).[17,18] This in turn enhances gonadotropin-stimulated steroid production in granulosa cells and theca cells resulting in increased ovarian androgen production and subsequently increased AMH.[19]

Follicle-stimulating Hormone

Follicle-stimulating hormone is produced by pituitary and its secretion is controlled gonadotropin-releasing hormone (GnRH) from the hypothalamus and by the negative feedback of estrogen **(Fig. 4)**. It acts on granulosa cells to produce estrogen. In the initial phases of the menstrual cycle, the estrogen level is low and the FSH level is raised. When the follicle size is <6 mm, these follicles are FSH independent. By the sensitizing effect of androgen, these follicles become FSH sensitive at 6–9 mm and beyond 9–10 mm these follicles become FSH dependent. AMH, produced by the granulosa cells of preantral and small antral follicles, inhibits factors affecting FSH sensitivity of the follicle. As AMH levels decrease with follicle growth, this inhibition would be removed.[20] This means that the follicular growth beyond 6-mm size suggests FSH action. Therefore, faster growth of the follicles indicates high FSH. Early follicular recruitment, fast growth of the follicle in early follicular phase, and follicle of >10 mm on the baseline scan indicate high-basal FSH levels. But it is important to remember that the follicle that is recruited early may grow fast on stimulation, but is less likely to produce good-quality follicle due to its shorter duration to maturity.

Whereas, a slow follicular growth rate indicates that the FSH level is lower than optimum. This is the situation in PCOS patients. Because of multiple follicular development and aromatization of excess androgen to estrogen, there is rise in estrogen level leading to negative feedback to FSH and therefore slow rise in FSH and therefore slow growth of follicles.

High-basal FSH—early recruitment of follicle is shown in **Figure 5)**.

Luteinizing Hormone

The LH is also produced by pituitary. Its secretion is controlled by GnRH from hypothalamus and by positive feedback of estrogen and acts on theca cells to produce androgen and progesterone from cholesterol. LH is also responsible for proliferation of theca cells.

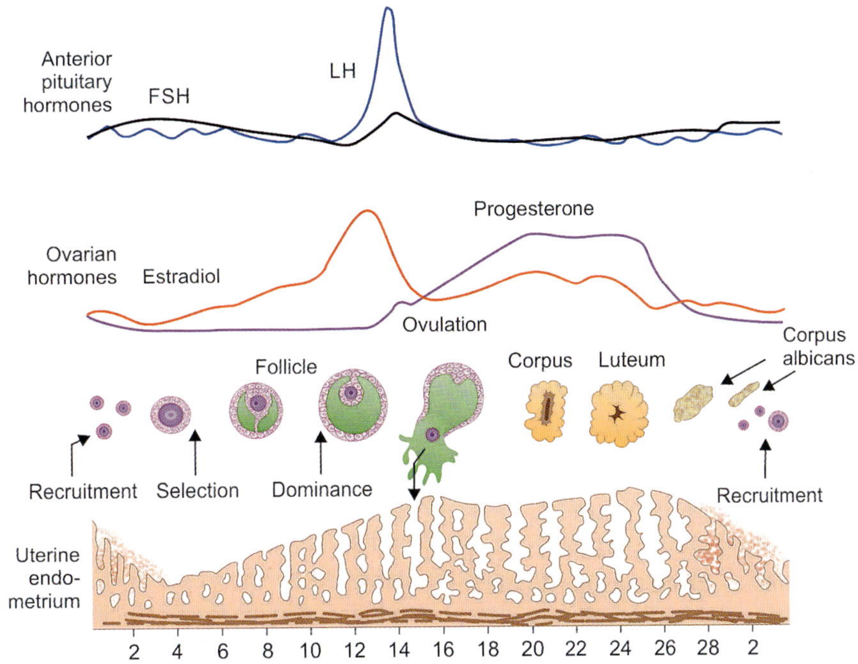

Fig. 4: Diagrammatic representation of hormonal and morphological changes occurring during the menstrual cycle. (FSH: follicle-stimulating hormone; LH: luteinizing hormone)

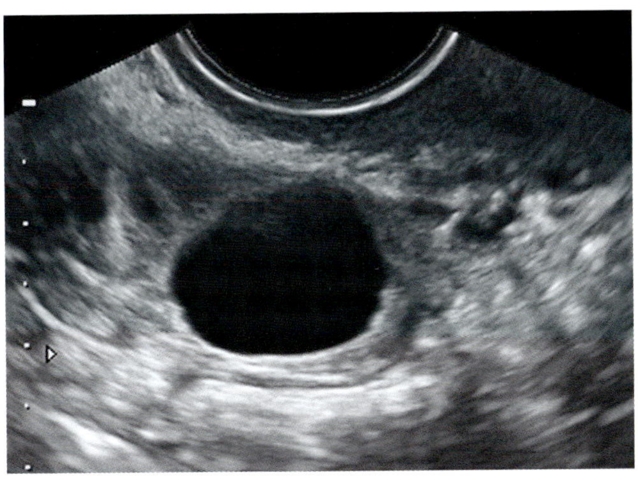

Fig. 5: Day 3 scan showing dominant follicle—early follicular recruitment.

Elevated LH levels may be responsible for increased stromal vascularization due to neoangiogenesis, catecholaminergic stimulation, and leukocyte and cytokine activation. This means LH is responsible for stromal vascularity.[21] This is the reason why PCOS patients have increased stromal vascularity as compared to the normal controls.

The vascular parameters of the ovarian stromal vessels **(Figs. 6A and B)** in PCOS and normal patients are given in **Table 1**.[22]

When assessed by 3D power Doppler, compared to the normal control women, PCOS women had higher AFC (median 16.3 vs. 5.5 per ovary), ovarian volume

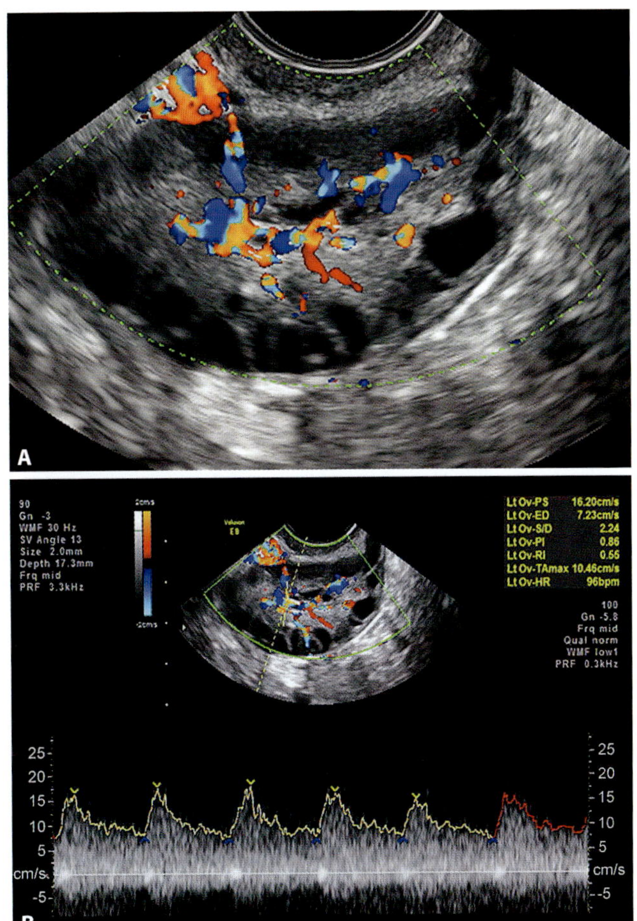

Figs. 6A and B: Stromal vascularity in polycystic ovary on color Doppler and pulsed wave Doppler.

(12.56 vs. 5.6 mL), stromal volume (10.79 vs. 4.69 mL), and stromal vascularization [vascularization index (VI) 3.85 vs. 2.79%, vascularization flow index (VFI) 1.27 vs. 0.85]. Though this study quotes that 2D power Doppler indices were not higher in PCOS than in controls.[23]

What is the Effect of High LH in PCOS?

It is known that PCOS is not a cause but a result of chronic anovulation. It is a process of evolution from adolescent-aged multicystic ovaries to polycystic ovaries. As a result of marginally high-androgen levels in early follicular phase in polycystic ovarian disease patients, there is recruitment of multiple antral follicles. But these follicles grow only up to 6–7 mm under the effect of androgen. These small follicles do secrete estrogen, and therefore, cumulative higher estrogen causes a negative feedback for FSH. Low FSH is not enough for follicular maturation and leads to chronic anovulation. But all these follicles do not become dominant due to high LH and/or AMH levels. These follicles, which were recruited but not matured, undergo atresia under the effect of LH and in the course of time become theca cells and contribute to stroma. This stroma tries to accommodate itself in the ovarian capsule and therefore starts becoming dense initially and then increases the ovarian volume. Polycystic ovarian morphology (PCOM) has been found to be a better discriminator than ovarian volume between PCOS and control women.[24] Patients having long-standing PCOS and long-standing anovulation have more dense stroma and this is a cardinal feature that has been shown as bright and highly echogenic stroma on transvaginal ultrasound.[25] In a study by Franks et al., it is also shown that PCOM in normal women is not a morphological variant of normal ovaries but rather represents a functional entity.[26] Lam et al. have concluded in their study that the current criteria of 10-cc ovarian volume will fail to identify a group of ovulatory, and normoandrogenic women still at risk of complications classically associated with PCOS such as ovarian hyperstimulation syndrome (OHSS), failed implantation, miscarriage, and hyperinsulinemia. To identify these women, further information, particularly about the ovarian stroma and the degree of vascularization, is required.[27]

TABLE 1: The vascular parameters of the ovarian stromal vessels in polycystic ovarian syndrome (PCOS) and normal patients.

Parameter	*PCOS*	*Normal*
RI	0.54 ± 0.04	0.78 ± 0.06
PI	0.89 ± 0.04	1.87 ± 0.38
PSV	11.9 ± 3.2	9.6 ± 2.1

(PI: pulsatility index; PSV: peak systolic velocity; RI: resistance index)

This means that high LH in PCOS patients can be identified by increased stromal vascularity and stromal abundance in the form of increased stromal echogenicity or increased stromal volume **(Figs. 7A and B)**.

It has been observed that the poor responders have poor ovarian stromal flows. Measurement of ovarian stromal flow in early follicular phase is related to subsequent ovarian response in in vitro fertilization (IVF) treatment. Those who had low-stromal peak systolic velocity (PSV) in the early follicular phase were poor responders.[28] VI, FI, and VFI of the ovary were significantly related to ovarian response to stimulation.[29] Total ovarian VI and VFI were significantly lower in women aged ≥41 years.[30] And according to the Poseidon criteria, it is the group of patients in whom LH needs to be added.[31] The explanation here may be that these patients have less flow and therefore may have less bioactive LH and the supplementation of LH therefore can be helpful for better response.

Less ovarian stromal flow indicates poor response to stimulation and needs for LH supplementation.

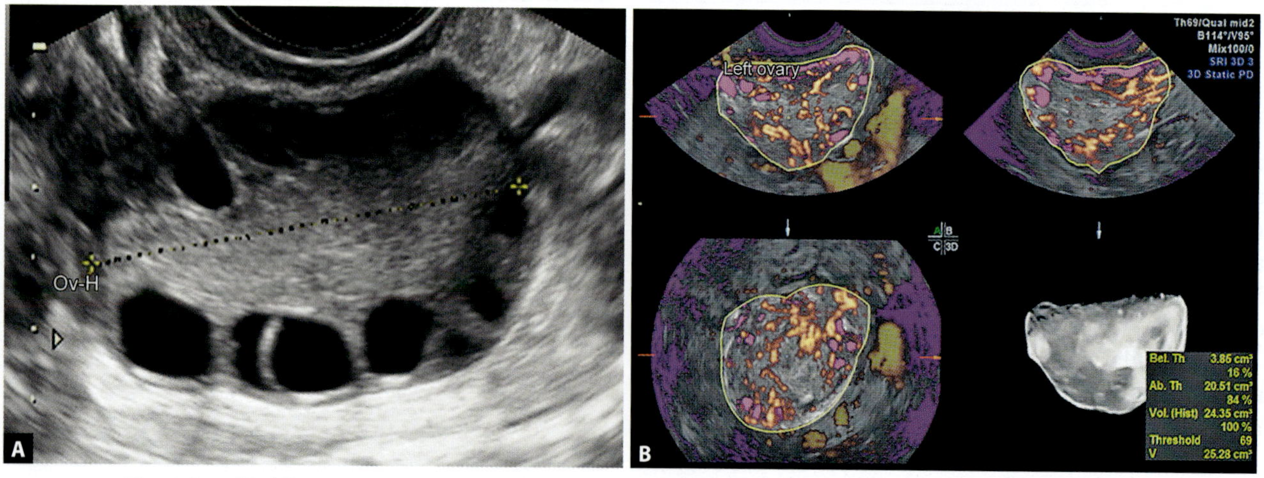

Figs. 7A and B: (A) Hyperechoic stroma seen on B-mode scan as an ultrasound feature for stromal abundance; (B) 3D ultrasound assessment of the stromal volume done by vocal software.

Estrogen

It is known that the granulosa cells of follicle are responsible for estrogen secretion and therefore increasing follicular size is associated with rising estrogen levels. Therefore, the simplest evidence that the estrogen level is rising is the follicular growth. It is worthwhile mentioning here that FSH is the cause and estrogen is the result of follicular growth.

This endometrial thickness can be used as a guide to estrogen levels on the baseline scan also. Thin linear endometrium on baseline scan suggests adequate downregulation and low-basal estrogen levels. For the patients on downregulation for IVF, if the baseline scan shows an endometrial thickness of >3 mm, it is an indicator of inadequate downregulation.[32] This endometrial thickness usually correlates with 30–50 pg/mL of estrogen.

Progesterone

In some cases, thick endometrium on baseline scan may be because of continuing activity of corpus luteum that may be confirmed by the corpus luteum with pericorpus luteal low-resistance flow in either ovary.

PREOVULATORY PERIOD

The hormonal assessments that may be indicated in this phase are estrogen, progesterone, and LH. These are to assess follicular maturity, endometrial receptivity, and possibility of premature LH surge.

Follicular maturity biochemically is assessed by estrogen level, and on ultrasound by B-mode and Doppler assessment of the follicle. Estrogen is responsible for perifollicular vascularity. It is known that the estrogen level gradually starts rising after fifth day of the menstrual cycle, when the dominant follicle is selected. Increase in perifollicular vascularity of dominant follicle in theca layer starts developing as early as eighth day of a normal length cycle. Fall in perifollicular resistance index (RI) starts 2 days before ovulation.[33] This is the time when the shoot up is seen in the estrogen level. At ovulation, when estrogen level has just passed the peak, the RI is the lowest. This means that the RI of the perifollicular vessels can be inversely correlated with the estrogen levels. Increase in PSV starts 29 hours before ovulation and continues for at least 72 hours after ovulation.[34,35] This can be explained by the fact that LH is responsible for the influx of blood in the ovary and neoangiogenesis that is essential for the follicular and in turn ovum oxygenation. The increase in perifollicular PSV can be correlated with the increase in the LH levels at the time of surge. It is the combined action of estrogen and LH surge that leads to these final circulatory changes before ovulation. Vascular changes at the time of impending ovulation include increased vascularity of the inner wall of the follicle and a coincident surge in blood velocity just prior to eruption.[36] A marked increase in the PSV around the follicle, in the presence of a relatively constant pulsatility index (PI), could be a sign of follicle maturity and impending ovulation.[37] In stimulated cycles, the surge is surrogate and that is by hCG. The influx of blood flow surrounding the follicle therefore follows hCG.

Thus, the increasing perifollicular blood flow and lowering resistance can be correlated with the rising estrogen levels. Whereas, increasing LH level correlates with the rising perifollicular PSV.

But, it is known that after the peak of LH surge, either natural or surrogate, there is a sudden downfall in the estrogen level, but the rise in the progesterone level is slow and reaches peak only in the mid-luteal phase. It is because of this that the uterine artery resistance increases after the LH surge[38,39] and the endometrial flow also decreases for 3–4 days, which then increases to reach the low-resistance flow in the mid-luteal phase. Histological and embryological data suggest that relatively low partial pressure of oxygen (pO_2) environment may be necessary for successful implantation of human blastocyst.[40] Low-endometrial VI and VFI are seen in pregnant group on the day of oocyte retrieval are considered a positive sign for endometrial receptivity. A nonsignificant trend of higher implantation and pregnancy rates is observed in patients with absent subendometrial and endometrial flow.[41]

It is known, according to two-cell-two-hormones theory,[42,43] that LH is responsible for conversion of granulosa cells to theca cells. In the preovulatory phase, this action of LH is seen whenever any follicle is exposed to LH. This means that if a mature follicle is exposed to LH, it leads to conversion of the granulosa cells of this follicle into theca cells and progresses it toward rupture leading corpus luteal formation. Instead, if an immature follicle that is dominant is exposed to LH, the granulosa cells of this follicle are converted into theca cells, and the follicle is converted into a luteinized unruptured follicle (LUF), which produces progesterone but not as much as corpus luteum; and if a follicle, which is still not dominant, may be only an antral follicle, the follicle undergoes atresia and the theca cells of this follicle also contribute to stroma.

This means a correct time to use the surrogate LH surge (hCG or GnRH agonist) is of utmost importance. And the ultrasound features, which would decide the follicular maturity on the pre-hCG scan, are as follows **(Figs. 8A and B)**:

- Follicular size of at least 18 mm
- Perifollicular vascularity covering three-fourths of the follicular circumference[44]
- Perifollicular RI 0.4–0.48[21] and PSV >10 c/s.[45]

Follicular RI and PSV are more important in decision making than the size of the follicle.[46] Ovarian flow correlates well with oocyte recovery rates and hence may be useful in determining the most appropriate time to administer hCG

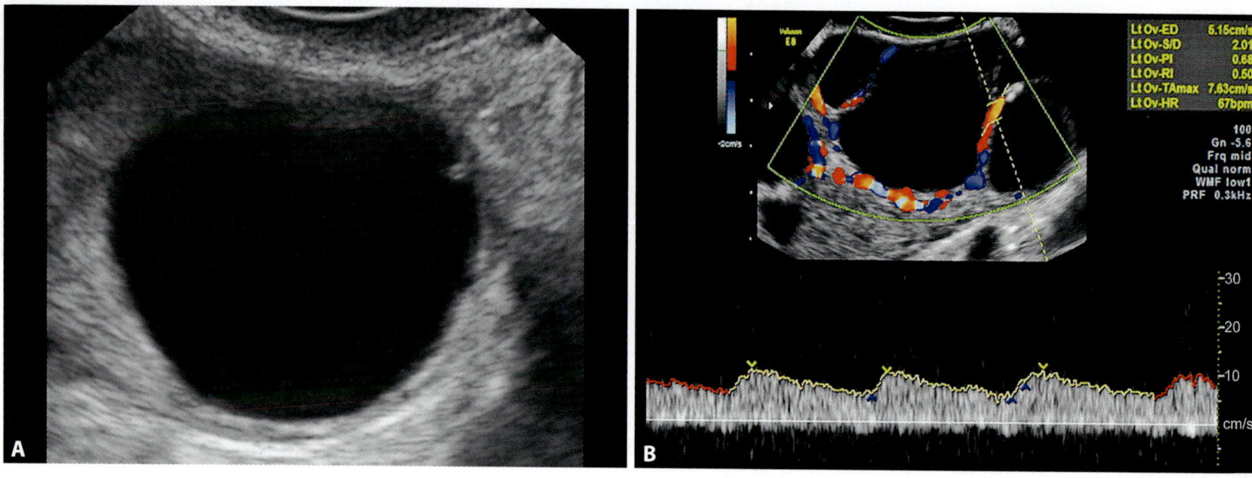

Figs. 8A and B: B-mode and Doppler ultrasound parameters of a mature follicle.

to optimize recovery rate. Oocytes from severely hypoxic follicles are associated with high frequency of abnormalities of organization of chromosomes on metaphase spindle and may lead to segregation disorders and catastrophic mosaics in embryo.[47]

Variation in these parameters may be of help in deciding the time of intrauterine inseminations (IUIs). At the LH surge, the perifollicular PSV is 10 cm/s. According to certain studies, perifollicular PSV goes as high as 45 cm/s before an hour of ovulation[36] under the effect of rising LH. This means that if the follicle is said to be functionally mature when PSV is 10 cm/s, that is the time when the LH surge starts and under the effect of that LH, the perifollicular PSV keeps on rising constantly. Rising PSV with steady low RI suggests that LH surge has already established and the follicle is close to rupture.[37] Steady or decreasing PSV with rising RI suggests that LH surge is either inadequate or has started before the follicle was mature and the follicle is proceeding toward LUF. Therefore, in patients with high pre-hCG perifollicular PSV, early IUI would improve the conception rates.

Preovulatory Findings and Luteinizing Hormone

- Fall in perifollicular RI suggests start of LH surge
- Rise in perifollicular PSV suggests fast-rising LH level and impending rupture
- Rising RI with steady or falling PSV suggests falling or inadequate LH levels and therefore is an indicator of follicle proceeding towards LUF.
- Fluffy outer margins of the endometrium.

ESTROGEN AFFECTS ENDOMETRIUM

The pre-hCG perifollicular ultrasound parameters mentioned earlier in this chapter are the parameters of a follicle that is producing sufficient estrogen. Estrogen is produced by the granulosa cells of the follicle, but uterus is the receptor organ for estrogen. Evidently therefore, assessment of the uterus and endometrium should give the clue to adequacy of estrogen levels and in turn of the functional maturity of the follicle. Increasing endometrial thickness and changing endometrial morphology to multilayered correlate with follicular growth and increasing estrogen levels.[48] Endometrium is the receptor organ for both estrogen and progesterone. Following the endometrium can also be a guide to predict estrogen and progesterone dominance. At the baseline scan, the endometrium is thin or the cavity contains blood **(Figs. 9A and B)**, but as the estrogen level starts rising with the growth of the follicle, the endometrium becomes multilayered and starts increasing in thickness. This means that when the patient is on ovulation induction treatment, if the endometrium is growing even when follicle size is not increasing, it means that the estrogen level is increasing that means the stimulation is working. As the estrogen level rises and the multilayered endometrium grows, it changes in morphology. Initially it is grade B **(Fig. 10A)**,[48] when it is multilayered with sharp outer margin and hypoanechoic intervening area, then it becomes multilayered with sharp outer margin and the intervening area grade A **(Fig. 10B)**, isoechoic to the myometrium and when the estrogen level rises to supraphysiological levels, the endometrium becomes homogeneous and isoechoic to the myometrium[48]—grade C **(Fig. 10C)**. If the LH surge starts, there is a minimal rise in progesterone even before ovulation. LH rise leads to fluffiness of the outer margin of the endometrium **(Fig. 11)** and when the progesterone exposure starts, the outer margin starts becoming hyperechoic **(Fig. 12)**. This hyperechogenicity progresses from periphery to the central line of the endometrium, to make it completely hyperechoic in the mid-luteal phase **(Fig. 12)**. This means that the fluffy endometrium should normally be found only close to ovulation normally. If it is seen when the follicle is not seen, check for a corpus

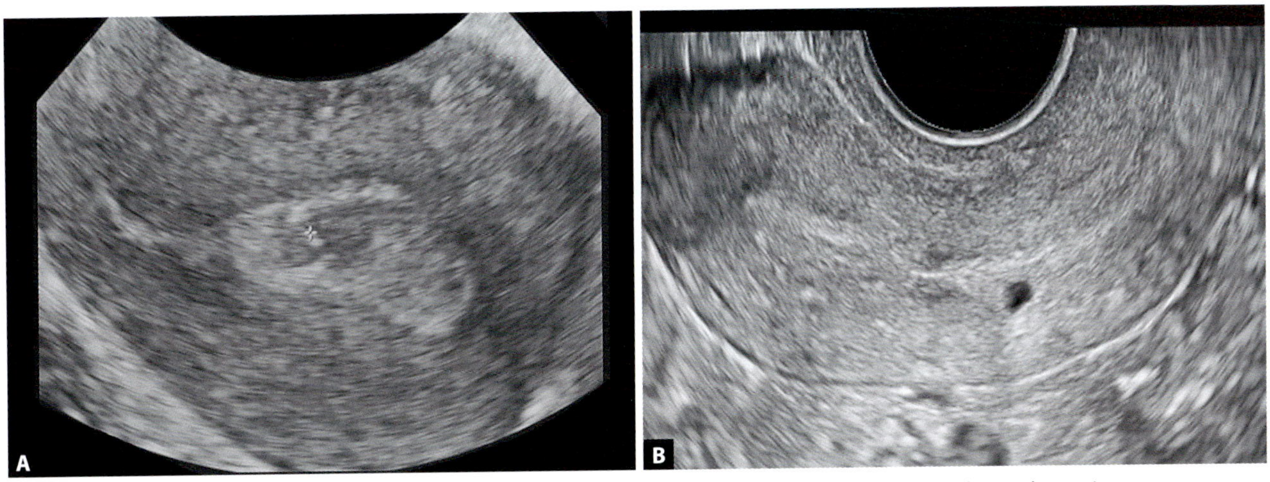

Figs. 9A and B: Endometrium during menstruation: (A) Blood in endometrial cavity; (B) Thin endometrium.

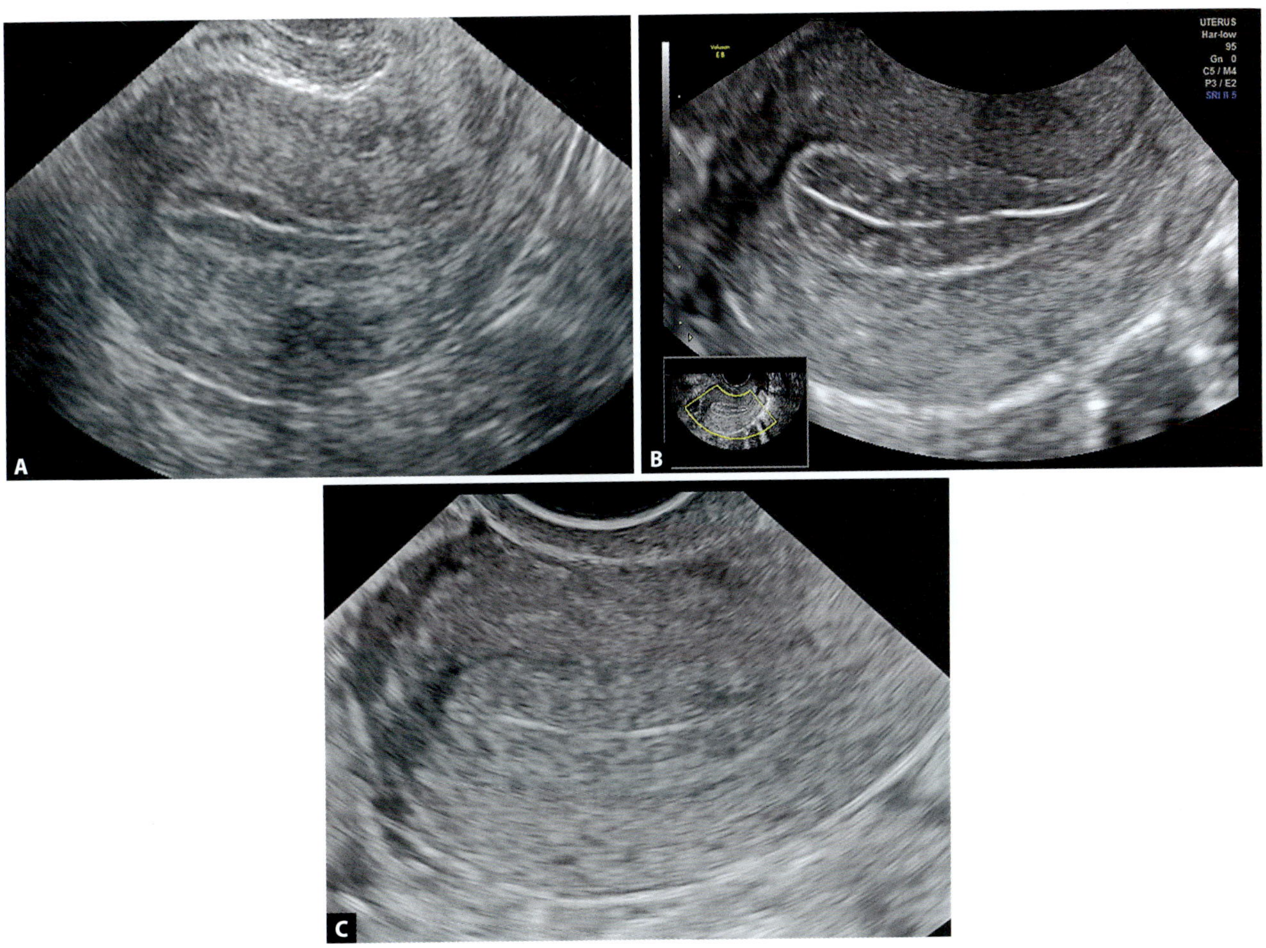

Figs. 10A to C: A, B, and C, respectively, are grade B, A, and C endometrium.

luteum in one of the ovaries, and if it is present, this scenario represents a very recent rupture of the follicle.

Cervical mucus **(Fig. 13)** was earlier assessed on postcoital test can now be seen on ultrasound as fluid in cervical canal and this again is the indicator of estrogen levels comparable to a mature follicle.

The vascularity of the endometrium also correlates with the estrogen levels also. There are several reports by different groups[35,39,49] that agree on the fact that implantation rates can be more correlated to the vascularity of the endometrium rather than the thickness and morphology of the endometrium. Endometrial and subendometrial flow increase in the

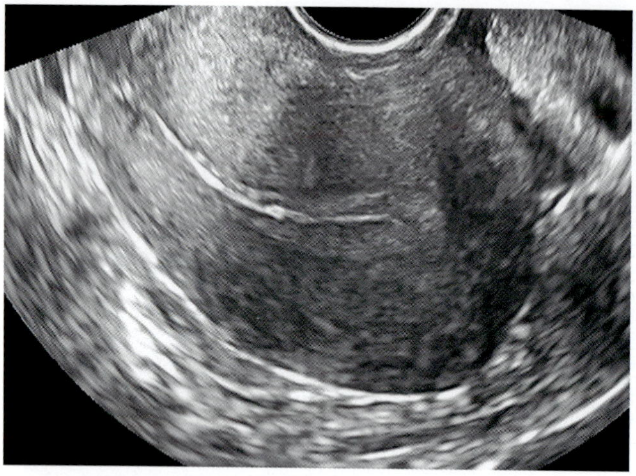

Fig. 11: Fluffy outer margin of the endometrium.

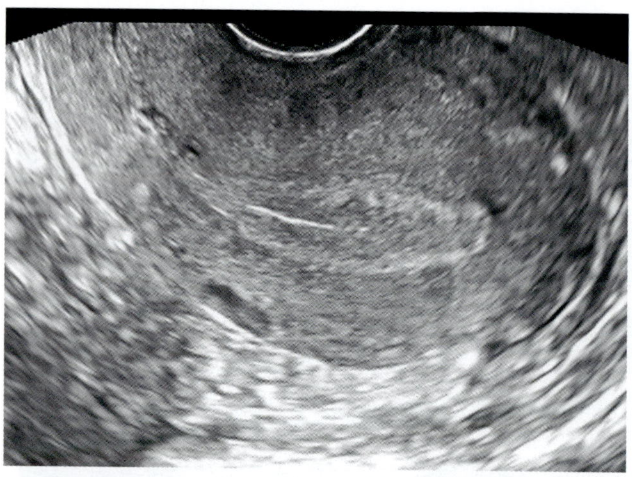

Fig. 12: Hyperechogenicity starting from the outer margin of the endometrium.

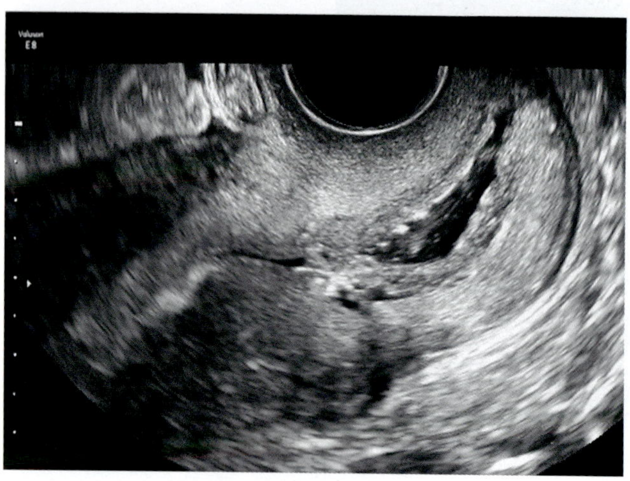

Fig. 13: Cervical mucus.

follicular phase and reach its maximum approximately 3 days prior to ovulation **(Figs. 14A to C)**. This is the time when estrogen level starts rising fast for the final peak. The spiral vessels grow toward the endometrium and penetrate the endometrium. Vascularization of the endometrium is

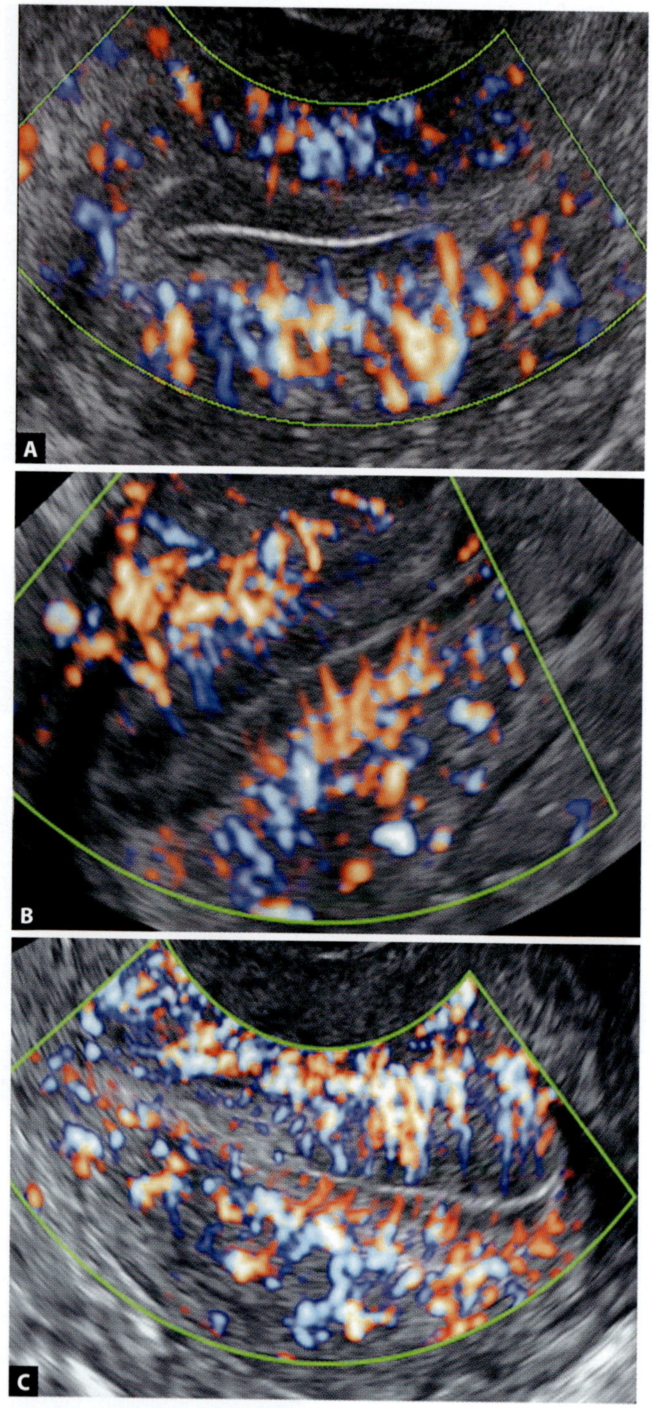

Figs. 14A to C: Endometrial vascularity growing toward the inner layers of endometrium as estrogen increases and the endometrial receptivity improves.

very important for pre-hCG evaluation of the endometrium and implantation. Endometrial thickness and vascularity are indicators of estrogen receptors in endometrium.

Spiral arteries are branches of uterine arteries and therefore if the resistance in uterine artery is high, evidently, resistance in spiral arteries is also high, so assessment of the uterine artery resistance may also be a clue to implantation potential of the endometrium. Just before ovulation, the uterine artery resistance rises due to fall in estrogen. Uterine artery resistance is affected by androgen levels also as discussed earlier, and so in patients with hyperandrogenemia (PCOS), uterine artery resistance remains higher throughout the cycle. This may be one of the reasons for implantation failure or early abortions in patients with PCOS. It has been shown in several studies that when uterine artery PI >3.2, implantation rates are extremely low and ET or IUI should be withheld.[50-52] If the upper limit of cut for uterine artery PI is established at 3-3.3, prediction of nonreceptive uterus has specificity of 96–100%, positive predictive value (PPV) of 88–100%, sensitivity of 13–35%, and negative predictive value (NPV) of 44–56%.[53] As has been discussed earlier, if with the start of the surge, there is increase in perifollicular PSV beyond 10 cm/s and this start of the surge also leads to increased resistance in uterine artery. Both together means that the surge has started but when the follicular PSV is low and the uterine artery resistance is high, it means that the follicle is not yet mature.

SECRETORY PHASE ASSESSMENT

Rupture of the follicle leads to formation of corpus luteum. Corpus luteum is responsible for progesterone production. The functional efficacy of the corpus luteum can be assessed by Doppler by assessing the pericorpus luteal vascularity.

Segmental uterine and ovarian artery perfusion demonstrates a significant correlation with histological and hormonal markers of uterine receptivity and may aid assessment of luteal phase defect.[54] A clear correlation between RI of corpus luteum and plasma progesterone levels has been seen in natural cycle. RI of the corpus luteum can therefore be used as an adjunct to plasma progesterone assay as an index of luteal function.[55] A corpus luteum that is functionally normal and produces adequate amount of progesterone shows corpus luteal flow—RI 0.35–0.50 and PSV 10–15 **(Fig. 15)**.

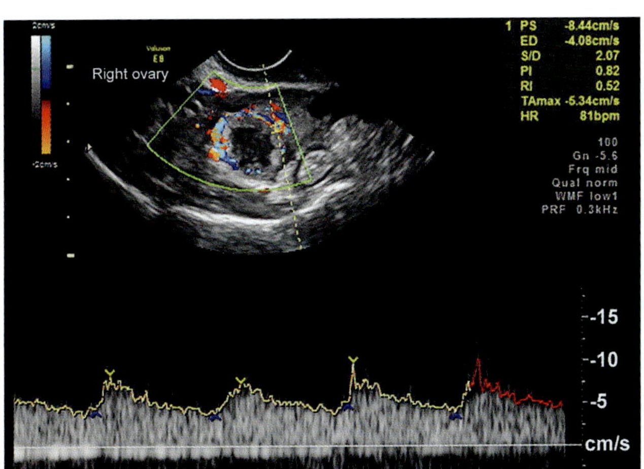

Fig. 15: Normal corpus luteal flow.

The receptor organ for progesterone also (like estrogen) is endometrium and its vascular studies can be a reliable clue to adequate progesterone production. Endometrial also becomes hyperechoic in the mid-luteal phase **(Figs. 16A and B)** as a result of progesterone exposure. With adequate progesterone levels that are achieved in the mid-luteal phase, the spiral arteries show RI 0.48–0.52 (low-resistance flow) **(Fig. 17)** and uterine artery shows PI of 2.0–2.5. This PI is lower than in the preovulatory phase because of smooth muscle relaxing effect of progesterone. Inadequate progesterone production and therefore corpus luteal inadequacy is suggested by high resistance flow in corpus luteal vessels.[55] Whereas, high spiral artery resistance would suggest inadequate response of endometrium to progesterone. This is because of inadequate progesterone receptors in the endometrium or because of local endometrial cause, like endometrial injury or chronic endometritis.

In luteal phase defect, because of low-progesterone levels, the resistance in the pericorpus luteal vessels is high. Because of low-progesterone levels, there is inadequate relaxation of the muscularis of the uterine artery and therefore the uterine artery resistance is high along with higher resistance in its branches—the spiral vessels.

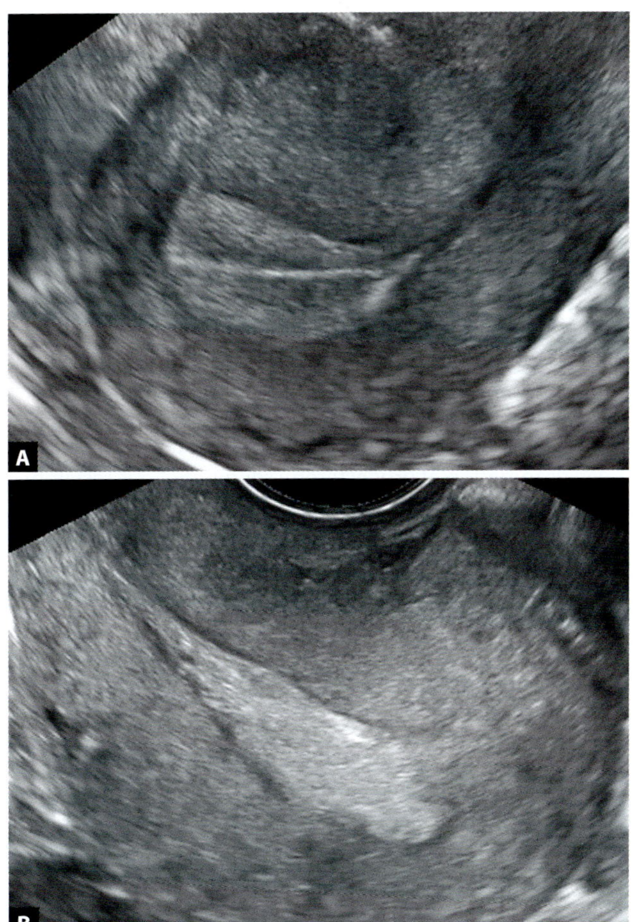

Figs. 16A and B: Secretory endometrium on B mode as it progresses from early luteal to late luteal phase.

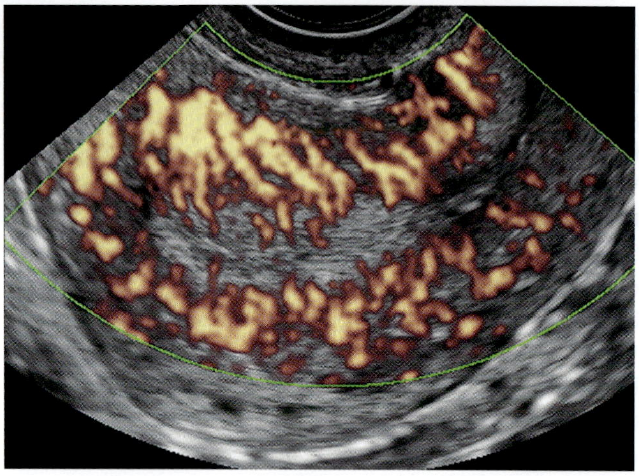

Fig. 17: Endometrial vascularity in mid-luteal phase.

TABLE 2: Corpus luteal flow and spiral artery flow in normal cycle and luteal phase defect (LPD).

	Normal	*LPD*
Perifollicular	0.56 ± 0.06	0.58 ± 0.04
LH peak day	0.44 ± 0.04	0.58 ± 0.04
Mid-luteal phase	0.42 ± 0.06	0.58 ± 0.04
Late-luteal phase	0.50 ± 0.04	0.58 ± 0.04
Phase	*Control RI*	*LPD RI*
Periovulatory	0.53 ± 0.04	0.70 ± 0.06
Mid luteal	0.50 ± 0.02	0.72 ± 0.06
Late luteal	0.51 ± 0.04	0.72 ± 0.04

(LH: luteinizing hormone; RI: resistance index)

Corpus luteal flow and spiral artery flow in normal cycle and luteal phase defect[55] are described in **Table 2**.

CORRELATION OF PROGESTERONE TO ULTRASOUND FINDINGS

Blurring of outer margin of multilayered endometrium suggests initiation of progesterone secretion. Low-resistance flow in corpus luteum with echogenic endometrium and low-resistance endometrial vascularity in mid-luteal phase suggests normal luteal phase. High-resistance corpus luteal flow suggests corpus luteal inadequacy. High-resistance endometrial flow in mid-luteal phase suggests either inadequate progesterone levels or inadequate progesterone receptors in endometrium.

The entire cycle monitoring can be summarized as:

- *On baseline scan:*
  - Early recruitment of the follicle—increased FSH
  - Increased endometrial thickness—high estrogen or progesterone
  - Increased stromal flow—high LH for a short period
  - Increased stromal echogenicity—high LH and anovulation
  - More antral follicles—high androgen
  - High-uterine artery resistance—high androgen
- *Pre-hCG scan:*
  - Good perifollicular flow—good estrogen production
  - Good endometrium with good endometrial flow, cervical mucus—adequate estrogen receptors in endometrium
  - Fluffy endometrial margins—early exposure to progesterone
  - Increasing echogenicity of the follicle wall and increased RI—premature LH surge
- *Luteal phase:*
  - Low-corpus luteal RI—normal progesterone production
  - High-endometrial vascularity—adequate progesterone receptors
  - Low-corpus luteal vascularity—luteal phase defect
  - Low-endometrial vascularity—inadequate progesterone or inadequate progesterone receptors.

CONCLUSION

Ultrasound is the modality of choice to monitor natural or stimulated cycle and understand the hormonal changes. High Androgen leads to more antral follicle cound and raised uterine artery resistance. AMH also can be correlated to AFC. Early recruitment of the follicle represents early fpllicle recruitement, high LH on baseline scan can be diagnosed by increase stromal vascularity and increased stromal vascularity. More antral follicles lead to high oestrogen and also as increased endometrial thickness with multilayered endometrium. High Progesterone also present as thick endometrium but is hyperechoic and the source is residual active.

Adequate oestrogen level and start of the LH surge can be diagnosed by follicular vascularity and its bioeffect can be judged by follicular and endometrial morphology and doppler assessment.It can also judge the approximate time of ovulation that helps to decide the time of IUI. Luteal phase scan can diagnose corpus luteal and endometrial abnormaliites to progesterone.

KEY POINTS

- Ultrasound is an excellent tool for assessment of the menstrual cycle.
- Hormonal changes occurring day-to-day during the menstrual cycle reflects as morphological and vascular changes in the ovary and the uterus.
- Assessing these changes by transvaginal ultrasound and Doppler and correctly interpreting can explain the hormonal basis of these changes.
- Ultrasound with Doppler can thus be used as the only modality for cycle assessment in patients undergoing assisted reproduction technology and may be of help to reduce the cost of the cycle by avoiding certain hormonal

assessments and still maintaining close and accurate watch on the hormonal changes occurring during treatment cycle.

REFERENCES

1. Jonard S, Robert Y, Cortet-Rudelli C, Pigny P, Decanter C, Dewailly D. Ultrasound examination of polycystic ovaries: is it worth counting the follicles? Hum Reprod. 2003;18(3): 598-603.
2. Chen MJ, Yang WS, Chen CL, Wu MY, Yang YS, Ho HN. The relationship between anti-Mullerian hormone, androgen and insulin resistance on the number of antral follicle in women with polycystic ovary syndrome. Hum Reprod. 2008;23(4):952-7.
3. Battaglia C, Battaglia B, Morotti E, Paradisi R, Zanatti I, Meriggiola MC. Two- and three- dimensional sonographic and color Doppler techniques for diagnosis of polycystic ovary syndrome. The stromal/ovarian volume ratio as a new diagnostic criterion. J Ultrasound Med. 2012;31(7):1015-24.
4. Ozkan S, Vural B, Caliskan E, Bodur H, Turkoz E, Vural F. Colour Doppler sonographic analysis of uterine and ovarian artery blood flow in women with PCOS. J Clin Ultrasound. 2007;35(6):305-13.
5. Haadsma ML, Bukman A, Groen H, Roeloffzen EMN, Groenewoud ER, Heineman MJ, et al. The number of small antral follicles (2-6 mm) determines the outcome of endocrine ovarian reserve tests in a subfertile population. Hum Reprod. 2007;22(7):1925-31.
6. Gruijters MJ, Visser JA, Durlinger AL, Themmen APN. Anti-Mullerian hormone and its role in ovarian function. Mol cell Endocrinol. 2003;211(1-2):85-90.
7. Van Rooij IA, Broekmans FJ, te Velde ER, Fauser BCJM, Bancsi LFJMM, de Jong FH, et al. Serum anti-Mullerian hormone levels: a novel measure of ovarian reserve. Hum reprod. 2002;17(12):3065-71.
8. Hehenkamp WJ, Looman CW, Themmen AP, de Jong FH, Te Velde ER, Broekmans FJM. Anti-Mullerian hormone levels in the spontaneous menstrual cycle do not show substantial fluctuation. J Clin Endocrinol Metab. 2006;91(10): 4057-63.
9. La MArca A, Stabile G, Artenisio AC, Volpe A. Serum anti-Mullerian hormone throughout the human menstrual cycle. Hum Reprod. 2006;21(12):3103-7.
10. te Velde ER, Pearson PL. The variability of female reproductive ageing. Hum Reprod Update. 2002;8(2):141–54.
11. Hendriks DJ, Mol BW, Bancsi LF, Te Velde ER, Broekmans FJM. Antral follicle count in the prediction of poor ovarian response and pregnancy after in vitro fertilization: a meta-analysis and comparison with basal follicle-stimulating hormone level. Fertil Steril. 2005;83(2):291-301.
12. Broer SL, Dolleman M, Opmeer BC, Fauser BC, Mol BW, Broekmans FJM. AMH and AFC as predictors of excessive response in controlled ovarian hyperstimulation: a meta-analysis. Hum Reprod Update. 2011;17(1):46-54.
13. Aflatoonian A, Oskouian H, Ahmadi S, Oskouian L. Prediction of high ovarian response to controlled ovarian hyperstimulation: anti-Mullerian hormone versus small antral follicle count (2-6 mm). J Assist Reprod Genet. 2009;26(6):319-25.
14. Panchal S, Nagori C. Comparison of AFC and AMH for assessment of ovarian reserve. JHRS. 2012;5(3):274-8.
15. Broer SL, Mol BW, Hendriks D, Broekmans FJM. The role of antimullerian hormone in prediction of outcome after IVF: comparison with the antral follicle count. Fertil Steril. 2009;91(3):705-14.
16. Loverro G, Vicino M, Lorusso F, Vimercati A, Greco P, Selvaggi L. Polycystic ovary syndrome: relationship between insulin sensitivity, sex hormone levels and ovarian stromal blood flow. Gynecol Endocrinol. 2001;15(2):142-9.
17. El Behery MM, Diab AE, Mowafy H, Ebraheim MA, Shehata AE. Effect of laparoscopic ovarian drilling on vascular endothelial growth factor and ovarian stromal blood flow using 3 dimensional power Doppler. Int J Gynecol Obstet. 2011;112(2):119-21.
18. Abd El Aal DEM, Mohamed SA, Amine AF, Meki ARMA. Vascular endothelial growth factor and insulin like growth factor-1 in polycystic ovary syndrome and their relationship to ovarian blood flow. Eur J Obstet Gynecol Reprod Biol. 2005;118(2):219-24.
19. Willis DS, Mason HD, Gilling-Smith C, Franks S. Modulation by insulin of follicle stimulating hormone actions in human granulosa cells of normal and polycystic ovaries. J Clin Endocrinol Metab. 1996;81(1):302-9.
20. Pellatt L, Rice S, Dilaver N, Heshri A, Galea R, Brincat M, et al. Anti-Müllerian hormone reduces follicle sensitivity to follicle-stimulating hormone in human granulosa cells. Fertil Steril. 2011;96(5):1246-51.
21. Battalgia C, Artini PG, Salvatori M, Guilini S, Petraglia F, Maxia M, et al. Ultrasonographic patterns of polycystic ovaries; color Doppler and hormonal correlations. Ultrasound Obstet Gynecol. 1998;11(5):332-6.
22. Battalgia C, Artini PG, D'Ambrogio G, Genazzani AD, Genazzani AR. The role of color Doppler imaging in the diagnosis of polycystic ovarian syndrome. Am J Obstet Gynecol. 1995;172(1 Pt 1):108-13.
23. Lam PM, Jhonson IR, Rainne-Fenning NJ. Three dimensional ultrasound features of the polycystic ovary and the effect of different phenotypic expressions on these parameters. Hum Reprod. 2007;22(12):3116-23.
24. Legro RS, Chui P, Kunselman AR, Bentley CM, Dodson WC, Dunaif A. Polycystic ovaries are common in women with hyperandrogenic chronic anovulation but do not predict metabolic or reproductive genotype. J Clin Endocrinol Metab. 2005;90(5):2571-9.
25. Buckett WM, Bouzayen R, Watkin KL, Tulandi T, Tan SL. Ovarian stromal echogenicity in women with normal and polycystic ovaries. Hum Reprod. 1999;14(3):618-21.
26. Franks S, Webber LJ, Goh M, Valentine A, White DM, Conway GS, et al. Ovarian morphology is a marker of heritable biochemical traits in sisters with polycystic ovaries. J Clin Endocrinol Metab. 2008;93(9):3396-402.
27. Lam PM, Raine-Fenning N. The role of three-dimensional ultrasonography in polycystic ovary syndrome. Hum Reprod. 2006;21(9):2209-15.
28. Zaidi J, Barber J, Kyei-Mensah A, Bekir J, Campbel S, Tan SL. Relationship of ovarian stromal blood flow at the baseline ultrasound scan to subsequent follicular response in an in vitro fertilization program. Obstet Gynecol. 1996;88(5): 779-84.

29. Merce LT, Barco MJ, Bau S, Troyano JM. Prediction of ovarian response and IVF/ICSI outcome by three-dimensional ultrasonography and power Doppler angiography. Eur J Obstet Gynecol Reprod Biol. 2007;132(1):93-100.
30. Ng EH, Chan CC, Yeung WS, Ho PC. Effect of age on ovarian stromal flow measured by three-dimensional ultrasound with power Doppler in Chinese women with proven fertility. Hum Reprod. 2004;19(9):2132-7.
31. Humaidan P, Alviggi C, Fishcer R, Esteves SC. The Novel Poseidon stratification of 'low prognosis patients in assisted reproductive technology' and its proposed marker of successful outcome. Version 1. F1000Res. 2016;5:2911.
32. Dogan MM, Uygur D, Alkan RN, Batioglu S, Mollamahmutoglu L. Prediction of pituitary down-regulation by evaluation of endometrial thickness in an IVF programme. Reprod Biomed Online. 2004;8(5):595-9.
33. Jokubkeine L, Sladkevicius P, Rovas L, Valentin L. Assessment of changes in volume and vascularity of ovaries during the normal menstrual cycle using three dimensional power Doppler ultrasound. Hum Reprod. 2006;21(10):2661-8.
34. Campbell S, Bourne T, Waterstone J, Reynolds KM, Crayford TJ, Jurkovic D, et al. Transvaginal color blood flow imaging of the preovulatory follicle. Fertil Steril. 1993;60(3):433-38.
35. Kupesic S, Kurjak A. Uterine and ovarian perfusion during the periovulatory period assessed by transvaginal color Doppler. Fertil Steril. 1993;60(3):439-43.
36. Bourne TH, Jurkovic D, Waterstone J, Campbell S, Collins WP. Intrafollicular blood flow during human ovulation. Ultrasound Obstet Gynecol. 1991;1(1):53.
37. Tan SL, Zaidi J, Campbell S, Doyle P, Collins W. Blood flow changes in the ovarian and uterine arteries during the normal menstrual cycle. Am J Obstet Gynecol. 1996;175(3 Pt 1):625-31.
38. Bassil S, Magritte JP, Roth J, Nisolle M, Donnez J, Gordts S. Uterine vascularity during stimulation and its correlation with implantation in IVF. Hum Reprod. 1995;10(6):1497-501.
39. Ng EH, Chan CC, Tang OS, Yeung WSB, Ho PC. Relationship between uterine blood flow and endometrial and subendometrial blood flows during stimulated and natural cycles. Fertil Steril. 2006;85(3):721-7.
40. Graham CH, Postovit LM, Park H, Canning MT, Fitzpatrick TE. Adriana and Luisa Castellucci award lecture 1999: role of oxygen in the regulation of trophoblast gene expression and invasion. Placenta. 2000;21(5-6):443-50.
41. Yu Ng EH, Chan CC, Tang OS, Yeung WSB, Ho PC. The role of endometrial and subendometrial blood flows measured by three-dimensional power Doppler ultrasound in prediction of pregnancy during IVF treatment. Hum Reprod. 2006;21(1):164-70.
42. Fevold HL. Synergism of follicle stimulating and luteinising hormone in producing oestradiol secretion. J Clin Endocrinol Metab. 1941;21:33-6.
43. Short RV. Steroids in the follicular fluid and the corpus luteum of the mare. A 'two-cell type' theory of ovarian steroid synthesis. J Endocrinol. 1962;24:59-63.
44. Chui D, Pugh N, Walker S, Gregory L, Shaw RW. Follicular vascularity— the predictive value of transvaginal power Doppler ultrasonography in an in vitro fertilization program: A preliminary study. Hum Reprod. 1997;12(1):191-6.
45. Nargund G, Doyle PE, Bourne TH, Parsons JH, Cheng WC, Campbell S, et al. Ultrasound-derived indices of follicular blood flow before hCG administration and prediction of oocyte recovery and preimplantation embryo quality. Hum Reprod. 1996;11(11):2512-17.
46. Nargund G, Bourne TH, Doyle PE, Parsons J, Cheng W, Campbell S, et al. Association between ultrasound indices of follicular blood flow, oocyte recovery and preimplantation embryo quality. Hum Reprod. 1996;11(1):109-13.
47. Van Blerkom J, davis P, Alexander S. Inner mitochondrial membrane potential, cytoplasmic ATp content and free Ca^{+} levels in metaphase II mouse oocytes. Hum Reprod. 2003;18(11):2429-40.
48. Smith B, Porter R, Ahuja K, Craft I. Ultrasonic assessment of endometrial changes in stimulated cycles in an in vitro fertilization and embryo transfer program. J In Vitro Fertil Embryo Transf. 1984;1(4):233-8.
49. Zaidi J, Campbell S, Pittrof FR, Tan SL. Endometrial thickness morphology, vascular penetration and velocimetry in predicting implantation in an IVF program. Ultrasound Obstet Gynecol. 1995;6(3):191-8.
50. Coulam CB, Stern JJ, Soenksen DM, Britten S, Bustillo M. Comparison of pulsatility indexes on the day of oocyte retrieval and embryo transfer. Hum Reprod. 1995;10(1):82-4.
51. Tsai YC, Chang JC, Tai MJ, Kung FT, Yang LC, Chang SY. Relationship of uterine perfusion to outcome of intrauterine insemination. J Ultrasound Med. 1996;15(9):633-6.
52. Cacciatore B, Simberg N, Fusaro P, Tiitinin A. Transvaginal Doppler study of uterine artery blood flow in in vitro fertilization embryo transfer cycles. Fertil Steril. 1996;66(1):130-4.
53. Salle B, Bied-Damon V, Benchaib M, Desperes S, Gaucherand P, Rudigoz RC. Preliminary report of an ultrasonography and colour Doppler uterine score to predict uterine receptivity in an IVF programme. Hum Reprod. 1998;13(6):1669-73.
54. Kupesić S, Kurjak A, Vujisić S, Petrovic Z. Luteal phase defect: comparison between Doppler velocimetry, histological and hormonal markers. Ultrasound Obstet Gynecol. 1997;9(2):105-12.
55. Glock JL, Brumsted JR. Colour flow pulsed Doppler ultrasound in diagnosing luteal phase defect. Fertil Steril. 1995;64(3):500-4.

CHAPTER 38

Transvaginal Ultrasound and Doppler in Infertility

Sonal Panchal, Chaitanya Nagori

INTRODUCTION

Transvaginal ultrasound (US) is a modality of choice for assessment of female genital tract and management of infertile female. Doppler further increases its value as it assesses vascular changes which are representatives of hormonal changes occurring throughout the menstrual cycle.

Applications of transvaginal US and Doppler in an infertile female can be divided under two main headings:

1. Diagnosis of abnormalities causing subfertility
2. Cycle assessment.

DIAGNOSIS OF ABNORMALITIES CAUSING SUBFERTILITY

- *Uterine abnormalities:* Congenital and acquired
- Ovarian abnormalities
- Tubal lesions.

Uterine Abnormalities

Congenital Uterine Abnormalities

Incidence of congenital uterine abnormalities is 0.1–3.8% in normal fertile females but reaches 6.7% in infertile patients.[1]

Sensitivity and specificity of various US methods for diagnosis of congenital uterine abnormalities have been given in **Table 1**.[2]

TABLE 1: Sensitivity and specificity of various ultrasound (US) methods for diagnosis of congenital uterine abnormalities.

Ultrasound	*Sensitivity (%)*	*Specificity (%)*
TVS	95.21	92.21
TVCD PD	99.29	97.23
Volume US	98.38	100
Sonohysterography	98.18	100

(PD: power Doppler; TVCD: transvaginal color Doppler; TVS: transvaginal sonography)

Uterine aplasia: It is suspected in patients with primary amenorrhea. Transabdominal scan with full bladder shows convex base with no dimple. This indicates complete absence of uterus and karyotyping is essential in these patients.

If rudimentary horns or uterus is seen anywhere in pelvis, it is not uterine aplasia, but is hypoplastic uterus. It is identified by pear-shaped isoechoic structure with or without thin echogenic line in the center. Ovaries may be seen in close vicinity to these horns.

Unicornuate uterus [the American Fertility Society (AFS) classification]:[3] Aplasia or severe hypoplasia of one of the Müllerian ducts leads to unicornuate uterus. When hypoplastic horn is present it may or may not communicate with the other horn. On transvaginal sonography (TVS), in most of the cases, uterus is not seen in midline, but a normal looking long axis of uterus is seen on one side in the pelvis. No uterine shadow or a rudimentary horn is seen on other side. Rudimentary or severely hypoplastic horn is seen as an isoechoic pear-shaped structure with or without a central thin echogenic endometrial line. Ovary is seen near the respective horn.

On transverse scan at the level of uterine fundus a beak-like projection from the endometrial shadow—cornu is seen only on one side. Three-dimensional (3D) US is ultimate and clearly shows a banana-shaped uterine cavity **(Figs. 1A to C)**. According to the European Society of Human Reproduction and Embryology (ESHRE)-the European Society for Gynecological Endoscopy (ESGE)[4] classification, this is called hemiuterus.

Duplication abnormalities: Differential diagnosis of these abnormalities is important as management and prognosis as far as fertility is concerned vary with different conditions. Uterus didelphys, bicornuate uterus, septate uterus, and arcuate uterus are the grades of duplication abnormalities from the most severe one to the least severe one according to AFS classification for Müllerian duct abnormalities. Uterus didelphys and bicornuate are similar to bicorporeal uterus

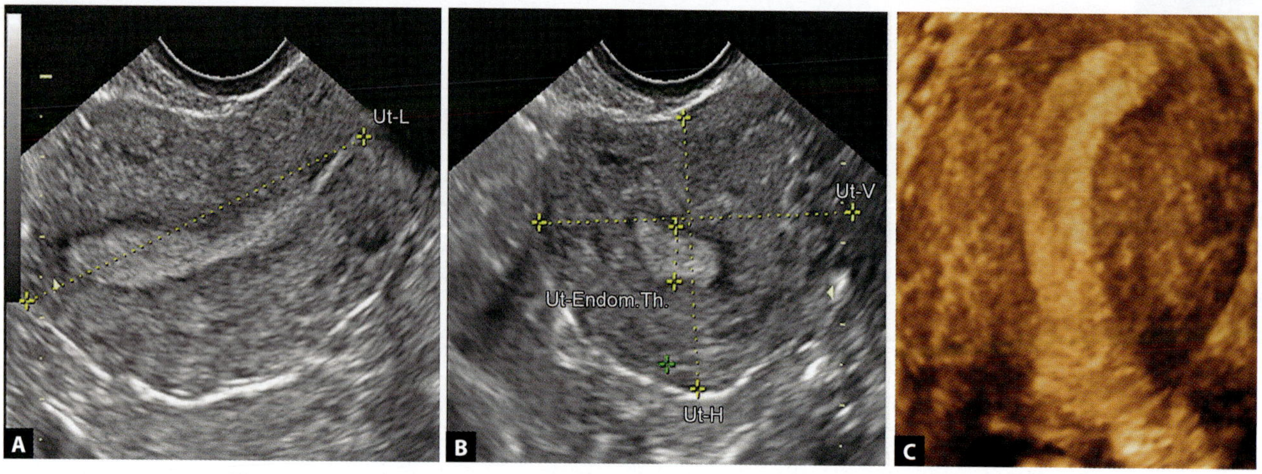

Figs. 1A to C: Unicornuate uterus: (A) Long axis two-dimensional (2D) ultrasound (US); (B) Transverse 2D US; (C) Three-dimensional (3D) US.

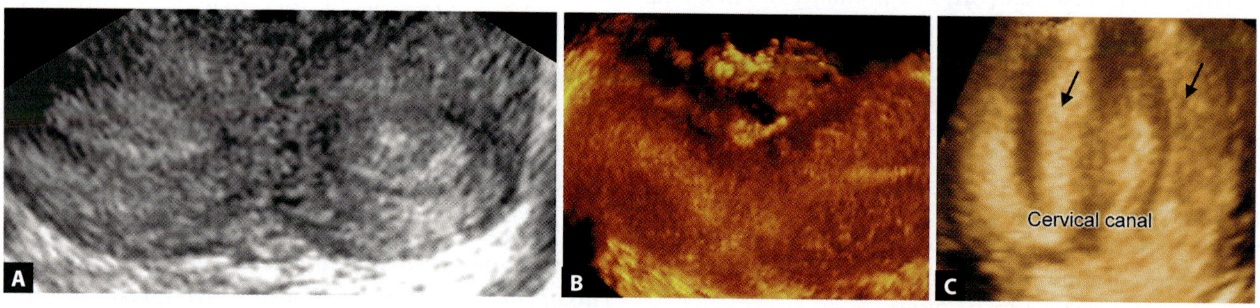

Figs. 2A to C: (A) Transverse section duplication abnormality; (B) Uterus didelphys; (C) Two separate corpus uteri and two cervices (arrows).

on ESHRE-ESGE classification and arcuate uterus, this entity does not exist in this classification.

Uterus didelphys: Uterus didelphys has two separate uteri and two cervices **(Figs. 2A to C)**. Two separate vaginas may be seen on per speculum examination. It has best prognosis of all malformations—fetal survival of 64%. Premature deliveries are common.

On US both cornu of uteri may be closely placed in the center of pelvic cavity and look like any duplication abnormality on transverse section, or may be placed far lateral on the lateral pelvic walls and look like unicornuate uterus one on each side. Two horns may show symmetrical or asymmetrical development. Always look for the ovaries in vicinity of the uterus.

Bicornuate uterus: On B-mode on transverse section tracing the uterus from the cervix to the fundus will show widening and division of the endometrial cavity toward fundus, with indentation on the fundus, looking like a figure of eight.

On color Doppler, blood vessels are seen in between the two endometrial cavities and have same resistance index (RI) as myometrium, between 0.58 and 0.84. The uterine arteries on two sides may or may not show a difference in RIs depending on the amount of unification.

Volume US has a very important role to play in the diagnosis of bicornuate uterus as it shows uterus in coronal view. According to AFS classification:

- Fundus of the uterus shows a dimple **(Fig. 3A)**.
- If a straight line is drawn joining the top of the endometrial cavities, the fundus dimple is <5 mm above this line **(Fig. 3B)**.
- Endometrial cavities appear convex medially, meaning they are leaf-shaped **(Fig. 3C)**.[5]
- Angle between the two cavities is >90° **(Fig. 3D)**.
- One more feature seen on 3D US is that myometrial layers can be seen dipping in between the endometrial cavities **(Fig. 3A, arrows)**.

According to ESHRE-ESGE classification a bicorporeal uterus is identified by: Fundal notch, the depth of which is >50% of the myometrial wall thickness with endometrial division **(Fig. 3E)**. Myometrial wall thickness is the longest vertical distance between the intercornual line to the highest point of the myometrium **(Fig. 3F)**.

Septate-subseptate uterus: A septum of the uterus is complete only when it divides the whole uterine cavity up to internal os **(Fig. 4A)** and then it is septate uterus. All other septa are incomplete and the uterus is subseptate.

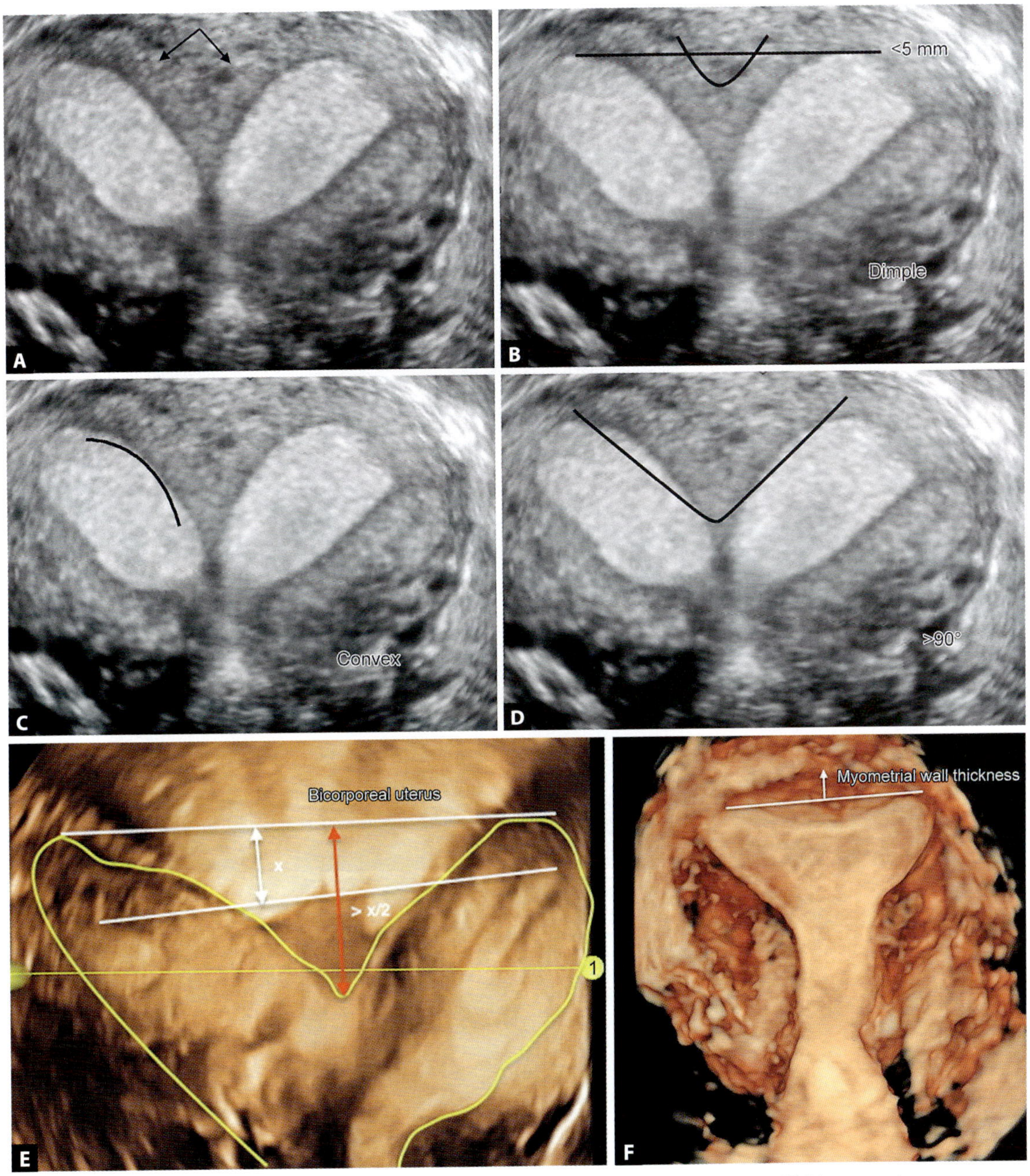

Figs. 3A to F: (A to D) Three-dimensional (3D) ultrasound (US) of bicornuate uterus; (E) Bicorporeal uterus; (F) Measuring myometrial wall thickness.

On B-mode, it is difficult to differentiate between duplication abnormalities of uterus, viz. bicornuate, septate/subseptate, and arcuate. But 3D US is conclusive. Preovulatory or secretory phase are the best phases to diagnose congenital uterine abnormalities especially on 3D US. Sonohysterography and 3D US have 100% sensitivity for diagnosis of septate/subseptate, bicornuate, and arcuate uterus.

Ultrasound features:

- No/minimal indentation on the fundus **(Fig. 4A)**
- At least 5 mm of uterine wall can be seen above the line joining tips of two endometrial cavities **(Fig. 4B)**
- The distance between this line and deepest point between endometrial cavities is >10 mm **(Fig. 4D)**
- Angle between cavities is <90° **(Fig. 4C)**
- Medial margins of the endometrial cavities are more often straight **(Fig. 4C)**
- It has been described in several studies that septa are avascular. But there are controversies regarding this. Vascularity may be seen in 71.22% of septae with RI between 0.68 and 1.00 (0.84) **(Fig. 4E)**.[6]

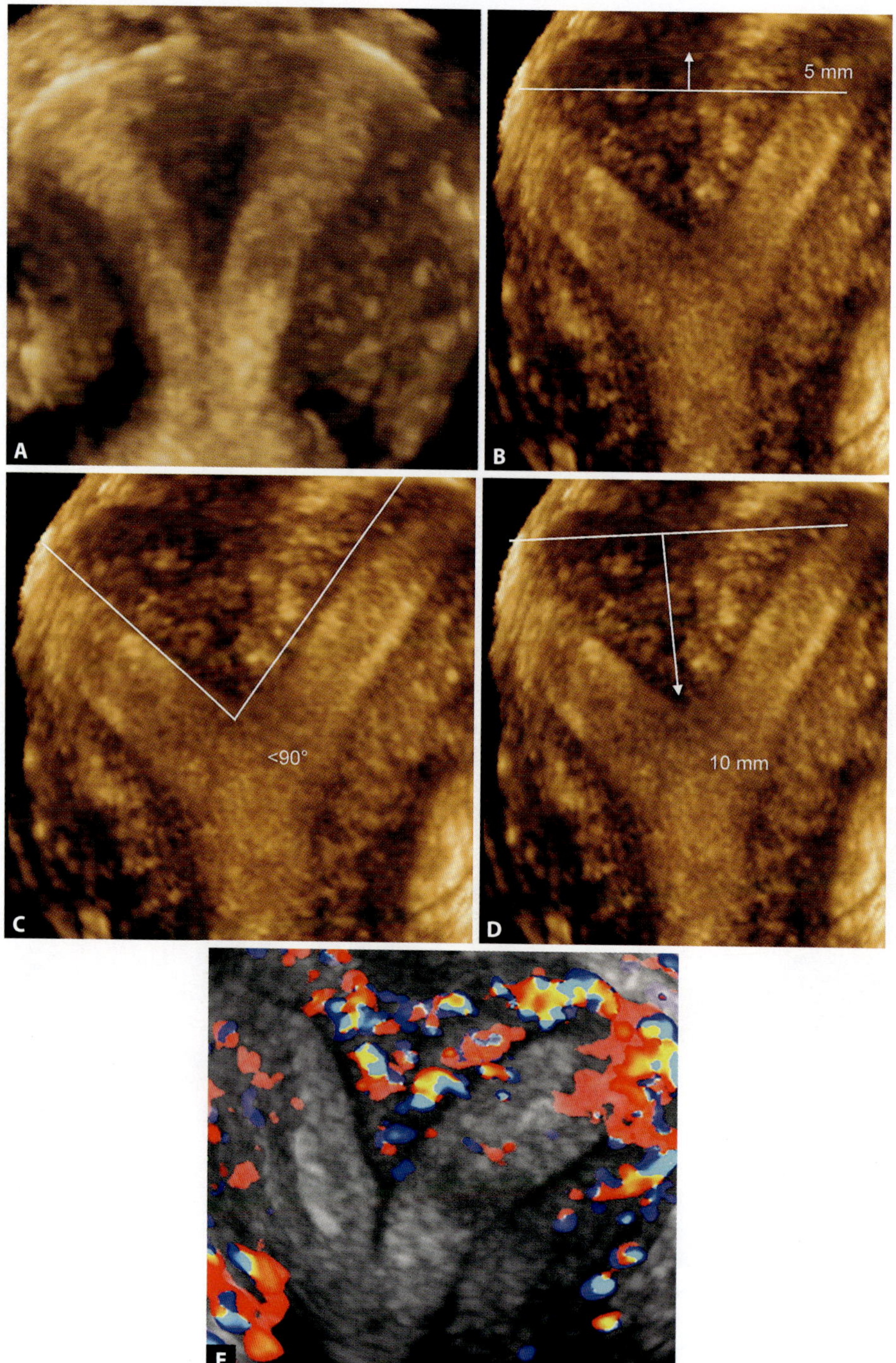

Figs. 4A to E: Septate uterus. (A) Complete septum; (B) Partial septum; (C) Bicornuate uterus with measurement of angle between two horns; (D) Bicornuate uterus with the perpendicular line drawn from the level of cornua to the fundus; (E) Vascularity in septum seen on 3D power Doppler.

According to ESHRE-ESGE classification a septate uterus is identified by:

- Fundal dip, if present, its depth is <50% of the myometrial wall thickness.
- Depth of the endometrial dip is >50% of the myometrial wall thickness **(Fig. 5A)**.
- There is still a third definition according to CUME (congenital uterine malformation by experts)[7] classification. According to this, a fundal notch if present of <1 cm and an endometrial notch of >1 cm is a septate uterus **(Fig. 5B)**.

Size of septum and implications: It was thought that if the septum divides at least two-thirds of the endometrial cavity **(Figs. 6A and B)**, it was more likely to cause complications but studies have shown that there is no correlation between the septal height and thickness and the incidence of abortions.[6] But still there are other studies that show that whether septate or arcuate uterus, the length of

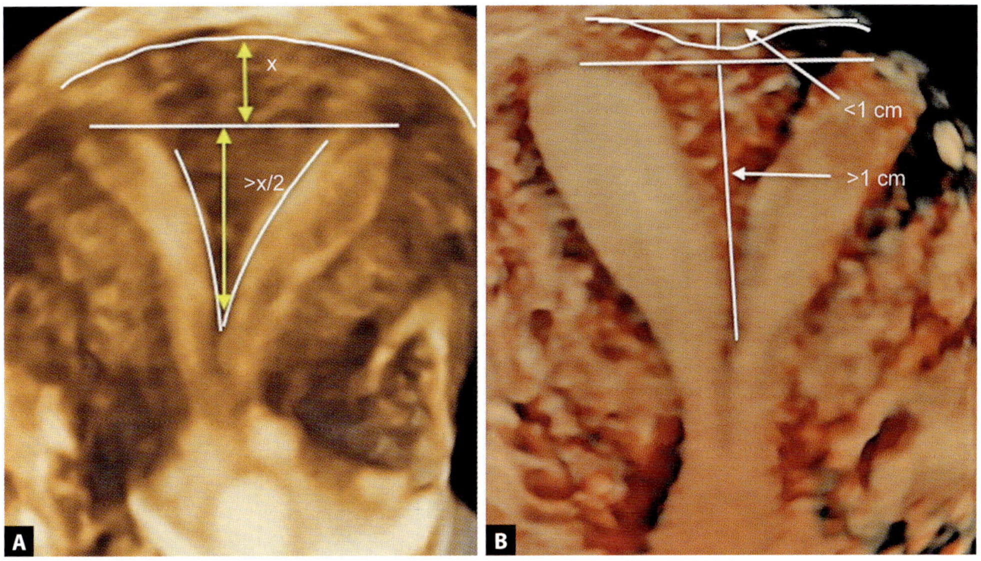

Figs. 5A and B: (A) Septate uterus [European Society of Human Reproduction and Embryology (ESHRE)-(European Society for Gynecological Endoscopy (ESGE)]; (B) Septate uterus: CUME (Congenital Uterine Malformation by Experts) classification.

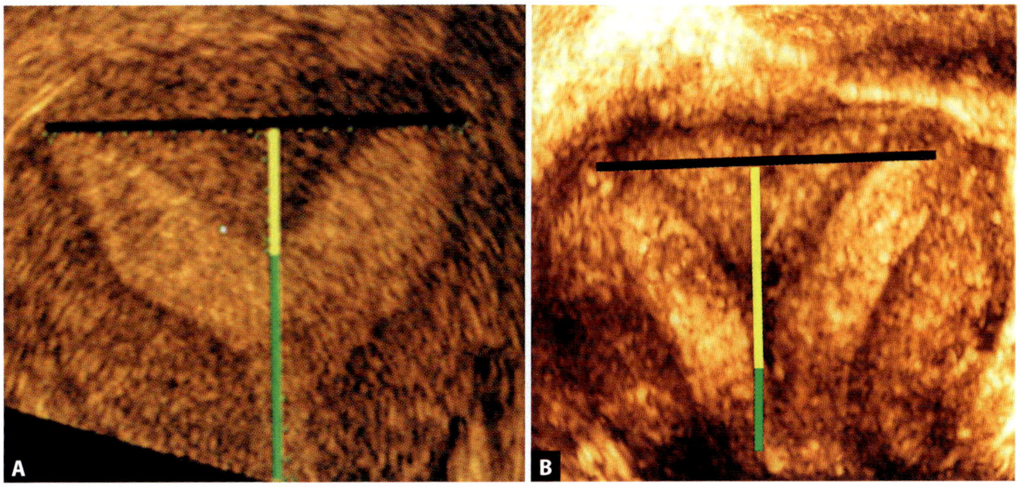

Figs. 6A and B: (A) Septum dividing one-third endometrial cavity; (B) Septum dividing two-thirds endometrial cavity.

remaining uterine was significantly shorter and distortion ratio was significantly higher in patients with recurrent miscarriage.[8]

Pitfalls in US-based differential diagnosis: The reliability of color and pulse Doppler for diagnosis of septum is reduced if there is another intracavitary lesion like polyp or submucous leiomyoma or fundal fibroid. Small uterine cavity due to adhesions, shadowing due to fibroids, may affect 3D US diagnosis.

Arcuate uterus: It can be diagnosed on coronal section.

- On 3D US, endometrial cavity is concave at fundus **(Fig. 7A)**.
- External fundal contour is flat or convex **(Fig. 7A).**
- Distance between line touching the tips of cornu and the deepest point between the endometrial cavities is <10 mm **(Fig. 7A)**.
- Angle between the cavities is >90° **(Fig. 7A)**.

Differential diagnosis of duplication abnormalities of uterus (bicornuate uterus vs. septate uterus vs. arcuate uterus) has been discussed in **Table 2**. According to ESHRE-ESGE classification, depth of the endometrial cavity notch of <50% of myometrial wall thickness till fits into a normal uterine shape **(Fig. 7B)**.

Hypoplastic uterus: Uterine body to cervix ratio is 2:1 in adults but in hypoplastic uterus, it is infantile type, i.e., uterus:cervix = 1:1. The 3D US shows a very small uterine cavity with long cervix.

T-shaped uterus: Though rarely seen now, this uterus was earlier seen due to diethylstilbestrol (DES) toxicity **(Fig. 8A)**. A narrow endometrial cavity is usually documented as T shaped uterus. But according to ESHRE-ESGE classification, a uterus with normal uterocervical ratio with increased lateral wall thickness is a T-shaped uterus. Increased lateral wall thickness is documented by drawing a line from cornu

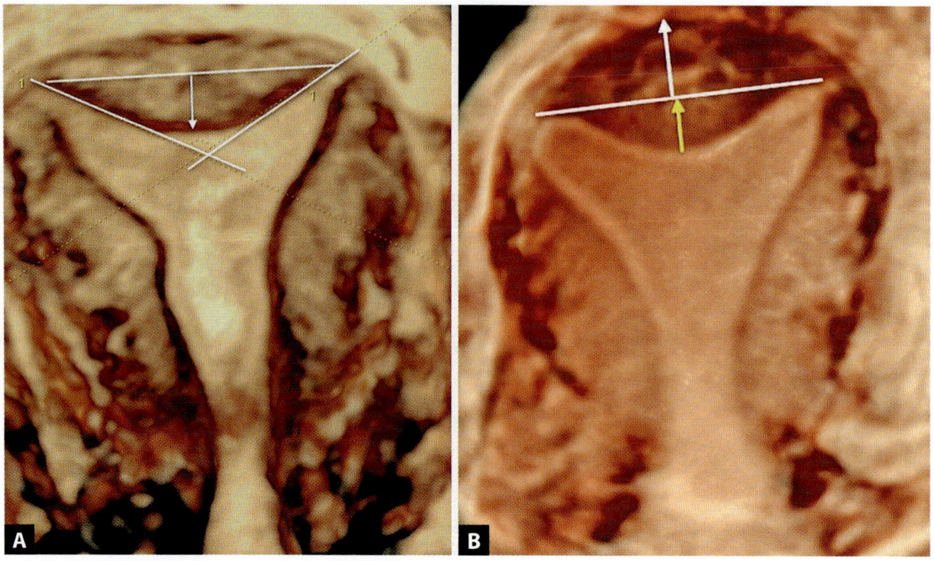

Figs. 7A and B: (A) Three-dimensional (3D) ultrasound (US) of arcuate uterus; (B) ESHRE (European Society of Human Reproduction and Embryology)-ESGE (European Society for Gynecological Endoscopy) classification, normal uterus with concave endometrial contour.

TABLE 2: Differential diagnosis of duplication abnormalities of uterus.

Characteristics	*Bicornuate*	*Septate/ subseptate*	*Arcuate*
External contour	Concave	Flat/convex	Flat/convex
Fundus tip to intercornual line distance	<5 mm	>5 mm	>5 mm
Angle	>90°	<90°	>90°
Endo. intercornual line to endometrial pit distance	—	>10 mm	<10 mm
Medial endo. shape	Convex	Flat	Flat
Myometrial dipping	Present	Absent	—

to internal os. Draw a perpendicular on this line from the deepest point on the lateral endometrial wall. The lateral part of this later line measures the lateral wall thickness. If it is >1.4 times the myometrial wall thickness, it is a T-shaped uterus **(Fig. 8B)**.

The definition of T-shaped uterus by CUME classification is much more simple to understand and use. If the cornual angle of endometrial cavity is <40°, the outer lateral angle is >130° and the distance from the deepest point on the lateral wall of the endometrium to the line joining cornu to internal os is >7 mm, it is a T-shaped uterus **(Fig. 8C)**.

Though it is very immature at this stage to commit, which of these classification systems is best or most accurate. In spite of the fact that there are studies that have claimed that ESHRE-ESGE is a better classification system, there are studies that have also mentioned that this system overdiagnoses septate uterus.

Congenital uterine abnormalities are commonly associated with congenital renal abnormalities like ectopic kidney or unilateral absent kidney. Therefore, an abdominal scan is essential in all patients with congenital uterine malformations.

Acquired Uterine Abnormalities

- Myometrial lesions
- Endometrial lesions
- Cervical lesions.

Myometrium: It is normally homogeneously hypoechoic and serosal surface is smooth and regular. Distortion in any of these two suggests myometrial lesion. Myometrial lesions most often seen are fibroids, adenomyosis, adenomyomas, and leiomyosarcomas.

Fibroid:[9] Fibroids are found in 20–40%of women from age 30 onward and are more common in nulliparous.

- Well defined, hypoechoic, homogeneous, round/oval/lobular, solid lesions, with peripheral hypoechoic rim due to displacement of myometrial fibers
- May also show whorled appearance
- Typically shows acoustic shadowing at the margins along with alternate hyper and hypoechoic vertical shadows seen posterior to larger lesions, respectively called edge shadows and fan shadows **(Fig. 9A)**
- Echogenicity increases with amount of fibrous tissue and vascularity.
- Calcification may be seen **(Fig. 9B)**.
- Cystic areas are also seen in fibroid-cystic degeneration **(Fig. 9C)**
- Degeneration in fibroids causes heterogenicity of texture.
- Fibroids typically show peripheral vascularity on Doppler **(Fig. 9D)**
- Vascularity increases with degeneration or necrosis. This vascularity is confined to the fibroid only and is called intralesional vascularity.

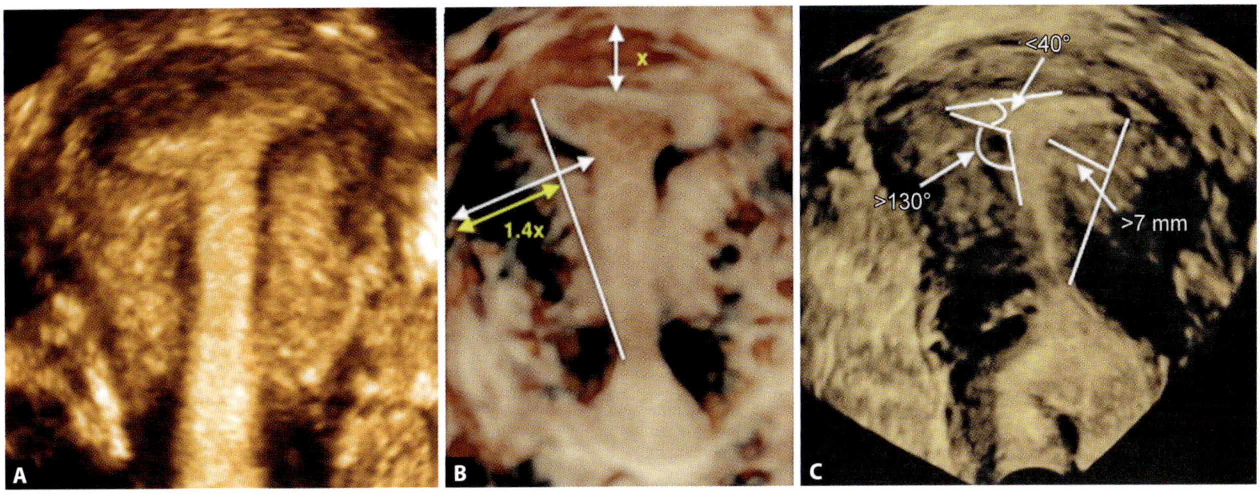

Figs. 8A and C: (A) Three-dimensional (3D) ultrasound (US) of T-shaped uterus; (B) T-shaped uterus according to the ESHRE (European Society of Human Reproduction and Embryology)-ESGE (European Society for Gynecological Endoscopy) definition; (C) Attributes of T-shaped uterus using CUME classification.

On color Doppler, peripheral vascularity is typical of a fibroid. These vessels are vessels of displaced muscle fibers and therefore show resistance similar to that of myometrium.[10] Resistance is higher in submucosal fibroids and deep intramural fibroids and lower in subserosal fibroids. When degenerated, the fibroids show lower resistance with internal vascularity in addition to the peripheral vascularity. Amount of vascularity decides the activity or growth potential of fibroid. Uteri with fibroids also show higher uterine artery peak velocity and lower RI (mean: 0.74 ± 0.09).

Fibroids are classified according to their location as subserosal, intramural, and submucosal But their penetration is best described according to FIGO classification[11] **(Fig. 10)**.

Volume US: It is a perfect tool to assess the invasion or distortion of endometrial cavity **(Fig. 11A to C)**. 3D power Doppler (PD) indices are especially useful for follow-up of fibroids in patients who are on GnRh-a therapy, menopausal, or pregnant.

Fibroids affect fertility because of:
- Distortion of endometrial cavity due to submucous fibroid.
- Pressure of the fibroid and stretching of endometrium overlying it causing atrophy of endometrial glands and stroma.
- Low flow due to stretching of vessels and less delivery of hormones.

Diffuse leiomyomatosis is a rare condition in which there is diffuse and uniform involvement of entire myometrium by multiple fibroids.

Fibroids are also seen arising from the cervix and show similar appearances as fibroid in the uterus.

Adenomyosis: Adenomyosis is common in multiparous women.

- It is an invasive lesion and so has indistinct margins.
- It may be generalized involving the whole uterus or localized to one wall or a part of one of the walls. It causes asymmetrical thickening of myometrium.
- It shows heterogeneous echogenicity.
- Pressing the uterus with probe may cause pain.
- Alternate hyperechoic and hypoechoic zones in myometrium are typically described as rain in forest appearance or venetian blind appearance **(Fig. 12A)**. But these are also described as fan shadows.
- Echogenic spots and anechoic areas (myometrial cysts) are commonly seen close to junctional zone **(Fig. 12B)**.
- Typically the myometrium shows alteration in the echogenicity depending on the phase of the menstrual cycle. Isoechoic in the follicular phase and mildly hyperechoic in secretory phase.
- Depending on the severity of the adenomyosis the uterus may or may not appear bulky.

On color Doppler, affected myometrium shows markedly increased vascularity with vascular clumps **(Fig. 12C)**. The normal vascular architecture of spiral arteries is disturbed. Vessels traverse across the lesion-translesional vessels, and have larger diameter than normal spiral vessels.

Decreased uterine artery resistance and increased velocity may be seen with large areas of adenomyosis. Though sonohysterography is not a routine investigation for adenomyosis, it shows contrast (negative or positive), percolating into the myometrium.

More difficult situation is the adenomyoma. This is a localized adenomyosis. When seen in the follicular phase, it appears hypoechoic like a fibroid and if fibroid is degenerated it looks like adenomyoma. But like generalized adenomyosis it alters its echogenicity with the phase of the cycle. The main differentiating point between the adenomyoma and the fibroid is the capsular vascularity that is seen in fibroid

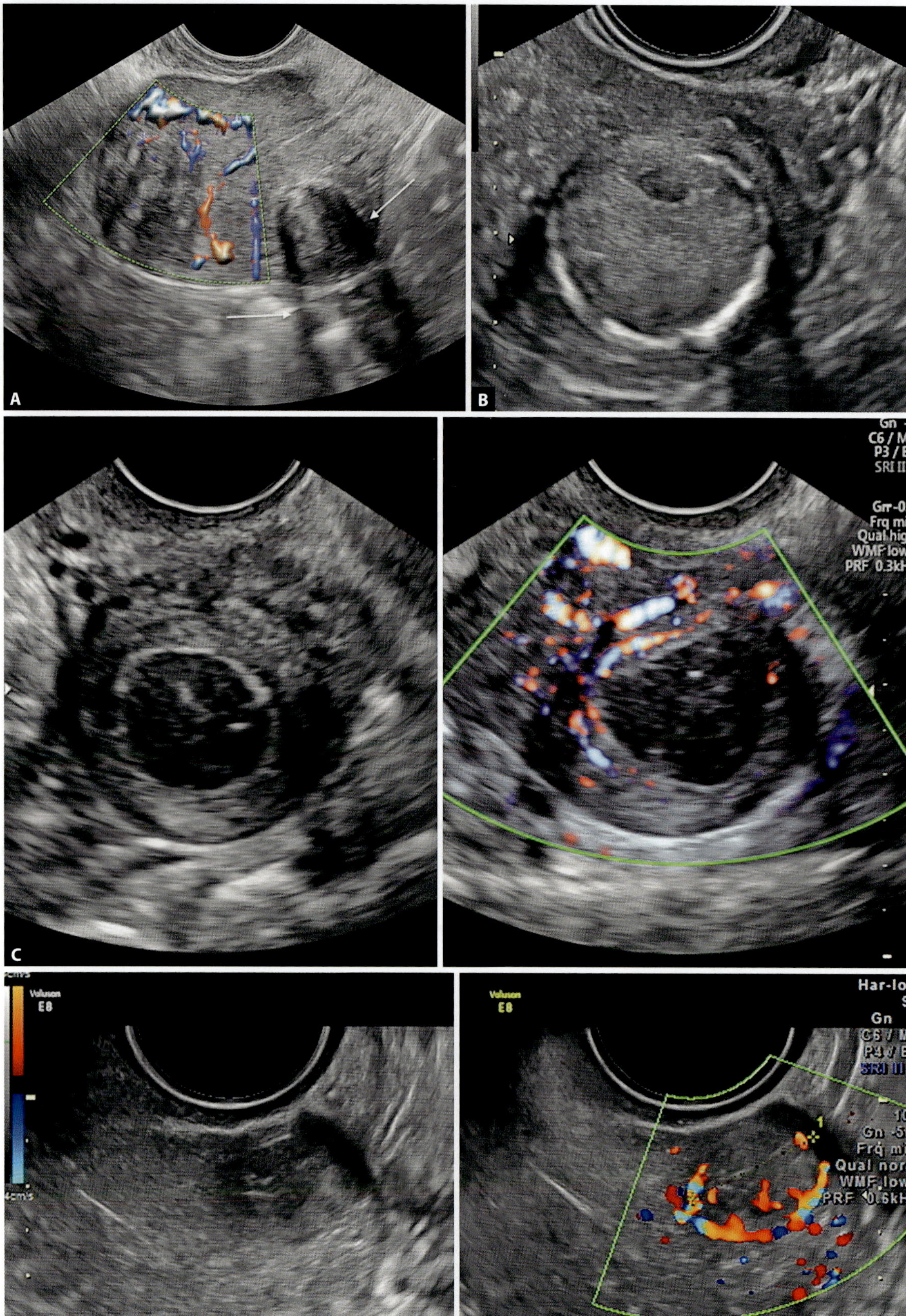

Figs. 9Ato D: (A) Fibroid uterus 2D ultrasound (US) with edge shadows; (B) Fibroid with calcification; (C) Cystic degeneration of fibroid; (D) Doppler showing peripheral vascularity of fibroid.

Leiomyoma subclassification system

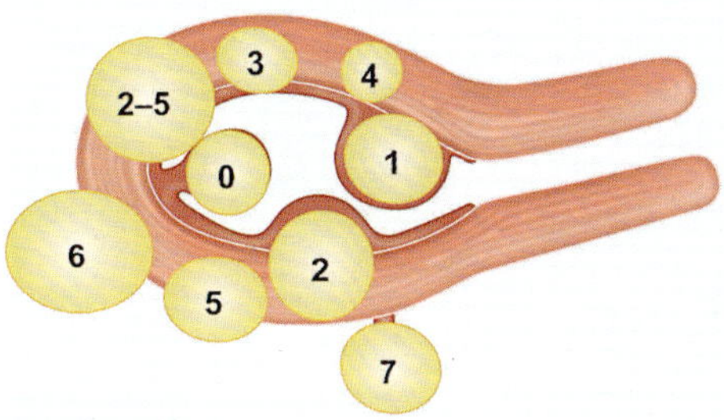

SM–Submucosal	0	Pedunculated intracavitary
	1	<50% intramural
	2	≥50% intramural
O–Other	3	Contacts endometrium: 100% intramural
	4	Intramural
	5	Subserosal ≥50% intramural
	6	Subserosal <50% intramural
	7	Subserosal pedunculated
	8	Other (specify, e.g., cervical, parasitic)

Hybrid leiomyomas (impact both endometrium and serosa)	Two numbers are listed separated by a hyphen. By convention, the first refers to the relationship with the endometrium while the second refers to the relationship to the serosa. One example is below	
	2–5	Submucosal and subserosal, each with less than half the diameter in the endometrial and peritoneal cavities, respectively

Fig. 10: Leiomyoma subclassification system (FIGO/Palm Coine classiciation).

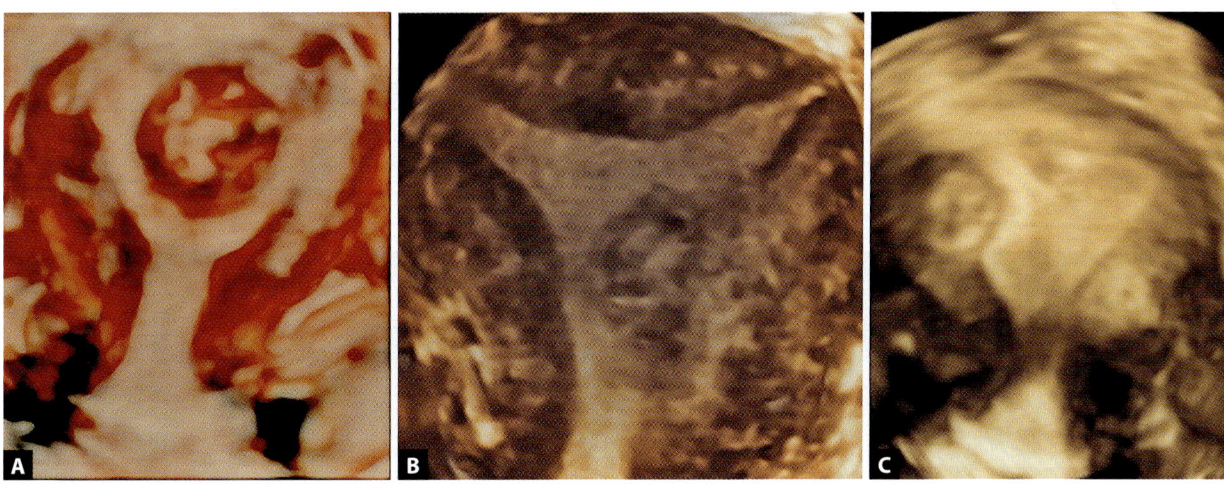

Figs. 11A to C: (A) Type 0 fibroid; (B) Type 1 fibroid; (C) Type 2 fibroid on 3D ultrasound (US)-rendered images.

but is never seen in adenomyoma. When seen on 3D PD also a vascular fibroid shows circumferentially arranged vessels while in adenomyoma the vascular arrangement is radial or penetrating **(Figs. 12D and 13)**. Endometrial strands extending into myometrium are also seen on 3D US **(Fig. 12E)**. Adenomyoma does not show edge shadow.

Endometrium: It is normally pear shaped and has an intact endometriomyometrial junction (junctional zone) **(Fig. 14A)**. Distortion of endometrial contour and disruption of junctional zone are signs of endometrial pathologies.

Common endometrial pathologies are endometritis, polyps, endometrial hyperplasia, endometrial malignancies, synechiae, and other miscellaneous conditions with residual products of conception in endometrial cavity.

- *Endometritis:* Acute endometritis presents as thick, isoechoic endometrium with disruption of junctional zone **(Fig. 14B)**, minimal fluid in endometrial cavity and increased vascularity, even in early follicular phase.

  Chronic endometritis presents as persistently thin avascular/severely hypovascularized endometrium with disrupted junctional zone. Calcified pelvic lymph nodes or calcified spots in the adnexa are also seen in chronic inflammatory lesions. Tuberculosis is one of the common causes of chronic endometritis, especially in developing countries. Though US is not diagnostic of tuberculous endometritis, but shows certain signs that may raise a suspicion of tuberculous pathology. These are persistently thin endometrium, irregular junctional zone,

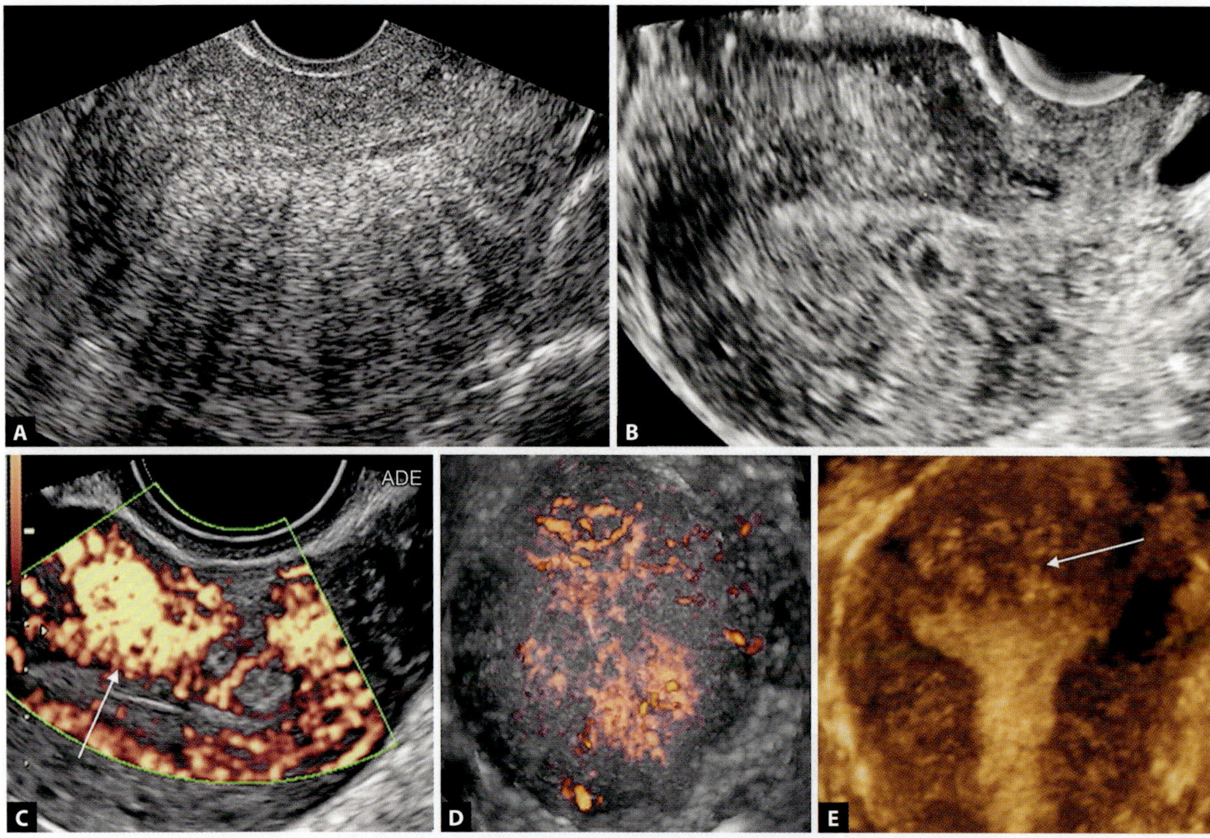

Figs. 12A to E: Adenomyosis uterus. (A) Swiss cheese appearance; (B) Heterogeneous echogenicity, myometrial cysts; (C) Adenomyosis (arrow); (D) 3D power Doppler; (E) 3D adenomyosis (arrow).

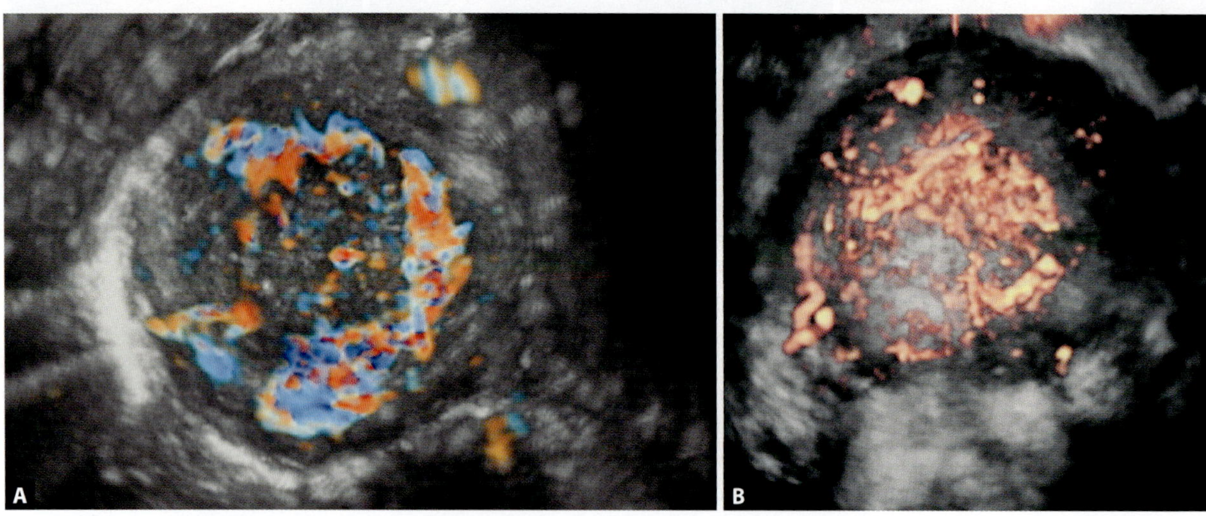

Figs. 13A and B: Three-dimensional (3D) power Doppler of (A) Degenerating fibroid; and (B) Adenomyosis uterus.

fluid in the endometrial cavity with hyperechoic inner margin, micropolyps, vertical orientation of interstitial part of the tube endometrial synechiae, contracted T-shaped endometrial cavity, myometrial cysts with no peripheral vascularity, endometrial, subendometrial, and myometrial calcifications **(Figs. 14C to F)**.

- *Endometrial hyperplasia:* This is a localized overgrowth of endometrium with normal histology, presenting as thick echogenic endometrium, in part or entirely. Endometrial thickness >14 mm in premenopausal patient and <5 mm in postmenopausal patients is hypertrophic. But endometrium thicker than this cut off is often seen

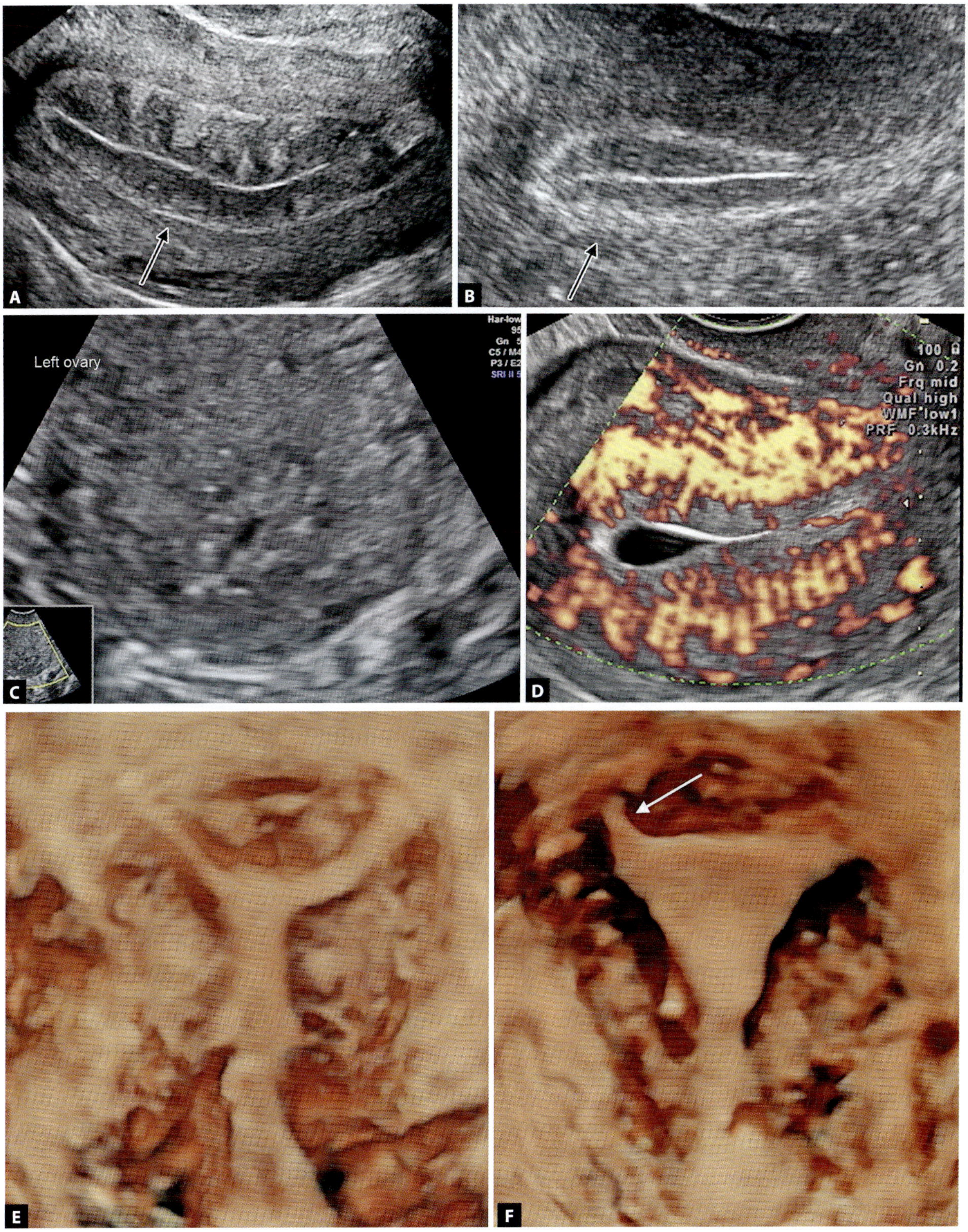

Figs. 14A to F: Endometritis. (A) Normal junctional zone (arrow); (B) Obliterated junctional zone (arrow); (C) Calcifications in junctional zone; (D) Hyperechoic inner endometrial margin with fluid in endometrial cavity and absent subendometrial vascularity; (E) Contracted endometrial cavity; (F) Vertical orientation of interstitial part of the tube.

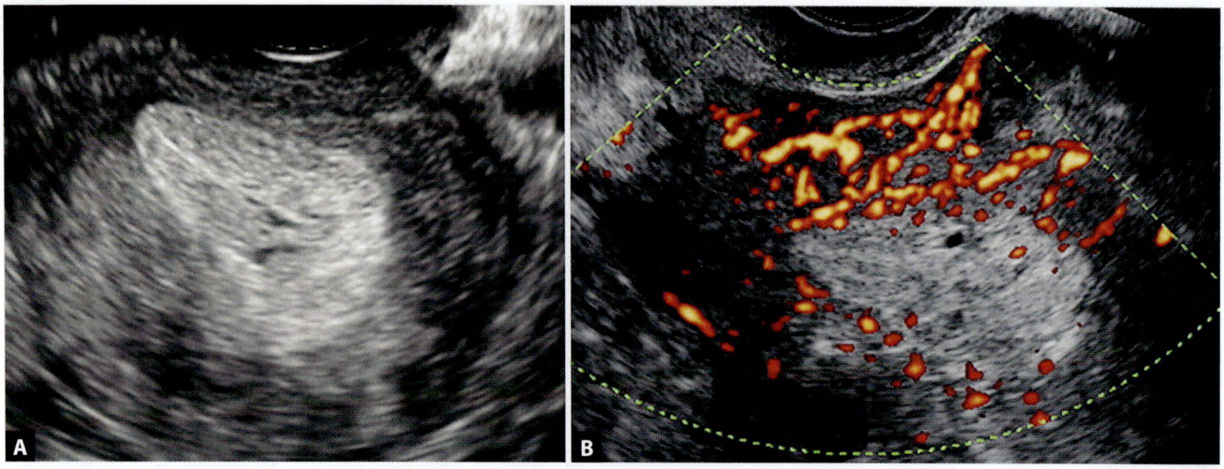

Figs. 15A and B: (A) Endometrial hyperplasia; (B) Mode and power Doppler.

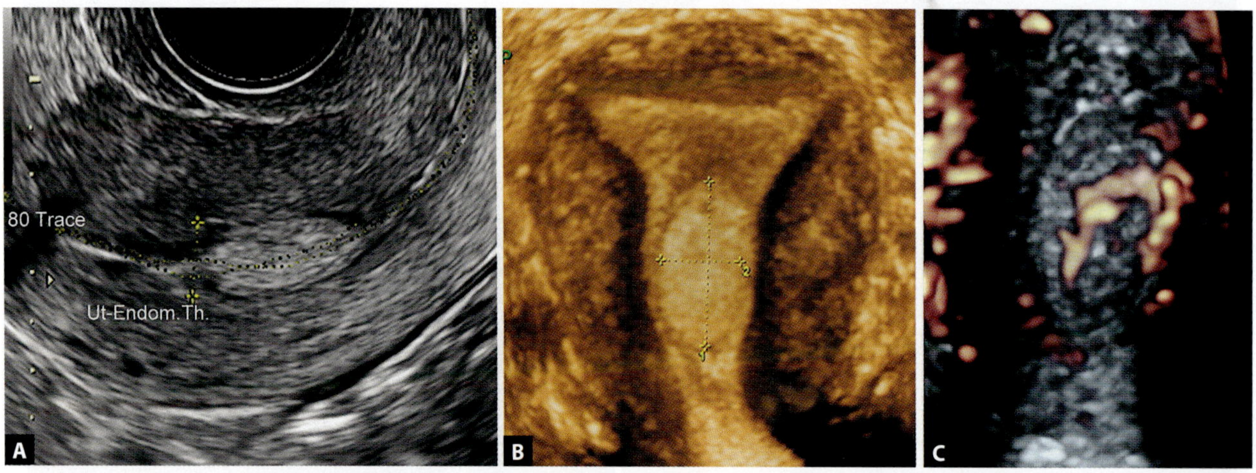

Figs. 16A to C: Endometrial polyp. (A) 2D ultrasound (US); (B) 3D US coronal view; (C) 3D color Doppler showing two closely placed vessels in pedicle of polyp.

patients on fertility treatment. As long as the morphology is normal, it may be considered normal according to our experience based opinion. Endometriomyometrial junction is well maintained. On color Doppler, it shows regularly placed vessels supplying it with normal branching pattern **(Figs. 15A and B)** and mean RI of 0.55 ± 0.05.

- *Polyps:* Endometrial polyps are projectile solid lesions from the endometrial walls into the endometrial cavity.

Sonographically, they are seen as solid echogenic lesions in the endometrial cavity **(Figs. 16A and B)**. Smaller lesions are easier to diagnose but larger lesions fill up the cavity and look like generalized endometrial thickening but color Doppler helps for differentiation.

On two-dimensional (2D) US, the polyps are best visible in periovulatory phase or in menstrual phase when there is fluid in endometrial cavity. On Doppler, polyp shows a single feeding vessel **(Fig. 16C)** or maximum two vessels very closely placed (pedicular vessels). Infection, necrosis, or atypia may show very low resistance. Vascular pattern has a high accuracy for differential diagnosis of endometrial lesions. Single-vessel pattern for polyp has been presented in **Table 3.**[12]

Polyps may arise in the cervix or may prolapse into cervix if these have long pedicle.

Endometrial fibroids are hypoechoic, well demonstrated in echogenic endometrium of secretory phase and have peripheral vascularity, typical of fibroids **(Figs. 17A to C)**. Rim-like vessel pattern for fibroids has been presented in **Table 4.**[12]

- *Synechiae:* When the endometrium is triple line or the cavity is distended with the fluid, synechiae are seen as lines bridging between layers of endometrium **(Figs. 18A to C)**. On 3D US, it helps in exact assessment of restriction of cavity **(Fig. 18B)** in case of bridging adhesions.

Sonohysterography has 100% sensitivity for the differentiation of all endometrial pathologies **(Fig. 18C)**.

TABLE 3: Single-vessel pattern for polyp.	
Sensitivity	81.2%
Specificity	88.2%
Positive-predictive value	92.9%
Negative-predictive value	71.4%

TABLE 4: Rim-like vessel pattern for fibroids.	
Sensitivity	70.6%
Specificity	100%
Positive-predictive value	100%
Negative-predictive value	86.5%

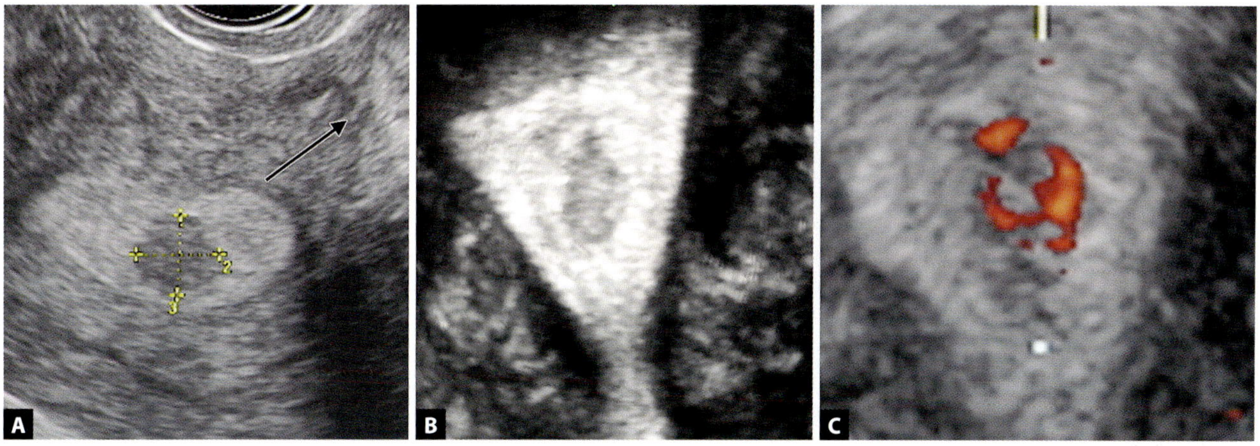

Figs. 17A to C: Endometrial fibroid. (A) 2D ultrasound (US); (B) 3D US coronal view; (C) 3D power Doppler showing peripheral vascularity.

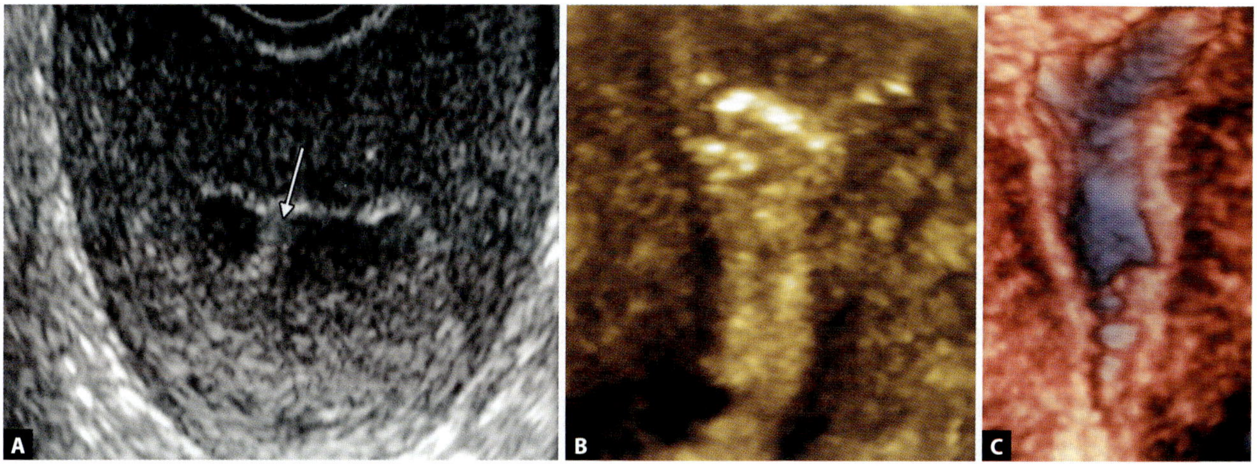

Figs. 18A to C: Synechiae. (A) 2D ultrasound (US) (arrow); (B) 3D US coronal view; (C) Sonohysterography.

Method:
- Lithotomy position
- A 6-French (external diameter 1.6 mm, internal diameter 1.1 mm) Foley's catheter is placed in cervix. Catheter balloon in cervical canal
- Distend balloon with 1.5–2 mL of fluid
- Slowly inject 5 mL of normal saline with 10 mL syringe to distend the uterine cavity
- Remove all metal instruments and introduce the probe into the vagina with catheter in situ
- Transvaginal sonography shows fluid-distended endometrial cavity
- Endometrial lesions will be clearly seen **(Figs. 19A and B)**.

Normal saline is a clear fluid, appears black on US and is therefore known as negative contrast. Positive contrast media like SonoVue (Bracco) is also available. This is an echogenic contrast and obscures solid endometrial lesions but is excellent for sonosalpingography.

Other endometrial lesions are postcurettage endometrial collection, missed abortion, incomplete abortion, etc. These are all avascular and show heterogeneous echogenicity. Clinical history guides to the diagnosis **(Figs. 20A and B)**.

Vesicular mole shows a thick echogenic endometrium with small anechoic areas **(Fig. 21A)**—snowstorm appearance. This echogenicity is higher than that of a normal secretory endometrium as it is because of decidual reaction. If it becomes malignant, it would break the endometriomyometrial interface. On color Doppler, it shows low resistance, low velocity vessels **(Fig. 21B)**. But in very early phase, Doppler will not fill up flow signals, due to very low velocities. Of course, beta-human chorionic gonadotropin (β-hCG) levels and its correlation with US findings are diagnostic. Vascularity is more evident in partial mole than in complete mole.

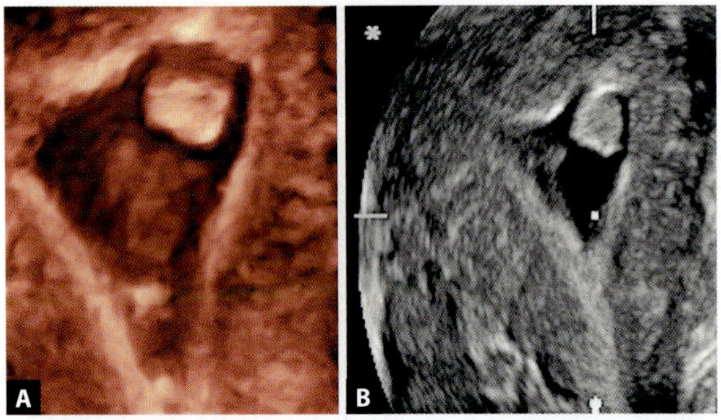

Figs. 19A and B: Sonohysterography showing polyp on (A) 3D rendering coronal view; (B) 3D volume, tomographic ultrasound imaging in coronal view showing pedicle of the polyp.

In patients with missed abortion, progressive disappearance of villous vascularity after embryonic death leads to villous hydrops and this condition is known as a pseudopartial hydatidiform (vesicular) mole. This is not actually a vesicular mole.

Endometrial calcifications are common after curettage and medical termination of pregnancy **(Figs. 22A and B)**.

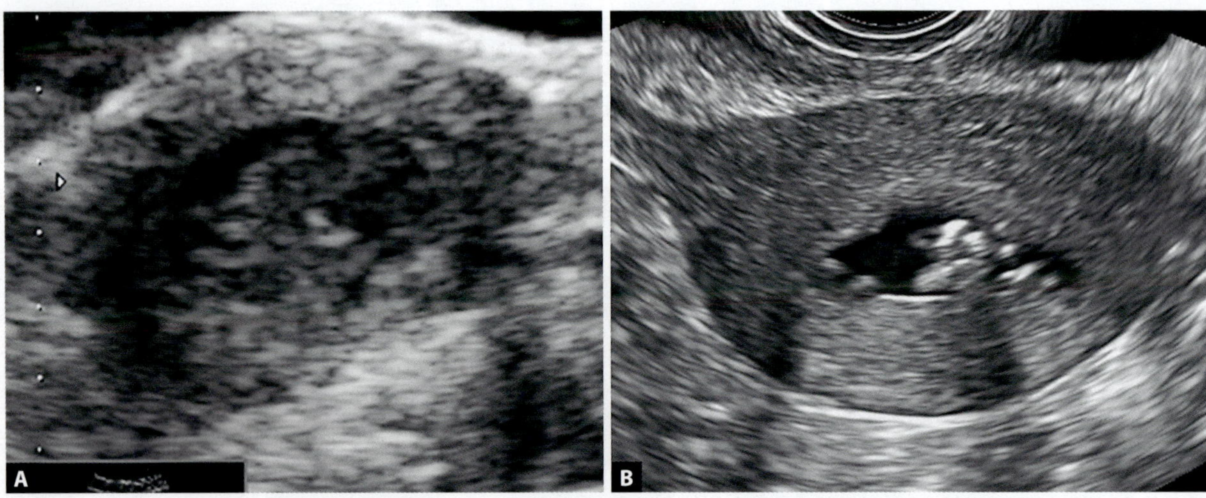

Figs. 20A and B: (A) Heterogeneous content in endometrial cavity: postcurettage; (B) Incomplete abortion.

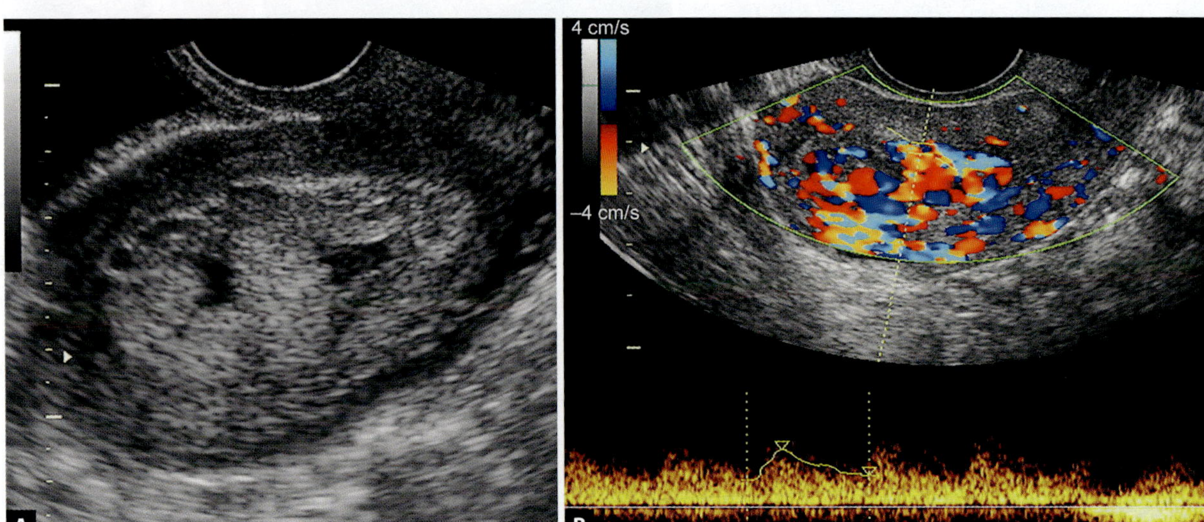

Figs. 21A and B: Vesicular mole. (A) 2D ultrasound (US); (B) Doppler.

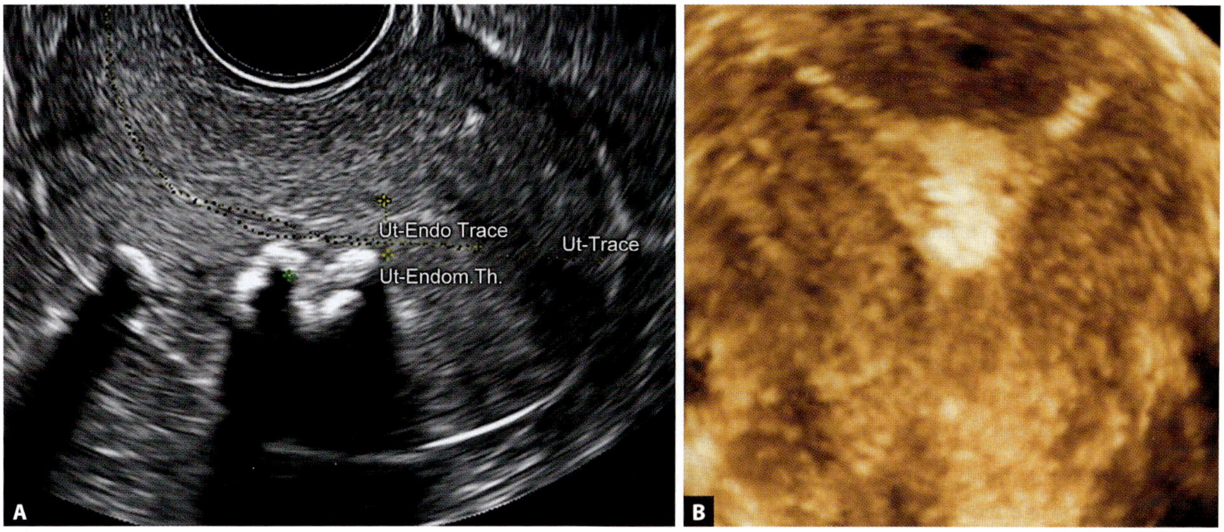

Figs. 22A and B: Endometrial calcification (A) 2D; and (B) 3D.

Adnexa

Adnexal lesions can be categorized as:

- Ovarian lesions
- Tubal/tubo-ovarian lesions
- *Miscellaneous lesions*: Paraovarian cysts, peritoneal inclusion cyst, and broad ligament fibroids.

Ovarian Lesions

Before describing a lesion, it is important to decide the origin of the lesion. The signs used to confirm the origin of the lesion from the ovary are:

- Place a probe in such a way that the lesion and the ovary are seen in the same frame on the screen. Apply pressure with the probe, to separate the two. If probe pressure can displace the two away from each other, the lesion is not arising from the ovary. If the two cannot be separated, the lesion is either adherent to the ovary or it is arising from the ovary.
- If the lesion is arising from the ovary, the lesion will be partially or completely covered by normal ovarian tissue and is typically described as a "rim sign" or "beak sign" **(Fig. 23)**.

Having confirmed the origin of the lesion from the ovary, the differential diagnosis of these lesions can be thought of. We would prefer to do this by dividing these lesions into different categories based on their US appearance.

Ultrasound-based classification of ovarian lesions:

- Nonseptated clear cysts
- Cysts with internal echogenicities and septae
- Solid lesions
- Complex lesions with cystic with solid areas.

Nonseptated clear cysts: These cysts are thin walled, have no internal echogenicities, no septae or no solid areas in it.

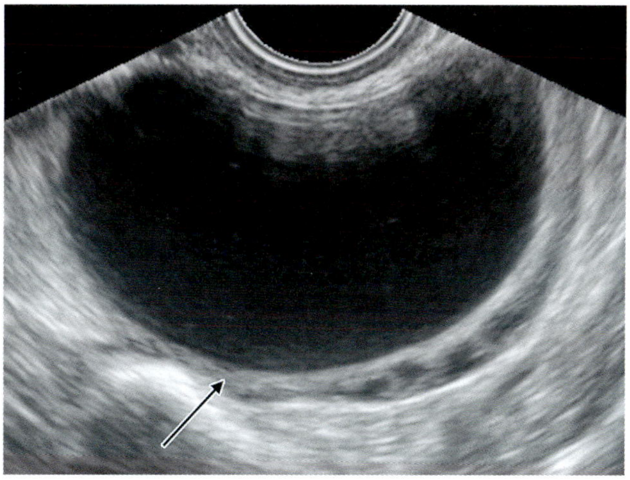

Fig. 23: Beak sign—intraovarian lesion.

The lesions/structures in this category are:

- Follicular cyst
- Simple cyst of the ovary.

Follicular cyst: Follicle starts growing in early follicular phase. It grows till 18–24 mm in diameter before it ruptures due to the surge of luteinizing hormone (LH) to release the ovum that it contains. If the surge is inadequate or does not occur, the follicle will not rupture and will result in a hormonally inactive/only minimally active structure. This is termed as a follicular cyst when it grows beyond 25 mm and persists in luteal phase of the cycle or even in the subsequent cycle. Contrary to the normal follicle, the follicular cyst shows scanty and high resistance flow. But it is ultimately a physiological cyst and would resolve on its own.

Simple cyst of the ovary: It is a thin-walled intraovarian cystic structure usually >5 cm. No internal echogenicities or septae seen. Doppler shows no flow. It does not resolve on its own and may require US-guided aspiration usually.

Cysts with internal echogenicities and septae:
The most common lesions in this category are:
- Corpus luteum
- Hemorrhagic cyst
- Luteinized unruptured follicle (LUF)
- Endometrioma.

All these structures have thick, shaggy walls, internal echogenicities and avascular septae. The appearance may vary, viz. absolutely isoechoic homogeneous, clear fluid, lace-like or cobweb pattern or ground glass appearance or debris seen as solid areas.

Corpus luteum: It has thick, crenulated walls. Contents of the cyst show heterogeneous echogenicity with or without septae. The echogenicity and appearance of the contents may change at different times. Doppler gives almost a complete ring of color with low resistance (RI <0.5). That is the most characteristic feature to separate it from other lesions with similar appearance on B-mode **(Figs. 24A to C)**.

Hemorrhagic cyst: It is a cyst containing blood. It is most of the times a result of unresolved corpus luteum but is hormonally inactive and therefore shows very scanty and high resistance blood flow. It changes echogenicity over the time due to fibrinolysis of the clot **(Fig. 25)**.

Luteinized unruptured follicle: It has thick, echogenic but not very shaggy walls, and does not contain blood or blood products. Therefore, it does show low level internal echogenicity but never lace-like or cobweb echogenicity **(Fig. 26)**.

The three above described lesions (corpus luteum, hemorrhagic cyst, LUF) are physiologic ovarian cysts and 53–89% of these show spontaneous regression on follow-up after 4–6 weeks.[13] To avoid confusing these with other lesions, two scans 2–3 weeks apart should be done so that assessment can be done in two different phases of menstrual cycle and complete or partial resolution of these lesions can be demonstrated.

Endometrioma: Endometriosis is detected in 15% of infertile women. It may cause acquired dysmenorrhea, dyspareunia, irregular bleeding, and infertility. One-third to one-half of the ovarian endometriotic cysts is bilateral. Most endometriomas are positioned medially or retrouterine. Features, typical of endometriomas, are thick shaggy walls with or without septae, internal echogenicities, ground glass appearance, fluid levels (with anechoic fluid anteriorly),

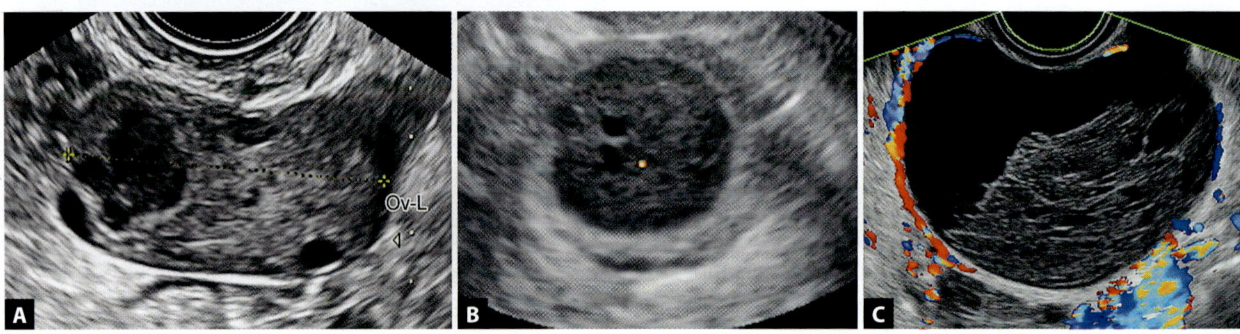

Figs. 24A to C: Different appearances of corpus luteum, also showing ring of color in the last frame.

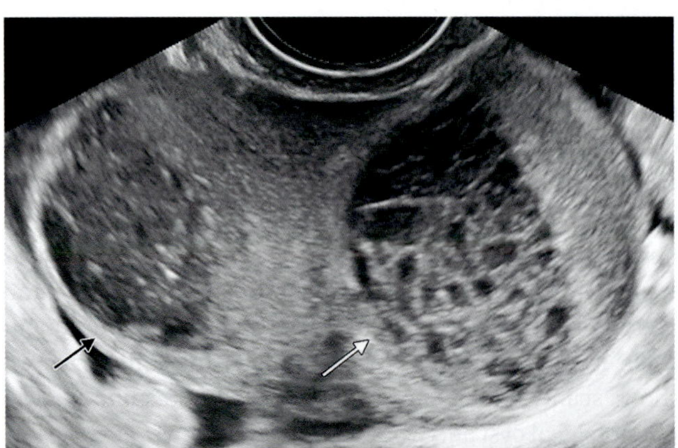
Fig. 25: Hemorrhagic cyst (white arrow) and endometrioma (black arrow).

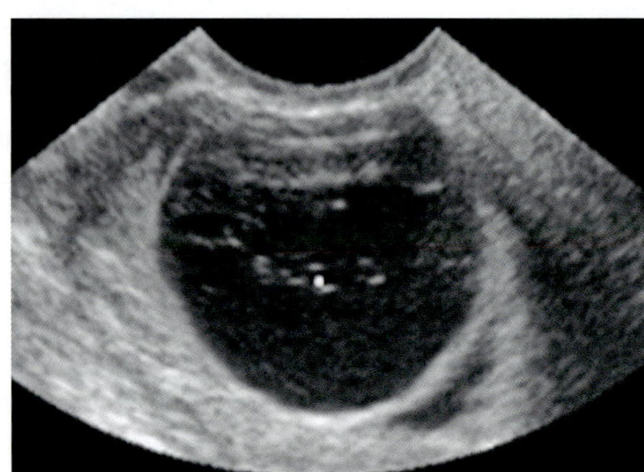
Fig. 26: Luteinized unruptured follicle (LUF): echogenic margins and internal echogenicity.

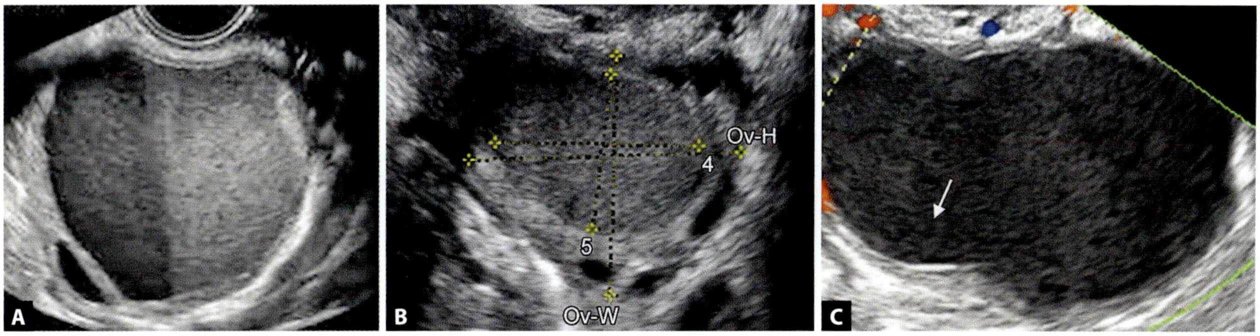

Figs. 27A to C: Endometrioma showing (A) Fluid level; (B) Ground-glass appearance, and (C) Echogenic flecks in wall.

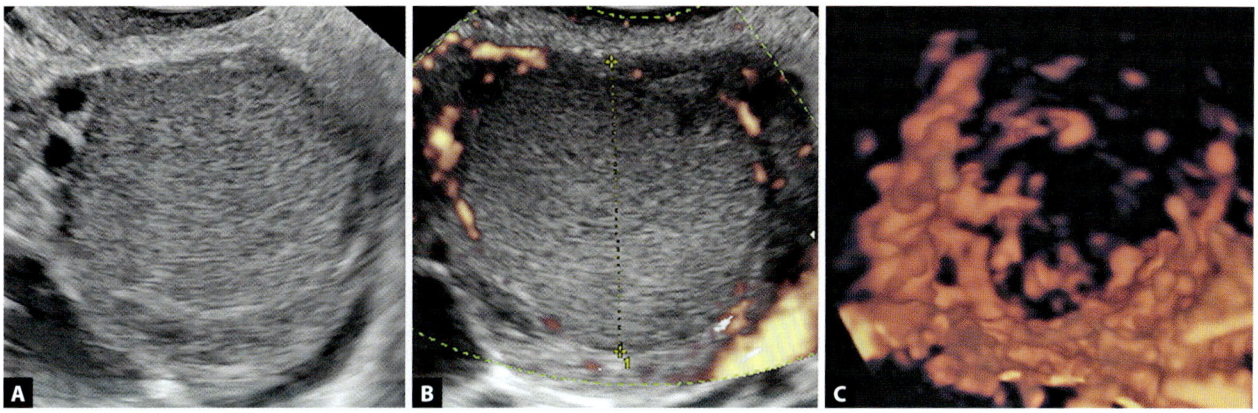

Figs. 28A to C: Endometrioma: (A) B-mode; (B) Power Doppler (PD) showing short-coursed peripheral vessels; and (C) 3D PD showing bird's nest appearance.

linear echogenic flecks in its walls **(Figs. 27A to C)**, and pain on pressure with the probe. Adhesions are very common. Solid areas may be sometimes seen. Streaming sign is often seen. This is slow downward movement of small low level echogenicities seen in endometrioma (chocolate cyst).

On Doppler: Scattered vascularity at ovarian hilus with moderate vascular impedance has been described in literature. Vascularity is higher during menstruation and in symptomatic patients.[14] Vascularity can be used as a means to decide the mode of therapy for endometriomas. Avascular lesions indicate scarification and are less convenient for delivery of medication and therefore should be considered for surgical therapy.[15]

Three-dimensional US allows detection of surface of the endometrioma, visualization of preserved ovarian tissue, and assessment of the ovarian relationship with neighboring pelvic structures. 3D PD typically shows multiple short-coursed regularly separated pericystic vessels giving a typical bird's nest appearance **(Figs. 28A to C)**.[16]

Kurjak et al. have shown a sensitivity of 83.9%, specificity of 97.1%, positive-predictive value (PPV) 82%, and negative-predictive value (NPV) 97.5% of vaginal sonography for characterization of endometriomas. If CA 125 > 35 IU/mL was added as a cutoff to these parameters, the sensitivity and specificity reached 99.04% and 99.64%, and PPV and NPV reached 98.10% and 99.82%, respectively.[15] Similar results were also confirmed by several other workers.

Solid lesions: Most common lesion in this group is fibroma. It is well-defined round/oval lesion with echogenicity like that of a fibroid—hypoechoic, homogeneous, but sometimes may be heterogeneous and may also show calcifications **(Figs. 29A and B)**. These may often be missed when small as fibroma is isoechoic to ovarian stroma. Like fibroids, fibromas also show peripheral vascularity.

Fibromas may also be pedunculated at times and may be confused with broad ligament fibroids and pedunculated subserosal uterine fibroids. Fibromas can be differentiated from fibroids by tracing the blood supply. Fibromas are often bilateral and may also be associated with ascites and pleural effusion. This complication is known as Meigs' syndrome.

Other lesions in this group are quite rare and may be thecoma, fibrothecoma, Brenner's tumor, etc.

Solid looking ovaries may also be seen in ovarian torsion. Stroma is hypoechoic with peripherally placed small follicles. Vascularity may or may not be present and that decides the viability of the ovary. Definitive sign is a whirlpool sign in adnexa due to twisting of vessels.[17]

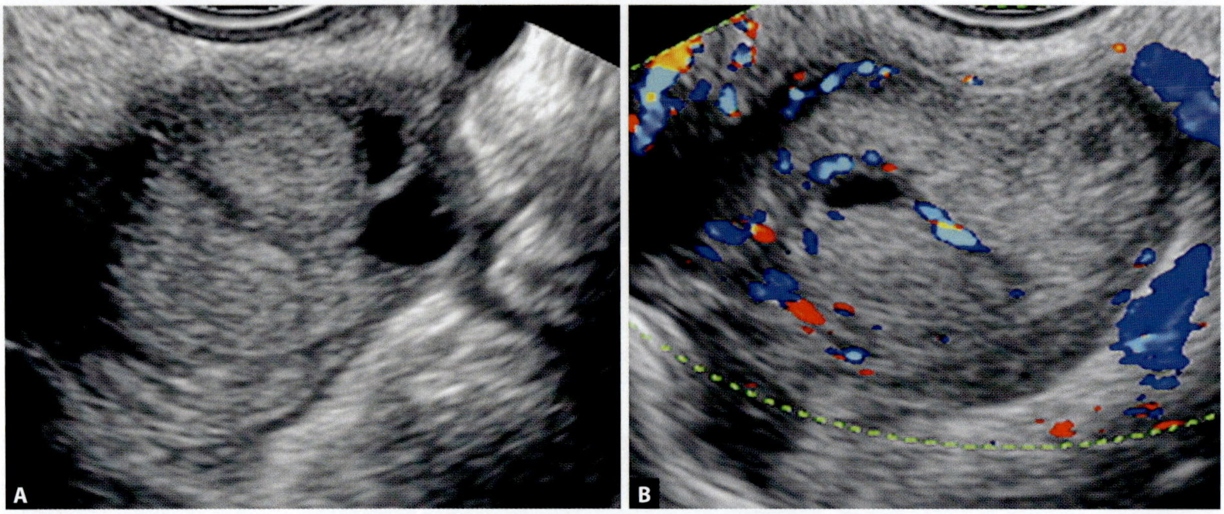

Figs. 29A and B: Ovarian fibroma with peripheral vascularity.

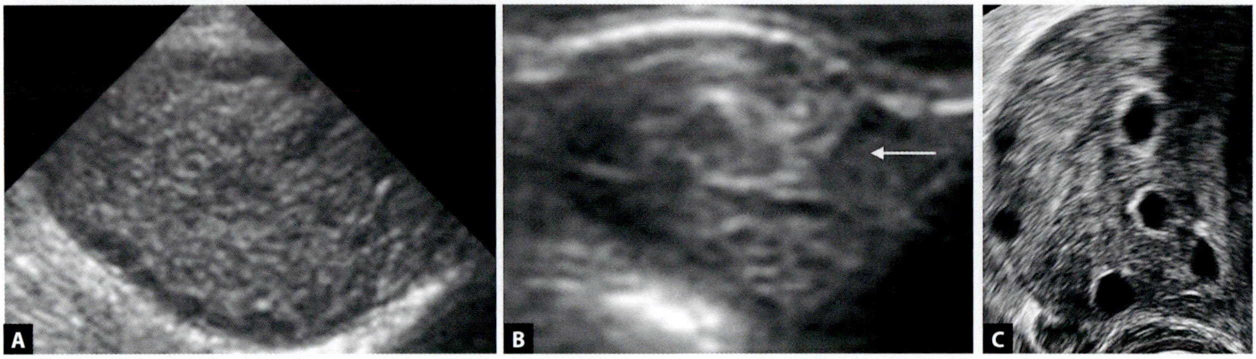

Figs. 30A to C: Enlarged ovary with (A) Peripherally placed follicles; (B) Whirlpool sign (arrow); and (C) Follicular ring sign.

Though this sign is not easy to pick up in patients of torsion due to the severe pain that they have.

Follicular ring sign has been claimed to be the earliest sign of ovarian torsion **(Figs. 30A to C)**.[18] This is a hyperechoic line surrounding the small follicles in the torsed ovary. It is a transient sign, only seen during early phase of torsion and is due to ovarian congestion and edema on occlusion of venous and lymphatic flow.

Complex lesions with cystic with solid areas: Lesions in this group have thick walls, with internal echogenicities and also solid projections arising from the walls. Lesions included in this group are:

- Dermoids
- Epithelial tumors
- Endometrioid tumors.

Dermoids: These are often an incidental finding. These are well-defined lesions with thick walls, low-level echoes, fluid-fluid level (with anechoic fluid posteriorly), hyperechoic lines and dots due to hair, hyperechoic/calcified echoes like teeth with posterior shadowing, regional diffuse bright echoes with or without acoustic shadowing due to hair clumps or fat in Rokitansky's protuberance **(Figs. 31A to E)**. 72% of cystic teratomas are avascular.

These features have been assigned for definite PPV:[10]

- 80% for shadowing echodensity
- 75% for regionally bright echoes
- 50% for hyperechoic lines and dots
- 20% for fluid-fluid level.

Positive-predictive value for more than two features is 100%.

Morphologic scoring system for dermoids by Kurjak et al. has sensitivity of 93.1% and specificity of 99.4%. Including color Doppler, sensitivity of 99% and specificity of 99.8% can be achieved.[19]

Epithelial tumors: Surface epithelial-stromal tumors account for 60% of ovarian neoplasms and 80–90% of ovarian malignancies. Of all these 46% are serous, 36.5% are mucinous, and 7.5% are endometrioid. These tumors are chiefly cystic, have septae, internal echogenicities, and projections arising from its walls. Benign and malignant counterparts of these tumors have a similar but overlapping US appearance. On US, therefore it is not possible to give

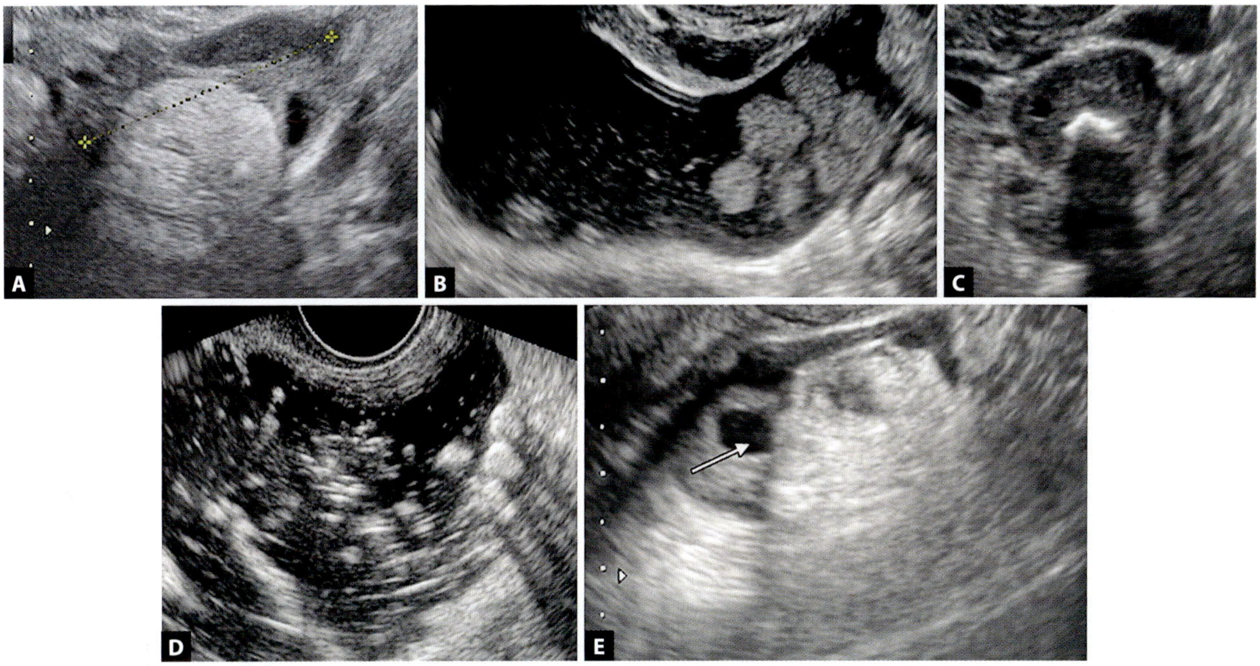

Figs. 31A to E: Dermoids: echogenic mass, hairballs in cyst, small echogenic area, teeth with posterior shadowing and echogenic lines and dots, large Rokitansky's tubercle (arrow).

a histopathological diagnosis. One can only doubt its malignant nature by US and we shall not discuss this here as malignancies are not common in infertile patients.

Tubal Lesions

Pelvic inflammatory disease (PID): Most common of tubal lesions are inflammatory in origin. These lesions are usually a part of PID and may also involve uterus and ovaries also to variable extent.

Inflammation of Fallopian tubes is known as salpingitis. Like inflammation anywhere in the body salpingitis leads to edema and hyperemia. On US, this is seen as thickened adnexa, >10 mm in transverse diameter or thickened tube walls if there is fluid surrounding may be appreciated with central hyperechoic mucosa. Normally, blood vessels are seen in adnexa on color Doppler and are parallel to the long axis of adnexa. But in acute salpingitis several small vessels are seen and these are not parallel to the long axis of adnexa but the run across. On pulse Doppler, these vessels show low resistance (RI < 0.45). In early phase of PID, ovarian parenchymal blood flow also shows low to moderate RI: 0.53 ± 0.09, but in chronic stage, it increases to 0.71 ± 0.09.[20] Regression of the infection on its own or in response to antibiotic, decreases the flow in tubes and ovaries. Salpingitis is usually associated with oophoritis. This is characterized by enlarged ovaries with hypoechoic stroma and increased vascularity. Salpingitis may lead to hydrosalpinx.

On US, extraovarian cystic lesion is seen in adnexa. On rotating the probe 90°, it changes its shape and becomes elongated **(Figs. 32A and B)**. It may typically show a retort, sausage or serpiginous shape. It can be differentiated from bowel by lack of peristalsis and from a blood vessel by Doppler which shows no flow.

It may show incomplete septae that are due to tubal haustra **(Figs. 32A and B)**. On transverse section, this tube gives a cogwheel appearance, due to fibrotic remnants of endosalpingeal tissue, or beads-on-a-string appearance on long axis.[21] The fluid may show low-level echoes if the collection becomes thicker and also at times purulent. 3D US with inversion mode rendering is a very good tool to demonstrate such lesions **(Figs. 33A and B)**.

Extension of the inflammatory process further may also involve the ovary and also sometimes bowel or omentum in vicinity and forms tubo-ovarian abscess **(Figs. 34A and B)**. It is seen as a complex lesion on US with low resistance (RI: 0.44 ± 0.04)[22] vascularity in its solid areas and wall.

Free fluid may be seen in pelvis. Abscess when heals still leaves a cyst behind or it causes fibrous scarring—tubo-ovarian adhesions and then shows high resistance vascularity (RI: 0.75 ± 0.04).

Timor-Tritsch et al. defined the sonographic markers for the tubal inflammation **(Table 5)**.[23]

Clinical correlation is very essential to differentiate inflammatory process from neoplastic process.

Saline infusion salpingography (SIS) and hysterosalpingo-contrast sonography (HyCoSy) are very useful investigations for assessment of tubal evaluation. Though, laparoscopy is a gold standard as these investigations do not give information about tubo-ovarian relations.

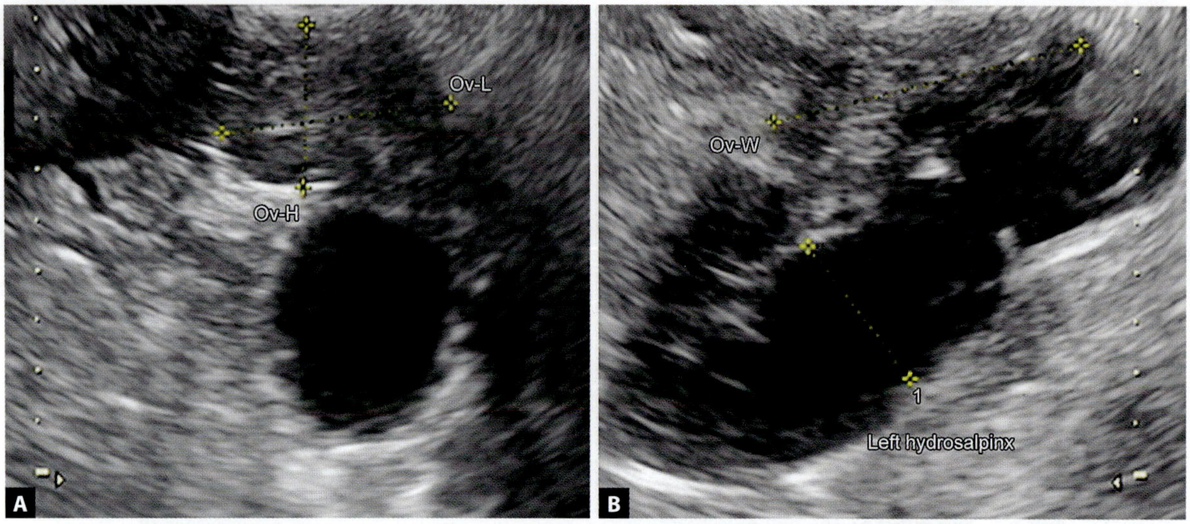

Figs. 32A and B: Hydrosalpinx: (A) Cystic roundish lesion in adnexa changes in (B) Shape on rotating the probe.

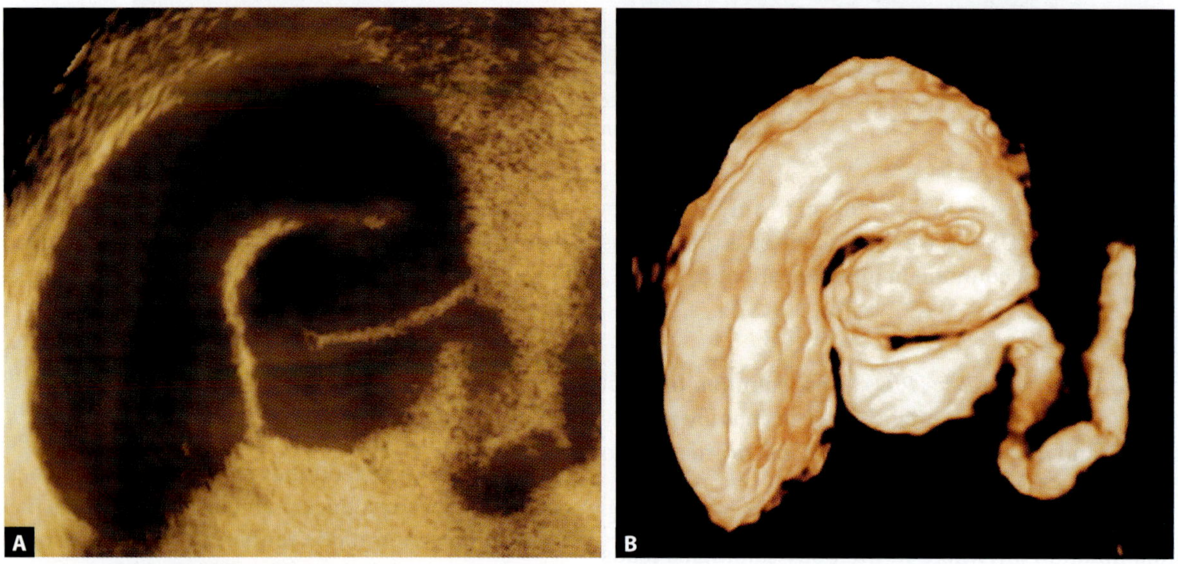

Figs. 33A and B: Hydrosalpinx: 3D ultrasound (US), surface rendering and inversion mode.

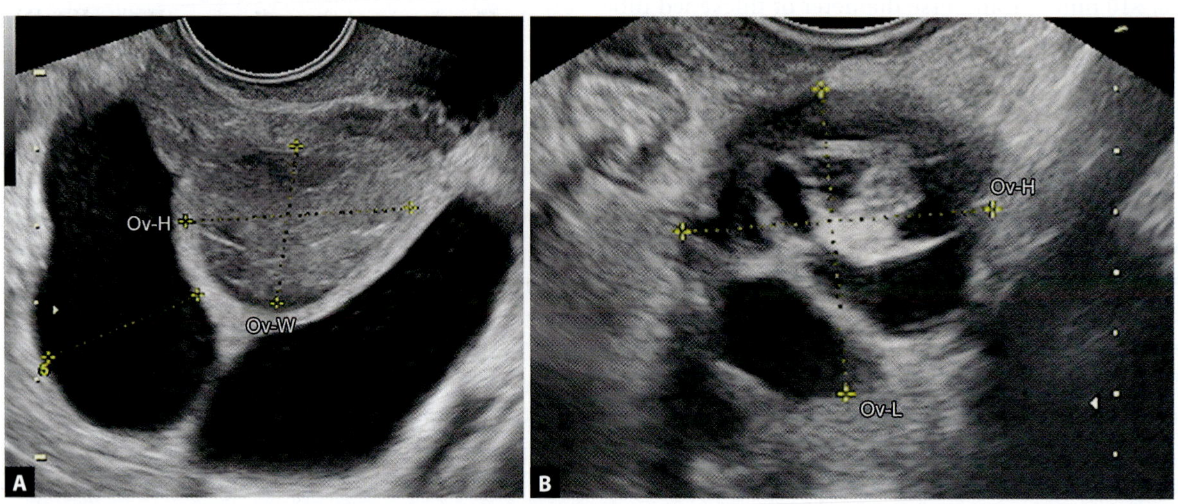

Figs. 34A and B: Pelvic inflammatory disease (PID): (A) Adherent ovary and distended tube; (B) Tubo-ovarian abscess where tube and ovary cannot be separately identified.

TABLE 5: Sonographic markers for the tubal inflammation.

	Acute	*Chronic*
Thickened tube wall ≥5 mm	100%	3%
Cogwheel sign	86%	3%
Incomplete septa (92%)	—	—
Beads-on-a-string appearance	00%	57%
(Flattened/fibrotic endosalpingeal folds 2–3 mm hyperechoic nodules on cross section of fluid-filled structure)		
Tubo-ovarian complex	36%	2%
Tubo-ovarian abscess	—	—
Fluid in cul-de-sac	50%	10%

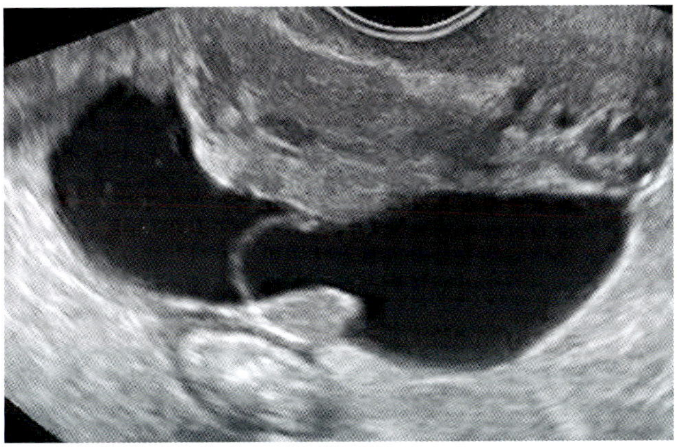

Fig. 35: Peritoneal inclusion cyst: irregular shape and lax septum.

Miscellaneous Lesions

- Broad ligament fibroid
- Peritoneal inclusion cyst
- Paraovarian cyst.

Broad ligament fibroid: On US, it is a well-circumscribed, usually round, hypoechoic lesion. It can be separated from both uterus and ovary by probe pressure and shows peripheral vascularity.

Peritoneal inclusion cyst: It is a fluid collection in the pelvic peritoneum with septations. This fluid collection is not under pressure and therefore changes shape on probe pressure. The septae inside move with respiration, pressure, or with pulsations of nearby vessel. These lesions typically do not show any vascularity **(Fig. 35)**.

Paraovarian cyst: Up to 20% of adnexal masses may be paraovarian cysts. These are benign, avascular lesions with thin walls and anechoic contents. The shape does not change with pressure but can be easily separated from ovary. Adhesions indicate infection and solid projections in it may raise a possibility of malignancy.

CYCLE ASSESSMENT

Cycle assessment consists of baseline scan, preovulatory scan, and secretory scan.

Hormonal changes occurring during the menstrual cycle are reflected as vascular changes and therefore color Doppler in this assessment is mandatory. 3D US is especially useful for volume measurements. 3D PD has given promising results in initial studies.

Baseline Scan

This scan is done on day 2–3 of the cycle. At this time of the cycle, ovaries have no active follicles or residual corpus luteum. This scan is differed to next cycle if the ovaries show any follicle larger than 9 mm or a residual corpus luteum. This scan consists of TVS, transvaginal color Doppler (TVCD), and volume US of ovaries and uterus. It is done to classify the ovary in one of the four categories: (1) polycystic ovaries (PCO), (2) normal ovaries, (3) low reserve ovaries, and (4) poorly responding ovaries. Or in other words to predict the ovarian reserve and response that can guide to decide the stimulation protocols for assisted reproductive technology (ART).

Ovaries

Two-dimensional US assessment of the ovaries consists of assessment of ovarian diameters and volume and counting of antral follicles as quantitative assessment and qualitative assessment of stromal density. Color or PD is used to see the presence of vessels in the stroma. If vascularity is present, pulse wave Doppler is used for quantitative assessment of the flows—intraovarian RI and peak systolic velocity (PSV). Then 3D and 3D PD volume of the ovary is acquired for ovarian volume and stromal volume, counting number of antral follicles. Global vascular indices—vascularity index (VI), flow index (FI), and vascularity flow index (VFI)—may be calculated, the values for these are not yet established but are likely to give promising results. Normal ovaries are 3–6 cc in volume with 512 antral follicles, and stromal flow with RI of 0.58–0.7 and PSV of between 5 and 10 cm/sec.

Ultrasound and Doppler Features for Polycystic Ovaries

Enlarged ovaries (>10 cc in volume) and multiple antral follicles (>20 antral follicles per ovary), according to Rotterdam criteria and dense stroma with or without asynchronous endometrium, are the features of PCO. But each of the features need elaborate discussion.

Enlarged ovaries: On 2D US, an ovary with the longest diameter of >3.5 cm is considered enlarged. Volume of the ovary is calculated by measuring three orthogonal diameters and applying the formula $(x \times y \times z) \times 0.523$. Calculation of ovarian volume by virtual organ computer-aided analysis (VOCAL) on 3D US is much more accurate **(Fig. 36)**.

According to the Rotterdam criteria, ovarian volume of 10 cc is a criterion for polycystic ovarian disease (PCOD).

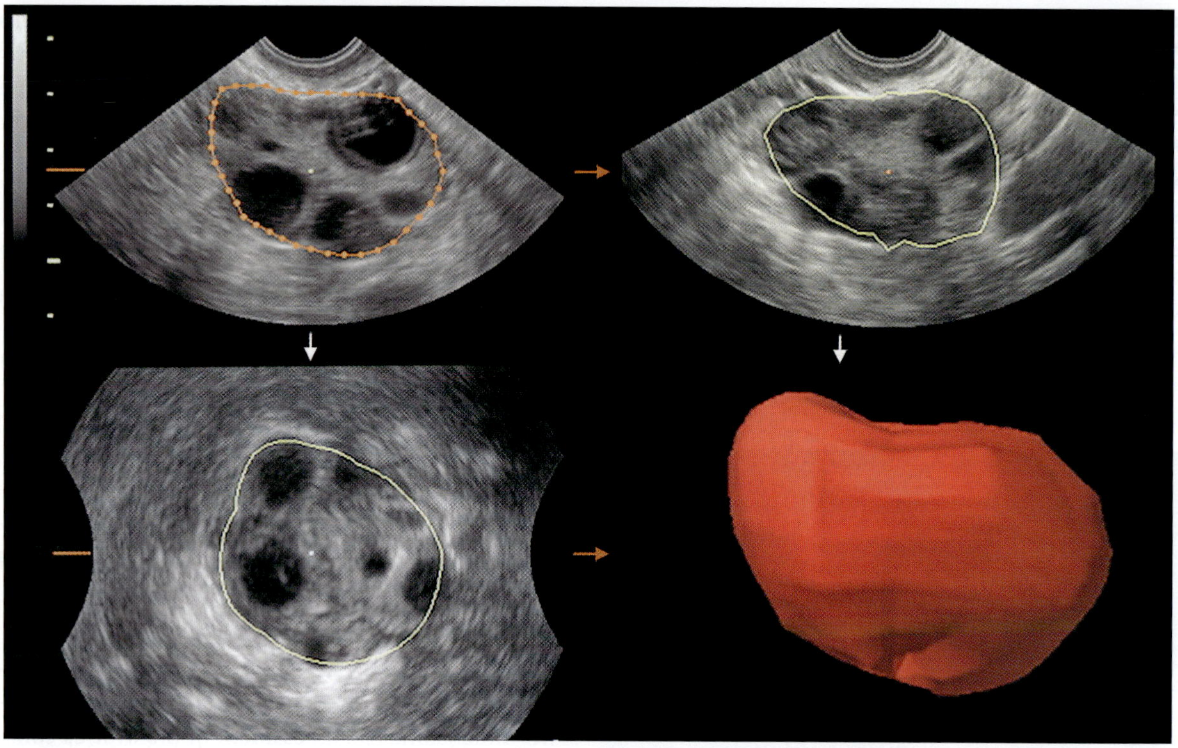

Fig. 36: Three-dimensional ultrasound with volume calculation of ovary by virtual organ computer-aided analysis (VOCAL).

"For an ovarian size of 10 cc, a good correlation has been shown between US diagnosis of polycystic morphology and histopathological criteria for PCO."[24] But reports have also shown that an ovarian size of 6.6 cc has 91% sensitivity and 91% specificity for polycystic ovarian syndrome (PCOS).[25] And yet another report says, "However, ovaries which are normal in volume can be polycystic as demonstrated by histological and biochemical studies (in 20%)".[26] This means ovarian volume cannot be used as the criteria for diagnosis of PCO.

Polycystic ovarian morphology has been found to be a better discriminator than ovarian volume between PCOS and control women.[27]

These morphological features are multiple antral follicles, their arrangement, atretic follicles and predominant stroma.

Multiple immature follicles: 20 or more antral follicles[61] of 2–9 mm size have also been quoted as one of the US features of PCOS. But this number has also been reported from 5 to 15 in different reports. Though setting the threshold at 12 for 2–9 mm follicle number per ovary (FNPO) offered the best compromise between specificity (99%) and sensitivity (75%).[28]

The more recent studies suggest FNPO of >19–20[29] antral follicles especially in PCO patients are difficult to count on 2D US. If 3D volume of the ovary is acquired and then is rendered in inversion mode or Sono-automatic volume calculation (Sono-AVC) is used, the antral follicle count is reliably done.

It is known that tonic elevation of LH in PCO patients in follicular phase leads to theca and stromal cell hyperplasia and increased androgen production. This leads to recruitment of multiple follicles in the ovaries. And altered LH:follicle-stimulating hormone (FSH) ratio in PCO does not allow maturation of small follicles, instead these become atretic. In the course of time, these atretic follicles get converted into theca cells and contribute to stroma.[30] In the early phase of the disease, the stroma becomes denser leading to a generalized cystic pattern (GCP) of PCO. As the disease progresses, not only the stromal density but also the stromal volume increases, leading to enlargement of the ovary. Along with this, the follicles are also pushed to the peripheral cystic pattern (PCP) of PCO. This means that from multicystic ovaries (ovaries normal in size having multiple follicles of various sizes and normal stroma) which is a normal appearance in adolescence to GCP PCO and PCP PCO is a process of evolution as a result of high basal androgen levels in these females **(Figs. 37A and B)**.[30] This explains not only the variability in the size of the ovaries but also the variability in the number of antral follicles in patients having oligo-ovulation and hyperandrogenism in patients with PCOS.

Predominant hyperechoic stroma: Polycystic ovaries show a hyperechoic stroma but assessment of this hyperechogenicity is subjective not only to the operator but also to equipment settings.[31,32] Therefore, a more objective or reproducible criteria would be ovarian area or stromal

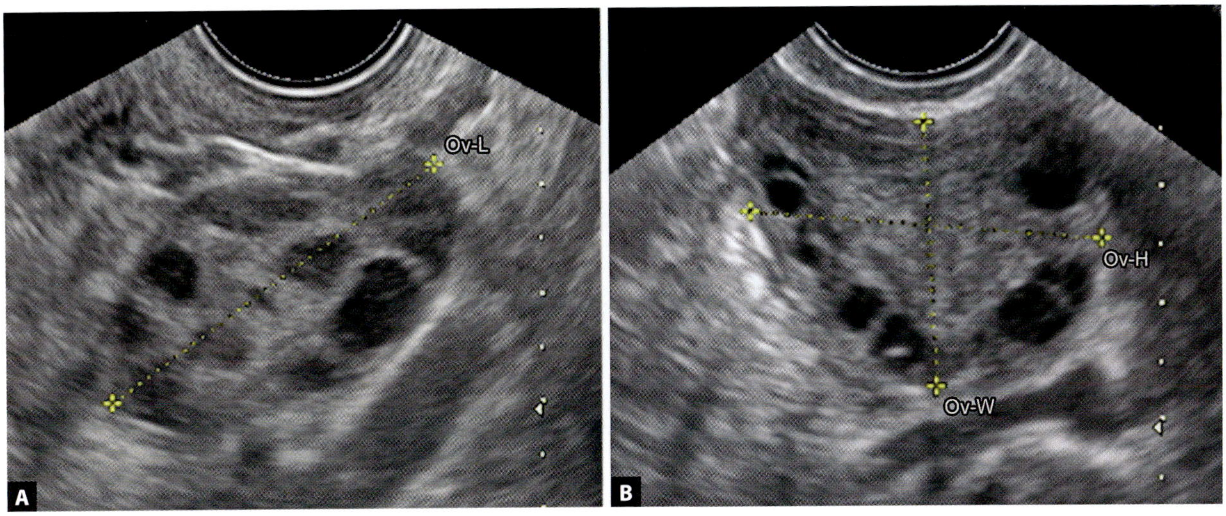

Figs. 37A and B: (A) Generalized cystic pattern; (B) Peripheral cystic pattern in polycystic ovaries.

TABLE 6: Sensitivity for diagnosis of polycystic ovary syndrome.

Ovarian volume	13.21 cc	21%
Ovarian area	7 cm^2	4%
Stromal area	1.95 cm^2	62%
Stromal/total area	0.34	100%

area. Ovarian area of 5.3 cm^2 on strict longitudinal ovarian section and stromal area of 4.6 cm^2 has high sensitivity for PCOS.[25]

Sensitivity for diagnosis of PCOS has been presented in **Table 6.**[33]

Ovarian volume and stromal volume can be calculated by acquiring a 3D volume of the ovary, calculating its volume by VOCAL and then using threshold volume, adjusting the threshold to exclude the follicles **(Fig. 38)**.

We have found stromal volume to ovarian volume ratio of >70% in an ovary that is larger than 6.6 cc or has >12 antral follicles in 95% of PCOS patients in a study of 800 PCOS patients studied (unpublished data).

Apart from these major features, PCOS patients show atypical endometrium or out of phase endometrium due to the hormonal derangements like high LH and early rise of estrogen due to multiple follicle recruitment and conversion of androgen to estrogen. It has also been observed by some workers that right to left ovarian volume ratio is reversed in PCOS patients. In control patients, left ovary is larger than right, and in PCOS patients right ovary is larger than left.[25]

These ovaries show increased and moderate resistance stromal flow on the baseline scan. Vessels close to the developing follicles are not stromal vessels. On pulse Doppler, these vessels show RI 0.50–0.58.[34] This is a reflection of high LH levels. If these blood vessels also show a PSV of >10 cm/sec, they are prone to hyperstimulation. High androgen levels in these patients also lead to high uterine artery pulsatility index (PI) **(Figs. 39A and B)**.

It is interesting to note here that higher uterine artery PI and lower ovarian stromal vessel resistance are seen in PCP ovaries than GCP ovaries, higher age, amenorrheic, rather than oligomenorrheic patients and in obese, hyperinsulinemic, and hirsute patients.

Second type of ovaries is poorly responding ovaries. These may be any size but have intraovarian stromal RI >0.70, and PSV <5 cm/sec. They have low vascularity and therefore respond to higher doses of stimulation.

Third type is low reserve ovaries which are small-sized ovaries with <2 cm in longest diameter or <3 cc in volume and have <3 antral follicles. They will produce very few follicles with any stimulation.

Based on this, predictors of ovarian response are:[35]

- Number of antral follicles
- Ovarian stromal FI
- Total ovarian stromal area
- Total ovarian volume.

In that order of importance, antral follicle count is a better marker than basal FSH for selection of older patients with acceptable pregnancy offer.[36] Antral follicle count and ovarian volume showed significant correlation with anti-Müllerian hormone (AMH), total testosterone, and free androgen index.[37]

Precise calculation of antral follicle count therefore can help in predicting the ovarian response. This can be done on 2D US by scanning across the whole ovary while counting the follicles. But this has high chances of error when follicles are multiple as in PCO. In these cases, counting the antral follicles by 3D US, using VOCAL, inversion mode **(Fig. 40A)** or Sono-AVC (GE Healthcare) is much more precise. Using this software, each follicle is coded by a different color and diameters and volumes of each are calculated separately.

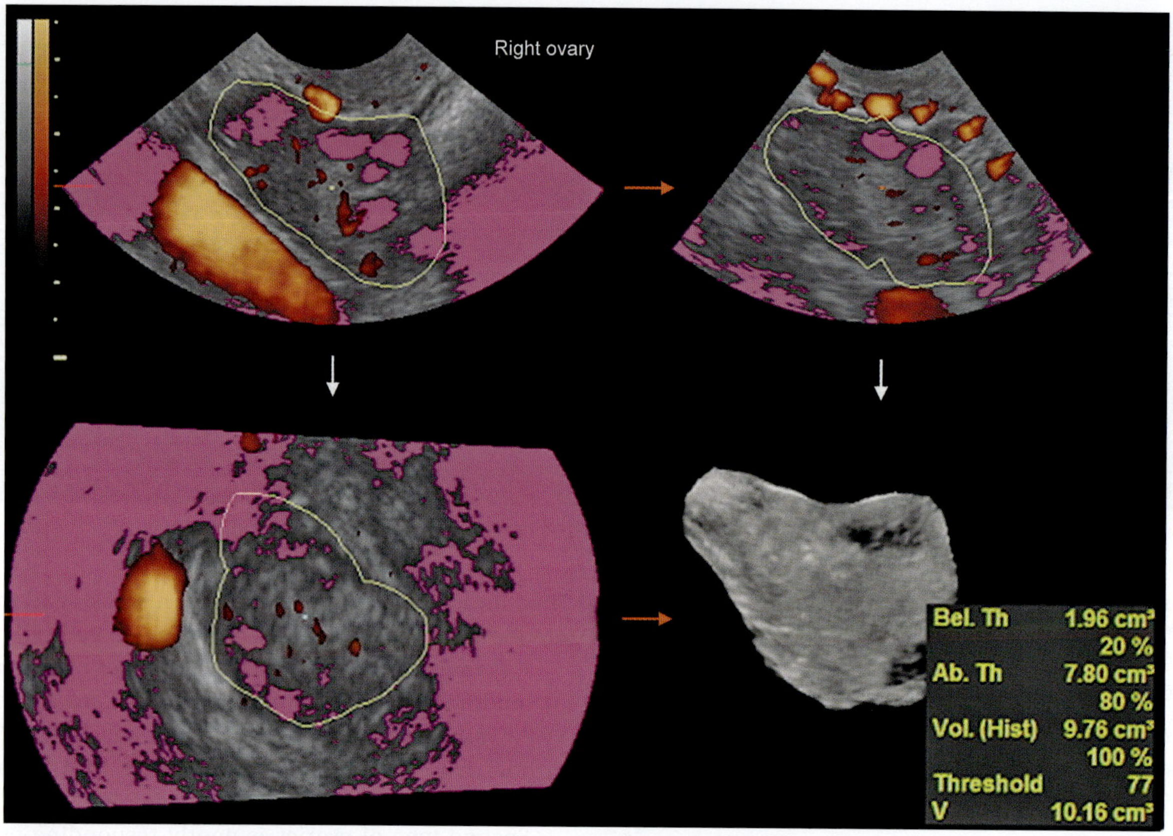

Fig. 38: Three-dimensional ultrasound of ovary with volume calculated by virtual organ computer-aided analysis (VOCAL) and stromal volume calculated by applying threshold volume to VOCAL calculated ovarian volume.

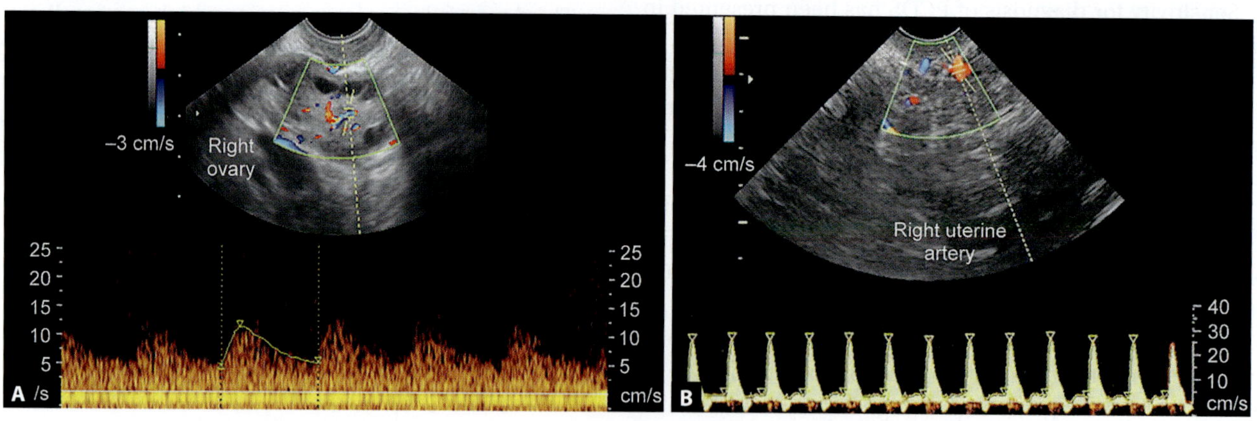

Figs. 39A and B: (A) Low resistance ovarian stromal flow; (B) High resistance uterine artery flow.

This is a more precise method as there is no overcounting of follicles. But to avoid undercounting, postprocessing is required **(Fig. 40B)**.

It has also been shown by Zaidi et al. that stromal blood flow velocity after pituitary suppression was an independent predictor of ovarian response.[28] Kupesic has shown correlation in the ovarian stromal FI and number of mature oocytes retrieved in an in vitro fertilization (IVF) cycles and pregnancy rates.[35]

Uterus

Baseline scan of the uterus is done to assess the uterocervical length by US. Longitudinal section of the uterus is imaged on the screen where whole of the uterus is seen with endometrial cavity starting from fundus to the internal os and external os. For all ART procedures may it be intrauterine insemination (IUI) or embryo transfer (ET), the uterocervical length is measured from the fundal end of the endometrium

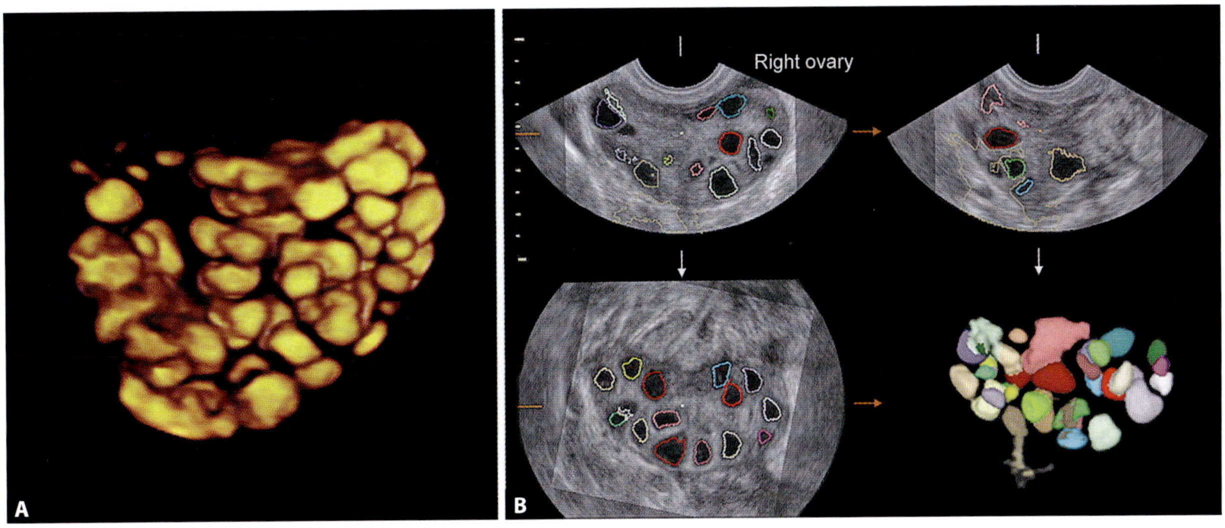

Figs. 40A and B: (A) Three-dimensional (3D) volume of polycystic ovary rendered in inversion mode; (B) 3D volume of polycystic ovary with Sono-automatic volume calculation (AVC).

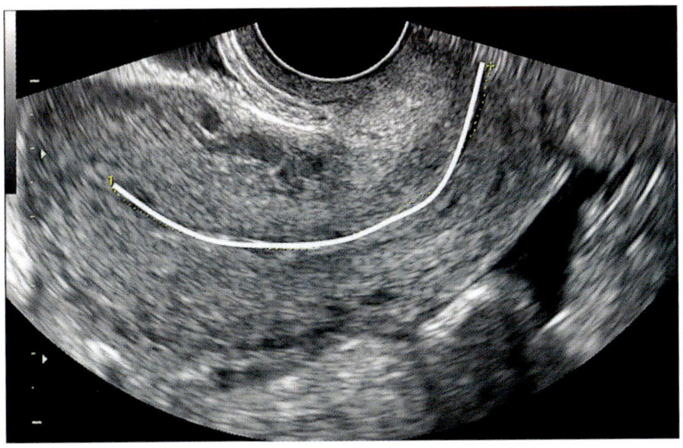

Fig. 41: Measuring functional uterocervical length.

to the external os and is known as functional/physiological uterocervical length **(Fig. 41)**. Doppler of the uterine artery is done. Uterine artery RI >0.79 indicates that high doses of stimulation will be required for endometrial maturation.[38,39] Subendometrial flow on day 2, if it is present, indicates a low receptive endometrium for implantation.

Preovulatory Scan

A follicle that grows to 10 mm is a dominant follicle and grows at a rate of 2–3 mm/day and ovulation occurs at 18–24 mm size. Follicular flow can be first detected when follicular size is 10 mm[40] and its RI starts falling 2 days prior to ovulation.

Features of a Mature Follicle

A rounded 16–18 mm sized follicle with thin walls and no internal echogenicity is seen. A sonolucent halo appears surrounding the follicle 24 hours prior to ovulation. Cumulus oophorus a small projection from wall in the follicular lumen may be seen.

On color Doppler, vascularity is seen covering three-fourth of the follicle. On pulse Doppler, these vessels show RI 0.4–0.48,[41] PSV > 10 cm/sec **(Figs. 42A and B)**. This means that if the follicle is said to be functionally mature when PSV is at least 10 cm/sec, i.e., the time when the LH surge starts and under the effect of that LH, the perifollicular PSV keeps rising constantly. The follicular PSV rises as high as 45 cm/sec before an hour of ovulation. We have done a study of 300 IUI cycles based on this. Single IUI was done between 36 and 38 hours and double IUI were done at 12–14 hours and 36–38 hours after hCG, in all patients in whom perifollicular PSV >15 cm/sec. When perifollicular PSV on the day of hCG was >20 cm/sec, and perifollicular RI was within normal range, double IUI has given higher pregnancy rates **(Fig. 43)**.[42]

Fertilization of a follicle with a PSV of <10 cm/sec has high chances of embryo with chromosomal abnormality.

Rising PSV with steady low RI suggests that the follicle is close to rupture.[40] Steady or decreasing PSV with rising RI suggests that the follicle is proceeding toward LUF.[43]

Application of 3D US for Follicular Assessment (Figs. 44A to D)

When there is multifollicular development as in PCO the follicular shapes become polygonal and therefore follicular diameter may not be a reliable parameter. Follicular volume by 3D is a more reliable parameter. Follicular volumes of between 3 and 7 cc are optimum for oocyte retrieval. The limits of agreement between the volume of the follicular aspirate and 3D volume of the follicle were +0.96 to –0.43 with 3D and +3.47 to –2.42 by 2D volume estimation.[44]

Cumulus can be seen in 80–90% of follicles using 3D US rendering. This is possible only in up to 30–40% follicles by 2D US. On the day of hCG, if cumulus like echo is not seen

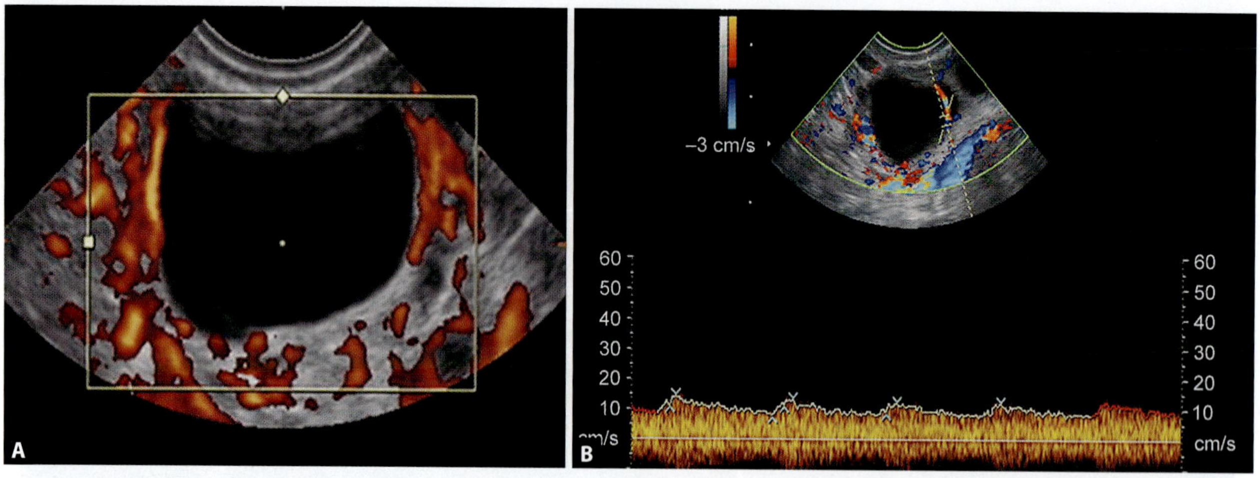

Figs. 42A and B: (A) Perifollicular flow on power Doppler; (B) Spectral Doppler of perifollicular flow.

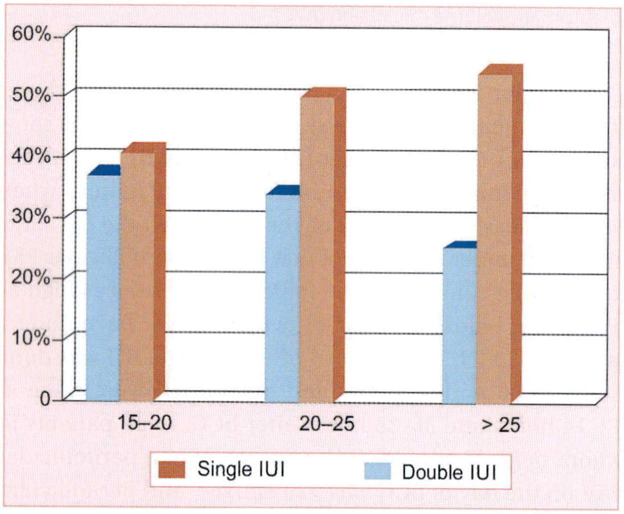

Fig. 43: Graphic representation showing increased pregnancy rates with double intrauterine insemination (IUI) in patients with perifollicular peak systolic velocity (PSV) >20 cm/sec.

in all three planes in the follicle, it is less likely to be mature fertilizable oocyte.[45] This information is especially useful in ART cycles where very few follicles are available. If cumulus is seen in the follicle and ovum is not retrieved, flushing of follicle may be recommended.

Three-dimensional PD gives idea about the global vascularity of the follicle. We have done a large study taking this into consideration. Based on study of >1,000 cycles, follicular volume of 3–7.5 cc, VI >6–20 and FI >35 if used as additional features of a mature follicle apart from the follicular features mentioned earlier in this chapter, these increased the pregnancy rates significantly.[46]

Features of a Mature Endometrium

On 2D US, endometrium should be 6 mm or more in thickness, preferably 8–10 mm. It should have an intact uniform endometriomyometrial junction and should be multilayered. But its morphological assessment is essential.

Endometrial grading:[47]

- *Grade A endometrium:* Multilayered with intervening area more echogenic than myometrium **(Fig. 45A)**
- *Grade B endometrium:* Multilayered with intervening area hypoechoic to myometrium
- *Grade C endometrium:* Homogeneous isoechoic endometrium

Two-dimensional US assesses the anatomy of the endometrium but its functional maturity can be assessed by Doppler of spiral arteries. Vascularity has been considered to be a better marker than morphology for endometrial receptivity.[48]

On color Doppler, the vascularity is classified by Applebaum as follows:[48]

- *Zone I:* Blood vessels reaching endometriomyometrial junction surrounding the endometrium
- *Zone II:* Blood vessels reaching hyperechoic endometrial edge
- *Zone III:* Blood vessels reaching internal endometrial hypoechoic zone
- *Zone IV:* Blood vessels reaching endometrial cavity **(Fig. 45B)**

On pulse Doppler, these blood vessels should show RI 0.49–0.59 and PI 1.1–2.3.

Even if TVCD of follicle is normal, endometrial and the uterine artery indices should be within normal limits for implantation. Absent subendometrial and intra-endometrial vascularization on the day of hCG, appears to be a useful predictor of failure of implantation in IVF, irrespective of morphological appearance.[49]

It has also been observed that when pregnancy is achieved in absence of endometrial and subendometrial flow on the day of ET, more than half of these pregnancies will finish as spontaneous miscarriage.[50]

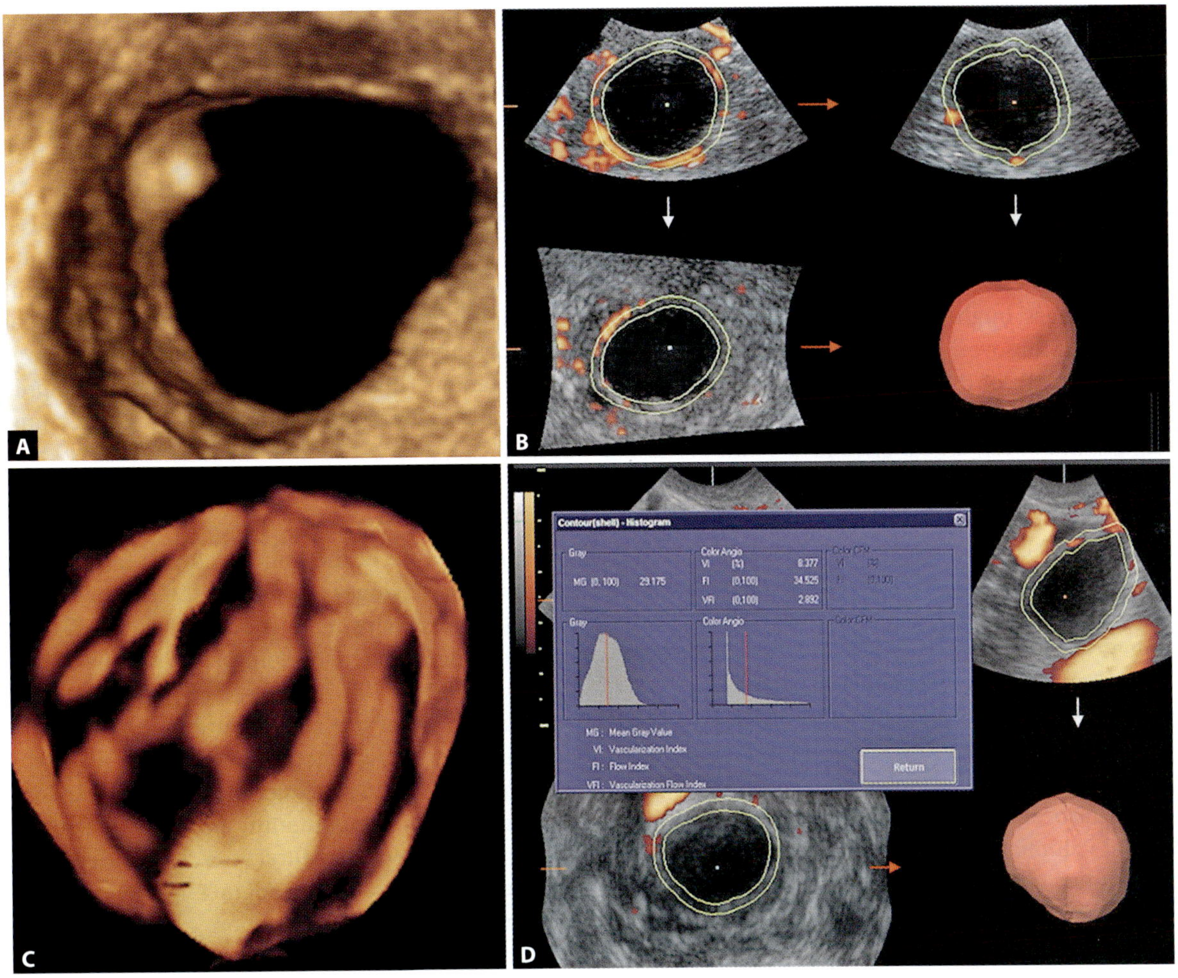

Figs. 44A to D: (A) Cumulus oophorus in follicle on 3D ultrasound (US) of follicle rendered view; (B) 3D power Doppler volume of follicle with virtual organ computer-aided analysis (VOCAL) and shell volume calculation; (C) 3D power angiography of perifollicular flow; (D) Calculation of 3D power Doppler vascular indices (volume histogram) after VOCAL and shell volume for perifollicular flow.

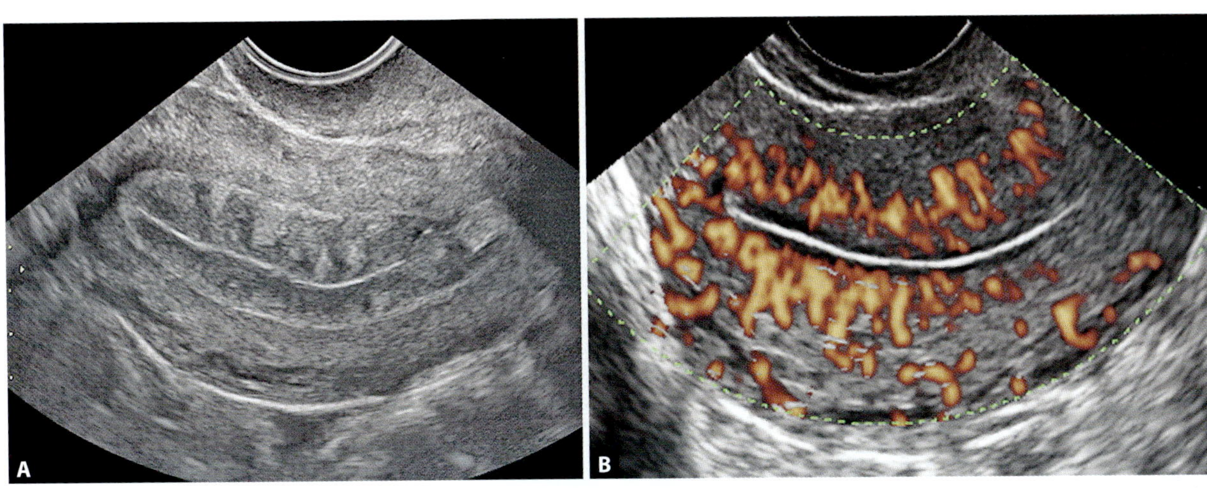

Figs. 45A and B: (A) Grade A endometrium on 2-D ultrasound (US); (B) Zone IV vascularity seen in endometrium on power Doppler.

Apart from endometrium and follicle, it is also essential to evaluate the uterine artery flow on the dominant side before hCG. The normal values of uterine artery are RI 0.60–0.80 and PI 2.22–3.16.[45] Even if TVCD of follicle is normal, endometrial and the uterine artery indices should be within normal limits for implantation. Doppler study for uterine receptivity should be done on the day of hCG. Embryo transfers in IVF cycles are also canceled if the uterine artery

PI >3.2.[51] hCG administration induces significant increase in the resistance of uterine artery for 48 hours and can affect its evaluation on the day of follicular aspiration/rupture therefore Doppler study for uterine receptivity should be done on the day of hCG.[37]

As for the follicle, the endometrium also, if evaluated by 3D and 3D PD, is more reliable. It gives endometrial volume instead of endometrial thickness. When we measure endometrial thickness, we measure it at the thickest part, and this thickness might not be uniform in the whole endometrium. Moreover, sometimes in spite of normal thickness the length of the endometrial cavity may be so little that the total endometrial volume is not enough for implantation. Moreover, 3D PD gives idea about the global vascularity of the endometrium not only in terms of quality but also in terms of quantity, which should be a more useful parameter than 2D Doppler where we can see vessels only in one plane at a time and also interrogate a few vessels not all. In our study, 25 3D PD studies that we have found reliable are endometrial volume >3 cc, FI >20 and VFI >5 **(Figs. 46A and B)**. There are several other people who have also worked on endometrial receptivity assessment by 3D and 3D PD. A study by Merce et al. of 40 IVF cycles has shown endometrial volume of 3–7 mL as most favorable for conception. Median values for a favorable endometrium are 4.28 ± 1.9 mL.[52] Endometrial volume of >2.0 mL has a significantly higher pregnancy rates and no pregnancies were recorded with endometrial volume of <1 mL.[53]

No pregnancy was documented when endometrial volume <3 mL and VI <10. Exceptionally better pregnancy rates were achieved with endometrial volume >7 ml and subendometrial VI between 10% and 35%.[51]

A study by Kupesic et al. shows lower RI of 0.49–0.57 in subendometrial vessels and FI of 11.0–15.4 in conception cycles as compared to 9.5–13.3 otherwise.[54]

Vascularity flow index on the day of trigger is more sensitive than volume, VI, and FI for prediction of pregnancy. VFI >0.24 has sensitivity of 83.3%, specificity of 88.9%, PPV 93.8%, and NPV 72.3% for prediction of pregnancy with 33% pregnancy rate.[55]

Scoring system has also been developed for endometrial receptivity, which apart from the endometrial thickness, morphology, vascularity, and uterine artery. Doppler also includes uterine contraction count. Calculating contractions/minute, >5 contractions/minute is considered bad for implantation and, 3–5 contractions/minute is considered good for implantation. This is purely based on the fact a uterus which is highly contractile, will not allow implantation. Though this scoring system is not practically applicable as even with full scores pregnancy might not occur.

Secretory Scan

With the rupture of the follicle, corpus luteum is formed and secretory changes are seen in the endometrium in the form of echogenicity of the endometrium which starts from outside, proceeding to the central line making a ring sign of the endometrium.[56]

Assessment of the corpus luteum endometrium and uterine artery by Doppler gives information about the luteal phase normalcy and progesterone levels. A clear correlation between RI of corpus luteum and plasma progesterone levels has been seen in natural cycle. RI of the corpus luteum can therefore be used as an adjunct to plasma progesterone assay as an index of luteal function.[57]

A healthy corpus luteum will show a vascular ring surrounding itself on color Doppler and on PD these vessels show RI 0.35–0.50, PI 0.70–0.80 **(Fig. 47A)**, and PSV 10–15 cm/sec.[43,58] This resistance starts increasing on day 23 of the cycle in a nonconception cycle. Endometrial Doppler shows branches of spiral arteries piercing the outer echogenic margins of the endometrium and better if vascularity reaches the central line with RI 0.48–0.52 **(Fig. 47B)**. Uterine artery at this time of the cycle is 2.0–2.5 and PSV 15–20 cm/sec.

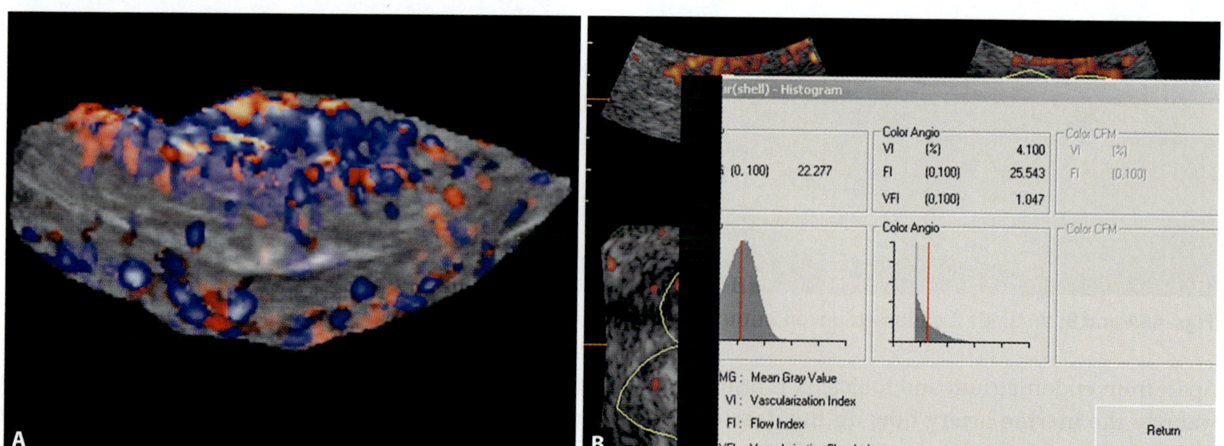

Figs. 46A and B: (A) Three-dimensional (3D) power angiography; and (B) Volume histogram of endometrium.

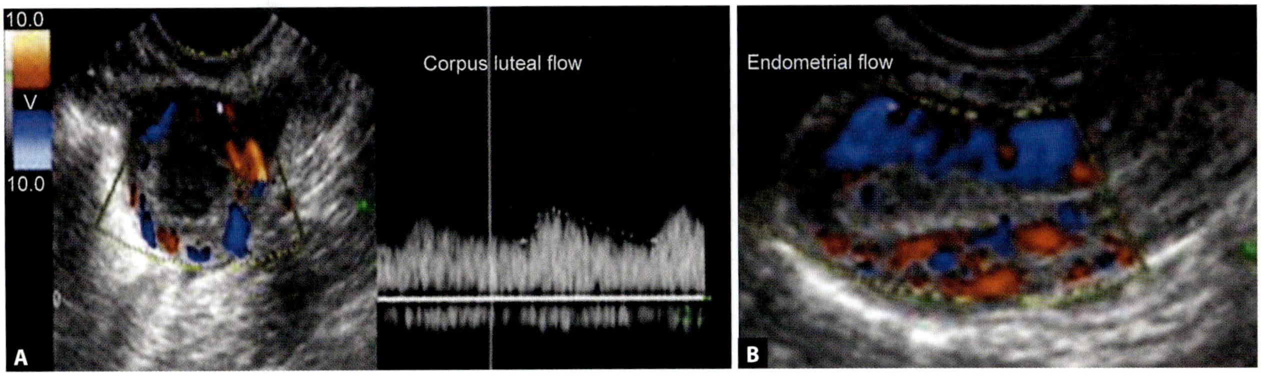

Figs. 47A and B: (A) Corpus luteum; and (B) Endometrial Doppler in secretory phase.

Based on these values, abnormal parameters indicate luteal phase problems like LUF or luteal phase defect.

Luteinized Unruptured Follicle

On 2D US, LUF is seen as persistent follicle with thick walls and progressive loss of cystic appearance which is difficult to differentiate from corpus luteum. Endometrium is thick and echogenic and no fluid is seen in pouch of Douglas (POD). On Doppler, perifollicular RI is 0.51–0.59, which is higher than normal and remains almost steady till the end of the cycle. Nondominant ovary also shows similar Doppler indices. Endometrial flow is also absent.[43]

Luteal Phase Defect

On Doppler, corpus luteum shows high resistance RI 0.58 ± 0.04. Bilateral ovarian RI shows no difference. Increased resistance is also seen in spiral arteries RI 0.72 ± 0.06.[59]

Increased resistance to uterine blood flow in the midluteal phase may be an important contributing factor to some causes of infertility and the cause of some previously "unexplained" infertility.[60] Segmental uterine and ovarian artery perfusion demonstrates a significant correlation with histological and hormonal markers of uterine receptivity and may aid assessment of luteal phase defect.

As quoted by Golan et al., Shoham et al., and Tan SL et al.:

"In the hands of experienced operators, ultrasound alone suffices for cycle monitoring, with no necessity for additional hormonal estimations."

CONCLUSION

Though follicle size and endometrial thickness assessment that are commonly used as monitoring tools for managing treatment cycles, this is grossly inadequate information for the same. Study of the blood flows by doppler helps to monitor the cycles more closely as these reflect the hormonal changes and allows the functional assessment of the follicle and endometrium through out the cycle.

KEY POINTS

- Three-dimensional US is a modality of choice for differential diagnosis of congenital uterine abnormalities.
- Sonohysterography is a modality of choice for differential diagnosis of endometrial pathologies.
- Color Doppler helps for differential diagnosis of myometrial and endometrial lesions.
- Ovarian lesions must be assessed at least twice, 2–3 weeks apart before stamping the diagnosis.
- For complex adnexal masses, clinical correlation is important.
- Baseline scan is a must before starting ART.
- Stromal morphology and vascularity assessment are must to diagnose PCO.
- Timing of hCG should never be decided without color Doppler assessment of follicle and endometrium.
- Luteal phase Doppler is a key to diagnose luteal phase problems.

REFERENCES

1. Raga F, Bonilla-Musoles F, Blanes J, Osborne NG. Congenital Müllerian anomalies: diagnostic accuracy of three-dimensional ultrasound. Fertil Steril. 1996;65(3):523-8.
2. Richman TS, Viscomi GN, deCherney A, Polan ML, Alcebo LO. Fallopian tubal patency assessed by ultrasound following fluid injection. Radiology. 1984;152(2):507-10.
3. The American Fertility Society classification of adnexal adhesions, distal tubal occlusion secondary to tubal ligation, tubal pregnancies, Mullerian anomalies and intrauterine adhesions. Fertil Steril 1998;49(6):944-55.
4. Grimbizis GF, Gordts S, Sardo ADS, Brucker S, Angelis CD, Gergolet M, et al. The ESHRE/ESGE consensus on the classification of female genital tract congenital anomalies. Human Reproduction. 2013;28(8):2032-44.
5. Barbot J. Hysteroscopy and hysterography. Obstet Gynecol Clin North Am. 1995;22(3):591-603.
6. Kupesic S, Kurjak A. Septate uterus: detection and prediction of obstetrical complications by different forms of ultrasonography. J Ultrasound Med. 1998;17(1):631-6.
7. Ludwin A, Martins WP, Nastri CO, Ludwin I, Cohelho Neto MA, Leitao VM, et al. Congenital uterine malformation by

Experts(CUME): Better criteria for distinguishing between normal, arcuate and septate uterus. Ultrasound Obstet Gynecol 2018;51(1):101-9.
8. Salim R, Woelfer B, Backos M, Regan L, Jurkovic D. Reproducibility of three- dimensional ultrasound diagnosis of congenital uterine anomalies. Ultrasound Obstet Gynecol. 2003;21(6):578-82.
9. Wamsteker K, de Blok S. Resection of intrauterine fibroids. In: Lewis BV, Magos AL (Eds). Endometrial Ablation. Edinburgh, UK: Churchill Livingstone; 1993.
10. Kurjak A, Kupesic-Urek S, Miric D. The assessment of benign uterine tumor vascularization by transvaginal color Doppler. Ultrasound Med Biol. 1992;18(6-7):645-9.
11. Munro MG, Critchley HOD, Broder MS, Fraser IS, FIGO working group on menstrual disorders. FIGO classification system (PALM-COEIN) for causes of abnormal uterine bleeding in nongravid women of reproductive age. Int J Gynecol Obstet. 2011;113(1):3-13.
12. Cil AP, Tulunay G, Kose MF, Haberal A. Power Doppler properties of endometrial polyps and submucosal fibroids: a preliminary observational study in women with known intracavitary lesions. Ultrasound Obstet Gynecol. 2010; 35(2):233-7.
13. Osmers R. Sonographic evaluation of ovarian masses and its therapeutical implications. Ultrasound Obstet Gynecol. 1996;8(4):217-22.
14. Alcázar JL. Transvaginal colour Doppler in patients with ovarian endometrium as and pelvic pain. Hum Reprod. 2001;16(12):2672-5.
15. Kurjak A, Kupesic S. Scoring system for prediction of ovarian endometriosis based on transvaginal color and pulsed Doppler sonography. Fertil Steril. 1994;62(1):81-8.
16. Raine-Fenning N, Jayaprakasan K, Deb S. Three-dimensional ultrasonographic characteristics of endometriomata. Ultrasound Obstet Gynecol. 2008;31(6):718-24.
17. Vijayaraghavan SB. Sonographic whirlpool sign in ovarian torsion. J Ultrasound Med. 2004;23(12):1643-9.
18. Sibal M. Follicular ring sign: a simple sonographic sign for early diagnosis of ovarian torsion. J Ultrasound Med. 2012;31(11):1803-9.
19. Kurjak A, Kupesic S, Babic MM, Goldenberg M, Illijas M, Kosuta D. Preoperative evaluation of cystic teratoma: what does color Doppler add? J Clin Ultrasound. 1997;25(6):309-16.
20. Kupesic S, Kurjak A, Pasalic L, Benic S, Elijas M. The value of transvaginal color Doppler in the assessment of pelvic inflammatory disease. Ultrasound Med Biol. 1995;21(6):733-8.
21. Timor-Tritsch IE, Rottem S, Lewitt N. The Fallopian tube. In: Timor Tritsch IE, Rottem S (Eds). Transvaginal Sonography, 2nd Edition. New York: Chapman and Hall; 1991. pp. 131-44.
22. Zalel Y, Soriano D, Lipitz S, Mashiach S, Achiron R. Contribution of color Doppler flow to the ultrasonographic diagnosis of tubal abnormalities. J Ultrasound Med. 2000;19(9):645-9.
23. Timor-Tritsch IE, Lerner JP, Monteagudo A, Murphy KE, Heller DS. Transvaginal sonographic markers of tubal inflammatory disease. Ultrasound Obstet Gynecol. 1998;12(1):56-66.
24. Wu MH, Tang HH, Hsu CC, Wang ST, Huang KE. The role of three-dimensional ultrasonographic images in ovarian measurement. Fertil Steril. 1998;69(6):1152-5.
25. Kupesic S, Kurjak A, Bjelos D. Sonographic imaging in infertility. In: Kurjak A, Arenas JB (Eds). Donald School Textbook of Transvaginal Ultrasound, 1st edition. New Delhi, India: Jaypee Brothers Medical Publishers (P) Ltd.; 2005. pp. 357-83.
26. Legros RS, Chiu P, Kunselman AR, Bentley CM, Dodson WC, Dunaif A. Polycystic ovaries are common in women with hyperandrogenic chronic anovulation but do not predict metabolic or reproductive phenotype. J Clin Endocrinol Metab. 2005;90(5):2571-9.
27. Jonard S, Robert Y, Cortet-Rudelli C, Pigny P, Decanter C, Dewaily D. Ultrasound examination of polycystic ovaries: is it worth counting the follicles. Hum Reprod. 2003;18(3): 598-603.
28. Zaidi J, Campbell S, Pittrof R, Kyei-Mensah A, Shaker A, Jacobs SH, et al. Ovarian stromal blood flow in women with polycystic ovaries—a possible new marker for diagnosis? Hum Reprod. 1995;10(8):1992-6.
29. Dewailly D, Gronier H, Poncelet E, Robin G, Leroy M, Pigny P, et al. Diagnosis of polycystic ovarian syndrome. Revisiting the threshold values of follicle count on ultrasound and of serum AMH level for the definition of polycystic ovaries. Hum Reprod. 2011;26(11):3123-29.
30. Takahashi K, Ozaki T, Okada M, Uchida A, Kitao M. Relationship between ultrasonography and histopathological changes in polycystic ovarian syndrome. Hum Reprod. 1994;9(12):2255-8.
31. Ardaens Y, Robert Y, Lemaitre L, Fossati P, Dewaily D. Polycystic ovarian disease: contribution of vaginal endosonography and reassessment of ultrasonic diagnosis. Fertil Steril. 1991;55(6): 1062-8.
32. Robert Y, Dubrulle F, Gaillandre L, Ardaens Y, Lemaitre L, Dewaily D, et al. Ultrasound assessment of ovarian stroma hypertrophy in hyperandrogenism and ovulation disorders: visual analysis versus computerized quantification. Fertil Steril. 1995;64(2):307-12.
33. Fulghesu AM, Ciampelli M, Belosi C, Apa R, Pavone V, Lanzone A. A new ultrasound criterion for the diagnosis of polycystic ovarian syndrome: the ovarian stroma/total area ratio. Fertil Steril. 2001;76(2):326-31.
34. Matsunaga I, Hata T, Kitao M. Ultrasonographic identification of polycystic ovary. Asia-Oceania J Obstet Gynecol. 1985;11(2):227-32.
35. Kupesic S, Kurjak A. Predictors of IVF outcome by three-dimensional ultrasound. Hum Reprod. 2002;17(4):950-5.
36. Klinkert ER, Broekmans FJ, Looman CW, Habbema JDF, te Velde ER. The antral follicle count is a better marker than basal follicle-stimulating hormone for the selection of older patients with acceptable pregnancy prospects after in vitro fertilization. Fertil Steril. 2005;83(3):811-4.
37. Chen MJ, Yang WS, Chen CL, Wu MY, Yang YS, Ho. The relationship between anti-Müllerian hormone, androgen and insulin resistance on the number of antral follicles in women with polycystic ovary syndrome. Hum Reprod. 2008;23(4):952-7.
38. Tan SL. Clinical applications of Doppler and three-dimensional ultrasound in assisted reproductive technology. Ultrasound Obstet Gynecol. 1999;13(3):153-6.
39. Bassil S, Magritte JP, Roth J, Nisolle M, Donnez J, Gordts S. Uterine vascularity during stimulation and its correlation with implantation in in vitro fertilization. Hum Reprod. 1995;10(6):1497-501.

40. Bourne T, Jurkovic D, Waterstone J, Campbell S, Collins WP. Intrafollicular blood flow during human ovulation. Ultrasound Obstet Gynecol. 1991;1(1):53-9.
41. Kupesic S, Kurjak A. Ulterine and ovarian perfusion during the periovulatory period assessed by transvaginal color Doppler. Fertil Steril. 1993;60(3):439-43.
42. Nagori CB, Panchal SY. Double IUI in cases with high pre-hCG perifollicular PSV for better pregnancy rates: a randomized study of 350 IUI cycles. Presented at 16th World Congress on Ultrasound in Obstetrics and Gynecology, 2006, London. J Ultrasound Obstet Gynecol. 2006;28(4):612.
43. Kupesic S, Kurjak A. The assessment of normal and abnormal luteal function by transvaginal color Doppler sonography. Eur J Obstet Gynecol Reprod Biol. 1997;72(1):83-7.
44. Kyei-Mensah A, Zaidi J, Pittrof R, Shaker A, Campbell S, Tan SL. Transvaginal three-dimensional ultrasound: accuracy of follicular volume measurements. Fertil Steril. 1996; 65(2):371-6.
45. Feichtinger W. Transvaginal three-dimensional imaging for evaluation and treatment of infertility. In: Merz E (Ed). 3D Ultrasound in Obstetrics and Gynecology. Philadelphia: Lippincott Williams and Wilkins; 1998. pp. 37-43.
46. Panchal SY, Nagori CB. Can 3D PD be a better tool for assessing the pre-hCG follicle and endometrium? A randomized study of 500 cases. Presented at 16th World Congress on Ultrasound in Obstetrics and Gynecology, 2006, London. J Ultrasound Obstet Gynecol. 2006;28(4):504.
47. Gonen Y, Casper RF. Prediction of implantation by the sonographic appearance of the endometrium during controlled ovarian stimulation for in vitro fertilization (IVF). J In Vitro Fert Embryo Transf. 1990;7(3):146-52.
48. Applebaum M. The 'steel' and 'teflon' endometrium—ultrasound visualization of endometrial vascularity in IVF patients and outcome. Presented at the third World Congress of Ultrasound in Obstetrics and Gynecology. Ultrasound Obstet Gynecol. 1993;3(Suppl 2):10.
49. Zaidi J, Campbell S, Pittrof R, Tan SL. Endometrial thickness, morphology, vascular penetration and velocimetry in predicting implantation in an in vitro fertilization program. Ultrasound Obstet Gynecol. 1995;6(3):191-8.
50. Chien LW, Au HK, Chen PL, Xiao J, Tzeng CR. Assessment of uterine receptivity by the endometrial-subendometrial blood flow distribution pattern in women undergoing in vitro fertilization-embryo transfer. Fertil Steril. 2002;78(2): 245-51.
51. Coulam CB, Stern JJ, Soenksen DM, Britten S, Bustillo M. Comparison of pulsatility indices on the day of oocyte retrieval and embryo transfer. Hum Reprod. 1995;10(1):82-4.
52. Merce LT, Barco MJ, Santiago B, Jose JB (Eds). 2D and 3D power Doppler Ultrasound study of endometrium as implantation marker. In: Kurjak A, Arenas JB (Eds). Donald Textbook of Transvaginal Sonography. New Delhi: Jaypee Brothers Medical Publishers; 2005. pp. 232-4.
53. Raga F, Bonilla-Musoles F, Casañ EM, Klein O, Bonilla F. Assessment of endometrial volume by three-dimensional ultrasound prior to embryo transfer: clues to endometrial receptivity. Hum Reprod. 1999;14(11):2851-4.
54. Kupesic S, Bekavac I, Bjelos D, Kurjak A. Assessment of endometrial receptivity by transvaginal color Doppler and three-dimensional power Doppler ultrasonography in patients undergoing in vitro fertilization procedures. J Ultrasound Med. 2001;20(2):125-34.
55. Wu HM, Chiang CH, Huang HY, Chao AS, Wang HS, Soong YK. Detection of subendometrial vascularization blood flow by three-dimensional ultrasound may be useful for predicting pregnancy rate for patients undergoing in vitro fertilization-embryo transfer. Fertil Steril. 2003;79(3):507-11.
56. Bald R, Hackeloer BJ. U ltraschall-darstellung verschiendener endometrium for men. In: Otto R, Jan FX (Eds). Ultraschalldiagnostik 1982. Stuttgart: Thieme; 1983. pp. 187.
57. Glock JL, Brumsted JR. Colour flow pulsed Doppler ultrasound in diagnosing luteal phase defect. Fertil Steril. 1995;64(3):500-4.
58. Salim A, Kurjak A, Zalud I. Ovarian luteal flow in normal and abnormal early pregnancies. J Maternal Fet Invest. 1992;2:119.
59. Kupesic S, Kurjak A, Vujisic S, Petrovic Z. Luteal phase defect: comparison between Doppler velocimetry, histological and hormonal markers. Ultrasound Obstet Gynecol. 1997; 9(2):105-12.
60. Steer CV, Tan SL, Mason BA, Campbell S. Midluteal-phase vaginal color Doppler assessment of uterine artery impedance in a subfertile population. Fertil Steril. 1994;61(1):53-8.
61. PCOS guideline: Human Reproduction. 2018 Sep 1;33(9):1602-1618. doi: 10.1093/humrep/dey256. Epub 2018 Jul 19.

CHAPTER 39

Polycystic Ovary Syndrome

Gotte Jhansi, Vyshnavi A Rao

INTRODUCTION

Polycystic ovary syndrome (PCOS) is a complex heterogeneous endocrine disorder, occurring due to synergistic interaction of genetic, epigenetic, and environmental factors, associated with both reproductive and metabolic abnormalities resulting in short- and long-term consequences in women's health.[1]

Anovulatory disorders account for about 30–40% of female infertility, with PCOS accounting for 80–90% of World Health Organization (WHO) group 2, normogonadotropic, normoestrogenic anovulation (hypothalamic-pituitary-ovarian dysfunction).[2]

The first description was given by Stein and Leventhal (1935) in seven women with variable clinical characteristics (i.e., obesity, hirsutism, acne, amenorrhea, sterility, and occasional menometrorrhagia) associated with bilateral enlarged polycystic ovaries (PCO) with thickened capsules and designated their name for the syndrome.[3] Later in the1960s, the term "polycystic ovary syndrome" and its abbreviation PCOS appeared, gradually replacing the Stein-Leventhal syndrome designation.

It is now well-recognized that PCOS is not necessarily a disease [earlier known as a polycystic ovarian disease (PCOD)], but rather a cluster of features that may predispose to various diseases in different stages of life, such as anovulatory infertility, type 2 diabetes mellitus (T2DM), and metabolic syndrome (MebS).[4] PCOS is known now as an endocrine, metabolic, and chronic inflammatory disorder, with hyperandrogenemia, insulin resistance (IR), and obesity as the key factors that influence the expression and symptoms of the condition.[5] The syndrome is associated with a heterogeneous collection of signs and symptoms forming a spectrum, with a mild presentation in some at one end, to the other end of the spectrum causing severe disturbance of reproductive, endocrine, and metabolic function.

This chapter reviews the diagnostic criteria, etiopathophysiology, clinical manifestations, evaluation, management in adolescents, women of reproductive age, pregnancy and menopause, and the long-term sequelae of this disorder.

DIAGNOSIS—EVOLUTION OF THE DIAGNOSTIC CRITERIA

- The diagnosis of PCOS has remained controversial for many years, as the symptoms and signs are heterogeneous, depending on the population and life stage of the women affected.
- For many years, PCOS was only diagnosed in those with increased luteinizing hormone (LH) or altered LH/follicle-stimulating hormone (FSH) ratio[6] and in those with chronic anovulation. However, these excluded many patients with full-blown disorders.
- Later, the diagnosis was based on the finding of hyperandrogenism (HA) and chronic anovulation after the National Institutes of Health consensus conference in the United States (NIH criteria)[7] **(Table 1)**. Again this criterion excluded many subjects, previously diagnosed with PCOS, as in the United Kingdom and other parts of Europe, NIH criteria were never used and the diagnosis was based on ultrasound morphology (and HA).
- Also, few ovulatory women present with all the features of PCOS, including HA and hyperinsulinemia (HI), and hence there is no reason to make the diagnosis of PCOS only in those with chronic anovulation.[8]
- Finally, the Rotterdam criteria[9] was adopted, and both NIH and the Endocrine Society have endorsed the Rotterdam criteria, which is the most widely adopted criteria **(Table 1)**.
- While the Rotterdam criteria are simple and easier to follow, problems in diagnosing PCOS using these criteria often occur because of:
    - Changing ultrasound criteria for the definition of PCO
    - Polycystic morphology on scan is seen in about 25–30% of normal women without any clinical features of PCOS.[10]
    - Low sensitivity (68–72%) of assessment of ovarian volume (OV) by ultrasound[8]

TABLE 1: Defining polycystic ovary syndrome (PCOS)—the evolution of the diagnostic criteria.

Parameter	*NIH Consensus 1990*[7]	*ESHRE/ASRM/Rotterdam Consensus 2003*[9]	*AEPCOS definition 2009*[11]	*NIH 2012 extension of ESHRE/ASRM 2003*[12]
Criteria	• Clinical and/or biochemical HA • Oligo/amenorrhea, anovulation	• Clinical and/or biochemical HA • Oligo/amenorrhea, anovulation • PCO appearance on ultrasound	• Clinical and/or biochemical HA • Oligo/amenorrhea, anovulation • PCO appearance on ultrasound	• Clinical and/or biochemical HA • Oligo/amenorrhea, anovulation • PCO appearance on ultrasound
Limitations	Two of two criteria required	Two of the three criteria required	Androgen excess and one other criterion	Two of three criteria are required; and identification of specific phenotypes **(Table 2)**

(AEPCOS: Androgen Excess and PCOS Society; ESHRE/ASRM: European Society for Human Reproduction and Embryology/American Society for Reproductive Medicine; HA: hyperandrogenism; Excluding all causes for androgen excess and anovulation; NIH: National Institutes of Health; PCO: polycystic ovaries)

- Low sensitivity of commercially available androgen assays
- Leads to significant increase in the number of subjects diagnosed with PCOS, as well as broadens the heterogeneity of PCOS phenotypes when compared with the NIH definition[4]

- However, the Androgen Excess Society (AES) has proposed that HA should be mandatory for the diagnosis of PCOS.[11]
- The global use of varying diagnostic criteria raised issues of compatibility for PCOS research worldwide and confusion within clinical practice. Therefore, the NIH 2012 undertook an Evidence-Based Methodology PCOS Workshop to address the "benefits and drawbacks" of existing diagnostic criteria.[12] The panel then recommended the use of the broader European Society of Human Reproduction and Embryology (ESHRE) or American Society for Reproductive Medicine (ASRM) 2003 criteria, but with the description of the PCOS phenotype as proposed by Azziz et al. **(Table 1)**.[13]

TABLE 2: Classification of polycystic ovarian syndrome phenotypes.[13,17]

Parameter	*Phenotype A*	*Phenotype B*	*Phenotype C*	*Phenotype D*
PCOS features	HA/OD/PCOM	HA/OD	HA/PCOM	OD/PCOM
HA	+	+	+	–
OD	+	+	–	+
PCOM	+	–	+	+
NIH 1990 criteria	X	X		
Rotterdam 2003 criteria	X	X	X	X
AEPCOS 2006 criteria	X	X	X	

(AEPCOS: ANDROGEN Excess and PCOS Society; HA: hyperandrogenism; NIH: National Institutes of Health; OD: ovulatory dysfunction; PCOM: polycystic ovarian morphology)
Source: Lizneva, et al.[17]

PREVALENCE

- The prevalence of PCOS is determined by the diagnostic criteria used, ethnic origin, and population of women studied. The overall incidence varies from 8% to 10%.[14]
- The prevalence among women of fertile age is 6–10% using the NIH criteria, 10% using the Androgen Excess and PCOS Society (AEPCOS) criteria, and 14–20% using the broader Rotterdam criteria.[15]
- The incidence is higher in the South Asian population which is about 50%, as against the Caucasian population, where the incidence is 5–25%.[16]

POLYCYSTIC OVARY SYNDROME—PHENOTYPES

- Four phenotypes have been identified, which may be influenced by genes, nutrients, physical activity, pollutants, psychological stress, and androgen excess and act to program and modify epigenome leading to PCOS **(Table 2)**.[13]
- Approximately, 75% of PCOS have the classic type and the remaining 25% are evenly divided between ovulatory and nonhyperandrogenic PCOS phenotypes.[13]
- Phenotypes A and B (classic or hyperandrogenic PCOS) have greater menstrual irregularity, HA, total and abdominal obesity, and IR, and are at risk for T2DM, MebS, and cardiovascular disease (CVD).[13]
- Phenotype D (nonhyperandrogenic PCOS), who do not demonstrate overt evidence of androgen excess, have little risk of metabolic dysfunctions.[17]
- Phenotype C (ovulatory PCOS) have lower body mass index (BMI), lesser degrees of HA and HI, milder forms of dyslipidemia, and reduced incidence of MebS.[17]

Pathophysiology

Genetics: Familial with clustering of cases, more common in monozygotic identical twins than in dizygotic or non-identical twins[18]

- Mode of inheritance could be oligogenic or polygenic.[18]
- Autosomal dominant, with variable penetrance or X-linked[18]
- Mutations in the candidate genes involved in any of the metabolic and reproductive pathways **(Table 3)**[18,19]
- Genome-Wide Association Studies (GWAS) identify susceptibility loci for PCOS on chromosomes 2p16.3, 2p21, and 9q33.3, and it is known that LH or chorionic gonadotropin receptor (LHGCR) and FSH receptor are both located on 2p21.18.18.

Various hypotheses have been implicated:

- *Fetal origin:* In utero programming
- *LH hypothesis:* Neuroendocrine defect with an increase in both the amplitude and pulse frequency of LH secretion
- *Ovarian hypothesis:* Primary defect of sex steroid synthesis resulting in hyperandrogenemia
- *Adrenal hypothesis:* Alteration in cortisol metabolism
- *Insulin hypothesis:* Defect in insulin action resulting in HI
- *Altered sympathetic tone:* High sympathetic activity.

TABLE 3: Candidate genes involved in polycystic ovary syndrome.

Steroidogenesis and metabolism	• *CYP11a (P450scc)* • *CYP17 (P450c17)* • *CYP19 (P450arom)*
Insulin receptors and substrates	• Beta-cell function: *TCF7L2, KCNJ11* • Insulin resistance: *IR, PPARȲ*
Ovary	• *Follistatin* • *Fibrillin-3* gene
Androgen action	*Androgen receptor*
Obesity	*Fat mass and obesity-associated gene (FTO)*
• Genes involved in gonadotropin release, regulation, and action • Genes encoding inflammatory cytokines	

Fetal Origin: In Utero Programming

- *Barker's hypothesis (fetal origin of adult disease):* Exposure to in utero HA may disturb the epigenetic reprogramming in the fetal reproductive system, thereby resulting in PCOS phenotype after birth.[20,21]
- However, it is unlikely that maternal androgen excess has a significant impact on fetal testosterone levels because of the efficient "buffering" by high circulating concentrations of sex hormone-binding globulin (SHBG), which reduces the biologically available fraction of testosterone and by placental aromatase activity which converts androgen to estrogen.
- An increased prevalence is seen in women with fetuses having androgen excess disorders such as classical congenital hyperplasia (21-hydroxylase deficiency) and congenital adrenal virilizing tumors.
- The fetal ovary and/or the fetal adrenal are genetically predisposed to secrete an excess of androgen **(Fig. 1)**.[4]
- The fetal ovary shows increased protein expression of P450c17 and an abundance of androgen receptors during follicle formation.

Neuroendocrine Dysfunction

- Increased LH pulse frequency and amplitude with relative FSH deficiency.[22,23]
- The term normogonadotropic anovulation does not apply to all PCOS, as about 60–75% showed elevated basal LH levels.[9,11] However, the LH/FSH ratio may be elevated in up to 95% of individuals.[9]
- More gonadotropin-releasing hormone (GnRH) neurons and/or greater GnRH neuronal connectivity leads to increased GnRH drive.[4]

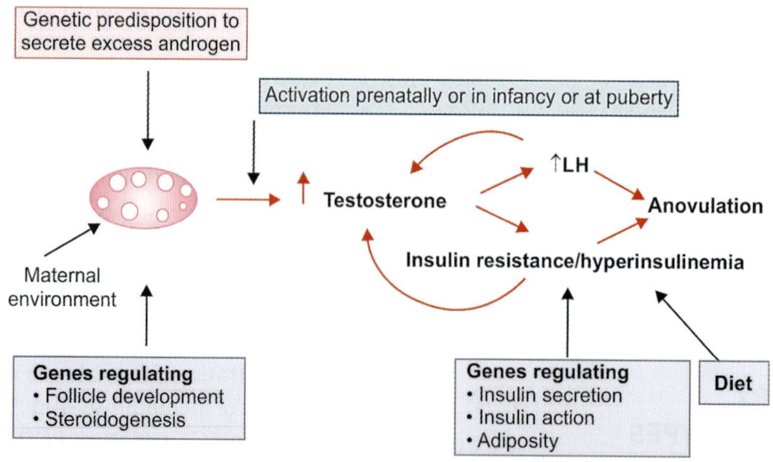

Fig. 1: The proposed developmental origin of polycystic ovary syndrome. (LH: luteinizing hormone)
Source: Franks S, et al.[4]

- Impaired inhibition of hypothalamic GnRH pulsatility, rather than acceleration of the GnRH pulse generator due to:[22,23]
    - HA (prenatal or prepubertal): Androgens block the inhibitory effect of progesterone on the hypothalamus.
    - Estrogen-progesterone feedback: Reduced sensitivity of the GnRH pulse generator to the negative feedback effects of sex steroids (progesterone and estrogen).
    - Anovulation and absence of luteinization → decrease progesterone levels → decrease negative feedback (hypothalamic/pituitary) → pituitary LH
    - HI
    - Estrone hypothesis: Peripheral aromatization of androstenedione (ASD) → estrone → pituitary LH secretion
    - Other neuroendocrine signals such as gamma-aminobutyric acid (GABA), serotonin, dopamine, opioids, anti-Müllerian hormone (AMH), and adiponectin may alter GnRH signalling.[4]
- Rapid GnRH pulse frequency without the normal cyclic variation seen in ovulatory women ~1 pulse/h → pituitary LH secretion → stimulates ovarian theca cells → androgens.
- It is a matter of debate whether the hypothalamic defect is primary or secondary.
- It has been reported that altered kisspeptin signaling could lead to disruption in the GnRH pulse generator. However, the exact role is still to be determined.[24]

Ovarian Hypothesis

The basic dysfunction lies within the ovary causing exaggerated androgen production. There is increased thickness of ovarian stroma, due to theca cell hyperplasia with deposition of collagen, manifesting as stromal echogenicity on ultrasound imaging and increased vascularity due to transforming growth factor (TGF) and vascular endothelial growth factor (VEGF) hyperactivity.

Alterations in both theca and granulosa cell function:

- Development of HA: Two-hit hypothesis—First "hit", one or more of the different mechanisms causing excess androgen production[23] **(Flowchart 1)**. For the second "hit", the preexisting HA reduces the sensitivity of the GnRH pulse generator to progesterone-mediated slowing during pubertal maturation sustaining HA, resulting in a vicious cycle.[23]
- Dysregulation of 17-hydroxylase and 17, 20-lyase activities, both properties of P450c17 (the rate-limiting enzyme in androgen biosynthesis) resulting in androgen activity.[23]

Flowchart 1: Development of hyperandrogenism.

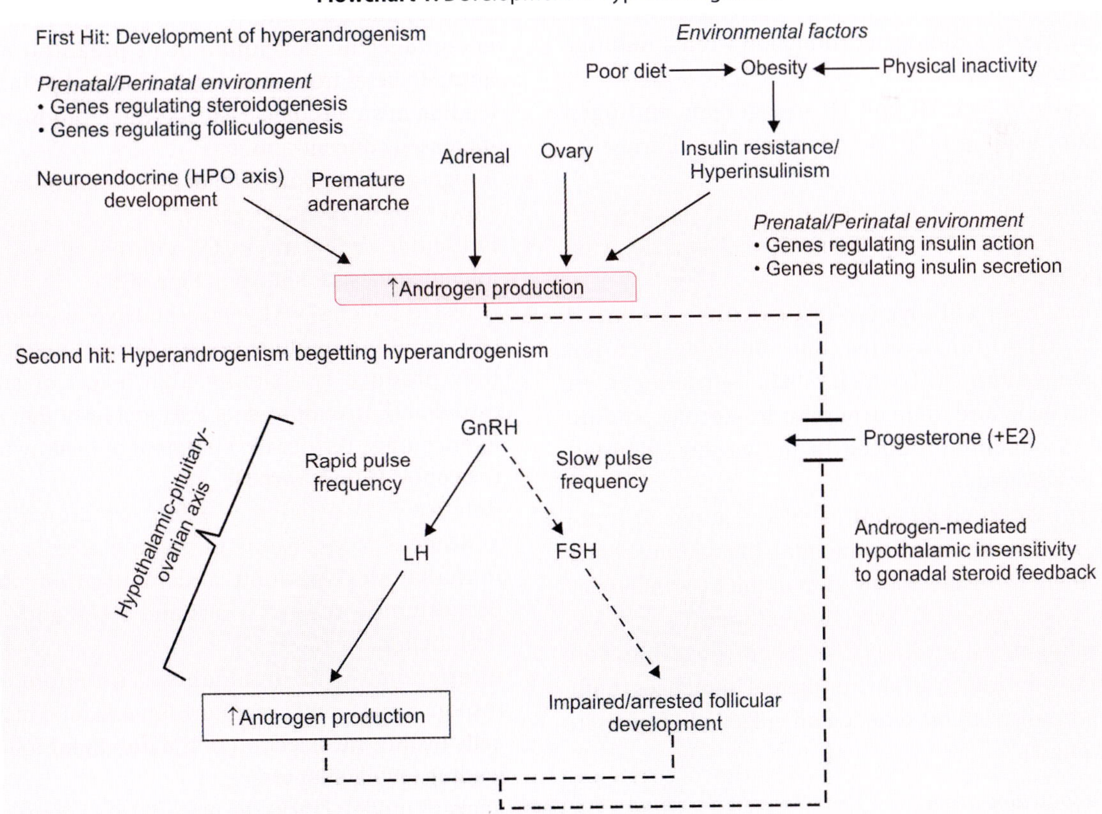

(E2: estradiol; FSH: follicle-stimulating hormone; HPO: hypothalamic-pituitary-gonadal; LH: luteinizing hormone)
Source: Bremer AA.[23]

Flowchart 2: Altered endocrine milieu in polycystic ovary syndrome.

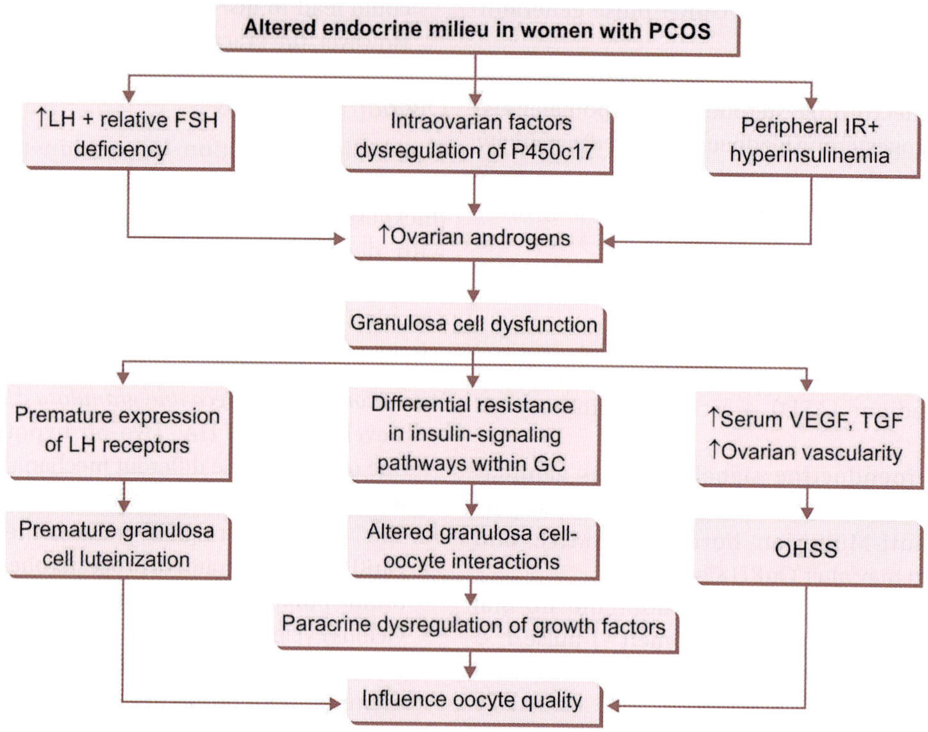

(FSH: follicle-stimulating hormone; GC: granulosa cell; IR: insulin resistance; LH: luteinizing hormone OHSS: ovarian hyperstimulation syndrome; TGF: transforming growth factor; VEGF: vascular endothelial growth factor)

- Intraovarian factors—inhibins, retinoids, and AMH increase ovarian androgen production while inhibiting aromatase activity.[25]
- Androgens induce HI and HI exaggerates androgen secretion, leading to a "vicious circle" of androgens-insulin-androgens.[21]
- As a result of all these, the endocrine milieu is altered in PCOS causing dysfunction of granulosa cells as depicted in **Flowchart 2**.
- All three main androgens—testosterone (produced equally from the ovaries and adrenal glands), androstenedione [(of which >90% is produced in the ovaries), and dehydroepiandrosterone sulfate [(DHEAS—mainly produced in the adrenal glands)] could be elevated.[11]
- Androgen excess could exert its effects, at one or more stages of development from fetal life, adolescence [when there is transient activation of the hypothalamic-pituitary-gonadal (HPO) axis], or adulthood.[4]
- The evolution and severity of its phenotypic expression result from the impact of environmental influences (both pre- and postnatal) on genetic and epigenetic factors in utero **(Fig. 2)**.[23]

Disordered folliculogenesis:

- Excess androgens and reduced levels of oocyte-secreted growth factors, mainly growth differentiation factor-9 (GDF-9) and bone morphogenetic protein 15 (BMP-15) encourage the development of preantral and small antral follicles from their primordial and primary stages, leading to small-follicle excess which produces AMH in increased concentrations.
- A higher initial population of primordial follicles and/or slower atresia could also exist.[25]
- Follicular defect in PCOS compared with normal folliculogenesis is shown in **Figure 3**.
- Arrested follicles are hyperresponsive to gonadotropins (GTs) and prematurely reach a level of maturity where they produce sufficiently high levels of circulating estradiol (E2), suppressing FSH to a level that is too low to encourage further development of healthy follicles in the cohort **(Flowchart 3)**.
- Relative FSH deficiency → impairs aromatization of androgens to estrogens in granulosa cells → impairs follicular development and maturation and luteal progesterone release → sustained HA and ovulatory dysfunction.[21]
- Interference with dominance: The attenuated FSH responsiveness and premature luteinization of granulosa cells distort the selection of the dominant follicle (DF), leading to follicular arrest.
- Lacker's model: Tracks the maturity of a cohort of follicles as a function of time through the selection phase. If all follicles are of "low sensitivity", then normal ovulatory

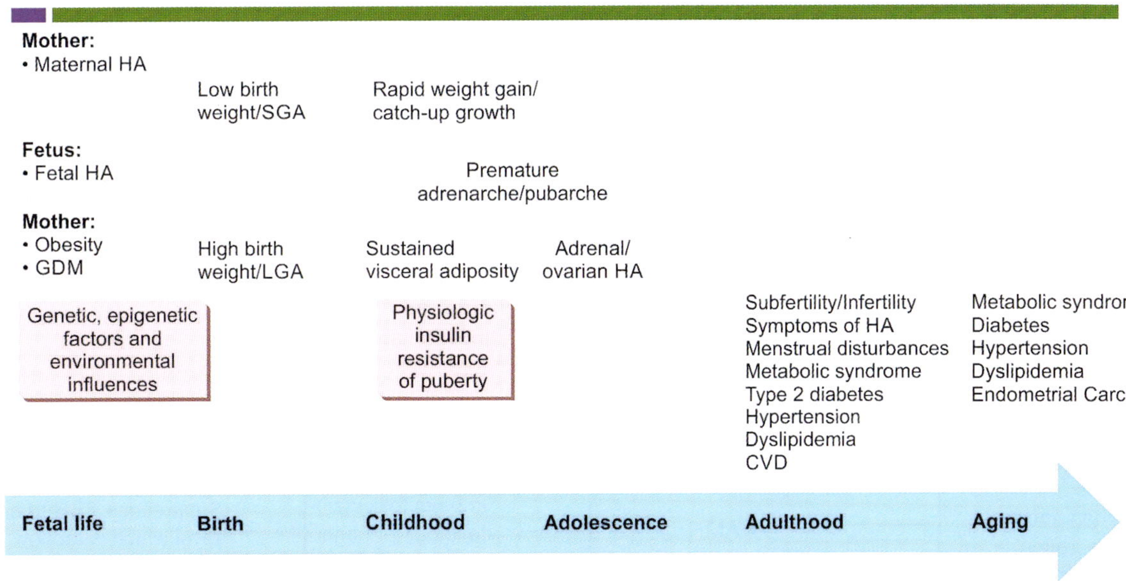

Fig. 2: Proposed evolution of PCOS from fetal life to adulthood. (CVD: cardiovascular disease; GDM: gestational diabetes mellitus; HA: hyperandrogenism; LGA: large for gestational age; SGA: small for gestational age)

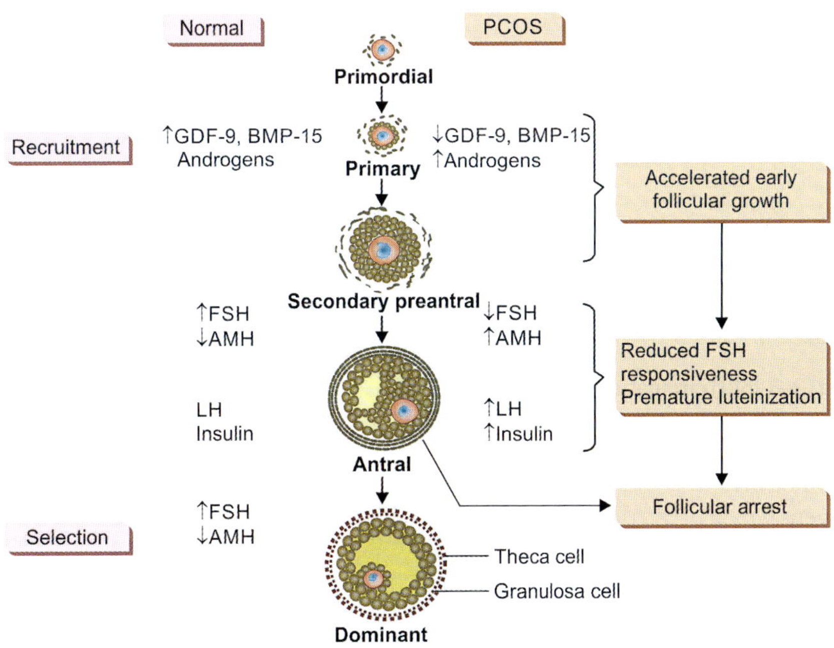

Fig. 3: Normal folliculogenesis and follicular defect in polycystic ovary syndrome (PCOS).
(AMH: anti-Müllerian hormone; BMP-15: bone morphogenetic protein 15; FSH: follicle-stimulating hormone; GDF-9: growth differentiation factor 9; LH: luteinizing hormone)
Source: Diamanti-Kandarakis E.[25]

cycles occur and if the majority of follicles are of "high sensitivity" then it results in a follicular arrest.[26]

Abnormalities of estrogen secretion:

- Estrogen secretion, especially E2, is usually low-to-normal without midcyclic increase due to arrested folliculogenesis.[26]
- High production of testosterone results in high estrone levels, further increasing LH levels, which in turn results in hyperplasia of the ovarian stroma and theca cells, leading to increased androgens, thus perpetuating the vicious cycle of excessive androgen and LH production.

Role of anti-Müllerian hormone:

- Anti-Müllerian hormone, a member of the TGF-beta superfamily, is derived specifically from the granulosa cells of early developing preantral and antral follicles.

Flowchart 3: Defective folliculogenesis.

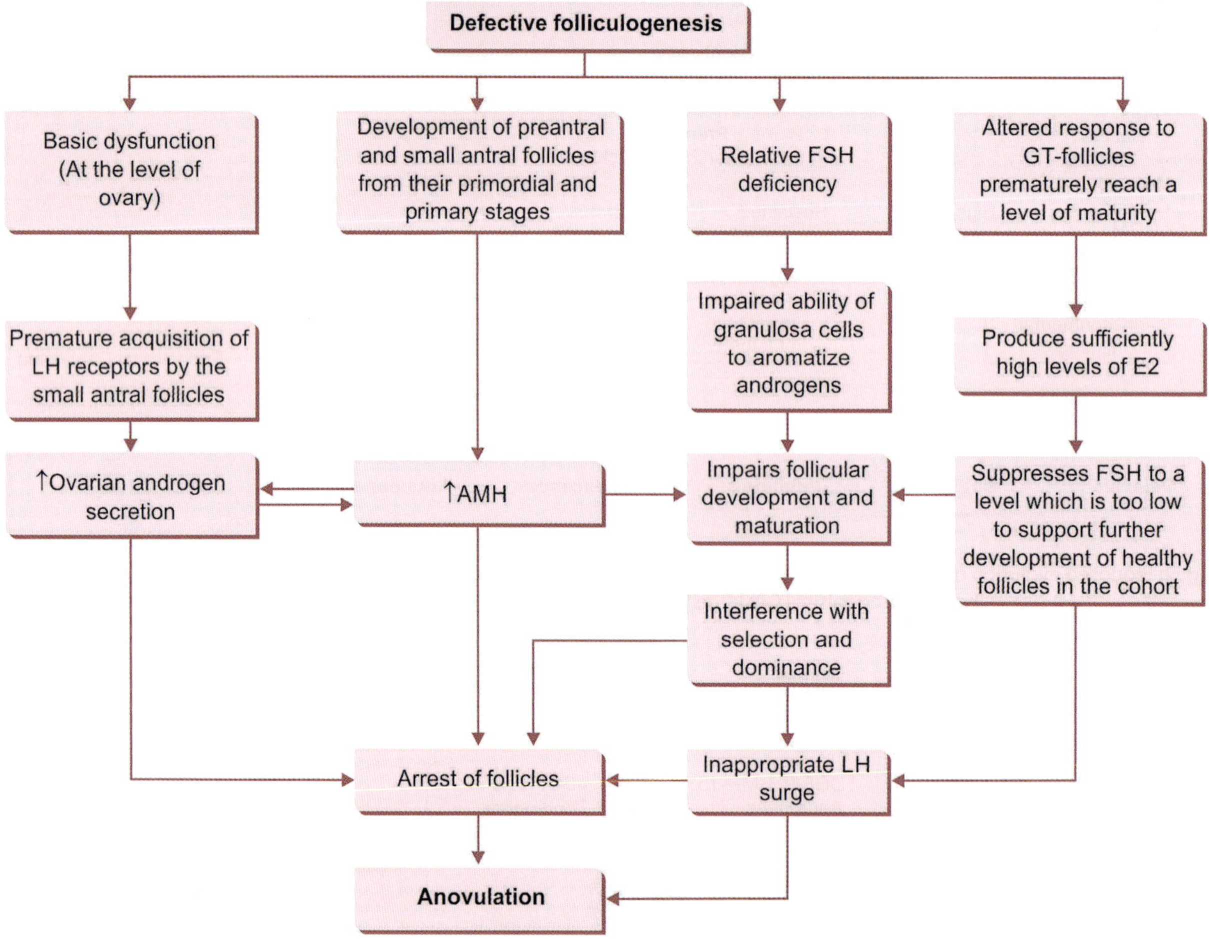

(AMH: anti-Müllerian hormone; E2: estradiol; FSH: follicle-stimulating hormone; GT: gonadotropin; LH: luteinizing hormone;)

- PCOS has increased (2–3-fold) circulating concentrations of AMH due to:[27,28]
  - Increased AMH production by individual follicles
  - Abnormally elevated LH
  - Elevated androgens
  - - HI
  - Advanced glycation end products (AGEs), or decreased soluble receptor for AGE (sRAGE)
  - Genetic factors such as variants of *ACVR1* gene 3
  - Increased follicular number (FN) with increased granulosa cell mass
- Increased AMH levels inhibit FSH-stimulated follicular activation and growth resulting in the arrest of follicles
- AMH also inhibits the action of FSH-induced aromatase production which is likely to contribute to HA.[21]
- AMH has a paracrine effect on theca interna cells, leading to theca cell dysregulation, resulting in increased androgen production.
- Stockpiling effect: AMH Hypothesis **(Flowchart 4)**.[21]
- AMH has good predictive accuracy for PCOS and correlates with the severity, making it a good candidate as an additional criterion for the diagnosis of this syndrome.[29]

Flowchart 4: Stockpiling effect: AMH hypothesis.

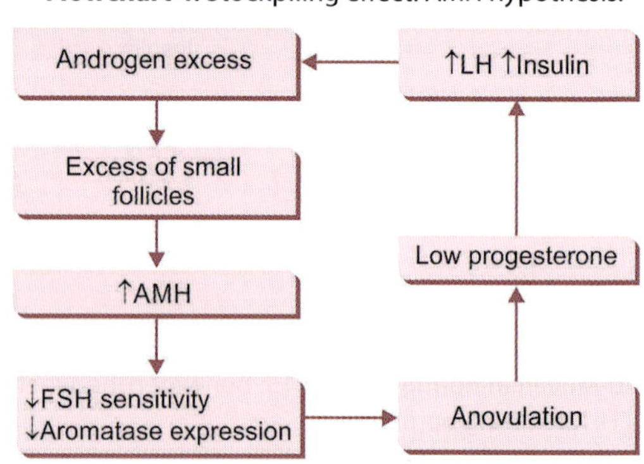

(AMH: anti-Müllerian hormone; LH: luteinizing hormone; FSH: follicle-stimulating hormone)

- Elevated serum AMH concentrations are predictive of poor response to various therapies of PCOS including weight loss, ovulation induction (OI), metformin therapy, and laparoscopic ovarian drilling (LOD), while responders to treatment were found to have a decline in AMH levels.[28]

Adrenal Hyperandrogenism

- Increased adrenal activity of P450c17.[23]
- Insulin indirectly enhances hypothalamic corticotropin-releasing hormone (CRH) secretion.[23]
- Adrenal hyperresponsiveness to adrenocorticotropic hormone (ACTH)
- Accelerated cortisol turnover secretion.

Insulin Hypothesis

- Insulin resistance is defined as "a state (of a cell, tissue, or organism) in which a greater than normal amount of insulin is required to elicit a quantitatively normal response" and maintain glucose levels within the normal range.[30,31]
- HI occurs secondary to resistance at the insulin receptor, decreased hepatic clearance of insulin, and/or increased pancreatic sensitivity.
- Overall IR is seen in 50–70% of PCOS (approximately 80–95% of obese PCOS and 40–75% of lean PCOS).[30,31]
- Insulin acts through its receptor to initiate a cascade of post-receptor events within the target cell. Phosphorylation causes insulin receptor substrates 1–4 (IRS1–4) to promote glucose uptake via the transmembrane glucose transporter type 4 (GLUT4), and also intracellular protein synthesis.
- In PCOS, the binding of insulin to the receptor induces serine phosphorylation instead of tyrosine autophosphorylation. Serine phosphorylation increases the activity of P450c17 in both the ovary and adrenal, thus promoting androgen synthesis.
- Individuals with IR may be overtly diabetic or merely have IR detected by testing.
- Methods for detecting IR:[31]
  - Euglycemic hyperinsulinemic clamp technique is the gold standard test and measures insulin-mediated glucose disposal in vivo. However, it has no clinical application, as it is invasive, expensive, and time-consuming, and requires experienced personnel.
  - Determination of insulin levels—fasting state or after oral glucose tolerance test (OGTT) and measurement of fasting glucose/insulin ratio
  - HOMA—homeostasis model assessment index
  - QUICKI—quantitative insulin sensitivity check index
  - Insulin tolerance test—assessment of sequential plasma glucose levels after administration of intravenous insulin.
  - FSIVGTT—estimation of an index of insulin sensitivity, by applying the minimal model technique to data obtained from the frequently sampled intravenous glucose tolerance test (FSIVGTT).
- All of the above measures have limitations, primarily the lack of a standardized universal insulin assay, changes in beta-cell function with the development of diabetes (which alters the sensitivity of the tests), and normal physiological fluctuation in insulin levels.[31]

Flowchart 5: Insulin resistance leading to PCOS.

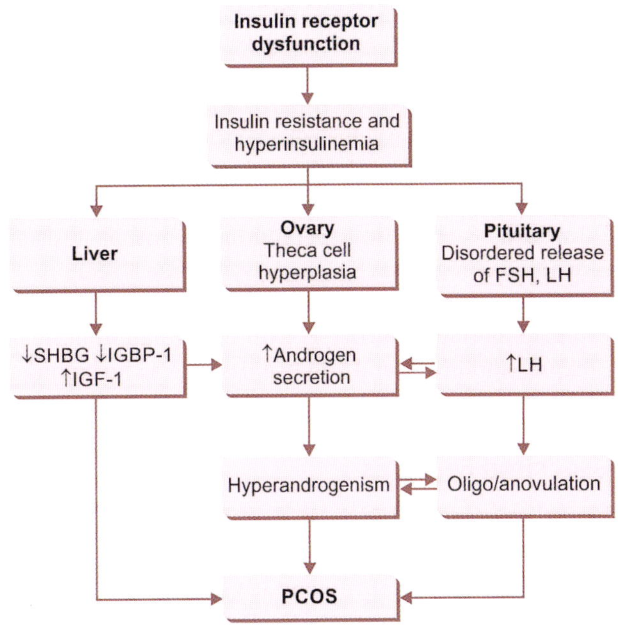

(FSH: follicle-stimulating hormone; IGBP-1: insulin growth factor-binding protein; IGF: insulin growth factor; IR: insulin resistance; LH: luteinizing hormone; PCOS: polycystic ovary syndrome; SHBG: sex hormone-binding globulin)

- The degree of HI correlates with the syndrome's severity.[30]
- Specifically, resistance to the metabolic actions of insulin has been reported in the liver, skeletal muscle, and adipose tissue, whilst the adrenal gland and ovary are insulin-sensitive.
- HI suppresses hepatic SHBG production and exacerbates HA **(Flowchart 5)**.[32]
- Although IR and HI are central to the pathophysiology, it is not a part of the diagnostic criteria.
- It is still been debated whether HA results from HI or HI results from HA or they are independent variable.[33]

Altered Sympathetic Nervous System

There is evidence of high sympathetic activity in PCOS, independent of BMI, with animal models to support increased sympathetic innervation in the appearance of cysts.[34]

AT THE PERIPHERAL COMPARTMENT (SKIN AND ADIPOSE TISSUE)

- In the skin, HI increases the activity of the enzyme 5-alpha (α)-reductase which converts testosterone to the stronger androgen dihydrotestosterone (DHT) causing hirsutism and acne.

- HI stimulates insulin-like growth factor receptor 1 (IGFR-1) present in the epidermis which leads to stimulation of tyrosine kinase growth factor-signaling pathways, causing proliferation of keratinocytes and fibroblasts, leading to skin thickening, resulting in acanthosis nigricans. Histopathology of acanthosis nigricans shows hyperkeratosis, acanthosis, and papillomatosis with or without basal hyperpigmentation.
- In cases of severe IR, hyperandrogenic insulin-resistant acanthosis nigricans (HAIRAN) syndrome is seen.
- In adipocytes, testosterone appears to induce serine phosphorylation of IRS-1, with upregulation of lipase expression in visceral adipose tissue (VAT) resulting in visceral adiposity and associated health disorders.

Associated Features

Inositol Deficient State

- Inositol (InS) is a member of the vitamin B-complex family. It is not an essential vitamin, as it can be manufactured by the body, but it tends to be deficient in women with PCOS.
- Free InS is transported actively across the intestinal wall by a sodium-dependent active mechanism, a process that can be inhibited by glucose. Circulating InS is then taken up by tissues by a membrane-associated sodium-InS cotransport mechanism.
- InS is incorporated into cell membranes as phosphatidyl myo-inositol (MI), the precursor of inositol phosphatidyl phosphate (IP3), which acts as a second messenger for both insulin and FSH, causing glucose uptake and FSH signaling.
- In human ovaries, 99% of the intracellular pool of InS comprises MI and the remaining consists of D-chiro-inositol (DCI). DCI is synthesized from MI through the epimerase enzyme in the theca cells, which in turn is stimulated by insulin.
- In PCOS, there occurs a defect in tissue availability or altered metabolism of inositol phosphoglycans (IPGs) or IPG mediators and increased epimerase activity, all leading to deficiency of MI, which decreases phosphatidylinositol-3-kinase (PI3K) activity and IP3 **(Fig. 4)**.[35]
- MI causes the release of calcium in the oocyte through IP3 and thereby promotes both nuclear and cytoplasmic maturity of the oocytes. A correlation between MI concentration in the follicular fluid and high oocyte quality has been reported in a few studies.[36]
- In PCOS, MI deficiency and increased DCI/MI ratio may adversely affect glucose uptake and metabolism of both the oocytes and follicular cells, probably compromising the oocyte quality.

Leptin Resistance

- Both obese and lean PCOS have higher circulating concentrations of leptin. However, leptin resistance is more commonly seen in insulin-resistant and obese PCOS as compared to lean PCOS.[37]
- Abnormalities of leptin secretion causes defective suppression of appetite, which perpetuates obesity in PCOS.
- Hyperleptinemia is inversely related to the degree of fertility.

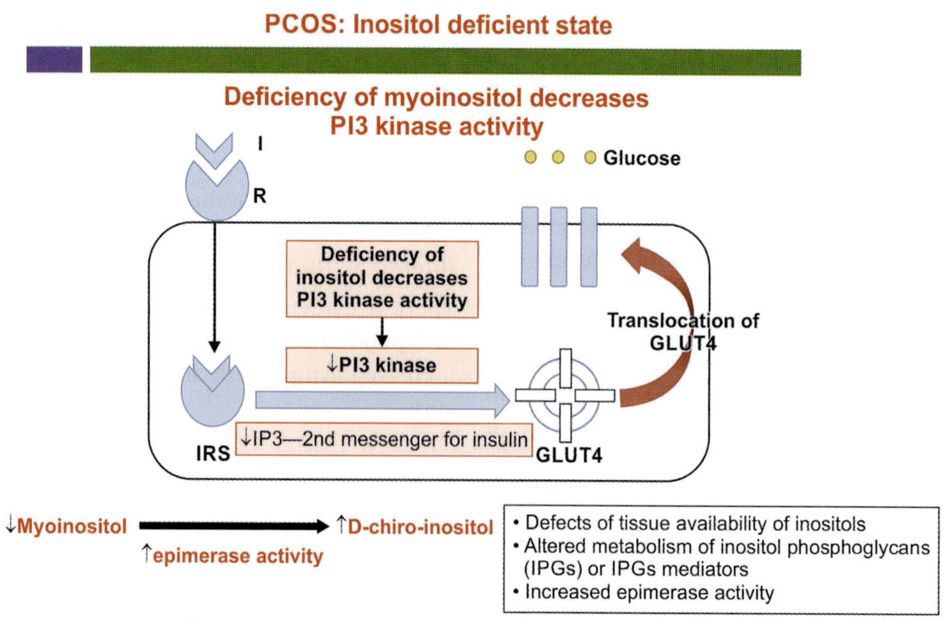

Fig. 4: Inositol deficiency.
(GLUT4: glucose transporter type 4; IP3: inositol phosphatidyl trisphosphate; IRS: insulin receptor substrates; PI3K: phosphatidylinositol-3-kinase)

- At the level of the ovary, deficiency of leptin or of its receptors and hyperleptinemia impairs the selection of DF causing the arrest of follicular development. It also decreases oocyte maturity and fertilization contributing to poor quality embryos and endometrial dysfunction, all resulting in lower pregnancy rates (PRs).[31,37]

Obesity and Polycystic Ovary Syndrome

- Obesity is seen in about 50–65% of women with PCOS.[37]
- Rather than PCOS leading to obesity, obesity amplifies the clinical severity of PCOS, thereby increasing the risk of metabolic dysfunction.[37]
- Obesity is associated with a reduction in SHBG, and a consequent increase in free testosterone.[36]
- There is an increased number of adipocytes that amplifies IR and HI, exacerbating HA.[3]
- Increased 5α-reductase activity and an increase in ACTH drive associated with obesity also contributes to HA.[37]
- The "adipose tissue expandability hypothesis" may also account for the pathogenesis of PCOS in some individuals.[38] An individual's metabolic set-point determines the caloric load which can be stored safely in the adipose tissues. A caloric load which exceeds this set-point results in lipotoxicity [condition with elevated free fatty acids, hypertriglyceridemia, low adiponectin levels, and high interleukin-6 (IL-6) and tumor necrosis factor alpha (TNF-α)], and the potential for ectopic fat deposition (fat in nonadipose tissues such as liver, skeletal muscle, and pancreas), all of which contribute to IR and its consequences.[38]
- Apple-shaped (android) obesity with visceral adiposity, typically seen in PCOS is associated with a more adverse metabolic risk profile than pear-shaped (gynecoid) obesity.
- It has been observed that ovulatory women as compared to anovulatory women with PCOS have lesser visceral obesity and exhibit lesser adipocyte dysfunction.[39]
- Measurement of waist circumference, therefore correlates more closely with metabolic risk than BMI.
- Circulating concentrations of adiponectin were found to be lower in both lean and obese PCOS, when compared to women without PCOS.[40] It is known that adiponectin is protective against IR, diabetes, and CVD, and also inhibits androgen production by theca cells.
- Obesity negatively affects fertility, reduces the response to GTs, and adversely affects both implantation and PR.[41]
- In adipose tissue, relatively inert androgens undergo aromatization into estrogens, predominantly estrone, causing menstrual dysfunction more so in obese women and it is this group, who are at risk of endometrial carcinoma by the unopposed estrogenic stimulation.
- The metabolic phenotype of PCOS (obesity, acanthosis nigricans, and IR) is predominantly seen in South Asians.[15]
- Obese PCOS has a higher incidence of IR, which predisposes to both impaired glucose tolerance (IGT) and T2DM.[42]
- *Oxidative stress and low-grade inflammation:* These are two features shared by both obese and nonobese PCOS due to:
- Advanced glycation end products: Hyperglycemia with induction of alternate pathways—hexosamine, polyol, and protein kinase C pathways causes oxidative damage with the release of free radicals, reactive oxygen species (ROS), and AGE, resulting in endothelial dysfunction. They increase vascular permeability and arterial stiffness, inhibit vascular dilatation by interfering with nitric oxide (NO), and also bind macrophage, endothelial, and mesangial cells to induce the release of a variety of cytokines.[43]
- AGE–RAGE system interaction: AGEs circulate and act on cell surface receptors, such as the receptor for AGE (RAGE). AGE receptors in circulating blood, called soluble RAGEs (sRAGE) can bind their ligands (AGEs) in the circulation, thus preventing the adverse intracellular events of the AGE–RAGE axis. The AGE–RAGE system interaction leads to activation of secondary messenger, activating nuclear factor-kappa B leading to the development of a proinflammatory state, cellular toxicity, and damage. In PCOS, there is an increased activity of this system at the serum, adipose tissue, and ovary levels **(Flowchart 6)**.
- In PCOS, numerous biochemical inflammatory and thrombotic markers of CVD risk circulate in excess like TNF-α, IL-6, IL-18, IL-17, factor VIIc, tissue plasminogen activator (tPA), fibrinogen, plasminogen activator inhibitor-1 (PAI-1), thrombomodulin, D-dimers, antithrombin III (ATIII), asymmetric dimethylarginine (ADMA), AGEs, malondialdehyde (MDA), and NO compared with non-PCOS controls.[44,45]

Vitamin D Deficiency

- Vitamin D binds to the vitamin D receptor, activates the peroxisome proliferator activator receptor-γ, and stimulates the expression of insulin receptors, thereby enhancing insulin-mediated glucose uptake.[46,47]
- Vitamin D deficiency in PCOS contributes to IR, HA, ovulatory dysfunction, and MebS.[46,48]

Role of Melatonin in PCOS

- Melatonin is a hormone of the pineal gland which maintains normal circadian rhythms and governs the release of pituitary GTs.

Flowchart 6: Relationship of the AGE–RAGE system with PCOS and infertility.

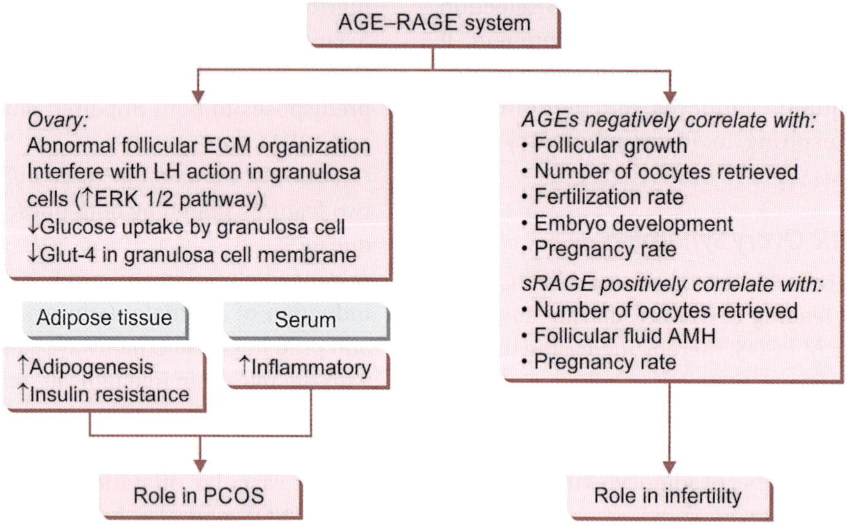

(AGE: advanced glycation end products; AMH: anti-Müllerian hormone; RAGE: receptor for AGE; ECM: extracellular matrix; ERK: extracellular signal-regulated kinase; sRAGE: soluble RAGE; GLUT-4: glucose transporter type 4)
Source: Merhi Z.[44]

- ROS produced within the follicles, especially during ovulation are scavenged by melatonin, thereby reducing the oxidative stress involved in oocyte maturation and embryo development.
- In PCOS, even if there are high concentrations of melatonin in serum, there is a deficiency of this indoleamine within the follicles resulting in low intrafollicular melatonin levels, affecting follicular growth, ovulation, and oocyte quality.[49]
- Melatonin can also alter the leptin levels, contributing to the pathophysiology of PCOS.[49]

Environmental Factors

It has been observed that serum levels of bisphenol A (BPA) are elevated and associated with hormonal and metabolic abnormalities in PCOS compared with BMI-matched healthy controls.[50] However, this needs to be further evaluated.

Immune Dysfunction

- Those with shorter leukocyte telomere lengths were found to have a higher risk of PCOS than those with longer telomere lengths, after adjustment of age.[51]
- All PCOS phenotypes have increased CD^4+$CD28^{null}$ T lymphocytes compared to controls, with the nonhyperandrogenic phenotypes showing the highest levels. $CD4^+CD28^{null}$ exerts proinflammatory, proatherogenic activity, by producing high levels of interferon (IFN)-γ, TNF-α, IL-2, and cytolytic enzymes, all of which increase the risk of cardiovascular (CV) events. Hence, CV risk evaluation should be performed in all PCOS phenotypes.[52]

Follicle-stimulating Hormone Receptor Polymorphism

- The FSH receptor variants Alanine–Threonine change at position 307 (Ala/Thr 307) and serine–serine at position 680 (Ser/Ser 680) were found to be significantly more prevalent among anovulatory women.[53,54]
- The FSH receptor polymorphism homozygous of Ser/Ser 680 allelic variant was associated with higher basal FSH and LH levels, higher frequency of HA, decreased FSH sensitivity, decreased ovarian responsiveness, requiring a significantly higher GT dose compared with Asn/Asn 680 and Asn/Ser 680 variants.[54,55]
- Also, in a few studies, the genotype asparagine—Asn68054 and alanine—Ala307 of the FSH receptor has been correlated with the risk of developing ovarian hyperstimulation syndrome (OHSS).[55]

Lean versus Obese Polycystic Ovary Syndrome

- About 20–50% of women with PCOS are of normal weight or thin.[56]
- HI is a common finding in both obese and nonobese PCOS populations. However, lean PCOS tends to have comparatively lower HI and IR.[57]
- The degree of HI- and HA-related clinical features is more pronounced in obese as compared to lean PCOS.
- HI in lean PCOS is due to increased pancreatic β-cell activity and reduced hepatic clearance of insulin.[56]
- Leptin resistance and adipokines inhibit GnRH secretion, hence lower LH levels in obese women, compared to lean PCOS, who tend to have higher LH levels.
- Differences between lean versus obese PCOS are shown in **Table 4**.

- Lean PCOS treated with metformin for 4–6 weeks demonstrated a decrease in insulin concentrations, a decrease in free and total testosterone concentrations, with the restoration of menstrual cycles.[57]

Management of Lean Polycystic Ovary Syndrome[58]

Management of lean PCOS is depicted in **Flowchart 7**.

TABLE 4: Differences between obese versus lean polycystic ovary syndrome (PCOS).

	Obese	*Lean*
LH/FSH	↑	↑↑ Defect in HPO axis
↑Androgen secretion	↑IGF-1 ↓IGFBP-1 ↓SHBG	↑GH
Hyperinsulinemia	IR	↑β-Cell function Decreased hepatic clearance of Insulin
IR	+++	+
Androgens	Testosterone + DHEAS	Testosterone
Hypertension	↑↑	↑
IGT	↑↑(about 30–35%)	↑(about 10%)
Diabetes mellitus	↑↑ (about 7–10%)	↑(3%)
Endometrial hyperplasia	↑↑	↑

(DHEAS: dehydroepiandrosterone sulfate; FSH: follicle-stimulating hormone; GH: growth hormone; HPO: hypothalamic-pituitary-gonadal ; IGF-1: insulin-like growth factor 1; IGFBP-1: insulin-like growth factor–binding protein 1; IGT: impaired glucose tolerance; IR: insulin resistance; LH: luteinizing hormone; SHBG: sex hormone-binding globulin)

Metabolic Complications

- Women with PCOS have an estimated 2.2-, 2.5-, and 4-fold increased prevalence of metabolic dysfunctions, IGT, and T2DM, respectively in both BMI and non-BMI-matched studies.[42,59]
- Dyslipidemia is the most common metabolic dysfunction in PCOS,[58] and PCOS is the leading cause of dyslipidemia among women of reproductive age.[61]
- Classic PCOS demonstrates 75–85% of IR, some form of metabolic dysfunction, and is at increased risk of IGT and diabetes.[15,62]
- Oxidative stress caused by ROS production in immune cells plays a fundamental role in the genesis and progression of endothelial dysfunction, which leads to the development of arterial hypertension and CVD.[63]
- Cross-talk between IR and chronic inflammation generates an environment conducive to the development of cardiometabolic disorders.
- MEbS or the IR syndrome or "syndrome X", first described in 1988 is a constellation of risk factors, identified as a "common soil" for the development of both CVD and T2DM.[64]
- Two classifications are used to define MebS. Firstly, under the National Cholesterol Education Program
- Adult Treatment Panel (NCEP ATP) III criteria[64] modified for the Asian population,[65] MebS is present, if at least three out of five criteria are present **(Table 5)**. Secondly, according to International Diabetes Federation,[66] the diagnosis of MebS requires WC >80 cm, and additionally two of the criteria as mentioned in **Table 5**.
- Prevalence of MebS varies, based on age, gender, and ethnicity, from 7% to 50%, with South Asians having a high prevalence of about 50% and in India being 7.9–46.5%.[67]
- The prevalence of MebS, hypertension, and dyslipidemia was observed to be increased in mothers, fathers, sisters,

Flowchart 7: Management algorithm for Lean polycystic ovary syndrome.

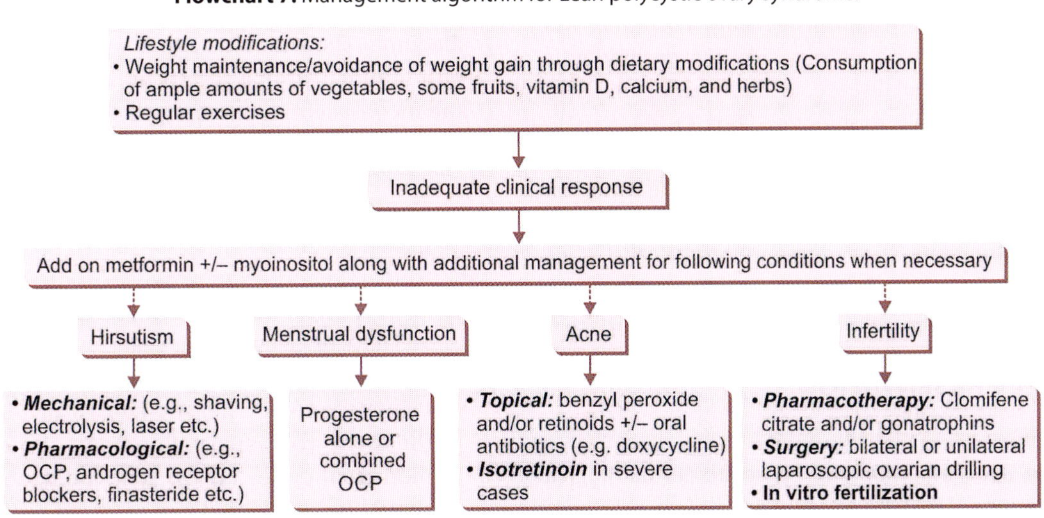

(OCP: oral contraceptive pill)

TABLE 5: Diagnostic criteria for the metabolic syndrome according to NCEP ATP III.[60]

Three of the following conditions:	
I. Central obesity (waist circumference in cm): • Male • Female	 ≥102 ≥88
II. Elevated triglycerides (mg/dL)	≥150
III. Decreased HDL cholesterol (mg/dL): • Male • Female	 <40 <50
IV. Elevated arterial blood pressure (mm Hg)	≥130/85
V. Elevated fasting blood glucose (mg/dL)	≥110

Source: Third Report of the National Cholesterol Education Program (NCEPIII) Expert Panel on Detection, Evaluation and Treatment of High Blood Cholesterol in Adults (Adult Treatment Panel III, ATP III).

BOX 1: Polycystic ovary syndrome (PCOS) who are at risk of metabolic dysfunction and cardiovascular disease (CVD).[63]

At high risk, if:
- Metabolic syndrome
- Type 2 diabetes mellitus
- Overt vascular or renal disease

At risk, if:
- Obesity (especially abdominal)
- Smoking
- Dyslipidemia
- Impaired glucose tolerance
- Hypertension
- Subclinical cardiovascular disease
- Family history of premature CVD

Source: Wild RA, et al.[63]

and brothers of PCOS women as shown in a recent systematic review.[61]

- Genetics, lifestyle, obesity, and IR are all etiological factors in the development of MebS.[61]
- PCOS individuals with a BMI > 30kg/m^2, and high-risk ethnic groups including South Asian, Hispanic, and Polynesian women with a BMI >25 kg/m^2, dyslipidemia, overt vascular or renal disease, or family history of T2DM are at risk of metabolic dysfunction **(Box 1)**.[68,69]
- The presence of MebS is one of the strongest and earliest predictors of CVD **(Box 1)**.[63] Hence, both the American College of Obstetricians and Gynecologists (ACOG) and the AEPCOS guidelines recommend that PCOS patients should have a complete fasting lipid profile evaluation as a part of CV risk assessment.[13,63]

CLINICAL PRESENTATION

Symptoms

- *Hirsutism, acne, and alopecia*: These are dermatological manifestations of HA which vary widely between different ethnic groups.
  - *Hirsutism*, excessive growth of thick, terminal, coarse hairs in androgen-dependent areas of the face and/or body in females in a male-type pattern, is seen in about 75–80% of PCOS. The modified Ferriman-Gallwey score is used to grade hirsutism.[11] A score of 0 (none) to 4 (severe) in nine areas of the body is assigned a maximum score of 36. Scores of <4 indicate mild, 4–7 moderate, and ≥8 severe hirsutism.[11]
  - *Acne*, a pilosebaceous unit disorder occurring predominantly on the lower face, neck, chest, and upper aspect of the back, occurs in about 20–40% of PCOS.[11]
  - *Androgenic alopecia* or male pattern balding is seen in severe cases of androgen excess and is relatively less common in PCOS. Diffuse loss of hair occurs from the anterior mid-vertex area extending to the crown with preservation of the frontal anterior hairline, and is seen in about 10% of PCOS cases.[11] It is graded according to the Ludwig's visual score.
- *Menstrual disturbances* are seen in about 60–85%.[69] The degree of ovarian dysfunction, the amount of follicular activity, and the circulating concentration of estrogens stimulating endometrial development will determine whether women would have amenorrhea or oligomenorrhea (cycle length more than 35 days). Sporadic anovulatory cycles do occur among regularly menstruating women. About 47% will have oligomenorrhea (8 or fewer cycles per year), amenorrhea in about 51%, and polymenorrhea (frequent cycles occurring at intervals of <26 days in length) in about 1.5–2.7%.[69]
  - *Normal menstrual cycles* are seen in about 12–20%.[11,30,31]
  - *Abnormal uterine bleeding (AUB)*:[30,36] AUB is due to chronic unopposed action of estrogen on the endometrium, seen in about 29% of cases.
- In the absence of ovulation, there is continued endometrial proliferation without progesterone-induced shedding. The endometrium being fragile, and vascular with minimal stroma results in bleeding that is erratic, and inconsistent in duration, cycle, and amount of flow. The ESHRE 2018 guidelines on PCOS define irregular menstrual cycles as follows:
  - Normal in the first year post menarche as part of the pubertal transition
  - >1 to <3 years post menarche: <21 or >45 days
  - >3 years post menarche to perimenopause: <21 or >35 days or <8 cycles per year
  - >1 year post menarche >90 days for any one cycle
  - Primary amenorrhea by age 15 or >3 years post thelarche (breast development). When irregular menstrual cycles are present, a diagnosis of PCOS should be considered and assessed according to the guidelines.[2]

- *Obesity:* 50–76%[30,37,69]
- *Asymptomatic*: 20%
- *Subfertility or infertility*: In about 74% of cases (50% with primary infertility and 25% with secondary infertility), due to oligo/anovulation and the combined effects of obesity, metabolic, inflammatory, and endocrine abnormalities on oocyte quality.[69]

Clinical Signs

- *Acanthosis nigricans:* Presents as dark brown, velvety, thickened cutaneous plaques, most often seen on the back of the neck, axillae, beneath the breasts, and exposed areas (elbows, knuckles). It has been reported in 5–10% of PCOS and in about 50% of obese PCOS.[69] Occurs as a result of IR, with an increased risk of diabetes, and lipid abnormalities. Management involves treating the underlying disorder and laser or surgical excision of the lesion. Although, topical tretinoin and calcipotriol have been used with limited success.
- *Clinical signs of HA*—hirsutism, acne, or alopecia
- *Obesity and central abdominal obesity.*

Signs of Polycystic Ovarian Morphology on Ultrasound

- *Polycystic ovarian morphology (PCOM):* Finding of increased follicle number per ovary [(FNPO) of ≥12] measuring 2–9 mm and/or increased ovarian size (OV ≥10 cc) in one or both ovaries on transvaginal sonography (TVS) as per the Rotterdam criteria **(Fig. 5)**[9,69]
  Recently ESHRE has updated the transvaginal ultrasound criteria as a FNPO of >20 and/or an OV ≥10 mL, ensuring no corpora lutea, cysts or DFs are present.[11]
- The AEPCOS task force observed that 70–90% of women with PCOS would demonstrate PCOM, although the false-positive rate was as high as it was seen in up to one quarter of unselected reproductive-aged women.[11] However, the observed frequency of PCOM in the PCOS population in a recent systematic review was found to be 28–40%. Depending on the age and ethnicity of the study population:[15]
  - FN thresholds do not apply to women <18 and >35 years.
  - Stromal hyperechogenicity is due to stromal abundance.
  - Arrangement of antral follicles may have a generalized or peripheral distribution.
  - Arrangement of follicles and stromal echogenicity, however, is not relevant to making a diagnosis.[9]
  - Unilateral PCOM is also diagnostic.[9]
  - PCO can also be observed during pubertal development, in about 25–30% of normal women and in those using oral contraceptive pills (OCPs) (about 14%), and in about 30–50% of patients with functional hypothalamic anovulation.[13,30]
  - FNPO ≥12 threshold leads to overdiagnosis of both PCOM and PCOS. Therefore, with the availability of better ultrasound resolution (i.e., transducer frequency ≥8 MHz) to identify even follicles smaller than 2 mm, the FNPO threshold was raised to 19 and subsequently ≥25, which gave a sensitivity of 81% and specificity of 92% for making a diagnosis of PCOS.[70] However, there is no consensus on the precise number.[68]
  - FNPO is recommended over OV, since FNPO has been shown to have greater predictive power for PCOS and less variability among populations aged 18–35 years. OV may have a role in instances when image quality does not allow for reliable estimates of FNPO, especially when the transvaginal route is not feasible.[70]

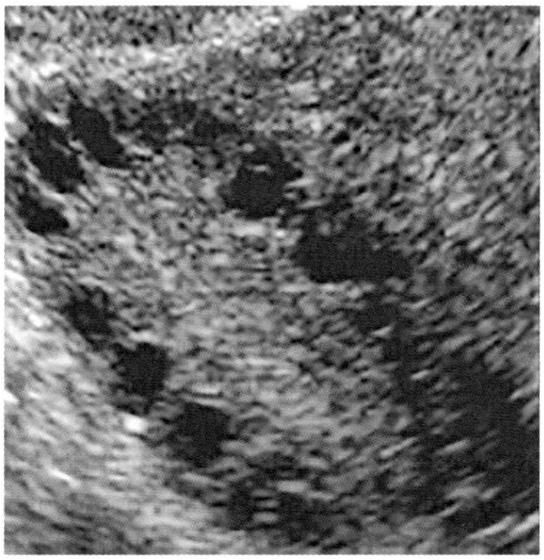

Fig. 5: Polycystic ovarian morphology on transvaginal sonography.

- *Differential diagnosis of PCOM—multicystic ovaries:* Fewer cysts (6–10/ovary), larger (up to 10 mm), and distributed throughout the ovary with no stromal hypertrophy; seen in mid-late normal puberty, hyperprolactinemia, hypothalamic anovulation, and weight-related amenorrhea
- Three-dimensional ultrasound has allowed a better and more objective assessment of ovarian morphology, considerably reducing intra and interobserver variability of 2D imaging.
- *Other imaging variables used to define PCOM:*
  - *Assessment of ovarian stroma*: By 3D ultrasonography, stromal volume can be measured through calculation and subtraction of total follicular volume from the total OV. The ratio of ovarian stroma to the total ovarian size of 0.32 indicates an association with hyperandrogenaemia.[70]
  - *Ovarian vascularization:* A higher ovarian stromal blood flow and reduced uterine perfusion on 3D power Doppler is seen in PCOS. However, the lack of uniform data and absence of cut-off values make vascular indices impractical for discriminating between polycystic and normal ovaries.[70]

Possible Late Sequelae[62]

- Impaired glucose tolerance
- DM
- Dyslipidemia
- Hypertension
- CVD
- Nonalcoholic fatty liver disease
- Obstructive sleep apnea
- Quality of life (QoL) affected with manifestations of anxiety, depression, psychological, and behavioral disorders
- Endometrial hyperplasia
- Endometrial carcinoma—2.7–2.9-fold risk
- (?) Ovarian cancer and breast cancer.

EVALUATION

- Patient history of any predisposing factors to PCOS (low birth weight with excessive catch-up growth, history of large for baby syndrome, or premature adrenarche/pubarche) to be noted.
- *Family history:* Approximately 35% of mothers and 40% of sisters of women with PCOS are affected.[11] However, the phenotypic and genetic heterogeneity in the family, inconsistent diagnostic criteria, and relative infertility make linkage analyses difficult. Family history of T2DM to be noted.
- *Menstrual history:* Menarche and nature of menstrual cycle to be enquired about. Irregular cycles (>35 or <21 days) continuing for more than 2 years after the onset of menarche are likely to reflect oligoovulation or anovulation.[68]
- Psychological issues, depression, and/or anxiety should be routinely screened for and, if present, appropriate counseling and intervention should be offered by a qualified professional.
- Given that PCOS is a diagnosis of exclusion, the clinical evaluation of the syndrome is aimed at excluding other causes of androgen excess and menstrual dysfunction **(Box 2 and Table 6)**.

BOX 2: Differential diagnosis of polycystic ovary syndrome.

- Nonclassic or late-onset congenital adrenal hyperplasia (NC-CAH)-21-hydroxylase deficiency
- Androgen-secreting tumor
- Primary hypothalamic amenorrhea
- Primary ovarian failure
- Thyroid disorder
- Prolactin disorder
- Exogenous androgens
- Cushing syndrome
- Acromegaly
- Idiopathic hirsutism
- Genetic defects in insulin action

- *Evaluation of HA:* HA, detected in about 60–80% of PCOS, is yet challenging to diagnose. Either clinical evidence or biochemical assessment of HA should suffice to define HA in PCOS as the degree of hirsutism or acne that correlates poorly with circulating androgen concentrations.
- Virilization (masculinization of body musculature, severe or extreme male-pattern balding or hirsutism, clitoromegaly), rarely a sign of PCOS, suggests disorders of androgen-secreting tumors, or androgenic substance abuse or severe IR (i.e., mutations in the insulin receptor gene).[11]
- *Physical examination:* Blood pressure (BP), BMI, WC, signs of HA (hirsutism, acne, and/or alopecia), and signs of IR (acanthosis nigricans)
- *Measurement of waist circumference:* Ethnic-specific BMI cut-off points should include WC measurement to identify those at risk and apply secondary prevention despite a "lower" BMI in high-risk groups.
- Waist-to-hip ratio (WHR) can be used as a surrogate marker for central fat accumulation, with a value of >0.8 suggestive of visceral adiposity.[69]
- *Biochemical assessment of HA:* The total testosterone is generally more markedly elevated in PCOS and is a good screening tool to exclude other of androgen excess.[11]
- Since the existing assays for measurement of androgens lack accuracy, recently, liquid chromatography-mass spectrometry has been adopted as the gold standard by many of laboratories, although expensive and normal ranges for different populations are yet to be formulated.
- *Screening for glucose intolerance and HI:* 75 g OGTT is regarded as the "gold standard" to screen and detect abnormal glucose tolerance in PCOS who are at high-risk (obese) and in high-risk ethnic groups (South Asian, Hispanic, Polynesian) to be performed at initial evaluation.[68]
- PCOS up to 35% exhibits IGT (140–199 mg/dL) and up to 10% have noninsulin-dependent DM
- Women with PCOS who are overweight (BMI ≥25 kg/m^2) and who are not overweight (BMI <25 kg/m^2), but with additional risk factors such as advanced age (>40 years), personal history of gestational diabetes, or family history of type 2 diabetes (T2D), should have a two-hour post 75 g OGTT performed (*RCOG Green-Top Guideline*).[71]
- In those with impaired fasting glucose or IGT after a two-hour OGTT, an OGTT should be performed annually (*RCOG Green-Top Guideline*).[71]
- A serum HbA1c may be performed, if the patient is unable to complete the OGTT.[68] The American Diabetes Association (ADA) defines raised HbA1c as >5.7%, and as diagnostic for T2DM at >6.4%. However, this has not been validated as in PCOS, the intrinsic IR is primarily at the level of the skeletal muscle, rather than at the liver, and fasting glucose and HbA1c may not reflect post-OGTT hyperglycemia.[72]

TABLE 6: Investigational profile in polycystic ovary syndrome (PCOS).

Test	*Normal (N) and values in PCOS (may vary with local laboratory assays)*	*Additional points*
Pelvic ultrasound	• *B-mode ultrasound:* To assess: – Polycystic ovarian morphology (PCOM) – Endometrial thickness – Stromal echogenicity: Hyperechoic, more than the echogenicity of the myometrium – Stromal/ovarian area >0.32, in HA PCOS[70] • *Doppler*: Stromal vascularity: increased	• As per the Rotterdam criteria, follicular number per ovary (FNPO) for the definition of PCOM is ≥12 • The AEPCOS Task Force recommends FNPO with a threshold of ≥25, but only when using maximal resolution with transducer frequency ≥8 MHz[70] • Subjective with intraobserver and interobserver variability
Testosterone (T)	• Total T (N): 20–80 ng/dL (0.5–3.5 nmol/L); PCOS: >60 ng/dL ≤150 ng/dL (>2.5 but ≤5 nmol/L) • PCOS: free T >0.75 ng/dL • Elevated free T levels is observed in about 70% PCOS[11] • About 20% and 40% of PCOS will have androgen levels within the "normal" range[11] • DHEAS—(N): 100–360 mg/dL • PCOS—moderately elevated	• Total T ≥150–200 ng/dL (≥6.94 nmol/L) warrants further evaluation • Most commercial androgen assays are highly variable, inaccurate with little specificity • A total testosterone is adequate for general screening, preferably early morning sample[37] • The assay of minor androgens, like ASD or DHEAS, does not add much value and is primarily indicated in women with rapidly progressive virilization or severe clinical HA • DHEAS is elevated in 25–35% of PCOS[11] • Majority of those with elevated DHEAS, the free and total testosterone is also elevated[73] • Existing laboratory assays do not evaluate the hormonal bioactivity, explaining the poor correlation between circulating androgen levels and clinical symptoms
Free androgen index (FAI): T×100/SHBG	• FAI >8.5—PCOS • SHBG (N): 16–119 nmol/L; PCOS <5 nmol/L	• Insulin suppresses SHBG, resulting in a high FAI in the presence of normal total T • FAI is thought to be the most sensitive indicator of hyperandrogenism • Measurement of SHBG assists in calculating FAI, may have a role in metabolic assessment as a surrogate marker for IR in PCOS[68] • Limitation: expensive
• FSH • LH E2	• N: 2–8 IU/L • N: 2–10 IU/L • N: 50–80 pg/mL	• Measured in early follicular phase on days 1–5 of cycle or at random in those with amenorrhea or oligomenorrhea[68] • To rule out WHO 1 and 3 anovulatory disorders 70–75% of PCOS show elevated basal LH levels[9,11]
LH:FSH ratio		• ↑LH: FSH ratio (>2:1) has been regarded as a marker of PCOS, more so in lean than in obese PCOS • Ratio varies with assays used to measure. • Hence, not a reliable diagnostic criterion
AMH	• N: 1.1–3.5 ng/mL or 5–15 pmol/L • PCOS: >5 ng/mL or >35 pmol/L	• Serum AMH ≥35 pmol/L showed 92% sensitivity and 97% specificity in the diagnosis of PCOM. • Serum AMH level-surrogate marker, as a substitute for antral follicle count (AFC) in PCOS diagnosis.[74] • The lack of standardization of AMH assay makes it unreliable.

Contd…

Contd...

Test	*Normal (N) and values in PCOS (may vary with local laboratory assays)*	*Additional points*
• Prolactin • Thyroid-stimulating hormone (TSH)	• N: 25–30 ng/mL • b N: 0.5–2.5 mLU/L	• Measure if oligo-/amenorrheic • To rule out WHO 4 anovulatory disorders (hyperprolactinemic anovulation)
Assessment of ovulation: a. Progesterone (P4) b. Ultrasound (US)	a. Measure mid-luteal P4 levels 7 days before anticipated menses in two consecutive cycles	• A single mid-luteal phase (day 21) P4 >10 ng/mL or 30 nmol/L confirms ovulation • Limitation: Peak P4 levels remain only for a short time. Hence, sample not taken at appropriate time might result in a low value • The "gold standard" would be US confirmation of follicular development and subsequent evolution of the follicle to a corpus luteum, combined with biochemical evidence of ovulation[68] • Additionally, US assessment of the endometrium benefits
a. 17-Hydroxyprogesterone: 17-OHP b. 24-hour urine free cortisol c. Overnight dexamethasone suppression test	• 17-OHP >200 ng/dL—to do Corticotropin stimulation test • 17-OHP >800 ng/dL establishes the diagnosis of late onset congenital adrenal hyperplasia	a. To rule out nonclassical/late onset congenital adrenal hyperplasia and c. To rule out Cushing syndrome
a. Fasting insulin (FI) b. 2-hour post-prandial insulin (PPI) c. Fasting glucose/insulin (FG/FI) ratio	a. FI (N): <30 µU/mL; IR: >20–30 µU/mL b. PPI (N): <80–100 µU/ml; IR: >100 µU/mL c. FG/FI (N) >4.5; IR <4.5	Not routinely measured due to lack of standardized insulin assay Instead OGTT done
OGTT	2-hour 75 g glucose	a. Fasting values:[72] • Normal: <100 mg/dL • Impaired: 100–125 mg/dL • Type 2 DM: >126 mg/dL b. 2-hour glucose values:[72] • Normal: <140 mg/dL • Impaired: 140–199 mg/dL • Type 2 DM: 200 mg/dL IGT: in 35–45% of PCOS[62,75] Type 2 DM: Prevalence is 10–15%, increases by 2% annually[62] For 6.2 years, the conversion rate, from IGT to diabetes was 54%[75]
Others: a. Serum homocysteine (SH) b. Lipid profile c. Endometrial sampling	a. SH (N): 5–11 µmol/L; PCOS: >11 µmol/L[76] b. Triglycerides ≥150 mg/dL HDL cholesterol ≤40 mg/dL	c. Endometrial sampling in women with potential long-term exposure to unopposed estrogen stimulation

(AEPCOS: Androgen Excess and PCOS Society; AMH: anti-Müllerian hormone; ASD: androstenedione; DHEAS: dehydroepiandrosterone sulfate; DM: diabetes mellitus; FG: fasting glucose; FSH: follicle-stimulating hormone; HA: hyperandrogenism; IGT: impaired glucose tolerance; IR: insulin resistance; LH: luteinizing hormone; OGTT: oral glucose tolerance test; OHP: hydroxyprogesterone; SHBG: sex hormone-binding globulin)

BOX 3: Screening strategy for PCOS: Recommendations by the ESHRE Capri Workshop Group.[69]

- Measure BMI and waist circumference at every visit
- Complete lipid profile and repeat every 2 years if normal
- 2 hour 75-g oral glucose tolerance test (OGTT): Repeat every 2 years if normal, and sooner in those with the below mentioned risk factors. Consider using HbA1c
  - Age >40 years
  - BMI >25 kg/m^2 (Asian population)
  - Waist to hip ratio >0.85
  - Hyperandrogenemia with anovulation
  - Acanthosis nigricans-stigmata of IR
  - History of gestational diabetes mellitus (GDM)
  - Family history of DM
- Measure the clinical blood pressure at each visit.
- Suggestion: Assess for depression, anxiety and quality of life

(BMI: body mass index; DM: diabetes mellitus; ESHRE: European Society for Human Reproduction and Embryology; HbA1c: hemoglobin A1c; PCOS: polycystic ovary syndrome)

- Screening strategy for PCOS as per the *Recommendations by the ESHRE Capri Workshop Group* **(Box 3)**.[69]
- TVS in those with AUB or oligomenorrhea (intervals between menstruation of more than 3 months corresponding to fewer than four periods each year) to evaluate the endometrial thickness and if evidence of hyperplasia, to consider endometrial sampling or hysteroscopic directed endometrial biopsy.

MANAGEMENT

It depends on the age, clinical manifestations of the disorder, and concern for fertility. Treatment is a multidisciplinary approach involving a gynecologist, pediatrician, endocrinologist, dermatologist, cardiologist, diabetologist, and geriatrician.[62] Management of polycystic ovarian syndrome is shown in **Table 7**.

TABLE 7: Management of polycystic ovarian syndrome.

Lifestyle modification	Healthy diet and exercises to achieve and maintain optimal BMI
Manage dermatological manifestations	• OCPs • Antiandrogens
Manage menstrual dysfunctions	Regulation of menstrual cycle and induction of withdrawal bleeds: • OCPs • Progestins
Manage infertility	• Ovulation induction—oral ovulogens, gonadotropins • Laparoscopic ovarian drilling • Intrauterine insemination • In vitro fertilization
Manage adverse metabolic dysfunctions	• Improve insulin sensitivity—insulin sensitizers • Statins • Antioxidants

(BMI: body mass index; OCP: oral contraceptive)

First-line Treatment: Lifestyle Modifications

- *First-line therapy for all PCOS women:* Lifestyle modifications targeting weight loss in those obese and overweight and prevention of weight gain in lean women.[64-68]
- To optimize adherence with lifestyle interventions, psychosocial factors be considered and necessary support provided.

Weight Loss

About 5–10% of weight loss is found to be effective to decrease testosterone levels, increasing SHBG levels, attenuating IR and other metabolic aberrations, with a 30% reduction in visceral fat, normalizing cycles in 44% of patients, and thereby improving fertility.[69-77]

Methods:
- Diet: Atkins diet;[77] intakes of low-glycemic index diet such as vegetables, fruit, fiber, wholegrain foods, and high protein from vegetable sources. To avoid refined carbohydrates and transfat-containing hydrogenated oils. A low-calorie diet of ~1,000–1,200 kcal/day with a calorie restriction of 500 kcal/day restriction typically reduces total body weight by ~10% over 6 months.[77]
- Exercise: Aerobic exercises 3–4 times/week for 20–30 minute sessions burn 100–200 kcal with 40% improvement in insulin sensitivity in 48 hours.[78] The US Department of Health and Human Services (DHHS) guidelines recommend either 150 minutes of moderate-intensity exercise per week or 75 minutes of vigorous-intensity exercise.[78] PCOS patients should be encouraged for vigorous physical activity as it has been demonstrated that every hour of vigorous exercise reduced a patient's odds of MebS by 22%.[79]

Pharmacological agents:
- Amphetamines, rimonabant, and sibutramine licenses as antiobesity drugs have been withdrawn because of their adverse effects.
- Orlistat is a lipase inhibitor that acts by reducing intestinal absorption of fats. An oral dose of 120 mg three times a day with meals; also decreases the absorption of fat-soluble vitamins, especially vitamin D; mainly associated with gastrointestinal side effects and has been approved for long-term treatment of obesity.[80]
- Drugs recently approved by the United States Food and Drug Administration (US-FDA) are lorcaserin, phentermine plus topiramate extended-release,

naltrexone sustained-release, and liraglutide. However, the adverse effect profile of these pharmacological agents is yet to be understood and is not widely available for use in the majority of the countries.[81]

Bariatric surgery: Bariatric surgery may be an option for morbidly obese women with PCOS (BMI of 40 kg/m^2 or more or 35 kg/m^2 or more with a high-risk obesity-related condition) if standard weight-loss strategies have failed (RCOG Guideline 33).

Management of Hirsutism/Alopecia/Acne

Hirsutism

Antiandrogens:

- Spironolactone (aldosterone-antagonist diuretic): Mechanism of action—competitive antagonist for the androgen receptor, suppresses cytochrome P450, inhibits ovarian and adrenal steroidogenesis, and directly inhibits 5-α-reductase activity. Dosage—100–200 mg/day. Common side effects—numbness, muscle pain, nausea, hypotension, fatigue, dizziness, menstrual irregularity, and hyperkalemia; need to monitor potassium and creatinine levels
- Flutamide (androgen receptor antagonist): Inhibits androgen uptake. Dosage—250 mg/day; limited value because of its dose-dependent hepatotoxicity.
- Finasteride: Inhibitor of type II 5-α-reductase and blocks the conversion of testosterone to DHT. Dosage—5 mg daily. Adverse effects—hepatotoxicity. Contraindicated in women of reproductive age due to the risk of feminization of male fetuses and liver abnormalities; finasteride 0.05% as the gel has been used for the treatment of female pattern hair loss.
- Cyproterone acetate (CPA): It is the most commonly used antiandrogen with progestogenic activity. Mechanism of action—competition for 5-α-reductase and androgen receptors, and inhibits the action of testosterone and DHT and direct action suppressing ovarian androgen production. It can be used alone in the dose of 25–50 mg/day on cycle days 5–14 or combined with ethinylestradiol (EE) (CPA—2 mg + EE 20 μg/day on days 5–25) to provide cycle control in addition to amelioration of hyperandrogenic symptoms. Side effects—Headache, nausea, weight gain, decreased libido, fatigue, breast tenderness, and rarely hepatotoxicity.
- Antiandrogens should not be used without effective contraception due to the risk of teratogenicity (feminization of male infant) and to stop at least 6 months before pregnancy is planned.[62]
- Spironolactone and finasteride can be used as second-line treatments for the management of hirsutism in PCOS.

Combined hormonal OCP:

- Oral contraceptive pills with antiandrogenic progestins such as CPA, drospirenone, and desogestrel are used as the first-line agents for pharmacologic treatment of hirsutism in PCOS not willing to conceive.[82] OCPs act to reduce the androgen levels through these mechanisms:
  - Estrogen component increases hepatic SHBG production.
  - Suppression of LH secretion and thereby ovarian androgen production by progestogens
  - Competition for 5-α-reductase and androgen receptors by progestogens, thereby inhibiting the peripheral conversion of testosterone to DHT and binding of DHT to androgen receptors in the skin.
- Antiandrogenic progestogens such as CPA, chlormadinone acetate, desogestrel, and drospirenone can block the action of testosterone through competition on the androgen receptor at the tissue level.
- OCP containing CPA (2 mg CPA + 35 μg EE) and drospirenone (3 mg of drospirenone + 30 μg EE) and desogestrel (150 μg +30 μg EE) are more effective in reducing the growth of new terminal hair and acne formation. Further, drospirenone is a derivative of spironolactone (≈25 mg of spironolactone) and thus has direct antiandrogenic activity.[83]
- At least 6 months of medical therapy for hirsutism is necessary to see a therapeutic response.[62]

Dermatological interventions:

- Permanent methods of hair removal include electrolysis and photo epilation devices such as laser and intense-pulsed light. Temporary current hair removal methods include waxing, plucking, shaving, depilation, epilation, and bleaching.
- Topical treatment with eflornithine hydrochloride 1%, an inhibitor of ornithine decarboxylase, approved by US-FDA, is shown to be effective for decreasing the development of new unwanted facial hair.[84] However, it is expensive and needs to be used continuously to yield its desired effect.

Management of Acne

- Use of OCPs (containing CPA, drospirenone, or desogestrel as progestin component) as first-line therapy for the management of all types of acne lesions, in consultation with a dermatologist.
- Topical treatment with salicylic acid, benzoyl peroxide, clindamycin/benzoyl peroxide preparations, tretinoin, and clindamycin/tretinoin combinations can be used.

Management of Alopecia

- OCPs and androgen blockers are recommended as first-line therapy.

- Use of CPA + EE for 6–9 months demonstrated a marked improvement in androgenic alopecia.[85] Topical treatment of hair loss is with minoxidil, 2–5% twice daily.

Existing guidelines:

- The Endocrine Society clinical practice guidelines recommend the use of hormonal contraceptives and dermatological interventions as the first-line therapy for the management of hirsutism/acne in women with PCOS.[86] Further, the guidelines recommend screening guidelines for use of OCPs and OCPs containing CPA for more effective management of HA. Then, if at least 6 months of therapy with OCP has not significantly decreased the rate of hair growth, antiandrogens may be added.[86]
- However, when estrogen is contraindicated, drugs with an antiandrogen effect should be used in combination with effective contraceptives (nonhormonal methods or progesterone-only contraceptives).
- The AEPCOS recommends OCPs containing progestogens with a greater antiandrogen potential, such as cyproterone, chlormadinone, and drospirenone as the choice for treatment of hirsutism.[11]

Management of Menstrual Dysfunction

Combined Hormonal Oral Contraceptive Pills

- The approach to the management of menstrual dysfunction will depend on the type of menstrual dysfunction, life stage, medical history, and preferences of the woman concerned.
- OCP has a primary role in the management of AUB and in oligo/amenorrhea. In women who do not wish to conceive, OCP given cyclically will confer regular monthly withdrawal bleeds.
- *Rationale for use of OCP:*
    - The progestin component → LH secretion → ovarian androgen production. With a reduction in androgens, there is decreased substrate available for aromatization and overall decreased endogenous sex steroid production.
    - Estrogen component → hepatic SHBG production → in circulating bioavailable free testosterone levels.
    - The progestin component protects the endometrium from unopposed estrogen.
- The most widely prescribed OCPs contain EE at doses ranging from 20 to 35 μg and progestin with minimal androgenic activity.
- Although both second- and third-generation OCPs are equally effective in controlling menses, it is advisable to avoid OCPs with higher estrogen doses or those containing 19-nor-derived progestins.
- Increased risk of metabolic abnormalities, CV events and venous thromboembolism, worsening of IR due to OCPs in PCOS who are inherently at risk, particularly the obese ones.[62] However, in the absence of other risk factors, there is no evidence that PCOS are at increased risk of CVD compared with normal women.
- Overall, the benefits of OCPs outweigh the risks in most patients with PCOS.[62] However, all patients should be counseled on the potential risk of thrombotic events with the use of OCPs.
- Low-dose OCs are metabolically safe and ameliorate several CV risk markers.[87]
- OCs containing third-generation progestins as well as drospirenone and CPA have reduced metabolic side effects compared to OCs containing more androgenic progestins.[88]
- Absolute and relative contraindications to the use of OCP according to the WHO guideline to be followed.[89] Absolute contraindications include smoking (>15 cigarettes a day) over the age of 35, liver dysfunction, hypertension (>160/100 mm Hg), deep venous thrombosis, ischemic heart disease, stroke, and breast cancer.

Existing guidelines: The clinical practice guidelines from the Endocrine Society,[86] RCOG,[90] ACOG,[84] RCOG, ACOG, ASRM, and ESHRE[62] all recommend the use of OCPs as the first-line management for the amelioration of clinical and biochemical HA and menstrual irregularity in the absence of contraindications. However, the guidelines do not suggest any specific combination of compounds.

Alternatives to Oral Contraceptive Pills

Progestin therapy:

- Indicated in those women who are intolerant to estrogen-containing therapies or when contraindication to estrogen or multiple risk factors for CVD are present.
- Regular withdrawal of the endometrium with progestin, if administered on a regularly basis, without prolonged episodes of amenorrhea, will regulate menses and provide some protection against endometrial hyperplasia.[25]
- Given cyclically (micronized progesterone 100–200 mg daily or medroxyprogesterone acetate 10 mg daily for 10–14 days per month)[25]
- Those in need of contraception might be candidates for progestin-only contraceptives including long-acting injectables (depot medroxyprogesterone), etonogestrel-containing implants, or levonorgestrel-containing intrauterine systems. These methods provide effective protection against endometrial hyperplasia.
- Levonorgestrel-releasing intrauterine device (IUD): (1) for control of abnormal bleeding. The use of levonorgestrel IUD was found to be more effective than usual

medical treatment in reducing the effect of heavy menstrual bleeding on QoL;[91] (2) protects the endometrium from unopposed estrogens; and (3) provides contraception.

- Transdermal contraceptive patch contains:
  - Norelgestromin and 0.75 mg EE, weekly application, is also a treatment option. However, it may be associated with an increased risk for venous thromboembolism compared to OCPs.[25]
  - A transvaginal contraceptive ring releasing 15 µg EE and 120 µg etonogestrel per day over 3 consecutive weeks (monthly insertion) is yet another option.
- There is a paucity of data regarding the use of hormonal contraceptives other than OCPs in PCOS and the long-term risks and benefits remain largely unknown.[92]

Existing guidelines: The RCOG Green-top guidelines recommend in those oligomenorrheic or amenorrheic regular induction of withdrawal bleed at least every 3–4 months with cyclical gestogens for at least 12 days or OCPs or endometrial protection gained by exposure to gestogens by the IUD.[71]

Management of Infertility in PCOS

- About 74–80% of PCOS suffer from subfertility due to anovulation.[36,69]
- Women with PCOS desiring pregnancy should be evaluated for all other factors causing anovulation along with evaluation of the male partner.
- Management of infertility as per the Thessaloniki ESHRE/ASRM-Sponsored PCOS Consensus Workshop[77] is shown in **Table 8**.

Oral Ovulation Induction Agents

Clomiphene Citrate

- Clomiphene citrate (CC) is the first choice for OI in anovulatory PCOS.[93]
- Nonsteroidal selective estrogen receptor modulator (SERM) triphenylethylene derivative
- Racemic mixture of two stereoisomers: En (cis) clomiphene and zu (trans) clomiphene. Zu form exists in tissues for weeks and contributes to its metabolic life; En form is the more potent isomer and contributes to the ovulation-inducing action of CC.[94]

TABLE 8: Management of infertility—Thessaloniki ESHRE/ASRM PCOS Consensus Workshop.[77]

• First-line treatment for ovulation induction • Alternative agents	• Clomiphene citrate (CC) • Tamoxifen • Aromatase inhibitors (Letrozole)
Second-line intervention	• Exogenous gonadotropins • Laparoscopic ovarian drilling (LOD)
Third-line treatment	In vitro fertilization

- *Mechanism of action:* Binds to hypothalamic nuclear estrogen receptors → blocks the negative feedback mechanism of circulating estrogen → FSH and LH → follicular development.

Dosing and monitoring:

- *Starting dose*: 50 mg/day for 5 days from day 2/3 of the menstrual cycle; over-response, reduce to 25 mg, no ovulation—50 mg increments with the maximum dose of 150 mg/day. FDA recommends 750 mg/treatment cycle.[93]
- Selection of patients for treatment is based on age, BMI, normal baseline FSH levels, and assessment of other associated infertility factors.
- Monitoring by ultrasound is not mandatory, though monitoring of the first cycle would allow adjustment of the dose for the subsequent cycles.[93] ASRM recommends monitoring by the menstrual calendar, serum progesterone concentration, or urinary LH excretion to ensure its effectiveness in OI.[94]
- Human chorionic gonadotropin (hCG) triggers when the lead follicle is 18–22 mm, in those requiring intrauterine insemination (IUI) and in whom LH monitoring would be difficult or unreliable in the timing of intercourse.
- *Outcome:* [68,69,93]
  - Ovulation rate: 75–80%
  - Conception rate per cycle: 22–36%
  - Multiple pregnancy rate (MPR): 8%
  - Miscarriage rate: 10–20%
  - Live birth rate (following 6 months of CC): 20–29%.
- *Discrepancy between ovulation and PR:* Due to peripheral antiestrogenic action of CC on the endometrium, cervical mucus, decreased uterine blood flow, impaired endometrial placental protein 14 synthesis, probable detrimental effects on tubal transport, oocytes, and luteal phase defect.[93]
- *Duration of treatment:* Six ovulatory cycles and in the absence of pregnancy, second-line therapy to be considered.
- *CC resistance (ovulation failure):* Defined as failure to ovulate after receiving 150 mg of CC daily for 5 days per cycle, for at least three cycles, is seen in about 20–25% of cases.[93] Such patients are likely to be more obese, insulin resistant, and hyperandrogenic.
- *Options for CC resistance*:[93]
  - Use of insulin sensitizers concomitantly
  - Second line of management; either GT/LOD
  - Extended use of clomiphene: For 7 or more days in the dose of 100 mg/day, rarely 150 mg/day
  - Use of aromatase inhibitors (AIs)
  - Addition of glucocorticoids either dexamethasone 0.25–0.5 mg or prednisolone 5 mg
  - Pretreatment with OCPs.
- *Clomiphene citrate failure:* Those who ovulate but fail to conceive after three or more ovulatory cycles with CC. Failure to conceive after 3–4 successful CC-induced

ovulation cycles is an indication for further evaluation to exclude other contributing factors of infertility, particularly in women more than 35 years of age.[94]

- *Side effects:* Vasomotor flushes, mood swings, bloating, abdominal distension, breast tenderness, visual symptoms (scotomas, light sensitivity, blurred/double vision), dryness of the vagina, headache, and ovarian hyperstimulation.
- *Clomiphene and ovarian malignancy:* With six CC cycles, the risk will not exceed that of other women, but with more than 12 cycles in a women's lifetime, there was a threefold increase in ovarian cancer.[93] However, a pooled analysis of 8 case–control studies concluded that neither fertility drug nor use for more than 12 months was associated with invasive ovarian cancer.[94]
- *Contraindications*: Ovarian cyst, pregnancy, liver disease, and visual disorders
- *Congenital anomaly:* The possibility of an association between CC exposure and anomalies included spina bifida occulta, hypospadias, cloacal exstrophy, ventricular septum heart defects, Dandy–Walker syndrome, and omphalocele.[68]

Tamoxifen

- Selective estrogen receptor modulator acts as potent estrogen antagonist on breast, blood vessel, and some peripheral sites, but as a partial agonist in uterus, bone, liver, and pituitary.
- *Mechanism of action:* Being structurally similar to CC, the mechanism of action is similar to CC, but may also involve a direct action on the ovary and improve folliculogenesis.[95]
- *Dose*: About 20–40 mg/day from day 2/3 of the menstrual cycle for 5 days.
- Ovulation and PRs similar in both CC and tamoxifen. However, better ovulation and PRs were reported in a few studies, maybe because of a higher score of the endometrium, cervical mucus, and better functioning of the corpus luteum.[95]
- Tamoxifen has shown reasonably good results in CC failure cases with beneficial effects on bone mineral density and serum lipids.[95]
- *Side effects:* Hot flushes, vomiting, anorexia, AUB, and endometrial hyperplasia.

Aromatase Inhibitors

- *Letrozole (LE):* It is the most commonly used AI as an ovulation-inducing agent.
- *Mechanism of action:* (1) Inhibits aromatase enzyme at the granulosa cells, prevents the conversion of androgens into estrogens → release of hypothalamo-pituitary axis (H-P axis) from E2-negative feedback → FSH → follicular development. (2) Transient in intraovarian androgenic environment → follicular sensitivity to FSH. (3) Induces intrafollicular high IGF-1 concentrations, which synergize with the action of FSH.
- *Advantages of AIs for ovulation induction:* (1) No antiestrogenic effect on the endometrium or cervical mucus. (2) LE is rapidly eliminated due to its short half-life (45 hours), leading to late follicular rise in circulating estrogen, with a shorter FSH window (mimicking the physiological cycle) resulting in mono-ovulation.[96] (3) Reduces the risks of ovarian hyperstimulation and multiple pregnancies.
- *Dose*: About 2.5–5 mg/day, from day 3/4 of the cycle for 5 days. The use of higher doses (5 and 7.5 mg), although might cause a shorter stimulation period, adds no advantage over 2.5 mg in terms of PRs. Moreover, the higher dose of 7.5 mg causes persistence of aromatase inhibition resulting in thin endometrium by the time of ovulation.[96]
- *Ovulation rate:* 75%; PR: 17–20%.[96]
- *Side effects:* Minimal and transient generally due to hypoestrogenemia, gastrointestinal disturbances, asthenia, headache, and back pain.
- *Safety*: Although an abstract (Biljan, ASRM abstract, 2005) raised the concern for the potential of teratogenicity suggesting a higher risk (4.7%) of congenital cardiac and musculoskeletal malformations in newborns,[97] the methodology was criticized and a peer-reviewed paper did not result from the presented abstract. Subsequent publications found LE to be safe[98,99] and the incidence of major malformation was 2.5% in babies in the LE group, 2.9% in babies conceived naturally, and 3.9% in babies in CC.[98]
- *Anastrozole:* There have been few studies on the use of anastrozole as an OI agent. Used in the dosage of 1 mg daily from day 3 for 5 days.

Existing guidelines: ACOG recommends LE as the first line of drug for ovulation-induction in PCOS with BMI of >30 kg/m^2 because of increased live birth rate when compared with CC.[99]

CC or LE (when available and permissible) should be the first-line pharmacological therapy to improve fertility outcomes in PCOS, with no other infertility factors.[68] Endometrial receptivity during the implantation window of LE is superior to CC in PCOS women, which may be related to higher clinical pregnancy and ongoing PRs.

Gonadotropins

- *Indications:*
  - Clomiphene/tamoxifen/LE resistance
  - Clomiphene/tamoxifen/LE failure
  - Persistent LH hypersecretion
  - IUI cycles
  - Assisted reproductive technology (ART) cycles
- GTs can be used alone or in combination with CC, LE, or tamoxifen.

- Initial dose depends on the age, BMI, AMH, and previous response to GTs with subsequent adjustment of dose based on follicular response.
- GT usage requires close monitoring with ultrasound and, if required, correlated biochemically with E2, LH, and progesterone levels, more so in ART cycles.
- Induction of ovulation in timed intercourse and IUI cycles, the difficulty is in achieving the desired monofollicular ovulation, due to the extreme sensitivity of the polycystic ovary to GTs. This is not due to a difference in FSH threshold levels but probably, the cohort contains twice the number of available FSH-sensitive antral follicles, compared to the normal ovary.[99]
- Any dose of FSH overstepping the threshold of the polycystic ovary will result in multifollicular development.
- Maximum of six cycles only (no response—resistance)
- *GTs used for OI*: Use of urinary FSH, highly purified FSH, recombinant FSH, or human menopausal gonadotropin (hMG) showed no difference in terms of pregnancy outcome and risks of OHSS.[99]
- *Complications*: OHSS and multiple pregnancies
- *Outcomes*: PR 20–25% per cycle, cumulative PR 50–70%, MPR 10–30%, OHSS rate 2%[93]
- Regimens for use of GT to fulfill two essential requirements for a successful outcome: (1) To allow a slow rise of FSH to just above the FSH threshold level (which is high in PCOS) and (2) to avoid an explosive ovarian response because of the exquisite sensitivity of PCO to exogenous GT.[93]

Step-up regimens:

- *Conventional step-up protocol:*
  - Principle: Supraphysiological dose of FSH provokes initial development of a large cohort, rescuing those follicles destined for atresia.
  - The classical protocol used in the 1970s for PCOS, included stimulation with 150 IU of hMG (containing 75 U FSH and 75 U LH), which was increased every 3–5 days by 50% until an ovarian response occurred.[36]
  - Although here the ovulation rate is 70% and cumulative PR as high as 21–75%, there is a high incidence of OHSS of 7–14% and multiple PRs of 36%.[99]
- *Low-dose step-up protocol:*
  - Principle: Increasing FSH in a gradual step-wise fashion allows rescue of a limited number of follicles mirroring that of the normal hormonal cycle.
  - GT is started in the dose of 75 IU, the first increment being done on day 7 of stimulation either by 50% or 100%, depending on the follicular growth **(Fig. 6)**.
  - Once follicle growth is observed, the same FSH dose is maintained until the DF is achieved.
  - With this, one can reduce the risk of OHSS and multiple pregnancies.

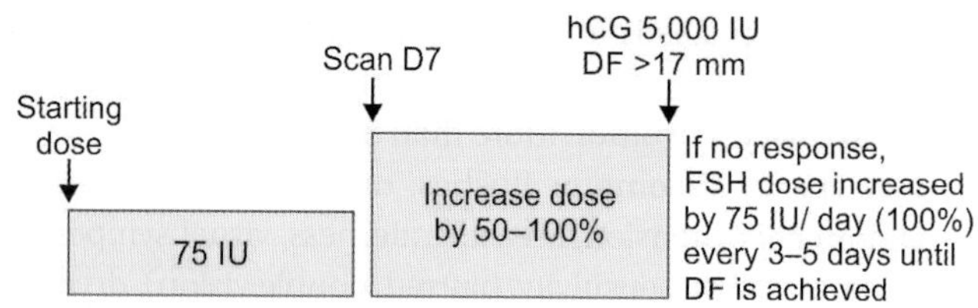

Fig. 6: Low-dose step-up protocol.
(DF: dominant follicle; FSH: follicle-stimulating hormone; hCG: human chorionic gonadotropin).

- *Chronic low-dose regimen:*
  - To further reduce the risk of ovarian hyper-responsiveness, the duration of the initial dose of FSH was extended (from 7 to 14 days) and the weekly dose increment was reduced (from 100% to 50% of the dose usually 37.5 IU) **(Flowchart 8)**.[100,101]
  - *Principle:* "Threshold theory", the attainment and maintenance of follicular development with exogenous FSH without exceeding the threshold requirement, aiming to achieve the development of a single DF.[102]
  - Safer in terms of monofollicular development.[101]
  - Avoids complications of OHSS and multiple pregnancies
  - *Drawback:* Long treatment cycles of 28–35 days.
  - Outcome:[101,102]
    - Mono-ovulatory cycles (70%)
    - PR: 20–40% per cycle
    - OHSS incidence: Very low (0.14%)
    - MPR: Less than 6% (88% twins).

Step-down regimen:

- Principle: To achieve FSH threshold through a loading dose of FSH, followed by subsequent stepwise reduction with the dominance of the follicle[103]
- Physiological as it mimics the natural intercycle FSH rise with a subsequent decrease in dependence of the developing DF to FSH than the smaller follicles, achieving monofollicular development
- In conventional step-down protocol in PCOS, FSH was started at the dose of 150 IU daily from day 2/3 of the cycle, decreasing the dose by 37.5 IU every 3 days till optimal follicular growth **(Flowchart 9)**.[102]
- In low-dose step-down, the starting dose is reduced to 100–112.5 IU/day, decreased by 25/37.5 IU every 3–5 days, respectively, decreasing to 75 IU, which is continued until hCG is administered to induce ovulation.[103]
- PR are comparable with those reported for step-up regimens. However, the French multicenter study demonstrated the superiority of the step-up regimen with regard to the rates of monofollicular development (88% of cycles), ovulation, and OHSS.[103]

Flowchart 8: Chronic low-dose step-up protocol.

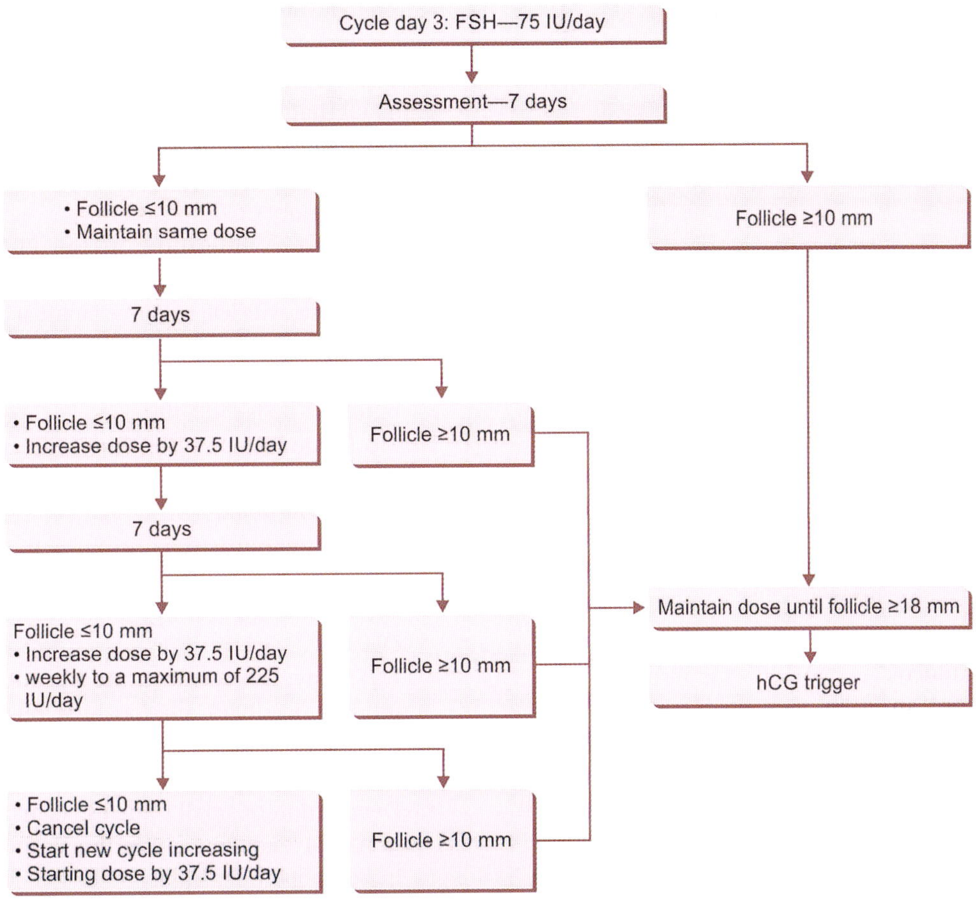

(FSH: follicle-stimulating hormone; hCG: human chorionic gonadotropin)

Source: Gardner DK, Wessman A (Eds).[101]

Flowchart 9: Step-down protocol.

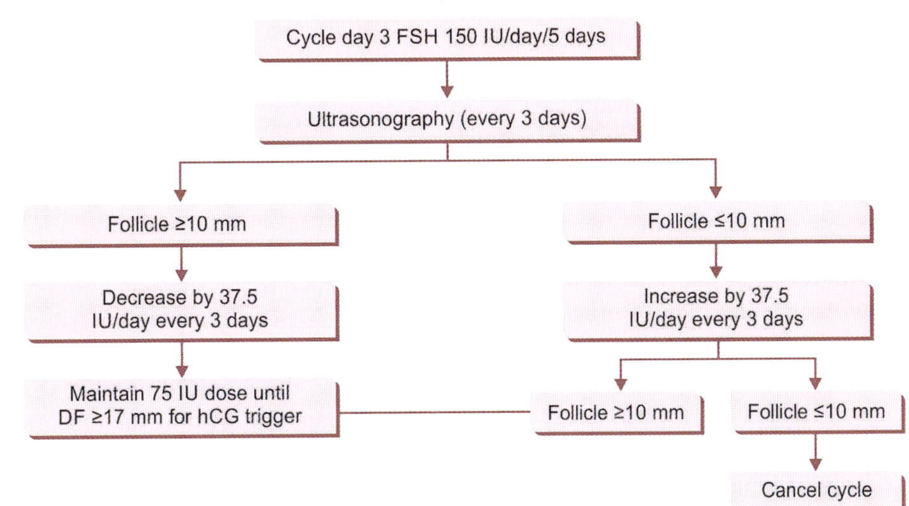

(DF: dominant follicle; FSH: follicle-stimulating hormone; hCG: human chorionic gonadotropin)

Flowchart 10: Sequential protocol.

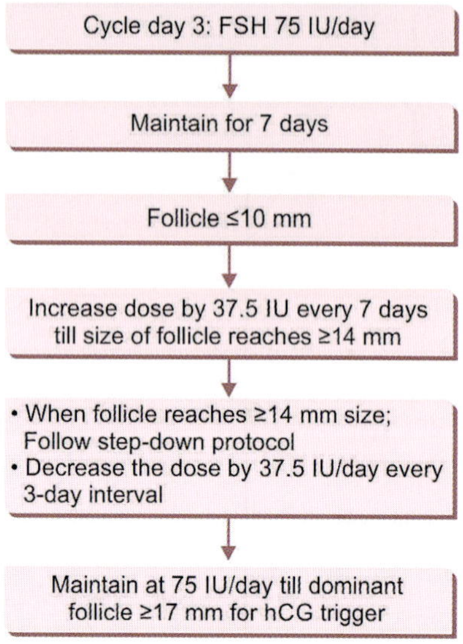

(FSH: follicle-stimulating hormone; hCG: human chorionic gonadotropin)

- Sequential protocol:
    - It combines an initial step-up GT administration followed by a step-down regimen after follicular selection.[104]
    - Reduces the risk of ovarian hyperstimulation by narrowing the follicular selection window due to atresia of the smaller follicles, with declining levels of FSH **(Flowchart 10)**[104]
- Combining GTs with GnRH analogs:
    - Hypersecretion of LH in PCOS may cause premature luteinization of the granulosa cells, premature oocyte maturation through inhibition of oocyte maturation inhibitor, and deleterious effects on granulosa cell steroidogenesis.[104]
    - To suppress LH hypersecretion, concomitant use of a GnRH agonist (GnRHa) is not justified, as this is associated with an increased risk of OHSS, additional inconvenience, cost, and multiple pregnancies.[77]
    - The benefit of LH suppression by GnRH antagonist during OI with GTs needs to be addressed by large-scale studies.[77]

Recommendations for gonadotropin: Anovulatory CC-resistant PCOS with no other infertility factors, where suitable to use GT, with consideration to provide a low-dose protocol and appropriate monitoring to minimize complications.[68]

Laparoscopic Ovarian Drilling

- The first description of laparoscopic drilling was by Gjonnaess in 1984 to reproduce the beneficial effects of the ancient ovarian wedge resection, performed by laparotomy, while avoiding its main complication, pelvic adhesions.[105]
- LOD is the creation of multiple ovarian punctures through the ovarian capsule, electrosurgical or with laser energy by a minimally invasive route, laparoscopically.
- Alternative routes for ovarian drilling are culdoscopy, transvaginal hydrolaparoscopy, and fertiloscopy, although uncommonly used.[106]
- *Indications:*[93]
    - Anovulatory CC/LE resistance
    - Anovulatory infertility in lean PCOS with raised serum LH (>10 IU/L) levels.
    - Anovulatory PCOS requires laparoscopic assessment of the pelvis.
    - Intensive monitoring is not feasible as in GT treatment or follow-up is difficult.
- Not to be done for nonfertility indications (irregular cycles, HA)[93]
- *How does LOD work*?
    - Exact mechanism is unknown. Probably, the destruction of androgen-producing stroma reduces the circulating androgens (testosterone, ASD, and DHEA).[106]
    - LOD may also result in modifications of ovarian-pituitary feedback relationships, releasing the ovary from some inhibitory process, thereby decreasing the LH levels.[106]
    - Destruction of small follicles (which are the source of AMH) leads to a fall in the serum AMH, thereby increasing the sensitivity of the follicles to circulating FSH resulting in ovulation.[107]
- *Predictors of success*: Higher likelihood of LOD success in those with young age, less than 3 years of infertility, elevated LH concentrations (>10 IU/L), lean PCOS, AMH ≤7.7 ng/mL, and no other associated infertility factors
- *Methods:*[108] (1) *Electrocautery:* insulated monopolar or bipolar electrode, preferably monopolar; (2) Laser energy [CO_2, argon, Nd: YAG (neodymium-doped yttrium aluminum garnet), KTP (potassium titanyl phosphate)]
- Armar's rule of 4:4 punctures/ovary with 40 W, 4 seconds, 4-mm depth, and 640 J/ovary (4 punctures × 4 seconds × 40 W = 640 J), fixed effective thermal dose.[108]
- However, an adjusted diathermy dose based on OV has been found to have a better reproductive outcome compared to the abovementioned fixed thermal dosage. The effective adjusted thermal dosage was found to be 60 J/cm^3 of ovarian tissue.[109]
- Ideally, the required number of punctures should be calculated by dividing the total individual ovarian dose based on OV by the dose delivered at each puncture point.[109]
- *Procedure:* Initially, the pelvis is examined, and a dye test is performed. The monopolar diathermy is set at 30 W, through cutting mode, the ovarian capsule is penetrated by an insulated monopolar electrode of

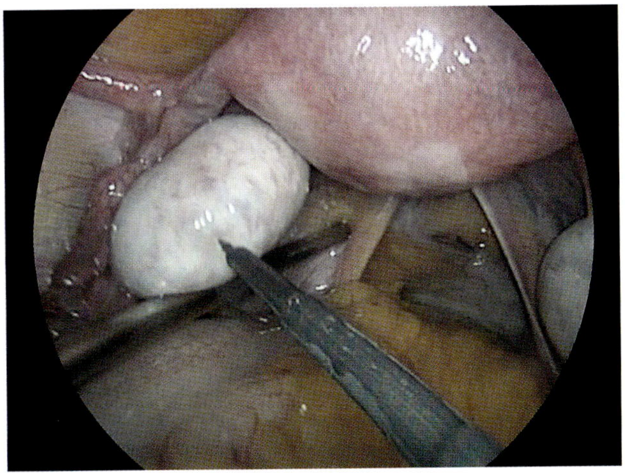

Fig. 7: Laparoscopic ovarian drilling.

1.5–2 mm in diameter with a conical tip. The denuded tip of the electrode is inserted perpendicular to the ovary, to a depth of 4–5 mm, and then the coagulation mode is activated for about 3–5 seconds **(Fig. 7)**. The instillation of 500–1,000 mL of isotonic solution into the pouch of Douglas cools the ovaries and prevents heat injury to the adjacent tissues, and thereby reducing the risk of adhesion formation. The procedure is ensured by the presence of appropriate hemostasis and a pelvic lavage.

- *Precautions to be taken in LOD:*
  - Away from the hilar area
  - Wash ovarian surface with crystalloid solution
  - Seven or more punctures per ovary discouraged—concern about excessive destruction of ovary without additional benefit[108]
  - Unilateral LOD is effective, less time-consuming, and probably with fewer complications.

Adhesions (10–20%), more with laser [(laser 41.5%, electrocautery 31%) (CO laser >Nd:YAG laser)[108]

- *Advantages of LOD over medical treatment:*
  - Correction of hormonal milieu (¯ androgens, ¯ LH)
  - Assessment of tubal patency and pelvic pathology simultaneously
  - One-time procedure (safe and effective)
  - No intense monitoring is required.
  - Cost-effective
  - Monofolliculogenesis
  - No multiple pregnancies
  - No OHSS complications are rare (premature ovarian failure/adhesions)
  - CC-resistant PCOS may respond as LOD improves the sensitivity to GTs.
  - The beneficial effects of LOD on reproductive outcomes appear to be sustained for about 9 years.[110]
- *Complications:*
  - Complications of anesthesia
  - Establishment of surgical access
  - Bleeding from the drilling site
  - Laceration of utero-ovarian ligament
  - Deep desiccation of hilar vessels—ovarian failure
  - *Adhesions:* Mechanical infertility, more with laser.[111] Abdominal lavage with the use of an insulated needle for cautery may decrease its incidence.
  - Damage to ovarian reserve, and risk of premature ovarian failure with multiple punctures
- LOD is usually effective in generating ovulation in about 50% of anovulatory PCOS, and in the remainder, additional OI agents would be required.[69]
- *Outcome:*[106] Ovulation rate: 70–80%, spontaneous PR: 20–64%.

Recommendations

- Laparoscopic ovarian drilling could be second-line therapy in CC-resistance or first-line therapy, if laparoscopy is indicated for another reason in infertile PCOS.[68]
- Minimal effective intervention dose should be applied to achieve ovulation and minimize complications, with consideration given to increased perioperative risks in those overweight or obese.[68]

Evidence

The Cochrane database compared GTs with LOD in CC-resistant PCOS and concluded that no difference exists in miscarriage rates, the live birth rate per patient, long-term cost, and QoL. However, LOD was better than GTs in reducing MPR [odds ratio (OR): 0.13 (95% confidence interval (CI): 0.03–0.52) I2 = 0%, $P = 0.004$; five studies, 166 participants] and short-term cost ($P < 0.00001$; two studies, 203 participants).[112]

Role of Intrauterine Insemination

- Ovulation induction with IUI in those with associated male factor infertility or any other associated risk factors and failure to conceive despite multiple successful inductions of ovulation
- Single IUI around the time of ovulation, at 36 ± 2 hours following hCG administration would provide a better cycle outcome compared to double insemination.[113]
- The clinical PRs per cycle: 16–20%; MPR (all protocols)—4–10%.[93]

Assisted Reproductive Technology in Polycystic Ovary Syndrome

- Anovulation is not an indication of in vitro fertilization (IVF).
- *Indications:*
  - Failure to conceive despite 6 ovulatory cycles with IUI
  - *Coexistent infertility factors:* Advanced maternal age, tubal factor infertility, severe endometriosis, male

factor infertility, need for preimplantation genetic screening/diagnosis (PGS/PGD)

- Relative GT resistance and increased GT consumption, may be related to obesity and IR.[114]
- Cycle cancellation is due to absent/limited ovarian response or OHSS.
- *Complications:* Hyper-response to GTs leading to the risk of OHSS. In IVF cycles, the incidence of moderate-to-severe OHSS is 3–8% which increases to 10–20% in high-risk PCOS population.[115]
- GnRH antagonist protocol should be the protocol of choice in PCOS, as it is associated with a shorter duration of stimulation, a lower total dose of GTs, and a significantly lower risk of moderate-to-severe OHSS.[116]
- *Individualized controlled stimulation (ICOS):* Dosage of GT based on age, BMI, AMH, and previous response to stimulation reduces the risk of OHSS in PCOS.[117]
- *Use of GTs:* With use of urinary or recombinant FSH, there was no significant difference in the number of oocytes retrieved, live birth rates, miscarriage, multiple pregnancy, or OHSS.[118]
- Trigger for follicular maturation: Use of GnRHa trigger instead of traditional hCG, which is feasible in a GnRH-antagonist protocol nearly eliminates the risk of OHSS.[119]
- *For prevention of OHSS, segmentation strategy[120] to be followed:* (1) *Segment A:* Optimization of ovarian stimulation, use of GnRH antagonist protocol with GnRHa trigger; (2) Segment B: Cryopreservation of all embryos by vitrification; (3) Segment C: Frozen embryo transfer in the subsequent cycle.
- However, the use of GnRHa as a trigger causes drastic luteolysis and is associated with luteal phase defect, presumably because of excessive negative steroid feedback resulting in suppressed pituitary LH release.[121] To circumvent this issue, there are two options: (1) intensified or modified luteal phase support in case of fresh transfer;[122] (2) cryopreservation of all oocytes/embryo by vitrification.
- Deferring fresh embryo transfer and following a freeze-all strategy would be beneficial due to these reasons: (1) To prevent early-onset OHSS; (2) To avoid the possibility of late-onset OHSS, in case of pregnancy by early embryonic hCG; (3) Impaired endometrial receptivity due to supraphysiologic steroid levels;[123] (4) To avoid embryo exposure to extremely high steroid levels, being embryo-toxic, following a high-ovarian response to ovarian stimulation.
- Performing single embryo transfer (SET) with blastocyst, the risk of multiple pregnancies and their complications are markedly reduced.[93]
- *IVF outcome:*
  - A greater number of oocytes were retrieved.[124]
  - Obese PCOS, independent of HI, was found to have an increased GT requirement and a lower oocyte yield.[124]
  - Impaired oocyte competence due to:
    - Abnormal follicular development[125] **(Fig. 3 and Flowchart 3)**
    - Altered granulosa cell–oocyte interactions, with impaired cytoplasmic and/or nuclear maturation of the oocyte due to paracrine dysregulation of growth factors[125] **(Flowchart 2)**
    - Premature granulosa cell luteinization due to HA and HI
  - An increased expression of TNF-α and epidermal growth factor receptors[125]
  - Reduced expression of GDF9 and BMP-15 mRNA in the cytoplasm of the oocytes[126]
  - Elevated follicular testosterone levels, especially in meiotically incompetent oocytes[125]
  - Increased follicular fluid homocysteine levels[76]
  - Nondisjunction and predivision of sister chromatids due to altered expression of key genes associated with chromosome alignment and segregation during mitosis and/or meiosis due to hyperandrogenemia[127]
  - Altered metabolic milieu throughout oogenesis, leading to reduced expression of genes encoding oxidative phosphorylation,[128] with increased pyruvate consumption due to impaired insulin signaling and glucose metabolism[129]
  - Lower fertilization and delayed cleavage kinetics from fertilization to 8-cell stage[130]
  - Poor embryo quality is due to poor quality oocytes and increased oxidative stress[128]
  - Endometrial dysfunction due to:
    - HA and HI cause suppression of uterine placental protein (PP14, also known as glycodelin), homeobox *A10 (HOXA10)* genes, insulin-like growth factor-binding protein 1 (IGFBP-1) and b3 integrins, and high plasma endothelin-1, all possibly impairing endometrial receptivity.[131]
    - Supraphysiological levels of E2
    - Inadequate endometrial blood flow[131]
- However, these features are not universal, and oocyte quality, fertilization, and implantation rates in women with PCOS may be normal.[92]
- It has been reported that the clinical pregnancy rate (CPR) following fresh embryo transfer in phenotypes A, B, C, and D was 32.5%, 26.4%, 36.8%, and 53.3%, respectively. Phenotypes A and B were associated with a decreased CPR compared with the control group, probably due to associated HA and chronic anovulation.[132]
- A randomized controlled clinical trial showed a statistically significant 7.3% absolute increase in live births following frozen embryo transfer and an increased

pregnancy loss in the fresh transfer group, which may involve the process of placentation as well as potential effects of aspects of PCOS on the endometrium or on the maternal response to pregnancy.[133]

Evidence

- Use of GnRH antagonist protocol in PCOS significantly lowers the incidence of OHSS (Cochrane analysis by Al-Inany).[116]
- GnRH agonists trigger for final follicular maturation seems to be safer than traditional hCG triggers due to the lower risk of OHSS (Cochrane 2015).[134]

SUMMARY OF EVALUATION AND MANAGEMENT OF PCOS (DEPICTED IN THE FORM OF FLOWCHART 11)

In Vitro Maturation

- Immature oocytes are retrieved transvaginally from antral follicles measuring 2–12 mm in diameter, either unstimulated or minimally stimulated ovaries and matured in vitro for 24–48 hours before fertilization.
- *Clinical protocol:*[135]
    - Priming with FSH and hCG has been shown to improve the maturity, fertilization, and implantation rates.

Flowchart 11: Evaluation and management of PCOS.

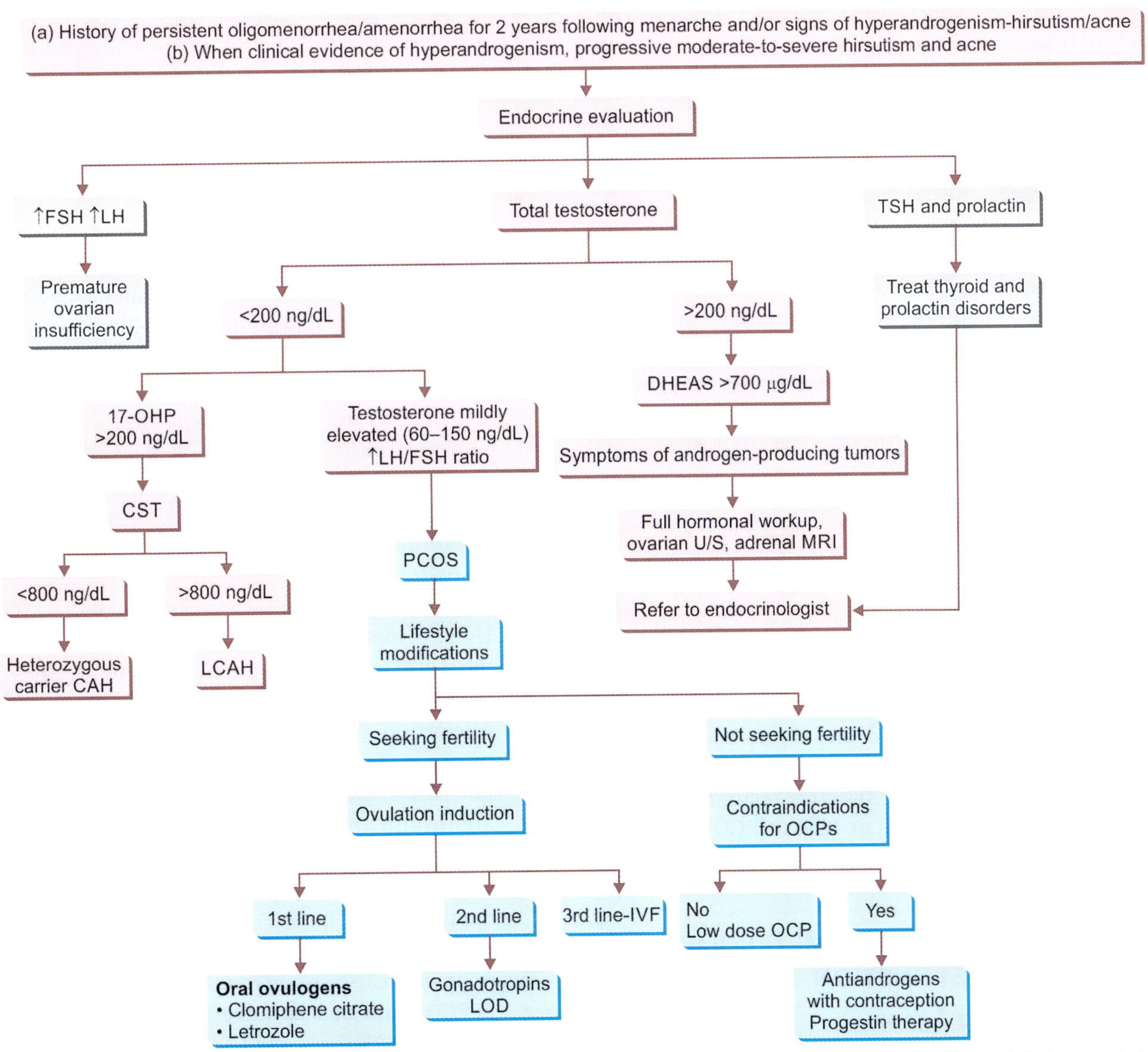

(CAH: congenital adrenal hyperplasia; CST: corticotropin stimulation test; DHEAS: dehydroepiandrosterone sulfate; FSH; follicle-stimulating hormone; LCAH: late-onset congenital adrenal hyperplasia; LH: luteinizing hormone; LOD: laparoscopic ovarian drilling; OCP: oral contraceptive pill)

- Unstimulated follicles are mobile and technically difficult to aspirate. A newly designed in vitro maturation (IVM) needle, composed of two needles, one for puncturing (21 G) and one for holding (17 G), facilitates easier puncture of small follicles.
- Aspiration pressure of 180 mm Hg yielded a higher retrieval rate compared to 300 mm Hg.
- Use heparinized media for flushing and rinsing the needle.
- Retrieved cumulus oophorus complexes (COCs) were cultured in IVM medium for 24–26 hours, and later assessed for maturity after denudation of cumulus cells.
- *Mode of fertilization:* Intracytoplasmic sperm injection (ICSI) is better than IVF.

- *Advantages:* Avoids/minimal use of GTs, patient-friendly, cost-effective, less monitoring, and avoids OHSS
- *Disadvantages:*
  - IVM when compared with conventional IVF, yields significantly fewer mature oocytes (7.8 vs. 12.0) and embryos (6.1 vs. 9.3), respectively.[136]
  - Lower CPRs per cycle in comparison to IVF (IVM 32.4% vs. IVF 45.8%) and lower live birth rate (IVM 23.5% vs. IVF 40.7%).[137]
  - The possible causes for lower implantation and CPRs:[136,137] (1) Reduced oocyte development potential (suboptimal culture conditions or defective oocytes due to inadequate cytoplasmic maturation); (2) Higher frequency of abnormal meiotic spindles and chromosomal alignment; (3) Nuclear, cytoplasmic asynchrony; (4) Failure of embryonic gene expression; and (5) Asynchronous endometrium or reduced endometrial receptivity
  - Concerns of epigenetic disorders in the offsprings.

Evidence

- This technique first offered in PCOS as an alternative to conventional IVF for the prevention of OHSS cannot be recommended now because of poor results and as GnRH antagonist with agonist-trigger protocols effectively prevent OHSS.[136]
- In a Cochrane systematic review, Siristatidis et al. concluded that no randomized controlled trials (RCTs) exist upon which to base practice recommendations regarding IVM before IVF or ICSI in PCOS. IVM as a treatment has yet to be adopted as a routine clinical entity, and may remain a research interest.[138]

ADJUVANTS TO IMPROVE METABOLIC AND REPRODUCTIVE FUNCTION

Insulin Sensitizing Agents

Metformin

- Metformin is an oral biguanide that lowers blood glucose levels in hyperglycemic individuals with T2DM but has no effect on glucose levels in normal subjects.[31]
- *Mechanism of action:*[31,139]
  - Inhibits hepatic glucose production
  - Improves insulin-stimulated peripheral glucose uptake by the liver, skeletal muscle, and adipose tissue
  - Reduces absorption of glucose uptake from the gastrointestinal tract
  - Reduces substrate availability for gluconeogenesis by lowering serum lipid levels
- *Pharmacokinetics:* Bioavailability of 50–60%, mean plasma elimination half-life of 4.0–8.7 hours, excreted renally
- *Dosage:* Orally in the dose of 500 mg/day and then increased gradually every week up to a total dose of 1,500 mg/day, after confirming normal renal and liver function tests
- Category B drug in pregnancy.
- *Side-effects:* Dose-dependent includes diarrhea (53%), nausea/vomiting (25.5%), flatulence (12.1%), asthenia (9.2%), indigestion (7.1%), abdominal discomfort (6.4%), headache (5.7%), and lactic acidosis (rare and fatal, but almost all patients who develop acidosis have impaired renal function).
- *Contraindications:* Renal disease, creatinine >1.4 mg/dL, cardiac failure, acute or chronic metabolic acidosis, sepsis, active liver disease alcoholism, should be stopped before intravenous contrast use and before surgery.
- *Advantages:*
  - Metformin has been shown to increase the frequency of ovulation in PCOS, although this impact may be mediated partly by weight loss, because of a slight anorectic effect and with some evidence of benefit on parameters of the MebS.[31]
  - Metformin has been observed to reduce serum testosterone concentration and free androgen index.[140]
  - Usage of metformin for 12 weeks prior to IVF, reduces the risk of moderate-to-severe OHSS by ameliorating the expression of VEGF.[141]
  - Alleviation of HA and IR at the ovarian level may improve folliculogenesis, the developmental potential of the embryo, and therefore the CPR.[140]
  - Metformin in combination with CC had better ovulation rates versus CC or metformin alone (60.4% vs. 49.0% vs. 29.0%) as shown by Legro et al. in a multicentric RCT.[142]
- *Uses:*
  - Adjunct in CC-resistant cases
  - In PCOS with glucose intolerance and T2DM
  - Obese PCOS for weight loss along with lifestyle modifications[143]
  - Adjuvants in IVF cycles may enhance ongoing PRs and reduce the incidence of OHSS.[144]

Evidence:

ASRM 2017 recommendations:[31]

- Metformin alone versus placebo increases the ovulation rate in PCOS (Grade A).
- Metformin in combination with CC improves ovulation and CPRs but does not improve live birth rates compared with CC alone (Grade A).
- Insufficient evidence to recommend metformin during pregnancy to reduce the chance of miscarriage (Grade C).

Cochrane: Recent Cochrane published in 2017 has concluded that metformin may improve menstrual frequency and ovulation rate, which may result in a marginal improvement in live birth rate when compared with placebo. Further, combined therapy with metformin and CC in CC resistance, in both obese and nonobese patients, improved clinical pregnancy and ovulation rates versus CC alone, although it did not improve live birth rates. Insufficient evidence to show any beneficial effect of metformin on multiple pregnancy and OHSS rates.[145]

Thiazolidinediones

- They are peroxisome proliferator-activated receptor gamma (PPAR-γ) agonists, approved for the treatment of T2D.
- They decrease IR at the periphery and liver and increase insulin-dependent glucose disposal. Because of this improvement in IR, they have been used in the treatment of PCOS with modest improvement in menstrual patterns.[146]
- Actively metabolized by the liver; half-life 3–7 hours.
- Rosiglitazone and pioglitazone are the two prescribed drugs, as they are relatively free of liver toxicity; however monitoring of liver function every 2 months is recommended.[146,147]
- Troglitazone, though has been shown to improve ovulation and PRs has been withdrawn from the market, due to its hepatotoxic effect.[147]
- Rosiglitazone: Initial dose of 4 mg/day; increased to 8 mg/day after 8–12 weeks. Pioglitazone: Used in the dose of 15–30 mg once a day.
- Side-effects: Gastrointestinal, hepatic effects, weight gain, edema, congestive heart failure, and bladder cancer risk with pioglitazone.
- Contraindications: Hypersensitivity to drugs, pregnancy, lactation, heart failure, and liver failure.
- FDA category C drugs, owing to the potential for fetal growth restriction.[146] Hence, must be discontinued as soon as pregnancy is established.

Inositol

- Myo-inositol is an insulin sensitizer. MI acts at the level of the ovary to reduce hyperandrogenemia, regularizes the cycle with spontaneous ovulation, improves ovarian response, induces nuclear and cytoplasmic maturation, thereby improving oocyte competence.[35,147]
- DCI acts at the level of the periphery to reduce IR, improves glucose metabolism, improves lipid profile, and thereby reduces CV and metabolic complications.[35]
- Hence, administration of both MI and DCI, in the physiological plasma ratio (40:1), ensures better clinical results.[147]
- Dose: 2–4 g/day

Vitamin D

- There is controversy regarding the efficacy of vitamin D3 supplementation to improve the various features of the syndrome.
- However, vitamin D supplementation has shown beneficial effects on IR, HA, follicular maturation, menstrual regularity, and ovulation.[47] It might also exert a protective effect against the inflammatory action of AGEs by increasing circulating soluble sRAGE.[44]
- Given orally in the form of vitamin D2 or D3 at a dose of 1,000–2,000 units/day or 50,000 units/week depending on the severity of deficiency to achieve a serum level of 25-hydroxyvitamin D more than 20 ng/mL
- Adverse effects are related to hypercalcemia which includes headache, nausea, vomiting, dizziness, loss of appetite, and dry mouth.
- Supplementation with vitamin D3 (400 IU/day) and calcium (1,000 mg/day) for 3 months can reduce the androgens, with a positive effect on follicle maturation and menstrual disorders.[47]

L-Methylfolate

- It is a natural and active form of folic acid, helps DNA synthesis, and reduces homocysteine levels and thereby improving endothelial function, preventing CV risk factors.[47]
- Dose: 1–5 mg/day for 3 months
- Also, high follicular fluid levels of homocysteine, an amino acid whose metabolism is facilitated by folic acid and other B vitamins, are negatively associated with embryo quality.[148] Thus, higher serum concentrations of folate and vitamin B12 were found to be associated with lower follicular fluid homocysteine levels, resulting in better fertilization and clinical pregnancy.[149]

Antioxidants

N-Acetyl cysteine (NAC):

- *N*-acetyl cysteine, the precursor of glutathione, is an antioxidant.
- It has effects on insulin receptor activity and insulin secretion, thereby increasing glucose utility.[150]

- Decreases total cholesterol, LDL, homocysteine, and oxidative stress and increases HDL levels.
- Antiapoptotic activity and aids healthy cervical secretions.
- Combination of NAC and CC enhances ovulation and PR in CC-resistant PCOS.[150]
- Dose*:* 600 mg twice a day for 6 weeks
- Melatonin: Melatonin administration reduces intrafollicular oxidative damage, prevents DNA damage, and lipid peroxidation and acts as a free radical scavenger, reducing ROS, thereby improving follicular growth and maturation, ovulation, oocyte quality, fertilization rates, and PRs. However, there needs more clarity regarding the benefit of adding melatonin in all PCOS.[151]
- L-Carnitine: Administration of 3 g/day over 8–12 weeks reduces IR, with improvement in lipid profile. In CC-resistant cases, the use of L-Carnitine throughout the cycle was shown to improve the ovulation and PR.[152]
- Omega-3 fatty acids*:* In the dose of 4 g/day for 8 weeks reduces IR, total cholesterol (TC), triglycerides, LDL, TC/HDL, LDL/HDL ratios, and MDA levels.[46]
- Soybeans: Soy phytoestrogen (Genistein) in the dose of 18 mg/day for 3 months reduces oxidative lipid damage, decreases triglycerides, low-density lipoprotein, LDL/HDL ratio, and testosterone levels. Useful for CV and metabolic disorders prevention in PCOS.[46]
- Coenzyme Q10: As an adjuvant to oral ovulatory agents in CC-resistant PCOS[153]
- Zinc: 50 mg of zinc or 220 mg/day of zinc sulfate supplementation for 8 weeks reduces IR, total cholesterol, LDL, triglyceride, and testosterone levels, resulting in beneficial effects on metabolic risk factors.[46]
- Chromium picolinate: In the dose of 200–1,000 µg for 4–6 months improved IR, fasting insulin level, and body weight; induced ovulation and regular menstrual cycles in obese PCOS[154]
- Selenium: 200 mg/day decreases serum insulin and triglycerides[46]
- Multiple micronutrients (vitamins, L-arginine, glutathione) and minerals (iron, Zn, magnesium) supplementation in PCOS undergoing OI reduces the ROS levels and maintains the cellular oxidant-antioxidant balance trace and thereby improves the reproductive outcome.

Corticosteroids

- Indication: PCOS with high DHEAS levels, which is seen in about 20–33% and in CC-resistant cases along with CC.[33]
- Mechanism of action: (A) Decrease in adrenal androgen secretion; (B) Indirect action, serum GH, serum IGF-1 → follicular fluid IGF-1 concentrations, thereby facilitating development of follicles; (C) Improves ovarian response to GTs
- Dose: Dexamethasone 0.25–0.5 mg/day; prednisone 5 mg/day from day 2 to 6 or for 10 days or throughout the follicular phase or from the mid-luteal phase of the previous cycle.
- Addition of 2 mg of dexamethasone in CC-resistant cases from days 5 to 14 was shown to be associated with a higher ovulation rate and cumulative PR.[155] However, prolonged use should be discouraged.

Oral Contraceptive Pill Pretreatment

It causes suppression of the HPO axis, and reduces LH and androgen levels, thereby improving folliculogenesis.[156] However, pretreatment with OCP results in more days of GT therapy and a higher amount of GTs.[157]

Statins

- Statin includes simvastatin and atorvastatin
- Selective inhibitor of the enzyme hydroxymethylglutaryl coenzyme A (HMG-CoA) reductase, decreases the production of cholesterol, the precursor to sex steroids, and thus, improves HA by decreasing ASD and testosterone biosynthesis.[146]
- Metabolized rapidly by the liver; half-life of 2 hours
- Improves lipid profile, decreases systemic inflammation (C-reactive protein), endothelial inflammation, and homocysteine levels[158]
- *Side-effects:* Myopathy, liver dysfunction, rhabdomyolysis, impairment of glucose metabolism, and teratogenicity
- It is a *category* X drug. Hence effective contraception is essential and not recommended as an adjunct to OI.
- Can be considered for the treatment of dyslipidemias in PCOS who are not trying to conceive[146]

Glucagon-like Peptide 1 Receptor Agonists

- Glucagon-like peptide 1 (GLP1) augments insulin secretion in response to oral glucose intake, inhibits glucagon secretion, slows gastric emptying, and reduces appetite and food intake.[146]
- Includes exenitide and liraglutide
- Liraglutide is long-acting and US-FDA approved.
- *Side-effects:* Nausea, vomiting, diarrhea, headache, risk of pancreatitis, possible increased risk of thyroid tumors with liraglutide
- Combination treatment of liraglutide with metformin for 12 weeks facilitates weight loss in PCOS.[146]
- Category C drug
- Although, these agents are promising for the treatment of IR and obesity in PCOS, larger studies are needed.[146]

POLYCYSTIC OVARY SYNDROME IN ADOLESCENTS

- During puberty, the normal physiologic IR in response to growth hormone, which peaks at this time, may aggravate the symptoms and phenotypic expression of PCOS **(Fig. 8)**.[25]

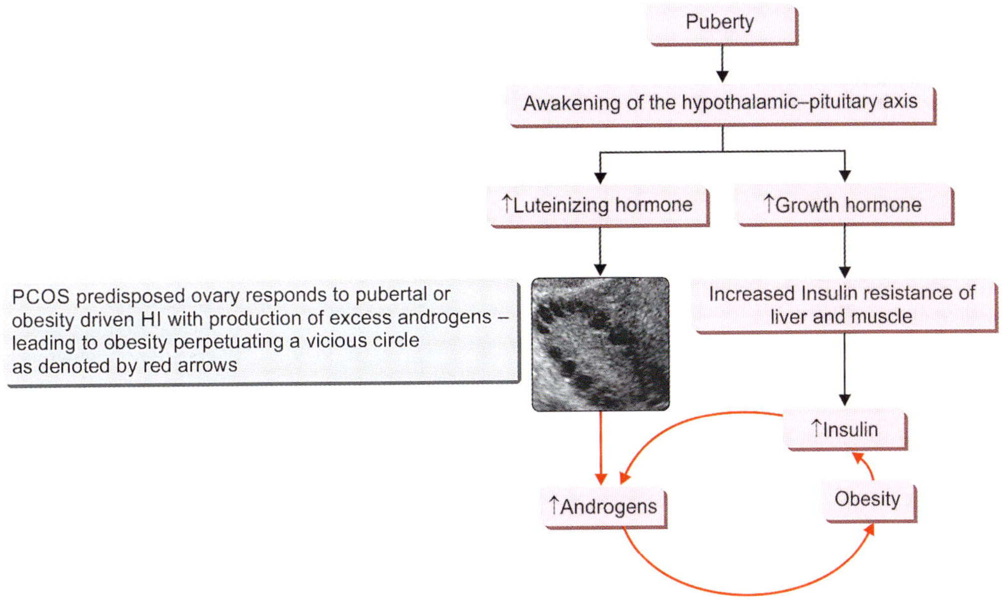

Fig. 8: Pathophysiology of PCOS in Puberty.

- Rapid weight gain in small for gestational age (SGA) girls and sustained adiposity in large for gestational age (LGA) girls accelerate the prepubertal appearance of PCOS **(Fig. 2)**.[25]
- Difficulties in diagnosing PCOS in adolescents, as several features suggestive of PCOS, may be transitory findings during the evolution of normal puberty to adulthood.[23,159]
  - A relatively higher rate of cycles being irregular and anovulatory during this period. About 85% of menstrual cycles are anovulatory during the first year following menarche, 59% in the third year, and 25% in the sixth year.
  - As acne and hirsutism are common during adolescence, there exist difficulties in interpreting clinical and biochemical evidence of HA.
  - PCOM on transabdominal sonography (TAS) has to be differentiated from multicystic ovaries, which is a normal variant feature of physiologic puberty. Hence ovary volume of more than 10 cm^3 is being considered a better marker for diagnosing PCOS in adolescents.
- Taking into account these problems, in an attempt to overcome the possibility of erroneous diagnoses, the diagnostic criteria differ in adolescents from those used for women of reproductive age **(Table 9)**.[75,159]
- *Evaluation for PCOS in adolescents:*
  - When persistent oligomenorrhea/amenorrhea for 2 years after menarche and/or primary amenorrhea by 16 years
  - When clinical evidence of HA, progressive moderate-to-severe hirsutism, and acne resistant to topical treatment
- Amenorrhea is defined when there are intervals between periods exceeding 199 days, whereas in oligomenorrheic patients the intercycle interval varies between 35 and 199 days.[75]
- Signs and symptoms of the disorder may appear in puberty, but may not be diagnosed until well into adulthood.
- Oligomenorrhea in adolescents does not require active treatment usually, but simple reassurance that with time, cycles will become regular. However, a regular follow-up to ensure that this does happen, if not further evaluation would be required.
- There has been evidence to show that low SHBG levels, HA and HI in the early teen years, predict subsequent development of class 3 obesity and MebS by mid-third decade.[23]

TABLE 9: Diagnostic criteria for PCOS in adolescents.

Parameter	*ESHRE/ASRM 2012*[62]	*Endocrine Society 2013*[86]
Criteria	1. Clinical or biochemical hyperandrogenism[a] 2. Oligo-/anovulation[b] 3. Polycystic ovarian morphology[c]	1. Clinical or biochemical hyperandrogenism[a] 2. Persistent oligo-anovulation[b]
Limitation	Three of three criteria required with exclusion of other etiologies	Two of two criteria required with exclusion of other etiologies

Note:
[a]Increased serum androgens and/or progressive hirsutism.
[b]Oligo-/amenorrhea for at least 2 years, or primary amenorrhea by the age of 16 years.
[c]Ovarian volume >10 cm^3

(ASRM: American Society for Reproductive Medicine, ESHRE: European Society for Human Reproduction and Embryology)

- A large study showed that about 26–35.3% of adolescents were at risk for MebS. Hence, screening for metabolic abnormalities in all adolescent PCOS, independent of body weight is required.[160] Menstrual irregularity and high free testosterone levels were associated with high MebS risk (OR: 3.00), the risk increased substantially with overweight or obesity.[160]
- *Screening test for IGT:* 2-hour OGTT with 75-g glucose load, interpreted using ADA guidelines. Although the most appropriate screening interval is not defined, the conversion from IGT to T2DM can occur within 5 years.[72]
- Although, routine ovarian imaging is not indicated for the diagnosis of PCOS in adolescents, TAS may be performed in those with high testosterone levels or rapidly progressive hirsutism or virilization to evaluate for malignancy.

The diagnostic value of serum AMH concentrations has also been studied since ultrasound is often unreliable to detect PCOM in this population. However, serum AMH concentrations were found to be a questionable surrogate marker of PCOM in adolescents.

- *Management:* Multidisciplinary approach, involving dietary and lifestyle modifications, symptomatic management of reproductive, metabolic, and cosmetic manifestations of the syndrome as discussed earlier
- Evaluation and management in adolescents is shown in **Table 10**.
- Lifestyle modification and OCPs significantly reduce androgens and increase SHBG in obese PCOS adolescents **(Table 11)**.
- There have been limited studies on the use of metformin in adolescents. Metformin, in combination with lifestyle modification and OCP, reduces central adiposity, reduces HA by increasing the levels of SHBG, reduces IR, and normalizes menstrual cycles. Also, indicated in those with glucose intolerance. However, it is not clear, as to for long it needs to be continued to result in long-term benefits and whether improvement in CV outcomes would occur, for which further larger longitudinal studies are required.[161]

TABLE 10: Diagnosis and management of adolescent PCOS.

Presentation	• Irregular menses more than 2 years post-menarche • Evidence of clinical androgen excess
Diagnosis	• A thorough medical history and physical examination • FSH, LH, prolactin, TSH, 17-OHP, total and free testosterone, SHBG, lipid profile and a random blood glucose level • If obese, OGTT • If unclear, define patient as at risk for PCOS but not definitive and reassess • TAS in indicated cases
Associated metabolic risk factors	Assess for hypertension (using the appropriate age- and height-percentile reference values), dyslipidemia, and impaired glucose metabolism
Hirsutism or severe acne	• Anti-androgens + OCP • OCPs containing CPA
Menstrual dysfunction	• OCPs • Progestin therapy
Obesity, glucose intolerance or diabetes, dyslipidemia	• Lifestyle modifications—diet and exercises • Metformin therapy

(CPA: cyproterone acetate; FSH: follicle-stimulating hormone; LH: luteinizing hormone; OCP: oral contraceptive pill; OGTT: oral glucose tolerance test; 17-OHP: 17-Hydroxyprogesterone; TSH: thyroid-stimulating hormone)

Recommendations by The Amsterdam ESHRE/ASRM-Sponsored 3rd PCOS Consensus Workshop Group[73]

- Adolescents at risk (e.g., obese, hirsute, irregular menses) should be identified, but be cautious of overdiagnosing PCOS.
- Individual PCOS manifestations in adolescents (e.g., obesity, hirsutism, and irregular menses) should be treated.
- OCPs—either containing or not containing an antiandrogen—may be safely used, following the contraindications to administration. Lipid patterns should be evaluated before and after a few months of treatment.

POLYCYSTIC OVARY SYNDROME AND PREGNANCY

- PCOS women may be at increased risk for adverse pregnancy outcomes, which may be exacerbated by obesity and/or IR. (Level B)[62]
- *Preconception management:* Folic acid supplementation, cessation of smoking, weight reduction, if obese and optimal control of sugars should be advised.[77] Assessment of serum homocysteine levels in those who have had repeated miscarriages.[76]
- Although data in relation to the risk of miscarriage in PCOS is conflicting, an increased risk of miscarriage has been observed (24–36% in PCOS vs. 15–18% in non-PCOS) due to:[36,162]
    - Obesity
    - Defective folliculogenesis
    - Developmental incompetence of the oocytes
    - Hyperandrogenemia
    - IR
    - Increased PAI-1
    - Hyperhomocysteinemia

TABLE 11: Lifestyle modification for polycystic ovary syndrome.

Intensity and measure[01]	*Description*	*Activities of daily living*
Light: 1.6–3† METs 40–55%* HRmax	• Aerobic activity that does not cause noticeable changes in breathing rate • An intensity that can be sustained for at least 60 minutes	Casual walking, cycling <8 km/h (5 mph), stretching, light weight training, dancing slowly, leisurely sports (playing catch) golf (using cart), light yard/house work
Moderate: 3–6† METs 55–70%* HRmax	• Aerobic activity that can be conducted whilst having an uninterrupted conversation • An intensity that may last between 30 and 60 minutes	Brisk walking (5–7 km/h, 3–4.5 mph), walking uphill, hiking, cycling (8–15 km/h, 5–9 mph), low impact or aqua aerobics, yoga gymnastics, weight training, moderate dancing, aerobic machines (stair climber, elliptical, stationary bike)—most competitive tennis, volleyball, badminton, recreational swimming, golf—carrying clubs, intense house/yard work or occupations with extended standing or walking
Vigorous: 6–9† METs 70–90%* HRmax	• Aerobic activity where an uninterrupted conversation generally cannot be maintained • Intensity that may last up to 30 minutes	Race walking, jogging/running, mountain climbing, cycling (>16 km/h, 10 mph), high impact aerobics, karate or similar, circuit weight training, vigorous dancing and aerobic machines, competitive basketball, netball, soccer, football, rugby, hockey, swimming, water jogging, downhill or cross country skiing, nonmotorized lawn mowing, occupations with heavy lifting or rapid movement

*Predicted maximal heart rate (HRmax) = 208 – [0.7 × AGE (years)]
†Metabolic equivalent (MET) where 1 MET is the O/kg body weight/min required to sustain ones resting metabolic rate (3.5 mL/kg/min)

- Altered serum leptin levels:
  - Endometrial glycodelin and IGFBP-I
- Decreased uterine vascularity and increased uterine vascular resistance.
- Recurrent miscarriage is found to be higher in PCOS (36–56%), in comparison to the general population (20–23%).[163]
- There is also a higher incidence of pregnancy complications such as gestational diabetes (40–50%), gestational hypertensive disorders (5%), and neonatal complications [(small-for-gestational-age babies (10–15%) and neonatal intensive care units admissions)], even in singleton pregnancies.[164,165]
- Pregnancy-related complications are greater in type A and B phenotypes due to impaired early decidual trophoblastic invasion and/or remodeling of spiral vessels and placentational defects.[166]
- Obese PCOS will have the additional risk of obstetric complications, such as shoulder dystocia and postpartum thromboembolism.[166]
- Metformin therapy lowers HI and may have a beneficial effect in reducing miscarriage rates and the risk of gestational diabetes.[167] Data supports their safety when used during pregnancy, with no major birth defects and no effect on social or motor development in infants followed up at 3 and 6 months of age.[167]
- *Evidence:* There is no evidence that the use of metformin either before conception or during pregnancy decreases pregnancy complications and improves the live birth rates (Level A).[167]
- Endometrial receptivity during the implantation window of LE is superior to CC in PCOS women, which may be related to higher clinical pregnancy and ongoing PRs. Endometrial FI examined by 3-D power Doppler, and integrin $\alpha v\beta 3$ in uterine secretion during the implantation window, could be preferable noninvasive predictor markers for pregnancy.[168]

POLYCYSTIC OVARY SYNDROME AND MENOPAUSE

- With age, many of the manifestations, including hirsutism, oligomenorrhea, testosterone levels, ovarian size, and morphology, may improve.[62]
- Diagnosis in postmenopausal first is based on the previous history of menstrual dysfunction (oligomenorrhea) and presence of HA during the reproductive period with PCOM, as formulated by the Endocrine Society (2013).[160]
- PCOS women will have a larger cohort of primary follicles than age-matched control women before menopause.
- Hirsutism, alopecia, and AUB are the presenting complaints of postmenopausal women with PCOS.
- Menopausal PCOS women have a higher incidence of obesity, hypertension, diabetes, CV complications, and stroke.
- Continuous unopposed estrogen-mediated endometrial proliferation leads to endometrial hyperplasia and carcinoma, with obesity and diabetes adding to the risk.
- It has been found the odds of PCOS developing endometrial carcinoma are almost three times higher (approximately 9%), as shown in a systematic review and

meta-analysis.[168] Further, in PCOS <50 years, there is a fourfold increased risk of developing endometrial cancer (EC).[169,170] When adjusted for BMI, this risk was reduced by half. Well-differentiated, endometrioid adenocarcinoma (a subtype of type-1 EC) is the most common.

- Women with PCOS may experience menopause on average 2 years later than healthy control women due to prolonged reproductive function as well as an increased ovarian reserve.[75]
- Although retrospective data suggest that they have higher rates of stroke and CVD, with mortality occurring at a similar rate and presumably at the same age, as in the general population, prospective data suggest they have increased CVD event rates and decreased survival.[75]

KEY POINTS

- Polycystic ovary syndrome is the most prevalent cause of anovulatory infertility accounting for 80–90% of WHO group 2, hypothalamic-pituitary-ovarian dysfunction.
- PCOS is an endocrine, metabolic, and chronic inflammatory disorder, with hyperandrogenemia, IR, and obesity being the key factors that influence the expression and symptoms of the condition.
- HA, like chronic anovulation, is a hallmark of PCOS, and its origin appears to be multifactorial; the evolution and severity of its phenotypic expression result from the impact of environmental influences (both pre- and postnatal) on genetic and epigenetic factors in utero.
- First-line therapy for all PCOS women is lifestyle modifications targeting weight loss in those obese and overweight and prevention of weight gain in lean women.
- CC or LE should be the first-line pharmacological therapy to improve fertility outcomes in PCOS, with no other infertility factors.
- Recommended second-line intervention should first-line fail to result in pregnancy is either exogenous GTs or LOD.
- Induction of ovulation great care must be taken to avoid multiple follicle development and its adverse consequences—OHSS and multiple pregnancy particularly with GTs.
- Metformin use in PCOS should be restricted to women with glucose intolerance and in combination with CC improves ovulation and CPRs but does not improve live birth rates.
- Screening by OGTT (75 g, 0- and 2-hour values) should be performed in the following conditions: obesity, women with a family history of T2D or GDM, HA with anovulation, and acanthosis nigricans.
- Women with PCOS have an estimated 2.2, 2.5, and 4-fold increased prevalence of metabolic dysfunctions, IGT, and T2DM, respectively in both BMI and non-BMI-matched studies.
- MebS is a cluster of risk factors, predisposing to both CVD and T2DM.
- PCOS with a BMI >30 kg/m^2, high-risk ethnic South Asian women with a BMI >25 kg/m^2, dyslipidemia, overt vascular or renal disease, or family history of T2DM are at risk of metabolic dysfunction.
- Recommended CVD risk assessment at any age: assessment for BP, glucose, lipid profile (cholesterol, triglycerides, HDL, and LDL), waist circumference, physical activity, nutrition, smoking, and psychosocial stress.
- During pregnancy, PCOS women should be followed closely as they may be at increased risk for the development of GDM, gestational hypertension, and neonatal complications, even in singleton pregnancies. This may be exacerbated by obesity and/or IR.
- Women with PCOS have a 2.7–2.9-fold increased risk for endometrial carcinoma. Most ECs are well differentiated and have good prognosis.

REFERENCES

1. Teede HJ, Misso ML, Costello MF, Dokras A, Laven J, Moran L, et al. Recommendations from the international evidence-based guideline for the assessment and management of polycystic ovary syndrome. Hum Reprod. 2018;33(9):1602-18.
2. Broekmans FJ, Knauff EA, Valkenburg O, Laven JS, Eijkemans MJ, Fauser BC. PCOS according to the Rotterdam consensus criteria: Change in prevalence among WHO-II anovulation and association with metabolic factors. BJOG. 2006;113(10):1210-7.
3. Stein IF, Leventhal ML. Amenorrhea associated with bilateral polycystic ovaries. Am J Obstet Gynecol. 1935;29(2):181-91.
4. Franks S, Berga SL. Does PCOS have developmental origins? Fertil Steril. 2012;97(1):2-6.
5. Diamanti-Kandarakis E, Piperi C, Spina J, Argyrakopoulou G, Papanastasiou L, Bergiele A, et al. Polycystic ovary syndrome: the influence of environmental and genetic factors. Hormones (Athens). 2006;5(1):17-34.
6. Rebar R, Judd HL, Yen SS, Rakoff J, Vandenberg G, Naftolin F. Characterization of the inappropriate gonadotropin secretion in polycystic ovary syndrome. J Clin Invest. 1976;57(5):1320-9.
7. Zawadzki JK, Dunaif A. Diagnostic criteria for polycystic ovary syndrome: towards a rational approach. In: Chang RJ, Heindel JJ, Dunaif A (Eds). Polycystic ovary syndrome. Massachusetts: Blackwell Scientific Publications; 1992. pp. 377-84.
8. Carmina E, Lobo RA. Polycystic ovaries in women with normal menses. Am J Med. 2001;111(8):602-6.
9. Rotterdam ESHRE-ASRM Sponsored PCOS Consensus Workshop Group. Revised 2003 consensus on diagnostic criteria and long-term health risks related to polycystic ovary syndrome. Hum Reprod. 2004;81(1):19-25.
10. Polson DW, Adams J, Wadsworth J, Franks S. Polycystic ovaries—A common finding in normal women. Lancet. 1988;1(8590):870-2.
11. Azziz R, Carmina E, Dewailly D, Diamanti-Kandarakis E, Escobar-Morreale HF, Futterweit W, et al; Task Force on

the Phenotype of the Polycystic Ovary Syndrome of The Androgen Excess and PCOS Society. The Androgen Excess and PCOS Society criteria for the polycystic ovary syndrome: the complete task force report. Fertil Steril. 2009;91(2): 456-88.

12. National Institutes of Health. (2012). Evidence-based Methodology Workshop on Polycystic Ovary Syndrome. Executive summary. [online] Available from https://prevention.nih.gov/sites/default/files/2018-06/FinalReport.pdf [Last accessed November, 2022].
13. Azziz R, Carmina E, Dewailly D, Diamanti-Kandarakis E, Escobar-Morreale HF, Futterweit W, et al. Positions statement: criteria for defining polycystic ovary syndrome as a predominantly hyperandrogenic syndrome: an Androgen Excess Society guideline. J Clin Endocrinol Metab. 2006;91(11):4237-45.
14. Azziz R, Woods KS, Reyna R, Key TJ, Knochenhauer ES, Yildiz BO. The prevalence and features of the polycystic ovary syndrome in an unselected population. J Clin Endocrinol Metab. 2004;89(6):2745-9.
15. Bozdag G, Mumusoglu S, Zengin D, Karabulut E, Yildiz BO. The prevalence and phenotypic features of polycystic ovary syndrome: a systematic review and meta-analysis. Hum Reprod. 2016;31(12):2841-55.
16. Rodin DA, Bano G, Bland JM, Taylor K, Nussey SS. Polycystic ovaries and associated metabolic abnormalities in Indian subcontinent Asian women. Clin Endocrinol (Oxf). 1998;49(1):91-9.
17. Lizneva D, Suturina L, Walker W, Brakta S, Gavrilova-Jordan L, Azziz R. Criteria, prevalence, and phenotypes of polycystic ovary syndrome. Fertil Steril. 2016;106(1):6-15.
18. Nam Menke M, Strauss JF 3rd. Genetics of polycystic ovarian syndrome. Clin Obstet Gynecol. 2007;50(1):188-204.
19. Chen ZJ, Zhao H, He L, Shi Y, Qin Y, Shi Y, et al. Genome-wide association study identifies susceptibility loci for polycystic ovary syndrome on chromosome 2p16.3, 2p21 and 9q33.3. Nat Genet. 2011;43(1):55-9.
20. Abbott DH, Barnett DK, Bruns CM, Dumesic DA. Androgen excess fetal programming of female reproduction: a developmental aetiology for polycystic ovary syndrome? Hum Reprod Update. 2005;11(4):357-74.
21. Homburg R. Androgen circle of polycystic ovary syndrome. Hum Reprod. 2009;24(7):1548-55.
22. Blank SK, McCartney CR, Helm KD, Marshall JC. Neuroendocrine effects of androgens in adult polycystic ovary syndrome and female puberty. Semin Reprod Med. 2007;25(5):352-9.
23. Bremer AA. Polycystic ovary syndrome in the pediatric population. Metab Syndr Relat Disord. 2010;8(5):375-94.
24. Pinilla L, Aguilar E, Dieguez C, Millar RP, Tena-Sempere M. Kisspeptins and reproduction: physiological roles and regulatory mechanisms. Physiol Rev. 2012;92(3):1235-316.
25. Diamanti-Kandarakis E. Polycystic ovarian syndrome: pathophysiology, molecular aspects and clinical implications. Expert Rev Mol Med. 2008;10:e3.
26. Franks S, Stark J, Hardy K. Follicle dynamics and anovulation in polycystic ovary syndrome. Hum Reprod Update. 2008;14(4):367-78.
27. Homburg R, Ray A, Bhide P, Gudi A, Shah A, Timms P, et al. The relationship of serum anti-mullerian hormone with polycystic ovarian morphology and polycystic ovary syndrome: a prospective cohort study. Hum Reprod. 2013; 28(4):1077-83.
28. Garg D, Tal R. The role of AMH in the pathophysiology of polycystic ovarian syndrome. Reprod Biomed Online. 2016;33(1):15-28.
29. Iliodromiti S, Kelsey TW, Anderson RA, Nelson SM. Can anti-Mullerian hormone predict the diagnosis of polycystic ovary syndrome? A systematic review and meta-analysis of extracted data. J Clin Endocrinol Metab. 2013;98(8):3332-40.
30. Fritz MA, Speroff L. Clinical Gynecologic Endocrinology and Infertility, 8th edition. Lippincott: Williams and Wilkins; 2011.
31. Practice Committee of the American Society for Reproductive Medicine. Role of metformin for ovulation induction in infertile patients with polycystic ovary syndrome (PCOS): a guideline. Fertil Steril. 2017;108(3):426-41.
32. Diamanti-Kandarakis E, Dunaif A. Insulin resistance and the polycystic ovary syndrome revisited: an update on mechanisms and implications. Endocr Rev. 2012;33(6):981-1030.
33. Tekin G, Tekin A, Kiliçarslan EB, Haydardedeoğlu B, Katircibaşi T, Koçum T, et al. Altered autonomic neural control of the cardiovascular system in patients with polycystic ovary syndrome. Int J Cardiol. 2008;130(1):49-55.
34. Unfer V, Carlomagno G, Dante G, Facchinetti F. Effects of myo-inositol in women with PCOS: a systematic review of randomized controlled trials. Gynecol Endocrinol. 2012;28(7):509-15.
35. Unfer V, Nestler JE, Kamenov ZA, Prapas N, Facchinetti F. Effects of Inositol(s) in Women with PCOS: A Systematic Review of Randomized Controlled Trials. Int J Endocrinol. 2016;2016:1849162.
36. Balen AH, Conway GS, Homburg R, Legro RS. Polycystic Ovary Syndrome: A Guide to Clinical Management. London: Taylor and Francis Group; 2005.
37. Vrbikova J, Hainer V. Obesity and polycystic ovary syndrome. Obes Facts. 2009;2(1):26-35.
38. Anderson AD, Burt Solorzano CM, McCartney CR. Childhood obesity and its impact on the development of adolescent PCOS. Semin Reprod Med. 2014;32(3):202-13.
39. de Zegher F, Lopez-Bermejo A, Ibáñez L. Adipose tissue expandability and the early origins of PCOS. Trends Endocrinol Metab. 2009;20(9):418-23.
40. Carmina E, Bucchieri S, Mansueto P, Rini G, Ferin M, Lobo RA. Circulating levels of adipose products and differences in fat distribution in the ovulatory and anovulatory phenotypes of polycystic ovary syndrome. Fertil Steril. 2009; 91(4 Suppl):1332-5.
41. Toulis KA, Goulis DG, Farmakiotis D, Georgopoulos NA, Katsikis I, Tarlatzis BC, et al. Adiponectin levels in women with polycystic ovary syndrome: a systematic review and a meta-analysis. Hum Reprod Update. 2009;15(3): 297-307.
42. Schulte MM, Tsai JH, Moley KH. Obesity and PCOS: the effect of metabolic derangements on endometrial receptivity at the time of implantation. Reprod Sci. 2015;22(1):6-14.
43. Moran LJ, Misso ML, Wild RA, Norman RJ. Impaired glucose tolerance, type 2 diabetes and metabolic syndrome in polycystic ovary syndrome: a systematic review and meta-analysis. Hum Reprod Update. 2010;16(4):347-63.

44. Merhi Z. Advanced glycation end products and their relevance in female reproduction. Hum Reprod. 2014;29(1):135-45.
45. Samy N, Hashim M, Sayed M, Said M. Clinical significance of inflammatory markers in polycystic ovary syndrome: their relationship to insulin resistance and body mass index. Dis Markers. 2009;26(4):163-70.
46. Amini L, Tehranian N, Movahedin M, Ramezani Tehrani F, Ziaee S. Antioxidants and management of polycystic ovary syndrome in Iran: A systematic review of clinical trials. Iran J Reprod Med. 2015;13(1):1-8.
47. Dunlop TW, Väisänen S, Frank C, Molnár F, Sinkkonen L, Carlberg C. The human peroxisome proliferator-activated receptor delta gene is a primary target of 1α, 25-dihydroxy vitamin D3 and its nuclear receptor. J Mol Biol. 2005;349(2):248-60.
48. He C, Lin Z, Robb SW, Ezeamama AE. Serum Vitamin D Levels and Polycystic Ovary Syndrome: A Systematic Review and Meta-Analysis. Nutrients. 2015;7(6):4555-77.
49. Tamura H, Nakamura Y, Korkmaz A, Manchester LC, Tan DX, Sugino N, et al. Melatonin and the ovary: physiological and pathophysiological implications. Fertil Steril. 2009;92(1):328-43.
50. Kandaraki E, Chatzigeorgiou A, Livadas S, Palioura E, Economou F, Koutsilieris M, et al. Endocrine disruptors and polycystic ovary syndrome (PCOS): elevated serum levels of bisphenol A in women with PCOS. J Clin Endocrinol Metab. 2011;96(3):E480-4.
51. Li Q, Du J, Feng R, Xu Y, Wang H, Sang Q, et al. A possible new mechanism in the pathophysiology of polycystic ovary syndrome (PCOS): the discovery that leukocyte telomere length is strongly associated with PCOS. J Clin Endocrinol Metab. 2014;99(2):E234-40.
52. Moro F, Morciano A, Tropea A, Sagnella F, Palla C, Scarinci E, et al. CD4 (+) CD28 (null) T lymphocyte frequency, a new marker of cardiovascular risk: relationship with polycystic ovary syndrome phenotypes. Fertil Steril. 2012;98(6):1609-15.
53. Laven JS, Mulders AG, Suryandari DA, Gromoll J, Nieschlag E, Fauser BC, et al. Follicle-stimulating hormone receptor polymorphisms in women with normogonadotropic anovulatory infertility. Fertil Steril. 2003;80(4):986-92.
54. Valkenburg O, van Santbrink EJ, König TE, Themmen AP, Uitterlinden AG, Fauser BC, et al. Follicle-stimulating hormone receptor polymorphism affects the outcome of ovulation induction in normogonadotropic (World Health Organization class 2) anovulatory subfertility. Fertil Steril. 2015;103(4):1081-8.e3.
55. LaMarca A, Sighinolfi G, Argento C, Grisendi V, Casarini L, Volpe A, et al. Polymorphisms in gonadotropin and gonadotropin receptor genes as markers of ovarian reserve and response in in vitro fertilization. Fertil Steril. 2013;99(4):970-8.e1.
56. Ciampelli M, Fulghesu AM, Cucinelli F, Pavone V, Caruso A, Mancuso S, et al. Heterogeneity in beta cell activity, hepatic insulin clearance and peripheral insulin sensitivity in women with polycystic ovary syndrome. Hum Reprod. 1997;12(9):1897-901.
57. Kumari AS, Haq A, Jayasundaram R, Abdel-Wareth LO, Al Haija SA, Alvares M. Metformin monotherapy in lean women with polycystic ovary syndrome. Reprod Biomed Online. 2005;10(1):100-4.
58. Toosy S, Sodi R, Pappachan, JM. Lean polycystic ovary syndrome (PCOS): an evidence-based practical approach. J Diabetes Metab Disord. 2018;17(2):277-85.
59. American Association of Clinical Endocrinologists Polycystic Ovary Syndrome Writing Committee. American Association of Clinical Endocrinologists Position Statement on Metabolic and Cardiovascular Consequences of Polycystic Ovary Syndrome. Endocr Pract. 2005;11(2):126-34.
60. Randeva HS, Tan BK, Weickert MO, Lois K, Nestler JE, Sattar N, et al. Cardiometabolic aspects of the polycystic ovary syndrome. Endocr Rev. 2012;33(5):812-41.
61. Yilmaz B, Vellanki P, Ata B, Yildiz BO. Metabolic syndrome, hypertension, and hyperlipidemia in mothers, fathers, sisters, and brothers of women with polycystic ovary syndrome: a systematic review and meta-analysis. Fertil Steril. 2018;109(2):356-64.e32.
62. Amsterdam ESHRE/ASRM-Sponsored 3rd PCOS Consensus Workshop Group. Consensus on women's health aspects of polycystic ovary syndrome (PCOS). Hum Reprod. 2012;27(1):14-24.
63. Wild RA, Carmina E, Diamanti-Kandarakis E, Dokras A, Escobar-Morreale HF, Futterweit W, et al. Assessment of cardiovascular risk and prevention of cardiovascular disease in women with the polycystic ovary syndrome: a consensus statement by the Androgen Excess and Polycystic Ovary Syndrome (AE-PCOS) Society. J Clin Endocrinol Metab. 2010;95(5):2038-49.
64. Expert Panel on Detection, Evaluation and Treatment of High Blood Cholesterol in Adults. Executive Summary of the Third Report of the National Cholesterol Education Program (NCEP) Expert Panel on Detection, Evaluation, And Treatment of High Blood Cholesterol In Adults (Adult Treatment Panel III). JAMA. 2001;285(19):2486-97.
65. Grundy SM, Brewer HB Jr, Cleeman JI, Smith SC Jr; Lenfant C; American Heart Association; National Heart, Lung, and Blood Institute. Definition of metabolic syndrome: Report of the National Heart, Lung, and Blood Institute/American Heart Association conference on scientific issues related to definition. Circulation. 2004;109(3):433-8.
66. Alberti KG, Zimmet P, Shaw J; IDF Epidemiology Task Force Consensus Group. International Diabetes Federation Epidemiology Task Force Consensus Group. The metabolic syndrome—a new worldwide definition. Lancet. 2005;366(9491):1059-62.
67. Cameron AJ, Shaw JE, Zimmet PZ. The metabolic syndrome: prevalence in worldwide populations. Endocrinol Metab Clin North Am. 2004;33(2):351-75.
68. Balen AH, Morley LC, Misso M, Franks S, Legro RS, Wijeyaratne CN, et al. The management of anovulatory infertility in women with polycystic ovary syndrome: an analysis of the evidence to support the development of global WHO guidance. Hum Reprod Update. 2016;22(6):687-708.
69. ESHRE Capri Workshop Group. Health and fertility in World Health Organization group 2 anovulatory women. Hum Reprod Update. 2012;18(5):586-99.
70. Dewailly D, Lujan ME, Carmina E, Cedars MI, Laven J, Norman RJ, et al. Definition and significance of polycystic ovarian morphology: a task force report from the Androgen Excess and Polycystic Ovary Syndrome Society. Hum Reprod Update. 2014;20(3):334-52.

71. Royal College of Obstetricians and Gynecologists. (2014). Long-term consequences of polycystic ovary syndrome: Green-top Guideline No. 33. [online] Available from https://www.rcog.org.uk/media/qmtlp2b0/gtg_33.pdf [Last accessed November, 2022].
72. ADA (American Diabetes Association). Standards of Medical Care in Diabetes—2015. Diabetes Care. 2015; 38(Suppl 1):S86-7.
73. Fauser BC, Tarlatzis BC, Rebar RW, Legro RS, Balen AH, Lobo R, et al. Consensus on women's health aspects of polycystic ovary syndrome (PCOS): the Amsterdam ESHRE/ASRM-Sponsored 3rd PCOS Consensus Workshop Group. Fertil Steril. 2012;97(1):28-38.e25.
74. Carmina E. Ovarian and adrenal hyperandrogenism. Ann N Y Acad Sci. 2006;1092:130-7.
75. Dewailly D, Gronier H, Poncelet E, Robin G, Leroy M, Pigny P, et al. Diagnosis of polycystic ovary syndrome (PCOS): revisiting the threshold values of follicle count on ultrasound and of the serum AMH level for the definition of polycystic ovaries. Hum Reprod. 2011;26(11):3123-9.
76. Berker B, Kaya C, Aytac R, Satiroglu H. Homocysteine concentrations in follicular fluid are associated with poor oocyte and embryo qualities in polycystic ovary syndrome patients undergoing assisted reproduction. Hum Reprod. 2009;24(9):2293-302.
77. Thessaloniki ESHRE/ASRM-Sponsored PCOS Consensus Workshop Group. Consensus on infertility treatment related to polycystic ovary syndrome. Fertil Steril. 2008;23(3): 462-77.
78. US. Department of Health and Human Services (DHSS). Physical Activity and Health: A Report of the Surgeon General. Atlanta: DHSS, Centers for Disease Control and Prevention, National Center for Chronic Disease Prevention and Health Promotion. [online] Available from https://www.cdc.gov/nccdphp/sgr/ [Last Accessed November, 2022].
79. Greenwood EA, Noel MW, Kao CN, Shinkai K, Pasch LA, Cedars MI, et al. Vigorous exercise is associated with superior metabolic profiles in polycystic ovary syndrome independent of total exercise expenditure. Fertil Steril. 2016;105(2):486-93.
80. Derosa G, Maffioli P. Anti-obesity drugs: a review about their effects and their safety. Expert Opin Drug Saf. 2012;11(3):459-71.
81. Krentz AJ, Fujioka K, Hompesch M. Evolution of pharmacological obesity treatments: focus on adverse side-effect profiles. Diabetes Obes Metab. 2016;18(6):558-70.
82. Badawy A, Elnashar A. Treatment options for polycystic ovary syndrome. Int J Womens Health. 2011;3:25-35.
83. Bhattacharya SM, Jha A. Comparative study of the therapeutic effects of oral contraceptive pills containing desogestrel, cyproterone acetate, and drospirenone in patients with polycystic ovary syndrome. Fertil Steril. 2012;98(4):1053-9.
84. ACOG Committee on Practice Bulletins–Gynecology. ACOG Practice Bulletin No 108: Polycystic ovary syndrome. Obstet. Gynecol. 2009;114(4):936-49.
85. Brzezinńska-Wcisło L. Assessment of efficacy of Diane-35 in androgenetic feminine alopecia. Wiad Lek. 2003;56(3-4): 202-5.
86. Legro RS, Arslanian SA, Ehrmann DA, Hoeger KM, Murad MH, Pasquali R, et al. Diagnosis and treatment of polycystic ovary syndrome: an Endocrine Society clinical practice guideline. J Clin Endocrinol Metab. 2013;98(12):4565-92.
87. Luque-Ramírez M, Mendieta-Azcona C, Alvarez-Blasco F, Escobar-Morreale HF. Effects of metformin versus ethinylestradiol plus cyproterone acetate on ambulatory blood pressure monitoring and carotid intima media thickness in women with the polycystic ovary syndrome. Fertil Steril. 2009;91(6):2527-36.
88. Sitruk-Ware R, Nath A. Characteristics and metabolic effects of estrogen and progestins contained in oral contraceptive pills. Best Pract Res Clin Endocrinol Metab. 2013;27(1):13-24.
89. World Health Organization. Medical Eligibility Criteria for Contraceptive Use. Switzerland: World Health Organization; 2009.
90. RCOG. (2007). Long-term Consequences of Polycystic Ovary Syndrome. Green-top Guideline No. 33. [online] Available from http://www.jsog.org/GuideLines/Long-term_consequences_of_polycystic_ovary_syndrome.pdf [Last accessed November, 2022].
91. Gupta J, Kai J, Middleton L, Pattison H, Gray R, Daniels J; ECLIPSE Trial Collaborative Group. Levonorgestrel intrauterine system versus medical therapy for menorrhagia. N Engl J Med. 2013;368(2):128-37.
92. Practice Committee of the American Society for Reproductive Medicine. Use of clomiphene citrate in infertile women: a committee opinion. Fertil Steril. 2013;100(2):341-8.
93. Steiner AZ, Terplan M, Paulson RJ. Comparison of tamoxifen and clomiphene citrate for ovulation induction: a meta-analysis. Hum Reprod. 2005;20(6):1511-5.
94. Casper RF, Mitwally MF. Review: aromatase inhibitors for ovulation induction. J Clin Endocrinol Metab. 2006;91(3):760-71.
95. Biljan MM, Hemmings R, Brassard N. The outcome of 150 babies following the treatment with letrozole or letrozole and gonadotrophins. Fertil Steril. 2005;84(Suppl. 1):S95.
96. Tulandi T, Martin J, Al-Fadhli R, Kabli N, Forman R, Hitkari J, et al. Congenital malformations among 911 newborns conceived after infertility treatment with letrozole or clomiphene citrate. Fertil Steril. 2006;85(6):1761-5.
97. American College of Obstetricians and Gynecologists. Committee opinion No. 663: Aromatase Inhibitors in Gynecological Practice. Obstet Gynecol. 2016;127(6):e170-4.
98. Homburg R. The management of infertility associated with polycystic ovary syndrome. Reprod Biol Endocrinol. 2003,1:109.
99. Weiss NS, Nahuis M, Bayram N, Mol BW, Van der Veen F, van Wely M. Gonadotrophins for ovulation induction in polycystic ovarian syndrome. Cochrane Database Syst Rev. 2015;(9):CD010290.
100. Hugues JN, Cédrin-Durnerin I, Howles CM, Amram M, Angelini A, Balen A, et al; FSH OI Study Group. The use of a decremental dose regimen in patients treated with a chronic low-dose step-up protocol for WHO Group II anovulation: a prospective randomized multicentre study. Hum Reprod. 2006;21(11):2817-22.
101. Gardner DK, Wessman A, Howles CM, Shoham Z (Eds). Textbook of Assisted Reproductive Techniques, 4th edition London: Informa Healthcare; 2012. pp. 75-98.
102. Christin-Maitre S, Hugues JN; Recombinant FSH Study Group. A comparative randomized multicentric study comparing the step-up versus step-down protocol in polycystic ovary syndrome. Hum Reprod. 2003;18(8):1626-31.

103. Hugues JN, Cédrin-Durnerin I, Avril C, Bulwa S, Hervé F, Uzan M. Sequential step-up and step-down dose regimen: an alternative method for ovulation induction with follicle-stimulating hormone in polycystic ovarian syndrome. Hum Reprod. 1996;11(12):2581-4.
104. Willis DS, Watson H, Mason HD, Galea R, Brincat M, Franks S. Premature response to luteinizing hormone of granulosa cells from anovulatory women with polycystic ovary syndrome: relevance to mechanism of anovulation. J Clin Endocrinol Metab. 1998;83(11):3984-91.
105. Gjoönnaess H. Polycystic ovarian syndrome treated by ovarian electrocautery through the laparoscope. Fertil Steril. 1984;41(1):20-5.
106. Fernandez H, Morin-Surruca M, Torre A, Faivre E, Deffieux X, Gervaise A. Ovarian drilling for surgical treatment of polycystic ovarian syndrome: a comprehensive review. Reprod Biomed Online. 2011;22(6):556-68.
107. Amer S, Li TC, Ledger WL. The value of measuring anti-Mullerian hormone in women with an ovulatory polycystic ovary syndrome undergoing laparoscopic ovarian diathermy. Hum Reprod. 2009;24(11):2760-6.
108. Amer SA, Li TC, Cooke ID. A prospective dose-finding study of the amount of thermal energy required for laparoscopic ovarian diathermy. Hum Reprod. 2003;18(8):1693-8.
109. Zakherah MS, Kamal MM, Hamed HO. Laparoscopic ovarian drilling in polycystic ovary syndrome: efficacy of adjusted thermal dose based on ovarian volume. Fertil Steril. 2011;95(3):1115-8.
110. Amer SA, Banu Z, Li TC, Cooke ID. Long-term follow-up of patients with polycystic ovary syndrome after laparoscopic ovarian drilling: endocrine and ultrasonographic outcomes. Hum Reprod. 2002;17(11):2851-7.
111. Mercorio F, Mercorio A, Di Spiezio Sardo A, Vincenzo Barba G, Pellicano M, Nappi C. Evaluation of ovarian adhesion formation after laparoscopic ovarian drilling by second-look minilaparoscopy. Fertil Steril. 2008;89(5):1229-33.
112. Farquhar C, Brown J, Marjoribanks J. Laparoscopic drilling by diathermy or laser for ovulation induction in an ovulatory polycystic ovary syndrome. Cochrane Database Syst Rev. 2012;6:CD001122.
113. Ghanem ME, Bakre NI, Emam MA, Al Boghdady LA, Helal AS, Elmetwally AG, et al. The effects of timing of intrauterine insemination in relation to ovulation and the number of inseminations on cycle pregnancy rate in common infertility etiologies. Hum Reprod. 2011;26(3): 576-83.
114. Fedorcsák P, Dale PO, Storeng R, Tanbo T, Abyholm T. The impact of obesity and insulin resistance on the outcome of IVF or ICSI in women with polycystic ovarian syndrome. Hum Reprod. 2001;16(6):1086-91.
115. Nastri CO, Teixeira DM, Moroni RM, Leitão VM, Martins WP. Ovarian hyperstimulation syndrome: pathophysiology, staging, prediction and prevention. Ultrasound Obstet Gynecol. 2015;45(4):377-93.
116. Al-Inany HG, Youssef MA, Aboulghar M, Broekmans F, Sterrenburg M, Smit J, Abou-Setta AM. Gonadotrophin-releasing hormone antagonists for assisted conception. Cochrane Database Syst Rev. 2011;(5):CD001750.
117. Fiedler K, Ezcurra D. Predicting and preventing ovarian hyperstimulation syndrome (OHSS): the need for individualized not standardized treatment. Reprod Biol Endocrinol. 2012;10:32.
118. Van Wely M, Kwan I, Burt AL, Thomas J, Vail A, Van der Veen F, et al. Recombinant versus urinary gonadotrophin for ovarian stimulation in assisted reproductive technology cycles. Cochrane Database Syst Rev. 2011;16(2):CD005354.
119. Humaidan P, Kol S, Papanikolaou EG; Copenhagen GnRH Agonist Triggering Workshop Group. GnRH agonist for triggering of final oocyte maturation: time for a change of practice? Hum Reprod Update. 2011;17(4):510-24.
120. Devroey P, Polyzos NP, Blockeel C. An OHSS-Free Clinic by segmentation of IVF treatment. Hum Reprod. 2011; 26(10):2593-7.
121. Kol S, Humaidan P, Alsbjerg B, Engmann L, Benadiva C, García-Velasco JA, et al. The updated Cochrane review 2014 on GnRH agonist trigger: repeating the same errors. Reprod Biomed Online. 2015;30(6):563-5.
122. Iliodromiti S, Lan VT, Tuong HM, Tuan PH, Humaidan P, Nelson SM. Impact of GnRH agonist triggering and intensive luteal steroid support on live-birth rates and ovarian hyperstimulation syndrome: a retrospective cohort study. J Ovarian Res. 2013;6(1):93.
123. Fatemi HM, Popovic-Todorovic B. Implantation in assisted reproduction: a look at endometrial receptivity. Reprod Biomed Online. 2013;27(5):530-8.
124. Beydoun HA, Stadtmauer L, Beydoun MA, Russell H, Zhao Y, Oehninger S. Polycystic ovary syndrome, body mass index and outcomes of assisted reproductive technologies. Reprod Biomed Online. 2009;18(6):856-63.
125. Dumesic DA, Abbott DH. Implications of polycystic ovary syndrome on oocyte development. Semin Reprod. Med. 2008;26(1):53-61.
126. Wei LN, Liang XY, Fang C, Zhang MF. Abnormal expression of growth differentiation factor 9 and bone morphogenetic protein 15 in stimulated oocytes during maturation from women with polycystic ovary syndrome. Fertil Steril. 2011;96(2):464-8.
127. Wood JR, Dumesic DA, Abbott DH, et al. Molecular abnormalities in oocytes from women with polycystic ovary syndrome revealed by microarray analysis. J Clin Endocrinol Metab. 2007;92(2):705-13.
128. Skov V, Glintborg D, Knudsen S, Jensen T, Kruse TA, Tan Q, et al. Reduced expression of nuclear-encoded genes involved in mitochondrial oxidative metabolism in skeletal muscle of insulin-resistant women with polycystic ovary syndrome. Diabetes. 2007;56(9):2349-55.
129. Harris SE, Maruthini D, Tang T, Balen AH, Picton HM. Metabolism and karyotype analysis of oocytes from patients with polycystic ovary syndrome. Hum Reprod. 2010;25(9):2305-15.
130. Wissing ML, Bjerge MR, Olesen AIG, Hoest T, Mikkelsen AL. Impact of PCOS on embryo cleavage kinetics. Reprod BioMed Online. 2014;28(4):508-14.
131. Mulders AG, Laven JS, Imani B, Eijkemans MJ, Fauser BC. IVF outcome in anovulatory infertility (WHO group 2)—including polycystic ovary syndrome—following previous unsuccessful ovulation induction. Reprod Biomed Online. 2003;7(1):50-8.
132. Ramezanali F, Ashrafi M, Hemat M, Arabipoor A, Jalali S, Moini A. Assisted reproductive outcomes in women with different polycystic ovary syndrome phenotypes: the

predictive value of anti-Müllerian hormone. Reprod Biomed Online. 2016;32(5):503-12.
133. Chen Z-J, Shi Y, Sun Y, Zang B, Liang X, Cao Y, et al. Fresh versus Frozen Embryos for Infertility in the Polycystic Ovary Syndrome. N Engl J Med. 2016;375(6):523-33.
134. Youssef MM, Abdelmoty HI, Ahmed MAS, Elmohamady M. GnRH agonist for final oocyte maturation in GnRH antagonist co-treated IVF/ICSI treatment cycles: Systematic review and meta-analysis. J Adv Res. 2015;6(3):341-9.
135. Gardner DK, Weissman A, Howles CM, Shoham Z Textbook of Assisted Reproductive Techniques. Volume 1: Laboratory Perspectives, 5th Edition. Informa Healthcare; 2018.
136. Ziegler DD, Streuli I, Gayet V, Frydman N, Bajouh O, Chapron C. Retrieving oocytes from small non-stimulated follicles in polycystic ovary syndrome (PCOS): in vitro maturation (IVM) is not indicated in the new GnRH antagonist era. Fertil Steril. 2012;98(2):290-3.
137. Das M, Son WY, Buckett W, Tulandi T, Holzer H. In vitro maturation versus IVF with GnRH antagonist for women with polycystic ovary syndrome: treatment outcome and rates of ovarian hyperstimulation syndrome. Reprod Biomed Online. 2014;29(5):545-51.
138. Siristatidis CS, Vrachnis N, Creatsa M, Maheshwari A, Bhattacharya S. In vitro maturation in subfertile women with polycystic ovarian syndrome undergoing assisted reproduction. Cochrane Database Syst Rev. 2013;(10):CD006606.
139. Palomba S, Falbo A, Zullo F, Orio F Jr. Evidence-based and potential benefits of metformin in the polycystic ovary syndrome: a comprehensive review. Endocr Rev. 2009;30(1):1-50.
140. Tang T, Glanville J, Orsi N, Barth JH, Balen AH. The use of metformin for women with PCOS undergoing IVF treatment. Hum Reprod. 2006;21(6):1416-25.
141. Tso LO, Costello MF, Albuquerque LE, Andriolo RB, Macedo CR. Metformin treatment before and during IVF or ICSI in women with polycystic ovary syndrome. Cochrane Database Syst Rev. 2014;2014(11):CD006105.
142. Legro RS, Barnhart HX, Schlaff WD, Carr BR, Diamond MP, Carson SA, et al; Cooperative Multicenter Reproductive Medicine Network. Clomiphene, metformin, or both for infertility in the polycystic ovary syndrome. N Engl J Med. 2007;356(6):551-66.
143. Naderpoor N, Shorakae S, de Courten B, Misso ML, Moran LJ, Teede HJ. Metformin and lifestyle modification in polycystic ovary syndrome: systematic review and meta-analysis. Hum Reprod Update. 2015;21(5):560-74.
144. Tang T, Glanville J, Hayden CJ, White D, Barth JH, Balen AH. Combined lifestyle modification and metformin in obese patients with polycystic ovary syndrome. A randomized, placebo-controlled, double-blind multicentre study. Hum Reprod. 2006;21(1):80-9.
145. Bordewijk EM, Nahuis M, Costello MF, Van der Veen F, Tso LO, Mol BW, et al. Metformin during ovulation induction with gonadotrophins followed by timed intercourse or intrauterine insemination for subfertility associated with polycystic ovary syndrome. Cochrane Database Syst Rev. 2017;1(1):CD009090.
146. Vitek OW, Alur S, Hoeger KM. Off-label drug use in the treatment of polycystic ovary syndrome. Fertil Steril. 2015;103(3):605-11.
147. Tang T, Lord JM, Norman RJ, Yasmin E, Balen JH. Insulin-sensitizing drugs (metformin, rosiglitazone, pioglitazone, D-chiro-inositol) for women with polycystic ovary syndrome, oligo amenorrhea and subfertility. Cochrane Database Syst Rev. 2012;(5):CD003053.
148. Ocal P, Ersoylu B, Cepni I, Guralp O, Atakul N, Irez T, et al. The association between homocysteine in the follicular fluid with embryo quality and pregnancy rate in assisted reproductive techniques. J Assist Reprod Genet. 2012;29(4):299-304.
149. Boxmeer JC, Brouns RM, Lindemans J, Steegers EA, Martini E, Macklon NS, et al. Preconception folic acid treatment affects the microenvironment of the maturing oocyte in humans. Fertil Steril. 2008;89(6):1766-70.
150. Badawy A, State O, Abdelgawad S. *N*-Acetyl cysteine and clomiphene citrate for induction of ovulation in polycystic ovary syndrome: a cross-over trial. Acta Obstet Gynecol Scand. 2007;86(2):218-22.
151. Seko LM, Moroni RM, Leitao VM, Teixeira DM, Nastri CO, Martins WP. Melatonin supplementation during controlled ovarian stimulation for women undergoing assisted reproductive technology: systematic review and meta-analysis of randomized controlled trials. Fertil Steril. 2014;101(1):154-61.e4.
152. Ismail AM, Hamed AH, Saso S, Thabet HH. Adding L-carnitine to clomiphene resistant PCOS women improves the quality of ovulation and the pregnancy rate. A randomized clinical trial. Eur J Obstet Gynecol Reprod Biol. 2014;180:148-52.
153. El Refaeey A, Selem A, Badawy A. Combined coenzyme Q10 and clomiphene citrate for ovulation induction in clomiphene-citrate-resistant polycystic ovary syndrome. Reprod Biomed Online. 2014;29(1):119-24.
154. Lydic ML, McNurlan M, Bembo S, Mitchell L, Komaroff E, Gelato M. Chromium picolinate improves insulin sensitivity in obese subjects with polycystic ovary syndrome. Fertil Steril. 2006;86(1):243-6.
155. Parsanezhad ME, Alborzi S, Motazedian S, Omrani G. Use of dexamethasone and clomiphene citrate in the treatment of clomiphene citrate-resistant patients with polycystic ovary syndrome and normal dehydroepiandrosterone sulfate levels: a prospective, double-blind, placebo-controlled trial. Fertil Steril. 2002;78(5):1001-4.
156. Goenka D, Goenka ML. Oral contraceptive pill pretreatment for clomiphene citrate resistant cases followed by repeat clomiphene citrate treatment. J Obstet Gynaecol India. 2006;56(2):159-61.
157. Griesinger G, Venetis CA, Marx T, Diedrich K, Tarlatzis BC, Kolibianakis BM. Oral contraceptive pill pretreatment in ovarian stimulation with GnRH antagonists for IVF: a systematic review and meta-analysis. Fertil Steril. 2008;90(4):1055-63.
158. Kaya C, Cengiz SD, Berker B, Demirtaş S, Cesur M, Erdoğan G. Comparative effects of atorvastatin and simvastatin on the plasma total homocysteine levels in women with polycystic ovary syndrome: a prospective randomized study. Fertil Steril. 2009;92(2):635-42.
159. Carmina E, Oberfield SE, Lobo RA. The diagnosis of polycystic ovary syndrome in adolescents. Am J Obstet Gynecol. 2010;203(3):201.e1-5.
160. Hart R, Doherty DA, Mori T, Huang RC, Norman RJ, Franks S, et al. Extent of metabolic risk in adolescent girls with features of polycystic ovary syndrome. Fertil Steril. 2011;95(7):2347-53.
161. Hoeger K, Davidson K, Kochman L, Cherry T, Kopin L, Guzick DS. The impact of metformin, oral contraceptives,

and lifestyle modification on polycystic ovary syndrome in obese adolescent women in two randomized, placebo-controlled clinical trials. J Clin Endocrinol Metab. 2008;93(11):4299-306.
162. Wang JX, Davies MJ, Norman RJ. Polycystic ovarian syndrome and the risk of spontaneous abortion following assisted reproductive technology treatment. Hum Reprod. 2001;16(12):2606-9.
163. Rai R, Backos M, Rushworth F, Regan L. Polycystic ovaries and recurrent miscarriage—a reappraisal. Hum Reprod. 2000;15(3):612-5.
164. Boomsma CM, Eijkemans MJ, Hughes EG, Visser GH, Fauser BC, Macklon NS. A meta-analysis of pregnancy outcomes in women with polycystic ovary syndrome. Hum Reprod Update. 2006;12(6):673-83.
165. Kjerulff LE, Sanchez-Ramos L, Duffy D. Pregnancy outcomes in women with polycystic ovary syndrome: a meta-analysis. Am J Obstet Gynecol. 2011;204(6):558.e1-6.
166. Palomba S, Falbo A, Chiossi G, Tolino A, Tucci L, La Sala GB, et al. Early trophoblast invasion and placentation in women with different PCOS phenotypes. Reprod Biomed Online. 2014;29(3):370-81.
167. Glueck CJ, Wang P, Goldenberg N, Sieve-Smith L. Pregnancy outcomes among women with polycystic ovary syndrome treated with metformin. Hum Reprod. 2002;17(11):2858-64.
168. Wang L, Lv S, Li F, Bai E, Yang X. Letrozole Versus Clomiphene Citrate and Natural Cycle: Endometrial Receptivity During Implantation Window in Women with Polycystic Ovary Syndrome. Front Endocrinol (Lausanne). 2021;11:532692.
169. Barry JA, Azizia MM, Hardiman PJ. Risk of endometrial, ovarian and breast cancer in women with polycystic ovary syndrome: a systematic review and meta-analysis. Hum Reprod Update. 2014;20(5):748-58.
170. Fearnley EJ, Marquart L, Spurdle AB, Weinstein P, Webb PM; Australian Ovarian Cancer Study Group and Australian National Endometrial Cancer Study Group. Polycystic ovary syndrome increases the risk of endometrial cancer in women aged less than 50 years: an Australian case-control study. Cancer Causes Control. 2010;21(12):2303-8.

CHAPTER

40 Assessment of Ovarian Reserve

Padma Rekha Jirge

INTRODUCTION

Ovarian reserve is the quantity and quality of the primordial follicle pool and is an important factor in determining the fertility potential of an individual.[1] Age-related decline in ovarian reserve has long been documented, noted as early as mid-twentieth century.[2] Two factors that necessitate the need for elaborate assessment of ovarian reserve are: wide variation in the age-related decline in fertility and absence of any clinical pointers for declining ovarian reserve, as majority of women continues to have regular menstrual cycles during this phase. It is believed that there is an accelerated decline in the follicle numbers when the critical figure reaches 25,000 and fertility remains for a relatively short period beyond this stage.[3,4] Hence, estimation of ovarian reserve would assist in making informed decisions about fertility, need for any active management, and fast tracking toward in vitro fertilization (IVF).

An ideal ovarian reserve test (ORT) should be easy to perform, easily reproducible, noninvasive and accurately measure the quantity and hence quality of the follicular pool; and predict the chances of pregnancy.[5] Over a period of time various static and dynamic tests have been introduced into clinical practice for evaluation of ovarian reserve. It has so far not been possible to estimate the primordial follicle pool and hence various indirect measures are used. These include direct ovarian assessment, including certain secretions from the ovarian follicles, various measurements of the ovaries, or indirect measurements of certain hormones, which reflect a declining ovarian follicular pool.

OVARIAN RESERVE TESTS

Ovarian reserve tests have been developed primarily with an aim to predict the ovarian response in IVF. However, it is not clear whether the decline in oocyte quality is dependent on chronological age or the changing hormonal environment with declining numbers of oocytes.[6] A list of these tests has been summarized in **Table 1**.

BIOLOGICAL AGE

Biological age remains the most important predictor of reproductive potential of an individual.[1] Fecundity is known to decline with maternal age and this is evident from ages as early as late 20s.[7-9] Despite wide variation within population and amongst different ethnicities, it is known that ovarian reserve declines rapidly after 37 years of age.[7,10,11] In those undergoing IVF, most of the embryos are found to be aneuploid by the age of 44 years.[12] It is interesting to note that even women with polycystic ovarian syndrome (PCOS) with high ovarian reserve do not appear to have an extended window of fertility.[13] However, it is generally believed that in women younger than 35 years of age despite poor ovarian response, risk of pregnancy loss with IVF cycles does not increase, due to euploid nature of most of the embryos obtained.[14] As there is a wide spectrum of response encountered in women undergoing IVF from normal to hyper-response, biological age alone cannot be used as

TABLE 1: Ovarian reserve tests.

Ovarian reserve tests	*Categories*	*Tests*
Biological	Biological age	–
Biochemical	• Static	• Baseline serum FSH (day 2–4) • Baseline serum estradiol • Serum inhibin B • AMH
	• Dynamic tests	• CCCT • EFFORT • GAST
Biophysical	Ultrasonological evaluation	• AFC • Ovarian volume • Ovarian Doppler
Histological	Ovarian biopsy	–

(AFC: antral follicle count; AMH: anti-Müllerian hormone; CCCT: clomiphene citrate challenge test; EFFORT: exogenous follicle-stimulating hormone ovarian reserve test; FSH: follicle-stimulating hormone; GAST: gonadotropin-releasing hormone agonist stimulation test)

a marker of ovarian reserve and hence efforts continue to identify a single or a set of markers of ovarian reserve to predict the ovarian response.

BASAL SERUM FOLLICLE-STIMULATING HORMONE

Basal follicle-stimulating hormone (FSH) has been the most widely used ORT to assess ovarian reserve for the past three decades. It is measured in the morning hours on days 2–4 of the cycle.[15] The measurement of FSH is easy and it is an inexpensive test. However, it has diurnal, intra- and intercycle variability.[16,17] Increasing levels of FSH occur due to progressive follicular depletion. There is no universally accepted cutoff value for FSH to predict poor ovarian response. However, most of the IVF clinics consider 10–12 IU/L as the upper limit of normal range. In women with regular menstrual cycles, FSH can predict poor ovarian response only at very high levels and consequently helpful to only a small number of women as a screening test for poor ovarian reserve. Considering that decline in ovarian reserve begins several years earlier to any elevation in serum FSH levels, a normal value cannot rule out a poor ovarian response.[18,19] In addition, significance of elevated basal FSH levels in young infertile women with regular menstrual cycles is unclear.[20,21] Hence, in the current clinical scenario with availability of more robust ovarian reserve markers, FSH cannot be used alone to predict ovarian reserve.

SERUM ESTRADIOL

The role of estradiol as an ORT has remained controversial. It is known that an elevated serum estradiol level may mask abnormal FSH levels and the ovarian reserve may be wrongly considered as normal.[22] Hence, addition of serum estradiol values on days 2–4 of the cycle with FSH values is considered to reflect ovarian reserve more precisely. Elevated basal estradiol in itself (>80 pg/mL) is considered as predictor of poor response.[23] However, a meta-analysis concluded that basal estradiol does not add to the predictive value of other ORTs and hence it should not be used in routine clinical practice as an ORT.[19]

SERUM INHIBIN B

Inhibin B is a glycoprotein produced in the granulosa cells of ovarian follicles. It is noted that serum inhibin B level of <45 pg/mL predicts poor response to ovarian stimulation for IVF.[23] Inhibin B was the first ORT used to predict hyper-response in IVF.[24] However, unreliability of the assays and availability of more robust markers of ovarian reserve such as anti-Müllerian hormone (AMH), to predict both ovarian response in IVF and occurrence of pregnancy, have limited the use of inhibin B as an ORT in recent years.[25,26]

SERUM ANTI-MÜLLERIAN HORMONE

Anti-Müllerian hormone is a dimeric glycoprotein exclusively produced by granulosa cells of preantral (primary and secondary) and small antral follicles (AFs) in the ovary.[27,28] AMH is produced by the granulosa cells of the follicles following their transition from primordial pool to the primary stage and continues till the follicles reach antral stage with diameters of 2–6 mm.[28-30] These small antral follicles reflect the size of the primordial pool. As the size of the follicular pool declines with age, AMH production diminishes and becomes undetectable at menopause.[31] It is considered as a regulator of follicular recruitment and with declining AMH levels, there is an accelerated recruitment of follicles from the primordial pool.[28]

Anti-Müllerian hormone exhibits certain advantages over other ovarian reserve markers:

- It exhibits little intra- and intercycle variability and hence can be measured on any day of the menstrual cycle.[32,33]
- It is the earliest marker to show decline in ovarian reserve. Levels below 1.26 ng/mL are considered to indicate poor ovarian response to ovarian stimulation. At levels of 0.5–1.26 ng/mL, AMH indicates perimenopausal transition within 3–5 years. Women with levels within this range still have a favorable outcome with IVF if the treatment is not delayed.[34]
- It is a very sensitive marker to predict hyper-response as well.[35]
- Serum AMH levels strongly correlate with antral follicle count (AFC) measured by transvaginal ultrasonography (TVS).[36]
- Age-related population nomograms are available for AMH[37,38] and this provides an opportunity to counsel young women with low AMH regarding prioritizing conception or for oocyte cryopreservation.[39]
- AMH has a unique place in that it may be applicable as a screening test in a general subfertile population.[39]
- AMH is the only ovarian reserve marker found to be reliable in assessing the residual ovarian reserve in young cancer survivors who have received gonadotoxic therapy previously.[40]
- Whether AMH can predict the occurrence of pregnancy is less clear. However, recent evidence suggests that AMH may be a better predictor of occurrence of pregnancy in young poor responders than age alone.[41]

Anti-Müllerian hormone assay technique has evolved over the past decade as well. From the initial enzyme-linked immunosorbent assay (ELISA), semiautomated assays, we now have fully automated assays. Original diagnostic systems lab (DSL) assay is considered as the benchmark for AMH assays. However, the fully automated assays have reduced the time consumed for performing the assay and made international comparison feasible.[42]

A comparison of three different ELISA assays and the two new automated assays have revealed certain important facts. All the three commercially available ELISA assays—Gen II (Beckman Coulter), EIA AMH/MIS (Immunotech, Beckman Coulter), and Ultrasensitive AL-105i (Anshlab) perform similarly.

The two new fully automated immunoassays are Access Dxi automatic analyzer (B13127, Beckman Coulter) and Cobas e instrument (Roche Diagnostics). Gen II and Cobas e assays use bovine AMH as calibrator whereas others use recombinant human anti-Müllerian hormone (rhAMH) as the calibrator. It is seen that even though all the assays have similar specificity of 91.7%, Cobas e has the highest sensitivity of 73.5% similar to Gen II assay.[43] As there is a shift toward use of fully automated assays in the recent years and as AMH is the most important deciding factor in individualizing the protocols and dosing, it is of importance to note that AMH values measured by Access assay are on an average 10% higher than that by Cobas e assay. This has led to concerns regarding incorrect dosing in up to 29% of women when Access assay used for AMH estimation.[44] However, current clinical experience is reassuring and suggest that the such differences little affect the calibration of FSH dose for ovarian stimulation.[45]

DYNAMIC TESTS

Three dynamic tests have been used in the past to assess ovarian reserve:[46]

1. *Clomiphene citrate challenge test (CCCT):* This involves estimating basal FSH level on day 3 followed by administration of 100 mg of clomiphene from day 5 to day 9 and estimation of FSH level on day 10. Either an abnormally high basal FSH or an abnormally high value of cumulative FSH (day 3 + day 10) is considered as evidence of poor ovarian reserve.
2. *Exogenous follicle-stimulating hormone ovarian reserve test (EFFORT):* This test involves estimation of basal FSH and estradiol on day 3 of the cycle followed by administration of 300 IU FSH on the same day. Serum estradiol concentration is rechecked 24 hours later. It was found to be of value in predicting hyper-response but has a high false positive rate.
3. *Gonadotropin-releasing hormone agonist stimulation test (GAST):* This test involves estimation of day 2 serum estradiol followed by administration of gonadotropin-releasing hormone agonist (GnRH-a) (triptorelin 100 µg) subcutaneously. The test is repeated 24 hours later and an elevation in estradiol is considered to indicate good ovarian reserve. It has been used in the past to identify poor responders.

The dynamic tests are time consuming, expensive, and are inferior to the more robust markers such as AMH and AFC.[46]

ANTRAL FOLLICLE COUNT

Antral follicles are all the small follicles seen in the ovary measuring 2–10 mm in diameter. The AFC is measured in the early follicular phase (day 2–4) using TVS with a 7.5 MHz probe. Two perpendicular measurements are taken of each of the follicles and the mean value is considered the diameter of the follicle. The follicles in both ovaries are added for the total AFC.[47] An AFC of 8–16 is considered to predict normal ovarian response in IVF whereas those below 8 are considered to predict poor ovarian response. An AFC of >16 is highly predictive of hyper-response. AFs of 2–6 mm and 2–9 mm are both considered to reflect AFC. However, the number of AFs of 2–6 mm diameter decline with age whereas those of 7–9 mm diameter remain constant and hence the former appears to be a more reliable marker of ovarian reserve.[48] There appears to be limited intercycle variability; however, interobserver variability in young women may be high. Use of 3D ultrasound does not have any advantage over 2D ultrasound in the assessment of ovarian reserve.[49]

Antral follicle count has a strong correlation to AMH and has similar sensitivity and specificity to predict both poor and hyper-response.[36] Current evidence does not support its ability to predict occurrence of pregnancy.[41]

OVARIAN VOLUME

Ovarian volume is measured by TVS using the formula for an ellipsoid. Even though increased ovarian volume is an important diagnostic criterion for PCOS, it does not add to the predictive value of AFC while assessing ovarian reserve.[50,51]

OVARIAN DOPPLER ASSESSMENT

Even though attempts have been made to utilize ovarian Doppler for assessing ovarian reserve, its role is currently limited to assessing perifollicular flow during ovarian stimulation with a view to select oocytes with best potential to achieve pregnancy.[52]

OVARIAN BIOPSY

Biopsy of ovarian cortex obtained during laparoscopy or laparotomy, have shown declining follicular density with age. However, the follicles are not uniformly distributed in the cortex and hence the biopsy may not represent the true follicular density.[53] In addition, any such invasive procedure has no place in the current clinical scenario in the presence of ovarian reserve markers such as AMH and AFC.

DISCUSSION

Historically, ORTs were thought to reflect oocyte quantity and were developed to provide prognostic information for IVF cycles.[1] Despite decades of research, controversy

TABLE 2: Role of ovarian reserve testing under various clinical scenarios.

ORT	Role
Prior to IVF	To individualize protocol and dosing; counseling regarding hyper- or poor response and their consequences
Subfertile women	To identify those with poor ovarian reserve and early recourse to IVF
General population	Informed decision regarding social egg freezing or prioritize conception
Young cancer survivors	To assess residual ovarian function and offer suitable fertility treatment

(IVF: in vitro fertilization; ORT: ovarian reserve test)

remains as to whether ORTs can also provide insight into oocyte quality and estimate an ovarian age. Over a period of four decades, various forms of ORTs have become available for clinical use.[54]

Table 2 highlights the role of ovarian reserve testing in various clinical situations commonly encountered. The primary role of any ovarian test has been prediction of ovarian response to ovarian stimulation in IVF. It is well understood that ovarian reserve declines with age. But clinical experience has also shown that there is a wide variation amongst young women of reproductive age in the rate of decline in ovarian reserve. Hence, the initial efforts were directed toward identifying poor responders. Basal FSH, estradiol, and various dynamic tests have been used to achieve this purpose,[18,19,23,46] and they are all found to have limited value in clinical use. However, AMH and AFC are the two markers of ovarian reserve found to have highest predictive value for not only for poor response but also for hyper-response.[35] They have made it possible to individualize the IVF protocols based on the ovarian reserve to improve both safety and efficacy of IVF.[55]

In the recent years, efforts have been directed at identifying poor responders in young women with infertility early enough and offer fast-tracking of treatment to maximize the chances of conception for such women with their own eggs. AMH is found to be the marker that declines earliest with age; and addition of AFC may not improve the predictive value.[34,36] AMH has also allowed exploration of an association between poor ovarian reserve and genetic factors such as *BRCA* mutations or environmental toxins such as bisphenol A and phthalate.[56,57]

Even though there is general consensus that ORTs predict the quantity of follicles reliably, there is controversy regarding their ability to predict the quality of oocytes and hence the occurrence of pregnancy. Age is generally considered the best measure of oocyte quality and young women with reduced quantity of oocytes still have a good pregnancy outcome.[14] However, recent evidence has challenged this view and low AMH and AFC in addition to predicting ovarian response may also be indicative of poor oocyte quality.[58-60]

Over the past two decades, there is a steady increase in the survival of children and young adults treated for various malignancies. This has also brought into focus the fertility issues in such young population treated previously with gonadotoxic chemotherapy and/or radiotherapy. AMH is found to be the only marker, which reflects the damage to the follicular pool during and immediately after such treatment and recovery of and residual ovarian reserve following treatment.[40] It plays an important role in decision-making process for suitable treatment in such young women who have not been offered or found ineligible for fertility preservation prior to cancer therapy.

One of the most important growing concerns in the field of reproductive medicine is the increasing global trend toward delaying pregnancy. This increases the need for usage donor oocytes in women with very poor ovarian reserve and those with advanced maternal age. AMH has been used to assess ovarian reserve in those who wish to delay fertility as it is known to be the earliest marker to show decline in ovarian reserve.[37-39] This helps in informed counseling of young women wishing to delay childbearing either for oocyte cryopreservation or to prioritize fertility based on the situation and individual's wish.

CONCLUSION

Ovarian reserve tests play an important role in the evaluation of infertile women. AMH and AFC have the best predictive value for ovarian reserve compared to all other markers. Age is considered to be most important factor in predicting the occurrence of pregnancy. However, recent evidence suggests that AMH and AFC may have better predictive value for euploid pregnancy in young women compared to age alone. AMH, in addition, is proven to be a good screening test for general population wishing to delay fertility and also to identify poor responders in the subfertile population to expedite and fast-track the treatment. The role of FSH in the current scenario for evaluation of ovarian reserve is limited.

REFERENCES

1. Testing and interpreting measures of ovarian reserve: a committee opinion. Fertil Steril. 2020;114(6):1151-7.
2. Block E. Quantitative morphological investigations of the follicular system in women; variations at different ages. Acta Anat (Basel). 1952;14(1-2):108-23.
3. Faddy MJ, Gosden RG, Gougeon A, Richardson SJ, Nelson JF. Accelerated disappearance of ovarian follicles in mid-life: implications for forecasting menopause. Hum Reprod. 1992;7(10):1342-6.
4. Nikolaou D, Templeton A. Early ovarian ageing: a hypothesis. Detection and clinical relevance. Hum Reprod. 2003;18(6):1137-9.

5. de Carvalho BR, Rosa e Silva AC, Rosa e Silva JC, dos Reis RM, Ferriani RA, Silva de Sá MF. Ovarian reserve evaluation: state of the art. J Assist Reprod Genet. 2008;25(7):311-22.
6. Massie JA, Burney RO, Milki AA, Westphal LM, Lathi RB. Basal follicle-stimulating hormone as a predictor of fetal aneuploidy. Fertil Steril. 2008;90:2351-5.
7. de Bruin JP, teVelde ER. Female reproductive ageing: Concepts and consequences. In: Tulandi T, Gosden RG (Eds). Preservation of Fertility. London UK: Taylor and Francis; 2004. p. 3.
8. Wood JW. Fecundity and natural fertility in humans. Oxf Rev Reprod Biol. 1989;11:61-109.
9. Piette C, de Mouzon J, Bachelot A, Spira A. In vitro fertilization (influence of woman's age on pregnancy rates) Hum Reprod. 1990;5(1):56-9.
10. Toner JP, Philput CB, Jones GS, Muasher SJ. Basal follicle stimulating hormone level is a better predictor of in vitro fertilization performance than age. Fertil Steril. 1991;55(4): 784-91.
11. Sharif K, Elgendy M, Lashen H, Afnan M. Age and basal follicle stimulating hormone as predictors of in vitro fertilization outcome. Br J Obstet Gynaecol. 1998;105(1):107-12.
12. Franasiak JM, Forman EJ, Hong KH, Werner MD, Upham KM, Treff NR. The nature of aneuploidy with increasing age of the female partner: a review of 15,169 consecutive trophectoderm biopsies evaluated with comprehensive chromosomal screening. Fertil Steril. 2014;101(3):656-63.
13. Kalra SK, Ratcliffe SJ, Dokras A. Is the fertile window extended in women with polycystic ovary syndrome? Utilizing the Society for Assisted Reproductive Technology registry to assess the impact of reproductive aging on live-birth rate. Fertil Steril. 2013;100(1):208-13.
14. Bishop LA, Richter KS, Patounakis G, Andriani L, Moon K, Devine K. Diminished ovarian reserve as measured by means of baseline follicle-stimulating hormone and antral follicle count is not associated with pregnancy loss in younger in vitro fertilization patients. Fertil Steril. 2017; 108(6):980-7.
15. Scott RT, Toner JP, Muasher SJ, Oehninger S, Robinson S, Rosenwaks Z. Follicle-stimulating hormone levels on cycle day 3 are predictive of in vitro fertilization outcome. 1989;51(4):651-4.
16. Scott RT, Jr Hofmann GE, Oehninger S, Muasher SJ. Intercycle variability of day 3 follicle-stimulating hormone levels and its effect on stimulation quality in in vitro fertilization. Fertil Steril. 1990;54(2):297-302.
17. Kwee J, Schats R, McDonnell J, Lambalk CB, Schoemaker J. Intercycle variability of ovarian reserve tests: Results of a prospective randomized study. Hum Reprod. 2004;19(3): 590-5.
18. Bancsi LF, Broekmans FJ, Mol BW, Habbema JD, teVelde ER. Performance of basal follicle-stimulating hormone in the prediction of poor ovarian response and failure to become pregnant after in vitro fertilization: Ameta-analysis. Fertil Steril. 2003;79(5):1091-100.
19. Broekmans FJ, Kwee J, Hendriks DJ, Mol BW, Lambalk CB. A systematic review of tests predicting ovarian reserve and IVF outcome. Hum Reprod Update. 2006;12(6):685-718.
20. Esposito MA, Coutifaris C, Barnhart KT. A moderately elevated day 3 FSH concentration has limited predictive value, especially in younger women. Hum Reprod. 2002;17(1):118-23.
21. Devranoğlu B, Özdamar Ö, Köle E, Eken MK, Bozdağ H, Doğer E. Do younger women with elevated basal follicular stimulating hormone levels undergoing gonadotropin-stimulated intrauterine insemination cycles represent compromised reproductive outcomes? Eur J Obstet Gynecol Reprod Biol. 2016;199:141-5.
22. Evers JL, Slaats P, Land JA, Dumoulin JC, Dunselman GA. Elevated levels of basal estradiol-17β predict poor response in patients with normal basal levels of follicle-stimulating hormone undergoing in vitro fertilization. Fertil Steril. 1998;69(6):1010-4
23. Seifer DB, Lambert-Messerlian G, Hogan JW, Gardiner AC, Blazar AS, Berk CA. Day 3 serum inhibin-B is predictive of assisted reproductive technologies outcome. Fertil Steril. 1997;67(1):110-4.
24. Dzik A, Lambert-Messerlian G, Izzo VM, Soares JB, Pinotti JA, Seifer DB. Inhibin B response to EFORT is associated with the outcome of oocyte retrieval in the subsequent in vitro fertilization cycle. Fertil Steril. 2000;74(6):1114-7.
25. Feyereisen E, Méndez Lozano DH, Taieb J, Hesters L, Frydman R, Fanchin R. Anti-Müllerian hormone: clinical insights into a promising biomarker of ovarian follicular status. Reprod Biomed Online. 2006;12(6):695-703.
26. Rosen MP, Johnstone E, McCulloch CE, Schuh-Huerta SM, Sternfeld B, Reijo-Pera RA. Characterization of the relationship of ovarian reserve markers with age. Fertil Steril. 2012;97(1):238-43.
27. Laven JSE, Mulders AGMGJ, Visser JA, Themmen AP, De Jong FH, Fauser BC. Anti-Müllerian hormone serum concentrations in normoovulatory and anovulatory women of reproductive age. J Clin Endocrinol Metab. 2004;89(1):318-23.
28. Weenen C, Laven JS, Von Bergh AR, Cranfield M, Groome NP, Visser JA. Anti-Müllerian hormone expression pattern in the human ovary: potential implications for initial and cyclic follicle recruitment. Mol Hum Reprod. 2004;10(2):77-83.
29. Durlinger AL, Visser JA, Themmen AP. Regulation of ovarian function: The role of anti-Mullerian hormone. Reproduction. 2002;124(5):601-9.
30. van Rooij IA, Broekmans FJ, teVelde ER, Fauser BC, Bancsi LF, de Jong FH, et al. Serum anti-Müllerian hormone levels: A novel measure of ovarian reserve. Hum Reprod. 2002;17(12):3065-71.
31. de Vet A, Laven JS, de Jong FH, Themmen AP, Fauser BC. Anti-Müllerian hormone serum levels: A putative marker for ovarian aging. Fertil Steril. 2002;77(2):357-62.
32. La Marca A, Stabile G, Artenisio AC, Volpe A. Serum anti-Mullerian hormone throughout the human menstrual cycle. Hum Reprod. 2006;21(12):3103-7.
33. Hehenkamp JK, Loomans CW, Themmen AP, de Jong FH, teVelde ER, Broekmans FJ. Anti-Mullerian hormone levels in the spontaneous menstrual cycle do not show substantial fluctuation. J Clin Endocrinol Metab. 2006;91(10):4057-63.
34. Gnoth C, Schuring AN, Friol K, Tigges J, Mallmann P, Godehardt E. Relevance of anti-Mullerian hormone measurement in a routine IVF program. Hum Reprod. 2005;23(6):1359-65.
35. Fraissinet A, Robin G, Pigny P, Lefebvre T, Catteau-Jonard S, Dewailly D. Use of the serum anti-Müllerian hormone

assay as a surrogate for polycystic ovarian morphology: impact on diagnosis and phenotypic classification of polycystic ovary syndrome. Hum Reprod. 2017;32(8): 1716-22.
36. Fleming R, Seifer DB, Frattarelli JL, Ruman J. Assessing ovarian response: antral follicle count versus anti-Müllerian hormone. Reprod Biomed Online. 2015;31(4):486-96.
37. Nelson SM, Messow MC, Wallace AM, Fleming R, McConnachie A. Nomogram for the decline in serum antimüllerian hormone: a population study of 9,601 infertility patients. Fertil Steril. 2011;95(2):736-41.
38. Nelson SM, Iliodromiti S, Fleming R, Anderson R, McConnachie A, Messow CM. Reference range for the anti-Müllerian hormone Generation II assay: a population study of 10,984 women, with comparison to the established Diagnostics Systems Laboratory nomogram. Fertil Steril. 2014;101(2):523-9.
39. Martyn F, O'Brien YM, Wingfield M. Review of clinical indicators, including serum anti-Müllerian hormone levels, for identification of women who should consider egg freezing. Int J Gynaecol Obstet. 2017;138(1):37-41.
40. Charpentier AM, Chong AL, Gingras-Hill G, Ahmed S, Cigsar C, Gupta AA, et al. Anti-Müllerian hormone screening to assess ovarian reserve among female survivors of childhood cancer. J Cancer Surviv. 2014;8(4):548-54.
41. Nelson SM, Fleming R, Gaudoin M, Choi B, Santo-Domingo K, Yao M. Antimüllerian hormone levels and antral follicle count as prognostic indicators in a personalized prediction model of live birth. Fertil Steril. 2015;104(2):325-32.
42. Li HW, Wong BP, Ip WK, Yeung WS, Ho PC, Ng EH. Comparative evaluation of three new commercial immunoassays for anti-Müllerian hormone measurement. Hum Reprod. 2016; 31(12):2796-802.
43. Pigny P, Gorisse E, Ghulam A, Robin G, Catteau-Jonard S, Duhamel A, et al. Comparative assessment of five serum antimüllerian hormone assays for the diagnosis of polycystic ovary syndrome. Fertil Steril. 2016;105(4):1063-9.
44. Iliodromiti S, Salje B, Dewailly D, Fairburn C, Fanchin R, Fleming R, et al. Non-equivalence of anti-Müllerian hormone automated assays-clinical implications for use as a companion diagnostic for individualised gonadotrophin dosing. Hum Reprod. 2017;32(8):1710-5.
45. La Marca A, Tolani AD, Capuzzo M. The interchangeability of two assays for the measurement of anti-Müllerian hormone when personalizing the dose of FSH in in-vitro fertilization cycles. Gynecol Endocrinol. 2021;37(4):372-6.
46. Maheshwari A, Fowler P, Bhattacharya S. Assessment of ovarian reserve-should we perform tests of ovarian reserve routinely? Hum Reprod. 2006;21(11):2729-35.
47. Broekmans FJ, de Ziegler D, Howles CM, Gougeon A, Trew G, Olivennes F. The antral follicle count: practical recommendations for better standardization. Fertil Steril. 2010;94(3):1044-51.
48. Haadsma MA, Bukman A, Groen H, Roeloffzen EM, Groenewoud ER, Heineman MJ, et al. The number of small antral follicles (2–6 mm) determines the outcome of endocrine ovarian reserve tests in a subfertile population. Hum Reprod. 2007;22(7):1932-41.
49. Jayaprakasan K, Hilwah N, Kendall NR, Hopkisson JF, Campbell BK, JohnsonI R, et al. Does 3D ultrasound offer any advantage in the pretreatment assessment of ovarian reserve and prediction of outcome after assisted reproduction treatment? Hum Reprod. 2007;22:1925-31.
50. Hendriks DJ, Kwee J, Mol BW, teVelde ER, Broekmans FJ. Ultrasonography as a tool for the prediction of outcome in IVF patients: a comparative meta-analysis of ovarian volume and antral follicle count. Fertil Steril. 2007;87:764-75.
51. Kwee J, Elting ME, Schats R, McDonnell J, Lambalk CB. Ovarian volume and antral follicle count for the prediction of low and hyper responders with in vitro fertilization. Reprod Biol Endocrinol. 2007;5:9.
52. Järvelä IY, Sladkevicius P, Kelly S, Ojha K, Campbell S, Nargund G. Quantification of ovarian power Doppler signal with three-dimensional ultrasonography to predict response during in vitro fertilization. Obstet Gynecol. 2003;102(4): 816-22.
53. Sharara FI, Scott RT. Assessment of ovarian reserve. Is there still a role for ovarian biopsy? First do no harm! Hum Reprod. 2004;19:470-1.
54. Jirge PR. Ovarian reserve tests. J Hum Reprod Sci. 2011;4(3): 108-13.
55. La Marca A, Sunkara SK. Individualization of controlled ovarian stimulation in IVF using ovarian reserve markers: from theory to practice. Hum Reprod Update. 2014;20(1): 124-40.
56. Turan V, Lambertini M, Lee DY, Wang E, Clatot F, Karlan BY, et al. Association of Germline BRCA Pathogenic Variants With Diminished Ovarian Reserve: A Meta-Analysis of Individual Patient-Level Data. J Clin Oncol. 2021;39(18):2016-24.
57. Park SY, Jeon JH, Jeong K, Chung HW, Lee H, Sung YA, et al. The association of ovarian reserve with exposure to bisphenol a and phthalate in reproductive-aged women. J Korean Med Sci. 2021;36(2):e1.
58. Grande M, Borobio V, Bennasar M, Stergiotou I, Mercadé I, Masoller N, et al. Role of ovarian reserve markers, antimüllerian hormone and antral follicle count, as aneuploidy markers in ongoing pregnancies and miscarriages. Fertil Steril. 2015;103(5):1221-7.
59. Gat I, AlKudmani B, Wong K, Zohni K, Weizman NF, Librach C, et al. Significant correlation between anti-müllerian hormone and embryo euploidy in a subpopulation of infertile patients. Reprod Biomed Online 2017;35(5):602-8.
60. Tal R, Seifer DB, Tal R, Granger E, Wantman E, Tal O. AMH highly correlates with cumulative live birth rate in women with diminished ovarian reserve independent of age. J Clin Endocrinol Metab. 2021;106(9):2754-66.

CHAPTER 41

Endometriosis

Nandita Palshetkar, Rohan Palshetkar, Erika Patel

INTRODUCTION

Endometriosis is a long-term, recurrent, and debilitating disease experienced by 5–10% women. It remains an everlasting challenge to the healthcare providers, one of the important reasons being a delay in its diagnosis.[1]

Endometriosis affects 1 in 10 women of reproductive age worldwide. The prevalence of endometriosis as reported is between 2% and 10% in the normal women, 20–50%[2,3] in the infertile population, and >60%[4] in women with chronic pelvic pain and dysmenorrhea. Maximum incidence is seen in the age group of 25–30 years.

Endometriosis is characterized classically by the presence of endometrial glands and stroma outside the endometrial cavity in ectopic locations like the pelvic peritoneum, ovaries, and retrocervical septum.[5,6]

The monthly fecundity rate (MFR) in a normal couple in the reproductive age group is around 30% in the first three cycles and <4% after 1 year. In endometriosis, MFR is reduced to 2–10% per month. Even minimal endometriosis may present with severe infertility.[7,8]

PATHOGENESIS OF ENDOMETRIOSIS

Flowchart 1 describes the pathogenesis of endometriosis.

PATHOGENESIS OF ENDOMETRIOSIS CAUSING INFERTILITY

Whether endometriosis causes subfertility or whether it is an incidental finding in subfertile women remains a controversial issue.

Various mechanisms are known to cause fertility impairment, which are discussed here.

Ovulatory Dysfunction

- Abnormal folliculogenesis
- Slow follicle growth with a decreased dominant follicle size
- Poor oocyte quality
- Decreased fertilization rate
- Low-grade embryo formation
- Reduced implantation
- Luteal phase defect (LPD)
- Luteinized unruptured follicle (LUF) syndrome.

Bacterial Contamination Hypothesis

Diagrammatic presentation of the lipopolysaccharide (LPS)/toll-like receptor-4 (TLR4) cascade in the bacterial contamination hypothesis of endometriosis is shown in **Figure 1**.

Flowchart 1: Pathogenesis of endometriosis.

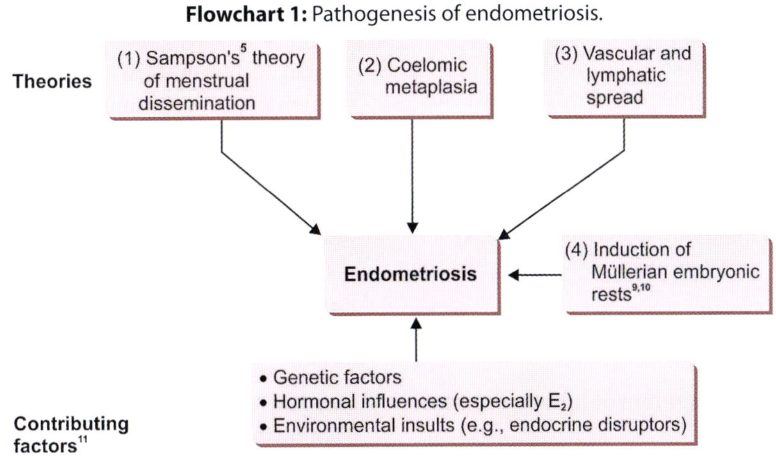

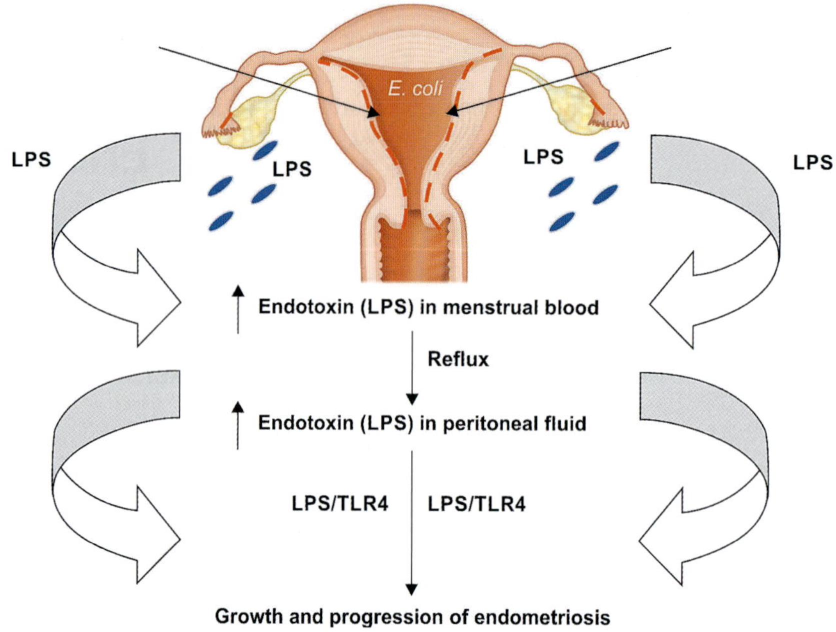

Fig. 1: Bacterial contamination hypothesis.
(*E. coli*: *Escherichia coli*; LPS: lipopolysaccharide; TLR: toll-like receptor)

The constant release of LPS from *Escherichia coli* (*E. coli*) contamination of the menstrual blood causes a higher endotoxin (LPS) concentration in the menstrual blood and consequently higher levels of endotoxin in the peritoneal fluid (PF) due to the retrograde flow of menstrual blood into the pelvis. Peritoneal macrophages, eutopic and ectopic endometrial epithelial cells, and epithelial stromal cells express TLR4, a receptor for LPS. The LPS/TLR4 complex induces pelvic inflammation and promotes the growth and progression of endometriosis via intracellular adaptor molecules and nuclear factor kappa-light-chain-enhancer of activated B-cells activation.[11]

Inflammation in the PF and at the follicular level is described in **Table 1.**

TABLE 1: Inflammation in peritoneal and follicular fluid.

In the peritoneal fluid (PF)	*In the follicular fluid*
↓	↓
• Increased cytokines (IL-1 beta, IL-6, TNF alpha, IL-10) promote adhesion • Decreased vascular endothelial growth factor (VEGF)[12] promotes follicular growth and vascularization • Increased matrix metalloproteinases (MMPs) promote invasion • Increased chemokines like IL-8, MCP, RANTES-1 which attract increased numbers of immune cells, thus increasing proliferation and angiogenesis	• Increased IL-6 which inhibits aromatase enzyme. This decreases estrogen (E2) causing subfertility[13] • Decreased VEGF thus hampering embryo quality and implantation rate[14]

(IL: interleukin; MCP: monocyte chemotactic peptide; RANTES: regulated on activation, normal T-cell expressed and secreted; TNF: tumor necrosis factor)

Oxidative Stress and Endometriosis

In women with endometriosis, expression of enzyme xanthine oxidase, which produces reactive oxygen species (ROS), is increased.[15] Also, large amounts of ROS are produced by macrophages and polymorphonuclear (PMN) leukocytes in PF and endometrial cells as well as apoptotic endometrioma cells.

Reactive oxygen species and elevated ROS produce oxidative stress, which has the following effects:

- Oocyte degeneration and apoptosis by damaging the meiotic spindle.
- Lipid peroxidation causing increased membrane and cell death.[16]
- Increased fragmentation at the time of intracytoplasmic sperm injection (ICSI).[16]
- Local inflammation resulting in increased cytokines, which in turn promote endometriosis.[17]
- Increased deoxyribonucleic acid (DNA) damage of the oocyte, sperm, and embryo thus adversely affecting the fertilization rate, implantation rate, and increasing the miscarriage rate.[18]
- Nitric oxide (NO) is a free radical which regulates apoptosis. Low levels of NO are crucial in ovarian function and implantation. However, increased amounts of NO and nitric oxide synthase (NOS) are seen in the endometrium of women having endometriosis.[19,20] Following effects of high levels of NO are seen:

- Deleterious effect on oviduct function and sperm motility
- Toxic to embryos
- Inhibits implantation.

[Corollary: In in vitro fertilization (IVF), contact of gametes with toxic peritoneal and oviductal factors (NO and ROS) is avoided, which increases pregnancy rate (PR)]

Endometriosis and Sperm Function

As discussed above, increased ROS production by activated macrophages can induce DNA fragmentation, lipid peroxidation in turn increasing membrane permeability, loss of membrane integrity, and enzyme inactivating the sperm.[16]

Also, severe ROS can negatively affect the acrosome reaction and sperm-oocyte fusion.[21]

In endometriosis, not only the sperm motility is affected, but also the tubal ampulla binds sperm more tightly, resulting in reduced quantity of free sperms available to travel through the lumen for fertilization.[22]

Endometriosis and Fertilization

There is reduced fertilization in endometriosis due to:[23-25]

- Poor oocyte quality
- Normal follicular fluid (FF) induces acrosome reaction and binding of sperms to zona pellucida (ZP). The PF and FF in endometriosis inhibit the Sperm—zona binding.[26-28]

Endometriosis and Implantation

Normally, during the window of implantation (WOI), the cellular adhesion molecule αVβ3 integrin expression is increased. But in endometriosis, the expression of αVβ3 is reduced or absent, thus decreasing the endometrial receptivity and hampering implantation.[29,30]

Also, delayed histologic maturation and biochemical disturbances may affect the endometrial receptivity.[29]

In a Nutshell

Factors causing infertility in endometriosis:
- Ovulatory dysfunction
- Immunological alterations
- Peritoneal factors
- Sperm inactivation—phagocytosis by macrophages
- Interference with implantation—endometrial dysfunction
- Interference with coital function—dyspareunia
- Mechanical factors:
  - Anatomical distortion of tubes
  - Altered tubal motility
  - Interference with ovum pickup
  - Peritubal adhesions.

The adverse effect of pelvic endometriosis on uterine cavity is seen not only before conception but even after, resulting in deep placentation and subsequently predisposing the woman to preeclampsia and antepartum hemorrhage in pregnancy.[31]

CLINICAL FEATURES[32]

The Guideline Development Group (GDG) recommends that the diagnosis of endometriosis should be considered in women with any of the following:

- Gynecological symptoms such as dysmenorrhea, chronic pelvic pain, deep dyspareunia, infertility, and fatigue.
- Nongynecological cyclical symptoms such as dyschezia, dysuria, hematuria, shoulder pain, or rectal bleeding in a woman of reproductive age.

DIAGNOSIS OF ENDOMETRIOSIS

Clinical examination must be performed in all women suspected to have endometriosis, although vaginal examination may not be appropriate for adolescents and women without any prior sexual intercourse. In some cases, rectal examination may be helpful, especially when rectal endometriosis or ovarian endometrioma is suspected.

When painful induration and/or rectovaginal wall nodules are felt and nodules are visible in the posterior vaginal fornix on clinical examination, the diagnosis of deep endometriosis may be considered **(Figs. 2 and 3)**.[33]

When adnexal masses are detected on clinical examination, the diagnosis of ovarian endometriosis may be strongly considered.

Sometimes even in presence of endometriosis, the clinical examination is normal.[34] Transvaginal sonography is a very good modality to diagnose or exclude ovarian endometrioma[35] and rectal endometriosis, but in the latter, a highly experienced operator is required.[1] Typical and atypical ultrasonography (USG) features of endometrioma are shown in **Table 2**.

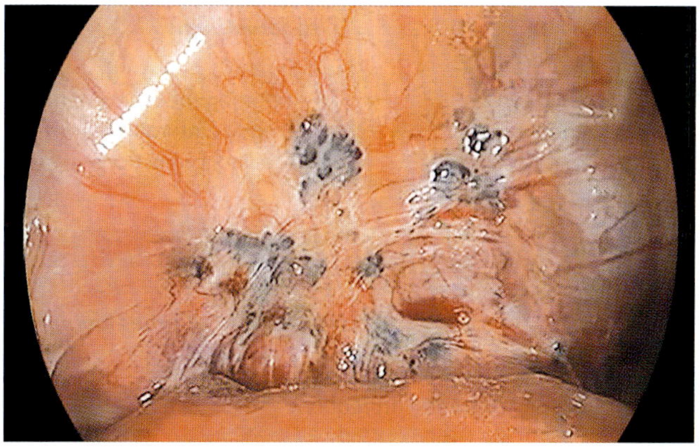

Fig. 2: Left ovarian cyst with endometriotic nodules in the pouch of Douglas with adhesions.

A monolateral, unilocular image <5 cm in the ovary, without septa or papillae with very sparse vascularization independent of its content's density, has very little possibility of being malignant. **Table 3** shows differential diagnosis of endometriotic cyst.

- Doppler ultrasound is of great help in the differential diagnosis, as most endometriomas show the typical peripheral vascularization, whereas others show the "hilus sign" described by Kurjak, which is the presence of vessels between the cyst capsule and the ovarian parenchyma.
- Three-dimensional USG to diagnose rectovaginal endometriosis is not a well established tool. Magnetic resonance imaging (MRI) is useful in diagnosis of extraovarian endometriosis.[36]
- Biomarkers in the endometrial tissue/follicles or menstrual blood and/or cancer antigen-125 (CA-125) should not be used to diagnose endometriosis.[37]

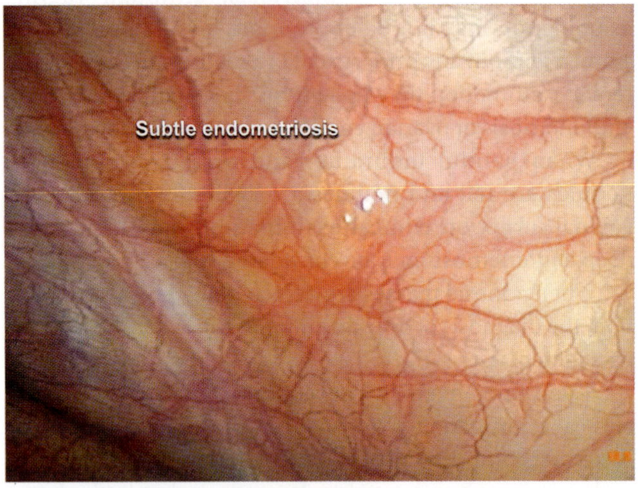

Fig. 3: Subtle endometriosis in the ovarian fossa.

TABLE 2: Typical and atypical ultrasonography (USG) features of endometrioma.

Typical USG features of endometrioma	*Atypical features of endometriomas*
• Oval mass • Hypoechoic content • Hyperechogenic wall • Absence of papillae	• Septae • Inhomogeneous content • Irregular internal wall • Papillary projections

Laparoscopy along with histological confirmation of endometriotic glands and/or stroma used to be the gold standard for diagnosis. However, according to the new European Society of Human Reproduction and Embryology (ESHRE) 2022 guidelines, laparoscopy is no longer the diagnostic gold standard and it is now only recommended in patients with negative imaging results and/or where empirical treatment was unsuccessful or inappropriate.

STAGING

Laparoscopy is essential for the definitive diagnosis of endometriosis. The American Society for Reproductive Medicine (ASRM) classification system is the most widely accepted staging system,[38] but unfortunately no staging system correlates adequately with the pregnancy chances following treatment **(Fig. 4)**.

MANAGEMENT OPTIONS

- Medical
- Surgical
- Combined medical and surgical
- Superovulation-intrauterine insemination (SO-IUI)/ IVF/ICSI
- Oocyte freezing.

Medical Treatment

Currently all the available treatment options for endometriosis are suppressive rather than curative. So, there is temporary relief of symptoms during the treatment and on discontinuation, recurrence is the rule. The most common indication for medical treatment is pain. The current treatment options for endometriosis-associated pain are contraceptive in nature by blocking the hypothalamic-pituitary-ovarian (HPO) axis.

A systematic review of 25 trials[39] showed that in subfertile women with endometriosis who wanted to conceive, there was no benefit of using ovulation suppression.

In women with endometriosis associated with pain, nonsteroidal anti-inflammatory drugs (NSAIDs) appear to be the only medical option. In a systematic review of three clinical trials,[40] pretreatment with a gonadotropin-releasing hormone (GnRH) agonist for 3–6 months before IVF/ICSI in endometriosis improved the clinical pregnancy rate (CPR) fourfold.

TABLE 3: Differential diagnosis of endometriotic cyst.

	Endometrioma	*Corpus luteum*	*Cystadenoma*	*Dermoid*	*Differential diagnosis of ovarian endometrioma*
Septae	Infrequent	No	Frequent	Infrequent	• Cystadenoma • Dermoid cyst • Hemorrhagic cyst • Luteinized unruptured follicle • Corpus luteum
Inhomogeneous content	Infrequent	Frequent	Rare	Frequent	
Posterior reinforcement	No	No	No	Frequent	
Hyperechogenic dots	Frequent	No	No	No	

AMERICAN SOCIETY FOR REPRODUCTIVE MEDICINE
REVISED CLASSIFICATION OF ENDOMETRIOSIS

Patient's Name ______________ Date ______________

Stage I (Minimal) - 1–5
Stage II (Mild) -6–15
Stage III (Moderate) 16-40
Stage IV (Severe) - >40
Total ______________

Laparoscopy__________ Laparostomy__________ Photography ______________
Recommended treatment ______________

Prognosis ______________

	ENDOMETRIOSIS	< 1 cm	1–3 cm	> 3 cm
PERITONEUM	Superficial	1	2	4
	Deep	2	4	6
OVARY	R Superficial	1	2	4
	Deep	4	16	20
	L Superficial	1	2	4
	Deep	4	16	20

POSTERIOR CUL-DE-SAC OBLITERATION	Partial	Complete
	4	40

	ADHESIONS	<1/3 Enclosure	1/3–2/3 Enclosure	>2/3 Enclosure
OVARY	R Filmy	1	2	4
	Dense	4	8	16
	L Filmy	1	2	4
	Dense	4	8	16
TUBE	R Filmy	1	2	4
	Dense	4*	8*	16
	L Filmy	1	2*	4
	Dense	4*	8*	16

*If the fimbriated end of the fallopian tube is completely enclosed, change the point assignment to 16.
Denote appearance of superficial implant types as red [(R), red, red-pink, flamelike, vesicular blobs, clear vesicles], white [(W), opacifications, peritoneal defects, yellow-brown], or black [(B) black, hemosiderin deposits, blue]. Denote percent of total described as R____%, W____% and B____% Total should equal 100%.

Additional Endometriosis: ______________

Associated Pathology: ______________

To be used with normal tubes and ovaries

L R

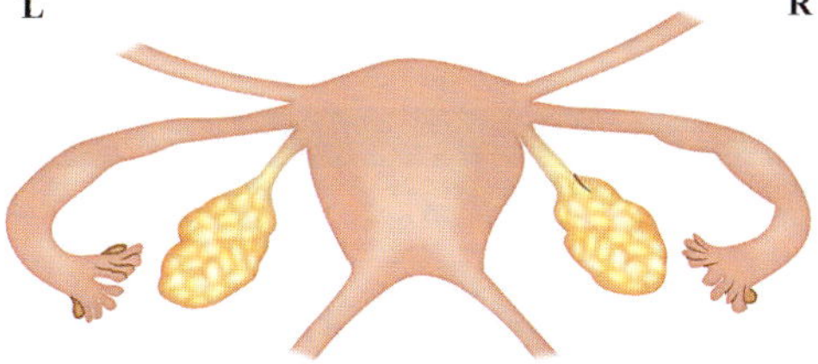

To be used with abnormal tubes and/or ovaries

L R

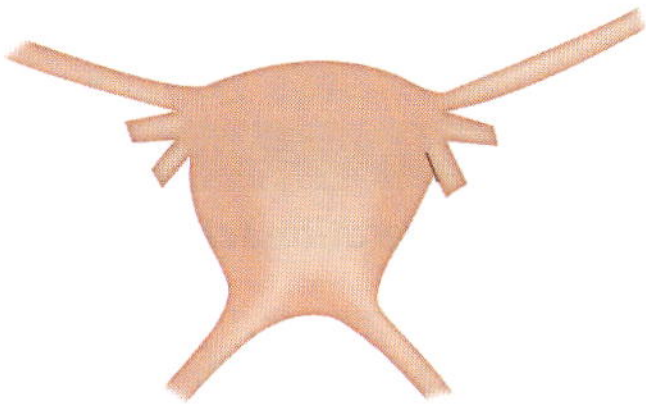

Fig. 4: The American Society for Reproductive Medicine (ASRM) staging system.

With aggressive disease, medical therapy may fail and consequently a large proportion of women may require multidisciplinary surgeries.

Medical Therapy

Refer **Table 4**.

Dienogest

Refer **Table 5**.

Gonadotropin-releasing Hormone Agonists

Refer **Table 6**.

Extrapelvic and Deep Infiltrating Endometriosis

Deep infiltrating endometriosis (DIE) involves the utero-sacral ligaments, rectovaginal septum, bowel, ureters, or urinary bladder. GnRH agonists are usually the first-line agents as they suppress ovarian hormone production and inhibit the growth of ectopic endometrial growth.[54]

TABLE 4: Medical treatment options for endometriosis.

Medical therapy[41]	
FDA approved therapies: • Three GnRH agonists: – Leuprolide – Goserelin – Nafarelin • Two progestins: – Depot medroxyprogesterone acetate 150 mg IM every 3 months. This may cause decrease in bone density with long-term use – Norethindrone acetate (oral) is the only oral progestin approved by the FDA. Dose—5 mg/day orally for 2 weeks, then increased by 2.5 mg/day every 2 weeks till 15 mg is reached for total 6–9 months • Danazol: – Antiestrogenic with weak androgen agonistic properties – Causes anovulation and suppression of menses by inhibiting gonadotropins, immunomodulatory action, and inhibition of cell proliferation – Category X drug	*Non-FDA approved therapies:* • Ovulation suppressing agents: – Combined hormonal contraceptives usually recommended as first-line therapy in adolescents with endometriosis and in those without contraindication to hormonal treatment – Progestins: - Oral medroxyprogesterone acetate 20–30 mg/day for 6 months - Dienogest (2 mg/day) – GnRH antagonists: - Cetrorelix acetate 3 mg subcutaneous weekly over a 8 weeks period - Elagolix (oral) • Anti-inflammatory agents: – *NSAIDs:* According to a Cochrane review[42] although NSAIDs are used as a first-line treatment in suspected endometriosis, there is little evidence for significant reduction in pain. No one NSAID is more effective than the other. Along with OCPs, usually given as first-line therapy[43] – *COX-2 inhibitors (Rofecoxib):* Inhibits PG synthesis—withdrawn from US market due to cardiovascular risk – *Peroxisome proliferator-activated receptor gamma (PPAR-γ) agonists (rosiglitazone and pioglitazone)* – *Pentoxifylline:* Not commonly used – *Antioxidants:* Role is speculative • Agents acting on endometriotic deposits directly: – Aromatase inhibitors (inhibition of estrogen formation in ovarian granulosa cells and also in endometriotic deposits) - Letrozole, anastrozole—concern is formation of functional cysts due to superovulation – Levonorgestrel intrauterine device (LNG-IUD) – Progesterone receptor antagonists/selective progesterone receptor modulators - Mifepristone – Selective estrogen receptor modulator (SERM)—raloxifene – Statins–e.g., simvastatin • Immunomodulators—e.g., infliximab, etanercept • Angiogenesis inhibitors—cabergoline, quinagolide • Gestrinone • Valproic acid • Melatonin • Phytoestrogens—isoflavones

(FDA: Food and Drug Administration; GnRH: gonadotropin-releasing hormone; NSAIDs: nonsteroidal anti-inflammatory drugs; OCP: oral contraceptive pills; PG: prostaglandin)

TABLE 5: Dienogest (DNG).

Type	***Fourth generation selective progestin steroid***
Route	Oral
MOA	Anovulation, antiproliferation, and inhibition of cytokine secretion from endometrial stromal cells
Additional effects	Antiandrogenic. Profound local effects on local endometriotic implants with minimal impact on metabolic parameters
Dose	2 mg daily is usually recommended
Comparison with other drugs	• When compared with norethisterone acetate (NETA) at 2.5 mg, DNG at 2 mg gave comparable symptomatic relief and health-related quality of life (QOL).[44] Due to high cost of DNG, it can be given in patients who do not tolerate NETA • In a recent systematic review of eight RCTs, comparing DNG with GnRH agonist which included 1,273 women with symptomatic endometriosis, DNG was superior to placebo but equivalent to GnRH agonists in controlling pain symptom in endometriosis[45]
Pharmacokinetics	Oral absorption rapid with 90% bioavailability, exclusively bound to albumin (90%), t1/2 10 hours, metabolism in liver[46]
Uses	In superficial and deep infiltrating endometriosis with or without visceral involvement
Safety profile	• Side effects though not common are mild to moderate—headache, breast discomfort, depressed mood, acne, nausea, vaginal bleeding • In a pooled analysis from four European RCTs, DNG at 2 mg dose was well tolerated and safe for up to 65 weeks[47]

(GnRH: gonadotropin-releasing hormone; MOA: mechanism of action; RCT: randomized controlled trial)

TABLE 6: Gonadotropin-releasing hormone agonists.

Route	***Intramuscular, subcutaneous or intranasal***	
Drug available	• Leuprolide acetate (parenteral) • Nafarelin acetate (intranasal) • Goserelin acetate (subcutaneous) • Triptorelin	
Manufacturing	Substitution of L-amino acid by D-amino acid at position 6 of the native GnRH, thus making it resistant to degradation and giving a longer half-life	
MOA	Administration of GnRH agonist ↓ Initial pituitary flare (FSH and LH) This may exacerbate endometriosis symptoms. This can be blunted by aromatase inhibitors for first 7–10 days of treatment or giving GnRH agonist in the luteal phase of the cycle[48] ↓ Downregulation of pituitary GnRH receptor ↓ Decrease in FSH and LH ↓ Ovarian suppression → ↓ ↓ E_2 and P. Within 1 month of GnRH use, the E_2 levels will be in the menopausal range	
Effects	Direct effects on endometriotic implants	
Efficacy	Second- or third-line medical treatment after COCs and progestin for endometriosis associated pain. Pain relief is between 50% and 90%. Combined surgical and medical treatment with GnRH agonists have the lowest recurrence rate and highest cure rate[49-51]	
Add back HT	• GnRH agonist therapy can lead to hypoestrogenic side effects like hot flushes, mood swings, vaginal dryness, decreased libido, bone loss, and headache. Therefore, add-back HT is used to treat these side effects and prevent any long-term sequelae. Only progesterone or a combination of estrogen/progesterone may be used. This does not affect the efficacy of GnRH agonist • Most commonly used is NETA 5 mg daily as add-back agent and is approved by the US-FDA • Typically, GnRH agonist is used for 3–6 months and could be extended to 1 year • Add-back therapy should be started along with GnRH-a therapy as this will reduce the vasomotor symptoms and bone density. According to "estrogen threshold hypothesis", E2 concentration of 30–45 pg/mL is required to maintain bone density • Also patients must be instructed to take adequate calcium and vitamin D along with HT • In those who cannot use HT as add-back they may benefit from herbal remedies, selective serotonin reuptake inhibitors (SSRIs), and serotonin/norepinephrine reuptake inhibitors • Alternatively, dose of GnRH agonist may be reduced or interval between doses may be increased[52,53]	
Doses	Leuprolide acetate	3.75 mg once a month or 11.25 mg every 3 months
	Nafarelin acetate	1 spray (200 µg) in the morning and evening. Total 400 µg/day for 6 months
	Goserelin acetate	3.6 mg every 4 weeks for 6 months in ≥18 years women
	Triptorelin	3.75 mg every 4 weeks

(COCs: combined oral contraceptives; E2: estrogen; FDA: Food and Drug Administration; FSH: follicle-stimulating hormone; GnRH: gonadotropin-releasing hormone; HT: hormone therapy; LH: luteinizing hormone; MOA: mechanism of action; NETA: norethisterone acetate)

Surgical Treatment

Surgery may be the first-line management in:[55]

- Highly symptomatic women
- Those with a normal ovarian reserve
- Unilateral and large cysts
- Those suspicious of malignancy.

After an initial surgery for infertility, performing any additional surgery will not increase the fecundability and such patients should be better subjected to assisted reproductive technology (ART).

Combined Medical and Surgical Treatment

Although theoretically beneficial, there is no evidence to support that combined medical and surgical therapy improves fertility. On the contrary, it may unnecessarily delay any further fertility therapy.

Assisted Reproductive Technology

Certain patient profiles may benefit from proceeding directly to IVF which are:

- Asymptomatic women
- Women with advanced reproductive age

- Bilateral endometriomas
- Prior surgical treatment as surgery may have a detrimental effect on the ovarian reserve and delay the initiation of treatment.

Endometriosis and Assisted Reproductive Technology

- There is almost up to 30% reduction in PR with controlled ovarian hyperstimulation (COH)-IUI in minimal/mild endometriosis.
- The GDG recommends ART in women with endometriosis when associated with tubal factor or male factor infertility and/or when other treatments have failed.
- Also, ART can be offered after surgery for endometriosis as controlled ovarian stimulation for IVF/ICSI does not increase the recurrence rate.[56]
- In a Cochrane review by Sallam et al. (2006), administration of GnRH agonist 3–6 months before ART in women with endometriosis increases the odds of clinical pregnancy by more than fourfold.[40]
- According to the new ESHRE 2022 guidelines, the extended administration of GnRH agonist prior to ART treatment to improve live birth rate (LBR) in infertile women with endometriosis (ultralong protocol) is no longer recommended due to unclear benefits.
- The Endometriosis Fertility Index (EFI) was added as a step in the treatment as it can support decision-making for the most appropriate option to achieve pregnancy after surgery.
- It is important to note that in women with endometriosis:
  - The ovarian response to COH is not decreased.
  - Stimulation protocol could be ultralong GnRH agonist or the GnRH antagonist protocol. Frozen embryo transfer may be performed after GnRH agonist depot suppression for 2 months.
  - There is no increase in size or rupture of endometriomas with COH.[57]
  - During oocyte retrieval, if one encounters endometrioma, avoid puncture and aspiration. Antibiotic prophylaxis may be used, but the risk of pelvic infection/abscess is low.[32]
  - There is no evidence to performing surgical excision in cases of deep nodular endometriosis prior to ART to improve PRs. Pain relief may be the only reason for their surgical removal.
  - There is no increase in the recurrence rate of endometriosis with ART.[32]

TREATMENT OF ENDOMETRIOSIS ASSOCIATED INFERTILITY

It is always important to weigh the risks against the benefits of surgery in endometriosis as here, the surgical procedure may neither be able to restore the pelvic anatomy completely nor it may inhibit the inflammatory process.

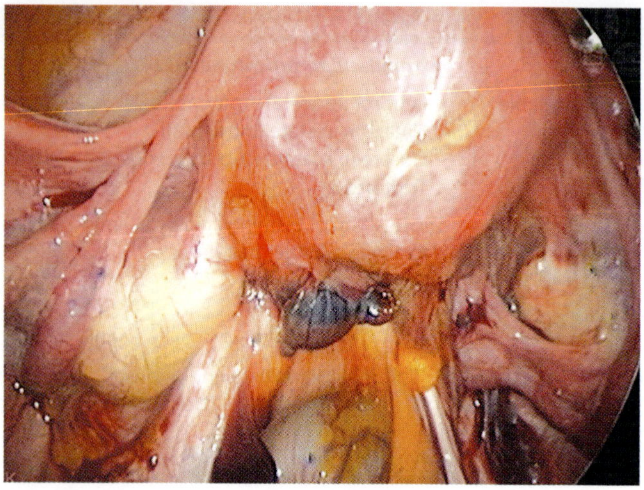

Fig. 5: Adhesions and endometriotic lesions between the bladder and anterior uterine surface.

American Fertility Society/American Society for Reproductive Medicine Stage I/II Endometriosis

In women <35 years of age with stage I/II endometriosis-associated infertility, expectant management or SO-IUI may be considered first-line therapy. In women >35 years, aggressive management like SO-IUI or ART may be considered.[58]

According to the ESHRE guidelines, in order to increase ongoing pregnancy rates (OPRs), one must perform operative laparoscopy [ablation or excision of endometriotic lesions, adhesiolysis rather than just performing diagnostic laparoscopy since there is an increase in LBR **(Fig. 5)** and OPR] [odd ratio (OR) 1.64; 95% confidence interval (CI) = 1.05–2.57].[32,59]

Also, instead of monopolar electrocoagulation, one may use CO_2 laser vaporization of endometriosis as it is associated with increased cumulative spontaneous PRs.[32,60] In minimal/mild endometriosis, COH-IUI increases LBR as compared to expectant management and increases the PR instead of only IUI.

Also, COH-IUI may be performed within 6 months after operative laparoscopy as PRs will be similar to that achieved in unexplained infertility.[32,61]

American Fertility Society/American Society for Reproductive Medicine Stage III/IV Endometriosis

There are no randomized controlled trials (RCTs) or meta-analysis to compare PRs after surgery and after expectant management in women with moderate to severe endometriosis. According to the ESHRE guidelines, it is a level B recommendation to consider operative laparoscopy rather than expectant management to increase spontaneous PRs.[32,62]

Women with stage III/IV endometriosis who do not conceive after conservative surgery or of advanced reproductive age must proceed with IVF/ICSI.[58]

Prognostic Tool for Pregnancy

The EFI was developed as a tool to predict PRs in patients with surgically documented endometriosis who attempt non-IVF conception **(Fig. 6)**.[63]

ENDOMETRIOSIS FERTILITY INDEX (EFI) SURGERY FORM

LEAST FUNCTION (LF) SCORE AT CONCLUSION OF SURGERY

Score	Description		Left		Right		
4	= Normal	Fallopian tube	☐		☐		
3	= Mild dysfunction						
2	= Moderate dysfunction	Fimbria	☐		☐		
1	= Severe dysfunction						
0	= Absent or nonfunctional	Ovary	☐		☐		
To calculate the LF score, add together the lowest score for the left side and the lowest score for the right side. If an ovary is absent on one side, the LF score is obtained by doubling the lowest score on the side with the ovary		Lowest score	☐	+	☐	=	☐
			Left		Right		LF Score

ENDOMETRIOSIS FERTILITY INDEX (EFI)

Historical factors			Surgical factors		
Factor	**Description**	**Points**	**Factor**	**Description**	**Points**
Age			LF Score	☐	
	If age is ≤35 years	2		If LF score = 7 to 8 (high score)	3
	If age is 36 to 39 years	1		If LF score = 4 to 6 (moderate score)	2
	If age is ≥40 years	0		If LF score = 1 to 3 (low score)	0
Years infertile			AFS Endometriosis score		
	If years infertile is ≤3	2		If AFS endometriosis lesion score is <16	1
	If years infertile is >3	0		If AFS endometriosis lesion score is ≥16	0
Prior pregnancy			AFS Total score		
	If there is a history of a prior pregnancy	1		If AFS total score is <71	1
	If there is no history of prior pregnancy	0		If AFS total score is ≥71	0
Total historical factors		☐	**Total surgical factors**		☐

EFI = Total historical factors + total surgical factors:	☐	+	☐	=	☐
	Historical		Surgical		EFI score

ESTIMATED PERCENT PREGNANT BY EFI SCORE

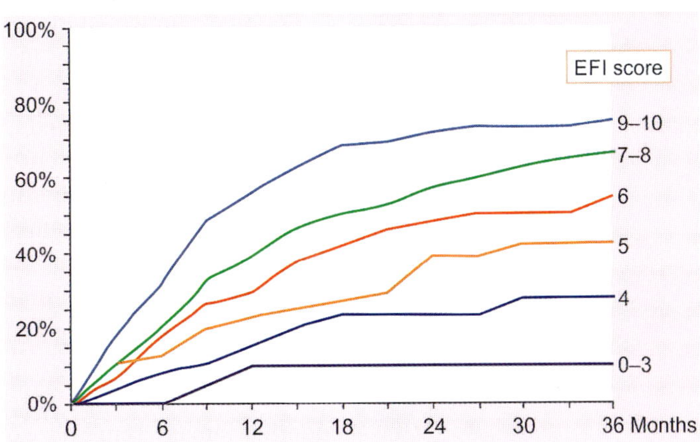

Fig. 6: Endometriosis fertility index.
Source: AFS—American Fertility Society

OVARIAN ENDOMETRIOMA[64,65]

Endometrioma is a pseudocyst originating from the ectopic endometrial tissue in the ovary and progresses by invaginating into the ovarian cortex.[66] It may be symptomatic or asymptomatic and is found in 17–44% of women with endometriosis. It can be diagnosed reliably by transvaginal USG **(Fig. 7)**.

Current medical treatment does not resolve an endometrioma. Also, surgical removal will diminish the ovarian reserve which has been seen in a systematic review.[67]

Risks and Benefits of Surgical Therapy of Endometrioma versus Expectant Management

Surgery[32]

Advantages:
- Facilitates access to oocyte retrieval
- Symptom relief
- Rules out malignancy
- Minimizes risk of cyst complications.

Disadvantages:
- Reduction of ovarian reserve and chances of ovarian failure as in 13% patients, normal tissue may be destroyed[68]
- Increased gonadotropin requirement
- Surgical risks
- Postoperative adhesions
- Recurrence.

Expectant Management

Advantages:
- No surgical risk
- Increased oocyte retrieval
- Ovarian reserve maintained
- May require comparatively lower dose of gonadotropins
- No delay in starting ART.

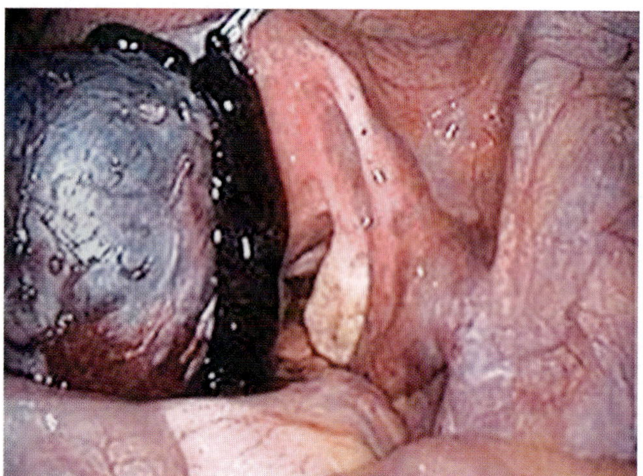

Fig. 7: An endometriotic cyst in the right ovary with drainage of chocolate-colored endometriotic fluid.

Disadvantages:
- Pain
- Small chance of pelvic infection following oocyte retrieval
- No tissue available for histopathological diagnosis
- Cyst rupture
- Difficulties in accessing the ovaries at the time of oocyte retrieval
- Contamination of FF
- Accelerated progression of the disease.

In a systematic review by Laursen et al.[69] where surgery versus conservative management of endometriomas in subfertile women was studied, very low quality evidence suggested no difference in the odds ratio of live birth between women who underwent surgery for endometriomas before IVF/ICSI compared with conservative management. They recommended to consider conservative treatment if subfertility was the only indication.

Brief surgical steps are as follows:
- Proper inspection of pelvis and upper abdomen
- Three laparoscopic working ports
- Peritoneal washings only in case of suspicious lesion or ascites
- Adhesiolysis after careful identification of ureter to prevent its damage
- A combined technique of both excision and ablation may be used to prevent ovarian tissue removal and bleeding.

Excision involves opening the endometriotic cyst with either scissors, electrosurgical, or laser. The cyst is opened and drained. The plane of cleavage between the cyst wall and ovarian tissue is then identified. Then the cyst wall is excised or stripped away by applying traction and counter traction with two grasping forceps. The edges may be sutured with suture ends being placed inside or inverted by minimal bipolar coagulation.[70]

A study by Donnez et al.[71] showed that combined technique of excision and laser ablation without suture is good for preserving ovarian reserve.

Endometrioma treated surgically have a high recurrence rate and using this option for women undergoing IVF has been challenged.[72] It has been reported that due to the technical difficulty involved in removal of endometriomas as they are usually adherent to the normal ovarian tissue, tissue rim containing primordial follicles is removed in >50% endometriomas.[73] This results in diminished ovarian reserve after its surgical removal.

The ESHRE guidelines state that there is no evidence that cystectomy before starting ART has any improvement in the PR.[32,74]

The GDG recommends cystectomy before ART or endometriomas >3 cm in size only to improve endometriosis associated pain and improving accessibility to the follicles for oocyte retrieval.

Also, the clinician must counsel the woman adequately about the risk of premature ovarian failure and the possible risk of loss of ovary after surgery. A cautioned decision must be taken if a woman has any previous ovarian surgery.

In a systematic review and meta-analysis which included 33 studies, women with an endometrioma undergoing IVF/ICSI had a similar LBR (OR 0.98; 95% CI = 0.71, 1.36) and a similar CPR (OR 1.17; 95% CI = 0.87, 1.58) but a higher cancellation rate compared to those without the disease. Surgical treatment of endometrioma did not affect the outcome of IVF/ICSI as compared to those without surgical management.[75]

Also a systematic review and meta-analysis by Tsoumpou et al.[65] concluded that surgical treatment of endometriomas did not have any significant effect on IVF PRs and also no effect on response to ovarian stimulation compared to expectant management.

Recurrent Disease

- In order for the treatment to be successful in curbing endometriosis, it must target to suppress endogenous estrogen synthesis which propagates endometriosis.[76]
- Rx → Suppression of ovulation

↓

Amenorrhea

↓

Hypoestrogenic environment

↓

Inhibition of ectopic endometrial growth

↓

Thus preventing disease progression.

- Hormone therapy acts by the above mechanism. Once hormone therapy is stopped there will be recurrence of symptoms due to growth of endometrial implants.
- The recurrence rate of endometriosis after medical or surgical therapy is up to 45% after 5 years, the rate reaching up to 56% in women <21 years.[77]
- Therefore, long-term therapy may be needed for this, frequently used are dienogest (DNG) and GnRH agonist with add back therapy.

ADOLESCENT ENDOMETRIOSIS

Early-onset endometriosis (EOE) starting around menarche or early adolescence may at times be severe, requiring early diagnosis, and proper treatment. Its origin may be different from its adult variant and is attributed to the neonatal uterine bleeding (NUB).[78]

Pathogenesis

Origin of Early-onset Endometriosis

In a small proportion of neonates

↓

Progesterone withdrawal bleeding occurs

↓

Secondary to the NUB is the reflux and seeding of endometrial stem and progenitor cells in the pelvic cavity. In a neonate, they quickly attach themselves to the peritoneum.[79]

↓

These may remain dormant for years and may get activated around the time of thelarche by factors known to develop endometriosis.

↓

This may then progress to highly angiogenic implants, recurrent ectopic bleeding, and endometrioma formation.

The above hypothesis provides explanation for the occurrence of endometriosis in the premenarcheal girl and severe endometriosis like ovarian endometrioma in an adolescent.

Clinical Features

The diagnosis in adolescents is usually delayed due to the nonspecific nature of symptoms, failure to give importance to these symptoms, and reluctance on the part of the clinician to subject an adolescent for invasive testing like laparoscopy. In adolescents, dysmenorrhea is a serious problem. An adolescent may present with severe primary dysmenorrhea usually resistant to NSAIDs and hormonal contraceptive pill. The younger the girls present at the time of diagnosis, more severe is the disease. It has been estimated that endometriosis or uterine anomalies may be seen in 10% adolescents with severe dysmenorrhea.[80] Symptoms include dysmenorrhea (most common), menorrhagia, abnormal or irregular uterine bleeding, and gastrointestinal and genitourinary symptoms.

Five practical ways to an early diagnosis in adolescents was suggested by Zannoni et al.,[81] which are as follows:

1. The pain should never be underestimated.
2. Endometriosis must always be considered as a possible cause of severe cyclical pain.
3. Detailed history must be obtained before performing clinical evaluation of USG.
4. Pain must be treated with hormonal therapies (combined oral contraceptive or progesterone-only pill) and analgesics (acetaminophen and NSAIDs).
5. Frequent follow-up visits must be planned for evaluating the patient.

Treatment

Medical/Surgical

Medical treatment: Same drugs are used in both adults and adolescents. Drugs commonly used are NSAIDs, combined estrogen-progesterone oral contraceptive pill, progesterone-only tablet [norethisterone acetate 15 mg/day

TABLE 7: Stepwise approach in managing adolescent endometriosis.

History ↓	• History of neonatal uterine bleeding • Maternal history of uteroplacental ischemia • Onset of menarche • Cycle length • Uterine anomaly

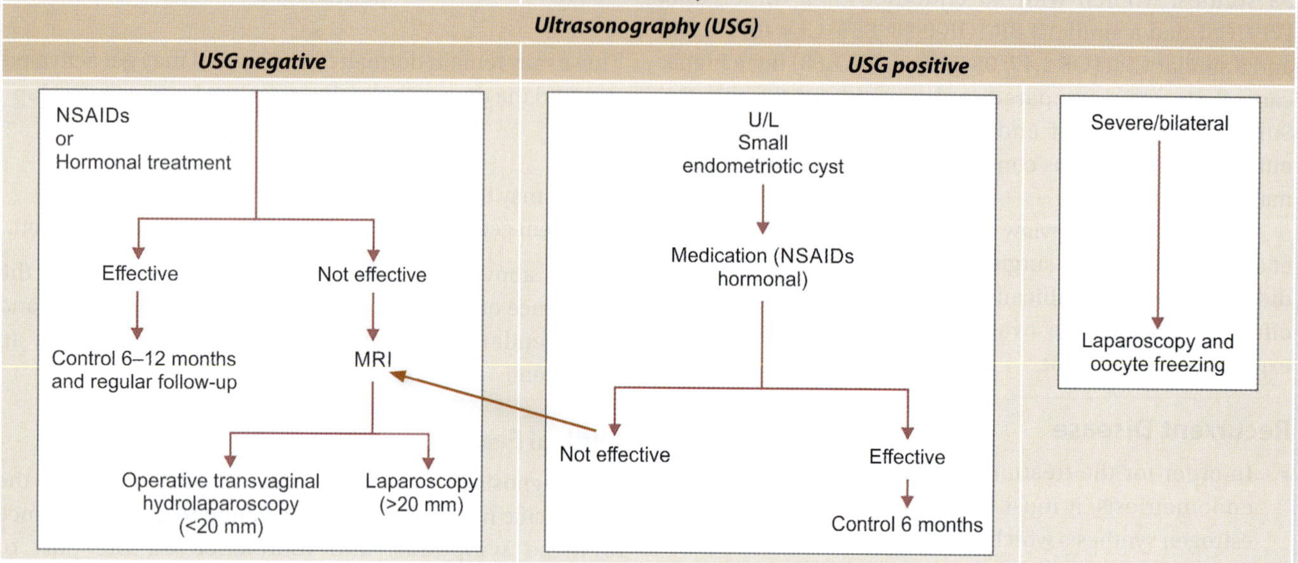

(NSAIDs: nonsteroidal anti-inflammatory drugs; MRI: magnetic resonance imaging; U/L: unilateral)

or medroxyprogesterone acetate (MPA) 50 mg/day] or MPA depot 150 mg intramuscular (IM) 3 monthly. Recent introduction of tablet DNG 2 mg/day in women >18 years is also a good option.82 GnRH agonists with add-back therapy to overcome hypoestrogenic side effects may also be considered.

If an adolescent's dysmenorrhea does not improve within 6 months of treatment with NSAIDs and oral contraceptive pill, laparoscopy is indicated to look for endometriosis.[83]

Surgical treatment: Surgical therapy in adolescents is like a double-edged sword. It may not only increase the risk of premature ovarian failure, but it itself may promote the development of endometriosis.84 Therefore, medical therapy forms a first-line therapy thus holding a special importance in treating adolescents.

Stepwise approach in managing adolescent endometriosis has been proposed, which is shown in **Table 7**.[78]

What is of paramount importance in adolescents is early diagnosis as endometriosis in these young women has a tendency to progress, endangering their reproductive potential.

ENDOMETRIOSIS AND CANCER

The ESHRE 2022 guidelines recommend that clinicians should inform women with endometriosis requesting information on their risk of developing cancer that endometriosis is not associated with a significantly higher risk of cancer overall.[85] Although endometriosis is associated with a higher risk of ovarian, breast, and thyroid cancers in particular, the increase in absolute risk compared with women in the general population is low.

In a systematic review by Kvaskoff et al., 2020, it was seen that the risk of ovarian cancer is 1.2% higher in women with endometriosis compared to all women and the risk of breast cancer and thyroid cancer by 0.5%.[86]

KEY POINTS

- Endometriosis is quite a common disease in women with infertility.
- Early diagnosis and appropriate management is crucial in managing early-onset endometriosis.
- One must consider the diagnosis of endometriosis even when the clinical examination is normal in the presence of symptoms.
- An adnexal mass with diffuse low-level internal echoes and absence of neoplastic features is highly suggestive of an endometrioma.
- While formulating a treatment plan for a particular patient, all factors like age, duration of infertility, symptoms, and stage of endometriosis must be considered.
- In infertile women having endometriosis, hormonal treatment like contraceptives, progestins, GnRH analogs, or danazol for suppressing ovarian function must not be prescribed to improve fertility.

- In minimal/mild endometriosis, medical management does not improve spontaneous PRs, but surgery is beneficial.
- The presence of an endometrioma does not appear to adversely affect IVF outcomes, and their surgical excision does not appear to improve IVF outcomes.
- There is no evidence that endometriosis causes cancer, nor there is an overall increase, but in these women incidence of some cancers like that of ovary and non-Hodgkin's lymphoma is slightly more.
- As compared to no management, ART improves the PRs.
- Women with endometriosis may benefit from a combination of medical, surgical, and ART therapy. Individualization of care is important.

REFERENCES

1. Hudelist G, Fritzer N, Thomas A, Niehues C, Oppelt P, Haas D, et al. Diagnostic delay for endometriosis in Austria and Germany: causes and possible consequences. Hum Reprod. 2012;27(12):3412-6.
2. Giudice LC, Kao L. Endometriosis. Lancet. 2004;364:1789-99.
3. Ilangavan K, Kalu E. High prevalence of endometriosis in infertile women with normal ovulation and normospermic partners. Fertil Steril. 2010;93(3):e10.
4. Guo SW, Wang Y. The prevalence of endometriosis in women with chronic pelvic pain. Gynecol Obstet Invest. 2006;62(3):121-30.
5. Burney RO, Giudice LC. Pathogenesis and pathophysiology of endometriosis. Fertil Steril. 2012;98(3):511-9.
6. Batt RE, Martin DC, Odunsi K. Endometriosis of the retrocervical septum is proposed to replace the anatomically incorrect term endometriosis of the rectovaginal septum. Hum Reprod. 2014;29(12):2603-5.
7. Strzempko Butt F, Chesla C. Relational patterns of couples living with chronic pelvic pain from endometriosis. Qual Health Res. 2007;17(5):571-85.
8. Guzick DS, Silliman NP, Adamson GD, Buttram Jr VC, Canis M, Malinak LR, et al. Prediction of pregnancy in infertile women based on the American Society for Reproductive Medicine's revised classification of endometriosis. Fertil Steril. 1997;67(5):822-9.
9. Sampson JA. Peritoneal endometriosis due to the menstrual dissemination of endometrial tissue into the peritoneal cavity. Am J Obstet Gynecol. 1927;14:422-69.
10. Bulun SE. Endometriosis. N Engl J Med. 2009;360(3): 268-79.
11. Khan KN, Fujishita A, Hiraki K, Kitajima M, Nakashima M, Fushiki F, et al. Bacterial contamination hypothesis: a new concept in endometriosis. Reprod Med Biol. 2018;17(2):125-33.
12. Lucena E, Cubillos J. Immune abnormalities in endometriosis compromising fertility in IVF-ET patients. J Reprod Med. 1999;44(5):458-64.
13. Yoshida S, Harada T, Iwabe T, Taniguchi F, Mitsunari M, Yamauchi M, et al. A combination of interleukin-6 and its soluble receptor impairs sperm motility: implications in infertility associated with endometriosis. Hum Reprod. 2004;19(8):1821-5.
14. Pellicer A, Albert C, Garrido N, Navarro J, Remohi J, Simon C. The pathophysiology of endometriosis-associated infertility: follicular environment and embryo quality. J Reprod Fertil Suppl. 2000;55:109-19.
15. Ota H, Igarashi S, Tanaka T. Xanthine oxidase in eutopic and ectopic endometrium in endometriosis and adenomyosis. Fertil Steril. 2001;75(4):785-90.
16. Agarwal A, Gupta S, Sikka S. The role of free radicals and antioxidants in reproduction. Curr Opin Obstet Gynecol. 2006;18(3):325-32.
17. Gupta S, Agarwal A, Krajcir N, Alvarez JG. Role of oxidative stress in endometriosis. Reprod Biomed Online. 2006;13(1):126-34.
18. Mansour G, Goldberg J, Agarwal A, Bareh G, Sharma RK, Falcone T. Correlation between sperm DNA damage, stage of endometriosis and the duration of infertility (ASRM 63rd annual meeting). Fertil Steril. 2007;90:247-57.
19. Chung HT, Pae HO, Choi BM, Billiar TR, Kim YM. Nitric oxide as a bioregulator of apoptosis. Biochem Biophys Res Commun. 2001;282(5):1075-9.
20. Khorram O, Lessey BA. Alterations in expression of endometrial endothelial nitric oxide synthase and alpha(v) beta(3) integrin in women with endometriosis. Fertil Steril. 2002;78(4):860-4.
21. Baker MA, Aitken RJ. The importance of redox regulated pathways in sperm cell biology. Mol Cell Endocrinol. 2004;216(1-2):47-54.
22. Reeve L, Lashen H, Pacey AA. Endometriosis affects sperm-endosalpingeal interactions. Hum Reprod. 2005;20(2):448-51.
23. Wardle PG, Mitchell JD, McLaughlin EA, Ray BD, McDermott A, Hull MG. Endometriosis and ovulatory disorder: reduced fertilisation in vitro compared with tubal and unexplained infertility. Lancet. 1985;2(8449):236-9.
24. Trinder J, Cahill DJ. Endometriosis and infertility: the debate continues. Hum Fertil (Camb). 2002;5(1 Suppl):S21-7.
25. Cahill DJ, Wardle PG, Maile LA, Harlow CR, Hull MG. Ovarian dysfunction in endometriosis-associated and unexplained infertility. J Assist Reprod Genet. 1997;14(10):554-7.
26. Qiao J, Yeung WS, Yao YQ, Ho PC. The effects of follicular fluid from patients with different indications for IVF treatment on the binding of human spermatozoa to the zona pellucida. Hum Reprod. 1998;13(1):128-31.
27. Coddington CC, Oehninger S, Cunningham DS, Hansen K, Sueldo CE, Hodgen GD. Peritoneal fluid from patients with endometriosis decreases sperm binding to the zona pellucida in the hemizona assay: a preliminary report. Fertil Steril. 1992;57(4):783-6.
28. Faber BM, Chegini N, Mahony MC, Coddington CC. Macrophage secretory products and sperm zona pellucida binding. Obstet Gynecol. 2001;98(4):668-73.
29. Lessey BA, Castelbaum AJ, Sawin SW, Buck CA, Schinnar R, Strom BL. Aberrant integrin expression in the endometrium of women with endometriosis. J Clin Endocrinol Metab. 1994;79(2):643-9.
30. Creus M, Balasch J, Ordi J, Fabregues F, Quinto L, Vanrell J, et al. Integrin expression in normal and out-of-phase endometria. Hum Reprod. 1998;13(12):3460-8.
31. Brosens I, Brosens JJ, Fusi L, Al-Sabbagh M, Kuroda K, Benagiano G. Risks of adverse pregnancy outcome in endometriosis. Fertil Steril. 2012;98(1):30-5.

32. Dunselman GA, Vermeulen N, Becker C, Calhaz George G, D'Hooghe T, De Bie B, et al. ESHRE guideline: management of women with endometriosis. Hum Reprod. 2014;29(3):400-12.
33. Bazot M, Lafont C, Rouzier R, Darai E, Roseau G, Thomassin-Naggara, et al. Diagnostic accuracy of physical examination, transvaginal sonography, rectal endoscopic sonography, and magnetic resonance imaging to diagnose deep infiltrating endometriosis. Fertil Steril. 2009;92(6):1825-33.
34. Chapron C, Dubuisson JB, Pansini V, Vieira M, Barakat H, Dousset B, et al. Routine clinical examination is not sufficient for diagnosing and locating deeply infiltrating endometriosis. J Am Assoc Gynecol Laparosc. 2002;9(2):115-9.
35. Moore J, Copley S, Morris J, Lindsell D, Golding S, Kennedy S. A systematic review of the accuracy of ultrasound in the diagnosis of endometriosis. Ultrasound Obstet Gynecol. 2002;20(6):630-4.
36. Pascual MA, Guerriero S, Hereter L, Barri-Soldevila P, Ajossa S, Graupera B, et al. Diagnosis of endometriosis of the rectovaginal septum using introital three-dimensional ultrasonography. Fertil Steril. 2010;94(7):2761-5.
37. May KE, Conduit-Hulbert SA, Villar J, Kirtley S, Kennedy SH, Bekker CM. Peripheral biomarkers of endometriosis: a systematic review. Hum Reprod Update. 2010;16(6):651-74.
38. American Society for Reproductive Medicine. Revised American Society for Reproductive Medicine classification of endometriosis: 1996. Fertil Steril. 1997;67(5):817-21.
39. Hughes E, Brown J, Collins JJ, Farquhar C, Fedorkow DM. Ovulation suppression for endometriosis. Cochrane Database Syst Rev. 2007(3):CD000155.
40. Sallam HN, Garcia Velasco JA, Dias S, Arici. Long-term pituitary down-regulation before in vitro fertilization (IVF) for women with endometriosis. Cochrane Database Syst Rev. 2006(1):CD004635.
41. Quaas AM, Weedin EA, Hansen KR. On-label and off-label drug use in the treatment of endometriosis. Fertil Steril. 2015;103(3):612-25.
42. Allen C, Hopewell S, Prentice A, Brown J, Crawford TJ, Hopewell S. Nonsteroidal anti-inflammatory drugs for pain in women with endometriosis. Cochrane Database Syst Rev. 2009;1(2):CD004753.
43. Giudice LC. Clinical practice. Endometriosis. N Engl J Med. 2010;362(25):2389-98.
44. Vercellini P, Bracco B, Mosconi P, Roberto A, Alberico D, Dhouha D, et al. Norethindrone acetate or dienogest for the treatment of symptomatic endometriosis: a before and after study. Fertil Steril. 2016;105(3):734-43.e3.
45. de Paula Andres M, Lopes LA, Baracat EC, Podgaec S. Dienogest in the treatment of endometriosis: systematic review. Arch Gynecol Obstet. 2015;292(3):523-9.
46. Bi-kowska M, Woro NJ. Progestogens in menopausal hormone therapy. Prz Menopauzalny. 2015;14(2):134-43.
47. Strowitzki T, Faustmann T, Gerlinger C, Schumecar U, Ahlers C. Safety and tolerability of dienogest in endometriosis: pooled analysis from the European clinical study program. Int J Womens Health. 2015;7:393-401.
48. Bedaiwy MA, Mousa NA, Casper RF. Aromatase inhibitors prevent the estrogen rise associated with the flare effect of gonadotropins in patients treated with GnRH agonists. Fertil Steril. 2009;91(4 Suppl):1574-7.
49. Alkatout I, Mettler L, Beteta C, Hedderich J, Jonat W, Salmassi A, et al. Combined surgical and hormone therapy for endometriosis is the most effective treatment: prospective, randomized, controlled trial. J Minim Invasive Gynecol. 2013;20:473-81.
50. Song JH, Lu H, Zhang J, Li B. Clinical study on the effectiveness and safety of combined laparoscopy and gonadotropin-releasing hormone agonist in the treatment of endometriosis. Zhonghua Fu Chan Ke Za Zhi. 2013;48(8):584-8.
51. Harada M, Osuga Y, Izumi G, Takamura M, Takemura Y, Tetsuya H, et al. Dienogest, a new conservative strategy for extragenital endometriosis: a pilot study. Gynecol Endocrinol. 2011;27(9):717-20.
52. Uemura T, Shirasu K, Katagiri N, Asukai K, Suzuki T, Suzuki N, et al. Low dose GnRH agonist therapy for the management of endometriosis. J Obstet Gynaecol Res. 1999;25(5):295-301.
53. Kang JL, Wang XX, Nie ML, Huang XH. Efficacy of gonadotropin- releasing hormone agonist and an extended-interval dosing regimen in the treatment of patients with adenomyosis and endometriosis. Gynecol Obstet Invest. 2009;69(2):73-7.
54. Korom S, Canyurt H, Missbach A, Schneiter D, Kurrer MO, Haller U, et al. Catamenial pneumothorax revisited: clinical approach and systematic review of the literature. J Thorac Cardiovasc Surg. 2004;128(4):502-8.
55. Jayaprakasan K, Becker C, Mittal M. The Effect of Surgery for Endometriomas on Fertility. Scientific Impact Paper No. 55. BJOG. 2017;125(6):e19-e28.
56. Benaglia L, Somigliana E, Santi G, Scardueli C, Ragni G, Fedele L. IVF and endometriosis-related symptom progression: insights from a prospective study. Hum Reprod. 2011;26(9):2368-72.
57. Koch J, Rowan K, Rombauts L, Yazdani A, Chapman M, Johnson M. Endometriosis and fertility—a consensus statement from a ACCEPT. Aust N Z J Obstet Gynaecol. 2012;52(6):513-22.
58. The Practice Committee of the American Society for Reproductive Medicine. Endometriosis and infertility: a committee opinion. Fertil Steril. 2012;98(3):591-8.
59. Marcoux S, Maheux R, Berube S. Laparoscopic surgery in infertile women with minimal or mild endometriosis. Canadian collaborative group on endometriosis. N Engl J Med. 1997;337:217-22.
60. Tummon IS, Asher LJ, Martin JS, Tulandi T. Randomized controlled trial of superovulation and insemination for infertility associated with minimal or mild endometriosis. Fertil Steril. 1997;68(1):8-12.
61. Werbrouck E, Spiessens C, Meuleman C, D'Hooghe T. No difference in cycle pregnancy rate and in cumulative live-birth rate between women with surgically treated minimal to mild endometriosis and women with unexplained infertility after controlled ovarian hyperstimulation and intrauterine insemination. Fertil Steril. 2006;86(3):566-71.
62. Adamson GD, Pasta DJ. Endometriosis fertility index: the new, validated endometriosis staging system. Fertil Steril. 2010;94(5):1609-15.
63. Vercellini P, Fedele L, Aimi G, Giorgi OD, Consonni D, Crosignani PG. Reproductive performance, pain recurrence and disease relapse after conservative surgical treatment for endometriosis: the predictive value of the current classification system. Hum Reprod. 2006;21(10):2679-85.

64. Gelbaya TA, Nardo LG. Evidence-based management of endometrioma. Reprod Biomed Online. 2011;23(1):15-24.
65. Tsoumpo I, Kyrgiou M, Gelbaya TA, Nardo LG. The effect of surgical treatment for endometrioma on in vitro fertilization outcomes: a systematic review and meta-analysis. Fertil Steril. 2009;92(1):75-87.
66. Hachisuga T, Kawarabayashi T. Histopathological analysis of laparoscopically treated ovarian endometriotic cysts with special reference to loss of follicles. Hum Reprod. 2002;17(2):432-5.
67. Raffi F, Metwally M, Amer S. The impact of excision of ovarian endometrioma on ovarian reserve: a systematic review and meta-analysis. J Clin Endocrinol Metab. 2012;97(9):3146-54.
68. Almog B, Sheizaf B, Shalom-Paz E, Shehata F, Al-Talib A, Tulandi T. Effects of excision of ovarian endometrioma on the antral follicle count and collected oocytes for in vitro fertilization. Fertil Steril. 2010;94(6):2340-2.
69. Brink Laursen J, Schroll JB, Macklon KT, Rudnicki M. Surgery versus conservative management of endometriomas in subfertile women. A systematic review. Acta Obstet Gynecol Scand. 2017;96(6):727-35.
70. Saridogan E, Becker CM, Feki A, Tanos V, Nisolle M, Hummelshoj L, et al. Recommendations for the surgical treatment of endometriosis—part 1: ovarian endometrioma. Gynecol Surg. 2017;14(1):27.
71. Donnez J, Lousse JC, Jadoul P, Donnez A, Squiflet J. Laparoscopic management of endometriomas using a combined technique of excisional (cystectomy) and ablative surgery. Fertil Steril. 2010;94(1):28-32.
72. Garcia-Velasco JA, Somigliana E, Management of endometriomas in women requiring IVF: to touch or not to touch. Hum Reprod. 2009;24(3):496-501.
73. Muzii L, Bianchi A, Croce C, Manci N, Panici PB. Laparoscopic excision of ovarian cysts: is the stripping technique a tissue-sparing procedure? Fertil Steril. 2002;77(3):609-14.
74. Benschop L, Farquhar C, van der Poel N, Heineman MJ. Interventions for women with endometrioma prior to assisted reproductive technology. Cochrane Database Syst Rev. 2010;(11):CD008571.
75. Hamdan M, Dunselman G, Li TC, Cheong Y. The impact of endometrioma on IVF/ICSI outcomes: a systematic review and meta-analysis. Hum Reprod Update. 2015;21(6):809-25.
76. Barbieri RL. Hormone treatment of endometriosis: the estrogen threshold hypothesis. Am J Obstet Gynecol. 1992;166(2):740-5.
77. Evers J, Dunselman G, Land J, Bouckeart PX. Is there a solution for recurrent endometriosis? Br J Clin Pract Suppl. 1991;72:45-53.
78. Benagiano G, Guo SW, Puttemans P, Gordts S, Brosens I. Progress in the diagnosis and management of adolescent endometriosis: an opinion. Reprod Biomed Online. 2018;36(1):102-44.
79. Arcellana RC, Robinson TW, Tyson RW, McKusick-Kaufman. Syndrome with legal complications of hydrometrocolpos and congenital endometriosis. J Perinatol. 1997;17 (3 Pt 1): 220-3.
80. Harel Z. Dysmenorrhea in adolescents. Ann N Y Acad Sci. 2008;1135:185-95.
81. Zannoni L, Forno SD, Paradisi R, Seracchioli R. Endometriosis in adolescence: practical rules for an earlier diagnosis. Pediatr Ann. 2016;45(9):e332-5.
82. Schindler AE, Henkel A, Moore C, Oettel M. Effect and safety of high-dose dienogest (20 mg/day) in the treatment of women with endometriosis. Arch Gynecol Obstet. 2010;282(5): 507-14.
83. Harel Z. Dysmenorrhea in adolescents and young adults: etiology and management. J Pediatr Adolesc Gynecol. 2006;19:363-71.
84. Zhang C, Yuan X, Zhang Y. The co-expression of GPER and Gankyrin in ovarian endometriosis and its correlation with the rASRM stages. Arch Gynecol Obstet. 2016;293(1): 133-41.
85. ESHRE 2022 Guidelines. https://www.eshre.eu/Guideline/Endometriosis.
86. Kvaskoff M, Mahamat-Saleh Y, Farland LV, Shigesi N, Terry KL, Harris HR, et al. Endometriosis and cancer: a systematic review and meta-analysis. Hum Reprod Update. 2021;27(2): 393-420.

CHAPTER 42

Endoscopy in Infertility

Nutan Jain, Tania G Singh, Vandana Jain, Shayari Jain

INTRODUCTION

Infertility is an emerging problem and affects one in eight patients. These significant proportions of patients tend to have structural or pathological causes. These factors that cause subfertility can be potentially treated by surgery. Data shows that in infertile woman, routine examinations and diagnostic procedures are of less use for the evaluation of pelvic pathology. Exploration of the peritoneal cavity and visualization of genital organs is important to diagnose any of the female pelvic pathologies especially in infertile patients. It also helps to evaluate any pelvic pain of non-specific etiology. Hysteroscopy and laparoscopic surgery have revolutionized gynecological surgery and are considered to be the gold standard in diagnosing tubal pathology and other intra-abdominal causes of infertility. It helps in providing a panoramic and magnified view of the pelvic and abdominal organs. It also gives the opportunity to perform extensive surgery in the same setting. This chapter aims to emphasize the management of infertility by advanced hysterolaparoscopy.

Indications for hysteroscopy-laparoscopy in infertility are manifold:

- Woman aged >25 years, married for 3 years with unprotected coitus
- Unexplained infertility
- Known pelvic factors:
    - Abnormal/suspicious hysterosalpingography (HSG)
    - Blocked tubes
    - Tubo-ovarian adhesions
    - Myoma
    - Endometriosis
    - Polycystic ovarian disease
    - Suspected/known Müllerian anomalies
    - Routinely before in vitro fertilization (IVF).

EQUIPMENT

- Veress needle
- Trocar and cannula
- Endoscope in 5 mm and 10 mm sizes and video camera
- Insufflation system
- Xenon cold light source
- Graspers
- Scissors
- Suction/irrigation system
- Electrosurgical equipment
- Harmonic scalpel
- Forceps
- Needle holder
- Uterine manipulator
- Morcellator
- Loop applicator
- Clip applicator
- Myoma screw
- Port closure needle (**Figs. 1A to D**).

LAPAROSCOPIC SURGERY ON UTERUS MYOMECTOMY

Fibroids are the most common pelvic tumors arising from the uterine smooth muscles. They are benign in nature. 70% of women are at risk of having them by the age of 45 years. However, most of these fibroids are small and do not produce any symptoms. Data analysis shows that they mainly are symptomatic in 25% of white and 50% of black women. Myomas can cause infertility as they lead to distortion of the endometrial cavity, defective implantation, pose a problem in sperm ascent, and embryo transport. They interfere with focal endometrial vascularity and cause endometrial inflammation. According to the statistics, removal of submucosal fibroids improves fertility, but removal of subserosal myomas has no role in improving fertility of the patient.[1] Great uncertainties exist about the relationship between intramural fibroids and fertility.[2] Benecke et al., have suggested that intramural fibroids should be removed, if they are close to the endometrium (<1 cm) and larger than 20 mm.[3] Semm and Mettler introduced laparoscopic myomectomy in 1980 for subserosal fibroids.[4] Minimal

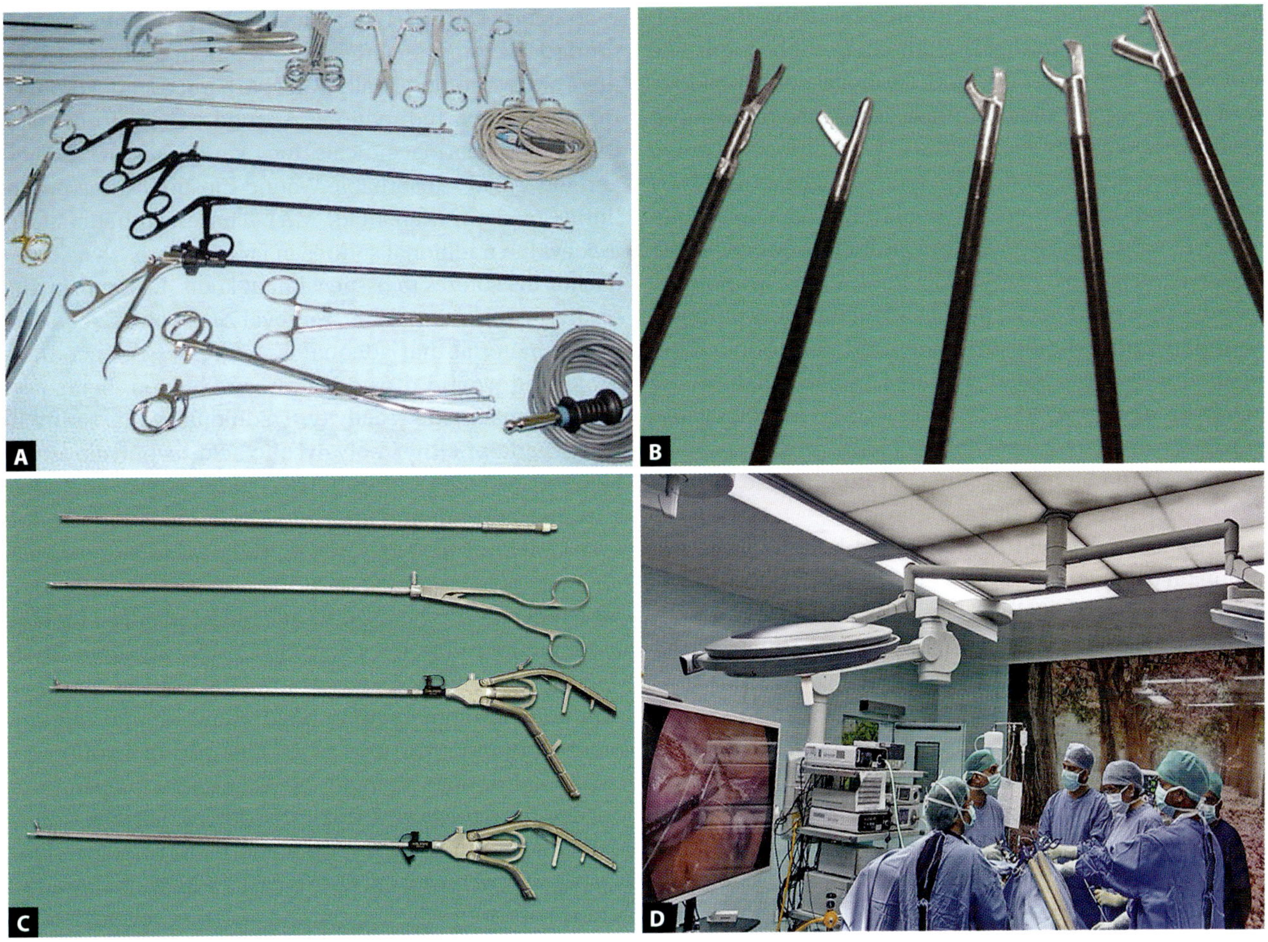

Figs. 1A to D: Basic laparoscopic instruments and setup.

access surgery since then is on a rising trend for treatment of uterine fibroids. The two main challenges associated with laparoscopic myomectomy are:

1. Control of bleeding during enucleation of myoma
2. Good closure technique to reduce postoperative adhesions.

Patient Selection Criteria

According to the old concepts, patient selection was dependent on number, size of myomas, and the uterine size. The limits were three myomas and a diameter of 8 cm or a uterus corresponding in size to 16 weeks gestation and a myoma measuring 12 cm, but now a days patient selection largely depends on the surgical expertise and backup operating staff and team.

Preoperative Use of GnRH Analogs

Preoperative use of gonadotropin-releasing hormone (GnRH) analogs should be avoided:

- delay in the diagnosis of leiomyosarcoma
- increase in hyalinization phenomena
- obliteration of the myoma-myometrium interphase
- difficulty in localizing the cleavage planes
- prolongation of duration of surgery
- increased rate of conversion to open surgery.

Procedure

Laparoscopic myomectomy requires a baseline preoperative evaluation. The patient should undergo routine blood investigations and transvaginal sonography to assess the uterine size. Mapping of fibroids using magnetic resonance imaging (MRI) is also done in order to specify the exact location of each myoma. Laparoscopy is performed under general anesthesia. Nitrous oxide is avoided as it causes bowel distension, which may hamper the operative field. Port placement is done according to surgeon's choice and expertise. After port insertion, the uterus is visualized. On peritoneal entry all pelvic and abdominal structures are inspected and if any pathology presents, it should be noted. Pitressin (8-arginine vasopressin), a derivative of vasopressin, is injected at the concentration of 20 units diluted in 400 mL normal saline between the serosa and pseudo capsule of myoma for hydro dissection and to obtain a bloodless field. Its duration of action is 20–30 minutes and dose can be repeated after 20–25 minutes, if required. It should be metabolized before the end of surgery. It is advisable to always inform the anesthetist before giving Pitressin, since strict vital monitoring is required. Complications like bradycardia, hypertension, and cardiovascular collapse have been reported. Hence, intravascular injection should be avoided and careful monitoring of vitals should be done. If there is persistent hypertension then nitroglycerine (NTG) infusion should be started. Anticholinergic (glycopyrrolate 0.2 mg IV) can be given before induction since it has protective role against bradycardia induced by vasopressin. Diluted NTG is also kept ready at hand for the same purpose. The radial pulse should be monitored continuously by palpation. 15% rise in blood pressure (systolic and diastolic) is tolerable, above this NTG is required. NTG (0.5 mg) when given intravenously causes fall in blood pressure within 2 minutes. If the blood pressure continues to rise, further NTG (0.5 mg) intravenously can be given.

Hysteroscopy should be performed before taking the incision on the myoma.

The harmonic scalpel is used and a transverse incision is given on the prominent part of the fibroid. The incision should not extend to the cornual ends. Transverse incision is preferred as it minimizes cutting of the radial arteries supplying the bulk of the uterus; however, oblique incision can also be given as it is easier to suture an oblique incision. The pseudo capsule and the myoma are separated by sharp dissection (*The Onion-Peel Appearance*) using harmonic scalpel. Application of myoma screw helps in traction and easy removal. Traction and counter traction help in easy enucleation of the myoma from its bed. It is preferred to do minimal bipolar coagulation of myoma bed after enucleation of the fibroid.

Suturing Myoma Bed—the Most Important and Determinant Step

Suturing of the myoma bed is done in multiple layers. The suture used is No. 1-0 vicryl. The taper cut needle is used with the length of the suture being 45–50 cm. The angle knot is taken by passing the suture from the upper and lower edges of the myoma bed, and an intracorporeal, tight, surgeon's knot is secured. From this point, continuous, nonlocking suturing is done, using needle holders in both hands, for a better grip. First, the layer of deep myometrium is completed and the same suture is used to take the second layer of superficial myometrium. The third layer of serosa is taken up using "one and half technique". In one and half technique of suturing innovated by us, a deep stitch is taken including the myometrium and then after going back a superficial stitch is taken in the serosa and no raw surface is left for formation of adhesions. A complete reconstruction is done with a single knot on the myoma bed giving the uterus its original shape. In order to prevent hematoma formation, it is advisable to take adequate tissue in every bite. Each suture should be at an equal distance thereby obliterating the dead space. In recent years, a new class of suture material, barbed suture has been introduced into the surgeon's armamentarium. Currently, there are two commercially available barbed suture products: the Quill™ SRS bidirectional barbed suture product line (Angiotech Pharmaceuticals, Inc., Vancouver, BC, Canada) and the V-Loc™ Absorbable Wound Closure Device product line (Covidien, Mansfield, MA). These synthetic sutures eschew the traditional sutures in favor of barbs that serve to anchor the sutures to tissue without knots. Reapproximation of the myometrium after removal of myomas requires a suture material that adequately addresses the need for a prolonged wound disruptive-force reduction, hemostasis, and minimal tissue reactivity. Traditionally, this suture has been made of either polyglycolic acid or polydioxanone. However, as noted earlier, braided sutures cause more tissue abrasion and inflammation than monofilaments and the transition from open to closed procedures has introduced the difficulty of laparoscopic suturing but when considerations for blood loss and hemostasis are added, the need for faster, more secure suture lines becomes readily apparent. To this end, barbed suture materials are an ideal solution. Their synthetic, monofilament configurations should minimize local inflammation and their absorption profiles and tissue pull-through strengths are well within the parameters needed for reduction of disruptive forces. Further, because barbed sutures allow for only minimal tissue recoiling, closing spaces such as myoma defects is easier with each subsequent suture pass exposed to less tension than the previous bite. The use of barbed suture reduces time of closure and blood loss significantly.[5] One of the serious complications from the use of barbed suture in surgery is bowel obstruction. Kindinger et al., 2012 reported a case of small bowel entanglement and obstruction involving an unraveled V-Loc suture 4 weeks following a laparoscopic myomectomy.[6] This complication could be avoided, if there is no exposure of the "free" barbed suture in the peritoneal cavity either through leaving no redundant suture material by cutting the suture flushed with the myometrium or to use the convention suture for repair of the seromuscular layer of the myometrium. Copious irrigation and lavage are done to obtain hemostasis. In the bag, morcellation is done to remove the myomas. It is important to remove all the myomatous fragments because leaving even a small piece of myoma can lead to the formation of "parasitic or wandering myoma", which can cause intestinal obstruction following formation of adhesions. About 2 L of ringer's lactate are left for hydroflotation. The patient is ambulated about within 6 hours of surgery, allowed orally and can be discharged after 24 hours **(Figs. 2A to H)**.

Jain's Backyard Theory for Broad Ligament and Cervical Fibroids

We have devised a novel way of taking care of the risk of injury to ureters when tackling broad ligament fibroids.

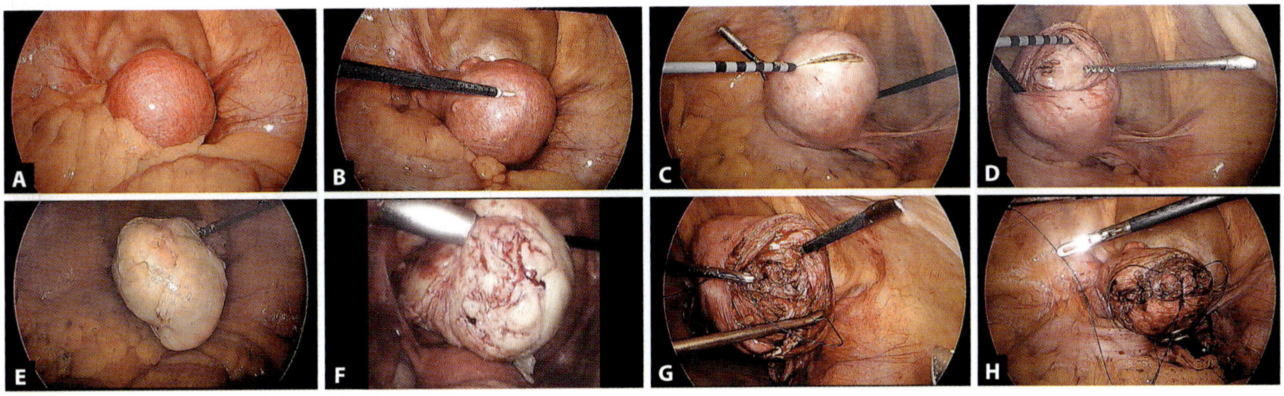

Figs. 2A to H: (A) Initial appearance of fundal myoma; (B) Blanched look of myoma after injecting diluted vasopressin; (C) Transverse incision given over the most bulging part of myoma with harmonic angiotensin-converting enzyme (ACE); (D) Showing onion-peel appearance. (E) Complete enucleation of myoma; (F) Morcellation of myoma (myoma brought close to the sleeve of morcellator); (G) Suturing of myoma and (H) Myoma bed sutured by continuous curve needle suturing.

Keeping in mind the risk of injury to ureter, especially in broad ligament and cervical myomas, we start with using 400 mL of diluted vasopressin to aid in hydrodissection. This helps in reducing the blood loss and getting the correct plane, especially in cases of broad ligament fibroids that attain large sizes. According to our "Backyard Theory", we prefer to give incision on the anterior aspect of the broad ligament myoma and even in posterior myomas, irrespective of its location. In such cases, an assistant pushes the posteriorly bulged myoma anteriorly with the help of a grasper. Myoma becomes prominent anteriorly and incision can be given on anterior aspect and enucleate the myoma with screw or spiral. Our technique has never failed us, thus now adhering to this "Backyard Theory" broad ligament and cervical myomas do not pose any challenges for us. They are taken up easily with a lot of vasopressin and anterior incision keeps ureters and the uterine arteries secured in their location just like we are operating in a living room and the rest of the stuff in the backyard does not bother us. In this endeavor, the myoma is brought out anteriorly and the ureter remains posteriorly and never comes across in field of surgery.

Degenerated Fibroid—A Diagnostic Challenge

Fibroids usually have a characteristic sonographic appearance. Degenerating fibroids can have variable patterns and pose a diagnostic challenge. Uterine leiomyoma with extensive cystic degeneration can masquerade as an ovarian tumor. Degeneration can be fatty, hyaline, calcified, cystic, and red degeneration. Nowadays a new entity has come up in which degeneration is due to medical management of fibroids (ulipristal, mifepristone, and GnRH analogues). Surgical management of these fibroids is a challenge as there is difficulty in finding the plane of cleavage, difficulty in traction making the myoma difficult to be held by a myoma screw or tenaculum. These fibroids are enucleated by using only scissors without using bipolar or harmonic angiotensin-converting enzyme (ACE).

Removal of Myoma

- Motorized (electromechanical) morcellator (Rotocut G1 morcellator, Karl Storz, Germany): Inserted in the abdomen with the help of trocar and cannula, usually via a 15 mm sleeve and in bag morcellation is done. This port site through which the morcellator is introduced requires closure, which is done with a port closure needle. This site also needs rectus sheath closure.
- By posterior colpotomy: A colpotomy incision can be made over, CCL vaginal extractor is placed in the vagina and the myoma can be removed by grasping with a 10 mm claw forceps, which is inserted through it. Incision is then sutured by endosuturing.
- By mini lap incision.

Future Pregnancy Rates

The pregnancy rates are 60–65% with no antepartum or intrapartum complications with multiple layer closure and of which several patients delivered vaginally. It should be mentioned in operation notes, if endometrial cavity has been opened and hence it is better to deliver these patients by cesarean section.

Advantages of Laparoscopic Myomectomy over Open Myomectomy

- Decrease postoperative pain
- Shorter hospital stay
- Early recovery
- Reduced febrile morbidity
- Decreased incidence of postoperative adhesion formation
- Cosmetically better

- Reduced fistula formation ileus, thromboembolic complications.

Rupture Uterus—A Grave Complication

Risk factors for uterine rupture after laparoscopic myomectomy can be:
- Hematoma formation.
- Deformed scar as a result of intraoperative thermal damage.
- Poor healing of wound due to improper approximation of the incision edges.

Risk of uterine rupture can be reduced by taking proper precautions during the surgery like reduced use of thermal devices and closure of myoma bed in multiple layers.

LAPAROSCOPIC TUBAL SURGERY

Surgeries for Tubal Infertility

Disease or damage to fallopian tube accounts for 25–35% of reported cases of infertility. A spectrum of severity of tubal disease exists from peritubal adhesions through damaged fimbriae and distorted anatomy to tubal occlusion, hydrosalpinges, and abnormal tubal mucosa. In tubal infertility, following factors have an important role:
- Role of the tubal mucosa.
- Tubal wall thickness.
- The mobility of the tube and ovary
- Any infective foci

Infections govern the results of tubal surgeries.

Surgery for Proximal Tubal Disease

Proximal tubal blockage accounts for 10–25% of tubal disease. It can be due to:
- Obstruction resulting from plugs of mucus and amorphous debris.
- Spasm of the intratubal ostium.
- Occlusion from fibrosis due to salpingitis isthmica nodosa (SIN), pelvic inflammatory disease (PID), or endometriosis.

A meta-analysis of studies suggests that 85% patients had bilateral proximal tubal occlusion (PTO) and half of the patients conceived after tubal cannulation.[7]

The meta-analysis also concluded that hysteroscopic cannulation has increased the pregnancy rates, although tubal patency rates are similar with fluoroscopic, and hysteroscopic techniques. Patients in which IVF is not advisable and there is failure of tubal cannulation, tubal microsurgery can be considered.

Surgical Approach to Distal Tubal Disease

Tubal repair or salpingectomy is performed based on intraoperative findings. It includes hydrosalpinges and fimbriae phimosis. Hydrosalpinges and fimbriae agglutination due to adhesions result in a narrow-phimotic tubal opening.

Both conditions can be due to:
- PID
- Peritonitis of any cause
- Previous surgery leading to tubal damage.

Good prognosis is associated with patients who have:
- Limited flimsy adnexal adhesions
- Mildly dilated (<3 cm) tubes with thin and pliable walls.
- A lush endosalpinx with preservation of mucosal folds.[8]

Salpingostomy improves the chances of conception in older woman. It is also considered a better option in those suffering from male factor infertility. It improves the success rate of IVF in patients suffering from mild hydrosalpinx. Women with both proximal and distal tube occlusions are generally not advised salpingostomy. Salpingectomy followed by IVF remains the mainstay of treatment for patients with severe hydrosalpinx. Postoperative reocclusions may occur necessitating an additional surgical procedure.

Alternatives include laparoscopic clipping of tubes and hysteroscopic occlusion of ostia; however, best results are achieved with salpingectomy followed by IVF.

Management of Hydrosalpinx

Hydrosalpinges refers to dilatation of fallopian tubes due to prior pelvic infection. According to the consensus the hydrosalpinx fluid reduces the success rate of ART. Hydrosalpinx fluid impairs implantation and decreases the endometrium receptivity. Two meta-analysis[9,10] of these studies noted that the pregnancy and delivery rates were approximately 50% lower and that the spontaneous abortion rate was higher in the presence of hydrosalpinges. The pregnancy rates were higher in patients who underwent laparoscopic salpingectomy before undergoing IVF **(Figs. 3A to D)**. In patients with sonographically diagnosed hydrosalpinges, salpingectomy is preferred to salpingostomy.[11]

Salpingoscopy

Salpingoscopy has become a very useful means of diagnosing diseased fallopian tubes. The mucosa of the ampullary segment, in normal cases, consisted of 3–5 major mucosal folds with secondary folds arising from them along with running vessels and several minor folds interspaced among them. The density of the mucosal folds increases toward the fimbriae end. Salpingoscopic mucosal appearance was graded according to Brosens and Puttemans classification (1989) as follows:
- Grade I: Normal mucosal folds (both major and minor)
- Grade II: The major folds are separated and flattened, but otherwise normal/dye staining of mucosa/minimal flattening
- Grade III: Focal adhesions between mucosal folds and variable flattening

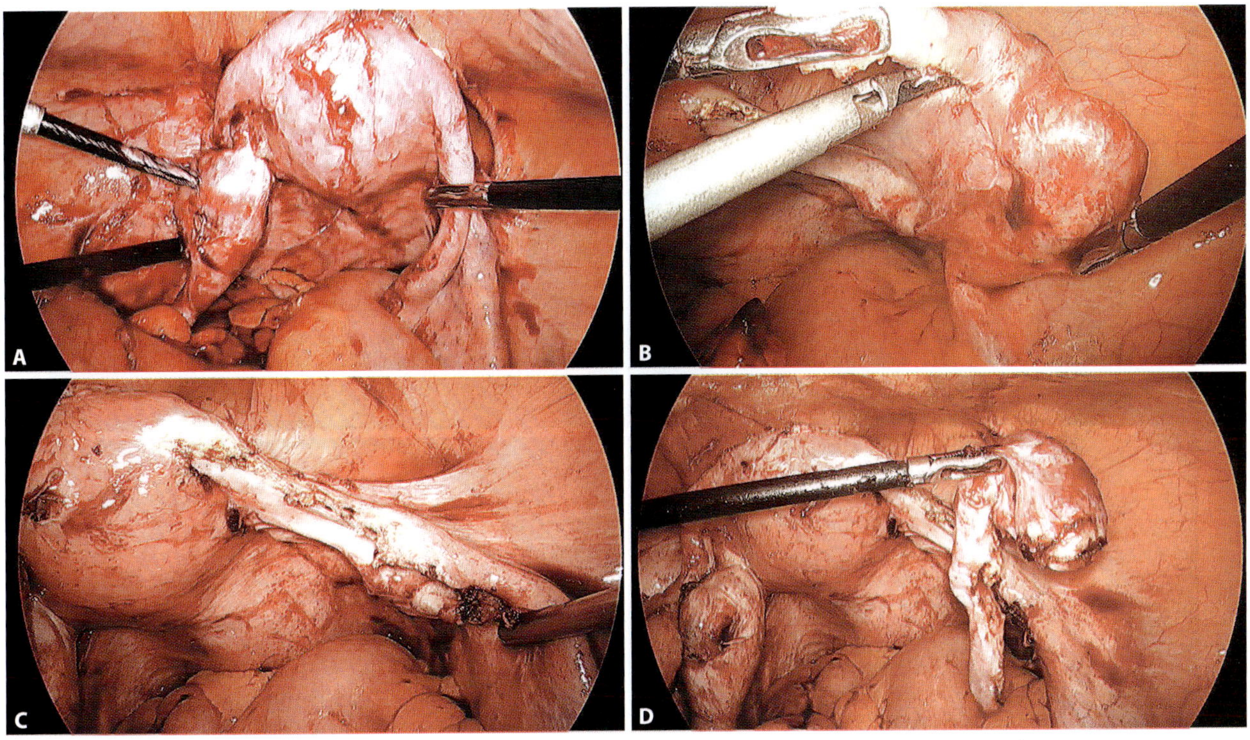

Figs. 3A to D: (A) Bilateral hydrosalpinx; (B) Salpingectomy with use of harmonic; (C) Uterus after salpingectomy; (D) Specimen of hydrosalpinx.

- Grade IV: Extensive adhesions between mucosal folds and disseminated flat areas
- Grade V: Complete loss of mucosal fold pattern.[12]

Nevertheless, salpingoscopy **(Figs. 4A to J)** is not routinely performed during laparoscopy. Salpingoscopy is a tedious process since it requires the use of a second telescope and additional devices. On the contrary, salpingoscopy is commonly practiced while performing fertiloscopy. Fertiloscopy is a simple technique. It requires stabilization of fimbria with grasping forceps introduced in the operative channel. A small telescope is used, which is pushed gently in the fimbria, which then enters the ampulla and reaches the isthmus-ampullary junction. It is important to continuously irrigate the tube throughout the procedure. A tap located on the sheath allows for inflow adjustment. Excessive pressure is avoided in the ampulla. The 30-degree lens enables us to examine each portion of the ampulla just by rotating the telescope on its axis. Any pathology in the ampulla is noted and corrected on a priority basis before performing any assisted reproductive technology (ART) procedure.

Tubotubal Reanastomosis by Laparoscopic Microsurgery

Tubal sterilization is currently the most popular form of birth control in India and is an everyday procedure. It is an important part of our National Family Planning Program. But due to unforeseen reasons, women may seek for reversal of sterilization. Nowadays, laparoscopic microsurgery is considered as the gold standard—derived from solid research and unchallenged dogma. Only surgeons who are very facile with laparoscopic suturing and who have extensive training in conventional tubal microsurgery should attempt this procedure.

Evolution of Microsurgery

Swolin in 1967 introduced microsurgery in the field of infertility for adhesiolysis and neosalpingostomy. After the introduction of microsuturing, the first series of microsurgical reversal of sterilization was published by Winston[13] (1977) and Gomel[14] (1977).

Why laparoscopic surgery and not open microsurgery?

Laparotomy itself exposes to:

- Desiccation
- Foreign body introduction.

In open laparotomy, adhesions and posterior pelvic organ lesions make the access difficult thereby making mobilization of the organs a must. Microsurgery can only be performed after the adnexa is elevated macro surgically.

- Restricted depth of field
- Small field of view
- Less scope of microsurgery via laparotomy in cases of cul-de-sac obliteration and severe pelvic sidewall endometriosis.

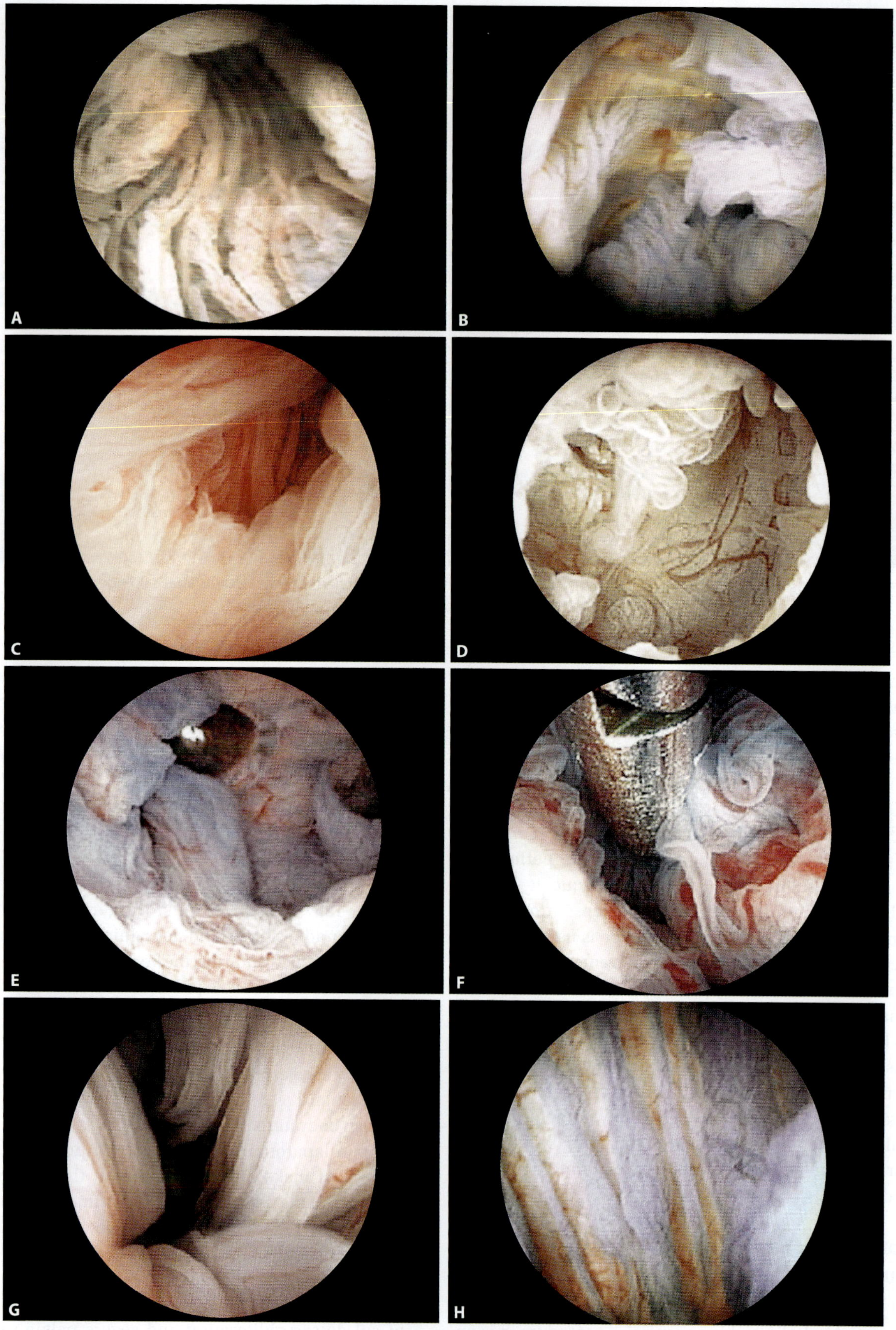

Figs. 4A to H

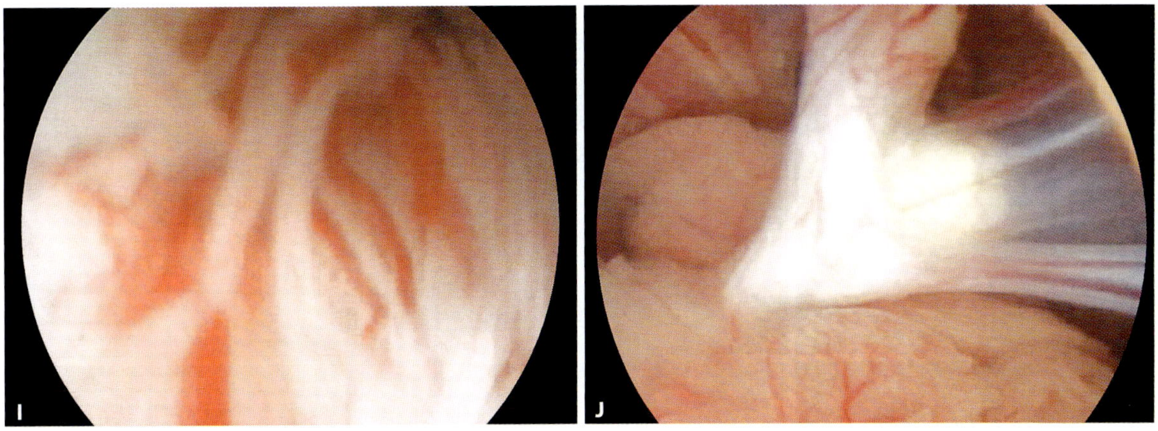

Figs. 4I and J

Figs. 4A to J: (A) Panoramic view; (B) Salpingoscopy; (C) Salpingoscopy (D) Salpingoscopy—flattened folds; (E) Ampulla; (F) Grasping the fimbrial; (G) Major folds; (H) Minor folds; (I) Intra-ampullary adhesions; (J) Intra-fimbrial adhesion.

Source: Watrelot A, Grudzinskas JG. Fertiloscopy. State of the Art Atlas of Endoscopic Surgery in Infertility and Gynecology, 1st edition. New Delhi: Jaypee Brothers Medical Publishers (P) Ltd; 2004. pp. 239-53.

Indications for Laparoscopic Tubal Anastomosis

- Reversal of sterilization
- Mid tubal block secondary to pathology
- Tubal occlusion secondary to ectopic pregnancy treatment
- Salpingitis isthmica nodosa
- Failed tubal cannulation for proximal block
- Failed previous macrosurgical sterilization reversal
- Tubal transposition for unicornuate uterus, discrepant tubo-ovarian anatomy.

Contraindications

- Final tubal length is less than 4 cm
- Significant tubo-ovarian adhesions
- Stage 3–4 endometriosis
- And/or there is more than a mild male factor.

Instruments Used

- Three-chip camera with digital enhancement
- High-resolution monitor
- Ultramicro instruments
- 6-0 vicryl suture and needles.

Procedure

It is done under general anesthesia and requires port placement. Tube on one side is held with atraumatic grasper. Diluted vasopressin is injected in mesosalpinx at the site of previous tubal ligation. With sharp scissors, the proximal and then the distal segments are cut. Scissors are always kept at right angles. Check the patency of both proximal segment (from uterine end) and distal segment (from fimbriae end). Take a bite at 6 O'clock position in proximal segment using 6–0 Vicryl in tubal muscularis and take inside out from 6 O'clock position in distal segment, so that knot is tied later. Take a mesosalpingeal suture beneath it to serve as a base for it, and then tie the knot of muscularis. Tubes come nicely together. Then a second suture is to be taken at 12 O'clock position in distal and then in proximal segment. The 6 O'clock and the 12 O'clock are the key sutures. Next, take two anchoring sutures at 3 O'clock and 9 O'clock positions. Thorough suction, irrigation, and lavage are done. Then take sutures through serosa-to-serosa. Again, check the tubal patency at the end of the procedure. Following points are to be kept in mind **(Figs. 5A to J)**:

- The 6 O'clock suture is tied after suture in mesosalpinx because 6 O'clock segment of the tube is then easily visualized and accuracy of stitch improves a lot.
- Preparation of the distal stump is the most important determinant of success. It is vital to avoid too large aperture.
- With proline, avoid entering the mucosa. With Vicryl, can be entered intraluminally.
- All principles of microsurgery, i.e.:
  - Closed internal environment
  - No tissue drying
  - Minimal tissue handling
  - Magnified vision.

Pregnancy Rates after Tubal Anastomosis

Woman's age plays an important role while considering tubal anastomosis as it is the most important prognostic factor. In women younger than 40 years of age, the cumulative rates of intrauterine pregnancy in 2 years are 70%, compared with more than 90% after microsurgical reversal of tubal sterilization.[15]

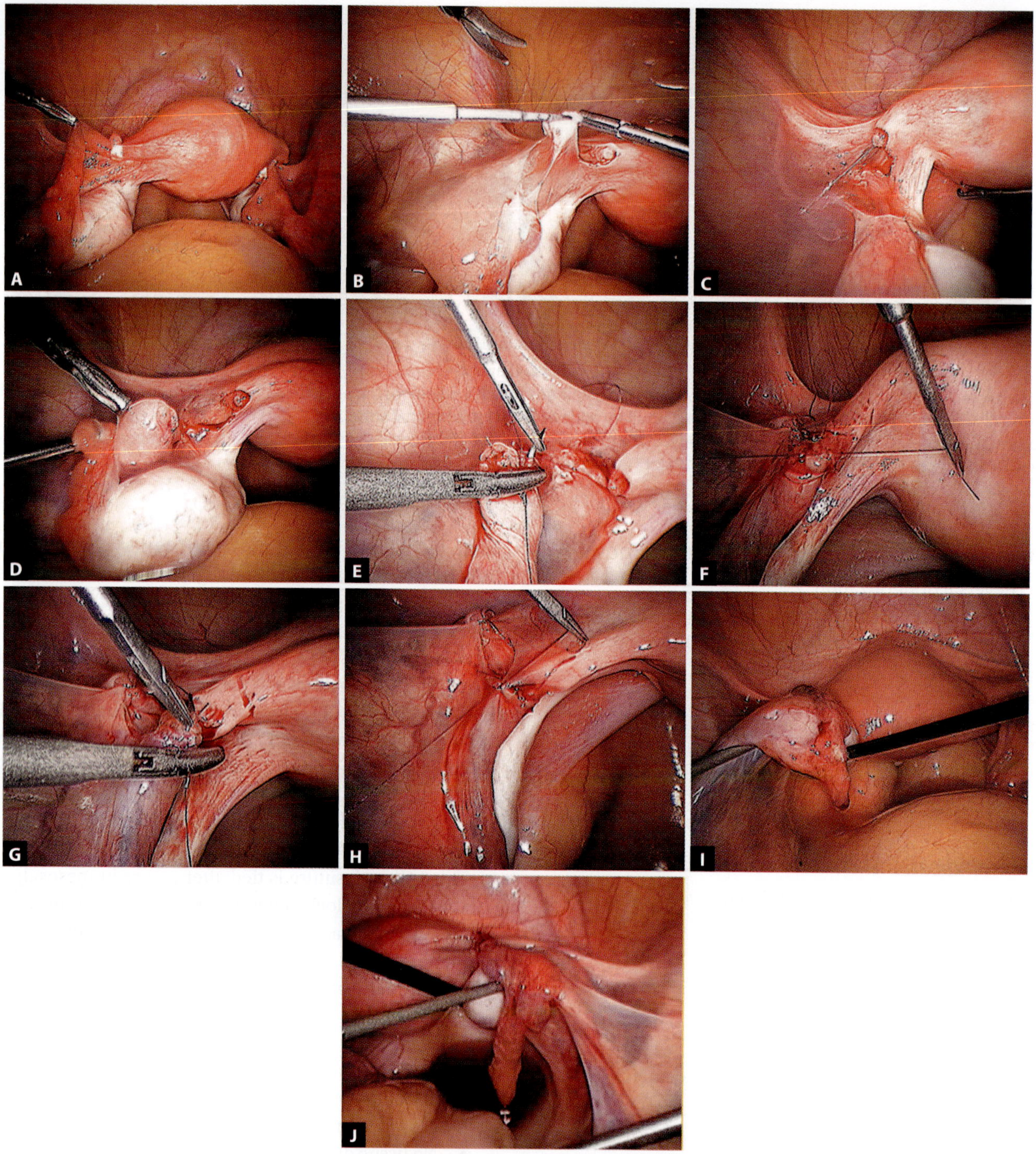

Figs. 5A to J: (A) Bilateral tubes with Falope rings; (B) Cutting and sectioning of Falope ring after injecting diluted vasopressin; (C) Patency of proximal end of tube; (D) Patency of distal end of tube; (E) Needle passed through 6 O'clock position; (F) 6 O'clock suture tied; (G) Passing suture through 12 O'clock position; (H) Serosal suture tied; (I) Left tube-free spill noted after anastomosis; (J) Right tube-free spill noted after anastomosis.

Salpingo-ovariolysis

Tubo-ovarian adhesions are commonly found in isthmic portions of the fallopian tubes. In the ampullary segment the adhesions are dense causing severe fimbriae stenosis.

Procedure

The thumb rule to achieve adhesiolysis **(Figs. 6A to F)** is to start by keeping close to the uterus initially. Adhesiolysis is achieved using scissors, thermal cauterization, or laser. Caution should be taken while dissecting between the ovary

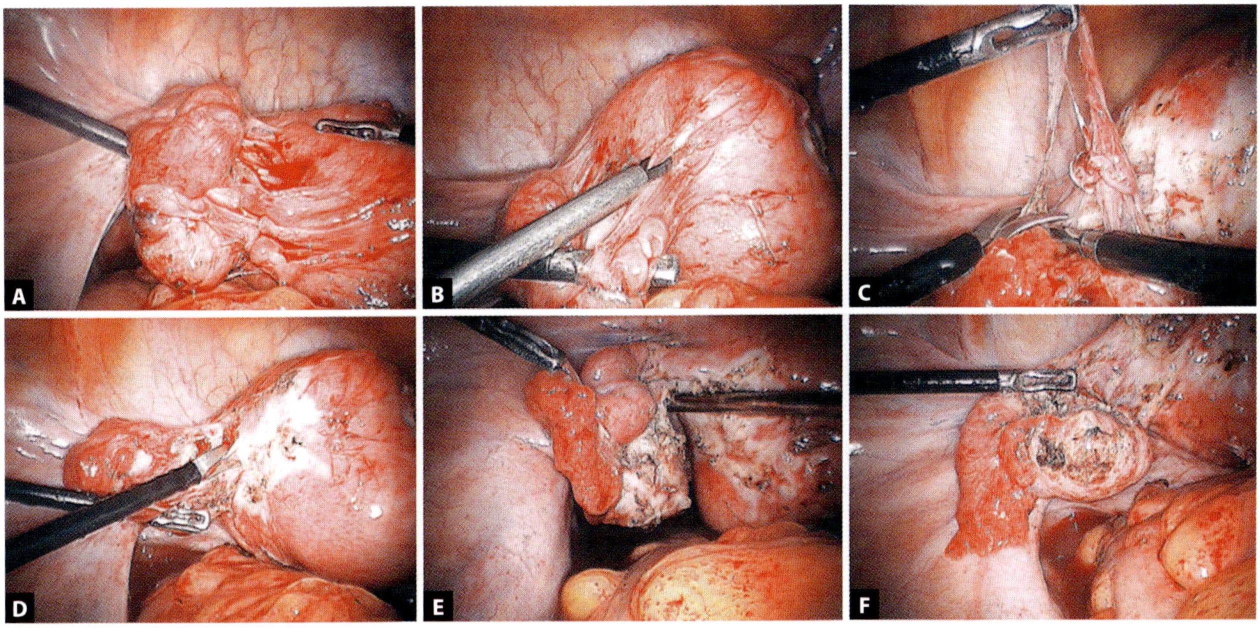

Figs. 6A to F: (A) Dense tubo-ovarian adhesion; (B) Micro-bipolar being used for prophylactic coagulation before sectioning the adhesion; (C) Adhesion put on a stretch and divided; (D) A sharp scissor used for division of adhesion; (E) Normal tubo-ovarian relationships restored with good fimbrial end noted and free spill of dye seen; (F) Normal tubo-ovarian relationship.

and fimbriae.[16] It should be done in continuation with tubo-ovarian adhesiolysis. The cleavage plane is generally easier to find posteriorly. Hemorrhage due to external tubal artery damage is common during adhesiolysis as adhesions can easily be confused with the end of mesosalpinx. Therefore, a neosalpingostomy is mandatory prior to adhesiolysis.

Neosalpingostomy

Neosalpingostomy is a procedure, which involves recreation of new ostia. It is mainly done in cases of hydrosalpinx or complete tubal occlusions with fimbrial adhesions. In cases of mild disease that are characterized by hydrosalpinges having a diameter less than 15 mm with few associated adhesions and recognizable fimbriae, pregnancy rates approach 80%. In contrast, severe disease, characterized by larger hydrosalpinges exceeding 30 mm in diameter with dense adhesions and no visible fimbriae, cumulative pregnancy rates are poor 10–15%. The extent of adhesions, macroscopic appearance of the endosalpingeal mucosa and tubal wall thickness also correlate with operative success.

Procedure (Figs. 7A to F)

After adhesiolysis and freeing of tubes, chromopertubation is done under high pressure to distend the hydrosalpinx. Bruhat's maneuver is carried out.[17] The most important point is to determine the opening point on the former ostium or else the incision should be made at the center of the hydrosalpinx. Periampullary portion of the tube is held with atraumatic forceps and presented to the laparoscopic scissors or CO_2 laser. A pinhole incision is made and enlarged in a star pattern over the four quadrants of hydrosalpinx. The opening is widened by pulling the peritoneum in opposite directions using atraumatic forceps. The avascular zones must be left intact. Microbleeding is managed by bipolar coagulation with continuous irrigation.

Fimbrioplasty

Fimbrioplasty is the procedure that involves reconstruction of fimbriae in a partially or completely occluded oviduct. Periadnexal adhesions are common in such cases and can be managed by doing salpingo-ovariolysis first. Agglutination of the fimbriae leads to stenosis giving a phimotic appearance to the terminal end. Complete occlusion can also occur in cases where the agglutinated fimbrial end gets covered with a fibrous layer. Therefore, the agglutinated fimbria should be completely exposed after excision of this fibrous layer. The excision can be done using laser energy or laparoscopic scissors.

Procedure (Figs. 8A to E)

Fimbrial deagglutination is achieved by using a closed 5 mm-curved atraumatic grasper, which is introduced into the fallopian tube through the phimotic end. The jaws of the grasper are opened within the tube and the forceps withdrawn with the jaws in the open position. This procedure is repeated several times, varying the direction of the jaws, until satisfactory fimbrial deagglutination is obtained. Copious irrigation and lavage are done.

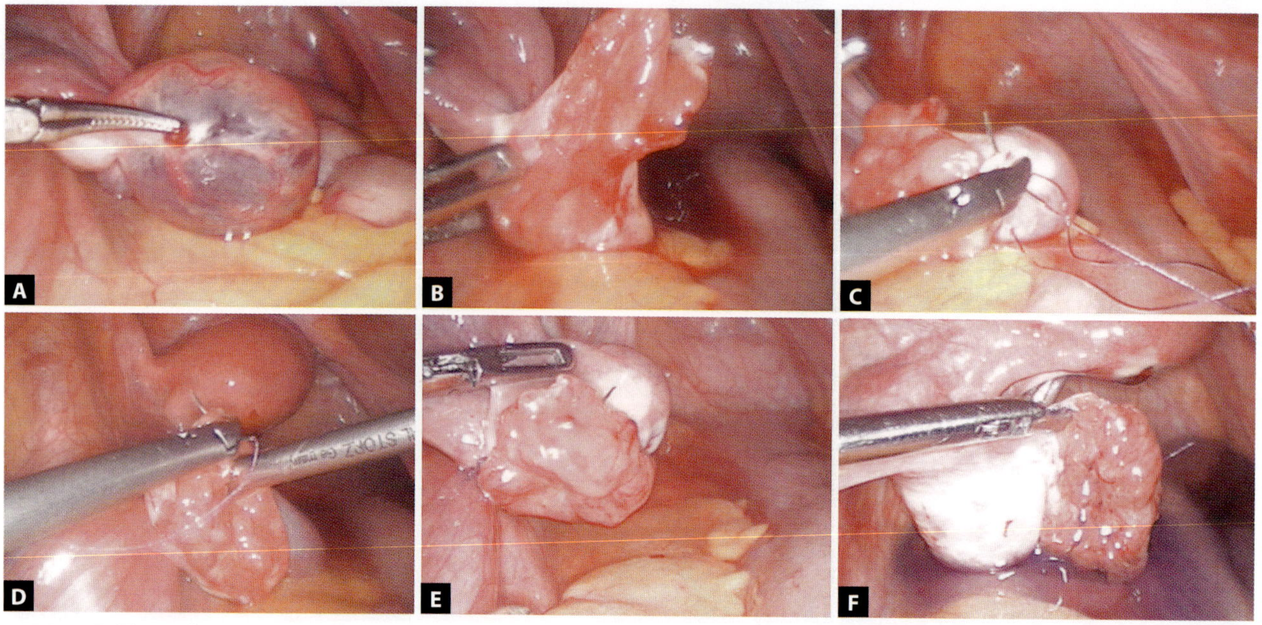

Figs. 7A to F: (A) Initial appearance of hydrosalpinx; (B) Appearance of normal fimbria after cruciate incision; (C) Passing the suture through 12 O'clock position; (D) Passing the suture through fimbria; (E) Final appearance after tubal reconstruction; (F) Chromopertubation at the end of procedure.

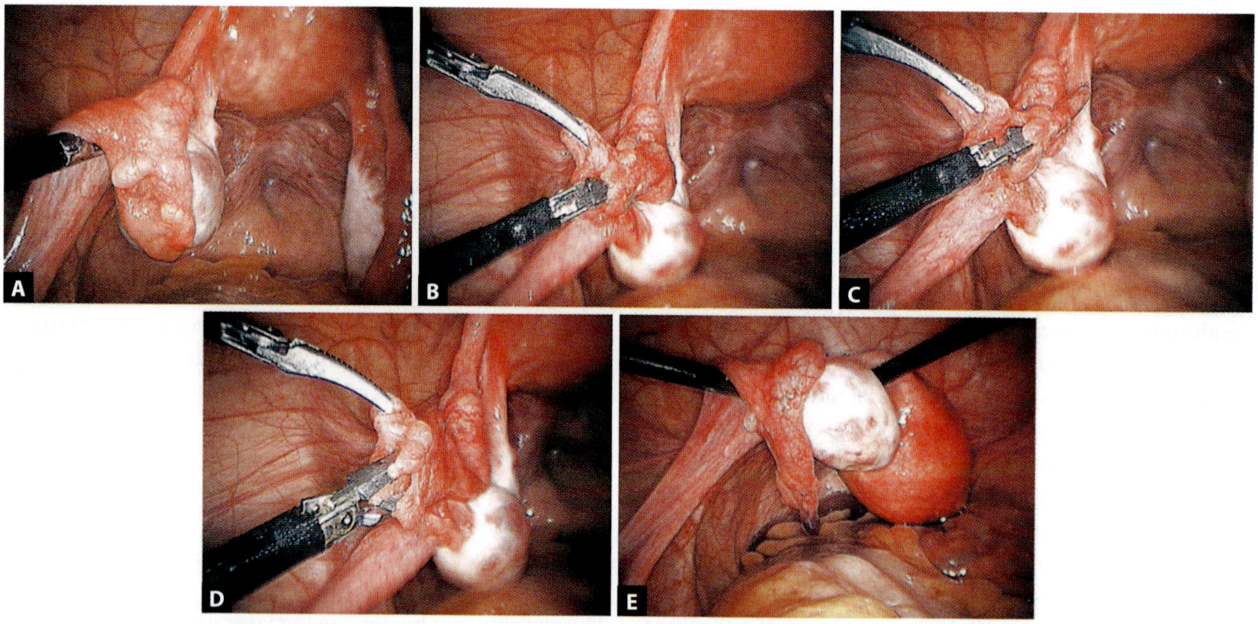

Figs. 8A to E: (A) Tube showing fimbrial agglutination; (B) Introducing a curved atraumatic grasper in the ampullary segment of tube in closed position; (C) Opening the jaws of the atraumatic grasper inside the ampullary end; (D) Taking out the grasper in an open jaw position; (E) Free spill of dye noted at end.

Adhesion Prevention

The chance of moderate and severe adhesion reformation after laparoscopic salpingo-ovariolysis was 40.2%. It has been claimed that second-look laparoscopy with adhesiolysis following pelvic reproductive surgery may increase the intrauterine pregnancy rate and decrease the ectopic pregnancy rate; however, a systematic review of RCTs has failed to show a significant benefit.[18] Various physical barriers like intercede, intergel, fluid barrier-like Adept, have been used and reported by various authors. Studies have also been done to evaluate efficacy of Adept and Ringer's lactate, and found fluid barrier to be more effective due to ease of universal distribution in pelvis and hydroflotation, which keeps various raw surfaces away by fluid interface.

ENDOMETRIOSIS

Endometriosis is a disease characterized by the presence of endometrial tissue outside the uterus. It is a chronic inflammatory condition resulting is formation of adhesions and fibrosis within the pelvis.

It is common among reproductive age women and causes chronic pelvic pain and infertility. According to the American Society for Reproductive Medicine, endometriosis may be found in up to 50% of infertile women. Endometriosis occurs in 6–22% of women of reproductive age undergoing tubal ligation,[19] 15–80% of women with chronic pelvic pain, and 21–65% of women evaluated because of infertility. Fecundity in normal couples is about 15–20% and decreases with age It is about 2–10% in age-matched women with untreated endometriosis and infertility. Pelvic examination may necessarily be normal. Sometimes enlargement of ovaries, mass in the ovary, thickened rectovaginal septum, and a retroverted fixed uterus may be present. Other finding may be indurations in the pouch of Douglas and nodules over uterosacral ligament. Vulval, vaginal, cervical, umbilical, and scar endometriosis are rare findings. Recent data suggests that endometriosis may also be associated with autoimmune disorders like multiple sclerosis, rheumatoid arthritis, hypothyroidism, hyperthyroidism, or systemic lupus erythematosus. Ovarian endometrioma are formed by the invagination of the ovarian cortex, as proposed by Hughesdon. They are usually associated with pelvic pain, infertility, or pelvic mass. Diagnosis can be made with reasonable accuracy by transvaginal sonography. Recently, transrectal sonography with a high frequency transducer has been used with 97% sensitivity for identification of vaginal and rectal wall infiltration. Ovarian endometriomas appear as round, hypoechoic, low level echo cyst with or without internal septa, or thin internal trabeculations with no or poor vascularization of the capsule and septa and bilateral endometrioma usually associated with adenomyoma. It has been reported that almost all patients with ovarian endometriomas have some amount of pelvic or intestinal endometriosis. By and large, laparoscopy has become the gold standard for diagnosis and treatment of endometriosis.

Management of Endometriomas

As in all laparoscopic procedures, first pneumoperitoneum is created using veress needle and then ports are made. Then size of the cyst, adhesions, if present, tubo-ovarian relationship, condition of contralateral tube and ovary, presence of peritoneal endometriosis, and implants and obliteration of pouch of Douglas are noted. Adhesiolysis is done by sharp dissection and ovary is freed from bowel and other surfaces like uterosacral ligament and rectosigmoid. In case of large cyst trocar and cannula are directly introduced in the intact cyst and all chocolate material is sucked out, which prevents peritoneal spillage of large quantities of chocolate material. Most of the cysts drain during antegrade adhesiolysis from the point of adherence, which is the weakest point and here ovarian cortex invagination has occurred in the process of forming an endometrioma. Thorough irrigation of the inside of the cyst is done and the cyst lining is inspected closely. To delineate the cleavage plane between the cyst lining and the outer ovarian cortex, the edge of the cyst is held with two graspers and a fresh cut is given with sharp cutting scissors. The cyst wall is held with a toothed grasper and ovarian cortex with an atraumatic grasper and by using the principle of traction-countertraction the cyst wall is stripped off from the ovarian cortex. Ease of enucleation and lack of bleeding confirm a good cleavage plane. Another way of finding a good plane of cleavage is use of diluted vasopressin (20 units diluted in 400 mL of normal saline), which is injected from inside the cyst wall into the space between the cyst wall and the cortex with an aspiration needle to achieve hydrodissection. When the injection is made into an appropriate layer, ballooning is visualized because of the hydrodissection effect. This also avoids damage to ovarian follicles and minimizes recurrence of endometriomas. Hemostasis is achieved using bipolar cautery, keeping it at minimum setting. Enucleated cyst lining is removed through a 10-mm port making cuts with sharp scissors at various segments of the cyst wall, so that it collapses while removing. Multiple cyst linings can also be removed using a 12-mm sleeve of morcellator. Once hemostasis is achieved, about 2 L of liquid adhesion barrier like 4% icodextrin solution or Ringer lactate is left inside the peritoneal cavity **(Figs. 9A to G)**.

Temporary Ovarian Suspension

Ovarian suspension surgery appears to be effective in decreasing adhesions after laparoscopy for endometriosis. This technique can ease the severity of pelvic pain, dysmenorrhea and dyspareunia to some extent. Ovarian suspension is done to anterior abdominal wall using non absorbable ethilon 1-0 on a straight needle or to round ligament with short-term resorbable suture for the prevention of periovarian adhesion formation. In case of big-sized ovary double ovarian suspension is done. The suture removal is done from anterior abdominal wall after 1 month.

Management of Future Fertility

Patients are immediately allowed active management of infertility in the postoperative phase. Only patients who seem to have an aggressive disease or very active endometriosis are given a shot of GnRh analog. Active management of infertility in the form of controlled ovarian hyperstimulation (COH) and intrauterine insemination (IUI) helps. Conception should be tried early because of progressive nature of the disease.

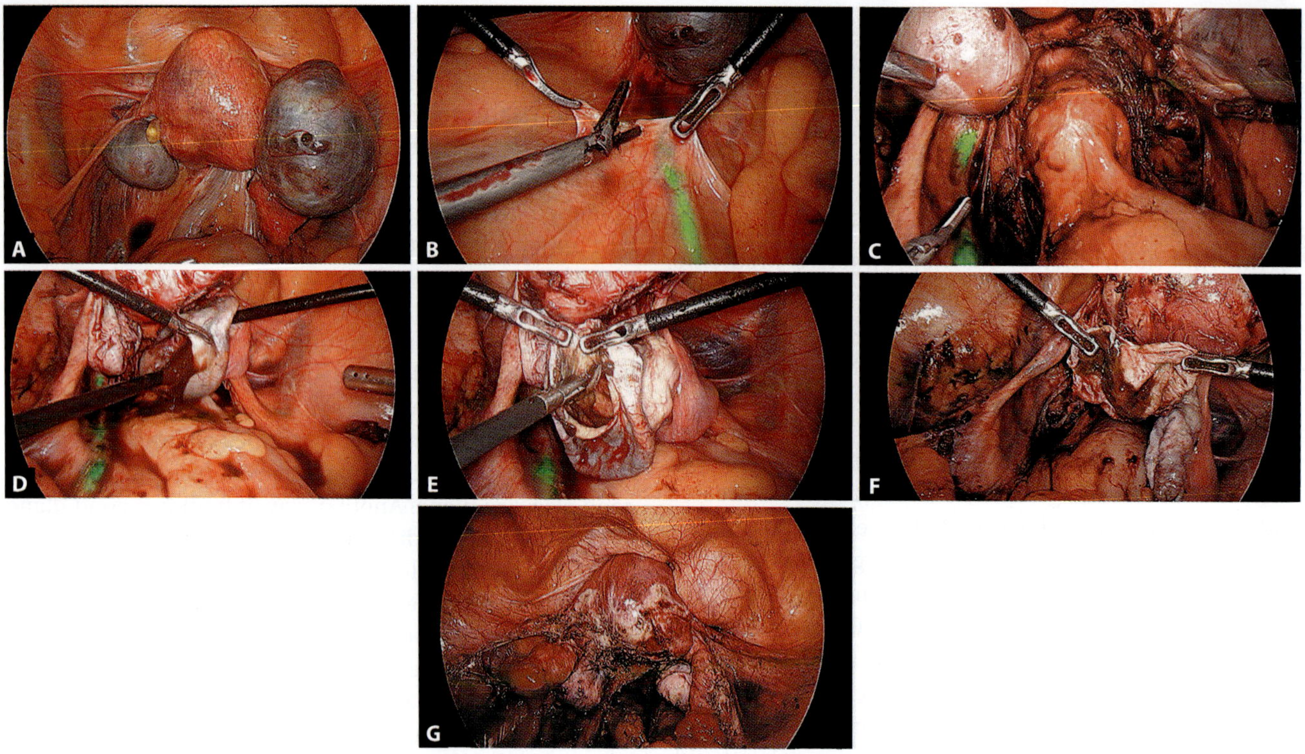

Figs. 9A to G: (A) Appearance of large endometrioma densely adherent to the back surface of uterus, obliterated pouch of Douglas; (B) Retroperitoneal dissection for ureterolysis under ICG illumination; (C) Complete rectovaginal space clearance; (D) Drainage of thick chocolate material during adhesiolysis from the endometrioma; (E) Ovarian cortex held by atraumatic grasper and cyst lining held by tooth grasper; (F) Cyst lining enucleated; (G) Normal looking bilateral ovaries after ovarian reconstruction.

LAPAROSCOPIC OVARIAN DRILLING

Polycystic ovarian syndrome (PCOS) is a fairly common condition in women of reproductive age. The incidence varies from 3 to 15% of women of reproductive age,[20] depending on the population studied and the diagnostic criteria applied.[21] The cause of PCOS is unknown. However, PCOS is thought to be a genetic disorder (autosomal dominant) meaning that each child has a 50% chance of inheriting the disorder from a parent who carries the gene. The gene can be inherited from either mother or father. The exact gene causing PCOS has not yet been identified. The condition was first described in 1935 by American gynecologists Irving F. Stein and Michael L. Leventhal, from whom its original name of *Stein-Leventhal syndrome* is taken.

The insulin resistance with compensatory hyperinsulinemia is a prominent feature of the syndrome and it seems to have a pathophysiologic role in the hyperandrogenism. It is a common hormonal disorder that is poorly understood and is characterized by lack of regular ovulation, irregular menstrual cycles, infertility, abnormal facial hair growth, obesity, and polycystic ovaries. Patients with PCOD are always at a higher risk of metabolic complications such as Type 2 diabetes mellitus, dyslipidemia, and cardiovascular disease.[22] The first line of management is given in the form of lifestyle modification, increase in physical activity, and loss of at least 10% of body weight. This may be combined with ovulation induction drugs like clomiphene citrate or aromatase inhibitors like letrozole. Insulin sensitizers like metformin may also be included in the first-line regimen. National Institute for Health and Clinical Excellence recommended in 2013, that women with PCOS and a body mass index more than 25 to be given metformin when other therapies have failed to produce results. Metformin treatment reduces hyperinsulinemia, LH levels and free testosterone concentrations in obese women with PCOS. Metformin improves menstrual regularity and increases the frequency of ovulation. Ovarian drilling is indicated in clomiphene resistant cases. Another approach in these cases may be gonadotropins. However, we prefer drilling over gonadotropins. This is because drilling appears to be equally effective with lesser chances of multiple pregnancies.

Mechanism of Action

The exact mechanism of induction of ovulation by ovarian drilling is not understood. Different theories were proposed by researchers. Stein and Leventhal postulated that bilateral ovarian wedge resection decreases the mechanical crowding of the cortex by cysts, which enables the progress of the normal Graafian follicles to the surface of ovary.

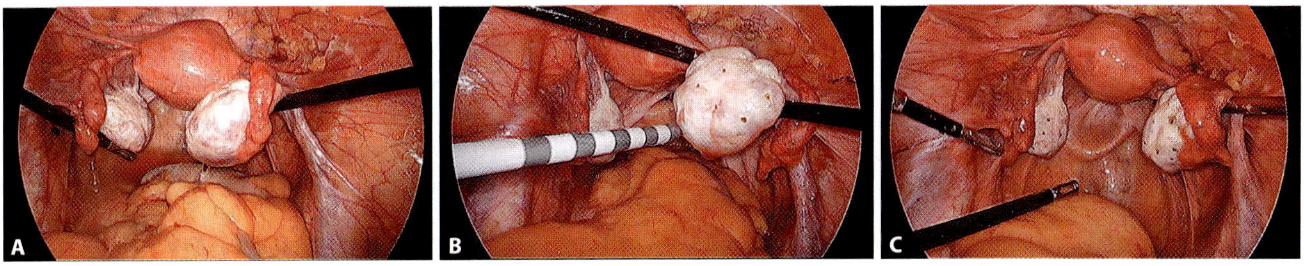

Figs. 10A to C: (A) Bilateral polycystic ovaries; (B) Holding the ovarian ligament with atraumatic grasping forceps and approaching the ovary with monopolar cautery needle at right angle to the ovarian surface and drilling done; (C) Bilateral polycystic ovaries after ovarian drilling.

Gjonnaess (1984) proposed that ovulation was initiated by either stromal destruction or extensive capsular destruction with discharge of the contents of multiple follicle cysts.[23] Daniell and Miller (1989) suggested that physical opening of subcapsular cysts led to the removal of androgen-containing follicular fluid from the ovarian environment, thus lowering the androgen content of the ovaries.

Changed Hormonal Milieu Following Ovarian Drilling

- The total and free testosterone is decreased by 40–50% of the preoperative levels
- LH levels also decrease following the procedure
- Change in FSH levels is less marked. Generally, they show a cyclical rise in keeping with the restoration of ovulation
- Normal inhibin pulsatility is restored.

The normalization of hormonal relationships leads to recruitment of a new cohort of follicles and resumption of ovarian function. These endocrine changes occur rapidly and are sustained for years.

Procedure of Ovarian Drilling

After inserting the scope, a general inspection of pelvis is carried out to look for any pathology. Fundus of the uterus is inspected as a wide fundus denotes a septal defect and is frequently associated with PCOS. Endometriosis and PID are infrequently associated with PCOS. RUMI uterine manipulator is inserted and uterus is anteverted and taken to contralateral side to stretch the ovarian ligament. A firm platform to ovary for drilling is provided by 5 mm suction irrigation cannula inserted through ipsilateral port between the fimbrial end of the tube and the ovary and wedging its lower end against the cervico uterine junction in pouch of Douglas. Ovaries must be kept static and monopolar needle is inserted from the contralateral lower port and ovary is approached at right angle to cauterize all visible bluish subcapsular follicles using 40 watts of pure cutting current. The number of holes depends on the size of the ovaries and the preoperative sonography. In moderately enlarged ovaries, about 10–12 holes are sufficient but more may be required in voluminous ovaries. Cooling of the ovaries is done using thorough irrigation. All attempts should be made to minimize bleeding from the punctures. An underwater examination is done to look for any bleeding point and if found, is cauterized. The depth of penetration of monopolar needle to just cauterize the capsule and puncture the follicle requires a depth of 2–3 mm and the monopolar cautery time of just 2 seconds. The instruments are changed to contralateral side once one ovary is done because it is better to approach the follicles at right angle, which is best achieved from the contralateral side. About 1000 mL of ringer lactate is left in the abdomen as adhesion barrier. Ovarian drilling is routinely followed by hysteroscopy and if a uterine septum (commonly associated with PCOS) is found, then hysteroscopic resection is done (**Figs. 10A to C**).

Precautions

- Ovary should be stabilized while drilling, because if ovary falls during drilling the charged monopolar needle can hit any vital structure and cause unintended damage.
- Avoid overenergetic drilling in terms of number of holes and electrosurgery as it may lead to premature ovarian failure.
- Cooling of the ovaries using irrigation after drilling should be done.

Future Fertility Management

Active management is done and patients are allowed to conceive immediately after the surgery. The couple is put on minimal required stimulation with clomiphene or letrozole as the ovaries are now receptive to lower dose. Pregnancy rates almost touching 80% as Gjonnaess et al., are achieved. Risk of hyperstimulation after drilling is avoided using ovulogens in moderation.

LAPAROSCOPY COMPLICATIONS

The final step in the infertility workup is diagnostic hysteroscopy laparoscopy, which involves evaluation of all the factors causing infertility. It rarely accounts for any complication and the risk is less than 1%. The most common complication, which can arise during this procedure, is while placing the laparoscope through the umbilicus. It may lead to injuries of the bowel, bladder, ureter, and injuries to the pelvic vessels. According to the American Society of

Reproductive Medicine, laparoscopic complications are observed only in 1–2%.

Few laparoscopic complications are:

- Damage to abdominal structures like bowel and bladder
- Hemorrhage due to abdominal and pelvic vessels injury
- Infection
- Anesthetic complications
- Cystitis after surgery
- Skin reactions at the site of incision
- Postoperative adhesions
- Abdominal wall hematomas
- Hypersensitivity reaction
- Nerve palsy
- Urinary retention
- Embolism
- Thermal injury.

Laparoscopic surgery—not a good choice in conditions such as:

- Patients with reduced ejection fraction and congestive heart failure
- Respiratory distress, COPD
- Presence of a distended bowel.

Laparoscopic surgery requires surgeon expertise in order to afford the best possible outcome for the patient. A good clinical acumen with an aptitude to manage all complications is essential for every surgeon.

HYSTEROSCOPY

The prevalence of uterine abnormalities in patients with infertility is as high as 50%. Therefore, evaluation of a couple with infertility should include assessment of the endometrial cavity. The first instrument known to illuminate the cavities of the human body was invented by Phillip Bozzini, some 200 years back, but his ingenious invention went unnoticeable. After Bozzini's invention Lichtleiter in 1807, Pantaleoni in 1869 successfully performed transcervical intrauterine evaluation and treatment with hysteroscopy. He used a 12 mm cystoscope, candlelight, and a concave mirror to treat polyps with silver nitrate in a 60-year-old woman. Later Nitze and Leiter added the optical lens to the endoscope in 1879, Heineberg used a water irrigation system in 1908, and Rubin used carbon dioxide (CO_2) in 1925.

HYSTEROSCOPIC MYOMECTOMY

Submucous fibroids are the most common types of leiomyomas. They account for 5–10% of all myomas. These submucous fibroids, along with endometrial polyps, are very commonly diagnosed during diagnostic hysteroscopy. Though transvaginal ultrasound and MRI remain the most sensitive techniques to detect the exact number, position, and size of different myomas. Diagnostic hysteroscopy remains the gold standard investigation for diagnosing a submucosal fibroid. It also helps in evaluation of the possibility of resection of the submucous myoma hysteroscopically **(Fig. 11)**.

Wamstekar's Classification[24]

- *Type 0:* Pedunculated; 100% within the cavity (fibroid polyp).
- *Type I:* Greater than 50% within the cavity (<50% is intramyometrial).
- *Type II:* Less than 50% within the cavity (>50% is intramyometrial).

Lasmar's Classification[25]

It includes:

- The penetration of the nodule into the myometrium.
- The extension of the base of the nodule with respect to the wall of the uterus:
    - *Score 0:* When the fibroid covers 1/3 or less of the wall
    - *Score 1:* When the base of the nodule occupies between 1/3 and 2/3 of the wall
    - *Score 2:* When it affects more than 2/3 of the wall.

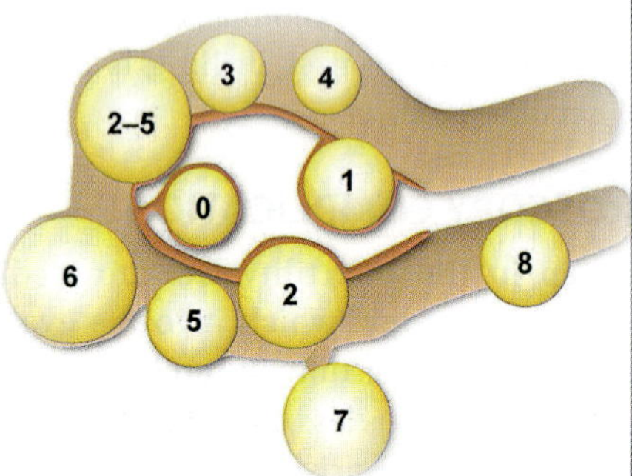

SM – Submucous	0	Pedunculated intracavitary
	1	<50% intramural
	2	≥50 intramural
O – Other	3	Contacts endometrium; 100% intramural
	4	Intramural
	5	Subserous ≥50% intramural
	6	Subserous <50% intramural
	7	Subserous pedunculated
	8	Other (specify e.g. cervical, parasitic)
Hybrid leiomyomas	2-5	Submucosal and subserosal, each with less than half the diameter in the endometrial and peritoneal cavities, respectively.

Fig. 11: FIGO classification of myomas.

Type 8 is fibroid that do not arise from myometrium but include cervical lesions, round or broad ligaments without direct attachment to the uterus, and other "parasitic" lesions.https://obgyn.onlinelibrary.wiley.com/doi/pdf/10.1002/ijgo.12666

- *Size:*
  - *Score 0:* When the nodule measures ≤2 cm
  - *Score 1:* When it is between 2 and 5 cm
  - *Score 2:* When it measures >5 cm
- *Topography:*
  - *Score 0:* When fibroid is in the lower third
  - *Score 1:* When in the middle third
  - *Score 2:* When fibroid is in the upper third
    - An extra point is attributed to lateral wall myomas
    - In case of multiple myomas, the myoma with the maximum points shall be taken into consideration. The maximum total score being 9 points.

Indications

- Symptoms, which are considered to be related to the presence of submucous fibroids.
- Subfertility due to submucous fibroids, when they interfere with the uniformity of the uterine cavity and implantation.
- Submucous fibroids less than 5 cm in diameter at the time of surgery.

Contraindications

- Resection of multiple submucous fibroids is time taking thereby increasing the risk of fluid overload and Asherman's syndrome.
- Large deep Type II fibroid

Others

- Pelvic Inflammation
- Carcinoma cervix and endometrial cancer
- Medical conditions like ischemic heart disease, coagulopathies, etc.

Different Methods to Remove Submucous Fibroids (Figs. 12 and 13)

Laser

Nd:YAG laser, which is an expensive device was popular in 1980s and 1990s. It can be used as a cutting tool for pedunculated Type 0 myomas or can be used for myolysis by burning numerous holes in the myoma, causing devascularization and shrinkage.

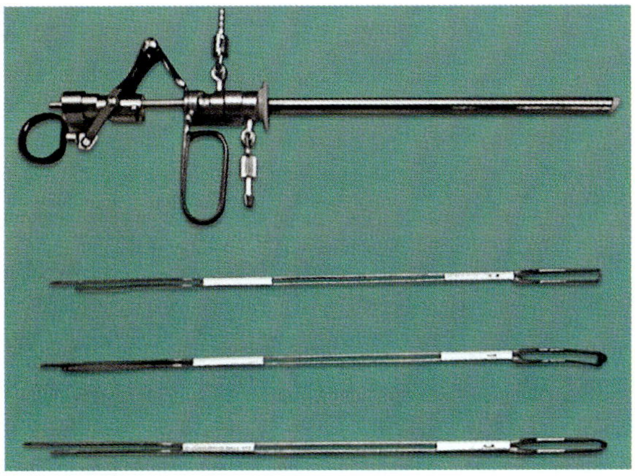

Fig. 12: Resectoscope with working element.

The only advantage is that it can be used in an isotonic fluid. Now a days, accurate fluid monitoring devices are available, the Nd: YAG laser is rarely used for this indication.

Vaporizing Electrode

It includes the bipolar and the monopolar electrodes using very high radiofrequency to vaporize fibroids. Advantage

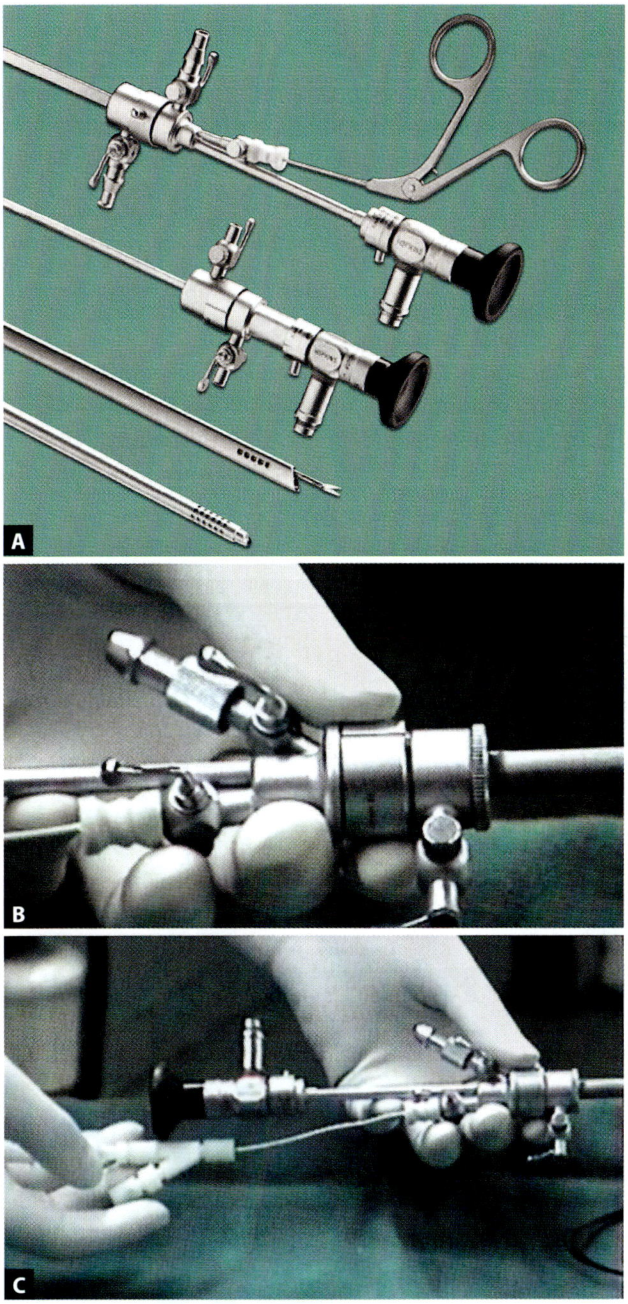

Figs. 13A to C: (A) Bettocchi hysteroscope, Karl Storz Tuttlingen, Germany; (B) Instrument channel of a number 7F operating hysteroscope through which cannulation system is introduced; (C) Instrument trolley showing the operative.

is that the fibroids are eradicated very quickly without any bothersome fibroid chips to remove.

Bipolar system can be used with isotonic fluid whereas monopolar requires nonelectrolyte containing distention media.

Disadvantages:
- Retrieval of tissue for histopathological examination cannot be carried out
- Due to the high power used, numerous gas bubbles are produced leading to air embolism.

Monopolar Loop Electrode

The instrument most commonly used to remove submucosal myomas is the monopolar loop electrode with a continuous-flow resectoscope. Fluid monitoring should be accurate.

The three most commonly used fluids for uterine distention are:
1. 1.5% glycine (hypotonic)
2. 3% sorbitol (hypotonic)
3. 5% mannitol (isotonic). All three lack electrolytes.

Serum sodium levels are kept in check as the levels of sodium approximately decrease 10 milliequivalents for every liter absorbed. Hence, it is important to monitor the fluid deficit rather than the total volume used.

Few serious but *avoidable* consequences of significant hyponatremia are:
- Pulmonary edema
- Transient blindness
- Cerebral edema.

The resectoscope remains the most efficient and widely used instrument for excising submucous fibroids.

Bipolar Versapoint

More recent alternative to resectoscope.

Technique of Hysteroscopic Resection (Figs. 14A to F)

Before commencing hysteroscopic myomectomy, adequate cervical dilatation needs to be achieved. Most gynecologists use a 26 or 27 Fr gauge resectoscope, with an outer diameter of 8.7–9 mm, so the cervix has to be dilated to Hegar 9 or 10. Over dilatation may cause inadequate uterine distention and difficulty in fluid monitoring, hence avoided.

A simple diagnostic hysteroscopy can be performed using normal saline, to inspect the cavity size, shape, and exact location of the myoma. Subsequently, the fluid can be changed to glycine before insertion of resectoscope. The excision of the fibroid is started medially and progressed toward the base. The loop is pushed beyond the fibroid under direct vision and is moved back and forth to continue

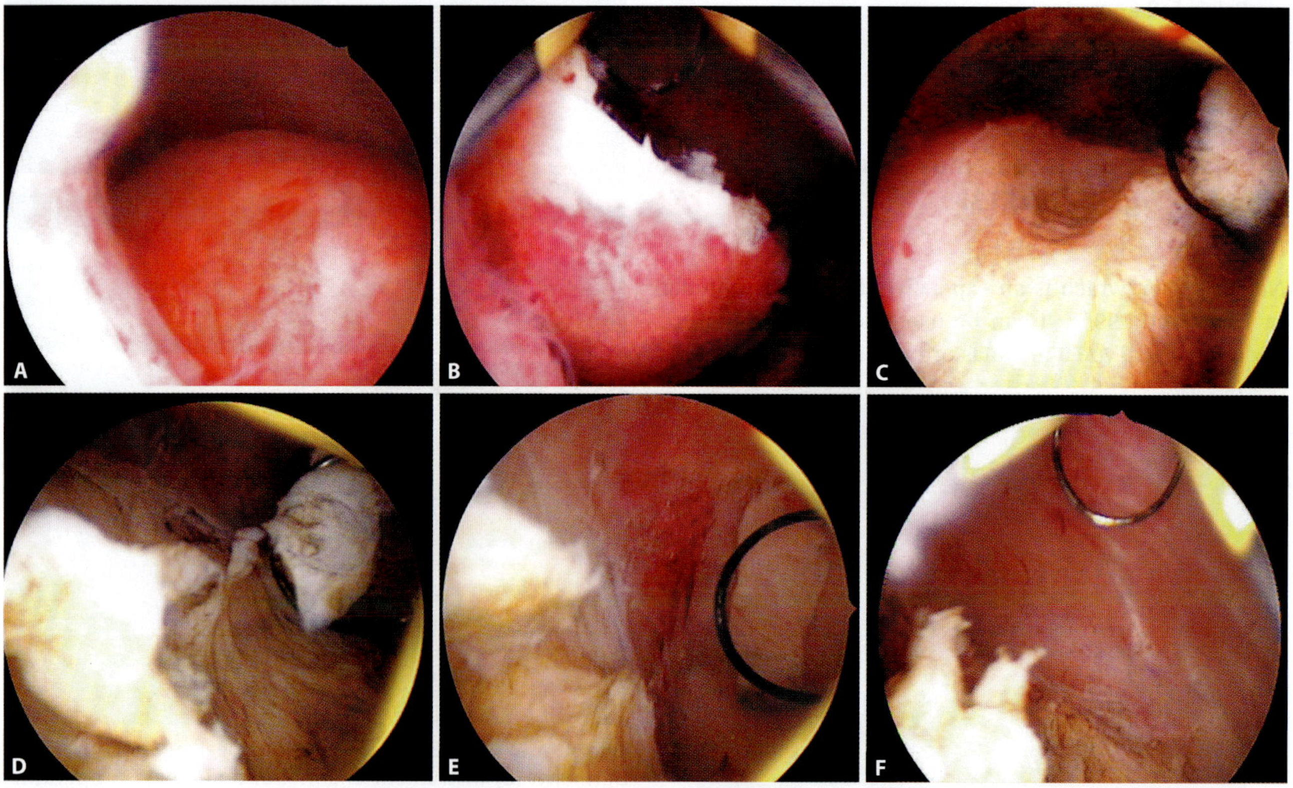

Figs. 14A to F: (A) Submucous myoma; (B) Resection of submucous myoma using forward angle loop; (C) Resection in progress; (D) Removing chip of myoma; (E) Almost completed resection done; (F) Normal uterine cavity noted at end.

the resection. The uterus is closely observed simultaneously from outside by a laparoscope. Only very large size fibroids may require the removal of the instrument from the uterine cavity. The resected chips are collected near the fundus and are removed using an ovum forceps or flushing curette at the end of the procedure. The resected specimen is sent for HPE. Type 0 and Type I fibroids can be resected using this technique. For Type II fibroids can be resected using a simple maneuver where after the resection of the superficial portion, the uterus is deflated and is rubbed bimanually to induce uterine contractions thereby making the deeper part of myoma protrude into the uterine cavity. The surgery shall be continued by redistension of the uterus thereafter. Resection should be avoided, if the residual fibroid remnant does not migrate toward the cavity as it is suggestive of a true transmural fibroid. Resection if continued can lead to dreaded complication like perforation. Glycine overload should be monitored.

Hysteroscopic Morcellation

The U.S. Food and Drug Administration in 2014 discouraged the use of power morcellators for the risk of spreading an unsuspected cancer. However, this Safety Communication does not affect Hysteroscopic Tissue Retrieval system (HTRs). HTRs consist of two metal, hollow, rigid, and disposable tubes with a wide range of diameters adaptable to the use of 5–9 mm hysteroscope. Different HTRs are commercially available: Truclear 8.0 (Medtronic, Minneapolis, Minnesota), Truclear 5C (Medtronic, Minneapolis, Minnesota), and MyoSure (Hologic, Marlborough, Massachusetts). As recently summarized by Noventa et al., Truclear 8.0 has a diameter of 8 mm and is introduced into the uterine cavity with a 9 mm rigid sheath. Truclear 5C hysteroscopy system incorporates a 2.9 mm rotatory-style blade through a 5 mm, 0-degree hysteroscope. MyoSure is introduced into the uterus through a 6 or a 7 mm, 0-degree, continuous-flow hysteroscope. All these devices work with saline solution as distension and irrigation media, instead of the electrolyte-free solutions used for monopolar high-frequency resectoscope.

Advantages of Morcellation

Morcellator uses a blade and a suction tube simultaneously to cut and remove tissue, which improves visibility and reduces the risk of perforations and gas embolus that are more likely with multiple insertions. There is no risk of thermal injury as no energy is used in uterine cavity. There is shorter operating time and the instrument is easy to use.

Disadvantages of Morcellation

Morcellator cannot cauterize blood vessels and have limited utility in cases of Type II myomas. Instrument is costly.

Complications and their Prevention

- *Cervical lacerations:* It can occur from the tenaculum site. They are easily controlled by pressure applied with a sponge forceps. Rarely, a suture is needed. Cervical tears can also result from difficult cervical dilatation, especially in postmenopausal/ nulliparous women or patients who previously received GnRH agonists.
- *Uterine perforation:* Incidence is 0.4–1.6%. If perforation is suspected, laparoscopy should be performed to evaluate the integrity of the abdominal viscera. An intrauterine balloon is not recommended, as it might enlarge the tear or divert bleeding into the peritoneal cavity.
- *Fluid overload and electrolyte imbalance:* Severe complications of operative hysteroscopy are pulmonary and cerebral edema, coagulopathy, and hyponatremia. Fluid management is essential. Careful monitoring of the patient and administration of intravenous furosemide might be needed. One should abandon the procedure, if the fluid deficit is greater than 1000 mL.
- *Incomplete removal*: The use of a preoperative GnRH agonists leads to a decrease in fibroid size and fluid loss, which facilitates complete removal of large fibroids. However, pretreatment with a GnRH agonist may render small myomas less visible and increases the probability of recurrence.
- *Bleeding:* Myometrial contraction is usually sufficient to control bleeding. However, in some patients, intravenous administration of uterotonic drugs or insertion of a Foley catheter balloon into the uterine cavity might be needed.
- *Postoperative uterine infection and intrauterine adhesions:* We use prophylactic antibiotics for hysteroscopic myomectomy.

HYSTEROSCOPIC TUBAL CANNULATION FOR PROXIMAL TUBAL BLOCK

Some 5–20% of hysterosalpingograms reveal PTO. There are two types of PTO. True occlusion can be due to salpingitis, endometriosis, or congenital malformations. Another type is apparent proximal occlusion due to tubal spasm at the time of HSG. Owing to the high incidence of false positives, a hysterosalpingographic finding of PTO must be followed by selective tubal catheterization. The cumulative pregnancy rate after tubal catheterization is 28% at 12-month follow-up. Approximately, 20% of tubes cannot be catheterized; such patients are best treated by in vitro fertilization.

Anatomy of Proximal Tubal Region

The fallopian tubes are 7–14 cm long and the intramural segment ranges 1.5–2.5 cm with an average diameter of 100 micron. Since the diameter of the proximal segment ranges from 0.8 to 1.2 mm, it allows easy passage of a cannula with a diameter of 1–1.2 mm without causing any epithelial injury. The intramural portion of the tube is divided into two segments (1) a proximal segment ≈1 cm in length, which follows a straight path and (2) a distal segment ≈1.5 cm in length, which is sinuous.

Using the hysteroscopic approach each ostium is visualized at the apex of the uterotubal junction. Therefore, a way of reaching respective tubal ostia is by passing flexible, smooth walled, and J-shaped cannula through the internal os along the uterotubal gutter of that side.

Gardner in 1856 first described the transvaginal approach of passing a wire probe through the intramural segment of the fallopian tube. The intramural bulge at about 1 cm beyond the ostia is a common location for less flexible cannulas and endoscopes to get stuck. Hence, it is important to have over the wire coaxial cannulation systems, which are preferable as they keep the lumen coaxially align with the lumen of the fallopian tube and aid the advancement of wire cannulas.

Cannulation Techniques

The most commonly used are

- Fluoroscopically guided selective salpingography and tubal catheterization.
- Hysteroscopic tubal cannulation. The fluoroscopic procedure is beyond the scope of this chapter.

Hysteroscopic Cannulation Methods

- Flexible guidewire through a catheter.
- Fluoroscopic-guided cannulation.
- Transcervical balloon cannulation with linear catheters

Flexible Guidewire through a Catheter

Procedure: We conduct the procedure in the follicular phase of the cycle. To exclude concomitant distal tubal disease, a laparoscopy is first performed. A second surgeon performs the hysteroscopy—ideally using a second light source and monitor. Cannulation is done with an operating hysteroscope. Guidewire is loaded into the inner cannula and this is loaded into the outer catheter. This whole system is loaded into outer channel of hysteroscope in such a way that its curve is at right angle to the optics of a 30-degree hysteroscope. The cannula is moved in the tube and this can be checked through the laparoscope. The laparoscopist can facilitate cannulation by manipulating the tube to decrease the angle between the cornua and the isthmus. If there is any resistance to the movement of the cannula, it is withdrawn and re-entry is made at a slightly different angle. Forceful negotiation is avoided as it may lead to tubal perforation. One needs to cannulate only 2–3 cm of the proximal tube and then the cannula is withdrawn under vision. Same procedure is repeated on the other side **(Figs. 15A to F)**.

Complications:

- Tubal perforation: Most common. Occurs in up to 6% of cases. Minor complication that does not need any treatment and it heals on its own.

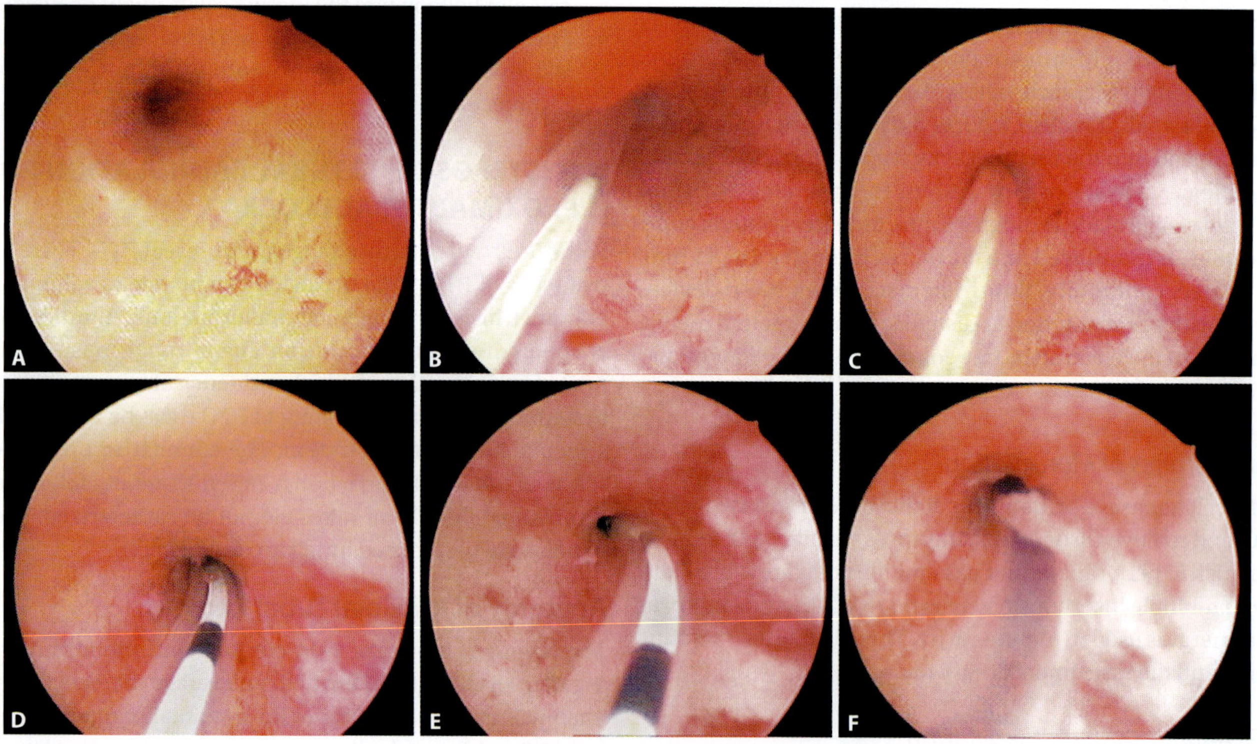

Figs. 15A to F: (A) Tubal ostia; (B) Novy's cannulation system outer catheter and J-shaped inner platinum guidewire; (C) Guidewire is advanced to negotiate the proximal tubal segment; (D) Inner cannula with centimeter markings is advanced over the platinum guidewire; (E) Inner cannula is further passed to negotiate proximal tubal segment up to 3 cm beyond the uterotubal junction; (F) Selective salpingografhy is carried out through outer cannula and flow of dye is monitored laparoscopically.

- Vasovagal reaction can occur in 0.5% of cases.
- We administer prophylactic antibiotics and rarely encounter infection. Infection can occur in the presence of undiagnosed hydrosalpinges.
- Ectopic pregnancy has been reported in 3.6–5.9% of cases following hysteroscopic tubal cannulation.

Contraindications: Women with distal tubal disease or previous tubal sterilization are not the candidates for tubal catheterization. A previous tubal catheterization is not a contraindication, as repeat procedure has led to pregnancies. Tubal catheterization is not indicated for women who are undergoing IVF treatment.

HYSTEROSCOPY FOR METROPLASTY

Congenital uterine malformations also called the Müllerian anomalies. They refer to the structural defects that affect the shape and size of the uterine cavity thereby having a poor reproductive outcome. They might be silent and do not cause any symptoms but, in few patients, they might be a significant cause of infertility or recurrent abortions. The uterine cavity is divided into two halves by a fibrous band, which is referred to as the uterine septum. Septate uterus occurs due to failure of resorption of the septum. This septum is formed when the two Müllerian ducts fuse together during the intrauterine life. A complete septum may involve the upper two-thirds of the vagina, cervix, and uterine cavity, whereas a partial septum only involves the uterine cavity. The highest rate of recurrent pregnancy loss and poor obstetric outcomes, such as preterm labor, intrauterine fetal growth restriction, fetal malpresentation, and retained products of conception is associated with a septate uterus.[26] Septate uterus has a higher incidence than bicornuate uterus as per the data available. Hysteroscopic metroplasty has significantly improved the reproductive outcome in patients with septate uterus.

Hysteroscopy does not cause excision or trauma to the uterine musculature, thereby allowing a shorter recovery time. Conception can be planned within 2 months after the procedure, and the patient can safely deliver vaginally. After hysteroscopic metroplasty, the rates of term delivery significantly improved and accounted for up to 80%, with a miscarriage rate of approximately 15%.

Preoperative Imaging

To assess the shape of the uterine cavity, the most common imaging modality is HSG. However, HSG cannot assess the contour of the uterine fundus or differentiate between different types of uterine anomalies. Office hysteroscopy is another imaging modality, but like HSG, it cannot assess the uterine contour accurately. Combined diagnostic hysterolaparoscopy is the gold standard technique for diagnosing congenital Müllerian anomalies. Transvaginal ultrasound is a good screening tool. Its sensitivity and specificity can be increased with saline-infused sonohysterography or 3D technology. Evaluation of thickness of bulge of uterine side wall or the height and depth of uterine septum should be done by sonography. Diagnosis of bicornuate uterus can be made, if the ultrasound is suggestive of a groove in the corner facing the posterior surface of the bladder between two half-uteri. The best nonsurgical technique for diagnosing and differentiating different types of uterine anomalies is MRI. This is particularly useful to differentiate septate, bicornuate, or didelphys uterus.

Timing of Surgery

- Early in the follicular phase or
- After preparation of the endometrium with progesterone or GnRH administration for a month.

Procedure

It can be performed using monopolar or bipolar system:

- *Monopolar:* Suction irrigation pump must be preset at flow rate of 250 mL/s, suction pressure should not be more than 0.2 bar and 45 watts of power. It is important to maintain an intrauterine pressure of less than 100 mm Hg during the procedure. The procedure should approximately take 45 minutes. Serious metabolic complications may occur, if there is difference between the suction and irrigation flow rates. These complications can be avoided by precise monitoring of the distension media.
- *Bipolar:* It is a newly developed system. The recommended suction irrigation settings are a flow rate of 150 mL/s, a preset pressure of 80 mm Hg, and a power of 100 watts or less.

Advantages of Using Bipolar

- No limitation to duration of the procedure.
- Reduced metabolic complications.
- Constant visibility of the bipolar system reduces the risk of perforation.

Steps of Procedure

Before starting the procedure, it is important to differentiate between uterus bicornis and uterine septum through laparoscopy. Bicornuate uterus is associated with high risk of perforation. Routine bimanual examination should be performed to evaluate the position and size of uterus before dilatation of the cervix. Hegar's dilators are used for progressive cervical dilatation, which should be performed with care. The hysteroscope with resectoscope is then introduced under visual guidance. Thorough visualization and exploration of the uterine cavity is done. The base of the septum is localized after visualization of the ostia on both sides. The division of the septum is then performed in a progressive manner using repetitive contact between the

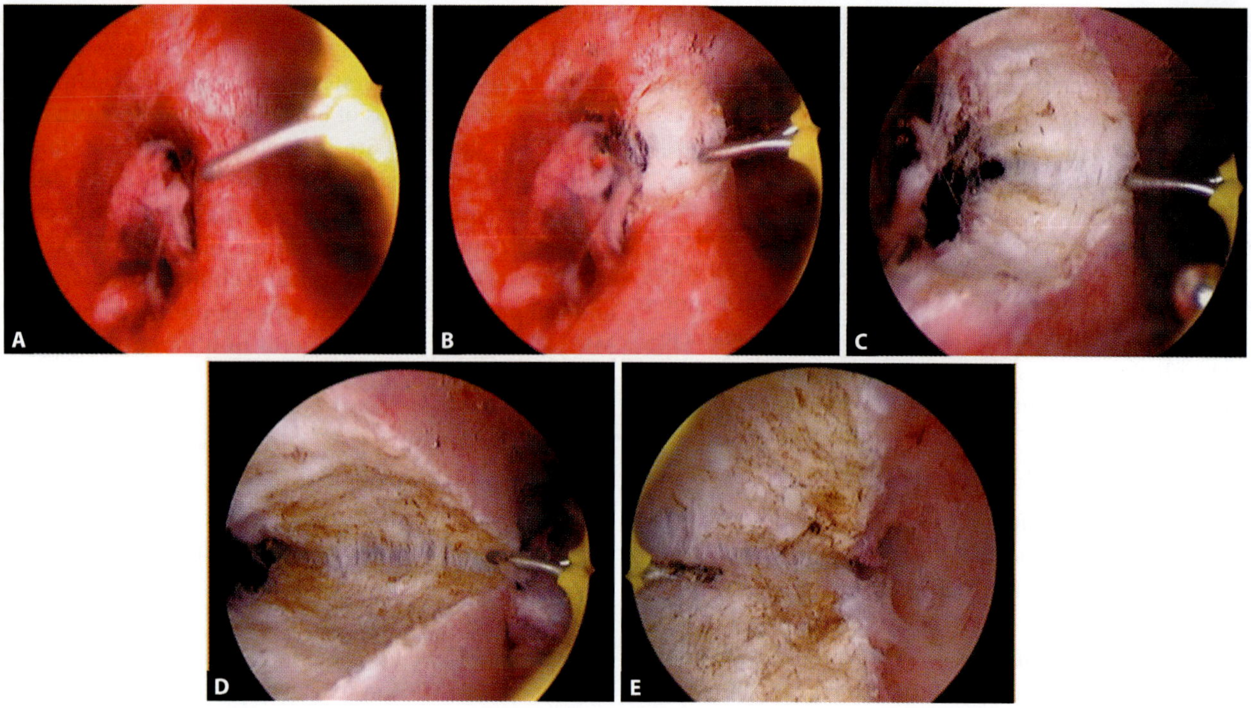

Figs. 16A to E: (A) Thick wide deep septum; (B) Septum resection being done using resectoscope; (C) Septum resection done using Collin's knife; (D) Septum resection done; (E) Septum resection done till ostia come in to view.

electrode and the septum **(Figs. 16A to E)**. The septum is divided transversely starting at its apex, halfway between its anterior and posterior surfaces, causing it to retract and become a part of the corresponding surface of the uterus. Distention of the uterus is progressively achieved as the septum is divided (the cavity opens like a book) and the cavity gradually acquires a normal shape. At the end of the procedure, it is preferable to leave a fundic spur of less than 1 cm in place to avoid weakening the fundic myometrium.

Golden Points to be Remembered

- The septal tissue is fibrous. It does not bleed. The septum ends where healthy myometrium is revealed by the occurrence of minimal bleeding and the procedure should be stopped where the two tubal ostia can be visualized in the same hysteroscopic field
- Septum should be divided but not removed in order to avoid destroying the endometrium.
- When septum extends down to the cervix, it is first divided with cold scissors or with a cutting probe. Resection begins at the level of the cervix and extends from external os toward uterus. Plane of tubal ostia should be preserved.
- When uterine septum is wide, division must be stopped as soon as any bleeding occurs. It is then performed in two phases with the second phase scheduled not before 2 months.

Follow-up after Metroplasty

There is no requirement for insertion of any intrauterine device postprocedure. Estrogen therapy is prescribed for 2 months. A diagnostic hysteroscopy can be done after a period of 2 months following estrogen therapy. If the remaining fundic spur is greater than 1 cm or new, fine adhesions have formed, it can be removed in the same sitting.

Metroplasty for Hypoplastic Uterus

Hypoplastic uterus with cylindrical uterine cavity and a bulging of the uterine side walls alone or in combination with adverse pregnancy outcomes in terms of primary infertility, recurrent pregnancy loss, or preterm delivery is an indication for metroplasty.

Procedure

General anesthesia is needed for induction of patient undergoing metroplasty. The cervix is grasped with vulsellum and progressive cervical dilatation is done using Hegar's dilators. Glycine is the media that is used for distension of the uterine cavity. The hook is introduced into the uterine cavity and the incision is performed under visual guidance. It extends from the fundus to the isthmus. The incision should be perpendicular to the lateral wall of the uterus and decreasing the depth of the incision as the section advances. Two incisions in the same groove are performed until a normal triangular and symmetric uterine

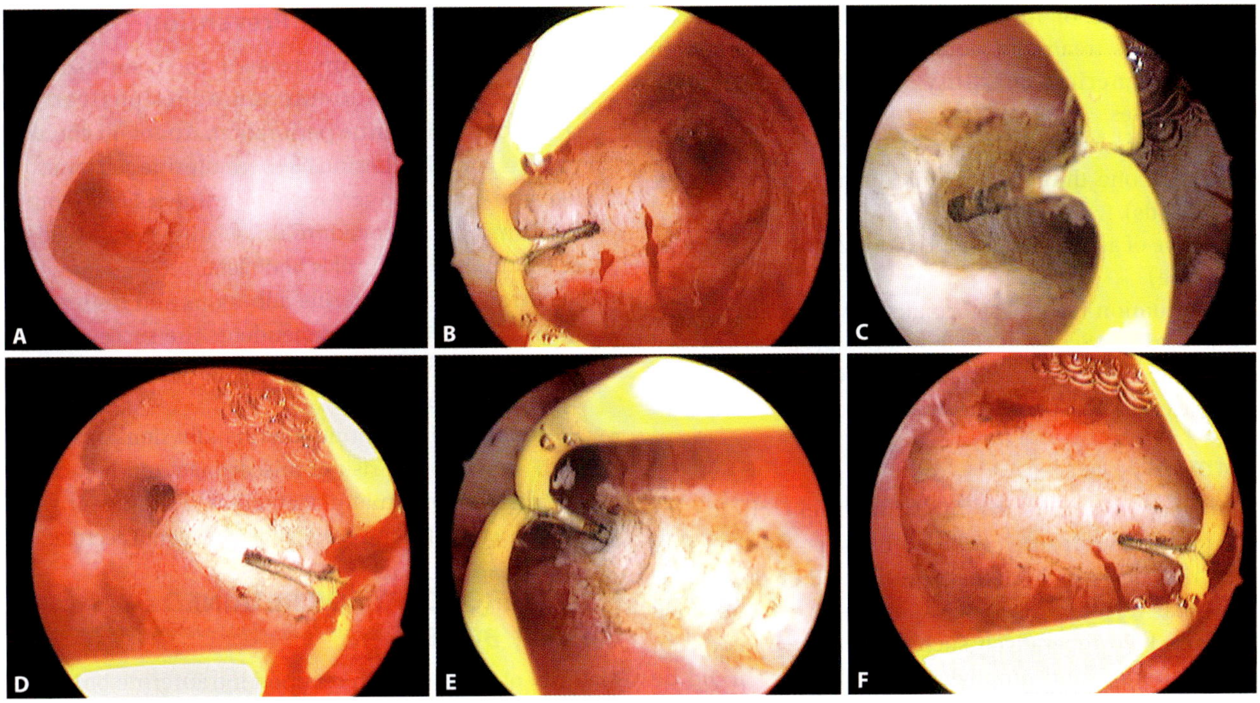

Figs. 17A to F: (A) Narrow tubular cavity; (B) Lateral metroplasty using Collin's knife started just below tubal ostia; (C) Successive cuts made by Collin's knife; (D) Lateral metroplasty on left side; (E) Lateral metroplasty incision made up to isthmus; (F) Fundal metroplasty incision between the two tubal ostia.

cavity is obtained **(Figs. 17A to F)**. The same incisions are repeated on the other lateral wall. Depth of incision should not exceed 5–7 mm.

Sequential use of estrogen/progesterone is prescribed for a period of 2 months and a repeat diagnostic hysteroscopy is performed thereafter.

Complications of Hysteroscopic Metroplasty

- *Mechanical complications:* Uterine perforation, which can lead to even visceral burns, if not timely detected.
- *Bleeding:* It occurs rarely. However, if the myometrium is disrupted, large venous sinuses can be encountered. To minimize intravasation, the intrauterine pressure should be reduced. Bleeding from small vessels can be controlled by laser or electrocautery. One can also perform bimanual compression of the uterus. An effective method is insertion of a Foleys catheter into the uterine cavity, with the balloon being filled with 15–30 cm^3 of normal saline. The catheter is left in situ for a few hours to overnight.
- *Postoperative infections:*
  - Endometritis occurs in few cases, hence the justification of giving postoperative antibiotics.
  - Intrauterine adhesion rarely occurs.
- *Metabolic complications:* The intravascular passage of a significant quantity of irrigation fluid can lead to hemodilution. Therefore, inflow and outflow of media used should be meticulously monitored.

INTRAUTERINE ADHESIONS (ASHERMAN'S SYNDROME)

Asherman described two different types of traumatic synechiae:

1. Stenosis or obliteration of the cervical canal in the vicinity of the internal os.
2. Partial or complete obliteration of the uterine cavity by conglutination of the opposing walls. Dilatation and curettage immediately after a delivery or a miscarriage are the main causes of intrauterine adhesions (75%). Infection might contribute to the development of intrauterine synechiae in 26% of cases. Other causes are cesarean or uterine surgery in nonpregnant uterus. The overall pregnancy rate after hysteroscopic adhesiolysis is 43%, with a live birth rate of 32%. The most severe form of intrauterine synechiae is related to endometrial tuberculosis, where the entire endometrial cavity may be completely lost, including the cornual regions. Its prognosis is poor.

Diagnosis

- Amenorrhea in the presence of ovulation suggests target organ defect such as intrauterine synechiae.
- Sonohysterography and HSG may show complete or partial obliteration of the uterine cavity. HSG is generally more sensitive and specific, especially if the adhesions are thin or not calcified.
- Diagnostic hysteroscopy allows accurate evaluation of the uterine cavity.

- Classification of intrauterine adhesions is critical, as it affects treatment outcome. The scoring system in the American Fertility Society classification incorporates
- The extent of the uterine cavity involvement (score 1: less than one-third; 2: one-third or two-thirds; 4: over two-thirds),
- The type of adhesions (score 1: filmy; 2: filmy and dense; 4: dense)
- Menstruation (score 0: normal; 2: hypomenorrhea; 4: amenorrhea). Scores of 1–4 indicate mild cases, scores of 5–8 indicate moderate cases, and scores of 9–12 indicate severe cases with poor outcome.

Treatment

Hysteroscopy remains the main treatment choice for Asherman's syndrome. Adhesiolysis is done using mechanical scissors hysteroscopically. Other modalities like bipolar needles, laser, or vaporizing electrodes may also be used. Postoperatively such patients are treated with estrogen therapy and prophylactic antibiotics should be given. The use of stents during the procedure also aid in complete removal of these adhesions **(Figs. 18A to D)**.

Complications and Their Prevention

- Besides complications related to hysteroscopy in general, lysis of intrauterine adhesions carries a specific risk of uterine perforation. Attention should be paid to lateral adhesions, where uterine perforation is likely to occur, if aggressive adhesiolysis is attempted. Performing the procedure under ultrasound guidance or laparoscopic control is beneficial.
- Recurrence of intrauterine adhesions and restoration of menstruation are case-dependent. The success rate can be increased with the use of intrauterine devices and estrogen postoperatively.
- Pregnancy after lysis of intrauterine adhesions is associated with an increased risk of miscarriage and hemorrhage because of abnormal placentation. The patient should also be warned of the possibility of placenta accreta.

HYSTEROSCOPY FOR RETAINED FETAL BONES

Majority of patients with retained intrauterine bones have an antecedent history of induced abortion and curettage. First trimester abortions, where fetal bone ossification

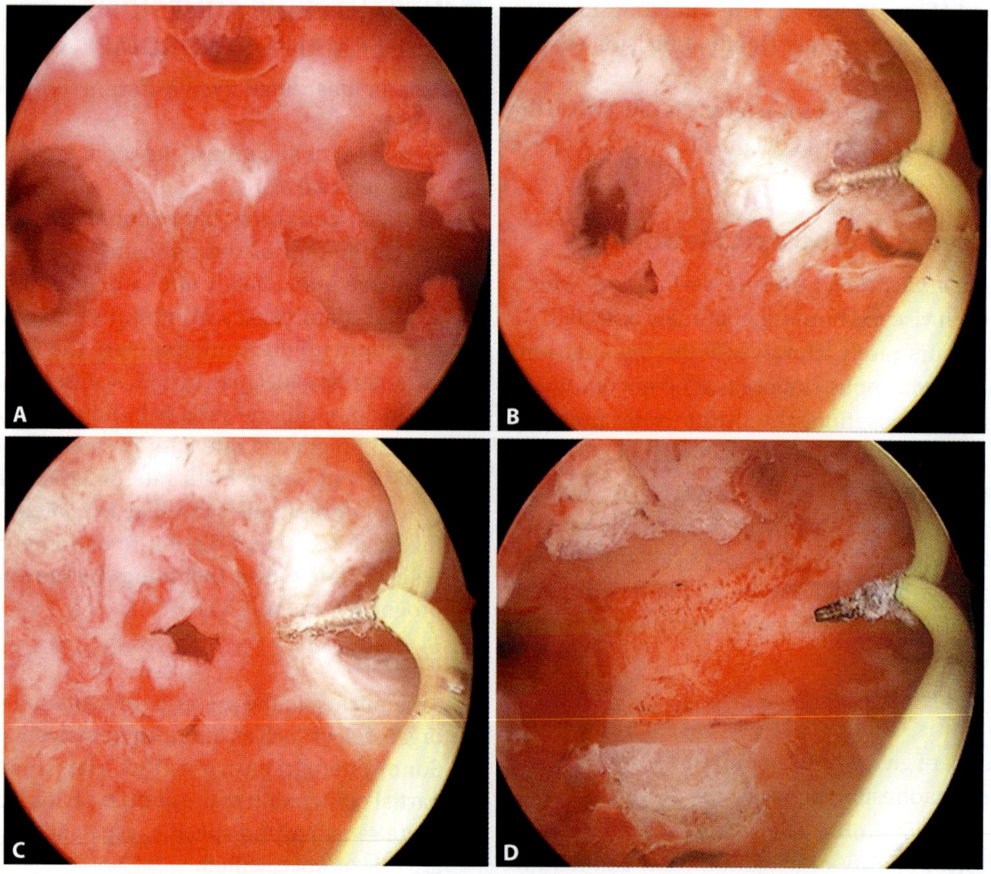

Figs. 18A to D: (A) Thick adhesions occluding uterine cavity; (B) Lysis of adhesion; (C) Hysteroscopic division of adhesion using Collin's knife; (D) Normal uterine cavity at end.

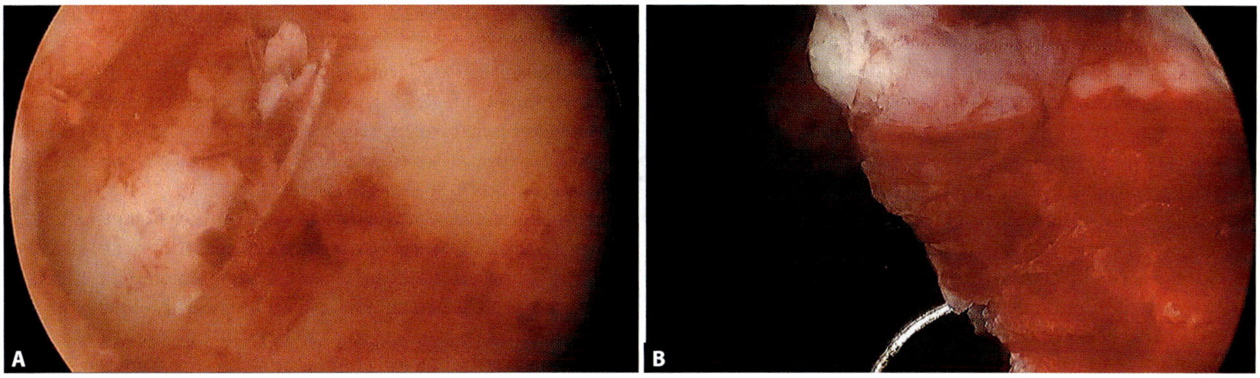

Figs. 19A and B: (A) Retained fetal bone visible in hysteroscopy; (B) Hysteroscopic removal of fetal bone.

has not completely occurred, lead to intrauterine bone formation by dystrophic calcification of retained products. Mid trimester abortion frequently require instrumentation and cause retention of fetal skull bones.[26] Incidence is more in anomalous uterus.[27] Bone formation may also be due to chronic endometritis and resulting osseous metaplasia of the endometrium. It can be distinguished from osseous metaplasia by the presence of tissue reaction. Metaplastic ossification following chronic inflammation affects it diffusely.

Diagnosis

- Ultrasonography—calcified specs in the endometrium
- Hysterosalpingography—may reveal filling defects of the uterine cavity
- Hysteroscopy—coral-like osseous fragments embedded within or projecting through the endometrium and confirms the diagnosis

These retained bones can be successfully retrieved with hysteroscopy or with a resectoscope **(Figs. 19A and B)**. Removal of bony fragments is associated with therapeutic success and correction of infertility. A spontaneous pregnancy rate of around 80% has been reported in one of the largest reviews of retained fetal bones and with most of the pregnancies occurring within 6 months of retrieval of fetal bones.

KEY POINTS

- Diagnostic hysterolaparoscopy is most effective and safe method of evaluation of female infertility, mainly in detecting endometriosis, intraperitoneal adhesions, and uterine malformations.
- These are all correctable abnormalities that can be missed by routine pelvic examination and usual imaging procedures.
- It is a very useful method that diagnoses and treats multiple tubal, ovarian, peritoneal, and uterine abnormalities in a single setting, especially in couples with normal hormonal profiles and male factor.
- Thus, hysterolaparoscopy may be considered as gold standard and definitive investigative daycare procedure for evaluation of female infertility.

REFERENCES

1. Eldar-Geva T, Meagher S, Healy DL, MacLachlan V, Breheny S, Wood C. Effect of intramural, subserosal, and submucosal uterine fibroids on the outcome of assisted reproductive technology treatment. Fertil Steril. 1998;70(4):687-91.
1. Pritts EA, Parker WH, Olive DL. Fibroids and infertility: an updated systematic review of the evidence. Fertil Steril. 2009;91(4):1215-23.
2. Benecke C, Kruger TF, Siebert TI, Van der Merwe JP, Steyn DW. Effect of fibroids on fertility in patients undergoing assisted reproduction. Gynecol Obstet Invest. 2005;59:225-30.
3. Semm K, Mettler L. Technical progress in pelvic surgery via operative laparoscopy. Am J Obstet Gynecol. 1980;138(2):121-7.
4. Alessandri F, Remorgida V, Venturini PL, Ferrero S. Unidirectional barbed suture versus continuous suture with intracorporeal knots in laparoscopic myomectomy: A randomized study. J Minim Invasive Gynecol. 2010;17(6):725-9.
5. Kindinger LM, Setchell TE, Miskry TS. Bowel obstruction due to entanglement with unidirectional barbed suture following laparoscopic myomectomy. Gynecol Surg. 2012;9(3):357-8.
6. AFS. The American Fertility Society classifications of adnexal adhesions, distal tubal occlusion, tubal occlusion secondary to tubal ligation, tubal pregnancies, Müllerian anomalies and intrauterine adhesions. Fertil Steril. 1988;49:944-55.
7. Zeyneloglu HB, Arici A, Olive DL. Adverse effects of hydrosalpinx on pregnancy rates after in vitro fertilization–embryo transfer. Fertil Steril. 1998;70(3):492-9.
8. Strandell A, Lindhard A, Waldenström U, Thorburn J, Janson PO, Hamberger L. Hydrosalpinx and IVF outcome: a prospective, randomized multicentre trial in Scandinavia on salpingectomy prior to IVF. Hum Reprod Oxf Engl. 1999;14(11):2762-9.
9. Camus E, Poncelet C, Goffinet F, Wainer B, Merlet F, Nisand I, et al. Pregnancy rates after in-vitro fertilization in cases of tubal infertility with and without hydrosalpinx: a meta-analysis of published comparative studies. Hum Reprod Oxf Engl. 1999;14(5):1243-9.

10. Kontoravdis A, Makrakis E, Pantos K, Botsis D, Deligeoroglou E, Creatsas G. Proximal tubal occlusion and salpingectomy result in similar improvement in in vitro fertilization outcome in patients with hydrosalpinx. Fertil Steril. 2006;86(6):1642-9.
11. Puttemans PJ, Brosens IA, Delattin P, Vasquez G, Boeckx W. Salpingoscopy versus hysterosalpingography in hydrosalpinges. Hum Reprod. 1987;2:535-40.
12. Winston RM. Microsurgical tubocornual anastomosis for reversal of sterilization. Lancet. 1977;1(8006):284-5.
13. Gomel V. The place of reconstructive tubal surgery in the era of assisted reproductive techniques. Reprod Biomed Online. 2015;31(6):722-31.
14. Yoon TK, Sung HR, Kang HG, Cha SH, Lee CN, Cha KY. Laparoscopic tubal anastomosis: fertility outcome in 202 cases. Fertil Steril. 1999;72(6):1121-6.
15. Alborzi S, Motazedian S, Parsanezhad ME. Chance of adhesion formation after laparoscopic salpingo-ovariolysis: is there a place for second-look laparoscopy? J Am Assoc Gynecol Laparosc. 2003;10(2):172-6.
16. Bruhat MA, Mage G, Pouly JL, Manhes H, Canis M, Wattiez A. Adhesions in Operatory Laparoscopy. Paris: Medsi/McGraw-Hill; 1989. p. 215.
17. Moen MH, Muus KM. Endometriosis in pregnant and non-pregnant women at tubal sterilization. Hum Reprod Oxf Engl. 1991;6(5):699-702.
18. Hughes EG, Fedorkow DM, Collins JA. A quantitative overview of controlled trials in endometriosis-associated infertility. Fertil Steril. 1993 May;59(5):963–70.
19. Vause TDR, Cheung AP. Reproductive endocrinology and infertility committee. Ovulation induction in polycystic ovary syndrome. J Obstet Gynaecol Can. 2010;32(5): 495-502.
20. Fauser BCJM, Tarlatzis BC, Rebar RW, Legro RS, Balen AH, Lobo R, et al. Consensus on women's health aspects of polycystic ovary syndrome (PCOS): the Amsterdam ESHRE/ASRM-Sponsored 3rd PCOS Consensus Workshop Group. Fertil Steril. 2012;97(1):28-38.e25.
21. American Association of Clinical Endocrinologists Polycystic Ovary Syndrome Writing Committee. American Association of Clinical Endocrinologists Position Statement on Metabolic and Cardiovascular Consequences of Polycystic Ovary Syndrome. Endocr Pract. 2005;11(2):126-34.
22. van Dongen H, de Kroon CD, Jacobi CE, Trimbos JB, Jansen FW. Diagnostic hysteroscopy in abnormal uterine bleeding: A systematic review and meta-analysis. BJOG Int J Obstet Gynaecol. 2007;114(6):664-75.
23. Wamsteker K, Emanuel MH, de Kruif JH. Transcervical hysteroscopic resection of submucous fibroids for abnormal uterine bleeding: Results regarding the degree of intramural extension. Obstet Gynecol. 1993;82(5):736-40.
24. Lasmar RB, Barrozo PRM, Dias R, Oliveira MAP de. Submucous myomas: a new presurgical classification to evaluate the viability of hysteroscopic surgical treatment--preliminary report. J Minim Invasive Gynecol. 2005;12(4):308-11.
25. Moon HS, Park YH, Kwon HY, Hong SH, Kim SK. Iatrogenic secondary infertility caused by residual intrauterine fetal bone after midtrimester abortion. Am J Obstet Gynecol. 1997;176(2):369-70.
26. Melius FA, Julian TM, Nagel TC. Prolonged retention of intrauterine bones. Obstet Gynecol. 1991;78(5 Pt 2):919-21.

CHAPTER 43

Reconstructive Surgeries Enhancing Fertility

Yehia Shawki, Osama Shawki, Amr Wahba, Zakiya Ahmed

INTRODUCTION

Conception is a complex and delicate process, the successful fulfillment of which requires normal anatomy and function of the female reproductive tract. Any factor, which might distort the normal anatomy of the female pelvis, or the uterine cavity could lead to the impairment of the fertility potential. Thanks to the advances that took place over the past decades in surgical techniques with the emergence and development of minimally invasive surgeries; namely laparoscopy and hysteroscopy, it has become now possible to reconstruct distorted pelvic anatomy and uterine cavity, and thus, restore fertility. Undoubtedly, comprehensive assessment of subfertile couples with detailed infertility workup is mandatory before proceeding with any reconstructive surgery to exclude other factors of infertility which might change the management plan. This chapter will focus on the factors that contribute in the distortion of pelvic and uterine anatomy and will highlight the surgical procedures used to correct this distortion aiming to increase fertility.

RECONSTRUCTION OF DISTORTED PELVIC ANATOMY

Pelvic Adhesions

Adhesions are bands of fibrous tissue that form as a result of the healing process which remain after the original inflammation or trauma has healed. Pelvic adhesions are one of the leading causes of female infertility. Almost 15–20% of female infertility is accounted for by adhesions.[1] The more extensive the adhesions are, the less likely it is for pregnancy to happen.[2] Peritoneal adhesions[3] can be the consequence of tissue trauma that may result from sharp, mechanical, or thermal injury; infection may result from a variety of causes including most commonly pelvic inflammatory disease (PID) especially if ignored or recurrent, endometriosis **(Fig. 1)**, history of an abdominal or pelvic surgery, complicated appendicitis, and inflammatory bowel disease.[4]

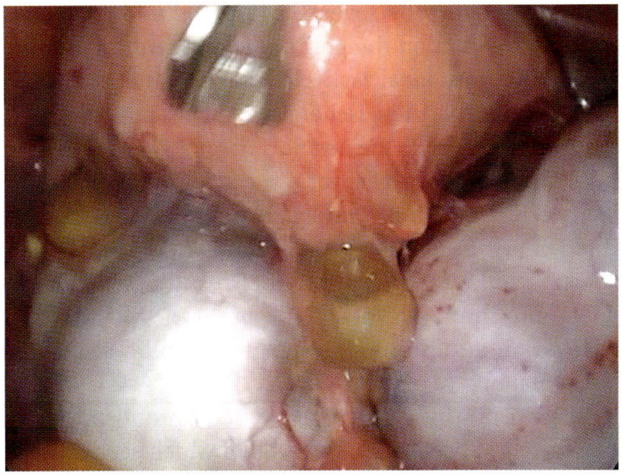

Fig. 1: Severe endometriosis with adhesions distorting the normal pelvic anatomy.

Less commonly, it can be caused by radiotherapy, bacterial peritonitis and foreign body reaction.

Such trauma triggers a cascade of events that begins with the disruption of stromal mast cells, which releases vasoactive substances such as histamine and kinins that increase vascular permeability. Oxidative stress is the result of tissue hypoxia. Free oxygen and nitrogen radicals enhance the inflammatory response that results in tissue injury. As a result, both large and small peritoneal defects heal relatively quickly. Fibrinous exudates form within 3 hours after injury. Most fibrinous exudates are transient and are broken down by fibrinolysis within 72 hours. Trauma-induced local suppression of peritoneal fibrinolysis leads to early fibrinous adhesions. The invasion of fibroblasts and blood vessels soon follows, resulting in permanent adhesions which can be vascular.

The most important potential consequences of adhesion formation are infertility, bowel obstruction, abdominal/pelvic pain, and injury to internal organs. Adhesions may affect fertility adversely by distorting adnexal anatomy and interfering with gamete and embryo transport.

Among infertile women with otherwise unexplained infertility diagnosed with adnexal adhesions at laparoscopy, pregnancy rates after subsequent adhesiolysis by laparotomy were 32% at 12 months and 45% at 24 months compared with 11% at 12 months and 16% at 24 months in women left untreated.

Intra-abdominal surgery is among the most important contributing factors for the development of peritoneal adhesions. The incidence of adhesions is higher after laparotomy rather than laparoscopy,[5] with increasing number of laparotomies[6] and midline incisions rather than suprapubic incisions.[5,6] Abdominal hysterectomy and myomectomy (especially after a posterior uterine wall incision) have high associations with pelvic adhesions.[7,8] The risk of formation of adhesions due to surgery may be predisposed to by several factors including excessive suturing, traction on the peritoneum, omentum, retained blood in the peritoneal cavity, lengthy operations, excessive tissue trauma, infection, ischemia, and latex powder.[9]

Adhesions distort the normal anatomy of the pelvis and can cause infertility by several ways. Peritubal adhesions may occlude the tube and may impair tubal motility which in turn leads to defective ovum pickup and embryo arrival into the uterus, thus, either resulting in infertility or ectopic implantation of the embryo into the tube. Periovarian adhesions prevent proper follicular growth and ovulation.[10]

Several scoring systems have been proposed for the assessment of pelvic adhesions, all of which seek to define a method to calculate the prognosis of adhesiolysis and whether or not the patient should seek in vitro fertilization (IVF). In 1982, Hulka suggested a scoring system based on two criteria; first is whether adhesions are filmy (A) or dense (B) and the second is the coverage of ovarian tissue. The study classified it into stage I, little or all of the ovarian surface is visible; stage II, over 50% of the ovary is visible; stage III, <50% of the ovary is visible; and stage IV, no ovarian surface is visible. Each adnexum should be described separately. Accordingly, the best prognosis was found in the stage I and the worst in stage IV.[11] In 1988, the American Fertility Society (AFS) [currently, the American Society for Reproductive Medicine (ASRM)] proposed a more detailed adhesion scoring system that also describes the site and extent of adhesions as shown in **Table 1**. Dense adhesions are given a score four times the filmy adhesions. The extent of organ involvement is classified into 1/3, between 1/3 and 2/3, and more than 2/3 enclosure. The score doubles with each class. Each adnexum should be described separately. Prognosis is based on the adnexum with the lesser pathology.[12]

According to this scoring system, the numbers are summed up and the adhesions are classified into *minimal* (0–5), *mild* (6–10), *moderate* (11–20), and *severe* (21–32). Several studies support the use of this scoring system to determine the prognosis and the plan of management of patients. Minimal and mild adhesions are associated with the highest pregnancy rates.[13-15] It was also found useful in predicting the rates of pregnancy, oocyte recovery, and embryo transfer for patients undergoing IVF where mild adhesions had higher rates compared to patients with severe adhesions.[16]

Measures to Reduce Adhesions

Formation of postoperative adhesions often may be minimized by careful surgical technique with adherence to microsurgical principles, including gentle tissue handling, meticulous hemostasis, excision of necrotic tissue, minimization of ischemia and desiccation, use of fine nonreactive suture materials, and prevention of foreign body reaction and infection. The larger the residual amount of blood and serosanguinous fluid, favors adhesion formation. Postoperative adhesions have been observed in up to 94% of patients after laparotomy. Laparoscopy does not necessarily result in fewer adhesions than laparotomy; the extent of tissue injury, note the surgical approach, is the determining factor. Risk for the development of de novo anterior abdominal wall adhesions is likely lower after laparoscopy than after laparotomy because the risk relates to the length of the abdominal incision(s).

TABLE 1: Adhesion scoring system, the American Fertility Society.[13]

		Extent		
Side and organ	***Adhesion severity***	***<1/3 Enclosure***	***1/3–2/3 Enclosure***	***>2/3 Enclosure***
Right ovary	Filmy	1	2	4
	Dense	4	8	16
Right tube	Filmy	1	2	4
	Dense	4	8	16
Left ovary	Filmy	1	2	4
	Dense	4	8	16
Left tube	Filmy	1	2	4
	Dense	4	8	16

The incidence of postoperative infection, another risk factor for adhesion formation, is lower after laparoscopy than after laparotomy. Pneumoperitoneum has a tamponade effect that may help to facilitate hemostasis during laparoscopy.

Evidence suggests that the incidence of adhesions at the site of closure after laparotomy is approximately 22% with peritoneal closure and 16% without peritoneal closure.

Adhesiolysis for Reconstruction of Pelvic Anatomy

Adhesiolysis is the surgical procedure in which adhesions are lysed to restore normal anatomy distorted by the adhesions. It is performed laparoscopically, usually through two or three punctures. Adhesion bands are put under tension using a grasper forceps to identify the limits of the adhesion bands. The bands are divided at their distal margins using either scissors, coagulation current, or laser. If adhesions are filmy and avascular, scissors are sufficient. If adhesions are vascular, coagulation or laser must be used to stop bleeding. When adhesions are near the ovaries, it is wise to cut about 1 mm away from the ovaries to avoid injury. Cohesive adhesions usually require plane dissection either using dissecting scissors, blunt dissection, or hydrodissection. Whenever possible, grasp the adhesions or the ovarian ligament instead of the ovary itself to reduce trauma. Adhesiolysis aims to restore tubo-ovarian relationship as much as possible. At the conclusion of surgery, irrigation of the pelvis by Ringer's lactate solution is needed to wash any blood clots or debris.

Does Adhesiolysis Improve the Fertility Outcome?

Evidence proved that adhesiolysis can improve pregnancy outcomes.[17] In one study, the cumulative pregnancy rate at 24 months follow-up was significantly higher in treated women, 45 versus 16% in the untreated group.[18] In another study, when patients who underwent laparoscopic adhesiolysis were followed up for 1 year, pregnancy occurred in 70.8%, 48.3%, and 21.6% patients in mild, moderate, and severe adhesions, respectively.[19] Some proposed the idea of second-look laparoscopy after pelvic reconstructive surgery. However, randomized controlled trials failed to prove its significance.[20]

ENDOMETRIOSIS AND INFERTILITY

The conundrum on how endometriosis affects fertility has long been debated with new studies changing the suggested course of action every few years. A measure of the issue lies with the number of afflicted patients; a diagnosis of endometriosis was considered "new" after verifying women had not been diagnosed in the previous 10 years. Incidence of endometriosis and adenomyosis in women aged 15–50 years is 0.14%. Prevalence estimated from incidence is 2.00%.[21] In the past, it has been suggested that endometriosis was not resulting in the tubal malfunction, nor endometrioma <5 cm was to be tackled prior to IVF. Revisiting the issue has led to the discovery of vital endometrial receptivity factors including HOXA 10 and HOXA 11 which are suppressed in cases of endometriosis and whose recovery, postsurgical intervention provide healthy additions to the fertility rate.[22] New technologies have also been introduced to tackle these pathologies with the growing concern of how coagulative damage to the ovaries may lead to decreased ovarian reserve compounded by the oxidative stress exerted by the disease progression already affecting ovarian reserve. Here is where the gray zone of risk versus reward of endometrioma surgery lies.[23,24]

Recent The European Society of Human Reproduction and Embryology (ESHRE) guideline recommends offering surgery as one of the options to reduce endometriosis associated pain. And when surgery is performed, clinicians may consider excision instead of ablation of endometriosis to reduce endometriosis-associated pain.[25] They have now concluded that laser uterine nerve ablation (LUNA) is not beneficial. When performing surgery in women with ovarian endometrioma, clinicians are advised to perform cystectomy instead of drainage and coagulation as it reduces recurrence of endometrioma and endometriosis-associated pain. They have also said that both cystectomy and CO_2 laser vaporization as both have similar recurrence rate beyond first year after surgery.[25]

Patients with deep endometriosis should be referred to a center of expertise. Clinicians may consider operative laparoscopy for the treatment of endometrioma associated infertility as it may increase chance of natural pregnancy; however, no data from comparative studies exist.

According to the ESHRE 2022 guideline, decision to perform surgery should be guided by the presence of absence of pain symptoms, patient's age and preferences, history of previous surgery, presence of other infertility factors, ovarian reserve, and estimated endometriosis fertility index (EFI).[25]

RECONSTRUCTION OF BLOCKED FALLOPIAN TUBES

Patency of the fallopian tube and normal function of its lining mucosa are mandatory for the transport of ovum, sperm, and embryo. It is in the ampulla of the fallopian tube where fertilization takes place. Blockage of this conduit will impair fertility and may cause ectopic pregnancy. The most common causes for tubal damage or occlusion are tubal infection and tubal sterilization. Tubal infection occurs as a part of PID secondary to sexually transmitted infections. The most common causative organism is usually *Chlamydia trachomatis*.[26]

Evaluation of Tubes

Hysterosalpingography (HSG) provides information on tubal patency, size, shape, and course along with the data on the shape of the uterine cavity **(Fig. 2)**. However, its accuracy in diagnosing pelvic adhesions is limited. Abnormal HSG must be offered laparoscopy. However, it is worth noting that 5% of patients with normal HSG will reveal a pathology after performing a laparoscopy.[27] Falloposcopy is a procedure which allows the transvaginal microendoscopic visualization of the whole interior of the fallopian tubes. It provides information about the tubal mucosa and the presence of any obstruction as well as the opportunity to cannulate the tube to overcome the obstruction. Its high expenses and technical difficulties limit its use in the clinical practice.[28,29]

Tubal Reconstructive Surgeries

Although several surgical procedures have been proposed to correct or enhance tubal patency, the new era of IVF made their use limited. However, properly selected subjects may still benefit from tubal reconstructive surgery, especially with selecting the proper procedure and optimum technique.

In cases of tubal infection, the resultant damage of the epithelial lining negatively affects the results of reconstructive surgery. On the other hand, reversal of sterilization is considered the most common indication for surgical reconstruction since most patients are young and only segmental damage is present. These factors denote high chances of conception afterwards. Sterilization using a Filshie clip is the most easily reversible as a small portion of the tube is damaged and it gives excellent results that could match an IVF trial. Pregnancy rates may reach 86%, while ectopic pregnancies are as low as 7%.[30]

The type of surgery used will depend on the *site* and *extent* of tubal damage. In cases of adhesions involving the tube and ovary, salpingo-ovariolysis can be performed laparoscopically. The reported pregnancy rates are from 51 to 62% for intrauterine pregnancies and 5 to 8% for ectopic pregnancies.[31] If the fimbrial end is agglutinated or shows fimbrial phimosis, fimbrioplasty can be performed with intrauterine pregnancies ranging from 40 to 48% and ectopic pregnancies from 5 to 6%.[26] On the other hand, distention of the tube with hydrosalpinx can be managed surgically by either tubal occlusion (disconnection), tubal removal (salpingectomy) or making a new tubal ostium (salpingostomy). In cases with mild hydrosalpinx, salpingostomy yields 40–60% pregnancy rates which decline to 20% with more severe affection.[31] Dilated tubes >3 cm with thick walls and damaged mucosa, will have a poor benefit from distal tubal surgeries and are best offered IVF treatment.[32] Disconnecting the tube before an IVF cycle is now the most accepted practice as it prevents spillage of toxic fluid into the uterine cavity which might kill the transferred embryos.[33] Occlusion can be done using Filshie clips or by bipolar diathermy and cutting the tube. In both cases, the site of occlusion must be medial to the proximal end of the hydrosalpinx and as close to the uterus as possible to avoid any residual part connecting to the uterus.

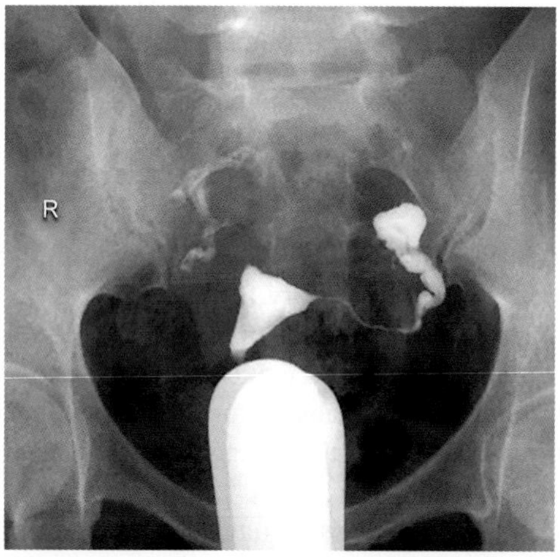

Fig. 2: Hysterosalpingography showing proximal block of right tube and distal block of the left tube.

Cases with proximal tubal block should be offered hysteroscopic tubal cannulation to overcome mild occlusions with mucous plugs.[34] However, true occlusions may be offered tubocornual anastomosis using microsurgical techniques. Intrauterine pregnancy rates may reach 56% and ectopic pregnancies up to 7%.[35] Combined proximal and distal diseases carry a poor prognosis after surgical repair. One study showed no live births after a 2-year follow-up.[30] Thus, such patients should be offered IVF.

Tubal Reanastomosis

When comparing open to laparoscopic approaches for reversal of sterilization, a meta-analysis reveals no significant difference in the rates of intrauterine and ectopic pregnancies. While laparoscopic approach is associated with less postoperative pain and rapid recovery, it took significantly longer operative time.[36] Robotic reanastomosis also had similar pregnancy rates as laparotomies but took longer and costed much higher.[37]

Chromopertubation of the tube may help identify the site of obstruction. The tube is transected using the microscissors just adjacent to the affected site. The incision should not reach the mesosalpinx as not to disrupt the vascular arcade of the adjacent segment. Throughout the procedure, meticulous hemostasis is essential. However, stoppage of unnecessary bleeders will devitalize the healthy tubal mucosa. If unhealthy mucosa is encountered, 1–2 mm thick segments are cut until the healthy mucosa is visible. The two ends are approximated in two layers: (1) musculosa and (2) serosa. The first suture is the most posterior at 6 o'clock. Usually four sutures are enough to hold both ends together. Then, the serosa is sutured in the same manner. The suture material used is usually 7-0 or 8-0 Vicryl or polydioxanone (PDS).[38,39] While some prefer using splint to facilitate tubal reanastomosis,[40] others recommend not using it as it might damage the tubal epithelium and reduce the success of the procedure. After finishing the procedure on both sides, chromopertubation is performed to ensure a watertight suture line. A more recent technique is called the sutureless laparoscopic reanastomosis where a 3-mm microclip is used to fix the seromuscularis with the addition of a biological glue. The 40-month cumulative clinical pregnancy rate was 74%, whereas the ongoing pregnancy rate was 59% and the ectopic pregnancy rates were 3.9%.[41]

Tubal reconstructive surgeries should follow the microsurgical principles. Microsurgery does not involve only the use of microscope, it is considered a surgical behavior with certain principles and approaches. The following are the important parameters in the microsurgery:[36]

- Delicate tissue handling with minimal injury and thorough hemostasis.
- Avoid foreign body contamination. Surgeons may wash their gloves before handling the cover sheets and may also change their gloves before handling the patient.
- Proper identification of anatomical plans and exact alignment of tissues.
- Proper tissue irrigation and peritoneal lavage using heparinized Ringer's lactate solution.
- The use of microscopic magnification to properly handle the tissues and surgical instruments.

Factors Affecting Surgery Outcome

Many factors were reported to have an impact on the success of tubal reconstruction. These include patient's age, length of fallopian tube, type of sterilization, and site of anastomosis. The older the woman undergoing reconstruction, the less likely she will conceive after having the surgery.[42,43] In one study, pregnancy rates after tubal reanastomosis decreased from 81% in patients below 36 years to 12.5% in patients above 43 years.[43] Pregnancy rates also decreased in cases with short fallopian tubes, especially below 4 cm in length.[40,42] Clip sterilization gave the best results after reversal followed by the ring sterilization, then coagulation, and Pomeroy sterilization.[43] The site of anastomosis influences the success of the surgery, and the best results in descending order were seen in the ampullo-ampullar, isthmo-isthmic, isthmo-cornual, isthmic-ampullary then ampullo-cornual anastomoses. In addition, ectopic pregnancy rates rise in the same order.[43] It appears that less the discrepancy between the diameters of both ends, the better the results.

Management of Hydrosalpinx

In the beginning of IVF era, tubal factor infertility was the sole indication for treatment. It is said that tubal factor infertility often yields worse results than other causes of infertility. Pregnancy rates were significantly lower (15%) in patients with visible hydrosalpinges compared with patients in whom the hydrosalpinges were not visible (31%). (CITE)

Treatment includes salpingectomy, tubal ligation, and transvaginal aspiration. Salpingectomy is the only method of prophylactic surgery in patients with hydrosalpinx that has been properly evaluated in a large randomized trial (CITE). Clinical pregnancy rates were 46 versus 22% in salpingectomized patients versus patients without any surgical intervention.

Other surgeries include laparoscopy with proximal ligation and salpingostomy. The procedure is currently recommended when pelvic adhesions are too extensive to perform a salpingectomy.

Salpingostomy is the method of choice if the tube is suitable for reconstructive surgery. However selection of patient is crucial. The selection of patients suitable for surgical repair has to be based on the evaluation of the tubal mucosa through an endoscopic technique, and tubes with more than half of the mucosa in a good condition may have a fair chance of spontaneous conception.

Transvaginal aspiration of hydrosalpinx is a simple method but leads to rapid recurrence of fluid (34%). To overcome the problem of the high recurrence rate after transvaginal aspiration of hydrosalpinx fluid, ethanol sclerotherapy has been introduced.

RECONSTRUCTION OF DISTORTED UTERINE CAVITY

Uterine cavity is the site where the embryo will implant and grow. Any distortion of this cavity will impair fertility and interfere with the completion of pregnancy. Uterine cavity can be distorted by many intracavitary lesions including endometrial polyps, submucous myomas, intrauterine synechia (Asherman syndrome) and uterine anomalies. Hysteroscopy provides a reliable modality not only for the diagnosis of these lesions but also for the reconstruction of the uterine cavity and treating such lesions.

UTERINE SEPTUM

A uterine septum is the most common uterine anomaly accounting for >50% of all uterine anomalies.[44] Its exact incidence in the general population cannot be determined accurately as many cases are asymptomatic. It results from failure of resorption of the part between the two Müllerian ducts during embryological development **(Fig. 3)**.

Several mechanisms have been postulated to explain the possible adverse impact of the uterine septum on reproduction. Based on the observation made by histopathology and color Doppler imaging that a uterine septum is made up of myometrial tissue and connective tissue, it was proposed that a septum creates irregular contractile patterns that expels an implanted embryo or

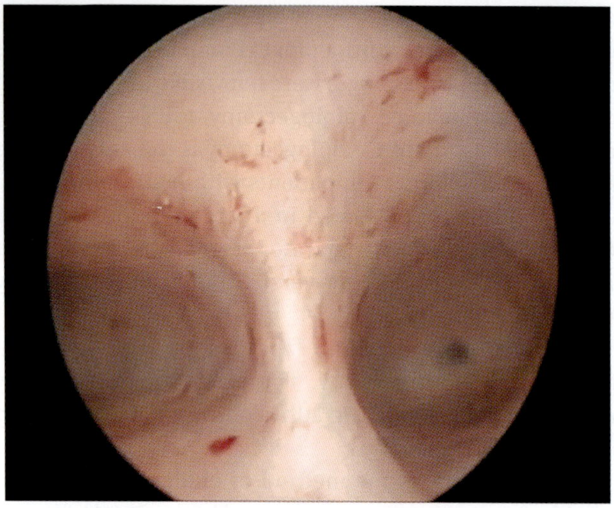

Fig. 3: Hysteroscopic view of a septate uterus.

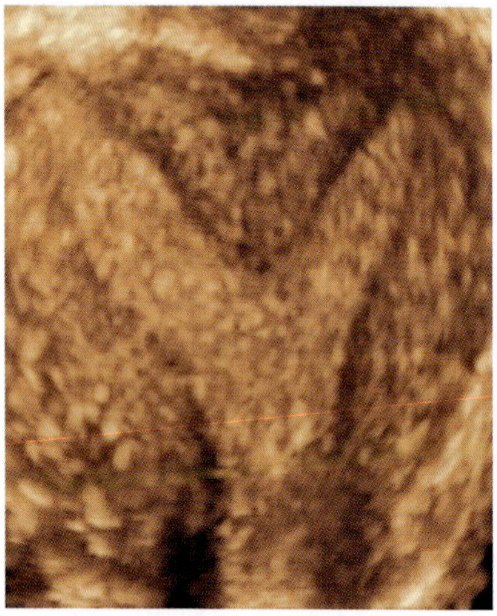

Fig. 4: 3D ultrasonography showing septate uterus.

prevents its implantation.[45] Another study showed that the endometrium overlying the septum is poor in hormonal receptivity which might waver its ability to accept embryos.[46] Being poor in blood supply may explain the cause of repeated spontaneous abortions.[47]

Diagnosis

Accurate diagnosis of a septate uterus is mandatory before considering treating it. The main challenge in diagnosing a septate uterus is differentiating it from bicornuate uterus which has a totally different plan of management. HSG is an easy and simple method for suspecting uterine anomaly. However, its accuracy reaches 55% only in differentiating between septate and bicornuate uterus as the fundus cannot be seen.[48] If a uterus is not well erected during an HSG, a small septum might be missed. More recently, 3D ultrasound was found to be extremely accurate in differentiating between septate and bicornuate uterus[49] and more accurate and cost-effective than HSG[50] **(Fig. 4)**. Before the availability of 3D ultrasound, laparoscopy used to be the gold standard for differentiating between a septate uterus and a bicornuate uterus.

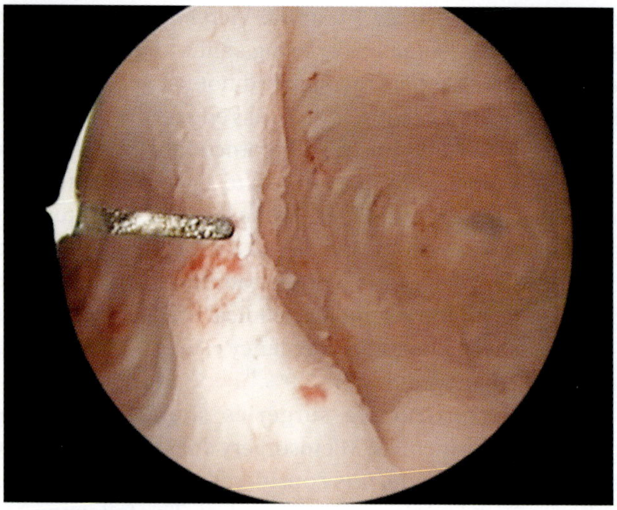

Fig. 5: Hysteroscopic septum resection by Collins knife electrode.

Septum Resection

Historically, Tompkins or Jones procedure was done which involved a laparotomy and excision of the septum, thus necessitating a cesarean section at delivery. Nowadays, hysteroscopy replaces such outdated operations. A hysteroscopic procedure merely incises the septum instead of resecting it. The septal tissues will then retract and the endometrium will heal over it within two cycles. A septum may be incised by scissors, laser, or electrosurgery. No evidence proves the superiority of one method over the other. However, a monopolar electrode requires an electrolyte-free medium which has its own drawbacks as hyponatremia and volume overload, while bipolar electrodes require an electrolyte-containing media which only causes volume overload in lengthy operations **(Fig. 5)**.

Postoperative Treatment

In the past, intrauterine devices were placed and estrogen therapy was given for several months after metroplasty to prevent formation of adhesions. Several studies proved that they have no role in preventing adhesions and do not improve pregnancy outcomes later on.[51,52] Follow-up is by ultrasound or hysteroscopy 1–2 months after metroplasty. The chance that a patient might need a second procedure to incise residual septum is 6%.[53]

Outcome

It has been proved that metroplasty improves the pregnancy rates, live birth rates (LBRs), and reduces abortion rates. In a recent retrospective cohort study over 1,501 women, pregnancy rates were 60% and a LBR was 45%.[49] Metroplasty improves pregnancy outcomes in patients with recurrent spontaneous abortions[53,54] and in unexplained infertility.[55,56] Incising a uterine septum improves the results of IVF or intracytoplasmic sperm injection (ICSI) cycles and makes them almost the same as an anomaly-free uterus.[57]

INTRAUTERINE ADHESIONS

Intrauterine adhesions (IUAs) or synechia are the bands of fibrous tissue that form within the uterine cavity resulting in distortion of the cavity with subsequent impairment of reproduction and menstrual patterns **(Fig. 6)**. >90% of IUA occurs following over curettage.[58,59] Usually, it occurs following postpartum or postabortive excessive bleeding. Curettage erodes the basal endometrial layer leaving it exposed which in turn heals by fibrous tissue formation. Other causes include abdominal metroplasties and myomectomies, but here misplaced sutures are more responsible for the adhesions rather than the procedure itself. Rarely, endometrial tuberculosis destroys the uterine lining which heals thereafter by secondary intention forming IUA. Another growing cause in the developing world is abuse of C-sections and misplaced sutures and infections resulting in IUA. The occurrence of amenorrhea following curettage for incomplete or missed abortion and postpartum hemorrhage has been described as Asherman syndrome.[59]

Diagnosis

Intrauterine adhesions should be suspected whenever a patient presents with amenorrhea, hypomenorrhea or infertility following a history of endometrial trauma after delivery or abortion. IUA may present with pregnancy morbidities, e.g., abortion, ectopic pregnancy, preterm labor, or even placenta accreta. HSG may show a small, fragmented, and distorted uterine cavity as a result of IUAs. Using ultrasonography, echogenic foci detected within endometrial lining may point to the presence of IUAs.[60]

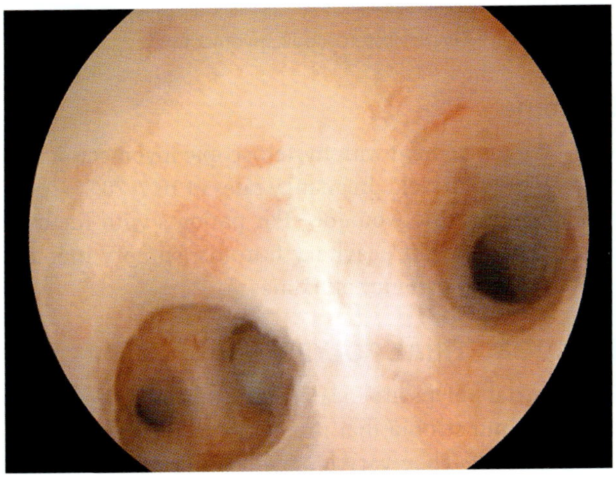

Fig. 6: Hysteroscopic view of intrauterine adhesions.

No worldwide consensus is made on the classification of IUAs. The ASRM[12] proposed a classification depending on the findings of HSG and hysteroscopy. Another classification divides IUA into central (Degree I), marginal (Degree II) and absent uterine cavity by HSG (Degree III).[61] IUAs can be classified as well into mild, moderate, and severe adhesions.[58]

- *Mild:* Filmy adhesions, partially or completely occluding the cavity
- *Moderate:* Fibromuscular adhesions (connective tissue covered by endometrial tissue), partially or completely occluding the cavity
- *Severe:* Connective tissue only (not covered by endometrial tissue), partially or completely occluding the cavity.

Hysteroscopic Adhesiolysis for Restoration of the Uterine Cavity

Historically, curettes, probes, dilator, and open hysterotomy were used to cut the adhesions but these methods had high morbidities and poor results. Currently, operative hysteroscopy is considered the gold standard approach. Filmy adhesions can be cut by the mere push of the hysteroscope. Division of more dense adhesions can be achieved with the use of semi-rigid scissors introduced through the operative sheath of hysteroscope with no risk of bleeding since most adhesions are avascular. Alternatively, resectoscope can be used to divide IUAs with loop, knife, or needle electrodes, though the effectiveness of the current on what remains of the endometrium is debatable and more studies are needed to prove if electrosurgery has a role in advanced Asherman syndrome. Fiberoptic lasers such as neodymium doped yttrium-aluminum-garnet (Nd:YAG), KTP/532, or argon can be used to divide IUAs. It can be used to selectively divide lateral and fundal adhesions due to its flexibility.[62] Laser can be used in electrolyte-containing media. Although, hemostasis is excellent with the use of electrocautery or laser, their use may cause damage to adjacent healthy endometrium. Also, they may lead to over division with increased risk of uterine perforation. Thus, some recommend the performance of concomitant laparoscope to guide the hysteroscopic division of IUAs. Following hysteroscopic adhesiolysis, the uterine wall should be kept separate from each other using either a pediatric 8F Foley catheter[9] or intrauterine devices.[63,64] Postoperative estrogen or estrogen and progesterone are given to promote growth of the endometrium.[9,63,64]

Outcome

Restoration of menses and reproductive outcome correlates well with the severity of IUA. Normal menstruation is restored in about 90% of cases.[58,65,66] Highest pregnancy rates are achieved after mild adhesions and lower in moderate and severe adhesions.[58,67,68]

SUBMUCOUS MYOMAS

The incidence of myomata in infertile women without any obvious cause of infertility is estimated to be between 1 and 2.4%[63] **(Fig. 7)**. Different theories have been suggested to explain how myomata can impair the fertility potential. The anatomical location of a myoma plays an important role with submucous myomata most commonly implicated followed by intramural and subserous myomas. Myomas may cause abnormal uterine contractility which may interfere with sperm migration and ovum transport.[69] Also, it has been postulated that myomata may be associated with implantation failure or gestation discontinuation due to focal endometrial vascular disturbance, endometrial inflammation, secretion of vasoactive substances, or an enhanced endometrial androgen environment.[70]

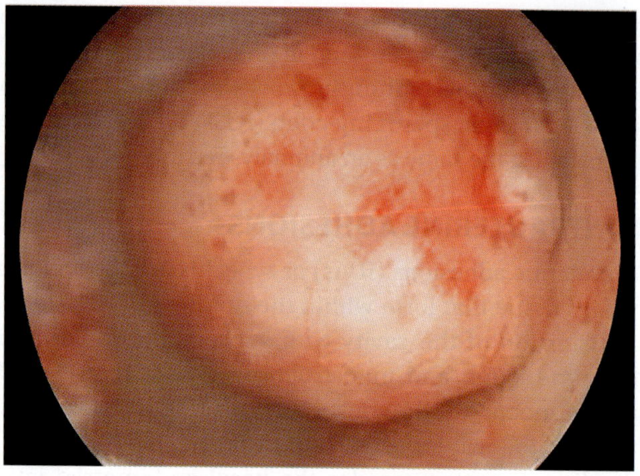

Fig. 7: Submucous myoma.

Preoperative Evaluation

The comprehensive preoperative evaluation of submucous myoma would entail the use of ultrasonography, sonohysterography, and hysteroscopy to determine the *number, size, location, degree of intramural extension of the submucous myomas* as well as *the distance between the myoma and the serosa*. Wamsteker et al.[70] classified submucous myomata according to the degree of intramural growth into three categories; (1) grade 0 (myoma with no intramural extension), (2) grade 1 (myoma with intramural part <50%), and (3) grade 2 (myoma with intramural part ≥50%). This classification was adopted by the European Society for Gynecological Endoscopy (ESGE) and is widely used by hysteroscopists **(Table 2)**.

TABLE 2: European Society for Gynecological Endoscopy classification of submucous myomas.

Grade	*Degree of intramyometrial growth*
0	No intramural extension (myoma is completely within the uterine cavity)
1	Intramural part <50%
2	Intramural part ≥50%

Hysteroscopic Myomectomy

Traditionally, symptomatic submucous myomata in infertile women were treated surgically by abdominal myomectomy. This approach requires an opening of the uterine cavity which may compromise any future parturition as it requires cesarean delivery; moreover, it may lead to the development of pelvic postoperative adhesions which may further reduce rather than enhance fertility.[71,72] Operative hysteroscopy has recently provided a better alternative for resection of submucous myomata transcervically, thus, avoiding the drawbacks of laparotomy and uterine incision. Many techniques have been described, however, the standard technique entails slicing of the submucous myoma from its top toward its base using the cutting loop of the resectoscope.

Using this technique, an intracavitary myoma is repeatedly and progressively shaved till its bases[73] **(Fig. 8)**. The resulting fragments can be pushed away from the myoma till they interfere with proper visualization, and then the fragments can be removed by withdrawing the resectoscope with its loop electrode grasping the loose fragment.

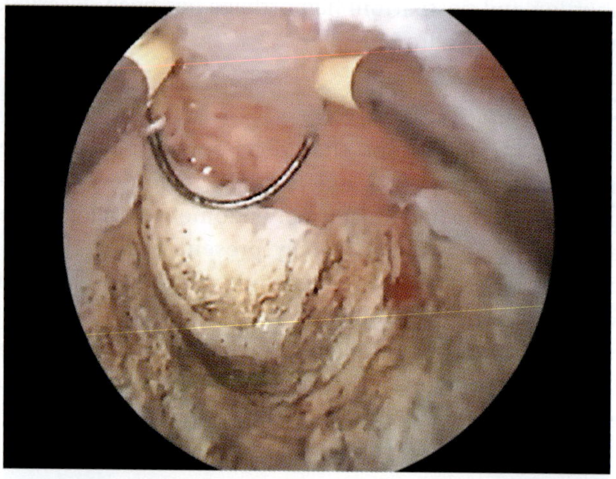

Fig. 8: Hysteroscopic myomectomy.

Outcome

Surgical management with hysteroscopic myomectomy has been reported to yield pregnancy rates of 16.7–76.9% (mean of 45%) in infertile women.[74] For patients with recurrent miscarriage and intracavitary fibroids, surgery increases rates of viable pregnancy outcomes.[75]

ENDOMETRIAL POLYPS

Endometrial polyps are localized hyperplastic overgrowths of glands and stroma that project form the surface of the endometrium. They vary in size from few millimeters to few centimeters and when large enough they can protrude

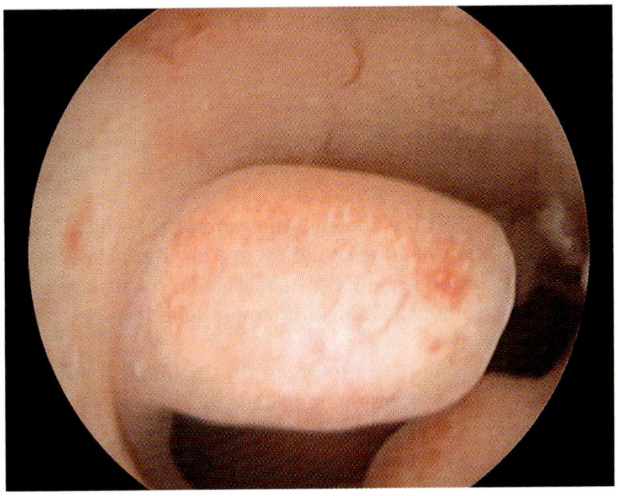

Fig. 9: Sessile endometrial polyp.

through the cervix. They may be single or multiple (polypoid endometrium), sessile or pedunculated, and may rarely include foci of neoplastic growth[2] **(Fig. 9)**. Endometrial polyps have been accused of causing infertility. Although the precise mechanism by which they do is unclear, it has been shown in a larger series that hysteroscopic polypectomy improves fertility and increases pregnancy rates, irrespective of the size, or the number of the polyps.[8] Hysteroscopy can precisely identify number, location, size of endometrial polyps, and presence of any suspicious features. It can also resect these lesions for pathological examination replacing the formal dilatation and curettage (D and C), as D and C has been reported that about 10% of polyps remain in situ after curettage.[16,17,76-82] Hysteroscopic resection currently represents the gold standard in the treatment of endometrial polyps[19] since it allows there complete removal under visual control preventing persistence or recurrence of these lesions. Resection of endometrial polyps under direct hysteroscopic visualization can be achieved with the use of different methods either using mechanical instruments or electrosurgery or more recently, intrauterine morcellator.

KEY POINTS

- Pelvic adhesions are commonly caused by PID and best treated by laparoscopy.
- AFS adhesion scoring system is a reliable method for choosing the management and predicting the outcome.
- Reversal of sterilization may give results similar to IVF while women with severe tubal damage are best offered IVF.
- While laparoscope is the golden standard for diagnosing a uterine septum, 3D ultrasound is as almost as accurate.
- Adhesiolysis is best done by scissors, and outcome depends on severity.
- Submucous myomas are divided into grades 0, 1, and 2, and are removed by resectoscope.
- Although the mechanism of infertility in endometrial polyps is not exactly known, their removal is important using hysteroscope instead of D and C.

MULTIPLE CHOICE QUESTIONS

1. Most common cause of pelvic adhesions is:
   a. Laparotomies   b. Endometriosis
   c. Chlamydia infection   d. Irradiation
2. Severe tubal disease is best managed by:
   a. IVF
   b. Adhesiolysis
   c. Tubal reanastomosis surgeries
   d. Tubal cannulation
3. Which of the following is not true concerning the adhesion scoring system of the American Fertility Society?
   a. Depends on the site and thickness of the adhesions
   b. Outcome depends on the pathology of the less affected side
   c. Not very accurate in predicting pregnancy rates
   d. The denser the adhesions, the higher the score
4. Which of the following is true about adhesiolysis?
   a. Open and laparoscopic approaches give almost the same results
   b. Has the same outcome regardless of the severity of the adhesions
   c. Second look laparoscopy after adhesiolysis improves pregnancy outcomes
   d. Mainly aims at restoring the anatomic relation between the tube and ovary
5. Concerning tubal blockage, the following are true except:
   a. A normal HSG cancels the benefit of a diagnostic laparoscope
   b. Highest rates of success of reconstructive surgery follow reversal of sterilization
   c. A remaining fallopian tube <4 cm usually carries a poor prognosis
   d. Laparoscopic reconstruction carries the same results as open reconstruction but takes more time to finish and learn
6. A uterine septum may cause abortion or infertility by all the following methods except:
   a. Low receptivity of the endometrium
   b. High vascularity on the septum
   c. Irregular contraction of the myometrial fibers of the septum
   d. Unknown mechanism
7. Which of the following is true about a uterine septum?
   a. 2D ultrasound can diagnose almost as accurate as 3D ultrasound
   b. Removed by excised instead of incised septum
   c. Hysteroscopic approach necessitates a cesarean delivery afterward
   d. Increases pregnancy rates as high as 60%

8. All of the following about intrauterine synechia is true except:
   a. Excessive curettage is the most common cause
   b. Best diagnosed by hysteroscopy
   c. Adhesiolysis best done by laser
   d. 9 out of 10 patients will regain menstruation after adhesiolysis
9. Concerning hysteroscopic myomectomy, which of the following is not true?
   a. Removed by shaving the myoma using a resectoscope
   b. Grade 2 myoma is the easiest in removal
   c. Care should be taken during long procedures to avoid volume overload
   d. Improves pregnancy rates as well as reduces rates of miscarriage
10. Concerning endometrial polyp, the following are false except:
   a. D and C is a method of management but 10% of the polyps may be missed
   b. Must be removed with scissors
   c. Considered a definite cause of infertility
   d. Only multiple polyps should be removed

ANSWERS

1. c	2. a	3. c	4. d
5. a	6. b	7. d	8. c
9. b	10. a		

REFERENCES

1. Luijendijk RW, de Lange DC, Wauters CC, Hop WC, Duron JJ, Pailler JL, et al. Foreign material in postoperative adhesions. Ann Surg. 1996;223:(3)242-8.
2. Caspi E, Halperin Y, Bukovski I. The importance of periadnexal adhesions in tubal reconstruction surgery for infertility. Fertil Steril. 1979;31(3):296-300.
3. Cheong YC, Laird SM, Li TC, Shelton JB, Ledger WL, Cooke ID. Peritoneal healing and adhesion formation/reformation. Hum Reprod Update. 2001;7(6):556-66.
4. Monk BJ, Berman ML, Montz FJ. Adhesions after extensive gynecologic surgery: clinical significance, etiology, and prevention. Am J Obstet Gynecol. 1994;170(5Pt1):1396-403.
5. Levrant SG, Bieber EJ, Barnes RB. Anterior abdominal wall adhesions after laparotomy or laparoscopy. J Am Assoc Gynecol Laparosc. 1997;4(3):353-6.
6. Dubuisson J, Botchorishvili R, Perrette S, Bourdel N, Jardon K, Rabischong B, et al. Incidence of intraabdominal adhesions in a continuous series of 1000 laparoscopic procedures. Am J Obstet Gynecol. 2010;203(2):111.e1-3.
7. Ellis H. The clinical significance of adhesions: focus on intestinal obstruction. Eur J Surg Suppl. 1997;577:5-9.
8. Stricker B, Blanco J, Fox HE. The gynecologic contribution to intestinal obstruction in females. J Am Coll Surg. 1994;178(6):617-20.
9. Nezhat C, Nezhat F, Nezhat C. Nezhat's Operative Gynecologic Laparoscopy and Hysteroscopy, 3rd edition. Cambridge: Cambridge University Press; 2008.
10. Mahadevan MM, Wiseman D, Leader A, Taylor PJ. The effects of ovarian adhesive disease upon follicular development in cycles of controlled stimulation for in vitro fertilization. Fertil Steril. 1985;44(4):489-92.
11. Hulka JF, Omran K, Berger GS. Classification of adnexal adhesions: a proposal and evaluation of its prognostic value. Fertil Steril. 1978;30(6):661-5.
12. American Fertility Society. The American Fertility Society classification of adnexal adhesions, distal tubal occlusion, tubal occlusion secondary to tubal ligation, tubal pregnancies, Mullerian anomalies and intrauterine adhesions. Fertil Steril. 1988;49:944-55.
13. Mage G, Pouly JL, de Joliniere JB, Chabrand S, Riouallon A, Bruhat MA. A preoperative classification to predict the intrauterine and ectopic pregnancy rates after distal tubal microsurgery. Fertil Steril. 1986;461:807-10.
14. Nagata Y, Honjou K, Shindou M, Kawarabayashi T, Shirakawa K. The effects of periovarian adhesions in human programs IVF-ET. J Fertil Implant (Tokyo). 1997;14:54-7.
15. Gomel V, Erenus M. Prognostic value of the American Fertility Society's (AFS) classification for distal tubal occlusion. Fertil Steril. 1990;64(Suppl l):97-106.
16. Nagata Y, Honjou K, Shindou M. Alternate prognostic classification for adnexal adhesions divided into peritubal adhesion and periovarian adhesion: Severe periovarian adhesions were the major cause of infertility. Fertil Steril. 1997;68(Suppl. l):90-135.
17. Nezhat C, Winer WK, Cooper JD, Nezhat F, Nezhat C. Endoscopic infertility surgery. J Reprod Med. 1989; 34(2):127-34.
18. Tulandi T, Collins JA, Burrows E, Jarrell JF, McInnes RA, Wrixon W, et al. Treatment-dependent and treatment-independent pregnancy among women with periadnexal adhesions. Am J Obstet Gynecol. 1990;162:354-7.
19. El Sahwi S. Laparoscopic pelvic adhesiolysis using CO_2 laser. J Am Assoc Gynecol Laparosc. 1994;1(4):10-1.
20. Johnson NP, Watson A. Cochrane review: post-operative procedures for improving fertility following pelvic reproductive surgery. Hum Reprod Update. 2000;6(3): 259-67.
21. Morassutto C, Monasta L, Ricci G, Barbone F, Ronfani L. Incidence and estimated prevalence of endometriosis and adenomyosis in Northeast Italy: a data linkage study. PLoS One. 2016;11(4):e0154227.
22. Celik O, Unlu C, Otlu B, Celik N, Caliskan E. Laparoscopic endometrioma resection increases peri-implantation endometrial HOXA-10 and HOXA-11 mRNA expression. Fertil Steril. 2015;104(2):356-65.
23. Streuli I, de Ziegler D, Gayet V, Santulli P, Bijaoui G, de Mouzon J, et al. In women with endometriosis anti-Müllerian hormone levels are decreased only in those with previous endometrioma surgery. Hum Reprod. 2012;27:3294-303.
24. Celik HG, Dogan E, Okyay E, Ulukus C, Saatli B, Uysal S, et al. Effect of laparoscopic excision of endometriomas on ovarian reserve: serial changes in the serum antimüllerian hormone levels. Fertil Steril. 2012;97(6):1472-8.
25. Coccia ME, Rizzello F. Impact of large ovarian endometriomas on the response to superovulation for in vitro fertilization: A retrospective study. Eur J Obstet Gynecol Reprod Biol. 2017;216:263-4.

26. Centers of Disease Control and Prevention. (2016). Sexually Transmitted Disease Surveillance 2016. [online] Available from: https://www.cdc.gov/std/stats16/CDC_2016_STDS_Report-for508WebSep21_2017_1644.pdf. [Last accessed November, 2022].
27. Swart P, Mol BW, van der Veen F, van Beurden M, Redekop WK, Bossuyt PM. The accuracy of hysterosalpingography in the diagnosis of tubal pathology: a meta-analysis. Fertil Steril. 1995;64(3):486-91.
28. Lundberg S, Rasmussen C, Berg AA, Lindblom B. Falloposcopy in conjunction with laparoscopy: possibilities and limitations. Hum Reprod. 1998;13(6):1490-2.
29. Rimbach S, Bastert G, Wallwiener D. Technical results of falloposcopy for infertility diagnosis in a large multicentre study. Hum Reprod. 2001;16(5):925-30.
30. Hanafi MM. Factors affecting the pregnancy rate after microsurgcal reversal of tubal ligation. Fertil Steril. 2003; 80(2):434-40.
31. Rock JA, Jones III HW. Te Linde's Operative Gynecology, 10th edition. Philadelphia: Lippincott Williams & Wilkins; 2008.
32. Hull MG, Fleming CF. Tubal surgery versus assisted reproduction: assessing their role in infertility therapy. Curr Opin Obstet Gynecol. 1995;7(3):160-7.
33. Johnson NP, Mak W, Sowter MC. Surgical treatment for tubal disease in women due to undergo in vitro fertilisation. Cochrane Database Syst Rev. 2004;(3):CD002125.
34. National Institute for Health and Clinical Excellence. Fertility: Assessment and Treatment for People with Fertility Problems. London, UK: RCOG Press; 2004.
35. Patton PE, Williams TJ, Coulam CB. Results of microsurgical reconstruction in patients with combined proximal and distal tubal occlusion: double obstruction. Fertil Steril. 1987;48(4):670-4.
36. la Grange J, Kruger TF, Steyn DW, van der Merwe JP, Siebert I, Matsaseng T, et al. Fallopian tube reanastomosis by laparotomy versus laparoscopy: a meta-analysis. Gynecol Obstet Invest. 2012;74(1):28-34.
37. Rodgers AK, Goldberg JM, Hammel JP, Falcone T. Tubal anastomosis by robotic compared with outpatient mini-laparotomy. Obstet Gynecol. 2007;109(6):1375-80.
38. Cha SH, Lee MH, Kim JH, Lee CN, Yoon TK, Cha KY. Fertility outcome after tubal anastomosis by laparoscopy and laparotomy. J Am Assoc Gynecol Laparosc. 2001; 8(3):348-5.
39. Gomel V. Tubal reanastomosis by microsurgery. Fertil Steril. 1977;28(1):59-65.
40. Kim SH, Shin CJ, Kim JG, Moon SY, Lee JY, Chang YS. Microsurgical reversal of tubal sterilization: a report on 1,118 cases. Fertil Steril. 1997;68(5):865-70.
41. Schepens JJ, Mol BW, Wiegerinck MA, Houterman S, Koks CA. Pregnancy outcomes and prognostic factors from tubal sterilization reversal by sutureless laparoscopical re-anastomosis: a retrospective cohort study. Hum Reprod. 2011;26(2):354-9.
42. Rouzi AA, Mackinnon M, McComb PF. Predictors of success of reversal of sterilization. Fertil Steril. 1995; 64(1):29-36.
43. Gordts S, Campo R, Puttemans P, Gordts S. Clinical factors determining pregnancy outcome after microsurgical tubal reanastomosis. Fertil Steril. 2009;92(4):1198-202.
44. Troiano RN. Magnetic resonance imaging of mullerian duct anomalies of the uterus. Top Magn Reson Imaging. 2003;14:269-79.
45. Sparac V, Kupesic S, Ilijas M, Zodan T, Kurjak A. Histologic architecture and vascularization of hysteroscopically excised intrauterine septa. J Am Assoc Gynecol Laparosc. 2001;8:111-6.
46. Fedele L, Bianchi S, Marchini M, Franchi D, Tozzi L, Dorta M. Ultrastructural aspects of endometrium in infertile women with septate uterus. Fertil Steril. 1996;65:750-2.
47. Burchell RC, Creed F, Rasoulpour M, Whitcomb M. Vascular anatomy of the human uterus and pregnancy wastage. Br J Obstet Gynaecol. 1978;85:698-706.
48. Reuter KL, Daly DC, Cohen SM. Septate versus bicornuate uteri: errors in imaging diagnosis. Radiology. 1989;172(3):749-52.
49. Faivre E, Fernandez H, Deffieux X, Gervaise A, Frydman R, Levaillant JM. Accuracy of three—dimensional ultrasonography in differential diagnosis of septate and bicornuate uterus compared with office hysteroscopy and pelvic magnetic resonance imaging. J Minim Invasive Gynecol. 2012;19(1):101-6.
50. Bocca SM, Oehninger S, Stadtmauer L, Agard J, Duran EH, Sarhan A, et al. A study of the cost, accuracy, and benefits of 3-dimensional sonography compared with hysterosalpingography in women with uterine abnormalities. J Ultrasound Med. 2012;31(1):81-5.
51. Dabirashrafi H, Mohammad K, Moghadami-Tabrizi N, Zandinejad K, Moghadami-Tabrizi M. Is estrogen necessary after hysteroscopic incision of the uterine septum? J Am Assoc Gynecol Laparosc. 1996;3(4):623-5.
52. Nawroth F, Schmidt T, Freise C, Foth D, Römer T. Is it possible to recommend an "optimal" postoperative management after hysteroscopic metroplasty? A retrospective study with 52 infertile patients showing a septate uterus. Acta Obstet Gynecol Scand. 2002;81(1):55-7.
53. Nouri K, Ott J, Huber JC, Fischer E-M, Stögbauer L, Tempfer CB. Reproductive outcome after hysteroscopic septoplasty in patients with septate uterus—a retrospective cohort study and systematic review of the literature. Reprod Biol Endocrinol. 2010;8:52.
54. Valli E, Vaquero E, Lazzarin N, Caserta D, Marconi D, Zupi E. Hysteroscopic metroplasty improves gestational outcome in women with recurrent spontaneous abortion. J Am Assoc Gynecol Laparosc. 2004;11(2):240-4.
55. Pabuccu R, Gomel V. Reproductive outcome after hysteroscopic metroplasty in women with septate uterus and otherwise unexplained infertility. Fertil Steril. 2004;81(6):1675-8.
56. Bakas P, Gregoriou O, Hassiakos D, Liapis A, Creatsas M, Konidaris S. Hysteroscopic resection of uterine septum and reproductive outcome in women with unexplained infertility. Gynecol Obstet Invest. 2012;73(4):321-5.
57. Tomaževič T, Ban-Frangež H, Virant-Klun I, Verdenik I, Požlep B, Vrtačnik-Bokal E. Septate, subseptate and arcuate uterus decrease pregnancy and live birth rates in IVF/ICSI. Reprod Biomed Online. 2010;21(5):700-5.
58. Valle RF, Sciarra JJ. Intrauterine adhesions: hysteroscopic diagnosis, classification, treatment, and reproductive outcome. Am J Obstet Gynecol. 1988;158(6Pt1):1459-70.
59. Asherman JG. Amenorrhea traumatica (atretica). J Obset Gynaecol Br Emp. 1948;55:23-30.

60. Confino E, Friberg J, Giglia RV, Gleicher N. Sonographic imaging of intrauterine adhesions. Obstet Gynecol. 1985;66: 596-8.
61. Neuwirth RS, Hussein AR, Schiffman BM, Amin HK. Hysteroscopic resection of intrauterine scars using a new technique. Obstet Gynecol. 1982;60:111-3.
62. Donnez J. Atlas of Operative Laparoscopy and Hysteroscopy, 3rd edition. London: Informa UK Ltd.; 2007.
63. Pabuccu R, Onalan G, Kaya C, Selam B, Ceyhan T, Ornek T, et al. Efficiency and pregnancy outcome of serial intrauterine device-guided hysteroscopic adhesiolysis of intrauterine synechiae. Fertil Steril. 2008;90(5):1973-7.
64. March CM, Israel R. Gestational outcome following hysteroscopic lysis of adhesions. Fertil Steril. 1981;36(4):455-9.
65. Preutthipan S, Linasmita V. Reproductive outcome following hysteroscopic lysis of intrauterine adhesions: a result of 65 cases at Ramathibodi Hospital. J Med Assoc Thai. 2000; 83(1):42-6.
66. Roy KK, Baruah J, Sharma JB, Kumar S, Kachawa G, Singh N. Reproductive outcome following hysteroscopic adhesiolysis in patients with infertility due to Asherman's syndrome. Arch Gynecol Obstet. 2010;281(2):355-61.
67. Verkauf BS. Myomectomy for fertility enhancement and preservation. Fertil Steril. 1992;58(1):1-15.
68. Vollenhoven BJ, Lawrence AS, Healy DL. Uterine fibroids: a clinical review. Br J Obstet Gynaecol. 1990;97(4):285-98.
69. Buttram VC Jr, Reiter RC. Uterine leiomyomata: etiology, symptomatology, and management. Fertil Steril. 1981; 36(4):433-45.
70. Wamsteker K, Emanuel MH, de Kruif JH. Transcervical hysteroscopic resection of submucous fibroids for abnormal uterine bleeding: results regarding the degree of intramural extension. Obstet Gynecol. 1993;82(5):736-40.
71. Ubaldi F, Tournaye H, Camus M, Van der Pas H, Gepts E, Devroey P. Fertility after hysteroscopic myomectomy. Hum Reprod Update. 1995;1:81-90.
72. Indman PD. Hysteroscopic treatment of submucous myomas. Clin Obstet Gynecol. 2006;49(4):811-20.
73. Di Spiezio Sardo A, Mazzon I, Bramante S, Bettocchi S, Bifulco G, Guida M, et al. Hysteroscopic myomectomy: a comprehensive review of surgical techniques. Hum Reprod Update. 2008;14(2):101-19.
74. Vercellini P, Zaina B, Yaylayan L, Pisacreta A, De Giorgi O, Crosignani PG. Hysteroscopic myomectomy: long-term effects on menstrual pattern and fertility. Obstet Gynecol. 1999;94(3):341-7.
75. Salm R. The incidence and significance of early carcinoma in endometrial polyps. J Pathol. 1972;108:47-53.
76. Stamatellos I, Apostolides A, Stamatopoulos P, Bontis J. Pregnancy rates after hysteroscopic polypectomy depending on the size or number of the polyps. Arch Gynecol Obstet. 2008;277(5):395-9.
77. Englund S, Ingelman-Sundberg A, Westin B. Hysteroscopy in diagnosis and treatment of uterine bleeding. Gynaecologia. 1957;143(3):217-22.
78. Word B, Gravlee LC, Wideman GL. The fallacy of simple uterine curettage. Obstet Gynecol. 1958;12(6):642-8.
79. Gebauer G, Hafner A, Siebzehnrübl E, Lang N. Role of hysteroscopy in detection and extraction of endometrial polyps: results of a prospective study. Am J Obstet Gynecol. 2001;184:59-63.
80. De Wit W, Gowrising CJ, Kuik DJ, Lens JW, Schats R. Only hydrosalpinges visible on ultrasound are associated with reduced implantation and pregnancy rates after in-vitro fertilization. Hum Reprod. 1998;13(6):1696-701.
81. Strandell A, Lindhard A, Waldenström U, Thorburn J, Janson PO, Hamberger L. Hydrosalpinx and IVF outcome: a prospective, randomized multicentre trial in Scandinavia on salpingectomy prior to IVF. Hum Reprod. 1999; 14(11):2762-9.
82. Gardner DK, Weissman A, Howles CM. Textbook of Assisted Reproductive Techniques. Fourth Edition, 2012.

SECTION

6 Intrauterine Insemination

CHAPTER

44 Intrauterine Insemination

Natchandra Chimote, Bindu Chimote

INTRODUCTION

About 15% couples, all over the world, have certain fertility problems that can be treated only with medical interventions. One of them is first-line treatment such as intrauterine insemination (IUI) with or without ovarian stimulation (OS) as recommended by World Health Organization (WHO).[1,2] The very first documentation of IUI was done in 1962 by Cohen MR.[3] Since then, IUI has evolved a lot through innovations such as sperm preparation, monitoring of follicular development using transvaginal sonography to determine preovulatory timing, and induction of ovulation with human chorionic gonadotropin (hCG). IUI also has been combined with OS using clomiphene citrate (CC)/letrozole or gonadotropins or combination of both. Though it has not been classified as an assisted reproductive technique (ART),[4,5] it is widely used, often as an empirical treatment, for a broad range of profertility indications.

The European IVF Monitoring Program in 2004 reported live birth rate (LBR) of 12.3% per cycle with 87% births of singletons 13% multiple births.[6] There is little evidence of the effectiveness of widely used IUI in male infertility,[7] and in stimulated IUI in the treatment of unexplained infertility.[8] The effectiveness of IUI across the range of methods and indications has to be evidence based. This includes the extent of IUI utilization, the indications for IUI, the optimal procedures for sperm preparation, insemination methods and timing, and the need, if any, to prevent premature luteinizing hormone (LH) surges and luteal deficiency in stimulated IUI cycles. Also, because IUI is often a stopgap treatment while waiting for, or instead of in vitro fertilization (IVF), a consideration of the evidence on IUI and IVF in treatment protocols is relevant to clinical practice.

INDICATIONS FOR IUI TREATMENT

Rationale

The rationale behind IUI is to increase this gamete density at the site of fertilization even when sperm or cervical mucus abnormalities are present. The increasing use of IUI in idiopathic and male infertility is mainly the result of the refinement of techniques for the preparation of washed motile spermatozoa, as used in IVF procedures.

In order to improve the quality and outcome of IUI procedures, there is a need for simple, inexpensive, reliable and safe sperm preparation techniques that isolate and select sperm cells with intact functional and genetic properties, including normal morphology, minimal DNA damage, and intact cell membranes with functional binding properties.[9] Seminal fluid acts as a transport medium for sperm, prostaglandins, ions, and antioxidants. Cells other than spermatozoa are also present in the ejaculate, including epithelial cells from the urinary tract, prostate cells, spermatogenic cells, and leukocytes. Reactive oxygen species, either produced by the different germ cells or by leukocytes, can be detrimental for the fertilizing potential of the spermatozoa.[10,11] The seminal plasma also contains decapitation factor(s) that need(s) to be removed for complete capacitation of the spermatozoa.[12] This process of capacitation is essential for both fertilization in vivo or in vitro, and hence spermatozoa to be used in IUI must be separated from the seminal plasma and its decapacitating factors such as spermine phosphate and prostaglandins. Preparation of human semen samples should also result in the removal of nonviable spermatozoa, leukocytes and/or bacteria, and other sources of contamination. Donor sperm is mainly cryopreserved and kept in quarantine for at least 6 months to prevent the transfer of infectious diseases. Thawed sperm is mostly used for IUI as compared to intracervical insemination, as supported by older evidence.[13]

CONTRAINDICATIONS

Intrauterine insemination is contraindicated in women with cervical atresia, cervicitis, endometritis or bilateral tubal obstruction, and in most cases of amenorrhea or severe oligospermia.

IUI IN A HISTORICAL PERSPECTIVE

Over the last centuries, the popularity of IUI has varied tremendously.[14] After the first description of spermatozoa by Antoni van Leeuwenhoek and his assistant Johannes Ham in 1678, it took >100 years before the first IUI was reported by John Hunter (1770) when he described the first case of human intravaginal insemination because of severe hypospadias. In the mid-1800s, J Marion Sims reported on 55 intravaginal inseminations. Only one pregnancy occurred, which is probably explained by the fact that Sims believed that ovulation occurred during menstruation. The first report on human IUI was documented by Guttmacher in 1943 and Kohlberg 1953.[15-17] This represents the start of a new era in assisted reproduction.

Dr Jerome K Sherman[18] introduced a simple method of preserving human sperm using glycerol and reported the first successful human pregnancy with frozen sperm in 1953. Due to the hostile climate for donor insemination (DI) at the time, nearly a decade passed before the first successful birth from frozen sperm was announcement in public in 1964.[19]

The renewed interest in sperm washing procedures owing to the introduction of IVF could be regarded as one of the most important milestones in the history of IUI.[20] Sunde et al.[21] reported the data of a European collaborative report on IUI describing 127 births in 20 clinics as a result of IUI with pretreated sperm. In 1989, the results of the first prospective controlled trials were published describing the value of IUI in case of cervical hostility and male factor infertility.[22,23] The evidence-based value of IUI as a treatment for cervical hostility, male factor, and unexplained infertility was first described in 2004.[24] Recent reports of Bensdorp et al.[25] and Tjon-Kon-Fat et al.[26] have shown that according to the results of a prospective multicenter trial, IUI–OS is recommended as the most cost-effective strategy for mild male factor or unexplained infertility with a poor prognosis of becoming pregnant with normal coitus. Insemination of semen in humans was originally developed to help heterosexual couples to become pregnant in case of severe male factor infertility of a physical or psychological nature; however, insemination with homologous semen nowadays is most commonly used for unexplained and mild male factor infertility. In the previous century, DI was mainly used for male infertility caused by azoospermia or very low-sperm count and for inherited genetic diseases linked to the Y chromosome. At present, DI is commonly used for individual women who desire a pregnancy.

Since IUI is a simple and noninvasive technique, it can be performed without expensive infrastructure resulting in IUI becoming the only treatment for male and unexplained infertility in resource-poor countries where IVF is either not available or not accessible for the majority of the population, owing to high costs.[27] In addition, it can be provided as a safe and simple treatment with minimal risks when appropriately monitored. These factors are responsible for high couple compliance in IUI programs when compared to IVF.[28]

It may be essential to mention that this chapter is based on comprehensive search using question-specific relevant search terms as per ESHRE draft recommendation (2018). For each PICO (population, intervention, comparison, and outcomes) drafted by WHO, specific search terms were used to find the available evidence in Medline (1950 to May, 2015) and the Cochrane Library (until May, 2015). The quality of the evidence was assessed using the GRADE system. The evidence and draft recommendation for each PICO question are summarized as follows. Women and men may have fertility problems that can only be resolved through medically assisted interventions. The WHO invited experts to help to develop and provide draft recommendations based upon the available evidence for six prioritized areas, including the fertility treatment IUI with or without OS. Prioritization of questions was accomplished and stakeholders considered global relevance that included the importance of cost-effectiveness, safety, and affordability. Thus, this chapter provides an overview of the process applied and the draft evidence-based recommendations generated.

What are the indications for IUI versus intercourse or expectant management in infertile couples and when should treatment be initiated?

- In couples with unexplained infertility with a prognosis of becoming pregnant without assistance within the next 12 months (estimate >30%), IUI could be postponed for at least 6 months.
- In couples with unexplained infertility and men with a total motile sperm count (TMSC) >10 million and a prognosis of spontaneous pregnancy <30% within a year, it is recommended that IUI plus OS is the treatment of first choice.
- In couples with solely a poor sperm quality (severe oligozoospermia, i.e., sperm count <5 million or astheno-zoospermia, i.e., Grade III and Grade IV motility <36%, or teratozoospermia, i.e., normal sperm morphology <4% as per strict criteria) in the male partner, it is not recommended either for or against use of IUI.

When is OS required in an IUI cycle?

In couples with unexplained infertility and men with a TMSC above 10 million, IUI should be combined with OS to improve LBRs would be a moderate statement.

What is the influence of sperm quality on IUI outcome? Can we define threshold levels for successful IUI?

It is not possible to define clear lower cut-off levels of pre- or postwash sperm parameters below which IUI should be withheld. A very few evidence about lower cut-off values of sperm parameters is available.

When is the best timing of insemination in an IUI cycle? What is the optimal method of timing in natural or stimulated IUI cycles?

Timing of trigger or insemination, whether in natural or stimulated cycles, cannot be exactly determined, as there is no concrete evidence for or against any particular method.

If an hCG injection is used, single IUI can be performed any time between 24 and 40 hours after hCG injection without compromising pregnancy rates.

Intrauterine insemination in a natural (not ovarian stimulated) cycle should be performed 1 day after LH rise.

What is the value of "fallopian sperm perfusion" (FSP) compared to IUI?

It is highly recommended that the intervention FSP, when compared to IUI, should not be the treatment of choice.

What is optimal number of inseminations per cycle?

In both unexplained and male infertility, there is insufficient evidence that the intervention, a double IUI, within the same cycle will lead to better pregnancy rates than a single IUI within a cycle.

Women undergoing IUI should be offered a single insemination per cycle.

Is there a benefit of bed rest after IUI?

Women undergoing IUI should have 10–15 minutes of bed rest after an insemination.

What is the ultimate number of consecutive IUI cycles per couple/woman in which pregnancy rates still increase significantly?

In couples with an indication for IUI, at least three consecutive IUI cycles should be performed. There is insufficient evidence to recommend a maximum number of IUI treatment cycles. However, most of the clinics withdraw IUI procedures after six procedures of IUI.

Which semen preparation technique used yields the best results (in terms of pregnancy rates) for IUI?

According to the available evidence, it is not possible to recommend any semen preparation technique over another (swim-up, gradient, wash and centrifugation).

What is the cost-effectiveness of IUI versus IVF/intracytoplasmic sperm injection (ICSI)?

In couples with unexplained infertility and men with a TMSC of >10 million and a prognosis of a pregnancy without assistance <30% within a year, at least three cycles of IUI–OS are the most effective option.

How can you prevent infections in an IUI laboratory?

Good practice point: Couples and individuals undergoing IUI and males providing semen samples for IUI should be screened for infectious agents based on local, regional, and national standards and regulations.

How can you prevent multiple pregnancies and ovarian hyperstimulation syndrome in an IUI program?

In order to prevent high rates of multiple gestation pregnancies in IUI–OS, IUI should be withheld when more than two dominant follicles of >15 mm or more than five follicles of >10 mm at the time of hCG injection or LH surge are present. When gonadotropins are used in IUI, regimens with 75 IU or lower should be used because higher doses have similar pregnancy rates but increase multiple pregnancy rates (MPRs).

Clomiphene citrate or tamoxifen is acceptable alternative to low-dose gonadotropins for low multiple pregnancy and birth rates and with lesser costs, although at a lower LBR than with gonadotropins.

Addition of gonadotropin-releasing hormone (GnRH) agonist to gonadotropins in IUI–OS is not recommended because there is no increase in pregnancy rate despite increased MPRs and increased costs.

Good practice point: As an alternative to cycle cancelation, aspiration of excess follicles at the time of hCG injection or LH surge might be additional options for reducing the risk of multiple pregnancy in IUI–OS.

Is there a different perinatal outcome for IUI pregnancies and how does this perinatal outcome differ from normal coitus and IVF/ICSI pregnancies?

Individuals with infertility undergoing treatment with IUI–OS should be informed about a possible increased risk for preterm birth and low-birth weight in singletons and twin pregnancies when compared to pregnancies in fertile couples not requiring assistance (IVF/ICSI outcome comparisons are assessed in the IVF/ICSI prioritized guideline).

Indications for IUI

After 36 years of publication of the first randomized controlled trial (RCT) by Kerin et al. in 1984, the indications for IUI remain a subject of debate. Widely used indications for IUI are:

- Unexplained infertility (including mild endometriosis)
- Male factor infertility
- Female cervical factor

Patients prefer IUI, with or without OS, over expectant management when their chance of spontaneous conception is <50 or 40%, respectively, and they prefer IUI over IVF up to six treatment cycles.[29,30]

Unexplained infertility from RBMO, 2012.

Possible reasons for unexplained infertility: The current knowledge of the reproductive system assessment is far from complete. There are many steps which are not routinely evaluated or unavailable, including cervical mucus, capacitation, or the ability of spermatozoa to negotiate the uterotubal junction. There is also a need for a test for the acrosome reaction and the ability to bind to and penetrate the zona pellucida. There is no infallible test which can provide fertilization profiles of spermatozoa. Similar limitations are also present in female fertility assessment. Defective oocytes, especially in aging patients, are an important cause of infertility which is difficult to assess. Tubal patency does not assess the characteristics of bidirectional tubal motility which is important for embryo transport. Tests for the evaluation of the chance for successful implantation are not available. Random delays in conception do not appear to account in a major way for unexplained infertility, whereas a nonrandom age effect is important. Therefore, the ideal definition for unexplained infertility should be a couple with a real but unobservable defect leading to infertility which may be prolonged and permanent.

Unexplained infertility and IUI: The diagnosis of unexplained infertility encompasses an important subset of couples seeking treatment for infertility. After evaluation of ovulatory function (baseline transvaginal ultrasonography/baseline hormone evaluation including serum AMH), tubal patency (HSG/sonosalpingography/diagnostic laparoscopy/hysteroscopy), and semen analysis (WHO, 2010; strict criteria which may include sperm function tests/DNA fragmentation index), no etiology is identified in 10–30% of couples seeking treatment for infertility.[31,32] Any treatment for unknown infertility is empiric by default, and the broad range of treatment, including expectant management, superovulation, and IVF, reflects the uncertainty with this diagnosis. However, there are limited data to support the efficacy of many of these treatments in the management of unexplained infertility, and no uniform protocol exists in clinical practice. One must take into account that, unexplained infertility is best characterized as 'subfertility'.[33] This nomenclature is significant, in that, some couples will conceive naturally without any fertility interventions. In one randomized trial of 253 patients with unexplained infertility, a 27% ongoing pregnancy rate was observed in the expectant management group.[8] Others observed a 13% spontaneous pregnancy rate in a group of patients awaiting IVF, although this cohort consisted of patients with unexplained subfertility of 2 years' duration or more and may represent a poorer prognostic subgroup.[34] Another cohort experienced only a 5.9% cumulative pregnancy rate over 12 months in an untreated group of patients awaiting IVF.[35] Despite this variability, it is evident that a proportion of couples will achieve pregnancy with no intervention.

Superovulation, which induces the development of more than one follicle per cycle, combined with either timed intercourse or IUI, is commonly used to treat unexplained infertility. The use of oral or injectable agents may increase the number of dominant follicles available for fertilization and correct subclinical ovulatory dysfunction.[36] Many argue that the addition of IUI ensures that sufficient numbers of sperm overcome any cervical barrier.[37] Disadvantages of treatment with gonadotropins and IUI include significant cost, ovarian hyperstimulation syndrome (OHSS), and higher rates of multiple pregnancies.[38] IVF has also been used to treat unexplained infertility. According to 2013 Society for Assisted Reproductive Technology data, LBRs per cycle of IVF ranged from 25 to 43% in patients with unexplained infertility aged <40 years.[39]

CC with timed intercourse versus expectant management: Bhattacharya et al.[37] in a high-graded quality trial of 580 patients (507 with unexplained infertility) found no benefit of therapy, with a 16% LBR with expectant management versus 13% after CC therapy. This trial randomized patients to one of three arms for a treatment period of 6 months:

1. Expectant management, consisting of no visits or interventions
2. CC at a starting dose of 50 mg on cycle days 2–6 with timed intercourse on cycle days 12–18 (initial cycle monitored with ultrasound and midluteal serum P, with subsequent cycles monitored only with midluteal progesterone)
3. IUI in the spontaneous cycle, with monitoring by urine LH kit starting on cycle day 12, with a single IUI performed at 20–30 hours after surge.

Patients in the study had a mean duration of infertility of 30 months and a mean age of 32 years. The median number of treatment cycles was five in the CC/timed intercourse group and four in the natural-cycle IUI group.

CC with IUI versus expectant management: Deaton et al.[40] examined CC with IUI in comparison with expectant management, and it found no significant difference. Of the 51 patients included in the data analysis of this trial, 24 patients had unexplained infertility, and 27 patients had endometriosis. This study had a crossover design whereby patients were randomized to either four treatment cycles or four control cycles and would then crossover to the other arm if pregnancy did not occur in the first four cycles. Mean age was 33 years, with a mean duration of infertility of 3.5 years. In the treatment cycles, patients received CC (50 mg) on cycle days 5–9 (or days 4–8 if the patient's average cycle length was <27 days), with hCG (10,000 IU) given when the lead follicle was 18 mm on ultrasound. IUI was performed 36 hours after hCG administration. In the control cycles, patients were instructed to have intercourse during the periovulatory period. The ongoing pregnancy rate in the treatment cycles (defined in this study as >20 weeks' gestation) was 10 of 46 (21%) and OPR in the control cycles was 5 of 40 (12%). Because of the crossover design of the study, some patients were counted twice in this analysis.

Gonadotropins with IUI versus expectant management: Steures et al.,[8] involving 253 patients, compared gonadotropins and IUI with expectant management, and it found no significant difference in ongoing pregnancy rate over the 6-month study period. In the treatment arm, patients received follicle-stimulating hormone (FSH) or human menopausal gonadotropin (hMG) (average 75 IU, range 37–150 IU) starting on cycle day 3 until the lead follicle measured 16 mm, when hCG was administered at a dose of either 5,000 or 10,000 IU, with IUI performed 36–40 hours later. If there were three or more follicles of >16 mm or five follicles of >12 mm, hCG was withheld. Patients' mean age was 33 years, with a mean duration of 2 years of infertility and baseline mean FSH of 7.0 and 6.7 IU/L in the gonadotropin and expectant management groups, respectively. Of the 127 patients assigned to the treatment arm, there were 29 ongoing pregnancies (23%) and 26 live births. In the expectant management arm, there were 34 ongoing pregnancies (27%) among 126 patients and 30 live births. There was no significant difference in OPR in the treatment arm compared with expectant management.

CC with IUI versus letrozole with IUI: Two trials examined CC with IUI versus letrozole with IUI. In a trial of 214 patients, Fouda et al.[41] demonstrated an improved ongoing pregnancy rate with letrozole plus IUI (33%) compared with CC plus IUI (19%), which was statistically significant. Mean age of patients was 26 years, with a mean duration of infertility of 3.7 years in the letrozole group and 3.4 in the CC group (no statistical difference); mean baseline FSH was 5.7 and 5.5 IU/L, respectively. Patients underwent up to three cycles of treatment. The letrozole arm consisted of an extended letrozole regimen of 2.5 mg daily on cycle days 1–9, and in the CC group, patients received CC (100 mg) on cycle days 3–7. Ultrasound monitoring was performed, and IUI was done 36–40 hours after administration of hCG (10,000 IU).

In the Diamond trial,[42] 900 patients were randomized to one of three treatment arms: (1) letrozole (5 mg) on cycle days 3–7; (2) CC (100 mg) on cycle days 3–7, and (3) FSH (150 IU) starting on cycle day 3 through the day of hCG administration. Mean age of patients in this trial was 32 years, and mean duration of infertility was 35 months. The mean anti-Müllerian hormone level was the same (2.6 ng/mL) and baseline FSH was similar at 7.0, 7.2, and 6.9 mIU/mL, respectively.[43] The oral intervention arms included a combined 599 patients and demonstrated a higher LBR in the clomiphene group (23.3%) compared with the letrozole group (18.7%), although the result was not statistically significant. Rates for ongoing clinical pregnancy and multiple gestations were also not significantly different between these two interventions, although this study was powered for a comparison of the letrozole group with the combined gonadotropin and clomiphene groups, not for individual comparisons.[43,44]

Gonadotropins with IUI versus CC with IUI: Three trials compared gonadotropins with clomiphene. The Berker et al. trial[45] with 93 patients reported ongoing pregnancy rate in 11.6% patients in the clomiphene arm versus 18% patients in the gonadotropin arm, which was not a statistically significant difference.

In the Dankert et al. trial,[46] a total of 138 patients (68 with unexplained infertility) were randomized to CC/IUI or FSH/IUI for up to four cycles. Mean age of the study population was 31 years, with a mean duration of infertility of 33 months. This trial, such as the Berker et al. study, showed no difference in these treatments, with a LBR of 31.4% in the CC group and 30.3% in the FSH group. Of note, neither of these studies achieved statistical power. The Diamond et al. trial[44] also directly compared these two interventions, however, showed a statistically significant difference in LBR, with 32.2% in the gonadotropin group compared with 23.3% in the clomiphene group. The rate of multiple gestations was also higher in the gonadotropin group, with 10 triplets and 24 twins, versus 0 and 8, respectively, in the CC group. One patient in the gonadotropin group developed OHSS, compared with none in the CC group.

Gonadotropins with IUI versus letrozole with IUI: Three trials assessed the efficacy of gonadotropins with IUI versus letrozole with IUI. Baysoy et al.[47] in a study involving 80 patients, reported that the efficacy of IUI using letrozole (5 mg daily from day 3 to day 7) was comparable with that using gonadotropins (75–150 IU per day). The primary outcome was clinical pregnancy rate, which was 18.4% for letrozole and 15.7% for gonadotropins. One triplet gestation occurred in the letrozole group, and a twin gestation in the gonadotropin group. One case of moderate OHSS occurred in the gonadotropin group. Gregoriou et al.[48] study (with 50 patients) similarly found no significant difference in the efficacy of letrozole (5 mg/day 3–7) after three cycles of CC/IUI failure versus gonadotropins (r-FSH 150 IU daily), with respect either to clinical pregnancy rate per cycle (the primary outcome) or LBR per couple. LBR in the gonadotropin group was 28%, compared with 20% in the letrozole group, which did not reach statistical significance, and there were no multiple gestations in either group. In contrast to the Baysoy and Gregoriou studies, the Diamond trial[44] showed a significantly higher LBR in the gonadotropin group (32.2%) compared with the letrozole group (18.7%). The letrozole group had nine twin pregnancies and no higher-order multiples, compared with 24 and 10, respectively, in the gonadotropin group.

These were the available evidence from clinical trials for the relative efficacy of various treatments for unexplained infertility with respect to the outcomes of clinical or ongoing pregnancy rate or LBR per couple.

Although there is considerable clinical heterogeneity among the studies mentioned above; the following significant findings are demonstrated:

- Clomiphene citrate with timed intercourse was more effective than expectant management in an older study,[33] although a larger, relatively more recent trial found no benefit.[37]

- When expectant management was compared either with CC with IUI[13] or with gonadotropins with IUI,[40] it was as effective as either intervention.
- Applicability of the Steures gonadotropin IUI trial[8] to clinical practice is limited, given its clear potential for underestimation of pregnancy due to a high cycle cancellation rate (14.9%), in addition to underestimation of multiple gestation rates due to the incidence of monofollicular recruitment (58%).
- When CC and letrozole (both with IUI) were compared, letrozole with IUI was superior in one study;[41] the larger, more recent Diamond trial[44] showed a higher ongoing pregnancy rate and LBR with CC, although the difference was not statistically significant. Two studies that examined letrozole with IUI versus gonadotropins with IUI showed these interventions to be equally effective,[47,48] as did two other studies that examined clomiphene with IUI versus gonadotropins.[45,46] However, Diamond trial demonstrated that gonadotropins were significantly more effective than either letrozole or clomiphene, despite a higher cycle cancellation rate of 6.9% versus 3.7% and 3.3%, respectively.
- Natural-cycle IUI was comparable to expectant management in Bhattacharya et al. study.[37] However, in the Goverde trial,[49] the per cycle pregnancy rate was higher for IVF than for IUI using gonadotropins.
- Additionally, an accelerated approach involving CC plus IUI followed by IVF seems to shorten the median time to pregnancy when compared with a conventional stepwise method of CC plus IUI, gonadotropins plus IUI, then IVF.[50]
- Any discussion of unexplained infertility must bear in mind that many of the reports contain treatment-independent pregnancies, highlighting the fact that "subfertility" is a better descriptor for this patient population.

Many of these individual studies had small sample sizes and lacked the statistical power to detect significant differences between interventions.

Conclusion: On the basis of the currently available literature—

- Expectant management may be comparable to treatment with CC and timed intercourse or IUI in patients with unexplained infertility.
- For patients who undergo superovulation with oral agents, clomiphene may be more effective than letrozole.
- Treatment with gonadotropins seems to be more effective than either oral agent, although its attendant risk of multiple gestations is an obvious disadvantage that should limit utilization.
- Despite its cost and widespread utilization, IVF was no more effective than gonadotropins with IUI but may accelerate the time to clinical pregnancy.
- Well-designed prospective trials with adequate sample size are needed to directly compare superovulation with oral agents and gonadotropins, as well as the role of IUI and IVF, with careful assessment of the risk and benefit profiles. Until such data are available, clinicians should individualize the management of unexplained infertility for each patient with appropriate counseling regarding the empiric nature of their treatment.

Male infertility and IUI: Intrauterine insemination for male infertility is still under debate. One of the major problems in male subfertility is the lack of validated definitions and strict cut-off values of sperm parameters to make a clear distinction between mild, moderate, and severe male infertility. A Cochrane systematic review by Bensdorp et al.[7] analyzed IUI (with or without OS) in patients with male infertility with various definitions of male infertility. The authors of this review concluded that there was insufficient evidence to recommend for or against IUI (with or without OS) in male infertility, mainly because large high-quality randomized trials are lacking. A recently published large RCT showed us that IUI–OS is noninferior to IVF in couples with unexplained and mild male infertility, defined as a TMSC of 3–10 million. However, the number of included couples in this study with mild male infertility was relatively low (only 10% of total inclusions).[25] Therefore, it is not possible to recommend for or against IUI in couples with solely poor sperm quality.

Over the past decades, the reported percentage of morphologically normal spermatozoa has decreased with the introduction of stricter criteria and the tendency toward lower reference values.[51] This is a disturbing factor in the use of sperm morphology as a prognostic factor for the probability of achieving a pregnancy. However, later, it was concluded that sperm morphology has no prognostic value in individual IVF and ICSI patients.[52]

However, it can be hypothesized that the role of sperm factors in IUI is different from their role in IVF and ICSI. Literature reviews reveal an ongoing debate on the value of sperm parameters as predictors of IUI outcome.[53-55] More specifically, conflicting results have been reported for the influence of sperm morphology assessment using strict criteria on pregnancy outcomes with IUI.[56-65] But these studies are characterized by a lack of standardization.

Besides sperm morphology, there is disagreement about the predictive value of the total progressively motile sperm count (TPMSC) to predict IUI outcomes.[55] In their review, Ombelet et al.[53] stated that the TPMSC has a substantial discriminative value. Others, however, have concluded that the TPMSC has poor sensitivity for selecting the couples most likely to conceive with IUI, but high specificity for identifying the couples unlikely to conceive with IUI.[55,66,67] The required number of inseminated progressively motile spermatozoa (NIPMS) is under discussion as well, although

Flowchart 1: Suggested unexplained infertility management protocol.

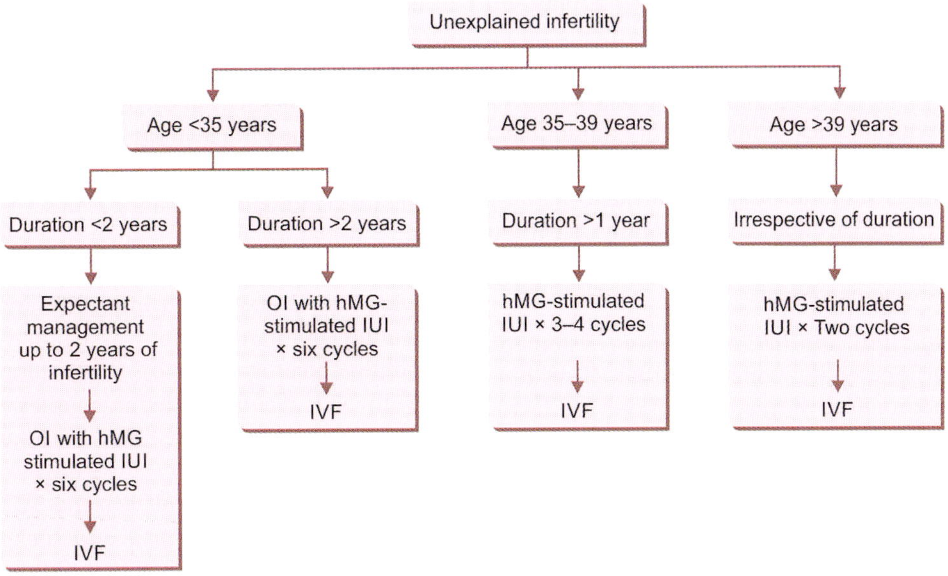

(hMG: human menopausal gonadotropin; IUI: intrauterine insemination; IVF: in vitro fertilization; OI: ovulation induction)
Courtesy: https://obgyn.onlinelibrary.wiley.com/doi/abs/10.1111/tog.12253

in general, a minimum of 5 million spermatozoa are stated as accurate.[51] This study reveals that couples with a lower percentage of morphologically normal spermatozoa (i.e., ≤4%) and a moderate NIPMS (i.e., 5-10 million) had the highest probability of becoming pregnant in the first finished IUI episode. In couples with a NIPMS of ≤1 million, this probability was lower. The TPMSC had no predictive value in this perspective.

In general, the predictive power of the semen parameters was limited, and it seems that especially female factors were critical for predicting the probability of becoming pregnant in individual couples.

Consequently, it is likely that the presence of female factors affects the relation between semen parameters and pregnancy outcome. When female factors are excluded, however, the probability of becoming pregnant based on semen parameters does not change in the opposite direction. Instead, the probability to become pregnant even increased in couples with ≤4% morphologically normal spermatozoa [OR: 1.58; 95% confidence interval (CI): 1.13–2.22]. These apparently contradictory results raise the question of whether sperm morphology is an adequate predictor for the outcome of IUI. This view is supported by many others.[61,65,68]

Note that it is also possible that the current WHO classification system may be inadequate (i.e., too strict criteria) but sperm morphology itself still could be an important parameter. It might be useful to consider the development of a new classification system. Another striking result is that the TPMSC showed no prognostic value to predict the probability of becoming pregnant in couples with IUI treatment. Other studies have shown that TPMSC is of great value when choosing between IUI and IVF or ICSI,[49,66,69,70] and TPMSC has been described as a relatively good indicator for male factor infertility in general.[70]

In contrast to TPMSC, NIPMS was relevant in predicting the ongoing pregnancy rate after IUI. This is in agreement with the literature.[51,53,55,59] Finally, the ongoing pregnancy rate in couples undergoing IUI was negatively influenced by a higher (>4%) percentage of morphologically normal spermatozoa, NIPMS of ≤1 million, higher female age, higher male age, and higher number of cycles within the episode. For most prediction models in reproductive medicine, the discriminatory performance is low to moderate.

Many factors of influence are taken into account. Along with the methodologically stable period with respect to semen analysis and adequate statistics, the influences of ejaculatory abstinence, type of ovulation induction, and the time interval between the fertility workup and IUI on the probability of becoming pregnant were checked. No effects were found. Still, it would be valuable to set up a prospective, multicenter study with clear inclusion of couples, sound statistics, and standardized and controlled protocols for semen analysis, semen preparation, fertility workup, and the IUI procedure in general. This will provide an opportunity to develop a better prognostic model. Accurate study design also would be helpful for reconsidering the accuracy of the percentage of morphologically normal spermatozoa as factor for sperm quality assessment.

The evidence based draft recommends that expectant management be attempted for at least 6 months in heterosexual couples with unexplained infertility and a prognosis of becoming pregnant without assistance within the next

12 months >30% prognosis. When this is <30%, IUI with OS is recommended in couples with unexplained infertility and men with a TMSC > 10 million as the first treatment option. The quality of the evidence found was graded as moderate to high.

In summary, with the lack of high-quality randomized trials investigating the effectiveness of IUI in male infertility, the question whether IUI should be applied in male infertility remains. Furthermore, a clear and generally accepted definition of mild, moderate, or severe male infertility terms often used in IUI studies is missing.

Cervical factor infertility and IUI: A Cochrane systematic review by Helmerhorst et al.[71] concluded that IUI with or without OS is not an effective treatment of cervical factor infertility. Although more recent studies were published on this subject, most clinicians no longer support performing postcoital testing as part of a fertility checkup. Therefore, cervical factor is less often diagnosed; however, it is recognized that good practice indicates that for heterosexual couples where the male partner refuses semen analysis (e.g., for personal or cultural reasons), the postcoital test can be used to suggest that further evaluation of male factor infertility is indicated (evidence-based consensus to support this draft recommendation is reviewed by the WHO evidence synthesis team which addressed female infertility diagnosis and management).

When is OS required in an IUI cycle?

- In couples with unexplained infertility with a prognosis of becoming pregnant without assistance within the next 12 months (estimate >30%), IUI could be postponed for at least 6 months. In couples with unexplained infertility and men with a TMSC above 10 million, IUI should be combined with OS to improve LBRs.
- In couples with unexplained infertility and men with a TMSC > 10 million and a prognosis of spontaneous pregnancy <30% within a year, it is recommended that IUI plus OS are the treatments of first choice.

The rationale of OS is to achieve multifollicular growth. van Rumste et al.[72] showed that multifollicular growth resulted in significantly higher pregnancy rates compared to monofollicular growth (15 versus 8.4%). Compared to one dominant follicle, pregnancy rates increased by a further 5, 8, and 8% when two, three, or four dominant follicles were present, respectively.[72] Cohlen et al.[73] conducted an RCT comparing IUI with or without OS in male infertility. In couples with a TMSC <10 million, OS did not improve pregnancy outcome, while it did in couples with a TMSC >10 million.

For unexplained infertility, the Cochrane systematic review of Veltman-Verhulst et al.[74] showed that IUI without OS does not positively influence pregnancy outcomes. Adding OS to IUI significantly increases LBRs in couples with unexplained infertility (OR: 2.07, 95% CI: 1.22–3.50, n = 396). However, when there is still a reasonable chance of becoming pregnant through normal intercourse with prognosis >30%,[75,76] expectant management for at least 6 months should be the first option because in these good prognosis couples, IUI in cycles with OS does not improve LBRs significantly [relative risk (RR): 0.85, 95% CI: 0.63–1.1, n = 253].[74] Furthermore, OS is well-known risks factor for (high order) multiple pregnancy as described above.

It is, therefore, recommended that expectant management can be attempted for at least 6 months in heterosexual couples with unexplained infertility and a prognosis of becoming pregnant without assistance within the next 12 months and prognosis >30%. When this prognosis is <30%, IUI with OS is recommended in couples with unexplained infertility and men with a TMSC > 10 million as the first treatment option.

Now that, it has become clear that IUI–OS is a first-line treatment option for mild male and unexplained infertility, the question arises whether IUI, with or without OS, is beneficial for moderate male infertility as well. Furthermore, as mentioned above, a clear definition of mild or moderate male infertility is mandatory.

What is the influence of sperm quality on IUI outcome? Can we define threshold levels for successful IUI?

It is not possible to define clear lower cut-off levels of pre- or postwash sperm parameters below which IUI should be withheld.

A recent systematic review and meta-analysis clearly presents the lack of robust evidence for clear lower cut-off levels of sperm parameters in IUI treatment. Based on very low quality evidence, it is recommended that IUI should be withheld below a TMSC count of 1 million and morphology <4%.[53] Van Weert et al.[55] found the postwash TMSC to be predictive for nonpregnancy but the lower cut-off levels varied tremendously between 0.8 and 5 million. So it cannot define clear lower cut-off levels of pre or postwash sperm parameters below which IUI should be withheld.

Because the lower cut-off level of semen parameters below which IUI is no longer cost-efficient has not been clearly identified, a randomized trial comparing IUI with either conventional IVF or IVF/ICSI to define these lower cut-off levels is required before any conclusion can be drawn.

When is the best timing of insemination in an IUI cycle? What is the optimal method of timing in natural or stimulated IUI cycles?

- Providers can determine the method of triggering in IUI stimulated with gonadotropins as there is no evidence to recommend for or against a method.
- Providers can determine the method of timing IUI in natural cycles (no OS) as there is no evidence to recommend for or against a method.

Flowchart 2: IUI with or without ovarian stimulation.

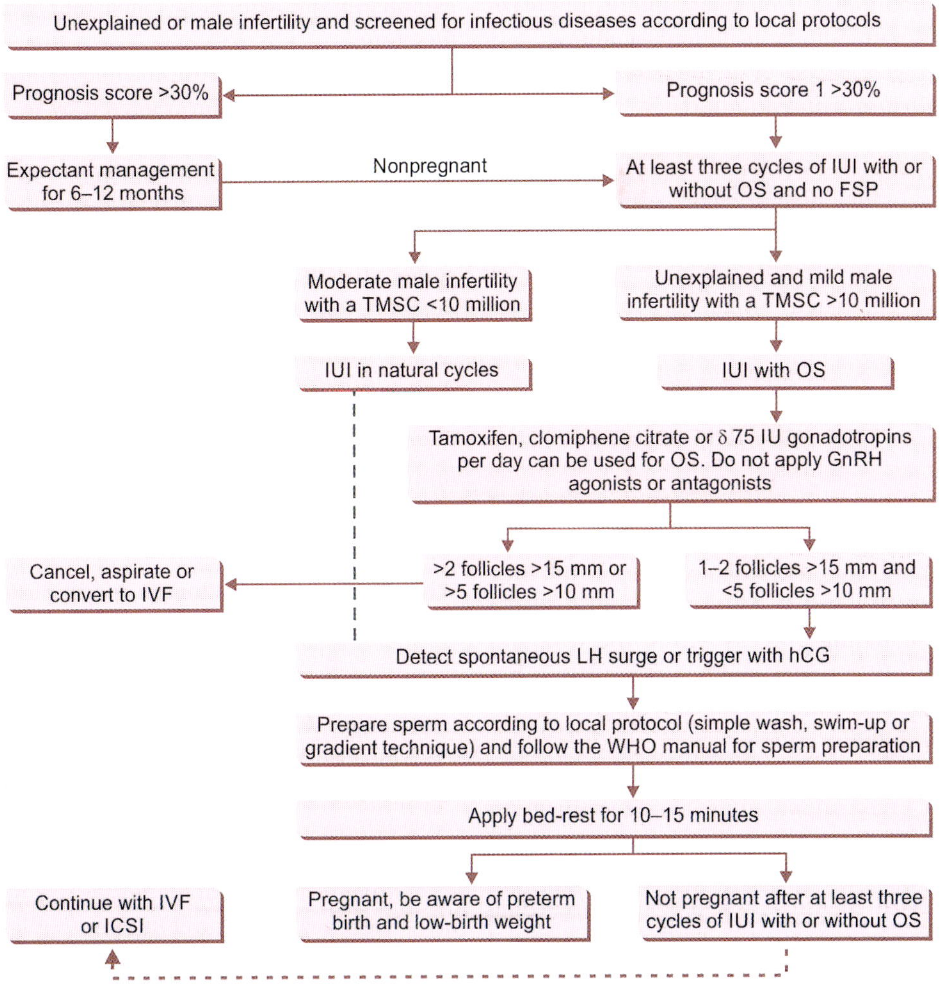

(GnRH: gonadotropin-releasing hormone; FSP: fallopian sperm perfusion; IUI: intrauterine insemination; ICSI: intracytoplasmic sperm injection; IVF: in vitro fertilization; LH: luteinizing hormone; TMSC: total motile sperm count)

- If an hCG injection is used, single IUI can be performed any time between 24 and 40 hours after hCG injection without compromising pregnancy rates.
- IUI in a natural (not ovarian stimulated) cycle should be performed 1 day after LH rise.

Age, indications of IUI, sperm preparation, and insemination methods are several important factors affecting the outcome of controlled ovarian hyperstimulation-IUI.[77-80] However, the timing of administration of IUI seems to be the most critical factor among them. It should be noted that medical regimens vary between centers and also between clinicians. Hence, the correct timing of insemination to improve pregnancy has been the subject of recent debate.

Huang et al.[81] compared 210 IUIs performed at 24 hours and 36 hours with different diagnostic and etiological categories including endometriosis, ovulation dysfunction, and unexplained infertility. The patients were divided into three subgroups who received FSH, hMG, and CC/hMG. Spermiogram parameters were all normal. Additionally, no significant difference in pregnancy outcomes was found between the two groups. Wang et al.[82] demonstrated the effects of different timings (24 hours and 36 hours) of IUI after hCG injection in the subgroups of patients who received CC, CC plus gonadotropin, and gonadotropin alone. The pregnancy rates were found to be similar between two groups. Similarly, Osuna et al.[83] performed a systematic review of the literature and they concluded that no significant differences were observed when two inseminations per cycle were performed, compared with one insemination. They also found great heterogeneity concerning ovarian management and insemination timing. The same group detected an improved pregnancy rate with two inseminations compared with one insemination when CC with or without gonadotropins and 5,000 IU of hCG were used. In another study, Ragni et al.[84] detected significant increases in pregnancy rates when the IUI procedure was performed during the preovulatory and periovulatory periods, but not the postovulatory period. According to another study, Kucuk[85] suggested that IUI should be withheld until follicular rupture is detected. He also claimed that monitoring of follicular rupture prior to IUI provides a pregnancy rate similar to natural fecundity.

In a Cochrane meta-analysis evaluating the effectiveness of different synchronization methods in natural and stimulated cycles for IUI in subfertile couples, the authors concluded that insufficient evidence exists to determine whether there is any difference in safety and effectiveness between different methods of synchronization of ovulation and insemination among subfertile patients.[86]

In our study, we compared the clinical pregnancy rates of patients with polycystic ovarian syndrome (PCOS) and unexplained infertility according to the timing of single IUI procedures. To homogenize the study groups, we excluded other possible causes of infertility. Clinical pregnancy rates per cycle were 22.9% in the PCOS group and 26.9% in the unexplained group. However, IUI procedures performed 24 hours following hCG trigger day were found to be related to better cycle outcomes among patients with unexplained infertility, unlike PCOS patients. This result can be related to the sperm capacitating process within the woman's genital tract. Intercourse performed before ovulation has been related to an increase in the fertilization potential and pregnancy establishment.

Primarily, the leading defect in pregnancy establishment for patients with unexplained infertility is fertilization defects.[77] This statement explains the importance of IUI procedure timing and the technique used for this group of patients who regularly menstruate and ovulate preceding the ovulation induction treatment cycle. Spermatozoa and oocytes have only a limited survival time (around 72 hours and 24 hours, respectively); therefore, correct timing of insemination is essential. Delaying the IUI procedure in couples with unexplained infertility theoretically decreases the fertilization potential of the inseminated sperm due to the short viability time of the oocyte. Also, in a prospective randomized controlled study, Blockeel et al.[87] demonstrated that significantly higher clinical pregnancy rates per IUI cycle were observed in patients undergoing IUI 1 day after the LH rise, when compared with patients undergoing IUI 2 days after the LH rise in natural cycles. This proves the clinical importance of IUI timing on pregnancy rates among subfertile patients.[87] The main problem for PCOS patients is anovulation. Accordingly, for PCOS patients, IUI timing is not as important as for patients with unexplained infertility. A significant relationship between the hCG trigger day of cycle and clinical pregnancy establishment was observed. This result can be a reflection of higher quality of oocytes in the later hCG/day trigger cycles than in earlier hCG day trigger cycles. Perhaps, clinicians trigger the preovulatory follicles earlier than physiologically needed, which decreases the fertility potential of an originally competent oocyte. In a study,[88] it was also found a significant relationship between hCG day endometrial thickness and clinical pregnancy establishment, which is consistent with the previous literature.

In conclusion, IUI performed at either 24 hours or 36 hours after ovulation triggered by hCG injection does not change the clinical pregnancy rates for PCOS patients. Contrarily, patients with unexplained infertility seem to benefit from earlier IUI procedures, which increase their fertility potential during ovulation induction with gonadotropins. However, avoiding artificial hCG triggering before IUI procedures earlier than physiologically needed results in improved pregnancy rates. Utilization of clinical interventions such as IUI during the treatment of infertile women necessitates rational applications, which increases the clinical usefulness of the procedure. Ultimately, large multicenter trials with increased patient numbers are necessary to elucidate the optimal timing of insemination among different infertile patient groups.

What is the value of fallopian sperm perfusion compared to IUI?

It is recommended that the intervention fallopian sperm perfusion (FSP), when compared to IUI, should not be the treatment of choice.

With regard to FSP, a technique that ensures the presence of higher sperm densities in the fallopian tubes at the time of ovulation, the recommendation of this PICO is clear. Based on a recent Cochrane systematic review,[89] without any more recent papers identified, the review was not able to show a beneficial effect of FSP on LBRs per couple compared to IUI (OR: 0.94, 95% CI: 0.59–1.49), therefore, IUI is the treatment of choice and the quality of this evidence was graded as high.

What is the optimal number of inseminations per cycle?

- In both unexplained and male infertility, there is insufficient evidence that the intervention, a double IUI, within the same cycle will lead to better pregnancy rates than a single IUI within a cycle.
- Women undergoing IUI should be offered a single insemination per cycle.

An assumption can be made that increasing the number of inseminations per cycle from one to two (or more) might increase the probability of a pregnancy in IUI treatment since more spermatozoa may be present at the moment of ovulation. One Cochrane systematic review and two additional relevant systematic reviews were identified after a systematic search. One additional RCT not included in one of these systematic reviews was also identified. The Cochrane systematic review[90] found a significant difference in favor of double insemination (OR: 1.8, CI 95%: 1.4–2.4) in heterosexual couples with unexplained or male infertility. This observed effect is largely due to the contribution of one study with a weight of 66.5%; however, this study yielded an unclear risk of bias because allocation concealment was not mentioned. Another systematic review[91] compared single versus double insemination in male infertility. This review showed a significant benefit of double IUI in male infertility but, again, this effect was largely due to the same dominant study.

A third systematic review[92] analyzed double versus single insemination in unexplained infertility. This meta-analysis showed that double IUI does not result in significantly higher pregnancy rates compared with single IUI in women with unexplained infertility. This was confirmed by a more recent RCT by Rahman et al.[93] The overall quality of evidence from systematic reviews was graded as moderate, mainly because of the dominating effect of one study, which did not clearly described allocation concealment.

Based upon our review, it can be concluded that there is insufficient evidence for a beneficial effect of double insemination in couples with unexplained infertility. Yet, in the case of male infertility, there might be a positive effect. However, this was only proven by one study with an unclear risk of bias. We, therefore, provide a draft recommendation that women undergoing IUI should be offered a single insemination per cycle.

The number of inseminations per cycle is not well defined. Future large prospective cohort studies or randomized trials for each indication separately might help clinicians to advise couples or individuals about the number of inseminations per cycle.

Is there a benefit of bed rest after IUI?

Women undergoing IUI should have 10–15 minutes of bed rest after an insemination. Studies on the intrauterine behavior of spermatozoa have shown that spermatozoa already reach the fallopian tubes within 5–10 minutes after insemination.[94] After vaginal intercourse, a large percentage of the semen is lost by "flowback" and no >1% of the spermatozoa are retained in the female reproductive tract. Thus, an assumed hypothesis is that immobilization in supine position after IUI could prevent direct loss of a large percentage of the spermatozoa and this action will improve fertility outcomes.

A systematic search resulted in the identification of two relevant articles[95] randomized 95 heterosexual couples to either direct mobilization after IUI or immobilization in supine position for 10 minutes. Groups were rather unbalanced with 40 couples in the mobilization group and 55 couples in the immobilization group. After three cycles, pregnancy rates per couple were significantly higher in the immobilization group. No information on LBRs was reported.[95] Custers et al.[96] performed a well-designed RCT in 391 heterosexual couples. They randomized between immobilization in a supine position for 15 minutes ($n = 199$) or immediate mobilization ($n = 192$) after IUI. LBRs after three cycles were significantly higher in the immobilization group: 27 versus 17%, respectively (RR = 1.6, 95% CI: 1.1–2.4).

Recently, results of a large RCT comparing immobilization for 15 minutes versus direct mobilization were published. In total, 498 patients with either unexplained or mild male infertility were included. No significant difference in cumulative ongoing pregnancy rate was found (RR = 0.81, 95% CI: 0.63–1.02).[97] Pooling the data of the last two studies mentioned here showed a nonsignificant difference between mobilization and immobilization (OR = 1.00, 95% CI: 0.74–1.33). However, a substantial statistical heterogeneity (I2 = 88%) was found. Conclusions should, therefore, be drawn with caution.

The data of van Rijswijk et al.[97] demonstrated that immobilization for 10–15 minutes after IUI has been determined to be an evidence-based draft recommendation.

What is the ultimate number of consecutive IUI cycles per couple/woman in which pregnancy rates still increase significantly?

- In couples with an indication for IUI, at least three consecutive IUI cycles should be performed.
- There is insufficient evidence to recommend a maximum number of IUI treatment cycles.

Three to six cycles of IUI have become common practice worldwide and the INeS trial from Bensdorp et al.[25] showed us that six cycles of IUI–OS are still cost-effective compared to direct IVF in patients with unexplained and mild male infertility.[25] But is there evidence to perform more cycles? Custers et al.[96] performed a retrospective cohort study among 3,714 women that had undergone 15,303 treatment cycles. Analysis was limited up to the ninth treatment cycle (15,245 cycles). There were 935 ongoing pregnancies, resulting in a mean ongoing pregnancy rate of 5.6% per cycle. The ongoing pregnancy rates were relatively high in the first two cycles, with 7.4 and 7.0%, respectively, compared with ~5% in higher order cycles. The cumulative clinical pregnancy rate after three cycles was 18%, which increases to 30 and 41% after six and nine cycles, respectively.[96] Aboulghar et al.[98] conducted an observational prospective study in 594 women with unexplained infertility. All participants had one to three cycles of treatment and 91 participants underwent four to six cycles of IUI–OS after failing to achieve pregnancy in the first three cycles. The clinical pregnancy rate per cycle was significantly higher in the first three cycles compared to the second three cycles ($p < 0.001$).[98] The overall quality of the evidence was graded as low to moderate mainly because of the retrospective and observational design of the studies. Based on this moderate quality evidence, a draft recommendation was developed to perform at least three cycles of IUI. There is insufficient evidence to recommend a maximum number of IUI treatment cycles.

The number of IUI cycles that couples or single woman should be offered is not well defined. Future large prospective cohort studies or randomized trials for each indication might help clinicians to advise couples or individuals when to switch to IVF.

Which semen preparation technique used yields the best results (in terms of pregnancy rates) for IUI?

- According to the available evidence, it is not possible to recommend any semen preparation technique over another (swim-up, gradient, wash, and centrifugation).

Currently, there are three semen preparation techniques that are routinely used worldwide: a simple dilution and washing technique, a swim-up technique, and use of density gradient centrifugation.

Whether one of these techniques is preferable was the subject of a Cochrane systematic review.[99] The Cochrane systematic review analyzed five RCTs comparing two or three techniques with each other. Concerns regarding heterogeneity might be suspected since they vary widely over the five studies or were not described clearly. The review found no significant difference in pregnancy rates among semen preparation techniques: swim-up versus gradient technique (OR = 1.57, 95% CI: 0.74–3.32), swim-up versus wash and centrifugation (OR = 0.41, 95% CI: 0.41–1.10), or gradient technique versus wash and centrifugation (OR = 1.76, 95% CI: 0.71–5.44).

Karamahmutoglu et al.[100] randomized 223 couples with unexplained and mild male infertility to either the swim-up technique or the gradient technique. They found a significantly higher ongoing pregnancy rate per patient after the gradient technique compared to swim-up: 23.4 versus 10.7%, respectively ($p < 0.05$). A subgroup analysis revealed that this difference was significant only in couples with unexplained infertility.[100] The overall quality was graded as low across all studies because of the suspected clinical heterogeneity, unclear descriptions of randomization and allocation in almost all included studies, and a low number of couples in the relevant comparisons. Therefore, according to review of evidence supporting IUI recommendations, it was not possible to recommend any semen preparation technique over another (swim-up, gradient, wash, and centrifugation).

It remains unclear that which semen preparation technique is superior (expressed as LBR per couple) in case of either unexplained or male infertility; therefore, a multicenter randomized trial comparing various techniques is recommended.

What is the cost-effectiveness of IUI versus IVF/ICSI?

- In couples with unexplained infertility and men with a TMSC of >10 million and a prognosis of a pregnancy without assistance <30% within a year, at least three cycles of IUI–OS are the most effective option.

The goal of research on cost-effectiveness is to maximize health outcomes with a minimum use of resources. As costs linked to fertility care in many countries are not covered by government or insurance companies, the relative cost-effectiveness of fertility treatments is a very important consideration.[101] Healthcare systems can become burdened by high costs associated with premature infants who are born from multiple gestations as a result from unregulated fertility treatments.[102] Therefore, cost-effectiveness studies in fertility are important not only to the individual and family but also to healthcare systems and society.

Large randomized trials evaluating the relative cost-effectiveness of different infertility treatments are scarce. Moreover, the outcome most often reported is the cost per delivery of at least one child and this outcome parameter does not include the substantial costs of caring for premature infants owing to the high rates of multiple gestations. On the other hand, there is the potential to consider twins as perhaps eliminating the need for future fertility treatments for some couples or individuals. However, this comes with a clear understanding of the maternal and perinatal morbidity and mortality outcomes of twin pregnancies in a local context. All of these factors have to be considered when studying the cost-effectiveness of IUI and IUI–OS.

Many retrospective cohort cost-effectiveness studies have compared IUI, IUI–OS, and conventional IVF in couples and individuals with differing causes of infertility. Most large cohort or randomized studies from individual centers have found IUI alone or IUI–OS to be the most cost-effective first-line therapy for heterosexual couples with infertility linked to cervical factor, endometriosis, unexplained infertility, and relatively mild male factor infertility,[103-105] but the retrospective designs make it difficult to draw firm conclusions.

For male factor infertility, several studies have been identified that support the concept of threshold values for sperm parameters below which IUI becomes significantly less effective.[53,69] Moolenaar et al.[69] studied the cost-effectiveness of interventions for male infertility according to the TMSC. A computer-simulated cohort of infertile women with a partner with a prewash TMSC of 0–10 million was investigated. They compared IUI with and without OS, conventional IVF, and IVF/ICSI. LBR was the main outcome parameter. Study results showed that above a prewash TMSC of 3 million, IUI is less costly than conventional IVF, and below a prewash TMSC of 3 million, IVF/ICSI is less costly. However, these findings need to be confirmed in a large randomized trial.

Contradictory results are published concerning the cost-effectiveness of IUI in heterosexual couples with unexplained infertility.[36,49,104-106] A multicenter RCT from Scotland (graded as high-quality evidence) compared the outcomes of 6 months of natural cycle IUI, CC stimulation followed by normal intercourse, and expectant management in couples with 2 years of unexplained infertility.[37] LBRs were not significantly different with 32/193 (17%) for expectant management,

26/192 (14%) for CC intercourse, and 43/191 (23%) for natural cycle-IUI. The authors recommended that IUI–OS should be the subject of future trials for unexplained infertility.

Most of the large retrospective cohort studies on cost-effectiveness tend to become "dated" as both costs and outcomes change over time. It is well known that IVF clinical pregnancy rates have increased steadily over time and high-order multiple births have declined, as there has been increased emphasis on the value of transferring less embryos. These changes have made conventional IVF a more attractive option from a cost-effective point of view when compared to IUI or IUI–OS. van Rumste et al.[72] stated in an economic analysis comparing IVF with elective transfer of a single embryo (eSET) with IUI–OS that when IVF–eSET would result in an ongoing pregnancy rate of >38%, IVF would be the preferred treatment.[72]

Only a few prospective randomized trials have compared natural cycle IUI, IUI–OS, and conventional IVF. In couples with male factor and unexplained infertility, Goverde et al.[49] compared three treatment arms—IUI alone, hMG–IUI, and conventional IVF, each performed for up to six cycles. The costs in this study were calculated through 12 weeks of pregnancy and neglecting the high costs associated with multiple gestations. According to this study, IUI was as effective as IVF, and IUI–OS did not yield higher pregnancy rates when compared with natural cycle IUI. They conclude that IUI was the most cost-effective first-line therapy for the infertile heterosexual couples. Furthermore, IUI was better tolerated by couples while IVF was associated with a higher dropout rate.[49] A big criticism against this study was an extremely low IVF pregnancy rate of 12.2% per cycle, a value that is clearly outdated. Even after careful monitoring and using low doses of FSH (75 IU/day), the MPR was 27% in the IUI–OS arm demonstrating the risky nature of this treatment.

In the prospective randomized Fast Track and Standard Treatment (FASTT) trial, graded as high quality, Reindollar et al.[50] addressed the important issue of time to pregnancy, both to alleviate the suffering and disappointment of infertile couples and to avoid the negative effects of aging on their reproductive potential. Only women between the ages of 21 and 39 years with unexplained infertility and a normal ovarian reserve were included in the study. Cost-effectiveness was calculated by summing all insurance charges divided by the number of women having at least one live birth. Out-of-pocket expenses (indirect costs) to the patient and the cost of multiple gestations as well as their associated increased hospital perinatal costs were included in the analysis. They concluded that CC–IUI seems to be the best first-line therapy for couples with unexplained infertility and, if not pregnant after three cycles, moving directly to conventional IVF was the most cost-effective approach.[50]

As mentioned before, in a recent multicenter randomized noninferiority trial in the Netherlands, the effectiveness of IVF with SET or IVF in a MNC was compared with the effectiveness of IUI–OS, with an outcome indicator of a healthy live birth.[25] The data of this trial showed that IUI–OS was noninferior as the two alternative strategies of IVF had a reasonably low multiple birth rate and was a more cost-effective strategy for heterosexual couples with mild male factor or unexplained infertility with a poor prognosis of becoming pregnant with expectant management. In another cost-effectiveness study on the same cohort of participants and investigating direct healthcare costs, it was concluded that both IVF strategies were significantly more expensive when compared with IUI–OS, without being significantly more effective.[26] Therefore, based on high-quality evidence, IUI–OS is recommended as the initial treatment for mild male factor and unexplained infertility with a poor prognosis of becoming pregnant through normal coitus. As mentioned before, there are no strict criteria for how to define mild male factor. Bensdorp et al.[25] used a TMSC of between 3 and 10 million although Cohlen et al.[73] showed that OS was only effective in couples with a TMSC above 10 million, which they defined as mild male infertility.

A significant increase in pregnancy rates has been observed with IVF and IVF/ICSI during the last decade; however, similar increases have not been reported with IUI treatments. If the singleton delivery rate per cycle can be improved, IVF or IVF/ICSI may become the favored first-line treatment for most causes of infertility.[72] On the other hand, it might be that a better selection of patients for IUI treatment and further improvement of the methodology of IUI may increase the success rates of IUI as well, and, hopefully not at the expense of increased multiple pregnancies. At present, the balance of all randomized trials still favors starting with a more conservative treatment regimen of IUI–OS before moving to IVF for the treatment of heterosexual couples with unexplained and mild male infertility.

Clear definitions of mild or moderate male infertility should be established before randomized trials can be started to define lower threshold levels of sperm parameters below which IUI with or without OS is no longer cost-effective and IVF or IVF/ICSI should be the first-line treatment option.

How can you prevent infections in an IUI laboratory?

- *Good practice point:* Couples and individuals undergoing IUI and males providing semen samples for IUI should be screened for infectious agents based on local, regional, and national standards and regulations.

In this era of semen preparation, infection is a lesser problem especially when managed in higher income settings. In some lower- and middle-income countries and settings, prevention of infections remains a critical issue. It is generally recommended that couples and individuals undergoing IUI and/or males providing semen samples for IUI should be screened for infectious agents based on local, regional, and national standards and regulations.

Furthermore, facilities for performing semen preparation for IUI should meet the criteria of the WHO laboratory safety manual for reducing the risk of infection.

Studies are lacking concerning the prevention and transmission of viral diseases in IUI treatment and thus these guidelines are, therefore, based upon best practice, guidelines associated with prevention of sexually transmitted infections, and local regulatory guidelines (good practice point).

It is recommended to compare various sperm preparation techniques in multicenter randomized trials both for success rates concerning the elimination of transmission of infectious diseases to both partners and to offspring.[107]

How can you prevent multiple pregnancies and OHSS in an IUI program?

- In order to prevent high rates of multiple gestation pregnancies in IUI–OS, IUI should be withheld when more than two dominant follicles of >15 mm or more than five follicles of >10 mm at the time of hCG injection or LH surge are present.
- When gonadotropins are used in IUI, regimens with 75 IU or lower should be used because higher doses have similar pregnancy rates but increase MPRs.
- Clomiphene citrate or tamoxifen is acceptable alternative to low-dose gonadotropins for low multiple pregnancy and birth rates and with lesser costs, although at a lower LBR than with gonadotropins.
- Addition of GnRH agonist to gonadotropins in IUI–OS is not recommended because there is no increase in pregnancy rate despite increased MPRs and increased costs.
- *Good practice point:* As an alternative to cycle cancellation, aspiration of excess follicles at the time of hCG injection or LH surge might be additional options for reducing the risk of multiple pregnancy in IUI–OS.

The most common side effects of IUI in cycles with OS are multiple pregnancies and OHSS. Multiple pregnancies carry increased risks of pregnancy complications and diminished neonatal outcome, such as preterm delivery, growth retardation, and preeclampsia. High MPRs are mainly caused by multifollicular growth following OS. Measures to prevent multiple pregnancies can be divided into primary and secondary measures. Primary measures include attempting to prevent the growth of more than two to three dominant follicles, as showed by van Rumste et al.[72] in a systematic review and meta-analysis including 14 studies (11,599 IUI cycles) (moderate quality of evidence). Multifollicular growth resulted in significantly higher pregnancy rates compared to monofollicular growth (15 vs. 8.4%). Compared with one dominant follicle, pregnancy rates increased by a further 5, 8, and 8%, respectively, when two, three, or four dominant follicles were present. Subsequently, the risk of multiple pregnancies after two, three, and four dominant follicles increased at 6, 14, and 10%, respectively.[72]

Another primary measure to prevent multiple pregnancies is to apply the appropriate drug and doses, and to individualize the doses when possible. CC (100 mg per day for 5 days) or tamoxifen is acceptable alternative to low-dose gonadotropins for low multiple birth rates and also results in lower costs, although at a lower LBR[108] (moderate quality of evidence). In this systematic review of Cantineau et al.,[108] significantly higher pregnancy rates were found with gonadotropins compared to antiestrogens (OR = 1.8, 95% CI: 1.2–2.7, n = 556, moderate quality of evidence). Two more recent high-quality evidence RCTs confirmed the outcomes of the Cochrane systematic review. In these trails, compared to CC, gonadotropins showed significantly higher LBRs and comparable, relatively low MPRs of between 3.6 and 12.5%.[109,110]

The Cochrane systematic review concluded also that there is no benefit in using letrozole compared to CC (pregnancy rate per couple: OR = 1.2, 95% CI: 0.64–2.1) based upon moderate-quality evidence. High-level evidence shows that when gonadotropins are used in IUI, regimens with 75 IU or lower should be used as higher doses have similar pregnancy rates while increasing MPRs.[108-110] Currently, an ongoing large multicenter trial is attempting to identify factors that might predict ovarian response with low-dose gonadotropin stimulation and thus might help to individualize stimulation doses in the future (PRORAILS study, NCT01662180). Based upon moderate-quality evidence, addition of GnRH agonist or antagonist is not recommended for our draft evidence-based guideline, because there is no increase in pregnancy rate despite increased MPRs and costs.[108] Cycles should be closely monitored by regular vaginal ultrasounds and when more than two to three follicles of >15 mm or when more than five follicles of >10 mm are seen, secondary measures can be advocated (moderate quality of evidence).[72] Of course, cycles can be cancelled and heterosexual couples should be advised to abstain from unprotected intercourse. As an alternative to cycle cancellation, aspiration of excess follicles at the time of hCG injection or LH surge, or conversion to IVF, might be additional options for reducing the risk of multiple pregnancy (good practice point). Finally, multifetal reduction can be proposed when a multiple pregnancy is observed.[111] However, multifetal reduction should be prevented at all costs with the above-mentioned measures for prevention of multiple pregnancies with IUI (good practice point). OHSS is very rare in IUI–OS treatment because the aim of the stimulation protocol should be two to three dominant follicles.[72] Regular ultrasound monitoring should identify any hyper-response early, such that hCG to induce ovulation can be withheld to avoid OHSS. With an adequate program to prevent multiple pregnancies, OHSS should be rarely encountered.

There is still debate regarding the most cost-effective drug for mild stimulation in IUI programs. Many randomized trials comparing gonadotropins with CC or letrozole have been published but the results are contradictory and often these trials are of (very) low quality. A large multicenter trial comparing gonadotropins with CC is ongoing in the Netherlands (SUPER trial NTR4057) and might be able to answer the question as to which strategy is the most cost-effective when addressing side effects and maternal and neonatal morbidity, and mortality associated with multiple pregnancies.

The majority of couples would prefer IUI with or without COH when the probability of a treatment-independent pregnancy in the next 12 months is 50% and 40%, respectively. The risk of a multiple pregnancy does not affect their preference for IUI, whereas IUI is rejected when the risk of OHSS exceeds 10%.[29]

Is there a different perinatal outcome for IUI pregnancies and how does this perinatal outcome differ from normal coitus and IVF/ICSI pregnancies?

- Individuals with infertility undergoing treatment with IUI–OS should be informed about a possible increased risk for preterm birth and low-birth weight in singletons and twin pregnancies when compared to pregnancies in fertile couples not requiring assistance (IVF/ICSI outcome comparisons are assessed in the IVF/ICSI prioritized guideline).

The perinatal outcome of pregnancies caused by ART and IUI is substantially worse when compared to pregnancies after normal coitus.[112] This is mainly attributed to a higher rate of multiple births. Few studies have been published reporting the obstetric and perinatal outcome after IUI in a direct comparison with medically unassisted pregnancies, with contradictory results. According to Nuojua-Huttunen et al.[113] using the data obtained from the Finnish Medical Birth Register, IUI treatment did not increase obstetric or perinatal risks compared with matched pregnancies through normal coitus or IVF pregnancies.[113] Wang et al.[114] examined preterm birth in 1,015 IUI/artificial insemination by donor (AID) singletons compared to 1,019 IVF/ICSI and 1,019 medically unassisted singletons. Singleton IUI/AID births were ~1.5 times more likely to be born preterm than medically unassisted singletons, whereas the IVF/ICSI group was 2.4 times more likely to be born preterm. They found no significant difference in the risk of preterm birth for IUI with partner or donor semen (7.0 vs. 7.5%, respectively).[114]

In a retrospective cohort study, Gaudoin et al.[115] described a poorer perinatal outcome of singletons born to infertile mothers through OS–IUI compared to matched medically unassisted pregnancies within the Scottish national cohort. The difference in perinatal outcome was caused by a higher incidence of prematurity and low-birth weight infants. The poor perinatal outcome of singletons after OS–IUI was associated with low-birth weight, but only when IUI was performed with partner's semen and not with donor semen.[115] In a matched case–control study, De Sutter et al.[116] did not observe a difference in pregnancy outcome in IUI versus IVF gestations.[116]

Two large cohort studies comparing the perinatal outcome after OS and/or IUI with medically unassisted pregnancies or IVF/ICSI pregnancies were performed in Flanders, Belgium.[117] Data were obtained from the Study Centre for Perinatal Epidemiology of Flanders. In the first study, the outcome from 661,065 births could be investigated. All women were matched for maternal age, parity, fetal sex, plurality, place, and year of birth. A significantly higher incidence of extreme prematurity (<32 weeks), very low-birth weight (<1,500 g), stillbirths, and perinatal death for OS–IUI singletons could be observed. Twin pregnancies resulting from OS–IUI showed a higher rate of neonatal mortality, assisted ventilation and respiratory distress syndrome when compared to medically unassisted twin pregnancies.

In the second study,[118] 1,039,415 singletons and 39,041 twins were available for analysis. Following logistic regression analyses, it was shown that IVF/ICSI singletons had a significantly worse outcome when compared to OS–IUI and medically unassisted pregnancies for almost all investigated perinatal parameters. OS singletons were also significantly disadvantaged for birth weight and prematurity when compared to pregnancies obtained through normal coitus. The outcome of twin pregnancies was similar for the three groups unless only unlike-sex twins were studied separately. Among this subgroup, IVF/ICSI carried a higher risk for low-birth weight when compared to medically unassisted pregnancies.

In a retrospective cohort study, Poon and Lian[119] also observed that perinatal outcomes after IUI/CC pregnancies represent an intermediate risk between IVF/ICSI and pregnancies obtained through normal coitus. A national cohort study in Denmark on 6,338 singletons born after IUI showed an increased risk of adverse perinatal outcomes compared with children born after normal coitus. Stimulation with CC was associated with higher risk of small for gestational age compared with natural cycle IUI.[120]

The reason why perinatal health problems occur more frequently after IUI is still unknown, but can be explained by the procedures itself, the endocrine changes caused by OS medication or the underlying reason for infertility.[121] In a structured review, Pinborg et al.[122] concluded that infertility is a major risk factor for adverse perinatal outcome for singletons, and even in the same mother, an ART singleton has a poorer outcome than the non-ART sibling. This could mean that factors related to the hormone stimulation and/or ART methods per se may play a role.

Both OS-IUI and IVF/ICSI are associated with an increased risk for multiple pregnancies.

It has been shown that spontaneous reduction of multiple pregnancies causes a higher risk for adverse obstetric and perinatal outcome compared to pregnancies without spontaneous reduction. >10% of IVF/ICSI singletons are the result of a vanishing twin, and the same can be expected after OS–IUI. Survivors of a vanishing co-twin have a higher risk for prematurity and low-birth weight compared to singletons from single gestations, the higher the gestational age at fetal demise, the higher the risk for the surviving co-twin.[123] This phenomenon can explain, at least partly, the worse perinatal health outcome after OS–IUI compared to singleton and twin pregnancies born without medical assistance.

Pregnancies in patients with diabetes insipidus (DI) carry no increased risk compared to pregnancies obtained through normal coitus.[114,115,124] In a large French population study, it was shown that after DI, the miscarriage and tubal pregnancy rate, the children's weight, and the prematurity rate were not different from that of the general French population.[125] The rate of birth defects was comparable to the figures reported in a general population. The chromosomal abnormality rate was normal and correlated not only to the mother's age but also to the sperm donor's age. In addition, not further elaborated upon here, according to the available literature, the use of frozen spermatozoa does not seem to affect the health of children. On the other hand, a clinical pregnancy resulting from IUI with donor sperm appears to increase the incidence of preeclampsia.[126] In a structured review and meta-analysis, it was shown that pregnancy using donor sperm was associated with an increased risk of preeclampsia (OR = 1.63, 95% CI: 1.36–1.95) compared with using partner's sperm. No difference was observed in any risk for gestational hypertension.[127]

Couples and single women undergoing treatment with IUI require counseling concerning the increased risk of perinatal mortality and morbidity in twins compared to singletons. They should also be informed about an increased risk for perinatal health problems if they become pregnant after IUI with homologous and donor sperm, even for singletons, although this draft recommendation is based upon low-quality evidence. A close follow-up of IUI pregnancies from the early beginning of pregnancy is mandatory to detect spontaneous reduction of multiple pregnancies, which might be very important for that particular pregnancy.

PROGNOSTIC FACTORS INFLUENCING IUI SUCCESS

Female age is the most relevant predictor of the probability of clinical pregnancy in IUI treatment and moderate-quality evidence-based data show that a sharp decline of IUI success rate is observed in women over the age of 40 years, which is presumably related to review of evidence supporting IUI recommendations oocyte quality.[2] In heterosexual couples with unexplained infertility, IUI treatment should be limited to women with female age <40 years, although IUI may be encouraged to continue up to 42 years when donor sperm is used.[74] Whether IVF or ICSI should be recommended as a first-line therapy when the female is in her late 30s or >40 years of age is still debatable and more studies are needed to examine the cost-effectiveness of such an approach.[2]

Male age seems to have no profound effect when the female partner or sperm recipient is <35 years but a synergistic adverse effect seems to exist when the woman is >35 years and the man as well.[128] A possible explanation may be a decline in sperm quality with increased male age, especially for semen volume, sperm motility, and sperm morphology, but not for sperm count.[129] Therefore, men in a heterosexual relationship (or identified as sperm donor) with a female partner >35 years should be informed that increasing paternal age (40 years and above) has a potential negative impact on IUI success rates.[130] Moreover, oxidative stress-induced mitochondrial DNA damage and nuclear DNA damage in aging men may put them at a higher risk for transmitting multiple genetic and chromosomal defects.[131]

Additional parameters can also influence the IUI success rates although well-organized prospective randomized trials are not available. In a structured review, Ombelet et al.[53] investigated which sperm parameter in the native and washed semen sample influences success rates after IUI. Their search indicated a lack of prospective studies, a lack of standardization in semen testing methodology, and a huge heterogeneity of patient groups and IUI treatment strategies. The review identified an urgent need for more and better prospective cohort trials investigating the predictive value of semen parameters on IUI success rates.

The four sperm parameters most frequently examined were—inseminating motile count after washing: cut-off value between 0.8 and 5 million; sperm morphology using strict criteria: cut-off value >4% normal morphology; TMSC in native sperm sample: cut-off value of 5–10 million; and total motility in native sperm sample: threshold value of 30%.

Several studies support the concept of threshold values for sperm parameters below which IUI becomes significantly less effective. Most important are sperm morphology with a threshold value of 4%[53,54] and the TMSC either in the ejaculate (an average of 10 million total motile sperm in at least two samples) or in the postwash inseminating motile count (between 0.8 and 5 million motile sperm).[53,55] When using these threshold values, a poor sensitivity for predicting pregnancy but high specificity for predicting failure to become pregnant with IUI could be observed.

Ultrasound parameters can also be used to provide important information on egg quality and endometrial receptivity that will optimize the chances of success in an IUI program. However, robust evidence is lacking and the role of Doppler assessment in the ovaries and endometrium needs to be studied in future randomized trials.[132,133] Endometrial thickness is another important factor predicting endometrial receptivity. It has been shown that endometrial thickness in stimulated IUI cycles is lower than in IVF cycles and is lower in cycles stimulated with CC compared with natural nonstimulated cycles.[134] A recent systematic review and meta-analysis on preovulatory endometrial thickness in IUI treatment (n = 3,846) showed that women treated with CC had a significantly thinner endometrial thickness than women treated with gonadotropins [n = 383, mean difference (MD): –0.33, 95% CI: –0.64 to –0.01]. However, pooling of seven relevant studies (n = 1,525) did not reveal an association between endometrial thickness and pregnancy rates (MD: 0.51, 95% CI: –0.05 to 1.07). Also, after a sensitivity analysis, the results remained nonsignificant.

The authors, therefore, concluded that endometrial thickness is not a good prognostic factor for IUI treatment success (low to moderate quality of evidence).[135] Studies on the influence of the body mass index (BMI) and obesity on IVF success rates are contradictory. A population-based cohort study[136] showed that an increased female and male BMI, both independently and combined, negatively influenced LBRs after IVF treatments.[136] In another prospective cohort study, weight status did not influence fecundity among heterosexual couples undergoing IVF treatment.[137] However, the influence of weight on IUI outcome remains unclear. Contradictory results were published in two retrospective analyses investigating the influence of BMI on IUI success: in one study, a BMI of 25 kg/m^2 or more in the woman was associated with higher success rates,[138] while in the second study, a BMI of <25 kg/m^2 was positively correlated with clinical pregnancy rates after IUI.[139] In most studies, it seems that a woman's BMI is not a determining factor for success rate after IUI although obese women require higher doses of medication. Once medication is adjusted to overcome the weight effect, the success rate is comparable for obese and normal weight women.[140-144] In addition, an underweight BMI may also be associated with poor fertility.[144] However, the advice to patients should be focused not only on ensuring optimal treatment outcomes, but also on promoting the best obstetrical outcomes because a high BMI is undoubtedly associated with adverse obstetrical and perinatal outcome.[145]

Studies on the influence of the smoking status on IUI success rates are almost nonexistent. It was shown that female smokers undergoing IUI-OS need significantly more gonadotropins than nonsmokers in order to achieve a comparable clinical pregnancy rate.[146] However, smoking was not significantly associated with a chance of becoming pregnant after secondary analyses of data from a prospective, randomized, multicenter "Assessment of Multiple Intrauterine Gestations from Ovarian Stimulation" (AMIGOS) clinical trial.[147] However, focus would need to be placed on obstetrical and perinatal outcome because of the detrimental effects of smoking.

EFFICACY AND SAFETY OF INTRAUTERINE INSEMINATION AND ASSISTED REPRODUCTIVE TECHNOLOGY IN POPULATIONS SERODISCORDANT FOR HUMAN IMMUNODEFICIENCY VIRUS

The controversy over whether the partners of patients infected with human immunodeficiency virus (HIV) should undergo procreative therapy was sparked in the 1980s when noninfected women were suspected to have contracted HIV through IUI.[148,149] Semprini et al.[150] subsequently demonstrated safe and effective sperm-washing techniques that could minimize the risk for transmission to the negative partner in 1992.[150] Though this has resulted in increased use of sperm processing and insemination for HIV-serodiscordant couples in Europe, it still is not commonly practiced in the United States. Couples who are HIV serodiscordant have both fertility desires and fertility needs. Infertility affects approximately 15% of the general population, and people with HIV have greater reproductive challenges secondary to sequelae from their HIV infection. Studies of the sperm quality of men with HIV who are on antiretroviral treatment have demonstrated significantly lower ejaculate volumes, lower sperm count, and lower progressive motility despite normal morphology.[151-153] This is consistent with HIV-associated hypogonadism, which can occur even without highly active antiretroviral therapy (HAART). Women with HIV have lower fertility rates across the world. The Joint United Nations Programme on HIV/AIDS (UNAIDS) estimated that the global age-specific fertility ratios for women with HIV in the reproductive-age group of 20–44 years are lower than that of women without HIV (ranging from 0.76 to 0.53).[154] These were suspected to be secondary to higher rates of gynecologic infections in women with HIV, with tubal factor infertility from pelvic inflammatory disease being an important obstacle to conception.[155,156] Many of these factors can be overcome via reproductive therapies, including insemination and assisted reproductive technology (ART).

The risk of transmission of HIV is 2.3 per 1,000 acts of receptive vaginal intercourse when a partner has a detectable viral load.[157] However, an undetectable viral load does not clearly translate to safety with unprotected intercourse, as almost 10% of men with undetectable viral load on HAART may still have detectable seminal virus.[158] Any ulcerative lesion in the genital tract and even seemingly benign conditions such as bacterial vaginosis can increase the risk of transmission of HIV several fold.[159,160] With no reported HIV transmission among serodiscordant couples identified in a systematic review,[161] with the upper 95% confidence limit for the risk of transmission from insemination therapy being fivefold less than the rate with coitus, and with the true value likely being even more favorable, this illustrates the potential value of using ART or IUI to reduce risk in couples committed to using their own gametes.

In terms of the balance of risk and benefits for procreation with IUI relative to ART, it appears that IUI in seropositive men results in approximately half the pregnancy rate per cycle. It does so at about 1/10th to 1/20th the cost and also has a lower risk for multiple gestations and miscarriage as well as a lower surgical risk. There were no detected cases of HIV transmission with either method. Finally, in the context of an increasing number of HIV-serodiscordant couples being counseled by their physicians to conceive through coitus while on antiretroviral therapy, we have to determine whether insemination-based approaches serve as a middle ground while more data are collected on the safety and efficacy of unassisted conception.

Serodiscordant couples with HIV who do not meet the criteria for AIDS have a reasonable chance of pregnancy through fertility therapy. Male and female candidates for insemination seem to have pregnancy rates comparable to the general fertility population. Miscarriage rates seem similar to those for HIV-seronegative subfertile couples for IUI but are higher for ART. Seropositive men with unaffected partners have pregnancy and live birth rates with ART comparable to seronegative couples. However, seropositive females undergoing ART were found to have lower pregnancy rates per cycle. This disparity may have multifactorial origins, and further studies will be needed to address this issue. For studies meeting inclusion criteria, there were no seroconversions of HIV-negative partners by either IUI or ART.

There certainly will be clinicians who believe any risk of HIV transmission is unacceptable, even if none are seen in our large meta-analysis. However, so that decisions are evidence based rather than emotional, the risks should be quantified and placed in the context of similar accepted risks.

Moreover, the procreative desires and needs of serodiscordant couples often mean that they may be exposing themselves to far greater risks when without medical alternatives. As clinicians striving to promote health, we need to reconsider the role of procreative therapy in HIV-serodiscordant couples.

FUTURE DEVELOPMENTS

Increasing success rates following IVF/ICSI with better implantation rates per embryo are reported year-on-year; however, similar increases have not been reported following IUI. This could eventually lead to an unacceptable high difference in cost-effectiveness between IVF/ICSI and IUI, subsequently encouraging those who prefer IVF above IUI in all cases. However, such a statement does not take into account the couple's or the individual woman's preference, and the difference in complications related to the various treatment strategies. Nevertheless, IUI will remain an effective first-line treatment in unexplained infertility and mild male factor infertility, as well as the use of donor sperm in same sex female couples and single women, if we succeed in increasing the delivery rate per cycle without increasing the risk for complications such as a higher MPRs and increased risk for OHSS.

A well-controlled mild OS with gonadotropins aiming for two dominant follicles is the most effective strategy when performing IUI for unexplained infertility, minimal-to-mild endometriosis, and moderate-to-mild male factor infertility. A standardized methodology for IUI taking into account evidence-based data on how to perform IUI as described in this chapter will likely increase IUI singleton pregnancy rates worldwide. Other methods to increase the delivery rate per IUI cycle will be a better selection of patients who have a reasonable prognosis with IUI. The evidence has identified several factors that might influence IUI outcome as presented and will require further confirmation by well-designed and adequately powered randomized trials. Prewashing the catheter with culture medium prior to IUI seems to increase the success rate per cycle and could be recommended in Good Laboratory Practice Guidelines, as is already the case for embryo transfer catheters. It is clear that more studies are needed examining the influence of certain infections, sperm DNA abnormalities, and other (unknown) factors on IUI outcome results. More evidence-based research is also needed to optimize IUI outcome in terms of a better selection of couples or individual women who are the best candidates for IUI.

CONCLUSION

After collecting and appraising the most recent evidence on IUI in infertility care, it is possible to conclude that most of the presented "evidence" does not stand up to modern quality parameters, and is of moderate or (very) low quality. Issues such as randomization method, allocation concealment, blinding, adequate power, and outcome measures are often not adequately dealt with and thus most evidence is often graded from moderate to low. Especially in an "old treatment option", as IUI is often viewed, many RCTs are published in the previous century and firm conclusions are hard to draw.

Nevertheless, recently published higher quality multicenter RCTs fail to devalue IUI in the world of more advanced medically assisted reproductive treatments. Therefore, IUI, often in combination with OS, remains a first-line treatment option for many heterosexual and same-sex infertile couples and single women as this strategy is supported by the results of cost-effectiveness trials. However, applied inappropriately, IUI–OS could be a harmful treatment. In the delivery of fertility care interventions and treatments, the prevention of multiple pregnancies should be as important as optimizing LBRs. In low- and middle-income countries and settings, the prevention of infections with a high risk of transmission, including review of evidence supporting IUI recommendations 315 endemic viral diseases such as HIV or hepatitis, is equally important.

This chapter presented several factors that might influence IUI outcome, such as women's age, BMI, and ultrasound parameters, and that need further confirmation by randomized trials so that in future, it might become possible to select those patients who would benefit most from IUI with a low risk of adverse events.

REFERENCES

1. World Health Organization. WHO Handbook for Guideline Development, 2nd edition. Geneva: World Health Organization; 2014.
2. Yarde F, Broekmans FJM. Factors influencing IUI outcome: female age. In: Cohlen BJ, Ombelet W (Eds). Intra-Uterine Insemination: Evidence-Based Guidelines for Daily Practice. Boca Raton, USA: CRC Press, Taylor & Francis Group; 2014. pp. 27-33.
3. Cohen MR. Intrauterine insemination. Int J Fertil. 1962; 7:235-40.
4. Zegers-Hochschild F, Nygren KG, Adamson GD, de Mouzon J, Lancaster P, Mansour R, et al. The ICMART glossary on ART terminology. Hum Reprod. 2006a;21:1968-70.
5. Zegers-Hochschild F, Nygren KG, Adamson GD, de Mouzon J, Lancaster P, Mansour R, et al. The International Committee Monitoring Assisted Reproductive Technologies (ICMART) glossary 1 on ART terminology. Fertil Steril. 2006b;86:16-19.
6. Andersen AN, Goossens V, Ferraretti AP, Bhattacharya S, Felberbaum R, de Mouzon J, et al. Assisted reproductive technology in Europe, 2004: results generated from European registers by ESHRE. Hum Reprod. 2008;23:756-71.
7. Bensdorp AJ, Cohlen BJ, Heineman MJ, Vandekerckhove P. Intra-uterine insemination for male subfertility. Cochrane Database Syst Rev. 2007;(3):CD000360.
8. Steures P, van der Steeg JW, Hompes PG, Habbema JD, Eijkemans MJ, Broekmans FJ, et al. Collaborative Effort on the Clinical Evaluation in Reproductive Medicine. Intrauterine insemination with controlled ovarian hyperstimulation versus expectant management for couples with unexplained subfertility and an intermediate prognosis: a randomised clinical trial. Lancet. 2006;368(9531):216-21.
9. World Health Organization. WHO Laboratory Manual for the Examination and Processing of Human Semen, 5th edition. Geneva: World Health Organization; 2010.
10. Aitken RJ, Clarkson JS. Cellular basis of defective sperm function and its association with the genesis of reactive oxygen species by human spermatozoa. J Reprod Fertil. 1987;81:459-69.
11. Aitken RJ, De Iuliis GN. On the possible origins of DNA damage in human spermatozoa. Mol Hum Reprod. 2010;16:3-13.
12. Mortimer D. Sperm preparation methods. J Androl. 2000;21: 357-66.
13. Besselink DE, Farquhar C, Kremer JAM, Marjoribanks J, O'Brien P. Cervical insemination versus intra-uterine insemination of donor sperm for subfertility. Cochrane Database Syst Rev. 2008;(2):CD000317.
14. Ombelet W, Van Robays J. (2010). History of human artificial insemination. [online] Available from https://fvvo.eu/assets/97/13-Ombelet_et_al.pdf. [Last accessed December, 2022].
15. Guttmacher AF. The role of artificial insemination in the treatment of human sterility. Bull NY Acad Med. 1943; 19:573-91.
16. Kohlberg K. Arzt und Samenübertragung. Dtsch Med Wochenschr. 1953a;78:855-6.
17. Kohlberg K. Die Praxis der Samenübertragung beim Menschen. Dtsch Med Wochenschr. 1953b;78:835-9.
18. Sherman JK, Bunge RG. Observations on preservation of human spermatozoa at low temperatures. Proc Soc Med Biol Med. 1953;84:686-8.
19. Sherman JK. Low temperature research on spermatozoa and eggs. Cryobiology. 1964;1:10329.
20. Steptoe PC, Edwards RG. Birth after the reimplantation of a human embryo. Lancet. 1978;2:366.
21. Sunde A, Kahn JA, Molne K. Intrauterine insemination: a European collaborative report. Hum Reprod. 1988;3:69-3.
22. Friedman A, Haas S, Kredentser J, Stewart E, Schiff I. A controlled trial of intrauterine insemination for cervical factor and male factor: a preliminary report. Int J Fertil. 1989;34:199-203.
23. te Velde ER, van Kooy RJ, Waterreus JJ. Intrauterine insemination of washed husband's spermatozoa: a controlled study. Fertil Steril. 1989;51:182-5.
24. Cohlen BJ. Should we continue performing intrauterine inseminations in the year 2004? Gynecol Obstet Invest. 2005;59:3-13.
25. Bensdorp AJ, Tjon-Kon-Fat RI, Bossuyt PM, Koks CA, Oosterhuis GJ, Hoek A, et al. Prevention of multiple pregnancies in couples with unexplained or mild male subfertility: randomised controlled trial of in vitro fertilisation with single embryo transfer or in vitro fertilisation in modified natural cycle compared with intrauterine insemination with controlled ovarian hyperstimulation. BMJ. 2015;35.
26. Tjon-Kon-Fat RI, Bensdorp AJ, Bossuyt PMM, Koks C, Oosterhuis GJE, Hoek A, et al. Is IVF-served two different ways-more cost-effective than IUI with controlled ovarian hyperstimulation? Hum Reprod. 2015;30:2331-9.
27. Ombelet W, Cooke I, Dyer S, Serour G, Devroey P. Infertility and the provision of infertility medical services in developing countries. Hum Reprod Update. 2008;14:605-21.
28. Homburg R. The case for initial treatment with intrauterine insemination as opposed to in vitro fertilization for idiopathic infertility. Hum Fertil (Camb). 2003;6:122-4.
29. Steures P, Berkhout JC, Hompes PG, van der Steeg JW, Bossuyt PM, van der Veen F, et al. Patients' preferences in deciding between intrauterine insemination and expectant management. Hum Reprod. 2005;20(3):752-5.
30. van Weert JM, van den Broek J, van der Steeg JW, van der Veen F, Flierman PA, Mol BWJ, et al. Patients' preferences for intrauterine insemination or in vitro fertilization. Reprod Biomed Online. 2007;15:422-7.
31. Athaullah N, Proctor M, Johnson NP. Oral versus injectable ovulation induction agents for unexplained subfertility. Cochrane Database Syst Rev. 2002;(3):CD003052.
32. Collins JA, Van Steirteghem A. Overall prognosis with current treatment of infertility. Hum Reprod Update. 2004;10:309-16.

33. Fisch P, Casper RF, Brown SE, Wrixon W, Collins JA, Reid RL, et al. Unexplained infertility: evaluation of treatment with clomiphene citrate and human chorionic gonadotropin. Fertil Steril. 1989;51:828-33.
34. Donderwinkel PF, van der Vaart H, Wolters VM, Simons AH, Kroon G, Heineman MJ. Treatment of patients with long-standing unexplained subfertility with in vitro fertilization. Fertil Steril. 2000;73:334-7.
35. Evers JL, de Haas HW, Land JA, Dumoulin JC, Dunselman GA. Treatment-independent pregnancy rate in patients with severe reproductive disorders. Hum Reprod. 1998;13:1206-9.
36. Guzick DS, Carson SA, Coutifaris C, Overstreet JW, Factor-Litvak P, Steinkampf MP, et al. Efficacy of superovulation and intrauterine insemination in the treatment of infertility. National Cooperative Reproductive Medicine Network. N Engl J Med. 1999;340:177-83.
37. Bhattacharya S, Harrild K, Mollison J, Wordsworth S, Tay C, Harrold A, et al. Clomifene citrate or unstimulated intrauterine insemination compared with expectant management for unexplained infertility: pragmatic randomized controlled trial. BMJ. 2008;337:a716.
38. Zeyneloglu HB, Arici A, Olive DL, Duleba AJ. Comparison of intrauterine insemination with timed intercourse in superovulated cycles with gonadotropins: a meta-analysis. Fertil Steril. 1998;69:486-91.
39. Society for Assisted Reproductive Technology. (2013). Society for Assisted Reproductive Technology National Summary, 2013. [online] Available from https://www.sartcorsonline.com/rptCSR_PublicMultYear.aspx?ClinicPKID=0. [Last accessed December, 2022].
40. Deaton JL, Gibson M, Blackmer KM, Nakajima ST, Badger GJ, Brumsted JR. A randomized, controlled trial of clomiphene citrate and intrauterine insemination in couples with unexplained infertility or surgically corrected endometriosis. Fertil Steril. 1990;54:1083-8.
41. Fouda UM, Sayed AM. Extended letrozole regimen versus clomiphene citrate for superovulation in patients with unexplained infertility undergoing intrauterine insemination: a randomized controlled trial. Reprod Biol Endocrinol. 2011;9:84.
42. Diamond MP, Mitwally M, Casper R, Ager J, Legro RS, Brzyski R, et al. Estimating rates of multiple gestation pregnancies: sample size calculation from the assessment of multiple intrauterine gestations from ovarian stimulation (AMIGOS) trial. Contemp Clin Trials. 2011;32:902-8.
43. Diamond MP, Legro RS, Coutifaris C, Alvero R, Robinson RD, Casson P, et al. Assessment of multiple intrauterine gestations from ovarian stimulation (AMIGOS) trial: baseline characteristics. Fertil Steril. 2015;103:962-73.e4.
44. Diamond MP, Legro RS, Coutifaris C, Alvero R, Robinson RD, Casson P, et al. Letrozole, gonadotropin, or clomiphene for unexplained infertility. N Engl J Med. 2015;373:1230-40.
45. Berker B, Kahraman K, Taskin S, Sukur YE, Sonmezer M, Atabekoglu CS. Recombinant FSH versus clomiphene citrate for ovarian stimulation in couples with unexplained infertility and male subfertility undergoing intrauterine insemination: a randomized trial. Arch Gynecol Obstet. 2011;284:1561-6.
46. Dankert T, Kremer JA, Cohlen BJ, Hamilton CJ, Pasker-de Jong PC, Straatman H, et al. A randomized clinical trial of clomiphene citrate versus low dose recombinant FSH for ovarian hyperstimulation in intrauterine insemination cycles for unexplained and male subfertility. Hum Reprod. 2007;22:792-7.
47. Baysoy A, Serdaroglu H, Jamal H, Karatekeli E, Ozornek H, Attar E. Letrozole versus human menopausal gonadotrophin in women undergoing intrauterine insemination. Reprod Biomed Online. 2006;13:208-12.
48. Gregoriou O, Vlahos NF, Konidaris S, Papadias K, Botsis D, Creatsas GK. Randomized controlled trial comparing superovulation with letrozole versus recombinant follicle-stimulating hormone combined with intrauterine insemination for couples with unexplained infertility who had failed clomiphene citrate stimulation and intrauterine insemination. Fertil Steril. 2008;90:678-83.
49. Goverde AJ, McDonnell J, Vermeiden JP, Schats R, Rutten FF, Schoemaker J. Intrauterine insemination or in-vitro fertilisation in idiopathic subfertility and male subfertility: a randomised trial and cost-effectiveness analysis. Lancet. 2000;355(9197):13-8.
50. Reindollar RH, Regan MM, Neumann PJ, Levine BS, Thornton KL, Alper MM, et al. A randomized clinical trial to evaluate optimal treatment for unexplained infertility: the fast track and standard treatment (FASTT) trial. Fertil Steril. 2010;94(3):888-99.
51. Tomlinson M, Lewis S, Morroll D, British Fertility S. Sperm quality and its relationship to natural and assisted conception: British Fertility Society guidelines for practice. Hum Fertil (Camb). 2013;16:175-93.
52. Van den Hoven L, Hendriks JC, Verbeet JG, Westphal JR, Wetzels AM. Status of sperm morphology assessment: an evaluation of methodology and clinical value. Fertil Steril. 2015;103:53-8.
53. Ombelet W, Dhont N, Thijssen A, Bosmans E, Kruger T. Semen quality and prediction of IUI success in male subfertility: a systematic review. Reprod Biomed Online. 2014;28:300-9.
54. Van Waart J, Kruger TF, Lombard CJ, Ombelet W. Predictive value of normal sperm morphology in intrauterine insemination (IUI): a structured literature review. Hum Reprod Update. 2001;7:495-500.
55. van Weert JM, Repping S, Van Voorhis BJ, van der Veen F, Bossuyt PM, Mol BW. Performance of the postwash total motile sperm count as a predictor of pregnancy at the time of intrauterine insemination: a meta-analysis. Fertil Steril. 2004;82:612-20.
56. Lee RK, Hou JW, Ho HY, Hwu YM, Lin MH, Tsai YC, et al. Sperm morphology analysis using strict criteria as a prognostic factor in intrauterine insemination. Int J Androl. 2002;25:277-80.
57. Ombelet W, Vandeput H, Van de Putte G, Cox A, Janssen M, Jacobs P, et al. Intrauterine insemination after ovarian stimulation with clomiphene citrate: predictive potential of inseminating motile count and sperm morphology. Hum Reprod. 1997;12:1458-63.
58. Burr RW, Siegberg R, Flaherty SP, Wang XJ, Matthews CD. The influence of sperm morphology and the number of motile sperm inseminated on the outcome of intrauterine insemination combined with mild ovarian stimulation. Fertil Steril. 1996;65:127-32.
59. Nikbakht R, Saharkhiz N. The influence of sperm morphology, total motile sperm count of semen and the number of motile sperm inseminated in sperm samples on the success of intrauterine insemination. Int J Fertil Steril. 2011;5:168-73.

60. Gauci MM, Kruger TF, Coetzee K, Smith K, van der Merwe JP, Lombard CJ. Stepwise regression analysis to study male and female factors impacting on pregnancy rate in an intrauterine insemination programme. Andrologia. 2001;33:135-41.
61. Karabinus DS, Gelety TJ. The impact of sperm morphology evaluated by strict criteria on intrauterine insemination success. Fertil Steril. 1997;67:536-41.
62. Sun Y, Li B, Fan LQ, Zhu WB, Chen XJ, Feng JH, et al. Does sperm morphology affect the outcome of intrauterine insemination in patients with normal sperm concentration and motility? Andrologia. 2012;44:299-304.
63. Hauser R, Yogev L, Botchan A, Lessing JB, Paz G, Yavetz H. Intrauterine insemination in male factor subfertility: significance of sperm motility and morphology assessed by strict criteria. Andrologia. 2001;33:13-7.
64. Lindheim SR, Barad DH, Zinger M, Witt B, Amin H, Cohen B, et al. Abnormal sperm morphology is highly predictive of pregnancy outcome during controlled ovarian hyperstimulation and intrauterine insemination. J Assist Reprod Genet. 1996;13:569-72.
65. Deveneau NE, Sinno O, Krause M, Eastwood D, Sandlow JI, Robb P, et al. Impact of sperm morphology on the likelihood of pregnancy after intrauterine insemination. Fertil Steril. 2014;102:1584-90.e2.
66. Van Voorhis BJ, Barnett M, Sparks AE, Syrop CH, Rosenthal G, Dawson J. Effect of the total motile sperm count on the efficacy and cost-effectiveness of intrauterine insemination and in vitro fertilization. Fertil Steril. 2001;75:661-8.
67. Tijani HA, Bhattacharya S. The role of intrauterine insemination in male infertility. Hum Fertil. 2010;13:226-32.
68. Lockwood GM, Deveneau NE, Shridharani AN, Strawn EY, Sandlow JI. Isolated abnormal strict morphology is not a contraindication for intrauterine insemination. Andrology. 2015;3:1088-93.
69. Moolenaar LM, Cissen M, de Bruin JP, Hompes PG, Repping S, van der Veen F, et al. Cost-effectiveness of assisted conception for male subfertility. Reprod Biomed Online. 2015;30:659-66.
70. Hamilton JA, Cissen M, Brandes M, Smeenk JM, de Bruin JP, Kremer JA, et al. Total motile sperm count: a better indicator for the severity of male factor infertility than the WHO sperm classification system. Hum Reprod. 2015;30:1110-21.
71. Helmerhorst FM, Van Vliet HAAM, Gornas T, Finken MJJ, Grimes DA. Intrauterine insemination versus timed intercourse for cervical hostility in subfertile couples. Cochrane Database Syst Rev. 2005;2005(4):CD002809.
72. van Rumste MME, Custers IM, van der Veen F, van Wely M, Evers JLH, Mol BWJ. The influence of the number of follicles on pregnancy rates in intrauterine insemination with ovarian stimulation: a meta-analysis. Hum Reprod Update. 2008;14:563-70.
73. Cohlen BJ, te Velde ER, van Kooij RJ, Looman CW, Habbema JD. Controlled ovarian hyperstimulation and intrauterine insemination for treating male subfertility: a controlled study. Hum Reprod. 1998;13:1553-8.
74. Veltman-Verhulst SM, Cohlen BJ, Hughes E, Heineman MJ. Intra-uterine insemination for unexplained subfertility. Cochrane Database Syst Rev. 2012;(9):CD001838.
75. Hunault CC, Habbema JDF, Eijkemans MJC, Collins JA, Evers JLH, te Velde ER. Two new prediction rules for spontaneous pregnancy leading to live birth among subfertile couple, based on the synthesis of three previous models. Hum Reprod. 2004;19:2019-26.
76. Hunault CC, Laven JSE, van Rooij IAJ, Eijkemans MJC, te Velde ER, Habbema JDF. Prospective validation of two models predicting pregnancy leading to live birth among untreated subfertile couples. Hum Reprod. 2005;20:1636-41.
77. Duran HE, Morshedi M, Kruger T, Oehninger S. Intrauterine insemination: a systematic review on determinants of success. Hum Reprod Update. 2002;8(4):373-84.
78. Khalil MR, Rasmussen PE, Erb K, Laursen SB, Rex S, Westergaard LG. Homologous intrauterine insemination: an evaluation of prognostic factors based on a review of 2473 cycles. Acta Obstet Gynecol Scand. 2001;80:74-81.
79. Kamath MS, Bhave P, Aleyamma T, Nair R, Chandy A, Mangalaraj AM, et al. Predictive factors for pregnancy after intrauterine insemination: a prospective study of factors affecting outcome. J Hum Reprod Sci. 2010;3:129-34.
80. Demir B, Dilbaz B, Cinar O, Karadag B, Tasci Y, Kocak M, et al. Factors affecting pregnancy outcome of intrauterine insemination cycles in couples with favorable female characteristics. J Obstet Gynaecol. 2011;31:420-3.
81. Huang FJ, Chang SY, Lu YJ, Kung FT, Tsai MY, Wu JF. Two different timings of intrauterine insemination for non-male infertility. J Assist Reprod Genet. 2000;17:213e7.
82. Wang YC, Chang YC, Chen IC, Cnien HH, Wu GJ. Comparison of timing of IUI in ovarian stimulated cycles. Arch Androl. 2006;52:371-4.
83. Osuna C, Matorras R, Pijoan JI, Rodríguez-Escudero FJ. One versus two inseminations per cycle in intrauterine insemination with sperm from patients' husbands: a systematic review of the literature. Fertil Steril. 2004;82:17-24.
84. Ragni G, Somigliana E, Vegetti W. Timing of intrauterine insemination: where are we? Fertil Steril. 2004;82:25-6.
85. Kucuk T. Intrauterine insemination: is the timing correct? J Assist Reprod Genet. 2008;25:427-30.
86. Cantineau AE, Janssen MJ, Cohlen BJ, Allersma T. Synchronised approach for intrauterine insemination in subfertile couples. Cochrane Database Syst Rev. 2014;(12):CD006942.
87. Blockeel C, Knez J, Polyzos NP, De Vos M, Camus M, Tournaye H. Should an intrauterine insemination with donor semen be performed 1 or 2 days after the spontaneous LH rise? A prospective RCT. Hum Reprod. 2014;29:697-703.
88. Yumusak OH, Kahyaoglu S, Pekcan MK, Isci E, Cinar M, Tasci Y. Does intrauterine insemination timing matter for achieving pregnancy during ovulation induction using gonadotropins? A retrospective cohort study. J Chin Med Assoc. 2017;80(6):366-70.
89. Cantineau AEP, Cohlen BJ, Heineman MJ, Marjoribanks J, Farquhar C. Intrauterine insemination versus fallopian tube sperm perfusion for non-tubal infertility. Cochrane Database Syst Rev. 2013;10:CD001502.
90. Cantineau AEP, Heineman MJ, Cohlen BJ. Single versus double intrauterine insemination (IUI) in stimulated cycles for subfertile couples. Cochrane Database Syst Rev. 2003;(1):CD003854.
91. Zavos A, Daponte A, Garas A, Verykouki C, Papanikolaou E, Anifandis G, et al. Double versus single homologous intrauterine insemination for male factor infertility: a systematic review and meta-analysis. Asian J Androl. 2013; 15:533-8.

92. Polyzos NP, Tzioras S, Mauri D, Tatsioni A. Double versus single intrauterine insemination for unexplained infertility: a meta-analysis of randomized trials. Fertil Steril. 2010;94:1261-6.
93. Rahman SM, Malhotra N, Kumar S, Roy KK, Agarwal A. A randomized controlled trial comparing the effectiveness of single versus double intrauterine insemination in unexplained infertility. Fertil Steril. 2010;94:2913-5.
94. Suarez SS, Pacey AA. Sperm transport in the female reproductive tract. Hum Reprod Update. 2006;12:23-37.
95. Saleh A, Tan SL, Biljan MM, Tulandi T. A randomized study of the effect of 10 minutes of bed rest after intrauterine insemination. Fertil Steril. 2000;74:509-11.
96. Custers IM, Flierman PA, Maas P, Cox T, Van Dessel TJ, Gerards MH, et al. Immobilisation versus immediate mobilisation after intrauterine insemination: randomised controlled trial. Br Med J. 2009;339:b4080.
97. van Rijswijk J, Caanen MR, Mijatovic V, Vergouw CG, van de Ven PM, Lambalk CB, et al. Immobilization or mobilization after IUI: an RCT. Hum Reprod. 2017;32:2218-24.
98. Aboulghar M, Mansour R, Serour G, Abdrazek A, Amin Y, Rhodes C. Controlled ovarian hyperstimulation and intrauterine insemination for treatment of unexplained infertility should be limited to a maximum of three trials. Fertil Steril. 2001;75:88-91.
99. Boomsma CM, Heineman MJ, Cohlen BJ, Farquhar C. Semen preparation techniques for intrauterine insemination. Cochrane Database Syst Rev. 2007;(4):CD004507.
100. Karamahmutoglu H, Erdem A, Erdem M, Mutlu MF, Bozkurt N, Oktem M, et al. The gradient technique improves success rates in intrauterine insemination cycles of unexplained subfertile couples when compared to swim up technique; a prospective randomized study. J Assist Reprod Genet. 2014; 31:1139-45.
101. Moolenaar LM, Mol BWJ, Van Voorhis BJ. Cost-effectiveness of IUI. In: Cohlen BJ, Ombelet W (Eds). Intra-Uterine Insemination: Evidence-Based Guidelines for Daily Practice. Boca Raton, USA: CRC Press, Taylor & Francis Group; 2014. pp. 105-110.
102. Chambers GM, Ledger W. The economic implications of multiple pregnancy following ART. Semin Fetal Neonatal Med. 2014;19:254-61.
103. Van Voorhis BJ, Sparks AE, Allen BD, Stovall DW, Syrop CH, Chapler FK. Cost-effectiveness of infertility treatments: a cohort study. Fertil Steril. 1997;67:830-6.
104. Pashayan N, Lyratzopoulos G, Mathur R. Cost-effectiveness of primary offer of IVF vs. primary offer of IUI followed by IVF (for IUI failures) in couples with unexplained or mild male factor subfertility. BMC Health Serv Res. 2006;6:80.
105. van den Boogaard NM, Bensdorp AJ, Oude Rengerink K, Barnhart K, Bhattacharya S, Custers IM, et al. Prognostic profiles and the effectiveness of assisted conception: secondary analyses of individual patient data. Hum Reprod Update. 2014;20:141-51.
106. Wordsworth S, Buchanan J, Mollison J, Harrild K, Robertson L, Tay C, et al. Clomifene citrate and intrauterine insemination as first-line treatments for unexplained infertility: are they cost-effective? Hum Reprod. 2011;26:369-75.
107. Zafer M, Horvath H, Mmeje O, van der Poel S, Semprini AE, Rutherford G, et al. Effectiveness of semen washing to prevent human immunodeficiency virus (HIV) transmission and assist pregnancy in HIV-discordant couples: a systematic review and meta-analysis. Fertil Steril. 2016;105:645-55.e2.
108. Cantineau AEP, Cohlen BJ, Heineman MJ. Ovarian stimulation protocols (anti-oestrogens, gonadotrophins with and without GnRH agonists/antagonists) for intrauterine insemination (IUI) in women with subfertility. Cochrane Database Syst Rev. 2007;(2):CD005356.
109. Erdem M, Abay S, Erdem A, Firat Mutlu M, Nas E, Mutlu I, et al. Recombinant FSH increases live birth rates as compared to clomiphene citrate in intrauterine insemination cycles in couples with subfertility: a prospective randomized study. Eur J Obstet Gynecol Reprod Biol. 2015;189:33-7.
110. Peeraer K, Debrock S, De Loecker P, Tomassetti C, Laenen A, Welkenhuysen M, et al. Low-dose human menopausal gonadotrophin versus clomiphene citrate in subfertile couples treated with intrauterine insemination: a randomized controlled trial. Hum Reprod. 2015;30:1079-88.
111. Dodd J, Dowswell T, Crowther C. Reduction of the number of fetuses for women with a multiple pregnancy. Cochrane Database Syst Rev. 2015;2015(11):CD003932.
112. Helmerhorst FM, Perquin DA, Donker D, Keirse MJ. Perinatal outcome of singletons and twins after assisted conception: a systematic review of controlled studies. Br Med J. 2004;328:261.
113. Nuojua-Huttunen S, Gissler M, Martikainen H, Tuomivaara L. Obstetric and perinatal outcome of pregnancies after intrauterine insemination. Hum Reprod. 1999;14:2110-5.
114. Wang JX, Norman RJ, Kristiansson P. The effect of various infertility treatments on the risk of preterm birth. Hum Reprod. 2002;17:945-9.
115. Gaudoin M, Dobbie R, Finlayson A, Chalmers J, Cameron IT, Fleming R. Ovulation induction/intrauterine insemination in infertile couples is associated with lowbirth-weight infants. Am J Obstet Gynecol. 2003;188:611-6.
116. De Sutter P, Veldeman L, Kok P, Szymczak N, Van der Elst J, Dhont M. Comparison of outcome of pregnancy after intra-uterine insemination (IUI) and IVF. Hum Reprod. 2005;20:1642-6.
117. Ombelet W, Martens G, De Sutter P, Gerris J, Bosmans E, Ruyssinck G, et al. Perinatal outcome of 12,021 singleton and 3108 twin births after non-IVF-assisted reproduction: a cohort study. Hum Reprod. 2006;21:1025-32.
118. Ombelet W, Martens G, Bruckers L. Pregnant after assisted reproduction: a risk pregnancy is born! 18-years perinatal outcome results from a population-based registry in Flanders, Belgium. Facts views Vis ObGyn. 2016;8:193-204.
119. Poon WB, Lian WB. Perinatal outcomes of intrauterine insemination/clomiphene pregnancies represent an intermediate risk group compared with in vitro fertilisation/intracytoplasmic sperm injection and naturally conceived pregnancies. J Paediatr Child Health. 2013;49:733-40.
120. Malchau SS, Loft A, Henningsen A-KA, Nyboe Andersen A, Pinborg A. Perinatal outcomes in 6,338 singletons born after intrauterine insemination in Denmark, 2007 to 2012: the influence of ovarian stimulation. Fertil Steril. 2014;102: 1110-6.e2.
121. Simpson JL. Birth defects and assisted reproductive technologies. Semin Fetal Neonatal Med. 2014;19:177-82.
122. Pinborg A, Wennerholm UB, Romundstad LB, Loft A, Aittomaki K, Soderstrom-Anttila V, et al. Why do singletons conceived after assisted reproduction technology have

adverse perinatal outcome? Systematic review and meta-analysis. Hum Reprod Update. 2013;19:87-104.

123. Pinborg A, Lidegaard O, Freiesleben NL, Andersen AN. Vanishing twins: a predictor of small-for-gestational age in IVF singletons. Hum Reprod. 2007;22:2707-14.
124. Hoy J, Venn A, Halliday J, Kovacs G, Waalwyk K. Perinatal and obstetric outcomes of donor insemination using cryopreserved semen in Victoria, Australia. Hum Reprod. 1999;14:1760-4.
125. Lansac J, Thepot F, Mayaux MJ, Czyglick F, Wack T, Selva J, et al. Pregnancy outcome after artificial insemination or IVF with frozen semen donor: a collaborative study of the French CECOS Federation on 21,597 pregnancies. Eur J Obstet Gynecol Reprod Biol. 1997;74:223-8.
126. Kyrou D, Kolibianakis EM, Devroey P, Fatemi HM. Is the use of donor sperm associated with a higher incidence of preeclampsia in women who achieve pregnancy after intrauterine insemination? Fertil Steril. 2010;93:1124-7.
127. Gonzalez-Comadran M, Urresta Avila J, Saavedra Tascon A, Jimenez R, Sola I, Brassesco M, et al. The impact of donor insemination on the risk of preeclampsia: a systematic review and meta-analysis. Eur J Obstet Gynecol Reprod Biol. 2014;182:160-6.
128. Mathieu C, Ecochard R, Bied V, Lornage J, Czyba JC. Cumulative conception rate following intrauterine artificial insemination with husband's spermatozoa: influence of husband's age. Hum Reprod. 1995;10:1090-7.
129. Kidd SA, Eskenazi B, Wyrobek AJ. Effects of male age on semen quality and fertility: a review of the literature. Fertil Steril. 2001;75:237-48.
130. De Brucker M, Tournaye H. Factors influencing IUI outcome: male age. In: Cohlen BJ, Ombelet W (Eds). Intra-Uterine Insemination: Evidence-Based Guidelines for Daily Practice. Boca Raton, USA: CRC Press, Taylor & Francis Group; 2014. pp. 35-8.
131. Desai N, Sabanegh E, Kim T, Agarwal A. Free radical theory of aging: implications in male infertility. Urology. 2010;75:14-9.
132. Bhal PS, Pugh ND, Gregory L, O'Brien S, Shaw RW. Perifollicular vascularity as a potential variable affecting outcome in stimulated intrauterine insemination treatment cycles: a study using transvaginal power Doppler. Hum Reprod. 2001;16:1682-9.
133. Nargund G, Sarafis V, Campbell S. Factors influencing IUI outcome: perifollicular flow and endometrial thickness. In: Cohlen BJ, Ombelet W (Eds). Intra-Uterine Insemination: Evidence-Based Guidelines for Daily Practice. Boca Raton, USA: CRC Press, Taylor & Francis Group; 2014. pp. 61-6.
134. Randall JM, Templeton A. Transvaginal sonographic assessment of follicular and endometrial growth in spontaneous and clomiphene citrate cycles. Fertil Steril. 1991; 56:208-12.
135. Weiss NS, van Vliet MN, Limpens J, Hompes PGA, Lambalk CB, Mochtar MH, et al. Endometrial thickness in women undergoing IUI with ovarian stimulation. How thick is too thin? A systematic review and meta-analysis. Hum Reprod. 2017;32:1009-18.
136. Petersen GL, Schmidt L, Pinborg A, Kamper-Jorgensen M. The influence of female and male body mass index on live births after assisted reproductive technology treatment: a nationwide register-based cohort study. Fertil Steril. 2013;99:1654-62.
137. Schliep KC, Mumford SL, Ahrens KA, Hotaling JM, Carrell DT, Link M, et al. Effect of male and female body mass index on pregnancy and live birth success after in vitro fertilization. Fertil Steril. 2015;103:388-95.
138. Soria M, Pradillo G, Garcia J, Ramon P, Castillo A, Jordana C, et al. Pregnancy predictors after intrauterine insemination: analysis of 3012 cycles in 1201 couples. J Reprod Infertil. 2012;13:158-66.
139. Yavuz A, Demirci O, Sozen H, Uludogan M. Predictive factors influencing pregnancy rates after intrauterine insemination. Iran J Reprod Med. 2013;11:227-34.
140. Dodson WC, Kunselman AR, Legro RS. Association of obesity with treatment outcomes in ovulatory infertile women undergoing superovulation and intrauterine insemination. Fertil Steril. 2006;86:642-6.
141. Souter I, Baltagi LM, Kuleta D, Meeker JD, Petrozza JC. Women, weight, and fertility: the effect of body mass index on the outcome of superovulation/intrauterine insemination cycles. Fertil Steril. 2011;95:1042-7.
142. Isa AM, Abu-Rafea B, Alasiri SA, Binsaleh S, Ismail KH, Vilos GA. Age, body mass index, and number of previous trials: are they prognosticators of intra-uterine insemination for infertility treatment? Int J Fertil Steril. 2014;8:255-60.
143. Thijssen A, Creemers A, Van Der Elst W, Creemers E, Vandormael E, Dhont N, et al. Predictive factors influencing pregnancy rates after intrauterine insemination with frozen donor semen: a prospective cohort study. Reprod Biomed Online. 2017a;34:590-7.
144. Thijssen A, Creemers A, Van Der Elst W, Creemers E, Vandormael E, Dhont N, et al. Predictive value of different covariates influencing pregnancy rate following intrauterine insemination with homologous semen: a prospective cohort study. Reprod Biomed Online. 2017b;34:463-72.
145. Petrozza JC, Dimitriadis I, Kumar P. Factors influencing IUI outcome: weight influences. In: Cohlen BJ, Ombelet W (Eds). Intra-Uterine Insemination: Evidence-Based Guidelines for Daily Practice. Boca Raton, USA: CRC Press: Taylor & Francis Group; 2014. pp. 39-42.
146. Farhi J, Orvieto R. Influence of smoking on outcome of COH and IUI in subfertile couples. J Assist Reprod Genet. 2009;26:421-4.
147. Hansen KR, He ALW, Styer AK, Wild RA, Butts S, Engmann L, et al. Predictors of pregnancy and live-birth in couples with unexplained infertility after ovarian stimulation-intrauterine insemination. Fertil Steril. 2016;105:1575-83.e2.
148. Centers for Disease Control (CDC). HIV-1 infection and artificial insemination with processed sperm. MMWR Morb Mortal Wkly Rep. 1990;39:249-56.
149. Wortley PM, Hammett TA, Fleming PL. Donor insemination and human immunodeficiency virus transmission. Obstet Gynecol. 1998;91:515-8.
150. Semprini AE, Levi-Setti P, Bozzo M, Ravizza M, Taglioretti A, Sulpizio P. Insemination of HIV-negative women with processed semen of HIV-positive partners. Lancet. 1992;340:1317-9.
151. White D, Mital D, Taylor S, St. John J. Sperm mitochondrial DNA deletions as a consequence of long term highly active antiretroviral therapy. AIDS. 2001;15:1061-2.
152. Bujan L, Sergerie M, Moinard N, Martinet S, Porte L, Massip P, et al. Decreased semen volume and spermatozoa motility

in HIV-1-infected patients under antiretroviral treatment. J Androl. 2007;28:444-52.
153. Nicopoullos JD, Almeida PA, Ramsay JW, Gilling-Smith C. The effect of human immunodeficiency virus on sperm parameters and the outcome of intrauterine insemination following sperm washing. Hum Reprod. 2004;19:2289-97.
154. Chen WJ, Walker N. Fertility of HIV-infected women: insights from demographic and health surveys. Sex Transm Infect. 2010;86(Suppl 2):ii22-7.
155. Sobel JD. Gynecologic infections in human immunodeficiency virus-infected women. Clin Infect Dis. 2000;31:1225-33.
156. Gilles C, Manigart Y, Konopnicki D, Barlow P, Rozenberg S. Management and outcome of cervical intraepithelial neoplasia lesions: a study of matched cases according to HIV status. Gynecol Oncol. 2005;96:112-8.
157. Gray RH, Wawer MJ, Brookmeyer R, Sewankambo NK, Serwadda D, Wabwire-Mangen F, et al.; Rakai Project Team. Probability of HIV-1 transmission per coital act in monogamous, heterosexual, HIV-1-discordant couples in Rakai, Uganda. Lancet. 2001;357:1149-53.
158. Vernazza PL, Gilliam BL, Flepp M, Dyer JR, Frank AC, Fiscus SA, et al. Effect of antiviral treatment on the shedding of HIV-1 in semen. AIDS. 1997;11:1249-54.
159. Rotchford K, Strum AW, Wilkinson D. Effect of coinfection with STDs and of STD treatment on HIV shedding in genital-tract secretions: systematic review and data synthesis. Sex Transm Dis. 2000;27:243-8.
160. Cohen CR, Lingappa JR, Baeten JM, Ngayo MO, Spiegel CA, Hong T, et al. Bacterial vaginosis associated with increased risk of female-to-male HIV-1 transmission: a prospective cohort analysis among African couples. PLoS Med. 2012;9:e1001251.
161. Barnes A, Riche D, Mena L, Sison T, Barry L, Reddy R, et al. Efficacy and safety of intrauterine insemination and assisted reproductive technology in populations serodiscordant for human immunodeficiency virus: a systematic review and meta-analysis. Fertil Steril. 2014;102(2):424-34.

CHAPTER 45

Optimizing Success in Intrauterine Insemination

Kamini A Rao, Jampana Pallavi

INTRODUCTION

The principle behind intrauterine insemination (IUI) is based on increasing sperm density at the time and site of fertilization.[1] The very first IUI dates back in 1770s when John Hunter performed IUI for women whose husbands had hypospadias. Since then various revolutions have happened in improving the success of IUI. Despite being easy to perform, inexpensive, and offers particular advantages such as the minimal equipment required, less stringent laboratory conditions, an easy technique to learn, being less invasive with a reduced psychological burden on the couple as compared to in vitro fertilization (IVF), or intracytoplasmic sperm injection (ICSI), the effectiveness of procedure is still controversial. The global success rate of IUI is 15–20%. This overview is to optimize the success of IUI, though the good quality evidence is still lacking.

Intrauterine insemination success depends on various factors **(Fig. 1)**.

PATIENT SELECTION AND WORKUP

One of the important factors for successful IUI is duration of infertility. Maximum success in IUI is noted in 5 years

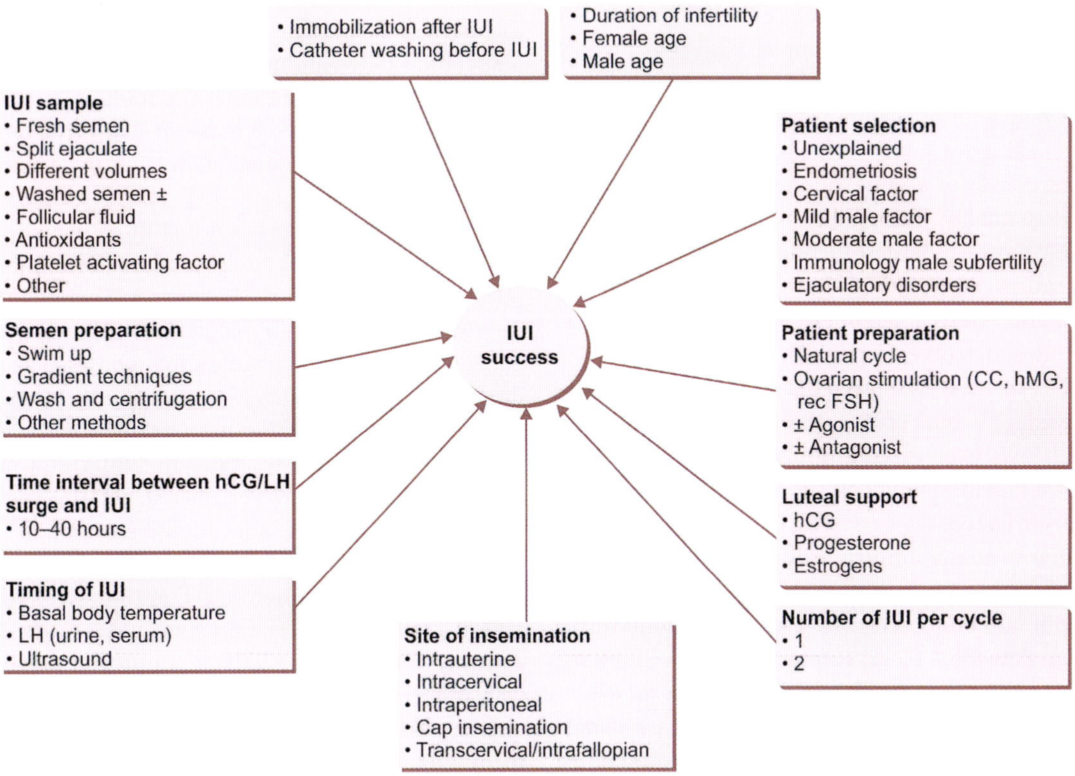

Fig. 1: Factors for intrauterine insemination (IUI) success.
(CC: clomiphene citrate; FSH: follicle-stimulating hormone; hCG: human chorionic gonadotropin; hMG: human menopausal gonadotropin; LH: luteinizing hormone)

suggested that IUI is not recommended in long duration infertility.[2,3] Although few studies such as Tay et al. found insufficient evidence of significant association of success of IUI with duration of infertility.[4]

Age of the couple, especially female age, has been found to be an important factor predicting success of IUI in many studies.[5,6] Increasing female partner age has adverse impact on oocyte number, oocyte quality, corpus luteal function, and endometrium and thus decreases the pregnancy rate.[2,7] Jayakrishnan et al. reported negative impact of >40 years of male partner age on IUI success.[8]

Evaluation of tubal factor and ovarian reserve must be done. At least one patent fallopian tube with healthy tubo-ovarian relationship is a good predictor of IUI success. In retrospective cohort study, with 3,217 IUI cycles, body mass index (BMI) between 25 and 29.99 did not have an inverse relationship with clinical pregnancy rate after IUI cycles; however, obesity may have higher chance of biochemical pregnancy.[9]

INDICATIONS OF INTRAUTERINE INSEMINATION

Way back in the 1770s, first IUI was done for hypospadias; the most common indications of IUI are mild male factor infertility, cervical factor, and unexplained infertility. Other indications include mild endometriosis, ovulatory dysfunction, and immunological factors. Cochrane review was inconclusive, there is no evidence of a difference in live birth or multiple pregnancy for couples with unexplained subfertility treated with IUI when compared with timed intercourse, both with and without ovarian hyperstimulation (OH).[10]

Different causes of an unexplained infertility are problems with egg quality, the inability of the sperm to fertilize the egg, undiagnosed tubal dysfunction, implantation failure, or genetic causes. Some studies have found that ovulatory dysfunction and unexplained infertility have better clinical pregnancy rates than other factors.[2,11]

Merviel P et al., results showed that pregnancy rates were greater in ovulatory and cervical factor infertility, but lower in endometriosis over varying numbers of cycles.[12] This implies that stimulation protocols successfully overcome the ovulatory disturbances.

According to many authors, endometriosis has been found beneficial in women younger than 35 years and with mild-to-moderate endometriosis.[13] Severe endometriosis, bilateral complete tubal block, severe male factor infertility, and ovarian insufficiency are absolute indications for IVF.

Though some authors find it unnecessary, in case of male infertility, sexual disorders such as erectile dysfunctions, ejaculatory failure, vaginismus, and hypospadias, IUI can be used as infertility treatment. Often subnormal semen parameters are accompanied by premature ejaculation, where use of IUI is absolutely justified.[14]

Donor insemination remains option in case of nonobstructive azoospermia, genetic hereditary diseases, homosexual couples, or single women willing for childbearing.[14] Selection of patients with ideal indication remains the key to optimize success of IUI.

PATIENT PREPARATION

Intrauterine insemination is done in the natural cycle and/or ovarian stimulation cycle with either oral ovulation agents or gonadotropins. The rationale behind the ovarian stimulation is to rectify the hidden ovulation disorders, to improve availability of oocyte number, to increase the steroid synthesis, and to time the ovulation so as to increase the chance of fertilization. Clomiphene citrate (CC) alone is not found to be efficacious in IUI in unexplained infertility.[15]

Although OH seems to result in higher pregnancy rates, it also increases the incidence of multiple pregnancy and ovarian hyperstimulation syndrome (OHSS). These both increase the risk and complications of both mother and baby's health.[16] Gonadotropins have been found to be the most efficient drugs when IUI is combined with OH.

Low-dose gonadotropins use is advised for ovarian stimulation as there is no difference in pregnancy rates with use of high-dose gonadotropins, instead complications from ovarian stimulation such as multiple pregnancy and OHSS are high with high-dose gonadotrophins.[17] A meta-analysis inclusive of 14 studies with 11,599 IUI cycles reported the association between multifollicular growth and increased pregnancy rates but at the cost of multiple pregnancy and hence no substantial increase in live birth rate. Hence, controlled ovarian stimulation for IUI is to be limited to one or two follicles only.[2,18]

Recently, there has been a shift of focus to letrozole (aromatase inhibitor) for ovulation induction in PCOS patients. According to European Society of Human Reproduction and Embryology (ESHRE), evidenced based guidelines on PCOS, letrozole should be used as a first-line drug for ovulation induction in anovulatory PCOS.

Cochrane review states that letrozole appears to improve live birth and pregnancy rates in subfertile women with anovulatory PCOS; however, the risk of OHSS seemed to be similar in both letrozole and clomiphene groups.[19]

In a pilot study, analysis was done for human chorionic gonadotropin (hCG) before IUI (228 cycles) versus hCG after IUI (104 cycles). The pregnancy rates were 10.9% and 19.6% (p = 0.040), respectively. Improved pregnancy rate was reported when hCG was given after IUI.[20] Similar analysis was done by Mustafa et al., he reported no difference in pregnancy rate between hCG injection immediately following IUI and standard hCG injection 24–32 hours before IUI.[21]

Ultrasound monitoring is better when ovarian stimulation is done to help to decide the timing of IUI and to cancel the IUI in cases of OHSS.

MONITORING OF INTRAUTERINE INSEMINATION

Different methods such as basal body temperature recording, luteinizing hormone (LH) kits, serum estradiol levels, and ultrasonography (USG) to time the IUI have been used. Although Ozkan et al. found the best results of IUI with serum estradiol levels >465 pg/mL, Marviel et al. found the best results of IUI with an estradiol concentration >500 pg/mL on the day of hCG administration, estradiol monitoring is costly.[22]

Perifollicular vascularity is an important factor modulating the success of IUI in stimulated treatment cycles. Study conducted on 601 follicles suggests that perifollicular vascularity has an important role to play in the success of IUI cycles, also power Doppler has the ability to improve the management of assisted reproduction treatment cycles.[23]

Growing follicle and corpus luteum require increased blood flow. A developed or mature follicle shows increased vascularity by >75% of its circumference. During this, the ovarian stromal arteries show peak systolic velocity of >10 cm/sec. This is the time where LH surge is started in natural cycles and this is the time to trigger in assisted reproductive cycles.[24]

Three-dimensional power Doppler ultrasound for evaluating endometrial and subendometrial neovascularization in IUI cycles may be useful predictors for pregnancy.[25] Elastography is another promising innovative tool for monitoring the IUI. The elasticity index is recorded for 5 minutes. The elasticity index can be calculated as the mean ratio of elastographic measurements between the subendometrial area (of interest) and the endometrial area (control). Uterine contraction frequency, endometrial thickness and volume, and subendometrial vascularization are other parameters helpful in predicting the success of IUI.[26] Correct timing of the insemination is essential as spermatozoa and oocytes have only limited survival time. Different techniques for timing IUI such as hCG, agonist, and LH surge and different time intervals are reviewed in Cochrane which concluded no evidence of any one technique to improve IUI success.[27]

TIME AND NUMBER OF INTRAUTERINE INSEMINATION

Among the different time intervals, IUI after hCG injection anywhere between 12 hours and 60 hours is recommended for management of infertility. A randomized controlled trial (RCT) was done on 125 cycles to evaluate the best time for IUI after hCG, comparing pregnancy rate of IUI after 24, 36, and 48 hours after hCG. Pregnancy rates were found similar between all groups.[28]

Blockleel et al. conducted an RCT, which showed significant higher pregnancy rates when IUI is performed one day after LH surge in natural cycles, compared to IUI being done after 2 days of the surge.[29]

Another study inclusive of 1,146 stimulated cycles concluded the better cycle pregnancy rate (CPR) with single postovulation IUI when compared with single preovulation IUI for non-male infertility, whereas for male factor infertility, double IUI gives a better CPR when compared with single IUI.[30,31] Other studies and recent meta-analysis too found no difference in single and double IUI though evidence in low quality.[32-35]

Cochrane review studied nine RCTs and concluded that benefit of live births and reduced miscarriage in double IUI over single IUI in subfertile couples is uncertain. The reported clinical pregnancy rate may be improved with double IUI, however results should be interpreted with caution.[36]

SITE OF INSEMINATION

Insemination of sperm can be done either cervical (CI) or intrauterine (IUI) routes. IUI has been found to be potentially more effective than CI as the sperm bypasses the cervical mucus and is deposited closer to the fallopian tubes.[37,38]

SEMEN

Sperm quality is of paramount importance in any assisted reproductive technique.

ABSTINENCE DURATION

The duration of sexual abstinence to provide maximum sperm quality is one of commonly discussed controversial issue. Eliahu et al. did analysis of 9,489 semen samples in relation to abstinence duration. Patients with male factor infertility should have abstinence of not >1 day to give best semen parameters.[39] The highest pregnancy rates per cycle were demonstrated with an ejaculatory abstinence period of ≥2 days before IUI when compared with longer intervals of ejaculatory abstinence.[40]

While in normospermic men, shorter duration of ejaculatory abstinence is not detrimental and it is a method of reducing DNA fragmentation.[41] A short period of abstinence leads to a significant improvement in the semen parameters on second day insemination. Hence, 2 days consecutive intercourses or inseminations maybe helpful for men with abnormal concentration or multiple abnormal semen parameters.[42] Whereas in men with normal basic semen parameters, a single-timed insemination and longer abstinence can be recommended because of reduction in semen quality is expected after 24 hours.[42]

TABLE 1: Correlation of processed TMC (total motile sperm count) and pregnancy rates.[47]

Processed total motile sperm		
Number of sperm recovered (×106)	**Numbers of men with indicated sperm count/ total number of men (%)**	**Pregnancy rate 1st/ pregnancy rate all cycle**
<5	168/1,768 (9.5%)	0 0
5–10	336/1,768	3.1 7.2
>10	1,264/1,768 (71.5%)	15.9* 13.7*

*p <0.001 vs. other groups by chi square analysis.

SEMEN PARAMETERS

Sperm parameters most frequently evaluated to achieve improved pregnancy rates are: (1) Inseminating motile count after washing: cut-off value between 0.8 million and 5 million; (2) sperm morphology using strict criteria: Cut-off value 5% normal morphology; (3) total motile sperm count (TMC) **(Table 1)** in the native sperm sample: Cut-off value of 5–10 million; and (4) total motility in the native sperm sample: Threshold value of 30%.[43] The postwash TMC more than or less than 5 million/mL at time of insemination can be a potential parameter used in counseling patients for either IUI or IVF.[44-46]

Recent retrospective cohort study done in 2019, which studied 655 IUI cycles, showed no live birth rates, whose prewash TMC is <2 million. However, prewash TMC is a poor predictor of pregnancy rate in IUI cycles.[48]

Taylor et al. performed a systematic review and meta-analysis to assess the effect of abnormal sperm morphology on pregnancy success for couples undergoing IUI. The thresholds of sperm morphology between >4% and 4% and 1% and <1% were not significant statistically or clinically to improve IUI success. Thus for couples with abnormal morphology, IUI must be tried before to advising significantly more expensive IVF.[49]

Branigan et al. evaluated the effect of total motile count of density gradient processed semen samples on IUI success. Although he suggested the processed TMC as useful prognostic factor of IUI, he did not find any significant relation between any of the basic semen parameters of concentration, motility, and morphology by World Health Organization (WHO) standards and pregnancy rates.[47]

DNA FRAGMENTATION INDEX

Altered DNA structure of sperm may also cause male infertility. These alterations are reflected by DNA fragmentation index (DFI). A study in 2019 evaluated the impact of DFI on the pregnancy outcomes by clinical pregnancy rates in IUI cycles and found no difference. DFI is not a part of evaluation before IUI cycles.[50,51]

PATERNAL AGE

A study with 901 IUI cycles showed reduced cumulative pregnancy rates in men aged >35 years compared to <30 years when maternal age, duration of infertility, ovulatory status, and teratozoospermia and asthenozoospermia in men are matched.[51]

COLLECTION TO INTRAUTERINE INSEMINATION TIME INTERVAL

The processing of semen specimens must be done just after liquefaction and within 30 minutes of collection, and IUI is to be performed immediately after processing and within 90 minutes of collection.[52] The prolonged incubation impairs the sperm parameters.[53]

SEMEN PREPARATION TECHNIQUE

The rationale of sperm preparation techniques (SPTs) is to isolate and select sperm cells with intact functional and genetic properties, including normal morphology, minimal DNA damage, and intact cell membranes with functional binding properties. To improve the quality and outcome of IUI procedures, simple, inexpensive, reliable, and safe SPTs are required. There is no specific evidence to recommend any specific semen preparation technique.[54] The WHO laboratory manual suggests the choice of the type of SPT is dictated by the nature of the semen sample. Swim-up generally produces a lower recovery of motile spermatozoa (<20%) than does density gradient concentration (>20%) though not supported by few studies.[55]

Cochrane review in 2019 studied six RCTs regarding the semen preparation techniques used in IUI, gradient versus, wash and centrifugation, there is uncertainty in clinical pregnancy rates in one technique over the other.[56]

Advanced techniques such as annexin V magnetic-activated cell sorting (MACS) based on the principle of separation nonapoptotic sperms from apoptic sperms.

Glass wool technique, separation technique based on electrical charge on sperm are still not validated. Integration of these techniques may help in improving the success of IUI.[57]

Frozen Semen Sample

The prefreezing progressive sperm motility is an important predictor for frozen sample IUI success.[58]

Pooled Semen Ejaculates

A recent retrospective study analyzed patients who underwent IUI in a single center between 2012 and 2019. All the participants with TMC <5 million were asked to ejaculate the second sample within an hour or two of the first sample. The pooled sample is used for processing and insemination.[59]

Combination of the first and consecutive ejaculates in oligoasthenoteratozoospermia men have higher inseminating motile count in the processed samples, which improves IUI success rates as in normozoospermic men. This simple intervention can help to overcome moderate male factor infertility and may be used in resource poor settings before referring for IVF.

TECHNIQUE OF INTRAUTERINE INSEMINATION

Intrauterine insemination success increases with use of abdominal USG with partially filled urinary bladder, no touch to fundus, slow injection of 0.3–0.5 mL of processed semen, and slow withdrawal of catheter.

Type of Catheter

Catheter technology has achieved a lot of importance in assisted reproductive technology (ART) with its proven benefit during embryo transfer technique. Catheters must be firm enough to negotiate the rigid curvature of the cervix, but soft enough to avoid any trauma to the endocervix and/or endometrium as it finds its way into the uterine cavity. Cochrane and other studies have found no evidence of flexible catheter over rigid catheter in IUI in regards to pregnancy rates.[60-62] In retrospective analysis of 1,038 cycles, the type of catheter used was correlated with differing pregnancy rates, 15.3% per cycle for soft catheter versus 7% for a hard catheter ($p < 0.02$).[12]

Volume of Insemination

The postwash inseminated semen volume between 0.3 mL and 0.5 mL has been found to be useful for successful pregnancy in IUI.[63]

Ultrasound-guided Insemination

A prospective RCT did not report benefit of ultrasound guidance in IUI.[64]

Whereas other studies noted improved pregnancy rate, reduced frequency of difficult IUI, and also higher success with use of ultrasound in hands of experienced personnel.[65,66]

Bed Rest

An RCT on 296 women recommended bed rest for 10–20 minutes after that showed positive effect on pregnancy outcome after IUI.[1,67]

Recently van Rijswijk et al. studied 498 patients in a RCT and found no significant difference in cumulative pregnancy rate between both immobilization and mobilization groups.[68,69]

Luteal Phase Support

Based on few studies and one meta-analysis, luteal support with vaginal progesterone appears to increase the pregnancy rate in gonadotropin-stimulated cycles where there is growth of more than one follicle.[70,71] While few studies recommend that a routine supplement of vaginal progesterone does not improve the pregnancy rate in normo-ovulatory women with CC stimulation or monofollicular growth.[72]

Number of Treatment Cycles

The maximum number of IUI required for successful pregnancy has been a controversial issue all the time. In a multicenter retrospective cohort analysis, 15,303 IUI cycles with controlled ovarian stimulation (COS) were analyzed. The cumulative ongoing pregnancy rates reported were 18% in the third cycle, 30% by seventh cycle, and 41% by ninth cycle. This study recommended not to abandon IUI treatment before nine cycles with mild COS, especially in young people (female age <35 years) and still have considerable time to conceive.[73] Maximum conception rate is reported in the first cycle, the decreasing trend toward second and third cycle.[7] Few studies reported no significant increase in pregnancy rates beyond four cycles.[2,8] Studies recommend that IVF-ICSI is a better plan of management after three cycles of IUI with COS for unexplained infertility.[74]

Premature Luteinizing Hormone Surge in Intrauterine Insemination Cycles

Final maturation and follicle rupture are under control of LH surge. Though the cause of premature luteinization is variable, it completely disturbs the treatment outcome. The premature luteinization occurs in almost 25–30% stimulated cycles of IUI, which ultimately leads to treatment failure or cancellation of cycles or interfere with timing of IUI which is of crucial importance.[75]

Gonadotropin-releasing hormone antagonist is a best technique to prevent premature luteinization but not cost-effective and not found to improve the pregnancy rates in IUI.[76]

Laboratory

According to the Assisted Reproductive Technology Bill 2014, Indian Council of Medical Research recommends the registration of IUI laboratories as mandatory. Ideal IUI laboratories should be isolated and should include a distinct area for diagnostic and therapeutic procedure with a sterile environment with the help of laminar airflow. Adequate space according to the number of tests done, air conditioning, air quality, and cleaning to be maintained. There should be separate space for liquid nitrogen cylinder and storage of disposables and media. Record maintenance and standard operating procedure should be meticulous.

According to Assisted Reproductive Technology Act 2022, all IUI centers should be registered under level 1 ART centers and need to be recognized by the authorities.

Personnel should have good laboratory skills and knowledge of the subject. Validation of all new equipment before use is must; it should be reliable in function and periodically monitored for efficiency.[77]

EUROPEAN SOCIETY OF HUMAN REPRODUCTION AND EMBRYOLOGY CAPRI WORKSHOP 2009

Intrauterine insemination is most widely and empirically used as stop gap treatment while waiting for or instead of IVF. ESHRE Capri group has tried to consider the evidences for IUI for best clinical practice.[75]

Recently, Cochrane and Capri studied three studies comparing three cycles of ovarian stimulation with IUI with IVF, no clear benefit was noted in either groups.[78]

KEY POINTS

- The live birth rate is better even without treatment in good prognosis couples.
- Most widely used treatment modality for infertility is IUI, except for bilateral tubal obstruction, severe male infertility, and severe ovulation defects.
- Success rate of IUI does not vary profoundly with different SPTs and IUI methodology.
- IUI with oral ovulation agents or gonadotropins is a relatively cheap, easy, convenient option before IVF, and many couples will conceive without need of IVF.
- A more number of placebo-controlled trials of CC/IUI required determining the optimal length, duration, and protocol of treatment.
- Higher-order multiple births are associated with ovarian stimulation which is effective in patients with >3 years' duration of infertility.
- The larger number of trials is required to confirm the good success rate recently associated with mild stimulated IUI cycles.
- Prevention of premature LH surges and luteal phase support are not mandatory for better success in IUI cycles.
- IVF is the most effective treatment for infertility even though IUI treatment is cheaper and less demanding for the patient.
- Requirement of management trials to evaluate the order of treatment and overall effectiveness of treatment strategies in more clinical and cost settings cannot be ruled out.

REFERENCES

1. Willem O. Evidence-based recommendations for IUI in daily practice. Middle East Fertil Soc J. 2013;18:74-7.
2. Azantee YW, Murad ZA, Roszaman R, Hayati MY, Norsina MA. Associated factors affecting the successful pregnancy rate of intrauterine insemination at International Islamic University Malaysia (IIUM) Fertility Centre. Med J Malaysia. 2011;66(3):195-8.
3. Zadehmodarres S, Oladi B, Saeedi S, Jahed F, Ashraf H. Intrauterine insemination with husband semen: an evaluation of pregnancy rate and factors affecting outcome. J Assist Reprod Genet. 2009;26(1):7-11.
4. Tay PY, Raj VR, Kulenthran A, Sitizawiah O. Prognostic factors influencing pregnancy rate after stimulated intrauterine insemination. Med J Malaysia. 2007;62(4):286-9.
5. Montanaro Gauci M, Kruger TF, Coetzee K, Smith K, Van Der Merwe JP, Lombard CJ. Stepwise regression analysis to study male and female factors impacting on pregnancy rate in an intrauterine insemination programme. Andrologia. 2001;33(3):135-41.
6. Hansen KR, He AL, Styer AK, Wild RA, Butts S, Engmann L, et al. Predictors of pregnancy and live-birth in couples with unexplained infertility after ovarian stimulation-intrauterine insemination. Fertil Steril. 2016;105(6):1575-83.
7. Ganguly I, Singh A, Bhandari S, Agrawal P, Gupta N. Pregnancy predictors after intrauterine insemination in cases of unexplained infertility: a prospective study. Int J Reprod Med. 2016;2016:5817823.
8. Jayakrishnan K, Abraham SA, Nambiar D. Factors affecting success of intrauterine insemination: a 3 year prospective study. Int J Reprod Contracept Obstet Gynecol. 2016;5(4):1077-83.
9. Whynott RM, Summers KM, Van Voorhis BJ, Mejia RB. Effect of body mass index on intrauterine insemination cycle success. Fertility and Sterility. 2021;115(1):221-8.
10. Veltman-Verhulst SM, Hughes E, Ayeleke RO, Heineman MJ. Intra-uterine insemination for unexplained subfertility. Cochrane Database of Syst Rev. 2016;2:CD001838.
11. Ahinko K (Ed). Successful Intrauterine Insemination Treatment. Finland: University of Tempere; 2009. pp. 24-25.
12. Merviel P, Heraud MH, Grenier N, Lourdel E, Sanguinet P, Copin H. Predictive factors for pregnancy after intrauterine insemination (IUI): an analysis of 1038 cycles and a review of the literature. Fertil Steril. 2010;93(1):79-88.
13. van der Houwen LE, Schreurs AM, Schats R, Heymans MW, Lambalk CB, Hompes PG, et al. Efficacy and safety of intrauterine insemination in patients with moderate-to-severe endometriosis. Reprod Biomed Online. 2014;28(5):590-8.
14. Putowski L, Kedzierski Z, Tkaczuk-Wlach J. Intrauterine insemination – current indications. Arch Perinatal Med. 2014;20(2):89-92.
15. Hughes E, Brown J, Collins JJ, Vanderkerchove P. Clomiphene citrate for unexplained subfertility in women. Cochrane Database Syst Rev. 2010;2010(1):CD000057.
16. Verhulst SM, Cohlen BJ, Hughes E, Heineman MJ. Intra-uterine insemination for unexplained subfertility. Cochrane Database Syst Rev. 2005;(9):CD001838.
17. Cantineau AEP, Cohlen BJ. Ovarian stimulation protocols (anti-oestrogens, gonadotrophins with and without GnRH agonists/antagonists) for intrauterine insemination (IUI) in women with subfertility. Cochrane Database Syst Rev. 2007;2:CD005356.
18. van Rumste MM, Custers IM, van der Veen F, van Wely M, Evers JL, Mol BW. The influence of the number of follicles on pregnancy rates in intrauterine insemination with

ovarian stimulation: a meta-analysis. Hum Reprod Update. 2008;14(6):563-70.
19. Franik S, Eltrop SM, Kremer JA, Kiesel L, Farquhar C. Aromatase inhibitors (letrozole) for subfertile women with polycystic ovary syndrome. Cochrane Database Syst Rev. 2018;5(5):CD010287.
20. Järvelä IY, Tapanainen JS, Martikainen H. Improved pregnancy rate with administration of hCG after intrauterine insemination: a pilot study. Reprod Biol Endocrinol. 2010;8:18.
21. Mostafa MS, El Huseiny AM, Soliman BS, Mohammed MM. Effect of postponing hCG injection after intrauterine insemination on pregnancy rate. Middle East Fertil Soc J. 2014;19:183-6.
22. Ozkan ZS, Ilhan R, Ekinci M, Timurkan H, Sapmaz E. Impact of estradiol monitoring on the prediction of intrauterine insemination outcome. J Taibah Univ Med Sci. 2014;9(1):36-40.
23. Bhal PS, Pugh ND, Gregory L, O'Brien S, Shaw RW. Perifollicular vascularity as a potential variable affecting outcome in stimulated intrauterine insemination treatment cycles: a study using transvaginal power Doppler. Hum Reprod. 2001;16(8):1682-9.
24. Sharma N, Saravanan M, Lakshmanan Saravanan MB, Narayanan S. The role of color Doppler in assisted reproduction: A narrative review. Int J Reprod Biomed. 2019; 17(11):779-88.
25. Kim A, Han JE, Yoon TK, Lyu SW, Seok HH, Won HJ. Relationship between endometrial and subendometrial blood flow measured by three-dimensional power Doppler ultrasound and pregnancy after intrauterine insemination. Fertil Steril. 2010;94(2):747-52.
26. Allahbadia GN. Intrauterine Insemination: Fundamentals Revisited. J Obstet Gynecol India. 2017;67(6):385-92.
27. Cantineau AEP, Janssen MJ, Cohlen BJ, Allersma T. Synchronised approach for intrauterine insemination in subfertile couples. Cochrane Database Syst Rev. 2014;12: CD006942.
28. Gheit SA. Pregnancy rates following three different timings of intrauterine insemination for women with unexplained infertility: A randomised controlled trial. Middle East Fertil Soc J. 2010;15:265-8.
29. Blockeel C, Knez J, Polyzos NP, De Vos M, Camus M, Tournaye H. Should an intrauterine insemination with donor semen be performed 1 or 2 days after the spontaneous LH rise? A prospective RCT. Hum Reprod. 2014;29(4):697-703.
30. Ghanem ME, Bakre NI, Emam MA, Al Boghdady LA, Helal AS, Elmetwally AG, et al. The effects of timing of intrauterine insemination in relation to ovulation and the number of inseminations on cycle pregnancy rate in common infertility etiologies. Hum Reprod. 2011;26(3):576-83.
31. Zavos A, Daponte A, Garas A, Verykouki C, Papanikolaou E, Anifandis G, et al. Double intrauterine insemination versus single intrauterine insemination for male factor infertility: a systematic review and meta-analysis. Asian J Androl. 2013;15(4):533-8.
32. Hill MJ, Richter KS, Zarek SM, Wu M, DeCherney AH, Osheroff JE, et al. Single and double donor sperm intrauterine insemination cycles for male factor infertility: does double IUI increase clinical pregnancy rates? Fertil Steril. 2014;102(3):739-43.
33. Polyzos NP, Tzioras S, Mauri D, Tatsioni A. Double versus single intrauterine insemination for unexplained infertility: a meta-analysis of randomized trials. Fertil Steril. 2010;94(4):1261-6.
34. Arab-Zozani M, Nastri CO. Single versus double intrauterine insemination (IUI) for pregnancy: a systematic review and meta-analysis. Eur J Obstet Gynecol Reprod Biol. 2017;215: 75-84.
35. Pathak B. Comparison of single versus double intra uterine insemination. Int J Reprod Contracept Obstet Gynecol. 2017;6(12):5277-81.
36. Rakic L, Kostova E, Cohlen BJ, Cantineau AE. Double versus single intrauterine insemination (IUI) in stimulated cycles for subfertile couples. Cochrane Database Syst Rev. 2021;7(7):CD003854.
37. Besselink DE, Farquhar C, Kremer JAM, Marjoribanks J, O'Brien P. Cervical insemination versus intra-uterine insemination of donor sperm for subfertility. Cochrane Database Syst Rev. 2008;2:CD000317.
38. Goldberg JM, Mascha E, Falcone T, Attaran M. Comparison of intrauterine and intracervical insemination with frozen donor sperm: a meta-analysis. Fertil Steril. 1999;72(5):792-5.
39. Levitas E, Lunenfeld E, Weiss N, Friger M, Har-Vardi I, Koifman A, et al. Relationship between the duration of sexual abstinence and semen quality: analysis of 9,489 semen samples. Fertil Steril. 2005;83(6):1680-6.
40. Marshburn PB, Alanis M, Matthews ML, Usadi R, Papadakis MH, Kullstam S, et al. A short period of ejaculatory abstinence before intrauterine insemination is associated with higher pregnancy rates. Fertil Steril. 2010;93(1):286-8.
41. Agarwal A, Gupta S, Plessis SD, Sharma R, Esteves SC, Cirenza C, et al. Abstinence time and its impact on basic and advanced semen parameters. Urology. 2016;94:102-10.
42. Lehavi O, Botchan A, Paz G, Yogev L, Kleiman SE, Yavetz H, et al. Twenty-four hours abstinence and the quality of sperm parameters. Andrologia. 2014;46(6):692-7.
43. Ombelet W, Nathalie D, Thijssen A, Bosmans E, Kruger T. Semen quality and prediction of IUI success in male subfertility: a systematic review. Reprod Biomed Online. 2014;28:300-9.
44. van Weert JM, Repping S, Van Voorhis BJ, van der Veen F, Bossuyt PM, Mol BW. Performance of the postwash total motile sperm count as a predictor of pregnancy at the time of intrauterine insemination: A meta-analysis. Fertil Steril. 2004; 82(3):612-20.
45. Kleppe M, van Hooff MH, Rhemrev JP. Effect of total motile sperm count in intra-uterine insemination on ongoing pregnancy rate. Andrologia. 2014;46(10):1183-8.
46. Hajder M, Hajder E, Husic A. The effects of total motile sperm count on spontaneous pregnancy rate and pregnancy after IUI treatment in couples with male factor and unexplained infertility. Med Arch. 2016;70(1):39-43.
47. Branigan E, Estes A, Walker K. The effect of processed total motile sperm counts and twenty four hour sperm survival on the efficacy of intrauterine insemination in male infertility. Andrology (Los Angel). 2017;6:191.
48. Mankus EB, Holden AE, Seeker PM, Kampschmidt JC, McLaughlin JE, Schenken RS, et al. Prewash total motile count is a poor predictor of live birth in intrauterine insemination cycles. Fertility and sterility. 2019;111(4):708-13.
49. Kohn TP, Kohn JR, Ramasamy R. Effect of Sperm morphology on pregnancy success via intrauterine insemination: A systematic review and meta-analysis. J Urol. 2018;199(3):812-22.

50. Yang H, Li G, Jin H, Guo Y, Sun Y. The effect of sperm DNA fragmentation index on assisted reproductive technology outcomes and its relationship with semen parameters and lifestyle. Translational andrology and urology. 2019;8(4):356.
51. Starosta A, Gordon CE, Hornstein MD. Predictive factors for intrauterine insemination outcomes: a review. Fertility Research and Practice. 2020;6(1):1-1.
52. Yavas Y, Selub MR. Intrauterine insemination (IUI) pregnancy outcome is enhanced by shorter intervals from semen collection to sperm wash, from sperm wash to IUI time, and from semen collection to IUI time. Fertil Steril. 2004;82(6):1638-47.
53. Koyun E, Okyay RE, Doğan OE, Kovalı M, Doğan SS, Gülekli B. The effect of intrauterine insemination time on semen parameters. J Turk Ger Gynecol Assoc. 2014;15(2):82-5.
54. Boomsma CM, Cohlen BJ, Farquhar C. Semen preparation techniques for intrauterine insemination. Cochrane Database Syst Rev. 2007;4:CD004507.
55. World Health Organization. WHO Laboratory Manual for the Examination and Processing of Human Semen, 5th edition. Geneva: WHO Press; 2010.
56. Boomsma CM, Heineman MJ, Cohlen BJ, Farquhar CM. Semen preparation techniques for intrauterine insemination. Cochrane Database Syst Rev. 2004;(3):CD004507.
57. Said TM, Agarwal A, Zborowski M, Grunewald S, Glander HJ, Paasch U. Utility of magnetic cell separation as a molecular sperm preparation technique. J Androl. 2008;29(2):134-42.
58. Guan HT, Zheng Y, Wang JJ, Meng TQ, Xia W, Hu SH, et al. Relationship between donor sperm parameters and pregnancy outcome after intrauterine insemination: analysis of 2821 cycles in 1355 couples. Andrologia. 2016;48(1):29-36.
59. Gurunath S, Gundlapalli S, Louis J. The use of pooled consecutive ejaculates in moderate male factor infertility to increase intrauterine insemination success. J Hum Reprod Sci. 2021;14(2):149-55.
60. Miller PB, Acres ML, Proctor JG, Higdon HL 3rd, Boone WR. Flexible versus rigid intrauterine insemination catheters: a prospective, randomized, controlled Study. Fertil Steril. 2005;83(5):1544-6.
61. Van der Poel N, Farquhar C, Abou-Setta AM, Benschop L, Heineman MJ. Soft versus firm catheters for intrauterine insemination. Cochrane Database Syst Rev. 2010;11:CD006225.
62. Abou-Setta AM, Mansour RT, Al-Inany HG, Aboulghar MA, Kamal A, Aboulghar MA, et al. Intrauterine insemination catheters for assisted reproduction: a systematic review and meta-analysis. Hum Reprod. 2006;21(8):1961-7.
63. Zhang E, Tao X, Xing W, Cai L, Zhang B. Effect of sperm count on success of intrauterine insemination in couples diagnosed with male factor infertility. Materia Socio-Medica. 2014;26(5):321-3.
64. Polat I, Ekiz A, Yildirim G, Sahin O, Ulker V, Alkis I, et al. Ultrasound-guided intrauterine insemination versus blind intrauterine insemination: a randomized controlled trial. Clin Exp Obstet Gynecol. 2015;42(5):657-62.
65. Oruç AS, Yılmaz N, Görkem U, Inal HA, Seçkin B, Gülerman C. Influence of ultrasound- guided artificial insemination on pregnancy rates: a randomized study. Arch Gynecol Obstet. 2014;289(1):207-12.
66. Oztekin D, Ozcinar E, Kose C, Gulhan I, Ozeren M, Tinar S. The use of ultrasound during intrauterine insemination in unexplained infertility may improve pregnancy outcomes. Med Princ Pract. 2013;22(3):291-4.
67. Orief YI, El-agwany AS, Elmoneem EA, Salim NM. The effect of bed rest after intrauterine insemination on pregnancy outcome. Middle East Fertil Soc J. 2015;20(1):11-5.
68. van Rijswijk J, Caanen MR, Mijatovic V, Vergouw CG, van de Ven PM, Lambalk CB, et al. Immobilization or mobilization after IUI: an RCT. Human Reproduction. 2017;32(11):2218-24.
69. Cohlen B, Bijkerk A, Van der Poel S, Ombelet W. IUI: review and systematic assessment of the evidence that supports global recommendations. Hum Reprod Update. 2018;24(3):300-19.
70. Miralpeix E, González-Comadran M, Solà I, Manau D, Carreras R, Checa MA, et al. Efficacy of luteal phase support with vaginal progesterone in intrauterine insemination: a systematic review and meta- analysis. J Assist Reprod Genet. 2014;31(1):89-100.
71. Gün I, Özdamar O, Yılmaz A. Luteal phase support in intrauterine insemination cycles. Turk J Obstet Gynecol. 2016;13(2):90-4.
72. Nilay K, Pinar O, Evrim KE, et al. Do women undergoing intrauterine insemination procedures critically require luteal phase support? A retrospective case-control study. 2016;01(01):006-011.
73. Custers IM, Steures P, Hompes P, Flierman P, van Kasteren Y, van Dop PA, et al. Intrauterine insemination: how many cycles should we perform? Hum Reprod. 2008;23(4):885-8.
74. Aboulghar M, Mansour R, Serour G, Abdrazek A, Amin Y, Rhodes C. Controlled ovarian hyperstimulation and intrauterine insemination for treatment of unexplained infertility should be limited to a maximum of three trials. Fertil Steril. 2001;75(1):88-91.
75. ESHRE Capri Workshop Group. Intrauterine insemination. Hum Reprod Update. 2009;15(3):265-77.
76. Dokuzeylül N. Antagonist use in intrauterine insemination (IUI) cycles. J Turk Ger Gynecol Assoc. 2009;10(4):226-31.
77. Olofsson JI, Banker MR, Sjoblom LP. Quality management systems for your in vitro fertilization clinic's laboratory: Why bother? J Hum Reprod Sci. 2013;6(1):3-8.
78. Bahadur G, Homburg R. Growing body of evidence supports intrauterine insemination as first line treatment and rejects unfounded concerns about its efficacy, risks and cost effectiveness. JBRA Assist Reprod. 2019;23(1):62-7.

SECTION

7 Ovarian Stimulation

CHAPTER 46

Drugs for Ovarian Stimulation

Duru Shah, Sabahat Rasool

INTRODUCTION

Drugs for ovarian stimulation are aimed at boosting the follicular growth and inducing ovulation. A number of drugs are available for stimulating the ovaries, the most commonly prescribed ones being clomiphene citrate (CC), tamoxifen, letrozole, and gonadotropins such as follicle-stimulating hormone (FSH) and luteinizing hormone (LH) **(Box 1)**. Human chorionic gonadotropin (hCG) and gonadotropin-releasing hormone (GnRH) analogs are used primarily for ovulation trigger and pituitary downregulation, respectively.

ORAL OVULOGENS

Clomiphene Citrate

Clomiphene citrate was synthesized in 1956 and introduced as a follicle stimulant in 1961 when Greenblatt and his group observed that it exerts a stimulatory effect on ovarian function in anovulatory women.[1] This synthetic nonsteroidal agent is a chlorotrianisene (TACE) analog consisting of three benzene rings. The molecular weight is 598.09 Daltons. CC is a white or pale yellow, odorless powder, unstable in air, and light. It is a racemic mixture of two stereochemical isomers, zuclomiphene (cis), and enclomiphene (trans).

The commercial preparations have these isomers in the ratio of 38% Zu and 62% En clomiphene. The En isomer is more estrogenic and potent, absorbed faster, and eliminated more completely than the Zu isomer. CC is metabolized by hepatic degradation, excreted through feces, with a small amount being cleared by kidneys. The drug can be detected in serum for up to 30 days if administered at a dose of 100 mg daily for 5 days.

BOX 1: Ovarian stimulation drugs.

Estrogen antagonists:
- Clomiphene citrate
- Tamoxifen
- Letrozole

Gonadotropins:
- Urinary-purified/highly purified FSH, LH, and hCG
- Recombinant—FSH, LH, CG, and FSH + LH

(CG: chorionic gonadotropin; FSH: follicle-stimulating hormone; hCG: human chorionic gonadotropin; LH: luteinizing hormone)

Action

Clomiphene citrate is a selective estrogen receptor modulator (SERM). It is a competitive estrogen receptor (ER) antagonist, exerting weak estrogenic activity in some tissues and moderate antiestrogenic activity in others. It acts on the ERs in hypothalamus, pituitary, ovary, endometrium, vagina, and cervix. CC blocks the negative feedback of endogenous estrogen primarily by prolonged depletion of hypothalamic and pituitary ERs. This causes a compensatory rise in GnRH release from the hypothalamus with a consequent rise in the release of pituitary gonadotropin.[2] To sum up, the antiestrogenic effect on the central nervous system increases FSH and LH pulse frequency and LH pulse amplitude, thereby moderately stimulating the ovaries with these gonadotropins.[3,4]

Clomiphene citrate is usually administered orally from early follicular phase of a natural or induced menstrual cycle in a dose of 50–150 mg daily for 5 days. This is aimed to coincide with the onset of gonadotropin-sensitive phase of follicle growth.

Indications

- Anovulatory infertility—polycystic ovary syndrome (PCOS)
- Unexplained infertility
- Luteal phase defect (CC induces LH receptors in corpora lutea)
- Coadministration with gonadotropin in in vitro fertilization (IVF) for poor responders.

Contraindications

- The WHO type I and III infertility
- Women with a defective hypothalamic pituitary axis like Sheehan's syndrome or Kallmann syndrome.

Clomiphene citrate is ineffective in hypogonadotropic hypogonadism because these women have a deficient estrogen signal to the hypothalamus.[5]

Efficacy

- *Ovulation rate*: 70–92%
- *Pregnancy rate*: 20–40%.

Treatment with CC is effective, safe, and economical. Low pregnancy rates are explained by the antiestrogenic effect of CC on tubal motility, cervical mucus and endometrium, decreased uterine blood flow, endometrium-embryo asynchrony, and detrimental effect on oocytes themselves.[6] CC gets accumulated within the body, leading to extended depletion of ERs and hostile effects on estrogen sensitive genital tissues.

Around 20–25% women are resistant to CC.[7] *CC resistance* is defined as failure to ovulate with 150 mg CC daily for 5 days for at least three cycles and occurs in 15–40% women with PCOS. Genetic predisposition, insulin resistance, hyperandrogenemia, and obesity all contribute to clomiphene resistance.[8] The treatment options for CC resistant patients include weight loss and lifestyle modifications, insulin sensitizers like metformin, oral contraceptive pill pretreatment, laparoscopic ovarian drilling, and use of gonadotropins.[9,10]

Clomiphene citrate failure is inability to get pregnant despite ovulating during three cycles with CC.

Side Effects

- Mood swings (64–78%)
- Hot flushes (10%)
- Abdominal distension (5%)
- Breast discomfort (2%)
- Nausea and vomiting (2%)
- Visual symptoms and headache (1.5%)
- Multiple pregnancy rate (5%)
- Adverse effects on cervical mucus (15%)
- Ovarian cysts (5%).

Tamoxifen

Tamoxifen is a nonsteroidal SERM widely used as adjunct therapy in breast cancer. It is structurally very similar to CC. Various studies have reported an ovulation rate of 50–90%, with pregnancy rates of 30–50%.[11] The drug is known to show good ovulation rates even in CC resistant cases. Since it acts as an agonist on ERs in vaginal mucosa and endometrium, there is a positive effect on endometrium and cervical mucus.[11,12] Side effects include headache and mild ovarian enlargement.

Aromatase Inhibitors

The conversion of androgen to estrogen occurs under the effect of a cytochrome P_{450}-dependent enzyme, aromatase. Aromatase inhibitors (AIs) are competitive inhibitors of aromatase enzyme **(Table 1)**. They lower the serum levels of estrone, estradiol as well as estrone sulfate, with maximum suppression achieved within 48–78 hours.[13] AIs were introduced for ovulation induction in 2001. AIs are also used for treatment of postmenopausal breast cancer.

TABLE 1: Generations of aromatase inhibitor.

Generation	Type I (steroid analogs)	Type II (nonsteroidal analogs)
First	–	Aminoglutethimide
Second	Formestane	• Fadrozole • Rogletimide
Third	Exemestane	• Anastrozole • Letrozole • Vorozole

Letrozole is a nonsteroidal competitive inhibitor of aromatase, with a half-life of 48 hours, and is mainly excreted through feces and urine.[14] It is administered orally in a dose of 2.5–5 mg per day for 5 days in early follicular phase.

Indications

- Obese PCOS
- PCOS with CC resistance and/or failure
- Unexplained infertility
- Coadministration with gonadotropin for poor responders.

Action

One of the most common causes of anovulation in PCOS (normogonadotropic anovulation) women is a static level of estrogen, either elevated or normal. Static level of estrogen, through negative feedback mechanism on hypothalamic–pituitary–adrenal axis (HPA), inhibits adequate release of pituitary FSH. Low level of FSH results in inadequate growth and development of follicles. Tonic elevated level of estrogen, through "positive feedback" effect on HPA, results in release of elevated tonic level of LH. There is no LH surge and therefore, no ovulation. AIs, by inhibiting estrogen synthesis temporarily, release hypothalamic-pituitary block, thereby normalizing the pulsatile release of pituitary FSH and ovulation. The hypoestrogenic state is quickly reversible due to the short half-life of letrozole (48 hours). There is no antiestrogenic effect on endometrium. Also, there is temporary elevation of testosterone to an optimum level, which is beneficial as it increases the follicular sensitivity to endogenous gonadotropins. Letrozole also increases the biosynthesis of endometrial receptivity markers such as integrin.

Efficacy

- *Ovulation rate*: 75%[15]
- *Pregnancy rate*: >25%.[15]

In a systematic review and meta-analysis of seven studies with 1,833 PCOS patients, live birth and pregnancy rates were statistically significantly better with letrozole compared to CC, with no differences in multiple pregnancy, miscarriage, and ovulation rates. It was concluded that letrozole was superior to CC when considering live birth and pregnancy rates in women with PCOS.[16] In yet another meta-analysis of 26 randomized controlled trails (RCTs), with 5,560 women, letrozole was found to improve live birth and pregnancy rates in subfertile women with PCOS compared to CC.[17] In a more recent double-blind RCT comparing letrozole 2.5 mg and CC 50 mg for anovulatory PCOS, women receiving letrozole achieved statistically higher pregnancy rate of 61%, compared to 43% in the CC group. Letrozole group showed a live birth rate of 48.8%, compared to 35.4% in the CC group. However, the live birth rates were not statistically different between the two treatment groups. This study implied that letrozole may be superior to CC as a primary ovulation induction agent in women with PCOS.[18] A recent systematic review and meta-analysis of 57 trials with 8,082 participants compared the effectiveness of first-line treatment options for anovulation in the WHO group II women.

It was found that compared to clomiphene alone, both letrozole and combination of clomiphene and metformin showed higher ovulation and pregnancy rates. Letrozole was the only treatment with significantly higher live birth rates compared to clomiphene alone.[19]

Side Effects

- Bone pain (20%)
- Hot flushes (18%)
- Back pain (17%)
- Nausea (15%)
- Dyspnea (14%)

Safety

There were safety concerns raised when letrozole was used for ovulation induction, the main being teratogenic and bone loss due to hypoestrogenism.

An abstract presented at the American Society for Reproductive Medicine (ASRM) meeting way back in 2005 eventually led to a ban on letrozole use for ovulation induction in India in 2011.[20] In the years following, good evidence suggested that letrozole is not associated with higher than normal teratogenic risk.

Tatsumi T et al. studied 3,136 natural cycles and 796 letrozole cycles for miscarriage and stillbirth rates, neonatal outcome, and congenital anomalies. The risk of miscarriage was found to be significantly lower in the letrozole cycles. No significant differences were observed in the overall risk of congenital anomalies between natural and letrozole cycles. The study concluded that letrozole reduces miscarriage rates, with no increase in the risk of major congenital anomalies or adverse pregnancy or neonatal outcomes when compared with natural cycles.[21]

Sharma S et al. studied 623 children born to infertile women who conceived naturally or following CC or letrozole induction. Congenital malformations and chromosomal abnormalities were found in 2.9% babies conceived naturally, in 2.5% babies in letrozole group and 3.9% babies in CC group. No statistical difference in overall rate of congenital malformations was found among children conceived naturally or after letrozole and CC induction.[22]

Gonadotropins

Historical Perspective

The word "gonadotropin" is derived from the Greek word, *trope*, which means turning on. In 1920s, with the surgical technique of hypophysectomy in animals, it was realized that removal of pituitary gland led to loss of reproductive function, and that it could be restored by administering exogenous pituitary gland extracts.[23] Zondek described the two gonadotropins extracted from the blood and urine of women as prolan A and B, which are now known to us as FSH and LH, respectively.[24] The first practice of exogenous gonadotropin for ovulation induction was achieved in 1950s with pituitary extracts from cows, swine, and sheep.[25] They were either used alone or in conjunction with pregnant mare serum gonadotropins (PMSGs). Follicular stimulation in women using PMSG was first attempted in 1931. Animal-origin gonadotropin, initially found to be effective, resulted in development of neutralizing antibodies, which rendered the ovaries unresponsive to these hormones over time. Human pituitary gonadotropins were isolated in 1958 and were successfully used to stimulate ovulation. They were forced off the market by mid-1980s after the unfortunate events of death and dementia caused by Creutzfeldt–Jacob disease (CJD).[26] Human menopausal gonadotropins (hMGs) were extracted from the urine of postmenopausal women in 1960s.[27] There was a continuous improvement in the extraction and purification techniques to remove impurities. Despite the best efforts, the active ingredients constituted only 1–2% of the final product. Finally, with the deoxyribonucleic acid (DNA) recombinant technology, recombinant gonadotropins were created, which are extremely pure, highly specific, and have a limitless supply. At present, both urinary and recombinant products are available for use **(Fig. 1)**.

Gonadotropins in Ovulation Physiology

A physiological ovarian cycle involves the growth of a cohort of synchronous primordial follicles to the preantral stage. With the rising FSH levels in the early follicular phase, the follicle most sensitive to FSH enlarges and becomes more and more receptive to FSH. Androgenic substrates are delivered to the granulosa cells, which convert them to estradiol. As the estradiol levels rise, FSH secretion from the pituitary is

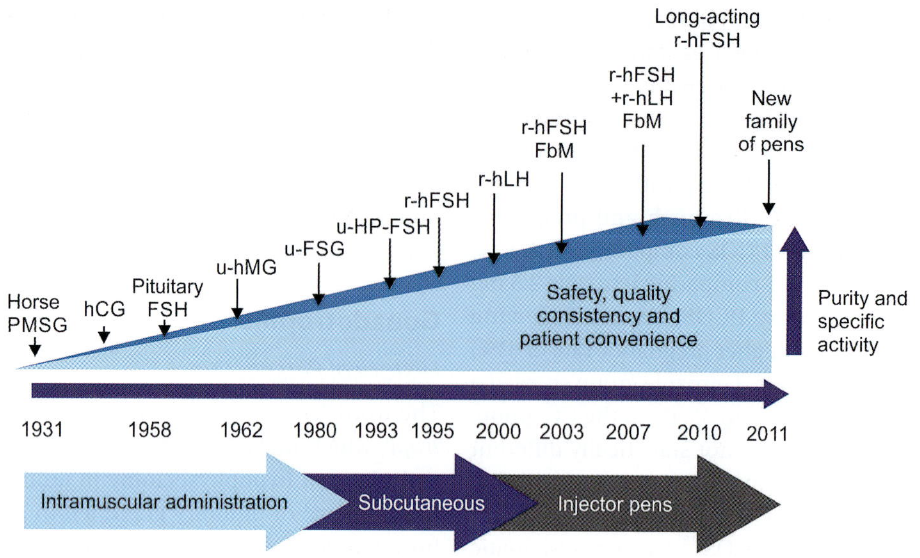

Fig. 1: Evolution of gonadotropins.
(PMSG: pregnant mare serum gonadotropin; hCG: human chorionic gonadotropin; FSH: follicle-stimulating hormone; u-hMG: urinary-human menopausal gonadotropin; u-HP-FSH: urinary-highly purified-follicle-stimulating hormone; r-hFSH: recombinant human follicle stimulating hormone; r-hLH: recombinant human leutinising hormone)

suppressed through a negative feedback. Despite the falling FSH concentrations, the "dominant" follicle continues to grow and develops LH receptors. The rest of the follicles, however, cannot keep pace and stop growing. The dominant follicle prevents the growth of its fellow follicles, maintaining a monovulatory cycle in humans. The use of gonadotropins in IVF, on the other hand, supports the growth of the entire cohort of developing preantral follicles. Of note, the earlier stages of follicle recruitment and development are gonadotropin-independent. Gonadotropins are either used to restore physiological monovulation or to induce superovulation or controlled ovarian hyperstimulation, where all the synchronized follicles are induced to grow to yield 6–10 oocytes.

Role of LH in ovulation: FSH and LH act in concert to complete follicle maturation and ovulation through a menstrual cycle. At 8–12 mm size, follicles develop LH receptors under the influence of FSH. Mid-cycle LH surge induces ovulation, resumption of meiosis, formation of corpus luteum, luteinization of theca and granulosa cells, and early production of progesterone **(Table 2)**.

TABLE 2: Role of luteinizing hormone in ovulatory cycle.

Early follicular phase	*Late follicular phase*
Steroidogenesis	• Steroidogenesis • Upregulates follicle-stimulating hormone (FSH) receptor expression sustains follicular growth and maturation ovulation

Urinary Menotropins or hMG: Gonadotropin treatment for ovulation induction in anovulatory women began in 1960s and for superovulation in 1980s.

Human menopausal gonadotropin or Menotropin was derived initially from the urine of postmenopausal women from a single nunnery in Italy. The collection was later expanded to various centers worldwide to meet the mounting demand. The earliest preparations were only 5% pure and contained FSH and LH in equal proportions with varying proportions of hCG. hMG preparations contain up to five different isomers of FSH and up to 9 LH isomers. Purification techniques led to the standardization of FSH and LH activity to 75 IU for each type of gonadotropin, but unfortunately, non-gonadotropin proteins such as tumor necrosis factor-binding protein I (TNF-BP-I), transferrin, Tamm–Horsfall protein, and epidermal growth factors (EGF) continued to exist. Despite all the extraction and purification methods, gonadotropin constituted only 1–2% of the final product.[28] The presence of non-gonadotropin proteins causes local side effects such as pain and allergic reactions.[29]

The LH activity of the gonadotropins extracted from menopausal urine is only about one-third of that of the FSH activity in terms of IU, and this makes it necessary to supplement LH activity through hCG derived from the urine of pregnant women to reach an LH:FSH ratio of 1:1. With time, it became clearer that most women needed FSH rather than LH for follicular growth, and consequently, there was a shift toward purer FSH products.

Purified and highly purified FSH: Removal of LH with antibodies resulted in a biologically pure urinary FSH preparation, urofollitropin. With the use of monoclonal antibodies specific to FSH, highly purified FSH (HP-FSH) was produced in 1990s with <0.1 IU LH and <5% of urinary proteins.[30] This HP-FSH was better suited for patients with high endogenous LH, as it was known by this time that FSH alone could induce folliculogenesis and that LH was also responsible for complications like ovarian stimulation.[31] The enhanced purity and specific bioactivity of HP-FSH made it possible to administer this gonadotropin through subcutaneous route.

Recombinant Gonadotropins

Recombinant DNA technology opened a new horizon for the production of recombinant human gonadotropin. Recombinant gonadotropin were developed by inserting the desired gene sequences for alpha and beta subunits of gonadotropin into expression vectors. These vectors are then transfected into immortalized Chinese hamster ovary (CHO) cell lines. Sereno laboratories produced the world's first recombinant follitropin alpha in 1988 and Organon laboratories produced the first follitropin beta in 1996. Though the names are different, both these FSH preparations contain one alpha and one beta chain. It is the post-translational glycosylation and purification that results in varied sialic acid residue compositions, and hence, different names. The clinical performance, nonetheless, is similar.[32] Follitropin alpha and beta are now available as prefilled pens which deliver a highly precise dose.[33] The FSH content of the recombinant FSH preparations can be quantified as mass in µg, contrary to urinary FSH, whose FSH content is quantified by bioactivity using Steelman–Pohley bioassay.

Recombinant LH (r-LH), Luveris, has been available for clinical use since 1993. It is used to enhance follicular growth with FSH in patients with profound LH deficiency, like that seen in hypogonadic hypogonadism. r-LH has also been found to improve implantation and clinical pregnancy rates when used in combination with r-FSH in patients older than 35 years and women with diminished ovarian reserve.[34]

A combination of recombinant FSH and LH in a ratio of 2:1 is also available as Pergoveris for use in suitable patients. Recombinant hCG is available as Ovitrelle or Ovidrel as 250 µg syringe, which is equivalent to 6,500 IU of hCG.[35]

Recombinant gonadotropins have some advantages over the urinary products in terms of purity, batch-to-batch consistency, limitless source and supply, predictable bioactivity, and safety. However, the pregnancy rates and reproductive outcomes are similar.[32]

Designer Recombinant Follicle-stimulating Hormone

Pushing the envelope of genetic engineering has led to the development of designer recombinant molecules. Long-acting formulation, corifollitropin alpha, or FSH-carboxy-terminal peptide (FSH-CTP) was created in 1992 by Fares FA et al.[36] Recombinant DNA technology was utilized to fuse the CTP of hCG beta-subunit to the FSH beta-subunit, resulting in a hybrid β chain. The resulting FSH analog has identical receptor-binding and biological activities as wild-type FSH (WT-FSH), but an increased circulating half-life. The serum elimination half-life of FSH-CTP is 65 hours, which is twice that of r-FSH.[36] FSH-CTP was designed with the idea of making stimulation more patient-friendly, as a single injection of FSH-CTP gives a sustained FSH level for 1 week.

The latest to be granted marketing authorization in the EU is follitropin-δ (FE 999049) which has been derived from human fetal retinal origin. The amino acid sequences of both subunits are the same as that of natural FSH but the sialic acid content is lower. It has a longer elimination life of 30 hours and induces stronger ovarian response. Follitropin-δ cannot be dosed according to bioactivity or specific bioactivity as other follitropins and is instead dosed by mass (µg).[37]

Orally active small peptides with FSH action are still a distant dream, but if realized, would be a big boon as it would avoid the need for painful injections altogether. One oral FSH agonist has been evaluated in females but it did not produce any follicular development.

Human Chorionic Gonadotropin

The most consistently used gonadotropin in assisted reproduction is hCG. It is used as a surrogate for mid-cycle LH surge. LH is necessary for final oocyte maturation, resumption of meiosis, development of corpus luteum, and production of progesterone. Because of 85% sequence similarity in the β subunit, both LH and hCG bind to the same receptor. Both have a molecular weight of approximately 30 kDa, identical α unit, and high cysteine content. CTP of the β subunit of hCG makes it different and confers a longer half-life due to slower metabolic clearance.[38] Long serum half-life of hCG, a sustained luteotropic effect, multiple corpora lutea development, leading to ovarian hyperstimulation syndrome (OHSS), supraphysiological levels of estradiol and progesterone synthesis leading to implantation failures and early pregnancy loss, and delayed ovulation of small follicles leading to multiple pregnancies are some of the disadvantages of hCG administration as a surrogate for LH surge **(Table 3)**.[39-42]

The minimal effective dose for triggering oocyte maturation and ovulation is 5,000–10,000 IU of hCG. There is no difference between r-LH, recombinant chorionic gonadotropin (r-CG), and urinary hCG in achieving final oocyte maturation, ovulation, pregnancy, and OHSS rates.[43] 5,000–6,000 IU of urinary hCG is equivalent to 250 µg of recombinant CG.[44] It takes around 36 hours for the completion of meiosis, and ovulation happens roughly 4 hours later **(Table 4)**.

Indications[45-50]

- Ovulation trigger
- Follicular stimulation along with FSH
- Luteal support
- hCG priming in in vitro maturation
- Hypogonadal hypogonadism.

TABLE 3: Luteinizing hormone (LH) versus human chorionic gonadotropin (hCG).

Characteristics	LH	hCG
Molecular weight (Daltons)	28,000	38,000
Secreted by	Pituitary	Embryo and placenta
Accumulation	Slight	Significant with LH receptor downregulation
Equivalence	6–8 IU of LH	1 IU of hCG
Physiological role	Support follicle development and induce ovulation	Support implantation and pregnancy
Potency and receptor affinity	Less	More
Sialic acid carbohydrate residues	1–2	20
β subunit	115 amino acids	145 amino acids
Circulatory half-life	38–60 minutes	6–8 hours

TABLE 4: Gonadotropins preparations.

Gonadotropin preparations	FSH activity (IU/ampoule)	LH activity (UI/ampoule)	% Protein contamination	Source	Route of administration
Urinary and highly purified urinary hCG	Negligible	5000 or 10,000	<5	Urine	IM
Recombinant hCG	0	250 g delivered	Unknown	Recombinant from transfected CHO cells	SC
Menotropins (hMG)	75 or 150	75 or 150	>95	Urine	IM
Urofollitropins (FSH)	75 or 150	Negligible	>95	Urine	IM
Highly purified urinary FSH	75 or 150	Negligible	<5	Urine	IM or SC
Follitropin alpha (FSH)	75, 450,300, 450, and 900	0	Unknown	Recombinant from transfected CHO cells	SC
Follitropin beta (FSH)	75, 150, 175, 350, 650, and 975	0	Unknown	Recombinant from transfected CHO cells	SC
Lutropin beta	0	75	Unknown	Recombinant from transfected CHO cells	SC

(CHO: chinese hamster ovary; FSH: follicle-stimulating hormone; hCG: human chorionic gonadotropin; hMG: human menopausal gonadotropin; IM: intramuscular; LH: luteinizing hormone; SC: subcutaneous; IU: international units)

Structure of Gonadotropins

Gonadotropins are composed of an α and a β chain. The α subunit is common to all three gonadotropins and thyroid-stimulating hormones (TSHs), and contains 92 amino acids (A/A) and 10 cysteine residues. It is the β subunit that actually differentiates the hormones.

Follicle-stimulating Hormone

The β subunit of FSH contains 111 A/A and 12 cysteine residues. The molecular weight of FSH is 34 kDa. The carbohydrate content of FSH determines its half-life, proper folding, secretion, target cell-binding, and signal transduction.[51] Human FSH circulates as a mixture of isoforms separated on the basis of charge. The various isoforms differ in their biological activity. The more acidic an isoform, the lower is the receptor-binding and bioactivity, but longer is the half-life.

Luteinizing Hormone

The β subunit of LH compromises of 121 A/A. The molecular weight of LH is 28 kDa.

The initial and terminal half-lives of endogenous LH are 0.6 and 10 hours, respectively and of r-LH are 0.8 and 11 hours, respectively. The pituitary LH is more sulfated and r-LH more sialylated.[52]

Human Chorionic Gonadotropin

The β subunit of hCG contains 145 A/A. hCG has a molecular weight of 38 kDa. The presence of CTP makes the subunit different form the β subunit of LH.

Success Rates and Complications of Using Gonadotropin[53-55]

- The cumulative live birth rates are of the order of 89% after six treatment cycles with gonadotropin.

- The incidence of severe OHSS is <1% and that of multiple pregnancies is 30%.
- The rate of major and minor malformations with the use of gonadotropin was found to be 54.3/1,000, which is similar to that of the general population.

Indications for Gonadotropin Use

- *Gonadotropin for ovulation induction (Fig. 2A)*: Gonadotropins are used for ovulation induction when other simpler, safer, and economical approaches such as CC, letrozole, ovarian drilling, and metformin have failed. Since our aim in ovulation induction is monovulation, low doses of FSH are used. Treatment must be individualized, monitored, and started with the lowest effective dose after a thorough patient counseling. A starting dose of 37.5–75 IU/day is given for at least 5–7 days, and dose increment done only after 7–14 days if ovarian response is not optimum. This is to ensure low rates of OHSS and multiple gestation.[53,56]
- *Gonadotropin for superovulation in intrauterine insemination and controlled ovarian stimulation (COS) in IVF/intracytoplasmic sperm injection (Figs. 2B and C)*: The goal of superovulation is to induce more than one follicular development. In COS, the entire cohort of preantral follicles is recruited and stimulated to yield 6–10 oocytes, while controlling the endogenous LH surge by pituitary downregulation. Starting doses of gonadotropin depend on patient's age, ovarian reserve, sensitivity to gonadotropin, and previous ovarian response, if any. Ovarian reserve-guided stimulation protocols significantly improve IVF outcome, while reducing cost and risks. Pretreatment counseling about the potential complications and multiple gestations is warranted.

For soft stimulation in IVF, starting doses of 150 IU/day are advocated.[57] La Marca et al. created a model for ovarian stimulation based on age, antral follicle count (AFC), and day 3 FSH. Using the normogram based on age, FSH, and AFC, the most appropriate gonadotropin dose for a woman of 30 years of age with normal day 3 FSH, AFC of 16, or AMH of 4 ng/mL (predicted hyper-responders) is 150 IU/day.[58] Older patients and those with diminished ovarian reserve may require higher doses of 300–450 IU/day.[59,60] Increasing gonadotropin dose beyond a particular limit in such patients does not make the oocyte yield better. On the contrary, high gonadotropin doses worsen the oocyte quality, endometrial receptivity, implantation, and pregnancy rates.[61] Gianaroli et al. found that the number of euploid oocytes is directly proportional to mature oocytes and establishment of clinical pregnancy and inversely proportional to age and the number of FSH units used per oocyte and per mature oocyte.[62]

Indications for Luteinizing Hormone Use in Assisted Reproduction Technology

- Hypogonadotropic hypogonadism
- *r-LH cotreatment with r-FSH for poor responders*: In a systematic review and meta-analysis of 14 trials with 2,612 women, r-LH supplementation to r-FSH was found to have a beneficial effect in poor responders and patients with history of pregnancy loss.[63]
  - *Patients with advanced reproductive age*: Hill MJ et al. evaluated the effect of r-LH in assisted reproduction technology (ART) cycles in patients of advanced reproductive age in a systematic review and meta-analysis. They concluded that implantation and clinical pregnancy rates were higher in the r-LH-supplemented group.[34]
  - *Poor responders*: The benefits of r-LH supplementation in specific subpopulations was confirmed in a large meta-analysis of 40 randomized controlled trials of 6,443 patients treated with either r-LH/r-FSH or FSH only, in women aged 18–45 years or older. Significantly, more oocytes were retrieved in poor responders in the r-LH supplemented group compared to r-FSH alone group. A significantly higher clinical pregnancy rate was seen with the r-LH/R-FSH group.[64]

Gonadotropin-releasing Hormone Analogs

Gonadotropin-releasing hormone, first discovered in 1971, is a decapeptide with a structure that is common to all mammals. Its action is similar in both males and females.

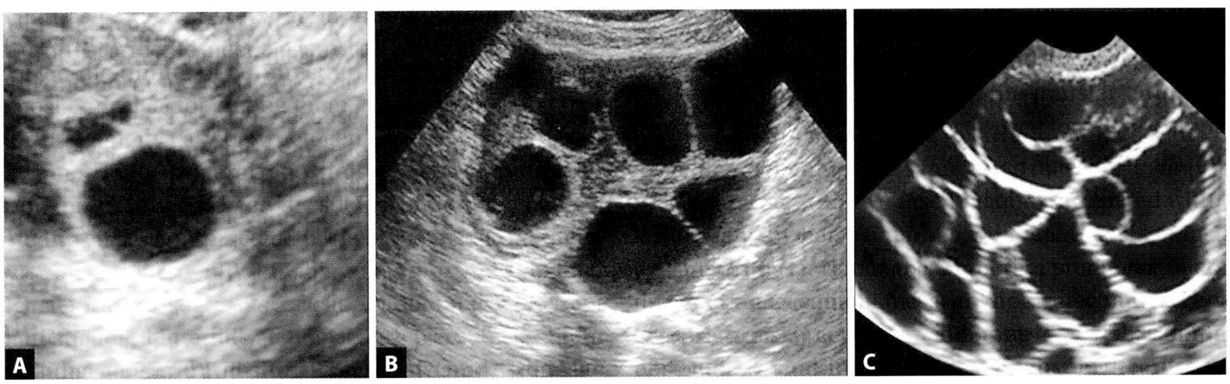

Figs. 2A to C: (A) Ovulation induction; (B) Superovulation; and (C) Controlled ovarian stimulation.

It is released from the hypothalamus in a pulsatile manner, with pulses ranging between 71 minutes in late follicular phase to 216 minutes in late luteal phase.[66,66]

Gonadotropin-releasing Hormone Agonist

Gonadotropin-releasing hormone agonists (leuprolide, triptorelin, and goserelin) are parenterally administered to prevent gastrointestinal degradation. Buserelin and nafarelin are available as extremely effective intranasal sprays, but require very frequent dosing due to rapid elimination. Long-term depot preparations are available for maintaining therapeutic levels for 28–35 days.[67]

Action: With the initial administration, there is an expected flare-up effect increasing gonadotropin secretion. With prolonged use, GnRH receptors are downregulated and internalized via receptor-mediated endocytosis and dissociated.[68] For achieving pituitary suppression, 7–14 days of daily administration is required.

Safety and side effects:[69,70]

- Hot flushes
- Vaginal dryness
- Loss of libido
- Reduced breast size
- Emotional instability
- Significant but reversible bone loss.

Gonadotropin-releasing Hormone Antagonist

Gonadotropin-releasing hormone antagonist (GnRH-ant) acts by directly blocking the receptors competitively and suppressing the gonadotropin secretion from the pituitary within 8 hours of administration. There is no initial flare-up as is seen with the use of agonists. The first- and second-generations of antagonists resulted in histamine release and consequent anaphylactic reactions. The third-generation antagonists that are being clinically used at present and include ganirelix, cetrorelix, abarelix, antarelix, and iturelix have not caused any major local or systemic reactions in thousands of treated patients worldwide. However, nausea, malaise, fatigue, and headache are reported with their use.[71] The highest pregnancy rates are achieved when a daily dose of 0.25 mg of the antagonist is used. Higher dose was found to lower implantation rates due to its possible direct effects on embryos.[72]

A meta-analysis of 45 RCTs with nearly 7,500 women comparing GnRH agonists and antagonists for COS in ART cycles did not show any difference in the live birth or ongoing pregnancy rates but significantly lower incidence of OHSS with the antagonist use.[73] GnRH antagonists are particularly beneficial in anticipated hyper-responders.

Long-acting GnRH antagonist, degarelix, was introduced for prostatic cancer treatment. Its use in ART seems to address the flexibility issue with the antagonist protocols.

TABLE 5: GnRH agonist versus GnRH antagonist.

GnRH agonist	*GnRH antagonist*
Receptor blockage	Initial activation followed by downregulation
Competitive inhibition	Desensitization
Dose-dependent immediate suppression	Initial flare-up
Rapid reversibility	Slow reversibility

(GnRH: Gonadotropin-releasing hormone)

A single injection in luteal phase is effective enough to promote LH suppression and maintain low estradiol levels.[74]

Differentiations between GnRH agonist and GnRH antagonist are depicted in **Table 5**.

Deep understanding of the physiology of reproduction and pharmacokinetics and pharmacodynamics of the ovulation stimulant drugs goes a long way in achieving optimum reproductive outcome. Individualized and patient-tailored treatment yields the best reproductive outcome with maximum safety.

Gonadotropins are the most essential and effective drugs for controlled ovarian hyperstimulation and superovulation in ART. The source of gonadotropin does not make much of a difference in the pregnancy rates. However, rational and judicious use of gonadotropins is important for patient safety and good results.

REFERENCES

1. Greenblatt RB, Barfield WE, Jungck EC, Ray AW. Induction of ovulation with MRL/41. Preliminary report. JAMA. 1961;178:101-4.
2. Clark JH, Peck EJ, Anderson JN. Oestrogen receptors and antagonism of steroid hormone action. Nature. 1974;251:446-8.
3. Kerin JF, Liu JH, Phillipou G, Yen SS. Evidence for a hypothalamic site of action of Clomiphene citrate in women. J Clin Endocrinol Metab. 1985;61(2):265-8.
4. Martikainen H, Ronnberg L, Ruokonen A, Kauppila A. Gonadotropin pulsatility in a stimulated cycle: clomiphene citrate increases pulse amplitudes of both luteinizing hormone and follicle-stimulating hormone. Fertil Steril. 1991;56(4):641-5.
5. Yeko TR, Khan-Dawood FS, Dawood MY. Luteinizing hormone and human chorionic gonadotropin receptors in corpora lutea from clomiphene citrate-induced cycles. Fertil Steril. 1990;54(4):601-5.
6. Out HJ, Coelingh Bennink HJ. Clomiphene citrate or gonadotropins for ovulation induction? Hum Reprod. 1998;13(9):2358-61.
7. Elnashar A, Fouad H, Eldosoky M, Saeid N. Letrozole induction of ovulation induction in women with clomiphene citrate-resistant polycystic ovary syndrome may not depend on the period of infertility, body mass index or the LH/FSH ratio. Fertil Steril. 2006;85(2):511-3.
8. Brown J, Farquhar C, Beck J, Boothroyd C, Hughes E. Clomiphene and anti-oestrogens for ovulation induction in PCOS. Cochrane Database Syst Rev. 2009;(4):CD002249.

9. Hoeger KM. Obesity and lifestyle management in polycystic ovary syndrome. Clin Obstet Gynecol. 2007;50(1):277-94.
10. Vaux TD, Cheung AP, Sierra S, Reproductive Endocrinology and Infertility Committee. Ovulation induction in PCOS. J Hum Reprod Update. 2004(10);3:267-80.
11. Borenstein R, Shoham Z, Yemini M, Barash A, Fienstein M, Rozenman D. Tamoxifen treatment in women with failure of clomiphene citrate therapy. Aust N Z J Obstet Gynaecol. 1989;29(2):173-5.
12. Williamsons JG, Ellis JD. The induction of ovulation by tamoxifen. J Obstet Gynecol. 1973;80(9):844-7.
13. Gross PE, Gwyn KM. Current perspectives on aromatase inhibitors in breast cancer. J Clin Oncol. 1994;12(11): 2460-70.
14. Lamb HM, Adkins JC. Letrozole. A review of its use in postmenopausal women with advanced breast cancer. Drugs. 1998;56(6):1125-40.
15. Mitwally MF, Casper RF. Use of an aromatase inhibitor for induction of ovulation in patients with inadequate response to clomiphene citrate. Fertil Steril. 2001;75(2): 305-9.
16. Roque M, Tostes AC, Valle M, Sampaio M, Geber S. Letrozole versus clomiphene citrate in polycystic ovary syndrome: systematic review and meta-analysis. Gynecol Endocrinol. 2015;31(12):917-21.
17. Franik S, Kremer JA, Nelen WLDM, Farquhar C. Aromatase inhibitors for subfertile women with PCOS. Cochrane Database Syst Rev. 2014;(2):CD010287.
18. Amer SA, Smith J, Mahran A, Fox P, Fakis A. Double-blind randomized controlled trial of letrozole versus clomiphene citrate in subfertile women with polycystic ovarian syndrome. Hum Reprod. 2017;32(8):1631-8.
19. Wang R, Kim BV, van Wely M, Johnson NP, Costello MG, Zhang H, et al. Treatment strategies for women with WHO group II anovulation: systematic review and network meta-analysis. BMJ. 2017;356:j138.
20. Al-Fadhli R, Sylvestre C, Buckett W, Tan SL, Tulandi T. A randomized trial of superovulation with two different doses of letrozole. Fertil Steril. 2006;85:161-4.
21. Tatsumi T, Jwa SC, Kuwahara A, Irahara M, Kubota T, Saito H. No increased risk of major congenital anomalies or adverse pregnancy or neonatal outcomes following letrozole use in assisted reproductive technology. Hum Reprod. 2017;32(1): 125-32.
22. Sharma S, Ghosh S, Singh S, Chakravarty A, Ganesh A, Rajani S, et al. Congenital malformations among babies born following letrozole or clomiphene for infertility treatment. PLoS One. 2014;9(10):e108219.
23. Smith PE. Hastening development of female genital system by daily homoplastic pituitary transplants. Proc Soc Exp Biol Med. 1926;24:131-2.
24. Lunenfeld B. Historical perspectives in gonadotropin therapy. Hum Reprod Update. 2004;10(6):453-67.
25. Gemzell CA, Diczfalusy E, Tillinger G. Clinical effect of human pituitary follicle-stimulating hormone (FSH). J Clin Endocrinol Metab. 1958;18(12):1333-48.
26. Lazarus L. Suspension of the Australian human pituitary hormone programme. Med J Aust. 1985;143(2):57-9.
27. Lunenfeld B. Development of gonadotropins for clinical use. Reprod Biomed Online. 2002;4(1):11-17.
28. Rosenburg E, Coleman J, Damani M, Garcia CR. Clinical effect of post menopausal gonadotropin. J Clin Endocrinol Metab. 1962;23:181-9.
29. Cook AS, Webster BW, Terranova PF, Keel BA. Variation in the biologic and biochemical characteristics of human menopausal gonadotropin. Fertil Steril. 1998;49:704-12.
30. Giudice E, Crisci C, Eshkol A, Papoian R. Composition of commercial gonadotropin preparations extracted from human post-menopausal urine: characterization of non-gonadotrophin proteins. Hum Reprod. 1994;9(12):2291-9.
31. Loumaye E, Engrand P, Shoham Z, Hillier SG, Baird DT. Clinical evidence for an LH 'ceiling' effect induced by administration of recombinant human LH during the late follicular phase of stimulated cycles in World Health Organization type I and type II anovulation. Hum Reprod. 2003;18(2):314-22.
32. Olijve W, de Boer W, Mulders JW, van Wezenbeek PM. Molecular biology and biochemistry of human recombinant follicle stimulating hormone (Puregon). Mol Hum Reprod. 1996;2:371-82.
33. Hugues JN, Durnerin IC. Gonadotropins filled-by-mass versus filled-by-bioassay. Reprod Biomed Online. 2005;10(3): 11-8.
34. Hill MJ, Levens ED, Levy G, Ryan ME, Csokmay JM, DeCherney AH, et al. The use of recombinant luteinizing hormone in patients undergoing assisted reproductive techniques with advanced reproductive age: a systematic review and meta-analysis. Fertil Steril. 2012;97(5):1108-14.
35. Practice Committee of the ASRM. Gonadotropin preparations: past, present and future perspectives. Fertil Steril. 2008;90:S13-S20.
36. Fares FA, Suganuma N, Nishimori K, LaPolt PS, Hsueh AJ, Boime I. Design of a long- acting follitropin agonist by fusing the C-terminal sequence of the chorionic gonadotropin β subunit. Proc Nat Acad Sci USA. 1992;89(10):4304-8.
37. Koechling W, Plaksin D, Croston GE, Jeppesen JV, Macklon KT, Andersen CY. Comparative pharmacology of a new recombinant FSH expressed by a human cell line. Endocr Connect. 2017;6:297-305.
38. Biome I, Ben-Menahem D, Olijve W. Studies of recombinant gonadotropins: intersection of basic science and therapeutics. In: Fauser BCJM (Ed.). Molecular biology in reproductive medicine. New York: Parthenon Publications; 1999. pp. 147-64.
39. Nader S, Berkowitz AS. Endogenous luteinizing hormone surge following administration of human chorionic gonadotropin: further evidence for lack of loop feedback in humans. J Assist Reprod Genet. 1992;9:124-7.
40. Golan A, Ron-el R, Herman A, Soffer Y, Weinraub Z, Caspi E. Ovarian hyperstimulation syndrome: an update review. Obstet Gynecol Surv. 1989;44(6):430-40.
41. Gidley-Baird AA, O'Neill C, Sinosich MJ, Porter RN, Pike L, Saunders DM. Failure of implantation in human in vitro fertilization and embryo transfer patients: the effects of altered progesterone/estrogen ratios in humans and mice. Fertile Steril. 1986;45(1):69-74.
42. Forman R, Fries N, Testart J, Belaisch-Allart J, Hazout A, Frydman R. Evidence for an adverse effect of elevated serum estradiol concentrations on embryo implantation. Fertil Steril. 1988;49:118-22.
43. Youssef MA, Al-Inany HG, Aboulghar M, Mansour R, Abou-Setta AM. Recombinant versus urinary chorionic

gonadotropin for final oocyte maturation triggering in IVF and ICSI cycles. Cochrane Database Syst Rev. 2011;(4):CD003719.
44. The European Recombinant Human Chorionic Gonadotrophin Study Group. Induction of final follicular maturation and early luteinization in women undergoing ovulation induction for assisted reproduction treatment-recombinant hCG versus urinary hCG. Hum Reprod. 2000;15(7):1446-51.
45. Ashrafi M, Kiani K, Ghaseni A, Rastegar F, Nabavi M. The effect of low dose human chorionic gonadotropin on follicular response and oocyte maturation in PCOS patients undergoing IVF cycles: a randomized clinical trial of efficacy and safety. Arch Gynecol Obstet. 2011;284(6):1431-8.
46. Gomaa H, Casper RF, Esfandiari N, Chang P, Bentov Y. Addition of low dose hCG to rFSh benefits older women during ovarian stimulation for IVF. Reprod Biol Endocrinol. 2012;10:55.
47. Beretsos P, Partsinevelos GA, Arabatzi E, Drakakis P, Mavrogianni D, Anagnostou E, et al. "hCG priming" effect in controlled ovarian stimulation through a long protocol. Reprod Biol Endocrinol. 2009;7:91.
48. Blockeel C, DeVos M, Verpoest W, Stoop D, Haentjens P, Devroey P. Can 200 IU of hCG replace recombinant FSH in late follicular phase in a GnRH antagonist cycle? A pilot study. Hum Reprod. 2009;24(11):2910-6.
49. van der Linden M, Buckingham K, Farquhar C, Kremer JA, Metwally M. Luteal phase support for assisted reproduction cycles. Cochrane Database Syst Rev. 2011;(10):CD009154.
50. Andersen CY, Fischer R, Giorgione V, Kelsey TW. Micro-dose hCG as luteal phase support without exogenous progesterone administration: mathematical modelling of the hCG concentration in circulation and initial clinical experience. J Assist Reprod Genet. 2016;33(10):1311-8.
51. Ulloa-Aguirre A, Timossi C, Damián-Matsumura P, Dias JA. Role of glycosylation in function of follicle stimulating hormone. Endocrine. 1999;11(3):205-15.
52. Amoresano A, Siciliano R, Orru S, Napoleoni R, Altarocca V, De Luca E, et al. Structural characterisation of human recombinant glycohormones follitropin, lutropin and choriogonadotropins expressed in Chinese Hamster Ovary cells. Eur J Biochem. 1996;242:608-18.
53. Fluker MR, Urman B, Mackinnon M, Barrow SR, Pride SM, Yuen BH. Exogenous gonadotropin therapy in World Health Organization groups I and II ovulatory disorders. Obstet Gynecol. 1994;83:189-96.
54. Tadokoro N, Vollengoven B, Clark S, Baker G, Kovacs G, Burger H, et al. Cumulative pregnancy rates in couples with anovulatory infertility compared with unexplained infertility in an ovulation induction programme. Hum Reprod. 1997; 12(9):1939-44.
55. Shoham Z, Zosmer A, Insler V. Early miscarriage and fetal malformations after induction of ovulation (by clomiphene citrate and/or human menotropins) in in vitro fertilization and gamete intra fallopian transfer. Fertil Steril. 1991;55(1):1-11.
56. Oelsner G, Serr DM, Mashiach S, Blankstein J, Snyder M, Lunenfeld B. The study of induction of ovulation with menotropins: analysis of results of 1897 treatment cycles. Fertil Steril. 1978;30(5):538-44.
57. Yates AP, Rustamov O, Roberts SA, Lim HYN, Pemberton PW, Smith A, et al. Anti-Mullerian hormone-tailored stimulation protocols improve outcomes whilst reducing adverse effects and cost of IVF. Hum Reprod. 2011;26(9):2353-62.
58. La Marca A, Grisendi V, Giulini S, Argento C, Tirelli A, Dondi G, et al. Individualization of the FSH starting dose in IVF/ICSI cycles using the antral follicle count. J Ovarian Res. 2013;6(1):11.
59. Nyboe Andersen A, Nelson SM, Fauser BC, García-Velasco JA, Klein BM, Arce J-C, et al. Individualized versus conventional ovarian stimulation for IVF: a multi-center, randomized controlled, assessor-blinded, phase 3 non inferiority trial. Fertil Steril. 2017;107(2):387-96.
60. Out HJ, Rutherford A, Fleming R, Tay CC, Trew G, Ledger W, et al. Randomized, double-blind, multicentre clinical trial comparing starting dose of 150 and 200 IU of recombinant FSH in women treated with the GnRH antagonist Ganirelix for assisted reproduction. Hum Reprod. 2004;19(1):90-5.
61. Friedler S, Meltzer S, San-Ryss B, Rabinson J, Lazer T, Liberty G. An upper limit of gonadotropin dose in patients undergoing ART should be advocated. Gynecol Endocrinol. 2016;32(12):965-9.
62. Gianaroli L, Magli MC, Cavallini C, Crippa A, Capoti A, Resta S, et al. Predicting aneuploidy in human oocytes: Key factors which affect meiosis process. Hum Reprod. 2010;25(9): 2374-86.
63. Mochtar MH, van der Veen, Ziech M, van Wely M. Recombinant Luteinizing Hormone (rLH) for controlled ovarian hyperstimulation in assisted reproductive cycles. Cochrane Database Syst Rev. 2007;(2):CD005070.
64. Lehert P, Kolibianakis EM, Venetis CA, Schertz J, Saunders H, Arriagada P, et al. Recombinant human follicle stimulating hormone (r-hFSH) plus recombinant luteinizing hormone versus r-hFSH alone for ovarian stimulation during assisted reproductive technology: systematic review and meta-analysis. Reprod Biol Endocrinol. 2014;12:17.
65. Schally AV, Arimura A, Kastin AJ, Matsuo H, Baba Y, Redding TW, et al. Gonadotropin-releasing hormone: one polypeptide regulates secretion of luteinizing and follicle stimulating hormones. Science. 1971;173:1036-8.
66. Reame N, Sauder SE, Kelch RP, Marshall JC. Pulsatile gonadotropin secretion during the human menstrual cycle: evidence for altered frequency of GnRH secretion, J Clin Endocrinol Metab. 1984;59(2):328-37.
67. Lemay A, Metha AE, Tolis G, Faure N, Labrie F, Fazekas AT. Gonadotropins and estradiol responses to single intranasal or subcutaneous administration of a luteinizing-hormone-releasing hormone agonist in the early follicular phase. Fertil Steril. 1983;39(5):668-73.
68. Schvartz I, Hazum E. Internalization and recycling of receptor-bound gonadotropin releasing hormone agonist in pituitary gonadotrophes. J Biol Chem. 1987;262:17046-50.
69. Wallach EE, Fogelman I. Gonadotropin-releasing hormone agonists and the skeleton. Fertil Steril. 1992;57(4):715-24.
70. Weissman A, Shoham Z. Favourable pregnancy outcome after administration of a long-acting gonadotropin-releasing hormone agonist in the mid-luteal phase. Hum Reprod. 1993; 8(3):496-7.
71. Borm G, Mannaerts B. Treatment with the GnRH antagonist Ganirelix in women undergoing ovarian stimulation with recombinant FSH is effective, safe and convenient: results of a controlled, randomized multicentre trial. The European Orgalutran Study group. Hum Reprod. 2000;15(7): 1490-8.

72. A double-blind randomized dose-finding study to assess the efficacy of the GnRH antagonist, Ganirelix, to prevent premature luteinizing hormone surges in women undergoing ovarian stimulation with recombinant follicle stimulating hormone. The ganirelix dose-finding group study. Hum Reprod. 1998;13(11):3023-31.
73. Al-Inany HG, Youssef MA, Aboulghar M, Broekmans F, Sterrenburg M, Smit J, et al. Gonadotropin-releasing hormone antagonists for assisted reproductive technology. Cochrane Database Syst Rev. 2011;5:CD001750.
74. Papanikolaou EG, Yarali H, Timotheou E, Gyrnberg M, Zafieratis O, Tournaye H, et al. Proof-of-concept clinical trial of a single luteal use of long-acting gonadotropin-releasing hormone antagonist degarelix in controlled ovarian stimulation for in vitro fertilization: long antagonist protocol. Front Endocrinol. 2018;9:25.

CHAPTER 47

Ovulation Induction and Ovarian Stimulation Protocols

Rutvij Dalal, Sonal Agarwal

OVULATION INDUCTION AND SUPEROVULATION

This section attempts to summarize the latest evidence regarding various agents currently used for ovulation induction. A brief review about the origin of ovulation induction and the relevant physiology is mentioned.

INTRODUCTION

Normal menstrual cycle is under the control of various paracrine and endocrine mechanisms through neuro-endocrine system via hypothalamic-pituitary-ovarian axis (HPO axis). Changes occur both in ovary and uterus, which result in egg production and preparation of endometrium, which is utmost important for reproduction.[1] Induction of ovulation in an-ovulatory women is a landmark achievement in the history of reproductive endocrinology. The last century has seen major advancement in the field of infertility and the discovery of various medical and surgical methods of ovulation induction has changed the face of treatment worldwide. Earlier women who had little hope of normal menstruation can now successfully ovulate and bear children. Ovulation induction is the treatment of choice in anovulatory infertility. Anovulation and oligo-ovulation are the etiological factors for almost 21% of infertile couples. Ovulation induction and superovulation terminology is used interchangeably quite often but these two have different concepts behind it. Ovulation induction is development of a follicle in an anovulatory patient. The aim is to combat any subtle fault in ovulatory function and luteal phase defect (LPD) that are not detected with recent investigations. Superovulation has been useful in conditions such as mild to moderate male factor infertility, transient anovulation, minimal-to-mild endometriosis, cervical factor, and unexplained infertility. It is done in women already ovulating with subtle defects.

CATEGORY OF PATIENTS BENEFITING FROM OVULATION INDUCTION

Patients belonging to WHO class 1 and 2 benefit the most. WHO classification of ovulatory disorders is enlisted in **Box 1**.

WHO type I ovulatory dysfunction (hypothalamic pituitary failure or hypothalamic amenorrhea or hypo-gonadotropic hypogonadism) are characterized by low gonadotropin levels, low estrogen levels, and normal prolactin levels and account for 10% of all ovulatory disorders. Amenorrhea is present which is un-responsive to progestin challenge test.

WHO type II ovulatory dysfunction (hypothalamo-pituitary dysfunction) comprises of women with gonado-tropin disorder and normal estrogen levels accounting for 85% of patients with ovulatory dysfunction. Other causes of anovulation include hyperprolactinemia, hypothyroidism, pituitary tumors, etc. In these conditions, it is always prudent to treat the cause first.

BOX 1: WHO classification of anovulation.[2]

Class 1: Hypogonadotropic hypogonadal anovulation
- FSH low/normal
- Estradiol low
- Pituitary is less or unresponsive to GnRH

Class 2: Normogonadotropic normoestrogenic anovulation
- Pituitary-ovarian dysfunction
- FSH normal
- Estradiol normal
- 70–80% are PCOS, rest are other hyperandrogenic disorders

Class 3: Hypergonadotropic hypoestrogenic anovulation
- FSH high
- Estradiol low
- Suggestive of ovarian failure/insufficiency

Class 4: Hyperprolactinemic anovulation
- High prolactin levels
- Normal FSH
- Low estradiol

Brief Review of Evolution of Ovulation Induction

Before 1960s, treatment of anovulatory infertility was restricted to psychological support and proper timing and frequency of intercourse. In 1961, Greenblatt and colleagues published their first experience of successful induction of ovulation and results with clomiphene. Sixty years have passed and clomiphene still remains the first-line treatment for polycystic ovary syndrome (PCOS) and this simple and inexpensive treatment has resulted in innumerable pregnancies. Gemzell in 1958 and Bettendorf in 1961 achieved a major leap forward with successful induction of ovulation using human pituitary gonadotropins. They were independently able to achieve successful pregnancies in hypophysectomized individuals. In 1963, Lunenfeld and coworkers isolated gonadotropins from urine of postmenopausal women and reached another landmark since this inexpensive source helped in isolating large quantities of the hormone for widespread use. Insler and Lunenfeld were able to achieve pregnancies in large number of amenorrheic women. Gonadotropin-releasing hormone (GnRH) was isolated and synthesized in the laboratory in 1978, but it was Knobil in 1980 who demonstrated its clinical efficacy by pulsatile administration of the drug. Though these were the foremost milestones in the history of ovulation induction, management has indeed come a long way today with advent of controlled ovarian stimulation (COS) and GnRH agonists (GnRHa) and antagonist protocols used in assisted reproduction.

PHYSIOLOGY OF OVULATION

Folliculogenesis and ovulation occur because of a complex interplay between cellular, endocrine, and paracrine factors.[3] Germ cells or oogonia that migrate from the genital ridge to the fetal ovary undergo mitosis and reach their maximum number of 6–7 million at midgestation. Onset of meiosis and follicular atresia result in decline in their number after birth and at puberty only about 300,000 oocytes are left. The final development of ovarian follicles begins about 3–6 months before ovulation. Over a period of 3–6 months these follicles acquire follicle-stimulating hormone (FSH) and luteinizing hormone (LH) receptors and the follicle forms antrum.[4] The antral follicles are dependent on gonadotropins as depicted in **Figure 1**. Oogonia are transformed into primary oocytes after the first meiotic division and are arrested at prophase of the first meiotic division until just before ovulation.

As the levels of estradiol, inhibin A, and progesterone decrease with regression of the corpus luteum in the latter part of the cycle, the concentrations of FSH and LH rise. When this intercycle rise of FSH exceeds the critical level, it activates the largest antral follicles (2–5 mm) present at this time. This activation involves induction of key enzymes like aromatase and appearance of LH receptors. LH stimulates the production of androstenedione from the thecal cells. Androstenedione diffuses into the granulosa cells and are here converted to estradiol by the action of aromatase, the production of which is stimulated by FSH. The emerging dominant follicle produces increasing amounts of estrogen and inhibin A and this induces a negative feedback of FSH. The fall in FSH prevents further recruitment of follicles.

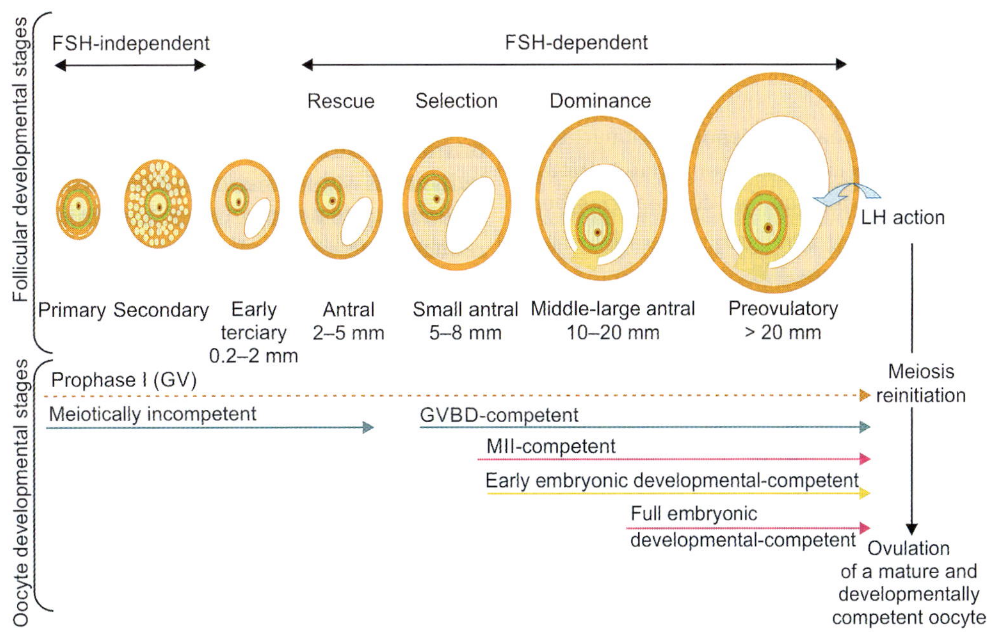

Fig. 1: Folliculogenesis and oogenesis.
(FSH: follicle-stimulating hormone; GV: germinal vesicle; GVBD: germinal vesicle breakdown; LH: luteinizing hormone; MII: metaphase II).

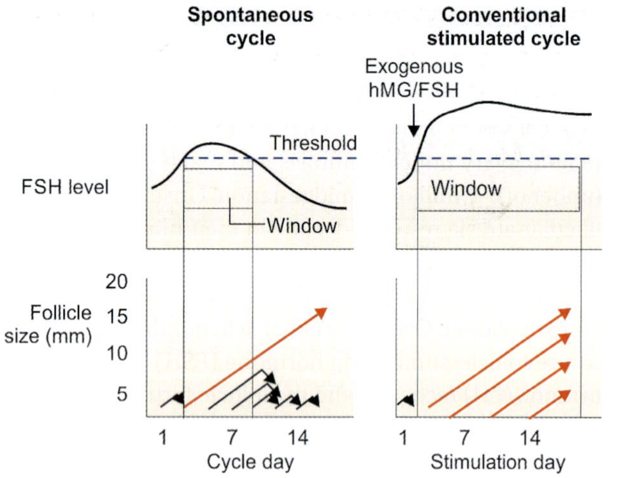

Fig. 2: Follicle-stimulating hormone threshold and window in spontaneous and stimulated cycle.
(FSH: follicle-stimulating hormone; hMG: human menopausal gonadotropin)

As the follicle further acquires LH receptors, it matures and at LH surge, the first meiotic division is completed and it transforms into a secondary oocyte. The two cell-two gonadotropin theory states that FSH concentration must exceed a certain threshold before follicular development will proceed. The duration for which the FSH level exceeds the threshold is called the "FSH window" and it is the short duration of this window in normal ovulation that permits monofollicular selection.

The physiological principles of ovulation induction include either increasing the number of antral follicles available in the ovary at the time of selection, releasing the ovary from inhibitory influences, or by maintaining the level of FSH above the threshold level for longer either by enhancing endogenous gonadotropins or administration of exogenous gonadotropins. This effect is illustrated in **Figure 2**.

Dominant follicle should have LH exposure for particular period of time and concentration for final follicular maturation. LH threshold and ceiling concept has been described in **Box 2**.

MANAGEMENT OPTIONS FOR OVULATION INDUCTION[6]

- Lifestyle modifications in form of diet and exercise
- Medical management with:
  - Antiestrogens
  - Aromatase inhibitors (AIs)
  - Insulin sensitizers
  - Gonadotropins
  - Dopamine agonists
  - Gonadotropin-releasing hormone
  - GnRH agonists and antagonists
- Surgery.

BOX 2: Concept of LH threshold and ceiling.[5]

- Suppression of granulosa cell proliferation
- Oocyte development compromised
- Follicular atresia
- Premature luteinization

LH ceiling

Normal follicular growth and development

- Paracrine signaling activated by FSH and LH] LH Window
- Adequate granulosa cell proliferation]
- Functional maturation
- Androgen and estrogen biosynthesis
- Oocyte maturation

LH threshold

No paracrine signaling between granulosa cells and theca cells
Androgen and estrogen biosynthesis hampered
Impaired oocyte maturation
Improper granulosa cell proliferation
Decreased activation of aromatase activity by LH.

Lifestyle Modification for Obesity-related Infertility

Obesity has been known to have an adverse effect on ovarian function and fertility.[7] Defined as a body mass index (BMI) of over 25 kg/m^2, obesity is associated with lower fertility rates, both at natural conception and ovulation induction; higher doses of ovulation inducing drugs, and higher miscarriage rates.[8] Obesity is also an important arm of the PCOS triad and is seen in 50% of women with PCOS. 80% of obese patients are insulin-resistant as well. These women have a higher tendency to multifollicular response even on low dose FSH and a greater tendency for cycle cancellation and ovarian hyperstimulation.

Obesity evidently expresses and exaggerates the signs and symptoms of insulin resistance. Weight loss can be achieved either through exercise, diet, or both. Studies have shown that a weight loss of just 5–10% through diet or exercise restores reproductive function in 55–100% of individuals within a period of 6 months. Reduction in weight results in a 30% fall in visceral fat restoring ovulation and reducing the markers for metabolic disease. Weight loss in patients with PCOS has been observed to decrease elevated androgen and LH levels, enhance insulin sensitivity, re-establish mono-ovulation, and improve response to ovulation inducing agents.[9]

Exercise helps in weight loss, improving insulin resistance, and restoration of reproductive function. Exercise burns visceral fat more than subcutaneous fat. Aerobic exercise should last for at least 20–30 minutes thrice a week sufficient to cause sweating to be effective. A diet that is low in calorie, fat, and carbohydrate with a low glycemic index is recommended.[10] Thus, weight loss is an intervention that is effective, inexpensive, and without adverse effects. It has an added advantage in decreasing the long-term complications of diabetes and cardiovascular disease. Since a minimal 5–10% reduction in weight is sufficient to reinstate ovarian function, it should be advised as the first line of treatment in obese subjects. In patients with a BMI more than 28–30 kg/m^2 who would respond poorly to ovulation induction, it is wise to advise weight loss prior to treatment.[11]

Medical Management

Antiestrogens

In normogonadotropic anovulation, administration of small amounts of FSH will induce ovulation. This can be achieved by antiestrogens, pulsatile GnRH or low-dose gonadotropins. Clomiphene citrate (CC) and tamoxifen are the two antiestrogens [SERM (selective estrogen receptor modulator)] used. It is the best treatment for ovulatory dysfunction and normal estrogen levels (WHO type II). Combined with intrauterine insemination (IUI), CC enhances fecundity in unexplained infertility.[12]

Chemical structure and pharmacokinetics: Clomiphene citrate is a nonsteroidal triphenylethylene derivative and a competitive nonselective estrogen receptor modulator. It has both agonistic and antagonistic actions at the level of estrogen receptors (ERs).[13] It binds to the nuclear ER in the hypothalamus for extended periods (weeks rather than hours) and depletes ER concentrations by interfering with the normal process of ER replenishment. It thus blocks the negative feedback effect of estrogen, alters the pulsatile release of GnRH, and stimulates gonadotropin secretion from the pituitary gland. In ovulatory women, it increases the GnRH pulse frequency and in anovulatory women, it increases the amplitude. LH surge occurs when estrogen is secreted from growing follicle.[14] Exogenous hCG is not given in CC- induced cycles.[15]

Pharmacokinetics: Clomiphene citrate has a low clearance rate and has a long half-life of 5 days.[16] It has two distinct isomers: (1) enclomiphene that is more potent and responsible for the ovulation inducing action of CC and (2) zuclomiphene that is less active, longer lasting, and cleared more slowly from the body. The euclomiphene levels rise rapidly and fall to insignificant levels after a few days (**Table 1**). The starting dose of CC is 50–100 mg and CC can be begun from day 2–5 of a normal period or a withdrawal bleed without any impact on outcome. If there is no response in three cycles, the dose is increased as women who do not respond to 50 mg, two-thirds will not do so in the first cycle. The maximum dose should not be more than 150 mg as higher doses do not enhance ovulation and pregnancy rates and only add to side effects. CC treatment generally should be limited to the minimum effective dose and to no more than six ovulatory cycles per attempt and not more than 12 total cycles. Failure to conceive after successful CC-induced ovulation is indication for further evaluation to exclude other contributing causes of infertility. CC is excreted through stools and cleared mainly by the liver.

TABLE 1: Differences between two isomers of clomiphene.[17]

Enclomiphene	*Zuclomiphene*
62% concentration	38% concentration
Antiestrogenic action is more	Less antiestrogenic and more estrogenic
Potency is more than zuclomiphene	Less potent
T1/2 of 2.5–11.8 hours	T1/2 of 14.2–33.4 hours

Caution has to be exerted as CC treatment is futile in women with elevated FSH values, hypogonadotropic hypogonadism, tubal factor, male factor, and uterine factor infertility. It is also prudent to confirm tubal patency before embarking on any ovulation induction regime.

Monitoring response: Response to treatment should be monitored by the measurement of basal body temperature, serum progesterone levels (day 21 and 28), urinary LH levels, or ultrasound.[18] No studies have evaluated the advantage of using more intensive monitoring methods like ultrasound to assess treatment response. But ultrasound when available should be used to monitor IUI cycles and preferably the first cycle to determine the minimum effective dose.[19]

About 20–25% of women fail to ovulate despite maximum doses of clomiphene and this is called "clomiphene resistance". This commonly occurs in obese, hyperandrogenic, and insulin-resistant women with high LH levels. Failure to conceive despite successful ovulation is called "clomiphene failure".[20]

Results with treatment: Ovulation rates following treatment with clomiphene in properly selected patients is usually 70–85% and conception rates are 40–50%.[21] The cycle fecundity in patients who respond to clomiphene is approximately 15%. Three-fourths of the pregnancies reportedly occur in the first three cycles. Cumulative pregnancy rates can be as high as 60% after six cycles and may reach almost 97% after 12 cycles. 20% of pregnancies that occur due to clomiphene may end in a spontaneous abortion and the estimated risk of multiple pregnancies is about 8–13%; majority being twins. The discrepancy between ovulation and pregnancy rates is commonly due to lack of persistence of therapy or other associated causes of infertility. The reasons for the relatively low pregnancy rate are unclear, but may be related to high LH levels, the antiestrogenic effects of clomiphene, and to adverse effects on the oocytes. Because of the long half-life of clomiphene isomers, they may exert an antiestrogenic effect on the quality and quantity of cervical mucus and growth and maturation of the endometrium. These effects are thought to occur with prolonged therapy and at larger doses. Traditionally the antiestrogenic effect of CC on the endometrium has been implicated to be responsible for the discrepancy in ovulation and pregnancy rates. Successful implantation depends on adequate endometrial thickness and a receptive endometrium. A reduction in endometrial thickness below the minimum, thought to be necessary for pregnancy to occur, was seen in 30% of patients on clomiphene. Another study found the endometrium to be deleterious to implantation in clomiphene-induced cycles because of having a reduction in glandular density and presence of vacuolated cells.[22] Due to the inability to define a minimum endometrial thickness necessary for pregnancy to occur and tremendous individual variability in the antiestrogenic effect of CC, the significance of these effects is difficult to quantify.[23] The antiestrogenic effect of CC on the cervix has been reported to occur in about 15% of cases, and if demonstrated, the adverse effect can be circumvented by IUI.[24]

A systematic review of four cross-over randomized controlled trials (RCTs), that compared CC with placebo in patients with PCOS, found that all doses of CC were associated with increased pregnancy rates per treatment cycle [odds ratio (OR) 3.41, 95% confidence interval (CI) 4.23–9.48] and increased ovulation (OR 4.6, 95% CI 2.84–7.45). Life-table analysis demonstrates upto 22% conception rate.[25-27]

Routine administration of hCG adds little to improving conception rates. It is indicated only when there is an absent or delayed LH surge or for timing IUI or intercourse. Both recombinant and urinary hCG are equally effective though urinary hCG is reported to have more local reactions. Steroids have been tried as adjunctive agents with CC in women with elevated dehydroepiandrosterone (DHEAS) levels (>200 μg/dL). Dexamethasone helps to decrease the adrenal production of androgens and increases ovulation rates by reducing the inhibitory effect of local androgens. It suppresses the action of estradiol on the pituitary gland and increases serum growth hormone and IGF-1 levels. It is usually administered at a dose of 0.5 mg at bedtime for 1 month (low dose), or prednisolone that is administered at a dose of 5 mg. Long standing use of oral steroids demands caution in view of their adverse effects. An increased appetite and weight gain would further deteriorate the metabolic profile of any patient with PCOS. High-dose, short-course regimen has also lately been tried in clomiphene-resistant women but with normal DHEAS levels with successful outcome.[28]

Clomiphene resistance: Failure to ovulate after three cycles of CC treatment with maximum dose of 150 mg is called clomiphene resistance. Resistance to CC treatment occurs in obese, hyperandrogenic, and insulin-resistant individuals with elevated LH levels. Alternatives to management include higher doses of CC, weight reduction, extended CC therapy for 8 days, pretreatment with oral contraceptive pills (OCPs) (to lower LH levels), concomitant use of GnRH agonist to suppress LH, and adjunctive therapy with dexamethasone or insulin-sensitizing agents. Alternative drugs such as AIs and gonadotropins can be tried.[29]

Clomiphene failure: Failure to conceive despite successful ovulation for six cycles calls for seeking other causes for infertility. Combinations and alternative strategies can be attempted. Lack of pregnancy, despite 12 successful ovulatory cycles, in the absence of other causes is usually an indication for assisted reproduction.

Indications of antiestrogens:[8]

- Anovulation
- Luteal phase deficiency
- Unexplained infertility
- Hypothalamic or pituitary dysfunction
- IUI or in vitro fertilization (IVF)—mild stimulation
- Endometriosis—stage 1 and 2.

Prerequisites for clomiphene citrate:

- Male partner evaluation
- History and physical examination
- Age, duration, and cause of infertility
- Normal thyroid and prolactin function
- Normal functioning of pituitary.

Adverse effects:

- Vasomotor flushes are temporary and seen in about 10% of patients. They cease once treatment ends
- Mood swings and nausea
- Blurred vision, double vision, scotoma, light sensitivity, and optic neuropathy (severe and persistent). Visual disturbances (<2%) are mostly uncommon and reversible. In the eventuality of persistent or severe complications, treatment needs to be stopped, and alternative methods should be considered.[12]
- Breast tenderness (2–5%)
- Pelvic discomfort
- Effect on endometrium and cervical mucus[30]
- Multiple pregnancies are lowest with CC. The incidence of multiple pregnancies can be further reduced by ultrasound monitoring and withholding hCG and IUI when there are more than two follicles more than 18 mm. The earlier notion that CC-induced successful pregnancies have a higher incidence of spontaneous abortions has not been proved in any study. Recent reports have shown that abortion rates are not increased compared to normal (20%).[15]
- *Ovarian cancer:* Some case reports and epidemiological studies have suggested an association between epithelial ovarian cancer and fertility drugs. But there is little evidence for an increased risk of invasive epithelial ovarian cancer in women exposed to fertility treatment. Those studies that have found higher rates of the disease report a two-fold increased risk at the most, although this has rarely been statistically significant.

These facts must be viewed in context of considerable methodological difficulties that frustrate these studies. There is a clear need for larger studies employing longer periods of follow-up, detailing precisely the types, doses, and duration of treatments patients have received, and controlling for potential confounding reproductive factors.
- *Ovarian hyperstimulation syndrome (OHSS):* Mild OHSS is relatively common but severe OHSS rarely occurs.

Contraindications:
- Suspected pregnancy
- Hypersensitivity to drug
- Liver failure and dysfunction
- Functional ovarian cysts
- Visual disorders.

Other selective estrogen receptor modulators:

Tamoxifen: Tamoxifen has been useful in patients with anovulation even in failed CC treatment cycles. One recent study has shown comparable results of ovulation and pregnancy rates when efficacy of tamoxifen with that of CC was tested. Some studies suggest superiority of tamoxifen as it has no effect on endometrium.[31] Raloxifene has recently been tried in trials but not in use presently.

Aromatase Inhibitors

The two compounds currently being used for ovulation induction are the selective nonsteroidal AIs namely—letrozole and anastrozole.[32] Aromatase is a microsomal cytochrome P450 hemoprotein-containing enzyme that catalyzes the rate-limiting step in estrogen biosynthesis. Aromatase enzyme activity is found in the ovary, adipose tissue, brain, muscle, liver, and breast tissue.

Three generations of AIs have been developed over the past three decades but the first two-generation drugs were clinically not found useful owing to significant adverse effects and low potency. Generations of AIs are given in **Table 2**. Till recently, they were approved for the use in treatment of postmenopausal breast cancer; but letrozole has been lately approved for use as an ovulation-inducing agent.

Classification:
- *Steroidal:* Competes with endogenous androstenedione and testosterone for P450 causing irreversible enzymatic inhibition.
- *Nonsteroidal:* Competes with endogenous substrates for cytochrome P450 forming a reversible bond.

TABLE 2: Classification of aromatase inhibitors.

Generation	Nonsteroidal/Reversible	Steroidal/Irreversible
First	Aminoglutethimide	None
Second	Fadrozole	Formestane
Third	Anastrozole/Letrozole/ Exemestane	Exemestane

Aromatase inhibitors are also classified as:
- *First generation of AI:* Induces hepatic enzymes and inhibits cortisol, aldosterone, thyroxine, and aromatase.
- *Second generation of AI:* Potency twice than first generation.
- *Third generation of AI:* Inhibits aromatase enzyme only. Potency is 3–4 times more than that of second-generation AI.

Mechanism of action:
- Aromatase inhibitors block conversion of androgens to estrogens and thus cause an increase in testosterone levels.
- Block inhibitory feedback of testosterone on hypothalamo-pituitary-gonadal (HPG) axis and converts into more potent estrogen without any increase in circulating estrogens and estradiol (E2) receptor modulators.[33]

Letrozole and anastrozole are competitive, potent, and reversible AIs and reduce estrogen levels by 97–99%. They inhibit release of estrogen from various sources, namely ovarian, adipose tissue, and locally produced estrogen in the brain and thus release the hypothalamo-pituitary axis from the negative feedback effect of estrogen.[34] The consequent increase in the release of gonadotropins stimulates follicular growth. Unlike CC, which has a prolonged duration of action and causes depletion of ERs, letrozole does not deplete ERs resulting in intact central feedback. As the dominant follicle grows, it produces estrogen that exerts negative feedback at the center and decreases FSH release. Suppression of FSH secretion results in atresia of smaller follicles and monofollicular growth. Studies have also proposed peripheral mechanisms of action. Inhibition of aromatase in the ovary would result in the temporary accumulation of androgens. It has been postulated that this increased androgen level stimulates follicular growth by increasing its sensitivity to FSH. By decreasing follicular estrogen levels, the ER levels in the endometrium are upregulated leading onto a rapid endometrial growth once the drug is stopped and estrogen secretion resumes. This results in a thicker and more receptive endometrium in patients receiving AIs. In patients with PCOS, FSH production in the early follicular phase may be blunted because of high androgen levels being aromatized to estrogen in the brain and exerting a negative feedback. Thus, AIs may be particularly useful in PCOS patients. A recent study has evaluated expression of HOXA10 and integrin $\alpha(v)\beta(3)$

in rat endometrium exposed to either letrozole or clomiphene. This study found that letrozole affects HOXA10 expression but not integrin in uterine endometrium and concluded that clomiphene suppresses endometrial receptivity more than letrozole.[35]

Pharmacokinetics: Letrozole is used in a dose of 2.5–5 mg orally from day 2–3 of the cycle for 5 days. These compounds are completely absorbed after oral administration with a

TABLE 3: To show various evidences on clomiphene and letrozole.

Author	Year	Study	Patient group	Follicles	Endometrial thickness	Ovulation rates	E2 level	Pregnancy rate
Casper[36]	2007	CC vs. letroz	PCOS	Similar				Similar
Badawy[37]	2007	CC vs. letroz*	PCOS	CC>L	CC>L	Not significant	CC>L	Similar
Bayar	2006	CC vs. letroz*	PCOS	Similar	Similar	Not significant	CC>L	Similar
Atay[38]	2006	CC vs. letroz*	PCOS	CC>L	L>CC	L>CC	L>CC	L>CC
Bayar	2006	CC vs. letroz *	Ovulatory		Similar	Similar	CC>L	Similar

(*: randomized trials; CC: clomiphene citrate; PCOS: polycystic ovary syndrome; L: letrozole)

mean terminal half-life of about 30–60 hours. It is eliminated from the circulation rapidly and do not continue to exert their action after cessation of the drug.

Evidence from controlled studies (Table 3): Theoretically and by earlier studies, evidence emerged that letrozole use is associated with monofollicular response, lower multiple pregnancy rates, thicker and more receptive endometrium, and consequently better pregnancy rates.

Though earlier studies did show a thicker endometrium and a trend toward higher pregnancy rates, evidence accumulating from recently published randomized studies is conflicting. Studies have shown greater follicular number and estradiol levels with CC on the day of hCG and no significant difference in pregnancy rates, endometrial thickness, and ovulation rates.

Aromatase inhibitors have been tried in patients with clomiphene failures either alone or in conjunction with gonadotropins. In patients with CC failures, letrozole alone has shown 75% ovulation rates and 20–25% pregnancy rates. In comparative studies with gonadotropins and letrozole in patients with CC failure or advanced age, gonadotropins have been found to have better pregnancy rates. When used in a sequential regime with gonadotropins, women who received letrozole and FSH had fewer follicles, and E2 levels on the day of hCG, similar or higher endometrial thickness, equivalent pregnancy rates, and lower multiple pregnancy. In comparison with gonadotropins alone, similar pregnancy rates could be achieved with 40–50% lower gonadotropin usage and lower multiple pregnancy rates. Recently one double-blinded randomized trial by Amer et al.,[39] has shown higher pregnancy rates with letrozole as compared to CC but live birth rates were not statistically significant among them.

Indications for use:
- Clomiphene failure cases[40]
- Persistent thin endometrium with clomiphene cases
- Ovarian stimulation in women having breast cancer as it does not cause high estrogen levels but give good oocyte yield.[41]

Advantages over clomiphene citrate:
- No antiestrogenic effect on endometrium and cervical mucus.
- Absence of ER depletion.
- Better uterine blood flow.
- Rapidly eliminated from body due to short half-life of 45 hours.
- Limited follicles.[42]
- Reduced multiple pregnancy rates.[43]
- Decreased chances of OHSS.[44]

Adverse effects:
- Vasomotor symptoms such as hot flushes.
- Nausea and fatigue.
- Alopecia.
- Vaginal bleeding after long-term use in cases of breast cancer.

Contraindications:
- Women at risk of endometrial hyperplasia and endometrial neoplasia.
- Osteoporosis.

Insulin Sensitizers

Insulin sensitizers are discussed in chapter on "Role of Adjuvants in Ovarian Stimulation".

Evidence: Metformin has been better than a placebo for ovulation rate and pregnancy rate in PCOS women, but there was significant statistical heterogeneity in that.[45] Combined analyses of all women demonstrated a benefit of metformin over placebo without statistical heterogeneity for pregnancy rate. Metformin induced more minor gastrointestinal-related adverse events compared to placebo. Metformin therefore improves ovulation and pregnancy rates, but there is currently inadequate data for an effect on live birth rates. It is generally recommended, if using metformin, that doses are initiated at 500 mg daily and increased by 500 mg daily every 2 weeks. There is considerable controversy over when metformin should be ceased, if pregnancy occurs. In general, there is inadequate evidence to support continuing metformin following conception with more research needed. There was no benefit of metformin over CC for live birth rate, and CC was better than metformin for live birth rate in those with a BMI more than or equal to 30 kg/m^2. Metformin, therefore, did not result in improved reproductive outcomes compared to CC.

Current evidence-based guidelines recommend intensive lifestyle modification, particularly in those with a BMI more than or equal to 30 kg/m^2, including frequent multidisciplinary engagement for 3–6 months as first-line therapy—level of evidence 1B. This recommendation was underpinned by RCTs, which found that there was no benefit of metformin over lifestyle.

Gonadotropins

Exogenous gonadotropins are used in the treatment of WHO type-I infertility and WHO type-II infertility who have failed to conceive with antiestrogens despite ovulation (clomiphene failure) or have failed to ovulate with CC (clomiphene resistance). Gonadotropins are more effective than CC but are expensive, require parenteral administration, and have higher risk for ovarian hyperstimulation and multiple pregnancies. The principle of gonadotropin induction of ovulation is to mimic the normal physiological cycle of follicular selection, maturation, and ovulation. To use gonadotropins successfully for ovulation induction requires a sound knowledge of the normal endocrinologic processes that govern ovulation. Ovarian hyperstimulation, multiple follicular developments, and multiple pregnancies are serious complications that could occur with uncontrolled stimulation.

As mentioned earlier, it is the duration of the "FSH window" during which the FSH levels are above the threshold required to stimulate the growing follicles that determines the number of follicles that will be recruited. The essence of monofollicular achievement in gonadotropin induction of ovulation is to identify that FSH threshold dose that results in the selection of a single follicle. Administration of an FSH dose higher than the threshold for a period of time inevitably results in multifollicular recruitment. Earlier higher dose conventional gonadotropin stimulation was in vogue but had associated with it a higher incidence of hyperstimulation and multiple pregnancies. It involved starting with a dose of 2 ampoules (150 IU) of gonadotropins and increasing the dose every 3–5 days by 75 IU. Though ovulation rates were high, this regime was associated with high complication rates. Currently used protocols are—low-dose step-up regime, step down, or sequential regimen.

These aim to increase the FSH concentrations gradually to reach the threshold level and at the same time avoid an explosive ovarian response.

Low-dose step-up protocol: This has been the preferred method of gonadotropin induction in PCOS patients. This is based on a threshold concept that initiation of follicular growth requires only a 10–30% increase in dose of exogenous FSH. This small dose increase is done at weekly intervals. This protocol begins with 75IU daily for 7 days as low starting dose.[46] An ultrasound is done at the end of 1 week and if the dominant follicle is more than 10 mm in diameter, the same dose is continued and if it is less than 10 mm, the same dose is maintained for another week. At the end of the second week, if the follicular size is still less than 10 mm, the dose of gonadotropin is increased by half ampoule weekly up to a maximum of 225 IU/day **(Flowchart 1)**. This regime has the disadvantage that it is prolonged and requires multiple injections. But studies have shown that it maintains fair pregnancy rates (20%) and incidence of complications like multiple pregnancies (6%) and OHSS (0.14%) are low.

Step down protocol: This protocol aims to mimic the normal physiological rise of FSH in the early follicular

Flowchart 1: Chronic low-dose step-up protocol.

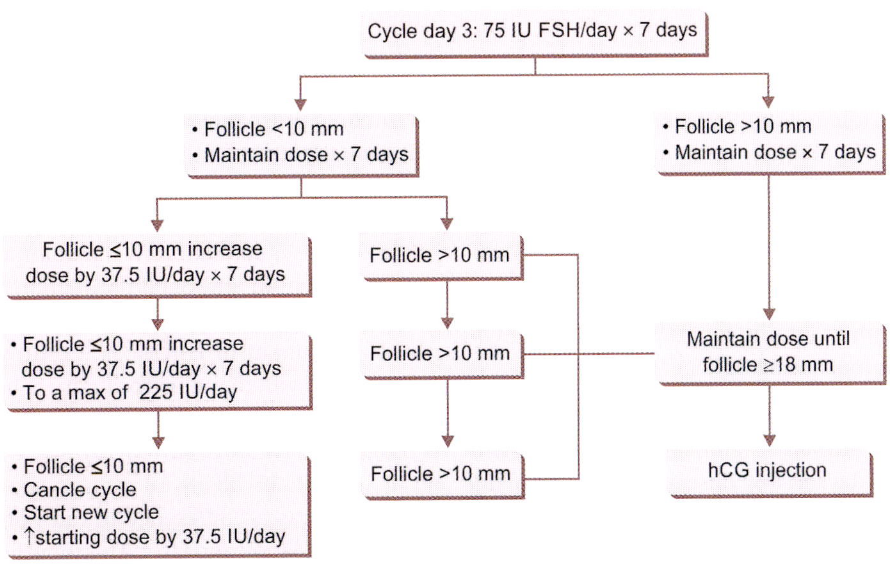

(FSH: follicle-stimulating hormone; hCG: human chorionic gonadotropin)

Flowchart 2: Step down protocol.

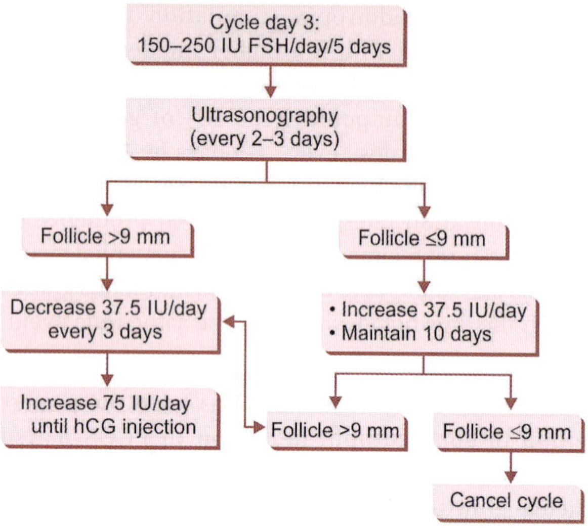

(FSH: follicle-stimulating hormone; hCG: human chorionic gonadotropin)

phase and subsequent decreasing dependence of the dominant growing follicle toward FSH. The starting dose is higher than the step up protocol and once a follicular response is seen on ultrasound, the dose is reduced to a baseline level that is persisted with till it reaches 18 mm. This protocol warrants experience and judgment to determine the effective starting dose that should neither be administered high or long enough to stimulate multi-follicular growth. It thus calls for more stringent monitoring. The duration of treatment is smaller. It is depicted in **Flowchart 2**.

Oral ovulogens when used with gonadotropins, they result in almost equivalent pregnancy rates as gonadotropins alone and have the advantage of reducing gonadotropin use by 45–55%, lower cost per cycle, and no antiestrogenic side effects.[47]

Dopamine Agonists

Study and understanding of pathophysiology of OHSS has explained the use of cabergoline as dopamine agonist. It reduces vascular permeability, hemoconcentration, and ascites. With proper informed consent, it can be used in high risk situations.[48]

Mechanism of action: Dopamine agonists decrease receptor expression for vascular endothelial growth factor (VEGF) which is responsible for causing OHSS.[49]

Dosage and risks: It should start on day of trigger at a dose of 0.5 mg daily for 8 days. No significant risk is seen with administration for 8 days at low dose. Most common side effects are headache, nausea, and dizziness. With long-term treatment, valvular heart disease was rarely observed with doses higher than 0.5 mg with incidence of 3/1,000 cases.

Gonadotropin-releasing Hormone

Pulsatile GnRH therapy can be given when pituitary gland is present in women, idiopathic hypogonadotropic hypogonadism, and weight loss-related amenorrhea. It can be given with computerized mini-pump at pulse intervals of 60–180 minutes. More than 90% ovulation rates can be achieved after six cycles. Incidence of multiple pregnancy rates is about 17.4%.

Disadvantages:
- Pump needs to be connected to the body at all times.
- Development of antibodies.
- Allergic skin reactions.

Gonadotropin-releasing Hormone Analogs

Structure, preparations, and mechanism of action is been dealt in the chapter on "Gonadotropin-releasing Hormone Analogs". They are seldom used for ovulation induction treatment.

Surgical Methods

Stein and Levinthal in 1935 first performed ovarian wedge resection in infertile patients with PCOS. Though it was followed by promising results, the procedure was soon abandoned in view of extensive postoperative adhesions, tissue loss, and emergence of easier medical methods for ovulation induction. The introduction of minimally invasive surgery or laparoscopy created resurgence of interest in surgical methods. The process of laparoscopic ovarian drilling has been controversial and evolving and its current status must be evaluated in the context of newer theories of pathogenesis of PCOS, newer definition of the disease, and the growing popularity of insulin sensitizers.

The first-line of treatment in PCOS still remains CC or letrozole. Options to treat women who are clomiphene resistant are insulin sensitizers, ovarian drilling, and gonadotropic induction. Ovulation induction with gonadotropins is expensive, requires experience since response can be explosive in later stages and is associated with higher rates of multiple pregnancies. Ovarian drilling relatively is a more invasive procedure and is associated with irreversible complications like adhesion formation and poor ovarian reserve.

Laparoscopic ovarian drilling with either electrocautery or laser causes reduction in the volume of ovarian stroma and reduction in androgen production. This leads to lesser peripheral aromatization and elevated FSH levels and re-establishment of HPO axis. Controversies continue to persist as to whether electrocautery is better than laser; the type of laser preferred the number of holes per ovary, duration, strength, and nature of current to be used. In a review by Saleh et al., in 2004 involving 18 articles, the authors concluded that there was no difference in rates of ovulation between electrocoagulation and laser. This topic has been explained in detail in chapter on "Polycystic Ovarian Syndrome".

STIMULATION PROTOCOLS IN ART

INTRODUCTION

The first successful human IVF was a natural cycle IVF. Soon, there was a shift to ovarian stimulation to get an increased number of oocytes, embryos, and thus improve the pregnancy rates. The goal of assisted-reproductive technique (ART) is mainly to achieve a live birth safely in a patient friendly but at the same time in a cost-effective manner.

The concept of COS for multiple follicular developments is to generate multiple embryos and increase pregnancy rates.[6] Number of oocytes directly correlates with ongoing pregnancy rates but patients may not respond similar to each other with same protocol. This has brought the concept of individualized controlled ovarian stimulation (i-COS).[50]

INDIVIDUALIZING APPROACH TOWARD PATIENT FOR COS

Recently, a joint venture of discussion amongst American Society for Reproductive Medicine and the European Society of Human Reproduction and Embryology (ESHRE) has given the concept of "patient-tailored stimulation". It should be a result of shared-decision making (SDM) process. In expert committee opinion, Dr Politi[51] told that SDM is important in situations where decisions are being made between treatment options with "similar outcomes from a medical standpoint" and patients' preferences for the possible risks and benefits. Decision making help is provided to assist patients decide their treatment regarding number of embryos to be transferred but no such aids are still there for deciding the approach to COS.[52]

Objectives of I-COS

- Tailoring of protocol for each woman separately with no compromise on the quality.
- To achieve a sufficient number of fertilizable oocytes of good quality so that at least two or three superior quality embryos can be selected for transfer and the remaining embryos can be cryopreserved for a subsequent freeze-thaw cycle.
- To avoid multiple pregnancy.
- Eliminate risk of OHSS as it is iatrogenic cause.
- Reduce risk of cycle cancellation to minimal rate.[53]
- Increase the pregnancy rate.
- Endometrial environment should be suitable for implantation.
- Appropriate plan and calculation of dosage for expected poor responders.
- Drop-out rates and costs should be as less as possible to reduce financial burden of patients.

In this era of personalized medicine, moderate ovarian stimulation targeting 8–15 oocytes is the best way to optimize IVF outcome safely.

TABLE 4: Markers of ovarian response.

Clinical	*Investigational*
Age	FSH
Smoking status	AMH[54]
Menstrual cycle	AFC[55]
BMI	Ovarian volume
Previous response to stimulation	
PCOS	

(AFC: antral follicle count; AMH: anti-Müllerian hormone; BMI: body mass index; FSH: follicle-stimulating hormone; PCOS: polycystic ovary syndrome)

Factors which decide personalized approach are:

- Availability of different drugs and options of making small changes of even 12.5 IU for decision of optimum dosage for a patient.
- Embryology laboratory conditions.
- Endocrine and clinical profile of the couple.
- Ovarian response markers **(Table 4)**.

The International Society for Mild Approaches in Assisted Reproduction (ISMAAR) has given a physiological, lower risk, lesser drug-oriented and more patient friendly approach. Main emphasis in this classification has been given on clinical aspects of assisted reproduction.[56] Recent trials have shown comparable results of mild stimulation versus conventional stimulation protocols. This approach will help to promote mild, affordable, and safe techniques.[57] Concerns related to poor oocyte and embryo quality with conventional stimulation and its effect on endometrial function can be dealt in a better way. The ISMAAR consensus on terminology of stimulation for IVF is given in **Table 5**.

Classification of Patients According to Their Ovarian Response

- *Normal responder:* 8–15 follicles/eggs.
- *Poor responder:* 1–4 follicles/eggs.
- *Hyper-responder:* Not more than 15 follicles/eggs.

Number of eggs in IVF is a surrogate for clinical success. Results in study by Sunkara et al.,[58] has shown a nonlinear relationship between the number of eggs and live birth rates. The number of eggs to maximize the live birth rate is ~15, plateaus between 15 and 20, and declines beyond 20 eggs. Depending on clinical characteristics and ovarian response,[59] they can be divided into three types **(Table 6)**.

Two separate consensuses are there for poor responders. ESHRE consensus gave Bologna criteria for poor responders having following features:[60]

Two of the following three features must be present:

1. Advanced maternal age more than or equal to 40 years or any other risk factor for poor ovarian response.
2. A previous poor ovarian response less than or equal to three oocytes with a conventional stimulation protocol.

TABLE 5: ISMAAR consensus on stimulation for in vitro fertilization.

Terminology	*Aim*	*To replace*	*Method used*
Natural cycle IVF	1 oocyte	No stimulation	No medication
Modified natural cycle IVF	1 oocyte	Semi-natural, controlled natural cycle IVF	hCG only
Mild IVF	2–7 oocytes	Soft minimal stimulation, "friendly" IVF	Low dose Gn, oral ovulogens and GnRH antagonist
Conventional IVF	>/=8 oocytes	Standard, routine IVF, COS IVF	GnRH agonist or antagonist with conventional hMG/FSH dose

(COS: controlled ovarian stimulation; FSH: follicle-stimulating hormone; hCG: human chorionic gonadotropin; GnRH: gonadotropin-releasing hormone; hMG: human menopausal gonadotropin; IVF: in vitro fertilization)

TABLE 6: How to identify different types of ovarian response.

Poor responder	*Normal responder*	*Hyper responder*
Regular or short cycles Obese/thin Age >37 years FSH >12 mIU/mL AMH <5–1.4 ng/mL AFC <8 Previous poor response to stimulation	Regular cycles Normal built Age <37 years FSH <12 mIU/mL AMH 1.5–3.5 ng/mL AFC 8–15 Previous normal response to stimulation	Regular/irregular cycles Thin or obese built Age <37 years LH/FSH >2 mIU/mL AMH >3.5 ng/mL AFC >15 Previous hyper-response to stimulation

(AFC: antral follicle count; AMH: anti-Müllerian hormone; FSH: follicle-stimulating hormone; LH: luteinizing hormone)

3. An abnormal ovarian reserve test [antral follicle count (AFC) <5–7 follicles or anti-Müllerian hormone (AMH) <0.5–1.1 ng/mL].

But this criterion had many shortcomings[61] and pitfalls **(Flowchart 3)**. After years of criticism, the Bologna criteria was not appropriate and thus came the second stratification by Patient-Oriented Strategies Encompassing IndividualizeD Oocyte Number (POSEIDON) group in patients with reduced ovarian reserve or unexpected sub-optimal ovarian response to exogenous gonadotropins.[62] Four groups have been made based on both qualitative and quantitative parameters **(Fig. 3)**. Management of all four groups based on their parameters is given in detail in chapter on "Poor Responders".

Identification of protocols based on reserve parameters is described in **Table 7**.

Flowchart 3: Criticism of Bologna criteria.

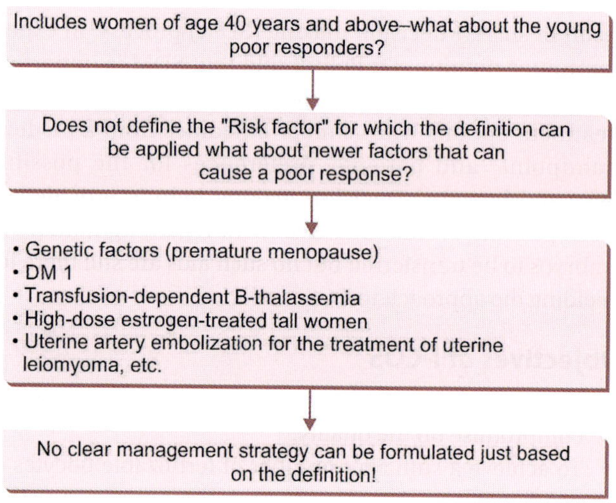

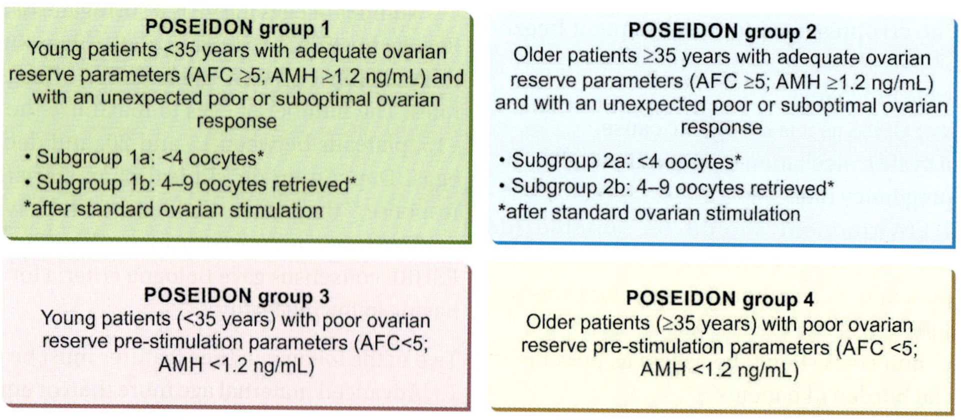

Fig. 3: Four groups of "low prognosis patients" in assisted reproductive technology according to the POSEIDON's stratification based on oocyte quantity and quality.
(AFC: antral follicle count; AMH: anti-Müllerian hormone)

TABLE 7: Identification of protocol based on reserve parameters.

Parameters	*Principle*	*Protocol/adjuvants*	*Gonadotropin dosage*	*Advantages/disadvantages*
AMH</-0.1 AFC 0–2	Very low reserve so less chances of follicles	Minimal/mild Pretreatment with: • Androgens (DHEA 75 mg/day 3 months before) • Testesterone gel previous month 12.5 mg. Sunkara meta-analysis.[63] Both these interventions do not improve outcome • E2 priming or antagonist in previous luteal phase (crash protocol) for synchronous cohort in a systematic review and meta-analysis by Bosdou et al.[64] Transdermal testosterone pretreatment seems to increase clinical pregnancy and live birth rates in poor responders undergoing ovarian stimulation for IVF. There is insufficient data to support a beneficial role of rLH, hCG, DHEA, or letrozole administration in the probability of pregnancy in poor responders undergoing ovarian stimulation for IVF. Growth hormone supplementation (Cochrane Duffy et al)[65] Increases pregnancy rate OR: 5; Dose: 4–8 IU daily from day 2 till hCG	150–225 IU	• Less cost • Better quality as compared to quantity • Better compliance • Less success
AMH 0.7–1.3 AFC 5–7	• Downregulation may cause profound suppression • Self phase FSH and LH to be utilized	Antagonist/short flare	300 IU	• Higher success rates with antagonist protocol • Substantial reduction in cancellation rates • Agonist trigger can be used • Increased yield • Compliance good
AMH 1.4–3.5 AFC 8–14	As reserve is good, will respond to either of the protocol	GnRH downregulation/antagonist	225 IU	• Good yield • Decision depends on patient compliance
AMH >3.5 AFC >15	Risk of OHSS, so to keep the option of agonist trigger open	Antagonist • Metformin (1500–2000 mg/day)— increased clinical pregnancy rates and decreased risk of OHSS (Tso, 2014)[66] • Addition of dopamine agonist in the luteal phase	150 IU	• Less days of stimulation • Decreased chances of OHSS • Higher pregnancy rates

(AMH: anti-Müllerian hormone; AFC: antral follicle count; DHEA: dehydroepiandrosterone; E2: estradiol; rLH: recombinant luteinizing hormone)

INDIVIDUALIZATION OF GONADOTROPIN PREPARATION AND DOSAGE

Different preparations of gonadotropins are given in **Table 8**.

- *Normoresponders:* Highly purified (Hp) human menopausal gonadotropin (hMG) or recombinant (r) FSH should be used.
  - Less than 30 years: 75 IU
  - 30–35 years: 150 IU
  - More than 35 years: 225 IU
- *Poor responders:* Hp hMG or rFSH + rLH should be used.
  - Less than 30 years: 225 IU
  - 30–35 years: 300 IU
  - More than 35 years: 300–450 IU

TABLE 8: Gonadotropin preparations.[67]

Gonadotropin preparations	*Contents and properties*
hMG	FSH and LH are present in equal proportion
uFSH	FSH with nongonadotropin protein content of >95%
Pure FSH	FSH with nongonadotropin protein content of <5%
Recombinant FSH	High purity and does not have LH activity
Recombinant LH	High purity and greater specific LH activity
Corifollitropin alfa[66]	Subcutaneous depot preparation, sustained long half-life

(FSH: follicle-stimulating hormone; hMG: human menopausal gonadotropin; LH: luteinizing hormone)

- *Hyper-responders:* rFSH should be used.
  - Less than 30 years: 75 IU
  - 30–35 years: 75 IU
  - More than 35 years: 150 IU

To start or add LH in the following circumstances:
- Advance age more than 35 years
- Poor responder
- Plateau response on day 6.

After the introduction of GnRH antagonists and strategies to reduce multiple births such as single embryo transfer, now there is a developing interest in natural cycle and mild stimulation in IVF. Natural and mild IVF are patient friendly, cost-effective, and reduce patient discomfort and multiple pregnancies.

Models for Predicting Dose of Gonadotropins

Many models are there which combine different parameters of age, ovarian reserve, hormonal parameters, ultrasound findings, BMI, and smoking status. Popovic-Todorovic et al., model included age, AFC, smoking status, and ovarian stromal blood flow. La Marca et al., model has used age, AFC, and AMH to predict response to gonadotropin dose. Pivot et al., model has included AMH, AFC, age, BMI, and smoking habits. This normogram has helped in making even very small dose changes in the stimulation protocols.

Which Gonadotropin is Better?

The rFSH is more potent than urinary hMG or FSH preparations.[68] The rFSH produces significantly more oocytes than urinary with lower doses and shorter time.[69] In a study by Peter Plateau et al. (merit study), the findings of this integrated analysis demonstrated that ovarian stimulation with Hp-hMG, following a long downregulation protocol, in IVF cycles results in significantly more live births than stimulation with rFSH alone. In the Cochrane review by Van Wely M,[70] there was no evidence of a difference in live births when rFSH was compared with FSH-P or when rFSH was compared with FSH-Hp. Thus, the clinical choice of gonadotropin should depend on availability, convenience, and costs. Differences between urinary gonadotropins were considered unlikely to be clinically significant.

DIFFERENT PROTOCOLS FOR STIMULATION

- *Agonist protocols:*
  - Long protocol
  - Stop protocol
  - Short protocol
  - Ultrashort protocol
  - Microflare
- *Antagonist protocol:*
  - Fixed
  - Flexible
- *Mild stimulation protocol*
- *Special cases:*
  - Ultra long protocol
  - Double stimulation protocols
  - Stair step and chronic low-dose step-up protocols.

GONADOTROPIN-RELEASING HORMONE AGONIST

The introduction of GnRHa in the late 1980s was a great boon in the field of ovarian stimulation in ART. They provided the ability to downregulate endogenous pituitary gonadotropin secretion and thereby prevent a premature LH surge during exogenous gonadotropin stimulation.

Mechanism of Action

The GnRHa molecule is derived from the native GnRH by amino acid substitution at 6th and 10th position, which leads to an increase in FSH and LH. It has a flare effect lasting for 5–7 days and on continuous administration, there is suppression of the HPO axis because of receptor downregulation and desensitization, thus decreasing the circulating levels of gonadotropins and sex steroids and finally receptor internalization occurs.

Route

They are available as daily injections, depot preparation (monthly or 3 monthly), and nasal sprays (multiple daily doses, which mimic the natural pulses). They can be administered intramuscular (IM), subcutaneous (SC), or intranasal. SC route is the most commonly used. Daily SC injections are preferred for use in IVF. However, depot preparations (leuprolide 3.75 mg, goserelin 3.6 mg or 11.8 mg) are used in patients with endometriosis prior to IVF for downregulation. **Tables 9 and 10** illustrate various preparations and their half-lives.

Uses

- Pituitary suppression prior to ovarian stimulation
- Used as trigger in antagonist protocol or in modified natural protocol.

TABLE 9: Gonadotropin-releasing hormone agonist preparation.

Nonapeptides	*Decapeptides*
Leuprolide[71]	Nafarelin
Buserelin	Triptorelin (Decapeptyl)
Goserelin (Zoladex)—only available as a depot	
Histrelin	
Deslorelin (not been used in human in vitro fertilization)	

TABLE 10: Bioavailability and half-life of different agonist preparations.

Drug	*Bioavailability*	*T max*	*Half-life*
Leuprolide	94%	2–6 hours	3 hours
Decapeptyl	100%	45 minutes	3–5 hours
Cetrorelix	85%	1 hour	5 hours
Ganirelix	91%	1–2 hours	13 hours

- Prevention of premature LH surge
- Luteal phase support (LPS)
- Prevention of OHSS
- Breast cancer patients
- Central precocious puberty
- Endometriosis
- Fibroids
- Hirsutism.

Advantages

- Synchronization of follicular growth
- Flexibility in IVF programming
- Favors batch IVF
- *Abolition of spontaneous LH surge:* A meta-analysis of RCTs has shown that the use of GnRHa has not only reduced cancellation rates but has also increased the number of oocytes and embryos, allowing better selection so that, on an average, the outcome in terms of pregnancy rates was improved.
- Less expensive than antagonist.

Disadvantages

- Less "patient friendly"
- Stressful due to longer treatment cycles (3–4 weeks for GnRHa)
- Less safe
- Increased gonadotropin doses
- Only hCG can be used as trigger
- Increased risk of OHSS
- Overall costly due to increased gonadotropin usage
- Slow follicular growth
- Luteal phase defect.

Side Effects

- Hot flushes
- Vaginal dryness
- Transient frontal headaches
- Arthralgia
- Myalgia
- Insomnia
- Headaches
- Loss of libido
- Hypoestrogenic state
- Excessive suppression.

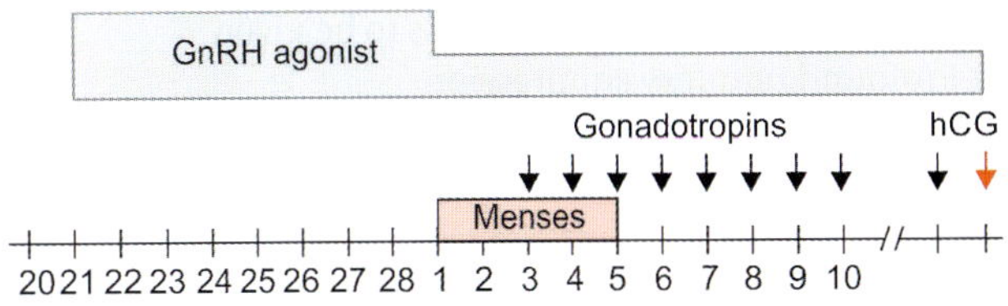

Fig. 4: Long protocol.

PROTOCOLS FOR AGONIST

Long Protocol (Fig. 4)

It is the first protocol used to prevent premature LH surge. It was the gold standard till the introduction of GnRH antagonist. The GnRHa is started in the midluteal phase of the preceding menstrual cycle or in the early follicular phase, but the time required to achieve pituitary downregulation is longer and the prevalence of cystic follicles is higher in the latter. No evidence of a significant difference between depot and daily GnRHa use for pituitary downregulation in IVF cycles using the long protocol is there, but substantial differences could not be ruled out.[72] Since depot GnRHa requires more gonadotropins and a longer duration of use, it may increase the overall costs of IVF treatment. Injection lupride 1 mg is started from midluteal phase of the preceding cycle for 10 days or until the onset of menses.

To confirm downregulation:

- Ultrasonography (endometrial thickness of less than 5 mm and no cysts more than 10 mm)
- Serum estradiol levels less than 50 pg/mL
- Serum LH less than 5 mIU/mL
- Serum progesterone less than 0.5 ng/mL.

Exogenous gonadotropins and GnRH agonists (reduced dose of GnRH agonists in mini dose long protocol) are continued till the day of hCG administration. The goal is to have at least two follicles measuring 17–18 mm in mean diameter, ideally with a few others in the 14–16 mm range when the hCG trigger of 10,000 IU is given to achieve final follicular maturation. A Cochrane review by Maheshwari et al.,[73] concluded that the number of oocytes retrieved and the pregnancy rate was higher in the long protocol. There was no difference in the live birth rate; however, this outcome is reported in only three studies. There was no evidence of a difference in the outcomes among various long protocols; nor that stopping or reducing GnRHa at the start of stimulation were associated with a reduced pregnancy rate. Comparison was long protocol versus short or ultrashort protocol.[74]

Disadvantages

- Increased dose of gonadotropins
- Increased overall cost
- Increased chances of OHSS in hyper-responder

- Luteal phase support also needs to be given
- Profound pituitary suppression
- Functional cyst formation—combined OCP and agonist prevents cyst formation.

Stop Protocols

It has two types of protocols namely menstrual early cessation and follicular early cessation protocols as depicted in **Figures 5 and 6**.

Short or Flare Protocol (Fig. 7)

Rationale

The flare effect of the agonist releases the stored FSH and LH, which augments the folliculogenesis, which has already been started. Main use is in poor responders.

Disadvantages

The flare effect causing the surge of LH in the initial phase of folliculogenesis may have adverse effects on the developing follicles. Also, this is commonly associated with significant increases in serum progesterone and androgen levels, which may be due to the late corpus luteal rescue. This may be deleterious to the oocyte and may hamper the fertilization and pregnancy rates.

Microdose Flare Protocol (Fig. 8)

Pretreatment with OCPs for 14–21 days should be done in the preceding cycle.[75] Injection leupride 40 μg twice a day from day 2 of withdrawal bleed is given till day of hCG trigger. Gonadotropin stimulation 300-450 IU/day started from day 3 of withdrawal bleed till day of hCG trigger (criteria for hCG trigger same as that for long protocol).

Advantages

No increase in serum progesterone or androgen because:
- Decreased GnRH agonist dose.
- The preliminary OCP pretreatment.

This protocol may be useful in previous poor responders in whom it has been observed to stimulate increase in serum FSH (not attributable to exogenous gonadotropin treatment)

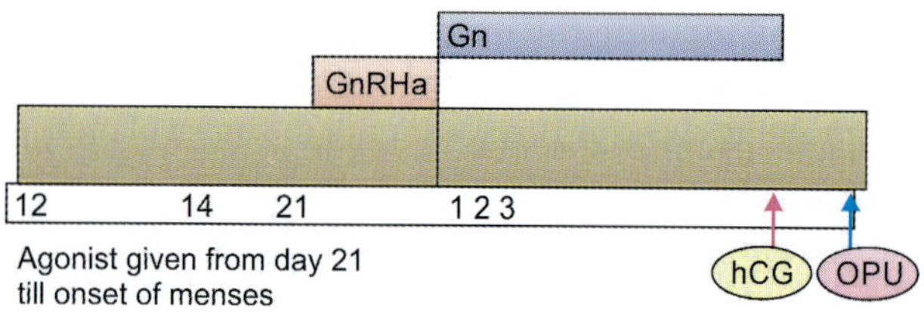

Fig. 5: Menstrual early cessation agonist protocol.

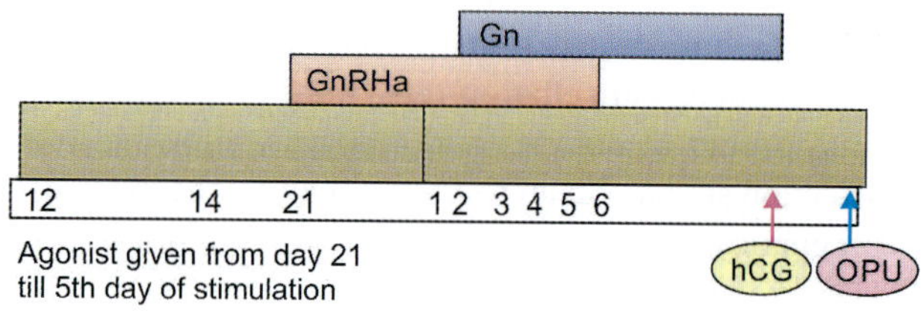

Fig. 6: Follicular early cessation agonist protocol.

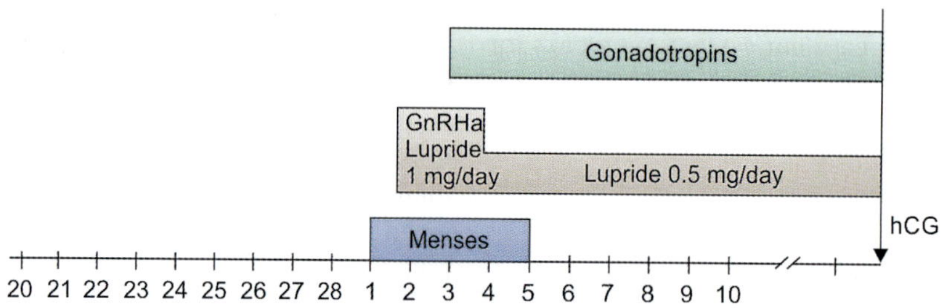

Fig. 7: GnRH agonist short protocol.
(GnRHa: gonadotropin-releasing hormone agonist; hCG: human chorionic gonadotropin)

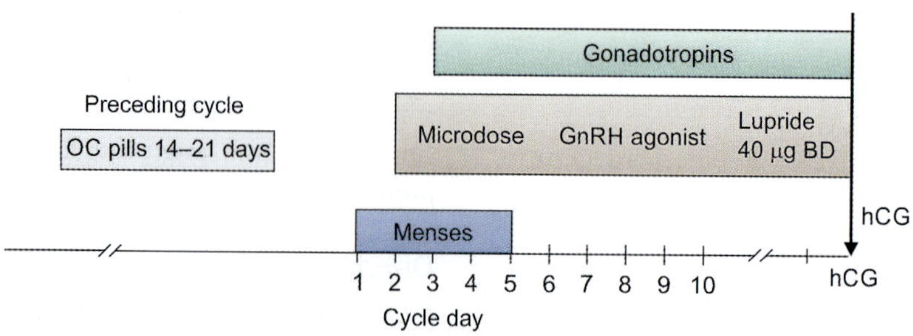

Fig. 8: Microdose Flare protocol.
(GnRH: gonadotropin-releasing hormone; hCG: human chorionic gonadotropin; OC: oral contraceptive)

and lower cancellation rates and good clinical and ongoing pregnancy rates. Long GnRH agonist and antagonist regimens offer a suitable choice for poor responders, whereas the short agonist regimen may be less effective because of fewer eggs retrieved.[76]

Ultrashort Protocol

In this protocol, the GnRHa is administered only for 3 days. The short regimens have the advantage of a shorter duration of stimulation, with the use of fewer ampoules of gonadotropins and therefore lower costs.[77]

Safety of GnRH Agonists

Lahat et al.,[78] reported a high incidence of attention deficit hyperactivity disorder (ADHD) in long-term follow-up of children inadvertently exposed to GnRH agonists in early pregnancy.[12]

GONADOTROPIN-RELEASING HORMONE ANTAGONISTS

The GnRH antagonists earlier were not very popular because of their histamine releasing capability and associated systemic edema.[79] However, the development of third generation antagonists—cetrorelix and ganirelix was a major breakthrough in the field of reproductive medicine because of their metabolic stability and histamine induced reduced allergic side effects.

Structure

Amino acids at 1, 2, 3, 6, and 10 positions play a significant role in structure and function of native GnRH molecule (decapeptide). Sixth position is involved in enzymatic cleavage. Positions 1, 6, and 10 are important for three-dimensional structure of the molecule and position 2 and 3 are important for gonadotropin release.[80]

Mechanism of Action

The antagonists block the GnRH receptor in a dose-dependent competitive fashion and they have no flare effect. There is immediate suppression of pituitary gonadotropin release. This is in contrast to the long-acting agonists, which first stimulate and later inhibit pituitary gonadotropin secretion by desensitization and receptor downregulation. After the GnRH antagonist is discontinued, there is a short recovery phase of 2–4 days.

Preparations

Third-generation GnRH antagonists: Cetrorelix and ganirelix.

Doses and Route

No adjustment in dose of obese women for cetrorelix. Half-life of cetrorelix 3 mg dose is 62.8 hours, 0.25 mg 20.6 hours, and ganirelix 0.25 mg is 16.2 hours.

PROTOCOL FOR ANTAGONIST PROTOCOL

- Single-dose antagonist protocol and multiple-dose antagonist protocol
- Fixed antagonist and flexible antagonist protocol.

Single-dose Antagonist Protocol (Fig. 9)

Cetrorelix 3 mg is given on day 7 in fixed protocol (French Protocol). A single injection prevents LH surge for 96 hours.

Multiple-dose Antagonist Protocol

Common protocol. Both cetrorelix/ganirelix can be used. In the *fixed protocol* **(Fig. 10)**, GnRH antagonist is started on day 6 of stimulation and is continued till the day of hCG trigger.[81] In the *flexible protocol* **(Fig. 11)**, GnRH antagonist is started once the leading follicle is more than 14 mm. Flexible protocol is a more cost-effective approach, as it avoids unnecessary injections. Statistically significant reduction found both in number of antagonist ampoules and amount of gonadotropin used in the flexible protocol. No statistically significant difference found in pregnancy rate between flexible and fixed protocols.[82]

Advantages

- More physiological
- More patient friendly
- Less stressful due to shorter treatment cycles
- Safer

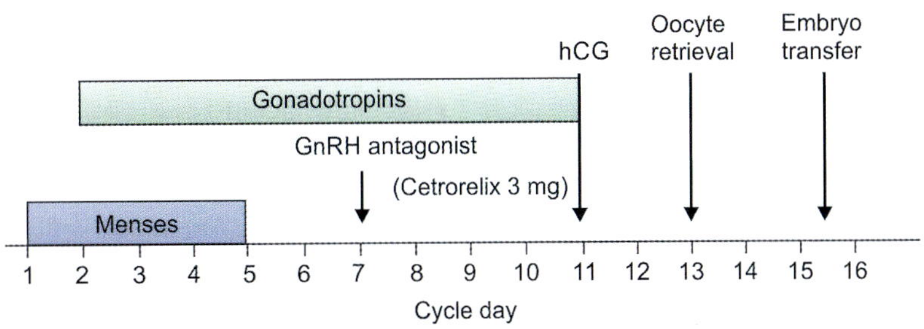

Fig. 9: Single dose antagonist protocol.
(GnRH: gonadotropin-releasing hormone; hCG: human chorionic gonadotropin)

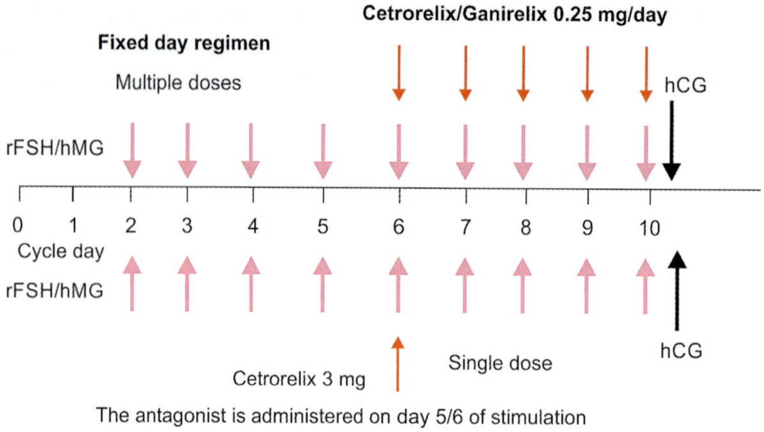

Fig. 10: Fixed dose antagonist protocol.
(rFSH: recombinant follicle-stimulating hormone; hMG: human menopausal gonadotropin; hCG: human chorionic gonadotropin)

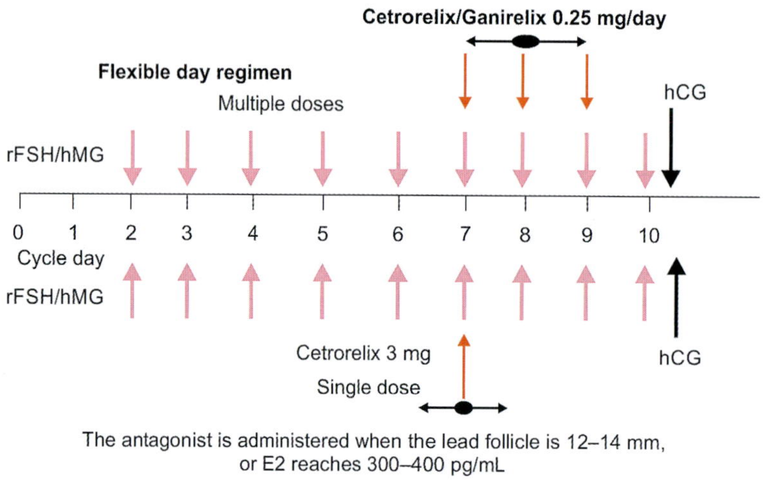

Fig. 11: Flexible dose antagonist protocol.
(rFSH: recombinant follicle-stimulating hormone; hMG: human menopausal gonadotropin; hCG: human chorionic gonadotropin; E2: estradiol)

- Decreased dose of gonadotropins
- Minimal ovarian stimulation
- Agonist trigger can be used
- Negligible chances of OHSS
- Cost friendly
- Flexible protocols.

Disadvantages

- Does not suppress raised LH levels in early phase of stimulation
- Does not allow flexibility in IVF programming
- Does not favor batch IVF
- Drug per se is more expensive than GnRH agonist.

GNRH AGONIST VERSUS ANTAGONIST[83]

Cochrane analysis suggests that there is significant reduction in the incidence of OHSS (by more than 50%) with the use of antagonists. However, this analysis has been criticized by Orvito et al. who say that GnRH agonist still have demonstrable superiority over antagonists in terms of ongoing pregnancy rates and live birth rates.

Differences between GnRH agonists and antagonists are given in **Table 11**.

TRIGGER

List of triggers:

- hCG: 5,000 IU SC or IM
- R hCG: 250 µg SC ↭ 6,000–7,000 IU hCG
- R GnRH agonists:
  - Leuprolide: 500–1,000 µg SC
  - Triptorelin: 200 µg SC
  - Buserelin: 500 µg SC

Youssef[84] concluded that urinary hCG remains the best choice for final oocyte maturation triggering in IVF and intracytoplasmic sperm injection (ICSI) treatment cycles due to availability and cost (Youssef 2011).

In high responder patients, avoiding hCG and using GnRH agonist (0.2 mg triptorelin) as the trigger almost eliminates OHSS. A meta-analysis showed lesser pregnancy rates in fresh embryo transfer with agonist trigger.[85] Griesinger G et al.,[86] proposed frozen thawed cycle.

In 2014, Youssef et al., found lower live birth rate and higher miscarriage rate in women who received a GnRHa with reduced OHSS rates.[87]

NATURAL CYCLE IN VITRO FERTILIZATION

In vitro fertilization is carried out in a spontaneous menstrual cycle. No medication is given with aim to collect one naturally selected oocyte at least expenses.[88]

TABLE 11: Comparison between GnRH agonist and antagonist.

Agonist	*Antagonist*
Initial flare followed by pituitary desensitization	Immediate Gn suppression by competitive block of GnRH receptors
More ampoules of gonadotropin needed	Lesser ampoules required
Longer duration of stimulation	Shorter duration of stimulation
Slow recovery of pituitary function	Quick recovery of pituitary function
hCG as trigger	GnRH agonist or hCG can be used as trigger
More oocytes for IVF and cryopreservation	Fewer oocytes, but also less OHSS
Risk of OHSS is more	Significantly lesser risk of OHSS
Symptoms of E2 deprivation are more	Symptoms of E2 deprivation are less
More programmable IVF procedures	Less programmable IVF, but greater patient convenience
Gold standard in normoresponders	Particularly advantageous in hyper and poor responders. Can also be used in normoresponders

(E2: estradiol; GnRH: gonadotropin- releasing hormone; hCG: human chorionic gonadotropin; IVF: in vitro fertilization; OHSS: ovarian hyperstimulation syndrome)

Protocol

It has high-cancellation rates and low success rates. It is used in cancer patients where gonadotropins cannot be given. The timing of oocyte collection may be based on an optimum level of serum E2 and LH and/or ultrasound measurement of follicular diameter and endometrial thickness.[89,90]

MODIFIED NATURAL CYCLE IN VITRO FERTILIZATION

The aim is to reduce chances of cycle cancellation.

- Human chorionic gonadotropin as trigger +/– luteal support.
- GnRHa +/– Gn. hCG injection and luteal support are given.

Recent evidence suggests that it may be useful in poor responders.[91]

MILD IN VITRO FERTILIZATION (FIG. 12)

Gonadotropin (FSH or hMG) are administered at lower doses or oral compounds (antiestrogens or aromatase inhibitors) are used along with it. hCG injection and luteal support are also given.[92] The criteria for administration of hCG, IVF, and embryo transfer techniques are similar to those applied in other IVF protocols. Luteal support is given either in the form of hCG or progesterone.[93]

Advantages

- Less complex
- Less time-consuming
- Cheaper
- Reduced chances for complications
- Reduced chances for discomfort
- Reduced chances for drop-out
- Effects on oocyte quality
- Effects on endometrial receptivity
- Emphasize on maximizing chances for healthy children born per treatment started at reasonable cost, less patient discomfort and fewer chances of complications.

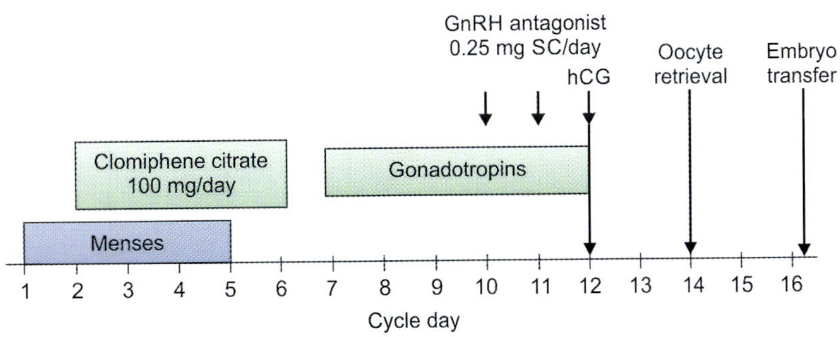

Fig. 12: Mild stimulation IVF.
(GnRH: gonadotropin-releasing hormone; hCG: human chorionic gonadotropin; SC: subcutaneous).

Disadvantages

- Lower pregnancy rates per cycle
- Lower success rates
- High-cycle cancellation rate
- Decreased number of oocytes and embryos
- Less margin for suboptimal laboratory performance
- Mild IVF not yet tested in women less than 38 years old
- Difficulty in programming the cycle.

KATO PROTOCOL

This minimal ovarian stimulation protocol **(Fig. 13)** has full advantage of the characteristics of CC. Administration of 50 mg CC is started on cycle day 3 and from day 8, patients receive 150 IU of FSH every other day. Once the size of the dominant follicle and the estradiol concentration reaches the predefined values, GnRH agonist is administered as the trigger. Oocytes are then retrieved 32–35 hours later.

Enclomiphene has a short half-life (24 hours) and therefore it is necessary to continue oral administration of CC until the day before maturation is triggered. In the large-scale retrospective study by Teramoto S and Kato O, of all 43,433 cycles initiated, the rates for oocyte retrieval and embryo cleavage were 83% and 64%, respectively.[94] The mean number of oocytes retrieved was 2.2. The rates for live births, miscarriages, and ectopic pregnancies, in relation to initiated cycles, including cases of frozen-thawed transfer, were 11.1, 3.4, and 0.2%, respectively. In view of this protocol being inexpensive and much more compatible, it can be expected to provide a huge benefit to infertile women especially in developing countries.

CONTROLLED OVARIAN STIMULATION WITH LETROZOLE SUPPLEMENTATION (COST-LESS PROTOCOL) (FIG. 14)

Day 2: Letrozole 5 mg/day till 48 hours before oocyte pick up.

Day 5: FSH 150–225 according to age, AFC, and weight. Antagonist to prevent LH surge along with agonist trigger.

After the oocyte retrieval, the patients restarted the letrozole regimen until their estradiol concentrations were less than 50 pg/dL.

Results: Patients had less E2 levels but similar oocyte yield as compared to conventional antagonist protocol. Letrozole versus anastrolzole versus tamoxifene, least peak E2 levels are seen with letrozole.[95]

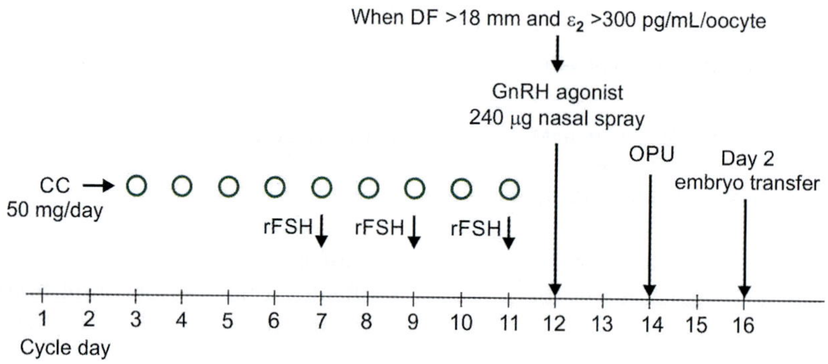

Fig. 13: Kato protocol.
(CC: clomiphene citrate; DF:dominant follicle; GnRH: gonadotropin-releasing hormone; OPU: oocyte pickup; rFSH: recombinant follicle-stimulating hormone).

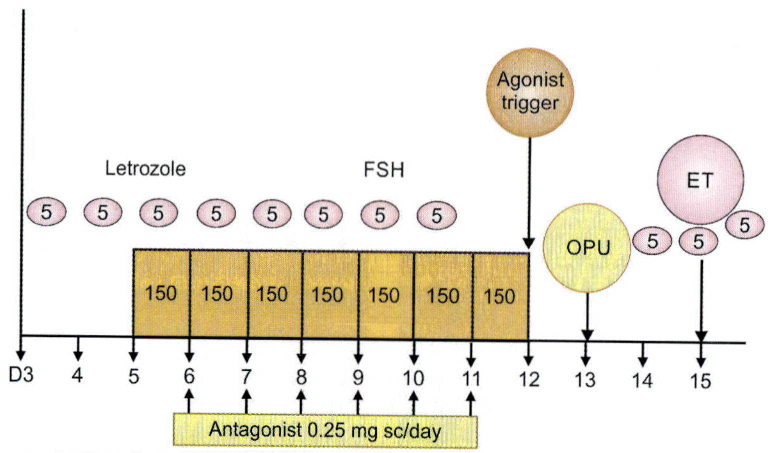

Fig. 14: Cost-less protocol with letrozole.
(ET: embryo transfer; FSH: follicle-stimulating hormone; OPU: oocyte pickup)

SHANGHAI PROTOCOL (KUANG ET AL.) (FIG. 15)

Double stimulations during the follicular and luteal phases of poor responders in IVF or ICSI programs in the same menstrual cycle provided more opportunities to retrieve oocytes with embryos of similar development potential. This approach is useful for cases with history of negative oocyte retrieval and also in cancer patients who need emergency fertility preservation.[96]

DUPLEX PROTOCOL (MOFFAT ET AL.)

It is also known as Dual ovarian stimulation. This protocol features dual stimulation, with the second stimulation starting immediately after the first oocyte retrieval. In this Duplex (DPX) protocol, both the first and second stimulations used a similar regimen consisting of a classical antagonist protocol using 300 IU of FSH per day, cetrorelix 0.25 mg starting on ovarian stimulation day 6, and GnRH trigger (triptorelin 0.2 mg) when follicular maturation was reached. The first and second stimulations provided a similar number of oocytes, zygotes, and blastocysts. The DPX protocol thus doubled the final blastocyst yield, compared with a classical single ovarian stimulation cycle. This approach can be used in fertility preservation and the desire to collect the largest number of oocytes can be possible.[97]

ULTRALONG PROTOCOL FOR ENDOMETRIOSIS (ESHRE 2013 GUIDELINES)

Depicted in **Figure 16**. It is discussed in detail in chapter on "Endometriosis".

Progestin-primed Ovarian Stimulation (PPOS)

Progestin-primed ovarian stimulation (PPOS) is a new protocol designed for ovarian stimulation **(Fig. 17)**. In this protocol instead of down-regulation with agonist or antagonist use, progesterone is used to prevent LH surge.[98] Meta-analysis by Guan et al., has showed that premature LH surge incidence, clinical pregnancy rate, live birth rate, and ongoing pregnancy rate in PPOS protocol is similar to nonPPOS cycles in all patient populations.[99] Another meta-analysis by Alexandru et al., also suggested effective role of progestins in prevention of LH surge.[100] PPOS protocol in PCOS patients have shown in lower incidence of OHSS as progestin reduces chances of OHSS in both follicular and luteal phase.[101] Retrospective study by Huang et al.,

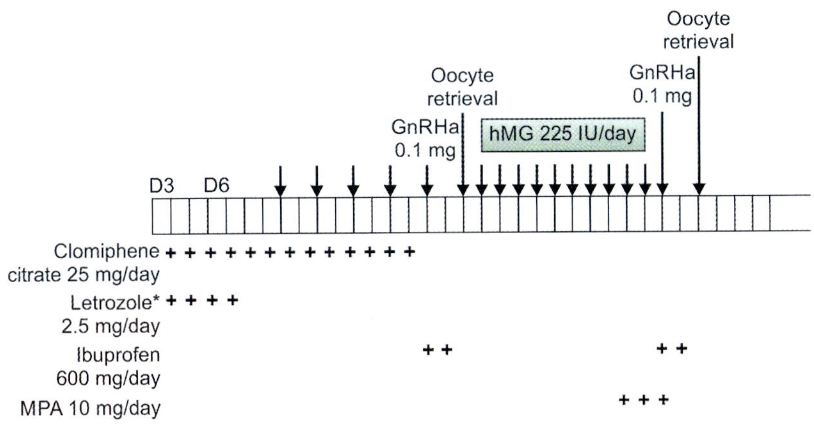

Fig. 15: Shanghai protocol.
(GnRHa: gonadotropin-releasing hormone agonist; hMG: human menopausal gonadotropin)

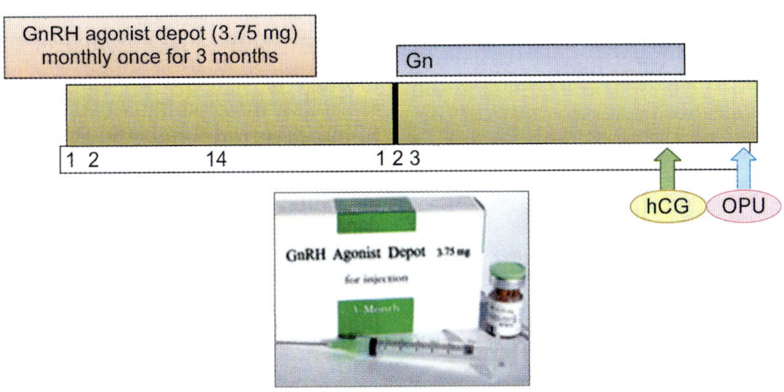

Fig. 16: Ultralong protocol for endometriosis.
(hCG: human chorionic gonadotropin; OPU: oocyte pickup)

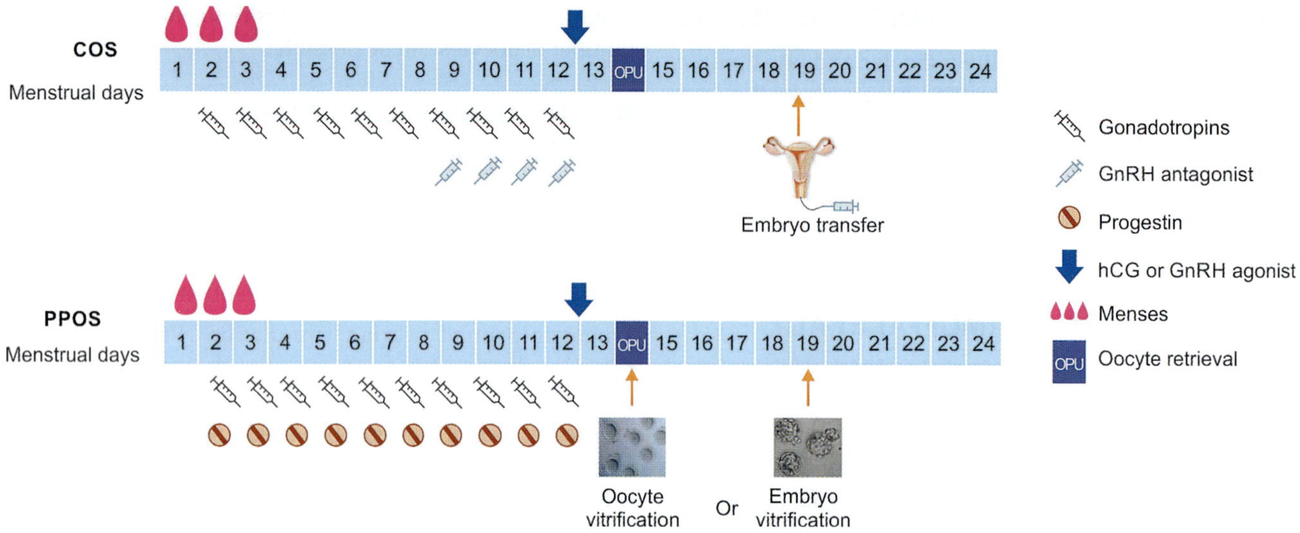

Fig. 17: Progestin-primed ovarian stimulation (PPOS) protocol.
(GnRH: gonadotropin releasing hormone; hCG: human chorionic gonadotropin)

have demonstrated similar neonatal outcomes when PPOS was compared to short antagonist protocol.[102] The only drawback so far is that fresh embryo transfer cannot be done as early exposure to progesterone results in endometrial advancement.[103]

ICMR Guidelines for Recommencing ART Services during COVID-19 Pandemic 2021

ICMR designed a step-wise module for ART clinic to be followed:[104]

(A) *Patient information and counseling:* COVID-19 pandemic might have effect on treatment and pregnancy outcomes in couples undergoing ART procedures, so couples should be properly counseled and informed about symptoms, social distancing, and situations where treatment may be stopped in between due to high-risk clinical situation.

(B) *Consent:* Specific consent form related to COVID-19 infection should be taken.

(C) *Risk Assessment triage:* Risk is assessed by following factors—clinical history and possibility of contact with suspected or positively infected individuals.

Group I: Couple low risk and asymptomatic: RTPCR test should be done before starting ART treatment and before oocyte retrieval or HCG trigger.

- If RTPCR negative: Continue the treatment
- If RTPCR positive: Postpone the treatment.

Group II: Couple recovered from COVID-19 infection: RTPCR test done prior to starting ART treatment and before oocyte retrieval or HCG trigger.

- If RTPCR negative: Continue the treatment
- If RTPCR positive: Postpone the treatment.

Group III: Any one partner with symptoms before starting ovarian stimulation for IUI/IVF: RTPCR test should be done prior to starting ART treatment

- If RTPCR negative: Continue the treatment
- If RTPCR positive: Postpone the treatment.

Group IV: COVID-19 symptoms arising during ovarian stimulation in IUI/IVF cycle: RTPCR test before further treatment like oocyte retrieval or HCG trigger.

- If RTPCR negative: Continue the treatment
- If RTPCR positive: Postpone the treatment.

Group V: COVID-19 symptoms arising after oocyte retrieval in IVF cycle: RTPCR test before further treatment.

- If RTPCR negative: Continue the treatment
- If RTPCR positive: Freeze all embryos, if positive after oocyte retrieval and before embryo transfer.

(D) *Modification of ART clinic layout and services:*

- Specific COVID-19 sanitization procedures, staff training, provision of PPE, and sanitation equipment.
- Use of Aarogya setu app.
- Limited persons at one time with division of staff into mini teams accompanying proper social distancing protocols.
- Follow up of patients 14 days after ART procedure to look for COVID-19 patients.
- Teleconsultations instead of direct interactions.
- Collaboration with nearby centers to refer patients in case own center gets closed due to any COVID-19 positive case detection or other emergencies.
- Adapt freeze all policy in suspected or COVID-19 positive patients during embryo culture.

(E) *Individualized treatment:*

- Individualized treatment.
- Telemedicine with avoidance of unnecessary visits.

- Provision of psychological counseling and education to couples as such patients are at increased risk of mental health deterioration and behavioral disorders during corona pandemic.

STUDIES DONE IN COVID-19 ERA

Orvieto et al.,[105] studied COVID-19 infection effect on IVF treatments in nine couples. They found that IVF treatment was resumed within 8–92 days after recovery from COVID-19 infection. All stimulation and embryological variables were similar before and after the infection with significantly lesser number of top-quality embryos recoveries. It is thereby suggested that IVF treatment should at least be delayed for 3 months after recovery from COVID-19 infection, so that recruitment of healthy gametes could occur.

Bhattacharya et al.,[106] used a prediction model to assess impact of COVID-19 infection on different age group women. It was noticed that older women with known cause of infertility had lesser live birth rates while couples with unexplained infertility even conceived naturally while waiting for the treatment.

Orvieto et al.,[107] assessed 36 couples who received IVF treatment within 7–85 days after receiving mRNA SARS-CoV-2 vaccine and concluded that the vaccine did not have any effect on either ovarian reserve or stimulation characteristics during the cycle.

KEY NOTES

- With recent evolution of various oral ovulogens, ovulation induction and superovulation has become easier and importance to occurrence of negligible or no complications is possible now.
- Concentration should be on the quality output and not only on quantity output so as to increase pregnancy rates.
- One size does not fit all. Our endeavor should be to customize the treatment as per our patient's individual needs.
- The goals of iCOS are to achieve optimum success, reduce complications like OHSS, and to achieve a singleton pregnancy.
- Recombinant versus urinary gonadotropin for ovarian stimulation in ART cycles: All available gonadotropins are equally effective and safe. The choice of the product will depend upon its availability, the convenience of its use, and the cost.[70]
- The short flare and the microdose flare GnRH agonist protocol can be used in patients with diminished ovarian reserve.
- The administration of GnRHa for a period of 3–6 months prior to IVF or ICSI in women with endometriosis increased the odds of clinical pregnancy by four-fold.[108]
- GnRH antagonists have rendered IVF, a patient friendly and safe procedure of high efficacy.
- One of the most important aspects of GnRH antagonist protocol is the option of triggering final oocyte maturation with GnRH agonist in high-responder patients, which thus helps in reducing the incidence of OHSS to practically zero.
- GnRH antagonists have stimulated thinking in developing new concepts in ovarian stimulation like modified natural cycle, mild IVF, agonist triggering, and cryopreservation of all 2PN oocytes, and re-initiation of antagonist in case of severe established OHSS.
- There was evidence of improved pregnancy outcomes with progestogen pretreatment and poorer pregnancy outcomes with a combined OCP pretreatment.[109]
- There was no evidence of a significant difference in pregnancy rates between natural cycle and standard IVF.[88]
- It is true that mild or minimal stimulation may not be the optimal treatment protocol for all patients but may be used in a certain group of patients like hyper-responders or in poor responders who have failed other treatments.
- Random start COS is as effective as conventional start COS in fertility preservation. This protocol would minimize delays and allow more patients to undergo fertility preservation and still proceed with cancer treatment within 2–3 weeks.
- COVID-19 era has impacted life of couples seeking treatment both physically and mentally. Future studies are required to understand the impact better.

REFERENCES

1. Baerwald AR, Adams GP, Pierson RA. Ovarian antral folliculogenesis during the human menstrual cycle: A review. Hum Reprod Update. 2012;18(1):73-91.
2. Santbrink EJV, Eijkemans MJ, Laven JSE, Fauser BCJM. Patient-tailored conventional ovulation induction algorithms in anovulatory infertility. Trends Endocrin Metab. 2005;16(8):381-9.
3. Oktem O, Urman B. Understanding follicle growth in vivo. Hum Reprod. 2010;25(12):2944-54.
4. Vegetti W, Alagna F. FSH and folliculogenesis: From physiology to ovarian stimulation. Reprod Biomed Online. 2006;12(6):684-94.
5. Balasch J, Fabregues F. LH in the follicular phase: Neither too high nor too low. Reprod Biomed Online. 2006;12(4): 406-15.
6. Ludwig M, Felberbaum RE, Diedrich K, Lunenfeld B. Ovarian stimulation: From basic science to clinical application. Reprod Biomed Online. 2002;5(Suppl. 1):73-86.
7. Derosa G, Maffioli P. Anti-obesity drugs: A review about their effects and their safety. Expert Opin Drug Saf. 2012;11(3): 459-71.
8. Homburg R, Insler V. Ovulation induction in perspective. Hum Reprod Update. 2002;8(5):449-62.
9. Macklon NS, Stouffer RL, Giudice LC, Fauser BC. The science behind 25 years of ovarian stimulation for in vitro fertilization. Endocr Rev. 2006;27:170-207.

10. ESHRE Capri Workshop Group. Mono-ovulatory cycles: A key goal in profertility programmes. Hum Reprod Update. 2003;9(3):263-74.
11. van Santbrink EJ, Fauser BC. Ovulation induction in normogonadotropic anovulation (PCOS). Best Pract Res Clin Endocrinol Metab. 2006;20(2):261-70.
12. ESHRE Capri Workshop Group. Health and fertility in World Health Organization group 2 anovulatory women. Hum Reprod Update. 2012;18(5):586-99.
13. Brown J, Farquhar C, Beck J, Boothroyd C, Hughes E. Clomiphene and anti- oestrogens for ovulation induction in PCOS. Cochrane Database Syst Rev. 2009;4:CD002249.
14. Kosmas IP, Tatsioni A, Fatemi HM, Kolibianakis EM, Tournaye H, Devroey P.. Human chorionic gonadotropin administration vs. luteinizing monitoring for intrauterine insemination timing, after administration of clomiphene citrate: a meta-analysis. Fertil Steril. 2007;87(3):607-12.
15. George K, George S, Chandy A, Raju R, Bala S. hCG administration offers no outcome benefit over spontaneous ovulation in anovulatory women treated with clomiphene citrate. Fertil Steril. 2007;87(4):985-7.
16. Goldstein SR, Siddhanti S, Ciaccia AV, Plouffe L. A pharmacological review of selective oestrogen receptor modulators. Hum Reprod Update. 2000;6(3):212-24.
17. Young SL, Opsahl MS, Fritz MA. Serum concentrations of enclomiphene and zuclomiphene across consecutive cycles of clomiphene citrate therapy in anovulatory infertile women. Fertil Steril. 1999;71:639-44.
18. Randall JM, Templeton A. Transvaginal sonographic assessment of follicular and endometrial growth in spontaneous and clomiphene citrate cycles. Fertil Steril. 1991;56:208-12.
19. Jirge PR, Patil RS. Comparison of endocrine and ultrasound profiles during ovulation induction with clomiphene citrate and letrozole in ovulatory volunteer women. Fertil Steril. 2010;93:174-83.
20. Eden JA, Place J, Carter GD, Jones J, Alaghband-Zadeh J, Pawson ME. The effect of clomiphene citrate on follicular phase increase in endometrial thickness and uterine volume. Obstet Gynecol. 1989;73:187-90.
21. Hughes E, Collins J, Vandekerckhove P. Clomiphene citrate for ovulation induction in women with oligo-amenorrhoea. Cochrane Database Syst Rev. 2000;(2):CD000056.
22. Sammour A, Biljan MM, Tan SL, Tulandi T. Prospective randomized trial comparing the effects of letrozole (LE) and clomiphene citrate (clomiphene citrate) on follicular development, endometrial thickness and pregnancy rate in patients undergoing super-ovulation prior to intrauterine insemination (IUI). Fertil Steril. 2001;76(Suppl 1):S110.
23. Badawy A, Elnashar A, Totongy M. Clomiphene citrate or aromatase inhibitors for superovulation in women with unexplained infertility undergoing intrauterine insemination: A prospective randomized trial. Fertil Steril. 2009;92:1355-9.
24. Mahani IM, Afnan M. The pregnancy rates with intrauterine insemination (IUI) in superovulated cycles employing different protocols (clomiphen citrate (CC), human menopausal gonadotropin (HMG) and HMG+CC) and in natural ovulatory cycle. J Pak Med Assoc. 2004;54:503-5.
25. Hammond MG, Halme JK, Talbert LM. Factors affecting the pregnancy rate in clomiphene citrate induction of ovulation. Obstet Gynecol. 1983;62(2):196-202.
26. Kousta E, White DM, Franks S. Modern use of clomiphene citrate in induction of ovulation. Hum Reprod Update. 1997;3(4):359-65.
27. Imani B, Eijkemans MJ, te Velde ER, Habbema JD, Fauser BC. Predictors of patients remaining anovulatory during clomiphene citrate induction of ovulation in normogonadotropic oligoamenorrheic infertility. J Clin Endocrinol Metab. 1998;83(7):2361-5.
28. Elnashar A, Abdelmageed E, Fayed M, Sharaf M. Clomiphene citrate and dexamethasone in treatment of clomiphene citrate resistant polycystic ovary syndrome: a prospective placebo-controlled study. Hum Reprod. 2006;21(7):1805-8.
29. Holzer H, Casper R, Tulandi T. A new era in ovulation induction. Fertil Steril. 2006;85(2);277-84.
30. Annapurna V, Dhaliwal LK, Gopalan S. Effect of two anti-estrogens, clomiphene citrate and tamoxifen, on cervical mucus and sperm-cervical mucus interaction. Int J Fertil Womens Med. 1997;42(3):215-8.
31. Boostanfar R, Jain JK, Mishell DR Jr, Paulson RJ. A prospective randomized trial comparing clomiphene citrate with tamoxifen citrate for ovulation induction. Fertil Steril. 2001;75(5):1024-6.
32. Franik S, Kremer JA, Nelen WL, Farquhar C. Aromatase inhibitors for subfertile women with polycystic ovary syndrome. Cochrane Database Syst Rev. 2014:CD010287.
33. Yasser E, Ibrahim F. Aromatase inhibitors in the treatment of male infertility. Human Androl. 2011;1(2):35-8.
34. Mitwally MF, Casper RF. Aromatase inhibition: a novel method of ovulation induction in women with polycystic ovary syndrome. Reprod Technol. 2000;10:244-7.
35. Bao SH, Sheng SL, Peng YF, Lin QD. Effects of letrozole and clomiphene citrate on the expression of HOXA10 and integrin alpha v beta 3 in uterine epithelium of rats. Fertil Steril. 2009;91:244-8.
36. Fisher SA, Reid RL, Van Vugt DA, Casper RF. A randomized double- blind comparison of the effects of clomiphene citrate and the aromatase inhibitor letrozole on ovulatory function in normal women. Fertil Steril. 2002;78(2):280-5.
37. Badawy A, Abdel Aal I, Abulatta M. Anastrozole or letrozole for ovulation induction in clomiphene resistant women with polycystic ovarian syndrome: A prospective randomized trial. Fertil Steril. 2008;89:1209-12.
38. Atay V, Cam C, Muchu M, Cam M, Karateke A. Comparison of letrozole and clomiphene citrate in women with polycystic ovaries undergoing ovarian stimulation. J Int Med Res. 2006;34:73-6.
39. Amer SA, Smith J, Mahran A, Fox P, Fakis A.. Double-blind randomized controlled trial of letrozole versus clomiphene citrate in subfertile women with polycystic ovarian syndrome. Hum Reprod. 2017;32(8):1631-8.
40. Legro RS, Brzyski RG, Diamond MP, Coutifaris C, Schlaff WD, Casson P, et al. Letrozole versus clomiphene for infertility in the polycystic ovary syndrome. N Engl J Med. 2014;371:119-29.
41. Geisler J, Haynes B, Anker G, Dowsett M, Lønning PE. Influence of letrozole and anastrozole on total body aromatization and plasma estrogen levels in postmenopausal breast cancer patients evaluated in a randomized, cross-over study. J Clin Oncol. 2002;20:751-7.
42. Mitwally MF, Casper RF. Aromatase inhibition reduces gonadotrophin dose required for controlled ovarian

stimulation in women with unexplained infertility. Hum Reprod. 2003;18(8):1588-97.

43. Palomba S, Orio F Jr, Zullo F. What is the best first-step therapeutic approach in treating anovulatory infertility in patients with polycystic ovary syndrome? Questions that are still unanswered. Gynecol Endocrinol. 2007;23: 245-7.
44. Mitwally MF, Biljan MM, Casper RF. Pregnancy outcome after the use of an aromatase inhibitor for ovarian stimulation. Am J Obstet Gynecol. 2005;192(2):381-6.
45. Sohrabvand F, Ansari Sh, Bagheri M. Efficacy of combined metformin-letrozole in comparison with metformin-clomiphene citrate in clomiphene-resistant infertile women with polycystic ovarian disease. Hum Reprod. 2006;21: 1432-5.
46. Thessaloniki ESHRE/ASRM-Sponsored PCOS Consensus Workshop Group. Consensus on infertility treatment related to polycystic ovary syndrome. Hum Reprod. 2008;23: 462-77.
47. Fields E, Chard J, James D, Treasure T; Guideline Development Group. Fertility (update): summary of NICE guidance. BMJ. 2013;346:f650.
48. Alverez C, Marti-Bonmati L, Novella-Maestre E, Sanz R, Gómez R, Fernández-Sánchez M, et al. Dopamine agonist cabergoline reduces hemoconcentration and ascites in hyperstimulated women undergoing assisted reproduction. J Clin Endocrinol Metab. 2007;92:2931-7.
49. Soares SR, Gomez R, Simon C, García-Velasco JA, Pellicer A. Targeting the vascular endothelial growth factor system to prevent ovarian hyperstimulation syndrome. Hum Reprod Update. 2008;14:321-33.
50. La Marca A, Sunkara SK. Individualization of controlled ovarian stimulation in IVF using ovarian reserve markers: from theory to practice. Hum Reprod Update. 2014;20(1): 124- 40.
51. Politi MC, Lewis CL, Frosch DL. Supporting shared decisions when clinical evidence is low. Med Care Res Rev. 2013;70(1 Suppl):113S-128S.
52. van Peperstraten AM, Hermens RP, Nelen WL, Stalmeier PF, Wetzels AM, Maas PH, et al. Deciding how many embryos to transfer after in vitro fertilisation: Development and pilot test of a decision aid. Patient Educ Couns. 2010;78(1): 124-9.
53. van Tilborg TC, Eijkemans MJ, Laven JS, Koks CA, de Bruin JP, Scheffer GJ, et al. The OPTIMIST study: optimisation of cost effectiveness through individualised FSH stimulation dosages for IVF treatment. A randomised controlled trial. BMC Womens Health. 2012;12:29.
54. Broer SL, Mol BW, Hendriks D, Broekmans FJ. The role of antimullerian hormone in prediction of outcome after IVF: comparison with the antral follicle count. Fertil Steril. 2009;91:705-14.
55. Broekmans FJ, Kwee J, Hendriks DJ, Mol BW, Lambalk CB. A systematic review of tests predicting ovarian reserve and IVF outcome. Hum Reprod Update. 2006;12:685-718.
56. Nargund G, Fauser BCM, Macklon NS. The Rotterdam ISMAAR Consensus Group on Terminology for Ovarian Stimulation for IVF. The ISMAAR proposal on terminology for ovarian stimulation for IVF. Hum Reprod. 2007;22: 2801-4.
57. Nargund G. ISMAAR: The International Society for Mild Approaches in Assisted Reproduction. Facts Views Vis Obgyn. 2011;3(1):5-7.
58. Sunkara SK, Rittenberg V, Raine-Fenning N, Bhattacharya S, Zamora J, Coomarasamy A.. Association between the number of eggs and live birth in IVF treatment: an analysis of 400 135 treatment cycles. Hum Reprod. 2011;26(7): 1768-74.
59. Hamoda H, Sunkara S, Khalaf Y, Braude P, El-Toukhy T. Outcome of fresh IVF/ ICSI cycles in relation to the number of oocytes collected: A review of 4,701 treatment cycles. Hum Reprod. 2010;25:147.
60. Ferraretti AP, La Marca A, Fauser BC, Tarlatzis B, Nargund G, Gianaroli L; ESHRE working group on Poor Ovarian Response Definition: ESHRE consensus on the definition of 'poor response' to ovarian stimulation for in vitro fertilization: the Bologna criteria. Hum Reprod. 2011;26(7):10.
61. Younis JS, Ben-Ami M, Ben-Shlomo I. The Bologna criteria for poor ovarian response: a contemporary critical appraisal. J Ovarian Res. 2015;8:10.
62. Alviggi C, Andersen CY, Buehler K, Conforti A, De Placido G, Esteves SC, et al. Poseidon Group Patient-Oriented Strategies Encompassing IndividualizeD Oocyte Number, A new more detailed stratification of low responders to ovarian stimulation: from a poor ovarian response to a low prognosis concept. Fertil Steril. 2016;105(6):10.
63. Sunkara SK, Pundir J, Khalaf Y. Effect of androgen supplementation or modulation on ovarian stimulation outcome in poor responders: A meta-analysis. Reprod Biomed Online. 2011;22:545-55.
64. Bosdou JK, Venetis CA, Kolibianakis EM, Toulis KA, Goulis DG, Zepiridis L, et al. The use of androgens or androgen modulating agents in poor responders undergoing in vitro fertilization: a systematic review and meta-analysis. Hum Reprod Update. 2012;18(2):127-45.
65. Duffy JMN, Ahmad G, Mohiyiddeen L, Nardo LG, Watson A. Growth hormone for in vitro fertilization (Review). Cochrane Database Syst Rev. 2010;(1):CD000099.
66. Tso LO, Costello MF, Albuquerque LET, Andriolo RB, Macedo CR. Metformin treatment before and during IVF or ICSI in women with polycystic ovary syndrome. Cochrane Database Syst Rev. 2014;(11): CD006105.
67. Practice Committee of American Society for Reproductive Medicine. Gonadotropin preparations: past, present, and future perspectives. Fertil Steril. 2008;90(5 Suppl): S13-20.
68. Platteau P, Andersen AN, Loft A, Smitz J, Danglas P, Devroey P. Highly purified HMG versus recombinant FSH for ovarian stimulation in IVF cycles. Reprod Biomed Online. 2008;17(2):190-8.
69. Devroey P, Boostanfar R, Koper NP, Mannaerts BM, Ijzerman-Boon PC, Fauser BC; A double-blind, non-inferiority RCT comparing corifollitropin alfa and recombinant FSH during the first seven days of ovarian stimulation using a GnRH antagonist protocol. Hum Reprod. 2009;24(12): 3063-72.
70. van Wely M, Kwan I, Burt AL, Thomas J, Vail A, Van der Veen F, et al. Recombinant versus urinary gonadotrophin for ovarian stimulation in assisted reproductive technology cycles. Cochrane Database Syst Rev. 2011;(2):CD005354.

71. Janssens RM, Lambalk CB, Vermeiden JP, Schats R, Bernards JM, Rekers-Mombarg LT, et al. Dose-finding study of triptorelin acetate for prevention of a premature LH surge in IVF: a prospective, randomised, double-blind, placebo-controlled study. Hum Reprod. 2000;15:2333-40.
72. Albuquerque TE, Tso LO, Saconato H, Albuquerque MC, Macedo CR. Depot versus daily administration of gonadotrophin-releasing hormone agonist protocols for pituitary down regulation in assisted reproduction cycles. Cochrane Database Syst Rev. 2013;2013(1): CD002808. Cochrane Database Syst Rev. 2013 Jan 31;2013(1): CD002808.
73. Maheshwari A, Gibreel A, Siristatidis CS, Bhattacharya S. Gonadotrophin- releasing hormone agonist protocols for pituitary suppression in assisted reproduction. Cochrane Database Syst Rev. 2011;(8):CD006919.
74. Coomarasamy A, Afnan M, Cheema D, van der Veen F, Bossuyt PM, van Wely M. Urinary hMG versus recombinant FSH for controlled ovarian hyperstimulation following an agonist long down-regulation protocol in IVF or ICSI treatment: a systematic review and meta-analysis. Hum Reprod. 2008; 23(2):310-5.
75. Berkkanoglu M, Ozgur K. What is the optimum maximal gonadotropin dosage used in microdose flare-up cycles in poor responders? Fertil Steril. 2010;94(2):662-5.
76. Sunkara SK, Coomarasamy A, Faris R, Braude P, Khalaf Y. Long gonadotropin-releasing hormone agonist versus short agonist versus antagonist regimens in poor responders undergoing in vitro fertilization: a randomized controlled trial. Fertil Steril. 2014;101(1):147-53.
77. Balasch J, Howles CM. GnRH agonist protocols: which one to use? In: Shoham Z, Howles CM, Jacobs JS (Eds). Female Infertility Therapy: Current Practice. London: Martin Duntiz; 1999. pp. 189-201.
78. Lahat E, Raziel A, Friedler S, Schieber-Kazir M, Ron-El R. L et al. Long-term follow-up of children born after inadvertent administration of a gonadotrophin-releasing hormone agonist in early pregnancy. Hum Reprod. 1999;14: 2656-60.
79. Al-Inany, Aboulghar M, Mansour RT, Serour GI. Optimizing GnRH antagonist administration: Meta-analysis of fixed versus flexible protocol. Reprod Biomed Online. 2005;10(5): 567-70.
80. Al-Inany HG, Youssef MA, Aboulghar M, Broekmans F, Sterrenburg M, Smit J, et al. Gonadotropin- releasing hormone antagonists for assisted reproductive technology. Cochrane Database Syst Rev. 2011;(5):CD001750.
81. Olivennes F, Fanchin R, Bouchard P, Taïeb J, Selva J, Frydman R. Scheduled administration of a gonadotrophin-releasing hormone antagonist (Cetrorelix) on day 8 of in vitro fetrilization cycles: A pilot study. Hum Reprod. 1995;10(6): 1382-6.
82. Al-Inany HG, Abou-Setta AM, Aboulghar M. Gonadotropin-releasing hormone antagonists for assisted conception. Cochrane Database Syst Rev. 2006;(3):CD001750.
83. Orvieto R, Patrizio P. GnRH agonist versus GnRH antagonist in ovarian stimulation: an ongoing debate. Reprod Biomed Online. 2013;26(1):4-8.
84. Youssef MAFM, Al-Inany HG, Aboulghar M, Mansour R, Abou-Setta AM. Recombinant versus urinary human chorionic gonadotrophin for final oocyte maturation triggering in IVF and ICSI cycles. Cochrane Database Syst Rev. 2011;(4): CD003719..
85. Griesinger G, Diedrich K, Devroey P, Kolibianakis EM. GnRH agonist for triggering final oocyte maturation in the GnRH antagonist ovarian hyperstimulation protocol: A systematic review and meta-analysis. Hum Reprod Update. 2006;12(2):159-68.
86. Griesinger G, Berndt H, Schultz L, Depenbusch M, Schultze-Mosgau A. Cumulative live birth rates after GnRH agonist triggering of final oocyte maturation in patients at risk of OHSS: A prospective clinical cohort study. Eur J Obstet Gynecol Reprod Biol. 2010;149(2):190-4.
87. Youssef MAFM, Van der Veen F, Al-Inany HG, Mochtar MH, Griesinger G, Nagi Mohesen M, et al. Gonadotropin-releasing hormone agonist versus HCG for oocyte triggering in antagonist assisted reproductive technology. Cochrane Database Syst Rev. 2014;(10): CD008046.
88. Allersma T, Farquhar C, Cantineau AE. Natural cycle in vitro fertilisation (IVF) for subfertile couples. Cochrane Database Syst Rev. 2013;8:CD010550.
89. Nargund G, Fauser BC, Macklon NS, Ombelet W, Nygren K, Frydman R; Rotterdam ISMAAR Consensus Group on Terminology for Ovarian Stimulation for IVF. The ISMAAR proposal on terminology for ovarian stimulation for IVF. Hum Reprod. 2007;22(11):2801-4.
90. Pelinck MJ, Hoek A, Simons AHM, Heineman MJ. Efficacy of natural cycle IVF: a review of the literature. Hum Reprod Update 2002;8:129-39.
91. Feldman B, Seidman DS, Levron J, Bider D, Shulman A, Shine S, Dor J. In vitro fertilization following natural cycles in poor responders. Gynecol Endocrinol 2001;15:328-34.
92. Fauser BC, Nargund G, Andersen AN, Norman R, Tarlatzis B, Boivin J, et al. Mild ovarian stimulation for IVF: 10 years later. Hum Reprod. 2010;25: 2678-84.
93. Baart EB, Martini E, Eijkemans MJ, Van Opstal D, Beckers NG, Verhoeff A, et al. Milder ovarian stimulation for in-vitro fertilization reduces aneuploidy in the human preimplantation embryo: a randomized controlled trial. Hum Reprod. 2007;22(4):980-8.
94. Teramoto S, Kato O. Minimal ovarian stimulation with clomiphene citrate: A large- scale retrospective study. Reprod Biomed Online. 2007;15(2):134-48.
95. Checa MA, Robles A. The effects of letrozole on ovarian stimulation for fertility preservation in cancer affected women. Reprod Biomed Online. 2012;24(6):606-10.
96. Kuang Y, Chen Q, Hong Q, Lyu Q, Ai A, Fu Y, et al. Double stimulations during the follicular and luteal phases of poor responders in IVF/ ICSI programmes (Shanghai protocol). Reprod Biomed Online. 2014;29:684-91.
97. Moffat R, Pirtea P, Gayet V, Wolf JP, Chapron C, de Ziegler D. Dual ovarian stimulation is a new viable option for enhancing the oocyte yield when the time for assisted reproductive technology is limited. Reprod Biomed Online. 2014;29: 659-61.
98. Ghasemzadeh A, Dopour Faliz M, Farzadi L, Navali N, Bahramzadeh B, Fadavi A, et al. Effect of oral utrogestan in comparison with cetrotide on preventing luteinizing hormone surge in IVF cycles: A randomized controlled trial. Int J Reprod Biomed. 2019;18:41-6.

99. Guan S, Feng Y, Huang Y, Huang J. Progestin-primed ovarian stimulation protocol for patients in assisted reproductive technology: A meta-analysis of randomized controlled trials. Front Endocrinol. 2021;12:702558.
100. Alexandru P, Cekic SG, Yildiz S, Turkgeldi E, Ata B. Progestins versuss GnRH analogues for pituitary suppression during ovarian stimulation for assisted reproductive technology: a systematic review and meta-analysis. Reprod BioMed Online. 2020;40:894-903.
101. Kuang Y, Chen Q, Fu Y, Wang Y, Hong Q, Lyu Q, et al. Medroxyprogesterone acetate is an effective oral alternative for preventing premature luteinizing hormone surges in women undergoing controlled ovarian hyperstimulation for in vitro fertilization. Fertil Steril. 2015;104:62-70.e63.
102. Huang JY, XieQ, Lin JY, LuXF, WangNL, GaoHY, et al. Neonatal outcomes and congenital malformations in children born after dydrogesterone application in progestin-primed ovarian stimulation protocol for IVF: A retrospective cohort study. Drug Des Dev Ther. 2019;13:2553-63.
103. Massin N. New stimulation regimens: Endogenous and exogenous progesterone use to block the LH surge during ovarian stimulation for IVF. Hum Reprod Update (2017) 23:211-20.
104. ICMR (2021). ICMR Guidelines 2021. [online] Available from https://main.icmr.nic.in/content/guidelines. [Accessed November, 2022].
105. Orvieto R, Segev-Zahav A, Aizer A. Does COVID-19 infection influence patients' performance during IVF-ET cycle?: an observational study. Gynecol Endocrinol. 2021;37(10): 895-7.
106. Bhattacharya S, Maheshwari A, Ratna MB, van Eekelen R, Mol BW, McLernon DJ. Prioritizing IVF treatment in the post-COVID 19 era: A predictive modeling study based on UK national data. Hum Reprod. 2021;36(3):666-75.
107. Orvieto R, Noach-Hirsh M, Segev-Zahav A, Haas J, Nahum R, Aizer A. Does mRNA SARS-CoV-2 vaccine influence patients' performance during IVF-ET cycle? Reprod Biol Endocrinol. 2021;19(1):69.
108. Sallam HN, Garcia-Velasco JA, Dias S, Arici A. Long-term pituitary down-regulation before in vitro fertilization (IVF) for women with endometriosis. Cochrane Database Syst Rev. 2006;2006(1):CD004635.
109. Smulders B, van Oirschot SM, Farquhar C, Rombauts L, Kremer JA. Oral contraceptive pill, progestogen or estrogen pre-treatment for ovarian stimulation protocols for women undergoing assisted reproductive techniques. Cochrane Database Syst Rev. 2010;(1):CD006109.

CHAPTER 48

Role of Adjuvants in Ovarian Stimulation

Mirudhubashini Govindarajan, Ramya Jayaram

INTRODUCTION

Controlled ovarian stimulation (COS) is the principal step of current assisted reproductive technology (ART) procedures. Gonadotropins are administered in ART in order to maximize the number of good quality oocytes obtained. Along with gonadotropins gonadotropin-releasing hormone (GnRH) analogs are used to prevent unwarranted luteinizing hormone (LH) surge during COS. In some women, the response to standard stimulation is abnormal, either poor response yielding very few or poor quality oocytes or very high, leading to ovarian hyperstimulation syndrome (OHSS). In order to optimize these adverse outcomes, various add-ons have been proposed. Adjuvants have been clinically used in poor responders to improve the number and quality of oocytes, and in hyper-responders to lessen the chances of hyperstimulation.

ADJUVANTS FOR OVARIAN STIMULATION IN POOR RESPONDERS

A poor responder is generally identified by factors such as age, abnormal ovarian response tests [anti-Müllerian hormone (AMH) and antral follicle counts (AFC)], previous ovarian surgery, and endometriosis. Poor ovarian response (POR) is still one of the major challenges in controlled ovarian hyperstimulation (COH). Incidence of POR is reported to range from 5.6 to 35.1% (Jenkins et al. 1991). "Bologna" criteria were proposed by The European Society of Human Reproduction and Embryology (ESHRE) in 2011 (Ferraretti and Gianaroli) to define poor responders. Humaidan et al. have modified and subclassified POR into "POSEIDON" (Patient-Oriented Strategies Encompassing Individualized Oocyte Number) subgroups in 2016. POSEIDON subgroups I and II are basically women with normal ovarian reserve and are more likely to respond to modifications in the stimulation protocols. POSEIDON subgroups III and IV have abnormal ovarian reserve tests and are less likely to respond. Numerous adjuvants have been tried in poor responders over the last few years to potentially optimize the quality and quantity of oocytes and thereby improve the pregnancy rates. However, majority of published studies so far have not classified their patients according to POSEIDON subgroups.

Growth Hormone

Probable Mode of Action

- Growth hormone (GH) enhances ovarian response to follicle-stimulating hormone (FSH) and thereby stimulates ovarian steroidogenesis and follicular development. This hypothesis was proposed as early as 1986.[1]
- GH and its intermediary insulin-like growth factor-1 (IGF-1) promote the health and proliferation of granulosa cells which are critical to the nourishment and health of the oocyte.[2]
- Both IGF-1 and IGF-2 are present in the follicular fluid and are believed to play a crucial role in cytoplasmic maturation and in potentiating the actions of FSH.[3,4]

Literature Evidence

- 2010 Cochrane review indicated that the addition of GH in ovarian stimulation of poor responders resulted in statistically significant difference in both live birth rates (25 vs. 8%) and pregnancy rates without increasing the adverse events. However, the results of this review needs to be interpreted with caution as the number of included trials were few and the sample size was small.[5]
- Meta-analysis by De Ziegler also concluded that GH supplementation improved pregnancy and live birth rates by threefold to fourfold, but did not increase the number of oocytes.[6,7]
- Network meta-analysis and systematic review published in Human Reproduction Update in 2020 by Zhang et al. shows that adjuvant treatment with GH was the optimal strategy in terms of outcome measures, i.e., oocyte and embryo numbers.

Dosage and Timing

- There is no consensus between majority of studies on the dosage and the timing of GH administration.[8]
- GH was started concomitantly with gonadotropins in most of the studies. In a study by Kucuk et al.,[9] it was initiated on day 21 of the previous cycle.

Conclusion

Current network meta-analysis suggests that the response to GH addition appears to be beneficial;[10,11] however, it may vary in different subgroups. Much larger studies may be necessary to accurately determine the treatment effect on different subgroups before recommending the *routine* use of GH in *all* poor responders undergoing *in vitro* fertilization (IVF).

Androgens and Androgenic Drugs

Testosterone

Mode of action:

- Testosterone (T) increases both antral follicle numbers and granulosa cell proliferation. It also reduces apoptosis in subhuman primates.
- Androgens act directly via the androgen receptors. Androgen receptor messenger ribonucleic acid (RNA) correlates positively with granulosa cell proliferation and negatively with granulosa cell apoptosis.[12]
- Androgens also have an indirect effect by their conversion to estrogens and 3-beta-diol that can activate the estrogen receptor.
- Testosterone has been shown to cause a marked increase of ovarian response in women who had a consistently poor response to repeated ovarian stimulation for IVF.[13]

Literature evidence:

- Testosterone increases follicular response by increasing FSH-receptor activity and by stimulating IGF-1.[14]
- Application of transdermal testosterone resulted in a significant improvement in number of follicles recruited, oocytes retrieved, implantation rates, clinical pregnancy rates, and a decrease in cycle cancellation rates.[15,16]
- Two meta-analyses showed that the transdermal testosterone significantly reduced the doses of FSH required and increased live birth rate.[16,17]
- Meta-analyses by Sunkara et al. however did not find the available evidence on androgens sufficient enough to support the use of androgen supplementation to improve live birth outcome in poor responders undergoing ART.[18]
- Current network meta-analysis by Zhang et al. using exogenous androgens [dehydroepiandrosterone (DHEA) and transdermal testosterone] had demonstrated beneficial effects. DHEA had the best clinical pregnancy rates while testosterone produced the highest numbers of embryos.

Conclusion: More evidence from randomized controlled trials (RCTs) with large sample size is required before advocating the *routine* use of testosterone in *all* poor responders.

Dehydroepiandrosterone

Mode of action:

- Oral DHEA has been used to increase ovarian androgens and thereby the ovarian response in poor responders. DHEA is the prohormone for follicular fluid testosterone. Circulating DHEA levels decrease by about 50% between ages 25 years and 45 years. 50% of follicular fluid testosterone is derived from circulating DHEA. Both serum testosterone levels and number of oocytes retrieved decrease with age. Using multivariate analysis, baseline testosterone levels were found to independently correlate positively with the number of oocytes retrieved.[19]
- Casson et al. in 2000 were the first to report positive effect on supplementation of DHEA in women with diminished ovarian reserve.[20]

Literature evidence:

- In a study using the patient's prior cycles as their own controls, the number of oocytes retrieved increased significantly from 3.4 to 4.4 after an average of 4 months of 25 mg three times daily of oral DHEA.[21]
- In a prospective randomized study, Wiser et al. found significantly increased live birth rates (23.1 vs. 4.0%) in patients with diminished ovarian reserve on DHEA supplementation. This study was criticized for severe methodological and statistical problems.[22]
- However, two meta-analyses[16,17] found no significant difference in clinical pregnancy and live birth rates between patients who received DHEA and those who did not, deserving further evidence.

Conclusion: In the current meta-analysis, adjuvant treatment using exogenous androgens (DHEA or transdermal testosterone) had beneficial effects. DHEA resulted in the best clinical pregnancy rate, and testosterone produced the highest number of embryos. Pretreatment with transdermal DHEA or testosterone has been proposed as a safe and effective means to increase the concentration of intraovarian androgens (Balasch et al., 2006; Casson et al., 2000). Theoretically, intraovarian androgens promote cellular sensitivity to FSH in growing follicles (Hillier and De Zwart, 1981; Vendola et al., 1998) and may thereby increase oocyte yield and oocyte maturity during ovarian stimulation, subsequently improving the pregnancy rate. Although estradiol levels on the human chorionic gonadotropin (hCG) day were low in the DHEA groups, the clinical pregnancy rate was highest, and the cycle cancelation rate was lowest. A previous meta-analysis review demonstrated that pretreatment with transdermal testosterone, but not DHEA, increased clinical pregnancy and live birth rates (Bosdou et al., 2012). Two papers included in the present review showed that testosterone significantly increased clinical pregnancy rates, although only DHEA had a better prospect for improving pregnancy probability.

Human Chorionic Gonadotropin-recombinant Luteinizing Hormone

Human chorionic gonadotropin and recombinant luteinizing hormone (rLH) have long been used as adjuvant agents for increasing the production of endogenous intraovarian androgens (through the addition of LH activity). In the only eligible study in the present network meta-analysis, hCG obtained the highest number of retrieved oocytes. However, neither rLH nor hCG was associated with better clinical outcomes, including the clinical pregnancy rate, the number of embryos, and the cycle cancelation rates. These results are consistent with those of several previous meta-analyses (Bosdou et al., 2012; Gizzo et al., 2015), although the RCTs included in those meta-analyses were very different. However, these results are inconsistent with the results obtained from studies on exogenous androgens (transdermal testosterone and DHEA). This inconsistency may be because the two different interventions have overall differential effects or because different adjuvant agents act through different molecular mechanisms.

Coenzyme Q

Coenzyme Q (CoQ) data is available from only one study, which has claimed that the addition of CoQ10 may have a beneficial effect on the ovarian response (Xu et al., 2018). In the current network meta-analysis, CoQ10 treatment had the lowest cycle cancelation rate and achieved the second highest clinical pregnancy rate, indicating that the prospects are possibly good for using CoQ10 in POR. However, these results need to be confirmed in further prospective studies.

Letrozole/Clomiphene as Adjuvants

Mild COS protocols combining clomiphene or letrozole with gonadotropins have been implemented as an effective alternative for conventional COS, in normal responders swell as in POR (Verberg et al., 2009). Clomiphene acts by blocking hypothalamic estrogen receptors, thereby blocking the negative feedback effect of circulating endogenous estrogen and subsequently increasing the release of GnRH, FSH, and LH (Dickey and Holtkamp, 1996). Letrozole reversibly binds and prevents aromatase from producing estrogens. With the growing demand for patient-friendly COS protocols for ART, there is a valid interest in milder protocols involving the addition of clomiphene or letrozole to COS with the aim of retrieving fewer and better quality oocytes without compromising endometrial receptivity. Based on the results in some meta-analysis earlier, a mild ovarian stimulation strategy involving clomiphene or letrozole addition obtained pregnancy outcomes similar to those of conventional COS protocols[23] (Bosdou et al., 2012; Song et al., 2016).

In the current network meta-analysis, although there were no significant differences compared with the control group, surface under the cumulative ranking curve (SUCRA) values showed that cotreatment using clomiphene or letrozole with gonadotropin, especially clomiphene, led to the worst clinical outcomes, including the lowest pregnancy rates, the lowest oocyte numbers, the lowest embryo numbers, and the highest cycle cancelation rates. Therefore, using clomiphene or letrozole for mild stimulation regimens as the first-line adjuvant treatment for patients with POR cannot be recommended.

Estrogens and Oral Contraceptives

Adjuvant hormonal drugs such as oral contraceptive pills (OCPs) and estrogens have been used for synchronization of follicular growth in poor responders. They are also utilized for scheduling of the ART cycles. The increased homogeneity of the follicular cohort induced by steroid pretreatment is thought to improve the synchrony of follicular growth during stimulation. This can result in an increase in both oocyte yield and gamete quality leading to an increase in pregnancy rates.[24]

Estrogen Pretreatment

Oral estrogen has been used to schedule ovarian stimulation cycles using 4 mg daily of estradiol-valerate beginning in the midluteal phase of the previous menstrual cycle. Ovarian stimulation was started on the day following discontinuation of estrogen.[25] No adverse events have been noted with usage of estrogen for cycle programming.

Previous studies have proposed that luteal phase estradiol priming may improve the synchronization of the pool of follicles available for COS, resulting in more favorable responses to COS (Fanchin et al., 2003, Fanchin et al., 2003b). In the current network meta-analysis, estradiol pretreatment increased the oocyte number significantly. As only one RCT was included in the present network meta-analysis, more rigorous RCT studies are still needed to determine whether adjuvant treatment with estrogen is beneficial.

Combined Oral Contraceptive Pills Pretreatment

Mode of action: Combined oral contraceptive (COC) pills suppress endogenous gonadotropins. COC when given prior to ovarian stimulation aids in synchronization of follicular development, reduces cyst formation, prevents spontaneous LH surge, and shortens the length of GnRH analog treatment.[26]

Literature evidence:

- Cochrane review on COC treatment prior to antagonist protocol for ovarian stimulation in unsegregated patients found fewer clinical pregnancies and higher amount of total gonadotropin dosage.[27]
- Some studies have found an increase in the miscarriage rates in antagonist cycles using OCP pretreatment.[28]

Conclusion: Combined oral contraceptives and estrogens are commonly used agents for programming ART cycles and obtaining uniform cohort of follicles. Decreased pregnancy rates and increased miscarriage rates have been noted with usage of OCPs in some studies. No adverse outcomes have been noted with usage of estrogens for programming.

ADJUVANTS FOR HYPER-RESPONDERS

Women with polycystic ovary syndrome (PCOS) are hyperinsulinemic with a large number of antral follicles, and higher incidence of OHSS when exposed to conventional protocols.

Metformin

- The use of metformin in PCOS improves insulin resistance and intraovarian hyperandrogenism thereby reducing the risk of OHSS. Meta-analysis of five RCTs with adjunctive use of metformin in PCOS have shown a dramatic reduction in OHSS [odds ratio (OR) 0.21, confidence interval (CI) 0.11-0.41, $p < 0.00001$).[29]
- Metformin appears to improve the odds of pregnancy in women with PCOS undergoing ovarian stimulation. Meta-analysis of 17 RCTs has shown both increased ovulation (OR 4.39, CI 1.94–9.96) and pregnancy rates (OR 2.67, CI 1.54–4.94) when metformin was added to clomiphene citrate. This effect of metformin was found to be statistically significant in obese women with PCOS (OR 10.9), whereas it failed to reach significance in nonobese PCOS women.[30]
- Palomba et al. conducted a randomized, double blind, placebo-controlled trial with metformin supplementation in patients who had previous cancelled IVF cycles due to a high risk of OHSS. The incidence of OHSS was significantly reduced by approximately 70% [relative risk (RR 2.9)] with a number needed to treat (NNT) of 5.[31]
- Metformin has also been associated with an improved pregnancy rate in PCOS women undergoing ART.[32,33] However when all RCTs were combined, the increase in pregnancy rate (29%) was not statistically significant.[33]

ADJUVANTS TO ORAL OVULOGENS

Dexamethasone

- Dexamethasone was found to improve response to ovarian stimulation when combined with clomiphene citrate. An RCT showed a higher rate of ovulation with clomiphene citrate when 0.5 mg of dexamethasone was given continuously.[34]
- In another two RCTs where women failed to ovulate with up to 150–250 mg of clomiphene citrate, adjunctive use of dexamethasone increased ovulation rate by 4–5-fold and pregnancy rate by 8–10-fold. In these studies, a higher dose of 2 mg of dexamethasone was given, but only during the 5 days of clomiphene citrate and for the following 5 days.[35,36]

Dexamethasone may enhance ovulation in situations of clomiphene citrate resistance in ovulation induction.

Conclusion

All adjuvant treatment groups used a lower dosage of gonadotropin for ovarian stimulation. Studies have shown that a higher dosage of FSH has a detrimental effect on egg and oocyte quality, increasing the incidence of chromosomaly abnormal embryos and significantly decreasing live birth rates (Baart et al., 2007). Moreover, a higher dosage of gonadotropins may increase the total consumption of ovarian follicles, which is not beneficial for patients with POR. Indeed, clinical studies have confirmed that higher dosages of FSH resulted in an increased number of follicle recruitments but low-quality embryos (Hohmann et al., 2003). The optimal COS protocol for patients with POR is most likely supplementation with appropriate adjuvant agents to improve clinical outcomes rather than simply increasing the FSH dosage.

Based on the available evidence, for patients with POR, COS protocols that used adjuvant treatment with DHEA, CoQ10, and GH produced better clinical outcomes in terms of pregnancy. A lower dosage of gonadotropin was required for ovulation induction than what was used in the control group. Adjuvant treatment using clomiphene led to the lowest pregnancy rates, even though the total dosage of gonadotropins was the most economical.

KEY POINTS

- Aggressive COS with higher dosage of gonadotropins in POR is associated with a variety of side effects, higher costs, and is less likely to succeed (Kailasam et al. 2004; Cheung et al. 2005). Higher dosage of FSH has detrimental effects on egg and oocyte quality, increasing the incidence of abnormal embryos and significantly decreasing live birth rates (Baart et al., 2007).
- Efficacy of natural cycle or minimal stimulation IVF for POR is also disappointing because of high cancellation rates.

- All adjuvant treatment groups use a lower dosage of gonadotropin for ovarian stimulation. The optimal COS protocol for patients with POR is most likely supplementation with appropriate adjuvant agents to improve clinical outcomes rather than just increasing the FSH dosage.
- Based on the available evidence, in poor responders, adjuvant treatment with DHEA, CoQ10, and GH produced better clinical outcomes in terms of pregnancy (OR 2.46, 95% CI 1.16–5.23) Zhang et al. HR update 2020.[37]
- CoQ10 supplementation resulted in lowest cancellation rates.

REFERENCES

1. Jia N, Kalmijn J, Hseuh A. Growth hormone enhances FSH induced differentiation of cultured rat granulosa cells. Endocrinology. 1986;118:1401-9.
2. Bencomo E, Perez R, Arteaga MF, Acosta E, Peña O, Lopez L, et al. Apoptosis of cultured granulosa-lutein cells is reduced by insulin-like growth factor I and may correlate with embryo fragmentation and pregnancy rate. Fertil Steril. 2006;85:474-80.
3. Fraser HM. Regulation of ovarian follicular vasculature. Reprod Biol Endocrinol. 2006;4:18.
4. Adashi EY, Resnick CE, Hurwitz A, Ricciarelli E, Hernandez ER, Roberts CT, et al. Insulin-like growth factors: the ovarian connection. Hum Reprod. 1991;6:1213-9.
5. Ahmad G, Brown J, Duffy JM. Growth hormone for *in vitro* fertilization. Cochrane Database Syst Rev. 2010;(4):CD000099.
6. de Zeigler D, Streuli I, Meldrum DR, Chapron C. The value of growth hormone supplements in ART for poor ovarian responders. Fertil Steril. 2011;96:1069-76.
7. Kolibiniakis EM, Veneti CA, Diedric K, Tarlatzis BC, Griesinger G. Addition of growth hormone to gonadotropins in ovarian stimulation of poor responders treated by *in vitro* fertilization: a systematic review and meta-analysis. Hum Reprod Update. 2009;15(6):613-22.
8. Kyrou D, Kolibianakis EM, Venetis CA, Papanikolaou EG, Bontis J, Tarlatzis BC. How to improve the probability of pregnancy in poor responders undergoing *in vitro* fertilization: a systematic review and meta-analysis. Fertil Steril. 2009;91:749-6.
9. Kucuk T, Kozinoglu H, Kaba A. Growth hormone co-treatment within a GnRH agonist long protocol in patients with poor ovarian response: a prospective, randomized, clinical trial. J Assist Reprod Genet. 2008;25:123-7.
10. Delitala G, Tomasi P, Virdis R. Neuroendocrine regulation of human growth hormone secretion. Diagnostic and clinical applications. J Endocrinol Invest. 1988;11:441-62.
11. Kim CH, Chae HD, Chang YS. Pyridostigmine co-treatment for controlled ovarian hyperstimulation in low responders undergoing *in vitro* fertilization-embryo transfer. Fertil Steril. 1999;71:652-7.
12. Vendola KA, Zhou J, Adesanya OO, Weil SJ, Bondy CA. Androgens stimulate early stages of follicular growth in the primate ovary. J Clin Invest. 1988;101:2622-9.
13. Balasch J, Fabregues F, Penarrubia J, Carmona F, Casamitjana R, Creus M, et al. Pre-treatment with transdermal testosterone may improve ovarian response to gonadotropins in poor-responder IVF patients with normal basal concentration of FSH. Hum Reprod. 2006;21:1884-93.
14. Nielsen ME, Rasmussen RA, Kristensen SG, Christensen ST, Møllgård K, Andersen EW, et al. In human granulosa cells from small antral follicles, androgen receptor mRNA and androgen levels in follicular fluid correlate with FSH receptor mRNA. Mol Hum Reprod. 2011;17:63-70.
15. Kim CH, Howles CM, Lee HH. The effect of transdermal testosterone gel pre-treatment on controlled ovarian stimulation and IVF outcome in low responders. Fertil Steril. 2011;95:679-83.
16. Gonzalez-Comadran M, Duran M, Sola I, Fabregues F, Carreras R, Checa MA. Effects of transdermal testosterone in poor responders undergoing IVF: systematic review and meta-analysis. 2012;25:450-9.
17. Bosdo JK, Venetis CA, Kolibianakis EM, Toulis KA, Goulis DG, Zepiridis L, et al. The use of androgens or androgen-modulating agents in poor responders undergoing *in vitro* fertilization: a systematic review and meta-analysis. Hum Reprod Update. 2012;18(2):127-45.
18. Sunkara SK, Pundir J, Khala Y. Effect of androgen supplementation or modulation on ovarian stimulation outcome in poor responders: a meta-analysis. Reprod Biomed Online. 2011;22:545-55.
19. Frattarelli JL, Gerber MD. Basal and cycle androgen levels correlate with *in vitro* fertilization stimulation parameters but do not predict pregnancy outcome. Fertil Steril. 2006;86:51-7.
20. Casson PR, Lindsay MS, Pisarska MD, Carson SA, Buster JE. DHEA supplementation augments ovarian stimulation in poor responders: a case series. Hum Reprod. 2000;15(10): 2129-32.
21. Barad D, Gleicher N. Effect of dehydroepiandrosterone on oocyte and embryo yields, embryo grade and cell number in IVF. Hum Reprod. 2006;21:2845-9.
22. Wiser A, Gonen O, Ghetler Y, Shavit T, Berkovitz A, Shulman A. Addition of dehydroepiandrosterone (DHEA) for poor responder patients before and during IVF treatment improves the pregnancy rate: a randomized prospective study. Hum Reprod. 2010;25(10):2496-500.
23. Goswami SK, Das T, Chattopadhyay R, Sawhney V, Kumar J, Chaudhury K, et al. A randomized single-blind controlled trial of letrozole as a low-cost IVF protocol in women with poor ovarian response: a preliminary report. Hum Reprod. 2004;19:2031-5.
24. Frattarelli JL, Hill MJ, McWilliams GDE, Miller KA, Bergh PA, Scott RT Jr. A luteal estradiol protocol for expected poor responders improves embryo number and quality. Fertil Steril. 2008;89:1118-22.
25. de Ziegler D, Jaaskelainen AS, Brioschi PA, Fanchin R, Bulletti C. Synchronization of endogenous and exogenous FSH stimuli in controlled ovarian hyperstimulation (COH). Hum Reprod. 1998;13:561-4.
26. Biljan MM, Mahutte NG, Dean N, Hemmings R, Bissonnette F, Tan SL. Pretreatment with an oral contraceptive is effective in reducing the incidence of functional ovarian cyst formation during pituitary suppression by gonadotropin-releasing hormone analogues. J Assist Reprod Genet. 1998; 15(10):599-604.
27. Smulders B, van Oirschot SM, Farquhar C, Rombauts L, Kremer JA. Oral contraceptive pill, progesterone or estrogen pretreatment for ovarian stimulation protocols for women

undergoing assisted reproductive techniques. Cochrane Database Syst Rev. 2010;(1):CD006109.
28. Kolibianakis EM, Papanikolaou EG, Camus M, Tournaye H, Van Steirteghem AC, Devroey P, et al. Effect of oral contraceptive pill pretreatment on ongoing pregnancy rates in patients stimulated with GNRH antagonists and recombinant FSH for IVF: A randomized controlled trial. Hum Reprod. 2006;21(2):352-7.
29. Costello MF, Chapman M, Conway U. A systematic review and meta-analysis of randomized controlled trials on metformin co-administration during gonadotropin ovulation induction or IVF in women with polycystic ovary syndrome. Hum Reprod. 2006;21:1387-99.
30. Creanga AA, Bradley HM, McCormick C, Witkop CT. Use of metformin in polycystic ovary syndrome: a meta-analysis. Obstet Gynecol. 2008;111:959-68.
31. Palomba S, Falbo A, Carrilo L, Villani MT, Orio F, Russo T, et al. Metformin reduces risk of hyperstimulation syndrome in patients with polycystic ovary syndrome during gonadotropin-stimulated *in vitro* fertilization cycles: a randomized controlled trial. Fertil Steril. 2011;96:1384-90.e4.
32. Stadtmauer LA, Toma SK, Riehl RM, Talbert LM. Metformin treatment of patients with polycystic ovary syndrome undergoing *in vitro* fertilization improves outcomes and is associated with modulation of the insulin-like growth factors. Fertil Steril. 2001;75:505-9.
33. Tang T, Glanville J, Orsi N, Barth JH, Balen AH. The use of metformin for women with PCOS undergoing IVF treatment. Hum Reprod. 2006;21:1416-25.
34. Daly DC, Walters CA, Soto-Albors CE, Tohan N, Riddick DH, et al. A randomized study of dexamethasone in ovulation induction with clomiphene citrate. Fertil Steril. 1984;41:844-8.
35. Parsanezhad ME, Alborzi S, Motazedian S, Omrani G. Use of dexamethasone and clomiphene citrate-resistant patients with polycystic ovary syndrome and normal dehydroepiandrosterone sulfate levels: a prospective double-blind, placebo-controlled trial. Fertil Steril. 2002;78:1001-4.
36. Elnashar A, Abdeelmageed E, Fayed M, Sharaf M. Clomiphene citrate and dexamethasone in treatment of clomiphene citrate resistant polycystic ovary syndrome: a prospective placebo-controlled study. Hum Reprod. 2006;21:1805-8.
37. Zhang Y, Zhang C, Shu J, Guo J, Chang H-M, Leung PCK, et al. Adjuvant treatment strategies in ovarian stimulation for poor responders undergoing IVF: a systematic review and network meta-analysis. Hum Reprod Update. 2020;26:247-63.

CHAPTER 49

Gonadotropin-releasing Hormone Analogs

Mamta Dighe

INTRODUCTION

Schally and coworkers first isolated and synthesized porcine gonadotropin-releasing hormone (GnRH) in 1971.[1-3] Since then the application of GnRH analogs has been used in various aspects of ovarian stimulation and newer analogs, both, agonists and antagonists, have been formulated.

The understanding of the molecular biology and mechanism of action of the GnRH analogs has proved its unique ability to both elicit the release and synthesis of gonadotropins with pulsatile administration or when administered in the initial phases as well as to downregulate the receptors and inhibit release of gonadotropins when administered over a prolonged period. This unique ability to both stimulate and inhibit gonadotropin release has permitted its use in ovulation induction, both for follicle development as well as to prevent luteinizing hormone (LH) surges. Its use has also been applied to treatment of diseases dependent on gonadal steroids.

Depending on its method of usage and the pharmacokinetics rationale behind, it could be used in different types of treatments as follows:

- *In ovulation induction:* It controls the effects of gonadotropin secretion in ovulation induction or in controlled ovarian hyperstimulation and in in vitro fertilization (IVF) techniques.
- *In hormone-dependent diseases:* By suppressing sex steroids in diseases where its progression is hormone-dependent, e.g., uterine fibroids, endometriosis, endometrial, and prostatic cancer.
- *In central precocious puberty:* To suppress the early appearance of GnRH pulsatility (central precocious puberty) or even to delay the normal onset of pubertal GnRH pulsatility, thus postponing epiphyseal closure and permitting bone growth to continue.

ENDOGENOUS GONADOTROPIN-RELEASING HORMONE

Gonadotropin-releasing hormone is originated and released from group of loosely connected neurons located in the medial basal hypothalamus. It is released in pulsatile fashion into the capillary system of the pituitary gland.[4] The GnRH binds selectively to highly specific receptors on the anterior pituitary gonadotropin cells leading to a cascade which causes release of gonadotropins from the anterior pituitary, thus helping in the process of ovulation. The GnRH pulse frequency alters throughout the menstrual cycle with pulses occurring less often in the luteal phase. Any alteration in the frequency or amplitude of the GnRH pulses causes disorder in the menstrual cycle.

Half-life of GnRH is 2–4 minutes as it is broken down by peptidase and cleared by glomerular filtration. Its rapid metabolic degradation and short half-life made it difficult to use native GnRH for therapeutic purposes. To stabilize the molecule against enzymatic degradation and increase its duration of action, various changes were made in its chemical composition leading to the development of GnRH analogs, both agonists, and antagonists.

GONADOTROPIN-RELEASING HORMONE AGONISTS

Development of Gonadotropin-releasing Hormone Agonists

Gonadotropin-releasing hormone agonists were evolved so as to put GnRH into clinical use. Replacement of glycine at number 10 at the C-terminus was the first major development leading to the increase in the potency of GnRH. Although 90% of biologic activity is lost doing this with the attachment of NH2–ethylamine to the proline of position 9, most of this activity is restored.[5] To slow down the enzymatic degradation, the next step was the substitution of the glycine at position 6 by D-amino acids. The combination of these two adaptations also exhibited higher receptor binding affinity. Introduction of larger and more hydrophobic and lipophilic D-amino acid at the position number 6 also prolonged the half-life. These changes in the chemical composition of the native GnRH protect the GnRH agonists against enzymatic degradation, stabilizing it, and increase its receptor binding capacity and affinity. Thus in all GnRH agonists, position 6 is substituted with a D-amino acid.

The leuprolide, goserelin, and histrelin contain either thylamide or aza-glycine at position 10. These substitutions increase metabolic stability and potency.[6] Leuprolide in the ovulation induction test in the rat was 50–80 times more potent than the parent hormone. In the test, nafarelin, which contains hydrophobic amino acid at position 6, was 200 times more active than the endogenous hormone[7] **(Table 1)**.

The GnRH agonists have great affinity for the GnRH receptors and bind to them strongly, exerting an initial flare effect. All GnRH agonists increase secretion of gonadotropins upon acute administration. This is known as the flare effect. However, with sustained administration the receptor is downregulated as it is internalized via receptor-mediated endocytosis,[8] thus resulting in suppression of both the gonadotropin, the LH:follicle-stimulating hormone (FSH) ratio, and sex steroids.[5]

Routes of Administration

All GnRH agonists are small polypeptide molecules that have to be given parenterally, as they would otherwise be susceptible to proteolysis in the gastrointestinal tract. Administration routes of GnRH agonists are intramuscular or subcutaneous depot injection, or daily intranasal or subcutaneous administration.

The subcutaneous route is very commonly used, assures good bioavailability, and there is less interindividual variation. The intranasal route may cause variations in bioavailability and also needs more frequent administration.

The sustained release method allows a constant exposure to the hormone and delivers a steady state of suppression. Also the frequency of administration is limited, making it more comfortable for the patient. The depot preparations are used as once a month or once in 3 months injections. Though no difference in the outcome of pregnancy has been observed with depot versus daily injections, there was an increase in the dose of gonadotropins required after the depot injection, and stimulation time was increased. Hence, depot injections are not the first choice in terms of cost-effectiveness except in cases of endometriosis where the ultra-long protocol increases pregnancy rates.[9]

GONADOTROPIN-RELEASING HORMONE ANTAGONISTS

Development of Gonadotropin-releasing Hormone Antagonists

The antagonist analogs have an immediate and direct suppressive effect on the gonadotropin secretion. This inhibition or suppression is reversible, getting corrected once the antagonist administration is stopped. The GnRH antagonists act by competitive blocking of pituitary GnRH receptors. The search for antagonists suitable for therapeutic use encountered two major hurdles—low potency and low safety. Over the last 20 years, three generations of GnRH antagonists have been developed. In the third generation of antagonistic analogs, the risk of histamine release and anaphylaxis was significantly reduced making it suitable for clinical use and compounds such as cetrorelix and ganirelix were deployed for the use in stimulation protocols. In GnRH antagonists, substitutions have been made at multiple positions.[10-12] The substitution in the first three amino acids is what makes these compounds antagonists rather than agonists. In the third-generation antagonists, the substitutions at amino acid positions 8 and 10 have resulted in the elimination of the histamine release seen in the early antagonists **(Table 2)**.

TABLE 1: Structure of gonadotropin-releasing hormone (GnRH) and its agonists.

Compound	*1*	*2*	*3*	*4*	*5*	*6*	*7*	*8*	*9*	*10*
GnRH	Glu	His	Trp	Ser	Tyr	Gly	Leu	Arg	Pro	Gly-NH2
Leuprolide						Leu				NH-Et
Buserelin						Ser				NH-Et
Goserelin						Ser				AzaGly-NH2
Histrelin						D-His				AzaGly-NH2
Nafarelin						2Nal				Gly-NH2
Triptorelin						Trp				Gly-NH2

TABLE 2: Structure of gonadotropin-releasing hormone (GnRH) and its antagonists.

Compound	*1*	*2*	*3*	*4*	*5*	*6*	*7*	*8*	*9*	*10*
GnRH	Glu	His	Trp	Ser	Tyr	Gly	Leu	Arg	Pro	Gly-NH2
Cetrorelix	Ac-D-Nal	D-Phe	D/Pal	Ser	Tyr	D/Cit	Leu	Arg	Pro	D-Ala-NH2
Ganirelix	Ac-D-Nal	D-Phe	D/Pal	Ser	Tyr	D-hArg	Leu	L-h Arg	Pro	D-Ala-NH2

CLINICAL USES OF GONADOTROPIN-RELEASING HORMONE ANALOGS

Due to its ability to cause rapid desensitization of the pituitary gland after continuous and prolonged nonpulsatile administration leading to inhibition of ovarian steroidogenesis, many clinical applications were derived. Also, stopping administration of the analog leads to reversal of this condition and normal functioning of the ovary was resumed. This reversible state of hypogonadotropic hypogonadism was also termed as "medical gonadectomy" or "medical hypophysectomy".

Initially, the agonists offered a major advantage that was the efficient termination of the spontaneous LH surge. Without the use of a GnRH agonist, the incidence of premature LH surges and subsequent luteinization in cycles with exogenous gonadotropin stimulation, lead to an increased cancelation rate.[13] A meta-analysis of randomized controlled trials has concluded that the use of GnRH agonist has reduced cancelation rates and has also increased the number of oocytes and embryos, allowing better selection and increasing pregnancy rates.[14]

Wide scale clinical use of commercially available GnRH agonists have proved their efficacy in treatment of metastatic prostatic cancer,[15] breast cancer,[16] uterine fibroids and precocious puberty, and endometriosis.[17] The physically, psychologically, and socially impairing syndrome of central or true isosexual precocious puberty is another condition where GnRH analogs have found wide application.

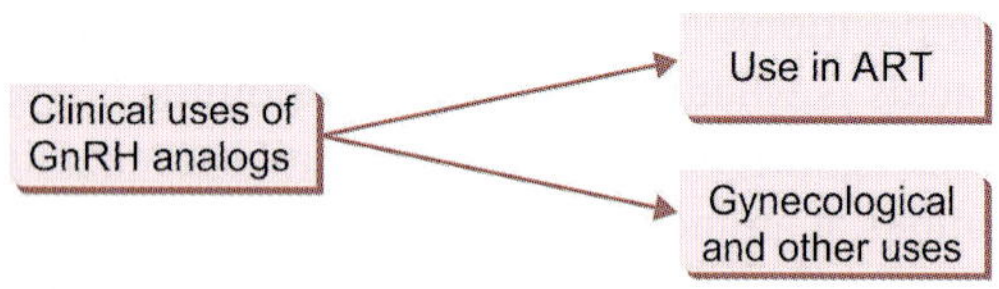

Use of Gonadotropin-releasing Hormone Analogs in Assisted Reproductive Technology

Gonadotropin-releasing Hormone Agonist

Dosage and protocols: The most commonly used GnRH agonist protocols during controlled ovarian hyperstimulation are:

- *Long agonist or the downregulation protocol:* GnRH analog is started in the midluteal phase usually as a daily dose and continued throughout the stimulation to achieve suppression of the LH surge. The cycle may be spontaneous or induced by progestogen and/or estrogen compounds. A long GnRH agonist protocol can be used in combination with oral contraceptive pills and may be advantageous in prevention of functional ovarian cysts and also for the programming of IVF cycles. The rare possibility of an early pregnancy being there during the administration of GnRH agonist is also prevented by this approach.
- The long agonist protocol is useful in programming cycles and the administration of human chorionic gonadotropin (hCG) as the trigger required for final maturation prior to oocyte retrieval can be delayed, without any detrimental effect on IVF outcomes.[18,19]
- *Short agonist protocol:* Here the GnRH analog is started on day 2 of the menstrual cycle and continued throughout the stimulation. The initial administration helps in providing the flare effect and the release of pituitary gonadotropins helps to add to the stimulatory effect.[20] Continuous administration later helps to suppress the LH surge but not as effectively as in the long protocol. The immediate stimulatory action of GnRH agonist serves as initial stimulus for follicular recruitment (so called flare-up). On other hand, this short protocol might increase gonadotropin in early phase which induces enhanced ovarian androgen release. This is associated with the decreased oocyte quality and declined ongoing pregnancy rates compared to long protocol.[21]
- *Ultra-short and microdose protocols:* In the ultra-short protocol, the GnRH analog is administered only for the initial 3 days of the stimulation protocol. The gonadotropins are started 1 day after the initiation of the GnRH analogs. In the microdose protocol, doses of 60–80 µg are administered twice daily along with gonadotropins and it is especially useful in poor responders.

A meta-analysis that compared ultra-short, and long IVF protocols suggested a higher number of oocytes retrieved and higher pregnancy rates in long protocol, however more ampoules of gonadotropins were needed.[22] Nevertheless each protocol has its place and choosing the right indication for a certain type of protocol becomes beneficial **(Fig. 1)**.

GnRH agonists for triggering ovulation: The GnRH agonists can be used as an alternative way for hCG to trigger the endogenous LH and FSH surges and subsequent final maturation of the oocyte and ovulation. This is especially useful in the cases at risk of hyperstimulation as using hCG in these cases can aggravate the problem of ovarian hyperstimulation syndrome (OHSS).

Both LH and FSH levels rose over 4–12 hours and were elevated for 24–34 hours after GnRH agonists in comparison to approximately 6 days of elevated hCG levels after 5,000 IU hCG administration. The definite effect of single administration of GnRH analogs to trigger rupture of follicle in anovulatory women or in controlled ovarian

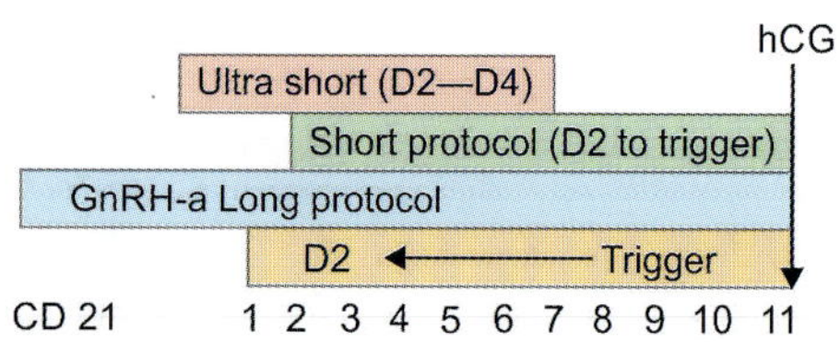

Fig. 1: Gonadotropin-releasing hormone agonist (GnRH-a) protocols. (hCG: human chorionic gonadotropin)

hyperstimulation is now well recognized.[23,24] However, use of GnRH agonist trigger leads to short luteal phases, in comparison to hCG cycles.[23-25]

The GnRH antagonists cause an immediate suppression of the LH surge and as long as sufficient antagonist is present, suppression of FSH and LH will continue. This property has helped in the development of various stimulation protocols that can utilize the effect of quick inhibition of the LH surge, right from the antagonist protocol to the minimal stimulation and luteal phase stimulation protocols.

GnRH agonists for luteal phase support: The concept of using GnRH agonist as luteal phase support (LPS) was introduced approximately in 2005. The hypothesis is that, GnRH agonist will amplify LH secretion from the anterior pituitary which supports the corpus luteum.

It has also been hypothesized to have effects on the endometrial GnRH receptors and even directly on the embryo.[26]

Routes of administration commonly used are single dose subcutaneous injection Decapeptyl 0.1 mg on day 5 or day 6 of oocyte retrieval or intranasal form with nafarelin 200 mg twice daily initiated on the evening of oocyte retrieval.

A Cochrane review by Van der et al. in 2015 suggested that there was an increased live birth rate and ongoing pregnancy rate with the use of GnRH agonist along with progesterone in the luteal phase, compared to using progesterone alone.[27]

Gonadotropin-releasing Hormone Antagonist

Dosage and protocols (**Fig. 2**):

- *Single high-dose protocol (French protocol):* Gonadotropins are started from day of the cycle and a single high-dose of antagonist (3 mg) is administered on day 8 or when the estradiol levels are around 200 pg/mL or when the leading follicle is 14 mm. This single dose is expected to suppress the LH surge for 3 days.[28] In case the criteria for trigger have not been reached by then a daily antagonist dose can be administered. This protocol is rarely used in the clinical practice nowadays.
- *The fixed daily dose protocol (Lubeck protocol):* In a dose-finding series with doses of 3 mg, 1 mg, and 0.5 mg, cetrorelix a dose of 0.25 mg was recognized as minimal effective dose in the multiple dose protocol.[29] In the fixed protocol, gonadotropins are started from the second day of the cycle and antagonist is added on a fixed day (day 6 of stimulation) in a daily dose of 0.25 mg till the hCG trigger.
- *The flexible daily dose protocol:* Daily dose of 0.25 mg is started when the leading follicle reaches a size of 14 mm till the day of hCG trigger.
- *Timing the hCG trigger:* In the long agonist protocol, delaying the time of hCG trigger has not shown any detrimental effect on cycle outcome. However, a prospective randomized study studied patients on antagonist cycles who were randomized to receive hCG (10,000 IU) on the day when follicle reached 17 mm in size or 2 days later.[30] Doing this, the authors observed a significant improvement in cycle outcome with a greatly improved implantation rate in the early hCG group and trend toward optimized ongoing pregnancy rates. Whether this leads to an improvement in embryo quality or endometrial quality is still a matter of debate. This is an important step in achieving an optimal cycle outcome in GnRH antagonist's cycles.

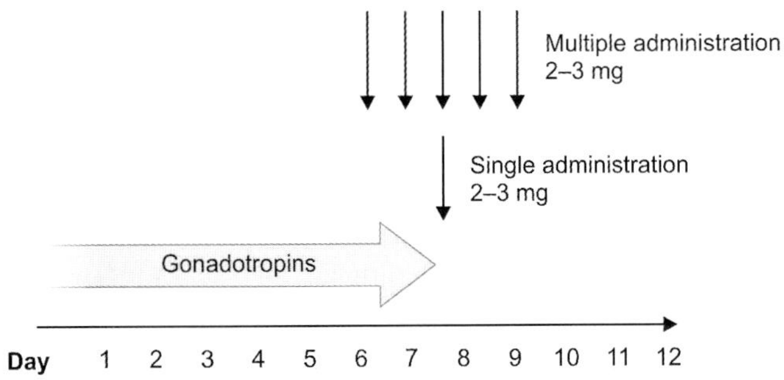

Fig. 2: Gonadotropin-releasing hormone (GnRH) antagonist dosage and protocols.

Newer treatments with antagonists: The advent of GnRH antagonists helped in formulating different protocols of ovarian stimulation where immediate suppression of LH surge could be applied when needed. Some examples are:

- *Modified natural cycle:* Here the antagonist is administered when follicle size reaches about 14 mm before hCG trigger. No stimulatory drugs are given prior to that; however, after addition of antagonist, FSH or LH could be given. It is used in poor responders, and if there is contraindication to stimulation.
- *Minimal and mild IVF:* The inception of GnRH antagonists has been a key to the development of these protocols. Here lower doses of FSH or human menopausal gonadotropin are used for stimulation at times along with oral ovulogens to obtain about eight or less oocytes.
- *Random start and luteal phase protocols:* Here the stimulation is started on any day of the menstrual cycle and the LH activity at that point is taken care of with the use of antagonists.

The introduction of GnRH antagonists in the field of ovarian stimulation has several advantages, such as:

- A more convenient method of ovarian stimulation with a shorter period of stimulation and no preceding pituitary suppression.
- A more physiologic way of ovarian stimulation integrated in a spontaneous menstrual cycle.
- Pituitary suppression is started when a prematuration LH surge threatens.

- The risk of OHSS can substantially reduce especially with the use of the GnRH antagonists cetrorelix.

The GnRH antagonists use differs in certain areas as compared to an analog, for example:

- Follicle cohort synchronization may be required so as to bring up good number of follicles.
- Timing of hCG may be a critical step and should happen at about 17–18 mm follicle size.
- LPS is necessary to achieve optimal outcome of the cycles.

The GnRH agonist trigger can be applied when at risk of OHSS or in donor stimulation and if freezing of all embryos is planned.

Clinical applications of GnRH analogs in the management of the infertile patients and in ovulation induction: In the management of the infertile patient, GnRH agonists can be used for various indications:

- To suppress the pituitary-ovarian axis before and simultaneously during ovarian stimulation and ovulation induction with exogenous gonadotropins.
- In endometriosis, for prolonged suppression of the pituitary-ovarian axis which is shown to improve IVF rates by fourfold.
- As an ovulation trigger, GnRH agonist trigger is used in IVF cycles using antagonist protocols. As mentioned previously, this is done in patients with polycystic ovary syndrome (PCOS) at the risk of hyperstimulation, in donor stimulation cycles and when freezing all embryos has been planned.
- The GnRH antagonists are used in combination with gonadotropins in many new stimulation protocols such as minimal and mild protocols, random start protocols, and the dual stimulation protocols where its ability to suppress LH immediately is utilized so that stimulation can be started at any point during the menstrual cycle.
- The choice of the GnRH analog to be used based on its delivery system, its mode of administration and its biological half-life, will determine the optimal gonadotropin treatment protocol.

With markers of ovarian reserve now available, patients are usually categorized into normal, poor or hyper-responders. Studies have identified protocols of GnRH analogs best suited for each of these categories in order to obtain optimal number of oocytes and prevent cycle cancellation or ovarian hyperstimulation.

Expected poor responders: In patients with an anti-Müllerian hormone (AMH) level of ≤0.1 and negligible antral follicles seen, no pregnancy was observed irrespective of the stimulation protocol used. These patients should be counseled regarding poor chances of success and using a modified natural cycle stimulation or minimal stimulation should be the goal in order to decrease the cost burden.

In patients with AMH levels between 0.5 and 1.3 ng/mL and antral follicles between 5 and 7, antagonist protocols were associated with a substantial fall in cycle cancellation and showed a trend toward higher pregnancy rates.[31] The short GnRH agonist protocols or the microdose flare protocols are also good options in these patients.

Advantages of antagonist protocol in poor responders are:

- The long downregulation protocol may have an unfavorable effect in poor responders as it may induce an excessive ovarian suppression that could result in decreased or absent follicular response.[32,33] The GnRH antagonists are not administered during the stage of follicular recruitment and hence suppression of endogenous gonadotropins secretion is not present at that time.
- The ovarian reserve is assessed by ultrasound on days 2–3 of the cycle to plan controlled ovarian stimulation (COS) and decide whether to initiate gonadotropins in the cycle, to predict and expect an optimal response.
- Second, with use of GnRH antagonist we can have recourse to a new gonadotropin, a hybrid molecule that has a prolonged half-life (corifollitropin alpha) and supports the cohort of follicle receptive to stimulation for 7 days.[34] The use of these long-acting gonadotropins causes a swift increase in the serum FSH concentration resulting in a remarkably higher exposure of the small antral follicles to constant high levels of FSH during the early follicular phase and significantly help in this category of patients.[35]

Expected normal responders: Women with AMH levels between 1.3 and 3.4 and antral follicle count (AFC) between 8 and 10 usually fall here. These patients would respond well to both the GnRH agonist downregulation protocol as well as the antagonist protocol. The aim would be to procure about 8–14 oocytes. The decision can be made depending on the patient compliance, time available for stimulation, and the comfort of the physician with the particular protocol.

Expected high responders: Recent studies have revealed that the use of antagonists is related to reduced occurrence of a high response and a significantly reduced incidence of OHSS or even of cycle cancellation because of the risk of OHSS.[36,37]

The days required for stimulation in an antagonist protocol were fewer in number than the GnRH agonist protocol (9 days vs. 13 days). It was also observed that in antagonist protocol there was reduced need for cryopreservation of embryos due to excess response and decline in hospitalization rate for OHSS (13.9% in the agonist group vs. 0.0% in the antagonist group).[38]

A significantly higher pregnancy rate was observed in antagonist protocol in higher responders (61.7 vs. 31.8%; *p*: 0.05).[38]

Finally, by using the GnRH antagonist protocol for COS, initiation of a LH surge when compared with that occurring physiologically at midcycle to trigger ovulation could be obtained by administering a single bolus of GnRH agonist.[39]

Gynecological and Other Uses of Gonadotropin-releasing Hormone Analogs

Clinical indications of use where gonadotropin suppression is desired are described here.

Endometriosis

Endometriosis is a complex disease and is characterized by the presence of ectopic endometrium. The growth and spread of endometriosis are established by the cyclic production of ovarian hormones. When the function of the ovary is suspended there is loss of cyclical hormone release, the uterine as well as ectopic endometria undergo atrophy, and endometriosis resolves. To control this course of the disease, temporary suppression of ovarian function is the principle of hormonal treatment in endometriosis. Endometriosis being a hormone-dependent condition, the possibility of selectively suppressing the ovarian secretion of estrogen by receptive GnRH administration causes reversible downregulation of gonadotropin secretion inducing a state of hypogonadotropic hypogonadism, pseudomenopause, or medical castration. Analogs are usually administered in monthly injections over 4–6 months. Undesirable symptoms of hypoestrogenism and decrease in bone density with long-term use can be tackled with the use of small doses of estrogen and progesterone. Several studies are underway to elicit the use of GnRH antagonists in endometriosis without the side effects of severe estrogen depletion. One study involved the use of 3 mg of cetrorelix administered weekly over 8 weeks. There was adequate control of symptoms and estradiol levels were maintained between 50 and 60 pg/mL preserving basic estrogen production.[40]

Recently an oral nonpeptide GnRH antagonist, elagolix, has been tried in women with endometriosis to reduce the symptoms of dysmenorrhea and pelvic pain. Elagolix has been tried in the dose of 15 mg daily (low dose treatment) and in the dose of 200 mg twice daily (high-dose treatment). However, both doses were associated with hypoestrogenic side effects.[41]

Uterine Fibroids

Fibroids are the most common tumors of female genital organs and probably the most common tumor in women. Fibroids may associate with infertility, menorrhagia, and/or dysmenorrhea. Management of patients who have sympathetic uterine fibroids has traditionally been myomectomy, i.e., surgical removal of the fibroid for those desirous of children or hysterectomy for women with large or multiple fibroids whose families are complete.

Luteinizing hormone-releasing hormone (LHRH) agonists, by creating a hypoestrogenic environment, have provided for the first time a medical treatment of uterine fibroids.[42] LHRH agonists significantly shrink these tumors in the majority of patients and cause their complete clinical disappearance in a majority of subjects.[43] In most cases, however, relief is temporary and regrowth to pretreatment size occurs within 3 months of cessation of therapy.

Preoperative treatment for 3 months may also help by improving the patient's preoperative status and providing concurrent symptom relief.[44] The 30–40% reduction in size may permit laparoscopic[45] or in cases of submucous myoma, hysteroscopic[46] removal of the myoma. However, the surgical plane may get altered making removal difficult.

The use of GnRH antagonists in fibroids is limited due to its short half-life and the nonavailability of the depot formulation, thus requiring repetitive dosing usually daily for most antagonists.

Precocious Puberty

The GnRH analogs remain the treatment of choice in central precocious puberty. The suppression of the pituitary-gonadal axis ceases sexual development, declines skeletal maturation, and decreases the growth rate without serious undesirable effects.

Benign Prostate Hyperplasia

Benign prostate hypertrophy affects males 60 years or older, and the treatment of choice is usually surgical removal. In patients with high surgical risk, the administration of GnRH agonists reduces the size of the prostate to 30% the original size, and improves the symptoms of urinary obstruction. GnRH antagonists can also be sued and its administration makes improvement last even after stopping medicine probably due to the direct effect of the antagonist on the prostatic epithelium or on some growth factors

Oncology

Cancers that depend on sex steroid hormones can be treated with GnRH analogs. These include prostate, breast, ovarian, and endometrial cancers. Prostate cancer, among all hormone-sensitive cancers, shows the best response to endocrine therapy. GnRH analogs can be used alone or in combination with antiandrogens such as flutamide. In breast cancer, GnRH agonists and antagonists have been tried both in pre- and postmenopausal women alone, or in combination with antiestrogens. GnRH receptors are located in the ovary; hence, GnRH antagonists may be of great value in the treatment of ovarian cancer by two mechanisms—through suppression of ovarian stimulation by gonadotropins and through direct inhibition of ovarian cells. In some cases of

TABLE 3: Comparison of gonadotropin-releasing hormone (GnRH) agonists and GnRH antagonists.

GnRH agonists	*GnRH antagonists*
Initial flare effect	No flare-up effect
Longer duration of stimulation	Shorter duration of stimulation
Increased gonadotropin requirement	Fewer ampoules of gonadotropin required
Small doses required	Need for higher doses
Pituitary response downregulated	Preserved pituitary response to GnRH
Asynchronicity of follicles rare	Asynchronous development may happen
Higher risk of OHSS	Lower risk of OHSS
Not used in mild or dual protocols	Used in natural, mild, and dual protocols
Slightly more oocytes obtained	Slightly less oocytes obtained

(OHSS: ovarian hyperstimulation syndrome)

recurrence of endometrial cancer, GnRH analogs provide prolonged relapse-free survival and better quality of life. This action can also be ancillary to steroid suppression or maybe due to an extrapituitary action of the analogs. The GnRH agonists and antagonists have also been known to preserve the gonad from the toxic effects of chemotherapy and radiotherapy on the germinal epithelium.

KEY POINTS

- The GnRH analogs are widely used in IVF to control the endogenous LH surge and achieve augmentation of multifollicular development. They also have widespread applications in many other areas as discussed above. The advent of GnRH antagonists has helped in devising newer stimulation protocols, making them more patient-friendly **(Table 3)**.
- The long GnRH agonist protocols give the highest pregnancy rates in the normal responders.
- There is some evidence that the short flare-up protocol is the treatment of choice for patients with diminished ovarian reserve (poor responders). Dose reduction might be the key point in optimizing pregnancy rates. Finally, GnRH agonists can be used to induce final maturation and ovulation as an alternative to hCG in assisted reproductive technology (ART).
- The GnRH-antagonist regimen (GnRH-ant) is effective in preventing a premature rise of LH and therefore results in a shorter and more cost-effective ovarian stimulation protocol compared to the long agonist protocol. However, there is a difference in the synchronization of follicular recruitment and growth in the GnRH-agonist (GnRH-a) and GnRH-antagonist regimens with better follicular growth and oocyte maturation seen with GnRH-a treatment.[47]

REFERENCES

1. Schally AV, Arimura A, Baba Y, Nair RM, Matsuo H, Redding TW, et al. Isolation and properties of FSH and LH-releasing hormone. Biochem Biophys Res Commun. 1971;43(2):393-9.
2. Baba Y, Matsuo H, Schally AV. Structure of porcine LH- and FSH-releasing hormone II: confirmation of the proposed structure by conventional sequential analysis. Biochem Biophys Res Commun. 1971;44(2):459-63.
3. Matsuo H, Arimura A, Nair RM, Schally AV. Synthesis of the porcine LH and FSH releasing hormone by the solid phase method. Biochem Biophys Res Commun. 1971;45(3):822-7.
4. Carmel PW, Araki S, Ferin M. Pituitary stalk portal blood collection in rhesus monkeys: evidence for pulsatile release of gonadotropin releasing hormone (GnRH). Endocrinology. 1976;99(1):243-8.
5. Karten MJ, Rivier JE. Gonadotropin-releasing hormone analog design. Structure-function studies towards the development of agonists and antagonists: rationale and perspective. Endocrinol Rev. 1986;7(1):44-66.
6. Fujino M, Shinagawa S, Yamazaki I, Kobayashi S, Obayashi M, Fukuda T, et al. (Des-Gly-Nh2-10, Proethylamide) LH-RH: a highly potent analog of luteinizing hormone releasing hormone. Arch Biochem Biophys. 1973;154:488-9.
7. Nestor JJ, Ho TL, Simpson RA, Horner BL, Jones GH, McRae GI, et al. Synthesis and biological activity of some very hydrophobic superagonist analogs of luteinizing hormone releasing hormone. J Med Chem. 1982;25(7):795-801.
8. Suarez-Quian CA, Wynn PC, Catt KJ. Receptor mediated-endocytosis of GnRH analogs: differential processing of gold labelled agonist and antagonist derivatives. J Steroid Biochem. 1986;24(1):183-92.
9. Surrey ES, Silverberg KM, Surrey MW, Schoolcraft WB. Effect of prolonged gonadotropin-releasing hormone against therapy on the outcome of in vitro fertilization embryo transfer patient with endometriosis. Fertil Steril. 2002;78(4):699-704.
10. Coy DH, Savary FLM, Coy EJ, Schally AV. LH releasing activity of potent LH-RH analogs in vitro. Biochem Biophys Res Commun. 1975;67(2):576-82.
11. Gordon K, Hodgen GD. GnRH agonists and antagonists in assisted reproduction. Balliere's Clinical Obstet Gynecol. 1992;6(2):247-65.
12. Felberbaum RE, Reissmann T, Kupker W, Bauer O, al Hasani S, Diedrich C, et al. Preserved pituitary response under ovarian stimulation with HMG and GnRH antagonists (cetrorelix) in women with tubal infertility. Eur J Obstet Gynecol Reprod Biol. 1995;61(2): 151-5.
13. Janssens RM, Lambalk CB, Vermeiden JP, Schats R, Bernards JM, Rekers-Mombarg LT, et al. Dose finding study of triptorelin acetate for prevention of premature LH surge in IVF: a prospective, randomized, double-blind, placebo-controlled study. Hum Reprod. 2000;15(11):2333-40.
14. Hughes EG, Fedorkow DM, Daya S, Sagle MA, Van de Koppel P, Collins JA. The routine use of gonadotropin-releasing hormone agonists prior to in vitro fertilization and gamete intrafallopian transfer: a meta-analysis of randomized controlled trials. Fertil Steril. 1992;58(5):888-96.
15. Schally AV. LH-RH analogues: I. Their impact on reproductive medicine. Gynecol Endocrinol. 1999;13(6):401-9.
16. Klijn JGM. LHRH-agonist therapy in breast cancer. Gynecol Endocrinol. 2003;17:8.

17. Conn PM, Crowley WF Jr. Gonadotropin releasing hormone and its analogs. N Engl J Med. 1991;324(2):93-103.
18. Chang SY, Lee Ml, Wang ML, Hu ML, Lai YM, Chang MY, et al. No detrimental effect in delaying initiation of gonadotropin administration after pituitary desensitization with gonadotropin-releasing hormone agonist. Fertil Steril. 1993;59(1):183-6.
19. Dimitry ES, Oskarsson T, Conaghan J. Beneficial effects of 24 h delay in human chorionic gonadotropin administration during in vitro fertilization treatment cycles. Hum Reprod. 1991;6(7):944-6.
20. Padilla SL, Dugan K, Maruchsak V, Shalika S, Smith RD. Use of the flare up protocol with high dose of follicle stimulation hormone and human menopausal gonadotropin for in vitro fertilization in poor responders. Fertil Steril. 1996;65(4):796-9.
21. Loumaye E, Coen G, Pampfer S, Vankrieken L, Thomas K. Use of gonadotropin releasing hormone agonist during ovarian stimulation leads to significant concentration of peptide in follicular fluids. Fertil Steril. 1989;52(2):256-63.
22. Daya S. Gonadotropin releasing hormone agonist protocol for pituitary desensitization in in vitro fertilization and gamete intrafallopian transfer cycles. Cochrane Database Syst Rev. 2002;(2):CD001299.
23. Emperaire JC, Ruffie A. Triggering ovulation with endogenous luteinizing hormone may prevent the ovarian hyper stimulation syndrome. Hum Reprod. 1991;6(4):506-10.
24. Lanzone A, Fulghesu AM, Villa P, Guida C, Guido M, Nicoletti MC, et al. Gonadotropin releasing hormone agonist versus human chorionic gonadotropin as trigger of ovulation in polycystic ovarian disease gonadotropin hyper stimulation cycles. Fertil Steril. 1994;62(1):35-41.
25. Romeu A, Monzo A, Peiro T, Diez E, Peinado JA, Quintero LA, et al. Endogenous LH surge versus hCG as ovulation trigger after low dose highly purified FSH in IUI: a comparison of 761 cycles. J Assist Reprod Genet. 1997;14(9):518-24.
26. Pirard C, Donnez J, Loumaye E. GnRH agonist as novel luteal support: results of a randomized, parallel group, feasibility study using intranasal administration of buserelin. Hum Reprod. 2005;20(7):1798-804.
27. van der Linden M, Buckingham K, Farquhar C, Kremer JAM, Metwally M. Luteal phase support for assisted reproduction cycles. Cochrane Database Syst Rev. 2015;2015(7):CD009154.
28. Olivennes F, Fanchin R, Bouchard P, Taïeb J, Selva J, Frydman R. Scheduled administration of a gonadotropin releasing hormone antagonist (Cetrorelix) on day 8 of in vitro fertilization cycles: a pilot study. Hum Reprod. 1995;10(6):1382-6.
29. A double-blind, randomized, dose-finding study to access the efficacy of the gonadotropin releasing hormone antagonist ganirelix (org37462) to prevent premature luteinizing hormone surges in women undergoing ovarian stimulation with recombinant follicle stimulating hormone (Puregon). The ganirelix dose-finding study group. Hum Reprod. 1998; 13(11):3023-31.
30. Kolibianakis E, Albano C, Tournaye H. Timing of hCG administration for ovulation triggering in GnRH antagonist cycles. A randomized controlled trial. Hum Reprod. 2003;18:2-2.
31. Marca A, Sunkara SK. Individualization of controlled ovarian stimulation in IVF using ovarian reserve markers: from theory to practice. Hum Reprod Update. 2014;20(1):124-40.
32. Yoshimura Y, Nakamura Y, Ando M, Shiokawa S, Koyama N, Nanno T, et al. Direct effect of gonadotropin-releasing hormone agonists on the rabbit ovarian follicle. Fertil Steril. 1992;57(5):1091-7.
33. Kowalik A, Barmat L, Damario M, Liu HC, Davis O, Rosenwaks Z, et al. Ovarian estradiol production in vivo. Inhibitory effect of leuprolide acetate. J Reprod Med. 1998;43(5):413-7.
34. van Schanke A, van De Wetering-Krebbers SF, Bos E, Sloot WN. Absorption, distribution, metabolism and excretion of corifollitropin alfa, a recombinant hormone with a sustained follicle-stimulating activity. Pharmacology. 2010;85(2):77-87.
35. Polyzos NP, Devos M, Humaidan P, Stoop D, Ortega-Hrepich C, Devroey P, et al. Corifollitropin alfa followed by rFSH in a GnRH antagonist protocol for poor ovarian responder patients: an observational pilot study. Fertil Steril. 2013;99(2):422-6.
36. Al-Inany HG, Abou-Setta AM, Aboulghar M. Gonadotrophin-releasing hormone antagonists for assisted conception. Cochrane Database Syst Rev. 2006;19(3):CD0001750.
37. Al-Inany HG, Youssef MA, Aboulghar M, Broekmans F, Sterrenburg M, Smit J, et al. Gonadotrophin-releasing hormone antagonists for assisted reproductive technology. Cochrane Database Syst Rev. 2011;(5):CD001750.
38. Nelson SM, Yates RW, Lyall H, Jamieson M, Traynor I, Gaudoin M, et al. Anti-Müllerian hormone-based approach to controlled ovarian stimulation for assisted conception. Hum Reprod. 2009;24(4):867-75.
39. Griesinger G, Diedrich K, Devroey P, Kolibianakis EM. GnRH agonist for triggering final oocyte maturation in the GnRH antagonist ovarian hyperstimulation protocol: a systematic review and meta-analysis. Hum Reprod Update. 2006;12(2):159-68.
40. Küpker W, Felberbaum RE, Krapp M, Schill T, Malik E, Diedrich K. Use of GnRH antagonists in the treatment of endometriosis. Reprod Biomed Online. 2002;5(1):12-6.
41. Taylor HS, Giudice LC, Lessey BA, Abrao MS, Kotarski J, Archer DF, et al. Treatment of endometriosis-associated pain with elagolix, an oral GnRH antagonist. N Engl J Med. 2017;377:28-40.
42. Healy DL, Lawsons SR, Abbot M, Baird DT, Fraser HM. Towards removing uterine fibroids without surgery: subcutaneous infusion of a luteinizing hormone-releasing hormone agonist commencing in the luteal phase. J Clin Endocrinol Metab. 1986;63(3):619-25.
43. Maheux R, Guilloteau C, Lemay A, Bastide A, Fazekas AT. Luteinizing hormone releasing hormone agonist and uterine leiomyoma: a pilot study. Am J Obstet Gynecol. 1985;152(8): 1034-8.
44. Stovall TG, Jenison EL, Memphis TN. A comparative study of adjuvant GnRH agonist (ZOLADEX) therapy vs immediate surgery in the treatment of uterine myoma. Endocrinol. 1993;7(Suppl 2):34.
45. Mettler L, Semm K. Laparoscopic approach of fibroid excision after treatment with GnRH Agonists. Gynecol Endocrinol. 1993;7(Suppl 2):30.
46. Donnez J. Large submucosal myoma. GnRH agonist and hysteroscopic myomectomy. Gynecol Endocrinol. 1993;7(Suppl 2):39.
47. Depalo R, Lorusso F, Palmisano M, Bassi E, Totaro I, Vacca M, et al. Follicular growth and oocyte maturation in GnRH agonist and antagonist protocols for in vitro fertilisation and embryo transfer. Gynecol Endocrinol. 2009;25(5):328-34.

CHAPTER

50 Monitoring of Ovarian Stimulation

Snehal Dhobale Kohale

INTRODUCTION

The basic functional unit of the ovary is "follicle", which undergoes different morphologic and hormonal changes in the menstrual cycle. The concept that "the mammalian oocyte was enclosed within the ovarian follicle" was first put forward by Karl Ernst von Baer in 1827.[1] During follicular development, antral follicle passes through various gonadotropin-dependent phases such as recruitment, selection, and dominance before ovulation.[2] Ovulation may need to be induced in anovulatory cycles (e.g., polycystic ovary disease) or during timed intercourse (TI), intrauterine insemination (IUI), and in vitro fertilization (IVF) cycles. The aim of ovulation induction (OI) can be monofollicular growth or multifollicular growth [controlled ovarian stimulation (COS)]. Ovulation-inducing agents (tablets and gonadotropins) cause follicular growth as well as hormonal changes in the ovary.

NEED FOR MONITORING

- To obtain the optimum outcome of stimulation by modifying drug dosages
- To avoid complications of stimulation such as ovarian hyperstimulation syndrome (OHSS) and multiple births.

METHODS OF MONITORING

There are two methods of monitoring given in **Table 1**:

1. Biochemical or hormonal monitoring
2. Clinical monitoring.

TABLE 1: Methods of monitoring.

Biochemical/hormonal monitoring	*Clinical monitoring (follicular growth and endometrial assessment)*
• Home monitoring: – Basal body temperature – Cervical mucus test – Salivary ferning assessment – Electronic resistance evaluation of salivary and vaginal secretions – Urinary LH test • Blood hormonal assays of AMH, FSH, LH, estradiol, progesterone, inhibin B, etc.	• Transvaginal ultrasound 2D, 3D, color Doppler • Self-operated endovaginal telemonitoring (SOET)

(AMH: anti-Müllerian hormone; FSH: follicle-stimulating hormone; LH: luteinizing hormone)

STAGES OF MONITORING

Before Stimulation

It involves baseline assessment that helps in choosing the appropriate stimulation protocol so as to avoid poor response, cycle cancellation, or hyperresponse.

- *Transvaginal ultrasound:* For antral follicle count (AFC) and for ruling out other pathologies
- *Hormonal profile:* Anti-Müllerian hormone (AMH), follicle-stimulating hormone (FSH), luteinizing hormone (LH), thyroid function test, and prolactin.

During Stimulation

- To confirm downregulation in gonadotropin-releasing hormone (GnRH) agonist long protocol
- To determine response to gonadotropins (poor response, hyperresponse, or no response)
- To determine the dose (step up and step down) and duration of gonadotropin therapy
- To detect premature LH surge
- To determine the optimal timing of trigger—human chorionic gonadotropin (hCG) administration
- To detect ovulation in OI or IUI cycles
- To assess the risk of OHSS in COS cycles so as to apply some strategies to prevent it (such as cabergoline use or GnRH agonist trigger instead of hCG in GnRH antagonist cycles).
- To determine the time of oocyte retrieval.

After Stimulation

- To establish ovulation
- To establish an optimal response to agonist trigger
- To identify complications of OI:
    - Luteinized unruptured follicle (LUF)
    - Retention or functional cyst
- To confirm pregnancy.

CHOOSING METHODS OF MONITORING

Monitoring should be easy, reliable, cost-effective, and patient-friendly.

Extent of monitoring will depend on:
- The aim of OI (monofollicular or multifollicular development)
- Drugs used for stimulation (oral medications or gonadotropins)
- Treatment planned (natural, IUI, or IVF) **(Table 2)**.

It is obvious that multifollicular development with gonadotropins in IVF cycles would need more intense and meticulous monitoring to avoid complications such as ovarian hyperstimulation.

TABLE 2: Optimum monitoring methods according to treatment planned.

Treatment planned	***Optimum monitoring***
Timed intercourse	Home monitoring (basal body temperature, cervical mucus assessment, salivary ferning assessment, urinary luteinizing hormone kits) or Transvaginal ultrasound
Intrauterine insemination	Transvaginal ultrasound
In vitro fertilization	Transvaginal ultrasound and blood hormonal assays

Home Monitoring

Basal Body Temperature

- *Principle:* Thermogenic property of progesterone causes a rise in basal body temperature (BBT) by 0.5°F when progesterone levels are >3–5 ng/mL, 1–5 days after mid-cycle LH surge.
- *Method:* Temperature has to be measured each morning, on awakening, before arising from the bed with a special thermometer having an expanded scale of 96.0–100.0°F marked in tenths of 1°.
- Ovulatory cycles have a "biphasic response" (follicular phase: 97–98°F; on day of ovulation: nadir; and 0.4–0.8°F rise in luteal phase) as shown in **Figure 1**.
- *Advantages:* It is a low-cost, easy, and noninvasive method.
- *Disadvantages:* It is a retrospective diagnosis of ovulation. BBT readings can be affected by factors such as illness, infection, anxiety, stress, fatigue, jet lag, nightmares, insomnia, smoking, alcohol, exercise, and electric blanket use.

Cervical Mucus Assessment (Figs. 2A and B)

- *Principle:* It is based on the change in the characteristics of cervical mucus due to preovulatory estrogen rise.
- *Method:* Insler scoring system—It is a semiquantitative assessment of cervical mucus. The assessment parameters are the appearance of cervical os, mucus quantity, spinnbarkeit, and ferning. In the modified

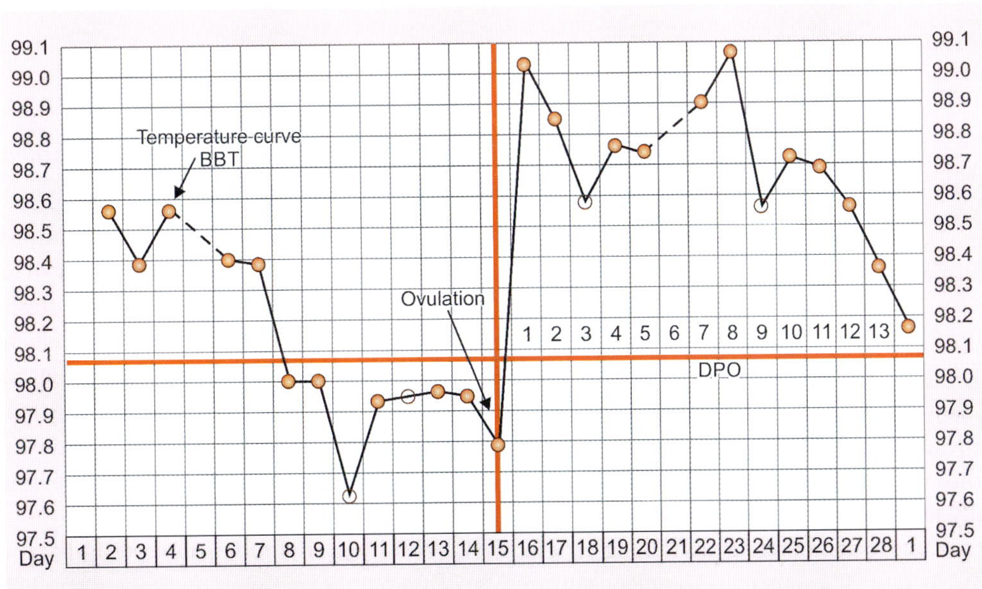

Fig. 1: Basal body temperature (BBT) chart in ovulatory cycle: Biphasic response. (DPO: days past ovulation)

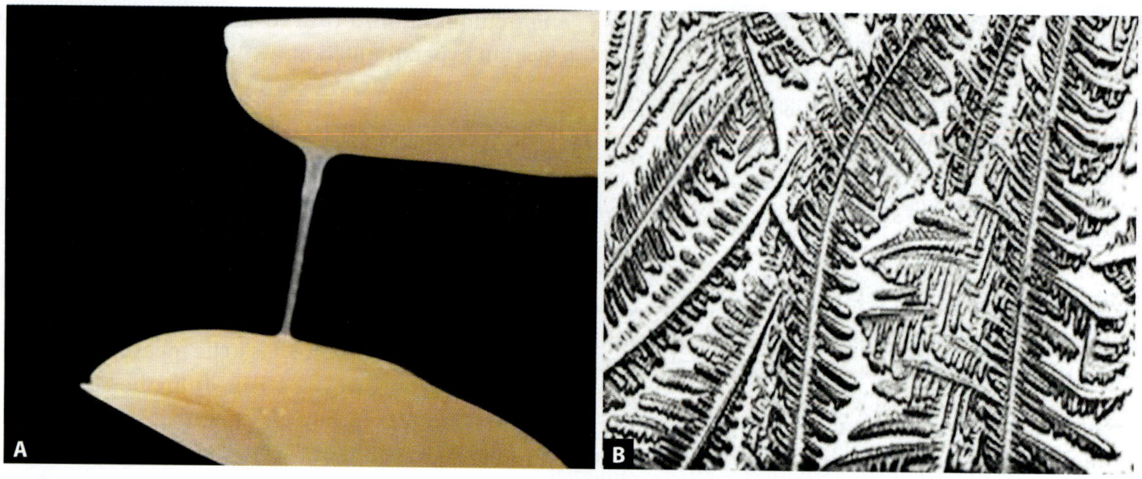

Figs. 2A and B: Cervical mucus: Spinnbarkeit and ferning patterns.

TABLE 3: Modified Insler scoring system.

Parameters	***Score***			
	0	***1***	***2***	***3***
Appearance of cervical os	Tightly closed, as pink as surrounding tissue	Beginning to open and redden	Intermediate between scores 1 and 3	Maximally dilated (6 mm diameter)
Mucus quantity	Not visible at external os and none aspirated (0 mL)	Not visible at external os but some aspirated (0.1 mL)	Visible at external os and can be aspirated (0.2 mL)	Definite cascade visible at external os (>0.3 mL)
Spinnbarkeit	No stretching	Stretches 1–4 cm before breaking	Stretches 5–8 cm before breaking	Stretches >8 cm before breaking
Ferning	Not visible	Less than half mucus starting to fern	More than half mucus showing good ferning (primary and secondary stem ferning)	All mucus showing good ferning (with tertiary and quaternary stem ferning)
Cellularity (leukocytes)	Full of leukocytes >20 per 40 × field or >1,000/mm	Many leukocytes 11–20 per 40 × field or 501–1,000/mm	Few leukocytes 1–10 per 40 × field or 1–500/mm	No leukocytes

Note: Score ≥12/15: Good ovulatory cervical mucus; score 10 or 11/15: Adequate ovulatory cervical mucus.

Insler scoring system, mucus cellularity is an additional parameter **(Table 3)**.

- *Disadvantages:* Less precision in determining exact ovulation time and individual variations in the response of the cervical glands to estrogen.

Salivary Ferning Assessment

During ovulation, with increased estradiol levels, saliva shows similar biochemical changes to cervical mucus. There is increase in salivary NaCl concentration, which results in crystallization, thus demonstrating a ferning pattern. There are commercially available kits that contain a handheld pocket mini microscope to demonstrate this ferning pattern. It has 78% specificity and 80% sensitivity to detect salivary ferning.

Electronic Resistance Evaluation of Salivary and Vaginal Secretions

The device called CUE Fertility Monitor provides a digital measurement of the electrical resistance of saliva (SER) and vaginal secretions (VL) using a computerized algorithm. Saliva and VL undergo NaCl and other electrolytic changes with LH rise; those can be measured by changes in electrical resistance by monitor. The data are stored and with computerized software, ovulatory window can be predicted with the use of oral probe for salivary assessment and vaginal sensor for VL.

- *Advantages:* Reusable monitors and easy to use at home
- *Disadvantages:* Costly device and conflicting data about the accuracy of this method.

Urinary Luteinizing Hormone Kit

- *Principle:* LH is having short half-life and is rapidly cleared in urine.
- Ovulation occurs 14–26 hours after LH surge detection, almost always within 48 hours.
- *Method:* Testing of late afternoon to early evening urine sample (4–10 PM).
- *Advantages:* It predicts ovulation in the next 24–48 hours of positive test result with >90% probability.
- *Disadvantages:* False-positive and false-negative results. Several diseases such as endometriosis, polycystic ovarian syndrome, premature ovarian failure, hyperthyroidism, renal failure, gonadotropin-producing neoplasia, and medications such as menotropins, danazol, clomiphene, hCG, hormone supplementation, and steroids can interfere with the accuracy of urinary LH test results. In women with irregular periods, LH surge can be missed even with daily testing. It cannot detect ovulation or complications such as LUF.

Ultrasound Monitoring

Real-time ultrasound is a frequently used method in the recent past for ovarian follicular development. "Follicular dynamics" is about the morphological and vascular response of the ovaries and uterus to the hormonal changes in the menstrual cycle.

- *Literature:* Visualization of follicles was first demonstrated by Kratochwil in 1972. A direct correlation between increasing follicular size and estradiol concentration in spontaneously ovulating women was demonstrated by Hackelöer et al. in 1979.[3,4] Several studies have demonstrated the correlation of follicle growth and changes in hormone levels in both stimulated and unstimulated cycles.[5,6]
- For real-time monitoring of ovarian function, the vaginal route is better than the abdominal route because of:
  - The smaller distance from the probe to the ovary
  - High resolution of the probes (5–7.5 MHz frequency)
  - The absence of a full bladder distorting pelvic organs
  - Improved convenience and patient compliance
  - The transvaginal scanning technique has been validated under normal, anovulatory, and gonadotropin-stimulated conditions.

Advantages of ultrasound for monitoring: Quick, easy, noninvasive method, and no known harmful effects to the oocyte or reproductive tract.

A few anatomical pelvic structures may look similar to the growing follicle on ultrasound. These include:

- Internal iliac artery and vein cross section
- Cross section of blood vessels around the uterus and ovary
- Bowel
- Hydrosalpinx
- Ovarian cysts.

Ultrasound provides information about:

- Uterus, ovary, and adnexa and their abnormalities
- Ovarian reserve (AFC and flow indices)
- Ovarian response (follicle and endometrial growth and blood flow)
- Time for trigger.

The qualitative information is assessed by color Doppler and the quantitative information by power Doppler.

Baseline scan: It is the first scan on day 2 or 3 of the cycle when no follicle is >9 mm. It demonstrates baseline pathology in ovary, uterus or adnexa, and ovarian reserve. Its purpose is to categorize the ovaries into a normal responder, poor responder, and hyperresponder and accordingly to choose the optimum stimulation protocol.

"*Ovarian reserve*" is assessed by AFC and ovarian volume. It is nothing but likely number of follicles that may develop or likely number of eggs that may be retrieved after stimulation.

"*Ovarian response*" is assessed by intraovarian flow indices. It is nothing but approximate doses required to produce dominant follicles.

Antral follicle count is the number of small antral follicles (2–10 mm) in both the ovaries **(Fig. 3)**.

Number of small antral follicles (2–6 mm) represents the "functional ovarian reserve" as it is significantly related to age. AFC correlates well with age, ovarian reserve, and response to stimulation. AFC is useful to predict the ovarian response, thus decreasing the chances of cycle cancellation.[7] A low AFC is considered to be total of 3–6 antral follicles [mean of 5.2 with standard deviation (SD) 2.11] and is associated with poor response to ovarian stimulation during IVF but does not reliably predict failure to conceive.[8] AFC >14 predicts hyperstimulation with sensitivity of 82% and specificity of 89%. AFC has good intercycle and interobserver reliability

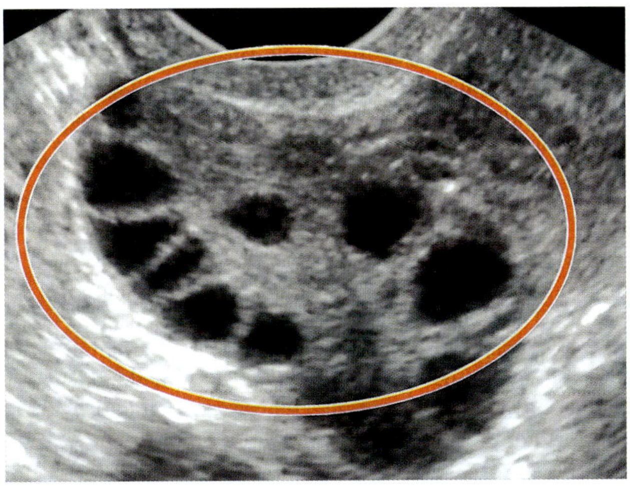

Fig. 3: Antral follicle count.

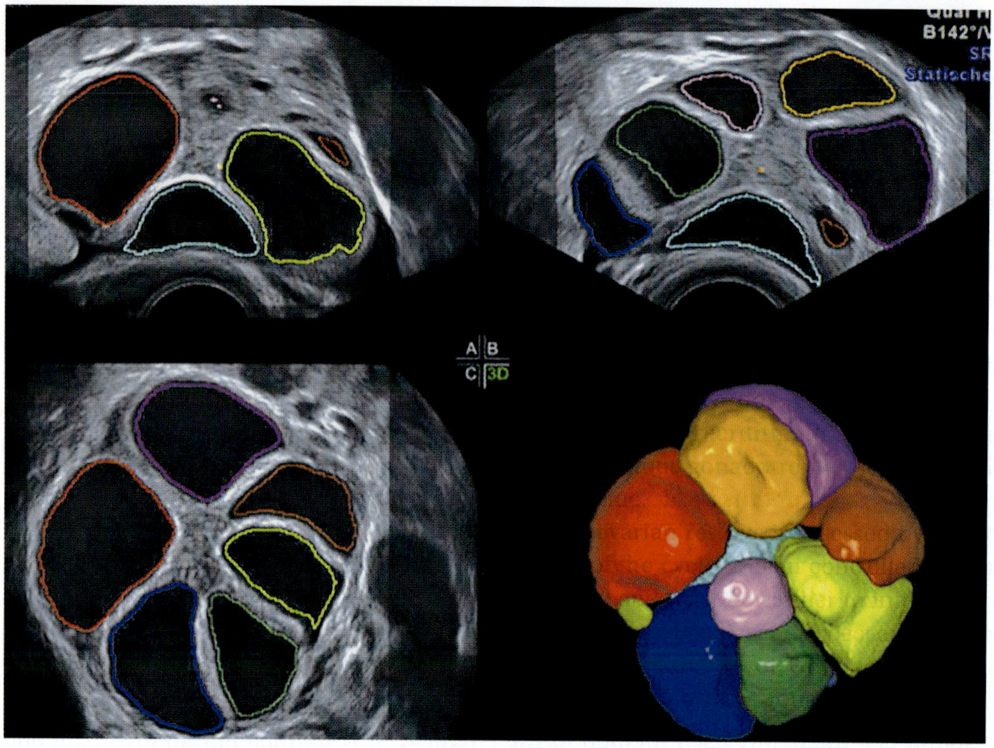

Fig. 4: Sonography-based automated volume calculation (SonoAVC).

in experienced centers.[9] Some variability is seen in younger women and those with high AFC. There is no impact of GnRH agonist used for pituitary downregulation on AFC, ovarian volume, and 3D power Doppler flow indices.[10] AFC can be evaluated by 2D, 3D, or 4D ultrasound.

Three-dimensional ultrasound is performed by manual measurement of follicle circumference through "virtual organ computer-aided analysis" (VOCAL) or by an automated ultrasound application, the "sonography-based automated volume calculation" (SonoAVC).[11,12] SonoAVC automatically identifies the boundaries of follicles. It measures the largest follicular diameters in "three orthogonal planes" **(Fig. 4)**.[11] A specific color is assigned to each follicle and it can be seen together with other follicles on the screen at the end. The "voxel" count within the identified hyperechoic area determines the follicular volume. It is the true measure of follicular volume even when its shape is irregular.[13,14] A good correlation has been demonstrated between the volume aspirated during oocyte retrieval and the SonoAVC calculated follicular volumes.[15] SonoAVC has more accuracy than traditional 2D measurements.[14] It also predicts the number of oocytes retrieved with a 60% retrieval rate.

Ovarian volume: Its is calculated by measuring each ovary in three planes with the formula of $D1 \times D2 \times D3 \times 0.52\ cm^3/mL$. The average volume of both ovaries gives mean ovarian volume. Poor response to stimulation is predicted by ovarian volume <3 mL, which has a high specificity of 80–90% and sensitivity of 11–80% **(Figs. 5A to C)**.[9]

Intraovarian flow indices **(Fig. 6)**: Ovarian stromal blood flow calculated at the time of starting stimulation shows good correlation with subsequent follicular response in IVF cycles.[16] Also, there is a good correlation between ovarian stromal flow index (FI) and the number of mature oocytes retrieved and pregnancy rate in the IVF cycle.[17]

Stromal flow index:

- *<11:* Poor responder
- *11–14:* Normal responder
- *>15:* Hyperresponder.

Stromal peak systolic velocity (PSV): Stromal PSV <10 after pituitary suppression is indicative of poor response. Stromal PSV >10 with unchanged resistance predicts the risk of hyperresponse.[18]

Uterine artery flow indices **(Fig. 7)**: Uterine artery resistance index (RI) >0.79 is associated with poor response and thus can predict the need of higher dosages of gonadotropins.[19] Lower uterine artery RI and higher PSV predict OHSS.

Ultrasound monitoring during ovarian stimulation includes assessment of:

- Follicular growth
- Endometrial thickness and patterns.

Assessment of Follicular Growth

Physiology: The first follicular structure that may be visualized on ultrasound is "secondary antral follicles" (2 mm), which

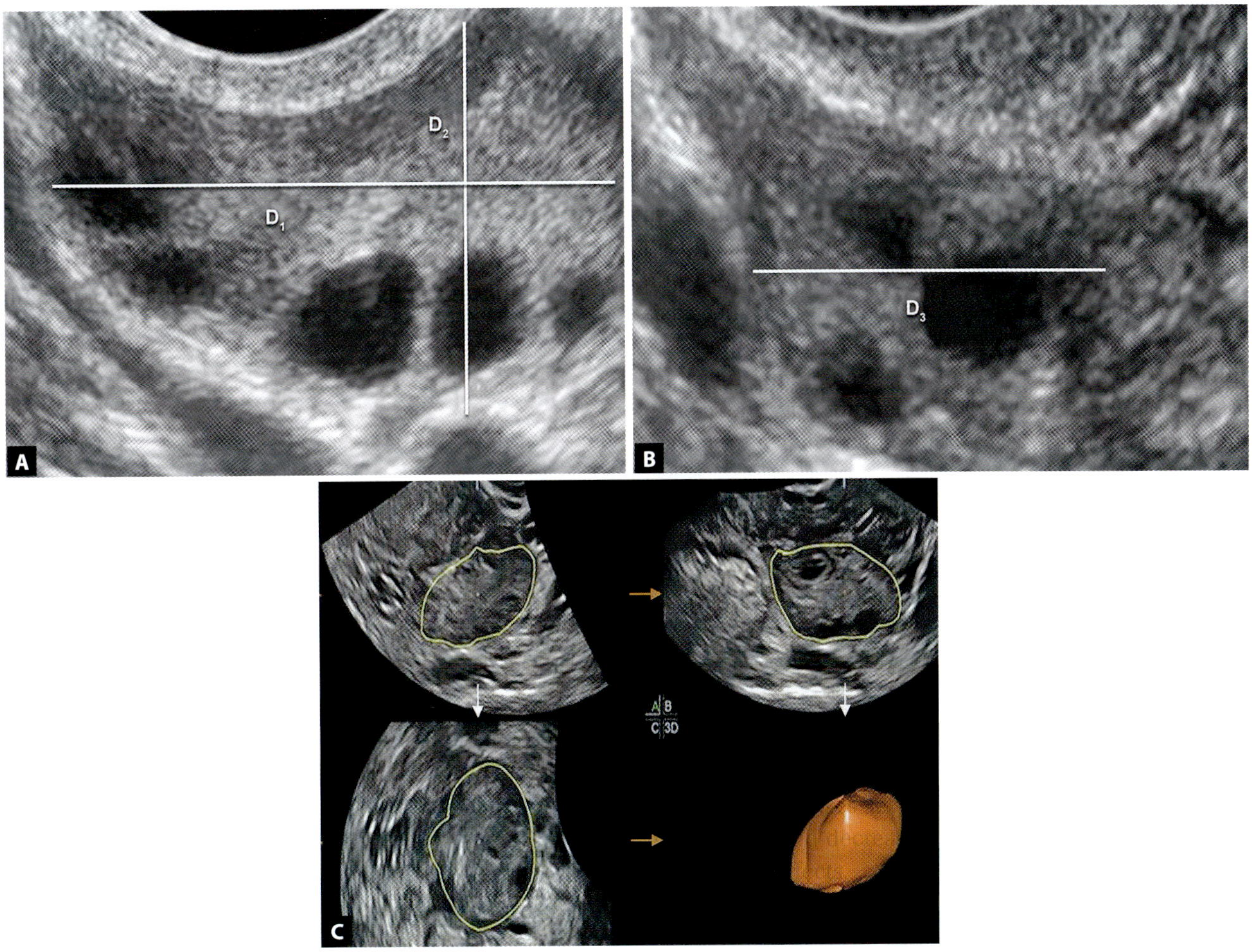

Figs. 5A to C: Ovarian volume 2D and 3D.

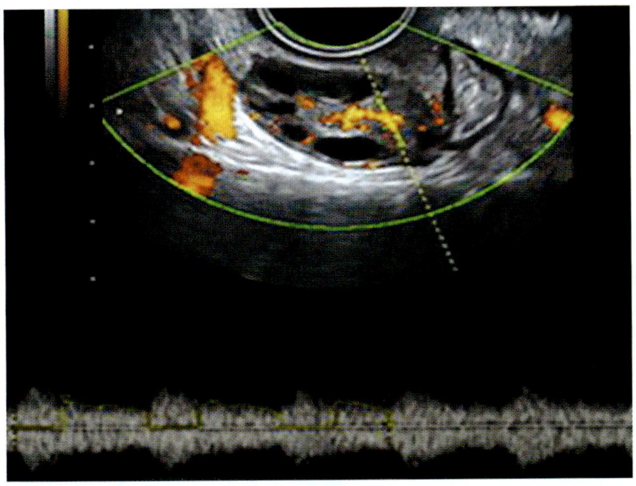

Fig. 6: Ovarian stromal flow index and peak systolic velocity.

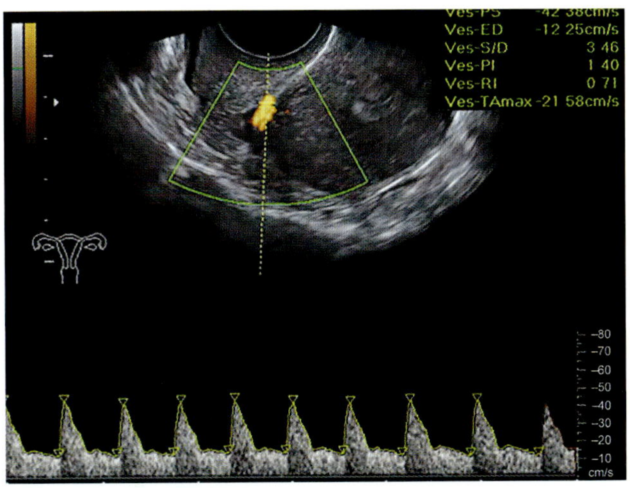

Fig. 7: Uterine artery flow indices.

are selected from the primordial follicular pool 80–90 days prior. There is a "selection" of dominant follicle by day 5. Between days 5 and 7, "dominance" of the follicle becomes apparent. Dominant follicle after 14 mm diameter has a growth rate of 1.5–2 mm/day until ovulation (20–25 mm diameter). Other follicles undergo atresia or developmental arrest.

Sonographically, the fate of the follicle can be decided by:

- Size
- Growth rate (as high as >2.3 mm/day in conception cycle)

- Wall thickness
- Internal echogenicity.

Prediction of ovulation:
- Increase in size (it is interesting to know that often the first largest follicle is not the largest follicle)
- Increase in granulosa cell thickness (growth rate 2–3 mm/day)
- Cumulus-like shadow 36 hours prior to ovulation[20]
- Sonolucent halo 24 hours prior to ovulation.[20] The vascularity of the theca cells is increased, and they become edematous after the LH surge. At the same time, separation starts between the granulosa cell and the theca cell layer. These changes are demonstrated as a line of decreased reflectivity around the follicle called "double contour" on ultrasound.
- Separation and folding of follicle lining 6–10 hours prior to ovulation.[20]

The "follicular growth pattern" rather than the follicular diameter has predictive value for anticipating the oocyte quality.[21] With the multifollicular growth in gonadotropin stimulation, it is difficult to identify changes in each follicle. The development of microvascular network around the follicle is responsible for proper follicular growth. The perifollicular blood flow (PFBF) indices are closely related to intrafollicular oxygen content and vascular endothelial growth factor (VEGF) concentrations **(Figs. 8A and B)**.[22] The oocytes retrieved from follicles with low oxygen content are frequently associated with mitochondrial dysfunction and abnormal chromosomal organization on metaphase spindle leading to segregation disorders and catastrophic mosaics in the embryos.[23] Thus, qualitative and quantitative analysis of PFBF by color Doppler and power Doppler is indicative of follicle competence. These ovarian flows also correlate well with the oocyte recovery rate.

By day 8 of the cycle, there is increase in the perifollicular vascularity in the theca cells of dominant follicle. The perifollicular RI starts falling from 2 days prior to ovulation and at the ovulation, it achieves the lowest value, which remains low for 4 days and then gradually starts rising to 0.5 by midluteal phase.

Perifollicular blood flow grading:
- *Grade 1:* Blood flow is <25% of follicle circumference
- *Grade 2:* Blood flow is ≥25% to <50% of follicle circumference
- *Grade 3:* Blood flow is ≥50% to <75% of follicle circumference
- *Grade 4:* Blood flow is ≥75% of follicle circumference.

Follicles having >75% of surface perfusion, ovarian stromal PSV >10 cm/s, and RI <0.4–0.48 usually contain good quality oocytes, which develop into good embryos.[22] Oocyte from follicle with PSV <10 cm/s has a high chance of developing into abnormal embryos.

Nargund et al.[24] demonstrated the probability of developing grades I and II embryos that is 75% when perifollicular PSV is >10 cm/s, 40% when PSV is <10 cm/s, and 24% when there is no PFBF. Rising PSV with steady low RI indicates impending follicular rupture (an hour before ovulation, PSV can be as high as 45 cm/s).

Steady or decreasing PSV with rising RI indicates impending LUF.

Changes in PFBF with ovarian stimulation:
- Clomiphene citrate use reduces ovarian, especially perifollicular vascularization.[25]
- Letrozole use does not alter PFBF.
- PFBF is demonstrated to be higher with the use of menotropins (urinary products) than that of recombinant FSH due to LH activity.[26]
- In IVF stimulations, cases with good ovarian PFBF in early follicular phase demonstrate good PFBF even in late follicular phase and are thus associated with higher clinical pregnancy rates.

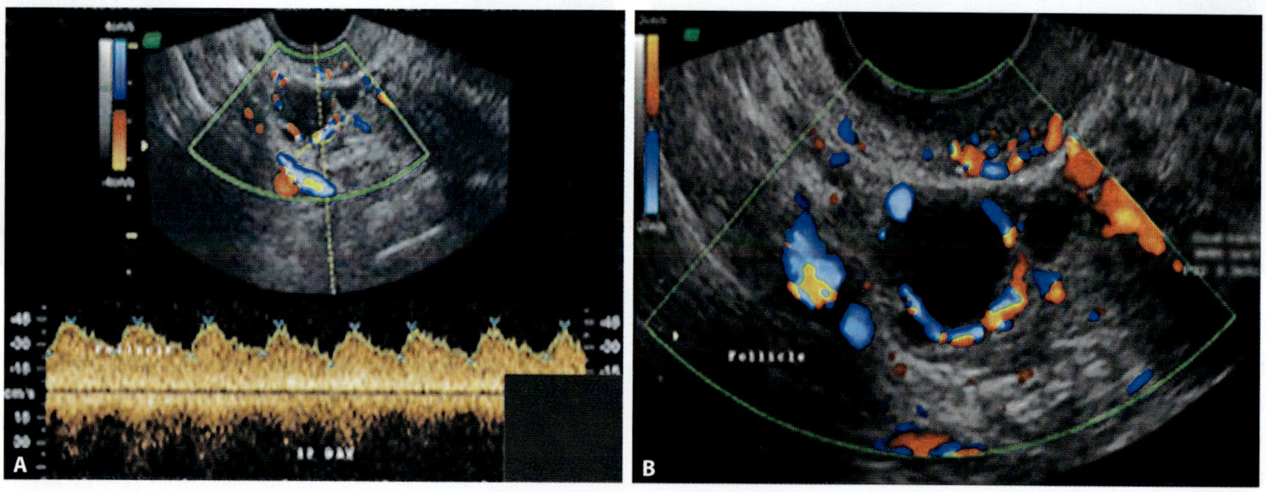

Figs. 8A and B: Perifollicular blood flow.

- Embryos derived from oocytes of highly vascularized follicles give higher clinical pregnancy rates. This has been demonstrated in the donor egg IVF cycles.[27]
- High perifollicular and uterine Doppler flow resistances are seen in poor responders.

Volume assessment of follicles by 3D ultrasound with Doppler consists of follicular volume, vascularization of cumulus, and perifollicular vascularization index (VI), FI, and vascularization flow index (VFI).

- 3D ultrasound is more accurate for assessment of the reliable parameter of follicle monitoring that is "follicular volume". In IVF cycles, follicles with a mean follicular diameter between 12 and 24 mm are associated with optimal oocyte recovery rate, fertilization rate, and cleavage rate, and it corresponds to the follicular volumes between 3 and 7 mL as stated by Wittmaack et al.[28]
- The chance of getting a mature oocyte from the follicle increases in the presence of cumulus, which can be detected by 3D ultrasound.[29]
- The perifollicular VI of 6–20 and FI >27 have higher pregnancy rates.[30]
- There is a strong correlation between 2D and 3D volume as well as 3D power Doppler angiography (PDA) indices as demonstrated in different studies.[31]

In practice, the follicular diameter is generally calculated by taking average of two or more measurements. Penzias et al.[32] found that the mean diameter of round and polygonal follicles accurately predicts the total follicular volume. But in cases of follicular crowding as may be seen in OI, especially with numerous ellipsoid follicles, the correlation between mean diameter and expected follicular volume and, presumably, oocyte maturity may be lacking.

Confirmation of ovulation: Although ultrasound does not allow precise timing or prediction of when ovulation will occur, it is an excellent technique for confirming ovulation once it has occurred. The ultrasound signs of ovulation are:

- Complete disappearance of the dominant follicle
- Decrease in the size of the follicle
- Irregularity of the follicular contour
- Central echoes within the follicle and formation of corpus luteum (echogenicity of the internal follicular area and that of the surrounding ovary becomes same)
- Presence of follicular fluid in the pouch of Douglas
- Hyperechogenic secretory endometrium.

Doppler of corpus luteum **(Fig. 9)**: It is the indicator of the functionality of corpus luteum. The normal value of RI of corpus luteum is 0.35–0.5. In the luteal phase deficiency (LPD), RI is 0.54–0.62, pulsatility index (PI) is 0.70–0.80, and PSV is 10–15.

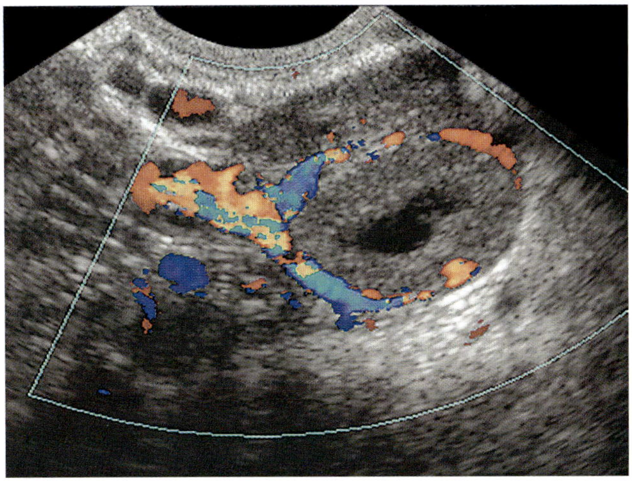

Fig. 9: Corpus luteum Doppler.

TABLE 4: Endometrial receptivity markers.

Conventional	*New*
Thickness	3D endometrial volume
Pattern	3D endometrial configuration
Peristalsis	3D endometrial vascularization indices
Uterine artery flow	

Assessment of Endometrium

The endometrium undergoes cyclical, morphological, and histological changes with typical sonographic patterns during the different phases of natural as well as stimulated cycles. These changes in the endometrium correlate with plasma estrogen and progesterone levels. Endometrial assessments have an important role in planning stimulation protocols, monitoring cycles, and predicting clinical outcomes **(Table 4)**.

Endometrial thickness is measured along the central longitudinal axis of the uterus. It is the maximum distance between the echogenic interfaces of the myometrium and the endometrium. The basal study of endometrial thickness should be started from cycle day 2 or 3 to look for proper shedding. The endometrium on this day should appear as a thin bright echogenic line or the cavity shows some blood with debris. A thick endometrium on basal scan (day 2) indicates improper endometrium shedding. The growth rate of endometrium in the proliferative phase is 0.5 mm/day and in the luteal phase, it is 0.1 mm/day. A thickness of >7 mm in the preovulatory period is associated with higher pregnancy rates **(Table 5)**.[33]

Smith's grading:

- *Grade A:* Bright endometrium—postovulation or the luteal phase
- *Grade B:* Endometrial reflectivity is similar to the myometrium—late follicular phase.

- *Grade C:* A solid area of reduced reflectivity appears as a darker area next to the lighter myometrium—mid-follicular phase.
- *Grade D:* Echoes are absent in the endometrium, but a bright central echo is seen, described as the triple line.

TABLE 5: Endometrial thickness and pattern in menstrual cycle.

Phase	*Thickness*	*Pattern*
Menstrual (days 1–5)	<5 mm	Thin
Early follicular (days 6–10)	7–9 mm	Distinct "triple line" hypoechogenic endometrium
Late follicular (day 11 to ovulation)	9–12 mm	Isoechogenic (similar to myometrium)
Luteal (postovulation)	10–14 mm	Bright, fluffy. Absence of triple line

In the late follicular phase, on trigger day, grade B pattern is associated with higher pregnancy rates.[34]

Nowadays, the endometrium pattern is classified into only two groups as multilayered and nonmultilayered **(Figs. 10A and B)**. Serafini et al.[35] have shown that a multi-layered pattern is more predictive of implantation than any other parameter measured.

Estrogen produces a vasodilatory effect on the uterine arteries. It has been seen that RI and PI of uterine artery drop with increasing estradiol levels. Steer et al.[36] have found that no pregnancy occurred if the PI of uterine was >3 and there was no spiral artery blood flow in the zones of endometrium. Depending on the vascularization of the endometrial layers, the late proliferative triple line endometrium is divided into four zones **(Figs. 11A to D)**:[37]

1. *Zone I:* 2 mm thick area surrounding zone II

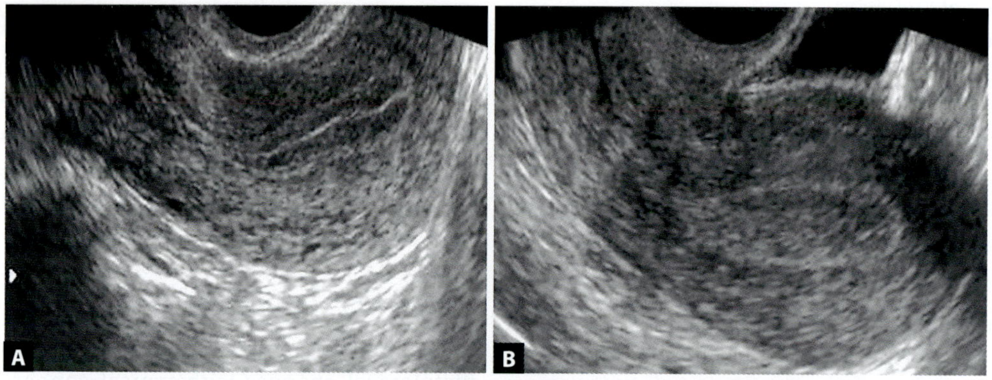

Figs. 10A and B: Multilayered and nonmultilayered endometrium.

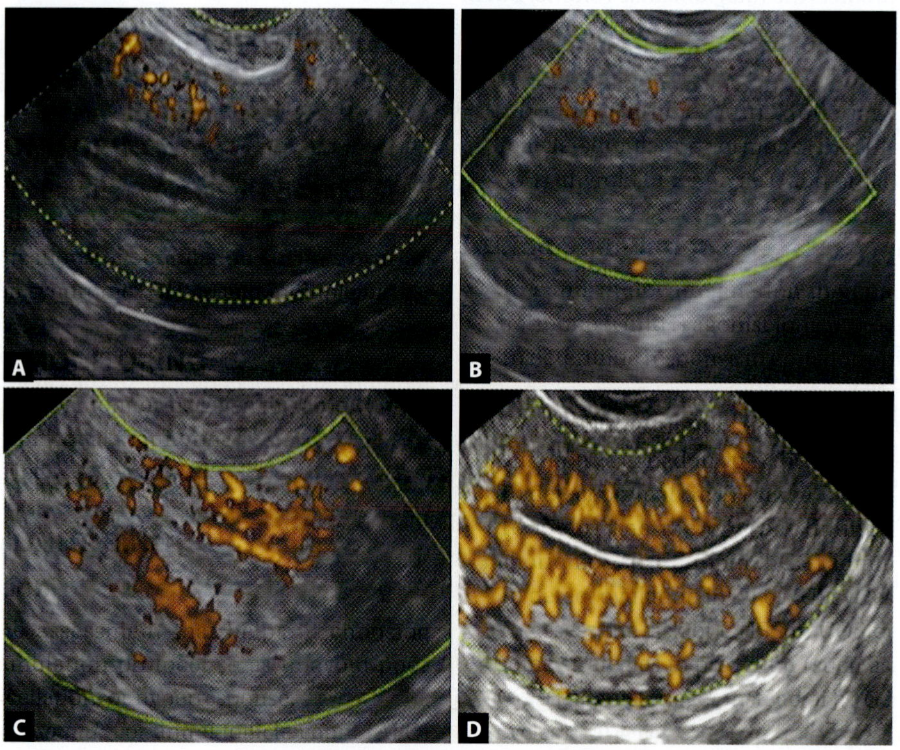

Figs. 11A to D: Endometrial vascularity zones.

TABLE 6: Applebaum's uterine scoring system for reproduction.

Parameter	Determination	Score
Endometrial thickness (mm)	<7	0
	7–9	2
	10–14	3
	>14	1
Endometrial layering	No layering	0
	Hazy five-line appearance	1
	Distinct five-line appearance	3
Endometrial motion (no. of myometrial contractions in 2 minutes—real time) **(Table 7)**	<3	0
	≥3	3
Myometrial echogenicity	Course, inhomogenous	1
	Relatively homogenous	2
Uterine artery Doppler flow (pulsatility index)	>3	0
	2.5–2.99	0
	2.2–2.49	1
	<2.19	2
Endometrial blood flow within zone 3	Absent	0
	Present but sparse	2
	Present multifocally	5
Myometrial blood flow (gray scale)	Absent	0
	Present	2

Note: The score of 13 or less was found to have no conception

2. *Zone II:* Hyperechoic outer endometrial edge
3. *Zone III:* Hypoechoic inner endometrial area
4. *Zone IV:* Endometrial cavity.

Applebaum's uterine scoring system for reproduction (USSR)–uterine biophysical profile (UBP): It is based on certain sonographic qualities of the uterus that are noted during the normal mid-cycle **(Table 6)**.[37]

Endometrial volume **(Fig. 12)**: 3D measurement of endometrial volume can predict outcomes, especially in intrauterine pathologies such as adhesions, uterine anomalies, and adenomyosis. Most of the pregnancies occur with a volume of 2–13 mL, but pregnancy has been reported at volume as low as 1.59 mL.[38]

Endometrial vascular flow indices **(Fig. 13)**: They are measured by the 3D power Doppler histogram analysis. For the calculations, VOCAL imaging program is used.

- *Vascularization index* represents the presence of blood vessels (vascularity) in the endometrium. It is measured as the ratio of the number of color voxels to the total number of voxels and is expressed as a percentage (%) of the endometrial volume.

TABLE 7: Uterine contractions during menstrual cycle.

Time of the menstrual cycle	Uterine contractions/min	Direction
Follicular phase	4–5	Retrograde
Luteofollicular transition phase	2–3	Anterograde
Luteal phase	<2.5	

5. *Flow index* is the mean power Doppler signal intensity inside the endometrium and represents the average intensity of flow.
   - VFI is a combination of vascularity and flow intensity.
   - *Flow vessel quotient (FVQ)* is FI divided by VI.

The endometrial and subendometrial blood flow was found to be significantly higher in women with pregnancies resulted in live birth than those with a miscarriage in the study by Ng et al.[39] Wu et al.[40] found that subendometrial VFI may be useful in predicting implantation and pregnancy rates in IVF.

- No pregnancy if VI is <1, FI is <31, and VFI is <0.25.
- In cases of low-volume endometrium, the flow indices are less. Such changes are not seen in cases with thin endometrium.[41]
- Flow indices are lower in stimulated cycles as compared to cycles without stimulation.[42]
- Use of clomiphene but not letrozole negatively affects endometrial vascularity.
- In IVF cycles, higher the estradiol (E2) levels, lower the flow indices.[43]

Timing of trigger: hCG is usually administered when there is a minimum of one follicle measuring 16–18 mm in diameter (usually three in IVF cycles), endometrial thickness around 8 mm, and serum E2 levels of 200–300 pg/mL per dominant follicle.

ABNORMAL RESPONSES IN OVARIAN STIMULATION

- *Poor response:* Less than two or three follicles on D7 of stimulation.
- *Hyperresponse:* It can be predicted by numerous small- and intermediate-sized follicles. The secondary follicles (<16 mm) constitute a heterogeneous group with variable endocrine function. Small follicles continue to grow after hCG administration, thus increasing estrogen secretion and contributing to the cascade of hyperstimulation syndrome. In cases of severe OHSS, ultrasound is useful in the treatment [ultrasonography (USG)-guided taping of ascetic and pleural fluid].
- *Premature luteinization:* Follicle with <15 mm with internal echoes in association with high progesterone levels.

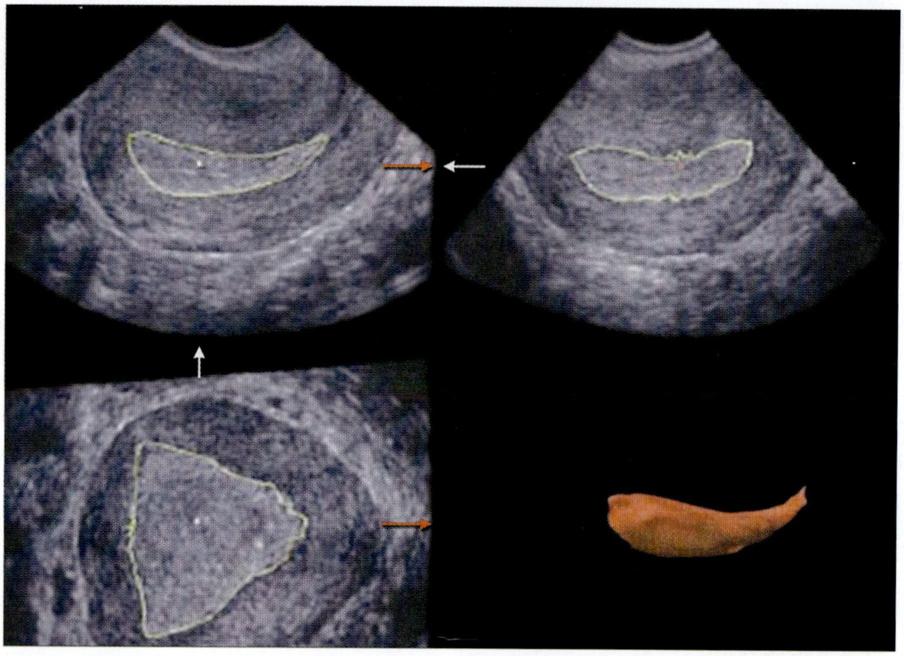

Fig. 12: Endometrial volume.

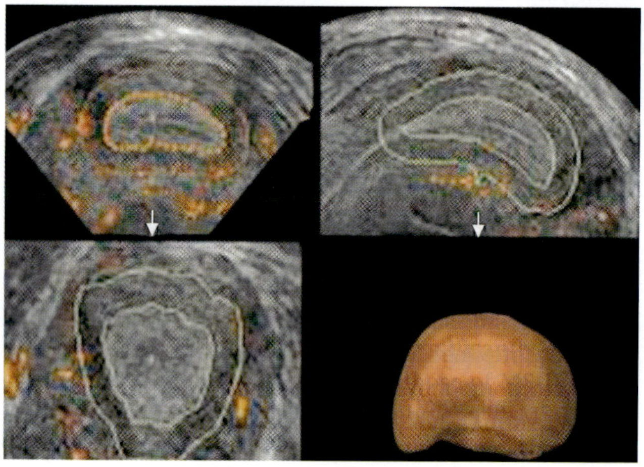

Fig. 13: Endometrial flow indices.

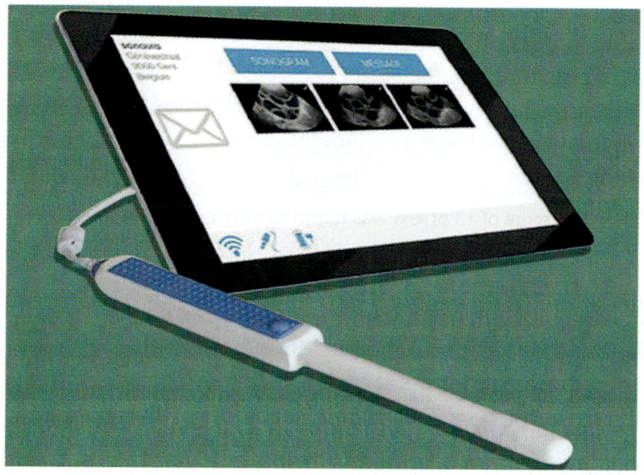

Fig. 14: Self-operated endovaginal telemonitoring (SOET) system.

- *LUF:* 34–36 mm thick-walled follicle with internal echoes persistent even after 48 hours of trigger, thick echogenic endometrium with no fluid in pouch of Douglas.
- *Endogenous LH surge:* Premature rupture of follicle at <16 mm diameter.
- *Functional cyst:* It is an anechoic structure with sharp edges. Present at baseline scan prestimulation as a result of initial high FSH levels. It requires either cycle cancellation or aspiration before starting stimulation.
- *Persistent or retention cyst:* Noticed at baseline scan. It can be a persistent corpus luteum or a cyst from previous cycle.

Self-operated endovaginal telemonitoring (SOET): It is the sonography performed by the patient and her partner at home. It is with the help of server-based communication and imaging software. Some studies showed that SOET reduced economic, logistic, emotional, and potential environmental costs and improved patient's participation and confidence without compromising conception and ongoing pregnancy rates as compared to routine ultrasound **(Fig. 14)**.[44]

HORMONAL MONITORING OF OVARIAN STIMULATION

The hypothalamus–pituitary–ovarian axis controls the ovarian and uterine cycles.[45] Hormones produced by each gland have various local and systemic effects. Bioassays of these various hormones are useful to assess ovarian reserve as well as response of ovary to stimulation.

In 1926, Zondek and Aschheim[46] described their ideas on the function of the human ovary and confirmed the involvement of hormones in the normal functioning of the ovary. Loewe and Lange[47] described the female sex hormone in the urine of menstruating women and the changes in their concentration with the phase of the menstrual cycle.

Hormonal tests for predicting ovarian reserve help to choose the treatment protocol and add prognostic information to the counseling. They are basal FSH, basal estradiol, AMH, and inhibin B.

- *Basal FSH:* Measured on day 2–4. It is less reliable as FSH assays show inter- and intracycle variability.[48,49] As per WHO Second International Standards, FSH assays with the cut point above 10 IU/L are associated with less than two to three follicles or four and less retrieved eggs. This cut point shows high specificity of 83–100% and low sensitivity of 10–80% to predict such poor response.[50] But it cannot predict total failure to conceive. Consistently, elevated FSH predicts poor response but, isolated single high FSH reading with age <40 years of age may not predict poor response.[51] It is suggested that women with fluctuating FSH levels should not wait for "ideal-normal FSH" cycles to initiate IVF cycle.[52]
- *Basal estradiol:* Measured on days 2–4. "Normal" basal FSH levels are correctly interpreted along with basal estradiol. Basal elevated estradiol >60–80 pg/mL with "normal" basal FSH indicates poor response, cycle cancellation, and poor pregnancy rate.[53-55] It has poor inter- and intracycle reliability.
- *Anti-Müllerian hormone:* It is produced by granulosa cells of preantral and early antral follicles. Serum AMH level is gonadotropin-independent, thus no intra- or intercycle variability.[56-59] Low AMH level has been associated with poor response to stimulation, poor egg, and embryo quality, and thus less pregnancy rates in IVF but it does not necessarily predict the same.[60] AMH predicts ovarian reserve more specifically and is thus considered as a more reliable ovarian reserve test. There is a strong positive correlation between serum AMH level and AFC. The use of AMH combined with AFC may improve ovarian reserve evaluation.[61] Low AMH cut points [0.2–0.7 ng/mL DSL enzyme-linked immunosorbent assay (ELISA)] have been found to have sensitivities from 40 to 97% and specificities from 78 to 92% for poor reserve and response (<3 follicles or ≤2–4 oocytes retrieved).[62-64]
- *Inhibin B:* It has high inter- and intracycle variability as the levels increase with stimulation. The levels are lower in poor responders (<45 pg/mL).[64]

Monitoring before stimulation helps to optimize IVF success rates by achieving individualized controlled ovarian stimulation (iCOS) where starting stimulation doses are adjusted considering different parameters as follows:

- *PIVET algorithm* based on age, AFC, AMH, body mass index, day-2 FSH, and smoking[65]
- *Ovarian response prediction index (ORPI)* based on AMH, AFC, and age[66]
- Only AMH.[67]

Hormonal monitoring during stimulation frequently involves assessment of levels of estradiol, LH, and progesterone.

Serum Estradiol

Serum estradiol is used to monitor ovarian activity. In unstimulated cycles, a linear response is observed between estrogen levels and growth of the dominant follicle. This correlation is disturbed with the development of multiple follicles during gonadotropin stimulation. Gonadotropin dose is adjusted every 3 days so that estradiol levels increase by 50% per day.[68] The total serum E2 is a function of the state of maturity of all follicles present at a given time. An equation to determine the expected serum E2 levels depending on the number and size of follicles in both ovaries is:[69]

$$\textit{E2 on trigger day} = 291\ \text{pg/mL} + 180\,(x) + 64\,(y) + 18.7\,(z)$$

where

x: Follicles measuring ≥17 mm
y: Follicles measuring 15–16 mm
z: Follicles measuring ≤14 mm

Estradiol level at the time of hCG administration is more critical than the rate of rise. Trigger is usually given when estradiol levels reach 200–300 pg/mL per large follicle.

Estradiol levels predict the IVF cycle prognosis:

- *Low E2 after first few days of stimulation:* Higher cycle cancellation rate and poor outcome[70-72]
- Higher pregnancy rate in cycles with a higher E2/oocyte ratio in the late follicular phase[73]
- *Optimum estradiol window:* 1,000–1,500 pg/mL[74]
- *Estradiol levels >3,000 pg/mL:* Significant risk of hyperstimulation[75-77]
- Very high E2 levels (>5,000 pg/mL) may diminish endometrial receptivity.[78]

The rate of E2 rise remains the same in natural and stimulated cycles as well as in the cycles which result in multiple pregnancies.[79]

Serum Luteinizing Hormone

Serum luteinizing hormone is monitored to detect the spontaneous premature LH surge and premature luteinization. Several literatures have demonstrated less pregnancy rates in the presence of premature LH surge during ovarian stimulation due to its effect on egg and embryo quality.[80] The incidence of premature LH surge in GnRH agonist cycles is negligible, but 1–2.5% in GnRH antagonist cycles.

Premature LH surge is nothing but an LH level of ≥10 mIU/mL and a progesterone level of ≥1.0 ng/mL demonstrated for at least 2 consecutive days before trigger.[81,82]

There are three types of premature LH rise:

1. *Sustained type:* LH release started during the stimulation and present till hCG administration.
2. *Transient type:* LH release started during the stimulation but normalized before hCG administration.
3. *Onset type:* LH was released only on the day of hCG administration.

Serum Progesterone

High serum progesterone on day 2 of the cycle predicts poor pregnancy outcomes.[83] It has been observed that 5–35% of GnRH agonist cycles and 20–38% of GnRH antagonist cycles will have subtle increases in serum progesterone levels at the end of the follicular phase.[84,85] This progesterone rise is not with LH rise; rather it reflects the granulosa cell response to high FSH stimulation.[85] Ongoing pregnancy rates are low when trigger day serum progesterone levels of 1.5 ng/mL or high irrespective of the GnRH analog are used for pituitary downregulation.[86] Elevated preovulatory progesterone mainly affects endometrial development, not the oocyte or embryo quality.[87] Embryo cryopreservation has been shown to be an effective means of circumventing disruptions caused by COS, including embryo-endometrium asynchrony.[88]

Criteria for Adequate Pituitary Suppression

- *Ultrasound markers:* No follicle ≥10 mm; endometrial thickness ≤5 mm, and absence of ovarian cyst
- *Hormonal markers:* LH <2 IU/L; E2 <50 pg/mL, and serum progesterone (P4) <1.2 ng/mL.

Protocol for the Monitoring of Ovarian Stimulation

- *Monitoring of ovarian stimulation in TI and IUI cycles:* In TI and IUI cycles, ovarian stimulation aims at unifollicular or maximum two or three follicle development. So usually, ultrasound monitoring alone would suffice to prevent complications. Sometimes, the LH kit method (urinary LH levels) is used to detect LH surge and thus to TI or IUI procedure accordingly. Serum monitoring of estradiol and LH levels is rarely required when there is hyperresponse, especially with gonadotropin use. As the follicular growth and endometrial thickness show a good correlation with serum estradiol levels in these cycles, serial transvaginal ultrasound examination alone is the most efficient and cost-effective way of monitoring.[89]
- *Monitoring of ovarian stimulation in IVF or intracytoplasmic sperm injection (ICSI) cycles:* Previously, combined use of USG and serum estradiol measurement was considered as optimum for monitoring of stimulation. Later in different studies, it was shown that E2 levels correlate well with the size of the dominant follicle, endometrial thickness, and uterine dimensions all of which can be easily measured by ultrasound. These USG parameters can be considered as "biological assays" of estrogen activity.[89] Thus, ultrasound can assess both morphology and function of the ovary. Currently, several trials are evaluating whether only ultrasound without hormonal assessment can be used for monitoring in IVF cycles.[90-93] As the incidence of premature luteinization is reduced with GnRH analogs use, merely USG without hormone monitoring is adequate in these cycles.

Cochrane review in 2014 by Kwan et al.[94] has found:

- No evidence from randomized trials to suggest that combined monitoring by transvaginal ultrasound and serum estradiol is more efficacious than monitoring by transvaginal ultrasound alone with regard to clinical pregnancy rates and the incidence of OHSS.
- The number of oocytes retrieved appeared similar for both monitoring protocols.
- The data suggest that both these monitoring methods are safe and reliable.
- A combined monitoring protocol including both transvaginal ultrasound and serum estradiol may need to be retained as precautionary good clinical practice and as a confirmatory test in a subset of women to identify those at high risk of OHSS.

With the increasing trend toward simplification of IVF and reduction of the costs involved, many centers now use ultrasound alone or in combination with minimal hormonal assays for the monitoring of COS.

CONCLUSION

- Some anatomical structures (such as internal iliac artery and vein cross section, cross section of blood vessels around the uterus and ovary, bowel, hydrosalpinx) will look similar to growing follicle, but they will change shape from circular to oblong when the probe is moved from transverse to longitudinal section.
- At the start of stimulation, 2D transvaginal ultrasound is the most commonly used clinical tool.
- AFC is the most commonly used ultrasound marker for ovarian reserve, which shows good correlation with AMH values and thus helps in determining gonadotropin dosages for iCOS.
- Endometrial thickness is measured by transvaginal ultrasound along the longitudinal axis of the uterus. It is the maximum distance between the echogenic interfaces of the myometrium and the endometrium.
- At the start of stimulation (day 2 of period), these readings indicate adequate pituitary suppression and give green signal to start gonadotropins:

- No follicle ≥10 mm, endometrial thickness ≤5 mm, and absence of ovarian cyst on USG
- LH: <2 IU/L, E2: <50 pg/mL, and P4: <1.2 ng/mL

- E2 levels are generally repeated on stimulation day 4, day 6, and trigger day with or without LH levels.
- E2 levels >250–300, along with one of the follicles >14 mm on scan is generally an indicator to start GnRH antagonist in the flexible antagonist protocol.
- Serum progesterone levels are generally done at the start of stimulation and on trigger day.
- Serum progesterone ≥1.5 ng/mL on trigger day is an indicator of cryopreservation of all the embryos and cancellation of fresh embryo transfer (ET).

KEY POINTS

- AFC shows a good correlation with age, ovarian reserve, and response to stimulation.
- AFC predicts the ovarian response and decreases the chances of cycle cancellation.[7]
- AFC has good intercycle and interobserver reliability in experienced centers.[9]
- There is a good correlation between the volume aspirated during oocyte retrieval and the SonoAVC calculated follicular volumes.[13]
- SonoAVC has more accuracy than traditional 2D measurements.[14]
- Follicles having >75% of surface perfusion, ovarian stromal PSV >10 cm/s, and RI <0.4–0.48 usually contain good-quality oocytes which develop into good embryos.[22]
- In TI and IUI cycles, serial transvaginal ultrasound examination alone is most efficient and cost-effective way of monitoring.[89]
- In IVF cycles, combined monitoring protocol, including both transvaginal ultrasound and serum estradiol, may need to be retained as precautionary good clinical practice.[94]

REFERENCES

1. Cobb M. Generation: The Seventeenth Century Scientists Who Unraveled the Secrets of Sex, Life, and Growth. New York: Bloomsbury Publishing; 2006.
2. Baerwald AR, Adams GP, Pierson RA. Ovarian antral folliculogenesis during the human menstrual cycle: a review. Hum Reprod Update. 2012;18(1):73-91.
3. Hackelöer BJ, Fleming R, Robinson HP, Adam AH, Coutts JR. Correlation of ultrasonic and endocrinologic assessment of human follicular development. Am J Obstet Gynecol. 1979;135(1):122-8.
4. Hackelöer BJ, Sallam HN. Ultrasound scanning of ovarian follicles. Clin Obstet Gynecol. 1983;10:603-20.
5. Vargyas JM, Marrs RP, Kletzky OA, Mishell Jr DR. Correlation of ultrasonic measurement of ovarian follicle size and serum estradiol levels in ovulatory patients following clomiphene citrate for in vitro fertilization. Am J Obstet Gynecol. 1982; 144(5):569-73.
6. Marrs RP, Vargyas JM, March CM. Correlation of ultrasonic and endocrinologic measurements in human menopausal gonadotropin therapy. Am J Obstet Gynecol. 1983;145(4):417-21.
7. Chang MY, Chiang CH, Hsieh TT, Soong YK, Hsu KH. Use of the antral follicle count to predict the outcome of assisted reproductive technologies. Fertil Steril. 1998;69(3):505-10.
8. Hendriks DJ, Mol BW, Bancsi LF, Te Velde ER, Broekmans FJ. Antral follicle count in the prediction of poor ovarian response and pregnancy after in vitro fertilization: a meta-analysis and comparison with basal follicle-stimulating hormone level. Fertil Steril. 2005;83(2):291-301.
9. McIlveen M, Skull JD, Ledger WL. Evaluation of the utility of multiple endocrine and ultrasound measures of ovarian reserve in the prediction of cycle cancellation in a high-risk IVF population. Hum Reprod. 2007;22(3):778-85.
10. Yu Ng EH, Chi Wai Chan C, Tang OS, Shu Biu Yeung W, Chung Ho P. Effect of pituitary downregulation on antral follicle count, ovarian volume and stromal blood flow measured by three-dimensional ultrasound with power Doppler prior to ovarian stimulation. Hum Reprod. 2004;19(12):2811-5.
11. Ata B, Tulandi T. Ultrasound automated volume calculation in reproduction and in pregnancy. Fertil Steril. 2011;95(7): 2163-70.
12. Tur-Kaspa I, Stadtmauer L. Ultrasonography in assisted reproduction. In: Gardner DK, Weissman A, Howles CM, Shoam Z (Eds). Textbook of Assisted Reproductive Techniques: Laboratory and Clinical Perspectives, 2nd edition. UK: Taylor & Francis; 2004.
13. Raine-Fenning N, Jayaprakasan K, Clewes J, Joergner I, Bonaki SD, Chamberlain S, et al. SonoAVC: a novel method of automatic volume calculation. Ultrasound Obstet Gynecol. 2008;31:691-6.
14. Raine-Fenning N, Jayaprakasan K, Chamberlain S, Devlin L, Priddle H, Johnson I. Automated measurements of follicle diameter: a chance to standardize? Fertil Steril. 2009;91: 1469-72.
15. Raine-Fenning N, Jayaprakasan K, Clewes J, Joergner I, Bonaki SD, Chamberlain S, et al. Establishing the validity of a new technique that facilitates automated follicular volume measurement. Ultrasound Obstet Gynecol. 2007;30(4):393.
16. Zaidi J, Barber J, Kyei-Mensah A, Bekir J, Campbell S, Tan SL. Relationship of ovarian stromal blood flow at the baseline ultrasound scan to subsequent follicular response in an in vitro fertilization program. Obstet Gynecol. 1996;88(5): 779-84.
17. Kupesic S, Kurjak A. Predictors of IVF outcome by three-dimensional ultrasound. Hum Reprod. 2002;17(4):950-5.
18. Engmann L, Sladkevicius P, Agrawal R, Bekir JS, Campbell S, Tan SL. Value of ovarian stromal blood flow velocity measurement after pituitary suppression in the prediction of ovarian responsiveness and outcome of in vitro fertilization treatment. Fertil Steril. 1999;71(1):22-9.
19. Battaglia C, Larocca E, Lanzani A, Valentini M, Genazzani AR. Doppler ultrasound studies of the uterine arteries in spontaneous and IVF stimulated ovarian cycles. Gynecol Endocrinol. 1990;4(4):245-50.
20. Picker RH, Smith DH, Tucker MH, Saunders DM. Ultrasonic signs of imminent ovulation. J Clin Ultrasound. 1983;11(1):1-2.

21. Nayudu PL. Relationship of constructed follicular growth patterns in stimulated cycles to outcome after IVF. Hum Reprod. 1991;6(4):465-71.
22. Mercé LT, Bau S, Barco MJ, Troyano J, Gay R, Sotos F, et al. Assessment of ovarian volume, number and volume of follicles and ovarian vascularity by three-dimensional ultrasonography and power Doppler angiography on the hCG day to predict the outcome in IVF/ICSI cycles. Hum Reprod. 2006;21(5):1218-26.
23. Van Blerkom J, Antczak M, Schrader R. The developmental potential of human oocyte is related to the dissolved oxygen content of follicular fluid: association with vascular endothelial growth factor levels and perifollicular blood flow characteristics. Hum Reprod. 1997;12(5):1047-55.
24. Nargund G, Doyle PE, Bourne TH, Parsons JH, Cheng WC, Campbell S, et al. Ultrasound derived indices of follicular blood flow before hCG administration and the prediction of oocyte recovery and preimplantation embryo quality. Hum Reprod. 1996;11:2512-7.
25. Palomba S, Russo T, Falbo A, Orio Jr F, Manguso F, Nelaj E, et al. Clinical use of the perifollicular vascularity assessment in IVF cycles: a pilot study. Hum Reprod. 2006;21(4):1055-61.
26. O'Leary AJ, Griffiths AN, Evans J, Pugh ND. Perifollicular blood flow and pregnancy in superovulated intrauterine insemination (IUI) cycles: an observational comparison of recombinant follicle-stimulating hormone (FSH) and urinary gonadotropins. Fertil Steril. 2009;92(4):1366-8.
27. Borini A, Maccolini A, Tallarini A, Bonu MA, Sciajno R, Flamigni C. Perifollicular vascularity and its relationship with oocyte maturity and IVF outcome. Ann NY Acad Sci. 2009;943:64-7.
28. Wittmaack FM, Kreger DO, Blasco L, Tureck RW, Mastroianni Jr L, Lessey BA. Effect of follicular size on oocyte retrieval, fertilization, cleavage, and embryo quality in in vitro fertilization cycles: a 6-year data collection. Fertil Steril. 1994;62(6):1205-10.
29. Poehl M, Hohlagschwandtner M, Doerner V, Dillinger B, Feichtinger W. Cumulus assessment by three-dimensional ultrasound for in vitro fertilization. Ultrasound Obstet Gynecol. 2000;16(3):251-3.
30. Panchal SY, Nagori CB. Can 3D PD be a better tool for assessing the pre hCG follicle and endometrium? A randomized study of 500 cases. Ultrasound Obstet Gynecol. 2006;28(4):504.
31. Pascual MA, Graupera B, Hereter L, Tresserra F, Rodriguez I, Alcázar JL. Assessment of ovarian vascularization in the polycystic ovary by three-dimensional power Doppler ultrasonography. Gynecol Endocrinol. 2008;24(11):631-6.
32. Penzias AM, Emmi AM, Dubey AK, Layman LC, DeCherney AH, Reindollar RH. Ultrasound prediction of follicle volume: is the mean diameter reflective? Fertil Steril. 1994;62(6):1274-6.
33. Rabinowitz R, Laufer N, Lewin A, Navot D, Bar I, Margalioth EJ, et al. The value of ultrasonographic endometrial measurement in the prediction of pregnancy following in vitro fertilization. Fertil Steril. 1986;45(6):824-8.
34. Smith B, Porter R, Ahuja K, Craft I. Ultrasonic assessment of endometrial changes in stimulated cycles in an in vitro fertilization and embryo transfer program. J In Vitro Fert Embryo Transf. 1984;1(4):233-8.
35. Serafini P, Batzofin J, Nelson J, Olive D. Sonographic uterine predictors of pregnancy in women undergoing ovulation induction for assisted reproductive treatments. Fertil Steril. 1994;62(4):815-22.
36. Steer CV, Campbell S, Pampiglione JS, Kingsland CR, Mason BA, Collins WP. Transvaginal colour flow imaging of the uterine arteries during the ovarian and menstrual cycles. Hum Reprod. 1990;5(4):391-5.
37. Applebaum M. The uterine biophysical profile (UBP). In: Allahabadia G (Ed). Endosonography in Obstetrics and Gynecology. Mumbai: Rotunda Medical Technologies Ltd; 1997. pp. 343-52.
38. Jokubkiene L, Sladkevicius P, Rovas L, Valentin L. Assessment of changes in volume and vascularity of the ovaries during the normal menstrual cycle using three-dimensional power Doppler ultrasound. Hum Reprod. 2006;21(10):2661-8.
39. Ng EH, Chan CC, Tang OS, Yeung WS, Ho PC. Endometrial and subendometrial vascularity is higher in pregnant patients with livebirth following ART than in those who suffer a miscarriage. Hum Reprod. 2007;22(4):1134-41.
40. Wu HM, Chiang CH, Huang HY, Chao AS, Wang HS, Soong YK. Detection of the subendometrial vascularization flow index by three-dimensional ultrasound may be useful for predicting the pregnancy rate for patients undergoing in vitro fertilization—embryo transfer. Fertil Steril. 2003;79(3):507-11.
41. Ng EH, Yeung WS, Ho PC. Endometrial and subendometrial vascularity are significantly lower in patients with endometrial volume 2.5 ml or less. Reprod Biomed Online. 2009;18(2):262-8.
42. Ng EH, Chan CC, Tang OS, Yeung WS, Ho PC. Comparison of endometrial and subendometrial blood flow measured by three-dimensional power Doppler ultrasound between stimulated and natural cycles in the same patients. Hum Reprod. 2004;19:2385-90.
43. Ng EH, Chan CC, Tang OS, Yeung WS, Ho PC. The role of endometrial and subendometrial blood flows measured by three-dimensional power Doppler ultrasound in the prediction of pregnancy during IVF treatment. Hum Reprod. 2006;21(1):164-70.
44. Gerris J, Delvigne A, Dhont N, Vandekerckhove F, Madoc B, Buyle M, et al. Self-operated endovaginal telemonitoring versus traditional monitoring of ovarian stimulation in assisted reproduction: an RCT. Hum Reprod. 2014;29(9):1941-8.
45. Marieb EN, Hoehn K. Human Anatomy & Physiology. San Francisco: Pearson Benjamin Cummings; 2007. pp. 1090-110.
46. Zondek B, Aschheim S. Zurfunktion des ovariums. Klin Wochenschr. 1926;10:400-8.
47. Loewe S, Lange I. Der gehalt des frauenharns an brunsterzengenden Stoffen in abhangigkeit von ovariellen zyklus. Klin Wochenschr. 1926;5:1038-9.
48. Scott Jr RT, Hofmann GE, Oehninger S, Muasher SJ. Intercycle variability of day 3 follicle-stimulating hormone levels and its effect on stimulation quality in in vitro fertilization. Fertil Steril. 1990;54(2):297-302.
49. Kwee J, Schats R, McDonnell J, Lambalk CB, Schoemaker J. Intercycle variability of ovarian reserve tests: results of a prospective randomized study. Hum Reprod. 2004;19(3):590-5.
50. Esposito MA, Coutifaris C, Barnhart KT. A moderately elevated day 3 FSH concentration has limited predictive value, especially in younger women. Hum Reprod. 2002;17(1):118-23.

51. Roberts JE, Spandorfer S, Fasouliotis SJ, Kashyap S, Rosenwaks Z. Taking a basal follicle-stimulating hormone history is essential before initiating in vitro fertilization. Fertil Steril. 2005;83(1):37-41.
52. Abdalla H, Thum MY. Repeated testing of basal FSH levels has no predictive value for IVF outcome in women with elevated basal FSH. Hum Reprod. 2006;21(1):171-4.
53. Evers JL, Slaats P, Land JA, Dumoulin JC, Dunselman GA. Elevated levels of basal estradiol-17beta predict poor response in patients with normal basal levels of follicle-stimulating hormone undergoing in vitro fertilization. Fertil Steril. 1998;69(6):1010-4.
54. Licciardi FL, Liu HC, Rosenwaks Z. Day 3 estradiol serum concentrations as prognosticators of ovarian stimulation response and pregnancy outcome in patients undergoing in vitro fertilization. Fertil Steril. 1995;64(5):991-4.
55. Smotrich DB, Widra EA, Gindoff PR, Levy MJ, Hall JL, Stillman RJ. Prognostic value of day 3 estradiol on in vitro fertilization outcome. Fertil Steril. 1995;64(6):1136-40.
56. Fanchin R, Taieb J, Lozano DH, Ducot B, Frydman R, Bouyer J. High reproducibility of serum anti-Müllerian hormone measurements suggests a multi-staged follicular secretion and strengthens its role in the assessment of ovarian follicular status. Hum Reprod. 2005;20(4):923-7.
57. Tsepelidis S, Devreker F, Demeestere I, Flahaut A, Gervy Ch, Englert Y. Stable serum levels of anti-Müllerian hormone during the menstrual cycle: a prospective study in normo-ovulatory women. Hum Reprod. 2007;22(7):1837-40.
58. La Marca A, Stabile G, Artenisio AC, Volpe A. Serum anti-Müllerian hormone throughout the human menstrual cycle. Hum Reprod. 2006;21(12):3103-7.
59. Hehenkamp WJ, Looman CW, Themmen AP, de Jong FH, Te Velde ER, Broekmans FJ. Anti-Müllerian hormone levels in the spontaneous menstrual cycle do not show substantial fluctuation. J Clin Endocrinol Metab. 2006;91(10):4057-63.
60. Ebner T, Sommergruber M, Moser M, Shebl O, Schreier-Lechner E, Tews G. Basal level of anti-Müllerian hormone is associated with oocyte quality in stimulated cycles. Hum Reprod. 2006;21(8):2022-6.
61. Barbakadze L, Kristesashvili J, Khonelidze N, Tsagareishvili G. The correlations of anti-Müllerian hormone, follicle-stimulating hormone and antral follicle count in different age groups of infertile women. Int J Fertil Steril. 2015;8(4):393-8.
62. Gnoth C, Schuring AN, Friol K, Tigges J, Mallmann P, Godehardt E. Relevance of anti-Müllerian hormone measurement in a routine IVF program. Hum Reprod. 2008;23(6):1359-65.
63. Peñarrubia J, Fábregues F, Manau D, Creus M, Casals G, Casamitjana R, et al. Basal and stimulation day 5 anti-Müllerian hormone serum concentrations as predictors of ovarian response and pregnancy in assisted reproductive technology cycles stimulated with gonadotropin-releasing hormone agonist—gonadotropin treatment. Hum Reprod. 2005;20(4):915-22.
64. Practice Committee of the American Society for Reproductive Medicine. Testing and interpreting measures of ovarian reserve: a committee opinion. Fertil Steril. 2015;103(3): e9-17.
65. Yovich JL, Alsbjerg B, Conceicao JL, Hinchliffe PM, Keane KN. PIVET rFSH dosing algorithms for individualized controlled ovarian stimulation enables optimized pregnancy productivity rates and avoidance of ovarian hyperstimulation syndrome. Drug Des Devel Ther. 2016;10:2561-73.
66. Oliveira JBA, Baruffi R, Petersen CG, Mauri AL, Nascimento AM, Vagnini L, et al. A new ovarian response prediction index (ORPI): implications for individualised controlled ovarian stimulation. Reprod Biol Endocrinol. 2012;10:94.
67. Nelson SM, Yates RW, Lyall H, Jamieson M, Traynor I, Gaudoin M, et al. Anti-Müllerian hormone-based approach to controlled ovarian stimulation for assisted conception. Hum Reprod. 2009;24(4):867-75.
68. Yovich JL. Assisted reproduction. In: Grossman A (Ed). Clinical Endocrinology. Blackwell Scientific: Oxford; 1992. p. 773.
69. Silverberg KM, Olive DL, Burns WN, Johnson JV, Groff TR, Schenken RS. Follicular size at the time of human chorionic gonadotropin administration predicts ovulation outcome in human menopausal gonadotropin-stimulated cycles. Fertil Steril. 1991;56(2):296-300.
70. Phelps JY, Levine AS, Hickman TN, Zacur HA, Wallach EE, Hinton EL. Day 4 estradiol levels predict pregnancy success in women undergoing controlled ovarian hyperstimulation for IVF. Fertil Steril. 1998;69(6):1015-9.
71. Hershlag A, Asis MC, Diamond MP, DeCherney AH, Lavy G. The predictive value and the management of cycles with low initial estradiol levels. Fertil Steril. 1990;53(6):1064-7.
72. Khalaf Y, Taylor A, Braude P. Low serum estradiol concentrations after five days of controlled ovarian hyper-stimulation for in vitro fertilization are associated with poor outcome. Fertil Steril. 2000;74(1):63-6.
73. Loumaye E, Engrand P, Howles CM, O'Dea L. Assessment of the role of serum luteinizing hormone and estradiol response to follicle-stimulating hormone on in vitro fertilization treatment outcome. Fertil Steril. 1997;67(5):888-99.
74. Haning Jr RV, Levin RM, Behrman HR, Kase NG, Speroff L. Plasma estradiol window and urinary estriol glucuronide determinations for monitoring menotropin induction of ovulation. Obstet Gynecol. 1979;54(4):442-7.
75. Asch RH, Li H, Balmaceda JP, Weckstein LN, Stone SC. Severe ovarian hyperstimulation syndrome in assisted reproductive technology: definition of high risk groups. Hum Reprod. 1991;6(10):1395-9.
76. Morris RS, Paulson RJ, Sauer MV, Lobo RA. Predictive value of serum oestradiol concentrations and oocyte number in severe ovarian hyperstimulation syndrome. Hum Reprod. 1995;10(4):811-4.
77. Mathur RS, Akanda AV, Keay SD, Hunt LP, Jenkins JM. Distinction between early and late ovarian hyperstimulation syndrome. Fertil Steril. 2000;73(5):901-7.
78. Ng EH. What is the threshold value for serum estradiol levels associated with adverse IVF outcomes? Fertil Steril. 2000;73(5):1071-2.
79. Wilson EA, Jawad MJ, Hayden TL. Rates of exponential increase of serum estradiol concentrations in normal and human menopausal gonadotropin-induced cycles. Fertil Steril. 1982;37(1):46-9.
80. Lee TH, Lin YH, Seow KM, Hwang JL, Tzeng CR, Yang YS. Effectiveness of cetrorelix for the prevention of premature luteinizing hormone surge during controlled ovarian stimulation using letrozole and gonadotropins: a randomized trial. Fertil Steril. 2008;90(1):113-20.

81. Engel JB, Ludwig M, Felberbaum R, Albano C, Devroey P, Diedrich K. Use of cetrorelixin combination with clomiphene citrate and gonadotrophins: a suitable approach to 'friendly IVF'? Hum Reprod. 2002;17(8):2022-6.
82. European and Middle East Orgalutran Study Group. Comparable clinical outcome using the GnRH antagonist ganirelix or a long protocol of the GnRH agonist triptorelin for the prevention of premature LH surges in women undergoing ovarian stimulation. Hum Reprod. 2001;16(4):644-51.
83. Kolibianakis EM, Zikopoulos K, Smitz J, Camus M, Tournaye H, Van Steirteghem AC, et al. Elevated progesterone at initiation of stimulation is associated with a lower ongoing pregnancy rate after IVF using GnRH antagonists. Hum Reprod. 2004; 19(7):1525-9.
84. Edelstein MC, Seltman HJ, Cox BJ, Robinson SM, Shaw RA, Muasher SJ. Progesterone levels on the day of human chorionic gonadotropin administration in cycles with gonadotropin-releasing hormone agonist suppression are not predictive of pregnancy outcome. Fertil Steril. 1990;54(5):853-7.
85. Bosch E, Valencia I, Escudero E, Crespo J, Simón C, Remohí J, et al. Premature luteinization during gonadotropin-releasing hormone antagonist cycles and its relationship with in vitro fertilization outcome. Fertil Steril. 2003;80(6):1444-9.
86. Bosch E, Labarta E, Crespo J, Simón C, Remohí J, Jenkins J, et al. Circulating progesterone levels and ongoing pregnancy rates in controlled ovarian stimulation cycles for in vitro fertilization: analysis of over 4000 cycles. Hum Reprod. 2010;25(8):2092-100.
87. Fanchin R, Righini C, Olivennes F, Taieb J, de Ziegler D, Frydman R. Computerized assessment of endometrial echogenicity: clues to the endometrial effects of premature progesterone elevation. Fertil Steril. 1999;71(1):174-81.
88. Shapiro BS, Daneshmand ST, Garner FC, Aguirre M, Hudson C, Thomas S. Embryo cryopreservation rescues cycles with premature luteinization. Fertil Steril. 2010;93(2):636-41.
89. Shoham Z, Di Carlo C, Patel A, Conway GS, Jacobs HS. Is it possible to run a successful ovulation induction program based solely on ultrasound monitoring? The importance of endometrial measurements. Fertil Steril. 1991;56(5): 836-41.
90. Barash A, Weissman A, Manor M, Milman D, Ben-Arie A, Shoham Z. Prospective evaluation of endometrial thickness as a predictor of pituitary down-regulation after gonadotropin-releasing hormone analogue administration in an in vitro fertilization program. Fertil Steril. 1998;69(3):496-9.
91. Wikland M, Hillensjo T. Monitoring IVF cycles. In: Gardner DK, Wiessman A, Howles CM, Shoham Z (Eds). Textbook of Assisted Reproductive Techniques: Laboratory and Clinical Perspectives. UK: Martin Dunitz Publisher; 2001. pp. 501-04.
92. Ben-Shlomo I, Geslevich J, Shalev E. Can we abandon routine evaluation of serum estradiol levels during controlled ovarian hyperstimulation for assisted reproduction? Fertil Steril. 2001;76(2):300-3.
93. Delvigne A, Rozenberg S. Preventive attitude of physicians to avoid OHSS in IVF patients. Hum Reprod. 2001;16(12): 2491-5.
94. Kwan I, Bhattacharya S, Kang A, Woolner A. Monitoring of stimulated cycles in assisted reproduction (IVF and ICSI). Cochrane Database Syst Rev. 2014;2014(8):CD005289.

CHAPTER 51

Ovulation Trigger

Vyshnavi A Rao, K Aruna Saradha

INTRODUCTION

Ovulation triggers are of many types. They are responsible for triggering the process of ovulation and also help in final maturation of the oocyte.

Couples are in tremendous psychological pressure while they attempt intercourse as their clinicians counsel them in detail about the most fertile period and the maximum chance of pregnancy would occur in this period.

Human chorionic gonadotropin (hCG) is responsible for producing progesterone which maintains the corpus luteum, which helps in maintaining pregnancy in the initial stages. It is also called a "trigger shot" **(Fig. 1)**.

Human chorionic gonadotropin was the most ideal ovulation trigger for the purpose of final oocyte maturation in assisted reproductive technology (ART) cycles. hCG has higher affinity for luteinizing hormone (LH) receptors and has a long half-life, being more prone for ovarian hyperstimulation syndrome (OHSS). With the advent of antagonist protocol, option of using gonadotropin-releasing hormone agonist (GnRHa) trigger for triggering the final oocyte maturation was instrumental in eliminating the risk of OHSS. Recombinant luteinizing hormone (r-LH) has also been used with some limitations. Kisspeptins (KPs) and combining small dose of hCG with GnRHa (dual trigger) in some patients have also been investigated. This chapter deals with the various agents available for triggering final oocyte maturation in ART cycles.

In a natural cycle, there is early rise in follicle-stimulating hormone (FSH) level which results in follicular growth thereby causing a rise in the level of serum estrogen **(Fig. 2)**. This initial increase in estrogen level initiates a negative feedback on the production of FSH from the hypothalamo-pituitary-ovarian (HPO) axis. The FSH level remains high which causes unifollicular development—"FSH window effect". Estrogen rises subsequently causing midcycle LH surge which begins oocyte maturation and release.

Ovulation occurs approximately 10–12 hours after LH peak and 24–36 hours after peak serum estradiol levels.

Onset of LH surge appears to be the most reliable indicator of ovulation occurring 34–36 hours prior to

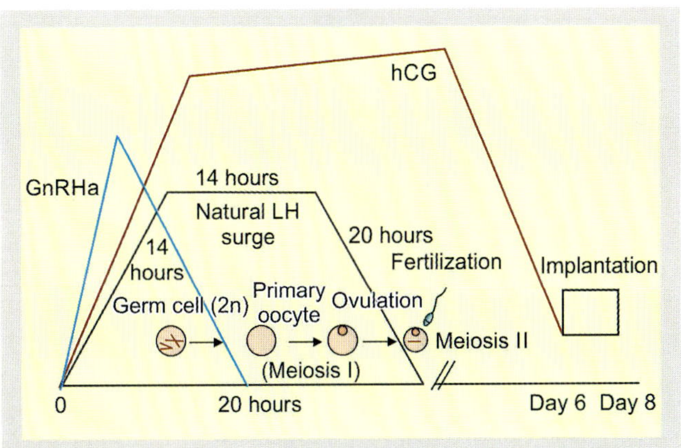

Fig. 1: The response shown by human chorionic gonadotropin (hCG) and gonadotropin-releasing hormone agonist (GnRHa) in final follicle maturation as surrogates for midcycle luteinizing hormone (LH) surge.

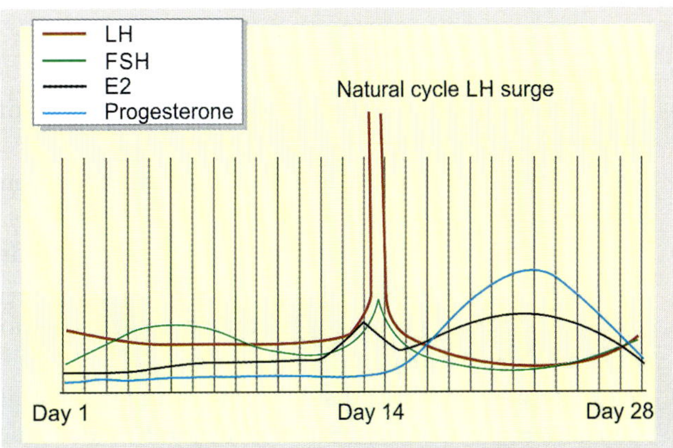

Fig. 2: Natural cycle luteinizing hormone (LH) surge. (E2: estradiol; FSH: follicle-stimulating hormone)

follicular rupture. The LH surge lasts for about 48–50 hours and comprises of three phases:
1. Ascending phase—14 hours
2. Plateau phase—14 hours
3. Descending phase—20 hours.

The midcycle LH surge is accompanied by a midcycle FSH surge, the influence of which is proven to be unclear, but plays a role in oocyte maturation, resumption of meiosis, and functioning of corpus luteum.

This gonadotropins surge initiates series of cascade of events which result eventually in ovulation, the physical release of oocyte, and its cumulus mass of granulosa cells.

OVULATION TRIGGER

Definition

A bioactive preparation which will trigger a cascade of events resulting in the maturation and release of developmentally competent oocyte from a preovulatory Graafian follicle. In a natural cycle, the physiological trigger is the midcycle surge of gonadotropins (LH and FSH surge) from the pituitary gland.

Physiology of Oocyte Maturation and Release

Luteinizing Hormone Surge

In an ovulatory cycle, LH surge is caused by estrogen released from preovulatory follicles, which causes luteinization of granulosa cells.[1]

Oocyte maturation and release occur as a result of positive feedback by high levels of estrogen (>300 pg/mL for >48 hours) which leads to LH surge from pituitary.[2]

Luteinizing hormone surge is characterized by three phases:
1. Ascending phase of 14 hours
2. Plateau phase of 14 hours
3. Descending phase of 20 hours.[3]

Luteinizing hormone surge is responsible for following events:
- Germinal vesicle breakdown
- Resumption of meiosis in oocyte
- Luteinization of granulosa cells and secretion of progesterone
- Expansion of cumulus and loss of gap junctions between cumulus cells and oocyte
- Secretion of prostaglandin and other eicosanoids essential for follicular rupture
- With LH surge, levels of progesterone in follicle rise up until the time of ovulation.
- Progesterone increases distensibility of follicular wall and causes preovulatory FSH surge by positive feedback mechanism from pituitary.

Follicle-stimulating hormone surge is known to help in cumulus expansion, promotion of nuclear maturation, and induction of LH receptors on granulosa and cumulus cells.[4,5]

Follicle-stimulating hormone, LH, and progesterone also stimulate the activity of proteolytic enzymes thereby causing digestion of collagen in follicular wall and increasing its distensibility, nuclear maturation (resumption of meiosis), cytoplasmic maturation, and release of the developmentally competent oocyte from follicle.
- Oocyte arrest in prophase 1 of meiosis is maintained by elevated levels of cyclic adenosine monophosphate (cAMP) in the oocyte which is transported inside oocyte from cumulus or somatic cells through gap junctions.[6]
- LH and FSH surge results in cumulus expansion and disruption of these gap junctions, resulting in low concentrations in cAMP in the oocyte. This results in the germinal vessel breakdown and resumption of meiosis **(Fig. 3)**.

Follicular Rupture

The process of follicular rupture consists of various events like:
- Changes in the cumulus and matrix
- Increase in plasminogen activator mediated by FSH and LH in granulosa cells to activate plasminogen to plasmin, which in turn activates collagenase to disrupt follicular wall
- Proteolytic digestion of tunica and basement membrane
- Follicular vascular and membrane remodeling
- Appearance of more inflammatory cells such as neutrophils in the follicular wall
- Prostaglandin being E2 and F2 α synthesized by cumulus cells, which causes cumulus expansion, resumption of oocyte meiosis, and extrusion of oocyte-cumulus complex from ruptured follicle by contraction of smooth muscle cells.

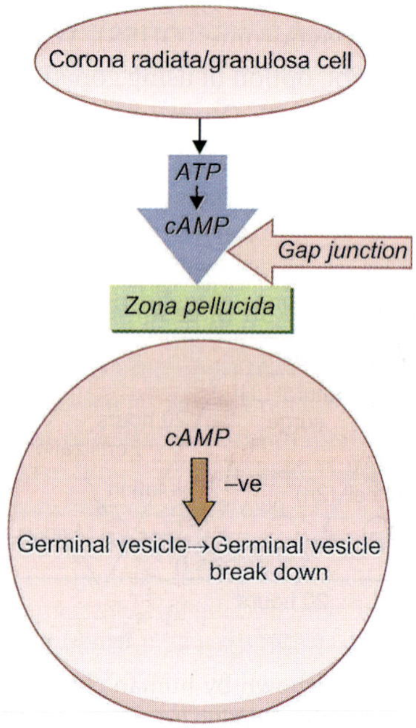

Fig. 3: Resumption of meiosis.
(ATP: adenosine triphosphate; cAMP: cyclic adenosine monophosphate)

Flowchart 1: Complex inter-related events in ovulation.

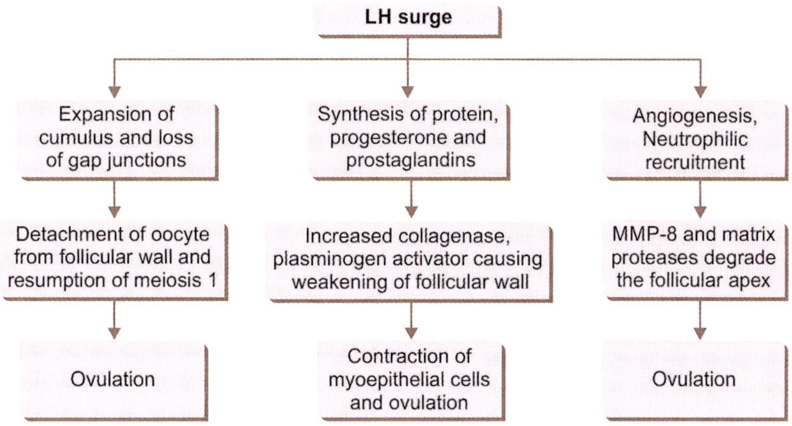

(LH: luteinizing hormone; MMP-8: matrix metalloproteinase-8)

- Apoptosis of the epithelial cells over the apex or stigma mediated by matrix metalloproteinases enzymes which are activated in response to LH
- Rise in intrafollicular pressure and contractions of the myoepithelial cells will result in the rupture of the follicle with extrusion of the mature oocyte[7] **(Flowchart 1)**.

Role of Ovulatory Triggers in Intrauterine Insemination and In Vitro Fertilization Cycles

In in vitro fertilization (IVF) cycles, mature oocytes are retrieved artificially around 34–36 hours after administration of ovulation trigger.

Since ovulation occurs 36 hours after ovulatory trigger, it enables correct timing of intrauterine insemination (IUI) and intercourse.

In natural cycle, midcycle LH surge induces follicular rupture and ovulation. In stimulated ART cycles, LH surge is deliberately suppressed by gonadotropin-releasing hormone (GnRH) analogs to prevent follicle rupture before oocyte retrieval. Hence, administration of trigger for final oocyte maturation is essential.

Various Pharmacological Options for Ovulation Trigger

- Urinary human chorionic gonadotropin (u-hCG)
- Recombinant human chorionic gonadotropin (r-hCG)
- Recombinant luteinizing hormone (r-LH)
- Gonadotropin-releasing hormone agonists (GnRH agonist)
- Dual trigger (hCG + GnRH Agonist)
- KPs.

Human Chorionic Gonadotropin

Chorionic gonadotropin (CG) is a heterodimeric glycoprotein comprising of α and β subunits. LH, thyroid-stimulating hormone (TSH), and FSH share a common 92-amino acid α subunit with CG.[8] The differences arise due to unique functions and receptor-binding capacity of all these hormones among the β subunits.

Human chorionic gonadotropin acts as surrogate for LH because of homology between these two hormones. Both are glycoproteins with molecular weight of 30 kDa and both have almost identical α subunits and high cysteine content. hCG is used for granulosa cells luteinization, resumption of meiosis, and final oocyte maturation of follicle 36 hours later and is proven to yield better clinical pregnancy rates compared to other ovulation triggering agents.

- As a result of structural differences and posttranslational modifications, hCG is more stable, has a longer half-life, and has greater receptor affinity than LH, thus making it more biologically active.[9]
- After subcutaneous administration, hCG has significantly longer half-life in comparison to LH.[10]
- Due to abovementioned pharmacokinetic properties and because of sustained luteotrophic effect, development of multiple corpus luteum, and supraphysiological levels of estradiol and progesterone synthesis, hCG is notorious in producing OHSS.
- Although hCG has LH-like activity, it does not reconstitute midcycle FSH surge.
- Minimal effective doses of u-hCG used to trigger oocyte maturation were studied as 2,000 IU, 5,000 IU, and 10,000 IU.
- In a randomized controlled trial (RCT) study involving 80 polycystic ovary syndrome (PCOS) patients stimulated with rFSH and antagonist being added on day 6 of stimulation, no significant difference was noted in terms of ongoing pregnancy rates, severe OHSS, or number of oocytes retrieved in 2,000 IU, 5,000 IU, and 10,000 IU groups.[11]
- Recombinant preparations are associated with higher serum progesterone and serum hCG levels postadministration and lower incidence of local adverse reactions.

- Urinary products still remain the first choice as they are cheap and easily available. A recent meta-analysis has found no difference in terms of follicular maturation, risk of OHSS, and pregnancy outcomes between two preparations.[12]
- 250 μg r-hCG = 5,000 IU u-hCG.[13]
- One RCT including 180 women comparing urinary hCG with recombinant hCG for triggering final oocyte maturation in long GnRH agonist protocol showed no difference in number of oocytes retrieved, occurrence of OHSS, and clinical pregnancy rates between two groups. However, 500 μg of r-hCG seemed to be more beneficial than 250 μg of r-hCG in this indication.[14]
- European Society of Human Reproduction and Embryology (ESHRE) guideline 2019 for ovarian stimulation for IVF/intracytoplasmic sperm injection (ICSI): Use of recombinant and urinary hCG is equally recommended for triggering final oocyte maturation during ovarian stimulation protocols.
- The use of other ovulatory triggers in anovulatory women treated with other ovulatory agents has not been properly evaluated.[15]

Recombinant Luteinizing Hormone

Recombinant luteinizing hormone has a shorter half-life and is very physiological **(Table 1)**. The European Recombinant LH Study Group, in a prospective multicenter dose finding study, found a single dose of r-LH of at least 15,000 IU (750 mg r-LH) or 30,000 IU (1,500 mg r-LH) equivalent to that of 5,000 IU u-hCG with safety superior to that of u-hCG, particularly with respect to the incidence of OHSS. However, in this dose finding study, it was also found that 30,000 IU LH yielded more metaphase 1 (M1) and germinal vesicle (GV) oocytes compared to u-hCG.

The research for using LH as trigger in literature is limited. Currently, recombinant luteinizing hormone (r-LH) is not routinely used as ovulation trigger. Hence, recombinant LH is not commercially available for ovulation triggering.[13]

The Cochrane meta-analysis reported no difference in live birth rate, moderate OHSS, and number of oocytes retrieved between r-LH and u-hCG when used for triggering final oocyte maturation.[12]

Another RCT done including 49 women with poor ovarian reserve to compare r-LH and u-hCG showed that there is no statistically significant difference in cycle cancellation rates, number of oocytes retrieved per cycle, fertilization rates, the number of embryos obtained per cycle, implantation, clinical pregnancy, and live birth rates.[16]

ESHRE guideline 2019 for ovarian stimulation for IVF/ICSI strongly recommends against administering r-LH for triggering final oocyte maturation as the available evidence to draw solid conclusions is lacking.

TABLE 1: Advantages and disadvantages of recombinant luteinizing hormone (r-LH).

Advantages	*Disadvantages*
• More physiological • Risk of ovarian hyperstimulation syndrome is almost nil	• Very high doses of r-LH is required to induce ovulation (15,000–30,000 IU) • Not cost-effective • Limited literature to support its use

Recombinant Human Chorionic Gonadotropin (Table 2)

The onset of spontaneous LH surge is usually sudden, the concentrations of which double within 2 hours between 100 IU/L and 200 IU/L, being elevated for 12–14 hours over a mean duration of 50 hours.[3]

The midcycle surge in addition to follicular rupture[17] aids in several periovulatory events which comprise the following events:

- Disruption of oocyte-cumulus oophorus cell contact and induction of resumption of meiosis[18]
- Cumulus oophorus mucification
- Luteinization of follicular granulosa cells[19]
- Secretion of progesterone.

Farrag et al. conducted a prospective randomized study in order to investigate the effect of r-hCG on oocyte nuclear and cytoplasm maturity compared to u-hCG, for inducing ovulation in women treated with ICSI for male factor infertility. Their results showed that r-hCG increases the rate of metaphase II (MII) oocytes with mature cytoplasm compared to u-hCG.[20]

However, many RCTs have shown that r-hCG and u-hCG are equally effective.[13]

Gonadotropin-releasing Hormone Agonist

Gonadotropin-releasing hormone agonist is an analog which activates GnRH receptors causing increase in the levels of FSH and LH. It mimics a natural midcycle FSH and LH surge following its administration. This is called "flare effect". This effect is used to obtain oocyte maturation.

TABLE 2: Luteinizing hormone (LH) and human chorionic gonadotropin (hCG) are not identical.

	LH	*hCG*
No. of AA beta subunit	121	145
Receptor-binding affinity	Low	High
Initial half-life (h)	0.6–1.3	3.9–5.5
Bioequivalency	6–8 IU	1 IU
Terminal half-life (h)	9–12	23–31
No. glycosylation sites	1	6

Source: Leao RB, Esteves SC, Choi J, Smitz J. (Androfert) Luteinizing hormone and human chorionic gonadotropin: origins of difference. Mol Cell Endocrinol. 2014.

TABLE 3: Gonadotropin-releasing hormone (GnRH) agonists.

Decapeptides	*Nanopeptides*
Native GnRH	Leuprolide
Nafarelin	Buserelin
Triptorelin	Goserelin
+	Histrelin

The capability of GnRH agonist to induce ovulation was first described by Nakano et al. in 1973.[21] The antagonist protocol has gained a lot of importance in recent years. Antagonist protocol not only is associated with low risk of OHSS but also allows clinicians to use an agonist trigger thereby reducing the risk of OHSS to be very minimal.

In antagonist protocol, antagonist blocks pituitary GnRH receptors by competitive inhibition. This prevents endogenous LH surge. GnRH agonist displaces antagonist from receptors and activates them to release gonadotropins from anterior pituitary.

- GnRH agonist is derived from native GnRH by substitution of amino acids at 6th and 10th positions.
- These modifications result in alteration of enzymatic cleavage and potency of the molecule.
- Native GnRH is a decapeptide **(Table 3)**.
- Dose of agonists as trigger: Triptorelin 0.2 mg, leuprolide 1–1.5 mg, and buserelin 0.5 mg.[22,23]
- Dose of leuprolide has been reported in literature for trigger as 0.5–4 mg.
- ESHRE guideline 2019 recommends choosing dosage of triptorelin ranging from 0.1 to 0.4 mg.
- Some studies have used higher dose (4 mg) and others two doses 12 hours apart.
- A single dose of 1 mg of leuprolide yields optimal mature oocyte yield.[24]
- The surge induced by a GnRH agonist is short-lasting and consists of two phases:
  1. A short ascending limb (4 hours)
  2. Long descending limb (20 hours), in total of 24–36 hours as compared to 48 hours in a natural cycle **(Fig. 4)**.[25]
- GnRHa trigger is as effective as hCG in inducing final follicular maturation and also has an additional theoretical advantage of inducing FSH surge which along with LH might help in bringing up better follicular maturation.
- There is no difference in oocyte and embryo quality when compared to hCG with almost elimination of OHSS.[25]
- But reduction in clinical pregnancy rates with GnRH agonist and conventional luteal support as compared to hCG in normal responders was noted in meta-analysis comparing 10,000 IU urinary hCG and 0.2 mg triptorelin.[26]
- The drawback of a GnRHa trigger is early corpus luteolysis and inadequate steroidogenesis due to lack of sustained endogenous LH in luteal phase which may result in decreased pregnancy rates and increased miscarriage rates.[27]
- ESHRE guideline 2019 strongly recommends against use of GnRH agonist for final oocyte maturation with conventional luteal phase support and fresh transfer in general IVF/ICSI population.

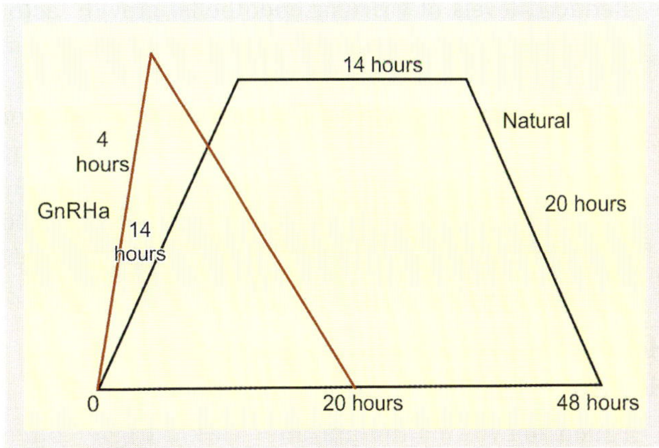

Fig. 4: Comparison of gonadotropin-releasing hormone (GnRH)-induced luteinizing hormone (LH) surge versus human chorionic gonadotropin (hCG)-induced LH surge.
(GnRHa: gonadotropin-releasing hormone agonist)

Intensive and optimal luteal support after GnRH agonist for fresh embryo transfers will improve pregnancy outcomes.

Indications for Gonadotropin-releasing Hormone Agonist Trigger

Any woman who is not planned for fresh embryo transfer can be triggered with GnRH agonist 28–30 like:

- Oocyte donors
- Fertility preservation
- Risk of OHSS
- Preimplantation genetic diagnosis
- Prematurely elevated progesterone prior to trigger.

Gonadotropin-releasing hormone agonist trigger is not preferred in patients with hypothalamic dysfunction and those with long-term hypothalamus and pituitary suppression as with oral contraceptive (OC) pill due to inability to mount sufficient surge of pituitary gonadotropins.[31]

Follicular Fluid and Granulosa/Luteal Cell Changes after Gonadotropin-releasing Hormone Trigger

- Combined higher levels of both FSH and LH than those after hCG trigger[32]
- Progesterone levels reduced by 25% due to lack of LH stimulus on luteal cells.[32,33]
- Levels of amphiregulin and members of epidermal growth factor like family are much lower in follicular fluid than hCG trigger.

- Reduced levels of vascular endothelial growth factor (VEGF) and angiopoietin-2, key factors in OHSS, help in preventing OHSS.[34]
- Higher levels of pigment epithelium derived factor (PEDF) and antiangiogenic factor help in preventing OHSS.
- The concerns of GnRH agonist trigger to be associated with empty follicle syndrome (EFS) have been abolished by recent studies.[35]

How to Predict Gonadotropin-releasing Hormone Agonist Trigger Failure?

- Failed oocyte maturation after GnRH trigger often detected with low serum LH on the day after trigger[36]
- GnRH agonist trigger needs to be avoided in patients with preexisting hypothalamus-pituitary axis dysfunction and also with a pretrigger LH <0.5 IU/L.
- Predicting probability of EFS after GnRH trigger is important as to decide whether to proceed with retrieval or whether rescue dose of hCG is needed.

Meyer et al.[31] aimed to identify risk factors in GnRHa trigger in IVF cycles who are known to be suboptimal responders. The main factors identified were: The prolonged use of contraception, very low levels of LH concentrations on the day of trigger, low serum levels of FSH and LH at the start of the cycle, and irregular menses at the baseline.

Using a Dual Trigger (GnRH Agonist with hCG)

- Shapiro et al.[37] retrospectively evaluated the administration of low-dose hCG (1,000–2,500 IU) in combination of GnRHa in order to induce final oocyte maturation in patients prone for OHSS, this combination was called "dual trigger".

The goal of dual trigger aided in oocyte maturation also provided sustained support for the corpus luteum, higher clinical pregnancy rates along with absence of OHSS, thereby concluding safety of this type of trigger in patients prone for OHSS **(Flowchart 2)**.

Kummer et al.[24] showed that there is no post-trigger progesterone cut-off that can be used to reliably predict the number of oocytes retrieved, but all patients with EFS after GnRH agonist trigger had low-serum LH and progesterone levels (<3.5 ng/mL).

Studies have shown that post-trigger LH and progesterone after GnRH agonist trigger strongly correlated with total oocytes and mature oocytes obtained.

- Serum LH and progesterone levels measured 12 hours after trigger can indicate failed endogenous response to trigger injection and need for intervention.
- If no LH surge and/or progesterone rise noted after GnRH trigger, repeat trigger with hCG and oocyte retrieval after 35 hours later is indicated.[24]

Flowchart 2: Algorithm to use gonadotropin-releasing hormone (GnRH) trigger to prevent ovarian hyperstimulation syndrome (OHSS).

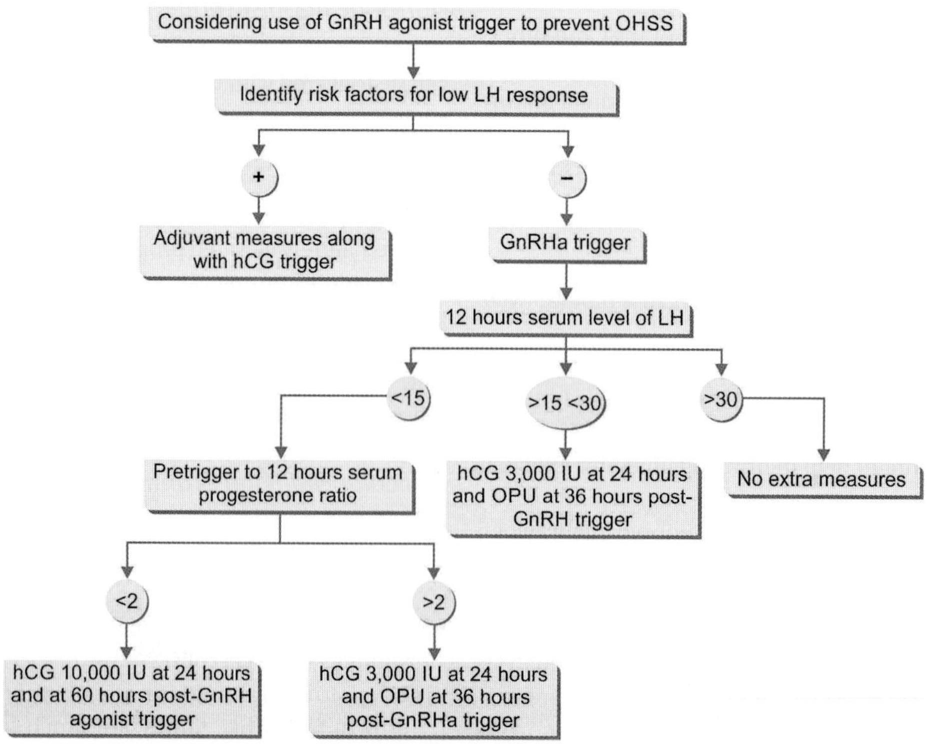

(GnRHa: gonadotropin-releasing hormone agonist; hCG: human chorionic gonadotropin; LH: luteinizing hormone; OPU: oocyte pick up)

- If suboptimal LH rise with value <15 IU/L is noted, repeat trigger with hCG as soon as possible and oocyte retrieval as planned or cancellation of cycle is indicated.
- Also, unilateral follicle aspiration and if no oocytes are obtained, hCG trigger and oocyte retrieval after 34 hours can be done.[36]

Luteal Phase Support after Gonadotropin-releasing Hormone Agonist Trigger

Luteinizing hormone acts as luteotropic hormone. It supports growth and function of corpus luteum and steroidogenesis after ovulation.

Gonadotropin-releasing hormone trigger luteal phase is shortened due to early luteolysis, partial downregulation of pituitary inhibiting LH secretion, and supraphysiological levels of estrogen and progesterone from ovarian stimulation suppressing LH secretion.

Average duration of luteal phase after GnRH agonist trigger may be as short as 9 days compared to 13 days after hCG trigger.[38]

Luteal Support with Progesterone and Estrogen

Serum levels of progesterone and estrogen throughout the luteal phase are significantly lower with GnRH agonist trigger than after hCG trigger.

Intense luteal phase support with estradiol and progesterone or low-dose hCG after GnRHa trigger have shown reasonable pregnancy rates after fresh transfer, in patients at risk of OHSS.

American approach is to supplement high dose of steroids in the luteal phase in the form of intramuscular progesterone 50 mg daily and transdermal estrogen patches three doses 0.3 mg alternate days. Engmann et al. described this approach.[22] Serum E2 and progesterone levels were evaluated on days 3 and 7 after oocyte retrieval and weekly thereafter and continuing intramuscular (IM) progesterone and transdermal estrogen till 10 weeks of gestation. Based on serum levels, doses of IM progesterone can be increased to maximum of 75 mg daily with addition of micronized vaginal progesterone daily as needed to maintain serum progesterone above 20 ng/mL. Similarly, estrogen patches can be increased to four 0.1 mg patches alternate days and adding oral micronized E2 (2–8 mg) daily if required to maintain serum E2 above 200 pg/mL.[39]

In this study, 53% ongoing pregnancy rate was reported after GnRH agonist with intensive luteal support compared to 48.3% in the hCG group with standard luteal phase support.

European approach relies on supplementing two small doses of hCG in the luteal phase which will rescue the corpus luteal function without increasing the incidence of OHSS. 1,500 IU hCG is given on the day of oocyte retrieval and 5 days after retrieval.[39]

Shapiro et al. in his study reported ongoing pregnancy rate of 50% in GnRH agonist trigger patients who received intensive luteal support compared to 25.3% ongoing pregnancy rate with standard luteal support.[40]

Intramuscular progesterone over vaginal progesterone in luteal support after GnRH agonist trigger improves pregnancy outcomes.[41]

Recombinant Luteinizing Hormone for Luteal Support

Luteinizing hormone supplementation in the luteal phase after agonist trigger can also be used to rescue luteal phase with good pregnancy rates[42] with less risk of OHSS due to shorter half-life.

Luteal Support with Human Chorionic Gonadotropin at the Time of Oocyte Retrieval

Human chorionic gonadotropin administration on the day of oocyte retrieval within 1 hour in addition to standard luteal support has been suggested in some studies after GnRH agonist trigger to support corpus luteal function.[43]

Radesic and Tremellen reported one case of severe OHSS among 71 women at risk of OHSS receiving 1,500 IU hCG within 1 hour of oocyte retrieval.[44]

Seyhan et al. evaluated 23 women at high risk of OHSS who had E2-4891 pg/mL on the day of trigger and received GnRH agonist trigger and hCG 1,500 IU administered within 1 hour of oocyte retrieval. OHSS rate reported in this study was 26%.[45]

Very Low-dose hCG for Luteal Support

This supports corpus luteum function. Additional progesterone or E2 support in luteal phase is not required.

Recombinant hCG 125 IU given daily starting from either the day 2 or 6 of stimulation and continued throughout luteal phase.[46,47]

This approach showed high luteal progesterone levels but pregnancy rates were similar.

This approach of luteal support is not currently used routinely and additional studies are needed.

LUTEAL COASTING

Kol et al. in a study of 21 patients at risk of OHSS no luteal phase supplementation was provided and serum progesterone levels were monitored and one bolus of 1,500 IU hCG was given if values dropped below significantly.[48]

By this method, luteal phase support was individualized and risk of OHSS was minimized.

FREEZING OF EMBRYOS

To avoid suboptimal luteal phase after GnRH agonist, trigger freezing of all embryos and transfer in subsequent cycles.

Garcia-Velasco study showed pregnancy rates of 50% who underwent freezing and transfer in subsequent natural cycles when compared to patients who had pregnancy rates of 29.5% who had coasting and fresh embryo transfer.[49]

PREDICTORS OF SUCCESS AFTER GONADOTROPIN-RELEASING HORMONE AGONIST TRIGGER

One study revealed that peak E2 >4,000 pg/mL and raised levels of LH on the day of trigger improved pregnancy rates after GnRH agonist trigger. Pregnancy rate in this group was 53.6% compared to 38.1% in the group that had E2 <4,000 pg/mL.[50]

In the group with E <4,000 pg/mL, dual trigger with GnRH agonist trigger and low-dose hCG 1,000 IU had higher pregnancy rates than GnRH agonist trigger alone.[51]

In all those with E >4,000 pg/mL, supplementation with E2 and progesterone alone is sufficient in luteal phase or freeze all embryos can be done. But in those with E <4,000 pg/mL, adjuvant low-dose hCG in luteal phase improves pregnancy rates.[51]

Number of follicles on the day of trigger will also determine if 1,500 IU of hCG has to be given on the day of oocyte retrieval after agonist trigger.[52]

Seyhan et al. suggested that all women with 10–14 mm follicles of >18 in number should not be given hCG bolus as the risk of OHSS is 26% and embryos should be cryopreserved.[45] Few other studies also suggested that women with >25 follicles of greater than 11 mm in diameter should not be given hCG bolus and cryopreservation of embryos should be done.[53]

OVARIAN HYPERSTIMULATION SYNDROME IN GONADOTROPIN-RELEASING HORMONE AGONIST TRIGGER

Because of short duration of LH surge and early corpus luteolysis, risk of OHSS is negligible after GnRH agonist trigger which has been shown in various studies.[54]

ESHRE guideline 2019 strongly recommends triggering with GnRH agonist for final oocyte maturation to reduce risk of early onset OHSS in patients at risk of OHSS.

Few cases of OHSS with use of GnRH agonist trigger have been reported which is thought to be due to low dose of hCG (dual trigger).

Very few cases of OHSS with use of GnRH agonist alone have been reported which has been attributed to activating mutations in GnRH or FSH receptor.[55]

Dual Trigger

Dual trigger which includes triggering of the final oocyte maturation by a combination of a GnRHa together with a low-dose hCG (1,000–2,500 IU) was first described by Shapiro.[37]

Dual trigger enables clinicians to lengthen time between ovulation triggering and oocyte pick up and also simultaneously adding a FSH component causing a FSH surge which can help overcome any impairment in granulosa cell function, oocyte meiotic maturation, or cumulus expansion.[56]

- Increase in the level of LH was found in the dual trigger soon after trigger along with a surge in FSH compared with hCG trigger. There was no major difference in the number of MII oocytes, or the number of two pronuclei oocytes.[57]
- The risk of OHSS was almost eliminated by using GnRHa trigger and proper luteal function was also modified by the added hCG when dual trigger was used.
- The combined surge of FSH and LH in dual trigger is particularly useful in patients with immature oocytes and EFS in the previous IVF cycles.[56]
- Dual trigger may aid in implantation, clinical pregnancy, and live birth rates when used in normal responder patients in an antagonist cycle.[56]

Haas et al. did a prospective control double-blinded RCT which inferred that the dual trigger helps in increasing the oocyte yield, mature oocytes, and the number of zygotes compared to triggering with hCG alone in patients who are normal responders. The increase in the number of mature oocytes may potentially benefit the outcome of the IVF cycle.[58]

Kisspeptins

Kisspeptins are recently discovered peptides which act on kisspeptin neurons located in the anteroventral periventricular nucleus, anterodorsal preoptic nucleus, and prearcuate nucleus in hypothalamus and are thought to play an important role of GnRH pulse generator in mammals. KP is an important regulator of onset of puberty, secretion of gonadotropins, and fertility. They bind to their specific receptor and result in release of GnRH from hypothalamus which in turn acts on pituitary to release LH and FSH. Many forms of endogenous KPs have been described which differ in length of amino acid chain. KP-10 and KP-54 are most studied for their potential applications.

After encouraging results from animal studies, now human studies are accumulating.

- Exogenously administering of KPs has been found to result in release of gonadotropins particularly in cases of hypothalamic amenorrhea.[59]
- When given in the periovulatory phase, exogenous KP has been shown to induce a 3–4-fold increase in LH secretion.[60]
- In women undergoing ART, KPs were capable of eliciting an effective LH surge that resulted in successful oocyte maturation and live birth.[61-63]
- KPs, therefore, may offer a completely different, "natural" concept for ovulation induction in ART without the risk of OHSS.

Ovulation Trigger Preferred in Oocyte Donors

Mourad et al.[64] did a study intervention for prevention of OHSS in ART cycles, that proved GnRHa trigger was better in donor oocyte or "freeze-all" programs. It included a total of 27 reviews in this Cochrane study, a study by Youssef et al.[27] included 17 RCTs which concluded that GnRH agonist trigger in donor recipient cycles would be the preferred trigger.

Several studies have showed that there is no difference in the number of oocytes retrieved, implantation, pregnancy, and live birth rates in donor cycles on comparison of GnRH agonist trigger with hCG trigger.[65,66] However, use of GnRH

TABLE 4: Differences between GnRH agonist trigger versus hCG trigger.[67]

Parameters	*GnRH agonist trigger*	*hCG trigger*
Basis of the Trigger	GnRH agonists induce LH endogenous surge by their flare up effect which is useful in ovulation triggering	A bolus dose of hCG induces ovulation in 24–36 hours. Longer half-life of more than 24 hours versus 60 minutes for endogenous surge of LH, is linked with prolonged stimulation of follicles and corpus luteum as well as increased serum estradiol levels
Half-life	Shorter half-life	Longer half-life
Risk of OHSS	Used for prevention of OHSS	Prolonged luteotrophic effect and increased VEGF expression with hCG is associated with higher risk of OHSS
Luteal phase support	Intensive luteal phase support is mandatory post GnRHa trigger as luteal phase is defective	Luteal phase support required modified according to individualized cases
Freeze all strategy	Usually employed	May or may not be employed

(GnRH: gonadotropin-releasing hormone; LH: luteinizing hormone; hCG: human chorionic gonadotropin; OHSS: ovarian hyperstimulation syndrome; VEGF: vascular endothelial growth factor)

TABLE 5: Advantages and disadvantages of various triggers.

Ovulation triggers	*Advantages*	*Disadvantages*
GnRH agonist	• GnRH agonist is an analog which activates GnRH receptors causing increase in the levels of FSH and LH. It mimics a natural midcycle FSH and LH surge following its administration. This is called "flare effect". This effect is used to obtain oocyte maturation • Significant reduction of OHSS using this type of trigger	The drawback of a GnRH agonist trigger is early corpus luteolysis and inadequate steroidogenesis due to lack of sustained endogenous LH in luteal phase which may result in decreased pregnancy rates and miscarriage rates. Intense luteal phase support with estradiol and progesterone or low-dose hCG after GnRH agonist trigger have shown reasonable pregnancy rates after fresh transfer, in patients at risk of OHSS
hCG trigger	• hCG acts as a surrogate LH. Used as an ovulation trigger for final maturation of oocyte 35 hours prior to oocyte pick up, yields better clinical pregnancy rate • More stability, longer half-life, greater affinity for LH receptors makes hCG biologically more active	In hyper responders, hCG is more prone for OHSS
Dual trigger	• Dual trigger which includes triggering of the final oocyte maturation by a combination of a GnRHa together with a low-dose hCG (1,000–2,500 IU) • Enables clinicians to lengthen time between ovulation triggering and oocyte pick up and also simultaneously adding a FSH component causing an FSH surge which can help overcome any impairments in granulosa cell function, oocyte meiotic maturation, or cumulus expansion[58] • Dual trigger is particularly useful in patients with immature oocytes and empty follicle syndrome in the previous IVF cycles • Dual trigger may aid in implantation, clinical pregnancy, and live-birth rates when used in normal responder patients in an antagonist cycle	The risk of OHSS was almost eliminated by using GnRHa trigger and proper luteal function was also modified by the added hCG when dual trigger was used
r-LH trigger	Shorter half-life and is physiological	Expensive; the research for using LH as trigger in literature is limited. Currently, r-LH is not routinely used as ovulation trigger
Kisspeptins	When given in the periovulatory phase, exogenous KP has been shown to induce a 3–4-fold increase in LH secretion	Not used as ovulation trigger in routine practice

(FSH: follicle-stimulating hormone; GnRH: gonadotropin-releasing hormone; GnRHa: gonadotropin-releasing hormone agonist; hCG: human chorionic gonadotropin; IVF: in vitro fertilization; KP: kisspeptin; LH: luteinizing hormone; OHSS: ovarian hyperstimulation syndrome; r-LH: recombinant luteinizing hormone) agonist trigger in donor cycles is associated with less risk of OHSS as shown in various studies. The differences between hCG trigger and GnRHa trigger are as shown in **Table 4**.

Advantages and disadvantages of each ovulation triggers are as shown in **Table 5**.

OVULATORY TRIGGER IN BREAST CANCER PATIENTS

In breast cancer patients, stimulation with aromatase inhibitor and gonadotropins helps in minimal estrogen exposure and use of GnRH agonist trigger is associated with less risk of OHSS and faster recovery.[29]

KEY NOTES

- In order to significantly reduce the risk of OHSS in ART cycles, using a GnRH agonist trigger in an antagonist protocol may be useful in most patients.
- Clinical pregnancy rates in fresh transfer after GnRH agonist trigger found to be less than with hCG trigger.
- Few clinicians may fear the use of GnRH agonist as a trigger due to its effects on the luteal phase which may be corrected by the use of hCG as a luteal phase support or with intensive luteal phase support.
- Adding 1,500 IU of hCG on the day of oocyte pick up has been useful in rescuing the luteal phase. Other alternatives such as increasing the progesterone and E2 are of vital importance.
- The possibility of performing a fresh embryo transfer following GnRH agonist trigger is high when the luteal phase support is modified accordingly.
- Vitrification of embryos thus obtained following a stimulated IVF cycle and subsequent transfer of the vitrified embryos in the next menstrual cycle has been found to be more effective.
- GnRH agonist trigger to be avoided in patients with hypothalamic dysfunction and those with low LH on the day of trigger (<0.5 IU/L).
- No difference in oocyte and embryo quality on comparison of GnRH agonist trigger with hCG trigger.
- Dual trigger is useful in patients with immature oocytes and empty follicle syndrome in previous cycles.
- No differences in oocyte maturation, quality, risk of OHSS and pregnancy, and live birth outcomes on comparison of r-hCG with u-hCG.
- No differences in clinical pregnancy rates, OHSS rates, and number of oocytes obtained in 2,000 IU, 5,000 IU, and 10,000 IU u-hCG dosages.
- GnRH agonist trigger preferred in donors due to reduced incidence of OHSS.

REFERENCES

1. Orvieto R. Triggering final follicular maturation—hCG, GnRH-agonist or both, when and to whom? J Ovarian Res. 2015;8:60.
2. Rodney R, Tanner GA. Medical Physiology, 2nd edition. US: Lippincott Williams & Wilkins; 2003. pp. 667-78.
3. Hoff JD, Quigley ME, Yen SS. Hormonal dynamics at midcycle: a reevaluation. J Clin Endocrinol Metab. 1983;57(4):792-6.
4. Eppig JJ. FSH stimulates hyaluronic acid synthesis by oocyte cumulus cell complexes from mouse preovulatory follicles. Nature. 1979;281(5731):483-4.
5. Zelinski-Wooten MB, Hutchison JS, Hess DL, Wolf DP, Stouffer RL. Follicle stimulating hormone alone supports follicle growth and oocyte development in gonadotrophin-releasing hormone antagonist-treated monkeys. Hum Reprod. 1995;10(7):1658-66.
6. Mehlmann LM. Stops and starts in mammalian oocytes: recent advances in understanding the regulation of meiotic arrest and oocyte maturation. Reproduction. 2005;130(6):791-9.
7. Yang WL, Godwin AK, Xu XX. Tumor necrosis factor-alpha induced matrix proteolytic enzyme production and basement membrane remodeling by human ovarian surface epithelial cells: molecular basis linking ovulation and cancer risk. Cancer Res. 2004;64(4):1534-40.
8. Bulun SE. Physiology and pathology of the female reproductive axis. In: Melmed S, Polonsky KS, Larsen PR, Kronenberg HM, (Eds). Williams Textbook of Endocrinology, 12th edition. Philadelphia: Elsevier Saunders; 2011. pp. 581-660.
9. Rahman NA, Rao CV. Recent progress in luteinizing hormone/human chorionic gonadotrophin hormone research. Mol Hum Reprod. 2009;15(11):703-11.
10. Ezcurra D, Humaidan P. A review of luteinising hormone and human chorionic gonadotropin when used in assisted reproductive technology. Reprod Biol Endocrinol. 2014;12:95.
11. Kolibianakis EM, Papanikolaou EG, Tournaye H, Camus M, Van Steirteghem AC, Devroey P. Triggering final oocyte maturation using different doses of human chorionic gonadotropin: a randomized pilot study in patients with polycystic ovary syndrome treated with gonadotropin-releasing hormone antagonists and recombinant follicle stimulating hormone. Fertil Steril. 2007;88(5):1382-8.
12. Youssef MA, Abou-Setta AM, Lam WS. Recombinant versus urinary human chorionic gonadotrophin for final oocyte maturation triggering in IVF and ICSI cycles. Cochrane Database Syst Rev. 2016;4:CD003719.
13. Induction of final follicular maturation and early luteinization in women undergoing ovulation induction for assisted reproduction treatment-recombinant hCG versus urinary hCG. The European Recombinant Human Chorionic Gonadotrophin Study Group. Hum Reprod. 2000;15(7):1446-51.
14. Madani T, Yeganeh LM, Ezabadi Z, Hasani F, Chehrazi M. Comparing efficacy of urinary and recombinant hCG on oocyte/follicle ratio to trigger ovulation in women undergoing intracytoplasmic sperm injection cycles: a randomized controlled trial. J Assist Reprod Genet. 2013;30(2):239-45.
15. George K, Kamath MS, Nair R, Tharyan P. Ovulation triggers in anovulatory women undergoing ovulation induction. Cochrane Database Syst Rev. 2014;(1):CD006900.
16. Mak SM, Wong WY, Chung HS, Chung PW, Kong GW, Li TC, et al. Effect of mid-follicular phase recombinant LH versus urinary HCG supplementation in poor ovarian responders undergoing IVF-a prospective double-blinded randomized study. Reprod Biomed Online. 2017;34(3):258-66.

17. Espey LL. Ovarian proteolytic enzymes and ovulation. Biol Reprod. 1974;10(2):216-35.
18. Lawrence TS, Dekel N, Beers WH. Binding of human chorionic gonadotropin by rat cumuli oophori and granulosa cells: a comparative study. Endocrinology. 1980;106(4):1114-8.
19. Brailly S, Gougeon A, Milgrom E, Bomsel-Helmreich O, Papiernik E. Androgens and progestins in the human ovarian follicle: differences in the evolution of preovulatory, healthy nonovulatory, and atretic follicles. J Clin Endocrinol Metab. 1981;53(1):128-34.
20. Farrag A, Costantini A, Manna C, Grimaldi G. Recombinant HCG for triggering ovulation increases the rate of mature oocytes in women treated for ICSI. J Assist Reprod Genet. 2008;25(9-10):461-6.
21. Nakano R, Mizuno T, Kotsuji F, Katayama K, Wshio M, Tojo S. "Triggering" of ovulation after infusion of synthetic luteinizing hormone releasing factor (LRF). Acta Obstet Gynecol Scand. 1973;52(3):269-72.
22. Engmann L, DiLuigi A, Schmidt D, Nulsen J, Maier D, Benadiva C. The use of GnRH agonist to induce oocyte maturation after cotreatment with GnRh antagonist in high risk patients undergoing in vitro fertilization prevents the risk of ovarian hyperstimulation syndrome: A prospective randomized controlled study. Fertil Steril. 2008;89(1):84-91.
23. Fauser BC, de Jong D, Olivennes F, Wramsby H, Tay C, Itskovitz-Eldor J, et al. Endocrine profiles after triggering of final oocyte maturation with GnRh agonist after cotreatment with GnRh antagonist ganirelix during ovarian hyperstimulation for in vitro fertilization. J Clin Endocrinol Metab. 2002;87(2):709-15.
24. Kummer NE, Feinn RS, Griffin DW, Nulsen JC, Benadiva CA, Engmann LL. Predicting successful induction of oocyte maturation after gonadotropin-releasing hormone agonist (GnRHa) trigger. Hum Reprod. 2013;28(1):152-9.
25. Itskovitz J, Boldes R, Levron J, Erlik Y, Kahana L, Brandes JM. Induction of preovulatory luteinizing hormone surge and prevention of ovarian hyperstimulation syndrome by gonadotropin-releasing hormone agonist. Fertil Steril. 1991;56(2):213-20.
26. Kolibianakis EM, Schultze-Mosgau A, Schroer A, van Steirteghem A, Devroey P, Diedrich K, et al. A lower ongoing pregnancy rate can be expected when GnRh agonist is used for triggering final oocyte maturation instead of hCG in patients undergoing IVF with GnRh antagonists. Human Reprod. 2005;20(10):2887-92.
27. Youssef MA, Van der Veen F, Al-Inany HG, Mochtar MH, Griesinger G, Nagi Mohesen M, et al. Gonadotropin-releasing hormone agonist versus HCG for oocyte triggering in antagonist-assisted reproductive technology. Cochrane Database Syst Rev. 2014;(10):CD008046.
28. Shapiro BS, Daneshmand ST, Garner FC, Aguirre M, Hudson C, Thomas S. Embryo cryopreservation recue cycles with premature luteinization. Fertil Steril. 2010;93(2):636-41.
29. Oktay K, Turkcuoglu I, Rodriguez-Wallberg KA. GnRh agonist trigger for women with breast cancer undergoing fertility preservation by aromatase inhibitor/FSH stimulation. Reprod Biomed Online. 2010;20(6):783-8.
30. Reddy J, Turan V, Bedoschi G, Moy F, Oktay K. Triggering final oocyte maturation with gonadotropin releasing hormone agonist (GnRHa) versus human chorionic gonadotropin (hCG) in breast cancer patients undergoing fertility preservation: An extended experience. J Assist Reprod Genet. 2014;31(7):927-32.
31. Meyer L, Murphy LA, Gumer A, Reichman DE, Rosenwaks Z, Cholst IN. Risk factors for a suboptimal response to gonadotropin releasing hormone agonist trigger during in vitro fertilization cycles. Fertil Steril. 2015;104:637-42.
32. Yding Andersen C, Westergaard LG, Figenschau Y, Bertheussen K, Forsdahl F. Endocrine composition of follicular fluid comparing human chorionic gonadotropin to gonadotropin releasing hormone agonist for ovulation induction. Human Reprod. 1993:8(6):840-3.
33. Anderson CY, Humaidan P, Ejdrup HB, Bungum L, Grøndahl ML, Westergaard LG. Hormonal characteristics of follicular fluid from women receiving either GnRh agonist or hCG for ovulation induction. Human Reprod. 2006;21(8):2126-30.
34. Cerrillo M, Rodrigues S, Mayoral M, Pacheco A, Martínez-Salazar J, Garcia-Velasco JA. Differential regulation of VEGF after final oocyte maturation with GnRh agonist versus hCG:A rationale for OHSS reduction. Fertil Steril. 2009;91 (4 Suppl):1526-8.
35. Castillo JC, Garcia-Velasco J, Humaidan P. Empty follicle syndrome after GnRHa triggering versus hCG triggering in COS. J Assist Reprod Genet. 2012;29(3):249-53.
36. Asada Y, Itoi F, Honnma H, Takiguchi S, Fukunaga N, Hashiba Y, et al. Failure of GnRH agonist-triggered oocyte maturation: Its cause and management. J Assist Reprod Genet. 2013;30(4):581-5.
37. Shapiro BS, Daneshmand ST, Garner FC, Aguirre M, Thomas S. Gonadotropin-releasing hormone agonist combined with a reduced dose of human chorionic gonadotropin for final oocyte maturation in fresh autologous cycles of in vitro fertilization. Fertil Steril. 2008;90(1):231-3.
38. Beckers NG, Macklon NS, Eijkemans MJ, Ludwig M, Felberbaum RE, Diedrich K, et al. Non supplemented luteal phase characteristics after administration of recombinant human chorionic gonadotropin,recombinant luteinizing hormone, or gonadotropin releasing hormone agonist to induce final oocyte maturation in vitro fertilization patients after ovarian stimulation with recombinant follicle-stimulating hormone and GnRh antagonist cotreatment. J Clin Endocrinol Metab. 2003;88(9):4186-92.
39. Humaidan P, Engmann L, Benadiva C. Luteal phase supplementation after gonadotropin-releasing hormone agonist trigger in fresh embryo transfer: the American versus European approaches. Fertil Steril. 2015;103(4):879-85.
40. Shapiro BS, Daneshmand ST, Garner FC, Aguirre M, Hudson C. Comparison of "triggers" using leuprolide acetate alone or in combination with low-dose human chorionic gonadotropin. Fertil Steril. 2011;95(8):2715-7.
41. Mitwally MF, Diamond MP, Abuzeid M. Vaginal micronized progesterone versus intramuscular progesterone for luteal support in women undergoing in vitro fertilization - embryo transfer. Fertil Steril. 2010;93(2):554-69.
42. Papanikolaou EG, Verpoest W, Fatemi H, Tarlatzis B, Devroey P, Tournaye H. A novel method of luteal supplementation with recombinant luteinizing hormone when a gonadotropin-releasing hormone agonist is used instead of human chorionic gonadotropin for ovulation triggering: a randomized prospective proof of concept study. Fertil Steril. 2011;95(3): 1174-7.

43. Humaidan P. Luteal phase rescue in high risk OHSS patients by GnRh agonist triggering in combination with low dose hCG: A pilot study. Reprod Biomed Online. 2009;18(5): 630-4.
44. Radesic B, Tremellen K. Oocyte maturation employing a GnRh agonist in combination with low dose hCG luteal rescue minimizes the severity of ovarian hyperstimulation syndrome while maintaining excellent pregnancy rates. Human Reprod. 2011;26(12):3437-42.
45. Seyhan A, Ata B, Polat M, Son WY, Yarali H, Dahan MH. Severe early ovarian hyperstimulation syndrome following GnRh agonist trigger with the addition of 1,500 IU hCG. Hum Reprod. 2013;28(9):2522-8.
46. Elbaek HO, Alsbjerg B, Laursen R, Povlsen BB, Mikkelsen AT, Anderson CY, et al. The exogenous progesterone free luteal phase in IVF-Exploring a new concept. Human Reprod. 2014;29(i326):P-502.
47. Andersen CY, Elbaek HO, Alsbjerg B, Laursen RJ, Povlsen BB, Thomsen L, et al. Daily low dose hCG stimulation during the luteal phase combined with GnRHa triggered IVF cycles without exogenous progesterone: a proof of concept trial. Human Reprod. 2015;30(10):2387-95.
48. Kol S, Breyzman T, Segal L, Humaidan P. "Luteal coasting" after GnRh agonist trigger - Individualized, HCG - based, progesterone-free luteal support in "high responders": a case series. Reprod Biomed Online. 2015;31(6):747-51.
49. Garcia-Velasco JA. Agonist trigger: What is the best approach? Agonist trigger with vitrification of oocytes or embryos. Fertil Steril. 2012;97(3):527-8.
50. Kummer N, Benadiva C, Feinn R, Mann J, Nulsen J, Engmann L. Factors that predict the probability of a successful clinical outcome after induction of oocyte maturation with a gonadotropin-releasing hormone agonist. Fertil Steril. 2011; 96(1):63-8.
51. Griffin D, Benadiva C, Kummer N, Budinetz T, Nulsen J, Engmann L. Dual trigger of oocyte maturation with gonadotropin - releasing hormone agonist and low - dose human chorionic gonadotropin to optimize live birth rates in high responders. Fertil Steril. 2012;97(6):1316-20.
52. Bodri D. Low dose hCG supplementation after GnRh agonist triggering: Don't be too quick on the trigger. Human Reprod. 2013;28(9):2315-7.
53. Humaidan P, Thomsen LH, Alsbjerg B. GnRHa trigger and modified luteal support with one bolus of hCG should be used with caution in extreme responder patients. Human Reprod. 2013;28(9):2593-4.
54. Humaidan P, Kol S, Papanikolaou EG, Copenhagen GnRH Agonist Triggering Workshop Group. GnRH agonist for triggering of final oocyte maturation: Time for a change of practice? Human Reprod Update. 2011;17(4):510-24.
55. Fatemi HM, Popovic-Todorovic B, Humaidan P, Kol S, Banker M, Devroey P, et al. Severe ovarian hyperstimulation syndrome after gonadotropin-releasing hormone (GnRh) agonist trigger and "freeze-all" approach to GnRh antagonist protocol. Fertil Steril. 2014;101(4):1008-11.
56. Haas J, Zilberberg E, Dar S, Kedem A, Machtinger R, Orvieto R. Co-administration of GnRH-agonist and hCG for final oocyte maturation (double trigger) in patients with low number of oocytes retrieved per number of preovulatory follicles-a preliminary report. J Ovarian Res. 2014;7:77.
57. Decleer W, Osmamagaoglu K, Seynhave B, Kolibianakis S, Tarlatzis B, Devroey P. Comparison of HCG triggering versus hCG in combination with a GnRH agonist: a prospective randomized controlled trial. Facts Views Vis Obgyn. 2014; 6(4):203-9.
58. Haas J, Bassil R, Cadesky K, Casper R. Dual trigger vs. HCG for final oocyte maturation. a prospective randomized controlled, double blinded study: preliminary results. Fertil Steril. 2017;108(3):e229.
59. Jayasena CN, Nijher GM, Abbara A, Murphy KG, Lim A, Patel D, et al. Twice-weekly administration of kisspeptin-54 for 8 weeks stimulates release of reproductive hormones in women with hypothalamic amenorrhea. Clin Pharmacol Ther. 2010;88(6):840-7.
60. Jayasena CN, Nijher GM, Comninos AN, Abbara A, Januszewki A, Vaal ML, et al. The effects of kisspeptin-10 on reproductive hormone release show sexual dimorphism in humans. J Clin Endocrinol Metab. 2011;96(12):E1963-72.
61. Jayasena CN, Abbara A, Comninos AN, Nijher GM, Christopoulos G, Narayanaswamy S, et al. Kisspeptin-54 triggers egg maturation in women undergoing in vitro fertilization. J Clin Invest. 2014;124(8):3667-77.
62. MacLean DB, Matsui H, Suri A, Neuwirth R, Colombel M. Sustained exposure to the investigational Kisspeptin analog, TAK-448, down-regulates testosterone into the castration range in healthy males and in patients with prostate cancer: results from two phase 1 studies. J Clin Endocrinol Metab. 2014;99(8):E1445-53.
63. Hancock K, Pereira N, Lekovich J, et al. The impact of estradiol drop after administration of ovulatory trigger on the success of donor oocyte-recipient cycles. Fertil Steril. 2017;108(3):e350-1.
64. Mourad S, Brown J, Farquhar C. Interventions for the prevention of OHSS in ART cycles: an overview of Cochrane reviews. Cochrane Database Syst Rev. 2017;(1):CD012103.
65. Hernandez ER, Gomez-Palomares JL, Ricciarelli E. No room for cancellation, coasting, or ovarian hyperstimulation syndrome in oocyte donation cycles. Fertil Steril. 2009;91 (4 Suppl):1358-61.
66. Bodri D, Guillen JJ, Galindo A, Mataró D, Pujol A, Coll O. Triggering with human chorionic gonadotropin or a gonadotropin releasing hormone agonist in gonadotropin-releasing hormone antagonist treated oocyte donor cycles: Findings of a large retrospective cohort study. Fertil Steril. 2009;91(2):365-71.
67. Taheripanah R, Zamaniyan M, Moridi A, Taheripanah A, Malih N. Comparing the effect of GnRH agonist and human chorionic gonadotropin on final oocytes for ovulation triggering among infertile women undergoing intrauterine insemination: an RCT. Int J Reprod Biomed (Yazd). 2017; 15(6):351-6.

CHAPTER 52

Individualized Controlled Ovarian Stimulation

Richa Sharma, Anindita Thakker

INTRODUCTION

Infertility can be due to various factors or can be multifactorial and can vary as per race, ethnicity, place, surrounding factors, etc., in different demographic areas. Childlessness has serious psychological, social, and health implications, and it affects not only an individual but also the whole family. The first successful in vitro fertilization (IVF) baby was born in 1978. Since then, science has undergone rapid advancement significantly,[1] so it was the beginning and not the end of medical evolution. Since that day, Louise Brown made a history; rather it was a stepping stone to an unraveled world of IVF. IVF technology has grown in leaps and bounds. Success rates have improved drastically. Besides, innovations in assisted reproductive technology (ART) laboratory supplemented with an individualized patient-directed approach have been a boon.

In vitro fertilization is an ever-evolving technology. There has been a sea change in technique in both the clinic and the laboratory and an improvement in drug quality and mode of administration. Despite these changes, there is still an immense physical and emotional burden attached to the treatment. The treatment involves daily injections, frequent ultrasounds and blood tests, and general or local anesthesia for oocyte retrieval. Among the complications, the most terrifying one is ovarian hyperstimulation syndrome (OHSS) which can be life-threatening.

Mild stimulation protocols resulted from a desire to make the procedure more safe and simple. The fact that there has been an immense improvement in the IVF laboratory gave courage to the physician to aim for fewer eggs reducing the dose of gonadotropins required and consequently the cost and complications. Unfortunately, the change was not universally accepted because the per-cycle pregnancy rates are lower, and the cumulative pregnancy rate (CPR), though projected to be similar, takes many more cycles of stimulation since there are less embryos available for cryopreservation. The cost too, though low per cycle, ultimately levels out.

The social scenario is also changing with an advanced age group of couples getting enrolled for IVF, especially due to more career orientation, delaying marriages with change in the patriarchal trend of society with more women empowerment enabling them to control their life, body, and future fertility. Increasing awareness and opting out of unmarried females for oocyte cryopreservation is one such example.

BASICS

Let us talk about the basics first. Treatment offered to a couple in ART can be:

- Timed intercourse with ovulation induction (fertile window utilization)
- Intrauterine insemination (IUI)
- IVF
- Intracytoplasmic sperm injection (ICSI)
- Third-party reproduction (gamete donation/surrogacy).

Irrespective of the kind of treatment, controlled ovarian stimulation (COS) protocols have been refined, focusing on multiple follicular development so as to extract the optimal number of mature (M2) oocytes per treatment cycle and to increase pregnancy rates.[2] Here comes the latest concept of individualized COS.[3-8]

How to Individualize Treatment and What are the Advantages?

- Individualized treatment optimizes success rate and improves the safety of IVF.
- Biomarkers help to individualize the treatment such that each couple will have a different treatment as per the clinical profile.
- Use of most reliable markers of ovarian reserve assessment
- Individualize expectations of oocyte yield
- Clinical workup supported by investigations—history, physical examination, and investigations have roles to

play in individualizing IVF treatment; the mainstay is individualized COS.
- Antral follicle count (AFC) and anti-Müllerian hormone (AMH) are the most specific of all prognostic factors.
- Categorization as per parameters—normal responders, high responders, and poor responders

PROGNOSTIC FACTORS FOR OVARIAN RESPONSE AND PROTOCOL RECOMMENDED

How to decide which protocol is for which patient? Definitely, that is a very routine common clinical query we face but practically it is very difficult to set fixed protocols [standard operating procedures (SOPs)] due to various confounding factors in ovarian stimulation, some of which are unpredictable/unexpected.

Grossly speaking, these factors can be:
- Genetic
- Nongenetic
- Demographic characteristics of patients
- Age of the female partner
- Presence of associated pathologies/factors such as endometriosis, polycystic ovaries, and a high body mass index (BMI)—all these can also affect the response of ovaries and the outcome.
- Physician experience, and SOPs and protocols of a fertility clinic play an important role. But definitely, at the end of the day, it is the success of an individual couple rather than of a clinic which depends a lot on their clinical profile besides the role of drugs and laboratory parameters.

It has been observed that in spite of similar parameters in two different patients, genetic differences may predispose some individuals to respond better as compared to other patients, though protocols may be the same. Tailoring of protocols is done based on all the above-mentioned factors.[9-15]

A study by Shahine et al. had compared Asian and Caucasian women and showed that even on transferring the highest quality embryos in both, Caucasian women had significantly higher implantation, clinical pregnancy, and live birth rates than Asian women.[16] Variable responses have been attributed to follicle-stimulating hormone (FSH) receptor gene polymorphisms in a study such that good responders more often carry the Asn/Ser allelic variant, which has a higher FSH sensitivity as compared to those with Ser/Ser allelic variant, which falls into the category of ovarian dysfunction.[14] To understand the utility of FSH receptor gene polymorphisms, more studies are needed.[17]

ROLE OF LUTEINIZING HORMONE AND RECEPTOR POLYMORPHISM

The need to add luteinizing hormone (LH) in some patients undertaking ovarian stimulation can vary due to the presence of common LH receptor polymorphisms, which is significantly higher in them. Such patients may also need high doses of recombinant FSH (r-FSH) for COS.[18-20] So we need to identify such patients for better results by following an individualized approach. Individualization can be based on AMH and AFC as depicted in **Figures 1 and 2.**

Clinical history with previous treatment records, more so if a patient had a previous IVF cycle, can be of help in

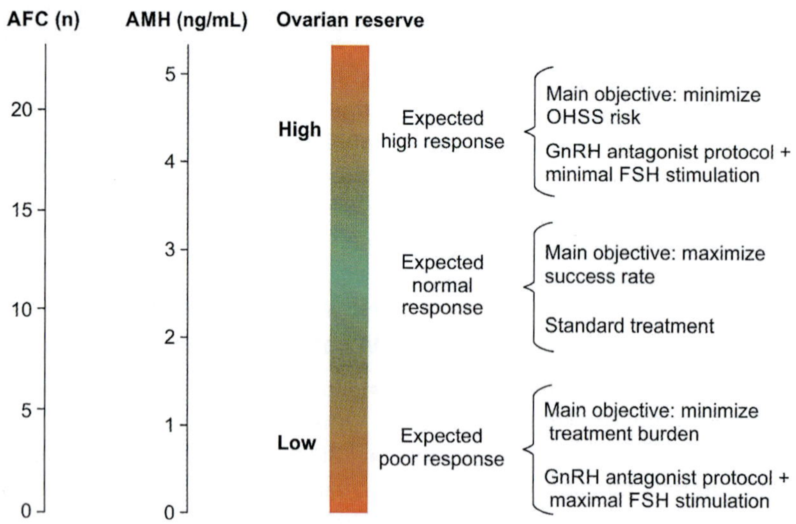

Fig. 1: Ovarian reserve testing before the first in vitro fertilization (IVF) cycle would permit categorizing patients as expected poor, normal, or hyper-responders. Since there is no evidence of superiority of one approach over another in the treatment of poor responders, the protocol associated with reduced discomfort and treatment burden should be preferred. In hyper-responder patients, one of the most important objectives of medical counseling is to prevent ovarian hyperstimulation syndrome (OHSS). Hence, the first-line protocol would be based on administration of low doses of follicle-stimulating hormone (FSH) in a GnRH antagonist-based scheme.[20]
(AFC: antral follicle count; AMH: anti-Müllerian hormone; GnRH: gonadotropin-releasing hormone)

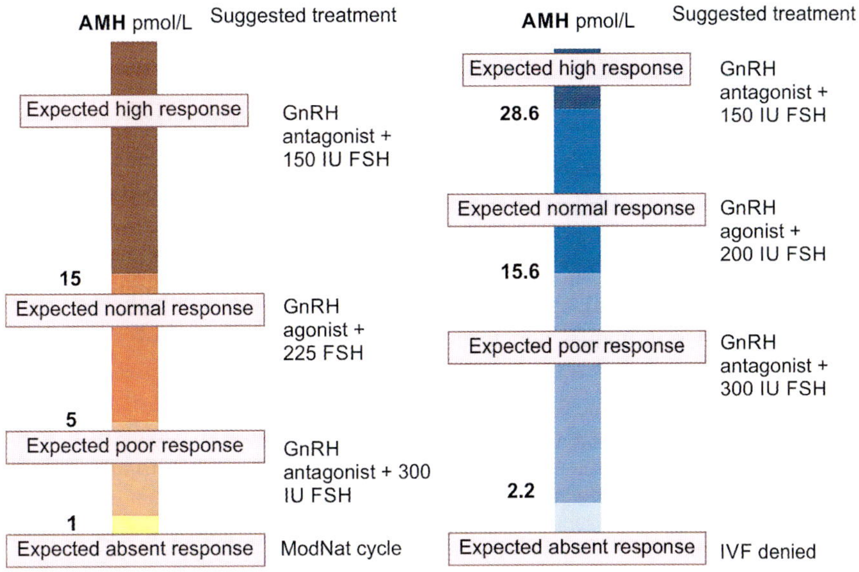

Fig. 2: Strategic (multiple models) modeling of controlled ovarian stimulation (COS) on the basis of ovarian reserve markers. The introduction of individualized anti-Müllerian hormone (AMH)-tailored COS utilizing agonist and antagonist protocols has been reported as associated with improved in vitro fertilization (IVF) cycle, i.e., increased pregnancy rate.[21]
(FSH: follicle-stimulating hormone, GnRH: gonadotropin-releasing hormone)

predicting response in the next cycle. For that, we need to extract the following information:

- Type of protocol used
- Type and dosage of stimulation drug
- Number of days on COS
- Number of oocytes retrieved
- Type of treatment (IVF/ICSI)
- Number of eggs retrieved and fertilized
- Day of embryo transfer and number of embryos transferred
- Any embryo freezing done
- Any history of cancellation of the cycle
- Any history of freezing all embryos with OHSS leading to ovarian suppression
- Luteal phase support—injectables/vaginal suppositories/gel form
- Outcome of IVF cycle.

Normal Responders

Favorable factors are:

- Age <35 years (younger age group)
- Normal BMI
- Adequate ovarian reserve [day 2/3 FSH <10 mIU/mL, estradiol (E2) <75 pg/mL]
- AFC between 6 and 10
- Short duration of infertility
- Previous live birth (secondary subfertility)
- Previous successful IVF
- Male factor as a predominant cause
- Tubal factor as a cause of infertility.

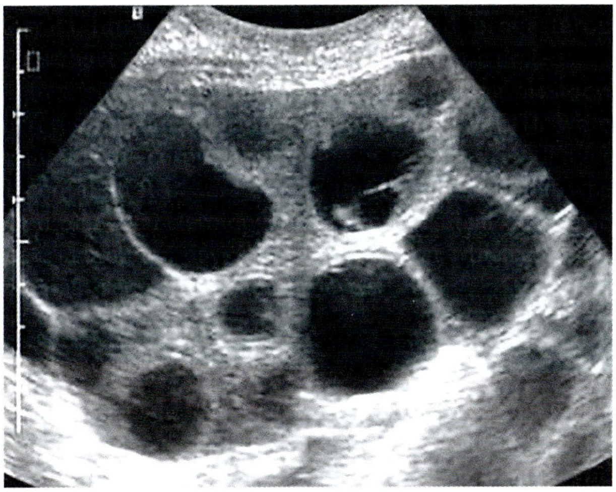

Fig. 3: Stimulated ovary in ovarian hyperstimulation syndrome (OHSS).

Protocols:

- Gonadotropin-releasing hormone (GnRH) agonist short or long protocols
- GnRH antagonist protocols.

High Responders

The greatest risk is OHSS, so we need to take precautions accordingly as depicted in **Figure 3**.

Factors that increase the risk of OHSS:

- Young age
- Polycystic ovaries on ultrasound
- Previous history of OHSS
- Lean polycystic ovary syndrome (PCOS)

- High dose of gonadotropins
- E2 levels >3,000 pg/mL on the day of ovulation trigger
- Rapidly rising E2 levels.

Why is individualized COS needed?

Each patient is different as etiology varies. The response of the body to medicines can also vary as per BMI or previous ovarian response.

Target on the number of oocytes in IVF is based on a study by Ben-Haroush et al. and Majumder et al. Appropriate ovarian reserve with a maximum of 8–12 mature oocytes is considered enough to achieve the highest CPRs. The quality of oocytes has more role than the number alone for a higher chance for a patient to become pregnant,[22,23] and a change in protocol may not always work.

ROLE OF AMH, AFC, AND OTHER BIOMARKERS IN INDIVIDUALIZED COS

- Various parameters, which include endocrine/paracrine biomarkers such as FSH, AMH, or inhibin B hormone levels, as well as sonological parameters such as AFC.[23]
- Day 3 FSH/LH, E2, and inhibin B—indicators of ovarian reserve.

Inhibin B: Inhibin levels are highest during the earliest and mid-stages of a menstrual cycle, and it is basically a protein produced by the granulosa cells of pre- and early antral follicles.[23]

Follicle-stimulating hormone and E2: They are more valid if done in the first 3–5 days of menstrual periods and their levels can vary from cycle to cycle besides being affected by factors such as presence of cysts and ovarian reserve. A patient with high levels of FSH in one cycle and having normal in another would behave differently on ovarian stimulation.[24,25]

Anti-Müllerian hormone: It can be used as an indicator of the quantity and quality of oocytes over a period of time. It is a member of the transforming growth factor beta family. It is the most specific of all parameters and is not affected by the day of the menstrual cycle but it definitely shows a decline with advancing age. Very rarely, especially in younger age groups, it may not correlate and in that case the final judgment is definitely by the clinical response of the patient after subjecting ovaries to stimulation by gonadotropins.[26,27]

Anti-Müllerian hormone plays an important role and is the most specific prognostic factor in predicting ovarian response, which can vary as per female age besides the inherent tendency to respond.[28]

It is likely that AMH cannot predict pregnancy, but it can predict probability, also predicting who will be poor responders and who will be prospective hyper-responders.

In a study by Nelson et al.,[29] they investigated the relationship between AMH levels and the success of different IVF treatment protocols and classified them as given in the following text.

High Responders

- Women with AMH levels >15 pmol/L
- Need a low starting dose of FSH in a GnRH antagonist protocol (to eliminate the need for complete cryopreservation of embryos due to excess response)
- These women have a higher fresh cycle clinical pregnancy rate.

Normal Responders

- Women with AMH levels of 5–15 pmol/L
- Generally treated with a traditional GnRH agonist long protocol
- Have a low incidence of excess response and poor response.

Poor Responders

- Women with low AMH of 1–5 pmol/L
- Also called reduced responders
- Generally show suboptimal response to COS and low pregnancy rates irrespective of the treatment protocol used.

INDIVIDUALIZED CONTROLLED OVARIAN STIMULATION AND DIFFERENT STIMULATION PROTOCOLS

Different ovarian stimulation protocols show variable success, and one single blanket treatment protocol would not work for all patients, which is why the concept of individualized COS exists **(Fig. 4)**. Individualized COS functions based on parameters such as AMH and AFC. The pregnancy rate depends on the quality and quantity of oocytes and embryos being produced per stimulated patient,

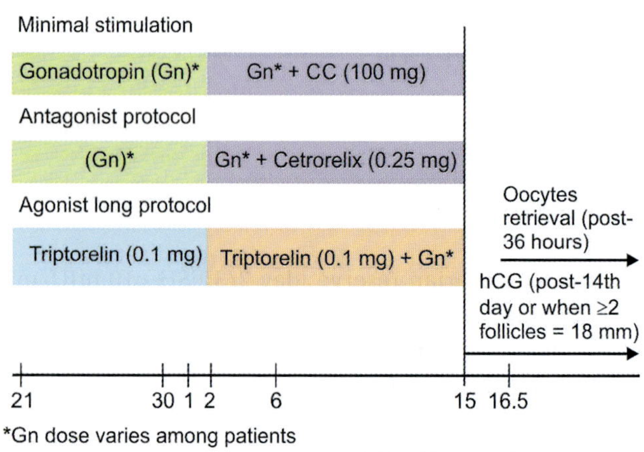

Fig. 4: Pictorial representation and comparison of different stimulation protocols.
(CC: clomiphene citrate, hCG: human chorionic gonadotropin)

TABLE 1: Summary of available conventional protocols for ovarian stimulation.

Protocol	*Agent*
Long, short, and microflare protocols	GnRH agonists and recombinant FSH, hMG, recombinant FSH plus recombinant LH, and other adjunctive agents
Standard, mild, and modified natural cycle protocols	GnRH antagonists and FSH, hMG, FSH plus LH, and other agents such as clomiphene citrate
Minimal and natural cycle protocols	No GnRH analogs and FSH, hMG, and FSH plus LH

(FSH: follicle-stimulating hormone; GnRH: gonadotropin-releasing hormone; hMG: human menopausal gonadotropin; LH: luteinizing hormone)

while the CPR is based on outcomes from fresh and frozen embryos from the same cycle of stimulation.

Various protocols are as follows:
Long protocol: It is the most common of all protocols and aims at complete pituitary suppression.

Short and ultrashort protocols: The initial "flare-up" of gonadotropins is used for ovarian stimulation.

- Conventional—step up/step down **(Table 1)**
- GnRH analogs—antagonist/short/microflare/flare/long protocols
- Mild/minimal/natural IVF cycles/modified natural protocols—what we call as patient-friendly protocols
- Accumulation and vitrification of embryos (ACCUVIT). Choices for COS according to possible combinations of GnRH agonist/antagonist and stimulation drugs:
  - GnRH agonist/antagonist protocol—standard, mild, modified natural, mini, natural
  - GnRH agonist—long, short, microflare, stop
- Agents used in stimulation can be:
  - Gonadotropins—FSH, human menopausal gonadotropin (hMG), FSH + LH
  - Others—clomiphene, letrozole, testosterone, estrogens.

Standard Long Protocol

A significant milestone in the development of COS was the implementation of GnRH agonists for pituitary suppression from the mid-luteal phase of the prior cycle until the completion of the COS process (long protocol). This approach allows IVF centers to manage patients more easily, thereby reducing cycle cancellation rates (as high as 35% before the introduction of GnRH agonists),[21,30] resulting in greater number of oocytes retrieved and producing better quality embryos and higher pregnancy rates than older protocols.[31]

Sub-variations of GnRH agonist protocols are:

- Short
- Ultrashort
- Microflare
- Stop

Basics

These protocols involve adjusting the timing and dose of GnRH agonist administration so that the patient benefits from the initial flareup of endogenous FSH and LH that may stimulate the follicles, in addition to the action of exogenous gonadotropins.

Disadvantages of Long Protocol

The protocol is time-consuming and involves complex regimens (at least 3 weeks of daily injections) that cause considerable patient discomfort and has important short-term complications, including OHSS and a high incidence of multiple pregnancies.

These negative aspects lead to a high rate of dropouts and increased costs.

Alternative Controlled Ovarian Stimulation Approaches: Mild and Minimal Ovarian Stimulation, Antagonist Protocol

Aim

The aim is to optimize the likelihood of achieving a healthy birth at a reasonable cost, while ensuring patient comfort and reducing the incidence of complications.

Principle of Action

It is based on two principles:

1. Use of GnRH antagonists, which cause immediate and dose-dependent gonadotropin suppression which may involve the use of clomiphene citrate.
2. Impact of r-FSH on follicular recruitment depends on the length of exposure above a threshold rather than the degree of FSH elevation.[32-34]

Advantages

- Less complex
- Less time-consuming
- Less expensive
- Lower dropout rates
- Have improved oocyte quality and endometrial receptivity with a higher proportion of chromosomally normal embryos.

Natural and Modified Natural Cycles

Natural cycles involve monitoring a patient's spontaneous cycle and retrieving a single oocyte prior to the LH peak, but it leads to a significantly lower pregnancy rate than is achieved with stimulated cycles. In modified natural cycles, a cumulative ongoing pregnancy rate of 30% after six

Flowchart 1: Soft protocol (mild stimulation).

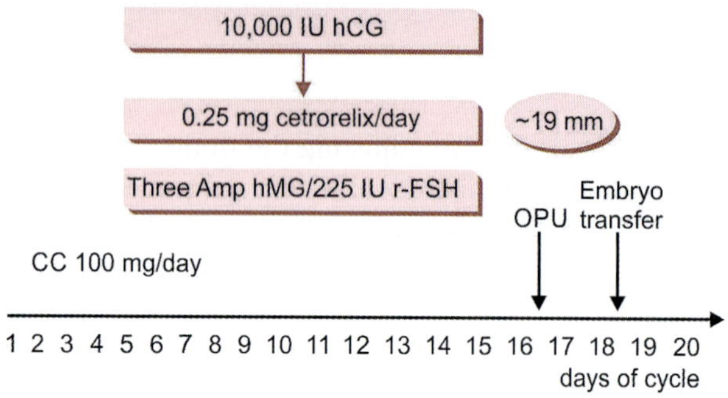

(CC: clomiphene citrate; hCG: human chorionic gonadotropin; hMG: human menopausal gonadotropin; OPU: oocyte pickup; r-FSH: recombinant follicle-stimulating hormone)

cycles has been reported and can be used before opting for conventional IVF.[5,35]

Soft Protocols (Flowchart 1)

Clomiphene citrate (100 mg) is administered orally from cycle days 2 to 8. From cycle day 6 onward, three ampoules of hMG or 225 IU r-FSH are administered, overlapping with clomiphene citrate for 3 days. Cetrorelix, in its minimal effective dose of 0.25 mg/day, is given from cycle day 6 onward until ovulation induction by 10,000 IU human chorionic gonadotropin (hCG) occurs.

Dosage Pattern

The dosage pattern of gonadotropins used also varies as per the criteria of the selection of patients. A list with starting dose of gonadotropins is given in **Table 2**.[36,37]

Treatment protocols in different situations will vary—individualized COS—mention individual protocols for each patient [as per the cause—PCOS/endometriosis/tubal factor/poor ovarian reserve/male factor/unexplained/frozen embryo transfer (FET)/donor embryo/donor egg/donor sperm/surrogacy/recurrent implantation failure (RIF)/recurrent pregnancy loss (RPL), etc.].

TABLE 2: Dosage of gonadotropins in different categories and age groups of patients.

Group of patients	*Starting dose of gonadotropins (IU)*
PCOS	100–112.5
First cycle <37 years	150
First cycle 37–39 years	225
First cycle >40 years	300
Previous normal response	150
Previous OHSS	75
Previous poor response	450
BMI > 30 kg/m^2	Increase by 75 IU (except in PCOS)
Severe endometriosis	Increase by 75 IU

(BMI: body mass index; OHSS: ovarian hyperstimulation syndrome; PCOS: polycystic ovary syndrome)

TABLE 3: Low prognosis groups—POSEIDON (Patient-Oriented Strategy Encompassing Individualize D Oocyte Number) classification.

Young	*Older*	*Ovarian reserve*
Group 1 Age <35 years AFC ≥5 AMH ≥1.2 ng/mL Subgroup 1a <4 oocytes Subgroup 1b 4–9 oocytes (in previous OS cycle)	Group 2 Age ≥35 years AFC ≥5 AMH ≥1.2 ng/mL Subgroup 1a <4 oocytes Subgroup 1b 4–9 oocytes (in previous OS cycle)	Adequate
Group 3 Age <35 years AFC <5 AMH <1.2 ng/mL	Group 4 Age ≥35 years AFC <5 AMH <1.2 ng/mL	Poor

(AFC: antral follicle count; AMH: anti-Müllerian hormone; OS: ovarian stimulation)

LOW PROGNOSIS GROUPS—POSEIDON (PATIENT-ORIENTED STRATEGY ENCOMPASSING INDIVIDUALIZED OOCYTE NUMBER) CLASSIFICATION

Low prognosis groups—POSEIDON (Patient-Oriented Strategy Encompassing IndividualizeD Oocyte Number) classification is shown in **Table 3**.

Management

- *Group 1 (good reserve, good quality)*
  - *Possible reasons:*
    - Asynchronous cohort
    - Starting dose of gonadotropin lower than required
    - Trigger issue
    - Polymorphism of FSH or LH receptors
  - *Suggestions:*
    - GnRH antagonist COS with E2/oral contraceptive pill (OCP)/progestin
    - r-FSH in preference to urinary FSH (uFSH)/hMG
    - Higher FSH dose + LH supplementation
  - *Measure of success:*
    - Minimum of five mature oocytes for one euploid embryo
- *Group 2 (good reserve, poor quality)*
  - *Possible reasons:*
    - Asynchronous cohort
    - Starting dose of gonadotropin lower than required
    - Trigger issue
    - Polymorphism of FSH or LH receptors

- *Suggestions:*
    - GnRH antagonist COS with E2/OCP/progestin priming
    - r-FSH in preference to uFSH/hMG
    - Higher FSH dose + LH supplementation
    - DuoStim
    - Dual/hCG trigger if not contraindicated
- *Measure of success:*
    - 10–12 mature oocytes for one euploid embryo

- *Group 3 (poor reserve, good quality)*
    - *Possible reasons:*
        - Poor ovarian reserve
        - Asynchronous cohort
        - Polymorphism of FSH or LH receptors
    - *Suggestions*:
        - Long GnRH agonist
        - GnRH antagonist with E2/OCP priming
        - Progestin-primed ovarian stimulation (PPOS) protocol[39]
        - Start r-FSH 300 units
    - *Measure of success:*
        - Four to seven mature oocytes for one euploid embryo
- *Group 4 (poor reserve, poor quality)*
    - *Possible reasons:*
        - Poor ovarian reserve
        - Asynchronous cohort
        - Polymorphism of FSH or LH receptors
    - *Suggestions:*
        - Long GnRH agonist
        - GnRH antagonist with E2/OCP priming
        - Start r-FSH 300 units
        - Add recombinant LH (rLH), androgens
        - DuoStim
        - PPOS protocol
    - *Measure of success:*
        - >12 mature oocytes for one euploid embryo.

ROLE OF LUTEINIZING HORMONE

Basics

The two-cell, two-gonadotropin model is a fundamental concept in ovarian physiology that establishes a role for both LH and FSH in hormone production. Androgen production and release during folliculogenesis are dependent on the stimulation of the theca cells by LH.

Follicle-stimulating hormone plays a crucial part in recruitment, selection, and dominance, while LH contributes to dominance, final maturation, and ovulation.

The amount of LH activity actually necessary for normal follicle and oocyte development, however, is not known but is likely to be very low since <1% of follicular LH receptors need to be occupied in order to elicit a maximal steroidogenic response and, accordingly, resting levels of LH (1–10 IU/L) should be sufficient to provide maximal stimulation to theca cells.[38-42]

Indications of the Use of Luteinizing Hormone in Ovulation Induction

Indications of the use of LH in ovulation induction include the following:

- Poor responders
- Poor ovarian reserve
- Advanced age of female
- Slow growth of the follicles
- Resistant response to FSH alone
- Low LH levels in blood
- Low E2 levels on ovarian stimulation.

INDIVIDUALIZATION FOR TIME CONSTRAINT

For fertility preservation before radiotherapy/chemotherapy, it is now accepted that ovarian stimulation can be done during both follicular and luteal phases of the same cycle, provided all embryos are frozen and no fresh transfer has been done, taking advantage of multiple waves of follicular recruitment in the same cycle.

- Protocols:
    - Duplex/DuoStim protocol
    - Random start protocol

Total oocyte yields of these protocols were found to be much more than only early follicular stimulations.

INDIVIDUALIZATION FOR NECESSITY OF LOW ESTROGEN

- Possible reasons:
    - Thrombosis-prone cases for COS [deep vein thrombosis (DVT) or another thrombotic event in the past]
    - Estrogen-sensitive malignancies such as estrogen receptor (ER)-positive breast and endometrial cancers
- Suggestions:
    - Serum E2 level is maintained at a level preferably lower than 200 pg/mL

Addition of letrozole up to maximum 10 mg/day with conventional doses of gonadotropins from the start of stimulation till the trigger day

CONCLUSION

- Individualized COS is the new modality to treat different patient groups as COS regimens are complex and cannot be optimal for all patients, so to get improved outcomes, we need to broaden our approach.
- Going to the basics and resorting to alternatives to standard COS protocols such as natural and mild cycles have shown some success. Also, we cannot negate

the negative effects of COS such as OHSS, multiple pregnancies, and ectopic pregnancy.

- Further development of objective biomarkers of response will be an important first step toward implementing personalized medicine in reproductive science.

REFERENCES

1. Trounson AO, Leeton JF, Wood C, Webb J, Wood J. Pregnancies in humans by in vitro fertilization and embryo transfer in the controlled ovulatory cycle. Science. 1981;212:681-2.
2. Steptoe PC, Edwards RG. Birth after the reimplantation of a human embryo. Lancet. 1978;2:366.
3. Mochtar MH, Van der Veen F, Ziech M, van Wely M, Musters A. Recombinant luteinizing hormone (rLH) for controlled ovarian hyperstimulation in assisted reproductive cycles. Cochrane Database Syst Rev. 2007;(2):CD005070.
4. Garcia-Velasco JA, Moreno L, Pacheco A, Guillén A, Duque L, Requena A, et al. The aromatase inhibitor letrozole increases the concentration of intraovarian androgens and improves in vitro fertilization outcome in low responder patients: a pilot study. Fertil Steril. 2005;84:82-7.
5. Schipper I, Hop WC, Fauser BC. The follicle-stimulating hormone (FSH) threshold/window concept examined by different interventions with exogenous FSH during the follicular phase of the normal menstrual cycle: duration, rather than magnitude, of FSH increase affects follicle development. J Clin Endocrinol Metab. 1998;83:1292-8.
6. Haouzi D, Mahmoud K, Fourar M, Bendhaou K, Dechaud H, De Vos J, et al. Identification of new biomarkers of human endometrial receptivity in the natural cycle. Hum Reprod. 2009;24:198-205.
7. FIVNAT 1996 report. French national register on in vitro fertilization. Contracept Fertil Sex. 1997;25:499-502.
8. Macklon NS, Stouffer RL, Giudice LC, Fauser BCJM. The science behind 25 years of ovarian stimulation for in vitro fertilization. Endocr Rev. 2006;27:170-207.
9. Coomarasamy A, Afnan M, Cheema D, van der Veen F, Bossuyt PMM, van Wely M. Urinary hMG versus recombinant FSH for controlled ovarian hyperstimulation following an agonist long down-regulation protocol in IVF or ICSI treatment: a systematic review and meta-analysis. Hum Reprod. 2008;23:310-5.
10. Verberg MFG, Eijkemans MJC, Macklon NS, Heijnen EMEW, Baart EB, Hohmann FP, et al. The clinical significance of the retrieval of a low number of oocytes following mild ovarian stimulation for IVF: a meta-analysis. Hum Reprod Update. 2009;15:5-12.
11. Detti L, Williams DB, Robins JC, Maxwell RA, Thomas MA. A comparison of three downregulation approaches for poor responders undergoing in vitro fertilization. Fertil Steril. 2005;84:1401-5.
12. Loutradis D, Vomvolaki E, Drakakis P. Poor responder protocols for in vitro fertilization: options and results. Curr Opin Obstet Gynecol. 2008;20:374-8.
13. Akerman FM, Lei Z, Rao CV, Nakajima ST. A case of spontaneous ovarian hyperstimulation syndrome with a potential mutation in the hCG/LH receptor gene. Fertil Steril. 2000;74:403-4.
14. Loutradis D, Patsoula E, Minas V, Koussidis GA, Antsaklis A, Michalas S, et al. FSH receptor gene polymorphisms have a role for different ovarian response to stimulation in patients entering IVF/ICSI-ET programs. J Assist Reprod Genet. 2006;23:177-84.
15. Huhtaniemi I, Pettersson K. Mutations and polymorphisms in the gonadotrophin genes; clinical relevance. Clin Endocrinol (Oxf). 1998;48:675-82.
16. Shahine LK, Lamb LD, Lathi RB, Milki AA, Langen E, Westphal LM. Poor prognosis with in vitro fertilization in Indian women compared to Caucasian women despite similar embryo quality. PLoS One. 2009;4:e7599.
17. Mohiyiddeen L, Nardo LG. Single-nucleotide polymorphisms in the FSH receptor gene and ovarian performance: future role in IVF. Hum Fertil (Camb). 2010;13:72-8.
18. Alviggi C, Clarizia R, Pettersson K, Mollo A, Humaidan P, Strina I, et al. Suboptimal response to GnRHa long protocol is associated with a common LH polymorphism. Reprod Biomed Online. 2009;18:9-14.
19. Lisi F, Rinaldi L, Fishel S, Lisi R, Pepe G, Picconeri MG, et al. Use of recombinant FSH and recombinant LH in multiple follicular stimulation for IVF: a preliminary study. Reprod Biomed Online. 2001;3:190-4.
20. La Marca A, Sunkara SK. Individualization of controlled ovarian stimulation in IVF using ovarian reserve markers: from theory to practice. Hum Reprod Update. 2014;20:124-40.
21. Nelson SM, Yates RW, Lyall H, Jamieson M, Traynor I, Gaudoin M, et al. Anti-Müllerian hormone-based approach to controlled ovarian stimulation for assisted conception. Hum Reprod. 2009;24:867-75.
22. Ben-Haroush A, Farhi J, Zahalka Y, Sapir O, Meizner I, Fisch B. Correlations between antral follicle count and ultrasonographic ovarian parameters and clinical variables and outcomes in IVF cycles. Gynecol Endocrinol. 2012;28:432-5.
23. Majumder K, Gelbaya TA, Laing I, Nardo LG. The use of anti-Müllerian hormone and antral follicle count to predict the potential of oocytes and embryos. Eur J Obstet Gynecol Reprod Biol. 2010;150:166-70.
24. Groome NP, Illingworth PJ, O'Brien M, Pai R, Rodger FE, Mather JP, et al. Measurement of dimeric inhibin B throughout the human menstrual cycle. J Clin Endocrinol Metab. 1996;81:1401-5.
25. Ravhon A, Lavery S, Michael S, Donaldson M, Margara R, Trew G, et al. Dynamic assays of inhibin B and oestradiol following buserelin acetate administration as predictors of ovarian response in IVF. Hum Reprod. 2000;15:2297-301.
26. Bancsi LFJMM, Broekmans FJM, Eijkemans MJC, de Jong FH, Habbema JDF, te Velde ER. Predictors of poor ovarian response in in vitro fertilization: a prospective study comparing basal markers of ovarian reserve. Fertil Steril. 2002;77:328-36.
27. Seifer DB, Scott Jr RT, Bergh PA, Abrogast LK, Friedman CI, Mack CK, et al. Women with declining ovarian reserve may demonstrate a decrease in day 3 serum inhibin B before a rise in day 3 follicle-stimulating hormone. Fertil Steril. 1999;72:63-5.
28. Hughes EG, Robertson DM, Handelsman DJ, Hayward S, Healy DL, de Kretser DM. Inhibin and estradiol responses to

ovarian hyperstimulation: effects of age and predictive value for in vitro fertilization outcome. J Clin Endocrinol Metab. 1990;70:358-64.

29. Nelson SM, Yates RW, Fleming R. Serum anti-Müllerian hormone and FSH: prediction of live birth and extremes of response in stimulated cycles—implications for individualization of therapy. Hum Reprod. 2007;22:2414-21.
30. Lee TH, Liu HC, Huang CC, Hsieh KC, Lin PM, Lee MS. Impact of female age and male infertility on ovarian reserve markers to predict outcome of assisted reproduction technology cycles. Reprod Biol Endocrinol. 2009;7:100.
31. Balasch J, Howles CM. GnRH agonist protocols: which one to use? In: Shoham Z, Jacobs HS, Howles CM (Eds). Female Infertility Therapy: Current Practice. London, UK: Martin Dunitz. 1998; pp. 89-203.
32. Bosch E, Labarta E, Crespo J, Simón C, Remohí J, Pellicer A. Impact of luteinizing hormone administration on gonadotropin-releasing hormone antagonist cycles: an age-adjusted analysis. Fertil Steril. 2011;95(3):1031-6.
33. Hughes EG, Fedorkow DM, Daya S, Sagle MA, Van de Koppel P, Collins JA. The routine use of gonadotropin-releasing hormone agonists prior to in vitro fertilization and gamete intrafallopian transfer: a meta-analysis of randomized controlled trials. Fertil Steril. 1992;58:888-96.
34. Verberg MF, Macklon NS, Nargund G, Frydman R, Devroey P, Broekmans FJ, et al. Mild ovarian stimulation for IVF. Hum Reprod Update. 2009;15:13-29.
35. Frydman R, Cornel C, de Ziegler D, Taieb J, Spitz IM, Bouchard P. Prevention of premature luteinizing hormone and progesterone rise with a gonadotropin-releasing hormone antagonist, Nal-Glu, in controlled ovarian hyperstimulation. Fertil Steril. 1991;56:923-7.
36. Rombatus L. Is there a recommended maximum starting dose of FSH in IVF? J Assist Reprod Genet. 2007;24(8):343-9.
37. Borini A, Dal Prato L. Tailoring FSH and LH administration to individual patients. Reprod Biomed Online. 2005;11(3):283-93.
38. Chappel SC, Howles C. Reevaluation of the roles of luteinizing hormone and follicle-stimulating hormone in the ovulatory process. Hum Reprod. 1991;6:1206-12.
39. Haahr T, Esteves SC, Humaidan P. Individualized controlled ovarian stimulation in expected poor-responders: an update. Reprod Biol Endocrinol. 2018;16:20.
40. Melo P, Eapen A, Chung Y, Jeve Y, Price MJ, Sunkara SK, et al. Controlled ovarian stimulation (COS) protocols for assisted reproduction: a cochrane systematic review and network meta-analysis. Hum Reprod. 2022;37(1).
41. Fiedler K, Ezcurra D. Predicting and preventing ovarian hyperstimulation syndrome (OHSS): the need for individualized not standardized treatment. Reprod Biol Endocrinol. 2012;10:32.
42. Silva ADR, Guimarães GB, de Castros EC. Individualization of controlled ovarian stimulation in vitro fertilization using markers of ovarian reserve: a systematic review. Reprod Climat. 2016;31:128-33.

CHAPTER 53

In Vitro Fertilization Lite

Adrija Kumar Datta, Stuart Campbell, Geeta Nargund, Anuradha Kumari

WHAT IS "IN VITRO FERTILIZATION LITE"?

In vitro fertilization (IVF) protocols, which involve reduced gonadotropin (Gn) stimulation, are various; called "IVF lite", "mild stimulation IVF", "minimal IVF", "mini IVF", or "gentle IVF". Essentially, all these terms mean the same thing. In this chapter, we will use the term mild stimulation IVF (MS-IVF) as defined by the International Society of Mild Approaches to Assisted Reproduction (ISMAAR) **(Table 1)**.[1]

Mild stimulation IVF entails the use of Gn or oral agents—clomiphene citrate (CC) or aromatase inhibitors (AI) either alone or in combination in an antagonist cycle with the intention of retrieving 2–7 oocytes. The standard dose of Gn is 150 IU from day 2 of the menstrual cycle, but this can rise to a maximum of 225 IU according to the woman's past history or body mass index (BMI). It is important to stress that MS-IVF is designed to elicit a mild response, which is in contrast with conventional controlled ovarian hyperstimulation (COH) that requires the maximum possible dose of Gn. MS-IVF should not be confused with natural IVF (N-IVF) or modified natural IVF (MN-IVF) which have distinct protocols and indications **(Tables 1 and 2)** and are not discussed in this chapter.

TABLE 1: Definitions of in vitro fertilization (IVF) protocols.

Types	*Definitions*
Natural cycle IVF	IVF is carried out with oocytes collected from a woman's ovary or ovaries in a spontaneous menstrual cycle without administration of any medication at any time during the cycle
Modified natural IVF with hCG	The use of hCG to induce final oocyte maturation in a natural cycle
Modified natural IVF with addition of GnRH-antagonist	The administration of GnRH-antagonist to block the spontaneous LH surge with or without FSH or hMG as add-back therapy
Mild stimulation IVF	A method when follicle FSH or hMG is administered at a lower dose and or for a shorter duration in GnRH-antagonist cotreated cycle, or when oral compounds: Antiestrogen or aromatase inhibitors are used either alone or in combination with gonadotropins with an aim to collect a fewer number of oocytes

(FSH: follicle-stimulating hormone; hCG: human chorionic gonadotropins; hMG: human menopausal gonadotropin; GnRH: gonadotropin-releasing hormone; LH: luteinizing hormone).
Source: Adapted from ISMAAR consensus statement.[1]

Mild stimulation IVF is being practiced by an enthusiastic but growing minority of IVF specialists and the reasons for this will be explored in this chapter.

EVOLUTION OF OVARIAN STIMULATION—RESURGENCE OF NATURAL OR MILD IVF

Mild approach to ovarian stimulation is not a new concept. We may recall that the first IVF baby was born from an oocyte collected in a natural cycle. Low dose of Gn with or without oral antiestrogen (mostly CC) were used in the early days of IVF, aiming to achieve multi follicular growth.[2] In course of time, as pituitary down regulation (desensitization) by gonadotropin-releasing hormone (GnRH)-agonist was introduced to prevent premature luteinizing hormone (LH) surge, COH with higher dose of Gn prevailed in the IVF world. The so-called "long down regulation" subsequently became the predominant protocol in "conventional" IVF (C-IVF) treatment. The intention of C-IVF is to collect as many eggs as possible, to allow selection of one or more embryos for transfer and cryopreservation of the remaining ones, from a decent cohort of embryos. The long down regulation protocol usually requires administration of Gn at a higher dose and or for a long duration, to develop follicles from completely shutdown ovaries.[3,4] However, side effects and risks of intense ovarian stimulation and multiple embryo transfer (ET) have now been well appreciated. The two major complications of IVF programs—ovarian hyperstimulation syndrome (OHSS) and multiple pregnancy are more commonly linked with C-IVF.[3-5] Considering these risks, in addition to physical discomfort, increasing emotional and

TABLE 2: In vitro fertilization (IVF) protocols.

Types	Protocols
Natural cycle IVF	The cycle is monitored from cycle day 4–6, by serial ultrasound scans ± serum LH and E2. Urine LH test is commenced once the dominant follicle reaches ≥12 mm in diameter. Optimal timing of oocyte retrieval is determined by hormone levels and follicular diameter. Indomethacin is usually added if there is a risk of premature ovulation. Luteal support is not necessary
Modified natural IVF with hCG	Elective "trigger" of final oocyte maturation by hCG, once the dominant follicle reaches ≥15 mm average diameter with satisfactory serum E2 levels. OR is scheduled 35–36 hours later. Triggering before endogenous LH surge reduces the incidence of premature ovulation. Luteal support is optional
Modified natural IVF with addition of GnRH-antagonist	The cycle starts with natural selection of the dominant follicle. Add-back FSH or hMG at 150 IU/day is started along with cetrorelix (antagonist), once the leading follicle is 13–14 mm size and serum E2 is >500 pmol/L. The hCG trigger is planned when the follicle reaches >16 mm in average diameter with a satisfactory serum E2 level and OR follows 35–36 hours later. The luteal phase support is required
Mild stimulation IVF	• *Low-dose Gn:* A fixed low dose of Gn (usually 150 IU of FSH), titrated with body mass index (BMI), is started in the early follicular phase (either on 2nd day or day 5 of a natural menstrual cycle). GnRH antagonist (e.g., cetrorelix) is commenced when the leading follicle is around 14 mm in diameter or if indicated by serum E2 level (usually >800 pmol/L). Ovulation is triggered when three follicles reach a diameter of 17 mm or greater. Oocyte retrieval is performed 35–36 hours after the ovulation trigger • Oral antiestrogen—selective estrogen receptor modulator (SERMs) or AIs with or without Gn top up: The SERM, commonly used is either CC (usually 100 mg/day) or rarely tamoxifen (40 mg/day). Letrozole (2.5 mg/day) is the most commonly administered AI. There are two different regimens for antiestrogen: – Antiestrogen are administered for 5 days—starting from 2nd or 3rd day of a natural menstrual cycle and low-dose (usually 150 IU) of FSH (± LH) is added from 5th day on either daily or alternate day, depending on the initial ovarian response. GnRH antagonist is commenced when the follicles are around 14 mm or as indicated by serum estradiol and LH levels – CC or tamoxifen is commenced from the 2nd or 3rd day of the cycle and continued until the day of ovulation trigger. FSH at a 150 IU daily dose may be added from 3rd–5th day and continued on alternate days or on a daily basis. SERMs, when administered in this way, effectively blocks the positive feedback action of E2 on the initiation of LH surge; therefore, no antagonist is usually required to suppress the surge

(AI: aromatase inhibitor; CC: clomiphene citrate; E2: estradiol; FSH: follicle-stimulating hormone; Gn: gonadotropin; GnRH: gonadotropin-releasing hormone; hCG: human chorionic gonadotropin; hMG: human menopausal gonadotropin; LH: luteinizing hormone; OR: oocyte retrieval)

Source: Adapted from ISMAAR consensus statement.[1]

financial burden associated with prolonged treatment cycles with aggressive hormonal manipulation, a safer and more "patient friendly" ovarian stimulation protocol was called for.[6] Recently, MS-IVF has been suggested as the way forward to make IVF more accessible and affordable globally.[7]

WHY ADOPT A MILDER APPROACH?

Several systematic reviews with meta-analysis have now demonstrated that mild ovarian stimulation significantly reduces the risk of OHSS.[3,4,8] MS-IVF allows administration of lower dose hCG for final oocyte maturation, which also lessens the risk of OHSS.[9] GnRH-agonist for ovulation trigger has recently been shown to be extremely effective in prevention of OHSS. Not a single patient developed OHSS in a very large cohort study (44,468 IVF cycles), by using a protocol comprising of CC plus Gn followed by a GnRH-agonist trigger.[10] A more recent study showed that, after a certain number of retrieved oocytes, the risk of OHSS rises in parallel with the number of oocytes, with no further increase in pregnancy rate (PR) or live birth rate (LBR).[11]

Elective single embryo transfer (SET) is the most effective way of reducing the chance of multiple births within an IVF program. A large randomized controlled trial (RCT) found significantly lower incidence of twin with similar cumulative LBRs when an MS-IVF with SET was compared with C-IVF and double embryo transfer (DET).[5] By applying strict SET policy in both MN-IVF and C-IVF cycles, a retrospective analysis of large database reported better cumulative LBRs (24% vs. 17.5%) with significantly fewer occurrence of OHSS and multiple pregnancy.[12] The aforementioned large Japanese study found the incidences of ectopic pregnancy (0.36%) and twin (0.9%) to be lower than those in general population by transferring single blastocyst following MS-IVF cycles.[10] High ovarian stimulation also increases the risk of venous thromboembolism (VTE) during the course of treatment, as well as in subsequent pregnancy.[13,14] To date, there is no published study that compares this particular risk between MS-IVF and C-IVF; however, by reducing the incidence of OHSS, the risk of VTE is also expected to be lowered.

Studies that assessed the psychological aspect of IVF treatment, often found the conventional down regulated protocol to be associated with treatment-related stress,[15] depression,[16] and anxiety[17] compared to those with MS-IVF. A systematic review identified physical and psychological stress to be the most common reason to discontinue IVF treatment.[18] Women undergoing MS-IVF are more likely to accept further treatment following a failed cycle and are less likely to drop out.[17,19] Getting the treatment "fitted" into a woman's natural cycles, the course of treatment tends to be shorter, with fewer clinic visits and less disruption to her working life. Thus, administration of lower dose of Gn for a short duration and its flexibility makes MS-IVF more tolerable and acceptable to the patients.[15,20] ISMAAR has taken a role in advocating the concept of "patient-centered" IVF worldwide.[21]

Apart from clinical safety and better tolerance, the mild approach is a way to make IVF treatment more affordable, by reducing the cost of medications. All the RCTs that compared the treatment cost found MS-IVF to be significantly less expensive than that of C-IVF, among normal responders,[12,22] as well as low responders.[23]

Despite the collection of fewer oocytes, comparable clinical outcomes may be achieved through a treatment cycle, which is less intense, less costly, safer, and more "patient friendly".[24] A recent study revealed that the dose of Gn actually inversely correlated with the LBRs, irrespective of women's age and other prognostic factors.[25] LBRs have been regarded as the benchmark of success in assisted reproduction. Currently, there is a trend of considering "a healthy singleton baby born at term" to be the yardstick of success with more emphasis on perinatal outcomes.[26] A study showed higher mean birth weight of the babies born out of MS-IVF.[27] An analysis of a large dataset of 63,686 singleton births has demonstrated an association between high number of recovered oocytes and higher incidence of perinatal complications, including preterm birth and low-birth weight babies.[28]

Is MS-IVF Clinically Effective?

There has been an ongoing skepticism on the clinical effectiveness of MS-IVF. The controversy has been fueled by publication of two meta-analyses that found the LBRs or ongoing pregnancy rates (OPRs) were lower with MS-IVF as compared to those with C-IVF.[4,29] However, a careful scrutiny of the meta-analyses revealed that predominant contribution to the pooled data came from a large RCT that undertook a policy of DET after conventional COH, while SET following mild stimulation.[5] Higher LBRs in this trial could be attributed to this differential ET policy. Several large adequately powered RCTs (which were not included in the above two meta-analyses) found no difference in the CPRs or LBRs between C-IVF and MS-IVF, whether in normal responders,[30,31] or poor responders.[23,32,33]

Cumulative LBRs of MS-IVF in normal responders have also shown to be comparable with C-IVF.[5,20]

A recent meta-analysis has shown that cumulative live birth rates were similar in poor, normal and hyper-responders following use of MS-IVF versus C-IVF. Risk of OHSS was significantly less with MS-IVF in both normal and hyper responders as compared to C-IVF.[34] A milder ovarian stimulation thus achieves a success, which is at least as good as that of C-IVF through a less intense process, making the approach more tolerable and affordable.

A milder ovarian stimulation thus achieves a success, which is at least as good as that of C-IVF through a less intense process, making the approach more tolerable and affordable.

How Does Mild IVF Hold Good Treatment Success?

High Proportion of Good Quality Oocytes or Embryos

Studies using C-IVF have found that an optimum of 13–15 oocytes needed to be retrieved to maximize the LBR.[35,36] However, these figures are not applicable for MS-IVF; it has been demonstrated that retrieval of only six oocytes optimize the LBR following MS-IVF cycles.[29] An RCT reported that six out of 10 women conceived when four or less oocytes were retrieved by MS-IVF, compared to none, when the similar numbers of oocytes were retrieved with long down regulation protocol.[37] A more recent RCT on good prognosis patients showed 46.7% top-grade embryos from mild IVF, compared to 42.1% from long protocol; however, the difference was not statistically significant.[20] A higher yield of oocytes in poor responders has been associated with higher proportion of morphologically as well as chromosomal abnormal embryos.[38] Indeed, one of the landmark RCTs found equal number of euploid embryos, whether mild or conventional IVF was undertaken, despite twice the number of embryos created in the latter.[39] In a more recent RCT, the doses of recombinant FSH was found to be strongly correlating with the number of recovered oocytes, but not with the number of blastocyst created.[40] The blastocyst-oocyte ratio and fertilization rate (FR) actually declined with the increasing dose of exogenous FSH in this study. This goes in the line with the aforementioned study by Baker et al. that identified a decline in LBRs with increasing Gn dose.[25] The emerging concept is that, low grade of stimulation encourages development of only healthier follicles with more competent eggs, strong ovarian stimulation may just force the growth of less competent follicles.[29]

Improved Endometrial Receptivity

There is increasing evidence that very high, supra-physiological serum estrogen levels may adversely affect implantation. A basic science study demonstrated progressively less adhesiveness of mouse embryos with human endometrium from fertile oocyte donors, as they were exposed to increasing high concentrations estrogen.[41] Endometrial gene expression has been found to be altered in COH cycles with high circulating estrogen as well as progesterone levels, when compared with those in natural cycles or treatment cycles with low-progesterone levels.[42,43] In practice, the implantation rates as well as PRs have been shown to be significantly lowered by high estradiol (E2) levels in normal or high responders.[44] Also, it has been shown that a "step-down" regimen with decreasing stimulation improved implantation.[29,45]

WHEN DO WE CONSIDER USING A MILD OVARIAN STIMULATION PROTOCOL?

Broadly speaking, there is hardly any clinical situation when MS-IVF should not be considered. Its effectiveness in treating the population in general has been demonstrated in large RCTs.[20,30,31] However, natural or mild stimulation is particularly advantageous in the following conditions:

- *Suspected or previous poor responders:* Treating women with poor ovarian reserve (POR) has always been a challenge; many strategies have been tried with no clear advantage. Until date, all the RCTs where one of MS-IVF protocols was judged against C-IVF, in women with POR found comparable to LBRs, OPRs, or PRs,[23,32,33] while the former was associated with significantly less use of medication and, hence the treatment cost.[23] Subsequently, two systematic reviews confirmed the advantages of MS-IVF in this clinical scenario.[8,46] Indeed, an RCT showed no difference in PRs among poor responders (according to Bologna criteria) whether 150, 300, or 450 IU daily dose of FSH was administered.[47] Natural IVF cycles, when compared with one of C-IVF protocols in women with POR, have also been reported to yield equivalent treatment outcomes.[48] Significant physical, emotional, and financial stress associated with high, often prolonged course of ovarian stimulation in C-IVF has made mild approach a preferred choice in this group of patients.
- *Older women undergoing IVF:* The changing socio-economic condition in the modern world has led women to delay in starting a family; therefore, increasingly more women in their late 30s or 40s are now seeking IVF to achieve a pregnancy. Data are limited on evaluation of mild IVF in older women. A study found no difference in PRs whether women were younger than or >35 years of age (26.6% vs. 35.0% per ET), when ovarian reserve was satisfactory.[49] The PR however was 6.2% among older women with POR in this study.
  An emerging option in treating poor responders or older women with POR is accumulation of oocytes and embryos through repeated cycles before embarking on ET. A retrospective study has demonstrated the benefit of this approach in poor responders.[50] Higher probability of obtaining good quality or euploid embryos from a larger pool of embryos, more likelihood of multiple embryos being available per ET or likelihood of more than one ET may raise the cumulative PR. Further studies are required to prove this unique concept.
- *Conditions where high doses of ovarian stimulation should be avoided:* A high serum estrogen level is not desirable while treating women with estrogen-sensitive breast cancer or early endometrial cancer. Some medical conditions, e.g., acute intermittent porphyria could be exacerbated by excess estrogen stimulation. The antiestrogen, tamoxifen, by virtue of its protective effect on the breast tissue and AI (e.g., letrozole), in conjunction with low gonadotropins may be considered for fertility preservation or treatment of women with breast cancer.[51,52] MS-IVF with AIs could be safer option for women with treated endometrial cancer[53] or porphyria. Other approaches for these clinical scenarios include conducting IVF through a purely natural cycle or in vitro maturation (IVM) of oocytes with little FSH priming.
- *Risk of OHSS:* Recently, the use of GnRH agonist as ovulation trigger, with or without freezing all embryos has been shown to almost eliminate the risk of OHSS in an IVF cycle. However, cases of primary OHSS have sporadically been reported.[54] Women with an extremely high risk of developing OHSS may choose to undergo an MS-IVF with oral agent or a delayed (day 5) start of Gn. Both these strategies tend to recruit fewer follicles. An IVM could also be an option for these women.[55]
- *Low-cost IVF:* Cost is an important consideration for IVF treatment, whether it is self or public funded, regardless of the economic status of the society. There is a drive to make IVF treatment more affordable and accessible to wider section of people by reducing the cost as much as possible.[7,21,26] As described earlier, all the studies that investigated the financial aspect of fertility treatment, found MS-IVF to be less expensive, with no compromise in its success. An MS-IVF protocol comprising of administration of CC or tamoxifen until ovulation trigger has been shown to be particularly inexpensive by avoiding relatively costly GnRH-antagonist injections.[56] There is an ongoing research on a "simplified culture media" that has the potential to reduce the laboratory expenses in IVF treatment. Preliminary results are encouraging.[57]

WHAT ARE THE LIMITING FACTORS IN MS-IVF?

Potential cycle cancellation: A treatment cycle is usually canceled either as a consequence of inadequate response or premature ovulation. The meta-analysis of three RCTs by Matsaseng et al. found an increased incidence of cycle cancellation before oocytes retrieval in MS-IVF, as compared to conventional IVF (16% vs. 9%; odds ratio 2.55, confidence interval 1.62–4.02).[4] The RCT by Revelli et al. on poor responders reported higher cycle cancellation with CC + Gn cycles, as compared to down regulated cycles (13% vs. 2.7%).[32]

In contrast, several other reports, including RCTs, failed to find an increased risk of cycle cancellation by mild approach, both in normal responders[20,58,59] and poor responders.[33,47] No cycle was canceled due to premature ovulation in the RCT by Lin et al.;[59] while a prospective study with CC + Gn protocol in normal responders reported a lower chance of cycle cancellation (4.7% vs. 34.0%).[60] Cancellation rates due to premature ovulation were between 2.1 and 2.8% by administration of CC up till ovulation trigger.[10] Interestingly, the Cochrane review by Gibreel et al., which compared COH with CC + Gn regimen, found an overall increased incidence of cycle cancellation with the latter, but there was no difference in the subgroup where a GnRH-antagonist was used.[3] Also, the majority of the studies, including RCTs adopted a criterion of canceling cycles if there are less than three dominant follicles for both C-IVF and MS-IVF; while the development of less than three dominant follicles is deemed a poor response for C-IVF, it could be actually a normal response for MS-IVF. Current evidence suggests that the risk of cycle cancellation rate with MS-IVF is low and comparable to that of C-IVF with appropriate use of GnRH-antagonist and close cycle monitoring.

Fewer embryos for cryopreservation: Sensibly, there is a concern that MS-IVF tends to generate fewer oocytes or embryos for transfer or cryopreservation.[61] In reality, the evidence is very conflicting—some RCTs showed the number of available oocytes or embryos not significantly different comparing cycles using C-IVF from those of MS-IVF[20,47,62] while others found fewer oocytes or embryos with MS-IVF.[33,63] However, a number of RCTs reported that the probability of obtaining good quality embryos or blastocyst was similar to,[33,40,63] if not higher with MS-IVF.[37,39,64] This finding may explain why the cumulative success (OPRs/LBRs) with MS-IVF has generally been found to be satisfactory and comparable with that of C-IVF, despite the disadvantage of obtaining fewer embryos for cryopreservation with the mild approach.[5,19,20]

Less flexible scheduling for the clinic and need for a high quality laboratory: Closer cycle monitoring and a high standard of embryology laboratory are the two essential prerequisites for MS-IVF. A successful vitrification program is vital for the success of cumulative outcomes. However, judicious administration of GnRH-antagonist or timely use of indomethacin to prevent ovulation, monitoring perifollicular blood flow, and serial measurement of serum E2 and LH levels may help flexibly scheduling treatment cycles avoiding weekend work.

Since the last 25 years, various literatures have been published suggesting a mild ovarian stimulation approach for all poor responders. Based on current evidence all poor responders are not same and should be managed on individualized basis rather than "one fits all" mild stimulation protocol.[65]

Mild approach is being practiced in different parts of the globe, and India is no exception. Does it fit the need, expectation, and financial situation of Indian couples? Studies from all over the world found MS-IVF overall to be as successful as C-IVF, with N/NM-IVF being a better option for poor responders. There is no reason why it will be different in an Indian population. The published evidence so far indicates an acceptable and comparable treatment outcome.[55,64] More importantly, a low-cost IVF may make this treatment more affordable to the vast section of people in the Indian subcontinent, where fertility treatment is predominantly self-funded. One of the few studies in the world literature, that did economic evaluation of a low-cost MS-IVF protocol (continuing CC until trigger day to avoid the use of more expensive GnRH antagonist) was conducted in Vellore, India.[55] Like Western society, more and more Indian women approaching 40 years or older are now seeking IVF to achieve a pregnancy. The use of MS-IVF in treating older women has become a burning topic among the specialists in India.[66,67] Conducting repeated mild cycles before transferring the embryos in poor responders has become increasingly adopted.[66] Patients' acceptance of undergoing repeated MS-IVF cycles and its cost implications are being investigated in Indian context— it would be interesting to follow future work in this regard.

FUTURE PROSPECTS

Today, the major deterrents to widespread practice of mild approach IVF are—lack of robust RCT data on its success rates, the clinicians' attitude of adhering to more convenient cycle scheduling, satisfaction in retrieving as many oocytes as possible, and variation in the standard of embryology laboratories and the public funding policies in some parts of the world.[68] Several adequately powered RCTs have been published in recent years; almost all the trials found MS-IVF to yield comparable treatment success, both in normal and poor responders. An updated meta-analysis and systematic review is now required to prove its effectiveness. Future research needs to look into its efficacy, especially among poor responders, in terms of LBR per cycle and cumulative success. Flexible cycle scheduling is possible by judicious cycle monitoring with ultrasound scans in combination with measurement of serum E2/LH, timely use of GnRH-antagonist. An effective vitrification technique, which is required for an MS-IVF, is an important goal for any successful IVF laboratory anyway.[68] Future research focusing on MS-IVF would help building up more robust protocols, taking patient's characteristics (age, BMI, etc.) into account. Further promotion of MS-IVF may be possible through education, training, and research.[69] Communication between the investigators and publishing research data on treatment success as well as patients' attitude and cost, would increase clinicians' acceptance of MS-IVF. Progress in this field may raise the hope that mild and natural IVF could replace C-IVF in all clinical circumstances.

KEY POINTS

- Mild stimulation IVF involves the use of gonadotropin (Gn) or oral agents—clomiphene citrate (CC) or aromatase inhibitors (AI) either alone or in combination in an antagonist cycle with the intention of retrieving 2–7 oocytes ISMAAR consensus.
- Mild stimulation protocols have been safer, less uncomfortable for patients, and at reduced costs when all the expenses are taken into account.

  However, concerns remain about the reduction in the per-cycle chance of pregnancy. Success rates should be evaluated with regard to safety, comfort, direct and indirect costs involved in treatment and management of OHSS.
- An individualized approach to controlled ovarian stimulation based on anti-Müllerian hormone and antral follicle count should be practiced to match patients with the most appropriate protocol.
- In women considered to be poor responders, there is fair evidence that clinical pregnancy rates after IVF are not substantially different when comparing mild ovarian stimulation protocols using low-dose gonadotropins (150 IU/d) to conventional-gonadotropins protocols [American Society for Reproductive Medicine (ASRM) 2018].
- Among poor responders, there is fair evidence to support the recommendation that mild ovarian stimulation is cost-effective, though live-birth rates are extremely low in both groups (ASRM 2018).

REFERENCES

1. Nargund G, Fauser BC, Macklon MS, Ombelet W, Nygren K, Frydman R, et al. The ISMAAR proposal on terminology for ovarian stimulation for IVF. Hum Reprod. 2007;22(11):2801-4.
2. Jones HW Jr, Jones GS, Andrews MC, Acosta A, Bundren C, Garcia J, et al. The program for in vitro fertilization at Norfolk. Fertil Steril. 1982;38(1):14-21.
3. Gibreel A, Maheshwari A, Bhattacharya S. Clomiphene citrate in combination with gonadotropins for controlled ovarian stimulation in women undergoing in vitro fertilization. Cochrane Database Syst Rev. 2012;11:CD008528.
4. Matsaseng T, Kruger T, Steyn W. Mild ovarian stimulation for in vitro fertilization: are we ready to change? A meta-analysis. Gynecol Obstet Invest. 2013;76(4):233-40.
5. Heijnen EM, Eijkemans MJ, De Klerk C, Polinder S, Beckers NG, Klinkert ER, et al. A mild treatment strategy for in-vitro fertilisation: a randomised non-inferiority trial. Lancet. 2007;369(9563):743-9.
6. Edwards RG, Lobo R, Bouchard P. Time to revolutionize ovarian stimulation. Hum Reprod. 1996;11(5):917-9.
7. Paulson RJ, Fauser BCJM, Vuong LTN, Doody K. Can we modify assisted reproductive technology practice to broaden reproductive care access? Fertil Steril. 2016;105(5):1138-43.
8. Figueiredo JB, Nastri CO, Vieira AD, Martins WP. Clomiphene combined with gonadotropins and GnRH antagonist versus conventional controlled ovarian hyperstimulation without clomiphene in women undergoing assisted reproductive techniques: systematic review and meta-analysis. Arch Gynecol Obstet. 2013;287(4):779-90.
9. Nargund G, Hutchison L, Scaramuzzi R, Campbell S. Low-dose HCG is useful in preventing OHSS in high-risk women without adversely affecting the outcome of IVF cycles. Reprod Biomed Online. 2007;14(6):682-5.
10. Kato K, Takehara Y, Segawa T, Kawachiya S, Okuno T, Kobayashi T, et al. Minimal ovarian stimulation combined with elective single embryo transfer policy: age-specific results of a large, single-centre, Japanese cohort. Reprod Biol Endocrinol. 2012;10:35.
11. Steward RG, Lan L, Shah AA, Yeh JS, Price TM, Goldfarb JM, et al. Oocyte number as a predictor for ovarian hyper-stimulation syndrome and live birth: an analysis of 256,381 in vitro fertilization cycles. Fertil Steril. 2014;101(4):967-73.
12. Groen H, Tonch N, Simons AH, van der Veen F, Hoek A, Land JA. Modified natural cycle versus controlled ovarian hyperstimulation IVF: a cost-effectiveness evaluation of three simulated treatment scenarios. Hum Reprod. 2013; 28(12):3236-46.
13. Hansen AT, Kesmodel US, Juul S, Hvas AM. Increased venous thrombosis incidence in pregnancies after in vitro fertilization. Hum Reprod. 2014;29(3):611-7.
14. Mor YS, Schenker JG. Ovarian hyperstimulation syndrome and thrombotic events. Am J Reprod Immunol. 2014;72(6):541-8.
15. Hojgaard A, Ingerslev HJ, Dinesen J. Friendly IVF: patient opinions. Hum Reprod. 2001;16(7):1391-6.
16. de Klerk C, Macklon NS, Heijnen EM, Eijkemans MJ, Fauser BC, Passchier J, et al. The psychological impact of IVF failure after two or more cycles of IVF with a mild versus standard treatment strategy. Hum Reprod. 2007;22(9):2554-8.
17. Verberg MF, Eijkemans MJ, Heijnen EM, Broekmans FJ, de Klerk C, Fauser BC, et al. Why do couples drop-out from IVF treatment? A prospective cohort study. Hum Reprod. 2008;23(9):2050-5.
18. Gameiro S, Boivin J, Peronace L, Verhaak CM. Why do patients discontinue fertility treatment? A systematic review of reasons and predictors of discontinuation in fertility treatment. Hum Reprod Update. 2012;18(6):652-69.
19. Ferraretti AP, Gianaroli L, Magli MC, Devroey P. Mild ovarian stimulation with clomiphene citrate launch is a realistic option for in vitro fertilization. Fertil Steril. 2015;104(2):333-8.
20. Casano S, Guidetti D, Patriarca A, Pittatore G, Gennarelli G, Revelli A. MILD ovarian stimulation with GnRH-antagonist vs. long protocol with low dose FSH for non-PCO high responders undergoing IVF: a prospective, randomized study including thawing cycles. J Assist Reprod Genet. 2012;29(12):1343-51.

21. Nargund G, Chian RC. ISMAAR: Leading the global agenda for a more physiological, patient-centred, accessible and safer approaches in ART. J Assist Reprod Genet. 2013;30(2):155-6.
22. Lou HY, Huang XY. Modified natural cycle for in vitro fertilization and embryo transfer in normal ovarian responders. J Int Med Res. 2010;38(6):2070-6.
23. Ragni G, Levi-Setti PE, Fadini R, Brigante C, Scarduelli C, Alagna F, et al. Clomiphene citrate versus high doses of gonadotropins for in vitro fertilisation in women with compromised ovarian reserve: a randomised controlled non-inferiority trial. Reprod Biol Endocrinol. 2012;10:114.
24. Ubaldi F, Rienzi L, Baroni E, Ferrero S, Iacobelli M, Minasi MG, et al. Hopes and facts about mild ovarian stimulation. Reprod Biomed Online. 2007;14(6):675-81.
25. Baker VL, Brown MB, Luke B, Smith GW, Ireland JJ. Gonadotropin dose is negatively correlated with live birth rate: analysis of more than 650,000 assisted reproductive technology cycles. Fertil Steril. 2015;104(5):1145-52 e1-5.
26. Frydman R, Nargund G. Mild approaches in assisted reproduction—better for the future? Fertil Steril. 2014; 102(6):1540-1.
27. Pelinck MJ, Keizer MH, Hoek A, Simons AH, Schelling K, Middelburg K, et al. Perinatal outcome in singletons after modified natural cycle IVF and standard IVF with ovarian stimulation. Eur J Obstet Gynecol Reprod Biol. 2010;148(1): 56-61.
28. Sunkara SK, La Marca A, Seed PT, Khalaf Y. Increased risk of preterm birth and low birthweight with very high number of oocytes following IVF: an analysis of 65 868 singleton live birth outcomes. Hum Reprod. 2015;30(6):1473-80.
29. Verberg MF, Eijkemans MJ, Macklon NS, Heijnen EM, Baart EB, Hohmann FP, et al. The clinical significance of the retrieval of a low number of oocytes following mild ovarian stimulation for IVF: a meta-analysis. Hum Reprod Update. 2009;15(1):5-12.
30. Grochowski D, Wolczynski S, Kuczynniski W, Domitrz J, Szamatowicz J, Szamatowicz M. Good results of milder form of ovarian stimulation in an in vitro fertilization/ intracytoplasmic sperm injection program. Gynecol Endocrinol. 1999;13(5):297-304.
31. Tummon IS, Daniel SA, Kaplan BR, Nisker JA, Yuzpe AA. Randomized, prospective comparison of luteal leuprolide acetate and gonadotropins versus clomiphene citrate and gonadotropins in 408 first cycles of in vitro fertilization. Fertil Steril. 1992;58(3):563-8.
32. Revelli A, Chiado A, Dalmasso P, Stabile V, Evangelista F, Basso G, et al. "Mild" vs. "long" protocol for controlled ovarian hyperstimulation in patients with expected poor ovarian responsiveness undergoing in vitro fertilization (IVF): a large prospective randomized trial. J Assist Reprod Genet. 2014;31(7):809-15.
33. Youssef MA, van Wely M, Al-Inahy H, Madani T, Jahangiri N, Khodabakhshi S, et al. A mild ovarian stimulation strategy in women with poor ovarian reserve undergoing IVF: a multicenter randomized non-inferiority trial. Hum Reprod. 2017;32(1):112-8.
34. Datta AK, Maheshwari A, Felix N, Campbell S, Nargund G. Mild versus conventional ovarian stimulation for IVF in poor, normal and hyper-responders: a systematic review and meta-analysis. Hum Reprod Update. 2021;27(2):229-53.
35. Sunkara SK, Rittenberg V, Raine-Fenning N, Bhattacharya S, Zamora J, Coomarasamy A. Association between the number of eggs and live birth in IVF treatment: an analysis of 400 135 treatment cycles. Hum Reprod. 2011;26(7):1768-74.
36. van der Gaast MH, Eijkemans MJ, van der Net JB, de Boer EJ, Burger CW, van Leeuwen FE, et al. Optimum number of oocytes for a successful first IVF treatment cycle. Reprod Biomed Online. 2006;13(4):476-80.
37. Hohmann FP, Macklon NS, Fauser BC. A randomized comparison of two ovarian stimulation protocols with gonadotropin-releasing hormone (GnRH) antagonist cotreatment for in vitro fertilization commencing recombinant follicle-stimulating hormone on cycle day 2 or 5 with the standard long GnRH agonist protocol. J Clin Endocrinol Metab. 2003;88(1):166-73.
38. Haaf T, Hahn A, Lambrecht A, Grossmann B, Schwaab E, Khanaga O, et al. A high oocyte yield for intracytoplasmic sperm injection treatment is associated with an increased chromosome error rate. Fertil Steril. 2009;91(3):733-8.
39. Baart EB, Martini E, Eijkemans MJ, Van Opstal D, Beckers NG, Verhoeff A, et al. Milder ovarian stimulation for in-vitro fertilization reduces aneuploidy in the human preimplantation embryo: a randomized controlled trial. Hum Reprod. 2007;22(4):980-8.
40. Arce JC, Andersen AN, Fernandez-Sanchez M, Visnova H, Bosch E, García-Velasco JA, et al. Ovarian response to recombinant human follicle-stimulating hormone: a randomized, antimüllerian hormone-stratified, dose-response trial in women undergoing in vitro fertilization/ intracytoplasmic sperm injection. Fertil Steril. 2014;102(6): 1633-40 e5.
41. Valbuena D, Martin J, de Pablo JL, Remohí J, Pellicer A, Simón C. Increasing levels of estradiol are deleterious to embryonic implantation because they directly affect the embryo. Fertil Steril. 2001;76(5):962-8.
42. Haouzi D, Assou S, Mahmoud K, Tondeur S, Rème T, Hedon B, et al. Gene expression profile of human endometrial receptivity: comparison between natural and stimulated cycles for the same patients. Hum Reprod. 2009;24(6):1436-45.
43. Labarta E, Martinez-Conejero JA, Alama P, Horcajadas JA, Pellicer A, Simón C, et al. Endometrial receptivity is affected in women with high circulating progesterone levels at the end of the follicular phase: a functional genomics analysis. Hum Reprod. 2011;26(7):1813-25.
44. Simon C, Cano F, Valbuena D, Remohí J, Pellicer A. Clinical evidence for a detrimental effect on uterine receptivity of high serum oestradiol concentrations in high and normal responder patients. Hum Reprod. 1995;10(9):2432-7.
45. Simon C, Garcia Velasco JJ, Valbuena D, Peinado JA, Moreno C, Remohí J, et al. Increasing uterine receptivity by decreasing estradiol levels during the preimplantation period in high responders with the use of a follicle-stimulating hormone step-down regimen. Fertil Steril. 1998;70(2):234-9.
46. Song D, Shi Y, Zhong Y, Meng Q, Hou S, Li H. Efficiency of mild ovarian stimulation with clomiphene on poor ovarian responders during IVF\ICSI procedures: a meta-analysis. Eur J Obstet Gynecol Reprod Biol. 2016;204:36-43.
47. Bastu E, Buyru F, Ozsurmeli M, Demiral I, Dogan M, Yeh J. A randomized, single-blind, prospective trial comparing three different gonadotropin doses with or without addition

of letrozole during ovulation stimulation in patients with poor ovarian response. Eur J Obstet Gynecol Reprod Biol. 2016;203:30-4.

48. Morgia F, Sbracia M, Schimberni M, Giallonardo A, Piscitelli C, Giannini P, et al. A controlled trial of natural cycle versus microdose gonadotropin-releasing hormone analog flare cycles in poor responders undergoing in vitro fertilization. Fertil Steril. 2004;81(6):1542-7.
49. Shaulov T, Velez MP, Buzaglo K, Phillips SJ, Kadoch IJ. Outcomes of 1503 cycles of modified natural cycle in vitro fertilization: a single-institution experience. J Assist Reprod Genet. 2015;32(7):1043-8.
50. Greco E, Litwicka K, Arrivi C, Varricchio MT, Zavaglia D, Mencacci C, et al. Accumulation of oocytes from a few modified natural cycles to improve IVF results: a pilot study. J Assist Reprod Genet. 2013;30(11):1465-70.
51. Azim AA, Costantini-Ferrando M, Oktay K. Safety of fertility preservation by ovarian stimulation with letrozole and gonadotropins in patients with breast cancer: a prospective controlled study. J Clin Oncol. 2008;26(16):2630-5.
52. Oktay K. Further evidence on the safety and success of ovarian stimulation with letrozole and tamoxifen in breast cancer patients undergoing in vitro fertilization to cryopreserve their embryos for fertility preservation. J Clin Oncol. 2005; 23(16):3858-9.
53. Azim A, Oktay K. Letrozole for ovulation induction and fertility preservation by embryo cryopreservation in young women with endometrial carcinoma. Fertil Steril. 2007;88(3):657-64.
54. Seyhan A, Ata B, Polat M, Son WY, Yarali H, Dahan MH. Severe early ovarian hyperstimulation syndrome following GnRH agonist trigger with the addition of 1500 IU hCG. Hum Reprod. 2013;28(9):2522-8.
55. Chian RC, Buckett WM, Abdul Jalil AK, Son WY, Sylvestre C, Rao D, et al. Natural-cycle in vitro fertilization combined with in vitro maturation of immature oocytes is a potential approach in infertility treatment. Fertil Steril. 2004;82(6):1675-8.
56. Aleyamma TK, Kamath MS, Muthukumar K, Mangalaraj AM, George K. Affordable ART: a different perspective. Hum Reprod. 2011;26(12):3312-8.
57. Van Blerkom J, Ombelet W, Klerkx E, Janssen M, Dhont N, Nargund G, et al. First births with a simplified culture system for clinical IVF and embryo transfer. Reprod Biomed Online. 2014;28(3):310-20.
58. Weigert M, Krischker U, Pöhl M, Poschalko G, Kindermann C, Feichtinger W. Comparison of stimulation with clomiphene citrate in combination with recombinant follicle-stimulating hormone and recombinant luteinizing hormone to stimulation with a gonadotropin-releasing hormone agonist protocol: a prospective, randomized study. Fertil Steril. 2002; 78(1):34-9.
59. Lin YH, Hwang JL, Seow KM, Huang LW, Hsieh BC, Tzeng CR. Comparison of outcome of clomiphene citrate/human menopausal gonadotropin/cetrorelix protocol and Buserelin long protocol—a randomized study. Gynecol Endocrinol. 2006;22(6):297-302.
60. D'Amato G, Caroppo E, Pasquadibisceglie A, Carone D, Vitti A, Vizziello GM. A novel protocol of ovulation induction with delayed gonadotropin-releasing hormone antagonist administration combined with high-dose recombinant follicle-stimulating hormone and clomiphene citrate for poor responders and women over 35 years. Fertil Steril. 2004; 81(6):1572-7.
61. Verberg MFG, Macklon NS, Nargund G, Frydman R, Devroey P, Broekmans FJ, et al. Mild ovarian stimulation for IVF. Hum Reprod Update. 2009;15(1):13-29.
62. Mohsen IA, El Din RE. Minimal stimulation protocol using letrozole versus microdose flare up GnRH agonist protocol in women with poor ovarian response undergoing ICSI. Gynecol Endocrinol. 2013;29(2):105-8.
63. Karimzadeh MA, Ahmadi S, Oskouian H, Rahmani E. Comparison of mild stimulation and conventional stimulation in ART outcome. Arch Gynecol Obstet. 2010;281(4): 741-6.
64. Dastidar SG, Maity S, Dastidar BG. Reappraisal of IVF stimulation in good prognosis patients—a prospective randomized study to compare mild versus standard long protocol. Fertil Steril. 2010;94(4):S28.
65. Polyzos NP, Popovic-Todorovic B. SAY NO to mild ovarian stimulation for all poor responders: it is time to realize that not all poor responders are the same. Hum Reprod. 2020;35(9):1964-71.
66. Allahbadia GN. Getting older women pregnant: contemporary thoughts. J Obstet Gynecol India. 2016;66(5):305-9.
67. Mahajan N. Should mild stimulation be the order of the day? J Hum Reprod Sci. 2013;6(4):220-6.
68. Fauser BC, Nargund G, Andersen AN, Norman R, Tarlatzis B, Boivin J, et al. Mild ovarian stimulation for IVF: 10 years later. Hum Reprod. 2010;25(11):2678-84.
69. Nargund G, Frydman R. Towards a more physiological approach to IVF. Reprod Biomed Online. 2007;14(5):550-2.

CHAPTER 54

Role of Luteinizing Hormone in Ovarian Stimulation

Nivedita Shetty, Shraddha Pol

INTRODUCTION

Normal follicular growth requires the complementary action of both follicle-stimulating hormone (FSH) and luteinizing hormone (LH). During controlled ovarian stimulation, exogenous FSH alone is usually adequate for optimal follicular growth, *if the endogenous LH activity is optimum.* However, in certain groups with inadequate or suppressed LH activity, the addition of LH may be necessary. This chapter attempts to understand the rationale behind LH supplementation during controlled ovarian stimulation, the specific groups that require LH and the various options available for adding LH activity.

PHYSIOLOGY OF THE ROLE OF LH IN FOLLICULOGENESIS

Two-cell–Two-gonadotropin Theory

Luteinizing hormone has a really important function in steroidogenesis. It has different roles during the early and the late folliculogenesis.[1,2]

Follicle-stimulating hormone receptors are present in the granulosa cells and the LH receptors are present in the theca cells in the *early follicular phase.* LH stimulates the theca cells to produce androgens, i.e., testosterone and androstenedione, from cholesterol. The androgens enter into the granulosa cells and are aromatized into estrogens.[3]

In the *late follicular phase*, when the follicular size is around 8–12 mm, LH receptors also appear in the granulosa cells. FSH and LH bring about the local production of inhibin B and insulin-like growth factor (IGF)-1 and -2, which have a role in promoting follicular maturation.[4] The final oocyte maturation, resumption of meiosis, and ovulation occur with the midcycle LH surge.

It can be concluded that both FSH and LH addition appear to be very pertinent for optimal follicular development.

Concept of LH Ceiling and Window

The ovarian follicle needs a certain minimum level of LH for optimal steroidogenesis, considered as the *LH threshold.* This concept is clearly reflected in hypogonadotropic hypogonadism patients, who require minimum LH supplementation during ovarian stimulation with FSH, for adequate steroidogenesis.[5]

However, excess amounts of LH also have been known to be linked with lower fertilization, lower implantation, and poorer pregnancy rates. The higher levels of LH may subdue aromatase activity and suppress cell growth. This is the concept of the LH ceiling.

The *LH window* is the range of LH level, between the LH threshold and LH ceiling, which is when optimal follicular growth occurs. The optimal range, i.e., the LH window, is considered to be between *1.2 and 5 IU/L.*

The LH ceiling may be higher in larger follicles and lower in smaller ones. An increasing LH level would result in growth of the leading follicle (being below its ceiling) and regression of the secondary follicles (by exceeding their ceiling).

Rationale of LH Supplementation during Controlled Ovarian Stimulation

The role of FSH, without any doubt, is very important to obtain adequate number of follicles, in controlled ovarian stimulation. The addition of LH during ovarian stimulation, however, is a controversy and there is no clarity as to which group would benefit and at what dose.

Most normogonadotropic women do not need exogenous supplementation with LH during controlled ovarian stimulation as the endogenous LH is usually sufficient to support multiple follicular growth. For adequate ovarian steroidogenesis, merely 1% of LH receptors need to be taken up. There is also the complex paracrine mechanism comprising inhibin B and IGF-1 and -2, which gets activated and contributes to the follicular growth.[4]

On the other hand, a meta-analysis by Lehert et al. found that in the group where ovarian stimulation was done with recombinant-FSH (rFSH) and recombinant-LH (rLH), the clinical pregnancy rate was slightly higher (estimate of 9%) as compared to the group treated with only recombinant human FSH (r-hFSH).[6]

Then the *MERIT* trial by Andersen et al. compared the clinical outcome following controlled ovarian stimulation with highly purified human menopausal gonadotropin (HP-hMG) or recombinant FSH, after downregulation with *long gonadotropin-releasing hormone (GnRH) agonist protocol.* They concluded that a higher number of oocytes were retrieved after rFSH stimulation (11.8) compared to HP-hMG (10.0). More importantly, a larger proportion of oocytes developed into top-quality embryos with HP-hMG (11.3%) than with rFSH (9.0%). The ongoing pregnancy rate per cycle was 27% with HP-hMG and 22% with rFSH [odds ratio (95% confidence interval): 1.25 (0.89–1.75)].[7]

In one study, the incidence of apoptosis was found to be higher in granulosa cells of follicles aspirated from patients who were not pregnant after IVF as compared to granulosa cells aspirated from patients who were pregnant.[8] Using the apoptosis rate in cumulus cells as an indicator of oocyte quality, a study investigated "low responder" patients undergoing ovarian stimulation with rFSH and recombinant LH versus rFSH alone. In the control group, controlled ovarian stimulation with rFSH from cycle day 3 was done for 42 patients. In the study group, from day 8 of stimulation, 150 IU of rLH was added to the rFSH. The cumulus cells in the control group had a higher rate of apoptosis than in the rLH group which could suggest that addition of rLH improves the chromatin quality of cumulus cells involved in the control of oocyte maturation.[9]

Another advantage with the addition of LH is the lesser risk of premature progesterone rise. FSH promotes the cholesterol conversion into progesterone while LH promotes the conversion of progesterone into androgens which get aromatized to estrogens. If the LH levels are inadequate, the progesterone that gets accumulated is secreted into the circulation. This can result in an endometrium that is advanced and hence resulting in asynchrony in embryo and endometrial development.[10,11]

Specific Groups that Require Luteinizing Hormone

- Hypogonadotropic hypogonadism to support FSH in development of follicles (levels of LH <1.2 IU/L; WHO group I anovulation)
- Deeply suppressed LH due to GnRH analogs
- In GnRH antagonists cycle
- In advanced reproductive age
- Women with low prognosis—Poseidon classification
- In women with a hypo response to exogenous FSH monotherapy.
- In prevention of ovarian hyperstimulation syndrome.

Hypogonadotropic Hypogonadism

The efficacy of recombinant human LH (r-hLH) was analyzed by the European Recombinant Human LH Study Group.[12] All patients were administered 150 IU of r-hFSH daily. They were then randomized to receive either nil or 25 IU or 75 IU or 225 IU/day of r-hLH. In the only FSH group, only 12.5% of patients developed follicles while 42.8% of patients who received 25 IU of recombinant LH developed follicles. However, in the group that received 75 IU of rFSH, 77.8% of patients and in patients who received 225 IU of rFSH, 80% developed follicles.

In conclusion, exogenous LH activity supplementation of at least 75 IU is necessary for follicles to develop in women with hypogonadotropic hypogonadism.

Deeply Suppressed LH Levels

Normogonadotropic women who undergo GnRH agonist downregulation and controlled ovarian stimulation, may demonstrate suppression of LH concentrations below the threshold needed for optimum steroidogenesis.

In a GnRH agonist downregulated cycle with FSH only ovarian stimulation, if the mid-follicular (day 7/8) serum LH levels are low (between 0.5 and 0.7 IU/L), the ovarian follicular response, oocyte yield, and outcome of the IVF cycle are also lower.

The number of patients having deeply suppressed mid-follicular LH suppression varied with the choice of GnRH analog. In one study, the pregnancy rate was similar in the low and normal LH groups (30% vs. 34% per started cycle, respectively). In the low LH group, however, a fivefold higher risk of early pregnancy loss was observed.[13]

However, few other studies have shown that low LH levels did not affect the follicular response, oocyte yield, and pregnancy outcome.

In GnRH Antagonist Cycles

The evidence concerning the clinical use of r-hLH in GnRH antagonist cycles is limited to women 35–39 years of age. In these women, a dosage of 75 IU r-hLH started on the first day of OS significantly improved the implantation rate. No effect was detected in studies that included women >40 years of age. Of note, although r-hLH did not exert a beneficial effect in infertile women <35 years of age undergoing IVF/ICSI, it improved the implantation rate and embryo quality in donor cycles from young good-prognosis women without infertility history.

In Advanced Reproductive Age Group

The available evidence suggests that r-hLH exerts a beneficial effect in terms of implantation rate in women aged 36–39 years, regardless of the pituitary suppression protocol. Nonetheless, no effect in terms of pregnancy rate was observed. No significant effect was observed in studies in which women aged ≥40 years were included in the groups receiving an agonist or an antagonist regimen.

Low Prognosis Women

The Poseidon group proposed a change, from the definition of *poor ovarian reserve* based on Bologna criteria,[14] to a concept of *low prognosis.*[15]

- *Group 1:* Patients below 35 years with good ovarian reserve parameters [antral follicle count (AFC) >5 and anti-Müllerian hormone (AMH) >1.2 ng/mL] and with an unexpected poor or suboptimal ovarian response—hyporesponders.
- *Group 2:* Patients >35 years with good ovarian reserve parameters (AFC >5 and AMH >1.2 ng/mL) and with an unexpected poor or suboptimal ovarian response.
- *Group 3:* Patients below 35 years with poor ovarian reserve (AFC <5 and AMH <1.2 ng/mL).
- *Group 4:* Patients above 35 years with poor ovarian reserve (AFC <5 and AMH <1.2 ng/mL).

Group 1—Hyporesponders: In 15% of normogonadotropic women, with normal AMH and AFC, an initial poor response to standard FSH doses is observed. This could be due to hyposensitivity to standard FSH doses resulting in "hyporesponse" identified by the absence of follicles over 10 mm on day 8 of stimulation with r-hFSH. It is also associated with low serum estradiol levels (below 180 pg/mL) and at least 6 follicles ranging between 6 mm and 10 mm.

Hyporesponders usually have a normal ovarian reserve and are young (<39 years). In spite of FSH requirement of hypo responders being higher (>2,500 IU total dose), the response is unexpectedly poor (i.e., <3 eggs retrieved) and IVF outcome is also poorer.

If hyporesponse is identified early (i.e., day 5–8 of COS), either r-hLH or increase in FSH dose are effective in rescuing and forming adequate numbers of follicles and good embryos. At least two genetic variations, one a polymorphic allele of the LH beta subunit gene (v-beta LH) and the other the FSH receptor (FSHR) *Ala/307 and Ser/680 variant, have been implicated in the resistance to* exogenous FSH.[16,17]

The FSHR gene can be used as a marker to predict ovarian response. The gene contains two important single-nucleotide polymorphisms (SNPs) in exon 10, wherein two amino acids at positions 307 and 680 can change. These women with 307 Ala and 680 Ser SNPs have been associated with a poorer ovarian response.

About 282 SNPs have been found to exist on the LH receptor gene. In 1991, Pettersson and Söderholm identified a common genetic LH beta variant or v-beta. Patients requiring LH addition, during ovarian stimulation, could be identified, if its role is confirmed, with further research.

De Placido et al. conducted a multicentric randomized control trial (RCT) of 117 in vitro fertilization/intracytoplasmic sperm injection (IVF/ICSI) cycles[17] analyzing the role of LH addition in high responders. These patients underwent downregulation and ovarian stimulation with r-hFSH of 225 IU for 8 days and were identified to be hyporesponders. They were randomized to either undergo the step-up protocol, wherein the daily dose of rFSH was increased by 150 IU and an equal number of patients were randomized to receive 150 IU/day of r-hLH addition ($n = 65$). "Normal responders" were selected as a control group ($n = 130$).

Significantly more oocytes were obtained in the rLH supplementation group (9.0 ± 4.3) compared with the group with increased dose of r-hFSH (6.1 ± 2.6; $p < 0.01$) while the highest number of oocytes were retrieved in the control group (10.49 ± 3.7; $p < 0.05$). The control group and the rLH supplemented group had similar implantation and ongoing pregnancy rates (14.2% and 32.5% vs. 18.1% and 40.2%, respectively), however, the group treated with the increase in FSH had the least pregnancy rates.[18]

Group 2—older women more than 35 years: Hill et al. analyzed seven trials comprising 902 assisted reproductive technology cycles in older women. They concluded that, in women more than 35 years old, it was beneficial to add LH as the clinical pregnancy rate was significantly higher.[19] A significant observation was that addition of LH did not increase the oocyte or M2 yield. This decrease is probably due to the fact that there was a decline in smaller developing follicles. The larger developing follicles may be yielding better quality oocytes and hence the better clinical pregnancy rate.

Also, a study which demonstrated lesser cumulus cell apoptosis in rLH supplemented cycles, suggested better oocyte quality.[9] The lower serum progesterone, on addition of LH, may also have a role to play in the better implantation rate.[10,11]

In older women the LH receptors become less sensitive and the serum androgen levels decline. The administration of LH enhances androgen levels and hence estrogen production is also increased.[20]

Current available evidence recommends that LH supplementation when started from day 1 of controlled ovarian stimulation has a better IVF outcome in women older than 35 years of age.

Groups 3 and 4—poor responders with poor ovarian reserve: A meta-analysis assessing the outcomes of r-hLH supplementation as compared to r-hFSH alone involved a total of 40 RCTs comprising of 6,443 women of which 14 studies (1,129 patients), specifically analyzed poor responders.

Significantly higher numbers of oocytes were retrieved and also significantly higher clinical pregnancy rates were observed with r-hFSH plus r-hLH, in the poor responders group as well.[6]

In women with hyporesponse to FSH monotherapy: It is important to know the distinction between hyporesponders and poor responders and analyze these groups separately. They defined hyporesponders as women with normal ovarian reserve tests (i.e., anti-Mullerian hormone and antral follicle count) and an adequate number of recruited oocytes, however they required higher doses of gonadotropins. In contrast, poor responders may have abnormal ovarian reserve tests but the number of oocytes retrieved is low irrespective of the amount of gonadotropin administered.

With the definition of hyporesponse in mind, current evidence indicates that in high responders: (1) r-hLH supplementation starting from day 7–10 of OS can rescue the ongoing cycle, thereby compensating for an initial slow response (stagnation); (2) administration of r-hLH is more efficient than increasing the dosage of r-hFSH; and (3) when a hyporesponse is retrospectively identified (i.e., history of excessive consumption of FSH, r-hLH supplementation from day 7 or 8 of stimulation seems to improve the outcome of IVF. Furthermore, it seems that 150 IU r-hLH results in more oocytes retrieved and a higher percentage of mature oocytes than does 75 IU r-hLH in a long GnRH agonist protocol. All of these findings were obtained with the use of a GnRH agonist long protocol. In contrast, the effect of r-hLH supplementation in high responders undergoing OS with the use of GnRH antagonists remains to be established. The mechanism by which r-hLH exerts its beneficial effect in hyporesponders is not fully understood. It is plausible that an excessively profound suppression of endogenous LH after downregulation with the use of GnRH analogs may create the need for exogenous LH supplementation.

In prevention of ovarian hyperstimulation syndrome: Caserta et al. investigated 999 infertile women ≤40 years of age with basal FSH levels ≤12 mIU/mL and no history of OHSS or polycystic ovary syndrome. The women were randomized to receive r-hFSH alone (n = 501) or r-hFSH þ r-hLH (n = 498). A daily dose of 150 IU r-hFSH was administered in both groups; r-hLH supplementation was given at a dose of 75 IU/d from stimulation day 7 onward. No differences in age or mean number of embryos transferred were observed between groups. Although the number of eggs retrieved was lower in the supplemented group than in the r-hFSH–alone group (6.1 ± 3 vs. 6.6 ± 3.8; $p < .05$), the clinical pregnancy rate was higher in the supplemented group than in the r-FSH–alone group (16.8% vs. 11.9%; $p < .05$). The proportion of canceled cycles owing to OHSS risk (8.3% vs. 2.4%; $p < .000001$) and the proportion of patients who developed clinical OHSS (1.6% vs. 0.2%; $p < .05$) were significantly higher in the r-hFSH–alone group than in the r-hFSH and r-hLH group.

Types of Luteinizing Hormone Activity

Luteinizing hormone activity containing gonadotropin preparations:

- Urinary hMG contains human chorionic gonadotropin (hCG) which has LH-like activity
- Recombinant LH
- Urinary and recombinant hCG, which have LH-like activity
- A combination of recombinant FSH and LH in a fixed ratio of 2:1.

Human Menopausal Gonadotropins

It is obtained from the urine of postmenopausal women and contains equal quantity of FSH and LH bioactivity (approximately 75 IU of each).

Disadvantages of hMG

- Local allergic reactions which may be due to protein contamination
- Batch-to-batch variations
- Difficulty in sourcing large quantities of urine of postmenopausal women
- Contamination with prion proteins which may be associated with transmissible spongiform encephalopathies.

In HP-hMG, it is hCG supplementation that provides 95% of LH bioactivity.[21] Urinary hMG undergoes a purification process but as the purity of an hMG preparation is increased, LH molecules get reduced[21] and in order to maintain the required FSH:LH ratio of 1:1 of the original hMG, more exogenous hCG needs to be added. This means that the longer terminal half-life of hCG being 32–34 hours leads to the possibility of drug accumulation. Patients treated with 50 IU/day of hCG showed increasing levels of hCG over the course of a treatment cycle to 16.2 ± 3.2 IU/L of hCG, which is equivalent to 113.4 IU/L of LH activity.[22] This is of importance since a threshold level of 1.2 IU/L of LH is required for optimal follicular development and there is a "ceiling" LH level (5 IU/L) above which granulosa cell proliferation is suppressed and atresia (of the nondominant follicles) and premature luteinization (of the preovulatory follicle) occur.

Noninferiority of hMG was established with the MERIT trial which compared the clinical outcome with HP-hMG and recombinant FSH following a long GnRH agonist protocol. The conclusion was that, although more oocytes were retrieved following ovarian stimulation with rFSH (11.8 oocytes vs. 10 oocytes, $p < 0.001$), the proportion of top quality embryos obtained with HP-hMG was higher (11.3% vs. 9%, $p = 0.044$). Lower levels of estradiol and higher levels of progesterone were noted on the day of hCG with rFSH. The ongoing pregnancy rates per cycle was 22% with rFSH and 27% with hMG [odds ratio (95% confidence interval): 1.25 (0.89–1.75)].[7]

The *Megaset* trial, by Paul Devroey et al., is a randomized trial including 749 women, wherein HP-hMG was compared with recombinant FSH in a *GnRH antagonist* cycle with compulsory single blastocyst transfer. They concluded that the ongoing pregnancy rate after a fresh cycle was 30% with HP-hMG versus 27% with rFSH for the per-protocol (PP) population and 29% versus 27% for the intention-to-treat

(ITT) population. When frozen cycles were considered, *the cumulative live birth rate was 40% and 38% for patients treated with HP-hMG and rFSH,* respectively. The results proved that HP-hMG is at least as efficient as rFSH in GnRH antagonist cycles.[23]

Recombinant Luteinizing Hormone[24-26]

A better safety profile and batch-to-batch consistency as compared to urinary gonadotropins is assured with rLH. Its shorter half-life allows for more precise dosing during controlled ovarian stimulation. On subcutaneous administration, the terminal half-life of recombinant LH is 21–24 hours. Hence, even if 150 IU of r-hLH is administered subcutaneously daily, it results in only a low level of 1.6 IU/L of LH.[27]

A meta-analysis of 40 RCTs[6] comparing the outcome of only rFSH as compared to r-hFSH supplemented with r-hLH demonstrated a minor increase (estimate of 9%) in clinical pregnancy rates with LH supplementation, although the number of oocytes obtained, were similar in both groups.

In the poor responders group, comprising 14 RCTs, significantly more oocytes were retrieved and significantly higher difference in clinical pregnancy rates was noted in the rLH supplemented group.

A meta-analysis by Oliveira et al. concluded that in *GnRH agonist* downregulated cycles, rLH supplementation with rFSH, resulted in shorter duration of stimulation ($p < 0.0001$), a lesser amount of rFSH used ($p < 0.0001$) and a greater serum E2 level on the day of hCG administration ($p < 0.0001$). However, the total number of oocytes retrieved, number of mature oocytes obtained, and the clinical pregnancy rate and miscarriage rates were similar.[28]

Another meta-analysis by Baruffi et al. concluded that with LH addition in *GnRH antagonist* cycles, the serum E2 level on the day of hCG was higher and also more oocytes were retrieved. However, there was no difference in the amount of rFSH used, duration of stimulation, total number of oocytes retrieved, the clinical pregnancy rate, and the miscarriage rate.[24,25]

Urinary and Recombinant hCG, Which have LH-like Activity

Human chorionic gonadotropin can be added during two different times of the follicular phase:

1. *Early follicular phase:* For ovarian priming.
2. *Late follicular phase:* When the LH receptors appear.

Early follicular phase: Between 200 and 1,250 IU hCG was used, for ovarian priming. It acts on the theca cells in preantral and small antral follicles and induces the formation of the androgens which are needed as a substrate for estradiol which in turn helps in follicular differentiation.

Late follicular phase: In both the GnRH agonist and antagonist cycles, hCG was administered at doses of 200 IU/day, when follicles reached 12–14 mm in diameter, i.e., in the late follicular phase. Even under physiological conditions, LH plays an important role in folliculogenesis in the late follicular phase as the FSH levels start decreasing. During ovarian stimulation, low-dose hCG may promote the growth of intermediate-sized follicles which have LH/hCG receptors and may be effective in ovarian stimulation until the final stages in the absence of FSH.

A meta-analysis by Checa et al. concluded that the use of hCG in the early and late follicular phase in controlled ovarian stimulation has the advantage of decreasing the consumption of FSH. The total dose of FSH required was decreased by over 800 IU, in patients in whom hCG was added. However, there was a slight decrease in the number of metaphase II (MII) oocytes retrieved.

Timing and Dosing of LH Supplementation

Exogenous LH activity supplementation of *at least 75 IU* is necessary for follicles to develop in women with hypogonadotropic hypogonadism.

In women >35 years of age, current available evidence recommends that LH supplementation gives a better IVF outcome, especially when *started from day 1* of controlled ovarian stimulation in GnRH antagonist protocol and on stimulation day 6 in a GnRH agonist protocol.

Controlled ovarian stimulation with an LH-to-FSH ratio of 0.30–0.60 resulted in the least risk of progesterone increase. Most risk of progesterone elevation >1.5 ng/mL was seen in patients where no LH was added during stimulation. This pattern of lowest risk in the 0.30–0.60 range held true for low, normal, and high response cycles. Hence, FSH and LH in a *ratio of 2:1* is recommended for ovarian stimulation.

The beneficial effect on implantation rate was for women between 36 and 39 years, but no effect was detected in women above 40 years.[29]

KEY POINTS

- Both FSH and LH appear to be important for optimal follicular development and pregnancy.
- The *LH window* is the range of LH level, between the LH threshold and LH ceiling which is when optimal follicular growth occurs. The optimal range, i.e., the LH window, is considered to be between *1.2 and 5 IU/L.*
- During controlled ovarian stimulation with FSH only, the endogenous LH is usually adequate to support multiple follicular growth. However, in certain groups, the addition of LH improves the IVF outcome.
- Addition of LH activity is recommended in *hypogonadotropic hypogonadism, poor responders, older women, and hyporesponders.*

- The LH activity can be added using gonadotropin preparations such as *urinary hMG, recombinant LH, and urinary and recombinant hCG.*

REFERENCES

1. Speroff L, Fritz MA. Regulation of the menstrual cycle. In: Speroff L, Fritz MA (Eds). Clinical Gynecologic Endocrinology and Infertility. Philadelphia: Lippincott Williams and Wilkins; 2005. pp. 348-83.
2. Speroff L, Fritz MA. Hormone biosynthesis, metabolism, and mechanisms of action: steroidogenesis. In: Speroff L, Fritz MA (Eds). Clinical Gynecologic Endocrinology and Infertility. Philadelphia: Lippincott Williams and Wilkins; 2005. pp. 109-16.
3. Hillier SG, Whitelaw PF, Smyth CD. Follicular oestrogen synthesis: the 'two-cell, two-gonadotrophin' model revisited. Mol Cell Endocrinol. 1994;100:51-4.
4. Chappel SC, Howles C. Reevaluation of the roles of luteinizing hormone and follicle-stimulating hormone in the ovulatory process. Hum Reprod. 1991;6:1206-12.
5. Raju GA, Chavan R, Deenadayal M, Gunasheela D, Gutgutia R, Haripriya G, et al. Luteinizing hormone and follicle stimulating hormone synergy: a review of role in controlled ovarian hyperstimulation. J Hum Reprod Sci. 2013;6:227-34.
6. Lehert P, Kolibianakis EM, Venetis CA, Schertz J, Saunders H, Arriagada P, et al. Recombinant human follicle-stimulating hormone (r-hFSH) plus recombinant luteinizing hormone versus r-hFSH alone for ovarian stimulation during assisted reproductive technology: systematic review and meta-analysis. Reprod Biol Endocrinol. 2014;12:17.
7. Andersen AN, Devroey P, Arce JC. Clinical outcome following stimulation with highly purified hMG or recombinant FSH in patients undergoing IVF: a randomized assessor-blind controlled trial. Hum Reprod. 2006;21:3217-27.
8. Oosterhuis GJ, Michgelsen HW, Lambalk CB, Schoemaker J, Vermes I. Apoptotic cell death in human granulosa-lutein cells: a possible indicator of in vitro fertilization outcome. Fertil Steril. 1998;70:747-9.
9. Giovanni R, Liana B, Antonina P, Morici G, Cittadini E, Roccheri MC. Lower apoptosis rate in human cumulus cells after administration of recombinant luteinizing hormone to women undergoing ovarian stimulation for in vitro fertilization procedures. Fertil Steril. 2007;87:542-6.
10. Bosch E, Labarta E, Crespo J, Simón C, Remohí J, Jenkins J, et al. Circulating progesterone levels and ongoing pregnancy rates in controlled ovarian stimulation cycles for in vitro fertilization: analysis of over 4,000 cycles. Hum Reprod. 2010;25:2092-100.
11. Venetis CA, Kolibianakis EM, Bosdou JK, Tarlatzis BC. Progesterone elevation and probability of pregnancy after IVF: a systematic review and meta-analysis of over 60,000 cycles. Hum Reprod Update. 2013;19:433-57.
12. European Recombinant Human LH Study Group. Recombinant human luteinizing hormone (LH) to support recombinant human follicle-stimulating hormone-induced follicular development in LH- and FSH-deficient anovulatory women: a dose-finding study. J Clin Endocrinol Metab. 1998;83:1507-14.
13. Westergaard LG, Laursen SB, Andersen CY. Increased risk of early pregnancy loss by profound suppression of luteinizing hormone during ovarian stimulation in normogonadotrophic women undergoing assisted reproduction. Hum Reprod. 2000;15:1003-8.
14. Ferraretti AP, La Marca A, Fauser BC, Tarlatzis B, Nargund G, Gianaroli L, et al. ESHRE consensus on the definition of 'poor response' to ovarian stimulation for in vitro fertilization: the Bologna criteria. Hum Reprod. 2011;26:1616-24.
15. Poseidon Group (Patient-Oriented Strategies Encompassing IndividualizeD Oocyte Number), Alviggi C, Andersen CY, Buehler K, Conforti A, De Placido G, Esteves SC, et al. A new more detailed stratification of low responders to ovarian stimulation: from a poor ovarian response to a low prognosis concept. Fertil Steril. 2016;105:1452-3.
16. Alviggi C, Pettersson K, Longobardi S, Andersen CY, Conforti A, De Rosa P, et al. A common polymorphic allele of the LH beta-subunit gene is associated with higher exogenous FSH consumption during controlled ovarian stimulation for assisted reproductive technology. Reprod Biol Endocrinol. 2013;11:51.
17. Alviggi C, Clarizia R, Pettersson K, Mollo A, Humaidan P, Strina I, et al. Suboptimal response to GnRHa long protocol is associated with a common LH polymorphism. Reprod Biomed Online. 2009;18:9-14.
18. De Placido G, Alviggi C, Perino A, Strina I, Lisi F, Fasolino A, et al. Recombinant human LH supplementation versus recombinant human FSH (rFSH) step-up protocol during controlled ovarian stimulation in normogonadotrophic women with initial inadequate ovarian response to rFSH. A multicentre, prospective, randomized controlled trial. Hum Reprod. 2005;20:390-6.
19. Hill MJ, Levens ED, Levy G, Strina I, Lisi F, Fasolino A, et al. The use of recombinant luteinizing hormone in patients undergoing assisted reproductive techniques with advanced reproductive age: a systematic review and meta-analysis. Fertil Steril. 2012;97:1108-14.
20. Bosdou JK, Venetis CA, Kolibianakis EM, Toulis KA, Goulis DG, Zepiridis L, et al. The use of androgens or androgen-modulating agents in poor responders undergoing in vitro fertilization: a systematic review and meta-analysis. Hum Reprod Update. 2012;18:127-45.
21. Wolfenson C, Groisman J, Couto AS, Hedenfalk M, Cortvrindt RG, Smitz JE, et al. Batch-to-batch consistency of human-derived gonadotrophin preparations compared with recombinant preparations. Reprod Biomed Online. 2005;10:442-54.
22. Le Cotonnec JY, Porchet HC, Beltrami V, Munafo A. Clinical pharmacology of recombinant human luteinizing hormone: Part II. Bioavailability of recombinant human luteinizing hormone assessed with an immunoassay and an in vitro bioassay. Fertil Steril. 1998;69:195-200.
23. Devroey P, Pellicer A, Nyboe Andersen A, Arce JC; Menopur in GnRH Antagonist Cycles with Single Embryo Transfer Trial Group. A randomized assessor-blind trial comparing highly purified hMG and recombinant FSH in a GnRH antagonist cycle with compulsory single-blastocyst transfer. Fertil Steril. 2012;97:561-71.
24. Werner MD, Forman EJ, Hong KH, Franasiak JM, Molinaro TA, Scott RT Jr. Defining the "sweet spot" for administered

luteinizing hormone-to-follicle- stimulating hormone gonadotropin ratios during ovarian stimulation to protect against a clinically significant late follicular increase in progesterone: an analysis of 10,280 first in vitro fertilization cycles. Fertil Steril. 2014;102: 1312-7.

25. Alviggi C, Conforti A, Esteves SC, Andersen CY, Bosch E, Bühler K, et al. Recombinant Luteinizing Hormone supplementation in assisted reproductive technology: a systematic review. Fertil Steril. 2018;109(4):644-64.
26. Caserta D, Lisi F, Marci R, Ciardo F, Fazi A, Lisi R, et al. Does supplementation with recombinant luteinizing hormone prevent ovarian hyperstimulation syndrome in down regulated patients undergoing recombinant follicle stimulating hormone multiple follicular stimulation for IVF/ET and reduce cancellation rate for high risk of hyperstimulation? Gynecol Endocrinol. 2011;27:862-6.
27. Ezcurra D, Humaidan P. A review of luteinising hormone and human chorionic gonadotropin when used in assisted reproductive technology. Reprod Biol Endocrinol. 2014;12:95.
28. Checa MA, Espinos JJ, Requena A. Efficacy and safety of human chorionic gonadotropin for follicular phase stimulation in assisted reproduction: a systematic review and meta-analysis. Fertil Steril. 2012;97:1343-50.
29. Maher JY, Segars J. When is Recombinant luteinizing hormone supplementation beneficial during ovarian stimulation? Fertil Steril. 2018;109(4):611-2.

CHAPTER 55

Anesthesia in Assisted Reproductive Techniques

Dorothy Dessa, Ravi Kumar IR

INTRODUCTION

In vitro fertilization (IVF), started first in the late 1970s, is now a common procedure—the answer to infertility due to both maternal and paternal disorders.[1,2] The 1980s witnessed a drastic change from follicle aspiration laparoscopically under general anesthesia to transvaginal ultrasound-guided oocyte retrieval.[3-6] Today, worldwide, almost all IVF techniques are performed under ultrasound guidance, transvaginally. IVF techniques include:

- Ovarian stimulation and monitoring
- Follicle aspiration or oocyte retrieval
- Fertilization in the embryology laboratory and transfer of the embryos into the uterus.

ANESTHETIC CONSIDERATIONS

Infertile couples, especially the female partner, are often anxious and in fear.[7-9] Although transvaginal oocyte retrieval (TVOR) is considered less invasive, it is one of the most painful and stressful components of the assisted reproductive treatment cycle. Pain during oocyte retrieval is due to the traction on the vaginal wall, ovarian capsule, and ligaments and also due to the puncture on the vaginal wall and the ovarian capsule by the aspiration needle.[10] Multiple attempts are usually needed according to the condition of the ovary and the follicles. Although oocyte retrieval can be done without anesthesia, adequate pain relief possesses more benefits during the procedure for both the patient and the surgeon.

In this 21st century, IVF procedures are performed as "day care procedures" based on the principle of "ambulatory or office-based anesthesia."[11]

IDEAL FEATURES OF THE ANESTHETIC TECHNIQUE FOR THE PROCEDURE OF IN VITRO FERTILIZATION[12]

The ideal features are as follows:

- Able to provide safe, effective, and adequate analgesia
- Rapid onset and recovery with minimum side effects and no effects on the oocytes
- Quick recovery time from anesthesia
- No changes in the follicular fluid and pH
- No effect on fertilization, early embryo development, and pregnancy rate.

GENERAL CONSIDERATIONS

Couples need to be evaluated for existing medical or surgical illnesses. In India, where tuberculosis is rampant and consists of a big chunk of infertile patients, it is important to know the drug interactions, especially antitubercular drugs with anesthetic drugs.

The hormonal manipulation during controlled ovarian stimulation causes variation in the serum estrogen level from baseline to supraphysiological level during oocyte pickup. The albumin and α-1 acid glycoprotein synthesis is affected by estrogen, which reduces drug binding and results in increased free fraction of the highly protein-bound drugs in the circulation. So, the selection of the drugs and appropriate dose is extremely important.

To prevent a hypercoagulable state due to prolonged gonadotropins use, some patients may be started on anti-coagulants (aspirin or heparin). Aspirin should be stopped 3 days prior to oocyte retrieval. If the patient is on heparin, it is wise to know the activated partial thromboplastin time (aPTT).

Infertility has a major psychological impact. Some of these patients may be on antidepressant drugs, antipsychotics, or antiepileptics. It is important to elicit this history during the preanesthetic evaluation. It is advised to take these drugs into consideration and anesthetic agents to be adjusted accordingly based on the expected interactions.[13,14]

Thyroid disorders, a common finding in the infertile population, also interfere with the anesthetic protocol. Therefore, appropriate anesthetic precautions should be taken. Special considerations are given for anesthesia in morbid obesity and severe pulmonary/cardiac or renal disease patients. A study conducted to evaluate the intravenous (IV) anesthesia for IVF in obese and normal body mass index (BMI) patients concluded that the visualization of the ovary during the procedure becomes difficult, leading to longer duration of the procedure and thus requiring additional dosage of anesthetic agent resulting in higher drug consumption and even frequent use of muscle relaxant (succinylcholine).[15]

Fertility preservation is an issue in patients undergoing chemotherapy or radiotherapy along with anesthetic implications of the basic malignancy. So, in cancer patients, oocyte retrieval is done prior to starting chemotherapy or radiotherapy.

Patients presenting to the IVF clinics are generally under psychological and social stress. This immense pressure, accompanied by hormonal manipulation during ovarian stimulation, makes them more susceptible to psychosomatic disorders. It is a challenge to the anesthetists to allay their anxiety and provide them with a conducive environment so as to extract complete medical and pharmacological history.

ANESTHESIA TECHNIQUES—OPTIONS AVAILABLE TO THE ANESTHETIST

- Conscious sedation or monitored anesthesia care (MAC)
- General anesthesia
- Regional anesthesia—spinal anesthesia and epidural anesthesia
- Local anesthesia—paracervical block and preovarian block
- Total intravenous anesthesia
- Patient-controlled anesthesia
- Acupuncture.

The most common procedure performed during an IVF cycle that requires anesthesia is oocyte retrieval. Occasionally, embryo transfer may be performed under anesthesia. Dilatation and curettage (D and C) is seldom encountered in an IVF unit. Very rarely, the urologist may incorporate percutaneous epididymal sperm aspiration (PESA) or testicular sperm aspiration (TESA) in the IVF anesthesia schedule.

According to Cochrane review 2013, no one method of anesthesia or technique is better over another during oocyte retrieval. However, conscious sedation is the most widely practiced method of anesthesia in IVF clinics.[16]

CONSCIOUS SEDATION

Conscious sedation ("twilight sleep") is a specific anesthesia technique for a diagnostic or therapeutic procedure done under local anesthesia along with sedation and analgesia. It is a drug-induced depression of consciousness where the patient remains calm while she is awake and responds to verbal commands or tactile stimulation. This is the most commonly used anesthesia technique in an IVF setting.[17]

Advantages

- No intervention is required for maintaining normal respiration and cardiovascular function
- Acts as a good anxiolytic, sedation, and analgesia effect
- The recovery post anesthesia is fast due to the quick metabolism—patients can be discharged fully awake because the post-anesthesia recovery is fast and also pain-free.
- Easily administered
- Well tolerated
- Minimal side effects.

Disadvantages

- Lack of airway control
- Risk of airway obstruction and aspiration.

Complications

- Due to the use of sedatives—cerebral hypoperfusion, hypoxia, and hypercarbia
- Due to local anesthesia toxicity:
  - Localized reactions—rash and urticaria
  - Systemic reactions—anaphylaxis, breathlessness, dysrhythmias, hypotension, and cardiac arrest

The commonly used drugs in conscious sedation are midazolam, fentanyl, propofol, ketamine, and dexmedetomidine.[18]

- *Midazolam:* It is a water-soluble benzodiazepine which is potent with a rapid onset and short duration of action. There is a low level of venous irritation after IV injection of midazolam. Midazolam causes anterograde amnesia. Dosage of 0.2 mg/kg is used for induction and 1 μg/kg/min for maintenance of anesthesia. Very low levels of midazolam have been reported in the follicular fluid, which has no detrimental effect on implantation or pregnancy rates.[11] The combination of midazolam with opioids increases the risk of apnea and hypoxemia. The addition of propofol has a synergistic effect causing cardiorespiratory depression.
- *Opioids (fentanyl, remifentanil, alfentanil, and meperidine):* Remifentanil and fentanyl are usually used during conscious sedation and in general anesthesia for oocyte retrieval due to the rapid onset and short duration of action. However, high doses of opioids may cause respiratory depression, muscle rigidity, and bradycardia. Opioids have been found to be safe during oocyte retrieval.[19,20] Fentanyl and alfentanil have the least penetration in the follicular fluid, i.e., 10:1 ratio in the serum and follicular fluid.[21] Among all opioids, remifentanil is the most preferred.[22,23]

- *Propofol:* The pharmacokinetic property of propofol makes it the first-choice drug for anesthesia. It is a lipophilic anesthetic agent. It rapidly distributes into the central nervous system (CNS) and is associated with reduced nausea and vomiting postoperatively. The administration of propofol causes a local burning sensation, which can be avoided by prior administration of IV lidocaine (10 mg). It is given in 2 mg/kg bolus dose or 150 μg/kg/min in titrated dose as an infusion. Monitoring is an important part while using this drug as it causes respiratory and myocardial depression.[24] There are controversial reports regarding propofol anesthesia on embryo quality, implantation, and pregnancy rates.[25-27] Propofol accumulates in the follicular fluid, which shows a rise in the concentration only with the increased duration of exposure.[28] Hence, propofol should be used with caution during oocyte retrieval by limiting the maximum dose administered to <4 mg/kg.
- *Ketamine:* It causes "dissociative anesthesia" (cataleptic state with eyes open and a slow nystagmic gaze). It belongs to the phencyclidine family. It is not a popular drug due to its postoperative psychological adverse effects like fear, vivid dreams, excitement, and illusions. A study showed reduced fertilization rate with ketamine as compared to propofol ($p = 0.013$) and in the combination group of propofol with ketamine ($p = 0.008$). An increased anesthesia duration (>30 minutes) was found to be associated with lower implantation and pregnancy rate.[29] Therefore, ketamine alone is not one of the good choices for assisted reproductive technology (ART), though there are reports of satisfactory outcomes when it is mixed with propofol or midazolam. Good analgesia is achieved with a bolus dose of 2 mg/kg.
- *Dexmedetomidine:* It is a centrally acting α-2 adreno-receptor agonist.[30] It has both analgesic and sedative properties with a lack of respiratory depression. Hence, it is also known as "cooperative sedation" because it induces a state similar to natural sleep and at the same time, the patient is easily arousable and cooperative.[31,32] It is rapidly absorbed, distributed, and metabolized in the body. Studies have shown that dexmedetomidine is a good alternative to midazolam for conscious sedation due to its better patient satisfaction, less opioid requirements, and minimal respiratory depression.[33-35] It is given in a dose of 1 μg/kg IV. The use of this anesthesia drug may be limited due to the reported increase of bradycardia, hypotension, and limited ability to achieve deep sedation.
- *Drugs to be avoided:* Majority of the studies have shown detrimental effects of halogenated fluorocarbons like nitrous oxide. These agents were found to have a negative effect on embryo quality and increased abortion rates.[36]

BOX 1: Sedation protocol for transvaginal oocyte retrieval (protocol followed by at Milann Infertility services).

- Confirm patient identification
- Preprocedure interview and documentation, informed consent
- Preparation in the procedure room:
  - Secure a peripheral intravenous (IV) line
  - Skin sensitivity test for local anesthesia—lignocaine and antibiotics
  - Pretreatment with antiemetic (Emeset) and ranitidine
- Check the availability of emergency equipment
- Place routine monitors
- Give oxygen via a nasal cannula or a mask
- Position patient in dorsal lithotomy position
- Start sedation with glycopyrrolate 0.2 mg bolus
- Give injection midazolam 0.2 mg/kg IV
- Give injection dexamethasone 8 mg IV—to prevent postoperative nausea and vomiting
- Give injection fentanyl 2–5 μg/kg body weight, injection propofol (1%) 10 mL IV slowly, and then titrate as per requirement
- Keep communicating with the patient
- Give reassurance during the retrieval
- Continuous monitoring of vitals

Monitoring of Conscious Sedation Anesthesia

- *Pulse oximetry*—for oxygen saturation. Other than sedatives, extremes of age, obesity, lithotomy position, respiratory disease, and preexisting upper airway obstruction predispose to hypoxia
- Electrocardiography (ECG), heart rate, respiratory rate, noninvasive blood pressure (NIBP)—ECG lead II should be continuously displayed. NIBP is measured and recorded at least every 5 minutes. Heart rate and respiratory rate should be recorded every 10–15 minutes.
- Temperature—external and core body temperature is measured to detect hypothermia or hyperthermia.

Response to communication—important for the titration of the anesthesia drug. Continuous evaluation of the response to tactile stimulation and verbal commands should be carried out **(Box 1)**.

ANESTHESIA IN EMBRYO TRANSFER

Sometimes, when the patient is anxious, uncooperative, or when a difficult embryo transfer is anticipated, conscious sedation may be used.[37] The use of sedation does not alter the outcome of the embryo transfer procedure.[38,39]

ANESTHESIA FOR SURGICAL SPERM RETRIEVAL

Majority of the sperm retrieval procedures can be performed under adequate local anesthesia. When the local anesthetic is performed well, the nonanxious patient will tolerate a TESA, PESA, testicular sperm extraction (TESE), and minimally invasive epididymal sperm aspiration (MIESA) with local anesthesia alone. Conventional microsurgical epididymal sperm aspiration (MESA) is usually performed under general anesthesia. Depending on patient factors, cost, patient, and surgeon preference, sperm retrieval techniques may require general anesthesia or preferably MAC, also known as conscious sedation or twilight anesthesia.[40]

For adequate local anesthesia during surgical sperm retrieval, a well-performed spermatic cord block must be used in addition to a peri-incisional and superficial pudendal block. A spermatic cord block is performed according to the initial technique described by Wakefield and Elewa.[41] Using a 10 mL syringe and 25-G, 1.5-inch needle, 1:1 mixture of lidocaine 1% and bupivacaine 0.25% is directly infiltrated into the high scrotal spermatic cord below the external inguinal ring. While fixating the cord in between the thumb and index finger, approximately three passes of the needle are made into the cord in a fan-like distribution, followed by subcutaneous infiltration lateral to the cord along the scrotal-inguinal plane to anesthetize the superficial branches of the pudendal nerve. A total of approximately 10 mL of anesthetic is used during the spermatic cord and superficial pudendal nerve block. After the initial cord block, a peri-incisional block along the planned skin incision is anesthetized using the same syringe, needle, and solution of lidocaine and bupivacaine as a subcutaneous skin block.

According to the American Urological Association Best Practice Policy Statement on Urologic Surgery Antimicrobial Prophylaxis, for a clean open case where the urinary tract is not entered, a single dose of a first-generation cephalosporin is recommended.[42] A randomized, double-blind, placebo-controlled trial of 34 patients who underwent open sperm retrieval demonstrated significant improvements in postoperative pain and narcotic use when twice-daily oral celecoxib 200 mg was initiated the day prior to surgery and continued for a total of 1 week versus placebo.[43] Hence for office-based sperm retrieval procedures, oral antibiotics and oral nonsteroidal anti-inflammatory drugs (NSAIDs) should be considered to be started the day prior to the scheduled procedure.

ANALGESIA FOR HYSTEROSALPINGOGRAPHY

Hysterosalpingography (HSG) is a minimally invasive day-care procedure to evaluate the fallopian tubes and uterine cavity. Patient experiences discomfort and lower abdominal pain during and after the procedure due to cervical manipulation, uterine distension, and stimulation of the peritoneum.

For effective pain relief during HSG, in addition to oral NSAID, local application of lidocaine cream to the posterior fornix of the cervix uteri and paracervical lidocaine injection into the cervix uteri appear to be the most effective methods.[44] Intravenous opioids (tramadol) may also provide effective pain relief, but their benefit must be weighed against their side effects and effect on recovery time.[45] However, there is no consensus concerning optimal analgesics or the timing of its administration. Immersive virtual reality (VR) is an emerging nonpharmacologic and noninvasive analgesic technique, being evaluated as an alternate option for analgesia during HSG.[46]

GENERAL ANESTHESIA

Occasionally, general anesthesia is used in an IVF clinic. It can be performed by the use of intravenous (fentanyl and propofol) or inhalational (nitrous oxide, isoflurane, and sevoflurane) agents with coadministration of sedatives and analgesic drugs. These drugs mainly act on the gamma-aminobutyric acid type A ($GABA_A$) receptors and *N*-methyl-D-aspartate glutamate receptors.[47] It is the technique of choice during laparoscopic follicular aspiration, transabdominal oocyte retrieval, laparoscopic gamete intrafallopian transfer (GIFT), and zygote intrafallopian transfer (ZIFT), and also has been used for TVOR in the past.[5,48,49] Invariably, all anesthetic agents have been detected in the follicular fluid and this raises concerns regarding their use.[28] However, fentanyl and propofol have been reported safe and effective.[50] The advantage with using general anesthesia is that the uterus becomes more relaxed, and therefore it is easier for the clinician to aspirate more number of follicles, unlike under sedation, where a contracted myometrium may interfere with the oocyte aspiration. With the proper relaxation of the walls, aspiration of even smaller ovarian follicles becomes simpler. However, it is important that the duration of general anesthetics should be kept to a minimum to avoid the negative effects of these drugs on the oocytes.[51,52]

REGIONAL ANESTHESIA

Regional anesthesia constitutes central neuraxial blockade or the peripheral neural block.

Paracervical and Preovarian Block

In the paracervical block, local anesthetic is injected into two to six sites along the vaginal portion of the cervix at a 3–7 mm depth. The principle of this block is that the nerve plexus lies laterally and posterior to the junction of the uterus and the cervix at the base of the broad ligament. It does not cover the ovarian walls, and the sensations from vaginal and ovarian pain fibers are incompletely blocked; thus, it needs to be supplemented with sedation. Lidocaine is the most common local anesthetic used and the drug acts within 5 minutes of injection. The common complications of this technique are broad ligament hematoma, sciatic nerve block, and neuropathy **(Fig. 1)**.

Preovarian block is a comparatively new technique where the drug is infiltrated into the vaginal wall under ultrasound guidance between the peritoneal surface of the ovary and the vaginal wall. The most commonly used agent is lidocaine at a dose of 50 mg. These techniques, in combination with an inhalational agent, such as remifentanil, are considered effective and safe.[53,54] There is no difference in pain experienced with either paracervical or preovarian blockade.[55] To improve the effectiveness of pain relief, electroacupuncture has also been used along with paracervical block.

Another local anesthetic used for oocyte retrieval is tetracaine. As a local anesthetic, it acts on the peripheral nerves to block nerve impulse transmission. It has been shown to decrease the total dose of propofol required when both of them are used in combination—propofol for sedation and tetracaine as a local anesthetic.[56,57]

Spinal Anesthesia

Drug is given at the L3–L4 level, into the subarachnoid space with a 27-G spinal needle, 0.5% hyperbaric bupivacaine (10–12 mg). The advantages of this technique are that the patient remains awake throughout the procedure and there is an increased comfort level of the gynecologist.[58] However, it is an invasive procedure with a delay in patient discharge from the hospital and urinary retention is common.[59]

Epidural Anesthesia

Epidural anesthesia is an alternative for IVF procedures. However, there is no advantage of this method over other anesthesia techniques.[60,61]

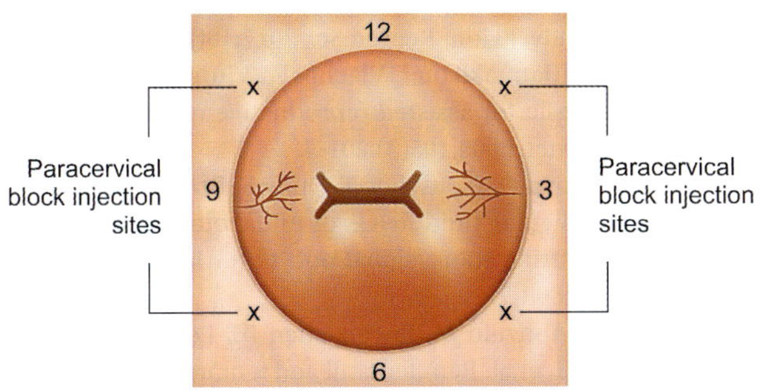

Fig. 1: Paracervical block injection sites—2, 4, 8, 10 o'clock positions. 3 and 9 o'clock positions are avoided due to the presence of blood vessels.

Acupuncture

Acupuncture is a traditional Chinese medicine which involves the insertion of fine needles into certain sites in the body. This method activates the endogenous opioid system by increasing the β-endorphin levels.[62] There is additional antidepressant, anxiolytic, and sympathoinhibitory effect with an increased uterine blood flow. It is usually used along with various conscious sedation regimens or peripheral neural block in order to enhance analgesia.[63,64] One study had reported that acupuncture on the day of embryo transfer had a positive effect on the reproductive outcome.[65] During oocyte retrieval, auricular acupuncture is performed and is believed to act as a pain-relieving method by stimulation of the A-delta fibers and the activation of descending inhibitory pain control systems, as well as psychological aspects.[66]

The electroacupuncture technique can be used along with paracervical block for TVOR, which utilizes the mechanism of neuropeptide release produced by electrical stimulation of different frequencies.[62]

Transcutaneous electrical acupoint stimulation (TEAS) is a user-friendly technique without the use of manual needles and electroacupuncture to reduce invasiveness. It can be used to reduce pain and discomfort during oocyte pickup procedures.[67]

Patient-controlled Analgesia

Patient-controlled analgesia is an alternative technique of analgesia with high levels of patient satisfaction by allowing women to control their drug administration. This method is very patient-compliant and was found to have very low levels of oversedation.[68,69]

Safety of Anesthesia Drugs

Majority of the anesthetic drugs used in the IVF setting have been found to be safe, especially for the gametes. Halogenated agents should be used with caution as they have been found to be associated with reduced reproductive outcomes.[50] The key to anesthesia in IVF is to aim for pharmacological exposure of the shortest duration with minimal penetration into the follicular fluid.

KEY DRUGS, DOSAGE AND SIDE EFFECT

Drug	*Class of drug*	*Dose*	*Significant side effects*
Midazolam	Benzodiazepine	*Induction:* 0.2 mg/kg *Maintenance:* 1 μg/kg/min	
Propofol	2,6-diisopropylphenol	2 mg/kg bolus or 150 μg/kg/min infusion (maximum <4 mg/kg)	Myocardial and respiratory depression
Ketamine (dissociative anesthesia)	Phencyclidine	2 mg/kg	Postoperative psychological adverse effects

Contd...

Contd...

Drug	Class of drug	Dose	Significant side effects
Dexmedetomidine (cooperative sedation)	α-2 adrenoreceptor agonist	1 μg/kg	Bradycardia and hypotension
Lidocaine (used in paracervical and preovarian blocks)		50 mg	
Bupivacaine (used in spinal anesthesia)		10–12 mg	Urinary retention and delay in discharge

KEY POINTS

- In conclusion, studies in different anesthetic techniques fail to give prominence to one specific technique.
- The role of the anesthetist is to provide relief and comfort to the patient to alleviate her fears and anxiety.
- Mild-to-moderate pain experienced during the oocyte retrieval can be relieved by conscious sedation.[70]
- However, the best sedation and anesthetic practice should be tailored to the patient and the provider needs.
- The impact of anesthetic agents on gametes needs to be continuously revisited.
- Majority of the sperm retrieval techniques can be performed under adequate local anesthesia.

REFERENCES

1. Kamel RM. Assisted reproductive technology after the birth of Louise Brown. J Reprod Infertil. 2013;14(3):96-109.
2. Brinsden PR, Brinsden PR. Thirty years of IVF: the legacy of Patrick Steptoe and Robert Edwards. Hum Fertil (Camb). 2009;12(3):137-43.
3. Feichtinger W, Kemeter P. Transvaginal sector scan sonography for needle guided transvaginal follicle aspiration and other applications in gynecologic routine and research. Fertil Steril. 1986;45(5):722-5.
4. Dellenbach P, Nisand I, Moreau L, Feger B, Plumere C, Gerlinger P. Transvaginal sonographically controlled follicle puncture for oocyte retrieval. Fertil Steril. 1985;44(5):656-62.
5. Torode HW, Picker RH, Porter RN, Robertson RD, Smith DH, O'Neill C, et al. Oocyte pickup by laparoscopy replaced by transvaginal aspiration in an in vitro fertilization program. J In Vitro Fert Embryo Transf. 1987;4(3):148-52.
6. Tanbo T, Henriksen T, Magnus O, Abyholm T. Oocyte retrieval in an IVF program. A comparison of laparoscopic and transvaginal ultrasound-guided follicular puncture. Acta Obstet Gynecol Scand. 1988;67:243-6.
7. Boivin J, Schmidt L. Infertility-related stress in men and women predicts treatment outcome 1 year later. Fertil Steril. 2005;83(6):1745-52.
8. Peterson BD, Newton CR, Feingold T. Anxiety and sexual stress in men and women undergoing infertility treatment. Fertil Steril. 2007;88(4):911-4.
9. Kitanovic B, Tulic L. Women coping strategies to infertility stress can impact IVF outcome. Eur Psychiatry. 2016;33:S624.
10. Kwan I, Bhattacharya S, Knox F, McNeil A. Pain relief for women undergoing oocyte retrieval for assisted reproduction. Cochrane Database Syst Rev. 2013;CD004829.
11. Fitzgerald J, Higgins N, Loughrey JPR. Infertility treatment: the role of anesthesia techniques. In: Goudra BG, Singh PM (Eds). Out of Operating Room Anesthesia, 1st edition. Springer International Publishing; 2017.
12. Yasmin E, Dresner M, Balen A. Sedation and anaesthesia for transvaginal oocyte collection: an evaluation of practice in the UK. Hum Reprod. 2004;19:2942-5.
13. Corrie K, Hardman JG. Mechanisms of drug interactions: pharmacodynamics and pharmacokinetics. Anaesth Intensive Care Med. 2011;12(4):156-9.
14. Ghafoor R, Rasool F. Antidepressants and antipsychotics: anaesthetic implications. Anaesth Intensive Care Med. 2017;18(7):340-3.
15. Videnovic N, Mladenovic J, Pavlovic A, Trpkovic S, Filipovic M, Markovic N, et al. Analysis of the applied technique of intravenous anesthesia for in vitro fertilization in obese and patients with normal body mass index. Srp Arh Celok Lek. 2019;147:588-94.
16. Elkington NM, Kehoe J, Acharya U. Intravenous sedation in assisted conception units: a UK survey. Hum Fertil (Camb). 2003;6:74-6.
17. Singhal H, Premkumar PS, Chandy A, Kunjummen AT, Kamath MS. Patient experience with conscious sedation as a method of pain relief for transvaginal oocyte retrieval: a cross sectional study. J Hum Reprod Sci. 2017;10(2):119-23.
18. Vlahos NF, Giannakikou I, Vlachos A, Vitoratos N. Analgesia and anesthesia for assisted reproductive technologies. Int J Gynecol Obstet. 2009;105(3):201-5.
19. Soussis I, Boyd O, Paraschos T, Duffy S, Bower S, Troughton P, et al. Follicular fluid levels of midazolam, fentanyl, and alfentanil during transvaginal oocyte retrieval. Fertil Steril. 1995;64(5):1003-7.
20. Achwal M, Abuzeid M, Bovenschen JL, Lawrence K, Jones ML, Verrill H, et al. Remifentanil and fentanyl concentrations in follicular fluid during transvaginal oocyte retrieval. Anesthesiology. 1999;90(Suppl):16A.
21. Schoeffler PF, Levron JC, Jany L, Brenas FJ, Pouly JL. Follicular concentration of fentanyl during laparoscopy for oocyte retrieval. Correlation with in vitro fertilisation results. Anesthesiology. 1988;69:A663.
22. Jarahzadeh MH, Davar R, Hajiesmaeili MR, Entezari A, Musavi F. Remifentanil versus fentanyl for assisted reproductive technologies: effect on hemodynamic recovery from anesthesia and outcome of ART cycles. Int J Fertil Steril. 2011;5(2):86-9.
23. Lier MC, Douwenga WM, Yilmaz F, Schats R, Hompes PG, Boer C, et al. Patient-controlled remifentanil analgesia as alternative for pethidine with midazolam during oocyte

retrieval in IVF/ICSI procedures: a randomized controlled trial. Pain Pract. 2014;15(5):487-95.

24. Nossair WS, Maaty AMA. Comparative study among ketamine, thiopental and propofol for sedation during in vitro fertilization procedures. SM J Gynecol Obstet. 2017;3(1): 1020.
25. Pierce ET, Smalky M, Alper MM, Hunter JA, Amrhein RL, Pierce Jr EC. Comparison of pregnancy rates following gamete intrafallopian transfer (GIFT) under general anesthesia with thiopental sodium or propofol. J Clin Anesth. 1992;4(5):394-8.
26. Beilin Y, Bodian CA, Mukherjee T, Andres LA, Vincent RD Jr, Hock DL, et al. The use of propofol probably does not affect pregnancy outcome following gamete intrafallopian transfer (GIFT). Anesthesiology. 1997;87(Suppl):884A.
27. Rosenblatt MA, Bradford CN, Bodian CA, Grunfeld L. The effect of a propofol-based sedation technique on cumulative embryo scores, clinical pregnancy rates, and implantation rates in patients undergoing embryo transfers with donor oocytes. J Clin Anesth. 1997;9(8):614-7.
28. Matsota P, Kaminioti E, Kostopanagiotou G. Anesthesia related toxic effects on in vitro fertilization outcome: burden of proof. Biomed Res Int. 2015;2015:475362.
29. Tola EN. The effect of anesthetic agents for oocyte pick-up on in vitro fertilization outcome: a retrospective study in a tertiary center. Taiwan J Obstet Gynecol. 2019;58:673-9.
30. Afonso J, Reis F. Dexmedetomidine: current role in anesthesia and intensive care. Brazil J Anesthesiol. 2012;62(1):118-33.
31. Weerink MAS, Struys MMRF, Hannivoort LN, Barends CRM, Absalom AR, Colin P. Clinical pharmacokinetics and pharmacodynamics of dexmedetomidine. Clin Pharmacokinet. 2017;56(8):893-913.
32. Kaur M, Singh PM. Current role of dexmedetomidine in clinical anesthesia and intensive care. Anesth Essays Res. 2011;5(2):128-33.
33. Elnabtity AM, Selim MF. A prospective randomized trial comparing dexmedetomidine and midazolam for conscious sedation during oocyte retrieval in an in vitro fertilization program. Anesth Essays Res. 2017;11(1):34-9.
34. Candiotti KA, Bergese SD, Bokesch PM, Feldman MA, Wisemandle W, Bekker AY, et al. Monitored anesthesia care with dexmedetomidine: a prospective, randomized, double-blind, multicenter trial. Anesth Analg. 2010;110(1):47-56.
35. Jakob SM, Ruokonen E, Grounds RM, Sarapohja T, Garratt C, Pocock SJ, et al. Dexmedetomidine vs midazolam or propofol for Sedation during prolonged mechanical ventilation. JAMA. 2012;307(11):1151.
36. Jennings JC, Moreland K, Peterson CM. In vitro fertilisation: a review of drug therapy and clinical management. Drugs. 1996;52:313-43.
37. Toth TL, Lee MS, Bendikson KA, Reindollar RH, American Society for Reproductive Medicine Embryo Transfer Advisory Panel. Embryo transfer techniques: an American Society for Reproductive Medicine survey of current society for assisted reproductive technology practices. Fertil Steril. 2017;107(4):1003-11.
38. Meyer L, Lekovic J, Reichman D, Chung P, Rosenwaks Z. The effect of anesthesia during embryo transfer on in vitro fertilization outcome. Fertil Steril. 2013;100(3):S526-7.
39. Gonen O, Shulman A, Ghetler Y, Shapiro A, Judeiken R, Beyth Y, et al. The impact of different types of anesthesia on in vitro fertilization-embryo transfer treatment outcome. J Assist Reprod Genet. 1995;12(10):678-82.
40. Coward RM, Mills JN. A step-by-step guide to office-based sperm retrieval for obstructive azoospermia. Transl Androl Urol. 2017;6(4):730-44
41. Wakefield SE, Elewa AA. Spermatic cord block: a safe technique for intrascrotal surgery. Ann R Coll Surg Engl. 1994;76:401-2.
42. Wolf Jr JS, Bennett CJ, Dmochowski RR, Hollenbeck BK, Pearle MS, Schaeffer AJ, et al. Best practice policy statement on urologic surgery antimicrobial prophylaxis. J Urol. 2008;179:1379-90.
43. Mehta A, Hsiao W, King P, Schlegel PN. Perioperative celecoxib decreases opioid use in patients undergoing testicular surgery: a randomized, double-blind, placebo controlled trial. J Urol. 2013;190:1834-8.
44. Unlu BS, Yilmazer M, Koken G, Arioz DT, Unlu E, Dogan Baki E, et al. Comparison of four different pain relief methods during hysterosalpingography: a randomized controlled study. Pain Res Manag. 2015;20(2):107-11.
45. Hindocha A, Beere L, O'Flynn H, Watson A, Ahmad G. Pain relief in hysterosalpingography. Cochrane Database Syst Rev. 2015;2015(9):CD006106.
46. Wang YL, Gao HX, Wang JS, Wang JH, Bo L, Zhang TT, et al. Immersive virtual reality as analgesia for women during hysterosalpingography: study protocol for a randomized controlled trial. Trials. 2020;21:102.
47. Lambert D. Mechanisms of action of general anaesthetic drugs. Anaesth Intensive Care Med. 2017;18(7):344-6.
48. Wikland M, Nilsson L, Hansson R, Hamberger L, Janson PO. Collection of human oocytes by the use of sonography. Fertil Steril. 1983;39(5):603-8.
49. Steptoe P, Webster J. Laparoscopy for oocyte recovery. Ann N Y Acad Sci. 1985;442:178-81.
50. Murthy T, Gupta P, Sharma RR. Anaesthetic issues in in-vitro fertilisation. Med J Armed Forces India. 2008;64(2):119-22.
51. Hayes MF, Sacco AG, Savoy-Moore RT, Magyar DM, Endler GC, Moghissi KS. Effect of general anesthesia on fertilization and cleavage of human oocytes in vitro. Fertil Steril. 1987;48:975-81.
52. Wilhelm W, Hammadeh ME, White PF, Georg T, Fleser R, Biedler A. General anesthesia versus monitored anesthesia care with remifentanil for assisted reproductive technologies: effect on pregnancy rate. J Clin Anesth. 2002;14(1):1-5.
53. Ng EH, Tang OS, Chui DK, Ho PC. Comparison of two different doses of lignocaine used in paracervical block during oocyte collection in an IVF programme. Hum Reprod. 2000;15(10):2148-51.
54. Ng EH, Tang OS, Chui DK, Ho PC. A prospective, randomized, double-blind and placebo-controlled study to assess the efficacy of paracervical block in the pain relief during egg collection in IVF. Hum Reprod. 1999;14(11):2783-7.
55. Cerne A, Bergh C, Borg K, Ek I, Gejervall AL, Hillensjö T, et al. Pre-ovarian block versus paracervical block for oocyte retrieval. Hum Reprod. 2006;21:2916-21.
56. Giordano D, Raso MG, Pernice C, Agnoletti V, Barbieri V. Topical local anesthesia: focus on lidocaine-tetracaine combination. Local Reg Anesth. 2015;8:95-100.
57. Shao X, Qin J, Li C, Zhou L, Guo L, Lu Y, et al. Tetracaine combined with propofol for painless oocyte retrieval: from a single center study. Ann Palliat Med. 2020;9:1606-13.

58. Endler GC, Magyar DM, Hayes MF, Moghissi KS. Use of spinal anesthesia in laparoscopy for in vitro fertilization. Fertil Steril. 1985;43:809-10.
59. Tsen LC, Schultz R, Martin R, Datta S, Bader AM. Intrathecal low-dose bupivacaine versus lidocaine for in vitro fertilization procedures. Reg Anesth Pain Med. 2001;26(1):52-6.
60. Botta G, D'Angelo A, D'Ari G, Merlino G, Chapman M, Grudzinskas G. Epidural anesthesia in an in vitro fertilization and embryo transfer program. J Assist Reprod Genet. 1995; 12:187-90.
61. Lehtinen AM, Laatikainen T, Koskimies AI, Hovorka J. Modifying effects of epidural analgesia or general anesthesia on the stress hormone response to laparoscopy for in vitro fertilization. J In Vitro Fert Embryo Transf. 1987;4(1):23-9.
62. Han JS. Acupuncture: neuropeptide release produced by electrical stimulation of different frequencies. Trends Neurosci. 2003;26:17-22.
63. Tsen L. Electro-acupuncture was as efficacious as i.v. alfentanil for pain control during oocyte retrieval for IVF. Evid Based Obstet Gynecol. 2004;6(3):131-2.
64. Stener-Victorin E. The pain-relieving effect of electro-acupuncture and conventional medical analgesic methods during oocyte retrieval: a systematic review of randomized controlled trials. Hum Reprod. 2005;20(2):339-49.
65. Westergaard LG, Mao Q, Krogslund M, Sandrini S, Lenz S, Grinsted J. Acupuncture on the day of embryo transfer significantly improves the reproductive outcome in infertile women: a prospective, randomized trial. Fertil Steril. 2006; 85(5):1341-6.
66. Sator-Katzenschlager SM, Wölfler MM, Kozek-Langenecker SA, Sator K, Sator PG, Li B, et al. Auricular electro-acupuncture as an additional perioperative analgesic method during oocyte aspiration in IVF treatment. Hum Reprod. 2006;21(8): 2114-20.
67. Tian L, Feng X, Zhang R, Wang S, Li R, Kong R, et al. Pain relief during oocyte retrieval by transcutaneous electrical acupoint stimulation: a single-blinded, randomized, controlled multi-center trial. Evid Based Complement Alternat Med. 2020; 2020:3285648.
68. Dell RG, Cloote AH. Patient-controlled sedation during transvaginal oocyte retrieval: an assessment of patient acceptance of patient-controlled sedation using a mixture of propofol and alfentanil. Eur J Anaesthesiol. 1998;15(2):210-5.
69. Lok IH, Chan MT, Chan DL, Cheung LP, Haines CJ, Yuen PM. A prospective randomized trial comparing patient-controlled sedation using propofol and alfentanil and physician-administered sedation using diazepam and pethidine during transvaginal ultrasound-guided oocyte retrieval. Hum Reprod. 2002;17(8):2101-6.
70. Esposito J, Qin S, Kovacs G. How much inconvenience and discomfort does modern IVF treatment cause? Glob J Reprod Med. 2017;1(2):555-7.

CHAPTER

56 Oocyte Retrieval

Sankalp Singh, Nivedita Ananth, Swati Singh, Mohammed Ashraf C

INTRODUCTION

Oocyte retrieval (OCR) can be defined as the process of the aspiration of follicular fluid and the oocytes contained therein, directly from the ovaries of a woman, before them being released spontaneously from the ovarian follicles. It is one of the most important steps of in vitro fertilization (IVF) procedure, since the success of IVF is directly related to the number and the quality of embryos, which in turn are dependent on the number and the quality of oocytes.

HISTORY

Miriam Menken and John Rock were the first to report retrieval of oocytes by laparotomy.[1] The procedure of laparotomy was associated with significant surgical risks to women including hemorrhage, wound infections and injury to abdominopelvic structures, and prolonged convalescence period. This led to the development of alternative surgical approaches for OCR. It took more than three decades from then to have the first birth after an assisted reproductive technology (ART) procedure.[2]

The first successful outcome of IVF was achieved on 25 July 1978 with the birth of Louise Brown in Manchester from a laparoscopic retrieval on the spontaneous cycle of a single ovarian follicle. In the years after that, following on from the excellent results achieved by Steptoe, oocyte pick-up was carried out using the laparoscopic technique, with hospitalization and general anesthesia (GA).[3]

After laparoscopic OCR, the transvesical approach for OCR was promoted by Lenz and Lauritsen in 1982. They showed that ultrasound could be used for operative rather than just a diagnostic tool. Danish gynecologists were the first to experiment with the efficiency of a new ultrasonically guided percutaneous aspiration method in reaching ovarian follicles and carrying out oocyte pick-up. During this procedure, the needle, attached to an abdominal transducer, was inserted percutaneously into the antral follicle, going through the abdominal wall and the urinary bladder. The harvest of oocytes collected was comparable to that of the laparoscopic approach, but with a lower rate of complications and with easier access to the ovaries. The procedure could not be conducted with short-lasting general anesthetic or local anesthetic in an outpatient capacity.[4]

One year later, another group from northern Europe, led by the gynecologists, Hamberger and Wikland, in Gothenburg, Sweden, described for the first time the possibility of using an echographic vaginal probe in OCR.

A needle was guided along the echographic vaginal probe to carry out a precise hole in the follicle and recover the follicular fluid.[5-7]

Once an initial fear relating to the danger of oocyte alteration and ultrasound was overcome, the transvaginal technique, thanks to its simplicity and efficacy, became widespread and now, having been carried out for >30 years, has become the default choice for the retrieval of oocytes for IVF.

VAGINAL PREPARATION BEFORE OOCYTE RETRIEVAL

Vaginal preparation is a common practice before any gynecological procedure. It is done with an aim to prevent infection and also to help improve IVF success rate. Theoretically, inserting a needle through the vaginal wall from essentially an unsterile environment, into the abdomen—a sterile field, increases the risk that intraperitoneal infection may occur. However, pelvic infection after transvaginal oocyte recovery is thankfully rare, irrespective of whether prophylactic antibiotics are used with an incidence of 0.6% as seen in a large series of 2,670 cases.[8]

The two most common agents used are povidone-iodine and normal saline. In a randomized controlled trial (RCT) comparing povidone-iodine (betadine) with a simple normal saline douche in 334 women undergoing OCR, no difference was found in the fertilization rates (45.5 vs. 47.8%) or cleavage rates (49.8 vs. 52.1%). However, the pregnancy rate was significantly lower in the betadine group (17.2 compared to 30.3%), indicating that betadine appeared to have an adverse impact on the outcome.[9] Likewise, even where betadine is removed by douching with normal saline, there was a higher biochemical pregnancy rate where betadine was employed.[10]

At our center, we do vaginal cleansing with saline a day prior and on the day of OCR.

ROLE OF PROPHYLACTIC ANTIBIOTICS

The benefit of prophylactic antibiotics for OCR is far from proven. The overall incidence of infection after an OCR is estimated to be about 0.4%.[11,12] In most instances, pelvic infections after OCRs have been noted in patients who have endometriosis, likely due to the presence of pelvic adhesions.[13,14]

Additionally, there is no convincing data to suggest improvement in IVF outcome by using antibiotics.

Until further data evaluating live birth is available, its use should be left at the discretion of the clinician and each clinic should have its own policy depending on local needs.

We, at our center, do give the combination of amoxicillin and clavulanic acid for a period of 5 days.

ANESTHESIA AND OOCYTE RETRIEVAL

Oocyte retrieval involves piercing the vaginal mucosa to aspirate the follicles. It is a physically and mentally stressful procedure for women. Women undergoing the procedure should be offered some form of anesthesia. Patient can feel the pain while the needle pierces the vaginal wall or the ovarian cortex. So, anesthesia should be offered to make it pain-free and comfortable for the patient. In cases where the patient is not cooperative during the procedure, there can be unwarranted movement of the patient with needle in situ causing trauma to vital structures or iliac vessels.

The ideal anesthetic modality should be safe for women, have effective pain relief, devoid of harmful effects to the oocytes, and easy to administer and monitor.

Prior to Ovum Pickup

Investigations for medical fitness should be done according to the local guidelines. Preanesthesia evaluation should be done to avoid any intraoperative mishaps. Taking accurate patient history before ovum pickup (OPU) is essential to highlight potential comorbidities and take actions to prevent any possible associated complications. Patients should at least be asked about the use of medications—more specifically the use of blood-thinning agents (aspirin and others), relevant previous surgeries, and any relevant disease or deficit of coagulation factors.

Monitoring

Noninvasive blood pressure and pulse oximetry must be used when drugs have been administered intravenously; electrocardiogram (ECG) and CO_2 monitoring are developmental standards for conscious sedation but are minimal monitoring standards for deep sedation and GA.

Various forms of anesthesia are:

- *Local or paracervical block:* Lidocaine 100 mg (10 mL of 1% lidocaine, xylocaine 10 mg/mL) is injected at two (3 and 9 o'clock) or four points around the cervix. It can be used alone or in conjunction with local sedation. Satisfaction with the procedure was higher when the blocks were used during a GA and postoperative pain was also lower.[15]
- *Conscious sedation:* In conscious sedation, the patient is able to communicate with personnel and be able to follow orders, for example "breathe deeply."

All respiratory and cardiovascular parameters remain intact. Agents such as midazolam, propofol, and ketamine are used for OCR.

Propofol has been shown to be devoid of any harmful effect on various IVF outcomes including live birth rates, thus making it a better anesthetic to use during OCRs. Along with the fact that it is short-acting, safe, and provides good pain relief which makes it an excellent choice for OCR procedures.

- Verbal anesthesia (VA) by the sedationist is a very important part of any OPU that is performed with conscious sedation and/or local anesthetics. VA is a conversational distraction associated with measures to ensure a calming environment, thereby reducing pain, anxiety, and stress.[16]

A Cochrane review which analyzed 21 RCTs performed to compare pain relief modalities during OCR found no difference between different modalities. It showed better pain relief if more than one method were used rather than single.[17]

In our center, 98% of retrievals are performed under conscious sedation with propofol/fentanyl.

The modality of providing anesthesia to a given patient should depend mainly on the patient's cooperation and anticipated difficulty in ovarian access. If the patient is comfortable, conscious sedation is a good option. However, in some cases, like ovaries above the pelvic brim needing abdominal retrieval, regional or GA may be required.

INSTRUMENTS FOR OOCYTE RETRIEVAL

The instruments needed for OCR include:

- Ultrasound machine with a transvaginal probe with a frequency of 5–7.5 mHz **(Fig. 1)**. The transvaginal probe has a groove near the tip where the needle guide could be firmly attached **(Fig. 1)**. Each machine has its corresponding probe which can be used. The ultrasound gel is applied and a nontoxic probe cover is attached over it.

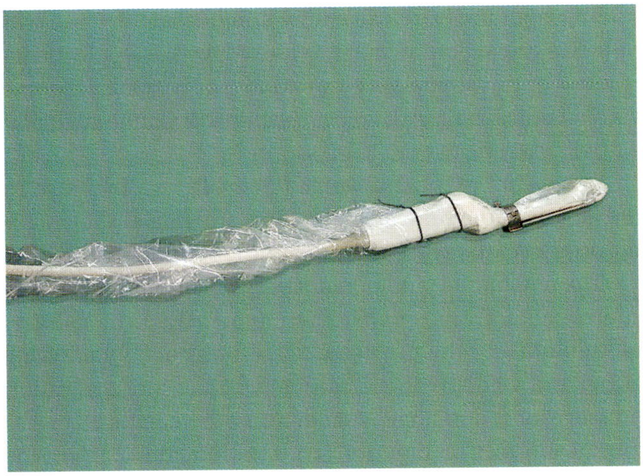

Fig. 1: Ultrasound probe with needle guide.

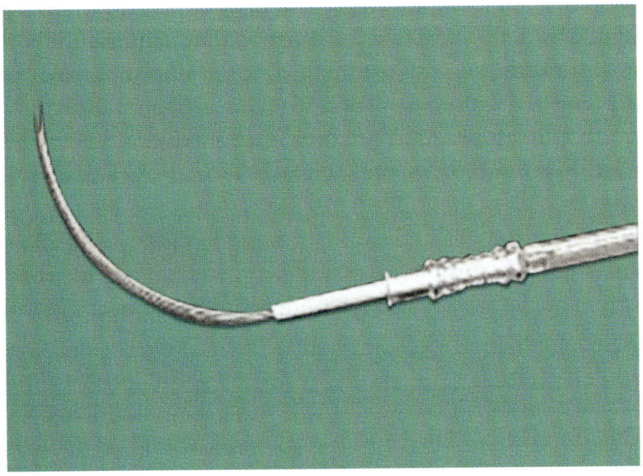

Fig. 2: Single lumen needle.

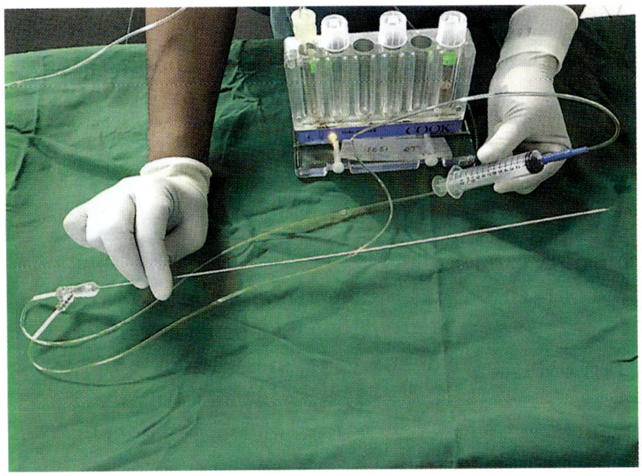

Fig. 3: Needle with connecting tube and stand.

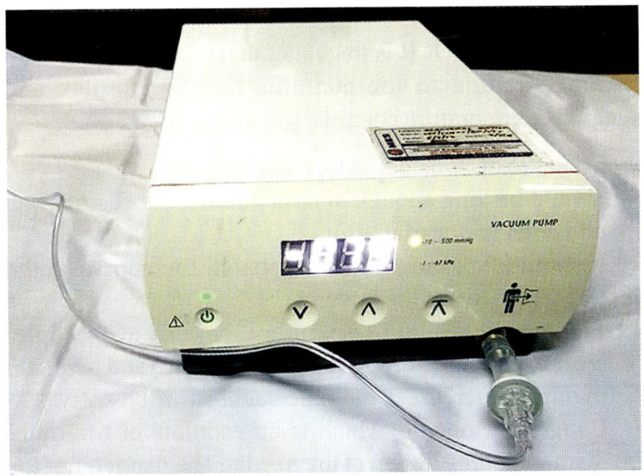

Fig. 4: Suction apparatus.

- *Aspiration needle:* The needle of either 17 or 18 gauge is inserted through the needle guide **(Fig. 2)**. The tip is kept inside the guide till the probe is inserted and the follicle has been brought into the view. The tip of the needle is beveled to facilitate aspiration in an irregular shaped follicle and easy insertion through the vagina and ovarian cortex. The hub or handle of the needle has the proximal portion of the tubing attached to it. The handle of the needle helps in the maneuvering of the needle. The distal end of tubing is fixed to the test tube with the help of a cork and the follicle fluid flows through the tubing into the test tube. Another tubing comes out of the cork and is attached to the suction apparatus tubing to maintain adequate suction pressure during OCR. The aspiration needles could be single lumen or double lumen. Double-lumen needles are usually used in case of follicular flushing or endometriotic cyst aspiration.
- *Test tube warmer stand:* The test tubes are placed in the test tube stand which helps in the maintenance of the temperature at 37°C **(Fig. 3)**.
- *Suction apparatus:* This helps in the formation and maintenance of the negative pressure inside the follicle necessary for aspirating the oocytes **(Fig. 4)**. The foot switch attached to the suction machine is used to apply pressure to suck the follicular fluid out.
- *Operation theater table:* Should have easy maneuverability to adjust the position of the patient **(Fig. 5)**. The patient needs to be in a lithotomy position using the stirrups attached to the table.

ASPIRATION SETUP

The ideal setup for OCR pertaining to the needle type, vacuum pressure, and culture media which can give optimal results is still unknown. Transvaginal ultrasound probe of frequency between 5 and 7.5 MHz is commonly used. The machine should have the option of color Doppler to distinguish the vessels. Also, they should have an option for biopsy line so as to have a marker for the needle entry.

Most commonly, we come across few basic questions:

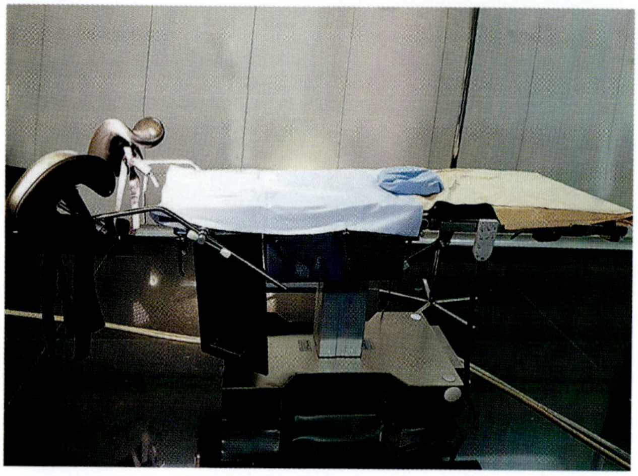

Fig. 5: Operation table.

What Size Needle to be Used for Aspiration

The main aim of OCR is to collect maximum follicles with minimal trauma to the cumulus oocyte complex and adequate temperature control.

Properties to be considered for a needle:

- Should be long enough to pass through the vaginal wall and enter the ovarian stroma
- It should be rigid enough to stay in the course of the tracer present on the screen
- The needle should be sharp and beveled at the tip to ensure easy entry through the ovarian tunica and maintain minimum increase in the follicular pressure on entry.
- Gauge of a needle, which is an estimate of the inner diameter of the lumen of the needle. The diameter of the needle is important as it needs to be great enough such that the inner channel is of a width to allow passage of the cumulus–oocyte complex intact, but small enough to minimize tissue trauma, diminishing the risk of serious bleeding if blood vessels are entered, and reducing pelvic discomfort.[18,19] The thinner the needle, the higher the aspiration pressure required to maintain the same flow rate. The dead space, which represents the volume of the cylinder created by the cross-sectional interior area of the needle and its length,[20,21] needs to be minimized, so collected oocytes pass into the collecting tube and do not remain in the tube.

A study comparing 15-, 17-, and 18-gauge single-lumen needles showed no difference in recovery rates, but a significant reduction in perceived pain when the smaller diameter needle was employed.[18] The needle is attached to a tubing system made of materials that are not toxic to gametes and can retain temperature well.

In our center, we use an 18G single-lumen needle for OCR.

Aspiration Pressure

Prior to the use of electric aspiration pump, hand-held syringes were used for aspiration.

The high pressure caused by a hand-held syringe was found to cause detrimental fracture of the zona pellucida.[22] In view of this, there was a need to find a suction source with a controlled aspiration pressure to drain the follicular without exerting too much pressure.

According to Hagen–Poiseuille's law, an increase in the length of the tube decreases the pressure at the end in proportion to the percentage that the length was increased.

The magnitude of the shear stress that a cumulus oocyte complex (COC) may experience depends on the velocity of the fluid and the diameter of the needle.[23,24] Increasing either the velocity of the fluid (by increasing aspiration pressure) or increasing the diameter of the needle increases the shear forces on the COC. The pressure at the exit of the aspiration device is different from the pressure experienced by the oocyte at the needle tip. Needle gauge, length of needle, connecting tube gauge, length of connecting tube, size of the collection tube, and size of the vacuum reservoir in the pump all play a role in determining the pressure experienced within the needle from the aspiration device.

In clinical practice, suction is applied just before the needle is inserted into the follicle so as to create a seal as to prevent leak of the follicular fluid (between the needle and the punctured follicular wall) and also to maintain the flow rate and avoid turbulence. If the vacuum is stopped too soon before the needle is removed from the follicle, there is risk of back flow, which could leave the oocyte in the follicle.

There was a study done in 537 patients between low aspiration pressure (150 mm Hg) and high pressure (300 mm Hg) for OCR and it was noted that the use of low aspiration pressure resulted in a significantly greater oocyte yield, maturity, and fewer oocytes with an empty zona pellucida compared to high aspiration pressure.

While aspiration pressure did not impact the pregnancy rate per transfer in this cohort, the higher number of usable embryos in the low-pressure group may result in a higher cumulative pregnancy rate.[25]

In our center, with a needle of 18 G, we use suction pressure of 120 mm HG in case of conventional aspiration.

Steps of Oocyte Retrieval (Box 1)

At the outset, the sterile operating room table, vaginal ultrasound probe with attached probe-specific needle guide, collecting tubes containing culture media in a warmer stand, and a working suction apparatus need to be prepared.

The suction apparatus should be checked before each procedure. The tubing should be checked for and the tubes should be tightly corked. After administration of the chosen anesthetic agent or paracervical block, the patient is placed in the dorsal lithotomy position and a sterile speculum is placed inside the vagina. The vagina is cleansed with saline. The vaginal speculum is then removed followed by placement of transvaginal ultrasound probe with already attached

BOX 1: Important steps in oocyte retrieval.

- Patient should be asked to empty the bladder before putting her in the lithotomy position
- Adequate anesthesia should be administered
- Cleansing of the vagina with normal saline
- Elbow support should be given while holding the vaginal probe
- Adequate pressure should be maintained on the probe
- Focus the maximum diameter of follicle after inserting the probe
- Insert the needle into the center of the maximum diameter of the follicle. The needle should be somewhere in the middle of the follicle
- Suction pedal should be switched on just before entry into the follicle
- Follicle collapse should be the focus of the eye rather than the drops in the tube
- Keep the needle surrounded by fluid at all times. If needed, gentle movement of the probe should be utilized
- Follicular curetting at the end of complete follicular collapse
- Anteroposterior movement of probe assisted by lateral movement when needed to focus next follicle
- Once all adequately grown follicles present in both ovaries are aspirated, the pouch of Douglas and both adnexa should be checked to rule out any blood collection

needle guide inserted into the vagina. Elbow support should be given while holding the vaginal probe inside the vagina by placing the elbow on the thigh of the clinician or on the stirrups. This will minimize unnecessary movements of the probe and allow better focusing. Adequate pressure should be maintained on the probe so that there is minimal distance between the vaginal probe and the ovary or follicle. Focus the maximum diameter of the follicle after inserting the probe. The follicle selected should be the one which is nearer to the probe. Warm culture media through the needle (we use 17- or 18-gauge) to stabilize the temperature inside the needle and the tubing. The needle is then passed through the needle guide piercing the vaginal wall and into the center of maximum diameter of follicle under ultrasound guidance. Care should be taken to avoid surrounding structures such as the iliac vessels, bowel, and bladder. The tip of the needle should be in the middle of the follicle, surrounded by fluid all around. The vacuum pump is activated using the footswitch at the entry of needle into the follicle and follicular fluid aspirated into prewarmed tubes placed in a tube warming rack containing culture media taking care to avoid overfilling leading to spillage into the tubing extending toward the suction apparatus. Follicular curetting is performed at the end of complete follicular collapse by gentle rotation of the needle. After completing one follicle, the next follicle should be focused. The movement which helps focus the next follicle better is often the anteroposterior movement of the probe rather than lateral movement. Preferably this follicle should be the one, which is adjacent to or just below the pricked follicle and the above-mentioned steps should be repeated. The tubes are then transferred carefully to the tube warming rack in the adjacent embryology laboratory. The embryologist then places the contents of the tubes into culture plates and the oocytes are identified using a microscope. We advise aspirating all follicles ≥10 mm in a non-in vitro maturation (IVM) OCR.

Postoperative Instructions

Details of following should be documented:

- Number of retrieved follicles, E2 level on the day of trigger, suction pressure, needle size and type used, anesthesia used, confirmed plan for either oocyte freeze or embryo freeze, ease of procedure. In case of any transmyometrial approach, it needs to be mentioned and also signs of premature ovulation should be documented for future reference.
- Any pelvic collection
- Postprocedure antibiotics is given in our center for 5 days.
- OHSS prophylaxis to be documented in specific cases
- In case of a pelvic collection, repeat ultrasonography (USG) after 2 hours to look for the collection.

TROUBLESHOOTING IN OOCYTE RETRIEVAL

ESHRE Guidelines (2019)

What to do when the Needle Tip is Not Visualized?

Withdraw the needle and ensure that the needle director/gauge is in place allowing the needle to move in the same sector as the ultrasound beam.

What to do When Suction Fails?

- Check for any discontinuity in the collection tubing leading to suction failure.
- Check if the needle tubing is properly attached to both the suction apparatus and collecting tube.
- Rotate the needle within the follicle to ensure that it is not blocked by follicular wall tissue.
- If there is still no suction, remove the needle and perform a "retrograde flush" to clear any blockage.
- Before reinserting the needle, recheck by aspirating some culture medium.
- It is always better to have an additional suction apparatus available in the operation theater.
- In case there is no other feasible option, then a manual suction with 20 mL syringe can be used by creating negative pressure.
- If premature ovulation is suspected, peritoneal fluid can be aspirated to recover some oocytes.

Presence of Endometriotic Cyst in Ovaries

Endometriomas should not be aspirated while OPU to prevent contamination of follicular aspirate and reduce risk of intra-abdominal infection. But sometimes they do get punctured inadvertently, so in such cases, intravenous (IV) antibiotics cover for 48 hours should be provided. Also, the needle should be immediately withdrawn and flushed with media and the collecting tube should be changed. The risk in such cases should be counseled to the patient preoperatively and necessary consent to be taken.[26-28]

ROLE OF FOLLICULAR FLUSHING

- Pregnancy rate is directly correlated to the number of oocytes retrieved.
- The more the number of oocytes, the more the quantity of embryos obtained.[29]
- To maximize the number of oocytes recovered, investigators have suggested follicular aspiration followed by a single 2-mL flush.[30]

There was a Cochrane review updated in 2018 which included 10 studies with total of 928 women to compare the role of follicular flushing and aspiration versus aspiration alone.[31-39]

All included studies reported outcomes per woman randomized.

The conclusion was as below.

- Comparing follicular flushing to aspiration alone revealed probably little or no difference in the live birth rate [odds ratio (OR) 0.95, 95% confidence interval (CI) 0.58–1.56; three randomized controlled trials (RCTs); $n = 303$; $I^2 = 30\%$; moderate-quality evidence]. This suggests that with a live birth rate of approximately 41% with aspiration alone, the equivalent live birth rate with follicular flushing is likely to lie between 29 and 52%.
- None of the included studies reported on the primary outcome of miscarriage rate.
- Six RCTs showed no difference in the oocyte yield following follicular flushing.[32-37]
- None of the studies showed any difference in the number of embryos or embryo cryopreserved or clinical pregnancy rate.

Mok-Lin et al. conducted an RCT comparing follicular flushing versus aspiration only in 50 extremely poor responders, including women with ≤4 follicles of ≥12 mm on the day of human chorionic gonadotropin (hCG) administration. There were no differences in the number of oocytes retrieved (4 vs. 3, $p = 0.41$). However, in flushing group, there were significantly fewer embryos for transfer (1.7 vs. 2.5, $p = 0.03$), lower implantation rate (5.3 vs. 34.2%, $p = 0.0006$), and lower clinical pregnancy rates (4 vs. 36%, $p = 0.01$) when compared to the flushing group. These differences remained significant even after adjusting for the number of embryos transferred. This was the first study to demonstrate a negative effect of follicular flushing on IVF outcomes.[37]

One study suggested that aspiration without flushing reduced operative time and decreased the amount of anesthetic required.[38,39]

Possible mechanisms quoted by authors were:

- Increased intrafollicular pressure generated by flushing could impact oocyte quality via mechanistic effects.
- Increased procedure and anesthesia times can be detrimental to oocyte quality.
- The presence of residual flushing fluid in the pelvis could have altered the uterine milieu at the time of implantation.
- Serial flushing could negatively impact granulosa cell number and function, thus impacting the luteal phase.

In our center, we do not advocate follicular flushing for any group of responders.

Temperature Control

The meiotic spindles of the human oocyte consist of microtubules and are extremely sensitive to temperature fluctuation, both up and down.[40,41] The spindle structure can dissemble relatively quickly on cooling, but takes longer to recover on rewarming.

The duration of the drop and the variation in the temperature to which the oocyte has been exposed will determine whether the spindle will recover.

The oocyte can tolerate drop in temperature from 37° to 33° for <10 minutes before rewarming. Further drop or for longer duration can lead to permanent damage to the spindle assembly.[42,43] The meiotic spindles are responsible for the chromosome alignment and separation of the maternal chromosomes during fertilization. Therefore, any disruption to the spindle may lead to abnormal chromosome distribution, leading subsequently to failed fertilization or aneuploidy.[44]

It is advisable to have closed workstations where temperature, oxygen concentration, and pH can be more reliably controlled to reduce these potential stresses.

Working with a closed isolator-based workstation may be technically more challenging but protects against ambient conditions, promoting the development of better-quality blastocysts and higher pregnancy rates.[45]

In Our Set-up

We have all the collecting tubes kept in a tube heater well-maintained at the temperature of 37°C.

The oocyte collecting system is flushed with media which was kept at 37°C before the onset of procedure. Each follicle is aspirated in turn and the collecting tube immediately given to the embryologist to identify the oocyte. There is a small connecting hatch through to the laboratory, where the embryologist is working in a grade A temperature-controlled workstation.

OOCYTE RETRIEVAL IN DIFFICULT CASES

Transvaginal approach is the most commonly used for OCR.

Studies comparing transvaginal, transabdominal, and laparoscopic approaches for OCR have found the transvaginal approach better in terms of safety, efficacy as well as time under anesthesia.

A study on a cohort of 85 infertile women comparing transmyometrial versus conventional approach showed that the transmyometrial retrieval did not significantly affect the pregnancy outcome.[46]

Transabdominal approach is mainly used in cases of women with radical hysterectomies, transposed ovaries, Müllerian agenesis as well as in cases of increased body mass index (BMI) where the poor image quality makes the ovaries unreachable.[47-49]

A study in 2014 was done comparing transabdominal versus transvaginal approach in 204 patients and concluded that in case with difficult transvaginal access due to previous surgery or high BMI, transabdominal approach can be a better alternative for OCR.[50]

Points to be remembered before opting for transabdominal approach:

- Expertise is required for performing the procedure to avoid inadvertent trauma to the vital structures or iliac vessels.
- Maintain stability and coordination of the probe and the operating hand.
- In case the ovaries are adherent to the posterior surface or fundus of the uterus, a transmyometrial approach rather than a transabdominal approach can be done.

COMPLICATIONS OF OOCYTE RETRIEVAL

Transvaginal ultrasound-guided OCR is a safe well-tolerated procedure, with a low risk of serious complications.

The most common problem encountered after USG-guided transvaginal OCR procedure is minor vaginal bleeding, which generally stops spontaneously or can be controlled with local compression. The incidence of vaginal bleeding is reported to be 8.6% of cases in literature.[8]

However, the risks associated with the procedure should not be underestimated because some complications, although rare, may be life-threatening (two deaths were reported in 2010).[51]

Most frequent complications noted are vaginal and peritoneal bleeding.

A retrospective analysis suggested that particularly in patients with ovarian endometriomas, complications, such as tubo-ovarian abscess, can occur even long after the completion of the assisted reproductive technology (ART) cycle, indicating that women with endometriosis are prone to develop infectious complications.[28] Other rarer complications, described as case reports, are ureterovaginal fistulas,[52] pseudoaneurysm of the iliac artery,[53,54] ureteral injury,[55,56] bladder injury with hematuria,[57,58] and ovarian abscess.[59]

Retrospective analysis was done over 10 years in a fertility center in Italy involving 23,827 consecutive transvaginal OCR procedures in 12,615 patients.[60]

A total of 96 complications related to OCR procedures (0.40%; 95% CI 0.33–0.49%) were encountered. A risk factor was present in 28 (29.17%) of the 96 cases experiencing complications. The complication rate for patient was 0.76% with no recurrence of a complication in the same patient. Hospital admission was necessary for 71 of 96 (73.96%) patients suffering complications, representing 0.29% (95% CI 0.23–0.38%) of the total retrievals and the average duration of a hospital stay was 2.77 days. In 54 cases, the complication was peritoneal bleeding (0.23%, 95% CI 0.17–0.30%). A total of 24 patients required surgery (0.1%, 95% CI 0.06–0.15%), of which 19 for peritoneal bleeding; in 18 (33.33%), a laparoscopy could evacuate the hemoperitoneum (volume >1,000 mL), whereas in one patient, an emergent laparotomy was necessary to repair a small laceration of the iliac vein. In one patient, the pelvic bleeding occurred 2 days after the OCR procedure; in another case, 15 days had elapsed between the OCR procedure. In another two cases, a laparoscopy had to be performed for infectious complications and in one patient, a laparotomy was necessary for severe sepsis. Pelvic pain was another retrieval complication and six patients required hospitalization (0.03%, 95% CI 0.009–0.055%). Vaginal lacerations were encountered in only two patients who required sutures (0.008%). Two cases of bladder trauma (0.008%) were noted and diagnosed by hematuria and vesical hematoma, but they did not require intervention.

Concerning anesthetic complications, a total of 14 patients were observed with 12 cases of circulatory shock and nausea. Two serious complications were atrial fibrillation and one case of cardiorespiratory insufficiency, agitation, and confusion.

28 of the 96 patients (29.17%) who suffered complications had pre-existing risk factors: History of endometriosis, history of pelvic surgery for benign reasons, previous pelvic inflammatory disease (PID), or hematologic disease (one was suffering from von Willebrand disease and one had chronic thrombocytopenia).

As some of the complications occur some days following the procedure, underreporting of cases is also possible.

Simple steps which can prevent complications:

- Empty the bladder prior to the procedure.
- Gentle movement of the probe and needle inside the ovary
- Avoid unnecessary lateral movement of the needle inside the ovarian stroma.
- Review any pelvic collection postprocedure to identify any intraperitoneal bleeding early.
- In case of any suspicion, put color Doppler to rule out presence of vessels in the path of the needle marker.

KEY POINTS

- Oocyte retrieval is a generally safe and well-tolerated procedure and is most often accomplished in the patient-friendly outpatient setting with conscious sedation and rarely requires GA.
- It is typically performed using transvaginal ultrasound guidance, but rarely may require transabdominal ultrasound-guided retrieval in case of abnormal anatomy. It is fairly simple to learn and master, if one keeps the basic things in mind.
- In common practice, prophylactic antibiotics are administered prior to the procedure and complications such as clinically significant bleeding or infection are extremely unusual.

REFERENCES

1. Menkin MF, Rock J. In vitro fertilization and cleavage of human ovarian eggs. Am J Obstet Gynecol. 1948;55(3):440-52.
2. Steptoe PC, Edwards RG. Birth after the reimplantation of a human embryo. Lancet. 1978;2(8085):366.
3. Steptoe PC. Laparoscopy in Gynecology. Edinburgh: Ed Livingstone; 1967.
4. Lenz S, Lauritsen JG. Ultrasonically guided percutaneous aspiration of human follicles under local anesthesia: a new method for collecting oocytes for in vitro fertilization. Palermo: Cofese Ed; 1982.
5. Gembruch U, Diedrich K, Welker B, Wahode J, van der Ven H, Al-Hasani S, et al. Transvaginal sonographically guided oocyte retrieval for in-vitro fertilization. Hum Reprod. 1988;3 Suppl 2:59-63.
6. Dellenbach P, Nisand I, Moreau L, Feger B, Plumere C, Gerlinger P, et al. Transvaginal sonographically controlled ovarian follicle puncture for egg retrieval. Lancet. 1984; 1(8392):1467.
7. Hamberger L, Wikland M. Clinical experience with ultrasound-guided follicle aspiration. In: Recent Progress in Human In Vitro Fertilization. Palermo: Cofese Ed; 1984.
8. Bennett SJ, Waterstone JJ, Cheng WC, Parsons J. Complications of transvaginal ultrasound-directed follicle aspiration: A review of 2,670 consecutive procedures. J Assist Reprod Genet. 1993;10(1):72-7.
9. Van Os HC, Roozenburg BJ, Janssen-Caspers HA, Leerentveld RA, Scholtes MCW, Zeilmaker GH, et al. Vaginal disinfection with povidine iodine and the outcome of in-vitro fertilisation. Hum Reprod. 1992;7(3):349-50.
10. Hannoun A, Awwad J, Zreik T, Ghaziri G, Abu-Musa A. Effect of betadine vaginal preparation during oocyte aspiration in in-vitro fertilisation cycles on pregnancy outcome. Gynaecol Obstet Invest. 2008;66(4):274-8.
11. Maxwell KN, Cholst IN, Rosenwaks Z. The incidence of both serious and minor complications in young women undergoing oocyte donation. Fertil Steril. 2008;90(6):2165-71.
12. Weinreb EB, Cholst IN, Ledger WJ, Danis RB, Rosenwaks Z. Should all oocyte donors receive prophylactic antibiotics for retrieval? Fertil Steril. 2010;94(7):2935-7.
13. Moini A, Riazi K, Amid V, Ashrafi M, Tehraninejad E, Madani T, et al. Endometriosis may contribute to oocyte retrieval-induced pelvic inflammatory disease: report of eight cases. J Assist Reprod Genet. 2005;22(7):307-9.
14. Romero B, Aibar L, Martínez Navarro L, Fontes J, Calderón MA, Mozas J. Pelvic abscess after oocyte retrieval in women with endometriosis: a case series. Iranian J Reprod Med. 2013;11(8):677-80.
15. Rolland L, Perrin J, Villes V, Pellegrin V, Boubli L, Courbiere B. IVF oocyte retrieval: prospective evaluation of the type of anesthesia on live birth rate, pain, and patient satisfaction. J Assist Reprod Genet. 2017;34(11):1523-8.
16. Gange SN, Baum NH. Verbal Anesthesia: How It's Used in Urologic Procedures. In Gonzalez CM. (ed). New York: Urology Times; 2017.
17. Kwan I, Bhattacharya S, Knox F, McNeil A. Pain relief for women undergoing oocyte retrieval for assisted reproduction. Cochrane Database Syst Rev. 2013;(1):CD004829.
18. Aziz N, Biljan MM, Taylor CT, Manasse PR, Kingsland CR. Effect of aspirating needle caliber on outcome of in-vitro fertilization. Hum Reprod. 1993;8(7):1098-100.
19. Wikland M, Blad S, Bungum L, Hillensjö T, Karlström PO, Nilsson S. A randomized controlled study comparing pain experience between a newly signed needle with a thin tip and a standard needle for oocyte aspiration. Hum Reprod. 2011;26(6):1377-83.
20. Rose BI. Follicle flushing for oocyte retrieval: targeted analysis for patients with few follicles. IVF Lite. 2014;1(2):75-80.
21. Rose BI. Approaches to oocyte retrieval for advanced reproductive technology cycles planning to utilize in vitro maturation: a review of the many choices to be made. J Assist Reprod Genet. 2014 Nov;31(11):1409-19. doi: 10.1007/s10815-014-0334-9. Epub 2014 Sep 12. PMID:25212532;PMCID: PMC4389947.
22. Lowe B, Osborn JC, Fothergill DJ, Lieberman BA. Factors associated with accidental fractures of the zona pellucida and multi-pronuclear human oocytes following in-vitro fertilization. Hum Reprod. 1988;3(7):901-4.
23. Mitroy J. Laminar and turbulent flows in pipes. Charles Darwin University, Australia. [online] Available from www.chu.edu.au/homepages/jmitroy/eng247/sec09.pdf. [Last accessed November 2022].
24. Sleigh PA. Fluid mechanics course, University of Leeds, England. [online] Available from www.efm.leeds.ac.uk/CIVE/CIVE1400/Section4/laminar_turbulent.htm. [Last accessed November 2022].
25. McQueen D, Boots CE, Jain T, Zhang JX, Robins J. Impact of aspiration pressure during oocyte retrieval. Fertile Steril. 2018;110(4):E241-2.
26. Benaglia L, Somigliana E, Iemmello R, Colpi E, Nicolosi AE, Ragni G. Endometrioma and oocyte retrieval-induced pelvic abscess: a clinical concern or an exceptional complication? Fertil Steril 2008;89(5):1263-6.
27. Kasapoglu I, Turk P, Dayan A, Uncu G. Does the presence of endometriosis cause a challenge for transvaginal oocyte retrieval? A comparison between patients with and without endometriosis. J Turk Ger Gynecol Assoc. 2018;19(3): 151-7.
28. Villette C, Bourret A, Santulli P, Gayet V, Chapron C, de Ziegler D. Risks of tubo-ovarian abscess in cases of endometrioma and assisted reproductive technologies are both under- and overreported. Fertil Steril. 2016;106(2):410-5.

29. Wood C, Trounson AO. Historical Perspectives of IVF. Handbook of In Vitro Fertilization, 2nd edition. New York: CRC Press; 2000. p. 4.
30. Hussein E, Balen AH, Tan SL. A prospective study comparing the outcome of oocytes retrieved in the aspirate with those retrieved in the flush during transvaginal ultrasound directed oocyte recovery for in-vitro fertilization. Br J Obstet Gynaecol. 1992;99(10):841-4.
31. Haines CJ, Emes AL, O'Shea RT, Weiss TJ. Choice of needle for ovum pickup. J In Vitro Fertil Embryo Transf. 1989;6(2): 111-2.
32. Haydardedeoglu B, Cok T, Kilicdag EB, Parlakgumus AH, Simsek E, Bagis T. In vitro fertilization-intracytoplasmic sperm injection outcomes in single- versus double-lumen oocyte retrieval needles in normally responding patients: a randomized trial. Fertil Steril. 2011;95(2):812-4.
33. Haydardedeoglu B, Gjemalaj F, Aytac PC, Kilicdag EB. Direct aspiration versus follicular flushing in poor responders undergoing intracytoplasmic sperm injection: a randomised controlled trial. Br J Obstet Gynaecol. 2017;124(8):1190-6.
34. Kara M, Aydin T, Turktekin N. Is follicular flushing really effective? A clinical study. Arch Gynecol Obstet.2012; 286(4):1061-4.
35. Kingsland CR, Taylor CT, Aziz N, Bickerton N. Is follicular flushing necessary for oocyte retrieval? A randomized trial. Hum Reprod. 1991;6(3):382-3.
36. Levens ED, Whitcomb BW, Payson MD, Larsen FW. Ovarian follicular flushing among low-responding patients undergoing assisted reproductive technology. Fertil Steril. 2009;91 Suppl 4:1381-4.
37. Mok-Lin E, Brauer AA, Schattman G, Zaninovic N, Rosenwaks Z, Spandorfer S. Follicular flushing and in vitro fertilization outcomes in the poorest responders: a randomized controlled trial. Hum Reprod. 2013;28(11):2990-5.
38. Tan SL, Waterstone J, Wren M, Parsons J. A prospective randomized study comparing aspiration only with aspiration and flushing for transvaginal ultrasound-directed oocyte recovery. Fertil Steril. 1992;58(2):356-60.
39. Georgiou EX, Melo P, Brown J, Granne IE. Follicular flushing during oocyte retrieval in assisted reproductive techniques. Cochrane Database Syst Rev. 2018;2018(4):CD004634.
40. Sun XF, Wang WH, Keefe DL. Overheating is detrimental to meiotic spindles within in vitro matured human oocytes. Zygote. 2004;12(1):65-70.
41. Wang WH, Meng L, Hackett R, Odenbourg R, Keefe DL. Limited recovery of meiotic spindles in living human oocytes after cooling-rewarming observed using polarized light microscopy. Hum Reprod. 2001;16(11):2374-8.
42. Almeida P, Bolton V. The effect of temperature fluctuations on the cytoskeletal organisation and chromosomal constitution of the human oocyte. Zygote. 1995;3(4):357-65.
43. Pickering SJ, Braude PR, Johnson MH, Cant A, Currie J. Transient cooling to room temperature can cause irreversible disruption of the meiotic spindle in the human oocyte. Fertil Steril. 1990;54(1):102-8.
44. Redding GP, Bronlund JE, Hart AL. The effects of IVF aspiration on the temperature, dissolved oxygen levels, and pH of follicular fluid. J Assist Reprod Genet. 2006;23:37-40.
45. Hyslop L, Prathalingam N, Nowak L, Fenwick J, Harbottle S, Byerley S, et al. A novel isolator-based system promotes viability of human embryos during laboratory processing. PLOS One. 2012;7(2):e31010.
46. Davis LB, Ginsburg ES. Transmyometrial oocyte retrieval and pregnancy rates. Fertil Steril. 2004;81(2):320-2.
47. Damario MA. Transabdominal-transperitoneal ultrasound-guided oocyte retrieval in a patient with müllerian agenesis. Fertil Steril. 2002;78(1):189-91.
48. Steigrad S, Hacker NF, Kolb B. In vitro fertilization surrogate pregnancy in a patient who underwent radical hysterectomy followed by ovarian transposition, lower abdominal wall radiotherapy, and chemotherapy. Fertil Steril. 2005;83(5): 1547-9.
49. Barton SE, Politch JA, Benson CB, Ginsburg ES, Gargiulo AR. Transabdominal follicular aspiration for oocyte retrieval in patients with ovaries inaccessible by transvaginal ultrasound. Fertil Steril. 2011;95(5):1773-6.
50. Weissbrot ES, Roman-Rodriguez C, Sung L. Transabdominal oocyte retrieval compared with the traditional transvaginal approach. Obstet Gynecol. 2014;123:190S.
51. Kupka MS, Ferraretti AP, de Mouzon J, Erb K, D'Hooghe T, Castilla JA, et al. Assisted reproductive technology in Europe, 2010: results generated from European registers by ESHRE. Hum Reprod. 2014;29(10):2099-113.
52. Von Eye Corleta H, Moretto M, D'Avila AM, Berger M. Immediate ureterovaginal fistula secondary to oocyte retrieval—a case report. Fertil Steril. 2008;90(5):2006.e1-3.
53. Pappin C, Plant G. A pelvic pseudoaneurysm (a rare complication of oocyte retrieval for IVF) treated by arterial embolization. Hum Fertil (Camb). 2006;9(3):153-5.
54. Bozdag G, Basaran A, Cil B, Esinler I, Yarali H. An oocyte pick-up procedure complicated with pseudoaneurysm of the internal iliac artery. Fertil Steril. 2008;90(5):2004.e11-3.
55. Grynberg M, Berwanger AL, Toledano M, Frydman R, Deffieux X, Fanchin R. Ureteral injury after transvaginal ultrasound-guided oocyte retrieval: a complication of in vitro fertilization-embryo transfer that may lurk undetected in women presenting with severe ovarian hyperstimulation syndrome. Fertil Steril. 2011;96(4):869-71.
56. Fiori O, Cornet D, Darai E, Antoine JM, Bazot M. Uro-retroperitoneum after ultrasound-guided transvaginal follicle puncture in an oocyte donor: a case report. Hum Reprod. 2006;21(11):2969-71.
57. Jayakrishnan K, Raman VK, Vijayalakshmi VK, Baheti S, Nambiar D. Massive hematuria with hemodynamic instability-complication of oocyte retrieval. Fertil Steril. 2011; 96(1):e22-4.
58. Modder J, Kettel LM, Sakamoto K. Hematuria and clot retention after transvaginal oocyte aspiration: a case report. Fertil Steril. 2006;86(3):720.e1-2.
59. Sharpe K, Karovitch AJ, Claman P, Suh KN. Transvaginal oocyte retrieval for in vitro fertilization complicated by ovarian abscess during pregnancy. Fertil Steril. 2006;86(1):219.e11-3.
60. Levi-Setti PE, Cirillo F, Scolaro V, Morenghi E, Heilbron F, Girardello D, et al. Appraisal of clinical complications after 23,827 oocyte retrievals in a large assisted reproductive technology program. Fertil Steril. 2018;109(6):1038-43.

CHAPTER 57

Embryo Transfer

Arya Rajendran, Akanksha Gautam Allahbadia, Swati Gautam Allahbadia, Gautam Allahbadia

INTRODUCTION

Embryo transfer (ET) is the final and most critical event in the success of a medically assisted reproduction (MAR) cycle. Very few advances have occurred in the last few decades with regard to this procedure and studies conducted thus far have focused on factors and interventions taking place before, during, and after this procedure. These factors are highly varied and range from methods to improve the psychological state of the patients to methods aimed at reducing uterine contractility and methods aimed at optimizing the precise transfer of the embryo.[1] Several factors preceding and during ET are instrumental in successfully performing an ET, including catheter type, degree of trauma, and ultrasound visualization.

There is good evidence to support an atraumatic transfer, ultrasound guidance,[2-7] the use of soft catheters[8] and echogenic catheters,[9-11] the significance of depth of transfer,[12-14] and the experience of the clinician performing ET,[15-17] in optimizing pregnancy and implantation rates. There has been improvement in different facets of assisted reproductive techniques such as in embryo culture and assessment of viability. With improved pregnancy and live birth rates (LBR), the onus has come on to reducing the complications including multiple gestations, leading to popularization of single ETs.[18-21] Technique of ET demands a detailed insight to optimize the pregnancy outcome. This chapter aims to elucidate clearly the various aspects regarding ET and the evidence to optimize the results.

DEFINITION OF EMBRYO TRANSFER

Embryo transfer is the accurate and atraumatic deposition of embryos by means of an ET catheter, into the uterine cavity at an area with maximum implantation potential.[22]

TYPES OF EMBRYO TRANSFER

Transvaginal Transcervical

- Embryos are passed through the ET catheter, which is inserted transcervically.
- *Advantage:* Most widely used method and also the simplest and least invasive.
- *Disadvantage:* In case of cervical stenosis, this method is not feasible.

Transvaginal Transmyometrial

- *Method:* A transvaginal ultrasound probe is inserted in the vagina and a "Towako" ET catheter (Cook, Queensland, and Australia) is used. The 18-gauge catheter needle with stylet is passed under transvaginal ultrasound guidance, passing through the anterior fornix and anterior myometrial wall, and stopping short of the myoendometrial junction. In case of retroverted (RV) uterus, the needle punctures through posterior fornix and posterior myometrial wall. After removal of stylet, preloaded inner catheter is threaded through the needle and the embryos are released.
- *Advantage:* This is performed in patients with extremely difficult or impossible transcervical ET.
- *Disadvantage:* Increased uterine manipulation triggers greater junctional zone contractions.[23]

Zygote Intrafallopian Transfer

- Involves laparoscopic delivery of embryos into the fallopian tube.
- *Advantages:*
  - Advocated in patients with nontubal infertility with repeated implantation failure (RIF). Since the fallopian tubes provide a more physiological environment for embryos to grow compared to in vitro culture systems.
  - No uterine manipulation, hence lesser myometrial contractions and less chances of embryo expulsion. Of special benefit in patients whose embryos consistently show poor in vitro development.
  - Higher pregnancy rates (PRs) have been documented in patients with RIF (25.5%).

- *Disadvantages:*
    - Surgical as well as anesthetic risks
    - Higher risk of tubal ectopic gestation[24]
    - No longer practiced.

Subendometrial Embryo Delivery

- *Method:* A light flexible tip hysteroscope is used to deliver embryos subendometrially (depth of 1 mm) at a favorable site (where the endometrium is thickest, at least 2 cm away from ostia). Nitrogen, an inert and non-embryotoxic gas, is used for uterine distension instead of CO_2.
- *Advantages:* Subendometrial deposition improves the chance for implantation, eliminates the possibility of ectopic gestation, prevents inadvertent excessive endometrial trauma that can happen in usual transcervical transfer, the mild endometrial injury can induce inflammation, and be favorable for implantation.
- *Disadvantage:* Inadvertent excessive endometrial injury.[25]

HOW TO PLAN A GOOD EMBRYO TRANSFER?

A good ET involves placement of a single good quality embryo in a primed endometrium, in the most atraumatic way, at the region of maximum implantation potential.

The optimal endometrial thickness has been described as 9–14 mm.[26] Following the achievement of optimal thickness, progesterone therapy is instituted, which can be either by vaginal or intramuscular route.

With timely progesterone level, a synchrony of activities is set in motion within the endometrium to optimize receptivity toward the embryo. The receptive period lasts only for a brief period of time known as the window of implantation (WOI).

Cleavage stage embryo is transferred on the 4th day of progesterone supplementation (P + 3 corresponds to the 3rd day of embryonic development) and blastocyst is transferred on the 6th day of progesterone supplementations (P + 5 corresponds to 5th day of embryonic development).

Steps of Embryo Transfer

Steps of ET are given in **Flowchart 1**.

FACTORS AFFECTING SUCCESS OF EMBRYO TRANSFER

Prior to Embryo Transfer

Uterine Cavity Evaluation

Cavity evaluation before ET would give an insight into cavitary abnormalities and provide opportunity to correct these. Hysteroscopy revealed 22.9% incidence of cavitary abnormalities and there is benefit for resection of submucosal fibroids, adhesions, and polyps. A three-dimensional (3D) saline sonohysterography is also useful in this regard.[27]

Uterine Position

Uterine position, anteverted (AV) or RV, should be known before the ET to prevent misdirecting the ET catheter. The uterine position is subject to changes between a mock transfer and the real ET.[28]

Mock Transfer

- ET aims to deposit the embryos gently with least trauma into the chosen portion of uterine cavity with maximum implantation potential.
- *Purpose:* Mock ETs are performed to assess the level of difficulty to be anticipated in the actual ET and modify the depth and direction of transfer accordingly. Anatomical deviations in cervix, cervical polyps, and fibroids, if any, can also be dealt with.
- *Timing:* The ideal timing to perform a mock transfer is just before the actual ET. Care must be taken to never go >0.5 cm beyond the internal os and this mock ET is always done under ultrasound guidance.
- *Cervical dilatation prior to ET:* Any unexpected cervical stenosis can be tackled prior to ET by cervical dilatation. Cervical dilatation done weeks prior to transfer can help in healing of any inadvertent endometrial injury caused by the same and has higher PRs than cervical dilatation during the hormone replacement therapy (HRT) cycle or during the procedure itself.[29] Hysteroscopic dilatation of the cervical canal results in easier ET in patients with cervical stenosis and history of difficult ET.[8]
- *Mock transfer at the time of ET:* The afterloading technique of ET can be also regarded as a form of mock transfer that is performed at the time of ET. The empty outer catheter is placed at or just beyond the internal os. The embryo loaded inner sheath is then introduced into the outer catheter. There is minimizing of the time that the embryo spends outside the incubator and till it is placed in uterus (ideally <120 seconds) and possibly reduced trauma to endometrium.
- *Pitfalls of mock transfers:* The uterine orientation can change from the time of mock transfer to the time of actual ET. For example, a RV uterus can become AV following heavy ovaries resting posterior to uterus following ovarian stimulation in cases of fresh ETs.

Borkar et al.'s very recent study concluded that mock embryo transfer (MET) prior to a first in vitro fertilization (IVF) cycle may not improve the success rate in young women without risk factors for a difficult ET.[30]

Embryo Quality

A significant factor that is pivotal in deciding whether to proceed with ET at all and its success thereafter is the embryo quality. Though a crude morphological assessment of the embryo does not give a sufficient insight into the viability and developmental potential of the embryo,

Flowchart 1: Steps of embryo transfer (ET).

Counseling and consent: The patient is informed about the fertilization rate, embryo stage, number and grading. Informed decision is taken regarding embryos to be transferred or frozen. After discussion between physician and the couple, informed consent forms (ICMR forms) are verified

↓

One milliliter syringe is used for ET, the nozzle of which is attached to ET catheter. The syringe is initially flushed with 500 microliters of transfer media, to ensure that there are no air bubbles

↓

The syringe is then attached with inner soft ET catheter, ensuring a tight seal. The inner catheter is again flushed with media to equilibrate the inner lining

↓

Embryos are selected from the cleavage plate. The selected embryos are transferred to well 1 of 4 well plates to remove oil. The embryos are quickly moved to well 2 and 3, followed by loading into the inner catheter

↓

The loaded inner catheter is held horizontally with gloved hands in a cupped fashion to prevent exposure to cold air currents

↓

The outer ET catheter is introduced through the cervix to stop short of the internal os under USG guidance and is stabilized with help of hypothenar eminence

↓

Embryologist brings the loaded inner catheter and then the inner catheter is introduced into the outer catheter and inserted up to mid-cavity of uterus and is stopped at 1–2 cm short of the fundus (For afterloading technique) (In case of preloading technique, syringe is attached to the inner catheter which is already placed within the outer catheter and embryos are loaded and handed over to physician for transfer)

↓

Catheter is left in situ for 30–60 seconds. Pressure is kept on the plunger of the syringe while slowly withdrawing the catheter out avoiding negative pressure

↓

The catheter is handed over horizontally to the embryologist. The inner catheter is flushed with culture media and the flushed fluid is observed for retained embryos. The outer catheter is withdrawn from cervix after the embryologist confirms that there is no retained embryo within the inner catheter

(ICMR: Indian Council of Medical Research; USG: ultrasonography)

nevertheless, it may be used as an index for further noninvasive evaluation.

Embryo selection is aided by morphological appearance of the embryos and various metabolic and protein markers present in culture media.[20] Computer-assisted scoring system (CASS) has the potential to overcome the disadvantages with standard embryo evaluation and can predict PR and LBR better than with the standard scoring system.[31] Time-lapse imaging makes it possible to know the timing of embryo cleavage and to predict the time of implantation.[31] Blastocyst culture is yet another means of evaluating the viability and developmental potential of the embryo. Blastocyst culture helps to achieve better uterine and embryonic synchronicity and natural selection of more viable embryos, culminating in higher implantation rates.[32] However, the use of prolonged culture hinges upon the number of available embryos, infrastructural facilities, and cost issues.

Selective single embryo transfer (SSET) cycle in women under 35 years is reported to yield higher rate of "healthy baby" per transfer compared to transfer of two embryos.[33] Trophectoderm biopsy and chromosome screening with array CGH (comparative genomic hybridization) reduce the miscarriage rates, thereby providing a way to eliminate multiple gestation without compromising on the LBR.[34]

Assessing the viability of a blastocyst is still empirical and was yet nonreproducible. Badiola et al. recently developed an algorithm based on artificial vision and machine learning (and other classifiers) that predicts pregnancy from both the morphology of an embryo and the age of the patients.[35] They created a system consisting of different classifiers that is fed with novel morphometric features extracted from the digital microphotographs, along with other non-morphometric data to predict pregnancy. It was evaluated using five different classifiers: Probabilistic Bayesian, support vector machines (SVMs), deep neural network, decision tree, and random forest (RF), using a k-fold cross validation to assess the model's generalization capabilities. Their results suggest that the system is able to predict a positive pregnancy test from a single digital image, offering a novel approach with the advantages of using a small database, being highly adaptable to different laboratory settings, and with easy integration into clinical practice.

Experience of the Physician

- The experience of the clinician in conducting an ET is among the most significant factors that influence the success rates of ART. For experienced physicians, choice of transfer catheter, difficult transfer, and blood on catheter do not cause significant reduction in pregnancy outcomes.[35] When different physicians used the same method of ET and similar number of embryos transferred, variation in PR was observed suggesting the importance of physician factor.[15] Hence, the resident physicians must be better monitored to avoid the lower PRs.[16]
- A cross-sectional survey was done by a specialized cell of the American Society for Reproductive Medicine (ASRM) to better understand practice patterns and opportunities for standardization of ET.[36] An anonymous 82-question survey was emailed to the Medical Directors of 286 IVF practices. A follow-up survey composed of three questions specific to the ET technique was emailed to the same Medical Directors. Descriptive statistics of the results were compiled. The survey assessed policies, protocols, restrictions, and specifics pertinent to the technique of ET. The study concluded that improved training and standardization based on outcomes data and best practices are warranted. A common practice procedure is suggested for validation by a systematic literature review.

Ramaiah et al. assessed the value of the American Society for Reproductive Medicine Embryo Transfer Certificate Course in confidence and skill-building for performing a live ET.[37] The main study outcomes included ET simulation scores of all exercises analyzed at various points of the training and self-assessed confidence before and after the completion of the Embryo Transfer Certificate Course based on a six-point Likert scale and association of both with the extent of prior live ET experience and year of their Reproductive Endocrinology and Infertility (REI) fellowship. The American Society for Reproductive Medicine Embryo Transfer Certificate Course data analysis demonstrated the effectiveness of simulator-based ET training for REI fellows across their 3 years of training, regardless of prior experience with live ET.

A recent study by McQueen et al. revealed striking differences between fellowship programs regarding the adequacy of ET training; nearly one-half of third-year fellows had performed fewer than 10 ETs.[38] The findings expounded that with appropriate supervision, there was no difference in LBR between ETs performed by fellows in training and attending physicians. Efforts should be made to set right barriers and set a compulsory minimum numbers of ETs for the trainees during their fellowship.

Continued performance analysis and the use of a digital simulator could help operators to test their expertise over time and either correct poor performance or avoid doing transfers.[39]

Role of Uterine Relaxants

Implantation failure is the main factor affecting the success rates of MAR. Studies have elucidated that uterine contractions (UCs) at the time of ET were inversely related to implantation and PR, hence bringing down PRs.

- Progesterone, beta-mimetics (ritodrine), and anti-prostaglandins (piroxicam, aspirin) have all been assessed for utility in depressing UCs. Only progesterone has been proven to have a uterine-relaxing effect.[40]
- Atosiban is vasopressin V1a and oxytocin receptor blocker that suppresses UCs. Routinely used in arresting preterm labor, it has found application during ET to prevent or ablate UCs. Studies have shown that in the general population of women undergoing IVF, atosiban enhances PRs but not LBR. In contrast, among women with recurrent implantation failure, atosiban improves both PR and LBR.[41-43]
  The findings of a recent study by Zarei et al. concluded that piroxicam administration before ET has no beneficial effects on PR among women undergoing IVF and frozen-thawed ET.[44] Various pharmacological agents, with the exception of calcium channel blockers, have been investigated to improve ET outcomes by reducing uterine activity. A double-blinded randomized, placebo-controlled trial was set up to determine whether nifedipine, a calcium channel blocker with potent smooth muscle relaxing activity and an excellent safety profile, can improve the outcome of patients undergoing ET.[45] 93 infertile women were recruited into one of two groups: placebo (n = 47) or nifedipine 20 mg (n = 46). The current double-blinded, randomized, and placebo-controlled trial clearly showed that the single use of 20 mg nifedipine given 30 minutes before ET did not improve implantation rates nor clinical PRs.
- *Role of adjuncts in ET*: Acupuncture is also used extensively as an adjunct during ET procedure. It involves passing several fine needles into the skin in a systematic pattern to alter the flow of energy in the body. A number of randomized controlled trials (RCTs) have been published to evaluate the role of acupuncture in ET with contradictory results. ASRM 2017 guidelines state that there is fair amount of evidence that acupuncture at the

time of ET does not improve LBR in IVF. Similarly, there is insufficient evidence to recommend massage therapy and transcutaneous electrical acupoint stimulation as adjuncts in ET.

Antibiotics Prior to Embryo Transfer

Vaginal or cervical microbial presence, especially *Enterobacteriaceae* and *Staphylococcus*, has been associated with reduced PRs, probably due to subclinical infection of endometrium.[46] Other isolated microorganisms do not impact the PRs significantly.[47] Though antibiotics (amoxicillin and clavulanic acid) prior to ET significantly reduce upper genital tract and catheter contamination rates, the routine use of antibiotics at ET did not translate into better outcomes such as clinical PRs.[48,49] Future research evaluating different antibiotic regimens and their impact on live birth and microbial colonization is warranted.

Hamdoun et al.'s study from Tunisia suggested that contamination of the transfer catheter by cervical passage decreases IVF results.[50] Prophylactic antibiotic prophylaxis should be used to reduce this negative impact.

During Embryo Transfer

- Anesthesia or analgesia is not routinely required for ET. Use of analgesics can improve patient comfort but are not beneficial in improving the PR (ASRM, 2017).
- *Position of patient:* In earlier days, position of patient during ET was based on uterine version. In case of AV uterus, knee chest position was practiced and dorsal position for RV uterus. However, the position of patient has not shown to influence the PRs and hence dorsal position with lithotomy is practiced commonly.[51]
- *Physician preparation:* Both powdered and non-powdered gloves are toxic to embryos when direct contact is established. The propensity for air-borne powder from gloves to harm embryos has been studied by a single RCT. There is fair evidence that powdered gloves do not impact embryos during ET. No particular glove is recommended as such for the ET procedure.[52]
- *Cervical mucus:* Removal of cervical mucus is an essential step in ET procedure since the presence of mucus can block the lumen of catheter and prevent the deposition of embryos in uterus as well as displace the embryos inadvertently within the cavity. Sterile gauze or cotton dipped in IVF media can be used to clean the cervical mucus. More persistent mucus especially from endocervix can be aspirated gently with a plastic syringe or by using a cytobrush. Alternatively, cervix can be flushed with culture medium. All manipulations should be of utmost care and gentleness in order to not to elicit UCs by excessive provocation. Removal of cervical mucus has been shown to have a higher PR.[53]

EMBRYO TRANSFER CATHETERS

The ET catheter has been shown in **Figure 1**.

What is an ideal catheter like?

- Soft and flexible:
  - Nontraumatic so as to not to produce any endometrial lesion. The reduction in success rate for a less experienced physician performing the transfer as compared to a well-experienced physician is directly correlated to endometrial lesions produced during the transfer. Hence, a nontraumatic catheter can reduce the endometrial lesions and improve the success rate.
  - Soft catheters induce less UCs especially when combined with the correct technique of not touching the fundus.
- Non-embryotoxic material
- Free of bacterial endotoxins
- Must be easy to maneuver inside the uterine cavity
- Must be clearly visible on ultrasound so that the depth of placement of embryos can be clearly assessed (desired depth being 15–20 mm from fundus).

Types of Embryo Transfer Catheters

Commercially available catheters can be divided into two major groups and are given in **Table 1**.

Meta-analysis of prospective RCTs compared soft versus rigid ET catheters and found statistically significant difference in clinical PR as well as birth rate in favor of soft

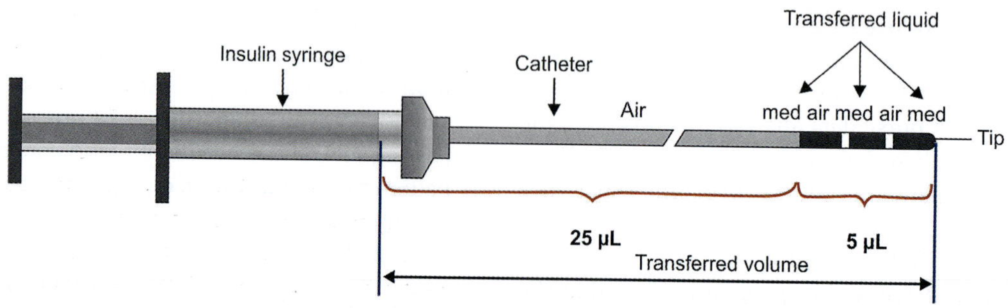

Fig. 1: Inner catheter with syringe.

TABLE 1: Types of embryo transfer catheters.

Soft ET catheters	*Firm (rigid) ET catheters*
(Including echogenic catheters)—Cook (Cook Ob/Gyn, Inc, Bloomington, OH) and Wallace catheters (Marlow Technologies, Willoughby, OH)	TDT (Laboratoire CCD, Paris), Frydman (Laboratoire CCCD), Tomcat (Kendell Healthcare, Hampshire, MA), Tefcat (Kendell Healthcare), and Rocket ET Catheters (Rocket Medical, Tyne and Wear, UK)

catheters.[54] Still rigid catheters cannot be overlooked as they often find use in difficult transfers where the os cannot be negotiated by a soft catheter.[55]

Components of embryo transfer catheter:

- Outer sheath or outer catheter also called guiding catheter—a thick hollow plastic tube (catheter) with a bulb, stopper, and markings (OD—2.5 mm).
  - Bulb—helps to bypass the blind endocervical crypts, which line the cervical canal and can cause the tip of the catheter to get trapped
  - Stopper—for depth adjustment
  - Markings—for easy positioning.
- Obturator or stylet also called mandrel—fits snuggly within the outer sheath allows to preshape the outer sheath—can negotiate the curvature of the endocervix. For difficult ET, OD—1 mm.
- Inner sheath also called transfer or loading catheter—a soft tube, with markings at distal end of the tip. Soft to minimize trauma to endometrium. The embryologist loads embryos into this sheath and then hands this to the doctor (OD—1.6 mm).
  - Handle with Luer lock fitting for secure connection to syringes
  - Total volume—0.2 mL
  - Sterilized with radiation.

POPULAR COMMERCIALLY AVAILABLE EMBRYO TRANSFER CATHETERS

- SureView **(Fig. 2)**:
  - Outer catheter—firm made of Teflon
  - 19 cm long
  - Inner catheter—23 cm long, made of polyethylene
  - External diameter of 1.6 mm (OD) with an open end
  - Visible under ultrasound from hub to tip
  - Highly visible in simulated uterine environment
  - Increased confidence of direction and position of the uterus
  - Optimal placement of catheter in the uterus
  - More accurate positioning for embryo expulsion.
- *Wallace-Smith Medicals:* Four types of Wallace-Smith Medicals are follows:
  - Classic **(Figs. 3A and B)**
  - SurePro **(Fig. 4)**
  - SurePro ultra **(Fig. 5)**
  - SureView.

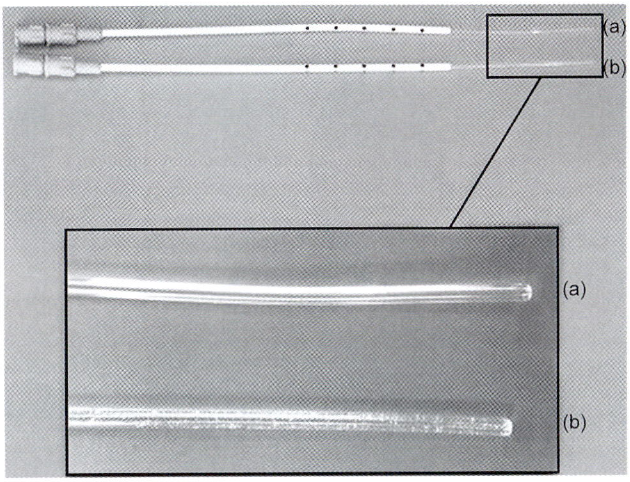

Fig. 2: Difference between standard and SureView Wallace catheters—small air bubbles are present in the wall of inner SureView catheter.

- Cooks catheter **(Fig. 6)**:
  - A double lumen catheter set
  - The guiding (outer) catheter is 19 cm long, has a polycarbonate hub, a bulb tip, and the distal end is angled.
  - The transfer (inner) catheter is 23 cm long and the tip is 2.8 French size.
  - The base of the transfer catheter fits onto a 1.0 mL plastic syringe.
  - Precurved guiding catheter facilitates catheter insertion.
  - Atraumatic bulb tip eases passage through cervix.
  - MicroVol® technology reduces medium volume required for ET.
  - Cervical stop comes set at 4 cm with additional stop at 5 cm.
- Gynetics **(Figs. 7A and B)**:
  - It uses a combination of a soft, flexible intrauterine catheter, and a solid cervix catheter.
  - *Types:* Emtrac—combination of soft and rigid catheters
  - Semtrac—soft catheters and Tulip—soft catheters with bulb at tip.
- Frydman rigid catheters **(Fig. 8)**:
  - The Frydman catheter is a polyethylene open-ended catheter with an external diameter of 1.6 mm.
  - It has a 4.5 cm soft distal part and a 12.5 cm more rigid proximal part, and is graduated at 5.5 and 6.5 cm distances from the tip.

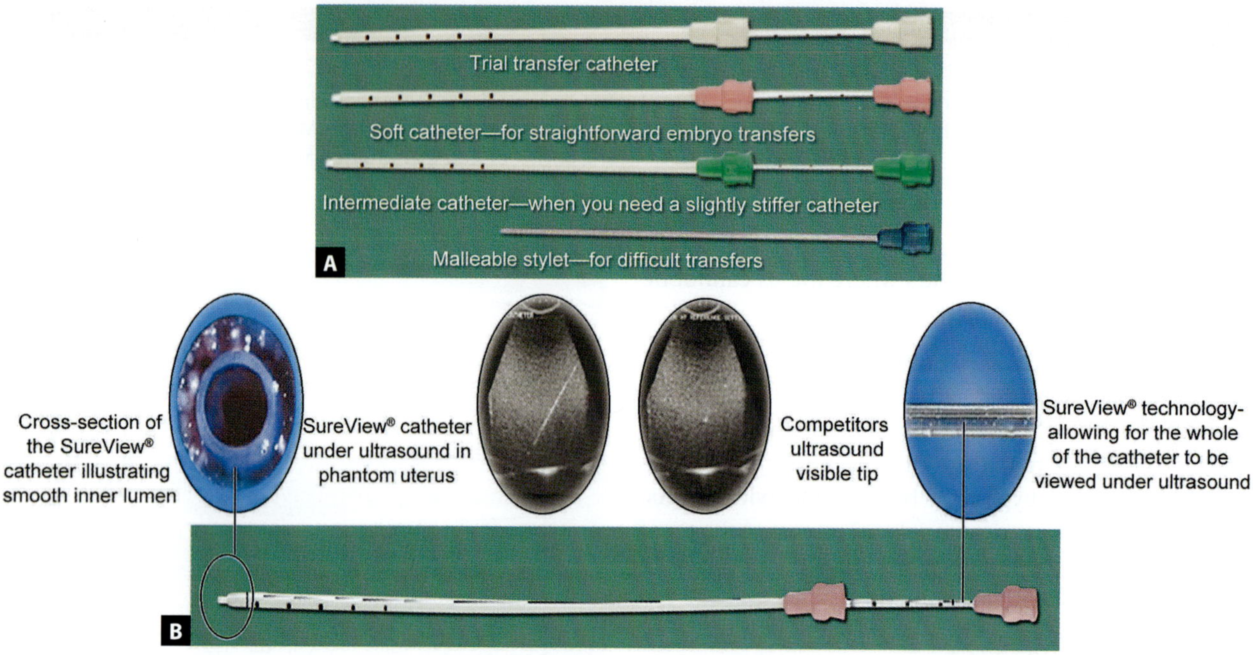

Figs. 3A and B: Classic Wallace–Smith medicals.

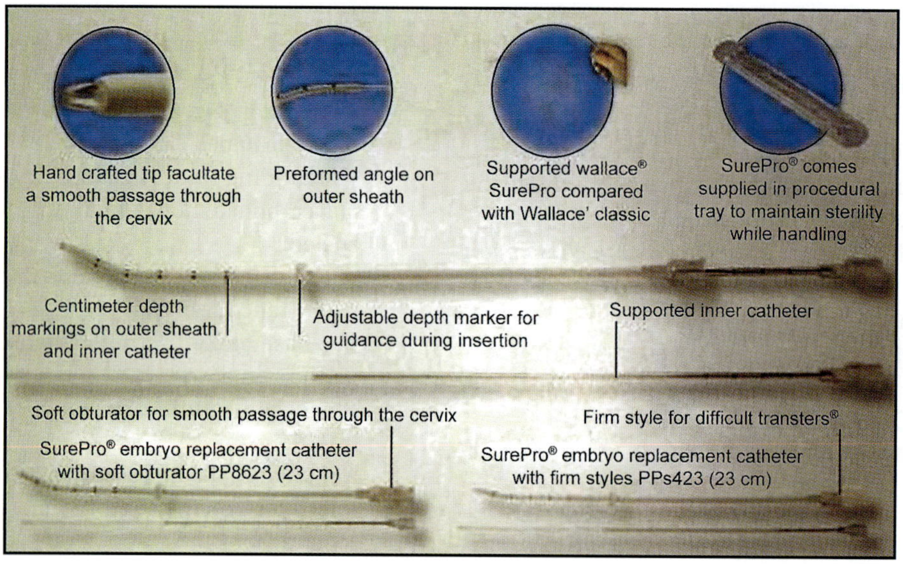

Fig. 4: Wallace SurePro medicals.

- There are several disadvantages for rigid catheters:
  - Bleeding due to disturbed endometrium
  - Trauma to cervical os
  - Incitement of UCs
  - Mucus plugging of catheter tip
  - Possibility of retained embryos.
- Labotect ET catheters **(Fig. 9)**:
  - Available in three lengths, i.e., 15, 19, and 23 cm
  - Labotect is an intermediate catheter.
  - It can be inserted without a malleable stylet.
  - Its unique curved stiff outer sheet with a ball-shaped spherical tip allows negotiation with difficult cervix more easily compared to soft ET catheters.
- Guardia™ proprotective ET catheter (**Figs. 10A and B**):
  - Designed to allow the controlled passage of embryos through cervical mucus and blood.
  - An outer sheath that protects the embryo through the cervix and then opens in petals to further advance the inner catheter and gently place the embryo.

An Egyptian study compared the use of semirigid and flexible catheters in terms of PR and level of difficulty of the ET procedure. The results suggested that a softer catheter may help with difficult ETs[56] and resulted in better implantation rates, while some authors reported significantly higher pregnancy and implantation rates with the ultrasoft catheter compared to the more rigid catheter.[8] The presence of blood

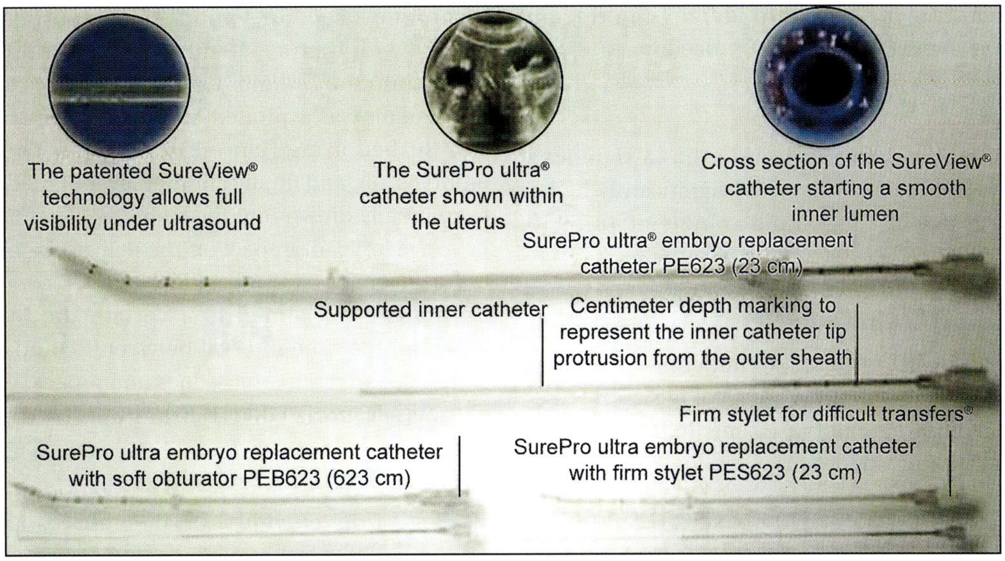

Fig. 5: Wallace SurePro ultra medicals.

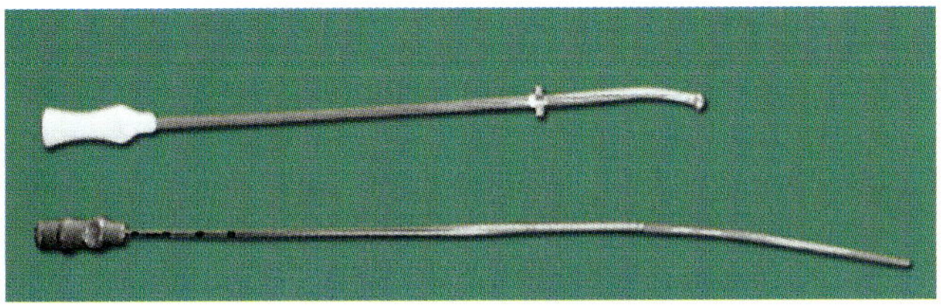

Fig. 6: Cooks catheter.

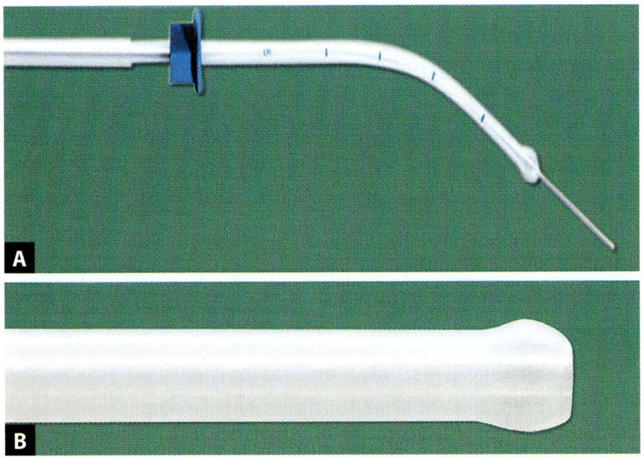

Figs. 7A and B: Gynetics.

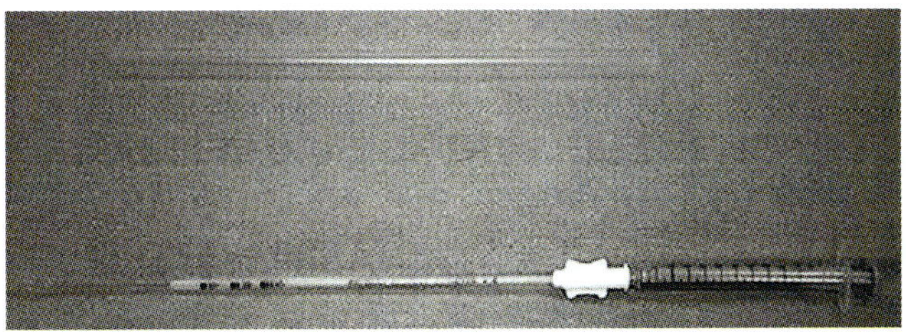

Fig. 8: Frydman rigid catheters.

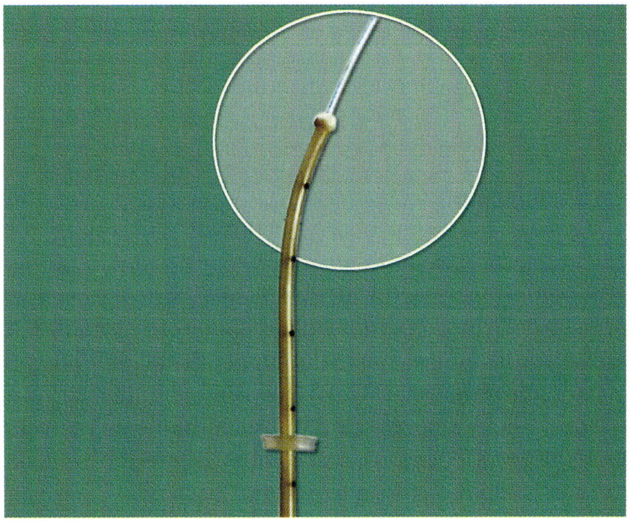

Fig. 9: Labotect embryo transfer catheters.

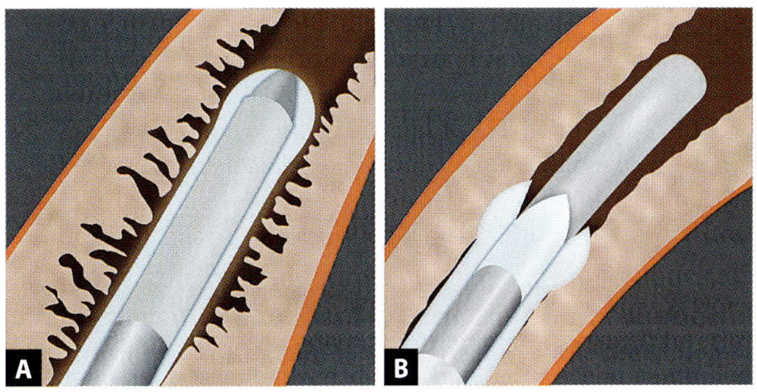

Figs. 10A and B: Guardia™ pro protective embryo transfer catheter.

on the catheter signaled severe endometrial injury. Severe endometrial lesions were less frequent when soft catheters were used. Echogenic catheters offer better visualization owing to the ultrasonic contrast properties, minimizing the need for catheter movement to identify the tip, and significantly shorter duration of the ET procedure.

Fluid Volume

The amount of fluid volume for transfer has a significant clinical impact. Montag et al. reported significantly higher PR following the use of a high-fluid volume of 40–50 μL compared to 15–20 μL.[57]

Embryo Loading Techniques (Fig. 11)

- Embryo loading (EL) is a stage immediately prior to ET and is performed by the embryologist. Preferred method is medium-air-embryo-air-medium, followed by medium in catheter with embryo, medium-air embryo, etc.
- There are several crucial choices in this procedure such as choice of syringe, the volume of transfer medium, the concentration of proteins, the catheter loading speed, the viscosity of the transfer medium, and embryo placement in the catheter. Among them, the volume of medium and the presence of an air bubble are very much debated.
- Meta-analysis has shown that the use of air brackets was neither beneficial nor detrimental when compared to the fluid—only technique of EL.[58]

Embryo loading probably affects the success of IVF. The study of Halvaei et al. compared the impact of two different techniques of EL on PR in IVF or ET cycles.[59] In Group A, the embryos were drawn directly into the ET catheter from culture microdrop under the oil. In Group B, the embryos were transferred from culture microdrop into G2 medium in center-well dish. Then, the embryos were drawn into the catheter and finally transferred into the uterus. Clinical pregnancy was higher in Group B compared to A, but the difference was insignificant, proving that there is no difference in the outcome by loading the embryo from microdrop or center-well dish.[59]

Omidi et al. compared two different EL techniques.[60] Two groups (A and B) were defined based on the EL technique used. In Group A, the entire catheter was flushed with Ham's F-10 medium. The embryos were then drawn into the catheter using one air bracket. In group B, 70 μL of air was aspirated into the syringe and the catheter was flushed using Ham's F10 medium. The medium, air, embryos, air, and finally another layer of medium were then sequentially drawn into the catheter. EL techniques did not have a significant impact on the delivery rate in either fresh or frozen embryo transfer (FET) cycles.[60]

Nouri et al. aimed to ascertain the influence of EL time and the time interval between EL and ET. The paper concluded that time to ET does not impact IVF or intracytoplasmic sperm injection (ICSI).[61]

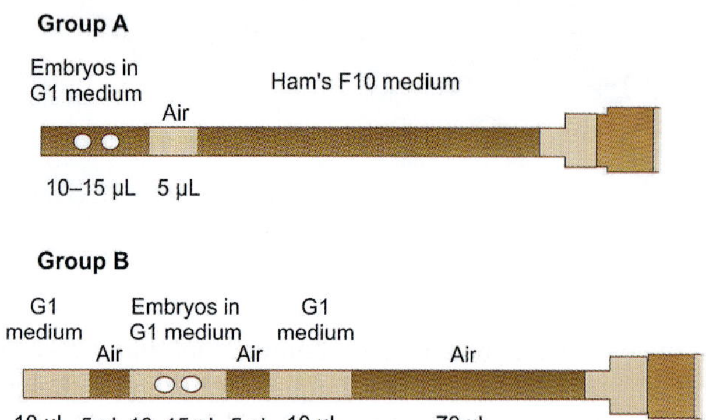

Fig. 11: Embryo loading techniques.

Embryo Transfer Techniques

- *Preloading of embryos:* The embryos are loaded into the transfer catheter by the embryologist by one of the methods described above and the loaded catheter is handed over to the physician. The embryos are deposited around 2.0 cm from the fundus under transabdominal scan (TAS) guidance. After approximately 5 seconds, the catheter is gently rotated 180° and removed, keeping the plunger of the catheter depressed until it has been entirely removed. The embryologist immediately flushes the catheter and checks for any retained embryo.
- *After loading of embryos:* This is a newer technique and was initially introduced in cases where difficult transfer is expected and also as a kind of mock transfer being performed at the time of actual ET. An empty Wallace catheter is passed to the level of the lower uterine segment under ultrasound guidance to a point just at the level of internal os, where the inner catheter enters the endometrial cavity, typically about 5 cm. The inner sheath is gradually removed, leaving the outer sheath just beyond the internal os. A second inner sheath already loaded with embryos by an embryologist is threaded into the catheter. The inner catheter is slowly advanced by the physician and the embryos are deposited 2.0 cm from the fundus. After approximately 5–10 seconds, the catheter is gently rotated and taken out.[62]
  - Advantages of after-loading of embryos:
    - It allows slow and gentle passage of catheter through the endocervix, reducing the duration of time that embryo remains in room condition (ideally this should be <120 seconds).
    - Embryos in the inner sheath are not exposed to the mucus in the cervix.

A very recent elegant study by Setti et al. suggested that the afterload technique seems to reduce the rate of difficult ETs.[63]

Ultrasound Guidance versus Clinical Touch

The ability to perform ET procedure under direct ultrasound visualization is a significant advancement in the field of

ART and an indispensable technology for ART practitioners. Both transabdominal (TA)[2-5] and transvaginal[6] ultrasound-guided transfers have been shown to increase PR and LBR in contrast to clinical touch method.[2-6]

A study measured the embryo-fundus distance (EFD) using transvaginal ultrasonogram performed immediately after ET. An EFD between 5 mm and 15 mm got significantly higher PR than an EFD above 15 mm. The abortion rate was much higher when EFD was below 5 mm than when it was between 5 mm and 15 mm. Ultrasound-guided ET could be advantageous compared to clinical-touch ET, as it allows to be more accurate in releasing embryos within the optimal EFD range.[64] PRs and ongoing PRs are higher if the embryos are replaced at a distance >10 mm from the fundal endometrial surface under ultrasound guidance. In addition, because significantly more embryos were replaced in cycles where the transfers occurred at a distance of >20 mm, a distance >10 mm to <20 mm seems to be the best site for ET to achieve higher PRs.[65]

The advantages of ultrasound-guided ET include:

- Facilitates placement of soft catheters leading to reduced requirement of use of tenaculum and less often presence of blood or mucus in the catheter tip[66]
- Avoids touching the fundus
- Enables evaluation of the uterine position, AV, or RV, during ET, thus facilitates catheter negotiation
- *Estimation of the cavity depth:* Pope et al.[12] suggest that the cavity depth by ultrasound is clinically useful to determine the depth beyond which catheter insertion should not occur.
- Confirms that the catheter is beyond the internal os in cases of an elongated cervical canal.
- Allows direction of the catheter along the contour of the endometrial cavity, thereby avoiding disruption of the endometrium, plugging of the catheter tip with endometrium, and instigation of bleeding.
- Full bladder required to perform TA ultrasound guidance is itself helpful in straightening the cervical uterine access and improving PRs.
- May facilitate an uncomplicated access through the cervix to access the uterine cavity, thus overcoming cervical stenosis.[5]

Both transvaginal ultrasound-guided ET and TA ultrasound-guided procedure yield similar pregnancy outcomes. Total time taken for transfer was significantly higher in the TVS group, whereas the TA-guided procedure reported increased patient discomfort due to the presence of bladder distension.[67]

3D ultrasound should not be currently recommended as a strategy to improve clinical outcomes in women undergoing ART treatment.[68]

Revelli et al. compared transvaginal ultrasound-guided uterine length measurement before transfer (ULMbET) with TA-UGET.[56] The ULMbET technique leads to IVF results comparable to those obtained with UGET and is better tolerated and easier to perform for a single physician.[69]

Depth of Embryo Transfer

Transfer distance from fundus (TDF) significantly affects PRs with 11% increase in PR for every millimeter that the embryos are deposited more away from the fundus.[12] Tiras et al. also reported higher pregnancy and ongoing PRs when embryos were replaced at a distance >10 mm from the fundal endometrial surface suggesting that a distance 10–20 mm seems to be the best site for ET to achieve higher PRs.[65] The objective of Santos et al.'s study was to determine the influence of the embryo placement depth on the endometrial cavity in relation to the reproductive outcomes, after frozen-thawed ET performed under transabdominal ultrasound guidance.[70] This retrospective cohort study evaluated the influence of the embryo placement depth in the endometrial cavity in relation to PRs. The patients were classified according to three variables: <10 mm, 10–15 mm, and >15 mm. Clinical and ongoing PRs were higher in the 10–15 mm and >15 mm groups, when compared to the <10 mm group; there was no statistical difference between the groups in terms of miscarriage and LBRs. They performed a subsequent analysis, using the same sample of patients, comparing only the <10 mm and ≥10 mm variables. The ≥10 mm group had better reproductive outcomes, with higher clinical and ongoing PRs. The authors concluded that PRs are influenced by the ET site, and better results can be achieved when the tip of the catheter is placed in the central area of the endometrial cavity, especially when the distance from the endometrial fundus is >10 mm. A study comparing the site of ET at 2 cm distance from the fundal endometrium (DFE) compared to the midpoint of the endometrial cavity length (ECL) revealed comparable results for both groups.[71]

Pacchiarotti et al.'s results also suggest that the depth of embryo replacement may be an important variable in ET technique. The authors recommend transferring at least >10 mm away from fundus.[72] In Ivanovski et al.'s study,[73] the transfer catheter was advanced to a defined distance from the uterine fundus, up to the point estimated for transfer: 10 +/– 2.5 mm and 15 +/– 2.5 mm, respectively in A and B groups. Analysis of their results demonstrated that PR was significantly influenced by transfer distance from the fundus where the PR decreases from 46.2% in group B to 28.8% in group A ($p < 0.05$).

A total of 180 consecutive patients undergoing ultrasound-guided ET were randomized to three study groups according to the distance between the tip of the catheter and the uterine fundus at the moment of the embryo deposition in the lumen of the endometrial cavity:

Group 1: 10 +/– 1.5 mm; group 2: 15 +/– 1.5 mm; group 3: 20 +/– 1.5 mm. Implantation rate was significantly higher ($p < 0.05$) in groups 2 (31.3%) and 3 (33.3%) compared with group 1 (20.6%). The depth of the embryo replacement into the uterine cavity may influence implantation rates, and thus it should be considered as an additional procedure among factors recently proposed as associated with successful ET after IVF.[74] Davar et al.'s recent study suggested that the depth of intrauterine embryo placement at a distance of 25 ± 5 mm below the fundal endometrial surface gives better IVF outcomes.[75]

Bakas et al. examined the accuracy of ET based on the previous measurement of cervical length and total uterine length.[76] All patients had transvaginal ultrasound measurement of cervical length and endometrial cavity length prior to ET and measurement of embryo distance (intrauterine air bubbles) from fundal surface of uterine cavity and internal cervical os immediately after ET. Primary outcome was to estimate the accuracy of ET based on the measurement of the embryo distance from middle of uterine cavity after ET and secondary outcome was to assess the effect of embryo distance from uterine fundus and internal cervical os to clinical PR. Multiple regression analysis showed that the embryo distance from middle of cavity was related to endometrial cavity length and to the embryo distance from the fundus and it was not related to Cx length, total uterine length, embryo distance from internal Cx os, and ET length. The study concluded that ET by a single operator with the previous measurement of total uterine length and estimation of ET length was very accurate.[76]

Pain during Embryo Transfer

In a prospective observational study, 284 women under 40 years undergoing IVF or ICSI cycles followed by fresh or frozen ETs were recruited. Pain was measured using a 100 mm visual analog scale. Several factors relating to both pain and also the nature of the ET procedure were recorded: Use of vulsellum, uterine contractility, depth of ET, duration of ET catheter insertion, urgency of micturition, psychological profile tests, salivary α-amylase, and salivary cortisol. Women who experienced pain during ET had a significantly lower clinical PR compared with women who did not (42.2% vs. 53.8%; $p = 0.03$).[77]

Injection Speed

Catheter injection speed determines the depth and positioning of the embryo into the cavity and is a highly varying factor during ET, even for the same physician. Caanen et al. developed automated pump-regulated embryo transfer (PRET) device.[78] Standardization of the injection speed and pressure with this PRET results in a better controlled positioning of the transferred embryo(s) with minimal variability. The ongoing PR was 21% in the PRET group versus 17% in the manual transfer group; frozen-thawed ETs resulted in 17.5 versus 10.9%, respectively. These findings need to be investigated in a multicenter trial for further validation.

Grygoruk et al. evaluated the impact of varying injection speed on embryo development and reported that a reduction of the ejection speed reduces injury to the embryos.[79] Embryos exposed to fast ET had the slowest development rate and a higher mean apoptotic index of embryos compared to the group exposed to the slow ET and the control group. It is advisable to transfer the embryos at the lowest possible speed.[79]

Prior Cesarean Delivery

Despite the apparently more difficult transfers, pregnancy outcomes were not different between cesarean delivered patients and those without prior cesarean delivery.[81] RCT showed that ETs took longer (approximately 30 seconds longer) in the CD group and were more likely to have mucus or blood on the catheter.

Temperature Control during Embryo Transfer

Twenty-nine simulated ET procedures were carried out across five clinics. A thermocouple probe was used for standardized measurements inside each of the ET catheters to record the changes in temperature that occur in the time period between loading the catheter and placing the catheter in the uterus. In all cases, the temperature at the loaded catheter tip fell rapidly to ambient temperature during transit from the ET workstation in the IVF laboratory to the ET procedure room. Considering the sensitivity of the preimplantation embryo to its immediate environment, the rapid and profound drop in temperatures observed at the catheter tip that houses the embryo during its transit from the IVF laboratory to the uterine environment may affect embryo viability and health. The authors suggested that the issue be addressed to ensure that the tight temperature control continues throughout the ET procedure, and could improve clinical outcomes.[81]

Difficult Embryo Transfer

There is no single definition for difficult ET. An easy procedure with no additional maneuvers required is assumed to be an easy transfer. Each additional instrument required such as holding of cervix with vulsellum, use of cervical dilators are associated with lowering PRs and are deemed as a difficult transfer. Other parameters include poor ultrasound visualization, touching the fundus of uterus, retained embryos, coiling of inner catheter inside the cavity, resistance to expulsion of embryos, and presence of blood on catheter tip. Poor ultrasound visualization of uterine cavity and inner catheter is associated with lower PRs. Other parameters mentioned above are not significantly correlated with poor outcome.[13]

The aim of a 2019 study was to determine whether a continuous visual analog scale (VAS) is a reliable tool to grade ET difficulty when assessing IVF outcomes.[82] ETs were stratified into three levels of ET "difficulty": (A) "easy"—no resistance; (B) "medium"—resistance overcome by advancing the catheter's outer sheath; and (C) "difficult"—a malleable stylet was required to overcome resistance; and these are compared to the VAS scores.

No significant relationship (p>0.05) was seen in clinical pregnancy or LBRs in either the standard difficulty or the VAS groupings suggesting the VAS is not itself a reliable enough tool to record ET difficulty in isolation.[82]

Alvarez et al. investigated the relationship between the difficult ET and LBR in frozen euploid (blastocyst) embryo transfers (FEET).[83] No significant reduction in LBR was observed after adjustment for confounders between difficult and easy FEET, or when use of stylet without or with a tenaculum was required for ET. The authors concluded that the lack of significance may be due to factors such as the sample size or the use of array comparative genomic hybridization analysis.[83]

Postembryo Transfer

Embryos transferred into the uterine cavity can be expelled due to many factors including uterine peristalsis and contractions, low site of deposition, and negative pressure generated when removing the transfer catheter. RCTs of interventions used to prevent post-transfer embryo expulsion in women undergoing IVF and ICSI[84] showed that there is insufficient evidence to support any specific length of time for women to keep lying down following ET nor is there evidence to recommend the use of fibrin sealants added to the ET fluid.

Catheter Rotation during the Exit Process after an Embryo Transfer

Literature suggested that catheter rotation during an ET could discharge mucus entrapped in the embryo to neutralize embryo displacement. The aim of Eftekhar et al.'s study was to compare the outcome of FET based on catheter rotation during withdrawal.[85] Patients were divided into two groups (n = 120/each), including (1) the rotation treatment group (360°) that underwent ET using catheter rotation and (2) the control group including the subjects who experienced ET with no catheter rotation. Their results demonstrated that catheter rotation during withdrawal increased the implantation rate and clinical pregnancy. On the other hand, Gurbuz and Yildiz's 2021 study found that 360° rotation while pulling catheter during ET had no effect on pregnancy and clinical pregnancy.[86]

Catheter Removal Time

Data on the timing of catheter removal technique following ET are quite limited. Cycles in which the transfer catheter was removed immediately were compared with those in which the catheter was removed after a delay period, to evaluate the impact that the time interval before removal of the catheter following embryo deposit may have on the pregnancy outcomes. The comparison of reproductive outcomes revealed no significant differences in pregnancy, clinical pregnancy, ongoing pregnancy, multiple pregnancy, and implantation rates between the groups. There appears no requirement to delay the withdrawal of the catheter to improve the outcomes in ICSI cycles.[84]

Blood on the Catheter

A significant decrease in the PRs, implantation rates, and LBRs follows the presence of blood on the catheter tip[55] or in the catheter[87] after the ET procedure. PRs were unaffected by mucus on the catheter that appeared to be a simple contamination, though the association between macroscopic or microscopic presence of blood or mucus and PRs has not found support from others.[80]

Plowden et al. attempted to estimate the effect of blood at the time of ET and the difficulty of ET on LBRs.[88] ETs were subjectively graded (easy, medium, or hard) by a physician at the time of transfer. The presence of blood at ET was associated with more difficult ETs, retained embryos, and presence of mucus in the catheter. ET with blood was not associated with live birth, while the degree of difficulty for ET had a negative impact on LBR.[88]

Retained Embryos

The retention of the embryo in the transfer catheter after ET during IVF is a fairly common feature, encountered by even the most experienced IVF physicians, and embryos retained in the ET catheter or within its sleeve require a repeat ET. The incidence and effect on PRs of having embryos retained in the transfer catheter, followed by immediate completion of transfer, were studied.[89] Immediate retransfer was found to not have any significant effect on clinical PRs.[89,90] The type of ET catheter used did not show any difference in terms of embryo retention.

The exact mechanism of embryo retention has not been explained. Therefore, Kozikowska et al.'s study aimed to investigate the mechanism of embryo retention in the catheter during ET by using a transparent uterus model equipped with pressure sensors and a video recorder.[91] Their results indicated that pressure changes in the uterine cavity during ET can influence the distribution of the transferred fluid containing the embryo. Under certain conditions, the transferred fluid can flow backward in the catheter, which may lead to retention of the embryo in the catheter.

Air Bubble Position

Does the air bubble (embryo flash) position and migration as visualized with ultrasound within 60 minutes of ET correlate with clinical outcome following fresh ART transfer cycles? Studies assessing the relation between the PR and the position of the catheter tip and/or the position of the air bubbles following ET show conflicting results to date. Air bubble location following ET is the presumable placement spot of embryos.[92] Confino et al. recorded the air bubble position immediately, 30 minutes later and when the patient stood up after embryo transfer.[93] Bubble migration analysis supported a rather random movement of the bubbles and possibly the embryos, suggestive of active UCs.

A study assessed the embryo flash position by 3D ultrasound at 1, 5, and 60 minutes after ET. The distance of the embryo flash from the fundus was measured at these time points. There was no significant association between the embryo position or movement and the PR at 1 and 5 minutes. At 60 minutes, however, the pregnancy and implantation rates among subjects with embryo flashes located <15 mm from the fundus were significantly higher than those with embryo flashes located >15 mm from the fundus.

Although the air bubbles seen at the time of ET are thought to represent the position of the embryo, they are in fact a surrogate marker of the embryo itself, as this cannot be directly visualized. These findings may challenge the traditional notion that the exact position of the embryo flash immediately following ET is related to clinical outcome.[94]

Speed of Embryo Injection at the Time of Embryo Transfer

Mo et al. set up a study to evaluate the location of transferred embryos under various parameters during ET in IVF by applying an in vitro experimental model for ET.[95] Mock ET simulations were conducted with a laboratory model of the uterine cavity. ET catheter was loaded with a sequence of air and liquid volumes as well as development-arrested embryos donated by patients. The transfer procedure was recorded using a high definition video camera. An orthogonal design, including three independent variables (uterine orientation, distance of the catheter tip to the fundus, and injection speed) and one dependent variable (final embryo position), was applied to the algorithm by the scientific team. The uterine cavity was divided into six regions and the distribution of the transferred embryos varied according to the uterine orientation. The medium speed-injected embryos were usually located in the static region while fast- and slow-speed injected embryos were mostly localized at the uterine fundus and the cervical region, respectively. The probability of embryo separation from the air-bubble interface increased from 11.1% in slow injection cases to 29.6% and 48.1% in the medium and fast injection cases, respectively. The authors suggested that faster injection of embryos into a retroverted uterus usually results in the embryo dissociating from the air bubble.[95]

Mechanical Pressure on Portio Vaginalis

Applying gentle mechanical pressure on the portio vaginalis of the cervix for few minutes post-ET by loosening the screws of vaginal speculum significantly improved the clinical pregnancy and implantation rates by reducing embryo expulsion from the uterus caused by UCs. Some authors, however, have expressed concern that this approach increases uterine contractility and may reduce the chances of successful ET.[96]

Bed Rest after Embryo Transfer

Bed rest for the variable durations of time is commonly advised after an ET carried out almost universally. This practice is based on beliefs that supine position and the reduction of physical activity—to the minimum—might prevent the risk of embryo expulsion once it is transferred to the uterus. Cozzolino et al.[97] designed a meta-analysis based exclusively on evidence from published RCTs, in the attempt to define the real effectiveness of bed rest after an ET to improve the PRs in IVF. The analysis of 1,002 women did not show any significant change in clinical PR between groups and the collated findings showed that immediate mobilization after an ET does not have a negative influence over the success rates of IVF.

RECENT ADVANCES

A recent meta-analysis by Yang et al.[98] evaluated the effects of intrauterine perfusion of peripheral blood mononuclear cells (PBMCs) on the pregnancy outcomes including clinical PRs, embryo implantation rates, LBRs, and miscarriage rates of infertile women who were undergoing IVF treatment. By searching Pubmed, Embase database, five articles meeting the inclusion criteria were included, and 1,173 women were enrolled (intrauterine PBMC group: $n = 514$; NO-PBMC group: $n = 659$). The paper summarized that current published evidence suggested that intrauterine perfusion of PBMC can significantly improve pregnancy outcomes in patients who have three or more IVF implantation failures.[98]

Abdallah et al. designed a parallel, RCT on 181 infertile women scheduled for fresh or vitrified-warmed ET, randomized in a 1:1 ratio to receive either human chorionic gonadotropin (hCG) (500 IU in 0.1 mL of tissue culture media) or culture media (0.1 mL of tissue culture media) via intrauterine injection 4 minutes before ET.[99] In both groups, an intrauterine insemination catheter was used for administering the medication. Primary outcome was live birth, with ongoing pregnancy and clinical pregnancy as secondary outcomes. Intrauterine injection of hCG before ET did not improve LBRs in women undergoing IVF. Laokirkkiat et al.'s recent study contrarily summarized that intrauterine infusion of a small volume of hCG at the time of ET can significantly improve the implantation rate, while the clinical PR may only be improved in younger patients (aged <40 years).[100]

Ochiai et al. studied the role of resveratrol, a polyphenolic compound in IVF-ET outcomes.[101] The outcomes of ET cycles in women receiving resveratrol supplementation (200 mg/day) continuously (RES group) with a control group (non-RES group) were studied. Their preliminary findings suggested that showed that resveratrol supplementation is strongly associated with a decrease in clinical PR [odds ratio (OR) 0.539, 95% confidence interval (CI) 0.341–0.853] and an increased risk of miscarriage (OR 2.602, 95% CI 1.070–6.325).[101]

Recent advances in the area of ET address the influence of the variation in injection speeds in manual ET and PRET that generate a standardized injection speed with the aim to standardize the ET process. Seven laboratory technicians performed simulated transfers, using the conventional ET technique, and compared their injection speeds with that of a PRET device.[102] The results indicated that in manually performed transfers, even after standardization of the protocol, there is still a large variation in injection speed, while a PRET device generates a reliable and reproducible injection speed and therefore brings new possibilities for further standardization of the ET procedure. Future research should reveal whether these experiments mimic real clinical circumstances and if a standardized injection speed results in more exact positioning of the transferred embryos and therefore higher PRs.

Ying et al. studied the effect of ET catheter contact with intravaginal progesterone preparations on mouse embryo development.[103] In a simulated ET model, ET catheters were loaded with culture medium, placed in contact with intravaginal progesterone gel (crinone 8%) or micronized progesterone intravaginal inserts (endometrin 100 mg), and the intracatheter culture medium flushed. Embryos were cultured in the flushed culture medium at variable dilutions for variable lengths of time. The contamination of ET catheter with intravaginal progesterone significantly impairs mouse embryo development, likely due in part to increased programmed cell death. The take home message is to absolutely avoid intravaginal progesterone dosing on the morning of the planned ET.[103]

Ultrasound elastography is a noninvasive medical imaging technique able to quantitatively characterize the stiffness of a given tissue. It has been shown to predict the risk for cervical insufficiency and preterm delivery, and to allow differentiation of malignancy from normal tissue. Cervical ultrasound elastography, by allowing the identification of cervical tissue dishomogeneity, may be of help in predicting the ET ease in infertile women candidates to IVF or ICSI.[104]

Riestenberg et al. compared the LBR between patients who undergo personalized embryo transfer (pET) after endometrial receptivity array (ERA) versus frozen embryo transfer (FET) with standard timing in first single euploid FET cycles.[105] Total of 228 single euploid FET cycles were included in their study. Of those patients, 147 (64.5%) were ERA/pET cycles, and 81 (35.5%) were standard timing FET cycles. Endometrial receptivity array was receptive in 60/147 (40.8%) and nonreceptive in 87/147 (59.2%) patients. Nonreceptive ERAs were prereceptive in 93.1% of cases. The LBRs were similar between patients who underwent FET with standard timing and patients who underwent ERA/pET, 45/81 (56.6%) and 83/147 (56.5%), respectively. The data from this study does not support the routine use of ERA in an unselected patient population undergoing first autologous single euploid programmed ET.[105]

Yenigul et al.[106] from Turkey published a study suggesting a scoring system by including all of the factors that are recommended for an ideal ET and to investigate its correlation with the beta human chorionic gonadotropin (β-hCG) results. The embryo grade, ET day, distance between the fundus to ET site measured via ultrasonography, endometrial thickness on ET day, and presence of mucus and blood in the catheter after transfer were the variables evaluated. Antral follicle count (13.3 ± 8 vs. 14.6 ± 8.2, p = 0,001), endometrial thickness on the ET day (9.9 ± 2 vs. 10.3 ± 2, p = 0.006), and number of mature oocytes (8.6 ± 6 vs. 9 ± 5.1, p = 0.003) were significantly higher in patients with positive β-hCG values. The total score in the β-hCG positive group was 9.8 ± 1.4 versus 8.9 ± 1.4 in the

BOX 1: ASRM 2017 guideline recommendations.

Grade A evidence:
- Transabdominal ultrasound-guided ET improves CPR and LBR
- Use of soft ET catheters improves CPR
- Bed rest after ET is not recommended

Grade B Evidence:
- Acupuncture does not increase LBR
- Routine use of prophylactic antibiotics such as amoxicillin is not recommended.
- Use of powdered gloves has no impact on pregnancy outcome
- There is benefit in removing cervical mucus
- ET catheter placement affects implantation and pregnancy rates.
- Immediate withdrawal of ET catheter is recommended
- Presence of mucus on ET catheter is not associated with lower CPR
- Retained embryos in catheter and immediate retransfer do not affect pregnancy rates

(ASRM: American Society for Reproductive Medicine; CPR: clinical pregnancy rate; ET: embryo transfer; LBR: live birth rate)

Flowchart 2: Problems in embryo transfer procedure.

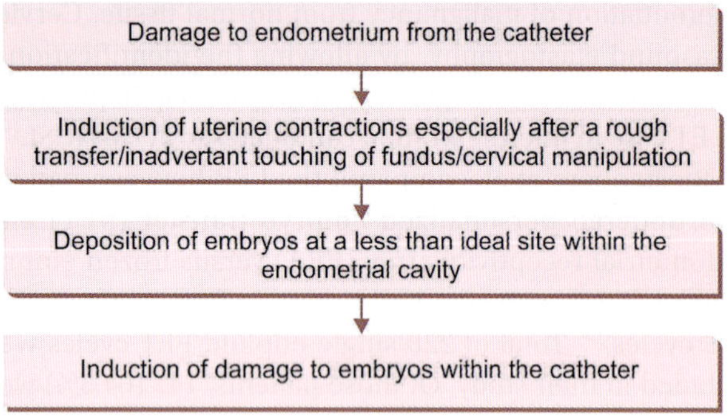

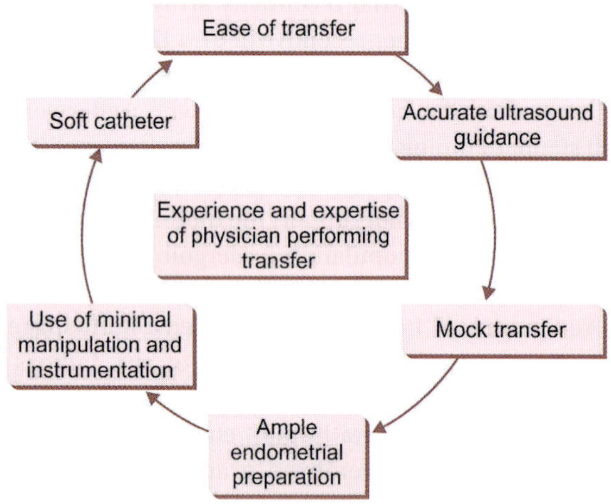

Fig. 12: Cornerstones of a perfect embryo transfer.

β-hCG negative group (p <0.001). The best ETSS cut-off value for predicting β-hCG positivity was 9.5, with 82% sensitivity and 67% specificity [area under curve (AUC): 0.808]. They concluded that their scoring system was an important step toward standardization, as it offered a new, practical, cost-free, and useful scoring system based on pre- and post-ET measurements and laboratory data.[106]

CONCLUSION

Many women undergoing an ART cycle will not achieve a live birth. Failure at the ET stage may be due to lack of good-quality embryo/s, lack of uterine receptivity, or the transfer technique itself. Standardization of the transcervical intrauterine transfer of embryos in larger randomized higher quality study with better explained methods, more specified inclusion, and exclusion criteria is needed to arrive at conclusion. Until more such properly designed studies are conducted, with the available evidence on the factors that are important in achieving an atraumatic ET and positively influencing the pregnancy outcome, we believe that the experience of the clinician performing the ET and adequate knowledge of the factors that are crucial to the success of the technique are paramount **(Box 1)**.

What can go wrong in an ET procedure (**Flowchart 2 and Fig. 12**)?

A poor ET technique accounts for up to 30% of all IVF failures.

REFERENCES

1. Saravelos SH, Li TC. Embryo transfer techniques. Best Pract Res Clin Obstet Gynaecol. 2019;59:77-88.
2. Eskandar M, Abou-Setta AM, Almushait MA, El-Amin M, Mohmad SE. Ultrasound guidance during embryo transfer: a prospective, single-operator, randomized, controlled trial. Fertil Steril. 2008;90(4):1187-90.
3. Porter MB. Ultrasound in assisted reproductive technology. Semin Reprod Med. 2008;26(3):266-76.
4. Buckett WM. A meta-analysis of ultrasound-guided versus clinical touch embryo transfer. Fertil Steril. 2003;80(4): 1037-41.
5. Matorras R, Urquijo E, Mendoza R, Corcóstegui B, Expósito A, Rodríguez-Escudero FJ. Ultrasound-guided embryo transfer improves pregnancy rates and increases the frequency of easy transfers. Hum Reprod. 2002;17(7):1762-6.
6. Anderson RE, Nugent NL, Gregg AT, Nunn SL, Behr BR. Transvaginal ultrasound-guided embryo transfer improves outcome in patients with previous failed in vitro fertilization cycles. Fertil Steril. 2002;77(4):769-75.
7. Allahbadia GN. Ultrasonography-guided embryo transfer: evidence-based practice. In: Rizk B (Ed). Ultrasonography in Reproductive Medicine and Infertility. UK: Cambridge University Press; 2010.
8. Poncelet C, Sifer C, Hequet D, Porcher R, Wolf JP, Uzan M, et al. Hysteroscopic evaluation of endocervical and endometrial lesions observed after different procedures of embryo transfer: a prospective comparative study. Eur J Obstet Gynecol Reprod Biol. 2009;147(2):183-6.
9. Allahbadia GN, Kadam K, Gandhi G, Arora S, Valliappan JB, Joshi A, et al. Embryo transfer using the SureView catheter-beacon in the womb. Fertil Steril. 2010;93(2):344-50.
10. Coroleu B, Barri PN, Carreras O, Belil I, Buxaderas R, Veiga A, et al. Effect of using an echogenic catheter for ultrasound-guided embryo transfer in an IVF programme: a prospective, randomized, controlled study. Hum Reprod. 2006;21(7):1809-15.
11. Karande V, Hazlett D, Vietzke M, Gleicher N. A prospective randomized comparison of the Wallace catheter and the Cook Echo-Tip catheter for ultrasound-guided embryo transfer. Fertil Steril. 2002;77(4):826-30.
12. Pope CS, Cook EK, Arny M, Novak A, Grow DR.. Influence of embryo transfer depth on in vitro fertilization and embryo transfer outcomes. Fertil Steril. 2004;81(1):51-8.
13. Kava-Braverman A, Martínez F, Rodríguez I, Álvarez M, Barri PN, Coroleu B. What is a difficult transfer? Analysis of 7,714 embryo transfers: the impact of maneuvers during embryo transfers on pregnancy rate and a proposal of objective assessment. Fertil Steril. 2017;107(3):657-663.e1.
14. Lambers MJ, Dogan E, Lens JW, Schats R, Hompes PG. The position of transferred air bubbles after embryo transfer is related to pregnancy rate. Fertil Steril. 2007;88(1):68-73.
15. Angelini A, Brusco GF, Barnocchi N, El-Danasouri I, Pacchiarotti A, Selman HA. Impact of physician performing embryo transfer on pregnancy rates in an assisted reproductive program. J Assist Reprod Genet. 2006;23(7-8):329-32.

16. Desparoir A, Capelle M, Banet J, Noizet A, Gamerre M, Courbière B. Does the experience of the provider affect pregnancy rates after embryo transfer? J Reprod Med. 2011;56(9-10):437-43.
17. De Placido G, Wilding M, Stina I, Mollo A, Alviggi E, Tolino A, et al. The effect of ease of transfer and type of catheter used on pregnancy and implantation rates in an IVF program. J Assist Reprod Genet. 2002;19(1):14-8.
18. Zander-Fox DL, Tremellen K, Lane M. Single blastocyst embryo transfer maintains comparable pregnancy rates to double cleavage-stage embryo transfer but results in healthier pregnancy outcomes. Aust N Z J Obstet Gynaecol. 2011;51(5):406-10.
19. Marsh CA, Farr SL, Chang J, Kissin DM, Grainger DA, Posner SF, et al. Trends and factors associated with the Day 5 embryo transfer, assisted reproductive technology surveillance, USA, 2001-2009. Hum Reprod. 2012;27(8):2325-31.
20. Kresowik JD, Stegmann BJ, Sparks AE, Ryan GL, van Voorhis BJ. Five-years of a mandatory single-embryo transfer (mSET) policy dramatically reduces twinning rate without lowering pregnancy rates. Fertil Steril. 2011;96(6):1367-9.
21. Wang SX. The past, present, and future of embryo selection in in vitro fertilization: Frontiers in Reproduction Conference. Yale J Biol Med. 2011;84(4):487-90.
22. Allahbadia GN. Embryo Transfer. New Delhi: Jaypee Brothers Medical Publishers; 2008. p. 558.
23. Ghazzawi IM, Al-Hasani S, Karaki R, Souso S. Transfer technique and catheter choice influence the incidence of transcervical embryo expulsion and the outcome of IVF. Hum Reprod. 1999;14(3):677-82.
24. Gat I, Levron J, Yerushalmi G, Dor J, Brengauz M, Orvieto R. Should zygote intrafallopian transfer be offered to all patients with unexplained repeated in-vitro fertilization cycle failures? J Ovarian Res. 2014;7:7.
25. Kamrava M, Yin M. SubEndometrial Embryo Delivery (SEED) with Egg Donation—Mechanical Embryo Implantation. New York: Intech Open Science; 2012.
26. El Toukhy T, Coomerasamy A, Khairy M, Sunkara K, Seed P, Khalaf Y, et al. The relationship between endometrial thickness and outcome of medicated frozen embryo replacement cycles. Fertil Steril. 2008;89(4):832-9.
27. Surrey ES. Should diagnostic hysteroscopy be performed before in vitro fertilization-embryo transfer? J Minim Invasive Gynecol. 2012;19(5):643-6.
28. Henne MB, Milki AA. Uterine position at real embryo transfer compared with mock embryo transfer. Hum Reprod. 2004;19(3):570-2.
29. Visser DS, Fourie FL, Kruger HF. Multiple attempts at embryo transfer: effects on pregnancy outcome in an in vitro fertilization and embryo transfer program. J Assist Reprod Genet. 1993;10:37-43.
30. Borkar A, Shah A, Gudi A, Homburg R. Outcome of mock embryo transfer before the first IVF cycle: A randomized control trial. Int J Reprod Biomed. 2020;18(11):951-960.
31. Meseguer M, Herrero J, Tejera A, Hilligsøe KM, Ramsing NB, Remohí J. The use of morphokinetics as a predictor of embryo implantation. Hum Reprod. 2011;26(10):2658-71.
32. Glujovsky D, Blake D, Farquhar C, Bardach A. Cleavage stage versus blastocyst stage embryo transfer in assisted reproductive technology. Cochrane Database Syst Rev. 2012;7:CD002118.
33. Forman EJ, Tao X, Ferry KM, Taylor D, Treff NR, Scott RT Jr. Single embryo transfer with comprehensive chromosome screening results in improved ongoing pregnancy rates and decreased miscarriage rates. Hum Reprod. 2012;27(4):1217-22.
34. Scriven PN, Ogilvie CM, Khalaf Y. Embryo selection in IVF: is polar body array comparative genomic hybridization accurate enough? Hum Reprod. 2012;27(4):951-3.
35. Chavez-Badiola A, Flores-Saiffe Farias A, Mendizabal-Ruiz G, Garcia-Sanchez R, Drakeley AJ, Garcia-Sandoval JP. Predicting pregnancy test results after embryo transfer by image feature extraction and analysis using machine learning. Sci Rep. 2020;10(1):4394.
36. Toth TL, Lee MS, Bendikson KA, Reindollar RH; American Society for Reproductive Medicine Embryo Transfer Advisory Panel. Embryo transfer techniques: an American Society for Reproductive Medicine survey of current Society for Assisted Reproductive Technology practices. Fertil Steril. 2017;107(4):1003-11.
37. Ramaiah SD, Ray KA, Reindollar RH. Simulation training for embryo transfer: findings from the American Society for Reproductive Medicine Embryo Transfer Certificate Course. Fertil Steril. 2021;115(4):852-9.
38. McQueen DB, Robins JC, Yeh C, Zhang JX, Feinberg EC. Embryo transfer training in fellowship: national and institutional data. Fertil Steril. 2020;114(5):1006-13.
39. Cirillo F, Patrizio P, Baccini M, Morenghi E, Ronchetti C, Cafaro L, et al. The human factor: does the operator performing the embryo transfer significantly impact the cycle outcome? Hum Reprod. 2020;35(2):275-82.
40. Fanchin R, Righini C, de Ziegler D, Olivennes F, Ledée N, Frydman R. Effects of vaginal progesterone administration on uterine contractility at the time of embryo transfer. Fertil Steril. 2001;75:1136-40.
41. Huang QY, Rong MH, Lan AH, Lin XM, Lin XG, He RQ, et al. The impact of atosiban on pregnancy outcomes in women undergoing in vitro fertilization-embryo transfer: A meta-analysis. PLoS One. 2017;12(4):e0175501.
42. Schwarze JE, Crosby J, Mackenna A. Atosiban improves the outcome of embryo transfer. A systematic review and meta-analysis of randomized and non-randomized trials. JBRA Assist Reprod. 2020;24(4):421-7.
43. Yuan C, Song H, Fan L, Su S, Dong B. The Effect of Atosiban on Patients With Difficult Embryo Transfers Undergoing In Vitro Fertilization-Embryo Transfer. Reprod Sci. 2019;26(12):1613-17.
44. Zarei A, Homayoon N, Hessami K, Hashemi A, Davoodi S, Razavi B, et al. Effect of piroxicam administration on outcome of frozen-thawed embryo transfer: A randomized, double-blinded, placebo-controlled trial. J Obstet Gynaecol Res. 2021;47(1):296-301.
45. Ng KKL, Rozen G, Stewart T, Agresta F, Polyakov A. Does nifedipine improve outcomes of embryo transfer?: Interim analysis of a randomized, double blinded, placebo-controlled trial. Medicine (Baltimore). 2019;98(4):e14251.
46. Egbase PE, al-Sharhan M, al-Othman S, al-Mutawa M, Udo EE, Grudzinskas JG. Incidence of microbial growth from the tip of embryo transfer catheter after embryo transfer in relation to clinical pregnancy rate following in-vitro fertilization and embryo transfer. Hum Reprod. 1996;11(8):1687-9.
47. Selman H, Mariani M, Barnocchi N, Mencacci A, Bistoni F, Arena S, et al. Examination of bacterial contamination at the

time of embryo transfer, and its impact on the IVF/pregnancy outcome. J Assist Reprod Genet. 2007;24(9):395-9.
48. Kroon B, Hart RJ, Wong BM, Ford E, Yazdani A. Antibiotics prior to embryo transfer in ART. Cochrane Database Syst Rev. 2012;3:CD008995.
49. Brook N, Khalaf Y, Coomarasamy A, Edgeworth J, Braude P. A randomized controlled trial of prophylactic antibiotics (co-amoxiclav) prior to embryo transfer. Hum Reprod. 2006;21(11):2911-5.
50. Hamdoun M, Braham M, Kacem K, Hannachi H, Zhioua F, Chakroun N, et al. Does bacterial colonization during embryo transfer have an impact on pregnancy rate in ICSI? : Tunisian preliminary results. J Gynecol Obstet Hum Reprod. 2021;50(2):101727.
51. Egbase PE, Al-Sharhan M, Grudzinskas JG. Influence of position and length of uterus on implantation and clinical pregnancy rates in IVF and embryo transfer treatment cycles. Hum Reprod. 2000;15(9):1943-6.
52. Hannoun A, Zeik TG, Ghaziri G, Abu Musa A, Awwad J. Effect of powdered gloves, worn at the time of embryo transfer, on the pregnancy outcome of IVF cycles. J Assist Reprod Genet. 2009;26(1):25-7.
53. Eskandar MA, Abou-setta AM, El-Amin M, Almushait MA, Sobande AA. Removal of cervical mucus prior to embryo transfer improve pregnancy rates in women undergoing assisted reproduction. Reprod Biomed Online. 2007;14(3):308-13.
54. Abou-Setta AM, Al-Inany HG, Mansour RT, Serour GI, Aboulghar MA. Soft versus firm embryo transfer catheters for assisted reproduction: a systematic review and meta-analysis. Hum Reprod. 2005;20(11):3114-21.
55. Ruhlmann C, Gnocchi DC, Cattaneo AR, Molina LG, Rivadeneira LR, Tessari L, et al. Embryo Transfer Catheters: Softer is Easier. JBRA Assist Reprod. 2015;19(4):204-9.
56. Sallam HN, Agameya AF, Rahman AF, Ezzeldin F, Sallam AN. Impact of technical difficulties, choice of catheter, and the presence of blood on the success of embryo transfer—experience from a single provider. J Assist Reprod Genet. 2003;20(4):135-42.
57. Montag M, Kupka M, van der Ven K, van der Ven H. Embryo transfer on day 3 using low versus high fluid volume. Eur J Obstet Gynecol Reprod Biol. 2002;102(1):57-60.
58. Ebner T, Yaman C, Moser M, Sommergruber M, Pölz W, Tews G. The ineffective loading process of the embryo transfer catheter alters implantation and pregnancy rates. Fertil Steril. 2001;76:630-2.
59. Halvaei I, Khalili MA, Razi MH, Agha-Rahimi A, Nottola SA. Impact of different embryo loading techniques on pregnancy rates in in vitro fertilization/embryo transfer cycles. J Hum Reprod Sci. 2013;6(1):65-9.
60. Omidi M, Halvaei I, Mangoli E, Khalili MA, Razi MH. The effect of embryo catheter loading technique on the live birth rate. Clin Exp Reprod Med. 2015;42(4):175-80.
61. Nouri K, Tempfer CB, Walch K, Promberger R, Dag S, Ott J. Predictive value of the time interval between embryo loading and transfer for IVF/ICSI success: a prospective cohort study. Reprod Biol Endocrinol. 2015;13:51-5.
62. Lindsay Mains, Van Voorhis BJ. Optimizing the technique of embryo transfer. Fertil Steril. 2010;94(3):785-90.
63. Levi Setti PE, Cirillo F, Morenghi E, Immediata V, Caccavari V, Baggiani A, et al. One step further: randomised single-centre trial comparing the direct and afterload techniques of embryo transfer. Hum Reprod. 2021;36(9):2484-92.
64. Rovei V, Dalmasso P, Gennarelli G, Lantieri T, Basso G, Benedetto C, et al. IVF outcome is optimized when embryos are replaced between 5 and 15 mm from the fundal endometrial surface: a prospective analysis on 1184 IVF cycles. Reprod Biol Endocrinol. 2013;11:114.
65. Tiras B, Polat M, Korucuoglu U, Zeyneloglu HB, Yarali H. Impact of embryo replacement depth on in vitro fertilization and embryo transfer outcomes. Fertil Steril. 2010;94(4):1341-5.
66. Mirkin S, Jones EL, Mayer JF, Stadtmauer L, Gibbons WE, Oehninger S. Impact of transabdominal ultrasound guidance on performance and outcome of trans cervical uterine embryo transfer. J Assist Reprod Genet. 2003;20(8):318-22.
67. Bodri D, Colodrón M, García D, Obradors A, Vernaeve V, Coll O. Transvaginal versus transabdominal ultrasound guidance for embryo transfer in donor oocyte recipients: a randomized clinical trial. Fertil Steril. 2011;95(7):2263-8.
68. Saravelos SH, Kong GW, Chung JP, Mak JS, Chung CH, Cheung LP, et al. A prospective randomized controlled trial of 3D versus 2D ultrasound-guided embryo transfer in women undergoing ART treatment. Hum Reprod. 2016;31(10):2255-60.
69. Revelli A, Rovei V, Dalmasso P, Gennarelli G, Racca C, Evangelista F, et al. Large randomized trial comparing transabdominal ultrasound-guided embryo transfer with a technique based on uterine length measurement before embryo transfer. Ultrasound Obstet Gynecol. 2016;48(3): 289-95.
70. Santos MMD, Silva AA, Barbosa ACP, Brum G, Nakagawa HM, Cabral I, et al. Embryo placement in IVF and reproductive outcomes: a cohort analysis and review. JBRA Assist Reprod. 2019;23(3):210-214.
71. Kwon H, Choi DH, Kim EK. Absolute position versus relative position in embryo transfer: a randomized controlled trial. Reprod Biol Endocrinol. 2015;13:78.
72. Pacchiarotti A, Mohamed MA, Micara G, Tranquilli D, Linari A, Espinola SM, et al. The impact of the depth of embryo replacement on IVF outcome. J Assist Reprod Genet. 2007;24(5):189-93.
73. Ivanovski M, Damcevski N, Radevska B, Doicev G. The influence of the depth of embryo replacement into the uterine cavity on in vitro fertilization outcome. Akush Ginekol (Sofiia). 2012;51(3):59-67.
74. Coroleu B, Barri PN, Carreras O, Martínez F, Parriego M, Hereter L, et al. The influence of the depth of embryo replacement into the uterine cavity on implantation rates after IVF: a controlled, ultrasound-guided study. Hum Reprod. 2002;17(2):341-6.
75. Davar R, Poormoosavi SM, Mohseni F, Janati S. Effect of embryo transfer depth on IVF/ICSI outcomes: A randomized clinical trial. Int J Reprod Biomed. 2020;18(9):723-32.
76. Bakas P, Simopoulou M, Giner M, Tzanakaki D, Deligeoroglou E. Accuracy and efficacy of embryo transfer based on the previous measurement of cervical length and total uterine length. Arch Gynecol Obstet. 2019;299(2):565-70.
77. Saravelos SH, Wong AW, Kong GW, Huang J, Klitzman R, Li TC. Pain during embryo transfer is independently associated with clinical pregnancy in fresh/frozen assisted reproductive technology cycles. J Obstet Gynaecol Res. 2016;42(6):684-93.
78. Caanen MR, van der Houwen LE, Schats R, Vergouw CG, de Leeuw B, Lambers MJ, et al. Embryo Transfer with Controlled

Injection Speed to Increase Pregnancy Rates: A Randomized Controlled Trial. Gynecol Obstet Invest. 2016;81(5):394-404.
79. Grygoruk C, Pietrewicz P, Modlinski JA, Gajda B, Greda P, Grad I, et al. Influence of embryo transfer on embryo preimplantation development. Fertil Steril. 2012;97(6):1417-21.
80. Patounakis G, Ozcan MC, Chason RJ, Norian JM, Payson M, DeCherney AH, et al. Impact of a prior cesarean delivery on embryo transfer: a prospective study. Fertil Steril. 2016; 106(2):311-6.
81. Macklon N, Delikari O, Lamanna G, Campbell A, Fishel S, Laiseca ZL, et al. Embryos are exposed to a significant drop in temperature during the embryo transfer procedure: a pilot study. Reprod Biomed Online. 2021;43(2):193-5.
82. Coats E, Carden H, Zujovic L, Maalouf W, Hopkisson J, Raine-Fenning N. Qualifying the difficulty of embryo transfer with a visual analogue scale and assessing its impact on IVF outcomes. Hum Fertil (Camb). 2019;22(3):177-81.
83. Alvarez M, Martínez F, Bourroul FM, Polyzos NP, Solé M, Parriego M, et al. Effect of embryo transfer difficulty on live birth rates studied in vitrified-warmed euploid blastocyst transfers. Reprod Biomed Online. 2019;39(6):940-46.
84. Abou-Setta AM, Peters LR, D'Angelo A, Sallam HN, Hart RJ, Al-Inany HG. Post-embryo transfer interventions for assisted reproduction technology cycles. Cochrane Database Syst Rev. 2014;(8):CD006567.
85. Eftekhar M, Saeed L, Hoseini M. The effect of catheter rotation during its withdrawal on frozen thawed embryo-transfer cycles outcomes: A Case-control study. Int J Reprod Biomed. 2019;17(7):481-6.
86. Gurbuz AS, Yildiz Y. Does rotation during catheter withdrawal in embryo transfer increase pregnancy rates? J Chin Med Assoc. 2021;84(12):1135-8.
87. Muñoz M, Meseguer M, Lizán C, Ayllón Y, Pérez-Cano I, Garrido N. Bleeding during transfer is the only parameter of patient anatomy and embryo quality that affects reproductive outcome: a prospective study. Fertil Steril. 2009;92(3):953-5.
88. Plowden TC, Hill MJ, Miles SM, Hoyt B, Yauger B, Segars JH, et al. Does the presence of blood in the catheter or the degree of difficulty of embryo transfer affect live birth? Reprod Sci. 2017;24(5):726-30.
89. Oraif A, Hollet-Caines J, Feyles V, Rebel M, Abduljabar H. Do multiple attempts at embryo transfer affect clinical pregnancy rates? J Obstet Gynaecol Can. 2014;36(5):406-7.
90. Lee HC, Seifer DB, Shelden RM. Impact of retained embryos on the outcome of assisted reproductive technologies. Fertil Steril. 2004;82(2):334-7.
91. Kozikowska M, Grusza M, Mrugacz G, Gagan J, Zbucka-Krętowska M, Grygoruk C. The influence of intrauterine pressure on embryo retention in a catheter after embryo transfer. Sci Rep. 2019;9(1):11969.
92. Spitzer D, Haidbauer R, Corn C, Stadler J, Wirleitner B, Zech NH. Effects of embryo transfer quality on pregnancy and live birth delivery rates. J Assist Reprod Genet. 2012;29(2):131-5.
93. Confino E, Zhang J, Risquez F. Air bubble migration is a random event post embryo transfer. J Assist Reprod Genet. 2007;24(6):223-6.
94. Saravelos SH, Wong AW, Chan CP, Kong GW, Cheung LP, Chung CH, et al. Assessment of the embryo flash position and migration with 3D ultrasound within 60 min of embryo transfer. Hum Reprod. 2016;31(3):591-6.
95. Mo J, Yang Q, Xia L, Niu Z. Embryo location in the uterus during embryo transfer: An in vitro simulation. PLoS One. 2020;15(10):e0240142.
96. Mansour R. Minimising embryo expulsion after embryo transfer : a randomized controlled study. Hum Reprod. 2005; 20(1):170-4.
97. Cozzolino M, Troiano G, Esencan E. Bed rest after an embryo transfer: a systematic review and meta-analysis. Arch Gynecol Obstet. 2019;300(5):1121-30.
98. Yang DN, Wu JH, Geng L, Cao LJ, Zhang QJ, Luo JQ, et al. Efficacy of intrauterine perfusion of peripheral blood mononuclear cells (PBMC) for infertile women before embryo transfer: meta-analysis. J Obstet Gynaecol. 2020;40(7): 961-8.
99. Abdallah KS, Makhlouf A, Badran E, El-Nashar IM, Al-Hussaini TK, Farghaly T, et al. Intrauterine injection of HCG before embryo transfer: a parallel, double-blind randomized trial. Reprod Biomed Online. 2021;43(4):663-9.
100. Laokirkkiat P, Thanaboonyawat I, Boonsuk S, Petyim S, Prechapanich J, Choavaratana R. Increased implantation rate after intrauterine infusion of a small volume of human chorionic gonadotropin at the time of embryo transfer: a randomized, double-blind controlled study. Arch Gynecol Obstet. 2019;299(1):267-75.
101. Ochiai A, Kuroda K, Ikemoto Y, Ozaki R, Nakagawa K, Nojiri S, et al. Influence of resveratrol supplementation on IVF-embryo transfer cycle outcomes. Reprod Biomed Online. 2019;39(2):205-10.
102. Groeneveld E, de Leeuw B, Vergouw CG, Visser OW, Lambers MJ, Heymans MW, et al. Standardization of catheter load speed during embryo transfer: comparison of manual and pump-regulated embryo transfer. Reprod Biomed Online. 2012;24(2):163-9.
103. Ying LY, Ying Y, Mayer J, Imudia AN, Plosker SM. Embryo Transfer catheter contamination with intravaginal progesterone preparations in a simulated embryo transfer model impairs mouse embryo development: are there implications for human embryo transfer technique? Reprod Sci. 2014;21(8): 1000-5.
104. Stanziano A, Caringella AM, Cantatore C, Trojano G, Caroppo E, D'Amato G. Evaluation of the cervix tissue homogeneity by ultrasound elastography in infertile women for the prediction of embryo transfer ease: a diagnostic accuracy study. Reprod Biol Endocrinol. 2017;15(1):64.
105. Riestenberg C, Kroener L, Quinn M, Ching K, Ambartsumyan G. Routine endometrial receptivity array in first embryo transfer cycles does not improve live birth rate. Fertil Steril. 2021;115(4):1001-06.
106. Yenigul NN, Dilbaz S, Ozelcı R, Aldemir O, Baser E, Kaplanoğlu İ, et al. Evaluation of embryo transfer through a scoring system: ETSS (Embryo transfer scoring system). J Gynecol Obstet Hum Reprod. 2022;51(1):102237.

CHAPTER 58

Troubleshooting in Assisted Reproductive Technology

Harpreet Kaur, Mir Jaffar

INTRODUCTION

There has been a significant increase in cases of infertility in the last decade which may be due to environmental factors, lifestyle factors such as obesity and stress, increase in late marriages, and postponement of first childbirth. This is paralleled with development in the treatment for infertility including in vitro fertilization (IVF).

In vitro fertilization involves the retrieval of oocytes after ovarian stimulation, their fertilization in vitro, growth of resulting embryos in the laboratory, and subsequent transfer of selected embryos back to the uterus and/or freezing of (excessive) embryos. The whole process is highly sophisticated and there can be mistakes at nearly every level throughout this procedure which can compromise the success rates in an IVF cycle. Troubleshooting is identifying the source of problems and finding the right solutions to get optimal IVF results with no complications. There has been tremendous development in the field of IVF in the last years, the same is accompanied by its associated complexities and problems as well. Maintaining a consistent and good success rate in an IVF program is a challenge.

Despite four decades of progress in reproductive medicine and technology, problems still occur. Our tools have increased in complexity and complex systems bringing problems that can be tackled with an in-depth knowledge of the associated scientific problems.

"Troubleshooting" is defined as a form of problem-solving, applied to repair failed products or processes. The assisted reproductive technology (ART) represents multiple complex systems and a single problem can have many possible causes.

Any changes in stimulation protocols, drug batches and doses, sperm characteristics, and oocyte quality can have negative effects on results. The same holds true for changes in culture conditions, incubators, temperature, pH, gasses, dishes, and culture media. When problems arise, it can be very difficult to know the source. Therefore, the process of troubleshooting can be simplified by a summary of steps:

- Define the problem.
- Produce a step-by-step process of analysis.
- Re-define the problem, find the root cause, and suggest a solution to the problem.

For any successful IVF unit, it is important to have a dedicated team of qualified staff with committed working hours and good team work. Standard operating procedures (SOPs), customized treatment protocols, and regular audits to evaluate performance are the key to success in an IVF program. Any adverse events should be discussed in detail and a root cause analysis is done without a blame culture so as to learn from incidences. Each laboratory should be prepared to encounter one or more of the problems and should have clear cut established systems to handle these problems.

It is important to report your success rates clearly.[1] Success in an ART cycle means birth of a healthy baby through a healthy mother. It is important to define success rate as live birth rate, clinical pregnancy rate, and implantation rate or biochemical pregnancy separately. Success rates should be compared with the national and international standards and the same conveyed to patients clearly.

Troubleshooting involves solving any problem related to clinical or laboratory parameters so as to get the optimum outcome from an IVF cycle.

CLINICAL PARAMETERS

Right from patient selection, choosing the appropriate stimulation protocol, a well-monitored stimulation, right choice of gonadotropins, right dose, timing of human chorionic gonadotropin (hCG) trigger quality control of drugs, and laboratory conditions—all put together finally affect the success rate of an IVF cycle.

Patient Selection

Today ART has become very individualized. One treatment does not suit all. Before starting an IVF cycle, it is very important to have proper patient selection to get optimal results.[2-4] Success of an IVF cycle depends on many variables.

It is important to consider the following factors *before starting an IVF cycle:*

- *Age:* Age of the female partner is the most important factor determining the success of an IVF cycle. It is very important to check ovarian reserve and take age into consideration while deciding the stimulation protocol and the amount of gonadotropins during an IVF cycle. Counseling the patient about success rate is important as chances of successful pregnancy decline with increasing age, especially after 35 years of age.
- *Body mass index (BMI):* If the patient has high BMI (i.e., >30), it is better to advice for weight reduction before embarking on to IVF as the dosage requirement of gonadotropins is higher in obese patients and the results of IVF are poor if BMI is >30 kg/m^2.
- *Medical disorders:* Any pre-existing medical disorders of the male or female partner need to be treated and in optimal condition before going ahead for IVF.
- *Screening for viral markers:* Rule out any infectious diseases such as hepatitis and HIV.
- Based on age, baseline scan, and anti-Müllerian hormone (AMH) of the female partner, make an assessment of ovarian reserve.[5] Women with advanced age and poor responders need to be dealt with separately. These women may need a higher dose of follicle-stimulating hormone (FSH) or addition of luteinizing hormone (LH) to stimulation and it has been seen that the antagonist cycle gives better pregnancy results in these select groups.
- *Records of previous IVF cycle:* This gives a lot of information regarding a patient's response to stimulation so that if needed, any changes can be made in this cycle.
- *Repeated implantation failures:* It is important to workup and find out any underlying cause, e.g., hydrosalpinx which should be removed before attempting further IVF, use of blastocyst transfer, and preimplantation genetic screening (PGS) in selected women may be helpful.[6]
- Rule out any contraindications such as active infection and current pregnancy before embarking on an IVF.
- *Thorough counseling:* Regarding procedure, success rate, failure rate, and alternative treatment, it is important to have psychological counseling particularly in cases of third-party reproduction. Dealing clinician should understand the emotional and interpersonal strain the couples undergo while taking treatment for infertility. A well-conducted IVF counseling allays anxiety and enables patient participation in the treatment.[7]
- *Consent forms:* Informed valid consent to be signed by the patient and where needed by the partner as well, in a language patient can understand.
- *It is always a good practice to have a checklist for all essentials before starting an IVF cycle including investigations, consents, and prior medications so as not to miss anything.*

During Stimulation

- *Cold chain maintenance for drugs:* The outcome of IVF cycle depends upon the quality of stimulation which in turn is influenced by the potency of gonadotropins. Therefore, it is very important to maintain the cold chain during transportation and storage of gonadotropins so as to ensure potency.
- *Selection of protocol:* Stimulation during IVF needs to be individualized, e.g., type of ovarian stimulation protocol, amount of gonadotropins, and type of gonadotropins administered. Nowadays, it is more or less individualized ovarian stimulation (iCOS) protocols which are used in IVF. Special care has to be taken in cases of polycystic ovary syndrome (PCOS) who are at high risk of ovarian hyperstimulation syndrome (OHSS) and poor responders where response may be suboptimal to conventional stimulation.[8,9]
- Dose titrations of gonadotropins have to be individualized. This depends upon BMI, ovarian reserve, prior ovarian response, and ovarian morphology.
- Be vigilant about OHSS—especially cases of PCOS, those who have had prior history of hyperstimulation. In this population, strategies proposed are—antagonist cycle, low-dose gonadotropins, agonist trigger, and no hCG for luteal support.[10]
- *Premature progesterone rise:* There is some evidence that premature progesterone rise during the follicular phase may affect the oocyte quality, endometrial receptivity, and finally success of an ART cycle. The effect is more pronounced in young good responders (i.e., the ideal patient) with large follicular response who is treated with gonadotropin-releasing hormone (GnRH) agonist and pure FSH.[11,12] The risk of premature progesterone rise appears to be associated with the number and size of follicles and the intensity of FSH stimulation. Various strategies proposed to prevent premature progesterone rise include—giving trigger early in these cases, to adopt mild stimulation protocol, and if progesterone levels on the day of hCG trigger are more than cutoff (1.5 ng/mL), then solution might be to vitrify all embryos and transfer subsequently in natural cycle.[13-15]
- *Trigger*: In cases of high risk of OHSS and undergoing antagonist cycle, it is safe to give GnRH agonist trigger which has been shown to give comparable results. Timings from trigger to oocyte pick-up (OPU) have to be specific, i.e., 34–36 hours.
- *Premature rupture of follicles:* The most common reason for premature rupture of follicles is ill-timed trigger. This needs to be looked at and there has to be a mechanism in place to ensure that OPU happens at the specified time after trigger. There should be sufficient gap between the cases or a provision for alternate operation theater (OT) in case of multiple OPU happening the same day. Special

care needs to be taken in case a patient gives such history in previous cycles.

- *Fluid in the endometrial cavity:* Presence of fluid in the endometrial cavity in the late follicular phase may compromise the success of ART cycle. In such cases, it is important to rule out infections, presence of hydrosalpinx, and if there is significant fluid, solution might be to vitrify embryos and transfer in the subsequent cycle.
- There has to be a frozen semen sample as a backup in case of any problems for semen collection on the day of OPU.

During Oocyte Pick-up

- *World Health Organization (WHO) Checklist:* Follow WHO safety checklist in all OT procedures. Always check the equipment, media, and scan machine are in order and there is adequate supply of disposables. Confirm the timings in relation to trigger. The WHO safety checklist should mention the timings and the date of trigger given and this should be signed off before shifting the patient to OT for OPU.
- *Empty follicle syndrome (EFS):* Problem of empty follicles can be frustrating to both the clinician and the patient where no oocytes are retrieved in spite of apparent normal mature follicles and normal estradiol levels. There may be many factors leading to all empty follicles, some still unknown, like genetic,[16] dysfunctional folliculogenesis,[17] and human errors.[18] It is important to check the timings and potency of hCG trigger which can be done by beta-human chorionic gonadotropin (bhCG) test. Various strategies proposed for EFS include—rule out any human errors, change the protocol, change batch of hCG, use of rhCG if not used earlier, rescue protocol by readministering second dose of hCG, and rescheduling OPU 24–36 hours later.[19]
- Problems during procedure:
  - Always check the pressure before starting OPU. It is important to use the specially designed pumps for OPU and the pressure should be maintained at 100–120 mm Hg to avoid damage to the oocytes. In case of suction pump failure, staff should be trained to use mechanical suction in case of emergency situations.[20]
  - *Connections:* Ensure all the connections are right. It is always wise to flush the media through the OPU needle to check all the connections before starting the procedure. If the system is not working, check for leakage—it may be due to broken tube, lid not tightly fitting, problem with the tubing, or the suction pump.
  - Tubes and other disposables should be prewarmed and checked for breakage. And there should be sufficient backup in case of damage during the procedure.
  - *Mobile ovary:* This can lead to difficulty in OPU. It is important to master the technique in such cases as the ovary is highly vascular and at risk of torsion as well when hyperstimulated. Sometimes gentle counter pressure from the abdomen may help.
  - *Excessive bleeding:* It is always important to know your patient in detail, rule out any bleeding disorders, and any medications which might increase the risk of bleeding. Always localize the iliac vessels before putting in the needle so as to avoid inadvertent injury to the major vessels. In case of excessive bleeding from the vault, vaginal packing with a roller gauge may be helpful.

Optimizing Embryo Transfer Technique

Finally, the success of an IVF cycle depends upon a meticulous embryo transfer (ET) procedure. ET with soft catheter and under ultrasonography (USG) guidance has been shown to give better pregnancy rates.[21] A mock ET before the actual ET may give valuable information, especially in cases of suspected cervical stenosis as it allows timely cervical dilatation. ET should be as atraumatic as possible and embryos placed in the mid-cavity under USG guidance.[22,23]

A variety of semirigid catheters or stylet should be available in cases of difficulty to negotiate the os during ET.

Appropriate Luteal Phase Support

Use of GnRH analogs and supraphysiological hormonal levels in ART cycles produce inherent luteal phase defect in all ART cycles. So it is important to give appropriate luteal phase support (LPS) in all IVF cycles. It is advisable to avoid use of hCG as LPS, especially in cases at high risk of OHSS and preferred agent for LPS is micronized progesterone either as tablets, vaginal gels, or suppositories. Estrogen support should be given wherever indicated.[24] One of the recent studies showed better LPS[39] in patients with reduced ovarian reserve, by stimulation with identical protocol in the follicular and luteal phase of the same menstrual cycle which resulted in similar number of blastocyst, thereby reducing the increased risk of aneuploidy when compared with standard stimulation.[1]

LABORATORY PARAMETERS

Troubleshooting in ART laboratory may be broadly categorized under the following headings:

- Environmental factors
- Equipment and instrument-related issues
- Culture conditions
- Technical aspects.

Environmental Factors

It is important to have a proper air purification system to avoid volatile organic compounds (VOCs) in the laboratory.

The gas supply to the incubators should go through the filters after purification and the filters should be changed on a regular basis. An unforeseeable rise in the VOC could be detected purely by smell and can be circumvented by increasing the room temperature and/or placing a dish with oil in the incubator or workstation to absorb hydrophilic VOC-sink in effect.[2]

Equipment and Instrument-related Issues

In case of incubator breakdown, there should be an alternate arrangement to store the embryos and media. Ideally, in a running IVF center, there should be more than one incubator. The incubator has to be fitted with an alarm system to raise an alert in case of interruption in power supply or any change in gas or temperature or humidity.

Culture Conditions and In Vitro Fertilization Culture Systems

The success of an ART cycle depends upon a good and well-maintained IVF laboratory.[40] By following the basic principles in the IVF laboratory, we can strive for a good outcome. Some good practice points include:

- Power backup in the form of UPS to ensure uninterrupted power supply
- *Asepsis:* Sterile precautions to be ensured in OT, laboratory, and semen preparation. The entire complex should be air-conditioned with filtered air under positive pressure and restricted entry of personnel to the laboratory.
- *Workstations:* It is important to maintain temperature, asepsis, and avoid vibrations.
- Standard operating procedures for the procedures.

In Vitro Fertilization Culture System[41,42]

Attention must be paid to any element in the culture system that might cause physiological stress to embryos, resulting in compromise to their potential viability.[28,29]

Gametes and embryos are maintained in a culture system in buffered media that provide a stable environment via complex interplays between physicochemical parameters of pH and temperature. These parameters are dependent upon the composition of media and its buffering systems as well as gas atmosphere and incubation conditions.[30,31]

Guidelines for handling the media:

- Ensure that the cold chain is not broken during transport of media.
- Check the production schedule of media so that media arrives with maximum shelf-life.
- Store the media continuously at the appropriate temperature.
- Media should be equilibrated for temperature and pH for 4–6 hours before use or by overnight incubation.
- Ensure that the media and disposables are checked for quality and proved to be nontoxic to the embryos by appropriate assay.

pH Regulation in Gamete and Embryo Culture Systems

Dishes that are used without an overlay are extremely sensitive to pH changes when placed in or removed from the incubator. Therefore, culture dishes with oil overlay are important. In this case, oil also requires equilibration in the CO_2 incubator up to 12 hours.[3] Do not expose the HEPES [4-(2-hydroxyethyl)-1-piperazineethanesulfonic acid]-buffered media to 5% CO_2 conditions, i.e., prepare dishes or tubes with tight lids which contain HEPES-buffered media.

pH is a critical parameter; in practice, it is not easy to monitor effectively. A standard glass probe pH meter can be used for solutions but it cannot measure pH under culture conditions. A number of devices are available for use in culture systems. Whatever device is used, careful validation and calibration are essential. Sample pH is measured after two-point calibration, with one buffer in an acid range and other in alkaline range.

Temperature Control in In Vitro Fertilization Laboratory

Control of temperature fluctuation is important to successful IVF culture. The optimal temperature range for human IVF culture is assumed to be between limits of 36.7 and 37°C. Temperature above 37°C may induce the formation of heat shock proteins, with detrimental effects on development.[32,33]

Two brief exposures of embryo/blastocyst culture dish to room temperature in a day show compromised development.[4]

Infections in In Vitro Fertilization Culture

In vitro fertilization culture systems are designed to promote and sustain cell metabolism and optimal cell growth and therefore also represent an ideal environment for microorganisms to thrive. Microbial growth has the potential to not only affect the health of gametes and embryos but also compromise the treatment of other patients via culture system.[34,35]

STRATEGIES TO MINIMIZE INFECTION

- Restrict access to the laboratory, only authorized personnel should be allowed into the IVF laboratory, wearing specific laboratory clothing and footwear in the sterile area of the laboratory.
- Wash and dry hands on entering the laboratory.
- Hair should be netted in surgical hats.
- Make sure that plastic sleeves containing dishes or tubes are clean before taking them to the culture environment.

- No eatables should be allowed in the sterile area.
- Laboratory must be cleaned and decontaminated. Separate waste materials according to hazard type, with sharps always discarded into sharps bins.
- Examine culture droplets on a regular basis for any evidence of gross bacterial or fungal infection. Incubators, centrifuges, and microscopes must be cleaned and serviced at regular timings.

TROUBLESHOOTING A CRYOPRESERVATION SYSTEM

Cryopreservation of oocytes, embryos, and reproductive tissue is an integral part of an ART service. But if vitrification results show consistently poor survival, then need to troubleshoot. Troubleshooting in cryopreservation requires an understanding of basic principles of cryobiology.[36-38]

Practical Tips for Vitrification

Pre-equilibrate all the media to the correct temperature and label each vitrification device fully prior to use because timing is crucial to effective vitrification and warming. Adhere to the correct timings strictly, use timers. Ensure that there are no air bubbles on the surface of the initial warming solutions as embryos tend to adhere to bubbles. The speed of warming is considered to be more important in avoiding lysis. If warming is too slow, the intracellular cyclopiazonic acid concentration is too low to prevent ice from recrystallizing and supercooled liquid forms lethal ice crystals. Embryo survival may not be immediately obvious after warming and survival is routinely assessed after a minimum period of 2 hours in culture. This is particularly important in blastocysts, which may appear collapsed immediately after warming but will re-expand within 2 hours when culture under optimal conditions.

Problems may arise if liquid N2 levels are not maintained, due to spillage, lack of proper labeling, and wrong freezing techniques.

TROUBLESHOOTING INTRACYTOPLASMIC SPERM INJECTION PROCEDURE

Make sure that all the controls are in the central position before starting a micromanipulation procedure. Coarse and fine controllers should be central. Keep all equipment clean, dust settling into joints can prevent further movement and create problems. Oil inside the tubing often remains in place for long periods, any change in color to yellow or brown is a sign of deterioration. Air bubbles in the oil will interfere with syringe pressure and should always be removed.

Sometimes when fitting a new injection pipette, a blockage in the pipette holder prevents full insertion, then undo the pipette holder and check for the presence of previously broken pipette. Remove that broken pipette and fit a new injection pipette. Angle of the injection pipette should be correctly set so that sperm can easily be trapped using injection needle.

Table 1 shows some practical tips to troubleshooting in the laboratory.

Finally, it is very important to review your performance and the areas of improvement and for that *audit your results regularly*.

Quality Management Systems

Essential elements of quality management systems (QMS) include process flowchart, SOPs, quality of all consumables and media in use, and contracts for service and documented calibration which are required for incubators, microscopes, manipulator stations, heated surface or microscope stages, centrifuge, refrigerators or freezers, and air filtration equipment.[25-27]

The staff working in the laboratory should be trained and there should be a clear policy to document any adverse incident and the actions taken after that.

The recordkeeping should be meticulous and all records pertaining to any ART-related procedure has to be maintained for 10 years as per Indian Council of Medical Research (ICMR) guidelines.

Tools to Understand and Minimize Risk

Double check for identity—witnessing to avoid accidents or mix-ups. Electron witnessing system is a step forward to ensure further that there is no mixing up of gametes and embryos and it saves time and increases patient's confidence level.[43,44]

CONCLUSION

The concept of benchmarking or key performance indicators (KPIs) is well known in many operations in science, medicine, and business. Systematic KPIs monitoring allows early detection of problems and the prompt adoption of corrective actions to prevent a clinical impact. Laboratory KPIs mainly cover the safety, effectiveness, efficiency, and timeliness dimensions of care. This can minimize adverse effects.

QUESTIONS

1. What is the threshold value of progesterone in the follicular phase of an IVF cycle and how to manage premature progesterone rise?
2. Highlight causes of EFS and how to manage it?
3. What should be the ideal temperature in an incubator and how to measure this?
4. How to check for contamination in the laboratory? What steps are important to prevent contamination in an IVF laboratory?
5. Your pregnancy rates have dropped consistently over the last 3 months. How to troubleshoot?

TABLE 1: Practical tips to troubleshooting in the laboratory.

Problem	*Which area best describes the problem?*	*Check*
A bottle of media appears cloudy when dishes are prepared	IVF culture system	• Refrigerator temperature • Media bottle capped? • Can clear media be sourced immediately?
All media in CO_2 incubator dishes are observed to be pink	pH	• Check incubator CO_2 level • Check CO_2 connection
Poor ICSI embryo quality since the ICSI station was moved to a different part of the laboratory, closer to air vents	Temperature	• Reset heated stage to compensate for any temperature loss • Consider relocating the ICSI station away from the air vent • ICSI should take place at the correct temperature
New fluorescent lighting installed in IVF laboratory. Pregnancy rates have dropped	Light	• Install a dimmer switch to control lighting level • Consider having fewer lights switched on • Light levels should be optimal for ART laboratory
Hissing sound noticed when new CO_2 cylinder is connected to the regulator indicating a leak	Gas	• Turn off the gas cylinder • Unscrew regulator, check, and clean thread • If still leaking, contact the gas company immediately • Check the regulator matches cylinder type
Bacteria are observed in a single dish from one patient on day 3 of embryo development	Infections	• Check infection is restricted to one couple only • Isolate the dish • Sample media to identify infection • Send culture for incubator
Vitrification results show consistently poor survival	Cryopreservation system	• Check SOP validation • Check nitrogen level in can • Check equilibration time in freezing solution • Check freezing media equilibrated at correct temperature • Check correct loading of embryos on straw
Sperm cannot be trapped using the injection pipette for ICSI	Micromanipulation	• Check the angle of injection pipette is correctly set • Remove air bubbles from tubing • Refill injector with oil
Poor fertilization after ICSI	Micromanipulation	• Check correct injection in cytoplasm • Check correct sperm immobilization • Select vital sperms • Check temperature of heating stage • Reduce exposure time for oocytes

(ART: assisted reproductive technology; ICSI: intracytoplasmic sperm injection; IVF: in vitro fertilization; SOP: standard operating procedures)

KEY POINTS

- The success of an IVF unit depends on both clinical and laboratory parameters.
- A well-selected patient with individualized stimulation protocol and ensuring quality control in an IVF laboratory can give the best results in ART cycles.
- It is very important to have SOPs and audit your results regularly and have in depth root cause analysis of any adverse events so as to learn lessons from such events.

REFERENCES

1. Saunders DM, Satchwell LJ. How can I improve 'success rates' and select the best for my patients? Textbook of Assisted Reproductive Technology. What The Doctor Should Know. Oxford: Taylor and Francis; 1995. p. 11.
2. Ben-Ami I, Raziel A, Friedler S, Gidoni Y, Ron-El R, Fauser BCJM. Indications for IVF treatment: from diagnosis to prognosis. In: Gardner DK, Weissman A, Howles CM, Shoham Z, (Eds). Textbook of Assisted Reproductive Technology: Clinical Perspectives, 4th edition. UK: Informa Healthcare; 2012. p. 18.
3. Norman RJ, Moran LJ, Robertson SA. Lifestyle, periconception and fertility. In: Gardner DK, Weissman A, Howles CM, Shoham Z, (Eds). Textbook of Assisted Reproductive Technology: Clinical Perspectives, 4th edition. UK: Informa Healthcare; 2012. p. 10.
4. Sharma R. Biedenharn KR, Fedor JM, Agarwal A. Lifestyle factors and reproductive health: taking control of your fertility. Reprod Biol Endocrinol. 2013;11:66.
5. American College of Obstetricians and Gynecologists Committee on Gynecologic Practice and Practice Committee of the American Society for Reproductive Medicine. Female age related fertility decline. Committee opinion No. 589. Obstet Gynecol. 2014;123(3):719-21.
6. Damario MA, Rosenwaks Z. Repeated implantation failure. In: Gardner DK, Weissman A, Howles CM, Shoham Z, (Eds). Textbook of Assisted Reproductive Technology: Clinical Perspectives, 4th edition. UK: Informa Healthcare; 2012. p. 208.
7. Fagan PG, Ponticas V. Psychological issues in IVF: Evaluation and care. In: Damewood MD, (Ed). The John Hopkins Handbook of an In Vitro Fertilization and Assisted

Reproductive Technologies. Boston, Massachusetts: Little, Brown and Company; 1990. pp. 27-36.
8. Weissman A, Howles CM. Treatment strategies in assisted reproduction in poor responder patient. In: Gardner DK, Weissman A, Howles CM, Shoham Z, (Eds). Textbook of Assisted Reproductive Technology: Clinical Perspectives, 4th edition. UK: Informa Healthcare; 2012. p. 162.
9. Nicholas S, Brewer C, Tang TH, Balen AH. PCOS and assisted reproduction. In: Gardner DK, Weissman A, Howles CM, Shoham Z, (Eds). Textbook of Assisted Reproductive Technology: Clinical Perspectives, 4th edition.UK: Informa Healthcare; 2012. p. 298.
10. Humaidan P, Quartaralo J, Papanaikolaou EG. Preventing ovarian hyperstimulation syndrome: guidance for the clinician. Fertil Steril. 2010;94(2):389-400.
11. Hugues JN, Cédrin-Durnerin I. Endocrine characteristics of ART cycles. In: Gardner DK, Weissman A, Howles CM, Shoham Z, (Eds). Textbook of Assisted Reproductive Technologies: Laboratory and Clinical Perspectives, 3rd edition. London, UK: Informa Healthcare; 2009. pp. 511-28.
12. Fleming R, Jenkins J. The source and implications of progesterone rise during the follicular phase of assisted reproduction cycles. Reprod Biomed Online. 2010;21(4):446-9.
13. Van Vaerenbergh I, Fatemi HM, Blockeel C, Van Lommel L, In't Veld P, Schuit F, et al. Progesterone rise on hCG day in GnRH antagonist/rFSH stimulated cycles affects endometrial gene expression. Reprod Biomed Online. 2011;22(3):263-71.
14. Kasum M, Radakovic B, Simunic V, Oreškovic S. Preovulatory progesterone rise during ovarian stimulation for IVF. Gynecol Endocrinol. 2013;29(8):744-8.
15. Fatemi HM, Kyrou D, Bourgain C, Van den Abbeel E, Griesinger G, Devroey P. Cryopreserved-thawed human embryo transfer: spontaneous natural cycle is superior to human chorionic gonadotropin-induced natural cycle. Fertil Steril. 2010;94(6):2054-8.
16. Zreik TG, Garcia-Velasco JA, Vergara TM, Arici A, Olive D, Jones EE. Empty follicle syndrome: evidence for recurrence. Hum Reprod. 2000;15(5):999-1002.
17. Ben-Shlomo I, Schiff E, Levran D, Ben-Rafael Z, Mashiach S, Dor J. Failure of oocyte retrieval during in vitro fertilization: a sporadic event rather than a syndrome. Fertil Steril. 1991; 55(2):324-7.
18. Ndukwe G, Thornton S, Fishel S, Dowell K, Aloum M, Green S. 'Curing' empty follicle syndrome. Hum Reprod. 1997;12(1): 21-3.
19. Deepika K, Rajashekar L, Patil M. Empty follicle syndrome-still an engima. J Hum Reprod Sci. 2008;1(2):86-9.
20. Kovacs G. Oocyte collection. In: Gardner DK, Weissman A, Howles CM, Shoham Z, (Eds). Textbook of Assisted Reproductive Technologies: Laboratory and Clinical Perspectives, 4th edition. London, UK: Informa Healthcare; 2009. pp. 145-52.
21. Brown J, Buckingham K, Buckett W, Abou-Setta AM. Ultrasound versus 'clinical touch' for catheter guidance during embryo transfer in women. Cochrane Database Syst Rev. 2010;1:CD006107.
22. Mains L, Van Voorhis BJ. Optimizing the technique of embryo transfer. Fertil Steril. 2010;94(3):785-90.
23. Mansour RT, Aboulghar MA. Optimizing the embryo transfer technique. Hum Reprod. 2002;17(5):1149-53.
24. Ziegler D, Streuli I, Gayet V, Bajouh U, Berdah J, Chapron C. Luteal support in ART. In: Gardner DK, Weissman A, Howles CM, Shoham Z (Eds). Textbook of Assisted Reproductive Technologies: Laboratory and Clinical Perspectives, 4th edition. London, UK: Informa Healthcare; 2009. p. 153.
25. Mortimer D, Mortimer ST. Quality and Risk Management in IVF Laboratory. UK: Cambridge University Press; 2007.
26. Go KJ, Patel JC, Dietz R. Troubleshooting in the clinical embryology laboratory: the art of problem-solving in ART. In: Nagy P, Varghese AC, Agarwal A, (Eds). Practical Manual of In Vitro Fertilization: Advanced Methods and Novel Devices. New York: Springer; 2012. pp. 631-7.
27. Boone WR, Higdon HL III. Quality control management. In: Nagy P, Varghese AC, Agarwal A, (Eds). Practical Manual of In Vitro Fertilization: Advanced Methods and Novel Devices. New York: Springer; 2012. pp. 33-9.
28. Biggers JD, Summers MC. Choosing a culture medium: making informed choices. Fertil Steril. 2008;90(3):473-83.
29. Lane M, Gardner DK. Embryo Culture: which is the best? Best Pract Res Clin Obst Gynaecol. 2007;21(1):83-100.
30. Quinn P (Ed). Culture Media, Solutions, and Systems in ART. UK: Cambridge University Press; 2014.
31. Conaghan J. pH control in the embryo culture environment. In: Quinn P, (Ed). Culture Media, Solutions, and Systems in ART. UK: Cambridge University Press; 2014.
32. Anifandis G. Temperature variations inside commercial IVF incubators. J Assist Reprod Genet. 2013;30(12):1587-8.
33. Bove R. Temperature measurement in the clinical laboratory. Good isn't good enough. Med Lab Obs. 2011;43:36-9.
34. Pomeroy KO. Contamination of human cultures by microorganisms: a review. J Clin Embryol. 2010;13(4):11-30.
35. Steyaert SR, Leroux-Roels GG, Dhont M. Infections in IVF: review and guidelines. Hum Reprod Update. 2000;6(5):432-41.
36. Byrd W. Cryopreservation, thawing, and transfer of human embryos. Semin Reprod Med. 2002;20(1):37-43.
37. Tucker M, Liebermann J (Eds). Vitrification in Assisted Reproduction: A User's Manual and Trouble-shooting Guide. Florida: CRC Press; 2007.
38. Leibo SP, Pool TB. The principal variables of cryopreservation: Solutions, temperature and rate changes, Fertil Steril. 2011; 96(2):269-76.
39. Ubaldi FM, Capalbo A, Vaiarelli A, Cimadomo D, Colamaria S, Alviggi C, et al. Follicular versus luteal phase ovarian stimulation during the same menstrual cycle (DuoStim) in a reduced ovarian reserve population results in a similar euploid blastocyst formation rate: new insight in ovarian reserve exploitation. Fertil Steril. 2016;105(6):1488-95.e1.
40. Consensus Group C. There is only one thing that is truly important in an IVF laboratory: everything. Cairo Consensus Guidelines on IVF Culture Conditions. Reprod Biomed Online. 2020;40(1):33-60.
41. Tarahomi M, de Melker AA, van Wely M, Hamer G, Repping S, Mastenbroek S. pH stability of human preimplantation embryo culture media: effects of culture and batches. Reprod Biomed Online. 2018;37(4):409-14.
42. Ramirez LB, Shi HL, Lvov E, Racowsky C, Bormann CL. Do thermal properties of a culture dish influence embryo development? Fertil Steril. 2015;104(3):e55.
43. Thornhill AR, Brunetti XO, Bird S, Bennet K, Rios LM, Taylor J. Reducing human error in IVF with electron witnessing. Fertil Steril. 2011;96(3):S179.
44. Holmes R, Wirka KA, Catherino AB, Hayward B, Swain JE. Comparison of electronic versus manual witnessing of procedures within the in vitro fertilization laboratory: impact on timing and efficiency. Fertil Steril. 2021;2(2):181-8.

CHAPTER 59

Luteal Phase Support

Sonal Agarwal, Neha Tyagi, Kamini A Rao

INTRODUCTION

Owing to the increasing incidence of infertility in the current era, assisted reproductive technology (ART) has seen a lot of advancements. The use of gonadotropin-releasing hormone (GnRH) analogs has achieved controlled ovarian stimulation (COS) by causing pituitary desensitization and reducing cycle cancellation rates. COS, however, impairs pulsatile release of luteinizing hormone (LH) from the anterior pituitary gland, which disrupts the function of corpus luteum. There is now a general consensus on luteal phase support (LPS) in in vitro fertilization (IVF) cycles to optimize outcomes.[1]

PHYSIOLOGY

The luteal phase is the time period between ovulation and either the establishment of a pregnancy or the onset of menses, which occurs 2 weeks later.[2] Corpus luteum is a unique endocrine gland that plays an important role in the regulation of menstrual cycle and early pregnancy. Corpus luteum is formed following follicular rupture causing theca and granulosa cells to separate from the basal lamina **(Fig. 1)**, thereby causing bleeding into the central cavity. The blood filled corpus luteum is known as "corpus hemorrhagicum". Corpus luteum secretes estrogen and progesterone **(Flowchart 1)**, which support the implantation process.

In a successful implantation, the growing blastocyst secretes human chorionic gonadotropin (hCG), which maintains the corpus luteum and its secretions until luteo-placental shift occurs during the fifth gestational week when placental steroidogenesis begins. Luteal vascularity, peaks at around 7 days following ovulation, which correlates with peak serum progesterone levels.[3]

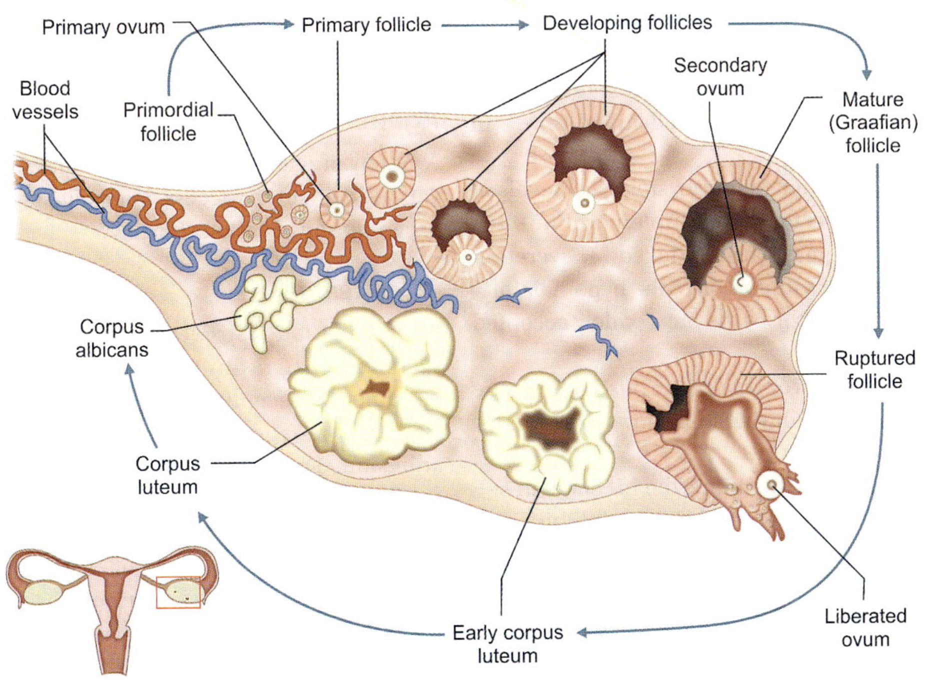

Fig.1: Physiology of corpus luteum.

Flowchart 1: Role of corpus luteum in luteal phase.

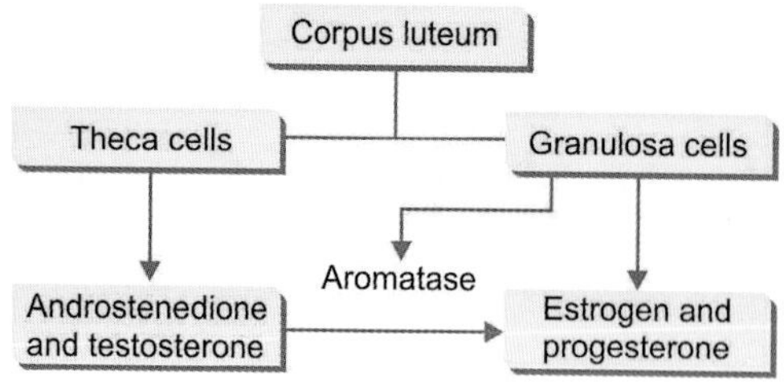

LUTEAL PHASE DEFECT

Luteal phase defect (LPD) can be described as failure to develop a receptive secretory endometrium due to disruption in the function of corpus luteum. Aberrant folliculogenesis results in defective neoangiogenesis leading to inadequate production of progesterone. Progesterone plays a pivotal role in the maintenance of endometrial integrity to sustain implantation. LPD presents clinically as short menstrual cycles, recurrent implantation failure or recurrent pregnancy loss (RPL).

Pathophysiology of Luteal Phase Defect

An intact functional hypothalamic-pituitary-ovarian (HPO) axis is essential for normal regulation of menstrual cycle and maintenance of early pregnancy **(Flowchart 2)**.

Flowchart 2: Pathophysiology of luteal phase defect.

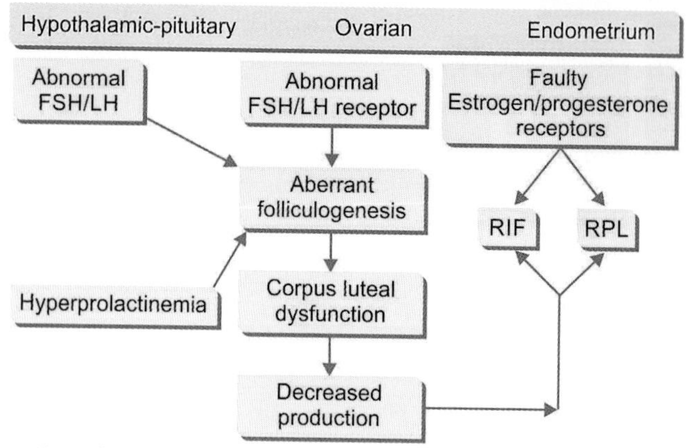

(FSH: follicle-stimulating hormone; LH: luteinizing hormone; RIF: re-current implantation failure; RPL: recurrent pregnancy loss)

LUTEAL PHASE SUPPORT IN ART: WHY IS IT NEEDED?

Many postulations have been described and studied as to why there is a LPD in the ART cycles.

- There is loss of pulsatile secretion of LH from the pituitary gland due to downregulation of LH receptors in GnRH agonist cycles.[4]
- It has been observed that there is premature luteolysis in GnRH antagonist treatment cycles leading to poor pregnancy rates and shortened luteal phase in unsupported cycles.[5]
- It has been postulated that supraphysiological levels of steroid hormones secreted by multiple corpora lutea in an IVF stimulation may cause reduced LH secretion due to negative feedback inhibition of the hypothalamic-pituitary axis. Currently, this is the most widely accepted theory of LPD in ART.[6]
- There is mechanical disruption of corpus luteum due to loss of granulosa cells during follicular aspiration for oocyte retrieval.[7]
- The administration of hCG to mimic the LH surge in IVF has been implicated as a cause of LPD by inhibition of endogenous LH secretion from the pituitary.[8]

LUTEAL PHASE SUPPORT

Luteal phase support may be defined as administration of pharmacological agents aimed at supporting implantation process to enhance the probability of pregnancy with a successful outcome.

Indications of Luteal Phase Support

- Recurrent pregnancy loss—LPD has been associated with RPL although causation is yet to be established. It is, however, a common practice to provide LPS to these patients.
- Controlled ovarian stimulation in IVF or intracytoplasmic sperm injection (ICSI) cycle.
- Frozen embryo transfer (FET) cycles—since there is no corpus luteum to support the pregnancy, there is a mandatory requirement of LPS.
- Ovulation induction with gonadotropins in intrauterine insemination (IUI) cycle.
- Luteal phase defect in cases of hyperprolactinemia, hypothyroidism, obesity, autoimmune disorders causing disruption of HPO axis.

Agents Used for Luteal Phase Support

A variety of agents have been used and studied so far, all with varying degrees of success. The mainstay of LPS still remains progesterone in various forms.

Progesterone

After adequate estrogen priming, progesterone causes secretory changes in the endometrium, which improves endometrial receptivity wherein endometrium acquires a transient ovarian steroid-dependent state favoring blastocyst adhesion. The endometrial glands become tortuous and secretory, and stromal vascularity increases which enhance the endometrial receptivity.[9] Progesterone induces nitric oxide synthesis in the decidua, which helps in promoting local vasodilatation and uterine musculature quiescence. Excessive uterine contractility has been found to play a role in causing ectopic pregnancies and miscarriages.[10] Hence, progesterone has been studied widely as an agent for LPS.

The two forms of progesterone that are used are natural or micronized progesterone and synthetic progesterone.

Micronized progesterone: It is available as oral, vaginal, rectal, and parenteral preparations.

- *Oral:* It is no longer recommended due to poor bioavailability (as less as 10%), owing to high first-pass hepatic metabolism. Hence, higher doses are required to reach an effective serum level, which causes sedative and anxiolytic central nervous system (CNS) side effects. Progesterone metabolites bind to gamma amino butyric acid (GABA), a receptor complex in CNS and cause headache, vertigo, and postural hypotension. According to a study oral doses of progesterone, even as high as 1 g/day have not been able to induce predecidual changes in the endometrium to help implantation.[11]
- *Transdermal:* Administration of progesterone through this route is not possible due to presence of an enzyme in the skin, 5α-reductase, which inactivates progesterone.
- *Intramuscular:* The use of intramuscular form of progesterone for LPS was first introduced during IVF in 1985.[12] It is associated with various side effects such as injection site pain, skin irritation, inflammatory reactions, and rarely abscess formation as these are oil-based preparations. Single daily dosing of 50 mg progesterone in oil produces physiological serum progesterone levels of 25 ng/24 hours. Intramuscular progesterone has been associated with highest serum levels compared to other routes.[13]

There have also been studies comparing the intramuscular route of progesterone administration versus vaginal route. A meta-analysis of such studies done in 2009 showed comparable results in terms of clinical pregnancy rates and ongoing pregnancy rates between vaginal and intramuscular preparations.[14]

A Cochrane review published in 2011 showed no difference in clinical pregnancy rate or live birth rate between intramuscular and vaginal route progesterone; however, it did find a difference favoring intramuscular progesterone in ongoing pregnancy rates.[15]

Although more randomized controlled trials (RCTs) are needed to confirm these findings, such studies hold particular promise in cultures where women feel uncomfortable using the vaginal route for drug administration.

- *Vaginal:* Vaginal preparations of progesterone have become the mainstay of LPS nowadays owing to the ease of use compared to daily painful injections and a comparable efficacy. Progesterone can be administered vaginally in various forms as tablet, suppository, 8% gel preparation, and vaginal spray.

The unique feature of 8% bioadhesive gel is its property of sustained-release delivery over time allowing for once daily administration. It comes with a prefilled applicator. Each applicator contains 1.125 g 8% (w/w) gel equivalent to

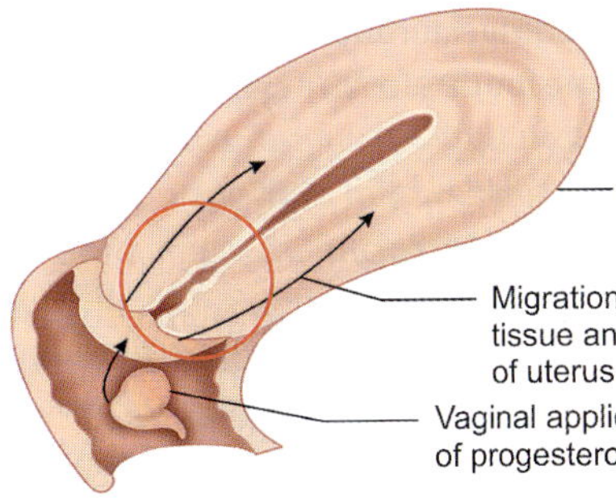

Fig. 2: Vaginal progesterone exhibiting first uterine-pass effect.

90 mg progesterone per dose. Vaginal preparations have an upper hand when compared to oral or parenteral route due to its first-pass uterine effect **(Fig. 2)**. Progesterone concentration in endometrial tissue is greater than would be expected based on serum levels.[16] However, a few patients report distress due to unavoidable vaginal discharge caused by these preparations.

According to a recent systematic review comparing different vaginal formulations for efficacy and safety in LPS during ART cycles, it was shown that there was no significant difference between them.[17]

- *Subcutaneous:* To avoid the painful intramuscular progesterone in oil injection, aqueous progesterone preparation was introduced. It is made by encapsulating progesterone in a starch residue called cyclodextrin, which increases the polarity, thus making it water-soluble. The aqueous form comes as 25 mg and 50 mg/day preparation, both found to reach serum progesterone levels resembling pulsatile progesterone levels in the luteal phase of menstrual cycle.[18]

According to an RCT, it was concluded that subcutaneous progesterone was well-tolerated and non-inferior to micronized vaginal progesterone as LPS in ART cycles.[19] Similar findings have been concluded by a meta-analysis, which showed that no statistically or clinically significant differences exist between subcutaneous and vaginal progesterone for LPS.[20]

Synthetic progesterone: Dydrogesterone was introduced to overcome the side effects of natural oral micronized progesterone and its less bioavailability. Its structure is closely related to progesterone and has a highly selective action on progesterone receptors. It lacks androgenic, estrogenic, and corticoid properties. It is available as 10 mg oral preparation.

According to a recent phase III multicenter RCT, dydrogesterone was shown to be non-inferior to micronized vaginal progesterone as an LPS in IVF cycles with respect to ongoing pregnancy rates (up to 12 weeks of gestation).[21] A meta-analysis done in 2016 comprising eight RCTs had also concluded that oral dydrogesterone seems to be as effective as vaginal progesterone for LPS in ART cycles, and appears to be better tolerated.[22]

Human Chorionic Gonadotropin

Human chorionic gonadotropin is similar to LH in its molecular structure, mode of action, and physiological effects. However, hCG has a longer half-life and potency owing to the presence of higher sialic acid residues. This formed the basis of its use as an agent for LPS. Two types of hCG have been in use:

- Intramuscular
- Subcutaneous—recombinant form.

Various studies have been done comparing the efficacy of hCG with respect to traditional progesterone preparations. Although luteal hCG has a similar efficacy to luteal progesterone in terms of pregnancy outcomes, hCG has rarely been used as a sole agent for LPS in ART clinics, and even this use has been declining. Human chorionic gonadotropin has been associated with increased rates of ovarian hyperstimulation syndrome (OHSS). More popularly, it is used in addition to progesterone preparations.[23,24]

Progesterone versus hCG with progesterone: According to a Cochrane review published in 2015, it was shown that there was no significant difference between the two groups in terms of live births and ongoing pregnancy rates. However, use of progesterone alone was associated with lower incidence of OHSS.[25]

Gonadotropin-releasing Hormone Agonist

Gonadotropin-releasing hormone was introduced as a new means of providing LPS in 2005. The concept behind its use was that it would increase LH secretion from the anterior pituitary, thereby supporting the corpus luteum. It was also hypothesized that it may have effects on the endometrial GnRH receptors or direct effects on the embryo.[29] It is available in three forms—subcutaneous, intramuscular, and intranasal. It has been used as either a single dose subcutaneous injection decapeptyl 0.1 mg on day 5 or day 6 of oocyte retrieval, or intranasal form with nafarelin 200 mg twice daily initiated on the evening after oocyte retrieval. As per a Cochrane review by van der et al. published in 2015, it was found that there was an increased live birth rate and ongoing pregnancy rate with the use of GnRH agonist along with progesterone in the luteal phase, compared to using progesterone alone.[25]

Despite promising early evidence, additional studies are needed given the lack of clear biologic mechanism before wide acceptance of this practice.

Estrogen

Estrogen pretreatment has a role in priming the endometrium in FET cycles, especially in donor egg recipients. Due to lack of endogenous estrogen production, there is inadequate endometrial priming, which hampers embryo implantation. It is available in various forms such as oral, transdermal, and intramuscular.

Oral dose of estradiol valerate is 4–8 mg/day. It has a high first liver-pass effect, hence it should be given with caution in patients at risk for venous thromboembolism. Transdermal gel or patch preparation should be considered in such patients. Transdermal preparations have been found to be less effective in hot and humid weather, and obese patients due to reduced absorption.

There has been no fixed protocol regarding dose and duration of estrogen administration in LPS. Scheffer et al. found no significant difference in pregnancy rates when either of oral or transdermal patch or transdermal gel of estrogen was used for LPS.[25]

However, according to the Cochrane review, there was no conclusive evidence of difference between patients using either progesterone alone or progesterone with oral estrogen for outcomes such as clinical pregnancy rate and ongoing pregnancy rates. It should be noted that there might be some benefit with the use of transdermal or oral with transdermal estrogen supplementation.[26]

Duration of 10–14 days of estrogen administration is usually sufficient in artificial protocol but for patients who do not respond,[27] it should not extend beyond 40 days, can lead to breakthrough bleeding.[28]

Optimal Timing of Luteal Phase Support

In ART cycles, there is substantial endogenous production of progesterone starting after the hCG trigger. Although it is important to give LPS in IVF cycles, it is equally important to time it correctly. LPS, if given early, might advance the endometrial maturation making it out of sync with the growing embryo, thus, hampering the implantation process.

It has been studied that administration of intramuscular progesterone early in the cycle, that is, prior to oocyte retrieval compared with within 24 hours after oocyte retrieval, will result in lower pregnancy rates.[30] According to an RCT, comparing the timing of onset of start of LPS in patient undergoing IVF cycles, there was no significant difference in the ongoing pregnancy rates between the three arms—starting LPS on the day of hCG administration, the day of oocyte retrieval, and the day of embryo transfer.[31] It may be concluded from the published data that there is an acceptable window of 24–48 hours of starting LPS after oocyte retrieval for optimum cycle results.

In a prospective study, it was shown that prolongation of progesterone supplementation beyond positive beta hCG test had no effect on miscarriage rate or delivery rate.[32] Another study randomized IVF patients into two groups comparing the impact of progesterone supplementation, beyond first ultrasound showing viable pregnancy. It concluded that there was no significant difference in miscarriage rates or bleeding in early pregnancy between the two groups.[33]

From the current available evidence, it has been found that continuation of progesterone supplementation beyond first viability ultrasound in patients undergoing IVF treatment is generally unnecessary.

Luteal Phase Support in Special Situations

Luteal Phase Support in IUI Cycle Using Various Ovulation Induction Protocols

Controlled ovarian stimulation in IUI cycles is similar to IVF or ICSI cycles with respect to multifollicular development. According to the published data available at present, it may be suggested to use LPS in gonadotropin-stimulated IUI cycles with multifollicular development.

In 2017, a large systematic meta-analysis was undertaken to evaluate the role of LPS in ovulation induction in IUI cycles and the conclusions from it were as follows:[34]

- Progesterone supplementation improves clinical pregnancy and live birth in gonadotropin ovulation induction–IUI (OI–IUI) cycles.
- There does not seem to be a benefit of exogenous progesterone in Clomiphene Citrate OI–IUI cycles.
- There is insufficient evidence that progesterone support improves outcomes in OI–IUI cycles using letrozole or clomiphene citrate plus gonadotropins.

Luteal Phase Support in IVF: Fresh Transfer Cycles Using GnRH Agonist as Trigger

With the advent of GnRH antagonist protocol to prevent premature LH surge in COS cycles, it became possible to use GnRH agonist as a trigger, thus reducing the risk of OHSS. However, it has a deleterious effect on the luteal phase of the IVF cycle compared to that of a natural cycle.[35,36]

There is a significant difference in the luteal phase of GnRH agonist trigger cycle compared to hCG trigger cycle owing to the shorter half-life of endogenous LH (~60 minutes) compared to that of hCG (>24 hours).[32] This leads to low circulatory levels of estrogen and progesterone throughout early or mid-luteal phase, causing premature luteolysis and implantation failure.

Modified Luteal Phase Support after GnRH Triggering

Earlier RCTs have shown high incidence of early pregnancy loss with the use of standard LPS with vaginal progesterone and oral estrogen in cycles where GnRH agonist was used as a trigger for final oocyte maturation.[37,38] This necessitated the use of modified LPS in such cycles:

- *hCG bolus:* Various RCTs have shown that hCG when used in small bolus (1,500 IU) after GnRH agonist trigger gives similar ongoing pregnancy rates and clinical pregnancy rates as compared to hCG triggered cycles, without increasing the risk of OHSS, thus allowing fresh embryo transfer.[39-42] A proof-of-concept study was conducted by Kol et al.[39] including women undergoing IVF or ICSI treatment with GnRH agonist trigger. The women were supplemented by two bolus doses of hCG (1,500 IU) on the day of ovum pick up and second dose 4 days later, with no exogenous progesterone support. The study reported an ongoing pregnancy rate of 47% with no incidence of OHSS. It may be said that a small dose of hCG rescues the luteal phase in GnRH agonist triggered cycles, however, more studies are needed to establish a protocol.
- *Recombinant LH (rLH):* According to a proof-of-concept study, similar reproductive outcomes were obtained using rLH as LPS in GnRH triggered cycles compared to hCG triggered cycles. rLH was used in doses of 300 IU on alternate days starting from the oocyte retrieval day along with daily vaginal progesterone. Larger studies are needed to establish the safety and efficacy of this protocol. Another drawback is the high cost associated with it.
- *Intensive progesterone and estrogen support*: Various studies have been performed using intensive LPS protocol consisting of estrogen and progesterone only, for GnRH agonist triggered cycles compared to cycles using hCG trigger. While some studies favored this protocol, others discouraged its use reporting a low reproductive outcome. There seems to be a need for larger RCTs to justify the use of intensive LPS.[43,44] Although, various protocols of modified LPS have shown promising reproductive outcomes after GnRH agonist triggering, without increasing the incidence of OHSS, the most optimal LPS still remains to be found out.[45]

Luteal Phase Support in Natural FET Cycles: Is there Any Role?

It is well-known that progesterone supplementation improves implantation rates in fresh embryo transfer cycles. It has also been observed that there is a positive role of luteal support in hormonally controlled frozen-thawed ET cycles. In general, endogenous production of progesterone is sufficient to support implantation in a natural ovulation cycle in a fertile female.

In a large retrospective cohort study involving 1,158 frozen-thawed ET cycles, it was concluded that vaginal progesterone supplementation significantly improves pregnancy rates in natural FET cycles.[46] This suggested that

TABLE 1: Adjuvants in luteal phase support.

	Adjuvant	*Rationale*	*Evidence*
1.	Intravenous immunoglobulin	Inhibiting (NK) cell production and/or activity correcting abnormal Th1:Th2 ratio	No convincing evidence for the use and safety of IVIg
2.	Anti-TNF alpha agents	Increased TNF-alpha:interleukin-4 ratio-role in RIF	Lack of evidence to support its use owing to adverse effects like lymphoma
3.	Intravenous lipids	Inhibits Th1 cytokines and reduces the cytotoxic effect of NK cells	Routine use not recommended
4.	Corticosteroids	• Anti-inflammatory and immunosuppressive activity • Improves intraendometrial milie	Limited evidence to improve pregnancy rate (PR) in women undergoing conventional IVF and in those with autoimmune disorders and unexplained RIF
5	Low-dose aspirin	Increases uterine blood flow, enhances endometrial receptivity and improves implantation rates	• Lack of evidence supporting routine use • Limited evidence to support use in RPL
6.	LMWH (Low molecular weight heparin)	• Anti-thrombotic effect • There is increased incidence of thrombophilia in women with RIF. LMWH reduces formation of microthrombi at implantation site	• Routine use not warranted • Should be considered in women with thrombophilia and RIF
7.	Metformin	Modulation of insulin like growth factors	Beneficial effects in PCOS patients undergoing IVF by reducing risk of OHSS and improving CPR
8.	Myo-Inositol[51]	Acts on insulin, FSH, and LH receptors	Pivotal role in the development of oocytes and embryos
9.	Probiotics[52]	Reduces IL-6 and hs-CRP and increases IL-10 level	Beneficial effects in PCOS patients undergoing IVF by improving CPR
10.	L-Arginine[53,54]	Activates immune system and increases uterine vascular flow	Role in patients with recurrent thin endometrium

(CPR: clinical pregnancy rate; FSH: follicle-stimulating hormone; IVF: in vitro fertilization; IVIg: intravenous immunoglobulin; LH: luteinizing hormone; OHSS: ovarian hyperstimulation syndrome; PCOS: polycystic ovary syndrome; RIF: recurrent implantation failure; RPL: recurrent pregnancy loss; NK: natural killer; IL: interleukins; hs: high sensitivity)

patients undergoing ART treatment and FET cycles have suboptimal endogenous progesterone production.

Di Guardo[47] et al. developed a web based questionnaire for 1,480 clinicians on when to start, route, dosage, and duration of progesterone in luteal phase supplementation. It was concluded that most common practice is to start progesterone on day of oocyte retrieval via vaginal/intramuscular route and continue until 12 weeks gestation. Ten-year follow-up done by Shoham[48] et al. has further proved that practice of starting progesterone on day of egg retrieval has not changed yet. Survey has shown gradual increase in use of vaginal progesterone for LPS instead of intramuscular or oral route. Drakopoulos[49] et al. studied the role of dydrogesterone as LPS and found high oral bioavailability and specificity for P receptors suggesting higher efficacy than micronized progesterone. Decreased incidence of preeclampsia has been found in this study after use of dydrogesterone in natural and IUI cycles.

Adjuvants in Luteal Phase Support

Endometrial receptivity is considered critical for successful implantation. Potential mechanisms implicated for embryo implantation failure include endometrial immune hostility, suboptimal uterine perfusion, inadequate LPS, and increased myometrial contractility.

Adjuvant therapies have been used in IVF cycles in order to counteract the reasons for recurrent implantation failure, and to optimize IVF outcomes.

Various adjuvants that have been studied so far are listed in **Table 1**.[50]

KEY POINTS

- Luteal phase support is mandatory in assisted reproductive technology (ART) cycles to optimize reproductive outcomes.
- Progesterone and human chorionic gonadotropin (hCG) use in the luteal phase confers benefit to infertile women undergoing in vitro fertilization (IVF) treatment.
- Use of hCG for trigger is associated with greater risk of ovarian hyperstimulation syndrome (OHSS).
- Natural micronized progesterone as a luteal phase agent is not effective if taken orally.
- Vaginal and injectable progesterone have similar implantation and clinical pregnancy rates.
- Synthetic progesterone, dydrogesterone, has been found to be equally effective as vaginal micronized progesterone for luteal phase support (LPS) in ART cycles.
- Concomitant use of estrogen with progesterone does not seem to enhance the probability of implantation and pregnancy rates.

- Gonadotropin-releasing hormone agonist along with progesterone may have a promising role in improving IVF outcomes but more studies are needed to adopt this approach.
- Optimal timing of LPS is important, the window of starting LPS being within 24–48 hours from the oocyte retrieval.
- According to the literature available, there is no role of continuation of LPS beyond first positive beta hCG or first ultrasound showing viability. Although, the common practice by clinicians is to continue LPS till 12 weeks.
- Modified LPS in GnRH agonist triggered cycles in the form of hCG bolus and rLH has shown positive effect on pregnancy outcomes, but more studies are needed to support its use.
- Despite widespread use of adjuvants in LPS, current evidence does not recommend their routine use in all IVF cycles.

REFERENCES

1. Yanushpolsky EH. Luteal phase support in in vitro fertilization. Semin Reprod Med. 2015;33(2):118-27.
2. Fatemi HM, Camus M, Kolibianakis EM, Tournaye H, Papanikolaou EG, Donoso P, et al. The luteal phase of recombinant follicle-stimulating hormone/gonadotropin-releasing hormone antagonist in vitro fertilization cycles during supplementation with progesterone or progesterone and estradiol. Fertil Steril. 2007;87:504-8.
3. Miyazaki T, Tanaka M, Miyakoshi K, Minegishi K, Kasai K, Yoshimura Y. Power and colour Doppler ultrasonography for the evaluation of the vasculature of the human corpus luteum. Hum Reprod. 1998;13:2836-41.
4. Albano C, Grimbizis G, Smitz J, Riethmüller-Winzen H, Reissmann T, Van Steirteghem A, et al. The luteal phase of nonsupplemented cycles after ovarian superovulation with human menopausal gonadotropin and the gonadotropin-releasing hormone antagonist Cetrorelix. Fertil Steril. 1998;70:357-9.
5. Penarrubia J, Balasch J, Fabregues F, Creus M, Casamitjana R, Ballescá JL, et al. Human chorionic gonadotrophin luteal support overcomes luteal phase inadequacy after gonadotrophin releasing hormone agonist-induced ovulation in gonadotrophin stimulated cycles. Hum Reprod. 1998;13:3315-8.
6. Beckers NG, Macklon NS, Eijkemans MJ, Ludwig M, Felberbaum RE, Diedrich K, et al. Nonsupplemented luteal phase characteristics after the administration of recombinant human chorionic gonadotropin, recombinant luteinizing hormone, or gonadotropin-releasing hormone (GnRH) agonist to induce final oocyte maturation in in vitro fertilization patients after ovarian stimulation with recombinant follicle-stimulating hormone and GnRH antagonist cotreatment. J Clin Endocrinol Metab. 2003;88(9):4186-92.
7. Garcia J, Jones GS, Acosta AA, Wright GL Jr. Corpus luteum function after follicle aspiration for oocyte retrieval. Fertil Steril. 1981;36:565-72.
8. Miyake A, Aono T, Kinugasa T, Tanizawa O, Kurachi K. Suppression of serum levels of luteinizing hormone by short- and long-loop negative feedback in ovariectomized women. J Endocrinol. 1979;80(3):353-6.
9. Kolibianakis EM, Devroey P. The luteal phase after ovarian stimulation. Reprod Biomed Online. 2002;5:26-35.
10. Bulletti C, de Ziegler D. Uterine contractility and embryo implantation, Curr Opin Obstet Gynecol. 2005;17: 265-76.
11. Fanchin R, De Ziegler D, Bergeron C, Righini C, Torrisi C, Frydman R. Transvaginal administration of progesterone. Obstet Gynecol. 1997;90:396-401.
12. Leeton J, Trounson A, Jessup D. Support of the luteal phase in in vitro fertilization programs: results of a controlled trial with intramuscular Prolusion. J In Vitro Fert Embryo Transf. 1985;2(3):166-9.
13. Cicinelli E, de Ziegler D. Transvaginal progesterone: evidence for a new functional "portal system" flowing from the vagina to the uterus. Hum Reprod Update 1999;5:365-72.
14. Zarutskie P, Phillips J. A meta-analysis of the route of administration of luteal phase support in assisted reproductive technology: vaginal versus intramuscular progesterone. Fertil Steril. 2009;92(1):163-9.
15. van der Linden M, Buckingham K, Farquhar C, Kremer JA, Metwally M. Luteal phase support for assisted reproduction cycles. Cochrane Database Syst Rev. 2011;(10):CD009154.
16. Miles RA, Paulson RJ, Lobo RA, Press MF, Dahmoush L, Sauer MV. Pharmacokinetics and endometrial tissue levels of progesterone after administration by intramuscular and vaginal routes: a comparative study. Fertil Steril. 1994; 62(3):485-90.
17. Child T, Leonard S, Evans JS, Lass A. Systematic review of the clinical efficacy of vaginal progesterone for luteal phase support in assisted reproductive technology cycles. Reprod Biomed Online. 2018;pii:S1472-6483(18)30055-5.
18. Sator M, Radicioni M, Cometti B, Loprete L, Leuratti C, Schmidl D, et al. Pharmacokinetics and safety profile of a novel progesterone aqueous formulation administered by the s.c. Route. Gynecol Endocrinol. 2013;29:205-8.
19. Baker VL, Jones CA, Doody K, Foulk R, Yee B, Adamson GD, et al. A randomized, controlled trial comparing the efficacy and safety of aqueous subcutaneous progesterone with vaginal progesterone for luteal phase support of in vitro fertilization. Hum Reprod. 2014;29(10):2212-20.
20. Doblinger J, Cometti B, Trevisan S, Griesinger G. Subcutaneous progesterone is effective and safe for luteal phase support in IVF: an individual patient data meta-analysis of the phase III trials. PLoS ONE. 2016;11(3):e0151388.
21. Tournaye H, Sukhikh GT, Kahler E, Griesinger G. A Phase III randomized controlled trial comparing the efficacy, safety and tolerability of oral dydrogesterone versus micronized vaginal progesterone for luteal support in in vitro fertilization. Hum Reprod. 2017;32(5):1019-27.
22. Barbosa MW, Silva LR, Navarro PA, Ferriani RA, Nastri CO, Martins WP. Dydrogesterone vs. progesterone for luteal-phase support: systematic review and meta-analysis of randomized controlled trials. Ultrasound Obstet Gynecol. 2016;48:161-70.
23. Daya S, Gunby J. Luteal phase support in assisted reproduction cycles. Cochrane Database Syst Rev. 2004;(3):CD004830.
24. Practice Committee of American Society for Reproductive Medicine in collaboration with Society for Reproductive Endocrinology and Infertility. Progesterone supplementation during the luteal phase and in early pregnancy in the treatment of infertility: an educational bulletin. Fertil Steril. 2008;90(5):S150-3.

25. Scheffer JB, Scheffer BB, Carvalho RF, Aguiar AP, Lozano DHM, Labrosse J, et al. A comparison of the effects of three luteal phase support protocols with estrogen on in vitro fertilization-embryo transfer outcomes in patients on a GnRH antagonist protocol. JBRA Assist Reprod. 2019;23(3):239-45.
26. van der Linden M, Buckingham K, Farquhar C, Kremer JAM, Metwally M. Luteal phase support for assisted reproduction cycles. Cochrane Database of Syst Rev. 2015;(7):CD009154.
27. Ying Y, Wu Y, Liu S, Huang Q, Liu H. The timing for initiating estrogen stimulation in artificial cycle for frozen-thawed embryo transfer can be flexible. Reprod Health. 2021;18(1):181.
28. Borini A, Dal Prato L, Bianchi L, Violini F, Cattoli M, Flamigni C. Effect of duration of estradiol replacement on the outcome of oocyte donation. J Assist Reprod Genet. 2001;18(4):185-90.
29. Pirard C, Donnez J, Loumaye E. GnRH agonist as novel luteal support: results of a randomized, parallel group, feasibility study using intranasal administration of buserelin. Hum Reprod. 2005;20(7):1798-804.
30. Sohn SH, Penzias AS, Emmi AM, Dubey AK, Layman LC, Reindollar RH, et al. Administration of progesterone before oocyte retrieval negatively affects the implantation rate. Fertil Steril. 1999;71(1):11-4.
31. Mochtar MH, Van Wely M, Van der Veen F. Timing luteal phase support in GnRH agonist down-regulated IVF/embryo transfer cycles. Hum Reprod. 2006;21(4):905-8.
32. Nyboe AA, Popovic-Todorovic B, Schmidt KT, Loft A, Lindhard A, Højgaard A, et al. Progesterone supplementation during early gestations after IVF or ICSI has no effect on the delivery rates: a randomized controlled trial. Hum Reprod. 2002;17:357-61.
33. Aboulghar MA, Amin YM, Al-Inany HG, Aboulghar MM, Mourad LM, Serour GI, et al. Prospective randomized study comparing luteal phase support for ICSI patients up to the first ultrasound compared with an additional three weeks. Hum Reprod. 2008;23(4):857-62.
34. Green KA, Zolton JR, Schermerhorn SM, Lewis TD, Healy MW, Terry N, et al. Progesterone luteal support after ovulation induction and intrauterine insemination: an updated systematic review and meta- analysis. Fertil Steril. 2017;107(4):924-33.
35. Humaidan P, Kol S, Papanikolaou EG, Copenhagen GnRH Agonist Triggering Workshop Group. GnRH agonist for triggering of final oocyte maturation: time for a change of practice? Hum Reprod Update. 2011;17(4):510-24.
36. Humaidan P, Ejdrup Bredkjaer H, Westergaard LG, Yding Andersen C. 1,500 IU human chorionic gonadotropin administered at oocyte retrieval rescues the luteal phase when gonadotropin-releasing hormone agonist is used for ovulation induction: a prospective, randomized, controlled study. Fertil Steril. 2010;93(3):847-54.
37. Kolibianakis EM, Schultze-Mosgau A, Schroer A, van Steirteghem A, Devroey P, Diedrich K, et al. A lower ongoing pregnancy rate can be expected when GnRH agonist is used for triggering final oocyte maturation instead of HCG in patients undergoing IVF with GnRH antagonists. Hum Reprod. 2005;20(10):2887-92.
38. Humaidan P, Papanikolaou EG, Kyrou D, Alsbjerg B, Polyzos NP, Devroey P, et al. The luteal phase after GnRH-agonist triggering of ovulation: present and future perspectives. Reprod Biomed Online. 2012;24(2):134-41.
39. Kol S, Humaidan P, Itskovitz-Eldor J. GnRH agonist ovulation trigger and hCG-based, progesterone-free luteal support: a proof of concept study. Hum Reprod. 2011;26(10):2874-7.
40. Humaidan P. Luteal phase rescue in high-risk OHSS patients by GnRHa triggering in combination with low-dose HCG: a pilot study. Reprod Biomed Online. 2009;18(5):630-4.
41. Humaidan P, Polyzos NP, Alsbjerg B, Erb K, Mikkelsen AL, Elbaek HO, et al. GnRHa trigger and individualized luteal phase hCG support according to ovarian response to stimulation: two prospective randomized controlled multi-centre studies in IVF patients. Hum Reprod. 2013;28(9):2511-21.
42. Iliodromiti S, Blockeel C, Tremellen KP, Fleming R, Tournaye H, Humaidan P, et al. Consistent high clinical pregnancy rates and low ovarian hyperstimulation syndrome rates in high-risk patients after GnRH agonist triggering and modified luteal support: a retrospective multicentre study. Hum Reprod. 2013;28(9):2529-36.
43. Engmann L, DiLuigi A, Schmidt D, Nulsen J, Maier D, Benadiva C. The use of gonadotropin-releasing hormone (GnRH) agonist to induce oocyte maturation after cotreatment with GnRH antagonist in high-risk patients undergoing in vitro fertilization prevents the risk of ovarian hyperstimulation syndrome: a prospective randomized controlled study. Fertil Steril. 2008;89(1):84-91.
44. Babayof R, Margalioth EJ, Huleihel M, Amash A, Zylber-Haran E, Gal M, et al. Serum inhibin A, VEGF and TNF alpha levels after triggering oocyte maturation with GnRH agonist compared with hCG in women with polycystic ovaries undergoing IVF treatment: a prospective randomized trial. Hum Reprod. 2006;21(5):1260-5.
45. Leth-Moller K, Hammer Jagd S, Humaidan P. The luteal phase after GnRHa trigger-understanding an enigma. Int J Fertil Steril. 2014;8(3):227-34.
46. Sun H, Lee K, Park I, Kim J, Chi H, Kim SG, et al. Does luteal phase support improve pregnancy outcome in natural frozen-thawed embryo transfer cycles? Fertil Steril. 2017;108(3):e357.
47. Di Guardo F, Midassi H, Racca A, Tournaye H, De Vos M, Blockeel C. Luteal Phase Support in IVF: Comparison Between Evidence-Based Medicine and Real-Life Practices. Front. Endocrinol. 2020;11:500.
48. Shoham G, Leong M, Weissman A. A 10-year follow-up on the practice of luteal phase support using worldwide web-based surveys. Reprod Biol Endocrinol. 2021;19(1):15.
49. Drakopoulos P, Roelens C, De Vos M, Mackens S, Racca A, Tournaye H, et al. The Future of Luteal Phase Support in ART and the Role of Dydrogesterone. Front. Reprod. Health. 2021;2:618838.
50. Nardo LG, El-Toukhy T, Stewart J, Balen AH, Potdar N. British Fertility Society Policy and Practice Committee: Adjuvants in IVF: Evidence for good clinical practice. Hum Fertility. 2015;18:2-15.
51. Russo M, Forte G, Montanino Oliva M, Laganà AS, Unfer V. Melatonin and Myo-Inositol: Supporting Reproduction from the Oocyte to Birth. Int J Mol Sci. 2021;22:8433.
52. Younis N, Mahasneh A. Probiotics and the envisaged role in treating human infertility. Middle East Fertil Soc J. 2020;25:33.
53. Takasaki A, Tamura H, Miwa I, Taketani T, Shimamura K, Sugino N. Endometrial growth and uterine blood flow: a pilot study for improving endometrial thickness in the patients with a thin endometrium. Fertil Steril. 2010;93:1851-8.
54. Nardo LG, El-Toukhy T, Stewart J, Balen H, Potdar N. British Fertility Society Policy and Practice Committee: Adjuvants in IVF: evidence for good clinical practice. Hum Fertil. 2015;18(1):2-15.

SECTION 8

Dilemma in ART

CHAPTER 60

Poor Responders

Madhuri Milind Patil

INTRODUCTION

The successful endpoint of any infertility treatment is a live birth. This depends on various factors, including adequate number of follicles being stimulated, adequate number of oocytes retrieved in an assisted reproductive technology (ART) cycle, and quality of oocytes, and this, in turn, depends on ovarian response. According to the Bologna criteria,[1] poor ovarian response (POR) is defined as the presence of any two of the following three criteria:

1. Advanced maternal age (≥40 years) or any other risk factor for POR.
2. A previous POR (≤3 oocytes with a conventional stimulation protocol).
3. An abnormal ovarian reserve test (ORT) [i.e., antral follicle count (AFC), 5–7 follicles or anti-Müllerian hormone (AMH), 0.5–1.1 ng/mL].

All patients above the age of 40 years with an abnormal ORT are also considered poor responders. Apart from the above any two points, episodes of POR even after maximal stimulation are also sufficient to diagnose poor response, in the absence of advanced maternal age or abnormal ORT. At least one stimulated cycle is considered essential for the diagnosis of POR.

There are eight subgroups of poor responders according to the Bologna criteria as shown in **Table 1**.

TABLE 1: Eight subgroups of the ESHRE (European Society of Human Reproduction and Embryology) Bologna criteria.

Categories	*Subgroups*	*ESHRE criteria fulfilled*
No previous IVF attempt	≥ years (+ risk factor for POR) + abnormal ORT	1 + 3
One previous IVF attempt with POR	≥ 40 years (+ risk factor for POR)	1 + 2
	Abnormal ORT	2 + 3
	≥ 40 years (± risk factor for POR) + abnormal ORT	1 + 2 + 3
Two previous IVF attempts with POR	No risk factor for POR and normal ORT	Supplemental criteria 4
	≥ 40 years (± risk factor for POR) but normal ORT	1 + supplemental criteria 4
	Abnormal ORT but no risk factor for POR	3 + supplemental criteria 4
	≥ 40 years (± risk factor for POR) and abnormal ORT	1 + 3 + supplemental criteria 4

(IVF: in vitro fertilization; ORT: ovarian reserve test; POR: poor ovarian response)

But Bologna criteria are not considered ideal, thus making it difficult to manage women with POR.

Why is the Bologna Criteria not Ideal?

Bologna criteria are not ideal due to:

- Heterogeneity of subgroups due to absence of homogeneous subgroups for live birth rates (LBRs) **(Fig. 1)**
- Specific profiles of abnormal ovarian response like hypo- and suboptimal response not being included **(Fig. 2)**.
- Age-related aneuploidies affecting the "oocyte quality": It was observed by Colls et al.[2] that euploidy rate is independent of the number of blastocysts obtained but not of the age. Thus, we may obtain good-quality blastocysts, but they still could be aneuploid.

Thus came the *new classification* of patients with poor prognosis by the Patient Oriented Strategies Encompassing IndividualizeD Oocyte Number (POSEIDON) working group.[3]

The patients were then classified into four groups as follows:

Group 1:

- Young patients <35 years with adequate ovarian reserve parameters (AFC ≥5; AMH ≥1.2 ng/mL) and with an unexpected poor or suboptimal ovarian response
- Subgroup 1a: <4 oocytes*
- Subgroup 1b: 4–9 oocytes retrieved*

*After standard ovarian stimulation.

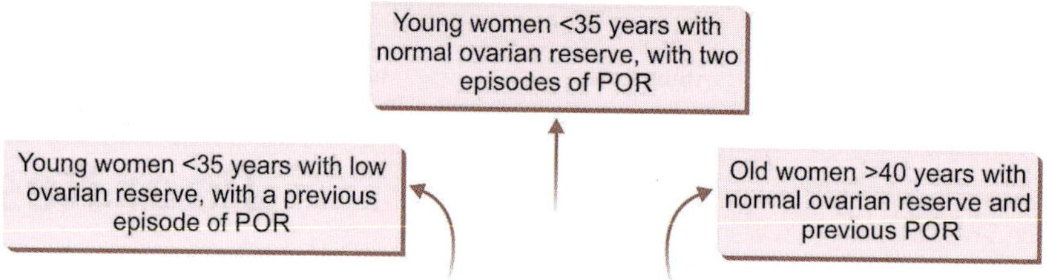

Fig. 1: Heterogeneity of subgroups for live birth rate. (POR: poor ovarian response)

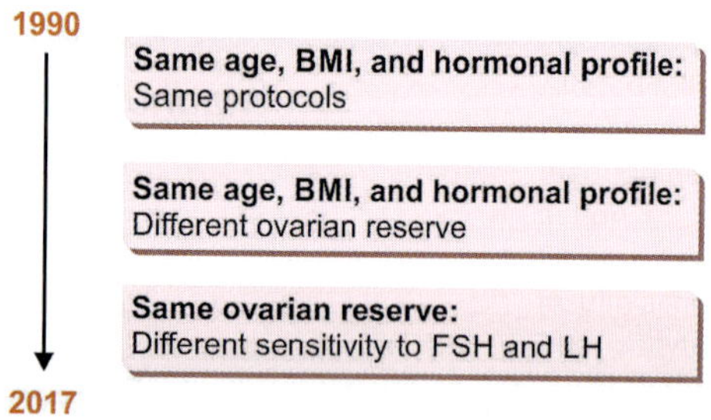

Fig. 2: Specific profiles and treatment over the last three decades. (BMI: body mass index; FSH: follicle-stimulating hormone; LH: luteinizing hormone)

Group 2:

- Older patients ≥35 years with adequate ovarian reserve parameters (AFC ≥5; AMH ≥1.2 ng/mL) and with an unexpected poor or suboptimal ovarian response
- Subgroup 2a: <4 oocytes*
- Subgroup 2b: 4–9 oocytes retrieved*

*After standard ovarian stimulation

Group 3: Young patients (<35 years) with poor ovarian reserve prestimulation parameters (AFC <5; AMH <1.2 ng/mL)

Group 4: Older patients (≥35 years) with poor ovarian reserve prestimulation parameters (AFC <5; AMH <1.2 ng/mL)

Thus, we must not only consider decreased ovarian reserve (DOR) patients as poor responders but also look at those patients with normal ovarian reserve who are hyporesponders. This is then based on the follicular output rate (FORT) after controlled ovarian stimulation (COS).[4] Thus, there could be women with good ovarian reserve but still having a poor response or vice versa where women with poor ovarian reserve have a good response to stimulation **(Fig. 3)**.

Thus, the first group of women are hyporesponders and have hyposensitivity to follicle-stimulating hormone (FSH) and show suboptimal or unexpected poor response to exogenous FSH. This response is in no way related to their ovarian reserve.[5] These women at times even when the ovarian response is normal (i.e., >5 eggs) tend to show an increase in the cumulative FSH dose (i.e., >2,500–3,000 IU) required and in the stimulation length (hyposensitivity to FSH).[6] These normo-ovulatory normogonadotropic young patients may have an initial slow (poor) response to recombinant human FSH (r-hFSH) characterized by normal follicular cohort with no follicle >10 mm on day 8 of stimulation or "stagnation" between day 7 and day 10.[7,8]

This phenomenon reflects hyposensitivity of granulosa cells to standard FSH dose and is associated with higher FSH consumption, low FORT, unexpected poor response (i.e., <3 eggs retrieved), and lower pregnancy rates (PRs). If hyporesponse is identified early (i.e., day 5–8 of COS), recombinant human luteinizing hormone (r-hLH)/human menopausal gonadotropin (hMG) is effective in rescuing follicle/oocyte number (FORT) and embryo competence.

The POSEIDON group[3] labeled patients with POR as low prognosis group and categorized women with POR by age and ovarian reserve **(Flowchart 1)**.

For this, the regulation of activation and growth of the antral follicles should be known though till date it stands unclear. It is postulated that the activation and growth of the primordial and preantral follicles may be due to local growth factor such as transforming growth factor-beta (TGF-β) and bone morphogenic protein (BMP), release of inhibitory signal or increase in stimulatory signals, local milieu of the neighboring follicles or stroma, and several sources still unknown.

Another new classification was coined by Yovich et al. and was called "PIVET poor-prognosis criteria".[9] The criteria used for classification of patients as poor prognosis were as follows:[9]

- All women aged 40 years and above.
- All women categorized as poor prognosis from previous in vitro fertilization (IVF), meaning cases of (≥3).
- All PORs (generating ≤4 oocytes despite FSH dosing maximized at 450 IU daily).
- All cases with "E" categorization according to PIVET FSH-dosing algorithms (AMH <5 pmol/L and AFC <5 follicles) matching ORT according to Bologna criteria.
- All cases where resultant embryo quality rated poor, meaning no suitable blastocysts for cryopreservation (good prognosis in IVF generates 8–12 oocytes resulting in ≥3 blastocysts with gradings 3BB or better).

PREDICTION OF POOR RESPONDERS

One can predict DOR but not poor responder with good ovarian reserve. The ORTs are illustrated in **Flowchart 2**.

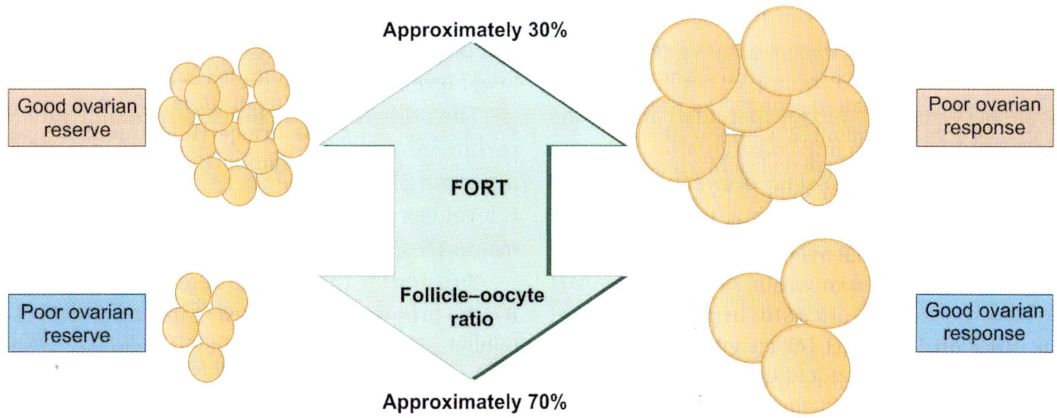

Fig. 3: Follicle–oocyte ratio. (FORT: follicular output rate)

Flowchart 1: Classification of poor responders by age and ovarian reserve.

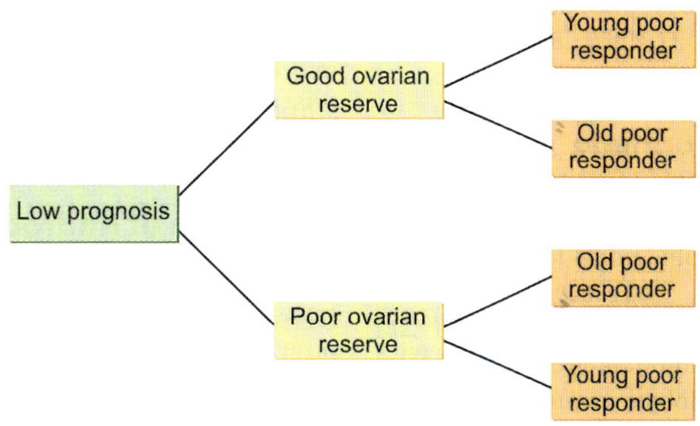

Flowchart 2: Ovarian reserve test.

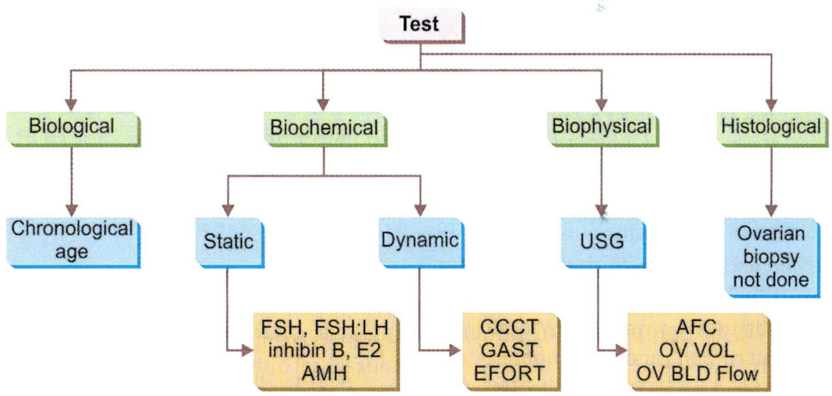

(AFC: antral follicle count; AMH: anti-Müllerian hormone; CCCT: clomiphene citrate challenge test; E2: estradiol; EFORT: exogenous FSH ovarian response test; FSH: follicle-stimulating hormone; GAST: gonadotropin agonist stimulation test; LH: luteinizing hormone; OV BLD: ovarian blood; OV VOL: ovarian volume; USG: ultrasonography)

Markers of Ovarian Reserve that will Predict Poor Response

- Age >40 years
- 4–6 months of oligomenorrhea
- Elevated FSH level of >25 IU/L at two occasions >4 weeks apart or once accompanied by low (<100 pmol/L) estradiol (E2) during COS
- AMH <0.35 ng/mL
- Day 3 inhibin B levels <45 pg/mL
- Low testosterone <0.51 nmol/L
- Transvaginal ultrasonography (USG) showing an AFC of <5–6 and ovarian volume of <3 cm.[3]

Of these, AFC and AMH have the best sensitivity and specificity. Both AMH and AFC decrease with age. Optimum cutoff value for AFC is ≤10 but the post-test probability was highest at cutoff levels of <8.[10]

Ovarian volume correlates with the number of growing follicles, but not with the number of oocytes retrieved.[11] Women with small ovaries with a volume <3 cm^3 have a high cancellation rate of IVF cycles[11] but are of limited prognostic value for IVF when LBR is taken into consideration.

There is a direct relationship seen between AMH and DOR. The optimum cutoff value for AMH to predict DOR is 0.99 ng/mL, but posttest probability was highest at cutoff levels of 0.59 ng/mL.[12] Evaluation of AFC and AMH as combined test did not significantly improve the level of prediction [area under curve (AUC) <0.946] of POR.[10] Though AMH gives information about the primordial follicular pool, it is not a panacea in determining DOR as there is significant discordance seen between AMH values and AFC. Moreover, AMH sample instability is one of the causes of nonreproducibility and sample storage is of utmost importance to obtain correct values for prediction of response.[13-17]

Day 3 Follicle-stimulating Hormone

Evaluation has several limitations for prediction of POR. This is because FSH is only an indirect measure of the size of follicle cohort and reflective of decreased granulosa cell function.[18] FSH does not diagnose DOR until high threshold values are reached[19] and high levels do not correlate with oocyte quality decline.[20] Moreover, intercycle and intersample variations may result in disparity in FSH measurements.[21]

Elevated day 3 FSH levels may also constitute a heterogeneous group where the women could have true reduced ovarian reserve or it could also be due to the presence of heterophilic antibodies or FSH receptor polymorphism in patients with otherwise normal ovaries.[22] It was seen that the PRs are significantly higher ($p < 0.05$) in women with normal FSH and age <36 years compared to those who are 36 years or more.[23] Elevated day 3 FSH/luteinizing hormone (LH) ratio is also supposed to be associated with inferior outcome in IVF treatment cycles and may be used as an additional predictor for decreased ovarian response.[24] With the three-variable model (FSH, AMH, and AFC), the proportion of patients misdiagnosed (11%) is almost halved when compared to the best single-variable model of AFC (20%).[25]

Day 2 Serum Estradiol

Elevated day 2 E2 levels of >75–80 pg/mL indicate an inappropriately advanced stage of follicular development, consistent with DOR and ovarian aging or simply reflect the presence of functional ovarian cysts. Prediction of ovarian reserve using E2 levels is still debatable[26] and no relationship has been found between serum E2 levels and PRs.[27]

Inhibin B

Inhibin B has a sensitivity of 87% and specificity of 49% in predicting DOR. Using 45 pg/mL as threshold for DOR,[28] the positive likelihood ratio of having DOR is 1.7. Inhibin B levels can be influenced by the amount of fat in an individual and lower levels are seen in obese women.[29]

The odds ratio for clinical pregnancy rate (CPR) (basal serum inhibin >45 vs. <45 pg/mL) was 6.8 [confidence interval (CI) 1.8–25.6]. It has been observed that inhibin B level is a better predictor for cancellation of cycles than ovarian response.

By using the three-variable model (AFC, FSH, and inhibin B), the proportion of patients misdiagnosed (11%) is almost halved when compared to the best single-variable model of AFC (20%).[25]

Of the dynamic test, one could use only the clomiphene citrate challenge test, which is of value in unmasking poor responders to COS who would not have been detected by basal FSH screening alone. Abnormal test is associated with a reduced chance of pregnancy. Exogenous FSH ovarian response test (EFORT) and gonadotropin agonist stimulation test (GAST) are only for research purpose and not used routinely in clinical practice.

Evaluation of Androgens in Diagnosis of Decreased Ovarian Reserve

Dehydroepiandrosterone sulfate (DHEAS) concentration was not significantly different between poor and normal responders or between pregnant and nonpregnant women. Lower basal testosterone was predictive, but with limited ability as a single marker for DOR. DOR for testosterone at cutoff point <0.51 nmol/L has a sensitivity of 88.6% and specificity of 98.3%, whereas for CPR at cutoff point ≤0.22 nmol/L has a sensitivity of 75% and specificity of 62.5%. Thus, we can conclude that apart from age, AMH and AFC had better predictive values for DOR.[30] But age still remains a better predictor of PR in women undergoing IVF.[31]

MANAGEMENT OF POOR RESPONDERS

Therapeutic strategies used to improve the success rate of ART in women with DOR and those with poor response in previous cycles have not helped much.

All types of empirical interventions are being tried, some with a hypothesis behind them, which might be biologically plausible, others with less plausibility but it is extremely difficult to establish criteria to define the population that should be treated and/or how to treat them. The different strategies that can be advocated to this group of women are to alter treatment protocols, improve the results with adjuvants, refuse treatment, or advise egg donation.

Once identified with DOR, we need to divide these women into two groups, one young that is <40 years and the other old that is >40 years, as different strategies may be applied for management. If women are >40 years, probably egg donation may be a better option as against those who are <40 years, where one could try new strategies to improve the outcome by focusing on oocyte competence since the number may be not be increased.

Interventions to enhance IVF outcome in women with DOR and poor responders are shown in **Table 2**.

Role of Adjuvants

Addition of Growth Hormone and Growth Hormone-releasing Factor

Growth hormone (GH) enhances the response of granulosa cells to gonadotropins[32] and basically acts by increasing the local production of insulin-like growth factor-1 (IGF-1), which modulates the action of FSH on granulosa cells, thus improving ovarian steroidogenesis.[33] GH is also known to induce LH receptor formation and also augment aromatase activity.[34] It is used in the dose of 8–12 IU/day starting on either day 2 or 3 of the menstrual cycle along with the gonadotropins and given till the day of human chorionic gonadotropin (hCG) injection. Initially, beneficial effects of GH were reported on the probability of live birth in women with DOR but as the sample size was small and statistical evidence was small, no firm conclusions could be drawn on its efficacy in improving ART cycle outcomes.

A recent publication by Bassiouny et al.[35] showed that GH co-treatment resulted in a higher number of oocytes collected, higher number of metaphase II (MII) oocytes retrieved with higher number of oocytes being fertilized, and higher number of embryos being transferred. The LBRs were also reported to be higher. Despite this, increase in the results did not reach statistical significance.[36] Therefore, it is mandatory for an individual clinician to decide on the use of GH according to their experience as one has to remember that the cost of treatment cycle increases considerably with the use of GH.

Ipsa et al. have shown that both GH and IGF have been demonstrated to promote steroidogenesis in granulosa and theca cells through alteration in metabolizing enzymes and work in synergy with gonadotropins. GH also promotes follicular selection and survival by decreasing follicular atresia through intracellular signaling pathways.[37] GH co-treatment increased the receptor density for granulosa follicle-stimulating hormone receptor (FSHR), bone morphogenetic protein receptor type 1B (BMPR1B), luteinizing hormone receptor (LHR), and growth hormone receptor (GHR) compared with the non-GH treated patients of the same age and ovarian reserve, which is supposed to increase GHR activity and result in a significant increase in PR.[38] GH supplementation reduced the cycle cancellation rate in women aged >40 years poor responders and promoted favorable ultrasonic endometrial pattern, with improved implantation and PR. This was related to the beneficial actions on embryo quality and endometrial receptivity.[39] Other publications have concluded that there is an increase in the number of oocytes retrieved but no difference was seen in the ongoing PR and LBR.[40,41] Two publications in 2020 have shown that the use of GH increases the CPR and LBR with an increased number of oocytes being retrieved with a lower cancellation rate.[42,43] Cozzolino et al. in a systemic review and meta-analysis showed a beneficial effect only on CPR, number of oocytes retrieved (mean difference 1.62), number of MII oocytes (mean difference 2.06), and number of embryos available to transfer but not on ongoing PR, LBR, or miscarriage rate.[44] Despite the evidence, European Society of Human Reproduction and Embryology (ESHRE) guidelines do not recommend the use of GH in poor responders.[45]

TABLE 2: Interventions to enhance IVF outcome.

Adjuvant therapy	*Change in OI protocols and ART*
• Growth hormone (GH) or GH-releasing factor (GHRF) • Pyridostigmine • Androgens: Transdermal testosterone, DHEA • Aspirin • L-arginine aromatase inhibitors • Antioxidants	• Modifications of long GnRH agonist protocol • Use of GnRH agonist short protocol • Use of GnRH antagonist protocol • Natural or mild cycle IVF • Modifications of ovarian stimulation • Use of LH in COS • Intracytoplasmic sperm injection • Day 2 versus day 3 ET

(ART: assisted reproductive technology; COS: controlled ovarian stimulation; DHEA: dehydroepiandrosterone; ET: embryo transfer; GnRH: gonadotropin-releasing hormone; IVR: in vitro fertilization LH: luteinizing hormone; OI: ovulation induction)

Growth Hormone-releasing Factor

Growth hormone-releasing factor (GHRF) results in a significant increase in GH and IGF-1 concentration, but no statistically significant differences were found in the number of oocytes retrieved, fertilization rate, and CPR.[46]

Pyridostigmine

Addition of pyridostigmine results in an increase in GH levels but has not shown to improve the ongoing PR or LBR in women with POR.

Initial studies which compared pyridostigmine with placebo reported lower number of ampoules used (38.4 vs. 48.3), higher number of oocytes collected (5.9 vs. 3.7), and improved PRs (25.7 vs. 11.4%) but did not improve the ongoing PR and LBR.[47,48] Thus, recent literature does not support the use of pyridostigmine as an adjuvant in poor responders.

Low-dose Aspirin

Addition of low-dose aspirin reported may improve gonadotropin responsiveness, implantation rates, and PRs due to enhanced blood flow to ovaries.[49] The evidence supporting the effect of a low dose of aspirin in women undergoing IVF is poor and controversial.[50,51] But beneficial effect is not currently supported by literature as no significant increase in implantation and PR was noted.[52] There was another study which looked into the combined effect of aspirin and prednisolone and did not find any beneficial effects.[53]

L-arginine

Addition of L-arginine results in increased number of oocytes being retrieved but no beneficial effect was seen on PRs.

Addition of Estradiol in the Luteal Phase

One meta-analysis has concluded that addition of E2 in the luteal phase decreases the risk of cycle cancellation and increases the chance of clinical pregnancy in poor responder patients[54] by improving the synchronization of the follicular pool available for COS.[55] This meta-analysis was strongly criticized because of methodological pitfall and not including any randomized controlled trial (RCT).[56]

Androgen Supplementation

Androgen supplementation being a simple and inexpensive method has been widely used in poor responders despite there being no adequate evidence in the view of lack of adequately powered RCTs. Garcia-Velasco et al. have shown that testosterone in vitro does increase the expression of the FSH receptor in granulosa cells thus increasing the responsiveness to gonadotropins.[57] It was also seen that androgens play a critical role in early follicular development and granulosa cell proliferation.[58] However, the hypothesis of androgen use in poor responders is weakened by the finding of similar intrafollicular androgenic concentrations in both normal and young or old poor responders.[59] It is also known that androgen excess stimulates early stages of follicular growth increasing the number of preantral and antral follicles, which in turn may deplete the ovarian reserve faster.[60,61]

Transdermal Testosterone

It is known that the use of transdermal testosterone is a safe and effective way of increasing intraovarian androgen concentration.[62,63] Transdermal testosterone pretreatment is also associated with decreased duration and total dose of gonadotropins and increased number of cumulus–oocyte complexes (COCs) retrieved which increases CPR by 15% and LBR by 11% in poor responders undergoing COS for IVF. It is used in the dose of 10–12.5 mg/day or 20 μg/kg/day starting from day 15 for a maximum of 2–3 weeks in the menstrual cycle preceding ovarian stimulation.[64,65] However, Bosdou et al.[66] concluded in their recent publication in 2016 that transdermal testosterone pretreatment at a dose of 10 mg/day for 21 days did not increase the number of COCs retrieved by >1.5. They also reported that there was no increase in LBR though it may be associated with reduced duration of gonadotropins stimulation and total dose of gonadotropins required. ESHRE guidelines also do not recommend the use of testosterone before ovulation induction.[45]

Dehydroepiandrosterone Pretreatment

The effect of dehydroepiandrosterone (DHEA) in the management of poor response is controversial with some studies reporting beneficial effects while others reporting no significant benefit. DHEA given in a dose of 75 mg/day for at least 6–8 weeks before stimulation (Wiser et al., 2010) has been shown to raise the IGF-1 concentration, and thus to enhance the gonadotropin effect.[58,67]

But most studies published had insufficient sample size, and therefore its use cannot be supported in poor responders to increase CPRs, LBRs, or the number of COCs retrieved. The Cochrane review in 2015[68] concluded that pretreatment with DHEA or testosterone may be associated with improved LBRs though the overall quality of the evidence is moderate due to small sample size of the studies published. Thus, androgen supplementation prior to ovarian stimulation is not supported by the best available evidence though it may be associated with a slight improvement in LBR. Definitive conclusions regarding the clinical role of either androgen await evidence from further well-designed studies. There is a need to identify a subgroup of poor responders that have theca cell failure but retain a relatively preserved granulosa cell function. Identifying this particular population and modulating their intrafollicular androgen environment may improve their ovarian response. Use of pretreatment androgens may be a useful approach for patients known to be poor responders but having normal basal FSH concentrations. It may be an option in patients for whom other modalities of treatment have failed till further decision on treatment like oocyte donation and adoption may be considered. ESHRE guidelines on ovarian stimulation also do not recommend the use of DHEA, before and/or during stimulation in poor responders.[45] But the network study concluded that the use of DHEA and CoQ10 treatments as compared to controls resulted in a significantly higher chance of clinical pregnancy and resulted in lower requirement of gonadotropin dose.[69]

Antioxidants

Oxidative stress may be one of the causative factors for female infertility due to increased level of reactive oxygen species (ROS).[70-72] The oxidative stress and increased ROS play an important role in oocyte maturation, ovarian steroidogenesis, formation of the corpus luteum and luteolysis, fertilization, embryo development, and pregnancy.[71,73,74] Oxidative damage can affect the oocyte quality and this is then accompanied by poor oocyte fertilization. Antioxidant therapy for 3 months before IVF cycles may decrease oxidative stress both in serum and in follicular fluid proteins and improve the follicular microenvironment and consequently increasing the number of good-quality oocytes.[75]

CHANGE IN PROTOCOL

Change in the Gonadotropin-Releasing Hormone Analog Protocol

Gonadotropin-releasing Hormone Agonists

Controlled ovarian stimulation strategies using gonadotropin-releasing hormone (GnRH) agonist and gonadotropins use GnRH agonist either in long, short, or ultrashort protocol. Microdose protocol has also been tried in women with poor response to ovarian stimulation.

Gonadotropin-releasing hormone agonist long protocol ***(Fig. 4A)****:* Here, GnRH agonist is started in the midluteal phase of the previous menstrual cycle in the dose of 500 μg and then the dose is reduced to half once the gonadotropins are started.[76] This protocol resulted in lower total gonadotropin dose, shorter stimulation time and increased number of oocytes retrieved, better quality of embryos obtained, and low cancellation rates.[77,78] Published data have reported conflicting outcomes, some reporting improvement while others not.[79-81]

"Stop" GnRH agonist protocols: This protocol involves stopping GnRH agonist once pituitary suppression has happened and COS has started. Two prospective RCTs did not show any statistical improvement in PRs or in cancellation rates.[82,83] But other prospective trials with historical controls have shown improved outcomes with an increased number of oocytes collected, high PRs, and lower cancellation rates.[84-86]

Gonadotropin-releasing hormone agonist flare or short protocol ***(Fig. 4B)****:* In this protocol, gonadotropins are started 2–3 days following the initiation of GnRH agonist. This protocol takes the advantage of the initial flare of gonadotropin secretion that occurs due to initial stimulatory effect on pituitary hormone levels once the GnRH agonist is started. This improves the ovarian response without excessive ovarian suppression.

The results of this protocol are also conflicting in the literature. Some publications have reported higher implantation and PRs, lower cancellation cycles, decreased miscarriage rates, and decreased total gonadotropin dose.[87-89] There are other studies which have reported poor outcome with GnRH agonist short protocol in women who are poor responders. The poor outcome is attributed to premature rise in the LH and progesterone levels in the follicular phase; these high levels could affect the oocyte quality, endometrial receptivity, or both.[90-97]

Modified flare protocol: High dose of GnRH agonist is administered for the first 4 days, followed by standard agonist dose for the rest of the period along with gonadotropins till the day of hCG administration. PRs reported with this protocol in one study were between 14 and 33.3%.[98,99]

Ultrashort GnRH agonist protocol ***(Fig. 4C)****:* Here, the oral contraceptive pills (OCPs) are given in the previous cycle and GnRH agonist in the dose of 500 μg is started on day 1 of menstrual cycle, and on day 4, gonadotropins are started in the dose of 300–450 IU. To prevent LH surge, GnRH antagonists are started once the dominant follicle is 14 mm and continued till the day of hCG administration. In this protocol, the incidence of high LH in the early follicular phase was higher with subsequent high progesterone levels in the early follicular phase and on the day of hCG.

Microdose flare regimen ***(Fig. 4D)****:* In 1994, the use of microdose flare protocol for poor responders was reported by Scott et al. In this protocol, the GnRH agonist is administered after pretreatment with OCPs for 12–21 days in the dose of 40 μg twice a day. It is started on the 3rd day after the OCP is stopped and then on day 5, the gonadotropins are started in

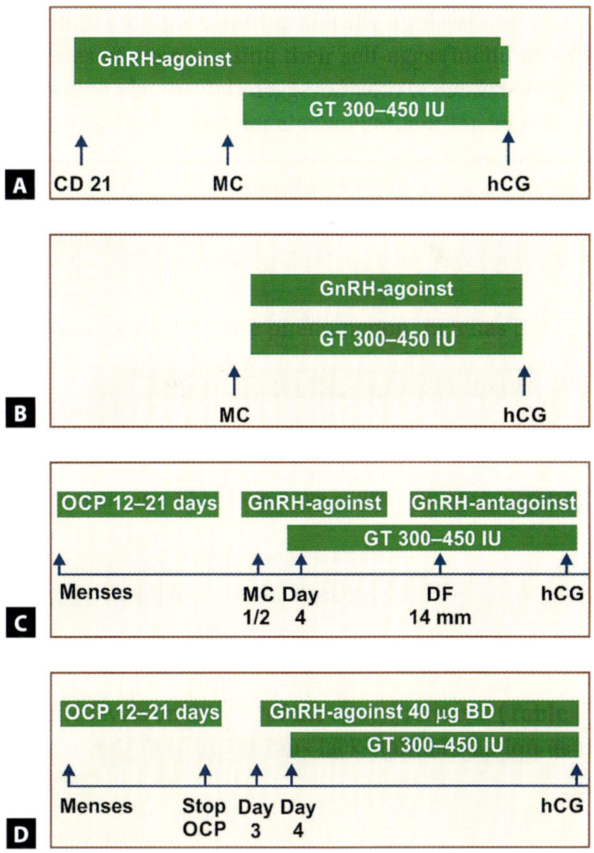

Figs. 4A to D: (A) Long protocol; (B) Short protocol; (C) Ultrashort protocol; (D) Microdose protocol. (CD: cycle day; DF: dominant follicle; GnRh: gonadotropin-releasing hormone; GT: gonadotropin; hCG: human chorionic gonadotropin; MC: menstrual cycle; OCP: oral contraceptive pill)

the dose of 300–450 IU.[100,101] Pretreatment with OCP prevents ovulation and thus the problem of persistent corpus luteum with high progesterone levels in the early follicular phase.[102] OCPs also reduce the early follicular phase LH levels.[102] Most published studies have shown significant improvement in peak E2, follicle recruitment, and number of mature oocytes at retrieval, fewer cycle cancellations, improved implantation rates, and ongoing PRs.[100,103]

When the microdose flare protocol was compared with a long luteal with decreasing dose of GnRH agonist, higher cancellation rates and lower clinical pregnancies were observed with the microdose protocol.[104] However, the choice between the different GnRH agonist protocols in poor responders remains controversial. Some investigators have shown improvement with the short protocol while others have not.[105,106]

In the study of Detti et al.,[107] when stop protocol, microdose flare protocol and short protocol were compared, it was concluded that the microdose flare protocol demonstrated a trend toward higher delivery rates.

Gonadotropin-releasing hormone antagonist regimens ***(Fig. 5)****:* The use of GnRH antagonists has given new hope in the management of poor responders as it prevents premature LH surge without minimizing the suppressive effect on pituitary as seen with GnRH agonist.[108] The GnRH antagonist protocol provides several advantages with shorter duration of stimulation, lower total doses of gonadotropins,

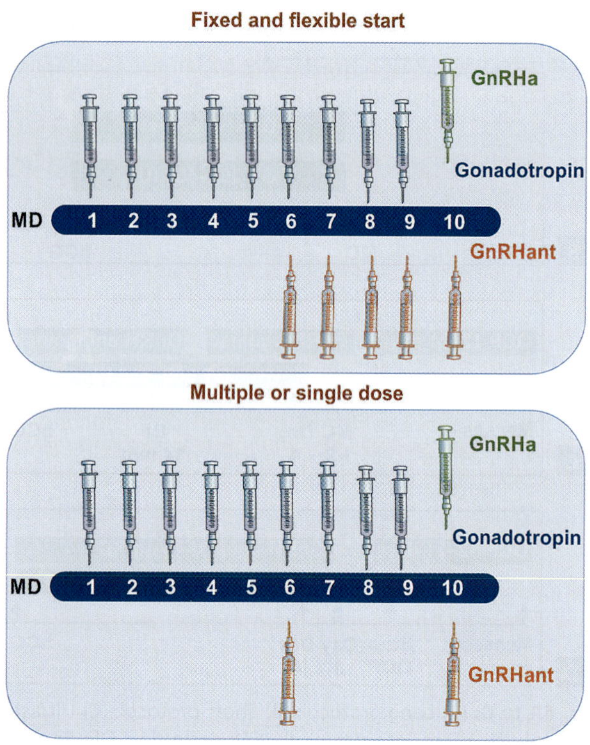

Fig. 5: GnRH antagonist protocol.
(GnRHa: gonadotropin-releasing hormone agonist; GnRHant: gonadotropin-releasing hormone antagonist; MD: menstrual day)

no increased risk of cyst formation, and no hormonal withdrawal symptoms.[109-111] However, GnRH antagonist cycles can result in lower E2 levels than agonist cycles[112] with consequent lower implantation and PRs.

Pretreatment with OCP in a GnRH antagonist cycle may help in scheduling flexibility with a more uniform cohort of follicular recruitment, but it is then associated with higher total doses of gonadotropins for ovarian stimulation.

Gonadotropin-releasing Hormone Antagonist versus Gonadotropin-releasing Hormone Agonist in Poor Responders

A meta-analysis[113] published in 2006 compared the efficacy of GnRH antagonist versus GnRH agonist in poor ovarian responders and did not show any difference in cycle cancellation rate, number of mature oocytes and CPR, per oocyte retrieval, or per embryo transfer (ET). The Cochrane review reported that the GnRH antagonist protocol produced a higher number of oocytes and used a lower dose of gonadotropins compared with the GnRH agonist long protocol. The GnRH agonist flare-up protocol had an increased frequency of IVF cancellation compared with the GnRH agonist long protocol.

A recent RCT by Sunkara et al. concluded that both the GnRH agonist long protocol and the GnRH antagonist protocol are equally efficient for COS in poor responders with a comparable number of oocytes retrieved.[33,105] The GnRH antagonist regimen is beneficial by reducing the burden of treatment as the number of days of gonadotropin stimulation and the dose required is much less with GnRH antagonist protocol. Moreover, as the cycle is not downregulated earlier, one can assess the ovarian reserve which gives the flexibility on whether or not to initiate COS. The cost of the cycle is also lower with lesser number of days of stimulation and lower total gonadotropin dose along with lesser incidence for cycle cancellation once stimulation is initiated in view of absent response. There were certain publications which showed conflicting and varied results when long GnRH agonist was compared with the GnRH antagonist regimen.[114-117]

Though the short and ultrashort GnRH agonist regimens are being used frequently due to their flare effect at the beginning of stimulation, they have been shown to be less effective than the GnRH agonist long protocol and GnRH antagonist protocol. The inferior outcome with the short agonist protocol is related to the elevated progesterone levels during the early follicular phase as a result of the initial flare effect of the GnRH agonist.[118] No relevant differences in PRs or oocyte numbers between GnRH agonist and GnRH antagonist protocols were also reported by Griesinger et al. in their meta-analysis.[119] ESHRE guidelines have concluded that GnRH antagonist and GnRH agonist are equally recommended for predicted low responders.[45]

Change in the Gonadotropin Type and Dose Increase the Dose of Follicle-stimulating Hormone

Most clinicians think that the oocyte yield will be better if the gonadotropin dose is increased. However, this increment in oocytes number and PR with increase of FSH dose was not seen in the studies published.[120-123] Berkkanoglu and Ozgur found no differences between the starting dose of 300, 450, and 600 UI of gonadotropins in terms of retrieved oocytes, number of embryos obtained, and PRs.[124]

Loutradis et al.[125] in their study concluded that FSH receptor gene polymorphisms may play a role in FSH response. Infertile women with ovarian dysfunction tend to carry the Ser/Ser allelic variant, whereas good responders carry the Asn/Ser allelic variant. It was observed that women with Asn/Ser allelic variant have a higher FSH sensitivity and respond with an increased number of follicles and oocytes. The Ser/Ser genotype variant requires a significantly higher gonadotropin dose.

Several clinicians use high doses of gonadotropins (450–600 IU) in the hope of getting a good response but a high-dose gonadotropin regimen using >450 IU has not shown to increase the number of oocytes retrieved or improved the probability of pregnancy in poor responders.[121,122,126]

Today, most clinics use a starting dose of 300–375 IU and a maximum daily dose of 450 IU. A worldwide survey of IVF clinics reported that 24% of the respondents said that their starting dose is >450 IU and when it came to the maximum daily dose that could be considered acceptable, about 93% of respondents reported to have used 600 IU, 5.9% reported to use 900 IU, and 1% would consider a dose as high as 1,200 IU.[127] According to the ESHRE guidelines on ovulation induction, a gonadotropin dose higher than 300 is not recommended for predicted poor responders.[45]

Use of Recombinant Follicle-stimulating Hormone

There is no conclusive evidence on using recombinant follicle-stimulating hormone (rFSH) instead of urinary FSH or hMG in poor responders.[128-132] In poor responders where the total dose of gonadotropins is going to be higher, using hMG is a more cost-effective option.[133] All randomized prospective trials have documented equivalence and similarity in results with both rFSH and hMG.[134,135]

Luteal Initiation of Follicle-stimulating Hormone

We know that follicular recruitment begins in the premenstrual period due to rise in intermenstrual FSH levels. Luteal initiation of FSH might increase the number of recruited follicles by opening the recruitment window in the late luteal phase of the preceding cycle.[136] In a prospective randomized trial,[137] the results with luteal initiation of FSH had high cancellation rates and lower PRs.

Use of Luteinizing Hormone in Controlled Ovarian Stimulation

Small doses of LH when used early in ovarian stimulation in IVF-ET cycles have beneficial effects in quality of oocytes, especially in poor responders.[138] We know that LH is necessary to have optimal levels of E2 during COS and levels <1.5 IU/L have shown to be detrimental.[139] Low periovulatory levels are associated with impaired fertilization and increased early pregnancy loss.[140,141] It was also observed in women with low ovarian reserve and poor responders that the number and quality of the embryos along with the developmental potential and embryogenesis is much better when the follicles are exposed to LH from the beginning of the stimulation protocol, rather than only during the later phase of the follicular stimulation.[142]

Addition of LH either in the form of hMG or recombinant LH (rLH) from the beginning of stimulation did not show a significant difference in the total dose of gonadotropin required for ovarian stimulation, in the duration of stimulation, or in the number of oocytes retrieved. There was also no significant increase in the CPR but there was a significant increase in the LBR.[8,143] A recent meta-analysis, however, showed higher implantation and CPRs in the rLH-supplemented group compared with rFSH alone.[144]

Addition of LH to POSEIDON groups 1, 2, and 3 has been shown to improve FORT and follicle-to-oocyte index (FOI) by overcoming hyposensitivity to FSH with a significant increase in CPR by 30%.[145-148] Poor Responder Outcome Prediction (PROsPeR) score is defined as the sum of two conditions: age over 40 years and fewer than two oocytes in a previous cycle or an AMH concentration <0.5 ng/mL.[149] The score can be used to categorize three levels (0, 1, and 2) of increasing baseline severity.[149] LH supplementation increases the cumulative LBR in moderate and severe POR groups.[149]

Low Human Chorionic Gonadotropin Dose in Early Stimulation Phase

Human chorionic gonadotropin can be used as an alternative to rLH or hMG. hCG can be used in the dose of 200 IU either for the first 5 days of stimulation, entire period of stimulation, or could be added in the late follicular phase. Addition of hCG was also associated with a lower number of gonadotropin ampoules used, higher fertilization rate, higher implantation rate, and better PR. It was also observed that the percentage of mature oocytes and the number and quality of embryos were comparable between rLH and hCG, as well as hMG and hCG. It was the longer plasma half-life of hCG (half-life of hCG is 33 hours while half-life of rLH is 10–12 hours) that resulted in a better and prolonged effect in the COS protocol. The longer half-life also permits highly effective and more stable occupancy of the LH/hCG receptors, which resulted in higher E2 levels.[150]

Addition of Clomiphene Citrate or Aromatase Inhibitors to Gonadotropin Therapy

Clomiphene Citrate

Clomiphene citrate results in the flare of endogenous gonadotropin secretion. When used with GnRH antagonist, it can prevent the premature rise of LH.

Using mild stimulation protocol which utilizes clomiphene citrate with gonadotropins in a GnRH antagonist protocol resulted in a higher number of oocytes being retrieved and a significantly lower cancellation rate with higher implantation and PRs.[151,152] When using clomiphene citrate, one needs to keep in mind the negative effect on endometrial receptivity because of its antiestrogenic effects and it is preferable to freeze all embryos and transfer them in a hormone replacement treatment (HRT) cycle.

There is insufficient evidence to recommend mild stimulation in normal or hyper-responders but it may be recommended in poor responders to decrease the burden of treatment (conditional low-quality evidence).[45] There is moderate- to high-quality evidence on pregnancy outcomes. There was no significant difference in the CPR and live birth rate despite high-grade embryos in the mild stimulation IVF in poor responders. Fewer oocytes and embryos were obtained with mild stimulation though the number and proportion of high-grade embryos were similar in both mild IVF and conventional IVF.[153,154] Mild IVF also resulted in reduced gonadotropin use and cost.[153,154] There were two papers published in 2021, which concluded that mild ovarian stimulation for IVF can be considered for poor responders without compromising pregnancy outcomes but reducing treatment burden and cost.[155,156] No difference was noted in the LBR, cumulative LBR, ongoing PR, cancellation rate, and proportion of high-grade embryos between mild and conventional stimulation.[155,156] With mild stimulation, the number of oocytes retrieved and embryos created were significantly less in the mild stimulation group.[155,156] The dose of gonadotropins required was also significantly less in the mild stimulation group.[155,156] ESHRE guidelines recommend the use of clomiphene citrate either alone or in combination with gonadotropins in poor responders.[45]

Aromatase Inhibitors

Aromatase inhibitors block estrogen synthesis and decrease its circulating levels, thus resulting in withdrawal of the negative feedback effects on the pituitary resulting in increased release of endogenous gonadotropins. Decrease in aromatase activity results in accumulation of follicular androgens, which may increase the follicular sensitivity through amplification of FSH receptor gene expression[157] or stimulate IGF-1 which may act in synergy with FSH.[158] Recent data suggest that letrozole when used in poor responders may improve ovarian response to FSH and also reduce gonadotropin dose required for stimulation.[159] It also increased the number of preovulatory follicles without having a negative effect on PRs.[160] Letrozole and other aromatase inhibitors have not been extensively used in women of reproductive age, so they have to be evaluated more carefully with larger randomized studies. Addition of letrozole to ovarian stimulation is not recommended in poor responders.[45] Polyzos et al. in their paper concluded that treatment in poor responders should be individualized rather than a "one fits all" mild stimulation approach where clomiphene citrate or letrozole is used with gonadotropins.[161]

Dual Stimulation (Fig. 6)

Dual stimulation protocol is based on the presence of multiple waves of follicle recruitment occurring regularly during a normal menstrual cycle. The follicles in each wave are similar, but not identical in diameter.[162]

Stimulation in the follicular and luteal phases of the same menstrual cycle resulted in the formation of a similar number of blastocysts in patients with POR. Blastocysts obtained from luteal phase stimulation contributed significantly to the final transferable blastocyst yield, thus increasing the number of patients undergoing ET per menstrual cycle.[163] Dual stimulation using corifollitropin alfa and a subsequent individualized FSH dose appears to be a valid alternative to conventional follicular stimulation, decreasing the risk of cycle cancellation.[164] The greatest benefit of dual stimulation is the accumulation of oocytes in a single cycle of stimulation, minimizing the time in which it will be performed. It also allows the production of a larger number of embryos, which can then be genetically evaluated, thus favoring the final clinical result.

But according to the ESHRE guidelines, dual stimulation in poor responders should be used only in the context of clinical research.[45] Nonconventional start of ovarian stimulation in the luteal phase is not recommended.[45]

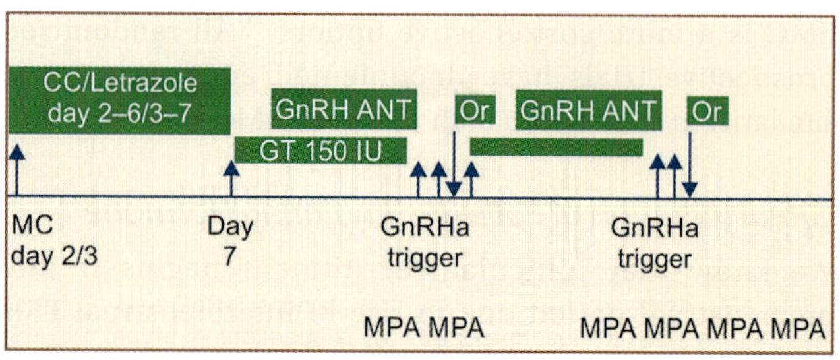

Fig. 6: Dual stimulation protocol.
(CC: clomiphene citrate; GnRHa: gonadotropin-releasing hormone agonist; GnRH ANT: gonadotropin-releasing hormone antagonist; GT: gonadotropin; MC: menstrual cycle; MPA: medroxyprogesterone acetate)

Natural Cycle

Though the first successful IVF treatment was performed in a natural cycle,[165] it was abandoned later due to the occurrence of the premature LH surge which resulted in high cancellation rates. Though the cancellation rates with a natural cycle are higher, it is postulated that a natural cycle can provide a single oocyte of a much better quality with a better fertilization and implantation rate as compared to the stimulated cycles. This will allow us the transfer of a healthy embryo into a more receptive endometrial environment which may not be the case in COS cycles due to high E2 levels.[166-169] Moreover, the cost of the cycle is also very low and more patient friendly.[170]

Gonadotropin-releasing hormone antagonists can be started once the follicle is 14 mm which will prevent premature LH surge and thus lower the risk of cycle cancellation.[171] The other option to prevent cycle cancellation is in vitro maturation (IVM), but the CPR and LBR are very low with it.[172] Natural cycle IVF should be avoided in those who have elevated FSH levels on day 2 of the cycle. There was a paper published in 2019, which looked at modified natural cycle IVF (MNC-IVF) and conventional high-dose ovarian stimulation (HDOS) in advanced-age Bologna poor responders. The authors concluded that in advanced-age Bologna poor responders, after adjustment for relevant confounders like number of oocytes retrieved and presence of at least one top-quality embryo, the ongoing pregnancy was similar in both groups. Thus, MNC-IVF may have a role in elderly poor responders who do not want to opt for oocyte donations and it may be more patient-friendly than conventional high-dose stimulation.[173] ESHRE guidelines do not recommend the use of natural cycle in poor responders.[45]

Trigger

Trigger maybe dual or double. Trigger may improve the results in a small subset of patients who are poor responders.

Dual Trigger

Gonadotropin-releasing hormone agonist and hCG were administered concomitantly at 35–37 hours prior to oocyte retrieval. A combination of recombinant hCG 250 µg (6,500 IU) or urinary hCG (5,000 IU) and 0.2 mg of triptorelin was administered.

Double Trigger

Gonadotropin-releasing hormone agonist (0.2 mg of triptorelin) and hCG (recombinant hCG 250 µg (6,500 IU) or urinary hCG (5,000 IU) administered 40 and 34 hours, respectively, prior to oocyte retrieval indicates double trigger.

When a dual or double trigger is used, GnRH agonist triggering mimics the natural cycle surge (endogenous LH and FSH) aiming to significantly improve outcome–oocyte maturity, fertilization rate, CPR, and LBR.[174-176]

Other studies did not demonstrate improved oocyte maturation, CPR, and ongoing PR with dual/double trigger.[177] According to the ESHRE guidelines, dual/double trigger in subgroups of patients with low maturation, recovery, or fertilization rate cannot be recommended until data on its efficacy and safety from RCTs are available.[45]

Laboratory Options in Poor Response Cycles

Intracytoplasmic Sperm Injection for Low Oocyte Yield

Intracytoplasmic sperm injection (ICSI) can be used instead of IVF in poor responders to prevent complete fertilization failure.[178] But several studies have shown similar fertilization, implantation, and PRs with ICSI and conventional IVF in women with POR without male factor.[179] Gabrielsen et al. found that most oocyte defects in poor responders are not overcome by ICSI.[180]

Preimplantation Genetic Screening for Poor Responders

As poor responder patients are either old or have low ovarian reserve, the chance of aneuploidy is higher in the embryo.[181] Therefore, preimplantation genetic screening (PGS) may have a role in identifying a euploid embryo for transfer, thus optimizing the treatment outcome. But studies have not shown increased LBR despite increased implantation rate.[182]

Ideal Day of Transfer—Day 2 Transfer Instead of Day 3 or 5[156-158]

We know that extending in vitro culture allows a better selection of embryos with higher implantation potential and CPR. Because of concerns regarding the impact of in vitro culture conditions on the limited number of developing embryos in poor responders, it has been proposed that shortening the duration of embryo culture might be associated with an improvement in PRs by increasing the number of embryos available for transfer. The ongoing pregnancy for day 2 versus day 3 ETs is 27.7 versus 16.3%.[183-185] The number of embryos transferred was also significantly more in the day 2 versus day 3 group (2.0 ± 0.8 vs. 1.7 ± 0.8 embryos).[183-185] Thus, shortening the duration of embryo culture is associated with an improvement in PRs probably by increasing the number of embryos available for transfer. Therefore, in poor responders where fewer oocytes and embryos are available for transfer, transferring embryos at an earlier stage of cleavage is beneficial.

Number of Embryos for Transfer

Today, when we are moving to single ET for optimal IVF outcome, increasing the number of embryos transferred in women with advanced reproductive age, poor ovarian reserve, and poor response may improve the outcome.

The guidelines by the American Society for Reproductive Medicine in 2009 for the number of embryos to transfer[186] suggest the transfer of up to two embryos in women aged <35 years, up to three embryos in women aged <38 years, and up to four embryos in women aged <41 years.

Donor Oocytes

In women who have repeated IVF failures, those with predicted poor prognosis, age >40 years or in patients with FSH over 15 mIU/mL or low AMH, oocyte donation may be an option.

Accumulation of Vitrified Embryos or Oocytes

Accumulation of vitrified embryos followed by frozen ET can be considered as a new strategy to improve PR in poor ovarian responders. Kwon et al. reported a significantly higher biochemical PR (31.6 vs. 11.9%; $p = 0.02$). Though the ongoing PR (15.8 vs. 8.7%; $p = 0.24$) and LBR (15.8 vs. 6.6%; $p = 0.1$) were higher, they did not reach statistical significance.[187] Accumulating vitrified oocytes over several stimulation cycles and fertilizing them later can give higher LBR per patient treated and potentially reduce the dropout rate in women with POR.[188] The advantages of accumulation of oocytes and embryos result in less cycle cancellations, reduce dropout rate, result in higher LBR per intention to treat, and reduce psychological distress caused by repeated failures. The disadvantage is that unnecessary stimulations are done if the pregnancy could be achieved from the first cycle. Multiple COS cycles with IVF and freezing increase the cost of the treatment.

ASSISTED REPRODUCTIVE TECHNOLOGY TREATMENT OUTCOME ACCORDING TO POSEIDON CLASSIFICATION

There was no statistical difference in LBR per ET following ART between POSEIDON groups 1 and 2 and women with a good prognosis, while the LBR was significantly lower in POSEIDON groups 3 and 4. Simple modifications, such as an increase in gonadotropin dosage and/or a protocol change, resulted in treatment outcomes that were comparable between POSEIDON groups 1 and 2 and the non-POSEIDON group.[189]

NEWER TREATMENT MODALITIES

Ovarian Fragmentation and in Vitro Activation (Flowchart 3)

Ovarian fragmentation and in vitro activation (IVA) promote follicle growth via different mechanisms. Kawamura et al. found that fragmentation of ovaries promoted actin polymerization and disrupted ovarian Hippo signaling, leading to increased expression of downstream growth factors, promotion of follicle growth, and generation of mature oocytes. They also reported additional follicle growth, when ovarian fragmentation was combined with Akt stimulator treatment followed by autografting.[190]

OUTCOME AFTER ASSISTED REPRODUCTIVE TECHNOLOGY IN POOR RESPONDERS

Poor response to COS for ART has been a therapeutic challenge to the clinician. Over the years, several treatment modalities have been suggested but have been in wane. Till date, there are hardly any publications on conception rates in poor responders who elect to undergo oocyte retrieval.

There was one study published by Blake et al. and Ulug et al.[183,191] who looked at the outcome of ART in poor responders. They reported PR of 15.9% in patients in whom four oocytes were retrieved and compared with patients in whom one or two oocytes were retrieved (2.3 and 4.3%, respectively). Younger patients <34 years had significantly higher PR (19.5%) as compared to older patients. Women <39 years had a PR of 7.2%, whereas those more than 39 years had a PR of 1.5%. The implantation and PRs when compared in poor responders and normal responders when three embryos were transferred were significantly lower (IR—6.6 vs. 15.3% and PR—16.6 vs. 37.3%). Patient age, number of oocytes retrieved, and number of embryos available for transfer determine prognosis for the success of

Flowchart 3: Ovarian fragmentation and in vitro activation treatment.

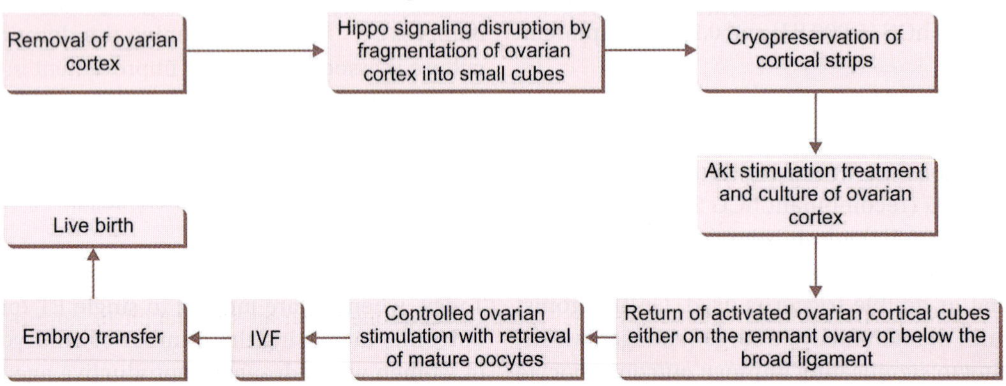

(IVF: in vitro fertilization)

IVF in patients who are subjected to assisted reproductive techniques and respond poorly to COS. There was another study by Moolenaar et al.[192] who looked at the response and LBR in the second cycle after an unexpected first cycle poor response. They correlated female age and basal FSH in the first cycle and IVF outcome in the second cycle. Poor response was seen in 5.7% of the total women subjected to COS for ART; of these 46.5% had a repeat poor response in the subsequent cycle.[192] An LBR of 21.8% was reported in the second cycle in women who had a good ovarian response.[192] So they concluded that unexpected poor response in the first COS cycle should not be a reason to discontinue further IVF treatment. Between the FSH and female age in the first cycle, only female age was a predictor of response and LBR in the second cycle, though the predictive value was very low.

Later in a retrospective study where the women were identified to be poor responders according to Bologna criteria they demonstrated very low LBRs, irrespective of age and treatment protocol used. An increase in the number of oocytes retrieved (>3 vs. 1–3 oocytes) is an independent variable related to LBRs. LBRs were similar in women <40 years and >40 years per cycle (7.1 vs. 5.2%) or per patient (11.6 vs. 8.8%).[193]

The most recent publication in 2017 by Bozdag et al., which was also a retrospective study of 821 patients, reported an LBR of <10%. Higher implantation (p = 0.024) and LBR per ET (p <0.001) or cycle (p = 0.001) were noted in group C (AFC <7 with a previous poor response). It was also noted in this study that the LBRs are not homogeneous and "young proven" poor responders have a more favorable pregnancy outcome.[194]

KEY POINTS

- Despite the numerous predictive tests for diminished ovarian reserve including age, the POR most times is diagnosed only when subjected to ovarian stimulation. No uniform definition of poor response makes the clinical trials incomparable till date. Moreover, majority of published trials on POR suffer from methodological flaws and are, thus, regarded as being at high risk for bias. This makes it very difficult to offer one particular management strategy or treatment protocol for optimal outcome in this group of women.[195]
- There is no evidence for any particular COS protocol to improve treatment outcome but GnRH antagonist protocols may reduce treatment burden.
- Addition of LH to COS protocols seems to increase the number of oocytes retrieved (+0.75) and the CPR (+30%).
- Natural and modified natural cycles may also improve the outcome in a small subset of women with poor response.
- There is insufficient evidence for most of the adjuvants to improve outcome in women who are poor responders.
- There may be a role for newer modalities of treatment such as oocyte and embryo accumulation, PGS to rule out aneuploidy, and IVA of ovarian cortical tissue. But before we bring them into routine clinical use, they need to be assessed in large-scale randomized controlled studies to assess the efficacy for poor responders.
- As poor responders are not homogeneous for pregnancy prospects, female age and number of oocytes retrieved will modulate the chances for pregnancy in current and subsequent cycles.[1,196]
- Management of poor ovarian responder still represents a therapeutic challenge for the clinician as it is heterogeneous group with no uniform protocols, and the prognosis for these patients may vary greatly depending on patient characteristics. One must also remember that one cannot recruit follicles that do not exist in a case of DOR and the egg quality cannot be fundamentally altered.

REFERENCES

1. Ferraretti AP, La Marca A, Fauser BCJM, Tarlatzis B, Nargund G, Gianaroli L, et al. ESHRE consensus on the definition of 'poor response' to ovarian stimulation for in vitro fertilization: the Bologna criteria. Hum Reprod. 2011;26(7):1616-24.
2. Colls P, Escudero T, Fischer J, Cekleniak NA, Ben-Ozer S, Meyer B, Damien M, Grifo JA, Hershlag A, Munné S. Validation of array comparative genome hybridization for diagnosis of translocations in preimplantation human embryos. Reprod Biomed Online. 2012 Jun;24(6):621-9. doi: 10.1016/j.rbmo.2012.02.006. Epub 2012 Feb 22. PMID: 22503275.
3. POSEIDON Group (Patient-Oriented Strategies Encompassing IndividualizeD Oocyte Number), Alviggi C, Andersen CY, Buehler K, Conforti A, De Placido G, et al. A new more detailed stratification of low responders to ovarian stimulation: from a poor ovarian response to a low prognosis concept. Fertil Steril. 2016;105(6):1452-3.
4. Gallot V, Berwanger da Silva AL, Genro V, Grynberg M, Frydman N, Fanchin R. Antral follicle responsiveness to follicle-stimulating hormone administration assessed by the Follicular Output RaTe (FORT) may predict in vitro fertilization-embryo transfer outcome. Hum Reprod. 2012;27(4):1066-72.
5. Alviggi C, Clarizia R, Pettersson K, Mollo A, Humaidan P, Strina I, et al. Suboptimal response to GnRHa long protocol is associated with a common LH polymorphism. Reprod Biomed Online. 2011;22:S67-72.
6. Shenfield F, Pennings G, De Mouzon J, Ferraretti AP, Goossens V, ESHRE Task Force 'Cross Border Reproductive Care' (CBRC). ESHRE's good practice guide for cross-border reproductive care for centers and practitioners. Hum Reprod. 2011;26(7):1625-7.
7. De Placido G, Alviggi C, Perino A, Strina I, Lisi F, Fasolino A, et al. Recombinant human LH supplementation versus recombinant human FSH (rFSH) step-up protocol during controlled ovarian stimulation in normogonadotrophic women with initial inadequate ovarian response to rFSH. A multicentre, prospective, randomized controlled trial. Hum Reprod. 2005;20(2):390-6.

8. Ferraretti AP, Gianaroli L, Magli MC, D'angelo A, Farfalli V, Montanaro N. Exogenous luteinizing hormone in controlled ovarian hyperstimulation for assisted reproduction techniques. Fertil Steril. 2004;82(6):1521-6.
9. Yovich JL, Ye Y, Regan SLP, Keane KN. The evolving concept of poor-prognosis for women undertaking IVF and the notion of growth hormone as an adjuvant; a single-center viewpoint. Front Endocrinol (Lausanne). 2019;10:808.
10. Jayaprakasan K, Campbell B, Hopkisson J, Johnson I, Raine-Fenning N. A prospective, comparative analysis of anti-Müllerian hormone, inhibin-B, and three-dimensional ultrasound determinants of ovarian reserve in the prediction of poor response to controlled ovarian stimulation. Fertil Steril. 2010;93(3):855-64.
11. Tomas C, Nuojua-Huttunen S, Martikainen H. Pretreatment transvaginal ultrasound examination predicts ovarian responsiveness to gonadotrophins in in-vitro fertilization. Hum Reprod. 1997;12(2):220-3.
12. Sharara FI, McClamrock HD. Ratio of oestradiol concentration on the day of human chorionic gonadotrophin administration to mid-luteal oestradiol concentration is predictive of in-vitro fertilization outcome. Hum Reprod. 1999;14(11):2777-82.
13. Hussain M, Cahill DJ, Akande V, Gordon U. Outcome of assisted reproduction treatment in women with extremely low antimullerian hormone (AMH) levels. Open J Obstet Gynecol. 2014;4(15):961-6.
14. Muzii L, Di Tucci C, Di Feliciantonio M, Marchetti C, Perniola G, Panici PB. The effect of surgery for endometrioma on ovarian reserve evaluated by antral follicle count: a systematic review and meta-analysis. Hum Reprod. 2014;29(10):2190-8.
15. Dewailly D, Andersen CY, Balen A, Broekmans F, Dilaver N, Fanchin R, et al. The physiology and clinical utility of anti-Müllerian hormone in women. Hum Reprod Update. 2014;20(3):370-85.
16. Raffi F, Metwally M, Amer S. The impact of excision of ovarian endometrioma on ovarian reserve: a systematic review and meta-analysis. J Clin Endocrinol Metab. 2012;97(9):3146-54.
17. Somigliana E, Berlanda N, Benaglia L, Viganò P, Vercellini P, Fedele L. Surgical excision of endometriomas and ovarian reserve: a systematic review on serum antimüllerian hormone level modifications. Fertil Steril. 2012;98(6):1531-8.
18. te Velde ER, Pearson PL. The variability of female reproductive ageing. Hum Reprod Update. 2002;8(2):141-54.
19. van Rooij IAJ, Bancsi LFJMM, Broekmans FJM, Looman CWN, Habbema JDF, te Velde ER. Women older than 40 years of age and those with elevated follicle-stimulating hormone levels differ in poor response rate and embryo quality in in vitro fertilization. Fertil Steril. 2003;79(3):482-8.
20. Van Blerkom J, Antczak M, Schrader R. The developmental potential of the human oocyte is related to the dissolved oxygen content of follicular fluid: association with vascular endothelial growth factor levels and perifollicular blood flow characteristics. Hum Reprod. 1997;12(5):1047-55.
21. Lambalk CB, de Koning CH. Interpretation of elevated FSH in the regular menstrual cycle. Maturitas. 1998;30(2):215-20.
22. Lambalk CB. Value of elevated basal follicle-stimulating hormone levels and the differential diagnosis during the diagnostic subfertility work-up. Fertil Steril. 2003;79(3):489-90.
23. Hugues JN, Barlow DH, Rosenwaks Z, Cédrin-Durnerin I, Robson S, Pidoux L, et al. Improvement in consistency of response to ovarian stimulation with recombinant human follicle stimulating hormone resulting from a new method for calibrating the therapeutic preparation. Reprod Biomed Online. 2003;6(2):185-90.
24. Shrim A, Elizur SE, Seidman DS, Rabinovici J, Wiser A, Dor J. Elevated day 3 FSH/LH ratio due to low LH concentrations predicts reduced ovarian response. Reprod Biomed Online. 2006;12(4):418-22.
25. Bancsi LF, Broekmans FJ, Eijkemans MJ, de Jong FH, Habbema JD, te Velde ER. Predictors of poor ovarian response in in vitro fertilization: a prospective study comparing basal markers of ovarian reserve. Fertil Steril. 2002;77(2):328-36.
26. Bukulmez O, Arici A. Assessment of ovarian reserve. Curr Opin Obstet Gynecol. 2004;16(3):231-7.
27. Scott RT, Toner JP, Muasher SJ, Oehninger S, Robinson S, Rosenwaks Z. Follicle-stimulating hormone levels on cycle day 3 are predictive of in vitro fertilization outcome. Fertil Steril. 1989;51(4):651-4.
28. Seifer R, Schiller M, Sameroff AJ, Resnick S, Riordan K. Attachment, maternal sensitivity, and infant temperament during the first year of life. Dev Psychol. 1996;32(1):12-25.
29. Tinkanen H, Bläuer M, Laippala P, Tuohimaa P, Kujansuu E. Correlation between serum inhibin B and other indicators of the ovarian function. Eur J Obstet Gynecol Reprod Biol. 2001;94(1):109-13.
30. Nardo LG, Gelbaya TA, Wilkinson H, Roberts SA, Yates A, Pemberton P, et al. Circulating basal anti-Müllerian hormone levels as predictor of ovarian response in women undergoing ovarian stimulation for in vitro fertilization. Fertil Steril. 2009;92(5):1586-93.
31. Chuang CC, Chen CD, Chao KH, Chen SU, Ho HN, Yang YS. Age is a better predictor of pregnancy potential than basal follicle-stimulating hormone levels in women undergoing in vitro fertilization. Fertil Steril. 2003;79(1):63-8.
32. Kucuk T, Kozinoglu H, Kaba A. Growth hormone co-treatment within a GnRH agonist long protocol in patients with poor ovarian response: a prospective, randomized, clinical trial. J Assist Reprod Genet. 2008;25:123-7.
33. Kyrou D, Kolibianakis EM, Venetis CA, Papanikolaou EG, Bontis J, Tarlatzis BC. How to improve the probability of pregnancy in poor responders undergoing in vitro fertilization: a systematic review and meta-analysis. Fertil Steril. 2009;91(3):749-66.
34. Erickson GF, Garzo VG, Magoffin DA. Insulin-like growth factor-I regulates aromatase activity in human granulosa and granulosa luteal cells. J Clin Endocrinol Metab. 1989;69(4):716-24.
35. Bassiouny YA, Rabie WA, Hassan AA, Darwish RK. Association of the luteinizing hormone/choriogonadotropin receptor gene polymorphism with polycystic ovary syndrome. Gynecol Endocrinol. 2014;30(6):428-30.
36. Bassiouny YA, Dakhly DM, Bayoumi YA, Hashish NM. Does the addition of growth hormone to the in vitro fertilization/intracytoplasmic sperm injection antagonist protocol improve outcomes in poor responders? A randomized, controlled trial. Fertil Steril. 2016;105(3):697-702.
37. Ipsa E, Cruzat VF, Kagize JN, Yovich JL, Keane KN. Growth hormone and insulin-like growth factor action in reproductive tissues. Front Endocrinol (Lausanne). 2019;10:777.

38. Regan SLP, Knight PG, Yovich JL, Arfuso F, Dharmarajan A. Growth hormone during in vitro fertilization in older women modulates the density of receptors in granulosa cells, with improved pregnancy outcomes. Fertil Steril. 2018;110(7):1298-310.
39. Lan KC, Lin PY, Chang YC, Chen YJ, Tsai YR, Mohamed ISI, et al. Growth hormone supplementation may improve the pregnancy rate and endometrial receptivity among women aged more than 40 years undergoing in vitro fertilization. Biomed J. 2019;42(6):411-6.
40. Choe SA, Kim MJ, Lee HJ, Kim J, Chang EM, Kim JW, et al. Increased proportion of mature oocytes with sustained-release growth hormone treatment in poor responders: a prospective randomized controlled study. Arch Gynecol Obstet. 2018;297(3):791-6.
41. Norman RJ, Alvino H, Hull LM, Mol BW, Hart RJ, Kelly TL, et al. Human growth hormone for poor responders: a randomized placebo-controlled trial provides no evidence for improved live birth rate. Reprod Biomed Online. 2019;38(6): 908-15.
42. Yang P, Wu R, Zhang H. The effect of growth hormone supplementation in poor ovarian responders undergoing IVF or ICSI: a meta-analysis of randomized controlled trials. Reprod Biol Endocrinol. 2020;18(1):76.
43. Li J, Chen Q, Wang J, Huang G, Ye H. Does growth hormone supplementation improve oocyte competence and IVF outcomes in patients with poor embryonic development? A randomized controlled trial. BMC Pregnancy Childbirth. 2020;20:310.
44. Cozzolino M, Cecchino GN, Troiano G, Romanelli C. Growth hormone cotreatment for poor responders undergoing in vitro fertilization cycles: a systematic review and meta-analysis. Fertil Steril. 2020;114(1):97-109.
45. The ESHRE Guideline Group On Ovarian Stimulation, Bosch E, Broer S, Griesinger G, Grynberg M, Humaidan P, et al. ESHRE guideline: ovarian stimulation for IVF/ICSI. Hum Reprod Open. 2020;2020(2):hoaa009.
46. Howles CM, Loumaye E, Germond M, Yates R, Brinsden P, Healy D, et al. Does growth hormone-releasing factor assist follicular development in poor responder patients undergoing ovarian stimulation for in-vitro fertilization? Hum Reprod. 1999;14(8):1939-43.
47. Delitala G, Tomasi P, Virdis R. Neuroendocrine regulation of human growth hormone secretion. Diagnostic and clinical applications. J Endocrinol Invest. 1988;11(6):441-62.
48. Kim CH, Chae HD, Chang YS. Pyridostigmine cotreatment for controlled ovarian hyperstimulation in low responders undergoing in vitro fertilization-embryo transfer. Fertil Steril. 1999;71(4):652-7.
49. Rubinstein M, Marazzi A, de Fried EP. Low-dose aspirin treatment improves ovarian responsiveness, uterine and ovarian blood flow velocity, implantation, and pregnancy rates in patients undergoing in vitro fertilization: a prospective, randomized, double-blind placebo-controlled assay. Fertil Steril. 1999;71(5):825-9.
50. Nardo LG, Granne I, Stewart J, Policy and Practice Committee of the British Fertility Society. Medical adjuncts in IVF: evidence for clinical practice. Hum Fertil (Camb). 2009;12(1):1-13.
51. Lok IH, Yip SK, Chung LP, Leung PHY, Haines CJ. Adjuvant low-dose aspirin therapy in poor responders undergoing in vitro fertilization: a prospective, randomized, double-blind, placebo-controlled trial. Fertil Steril. 2004;81(3):556-61.
52. Gelbaya TA, Kyrgiou M, Li TC, Stern C, Nardo LG. Low-dose aspirin for in vitro fertilization: a systematic review and meta-analysis. Hum Reprod Update. 2007;13(4):357-64.
53. Revelli A, Dolfin E, Gennarelli G, Lantieri T, Massobrio M, Holte JG, et al. Low-dose acetylsalicylic acid plus prednisolone as an adjuvant treatment in IVF: a prospective, randomized study. Fertil Steril. 2008;90(5):1685-91.
54. Reynolds KA, Omurtag KR, Jimenez PT, Rhee JS, Tuuli MG, Jungheim ES. Cycle cancellation and pregnancy after luteal estradiol priming in women defined as poor responders: a systematic review and meta-analysis. Hum Reprod. 2013;28(11):2981-9.
55. Fanchin R, Salomon L, Castelo-Branco A, Olivennes F, Frydman N, Frydman R. Luteal estradiol pre-treatment coordinates follicular growth during controlled ovarian hyperstimulation with GnRH antagonists. Hum Reprod. 2003;18(12):2698-703.
56. Polyzos NP, Tournaye H. Poor ovarian responders: to meta-analyse or not, that is the question. Hum Reprod. 2014;29:634-5.
57. Garcia-Velasco JA, Rodríguez S, Agudo D, Pacheco A, Schneider J, Pellicer A. FSH receptor in vitro modulation by testosterone and hCG in human luteinized granulosa cells. Eur J Obstet Gynecol Reprod Biol. 2012;165(2):259-64.
58. Vendola KA, Zhou J, Adesanya OO, Weil SJ, Bondy CA. Androgens stimulate early stages of follicular growth in the primate ovary. J Clin Invest. 1998;101(12):2622-9.
59. de los Santos MJ, García-Laez V, Beltrán D, Labarta E, Zuzuarregui JL, Alamá P, et al. The follicular hormonal profile in low-responder patients undergoing unstimulated cycles: is it hypoandrogenic? Hum Reprod. 2012;28(1):224-9.
60. Hillier SG, Tetsuka M, Fraser HM. Location and developmental regulation of androgen receptor in primate ovary. Hum Reprod. 1997;12(1):107-11.
61. Weil S, Vendola K, Zhou J, Bondy CA. Androgen and follicle-stimulating hormone interactions in primate ovarian follicle development. J Clin Endocrinol Metab. 1999;84(8):2951-6.
62. Casson PR, Lindsay MS, Pisarska MD, Carson SA, Buster JE. Dehydroepiandrosterone supplementation augments ovarian stimulation in poor responders: a case series. Hum Reprod. 2000;15(10):2129-32.
63. Balasch J, Fábregues F, Peñarrubia J, Carmona F, Casamitjana R, Creus M, et al. Pretreatment with transdermal testosterone may improve ovarian response to gonadotrophins in poor-responder IVF patients with normal basal concentrations of FSH. Hum Reprod. 2006;21(7):1884-93.
64. Massin N, Cedrin-Durnerin I, Coussieu C, Galey-Fontaine J, Wolf JP, Hugues JN. Effects of transdermal testosterone application on the ovarian response to FSH in poor responders undergoing assisted reproduction technique—a prospective, randomized, double-blind study. Hum Reprod. 2006;21(5):1204-11.
65. Kim CH, Howles CM, Lee HA. The effect of transdermal testosterone gel pretreatment on controlled ovarian stimulation and IVF outcome in low responders. Fertil Steril. 2011;95(2):679-83.
66. Bosdou JK, Venetis CA, Dafopoulos K, Zepiridis L, Chatzimeletiou K, Anifandis G, et al. Transdermal testosterone

pretreatment in poor responders undergoing ICSI: a randomized clinical trial. Hum Reprod. 2016;31(5): 977-85.
67. Hillier SG, De Zwart FA. Evidence that granulosa cell aromatase induction/activation by follicle-stimulating hormone is an androgen receptor-regulated process in-vitro. Endocrinology. 1981;109(4):1303-5.
68. Nagels HE, Rishworth JR, Siristatidis CS, Kroon B. Androgens (dehydroepiandrosterone or testosterone) for women undergoing assisted reproduction. Cochrane Database Syst Rev. 2015;(11):CD009749.
69. Zhang Y, Zhang C, Shu J, Guo J, Chang HM, Leung PC, et al. Adjuvant treatment strategies in ovarian stimulation for poor responders undergoing IVF: a systematic review and network meta-analysis. Hum Reprod Update. 2020;26(2):247-63.
70. Agarwal A, Gupta S, Sharma RK. Role of oxidative stress in female reproduction. Reprod Biol Endocrinol. 2005;3:28.
71. Agarwal A, Aponte-Mellado A, Premkumar BJ, Shaman A, Gupta S. The effects of oxidative stress on female reproduction: a review. Reprod Biol Endocrinol. 2012;10:49.
72. Gupta S, Ghulmiyyah J, Sharma R, Halabi J, Agarwal A. Power of proteomics in linking oxidative stress and female infertility. Biomed Res Int. 2014;2014:916212.
73. Ruder EH, Hartman TJ, Goldman MB. Impact of oxidative stress on female fertility. Curr Opin Obstet Gynecol. 2009;21:219-22.
74. Sugino N, Shimamura K, Takiguchi S, Tamura H, Ono M, Nakata M, et al. Changes in activity of superoxide dismutase in the human endometrium throughout the menstrual cycle and in early pregnancy. Hum Reprod. 1996;11:1073-8.
75. Luddi A, Capaldo A, Focarelli R, Gori M, Morgante G, Piomboni P, et al. Antioxidants reduce oxidative stress in follicular fluid of aged women undergoing IVF. Reprod Biol Endocrinol. 2016;14:57.
76. Kowalik A, Barmat L, Damario M, Liu HC, Davis O, Rosenwaks Z. Ovarian estradiol production in vivo. Inhibitory effect of leuprolide acetate. J Reprod Med. 1998;43:413-7.
77. Feldberg D, Farhi J, Ashkenazi J, Dicker D, Shalev J, Ben-Rafael Z. Minidose gonadotropin-releasing hormone agonist is the treatment of choice in poor responders with high follicle-stimulating hormone levels. Fertil Steril. 1994;62:343-6.
78. Olivennes F, Righini C, Fanchin R, Torrisi C, Hazout A, Glissant M, et al. A protocol using a low dose of gonadotrophin-releasing hormone agonist might be the best protocol for patients with high follicle-stimulating hormone concentrations on day 3. Hum Reprod. 1996;11:1169-72.
79. McKenna KM, Foster P, McBain J, Martin M, Johnston WI. Combined treatment with gonadotrophin releasing hormone agonist and gonadotrophins in poor responders to hyperstimulation for in vitro fertilization (IVF): clinical and endocrine results. Aust N Z J Obstet Gynaecol. 1989;29:428-32.
80. Horvath PM, Styler M, Hammond JM, Shelden RM, Kemmann E. Exogenous gonadotropin requirements are increased in leuprolide suppressed women undergoing ovarian stimulation. Fertil Steril. 1988;49:159-62.
81. Ashrafi M, Ashtiani SK, Zafarani F, Samani RO, Eshrati B. Evaluation of ovulation induction protocols for poor responders undergoing assisted reproduction techniques. Saudi Med J. 2005;26(4):593-6.
82. Garcia-Velasco JA, Isaza V, Requena A, Martínez-Salazar FJ, Landazábal A, Remohí J, et al. High doses of gonadotrophins combined with stop versus non-stop protocol of GnRH analogue administration in low responder IVF patients: a prospective, randomized, controlled trial. Hum Reprod. 2000;15:2292-6.
83. Dirnfeld M, Fruchter O, Yshai D, Lissak A, Ahdut A, Abramovici H. Cessation of gonadotropin-releasing hormone analogue (GnRH-a) upon down-regulation versus conventional long GnRH-a protocol in poor responders undergoing in vitro fertilization. Fertil Steril. 1999;72:406-11.
84. Schachter M, Friedler S, Raziel A, Strassburger D, Bern O, Ron-el R. Improvement of IVF outcome in poor responders by discontinuation of GnRH analogue during the gonadotropin stimulation phase—a function of improved embryo quality. J Assist Reprod Genet. 2001;18:197-204.
85. Pinkas H, Orvieto R, Avrech OM, Rufas O, Ferber A, Ben-Rafael Z, et al. Gonadotropin stimulation following GnRH-a priming for poor responders in in vitro fertilization-embryo transfer programs. Gynecol Endocrinol. 2000;14:11-4.
86. Wang PT, Lee RKK, Su JT, Hou JW, Lin MH, Hu YM. Cessation of low dose gonadotropin-releasing hormone agonist therapy combined followed by high-dose gonadotropin stimulation yields a favorable ovarian response in poor responders. J Assist Reprod Genet. 2002;19:1-6.
87. Katayama K, Roesler M, Gunnarson G, Stehlik E, Jagusch S. Short-term use of gonadotropin-releasing hormone agonist (leuprolide) for in vitro fertilization. J In Vitro Fert Embryo Transf. 1988;5:332-4.
88. Garcia J, Padilla S, Bargati J, Baramki TA. Follicular phase gonadotropin-releasing hormone agonist and human gonadotropins: a better alternative for ovulation induction in in vitro fertilization. Fertil Steril. 1990;53:302-5.
89. Padilla SL, Dugan K, Maruschak V, Shalika S, Smith RD. Use of the flare-up protocol with high dose human follicle stimulating hormone and human menopausal gonadotropins for in vitro fertilization in poor responders. Fertil Steril. 1996;65:796-9.
90. Cramer DW, Powers DR, Oskowitz SP, Liberman RF, Hornstein MD, McShane PM, et al. Gonadotropin-releasing hormone agonist use in assisted reproduction cycles: the influence of long and short regimens on pregnancy rates. Fertil Steril. 1999;72:83-9.
91. Kondaveeti-Gordon U, Harrison R, Barry-Kinsella C, Gordon AC, Drudy L, Cottell E. A randomized prospective study of early follicular or midluteal initiation of long protocol gonadotropin-releasing hormone in an in vitro fertilization program. Fertil Steril. 1996;66:582-6.
92. Karande V, Morris R, Rinehart J, Miller C, Rao R, Gleicher N. Limited success using the "flare" protocol in poor responders in cycles with low basal follicle-stimulating hormone levels during in vitro fertilization. Fertil Steril. 1997;67:900-3.
93. Loumaye E, Vankrieken L, Depreester S, Psalti I, de Cooman S, Thomas K. Hormonal changes induced by short-term administration of gonadotropin-releasing hormone agonist during ovarian hyperstimulation for in vitro fertilization and their consequences for embryo development. Fertil Steril. 1989;51:105-11.
94. Ron-El R, Herman A, Golan A, van der Ven H, Caspi E, Diedrich K. The comparison of early follicular and midluteal administration of long-acting gonadotropin-releasing hormone agonist. Fertil Steril. 1990;54:233-7.

95. Gindoff PR, Hall JL, Stillman RJ. Ovarian suppression with leuprolide acetate: comparison of luteal, follicular, and flare-up administration in controlled ovarian hyperstimulation for oocyte retrieval. J In Vitro Fert Embryo Transf. 1990;7:94-7.
96. Anserini P, Magnasco A, Remorgida V, Gaggero G, Testa D, Capitanio GL. Comparison of a blocking vs. a flare-up protocol in poor responders with a normal and abnormal clomiphene citrate challenge test. Gynecol Endocrinol. 1997;11:321-6.
97. San Roman GA, Surrey ES, Judd HL, Kerin JF. A prospective randomized comparison of luteal phase versus concurrent follicular phase initiation of gonadotropin-releasing hormone agonist for in vitro fertilization. Fertil Steril. 1992;58:744-9.
98. Serafini P, Yadid I, Motta ELA, Alegretti JR, Fioravanti J, Coslovsky M. Ovarian stimulation with daily late follicular phase administration of low-dose human chorionic gonadotropin for in vitro fertilization: a prospective, randomized trial. Fertil Steril. 2006;86(4):830-8.
99. Droesch K, Muasher SJ, Brzyski RG, Jones GS, Simonetti S, Liu HC, et al. Value of suppression with a gonadotropin-releasing hormone agonist prior to gonadotropin stimulation for in vitro fertilization. Fertil Steril. 1989;51(2):292-7.
100. Scott RT, Navot D. Enhancement of ovarian responsiveness with microdoses of gonadotropin-releasing hormone agonist during ovulation induction for in vitro fertilization. Fertil Steril. 1994;61:880-5.
101. Loutradis D, Stefanidis K, Drakakis P, Kallianidis K, El Sheikh A, Milingos S, et al. Does pre-treatment with micronized progesterone affect the ovarian response to a gonadotropin releasing hormone agonist flare-up protocol? Gynecol Endocrinol. 2003;17:101-6.
102. Cédrin-Durnerin I, Bulwa S, Herve F, Martin-Pont B, Uzan M, Hugues JN. The hormonal flare-up following gonadotrophin-releasing hormone agonist administration is influenced by a progestogen pretreatment. Hum Reprod. 1996;11:1859-63.
103. Surrey ES, Bower J, Hill DM, Ramsey J, Surrey MW. Clinical and endocrine effects of a microdose GnRH agonist flare regimen administered to poor responders who are undergoing in vitro fertilization. Fertil Steril. 1998;69:419-24.
104. Leondires MP, Escalpes M, Segars JH, Scott Jr RT, Miller BT. Microdose follicular phase gonadotropin-releasing hormone agonist (GnRH-a) compared with luteal phase GnRH-a for ovarian stimulation at in vitro fertilization. Fertil Steril. 1999;72:1018-23.
105. Sunkara SK, Coomarasamy A, Faris R, Braude P, Khalaf Y. Long gonadotropin-releasing hormone agonist versus short agonist versus antagonist regimens in poor responders undergoing in vitro fertilization: a randomized controlled trial. Fertil Steril. 2014;101(1):147-53.
106. Taşdemir M, Taşdemir I, Kodama H, Fukuda J, Tanaka T. Short protocol of gonadotropin releasing hormone agonist administration gave better results in long protocol poor-responders in IVF-ET. J Obstet Gynecol Res. 1996;22:73-7.
107. Detti L, Williams DB, Robins JC, Maxwell RA, Thomas MA. A comparison of three downregulation approaches for poor responders undergoing in vitro fertilization. Fertil Steril. 2005;84(5):1401-5.
108. Kenigsberg D, Littman BA, Williams RF, Hodgen GD. Medical hypophysectomy: II. Variability of ovarian response to gonadotropin therapy. Fertil Steril. 1984;42:116-26.
109. Diedrich K, Diedrich C, Santos E, Zoll C, al-Hasani S, Reissmann T, et al. Suppression of the endogenous luteinizing hormone surge by the gonadotrophin-releasing hormone antagonist cetrorelix during ovarian stimulation. Hum Reprod. 1994;9:788-91.
110. Albano C, Felberbaum RE, Smitz J, Riethmüller-Winzen H, Engel J, Diedrich K, et al. Ovarian stimulation with HMG: results of a prospective randomized phase III European study comparing the luteinizing hormone-releasing hormone (LHRH)-antagonist cetrorelix and the LHRH-agonist buserelin. Hum Reprod. 2000;15(3):526-31.
111. Olivennes F, Belaisch-Allart J, Emperaire JC, Dechaud H, Alvarez S, Moreau L, et al. Prospective, randomized, controlled study of in vitro fertilization-embryo transfer with a single dose of a luteinizing hormone-releasing hormone (LH-RH) antagonist (cetrorelix) or a depot formula of an LH-RH agonist (triptorelin). Fertil Steril. 2000;73:314-20.
112. European and Middle East Orgalutran Study Group. Comparable clinical outcome using the GnRH antagonist ganirelix or a long protocol of the GnRH agonist triptorelin for the prevention of premature LH surges in women undergoing ovarian stimulation. Hum Reprod. 2001;16:644-51.
113. Franco Jr JR, Baruffi RLR, Mauri AL, Petersen CG, Felipe V, Cornicelli J, et al. GnRH agonist versus GnRH antagonist in poor ovarian responders: a meta-analysis. Reprod Biomed Online. 2006;13(50):618-27.
114. Cheung LP, Lam PM, Lok IH, Chiu TT, Yeung SY, Tjer CC, et al. GnRH antagonist versus long GnRH agonist protocol in poor responders undergoing IVF: a randomized controlled trial. Hum Reprod. 2005;20:616-21.
115. Marci R, Caserta D, Dolo V, Tatone C, Pavan A, Moscarini M. GnRH antagonist in IVF poor-responder patients: results of a randomized trial. Reprod Biomed Online. 2005;11: 189-93.
116. Tazegül A, Görkemli H, Ozdemir S, Aktan TM. Comparison of multiple dose GnRH antagonist and minidose long agonist protocols in poor responders undergoing in vitro fertilization: a randomized controlled trial. Arch Gynecol Obstet. 2008;278:467-72.
117. Tehraninejad ES, Fazel A, Samiei A, Rashidi B, Kiani K. Flexible, multi-dose GnRH antagonist versus long GnRH agonist protocol in poor responders: a randomized controlled trial. Int J Fertil Steril. 2009;2:165-8.
118. Sims JA, Seltman HJ, Muasher SJ. Early follicular rise of serum progesterone concentration in response to a flare-up effect of gonadotrophin-releasing hormone agonist impairs follicular recruitment for in-vitro fertilization. Hum Reprod. 1994;9:235-40.
119. Griesinger G, Diedrich K, Tarlatzis BC, Kolibianakis EM. GnRH-antagonists in ovarian stimulation for IVF in patients with poor response to gonadotrophins, polycystic ovary syndrome, and risk of ovarian hyperstimulation: a meta-analysis. Reprod Biomed Online. 2006;13:628-38.
120. Land JA, Yarmolinskaya MI, Dumoulin JC, Evers JL. High-dose human menopausal gonadotropin stimulation in poor responders does not improve in vitro fertilization outcome. Fertil Steril. 1996;65(5):961-5.
121. Karande VC, Jones GS, Veeck LL, Muasher SJ. High-dose follicle-stimulating hormone stimulation at the onset of the menstrual cycle does not improve the in vitro

fertilization outcome in low-responder patients. Fertil Steril. 1990;53(3):486-9.

122. van Hooff MH, Alberda AT, Huisman GJ, Zeilmaker GH, Leerentveld RA. Doubling the human menopausal gonadotrophin dose in the course of an in-vitro fertilization treatment cycle in low responders: a randomized study. Hum Reprod. 1993;8(3):369-73.
123. Hofmann GE, Toner JP, Muasher SJ, Jones GS. High-dose follicle-stimulating hormone (FSH) ovarian stimulation in low-responder patients for in vitro fertilization. J In Vitro Fert Embryo Transf. 1989;6(5):285-9.
124. Berkkanoglu M, Ozgur K. What is the optimum maximal gonadotropin dosage used in microdose flare-up cycles in poor responders? Fertil Steril. 2010;94(2):662-5.
125. Loutradis D, Patsoula E, Minas V, Koussidis GA, Antsaklis A, Michalas S, et al. FSH receptor gene polymorphisms have a role for different ovarian response to stimulation in patients entering IVF/ICSI-ET programs. J Assist Reprod Genet. 2006;23:177-84.
126. Manzi DL, Thornton KL, Scott LB, Nulsen JC. The value of increasing the dose of human menopausal gonadotropins in women who initially demonstrate a poor response. Fertil Steril. 1994;62:251-6.
127. Patrizio P, Vaiarelli A, Levi Setti PE, Tobler KJ, Shoham G, Leong M, et al. How to define, diagnose and treat poor responders? Responses from a worldwide survey of IVF clinics. Reprod Biomed Online. 2015;30(6):581-92.
128. Ng EH, Lau EY, Yeung WS, Ho PC. HMG is as good as recombinant human FSH in terms of oocyte and embryo quality: a prospective randomized trial. Hum Reprod. 2001;16:319-25.
129. Westergaard LG, Erb K, Laursen SB, Rex S, Rasmussen PE. Human menopausal gonadotropin versus recombinant follicle-stimulating hormone in normogonadotropic women down-regulated with a gonadotropin-releasing hormone agonist who were undergoing in vitro fertilization and intracytoplasmic sperm injection: a prospective randomized study. Fertil Steril. 2001;76:543-9.
130. Gordon UD, Harrison RF, Fawzy M, Hennelly B, Gordon AC. A randomized prospective assessor-blind evaluation of luteinizing hormone dosage and in vitro fertilization outcome. Fertil Steril. 2001;75:324-31.
131. De Placido G, Mollo A, Alviggi C, Strina I, Varricchio MT, Ranieri A, et al. Rescue of IVF cycles by HMG in pituitary down-regulated normogonadotrophic young women characterized by a poor initial response to recombinant FSH. Hum Reprod. 2001;16:1875-9.
132. Eskandar M, Jaroudi K, Jambi A, Archibong EI, Coskun S, Sobande AA. Is recombinant follicle-stimulating hormone more effective in IVF poor responders than human menopausal gonadotrophins? Med Sci Monit. 2004;10:16-9.
133. Drakakis P, Loutradis D, Kallianidis K, Bletsa R, Milingos S, Dionyssiou-Asteriou A, et al. A comparative study of the effect of ovarian stimulation protocols with different gonadotropin preparations on the biological and clinical parameters of the outcome of intracytoplasmic sperm injection. Clin Exp Obstet Gynecol. 2002;29(4):286-9.
134. Andersen AN, Devroey P, Arce JC. Clinical outcome following stimulation with highly purified hMG or recombinant FSH in patients undergoing IVF: a randomized assessor-blind controlled trial. Hum Reprod. 2006;21(12):3217-27.
135. Al-Inany HG, Abou-Setta AM, Aboulghar MA, Mansour RT, Serour GI. Highly purified hMG achieves better pregnancy rates in IVF cycles but not ICSI cycles compared with recombinant FSH: a meta-analysis. Gynecol Endocrinol. 2009;25(6):372-8.
136. Gougeon A. Regulation of ovarian follicular development in primates: facts and hypotheses. Endocr Rev. 1996;17: 121-55.
137. Rombauts L, Suikkari AM, MacLachlan V, Trounson AO, Healy DL. Recruitment of follicles by recombinant human follicle-stimulating hormone commencing in the luteal phase of the ovarian cycle. Fertil Steril. 1998;69:665-9.
138. Drakakis P, Loutradis D, Kallianidis K, Liapi A, Milingos S, Makrigiannakis A, et al. Small doses of LH activity are needed early in ovarian stimulation for better quality oocytes in IVF-ET. Eur J Obstet Gynecol Reprod Biol. 2005;121:77-80.
139. Sullivan MW, Stewart-Akers A, Krasnow JS, Berga SL, Zeleznik AJ. Ovarian responses in women to recombinant follicle-stimulating hormone and luteinizing hormone (LH): a role for LH in the final stages of follicular maturation. J Clin Endocrinol Metab. 1999;84:228-32.
140. Esposito MA, Barnhart KT, Coutifaris C, Patrizio P. Role of periovulatory luteinizing hormone concentrations during assisted reproductive technology cycles stimulated exclusively with recombinant follicle-stimulating hormone. Fertil Steril. 2001;75:519-24.
141. Westergaard LG, Laursen SB, Andersen CY. Increased risk of early pregnancy loss by profound suppression of luteinizing hormone during ovarian stimulation in normogonadotrophic women undergoing assisted reproduction. Hum Reprod. 2000;15:1003-8.
142. Lévy DP, Navarro JM, Schattman GL, Davis OK, Rosenwaks Z. The role of LH in ovarian stimulation: exogenous LH: let's design the future. Hum Reprod. 2002;15:2258-65.
143. Bosdou JK, Venetis CA, Kolibianakis EM, Toulis KA, Goulis DG, Zepiridis L, et al. The use of androgens or androgen-modulating agents in poor responders undergoing in vitro fertilization: a systematic review and meta-analysis. Hum Reprod Update. 2012;18:127-45.
144. Hill MJ, Levens ED, Levy G, Ryan ME, Csokmay JM, DeCherney AH, et al. The use of recombinant luteinizing hormone in patients undergoing assisted reproductive techniques with advanced reproductive age: a systematic review and meta-analysis. Fertil Steril. 2012;97:1108-14.
145. Haahr T, Esteves SC, Humaidan P. Individualized controlled ovarian stimulation in expected poor-responders: an update. Reprod Biol Endocrinol. 2018;16(1):1-9
146. Alviggi C, Conforti A, Esteves SC, Andersen CY, Bosch E, Bühler K, et al. Recombinant luteinizing hormone supplementation in assisted reproductive technology: a systematic review. Fertil Steril. 2018;109(4):644-64.
147. Conforti A, Esteves SC, Di Rella F, Strina I, De Rosa P, Fiorenza A, et al. The role of recombinant LH in women with hypo-response to controlled ovarian stimulation: a systematic review and meta-analysis. Reprod Biol Endocrinol. 2019;17(1):1-2.
148. Marchiani S, Tamburrino L, Benini F, Pallecchi M, Bignozzi C, Conforti A, et al. LH supplementation of ovarian stimulation

protocols influences follicular fluid steroid composition contributing to the improvement of ovarian response in poor responder women. Sci Rep. 2020;10(1):1-2.
149. Arvis P, Massin N, Lehert P. Effect of recombinant LH supplementation on cumulative live birth rate compared with FSH alone in poor ovarian responders: a large, real-world study. Reprod Biomed Online. 2021;42(3):546-54.
150. Loutradis D, Drakakis P, Vomvolaki E, Antsaklis A. Different ovarian stimulation protocols for women with diminished ovarian reserve. J Assist Reprod Genet. 2007;24:597-611.
151. D'Amato G, Caroppo E, Pasquadibisceglie A, Carone D, Vitti A, Vizziello GM. A novel protocol of ovulation induction with delayed gonadotropin-releasing hormone antagonist administration combined with high-dose recombinant follicle-stimulating hormone and clomiphene citrate for poor responders and women over 35 years. Fertil Steril. 2004;81:1572-7.
152. Craft I, Gorgy A, Hill J, Menon D, Podsiadly B. Will GnRH antagonists provide new hope for patients considered 'difficult responders' to GnRH agonist protocols? Hum Reprod. 1999;14(12):2959-62.
153. Kamath MS, Maheshwari A, Bhattacharya S, Lor KY, Gibreel A. Oral medications including clomiphene citrate or aromatase inhibitors with gonadotropins for controlled ovarian stimulation in women undergoing in vitro fertilisation. Cochrane Database Syst Rev. 2017;11(11):CD008528.
154. Datta AK, Maheshwari A, Felix N, Campbell S, Nargund G. Mild versus conventional ovarian stimulation for IVF in poor responders: a systematic review and meta-analysis. Reprod Biomed Online. 2020;41(2):225-38.
155. Datta AK, Maheshwari A, Felix N, Campbell S, Nargund G. Mild versus conventional ovarian stimulation for IVF in poor, normal and hyper-responders: a systematic review and meta-analysis. Hum Reprod Update. 2021;27(2):229-53.
156. Montoya-Botero P, Drakopoulos P, González-Foruria I, Polyzos NP. Fresh and cumulative live birth rates in mild versus conventional stimulation for IVF cycles in poor ovarian responders: a systematic review and meta-analysis. Hum Reprod Open. 2021;2021(1):hoaa066.
157. Vendola K, Zhou J, Wang J, Bondy CA. Androgens promote insulin-like growth factor-I and insulin-like growth factor-I receptor gene expression in the primate ovary. Hum Reprod. 1999;14:2328-32.
158. Palter SF, Tavares AB, Hourvitz A, Veldhuis JD, Adashi EY. Are estrogens of import to primate/human ovarian folliculogenesis? Endocr Rev. 2001;22:389-424.
159. Mitwally MFM, Casper RF. Aromatase inhibition improves ovarian response to follicle-stimulating hormone in poor responders. Fertil Steril. 2002;77(4):776-80.
160. Healy S, Tan SL, Tulandi T, Biljan MM. Effects of letrozole on superovulation with gonadotropins in women undergoing intrauterine insemination. Fertil Steril. 2003;80:1325-9
161. Polyzos NP, Popovic-Todorovic B. SAY NO to mild ovarian stimulation for all poor responders: it is time to realize that not all poor responders are the same. Hum Reprod. 2020;35(9):1964-71.
162. Pierson RA, Ginther OJ. Ultrasonographic appearance of the bovine uterus during the estrous cycle. J Am Vet Med Assoc. 1987;190(8):995-1001.
163. Ubaldi FM, Capalbo A, Vaiarelli A, Cimadomo D, Colamaria S, Alviggi C, et al. Follicular versus luteal phase ovarian stimulation during the same menstrual cycle (DuoStim) in a reduced ovarian reserve population results in a similar euploid blastocyst formation rate: new insight in ovarian reserve exploitation. Fertil Steril. 2016;105(6):1488-95.
164. Alsbjerg B, Haahr T, Elbaek HO, Laursen R, Povlsen BB, Humaidan P. Dual stimulation using corifollitropin alfa in 54 Bologna criteria poor ovarian responders—a case series. Reprod Biomed Online. 2019;38(5):677-82.
165. Steptoe PC, Edwards RG. Birth after the reimplantation of a human embryo. Lancet. 1978;12:366.
166. Janssens RM, Lambalk CB, Schats R, Schoemaker J. Successful in-vitro fertilization in a natural cycle after four previously failed attempts in stimulated cycles: case report. Hum Reprod. 1999;14:2497-8.
167. Jenkins JM, Davies DW, Devonport H, Anthony FW, Gadd SC, Watson RH, et al. Comparison of 'poor' responders with 'good' responders using a standard buserelin/human menopausal gonadotrophin regime for in-vitro fertilization. Hum Reprod. 1991;6:918-21.
168. Fauser BC, Devroey P, Yen SS, Gosden R, Crowley Jr WF, Baird DT, et al. Minimal ovarian stimulation for IVF: appraisal of potential benefits and drawbacks. Hum Reprod. 1999;14:2681-6.
169. Paulson RJ, Sauer MV, Lobo RA. Embryo implantation after human in vitro fertilization: importance of endometrial receptivity. Fertil Steril. 1990;53:870-4.
170. Olivennes F, Frydman R. Friendly IVF: the way of the future? Hum Reprod. 1998;13:1121-4.
171. Elizur SE, Aslan D, Shulman A, Weisz B, Bider D, Dor J. Modified natural cycle using GnRH antagonist can be an optional treatment in poor responders undergoing IVF. J Assist Reprod Genet. 2005;22(2):75-9.
172. Morgia F, Sbracia M, Schimberni M, Giallonardo A, Piscitelli C, Giannini P, et al. A controlled trial of natural cycle versus microdose gonadotropin-releasing hormone analog flare cycles in poor responders undergoing in vitro fertilization. Fertil Steril. 2004;81:1542-7.
173. Drakopoulos P, Romito A, Errázuriz J, Santos-Ribeiro S, Popovic-Todorovic B, Racca A, et al. Modified natural cycle IVF versus conventional stimulation in advanced-age Bologna poor responders. Reprod Biomed Online. 2019;39(4):698-703.
174. Lin MH, Wu FS, Lee RK, Li SH, Lin SY, Hwu YM. Dual trigger with combination of gonadotropin-releasing hormone agonist and human chorionic gonadotropin significantly improves the live-birth rate for normal responders in GnRH-antagonist cycles. Fertil Steril. 2013;100(5): 1296-302.
175. Zhang J, Wang Y, Mao X, Chen Q, Hong Q, Cai R, et al. Dual trigger of final oocyte maturation in poor ovarian responders undergoing IVF/ICSI cycles. Reprod Biomed Online. 2017;35(6):701-7.
176. Lin MH, Wu FS, Hwu YM, Lee RK, Li RS, Li SH. Dual trigger with gonadotropin releasing hormone agonist and human chorionic gonadotropin significantly improves live birth rate for women with diminished ovarian reserve. Reprod Biol Endocrinol. 2019;17(1):1-7.
177. Eser A, Devranoğlu B, Ergen EB, Abide ÇY. Dual trigger with gonadotropin-releasing hormone and human chorionic gonadotropin for poor responders. J Turk Ger Gynecol Assoc. 2018;19(2):98-103.

178. Bhattacharya S, Hamilton MP, Shaaban M, Khalaf Y, Seddler M, Ghobara T, et al. Conventional in-vitro fertilisation versus intracytoplasmic sperm injection for the treatment of non-male-factor infertility: a randomised controlled trial. Lancet. 2001;357(9274):2075-9.
179. Moreno C, Ruiz A, Simón C, Pellicer A, Remohí J. Intracytoplasmic sperm injection as a routine indication in low responder patients. Hum Reprod. 1998;13(8):2126-9.
180. Gabrielsen A, Petersen K, Mikkelsen AL, Lindenberg S. Intracytoplasmic sperm injection does not overcome an oocyte defect in previous fertilization failure with conventional in-vitro fertilization and normal spermatozoa. Hum Reprod. 1996;11(9):1963-5.
181. Gianaroli L, Magli MC, Ferraretti AP, Munné S. Preimplantation diagnosis for aneuploidies in patients undergoing in vitro fertilization with a poor prognosis: identification of the categories for which it should be proposed. Fertil Steril. 1999;72(5):837-44.
182. Schoolcraft WB, Katz-Jaffe MG, Stevens J, Rawlins M, Munne S. Preimplantation aneuploidy testing for infertile patients of advanced maternal age: a randomized prospective trial. Fertil Steril. 2009;92(1):157-62.
183. Blake DA, Farquhar CM, Johnson N, Proctor M. Cleavage stage versus blastocyst stage embryo transfer in assisted conception. Cochrane Database Syst Rev. 2007;4:CD002118.
184. Shen S, Rosen MP, Dobson AT, Fujimoto VY, McCulloch CE, Cedars MI. Day 2 transfer improves pregnancy outcome in in vitro fertilization cycles with few available embryos. Fertil Steril. 2006;86(1):44-50.
185. Bahceci M, Ulug U, Ciray HN, Akman MA, Erden HF. Efficiency of changing the embryo transfer time from day 3 to day 2 among women with poor ovarian response: a prospective randomized trial. Fertil Steril. 2006;86(1):81-5.
186. Practice Committee of the American Society for Reproductive Medicine, Practice Committee of the Society for Assisted Reproductive Technology. Guidelines on number of embryos transferred. Fertil Steril. 2009;92(5):1518-9.
187. Kwon H, Choi DH, Kim EK, Kim EH, Lee SE. Accumulation of vitrified embryos followed by frozen embryo transfer in poor ovarian responders according to Bologna criteria. Gynecol Obstet (Sunnyvale). 2015;5:331.
188. Cobo A, Garrido N, Crespo J, José R, Pellicer A. Accumulation of oocytes: a new strategy for managing low-responder patients. Reprod Biomed Online. 2012;24(4):424-32.
189. Chinta P, Antonisamy B, Mangalaraj AM, Kunjummen AT, Kamath MS. POSEIDON classification and the proposed treatment options for groups 1 and 2: time to revisit? A retrospective analysis of 1425 ART cycles. Hum Reprod Open. 2021;2021(1):hoaa070.
190. Christian CA, Pielecka-Fortuna J, Moenter SM: Estradiol suppresses glutamatergic transmission to gonadotropin-releasing hormone neurons in a model of negative feedback in mice. Biol Reprod. 2009;80:1128-35.
191. Ulug U, Ben-Shlomo I, Turan E, Erden HF, Akman MA, Bahceci M. Conception rates following assisted reproduction in poor responder patients: a retrospective study in 300 consecutive cycles. Reprod Biomed Online. 2003;6(4):439-43.
192. Moolenaar LM, Mohiuddin S, Davie MM, Merrilees MA, Broekmans FJM, Mol BWJ, et al. High live birth rate in the subsequent IVF cycle after first-cycle poor response among women with mean age 35 and normal FSH. Reprod Biomed Online. 2013;27:362-6.
193. Polyzos NP, Nwoye M, Corona R, Blockeel C, Stoop D, Haentjens P, et al. Live birth rates in Bologna poor responders treated with ovarian stimulation for IVF/ICSI. Reprod Biomed Online. 2014;28:469-74.
194. Bozdag G, Polat M, Yarali I, Yarali H. Live birth rates in various subgroups of poor ovarian responders fulfilling the Bologna criteria. Reprod Biomed Online. 2017;34(6):639-44.
195. Papathanasiou A, Searle BJ, King NMA, Bhattacharya S. Trends in 'poor responder' research: lessons learned from RCTs in assisted conception. Hum Reprod Update. 2016;22(3):306-19.
196. Oudendijk JF, Yarde F, Eijkemans MJC, Broekmans FJM, Broer SL. The poor responder in IVF: is the prognosis always poor? A systematic review. Hum Reprod Update. 2012;18(1):1-11.

CHAPTER 61

Recurrent Implantation Failure

Divyashree PS

INTRODUCTION

Implantation is a highly complex process, which relies on the collaboration between two partners, i.e., the embryo and the endometrium. Failure of implantation is a consequence of embryo and/or uterine factors. The exact mechanism of implantation is far from clearly understood. Recurrent implantation failure (RIF) refers to failure to achieve a clinical pregnancy after transfer of at least four good-quality embryos in a minimum of three fresh or frozen cycles in a woman under the age of 40 years. RIF is a frustrating event for both patients and their clinicians. The aim of this chapter is to condense the reported etiologies for RIF, focus on the suggested investigations to be implemented, and analyze the suggested treatment strategies.

When a gestational sac is visible on ultrasound (US), which is usually 3 weeks after oocyte retrieval, implantation is said to be successful.[1,2]

Embryo implantation is the bottleneck for in vitro fertilization (IVF) success. Successful implantation involves two important players, a receptive endometrium and a normal and functional blastocyst, in association with a synchronized dialog between maternal and embryonic tissues.[1]

Recurrent implantation failure is a challenging and frustrating condition from both patient and clinician perspective. High rates of drop out (up to 50%) from IVF programs after fewer than three cycles is primarily because of the reason, failure to achieve pregnancy.[3,4]

DEFINITION OF RECURRENT IMPLANTATION FAILURE

Despite many publications on this topic,[5-8] there is no universally accepted definition till date. There are various definitions suggested for RIF, which are derivations of expert opinions and lack sound scientific evidence.

It is a matter of debate whether the diagnosis of RIF is based entirely on the number of embryos transferred or on the number of embryo transfer cycles. It is more logical and scientific to define RIF based on the number of embryos transferred, whereas it is difficult for the patients to comprehend. It is more practical and easily understood by patients if the RIF definition is based on the number of transfer cycles.

Various definitions suggested by different authors are given here.

Simon and Laufer[9] defined RIF as the failure to obtain a clinical pregnancy after three consecutive IVF attempts, in which one or two embryos of high-grade quality are transferred in each cycle.

Polanski et al.[10] defined RIF as the absence of a total implantation after two consecutive cycles of IVF, intracytoplasmic sperm injection (ICSI), or frozen embryo replacement cycles where the cumulative number of transferred embryos was no less than four for cleavage-stage embryos and no less than two for blastocysts, with all embryos being of good quality and of appropriate developmental stage.

Coughlan et al.[11] suggested the definition of RIF as the failure to achieve a clinical pregnancy after transfer of at least four good-quality embryos in a minimum of three fresh or frozen cycles in a woman under the age of 40 years.

Somigliana et al.,[12] however, have cautioned about overdiagnosis of RIF, if diagnosis of RIF is drawn after only two to three IVF cycles. Indeed, the rate of false-positive diagnosis remains above 50% in all sensitivity analyses, if diagnosis of RIF is considered after three IVF cycles.

It is after six cycles that the diagnosis of RIF becomes more reliable.

INCIDENCE

The actual prevalence of RIF is unidentified and randomly set at 10% (but then varied in sensitivity analysis from 5 to 25%). Even if an accurate estimation of this prevalence cannot be extrapolated from published research, data from studies reporting on the cumulative chance of pregnancy after seven to eight treatment cycles propose that the frequency of this condition is at least below 20%.[12]

IMPLANTATION

Human embryo implantation is a three-stage process (apposition, adhesion, and invasion) involving synchronized crosstalk between a receptive endometrium and a functional blastocyst.

A well-synchronized event, which includes cellular adhesion, invasion, and immune regulatory mechanisms, is required for embryo implantation. During most days of the menstrual cycle, endometrium is essentially hostile toward the embryo. To reverse this paradoxical condition, a major physiological endeavor is thus needed by the endometrium. During the first half of the menstrual cycle, rising estrogen levels cause endometrial cell proliferation. After ovulation, progesterone released by the corpus luteum causes secretory transformation. At this point, the endometrium is mature and primed for embryo implantation. This process is rigorously controlled both temporally and spatially. Prostaglandins control this fine-tuning of the window of implantation (WOI) timing. After entering the uterine cavity through the tubal ostia, blastocyst appears to move freely under the influence of selectins, which helps in suitable rolling. It is important for the blastocyst to attach to the endometrium in a polarized way and the "rolling" phenomenon will ensure that the blastocyst will settle in the proper area and in the correct orientation. Mucin-1 (MUC-1), by its repellent activity, prevents the blastocyst from adhering to the endometrium, which has got poor receptivity. Pinopods are the landing platforms for the blastocysts, which get attracted toward particular endometrial areas under the influence of chemokines and growth factors. Pinopods extend over the tips of the microvilli expressing the repellent MUC-1, and they are fully developed for only 1 or 2 days. To ensure adhesiveness between the endometrium and the embryo, adhesion molecules such as integrins and cadherins play an important role at this stage.

ASSUMED ETIOLOGIES FOR RECURRENT IMPLANTATION FAILURE

- Gamete and embryo factors
- Factors affecting endometrial receptivity (ER)
- Multifactorial effectors.

Gamete and Embryo Factors

Embryo quality is a very important variable for successful implantation. Embryo quality clearly depends on oocyte and sperm quality.

Oocyte quality is very important for the resulting embryo quality as it forms the majority of the volume of the embryo. Compromised oocyte quality as a cause of RIF can be suspected in following cases:

Oocyte yield in too extremes, i.e., too high and too low oocyte numbers, is associated with poor oocyte quality. High oocyte yield due to aggressive ovarian stimulation is associated with poor oocyte quality.[13]

Advanced maternal age, high follicle-stimulating hormone (FSH), low antral follicle count (AFC), low anti-Müllerian hormone (AMH) when it is associated with poor response to stimulation, fewer number of oocytes retrieved, high number of immature oocytes, reduced fertilization rate and embryo utilization rate, poor oocyte quality as a cause for RIF can be suspected.[14] Association between advanced maternal age and increased chromosomal nondisjunction, aneuploidy, increase mitochondrial damage, and decrease in mitochondrial membrane potential has been noted.[15]

Sperm quality is equally important to achieve fertilization, good embryo quality, and implantation. Conventional semen analysis may not reflect defects in sperm quality, which can give answers for RIF. There is a recent surge in interest in evaluating sperm DNA damage as cause for RIF. Association between DNA fragmentation and recurrent miscarriage has been proven, but its association with RIF is not very clear.[16]

Embryogenesis can be impaired by chromosomal abnormalities of the male or female partner, the gametes, or the developing embryo itself. Maternal cytoplasmic factors or mutations in cell cycle control genes can cause disruption of the normal sequence of chromosome replication and segregation in early human embryos, which can be a common cause for RIF. Despite good morphology and development rate, embryos fail to implant and it can be hypothesized that in RIF patients, majority of these embryos are chromosomally abnormal.[17]

To prevent polyspermy and to preserve the integrity of the preimplantation embryo, zona hardening is an essential process in mammalian fertilization. Factors such as aging, which is nonmodifiable and in vitro culture, which can be modified can induce zona hardening and thus affect hatching. Defective hatching due to zona hardening as a cause for RIF has been suggested by a few studies.[18,19]

Factors Affecting Endometrial Receptivity (Fig. 1)

Uterine Factors (Anatomical)

Congenital or acquired uterine abnormalities can affect ER.

Congenital uterine anomalies: It is well recognized that *Hox* genes, in particular *HOXA10* and *HOXA11*, play an important role not only in Müllerian duct development[20] but also in endometrial development in preparation for implantation.[21] Hence, it can be hypothesized that congenital uterine anomalies may be associated with RIF. There are studies supporting this hypothesis, one in which it was demonstrated that women who had undergone septal resection had better outcome following IVF treatment compared to women who were untreated.[22] Another study showed that the miscarriage rate was reduced to 30% after septal resection compared to 80% before septal resection.[23]

Acquired uterine abnormalities: Undiagnosed uterine pathology may be a cause for RIF. In patients with RIF, the frequency of undiagnosed intrauterine pathologies varies between 25% and 50%.[24] Repeat hysteroscopy revealed abnormalities such as myomas, adhesions, endometritis, polyps, and hyperplasia in 18–27% of women with RIF.[25] Various mechanisms by which these acquired uterine abnormalities could affect implantation are depicted in **Table 1**.

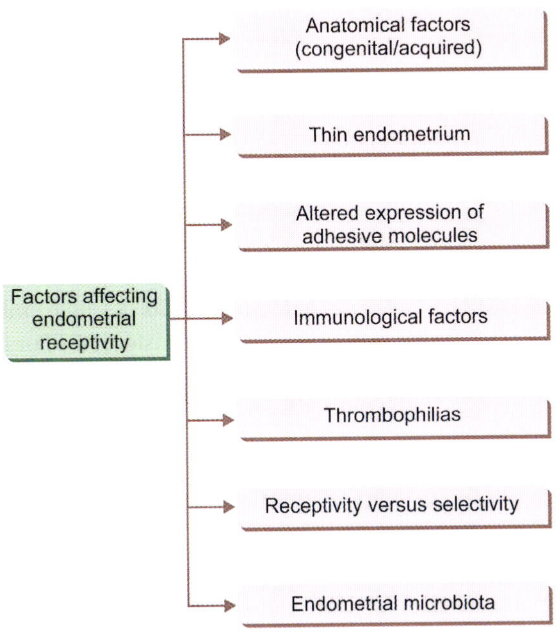

Fig. 1: Factors affecting endometrial receptivity.

Thin Endometrium

There is conflicting evidence regarding cutoff for endometrial thickness affecting implantation. Thin endometrium during embryo transfer did not influence the cumulative pregnancy rate, in a large prospective cohort study,[27] especially when transfer was done with high-quality embryos.[28] In tubal factor infertility, presence of thin or hyperechogenic endometrium or persistent fluid in cavity impaired IVF outcome whereas this did not affect outcome when same factors were present in polycystic ovary syndrome (PCOS).[29]

It was also noted that endometrial thickness predicted pregnancy outcome in IVF, but not for ICSI.[30] This is because thin endometrium was a prognostic indicator of pregnancy only in the case of a female indication for infertility (IVF). A thin endometrium in cases of female infertility may reflect a previous or present uterine pathology, whereas in indications of male infertility (i.e., cases using ICSI), in the absence of any associated uterine pathology, the presence of a thin endometrium is not predictive.

Altered Expression of Adhesive Molecules

Various cytokines are involved in implantation. Local dysregulation of normal expression or action of cytokines can cause implantation failure. Elevated endometrial natural killer (NK) cells, dysregulation of interleukin (IL)-12, -15, and -18, high IL-1β, and low interferon-γ and IL-10 were found in

TABLE 1: Uterine abnormalities and mechanism of disrupted implantation.

Uterine abnormality	*Anatomical*	*Physiological*	*Molecular*
Myoma	• Distorts endometrial lining • Disordered uterine contractility	• Altered uterine vascular perfusion • Increased uNK cells	• Decreased HOXA10, BTEB1, and LIF expressions • Altered TGF-β pathway • Decreased glycodelin and IL-10 in mid-luteal phase[26]
Polyps	Mechanical interference with embryo transport and implantation	• Increased cellular proliferation and apoptosis • Increased estrogen receptors	• Abnormal secretion of E2 and progesterone regulated implantation markers • Low IGFBP-1 and osteopontin levels • Impaired expression of HOXA10, HOXA11, and interferon-γ[26]
Adenomyosis	Disturbed endomyometrial junction	• Altered uterine vascular perfusion • Progesterone resistance • Alteration in PR-A to PR-B ratio	• Reduced αvβ3 - integrin and LIF expressions in the window of implantation • Absence of HOXA10 and HOXA11 peak in secretory phase[26]
Synechiae	Prevents the embryos from attaching to the luminal surface of the endometrium	Thought to impair ER by reducing pregnancy rates and increasing the risk of miscarriage	

(E2: estradiol; ER: endometrial receptivity; IGFBP-1: insulin-like growth factor binding protein 1; IL: interleukin; PR: progesterone receptor; TGF-β: transforming growth factor beta; uNK: uterine natural killer)

RIF. Failure of appearance of a specific integrin $\alpha\varpi\beta 3$ in the endometrium at the time of implantation was suggested as a cause of implantation failure. High levels of aromatase p450 messenger RNA (mRNA), changes in pinopode expression, and high matrix metalloproteinases have been suggested to be associated with RIF.[17]

Contribution of Immunology and Thrombophilia Toward Alteration in Endometrial Receptivity

Advances in reproductive medicine have allowed us to select euploid embryos for transfer, eliminating embryonic factors for failed implantation. However, even transfer of a euploid blastocyst does not lead to successful implantation and delivery in >30% of cases.[31] Apart from the above-mentioned causes for altered ER affecting implantation, the immune system has been the next possible and most debated cause. The three main players of immune system affecting implantation are as follows:

1. T helper (TH)1–TH2 balance
2. NK cells
3. Autoantibodies.

- *TH1–TH2 imbalance:* There are two broad classes of T helper lymphocytes, TH1 and TH2. Proinflammatory cytokines are released from TH1 cytokines, which include interferon-γ, tumor necrosis factor (TNF), and IL-1, -2, -12, -15, and -18. TH1 cytokines are counteracted by the TH2 cytokines, which are IL-4, -5, -6, -10, and -13 and granulocyte macrophage colony-stimulating factor. Depending on the type of immune challenge faced with, humans see variation in the balance of TH1 and TH2 cytokines.[32,33] Pregnancy is one such immunological change, where there is a shift toward TH2 dominance, which is very important to maintain pregnancy. In early pregnancy, following changes occur:[34,35]
    - Rising levels of progesterone
    - Increased secretion of TH2 cytokines such as IL-4 and -6
    - Decreased secretion of TH1 cytokines such as IL-2, -12, and interferon-γ
    - Even the embryo directly contributes to TH2 dominance by secreting IL-10 and transforming growth factor beta (TGF-β).

Several studies report association between loss of TH2 dominance and poor pregnancy outcomes such as an embryonic gestation and recurrent pregnancy loss (RPL). Whether this association is the cause or effect is not clearly understood.[34,35]

- *NK cells:* NK cells and their role in RIF are among the most debated and poorly understood topics. There are two types of NK cells, peripheral (pbNK) and uterine (uNK). pbNK and uNK are two different immune cells with different immunologic properties. pbNK cells are the first line of defense against tumor cells, viruses, and they are cytotoxic in nature. uNK cells are less cytotoxic in nature, unless they are posed with viruses such as cytomegalovirus (CMV). As previously misunderstood, they are not educated to reject or kill healthy embryos. There are conflicting evidences regarding association between NK cell parameters and pregnancy outcome.[36-39]

A systematic review and meta-analysis on pbNK and uNK, including 12 studies, failed to show any association between pbNK cell number or activity or uNK cell density and pregnancy outcome.[40] Hence, it is not just enough to know about quantity and activity of NK cells, it is important to understand the interaction between the maternal killer immunoglobulin-like receptors (KIRs), expressed on uNK, and their ligand human leukocyte antigen C (HLA-C), expressed by the extravillous trophoblast as shown in **Figure 2**. Various studies have proposed that this NK cell allorecognition mediates placentation process.[41,42] Accruing evidence suggests an important role of uNK KIR and HLA-C interaction in both normal and abnormal placentation. Further research should focus on determining the combination of maternal KIR haplotype and parental/donor HLA-C, which could segregate the benefits of single embryo transfer (SET) versus double embryo transfer (DET) or from donor selection according to HLA-C. This may increase the live birth rate (LBR) per cycle, which in turn would help to reduce the number of embryos transferred by promoting the increase in elective SET.[43]

Placentation is regulated by interactions between maternal KIRs, expressed by uNKs cells, and fetal HLA-C molecules, expressed by extravillous trophoblasts. Maternal and paternal HLA-C (HLA-Cm and HLA-Cp, respectively) are nonself (*foreign*).

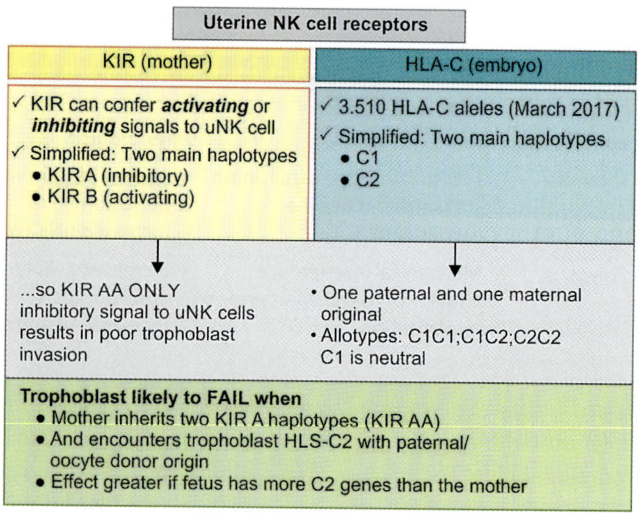

Fig. 2: Killer immunoglobulin-like receptor (KIR): human leukocyte antigen C (HLA-C) system.

(HLS: Human leukocyte system; NK: natural killer; uNK: uterine natural killer)

Source: Reproduced with permission from Alecsandru and García-Velasco (2017).[43]

- *Autoantibodies:* Another aspect of the immune system altering ER is related to autoimmunity. To understand this aspect, three meta-analyses will be highlighted here. In 2000, meta-analysis by Hornstein et al., analyzing, seven studies failed to show any difference in clinical pregnancy rate (CPR) or LBR in women undergoing IVF with or without antiphospholipid antibodies (APAs).[44] In 2008, the committee opinion of the American Society for Reproductive Medicine (ASRM) concluded that there is no statistically significant impact of the presence of APAs on IVF outcomes, after reviewing 12 studies with >2,000 patients in total.[45]

One more recent meta-analysis in 2011, involving 29 studies of >5,000 patients, concluded that the presence of one or more APAs was associated with increased risk of assisted reproductive technology (ART) failure. Further subgroup analyses showed that presence of lupus anticoagulant and antibodies antiphosphatidylserine, antiphosphatidylinositol, antiphosphatidic acid, and antiphosphatidylglycerol were more often present in women with ART failure and anticardiolipin antibodies, anti-β2 glycoprotein I antibodies, and antiphosphatidylethanolamine were less often associated with ART failure. However, the overall methodologic quality was poor due to inappropriate control group selection.[46]

At present, the association between autoantibodies and ART failure remains inconclusive, due to practical challenges faced in determining a more definitive answer. With an assumed 16% prevalence APAs, to prove the difference of 20% with 80% power in a cohort study, it is estimated that 1,300 patients with APAs and 8,200 controls would have to be enrolled.[46] At present, ASRM advises against the routine assessment of APAs in ART.[45]

Receptivity versus Selectivity

Recent studies have challenged the term endometrial "receptivity" as it denotes a more passive function of the endometrium. Decidual function is not only related to this passive act of receptivity but also has a more active role in biosensor function of selectivity, which has a key role in directing the maternal response to the implanting embryo. This biosensor function of the decidua is very important, when it comes to selection of the human embryos (unlike embryos of other species), which are characterized by their high rate of chromosomal abnormalities, the implantation of which can result in futile investment of maternal resources on these invasive but poorly viable embryos.[47] Impaired endometrial selectivity would result in superfertility but at the cost of recurrent early pregnancy loss. Conversely, an excessive biosensor function of the decidua would make the endometrium more choosy, decreasing recurrent miscarriage, but increases the likelihood of implantation delay or RIF[47] **(Fig. 3)**.

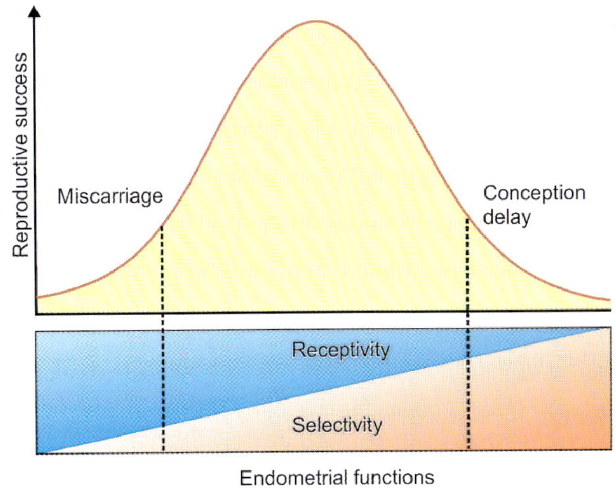

Fig. 3: Endometrial receptivity versus selectivity. Excessive receptivity and poor selectivity result in recurrent miscarriage and vice-versa result in recurrent implantation failure (RIF).
Source: Reproduced with permission from Macklon and Brosens (2014).[47]

Endometrial Microbiota

It was assumed that the uterus is sterile, and this was based on vaginal samples. *Lactobacillus* species is the predominant microbiome in the vagina;[48] however, this could vary according to the age and hormonal milieu.[49] Before puberty, vaginal flora is a mixture of both anaerobic and aerobic bacteria, while after puberty, vagina is predominantly colonized by *Lactobacillus* species, which is due to acidic environment created by rising glycogen.[50] Moreno et al. have analyzed the vaginal and endometrial microbiota in healthy nonpregnant women using next-generation sequencing (NGS) of the 16S ribosomal RNA (rRNA) gene and have identified bacterial communities in all the endometrial samples analyzed. *Lactobacillus* is the predominant microbiome, followed by *Gardnerella*, *Prevotella*, *Atopobium*, and *Sneathia*.[51] Study by the same group analyzed the endometrial fluid from 35 women with RIF and correlated between endometrial microbiome profiles with reproductive outcome. They found that non-*Lactobacillus* dominated microbiota correlated with adverse reproductive outcome such as failure of implantation and miscarriage.

Multifactorial Effectors

Multifactorial effectors include endometriosis, PCOS, and hydrosalpinx. The mechanism by which they cause implantation failure is summarized in **Table 2**.

INVESTIGATIONS

Recurrent implantation failure is not a diagnosis but a mere clinical presentation, which requires appropriate phenotyping and etiological investigations. We have various

TABLE 2: Mechanism of disrupted implantation in multifactorial effectors.

Pathology	*Anatomical*	*Physiological*	*Molecular*
Endometriosis	Impaired fertilization[26]	Altered folliculogenesis Poor oocyte quality[52]	• Reduced αvβ3 - integrin and LIF expressions in the window of implantation • Lack of IL-11 and IL-11Rα expressions in secretory phase • Absence of HOXA10 and HOXA11 peak in secretory phase • Elevated EMX2 expression • Progesterone resistance • Alteration in PR-A to PR-B ratio • Decreased HOXA10 expression due to hypermethylation of its promoter region[26]
PCOS		• Altered folliculogenesis • Defective ovulation • Inadequate progesterone action • Excessive androgen/ insulin action • Poor oocyte quality[26]	• Decreased αvβ3 - integrin, HOXA10 and IGFBP-1 during secretory phase • Overexpression of androgen receptors • Failure to downregulate estrogen receptor-α in the window of implantation • Overexpression of the steroid receptor coactivators such as nuclear receptor coactivator and transcriptional intermediary factor 2 (TIF2)[26]
Hydrosalpinx	Intermittent bathing of endometrial lining with hydrosalpinx fluid causing mechanical interference to apposition	Embryotoxic effect of the inflammatory hydrosalpinx fluid	• Reduced αvβ3 - integrin and LIF expressions • Decreased HOXA10 expression[26]

(IGFBP-1: insulin-like growth factor-binding protein 1; IL: interleukin; PCOS: polycystic ovary syndrome; PR: progesterone receptor)

Flowchart 1: Investigations in recurrent implantation failure (RIF).

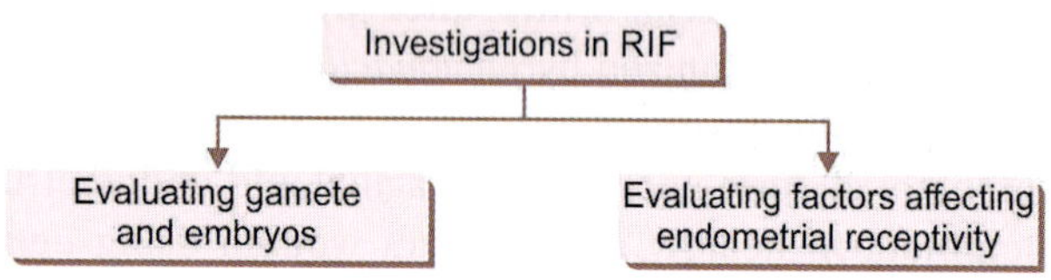

tools to detect the cause of RIF, whether it is at the level of embryo, endometrium, or it is multifactorial, as depicted in **Flowchart 1**.

Evaluating Gamete and Embryo Factors

Evaluating the Oocyte

Assessment of oocyte quantity and quality is through ovarian function tests. Women with RIF should be offered basal FSH, AFC, and AMH to diagnose extremes of ovarian reserve, which is associated with poor oocyte quality.

Assessment of Sperm DNA Damage

Evidence on association between sperm DNA damage with implantation failure or pregnancy failure is conflicting. Initial studies have shown that DNA fragmentation index (DFI) value of >27% is associated with pregnancy failure in ART,[53,54] although in later studies, the predictive value of this test is questioned.[55,56] A meta-analysis in 2015, evaluating the relationship between the extent of sperm DNA damage and LBR per couple and the influence of the method of fertilization on treatment outcome showed that high sperm DNA fragmentation in couples undergoing ART is associated with lower LBR; however, further sensitivity analysis showed no statistically significant difference in LBR between low and high sperm DNA fragmentation when ICSI was used.[57] At present, DFI should be offered to couple with RIF as a part of research program. Methods to assess sperm DNA damage are depicted in **Flowchart 2**.

Parental Karyotyping

The incidence of chromosomal abnormalities in couples with RIF is approximately 2.5%, which is still higher compared to the general population.[58] This higher incidence suggests that the karyotyping testing should be considered in couple with RIF.

Evaluating the Embryo

Evaluation of the embryo has been characterized in **Flowchart 3 and Table 3**.

Evaluation of Factors Affecting Endometrial Receptivity

Uterine Factors

Women with RIF should be investigated for uterine pathology (congenital/acquired), which can be a contributing cause for RIF.

Flowchart 2: Methods to assess DNA sperm damage.

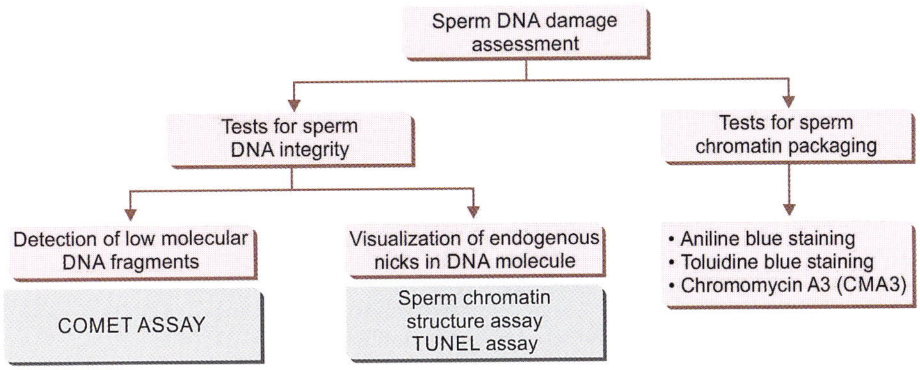

(TUNEL: terminal deoxynucleotidyl transferase dUTP nick end labeling)

Flowchart 3: Evaluation of the embryo.

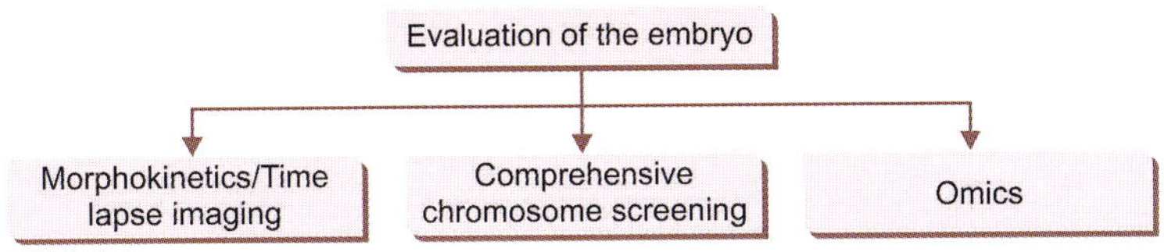

TABLE 3: Evaluation of the embryo.

Method	*Principle*	*Advantage*	*Disadvantage*	*Evidence*
Morphokinetics/ time-lapse imaging	• Analysis of embryo morphology and information about the dynamic changes in the embryo during peri-implantation period • Several studies have correlated time lapse with probability of selecting chromosomally normal embryos[59-61]	• No removal of the embryo from the incubator for evaluation, providing better culture environment • Better understanding of the poorly described concepts of embryology, such as duration of first three cell cycles[62]	• As with manual embryo morphology grading, inter- and intraobserver variability may impact time-lapse interpretation[63] • The risk of rejecting "viable embryos" based on suboptimal morphokinetic score[64]	• Can time-lapse parameters predict embryo ploidy? • A systematic review—2018 • No definitive conclusions can be drawn on the predictive value of morphokinetic evaluation for embryo aneuploidy • Time-lapse imaging cannot be used as a surrogate for preimplantation genetic screening (PGS)[65]
Comprehensive chromosome screening (CCS)	• Embryos with chromosomal abnormalities have lower implantation potential • PGS is used as a strategy to select normal embryos having higher implantation potential for transfer, thus eliminating embryos with low implantation potential from the cohort	• In poor prognosis patients such as advanced maternal age, RIF, genetic testing of the preimplantation embryo allows for selection • of chromosomally competent embryo, thus increasing the chance of conception[66-68]	• Mosaicism is an important variable to consider, especially when consistency in diagnosis has to be established[69] • Various studies have shown the frequency of mosaicism can be as low as 15.7% and as high as 32.4%[70-72] • Despite the efficacy and accuracy of CCS various studies have questioned its validity[73,74] • It is clear that not all euploid blastocysts will implant, suggesting that additional factors also determine the reproductive potential of an embryo such as "omics"	• CCS improves embryo selection: A meta-analysis (2015) • Three RCTs and eight observational studies included • PGS improves clinical implantation rates (IR) and sustained IR (beyond 20 weeks) particularly in patients with normal ovarian reserve • Results from ongoing RCTs conducted on different patient population are awaited

Contd...

Contd...

Method	Principle	Advantage	Disadvantage	Evidence
Omics	Analysis of "biomarkers" refers to measurement of proteins and metabolites that are associated pregnancy outcome, either positively or negatively	• Viability (ability of an embryo to implant and give rise to a healthy baby) is not just dependent on chromosome complement but with other factors such as inherent developmental potential • Embryo morphology does not alone suffice for assessment of embryo viability because morphology does not necessarily reflect physiology	• High cost involved • Very minimal sample available for analysis which affects the accuracy and sensitivity of the test • Biomarker levels are affected by various factors such as embryonic stage of development, sex of the embryo, medium composition, medium renewal frequency, • rate of ammonium accumulation, oxygen concentration, and stress[75]	Various studies have demonstrated that morphokinetics and omics are complementary approaches for the assessment of embryo viability[76-78]

(RCT: randomized controlled trial; RIF: recurrent implantation failure)

Diagnostic Modalities for Uterine Abnormalities

Hysteroscopy and laparoscopy, sonohysterography (SHG), and three-dimensional (3D) US are the most precise investigations and can be utilized as diagnostic tools. 3D-US offers the benefit of being noninvasive. SHG necessitates the introduction of fluid into the uterine cavity and this can usually be uncomfortable. Hysteroscopy and laparoscopy are both invasive procedures; however, they offer the advantage of simultaneous diagnosis and treatment. Hysteroscopy alone can identify the existence of an anomaly but cannot precisely differentiate between the different subtypes.

Two-dimensional US is the least accurate method of investigation; however, it is the most widely available and the easiest to perform. If used in combination with hysterosalpingogram (HSG), it can increase precision and aid as a valuable screening tool, especially in the absence of 3D-US, or where SHG is not practiced. Magnetic resonance imaging (MRI) seems to be more accurate than 2D-US or HSG alone, and could potentially be used for screening. However, its diagnostic accuracy remains unclear. Disadvantages are that it is more expensive than US and HSG, and is not available in the office setting.

Investigating Immunological and Thrombophilic Conditions in Implantation Failure

- *Testing TH1 and TH2 balance/imbalance:* As discussed previously, pregnancy is associated with TH2 dominance. Various studies have demonstrated an association between loss of TH2 dominance and poor pregnancy outcome.[34,35] There are several challenges to advise tests to measure TH1/TH2 balance as a routine in cases with RIF because of following reasons:
    - It is not known whether aberrations in the transition of TH2 dominance in poor pregnancy outcome is the cause or the effect.
    - In the peri-implantation interval, in fact, it is normal for a TH1 dominance.

  Therefore, no screening tests can be done in advance to predict TH1/TH2 imbalance in a future gestation.[31]
- *Testing of NK cells:* Disturbed population of uNK and/or pbNK cells has been suggested as one of the causes for implantation failure. NK cells can kill some cell lines in vitro but not decisively; but this terminology is often misleading, as it seems that these cells could harm or kill the embryos and thus associated with implantation failure.[79] A systematic review and meta-analysis failed to show any association between pbNK cell number or activity or uNK cell density and pregnancy outcome.[40] At present, routine testing of NK cell in women with RIF is not advised as there is no clear evidence of use and the potential adverse effect and cost of this therapy outweigh any benefits.[79]
- *Testing of autoantibodies:* Association between APAs and ART remains controversial. The ASRM currently recommends against the routine determination of APAs among couples undergoing ART.[45] However, there is some evidence to suggest that it is reasonable to test for thrombophilia in patients with RIF and consider treatment if a thrombophilic disorder is identified.[31]

Testing for Endometrial Receptivity

The end result is not always pregnancy, when a morphologically and/or chromosomally normal embryo is replaced into the uterus which is seemingly normal. It is the

TABLE 4: Various methods of assessing endometrial receptivity (ER).

Method	*Advantage*	*Disadvantage*
Histologic evaluation	In 1950s, in the absence of any objective means of assessing ER, Noyes criteria was widely used, but now it is obsolete	Its accuracy, reproducibility, and functional relevance as a predictor of ER has been questioned[80]
Transvaginal ultrasound	• When there are no structural abnormalities and the endometrium is thick enough with trilaminar pattern, ER is assumed • Low cost, high resolution, lack of radiation exposure, and widely used	Not sufficient to predict endometrial normalcy and implantation[81]
Hysteroscopy	• Gold standard for the diagnosis of intrauterine pathology • Minimally invasive procedure • Diagnostic as well as therapeutic at the same sitting	Not enough as it not informative about ER[82]
Transcriptomics	• For complex and multifactorial traits such as RIF and endometrial factor evaluation, genomic medicine provides a deeper understanding of diseases based on massive amounts of data generated by genomic technologies • Allows to practice more precise medicine	• Large variation in genes identified in different • studies • Variable expression of the genes • Differences in gene expression at RNA levels is not always reflected at protein levels • It is not the genes but the gene products that determine the phenotype

(RIF: recurrent implantation failure)

Flowchart 4: Transcriptomics in the assessment of pathology of endometrial receptivity.

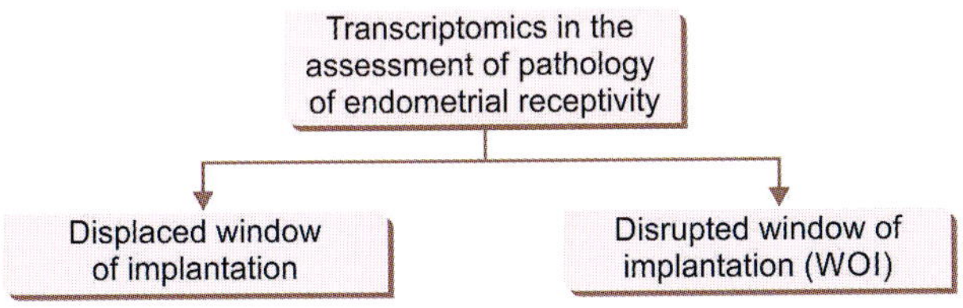

collaboration between the embryo and the endometrium, which decides success or failure. This is further dependent on the functionality and synchronization of both the partners, thus emphasizing that the embryo alone is not sufficient for successful implantation. All these point to the presence of endometrial pathology in some patients with RIF who produce seemingly normal embryos both morphologically and chromosomally. In recent years, there is a surge in interest in evaluating the role of endometrium in implantation and also the dysfunctions of endometrium that may underlie implantation failure **(Table 4 and Flowchart 4)**.

Transcriptomics to assess displaced WOI: In 1956, Hertig and Rock for the first time suggested the concept of ER and WOI.[83] Several studies following this have clearly demonstrated that the endometrium becomes receptive during 8–10 days post ovulation, with the same success during these 3 days regardless of whether it is a natural, stimulated, or hormone replacement cycle.[84-86] Díaz-Gimeno et al. (2011)[87] identified the transcriptomic signature of ER composed of 238 genes leading to the creation of the endometrial receptivity analysis (ERA). The ERA is a customized microarray now performed by NGS, coupled with a computational predictor, which enables to identify the receptivity of the endometrial sample, i.e., whether the endometrium is within the time frame of WOI or not, thus providing personalized WOI (pWOI) of a given patient facilitating personalized embryo transfer (pET). A biopsy of the endometrial tissue is taken at days luteinizing hormone (LH) +7 in the natural cycle and progesterone +5 in hormone replacement therapy (HRT) cycle. A state of nonreceptivity contemplates that the WOI is displaced. In this case, the process will be repeated according to data from the ERA predictor, which will give a new calculation of WOI (pWOI), which is depicted in **Flowchart 5**. Before beginning an ART treatment, performing an ERA can identify if the patient will need a pWOI and this could aid the clinical examination in modifying the timing of embryo transfer especially in cases of RIF. The ERA test is not sensitive to minor gene expression variations that might occur during normal reproductive life or to the effects of variability in experimental batches.

Transcriptomics to assess disrupted WOI: Endometrial gene expression has been shown to be sensitive to cyclical hormonal variation and exogenous hormone therapy.[88-91] But numerous studies have demonstrated that various factors can affect endometrial gene transcription, such as presence of endometriosis[92] and use of intrauterine device.[93] Hence, it is logical to think that although displaced WOI may be the cause in some RIF[94] patients, it may also originate as an effect of other causes and that these may include constitutive disruptions of endometrial function. The potential value of identifying a gene expression profile predictive of RIF is considerable because this would not only guide prognosis, but also could inform appropriate and effective therapeutic intervention. With regard to this hypothesis, study by Koot et al.[95] determined the transcriptomic differences between RIF patients and control subjects and demonstrated that RIF

Flowchart 5: Personalized embryo transfer (pET).

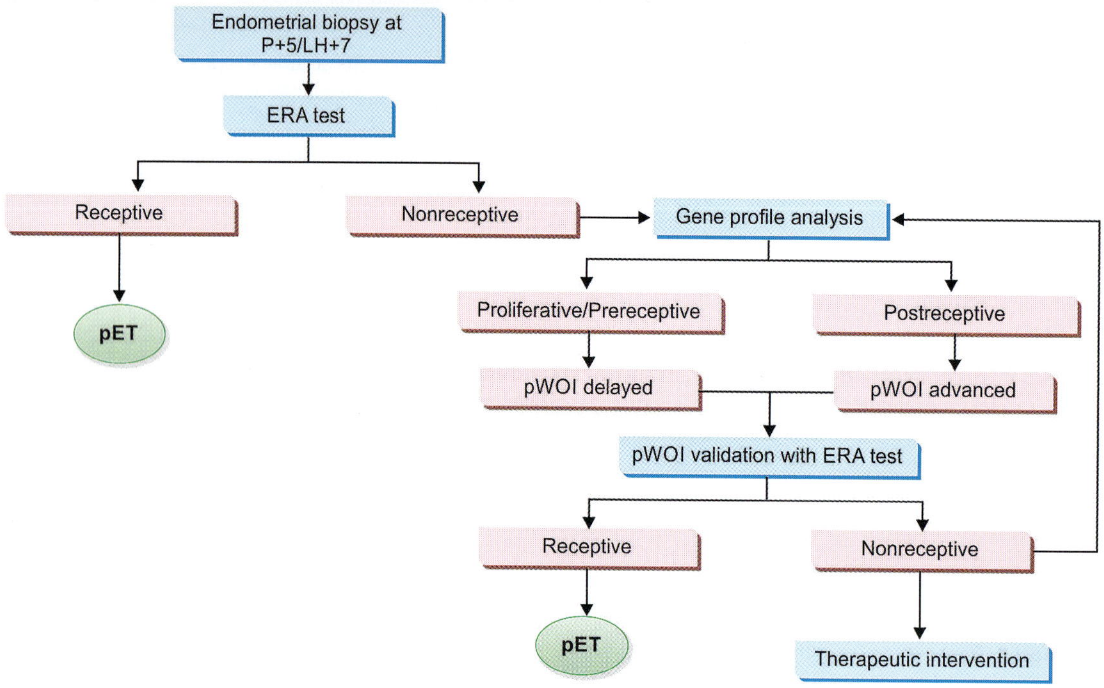

(ERA: endometrial receptivity analysis; LH: luteinizing hormone; P: progesterone; pWOI: personalized window of implantation)

may represent a pathology with a particular transcriptomic signature. Furthermore, Sebastian-Leon et al.[96] by analyzing 16 transcriptomic signatures have clearly predicted two causes of RIF: (1) a displaced WOI and (2) an on time but pathologically disrupted WOI.

Assessing endometrial microbiota: Although there are various studies regarding vaginal microbiome, there are only recent data supporting the presence of an indigenous endometrial microbiome. The endometrial cavity has long been considered to be sterile, but reports challenging this tenet support the existence of an endometrial microbiome comprising different microorganisms (specifically *Lactobacillus* spp., *Mycoplasma hominis*, *Gardnerella vaginalis*, and *Enterobacter* spp.) that affect reproductive outcomes.[97] Detection of bacteria with molecular techniques has enabled the study of low biomass microbiomes in tissues and organs. Subsequently, an abnormal endometrial microbiota has been associated with implantation failure, pregnancy loss, and other gynecological and obstetrical conditions. Further research on the reproductive tract microbiome will allow for a better realization of bacterial communities, role in physiology as well as pathophysiology, which in turn affects the ability to achieve pregnancy and maintain a healthy pregnancy.[98]

Hydrosalpinges: Hydrosalpinges as cause for RIF should be excluded, regardless of the initial infertility diagnosis. US does not always pick up hydrosalpinges; hence, HSG is preferred. Laparoscopy should be advised in women in whom HSG is inconclusive, to refute or confirm diagnosis.[11]

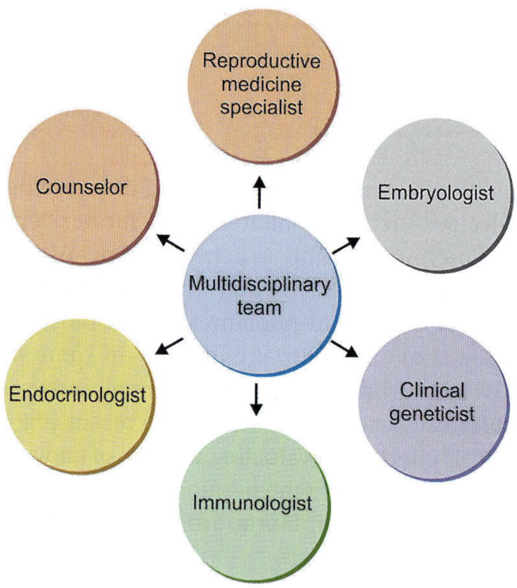

Fig. 4: Multidisciplinary team: Reproductive medicine specialist, embryologist, counselor, clinical geneticist, immunologist, and endocrinologist.

MANAGEMENT

Multidisciplinary Approach

The role of a multidisciplinary team in the management of RIF cannot be overemphasized. The multidisciplinary team should comprise reproductive medicine specialist, embryologist, counselor, clinical geneticist, immunologist, and endocrinologist **(Fig. 4)**. Couples with RIF should be

Flowchart 6: Management of recurrent implantation failure (RIF).

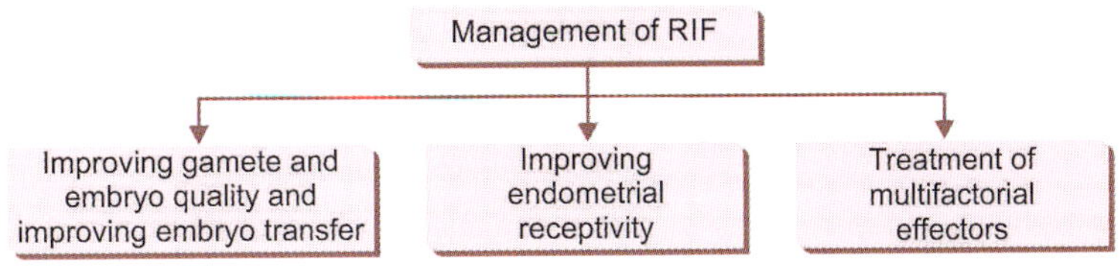

evaluated by this team. There should be a local protocol agreed upon by this team as to how to investigate these couples with RIF, which is based on robust evidence. During evaluation, the team should review all the details of the case that include cause of infertility, investigations done so far, treatment protocol adopted, response to ovarian stimulation, quality of oocytes and sperms, fertilization, cleavage, embryo quality, and any difficulties in embryo transfer. This consultation with the multidisciplinary team is "special" and should not be like any other routine outpatient consultation. The couple should be given ample time to discuss their problems and issues and the team should be empathetic with them. It is very important to explain in detail to the couple about the underlying cause of infertility, and also a possible explanation about why IVF did not work for them despite repeated attempts. Couple should also be explained about further plans of action and the scientific rationale behind this plan. It is very important to assess and explain the likelihood of success with further investigation and treatment. If likelihood of success is very low, they should be explained about alternative options including gamete donation, gestational surrogacy, or even adoption.

Recurrent implantation failure is a source of distress and dissatisfaction for both patients and clinicians. It is not uncommon to have the feeling of disgust with repeated failures. At times, it becomes very difficult to explain as to how the transfer of a euploid blastocyst failed to implant in a seemingly normal endometrium. In this situation, the clinicians can become illogical and begin to search for, and apply, unproven investigations and treatments based on just scientific hypotheses and anecdotal reports, with lack of robust evidence. At the same time, couples with RIF are such a vulnerable population that they are ready to do anything to achieve a pregnancy. Hence, it is very important to have this multidisciplinary approach, which can provide dedicated care and evidence-based treatment. In case such an evidence base is lacking, the patients should be counseled accordingly and, if the occasion arises, they might be invited to participate in a carefully designed clinical trial. They should not be exploited.

The role of a counselor is very crucial at this point of time. A counselor should help the couple to express their emotions, to identify the specific cause of stress, to enable coping strategies, and to facilitate decision making.

Before embarking on new investigation and treatment strategies, it should be emphasized about lifestyle modifications, which include maintaining a healthy body mass index (BMI), to quit smoking and alcohol. These lifestyle changes have shown to improve the probability of success to treatment **(Flowchart 6)**.[99-102]

Improving Gamete and Embryo Quality and Embryo Transfer

Treatment of Poor Oocyte Quality

In some patients, RIF might be because of compromised oocyte quality and this could be because of inherent problems in the oocyte quality or because of suboptimal ovarian stimulation, which is amenable for correction. As discussed previously, ovarian stimulation protocol must be reviewed as a part of RIF workup, and if previous ovarian stimulation is suboptimal in terms of number of oocytes obtained as compared to ovarian reserve, gonadotropin dosage can be increased. No particular protocol is superior to the other in this situation; however, few studies have suggested addition of LH is beneficial in hypo-responders and also in women older than 35 years.[103] In women with endometriosis, ultralong protocol with use of depot gonadotropin-releasing hormone agonists (GnRHa) 3–6 months prior to controlled ovarian stimulation is proven to increase pregnancy rate.[104] Cytoplasmic transfer as a method to improve oocyte competence has been demonstrated to be beneficial in a few studies,[105,106] but currently it is considered experimental.

Treatment of High DNA Fragmentation

Table 5 depicts the treatment of high DNA fragmentation.

Treatment of Poor Embryo Quality

Blastocyst transfer: Blastocyst transfer is superior to cleavage-stage embryos. Human embryos enter the uterine cavity 5 days after fertilization; hence, it is more physiological to transfer embryo at blastocyst stage. Although initial studies showed evidence in favor of blastocyst transfer,[112,113] meta-analysis by Glujovsky et al. (2016), which included 27 randomized controlled trials (RCTs) with 4,031 couples, concluded that blastocyst transfer is better than cleavage-stage embryo transfer; however, for LBR and CPR, the quality of evidence is low and moderate, respectively.[114]

TABLE 5: Methods to improve sperm quality.

Method	*Rationale*	*Evidence*
Oral antioxidants	Reduces oxidative stress on sperm	• Meta-analysis of 48 RCTs with a population of 4,179 subfertile men • Conclusion: Antioxidants could be considered for subfertile men; however, evidence is inconclusive[107]
Use of annexin-V columns and hyaluronic acid (HA) binding	Reduces the number of sperms with increased DNA fragmentation index (DFI)	• HA sperm selection method will likely reduce the potential genetic complications and adverse public health effects of intracytoplasmic sperm injection (ICSI)[108] • The selection of nonapoptotic sperm by magnetic cell sorting (MACS) may be used to enhance results of in vitro fertilization by increasing sperm–oocyte penetration[109]
Intracytoplasmic morphologically selected sperm injection (IMSI)	Morphologically selected sperms may improve reproductive outcome	Further trials are necessary to improve the quality of the evidence before recommending IMSI in clinical practice[110]
Testicular sperm retrieval (TSR)	Sperm DNA damage is lower in the seminiferous tubules as compared with the cauda epididymis and ejaculated spermatozoa	The use of TSR–ICSI in the absence of specific sperm DNA defects is still experimental[111]

(RCT: randomized controlled trial)

Assisted hatching (AH): Three possible mechanisms how AH could aid implantation:

- Procedures such as IVF, cell culture,[115] or cryopreservation[116] can cause hardening of zona, which could make hatching difficult and this issue can be solved with hatching.
- Women going through controlled ovarian stimulation with gonadotropins have prematurely displaced WOI,[117] this situation can be helped with AH, which causes anticipation of implantation.[118]
- For exchange of metabolites, growth factors, opening created through AH can serve as a channel.[119]

Three meta-analyses on AH have found a significant increase in CPR, but no difference in LBR. Martins et al. (2011) found a significant difference in CPR in frozen–thawed embryos in unselected women and also in women with repeated IVF failure. Limitation of this meta-analysis was that there were too few studies looking at LBR.[120] Cochrane review by Carney et al. (2012) analyzed 31 RCTs including 1,992 clinical pregnancies in 5,728 women, concluded that CPR was significantly higher following AH, just reaching statistical significance, but there was no effect on the "take-home baby rate."[121] Li et al. (2016) looked at 36 RCTs with 6,459 women and found that AH gave a significant increase in CPR and multiple pregnancy rate, but in the 15 RCTs that looked at LBR, there was no evidence of difference between the AH and control groups.[122]

Co-culture: Scientific hypothesis behind using co-culture include secretion of embryotrophic factors such as nutrients, growth factors, and cytokines and detoxification of free radicals.[123] Spandorfer et al. studied autologous endometrial co-culture in 1,030 patients with RIF and reported 49% pregnancy rate.[124]

Preimplantation genetic screening (PGS): In 1990s, thousands of IVFs were performed after biopsying a single blastomere from day 3 cleavage-stage embryo and analyzing the normalcy of five chromosomes through fluorescent in situ hybridization (FISH). Later on, RCTs showed that PGS did not increase CPR or LBR and in some cases decreased LBR.[125,126] It is due to following reasons that PGS with day 3 embryo may not be effective:

- Limited accuracy of FISH
- Limited number of cells available for analysis
- Day 3 embryos are at a peak of chromosomal abnormality and mosaicism.

With the advent of new technologies, comprehensive chromosome screening (CCS) is possible on day 5 embryos after biopsying trophectoderm cells. With this, there is a scientific hypothesis that CCS can increase implantation rates, decrease time to pregnancy, and decrease RPL and RIF. Three RCTs on this topic have been criticized because of poor study design. The pilot RCT by Yang et al. (2012) included a small sample size of 45 young good prognosis patients.[127] RCT by Scott et al. (2013) was on 72 good prognosis patients between 21 and 42 years, but the randomization was quite late and also the study failed to account for the difference between the unit of randomization (patients) and unit of analysis (embryos).[128] RCT by Forman et al. (2013) studied 89 women comparing PGS and SET, but the same methodological flaws were noted in this study and also a wide confidence interval for pregnancy did not demonstrate a beneficial effect.[129] Currently, two large RCTs are underway and the results are expected soon. The ESTEEM study (The Eshre Study into The Evaluation of Oocyte Euploidy by Microarray Analysis) recruits patients of advanced maternal age and involves analysis of polar bodies using array comparative genomic hybridization (CGH). The ESTEEM study has an intention to treat analysis and the outcome analysis will be of cumulative LBR. The other study is the STAR (Single Embryo TrAnsfeR of Euploid Embryo) study, which recruits all IVF patients and uses NGS on trophectoderm biopsies. The outcome analysis of STAR study is on ongoing pregnancy rate after one transfer. The results of these studies are much awaited to provide evidence of its use in various scenarios including RIF.

Mitochondrial DNA load measurement (mitoscore): It has been assessed that metaphase II oocytes contain ~10^5 mitochondrial DNA (mtDNA) copies, and it is these copies which get divided over the cleaving cells as replication of mtDNA does not occur up to blastocyst stage.[130] There are studies[131,132] reporting correlation between higher mtDNA level in blastocysts and lower implantation potential and this could be because of disturbed energy provision and higher metabolic stress in embryos with a higher mitoscore. Currently, there are no studies demonstrating lower mitoscore association with improved LBR; hence, it can only be recommended under research settings.

Time-lapse imaging and metabolomics: As mentioned previously, time-lapse imaging cannot be used as a surrogate for PGS[65] and various studies have demonstrated that morphokinetics and omics are complementary approaches for the assessment of embryo viability.[76-78]

Improving Embryo Transfer

Ultrasound-guided Embryo Transfer

Transabdominal ultrasound (TA-US)-guided embryo transfer technique is the one that is extensively studied, but its use to improve pregnancy rates has been debated.[133-136] This continuing debate could be because of bias involved in these systematic review and meta-analysis such as inclusion of meeting abstracts and observational or retrospective studies in data analysis. Moreover, the newer techniques such as transvaginal ultrasound (TV-US) guidance for embryo transfer, 3D-US, and uterine length measurement before embryo transfer (ULMbET) have not been studied. Systematic review and meta-analysis by Cozzolino et al. (2018) have addressed these issues and have concluded that there is moderate evidence to suggest TA-US embryo transfer over clinical touch in improving CPR, ongoing and LBR. No difference was found in CPR, ongoing and LBR between TV-US and TA-US. Larger RCTs are necessary to explore the possible benefits of TV-US, 3D-US, and ULMbET. Mature limitations of this analysis are: It provides only weak evidence about the ectopic pregnancy and miscarriage rates, potentially underestimating the possible beneficial effects of US application. Wide range of publication date from 1989 to 2013, and also the literature focus is mostly on day 2–3 embryo transfers, making the applicability of the results to day 5 transfers difficult.[137]

Embryo Glue and Adherence Compounds

The use of fibrin sealants to improve LBR and decrease ectopic pregnancy[138,139] was proposed in 1990s, but did not show significant improvement in clinical outcome. It is well reported that hyaluronic acid (HA) is naturally present in the female reproductive tract, and forms a viscous solution that could aid in implantation. Hence, recent studies have focused on the use of a specific embryo transfer medium enriched with HA. Cochrane review by Bontekoe et al. included 17 RCTs with 3,898 participants, demonstrating moderate-quality evidence for an improvement in CPR and LBR and an associated increase in multiple pregnancy rate.[140] RCT by Fancsovits et al. (2015) analyzed 581 cycles and did not show a benefit in implantation rate, CPR, or LBR, but found a higher birth weight in HA group.[141] In the presence of conflicting evidence, it is imperative to conduct further RCTs to evaluate the efficacy of HA as an adherence compound during embryo transfer.

Sequential Embryo Transfer

The rationale behind this strategy is to overcome the problem of embryo-endometrium asynchronicity as a potential cause of implantation failure. The possible disadvantage of this strategy is that the second insertion of the catheter can cause trauma to the endometrium or stimulate the secretion of prostaglandins, which could initiate uterine contractions. It could also cause additional microbial contamination and introduce more mucus into the uterine cavity thus affecting implantation. The possible advantage of sequential embryo transfer is that this interval embryo transfer could affect the endometrial cavity in a positive manner by inducing factors that enhance implantation. DET which happens with sequential embryo transfer can be beneficial in women with RIF. There are conflicting evidences with regard to sequential embryo transfers where a few studies support its use[142,143] and others do not.[144,145] Even though there appear preliminary evidence in favor of DET, further RCTs are required to confirm its use in women with RIF.

Freeze-all Strategy

A freeze-all strategy is a recently established methodology in which cryopreservation of all embryos after a conventional ICSI cycle is performed followed by successive fresh embryo transfer (FET) in expectations of refining the rate of implantation.[146] Currently, freeze-all strategy is adopted in hyper-responders, agonist trigger, along with PGS, etc.[147]

Magdi et al.[148] introduced RIF with FET as another indication for freeze-all strategy. It appears very likely that patients with repeated failed fresh transfers are a selected subgroup with significantly increased risk of impaired ER following ovarian stimulation, among other issues. In this study, 38.4% of patients in the freeze-all group attained ongoing pregnancy as did 20.7% of patients in the fresh transfer group. This difference was statistically significant. Assessments of secondary measures found significant differences in pregnancy rate, implantation rate, and CPR, all supporting the freeze-all group, but no significant difference in the rate of early pregnancy loss. The rate of multiple pregnancy in the freeze-all group was significantly higher than in the fresh group, indicating that, in regular clinical practice, the number of embryos transferred should be decreased in order to compensate for the higher implantation rate (40.0 vs. 16.0%) with thawed embryos than with fresh embryos in these patients.

Another strong indication for freeze-all strategy in RIF patients is when the embryos have been subjected to PGS. The fresh blastocyst transfer approach after PGS necessitates not only availability of expanded blastocysts on the morning of day 5, but also one of these being euploid, necessitating embryo transfer. Contrary to this, in freeze-all strategy, both day 5 and day 6 embryos can be biopsied, and the whole cohort of embryos can be cryopreserved, enabling patients to have their embryo transfer at a later date. Study by Kahraman[149] at Istanbul Hospital, Turkey, analyzed a total of 1,486 cycles and found that all positive outcomes, implantation, ongoing pregnancy rate, and LBR were significantly higher in the freeze-all group. In cases with advanced maternal age (38–43 years), ongoing pregnancy rate and LBR were significantly higher in the freeze-all group and this is possibly related to ER, as it is probable that in older women, the quiet endometrium is more crucial. Furthermore, it decreases the pressure in embryology laboratory as it permits more plasticity regarding the scheduling of embryo biopsy and also having the biopsy results of the whole cohort, at the same time permits inclusion of all blastocysts.

Zygote Intrafallopian Transfer

Human tubal fluid contains several growth factors and cytokines, which aid in the development of the embryo making it competent for implantation. This scientific hypothesis drives the rationale of following zygote intrafallopian transfer (ZIFT) technique in patients with RIF. However, meta-analysis by Habana and Palter[150] has reported similar pregnancy and implantation rates in ZIFT and intrauterine transfer groups (36.5 vs. 31.4% and 15 vs. 12%, respectively). At present, with improved culture conditions in ART, intrauterine transfer remains the technique of choice in women with RIF.

Improving Endometrial Receptivity

Treatment of Uterine Abnormalities

Treatment of factors affecting ER has been represented in **Table 6**.

TABLE 6: Treatment of uterine abnormalities—congenital and acquired.

Uterine abnormality	*Intervention*	*Rationale*	*Evidence*
Uterine septum	Operative hysteroscopy (HSC) and septal resection	• Increases implantation rate • Decreases MR • Increases term delivery rates	• Tomaževič et al. (2010) performed a retrospective matched-control study in IVF/intracytoplasmic sperm injection (ICSI) patients studying 289 embryo transfer before HSC and 538 embryo transfer following HSC. A control group consisted of 1,654 embryo transfers with normal uterus. However, in spite of these impressive results in favor of surgery before IVF/ICSI, pregnancy rate and LBR remained low (15–20% and ≤3%, respectively) and MRs were high (77%) in nonoperated patients compared with other published data, and therefore these results should be interpreted with caution.[151] Others have not observed lower pregnancy rates, but have detected increased miscarriage and reduced term delivery rates in women with uncorrected septate and bicornuate uterus undergoing IVF[152,153] • According to ASRM 2016, there is limited evidence to suggest septal resection would increase LBR in women with infertility or prior pregnancy loss[154]
Polyps	Hysteroscopic polypectomy	Improvement in pregnancy rate, both spontaneous and assisted	Meta-analysis supports a benefit with the hysteroscopic removal of polyps. If 28% of women become pregnant in the control group, the evidence suggests that between 50% and 76% of women will become pregnant after the removal of the endometrial polyps[155]
Submucosal fibroids and intramural fibroids protruding into the endometrial cavity	Myomectomy	Improvement in implantation rate, CPR, and LBR Decrease in MR	The presence of a submucous fibroid in women with RIF, regardless of the size, and fibroids protruding into the endometrial cavity should be removed as it is shown in various studies that removal improves reproductive outcome[156-159]

Contd...

Contd...

Uterine abnormality	*Intervention*	*Rationale*	*Evidence*
Intramural fibroids that do not affect the endometrial cavity	Myomectomy	Improvement in implantation rate, CPR, and LBR	Sunkara et al. (2010) published the most comprehensive systematic review and meta-analysis on this topic, including 6,087 and 11 studies, there was a statistically significant 21% relative reduction in LBR for women with non-cavity-distorting intramural fibroids compared with women without fibroids [relative risk (RR) 0.79, 95% confidence interval (CI): 0.70–0.88)]. When only studies with a prospective design were considered, the reduction in LBR was as high as 40% (RR 0.60, 95% CI: 0.41–0.87)[160]
			• Somigliana et al. (2011) studied 119 women with asymptomatic intramural or subserosal fibroids, 5 cm and compared these outcomes with 119 controls: The LBR were similar (18 vs. 13%, respectively), and the adjusted odds ratio (OR) was 1.45 (95% CI: 0.71–2.94). It was concluded that the presence of asymptomatic small fibroids did not affect ART outcomes[161] • Yan et al. (2014) included 249 women undergoing their first IVF/ICSI cycle with different types of fibroids and compared them with 249 controls without fibroids. After matching for several variables, delivery rates were 33.7% and 30.5% for controls and women with fibroids, respectively [adjusted OR 1.03 (95% CI: 0.95–1.11)]. A significant negative effect on delivery rate was noted when the largest tumor diameter was 2.85 cm[162]
Adenomyosis	Depot GnRHa alone or in combination with cytoreductive surgery	• GnRHa—regression of lesions through induction of hypogonadotropic status • Direct action on adeno-myotic lesions through types I and II receptors on the endometrium • Cytoreductive surgery reduces hypertrophy and subsequently improves function by bringing the uterine layers closer together • It also enhances blood supply, thereby facilitating GnRHa action	With respect to pregnancy outcomes with GnRHa, Wang et al. (2009) retrospectively studied two groups of women. In the first group, adenomyotic tissue was surgically removed and GnRHa was given for 6 months (n = 28). A second group (n = 37) only received 6 months of GnRHa. They noted uterine regrowth after the effect of GnRHa had disappeared in the GnRHa-only group. Cumulative spontaneous pregnancy rates after 36 months were significantly higher with the combined treatment of surgery plus GnRHa[163]
Synechiae	Hysteroscopic adhesiolysis with hysteroscopic scissors	Repair the impaired lining, restoring normal uterine cavity and fertility	Adhesiolysis permits the endometrium to re-establish its anatomy and function, depending on the degree of the adhesions and the preoperative appearance of the endometrium observed with TVS. Much more than other conditions, IUAs are associated with a high recurrence rate (3.1–62.5%), which is dependent on the severity of adhesions[164]

(ART: assisted reproductive technology; ASRM: American Society for Reproductive Medicine; CPR: clinical pregnancy rate; GnRHa: gonadotropin-releasing hormone agonist; IUAs: intrauterine adhesions; IVF: in vitro fertilization; LBR: live birth rate; MR: miscarriage rate; RIF: recurrent implantation failure; TVS: transvaginal sonography)

Treatment of Thin Endometrium

Treatment of thin endometrium has been depicted in **Flowchart 7 and Tables 7 to 9**.

Treatment of Thrombophilia and Immunological Factors

Treatment of thrombophilia and immunological factors has been explained in **Table 10**.

Flowchart 7: Treatment of thin endometrium.

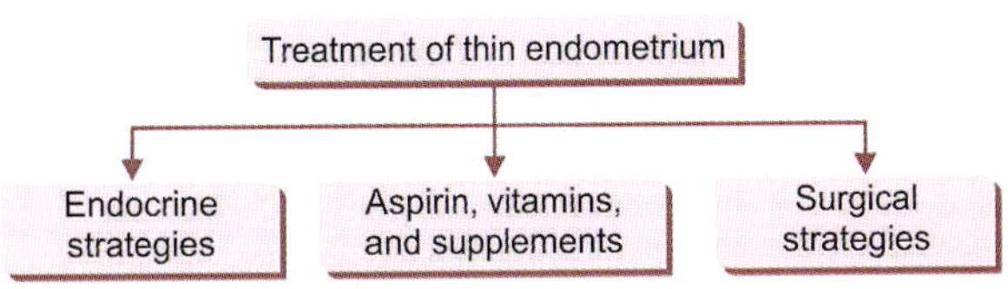

TABLE 7: Treatment of thin endometrium—endocrine strategy.

Strategy	***Rationale***	***Evidence***
High-dose oral E2	Estrogen helps endometrial proliferation by causing spiral artery contraction and reducing oxygen tension in the functional layer, which facilitates embryo implantation[165,166]	Different therapeutic approaches will most likely produce similar results, as exogenous estrogen administration compared with, or even combined with, endogenous estrogenic action from gonadotropin administration has not shown any superiority[11,167]
Intramuscular/ transdermal/vaginal E2	• Avoids first liver pass metabolism • Higher serum E2 concentrations • Better safety profile and longer mean t½ • Especially useful, when treating high-risk • patients, e.g., advanced maternal age	No clear benefit for one over another, and have achieved similar pregnancy rates[168]
GnRHa in luteal phase	Improved implantation and pregnancy rate, by supporting the corpus luteum	Luteal phase GnRHa (triptorelin 0.1 mg on the day of OPU, ET, and 3 days later) resulted in better pregnancy rate when compared with conventional luteal phase support. However, the quality of evidence in low[169]
Intrauterine G-CSF	G-CSF increases endometrial stromal cell decidualization mediated through cAMP by apocrine and paracrine action, and by inducing proliferation and differentiation of the human endometrium[170]	The only published RCT failed to show any impact on clinical outcome[171]
Autologous platelet-rich plasma (PRP)	Activates platelets by clotting, releases cytokines and growth factors, including VEGF, transforming growth factor, platelet-derived growth factor, and epidermal growth factor	Five patients with refractory endometrium received intrauterine PRP, along with high-dose E2 valerate. All five patients achieved endometrial thickness >7 mm, and they were all pregnant after embryo transfer (four ongoing pregnancy and one miscarriage).[172] However, no other study has validated these findings

(cAMP: cyclic adenosine monophosphate; E2: estradiol; ET: embryo transfer; G-CSF: granulocyte colony-stimulating factor; GnRHa: gonadotropin-releasing hormone agonists; OPU: oocyte pick up; RCT: randomized controlled trial; VEGF: vascular endothelial growth factor)

TABLE 8: Treatment of thin endometrium—with aspirin, vitamins, and supplements.

Strategy	***Rationale***	***Evidence***
Aspirin	• Decreasing subendometrial contractions • Inhibiting cyclo-oxygenase and prostaglandin biosynthesis • Improving uterine endometrial blood flow[173]	No beneficial effect on embryo implantation[174,175]
Nitroglycerine patches	• Nitric oxide (NO) is involved in endometrial cycle control and uterine preparation for pregnancy. Drugs that release • NO act as vasodilating agents, so they might be useful in women with thin endometrium	Ohl et al. (2002) administered nitroglycerin patches the day before embryo transfer in women with repeated implantation failure, but these authors were unable to demonstrate any effect.[176] There is no current evidence to support the use of nitroglycerin patches in women with a thin endometrium
Vitamin E ± pentoxifylline	Vitamin E—antioxidant and vasodilatory effect Pentoxifylline—inhibits phosphodiesterase by increasing intracellular cAMP—has a vasodilating effect and increases red cell membrane flexibility, while reducing blood viscosity by inhibiting red cell aggregation	Currently, only observational studies, no RCTs are available[177-179]
Sildenafil citrate	Enhances the vasodilator effect of NO by reducing cGMP degradation. It exerts its action at the endothelial smooth muscle level, and plays a relevant role in regulating vascular structure, growth and tone	Although biological plausibility exists, any evidence for the clinical benefit of sildenafil in women with a recurrent thin endometrium is weak, and very few publications[180,181] on nonrandomized studies have been found, with very few patients included
L-arginin	Arginin is an essential amino acid that plays an important role in regulating vasodilation and vascular flow. It is the main substrate for NO synthesis via NO synthase, and for ornithine and polyamines, which are key factors in placental angiogenesis and uterine flow regulation	Weak evidence to support its use in refractory endometrium,[182] solid data are still lacking to validate the usefulness of this approach

(cAMP: cyclic adenosine monophosphate; RCT: randomized controlled trial)

TABLE 9: Treatment of thin endometrium—surgical strategy.

Strategy	*Rationale*	*Evidence*
Hysteroscopy	Possible use could be to diagnose a previously unrecognized uterine pathology	Hysteroscopy in the preceding cycle has been reported to improve pregnancy outcomes in couples with three or more failed embryo transfer cycles,[183] but this evidence has recently been contradicted by a multicenter, randomized controlled trial that showed hysteroscopy to be of no value in RIF[184]
Endometrial scratch	The healing process following endometrial scratch may release cytokines and growth factors which encourages endometrial growth and facilitates implantation	• Meta-analysis including 14 trials and a total of 1,063 women concluded that moderate-quality evidence suggests that if 26% of women achieve live birth without endometrial injury, between 28% and 48% will achieve live birth with endometrial injury • A sensitivity analysis removing the studies at high risk of bias • showed no difference in effect[185]
Stem cells	Endometrial reconstruction based on the regenerative properties of the endometrium	• Three main sources of stem cells for endometrial cell reconstruction have been proposed, they are clonogenic multipotent mesenchymal stem/stromal cell, bone marrow derived stem cell, human embryonic stem cell • Till date, only one case of human endometrial regeneration • with reproductive success has been published[186]
Uterine transplantation	New therapeutic approach for women with absolute uterine factor infertility (AUFI), in whom adoption or surrogacy is not acceptable	• The first case of a healthy live birth after uterus transplantation[187] was published in 2014 in one of the nine women transplanted in Sweden[187] • Uterine transplantation as a promising clinical option for AUFI in the near future once experienced groups have settled the surgical, ethical, and social matters related to this technique

(RIF: recurrent implantation failure)

TABLE 10: Treatment of thrombophilia and immunological factors—immunomodulation.

Immunomodulator	*Rationale*	*Evidence*
Glucocorticoids	Glucocorticoids may mend the intrauterine environment by performing the action of as immunomodulation and reduce the uterine natural killer (NK) cell count and stabilize the cytokine expression profile in the endometrium and by decreasing of endometrial inflammation	14 studies (involving 1,879 couples) were included. Three studies reported LBR and these did not identify a significant difference after pooling the (preliminary) results (OR 1.21, 95% CI: 0.67–2.19). With regard to pregnancy rates, there was also no evidence that glucocorticoids improved clinical outcome (13 RCTs; OR 1.16, 95% CI: 0.94–1.44)[188]
Aspirin	Reduction of inflammation in the uterine cavity and improvement of uterine and ovarian perfusion, which might improve endometrial receptivity and ovarian responsiveness	13 trials (involving 2,653 couples) were included. There was no evidence of a difference between the aspirin group and the group receiving no treatment or placebo in rates of live birth (RR 0.91, 95% CI: 0.72–1.15, three RCTs, n = 1,053, I^2 = 15%, moderate-quality evidence). In addition, clinical pregnancy rates were also similar for the two groups (RR 1.03, 95% CI: 0.91–1.17, 10 RCTs, n = 2,142, I^2 = 27%, moderate-quality evidence). There was no evidence of a difference between groups in terms of multiple pregnancy, miscarriage, ectopic pregnancy, or vaginal bleeding. Data were lacking on other adverse effects[189]
Heparin	• The complex containing heparin-binding epidermal growth factor has been shown to enable an invasive phenotype of the trophoblast and hinder apoptosis[190] • Heparin also raises the free level of insulin-like growth factor (IGF) I and IGF II, which increase trophoblast invasion[191] • Heparin has been shown to encourage transcription of matrix metalloproteinases, which is known to control cell–cell interactions including breakdown of the decidua's basement membrane, helping trophoblast invasion	Two RCTs and one quasi-randomized trial were included in the meta-analysis. Pooled risk ratios in women with ≥3 RIF (N = 245) showed a significant improvement in the LBR (RR = 1.79, 95% CI = 1.10–2.90, p = 0.02) and a reduction in the miscarriage rate (RR = 0.22, 95% CI = 0.06–0.78, p = 0.02) with LMWH compared with controls. The IR for ≥3 RIF (N = 674) showed a nonsignificant trend toward improvement (RR = 1.73, 95% CI: 0.98–3.03, p = 0.06) with LMWH. However, the beneficial effect of LMWH was not significant when only studies with unexplained RIF were pooled. The summary analysis for the numbers needed to be treated with LMWH showed that approximately eight women would require treatment to achieve one extra live birth[192]

Contd...

Contd...

Immunomodulator	***Rationale***	***Evidence***
Intravenous immunoglobulin G (IVIG)	In ART, the proposed mechanism of action is by a reduction of peripheral cytotoxic NK cells,[193] enhancement of regulatory T cells, and downregulation of antibody producing B cells[194,195]	10 studies were included. The use of IVIG was significantly associated with a higher IR and RR was 2.708 (95% CI: 1.302–5.629) compared with the placebo. The clinical pregnancy rate and the LBR were significantly increased in patients randomized to IVIG; RR was 1.475 (95% CI: 1.191–1.825) for the clinical pregnancy rate and RR was 1.616 (95% CI: 1.243–2.101) for the LBR. Moreover, the miscarriage rate was significantly less in patients randomized to IVIG (0.352, 95% CI: 0.168–0.738), but the LBR per embryo transferred was not (2.893; 95% CI: 0.810–10.331) less
Anti-TNF-α	TNF-α is a cytokine produced by TH1 cells involved in the cell-mediated immune response. Anti-TNF-α interacts with and neutralizes TNF-α, thereby decreasing the inflammatory and cell-mediated immune response from TH1 lymphocytes	At present no RCTs have been reported investigating the effect of anti-TNF-α on pregnancy outcome from IVF or ICSI treatment
Intralipid	The therapeutic effect in the framework of IVF is proposed to be mediated by a decrease of peripheral blood NK cell activity and suppression of proinflammatory cytokines[196]	Only one RCT is available on this topic. No difference in chemical pregnancy was found between the two groups. The authors reported a borderline significant difference in ongoing pregnancy and live birth in favor of intralipid,[197] but the study was not sufficiently powered to enable differentiation of this from a chance observation

(ART: assisted reproductive technology; CI: confidence interval; ICSI: intracytoplasmic sperm injection; IR; implantation rate; IVF: in vitro fertilization; LBR: live birth rate; LMWH: low-molecular-weight heparin; OR: odds ratio; RCT: randomized controlled trial; RIF: recurrent implantation failure; RR: risk ratio; TNF-α: tumor necrosis factor alpha; TH: T helper)

Treatment of Multifactorial Effectors

Endometriosis

The administration of GnRHa for 3–6 months before ART in women with endometriosis significantly improves the ongoing pregnancy rate.[198] No harmful effect on ovarian response was observed. A meta-analysis of three RCTs showed that this treatment increased the odds of clinical pregnancy by fourfold.[104] Most investigators approve that there is no benefit in the removal of endometriomas before IVF,[154,155] whereas the role of laparoscopic treatment of nonovarian endometriosis in patients with failed IVF is controversial.[199,200] Furthermore, surgery might be deleterious for ovarian reserve.

Treatment of Hydrosalpinges

Treatment of hydrosalpinges has been explained in **Table 11**.

Gamete Donation and Surrogacy

Couples with RIF need help on the aptness of ensuing with further IVF attempts. If implantation fails to occur in spite of repeated treatment attempts or if the prognosis of further IVF treatment is measured to be poor, alternative treatment options should be reconnoitered. If the likely basis of the problem lies with the embryo, gamete donation should be recommended. On the other hand, if the problem lies in the uterus, e.g., multiple small fibroids or Asherman's syndrome, which has failed to react to surgical treatment, surrogacy must be discussed.

KEY POINTS

- There are a lot of controversial issues in the field of reproductive medicine, starting from the definition of infertility, which moves on to the diagnosis of unexplained infertility, which entitles the couple to an unproven treatment, IVF. And in those couples who do not conceive after three or more attempts of IVF, comes a fabricated diagnosis of RIF.
- A made up disease—infertility, refined by another refined diagnosis—unexplained infertility, and repeated failure with unproven treatment IVF, repeated failure of which leads to another new diagnosis—RIF, these are not diagnoses in themselves, but are mere clinical presentations.
- Until we understand and can accurately discern the underlying causes, the value of all proposed interventions is likely to be underestimated.
- William Watson rightly describes this as "The causes and treatment of non-disease". And JLH (Hans) Evers quotes in his prescient Editorial, "Perhaps the best course of action for a physician is to tell patients who have very little wrong with them that they do, indeed, have very little wrong with them, and then give them nothing for it".

TABLE 11: Treatment of hydrosalpinges.

Modality	*Advantage*	*Disadvantage*	*Evidence*
Salpingectomy	Improves implantation and live birth rate	May compromise ovarian response to stimulation during subsequent IVF treatment	• Strandell et al. (2005)[201] analyzed the cost-effectiveness of salpingectomy prior to IVF, for up to three IVF cycles. They found that the cost per live birth in the salpingectomy group was 22,823 Euros, which was significantly lesser than the cost per live birth in the control (no salpingectomy) group (29,517 Euros). The observation proposes that it is more cost-effective to routinely remove hydrosalpinges prior to IVF treatment • Meta-analysis159 of three RCTs involving prophylactic salpingectomy in 295 patients with hydrosalpinges, the pregnancy and live birth rates doubled following prophylactic salpingectomy
Salpingostomy	Salpingostomy not only "removes" the hydrosalpinges, but also produces the possibility of natural conception	The likely recurrence of hydrosalpinges after salpingostomy, which necessitates a further procedure to remove the tube, further delaying the treatment and suffering extra cost	• The intrauterine pregnancy rate following salpingostomy has been reported by a number of studies to be over 30%[202,203] • The results are likely to be higher if the damage to the Fallopian tubes is minimal[204]
Laparoscopic proximal tubal occlusion	Simpler operation and less likely to disturb ovarian blood supply and hence compromise ovarian response to stimulation by gonadotropins during IVF treatment	Occlusion of the proximal part of the tube leaves behind the dilated and blocked tube and increases the risk of future infection (pyosalpinx) and persistent pain, which necessitates salpingectomy in future	Meta-analysis[205] by Johnson et al. (2010) provides evidence that laparoscopic tubal occlusion is an alternative to laparoscopic salpingectomy in improving IVF pregnancy rates in women with hydrosalpinges
US-guided drainage of hydrosalpinx fluid	• Relatively simple • Less invasive • Less cost	The fluid may rapidly reaccumulate as the underlying pathology has not been altered risk of introducing infection	Studies have found no evidence of benefit for clinical pregnancy rate or live birth rate[206,207]

(IVF: in vitro fertilization; US: ultrasound)

- Couples with infertility belong to a very vulnerable group. They will do almost anything to achieve a pregnancy. They deserve our dedicated care and evidence-based treatment.
- In case such an evidence base is lacking, the patients should be counseled accordingly and, if the occasion arises, they might be invited to participate in a carefully designed clinical trial. They should not be exploited.

REFERENCES

1. Simon C, Martin JC, Pellicer A. Paracrine regulators of implantation. Baillieres Best Pract Res Clin Obstet Gynaecol. 2000;14:815-26.
2. Zegers-Hochschild F, Adamson GD, de Mouzon J, Ishihara O, Mansour R, Nygren K, et al. International Committee for Monitoring Assisted Reproductive Technology (ICMART) and the World Health Organization (WHO) revised glossary of ART terminology, 2009. Fertil Steril. 2009;92:1520-4.
3. Gameiro S, Boivin J, Peronace L, Verhaak CM. Why do patients discontinue fertility treatment? A systematic review of reasons and predictors of discontinuation in fertility treatment. Hum Reprod Update. 2012;18:652-69.
4. Gameiro S, Verhaak CM, Kremer JA, Boivin J. Why we should talk about compliance with assisted reproductive technologies (ART): a systematic review and meta-analysis of ART compliance rates. Hum Reprod Update. 2013;19:124-35.
5. Urman B, Yakin K, Balaban B. Recurrent implantation failure in assisted reproduction: how to counsel and manage. B. Treatment options that have not been proven to benefit the couple. Reprod Biomed Online. 2005;11:382-91.
6. Das M, Holzer HE. Recurrent implantation failure: gamete and embryo factors. Fertil Steril. 2012;97:1021-7.
7. Laufer N, Simon A. Recurrent implantation failure: current update and clinical approach to an ongoing challenge. Fertil Steril. 2012;97:1019-20.
8. Penzias AS. Recurrent IVF failure: other factors. Fertil Steril. 2012;97:1033-8.
9. Simon A, Laufer N. Repeated implantation failure: clinical approach. Fertil Steril. 2012;97:1039-43.
10. Polanski LT, Baumgarten MN, Quenby S, Brosens J, Campbell BK, Raine-Fenning NJ. What exactly do we mean by 'recurrent implantation failure'? A systematic review and opinion. Reprod Biomed Online. 2014;28:409-23.
11. Coughlan C, Ledger W, Wang Q, Liu F, Demirol A, Gurgan T, et al. Recurrent implantation failure: definition and management. Reprod Biomed Online. 2014;28:14-38.

12. Somigliana E, Vigano P, Busnelli A, Paffoni A, Vegetti W, Vercellini P. Repeated implantation failure at the crossroad between statistics, clinics and over-diagnosis. Reprod Biomed Online. 2018;36(1):32-8.
13. Verberg MFG, Eijkemans MJC, Macklon NS, Heijnen EMEW, Baart EB, Hohmann FP, et al. The clinical significance of the retrieval of a low number of oocytes following mild ovarian stimulation for IVF: a meta-analysis. Hum Reprod Update. 2009;15:5-12.
14. Ferraretti AP, La Marca A, Fauser BCJM, Tarlatzis B, Nargund G, Gianaroli L, et al. ESHRE consensus on the definition of 'poor response' to ovarian stimulation for in vitro fertilization: the Bologna criteria. Hum Reprod. 2011;26:1616-24.
15. Wang LY, Wang DH, Zou XY, Xu CM. Mitochondrial functions on oocytes and preimplantation embryos. J Zhejiang Univ Sci B. 2009;10:483-92.
16. Absalan F, Ghannadi A, Kazerooni M, Parifar R, Jamalzadeh F, Amiri S. Value of sperm chromatin dispersion test in couples with unexplained recurrent abortion. J Assist Reprod Genet. 2012;29:11-4.
17. Margalioth EJ, Ben-Chetrit A, Gal M, Eldar-Geva T. Investigation and treatment of repeated implantation failure following IVF-ET. Human Reprod. 2006;21:3036-43.
18. Cohen J, Inge KL, Suzman M, Wiker SR, Wright G. Video cinematography of fresh and cryopreserved embryos: a retrospective analysis of embryonic morphology and implantation. Fertil Steril. 1989;51:820-7.
19. De Vos A, Van Steirteghem A. Zona hardening, zona drilling and assisted hatching: new achievements in assisted reproduction. Cells Tissues Organs. 2000;166:220-7.
20. Du H, Taylor HS. Molecular regulation of Müllerian development by Hox genes. Ann N Y Acad Sci. 2004;1034: 152-65.
21. Daftary GS, Taylor HS. Implantation in the human: the role of HOX genes. Semin Reprod Med. 2000;18:311-20.
22. Lavergne N, Aristizabal J, Zarka V, Erny R, Hedon B. Uterine anomalies and in vitro fertilization: what are the results? Eur J Obstet Gynecol Reprod Biol. 1996;68:29-34.
23. Ban-Frangez H, Tomazevic T, Virant-Klun I, Verdenik I, Ribic-Pucelj M, Vrtacnik-Bokal E. The outcome of singleton pregnancies after IVF/ICSI in women before and after hysteroscopic resection of a uterine septum compared to normal controls. Eur J Obstet Gynecol Reprod Biol. 2009; 146:184-7.
24. Makrakis E, Pantos K. The outcomes of hysteroscopy in women with implantation failures after in-vitro fertilization: findings and effect on subsequent pregnancy rates. Curr Opin Obstet Gynecol. 2010;22:339-43.
25. Demirol A, Gurgan T. Effect of treatment of intrauterine pathologies with office hysteroscopy in patients with recurrent IVF failure. Reprod Biomed Online. 2004;8:590-4.
26. Cakmak H, Taylor HS. Implantation failure: molecular mechanisms and clinical treatment. Hum Reprod Update. 2011;17(2):242-53.
27. De Geyter C, Schmitter M, De Geyter M, Nieschlag E, Holzgreve W, Schneider HP. Prospective evaluation of the ultrasound appearance of the endometrium in a cohort of 1,186 infertile women. Fertil Steril. 2000;73:106-13.
28. Zhang X, Chen CH, Confino E, Barnes R, Milad M, Kazer RR. Increased endometrial thickness is associated with improved treatment outcome for selected patients undergoing in vitro fertilization–embryo transfer. Fertil Steril. 2005;83:336-40.
29. Akman MA, Erden HF, Bahceci M. Endometrial fluid visualized through ultrasonography during ovarian stimulation in IVF cycles impairs the outcome in tubal factor, but not PCOS, patients. Hum Reprod. 2005;20:906-9.
30. Rinaldi L, Lisi F, Floccari A, Lisi R, Pepe G, Fishel S. Endometrial thickness as a predictor of pregnancy after in-vitro fertilization but not after intracytoplasmic sperm injection. Hum Reprod. 1996;11:1538-41.
31. Franasiak JM, Scott RT. Contribution of immunology to implantation failure of euploid embryos. Fertil Steril. 2017;107:1279-83.
32. Wegmann TG, Lin H, Guilbert L, Mosmann TR. Bidirectional cytokine interactions in the maternal-fetal relationship: is successful pregnancy a TH2 phenomenon? Immunol Today. 1993;14:353-6.
33. Kalu E, Bhaskaran S, Thum MY, Vishwanatha R, Croucher C, Sherriff E, et al. Serial estimation of TH1:TH2 cytokines profile in women undergoing in-vitro fertilization–embryo transfer. Am J Reprod Immunol. 2008;59:206-11.
34. Raghupathy R. TH1-type immunity is incompatible with successful pregnancy. Immunol Today. 1997;18:478-82.
35. Del Prete G, Maggi E, Romagnani S. Human TH1 and TH2 cells: functional properties, mechanisms of regulation, and role in disease. Lab Investig J Tech Methods Pathol. 1994;70:299-306.
36. Emmer PM, Nelen WL, Steegers EA, Hendriks JC, Veerhoek M, Joosten I. Peripheral natural killer cytotoxicity and CD56(pos)CD16(pos) cells increase during early pregnancy in women with a history of recurrent spontaneous abortion. Hum Reprod. 2000;15:1163-9.
37. Quenby S, Kalumbi C, Bates M, Farquharson R, Vince G. Prednisolone reduces preconceptual endometrial natural killer cells in women with recurrent miscarriage. Fertil Steril. 2005;84:980-4.
38. Souza SS, Ferriani RA, Santos CMP, Voltarelli JC. Immunological evaluation of patients with recurrent abortion. J Reprod Immunol. 2002;56:111-21.
39. Wang Q, Li T-C, Wu Y-P, Cocksedge KA, Fu Y-S, Kong Q-Y, et al. Reappraisal of peripheral NK cells in women with recurrent miscarriage. Reprod Biomed Online. 2008;17:814-9.
40. Tang AW, Alfirevic Z, Quenby S. Natural killer cells and pregnancy outcomes in women with recurrent miscarriage and infertility: a systematic review. Hum Reprod. 2011;26: 1971-80.
41. Alecsandru D, Garrido N, Vicario JL, Barrio A, Aparicio P, Requena A, et al. Maternal KIR haplotype influences live birth rate after double embryo transfer in IVF cycles in patients with recurrent miscarriages and implantation failure. Hum Reprod. 2014;29:2637-43.
42. Morin SJ, Treff NR, Tao X, Scott 3rd RT, Franasiak JM, Juneau CR, et al. Combination of uterine natural killer cell immunoglobulin receptor haplotype and trophoblastic HLA-C ligand influences the risk of pregnancy loss: a retrospective cohort analysis of direct embryo genotyping data from euploid transfers. Fertil Steril. 2017;107:677-83.e2.
43. Alecsandru D, García-Velasco JA. Why natural killer cells are not enough: a further understanding of killer immunoglobulin-like receptor and human leukocyte antigen. Fertil Steril. 2017;107:1273-8.

44. Hornstein MD, Davis OK, Massey JB, Paulson RJ, Collins JA. Antiphospholipid antibodies and in vitro fertilization success: a meta-analysis. Fertil Steril. 2000;73:330-3.
45. Practice Committee of the American Society for Reproductive Medicine. Antiphospholipid antibodies do not affect IVF success. Fertil Steril. 2008;90(5 Suppl.):S172-3.
46. Di Nisio M, Rutjes AWS, Ferrante N, Tiboni GM, Cuccurullo F, Porreca E. Thrombophilia and outcomes of assisted reproduction technologies: a systematic review and meta-analysis. Blood. 2011;118:2670-8.
47. Macklon NS, Brosens JJ. The human endometrium as a sensor of embryo quality. Biol Reprod. 2014;92:98.
48. Ravel J, Gajer P, Abdo Z, Schneider GM, Koenig SSK, McCulle SL, et al. Vaginal microbiome of reproductive-age women. Proc Natl Acad Sci U S A. 2011;108(Suppl. 1):4680-7.
49. Gajer P, Brotman RM, Bai G, Sakamoto J, Schütte UME, Zhong X, et al. Temporal dynamics of the human vaginal microbiota. Sci Transl Med. 2012;4:132-52.
50. Huang B, Fettweis JM, Brooks JP, Jefferson KK, Buck GA. The changing landscape of the vaginal microbiome. Clin Lab Med. 2014;34:747-61.
51. Moreno I, Codoñer FM, Vilella F, Valbuena D, Martinez-Blanch JF, Jimenez-Almazán J, et al. Evidence that the endometrial microbiota has an effect on implantation success or failure. Am J Obstet Gynecol. 2016;215:684-703.
52. Barnhart K, Dunsmoor-Su R, Coutifaris C. Effect of endometriosis on in vitro fertilization. Fertil Steril. 2002;77:1148-55.
53. Larson-Cook KL, Brannian JD, Hansen KA, Kasperson KM, Aamold ET, Evenson DP. Relationship between the outcomes of assisted reproductive techniques and sperm DNA fragmentation as measured by the sperm chromatin structure assay. Fertil Steril. 2003;80:895-902.
54. Larson KL, DeJonge CJ, Barnes AM, Jost LK, Evenson DP. Sperm chromatin structure assay parameters as predictors of failed pregnancy following assisted reproductive techniques. Hum Reprod. 2000;15:1717-22.
55. Gandini L, Lombardo F, Paoli D, Caruso F, Eleuteri P, Leter G, et al. Full-term pregnancies achieved with ICSI despite high levels of sperm chromatin damage. Hum Reprod. 2004;19:1409-17.
56. Bungum M, Humaidan P, Axmon A, Spano M, Bungum L, Erenpreiss J, et al. Sperm DNA integrity assessment in prediction of assisted reproduction technology outcome. Hum Reprod. 2007;22:174-9.
57. Osman A, Alsomait H, Seshadri S, El-Toukhy T, Khalaf Y. The effect of sperm DNA fragmentation on live birth rate after IVF or ICSI: a systematic review and meta-analysis. Reprod Biomed Online. 2015;30:120-7.
58. Stern C, Pertile M, Norris H, Hale L, Baker HW. Chromosome translocations in couples with in-vitro fertilization implantation failure. Hum Reprod. 1999;14:2097-101.
59. Montag M. Morphokinetics and embryo aneuploidy: has time come or not yet? Reprod Biomed Online. 2013;26:528-30.
60. Swain JE. Could time-lapse embryo imaging reduce the need for biopsy and PGS? J Assist Reprod Genet. 2013;30:1081-90.
61. Davies S, Christopikou D, Tsorva E, Kragianni A. Delayed cleavage division and a prolonged transition between 2- and 4-cell stages in embryos identified as aneuploidy at the 8-cell stage by array-CGH. Hum Reprod. 2012;27:ii84-6.
62. Meseguer M, Herrero J, Tejera A, Hilligsøe KM, Ramsing NB, Remohí J. The use of morphokinetics as a predictor of embryo implantation. Hum Reprod. 2011;26:2658-71.
63. Chen AA, Tan L, Suraj V, Pera RR, Shen S. Biomarkers identified with time-lapse imaging: discovery, validation, and practical application. Fertil Steril. 2013;99:1035-43.
64. Stecher A, Vanderzwalmen P, Zintz M, Wirleitner B, Schuff M, Spitzer D, et al. Transfer of blastocysts with deviant morphological and morphokinetic parameters at early stages of in-vitro development: a case series. Reprod Biomed Online. 2014;28:424-35.
65. Reignier A, Lammers J, Barriere P, Freour T. Can time-lapse parameters predict embryo ploidy? A systematic review. Reprod Biomed Online. 2018;36:380-7.
66. Munne S, Sandalinas M, Escuredo T, Velilla E, Walmsley R, Sadowy S, et al. Improved implantation after preimplantation genetic diagnosis of aneuploidy. Reprod Biomed Online. 2003;7:91-7.
67. Kahraman S, Bahce M, Samli H, Imirzalioğlu N, Yakisn K, Cengiz G, et al. Healthy births and ongoing pregnancies obtained by preimplantation genetic diagnosis in patients with advanced maternal age and recurrent implantation failure. Hum Reprod. 2000;15:2003-7.
68. Kuliev A, Verlinsky Y. The role of preimplantation genetic diagnosis in women of advanced maternal age. Curr Opin Obstet Gynecol. 2003;15:233-8.
69. Taylor TH, Gitlin SA, Patrick JL, Crain JL, Wilson JM, Griffin DK. The origin, mechanisms, incidence and clinical consequences of chromosomal mosaicism in humans. Hum Reprod Update. 2014;20:571-81.
70. Capalbo A, Bono S, Spizzichino L, Biricik A, Baldi M, Colamaria S, et al. Sequential comprehensive chromosome analysis on polar bodies, blastomeres and trophoblast: insights into female meiotic errors and chromosomal segregation in the preimplantation window of embryo development. Hum Reprod. 2013;28:509-18.
71. Fragouli E, Alfarawati S, Daphnis DD, Goodall N-N, Mania A, Griffiths T, et al. Cytogenetic analysis of human blastocysts with the use of FISH, CGH and aCGH: scientific data and technical evaluation. Hum Reprod. 2011;26:480-90.
72. Northrop LE, Treff NR, Levy B, Scott Jr RT. SNP microarray-based 24 chromosome aneuploidy screening demonstrates that cleavage-stage FISH poorly predicts aneuploidy in embryos that develop to morphologically normal blastocysts. Mol Hum Reprod. 2010;16:590-600.
73. Gleicher N, Kushnir VA, Barad DH. Preimplantation genetic screening (PGS) still in search of a clinical application: a systematic review. Reprod Biol Endocrinol. 2014;12:22.
74. Mastenbroek S, Repping S. Preimplantation genetic screening: back to the future. Hum Reprod. 2014;29:1846-50.
75. Gardner DK, Meseguer M, Rubio C, Treff NR. Diagnosis of human preimplantation embryo viability. Hum Reprod Update. 2015;21(6):727-47.
76. Lee YS, Thouas GA, Gardner DK. Developmental kinetics of cleavage stage mouse embryos are related to their subsequent carbohydrate and amino acid utilization at the blastocyst stage. Hum Reprod. 2015;30:543-52.
77. Mitchell M, Cashman KS, Gardner DK, Thompson JG, Lane M. Disruption of mitochondrial malate-aspartate shuttle activity

in mouse blastocysts impairs viability and fetal growth. Biol Reprod. 2009;80:295-301.
78. Gardner DK, Wale PL. Analysis of metabolism to select viable human embryos for transfer. Fertil Steril. 2013;99:1062-72.
79. Moffet A, Shreeve N. First do no harm: uterine natural killer (NK) cells in assisted reproduction. Hum Reprod. 2015;30:1519-25.
80. Scott RT, Snyder RR, Strickland DM, Tyburski CC, Bagnall JA, Reed KR, et al. The effect of interobserver variation in dating endometrial histology on the diagnosis of luteal phase defects. Fertil Steril. 1988;50:888-92.
81. Kupesic Plavsic S. Ultrasound imaging of the endometrium. In: Simon C, Giudice LC (Eds). The Endometrial Factor: A Reproductive Precision Medicine Approach. Boca Raton: CRC Press; 2017. pp. 15-35.
82. Rambouts L. Invasive diagnosis. Hysteroscopy. In: Simon C, Giudice LC (Eds). The Endometrial Factor: A Reproductive Precision Medicine Approach. Boca Raton: CRC Press; 2017. pp. 36-42.
83. Hertig AT, Rock J, Adams EC. A description of 34 human ova within the first 17 days of development. Dev Dyn. 1956;98:435-93.
84. Navot D, Scott RT, Droesch K, Veeck LL, Liu HC, Rosenwaks Z. The window of embryo transfer and the efficiency of human conception in vitro. Fertil Steril. 1991;55:114-8.
85. Wilcox AJ, Baird DD, Weinberg CR. Time of implantation of the conceptus and loss of pregnancy. N Engl J Med. 1999;340:1796-9.
86. Direito A, Bailly S, Mariani A, Ecochard R. Relationships between the luteinizing hormone surge and other characteristics of the menstrual cycle in normally ovulating women. Fertil Steril. 2013;99:279-85.e3.
87. Díaz-Gimeno P, Horcajadas JA, Martínez-Conejero JA, Esteban FJ, Alamá P, Pellicer A, et al. A genomic diagnostic tool for human endometrial receptivity based on the transcriptomic signature. Fertil Steril. 2011;95:50-60.e15.
88. Talbi S, Hamilton AE, Vo KC, Tulac S, Overgaard MT, Dosiou C, et al. Molecular phenotyping of human endometrium distinguishes menstrual cycle phases and underlying biological processes in normo-ovulatory women. Endocrinology. 2006;147:1097-121.
89. Macklon NS, van der Gaast MH, Hamilton A, Fauser BCJM, Giudice LC. The impact of ovarian stimulation with recombinant FSH in combination with GnRH antagonist on the endometrial transcriptome in the window of implantation. Reprod Sci. 2008;15:357-65.
90. Horcajadas JA, Mínguez P, Dopazo J, Esteban FJ, Domínguez F, Giudice LC, et al. Controlled ovarian stimulation induces a functional genomic delay of the endometrium with potential clinical implications. J Clin Endocrinol Metab. 2008;93:4500-10.
91. Haouzi D, Assou S, Mahmoud K, Tondeur S, Rème T, Hedon B, et al. Gene expression profile of human endometrial receptivity: comparison between natural and stimulated cycles for the same patients. Hum Reprod. 2009;24:1436-45.
92. Kao LC, Germeyer A, Tulac S, Lobo S, Yang JP, Taylor RN, et al. Expression profiling of endometrium from women with endometriosis reveals candidate genes for disease-based implantation failure and infertility. Endocrinology. 2003;144:2870-81.
93. Horcajadas JA, Sharkey AM, Catalano RD, Sherwin JRA, Domínguez F, Burgos LA, et al. Effect of an intrauterine device on the gene expression profile of the endometrium. J Clin Endocrinol Metab. 2006;91:3199-207.
94. Ruiz-Alonso M, Blesa D, Díaz-Gimeno P, Gómez E, Fernández-Sánchez M, Carranza F, et al. The endometrial receptivity array for diagnosis and personalized embryo transfer as a treatment for patients with repeated implantation failure. Fertil Steril. 2013;100:818-24.
95. Koot YEM, van Hooff SR, Boomsma CM, van Leenen D, Koerkamp MJAG, Goddijn M, et al. An endometrial gene expression signature accurately predicts recurrent implantation failure after IVF. Sci Rep. 2016;6:19411.
96. Sebastian-Leon P, Garrido N, Remohí J, Pellicer A, Diaz-Gimeno P. Asynchronous and pathological windows of implantation: two causes of recurrent implantation failure. Hum Reprod. 2018;33(4):626-35.
97. Moreno I, Codoñer FM, Vilella F, Valbuena D, Martinez-Blanch JF, Jimenez-Almazán J, et al. Evidence that the endometrial microbiota has an effect on implantation success or failure. Am J Obstet Gynecol. 2016;215(6):684-703.
98. Moreno I, Franasiak JM. Endometrial microbiota—new player in town. Fertil Steril. 2017;108:32-9.
99. Klonoff-Cohen H, Natarajan L, Marrs R, Yee B. Effects of female and male smoking on success rates of IVF and gamete intra-fallopian transfer. Hum Reprod. 2001;16:1382-90.
100. Potts RJ, Newbury CJ, Smith G, Notarianni LJ, Jefferies TM. Sperm chromatin damage associated with male smoking. Mutat Res. 1999;423:103-11.
101. Wadden TA, Foster GD. Behavioral treatment of obesity. Med Clin North Am. 2000;84:441-61, vii.
102. National Institute for Health and Care Excellence. (2013). Fertility problems: Assessment and Treatment. Clinical Guidelines CG156. [online] Available from: https://www.nice.org.uk/guidance/cg156 [Last accessed December, 2022].
103. Hill MJ, Levens ED, Levy G, Ryan ME, Csokmay JM, DeCherney AH, et al. The use of recombinant luteinizing hormone in patients undergoing assisted reproductive techniques with advanced reproductive age: a systematic review and meta-analysis. Fertil Steril. 2012;97:1108-14.e1.
104. Sallam HN, Garcia-Velasco JA, Dias S, Arici A. Long-term pituitary down-regulation before in vitro fertilization (IVF) for women with endometriosis. Cochrane Database Syst Rev. 2006;2006(1):CD004635.
105. Glujovsky D, Blake D, Bardach A, Farquhar C. Cleavage stage versus blastocyst stage embryo transfer in assisted reproductive technology. Cochrane Database Syst Rev. 2012;(7):CD002118.
106. Cohen J, Scott R, Alikani M, Schimmel T, Munné S, Levron J, et al. Ooplasmic transfer in mature human oocytes. Mol Hum Reprod. 1998;4:269-80.
107. Showell MG, Mackenzie-Proctor R, Brown J, Yazdani A, Stankiewicz MT, Hart RJ. Antioxidants for male subfertility. Cochrane Database Syst Rev. 2014;(12):CD007411.
108. Jakab A, Sakkas D, Delpiano E, Cayli S, Kovanci E, Ward D, et al. Intracytoplasmic sperm injection: a novel selection method for sperm with normal frequency of chromosomal aneuploidies. Fertil Steril. 2005;84:1665-73.
109. Said T, Agarwal A, Grunewald S, Rasch M, Baumann T, Kriegel C, et al. Selection of nonapoptotic spermatozoa as a new tool

for enhancing assisted reproduction outcomes: an in vitro model. Biol Reprod. 2006;74:530-7.
110. Teixeira DM, Barbosa MAP, Ferriani RA, Navarro PA, Raine-Fenning N, Nastri CO, et al. Regular (ICSI) versus ultra-high magnification (IMSI) sperm selection for assisted reproduction. Cochrane Database Syst Rev. 2013;(7): CD010167.
111. Zini A, Bach PV, Al-Malki AH, Schlegel PN. Use of testicular sperm for ICSI in oligozoospermic couples: how far should we go? Hum Reprod. 2017;32:7-13.
112. Guerif F, Bidault R, Gasnier O, Couet ML, Gervereau O, Lansac J, et al. Efficacy of blastocyst transfer after implantation failure. Reprod Biomed Online. 2004;9:630-6.
113. Levitas E, Lunenfeld E, Har-Vardi I, Albotiano S, Sonin Y, Hackmon-Ram R, et al. Blastocyst-stage embryo transfer in patients who failed to conceive in three or more day 2–3 embryo transfer cycles: a prospective, randomized study. Fertil Steril. 2004;81:567-71.
114. Glujovsky D, Farquhar C, Quinteiro Retamar AM, Alvarez Sedo CR, Blake D. Cleavage stage versus blastocyst stage embryo transfer in assisted reproductive technology. Cochrane Database Syst Rev. 2016;(6):CD002118.
115. DeMeestere I, Barlow P, Leroy F. Hardening of zona pellucida of mouse oocytes and embryos in vivo and in vitro. Int J Fertil Womens Med. 1997;42:219-22.
116. Carroll J, Depypere H, Matthews CD. Freeze–thaw-induced changes of the zona pellucida explains decreased rates of fertilization in frozen–thawed mouse oocytes. J Reprod Fertil. 1990;90:547-53.
117. Nikas G, Develioglu OH, Toner JP, Jones Jr HW. Endometrial pinopodes indicate a shift in the window of receptivity in IVF cycles. Hum Reprod. 1999;14:787-92.
118. Liu HC, Cohen J, Alikani M, Noyes N, Rosenwaks Z. Assisted hatching facilitates earlier implantation. Fertil Steril. 1993; 60:871-5.
119. Cohen J, Alikani M, Trowbridge J, Rosenwaks Z. Implantation enhancement by selective assisted hatching using zona drilling of human embryos with poor prognosis. Hum Reprod. 1992;7:685-91.
120. Martins WP, Rocha IA, Ferriani RA, Nastri CO. Assisted hatching of human embryos: a systematic review and meta-analysis of randomized controlled trials. Hum Reprod. 2011;17:438-53.
121. Carney SK, Das S, Blake D, Farquhar C, Seif MMW, Nelson L. Assisted hatching on assisted conception [in vitro fertilisation (IVF) and intracytoplasmic sperm injection (ICSI)]. Cochrane Database Syst Rev. 2012;12(12):CD001894.
122. Li D, Yang DL, An J, Jiao J, Zhou YM, Wu QJ, et al. Effect of assisted hatching on pregnancy outcomes: a systematic review and meta-analysis of randomized controlled trials. Sci Rep. 2016;6:31228.
123. Simón C, Mercader A, Garcia-Velasco J, Nikas G, Moreno C, Remohí J, et al. Coculture of human embryos with autologous human endometrial epithelial cells in patients with implantation failure. J Clin Endocrinol Metab. 1999;84:2638-46.
124. Spandorfer SD, Pascal P, Parks J, Clark R, Veeck L, Davis OK, et al. Autologous endometrial coculture in patients with IVF failure: outcome of the first 1,030 cases. J Reprod Med. 2004;49:463-7.
125. Harper J, Coonen E, De Rycke M, Fiorentino F, Geraedts J, Goossens V, et al. What next for preimplantation genetic screening (PGS)? A position statement from the ESHRE PGD Consortium Steering Committee. Hum Reprod. 2010;25:821-3.
126. Geraedts J, Sermon K. Preimplantation genetic screening 2.0: the theory. Mol Hum Reprod. 2016;22:839-44.
127. Yang Z, Liu J, Collins GS, Salem SA, Liu X, Lyle SS, et al. Selection of single blastocysts for fresh transfer via standard morphology assessment alone and with array CGH for good prognosis IVF patients: results from a randomized pilot study. Mol Cytogenet. 2012;5:24.
128. Scott Jr RT, Upham KM, Forman EJ, Hong KH, Scott KL, Taylor D, et al. Blastocyst biopsy in CCS and fresh ET significantly increases IVF implantation and delivery rates; an RCT. Fertil Steril. 2013;100:687-703.
129. Forman EJ, Hong KH, Ferry KM, Tao X, Taylor D, Levy B, et al. In vitro fertilisation with single euploid blastocyst transfer: a randomized controlled trial. Fertil Steril. 2013;100:100-7.e1.
130. Fragouli E, Wells D. Mitochondrial DNA assessment to determine oocyte and embryo viability. Semin Reprod Med. 2015;33:401-9.
131. Fragouli E, Spath K, Alfarawati S, Kaper F, Craig A, Michel CE, et al. Altered levels of mitochondrial DNA are associated with female age, aneuploidy, and provide an independent measure of embryonic implantation potential. PLoS Genet. 2015;11:e1005241.
132. Diez-Juan A, Rubio C, Marin C, Martinez S, Al-Asmar N, Riboldi M, et al. Mitochondrial DNA content as a viability score in human euploid embryos: less is better. Fertil Steril. 2015;104:534-41.
133. Abou-Setta AM, Mansour RT, Al-Inany HG, Aboulghar MM, Aboulghar MA, Serour GI. Among women undergoing embryo transfer, is the probability of pregnancy and live birth improved with ultrasound guidance over clinical touch alone? A systemic review and meta-analysis of prospective randomized trials. Fertil Steril. 2007;88:333-41.
134. Brown J, Buckingham K, Buckett W, Abou-Setta AM. Ultrasound versus 'clinical touch' for catheter guidance during embryo transfer in women. Cochrane Database Syst Rev. 2016;3:CD006107.
135. Teixeira DM, Dassuncao LA, Vieira CV, Barbosa MAP, Coelho Neto MA, Nastri CO, et al. Ultrasound guidance during embryo transfer: a systematic review and meta-analysis of randomized controlled trials. Ultrasound Obstet Gynecol. 2015;45:139-48.
136. Sallam HN. Re: Ultrasound guidance during embryo transfer: a systematic review and meta-analysis of randomized controlled trials. Ultrasound Obstet Gynecol. 2015;45:757-8.
137. Cozzolino M, Vitagliano A, Di Giovanni MV, Lagana AS, Vitale SG, Blaganje M, et al. Ultrasound-guided embryo transfer: summary of the evidence and new perspectives. A systematic review and meta-analysis. Reprod Biomed Online. 2018;36:524-42.
138. Feichtinger W, Barad D, Feinman M, Barg P. The use of two-component fibrin sealant for embryo transfer. Fertil Steril. 1990;54:733-4.
139. Feichtinger W, Strohmer H, Radner KM, Goldin M. The use of fibrin sealant for embryo transfer: development and clinical studies. Hum Reprod. 1992;7:890-3.

140. Bontekoe S, Heineman MJ, Johnson N, Blake D. Adherence compounds in embryo transfer media for assisted reproductive technologies. Cochrane Database Syst Rev. 2014;2014(2):CD007421.
141. Fancsovits P, Lehner A, Murber A, Kaszas Z, Rigo J, Urbancsek J. Effect of hyaluronan-enriched embryo transfer medium on IVF outcome: a prospective randomized clinical trial. Arch Gynecol Obstet. 2015;291:1173-9.
142. Almog B, Levin I, Wagman I, Kapustiansky R, Schwartz T, Mey-Raz N, et al. Interval double transfer improves treatment success in patients with repeated IVF/ET failures. J Assist Reprod Genet. 2008;25:353-7.
143. Loutradis D, Drakakis P, Dallianidis K, Bletsa SR, Milingos S, Doumplis N, et al. A double embryo transfer on days 2 and 4 or 5 improves pregnancy outcome in patients with good embryos but repeated failures in IVF or ICSI. Clin Exp Obstet Gynecol. 2004;31:63-6.
144. Ashkenazi J, Yoeli R, Orvieto R, Shalev J, Ben-Rafael Z, Bar-Hava I. Double (consecutive) transfer of early embryos and blastocysts: aims and results. Fertil Steril. 2000;74:936-40.
145. Egbase PE, al-Sharhan M, al-Othman S, al-Mutawa M, Udo EE, Grudzinskas JG. Incidence of microbial growth from the tip of the embryo transfer catheter after embryo transfer in relation to clinical pregnancy rate following in-vitro fertilization and embryo transfer. Hum Reprod. 1996;11:1687-9.
146. Blockeel C, Drakopoulos P, Santos-Ribeiro S, Polyzos NP, Tournaye H. A fresh look at the freeze-all protocol: a SWOT analysis. Hum Reprod. 2016;31:491-7.
147. Shapiro BS, Daneshmand ST, Garner FC, Aguirre M, Hudson C. Clinical rationale for cryopreservation of entire embryo cohorts in lieu of fresh transfer. Fertil Steril. 2014;102:3-9.
148. Magdi Y, El-Damen A, Fathi AM, Abdelaziz AM, Abd-Elfatah Youssef M, Abd-Elmaged Abd-Allah A, et al. Revisiting the management of recurrent implantation failure through freeze-all policy. Fertil Steril. 2017;118:72-7.
149. Kahraman S. When to transfer? Fresh vs. deferred transfer. Reprod Biomed Online. 2018;36:e3.
150. Habana A, Palter SF. Is tubal embryo transfer of any value? A meta-analysis and comparison with the Society for Assisted Reproductive Technology database. Fertil Steril. 2001;76:286-93.
151. Tomaževič T, Ban-Frangež H, Virant-Klun I, Verdenik I, Požlep B, Vrtačnik-Bokal E. Septate, subseptate and arcuate uterus decrease pregnancy and live birth rates in IVF/ICSI. Reprod Biomed Online. 2010;21:700-5.
152. Marcus S, Al-Shawaf T, Brinsden P. The obstetric outcome of in vitro fertilization and embryo transfer in women with congenital uterine malformation. Am J Obstet Gynecol. 1996;175:85-9.
153. Jayaprakasan K, Chan YY, Sur S, Deb S, Clewes JS, Raine-Fenning NJ. Prevalence of uterine anomalies and their impact on early pregnancy in women conceiving after assisted reproduction treatment. Ultrasound Obstet Gynecol. 2011;37:727-32.
154. Practice Committee of the American Society for Reproductive Medicine. Uterine septum: a guideline. Fertil Steril. 2016;106:530-40.
155. Bosteels J, Kasius J, Weyers S, Broekmans FJ, Mol BWJ, D'Hooghe TM. Hysteroscopy for treating subfertility associated with suspected major uterine cavity abnormalities. Cochrane Database Syst Rev. 2015;(2):CD009461.
156. Hart R, Khalaf Y, Yeong CT, Seed P, Taylor A, Braude P. A prospective controlled study of the effect of intramural uterine fibroids on the outcome of assisted conception. Hum Reprod. 2001;11:2411-7.
157. Surrey ES, Minjarez DA, Stevens JM, Schoolcraft WB. Effect of myomectomy on the outcome of assisted reproductive technologies. Fertil Steril. 2005;83:1473-9.
158. Somigliana E, Vercellini P, Daguati R, Pasin R, De Giorgi O, Crosignani PG. Fibroids and female reproduction: a critical analysis of the evidence. Hum Reprod Update. 2007;13:465-76.
159. Pritts EA, Parker WH, Olive DL. Fibroids and infertility: an updated systematic review of the evidence. Fertil Steril. 2009;91:1215-23.
160. Sunkara SK, Khairy M, El-Toukhy T, Khalaf Y, Coomarasamy A. The effect of intramural fibroids without uterine cavity involvement on the outcome of IVF treatment: a systematic review and meta-analysis. Hum Reprod. 2010;25:418-29.
161. Somigliana E, De Benedictis S, Vercellini P, Nicolosi AE, Benaglia L, Scarduelli C, et al. Fibroids not encroaching the endometrial cavity and IVF success rate: a prospective study. Hum Reprod. 2011;26:834-9.
162. Yan L, Ding L, Li CH, Wang Y, Tang R, Chen ZJ. Effect of fibroids not distorting the endometrial cavity on the outcome of in vitro fertilization treatment: a retrospective cohort study. Fertil Steril. 2014;101:716-21.
163. Wang PH, Fuh JL, Chao HT, Liu WM, Cheng MH, Chao KC. Is the surgical approach beneficial to subfertile women with symptomatic extensive adenomyosis. Obstet Gynaecol. 2009;35:495-502.
164. Schlaff WD, Hurst BS. Preoperative sonographic measurement of endometrial pattern predicts outcome of surgical repair in patients with severe Asherman's syndrome. Fertil Steril. 1995;63:410-3.
165. Casper RF. It's time to pay attention to the endometrium. Fertil Steril. 2011;96:519-21.
166. Young SL. Oestrogen and progesterone action on endometrium: a translational approach to understanding endometrial receptivity. Reprod Biomed Online. 2013;27: 497-505.
167. Shen MS, Wang CW, Chen CH, Tzeng CR. New horizon on successful management for a woman with repeated implantation failure due to unresponsive thin endometrium: use of extended estrogen supplementation. J Obstet Gynaecol Res. 2013;39:1092-4.
168. Fanchin R, Righini C, Schönauer LM, Olivennes F, Cunha Filho JS, Frydman R. Vaginal versus oral E2 administration: effects on endometrial thickness, uterine perfusion, and contractility. Fertil Steril. 2001;76:994-8.
169. Qublan H, Amarin Z, Al-Qudah M, Diab F, Nawasreh M, Malkawi S, et al. Luteal phase support with GnRH-a improves implantation and pregnancy rates in IVF cycles with endometrium of ≤7 mm on day of egg retrieval. Hum Fertil (Camb.). 2008;11:43-7.
170. Jensen JR, Witz CA, Schenken RS, Tekmal RR. A potential role for colony stimulating factor 1 in the genesis of the early endometriotic lesion. Fertil Steril. 2010;93:251-6.
171. Barad DH, Yu Y, Kushnir VA, Shohat-Tal A, Lazzaroni E, Lee HJ, et al. A randomized clinical trial of endometrial perfusion

with granulocyte colony stimulating factor in in vitro fertilization cycles: impact on endometrial thickness and clinical pregnancy rates. Fertil Steril. 2014;101:710-5.

172. Chang Y, Li J, Chen Y, Wei L, Yang X, Shi Y, et al. Autologous platelet-rich plasma promotes endometrial growth and improves pregnancy outcome during in vitro fertilization. Int J Clin Exp Med. 2015;8:1286-90.
173. Wada I, Hsu CC, Williams G, Macnamee MC, Brinsden PR. The benefits of low-dose aspirin therapy in women with impaired uterine perfusion during assisted conception. Hum Reprod. 1994;9:1954-7.
174. Dentali F, Angeno W, Rezoagli E, Rancan E, Squizzato A, Middeldorp S, et al. Lose-dose aspirin for in vitro fertilization on intracytoplasmic sperm injection: a systematic review and a meta-analysis of the literature. J Thromb Haemost. 2012;10:2075-85.
175. Siristatidis CS, Dodd SR, Drakeley AJ. Aspirin for in vitro fertilisation. Cochrane Database Syst Rev. 2011;(8):CD004832.
176. Ohl J, Lefèbvre-Maunoury C, Wittemer C, Nisand G, Laurent MC, Hoffmann P. Nitric oxide donors for patients undergoing IVF. A prospective, double-blind, randomized, placebo-controlled trial. Hum Reprod. 2002;17:2615-20.
177. Letur-Konirsch H, Delanian S. Successful pregnancies after combined pentoxifylline-tocopherol treatment in women with premature ovarian failure who are resistant to hormone replacement therapy. Fertil Steril. 2003;79:439-41.
178. Lédée-Bataille N, Olivennes F, Lefaix JL, Chaouat G, Frydman R, Delanian S. Combined treatment by pentoxifylline and tocopherol for recipient women with a thin endometrium enrolled in an oocyte donation programme. Hum Reprod. 2002;17:1249-53.
179. Acharya S, Yasmin E, Balen AH. The use of combination of pentoxifylline and tocopherol in women with a thin endometrium undergoing assisted conception therapies—a report of 20 cases. Hum Fertil. 2009;12:198-203.
180. Firouzabadi RD, Davar R, Hojjat F, Mahdavi M. Effect of sildenafil citrate on endometrial preparation and outcome of frozen-thawed embryo transfer cycles: a randomized clinical trial. Iran J Reprod Med. 2013;11:151-8.
181. Sher G, Fisch JD. Effect of vaginal sildenafil on the outcome of in vitro fertilization (IVF) after multiple IVF failures attributed to poor endometrial development. Fertil Steril. 2002;78:1073-6.
182. Takasaki A, Tamura H, Miwa I, Taketani T, Shimamura K, Sugino N. Endometrial growth and uterine blood flow: a pilot study for improving gendometrial thickness in the patients with a thin endometrium. Fertil Steril. 2010;93:1851-8.
183. Shawki HE, Elmorsy M, Eissa MF. Routine office hysteroscopy prior to ICSI and its impact on assisted reproduction program outcome: a randomized controlled trial. Middle East Fertil Soc J. 2012;17:14-21.
184. El-Toukhy T, Campo R, Khalaf Y, Tabanelli C, Gianaroli L, Gordts SS, et al. Hysteroscopy in recurrent in-vitro fertilisation failure (TROPHY): a multicentre, randomised controlled trial. Lancet. 2016;387:2614-21.
185. Nastri CO, Lensen SF, Gibreel A, Raine-Fenning N, Ferriani RA, Bhattacharya S, et al. Endometrial injury in women undergoing assisted reproductive techniques. Cochrane Database Syst Rev. 2015;(3):CD009517.
186. Nagori CB, Panchal SY, Patel H. Endometrial regeneration using autologous adult stem cells followed by conception by in vitro fertilization in a patient of severe Asherman's syndrome. J Hum Reprod Sci. 2011;4:43-8.
187. Brännström M, Johannesson L, Dahm-Kahler P, Enskog A, Mölne J, Kvarnström N, et al. First clinical uterus transplantation trial: a six-month report. Fertil Steril. 2014;101: 1228-36.
188. Boomsma CM, Keay SD, Macklon NS. Peri-implantation glucocorticoid administration for assisted reproductive technology cycles. Cochrane Database Syst Rev. 2012;6: CD005996.
189. Siristatidis CS, Basios G, Pergialiotis V, Vogiatzi P. Aspirin for in vitro fertilisation. Cochrane Database Syst Rev. 2016;11: CD004832.
190. Nelson SM, Greer IA. The potential role of heparin in assisted conception. Hum Reprod Update. 2008;14:623-45.
191. Berker B, Taşkin S, Kahraman K, Taşkin EA, Atabekoğlu C, Sönmezer M. The role of low-molecular-weight heparin in recurrent implantation failure: a prospective, quasi-randomized, controlled study. Fertil Steril. 2011;95:2499-502.
192. Potdar N, Gelbaya TA, Konje JC, Nardo LG. Adjunct low-molecular-weight heparin two improve live birth rate after recurrent implantation failure: a systematic review and meta-analysis. Hum Reprod Update. 2013;19(6):674-84.
193. Ruiz JE, Kwak JY, Baum L, Gilman-Sachs A, Beaman KD, Kim YB, et al. Effect of intravenous immunoglobulin G on natural killer cell cytotoxicity in vitro in women with recurrent spontaneous abortion. J Reprod Immunol. 1996;31:125-41.
194. Ramos-Medina R, García-Segovia A, Gil J, Carbone J, de la Cruz AA, Seyfferth A, et al. Experience in IVIg therapy for selected women with recurrent reproductive failure and NK cell expansion. Am J Reprod Immunol. 2014;71:458-66.
195. Kwak JY, Kwak FM, Ainbinder SW, Ruiz AM, Beer AE. Elevated peripheral blood natural killer cells are effectively downregulated by immunoglobulin G infusion in women with recurrent spontaneous abortions. Am J Reprod Immunol. 1996;35(4):363-9.
196. Roussev RG, Ng SC, Coulam CB. Natural killer cell functional activity suppression by intravenous immunoglobulin, intralipid and soluble human leukocyte antigen-G. Am J Reprod Immunol. 2007;57:262-9.
197. Dakhly DMR, Bayoumi YA, Sharkawy M, Gad Allah SH, Hassan MA, Gouda HM, et al. Intralipid supplementation in women with recurrent spontaneous abortion and elevated levels of natural killer cells. Int J Gynecol Obstet. 2016;135:324-7.
198. Surrey ES, Silverberg KM, Surrey MW, Schoolcraft WB. Effect of prolonged gonadotropin-releasing hormone agonist therapy on the outcome of in vitro fertilization-embryo transfer in patients with endometriosis. Fertil Steril. 2002;78:699-704.
199. Garcia-Velasco JA, Mahutte NG, Corona J, Zúñiga V, Gilés J, Arici A, et al. Removal of endometriomas before in vitro fertilization does not improve fertility outcomes: a matched, case-control study. Fertil Steril. 2004;81:1194-7.
200. Wong BC, Gillman NC, Oehninger S, Gibbons WE, Stadtmauer LA. Results of in vitro fertilization in patients with endometriomas: is surgical removal beneficial? Am J Obstet Gynecol. 2004;191:597-606.

201. Strandell A, Lindhard A, Eckerlund I. Cost-effectiveness analysis of salpingectomy prior to IVF, based on a randomized controlled trial. Hum Reprod. 2005;20:3284-92.
202. Dubuisson JB, Chapron C, Morice P, Aubriot FX, Foulot H, de Jolinière JB. Laparoscopic salpingostomy: fertility results according to the tubal mucosal appearance. Hum Reprod. 1994;9:334-9.
203. Singhal V, Li TC, Cooke ID. An analysis of factors influencing the outcome of 232 consecutive tubal microsurgery cases. Br J Obstet Gynaecol. 1991;98:628-36.
204. Winston RM, Margara RA. Microsurgical salpingostomy is not an obsolete procedure. Br J Obstet Gynaecol. 1991;98:637-42.
205. Johnson N, van Voorst S, Sowter MC, Strandell A, Mol BWJ. Surgical treatment for tubal disease in women due to undergo in vitro fertilisation. Cochrane Database Syst Rev. 2010;2010(1):CD002125.
206. Sowter MC, Akande VA, Williams JA, Hull MG. Is the outcome of in-vitro fertilization and embryo transfer treatment improved by spontaneous or surgical drainage of a hydrosalpinx? Hum Reprod. 1997;12:2147-50.
207. Hammadieh A, Coomarasamy N, Ola A, Papaioannou S, Afnan M, Sharif K. Ultrasound-guided hydrosalpinx aspiration during oocyte collection improves pregnancy outcome in IVF: a randomized controlled trial. Hum Reprod. 2008;23:1113-7.

CHAPTER 62

Empty Follicle Syndrome

Ayesha Gupta, Kamini A Rao

INTRODUCTION

Empty follicle syndrome (EFS), a rare but frustrating complication of in vitro fertilization (IVF) leading to cycle cancellation, was first described by Coulam et al.[1] This rare event is responsible for substantial stress and anxiety to both the patients and the clinician during an assisted reproductive technology cycle.

DEFINITION

Empty follicle syndrome is a condition where no oocytes are retrieved despite repeated aspiration and flushing, after an apparently adequate ovarian response to stimulation, evidenced by serial ultrasound and adequate steroidogenesis. It was first described by Coulam et al. in 1986.[1]

INCIDENCE

Due to uncertainty of its existence and variability in the inclusion criteria across different studies, its prevalence varies over a wide range, from as low as 0.045 to 7% of IVF cycles.[2]

Also lack of the human chorionic gonadotropin (hCG) concentration threshold, to distinguish between genuine and false EFS, as well as the choice of the patient population are two key points responsible for this extreme variability in its incidence.

Considering only ovarian stimulation cycles with good ovarian response would underestimate the incidence of EFS, as in reality, the general IVF population includes at least about 30% of poor or suboptimal responders who are more likely to be affected with EFS than those with more than five well-developed follicles.

Kim and Jee (2012) in his study of 705 IVF cycles, excluding poor responders from the analysis, concentrated on the type of ovarian stimulation protocol, and demonstrated comparable EFS prevalence (2.4%) in both gonadotropin-releasing hormone (GnRH) antagonist and long GnRH agonist (GnRHa) protocols.[3]

More recently, in a study of 3,356 IVF cycles, Madani and Jahangiri (2015) reported a prevalence of 1.7%, with a slightly higher frequency with the miniflare GnRHa protocol,[4] as already known, this protocol is more often reserved for older women with a low ovarian reserve (Franco et al., 2006)[5] supporting the association of EFS with ovarian aging.

However contradicting this, Castillo et al. (2012)[6] compared 2,034 egg donor cycles (carried out among young high responders), receiving a GnRHa trigger, with 1,433 IVF cycles of women using their self-eggs (including poor responders of any age), triggered with recombinant hCG; and surprisingly, EFS prevalence was similar in both the patient populations, and higher overall than the prevalence reported in other studies (3.5% vs. 3.1%, respectively). This is the only study comparing EFS among egg donors and the general IVF patient population (women of any age and ovarian responsiveness).

In spite of being a rare phenomenon, EFS has profound implications for counseling about the future reproductive performance of the couple, especially when the chances of recurrence are high, especially in advanced age group patients. As per Velasco et al. study, it is estimated that patients with one EFS cycle have a 20% risk of recurrence in later IVF cycles.

CLASSIFICATION OF EMPTY FOLLICLE SYNDROME

Two classes of EFS can be defined as differentiated by the hormone levels on the day of the oocyte retrieval **(Table 1)**.

However, these definitions lack standardization as the threshold circulating level of hCG, in case of a hCG trigger to define a "correct trigger" is still uncertain, and a wide concentration range from 5 to 160 hCG IU/L after about 36 hours from exogenous hCG administration has been indicated by different investigators to differentiate between false (FEFS) and genuine empty follicle syndrome (GEFS).[4,7] Ndukwe et al. (1996) found a cut-off value of 10 mIU/L for

TABLE 1: Classification of empty follicle syndrome.

Genuine empty follicle syndrome	***False empty follicle syndrome***
It is defined as failure to retrieve oocytes from mature ovarian follicles, after triggering apparently normally developed follicles, in the presence of optimal beta hCG levels (in case of an hCG trigger) on the day of oocyte retrieval7 or in the presence of optimal LH levels 12 hours post agonist trigger	It is defined as failure to retrieve oocytes in the presence of low beta hCG levels, due to an error in administration or due to reduced bioavailability of the choriogonadotropin7 or inappropriately administered agonist trigger (e.g., hypogonadotropic hypogonadism group)
Rarest occurrence	Most common among EFS
Cycle cannot be rescued with a repeat trigger	Cycle can be rescued with a repeat trigger

(EFS: early follicle syndrome; hCG: human chorionic gonadotropin; LH: luteinizing hormone)

beta hCG in serum, 36 hours after an ovulatory dose of hCG, to have a 100% sensitivity and specificity for predicting EFS.

Similarly, post-agonist trigger serum luteinizing hormone (LH) and progesterone values defining an optimal trigger, to differentiate FEFS from GEFS are lacking currently. Some investigators have indicated an LH circulating level of 15 IU/L as the cutoff value,[8] but other studies have used different thresholds.[7]

In a review of EFS by Stevenson et al. (2008), incidence of GEFS and FEFS was 33% and 67%, respectively.[9]

ETIOPATHOPHYSIOLOGY

Empty follicle syndrome continues to be a rare condition of obscure etiology.

While some authors are totally skeptical about its existence,[2] various possible mechanisms have been attributed by others.

Pathophysiology of False Empty Follicle Syndrome Following hCG Trigger

Inadequate or Absent Luteinizing Hormone Surge

Throughout follicular development, the growing oocyte is surrounded by cumulus cells, and these are, in turn, linked to mural granulosa cells by cell-to-cell junctions. These junctions tightly bind the egg to the follicle wall. The physiological mid-cycle LH peak, mimicked by a bolus administration of hCG or GnRHa, brings about the rupture of these intercellular junctions and thus releases the cumulus-oocyte complex (COC) to freely float in the follicular fluid, and thereby be available for aspiration.[10]

The final triggering simulating the endogenous LH peak is a fundamental step of ovulation, and absence or any inadequacy of the LH or LH-like activity in IVF cycles, may result in failure to retrieve an oocyte (FEFS).

- *Errors in administration of the trigger:* False EFS is most likely associated with errors in the hCG administration, especially, when the patient or her partner has to self-administer the drug or, when it is administered by someone who lacks expertise. Urinary extract of hCG is available as a powder needing reconstitution before administration. Any errors in this step can deliver insufficient drug to the follicle and so FEFS can result.[11]
- *Error in timing of the injection:* Luteinizing hormone surge effect is fully displayed after 34–38 hours from injection, with a peak effect at about 36 hours.[12] Some patients may time the hCG injection incorrectly or some may refrain from informing nurses and physicians the actual hour at which they self-administered hCG.
- *Improper timing of the oocyte retrieval:* The effect of hCG may be impaired if oocyte retrieval is performed too early (before 34 hours from the injection), or too late (after 38 hours, when the largest follicles have already spontaneously ovulated).
- *Manufacturing defects and potency defects:* Such an event was described in a study showing the reduced in vivo biological activity of some batches of commercially available hCG.[13] Moreover, the manufacturers advise storing hCG medications away from direct light sources and at a temperature below 25°C; these conditions, if not met with, can alter the efficacy of the drug and hence can cause FEFS. *Poor metabolism of the bet-hCG trigger can also lead to FEFS.*
- *Low bioavailability due to variation in the absorption or clearance:* Subcutaneous administration of hCG injection in women with history of bariatric surgery may alter the absorption due to abdominal skin redundancy. In such patients intramuscular injections are preferred. In others, a very rapid clearance of hCG by the liver (desialylation of the hCG molecule subjects it to rapid clearance by the liver).[14]
- *Ovarian low bioavailability of hCG:* It may result in a unilateral EFS, as in ovarian torsion occurring between the time of trigger and follicular aspiration. Oocytes can be aspirated from the unaffected ovary.[15]
- For the above said reasons, FEFS can be rightly called—"the pharmaceutical industry syndrome".[13]

Pathophysiology of False Empty Follicle Syndrome Following GnRHa Trigger

- *Wrong trigger:* Gonadotropin-releasing hormone agonist trigger in a woman with hypogonadotropic

hypogonadism (WHO type 1 anovulation) or in an agonist protocol.
- *Inadequate response to agonist trigger:* Administering an agonist trigger in a woman with overly suppressed pituitary.

Pathophysiology of Genuine Empty Follicle Syndrome

Pathophysiology of GEFS is still poorly understood.

Recently, seven ZP1 mutations have been seen as the cause of genuine empty follicle syndrome. ZP1 encodes the ZP1 glycoproteins, these mutations are postulated to affect the secretion of zona pellucida proteins, this prevents zone pellucida formation.

Thus leading to defective oogenesis, folliculogenesis and subsequently impaired fertilization and implantation. In genuine empty follicle syndrome, the anti-ZP autoantibodies can induce GEFS.

Dysfunctional Folliculogenesis

It was observed that the granulosa cells of patients with recurrent EFS have an increased expression of some proapoptotic genes and a significant reduction in transcripts, whose products are responsible for normal follicular growth (e.g., PAPP-A, MAPK 3) than normal patients.[16] As a result, oocytes may be lost in the late folliculogenesis due to apoptosis.

- *Ovarian aging:*[17] A possible relationship exists between poor ovarian response and failure to retrieve oocytes, suggesting EFS may represent an advanced stage of ovarian aging, characterized by residual responsiveness of the granulosa cells while the oocytes fail to develop adequately.
- Faulty oocyte development and maturation[16]
- Strong attachment of the cumulus cell complexes to the follicular wall, dysfunctional signaling between the cumulus cells and the oocyte.[18]
- *Receptor polymorphism:* Novel mutation in LH/hCG receptor (LHCGR) was identified in two sisters with GEFS which is inherited as a recessive trait.[19] A mutation (p.N400S) in the gene coding for LHCGR was detected to be associated with GEFS and was inherited as a recessive trait. The mutation causes an irreversible block in the transmission pathway of LH signal, and so even repeat administration of hCG would be ineffective.[19]

A pericentric inversion in a fragile site of chromosome 2 (site 46, XX, inv(2) (p11q21) has been identified in a woman who had repeated GEFS.[20] Chromosome 2 has the genes coding for Inhibin βb, which are involved in the onset of premature ovarian insufficiency.[21] This may suggest a possible link between EFS and ovarian aging, precocious reduction of ovarian follicular reserve, or both.

Pathophysiology of EFS with Various Triggers

Physiology of EFS after triggering with hCG or a GnRHa is not the same.

Human Chorionic Gonadotropin Trigger

Human chorionic gonadotropin, when used as a surrogate for LH, as trigger, acts directly on the ovary. So, EFS in case of an hCG trigger can be said to be attributed to abnormal folliculogenesis or to the response of the ovary to the triggering stimulus or errors in administration of the trigger (dose, route, timing).

Gonadotropin-releasing Hormone Agonist Trigger

The pathology here may be the inability of the pituitary to release adequate LH sufficient to trigger ovulation or failure of the receptors on the ovary to mediate the action of LH or polymorphism of the LH β subunit gene.

Likely patients to have EFS with agonist trigger are:
- *Hypogonadotropic hypogonadism patients (WHO Type 1):* These patients are characterized by endogenous follicle-stimulating hormone (FSH) and LH <1.2 IU/L.
- The second is the possibility of EFS in a patient with borderline hypothalamic pituitary dysfunction, but with gonadotropin levels just above the hypogonadotropic hypothalamic level. The lower production of LH in these patients would allow for follicular development and initial luteinization, but would be insufficient to complete cumulus cell expansion and its loosening from the follicular wall. Hence, depending upon the degree of response of the pituitary to the agonist trigger, a GEFS or FEFS may occur.[6]
- A temporary state of hyposensitivity of the pituitary to the agonist trigger may exist in some cycles, so in such cases an hCG trigger may recover mature oocytes.
- *Patients with GnRH receptor polymorphism:* These women need a high dose of the agonist to activate the receptor.
- Women with a variant LH β gene polymorphism, especially the homozygous form, have the less bioactive LH molecule and so are at risk for a blunted response after an agonist trigger.

RISK FACTORS FOR EMPTY FOLLICLE SYNDROME

No definitive risk factors to predict the incidence of EFS before the start of controlled ovarian stimulation have been elicited.

However, the possible risk factors include:[17]
- Previous history of EFS
- Advanced age with poor ovarian reserve (37.7 ± 6 years vs. 34.2 ± 6 years, p <0.001).

- Ovarian resistance to various stimulations
- Obesity
- Longer duration of infertility (8.8 ± 10.6 years vs. 6.3 ± 8.4 years, p <0.05)
- Higher baseline FSH levels (8.7 ± 4.7 IU/L vs. 6.7 ± 2.9 IU/L, p <0.001)
- Lower estradiol levels on the day of trigger (499.9 ± 480.9 pg/mL vs. 1,516.3 ± 887.5 pg/mL, p <0.001).

DIAGNOSIS AND PREVENTION

At the time of oocyte retrieval, if no oocytes can be retrieved after aspirating a good number of follicles, EFS can be diagnosed by detecting hCG in urine or follicular fluid (using a rapid home pregnancy kit) or blood (>40 mIU/L), to exclude incorrect or inadequate trigger administration. Presence of hCG in these samples more likely suggests a GEFS and the absence or suboptimal values of hCG suggests FEFS.

For an agonist trigger, a 12-hour post-trigger LH concentration at or near 15 mIU/mL is used as a threshold between adequate and inadequate response to the GnRHa trigger.[22,23]

A 12 hour post-trigger progesterone concentration (progesterone level >3.5 ng/mL 8–12 hours after trigger) can be a complementary indicator of trigger response over LH alone.[24] Luteinization of the follicle releases progesterone. Patients with a higher number of follicles will have higher values of progesterone. An appropriately elevated post-trigger progesterone concentration associated with a borderline or even low LH concentration can still result in successful oocyte retrieval. But, conversely, low post-trigger progesterone concentration associated with LH concentration >15 mIU/mL might suggest an inadequate response.

When interpreting post-trigger LH and progesterone concentrations, considering the time interval between the trigger and the post-trigger assay is crucial, especially true for LH, as peak LH levels occur 4 hours after agonist trigger followed by a rapid decline,[25] making LH highly dependent on the time of measurement, in relation to the time of trigger. Shorter time intervals (e.g., 4–8 hours) will result in higher LH values and progesterone results. Longer post-trigger intervals (e.g., 12–15 hours) will result in lower serum LH values and higher serum progesterone values.

MANAGEMENT OF EFS IN THE CURRENT CYCLE

Though EFS can be a rare event, it can be a frustrating complication of IVF, leading to cycle cancellation. So, every attempt to rescue the cycle should be made **(Flowchart 1)**.

- *Re-administering hCG and reaspiration in a case of FEFS:* A repeat, rescue dose of hCG in cases of FEFS was first proposed by Ndukwe et al. in 1997, and this has remained as the consensus solution in the literature since that time.[11,14,26-28] During the second retrieval attempt, 24–36 hours later, follicles from the previously aspirated ovary

Flowchart 1: Management of empty follicle syndrome.

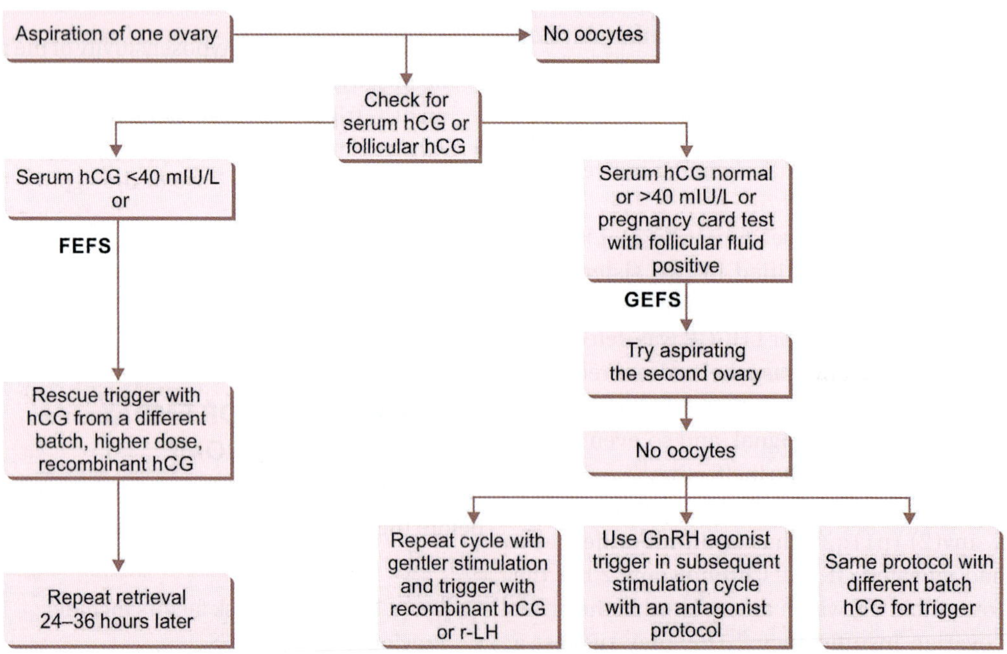

(FEFS: false empty follicle syndrome; GEFS: genuine empty follicle syndrome; hCG: human chorionic gonadotropin; r-LH: recombinant-luteinizing hormone)

should be reaspirated. Mucification of the cumulus cells in response to circulating hCG allows dissociation of the cumulus-oocyte complex, and collection with a second aspiration may be possible. The rescue dose may be of a higher dose or from a different batch of urinary hCG or switched to recombinant hCG. A recent review of literature has documented that 42.8% of cycles (6 out of 14) rescued with repeat hCG resulted in a healthy live born fetus.[9]

Contrary to the above findings, Reichman et al. in his large study, presented a less optimistic picture with rescue hCG trigger. The probable theories proposed for this included a 72 hour unintended "coasting" period, thereby resulting in the post maturity of some oocytes. However, the success rates should further be investigated and the patients should be thoroughly counseled.

- *Delayed retrieval if there was an error in timing:* It may be hypothesized that cumulus expansion, which allows the oocyte to detach from the follicular wall, may also require longer time periods in certain patients.

MANAGEMENT OF SUBSEQUENT CYCLES AFTER EMPTY FOLLICLE SYNDROME

- Check for possible risk factors before the start of the stimulation.
- Triggering the next cycle with recombinant hCG or recombinant LH
- Gonadotropin-releasing hormone agonist trigger (GnRHa trigger).

Agonist trigger to induce, the more physiological LH surge, in an antagonist cycle has been proposed as one of the strategies to prevent EFS.[29-31]

PROGNOSIS

Counseling of the couples who may be at risk for EFS is very important. Though EFS may be a sporadic event with a self-limiting phenomena, it may recur in 15.8–31% of cases.[17] This recurrence increases with increasing age suggesting the association of EFS with ovarian aging.

KEY POINTS

- EFS is a condition where no oocytes are retrieved despite repeated aspiration and flushing after apparently adequate response to stimulation.
- Prevalence varies from 0.45 to 7% of IVF cycles.
- Genuine EFS is failure to retrieve oocytes from mature ovarian follicles, after triggering apparently normally developed follicles. It is a rare phenomenon, cycle cannot be rescued with a repeat trigger.
- False EFS failure to retrieve oocytes in the presence of low beta hCG levels, due to an error in administration or due to reduced bioavailability of the choriogonadotropin or inappropriately administered agonist trigger.
- Cut-off value of 10 mIU/L for beta hCG in serum, 36 hours after an ovulatory dose of hCG, is found to have a 100% sensitivity and specificity for predicting EFS. Wide range of 5–160 hCG IU/L is documented.
- FEFS causes can be attributed to errors in HCG administration, its dosage, its bioavailability, error in timing of hCG administration, improper timing of oocyte administration, manufacturing defects, its potency or ovarian low bioavailability of hcG.
- *GEFS:* Recent studies attribute ZP1 mutation leading to poor zona pellucida formation as the cause, other causes could be ovarian aging, temporary pituitary hyposensitivity to agonist trigger, faulty oocyte maturation and development, strong cumulus cell complexes attached to the follicular wall, GnRH receptor polymorphism or variant LH Beta gene polymorphism.
- EFS with GnRHa trigger can be due to inadequate release of LH by pituitary. This can be found in hypogonadotropic hypogonadism cases, with borderline hypothalamic pituitary dysfunction, GnRH receptor polymorphism or variant LH Beta gene polymorphism.
- Attempt to rescue a cycle in GEFS by readministering hCG (rescue dose) of different batch/higher dosage/recombinant hcG and attempting ovum pick up after 24–36 hours.
- For subsequent cycles check for risk factors, trigger with recombinant hcG or recombinant LH or GnRHa trigger in an antagonist cycle.
- Counsel the couple for recurrence risk in GEFS, which is 15.8–31% of cases.

REFERENCES

1. Coulam CB, Bustillo M, Schulman JD. Empty follicle syndrome. Fertil Steril. 1986;46:1153-5.
2. Ben-Shlomo I, Schiff E, Levran D, Ben-Rafael Z, Mashiach S, Dor J. Failure of oocyte retrieval during in vitro fertilization: a sporadic event rather than a syndrome. Fertil Steril. 1991;55:324-7.
3. Kim JH, Jee BC. Empty follicle syndrome. Clin Exp Reprod Med. 2012;39:132-7.
4. Madani T, Jahangiri N. Empty follicle syndrome: the possible cause of occurrence. Oman Med J. 2015;30:417-20.
5. Franco JG, Baruffi RLR, Mauri AL, Toftager M, Pinborg A, Homburg R, et al. GnRH agonist versus GnRH antagonist in poor ovarian responders: a meta-analysis. Reprod Biomed Online. 2006;13:618-27.
6. Castillo JC, Garcia-Velasco J, Humaidan P. Empty follicle syndrome after GnRHa triggering versus hCG triggering in COS. J Assist Reprod Genet. 2012;29:249-53.
7. Stevenson TL, Lashen H. Empty follicle syndrome: the reality of a controversial syndrome, a systematic review. Fertil Steril. 2008;90:691-8.

8. Blazquez A, Guillen JJ, Colome C, Coll O, Vassena R, Vernaeve V. Empty follicle syndrome prevalence and management in oocyte donors. Hum Reprod. 2014;29:2221-7.
9. Kummer NE, Feinn RS, Griffin DW, Nulsen JC, Benadiva CA, Engmann LL. Predicting successful induction of oocyte maturation after gonadotropin-releasing hormone agonist (GnRHa) trigger. Hum Reprod. 2013;28:152-9.
10. Choi J, Smitz J. Luteinizing hormone and human chorionic gonadotropin: origins of difference. Mol Cell Endocrinol. 2014;383:203-13.
11. Quintans CJ, Donaldson MJ, Blanco LA, Pasqualini RS. Empty follicle syndrome due to human errors: its occurrence in an in vitro fertilization programme. Hum Reprod. 1998;13:2703-5.
12. Meniru GI, Craft IL. Evidence from a salvaged treatment cycle supports an aetiology for the empty follicle syndrome that is related to terminal follicular developmental events. Hum Reprod. 1997;12:2385-7.
13. Zegers-Hochschild F, Fernandez E, Mackenna A, Fabres C, Altieri E, Lopez T. The empty follicle syndrome: a pharmaceutical industry syndrome. Hum Reprod. 1995;10:2262-5.
14. Ndukwe G, Thornton S, Fishel S, Fabres C, Altieri E, Lopez T. Curing empty follicle syndrome. Hum Reprod. 1997;12:21-3.
15. Stefunidis K, Grammatis M, Pappas K, Haidopoulos D, Chronopoulos K, Pantos K, Diakomanolis E. Empty follicle syndrome associated with ovarian torsion in an in vitro fertilization program. JSLS. 2002;6(3):215-6. PMID: 12166759; PMCID: PMC3043427.
16. Inan MS, Al-Hassan S, Ozand P, Coskun S. Transcriptional profiling of granulosa cells from a patient with recurrent empty follicle syndrome. Reprod Biomed Online. 2006;13:481-91.
17. Baum M, Machtinger R, Yerushalmi GM, Maman E, Seidman DS, Dor J, et al. Recurrence of empty follicle syndrome with stimulated IVF cycles. Gynecol Endocrinol. 2012;28:293-5.
18. Tharasanit T, Colleoni S, Galli C, Colenbrander B, Stout TAE. Protective effects of the cumulus-corona radiata complex during vitrification of horse oocytes. 3(2009) Bioscientifica Reproduction 10.1530/rep-08-0333 http://dx.doi.org/10.1530/rep-08-033.
19. Yariz KO, Walsh T, Uzak A, Spiliopoulos M, Duman D, Onalan G, et al. Inherited mutation of the luteinizing hormone/choriogonadotropin receptor (LHCGR) in empty follicle syndrome. Fertil Steril. 2001;96:125-30.
20. Vujisic S, Stipoljev F, Bauman R, Dmitrovic R, Jezek D. Pericentric inversion of chromosome 2 in a patient with the empty follicle syndrome: case report. Hum Reprod. 2005;20:2552-5.
21. Shelling AN, Burton KA, Chand AL, van Ee CC, France JT, Farquhar CM, et al. Inhibin: a candidate gene for premature ovarian failure. Hum Reprod. 2000;15:2644-9.
22. Meyer L, Murphy LA, Gumer A, Reichman DE, Rosenwaks Z, Cholst IN. Risk factors for a suboptimal response to gonadotropin-releasing hormone agonist trigger during in vitro fertilization cycles. Fertil Steril. 2015;104:637-42.
23. Shapiro BS, Daneshmand ST, Restrepo H, Reichman DE, Rosenwaks Z, Cholst IN. Efficacy of induced luteinizing hormone surge after "trigger" with gonadotropin-releasing hormone agonist. Fertil Steril. 2011;95:826-8.
24. Kummer NE, Feinn RS, Griffin DW, Nulsen JC, Benadiva CA, Engmann LL. Predicting successful induction of oocyte maturation after gonadotropin-releasing hormone agonist (GnRHa) trigger. Hum Reprod. 2013;28: 152-9.
25. Fauser BC, de Jong D, Olivennes F, Wramsby H, Tay C, Itskovitz-Eldor J, et al. Endocrine profiles after triggering of final oocyte maturation with GnRH agonist after cotreatment with the GnRH antagonist ganirelix during ovarian hyperstimulation for in vitro fertilization. J Clin Endocrinol Metab. 2002;87:709-15.
26. Snaifer E, Hugues JN, Poncelet C, Sifer C, Pasquier M, Cedrin-Durnerin I. "Empty follicle syndrome" after human error: pregnancy obtained after repeated oocyte retrieval in a gonadotropin-releasing hormone antagonist cycle. Fertil Steril. 2008;90(3):850.
27. Quintans CJ, Donaldson MJ, Blanco LA, Pasqualini RS. Empty follicle syndrome due to human errors: its occurrence in an in vitro fertilization programme. Hum Reprod 1998;13:2703-5.
28. Reichman DE, Hornstein MD, Jackson KV, Racowsky C. Empty follicle syndrome—does repeat administration of hCG really work? Fertil Steril. 2010;94:375-7.
29. De Jong D, Van Hooren EG, Macklon NS, Mannaerts BM, Fauser BC. Pregnancy and birth after GnRH agonist treatment for induction of final oocyte maturation in a woman undergoing ovarian stimulation for ICSI, using a GnRH Antagonist to prevent premature LH surge: a case report. J Assist Reprod Genet. 2001;18(1):30-3.
30. Dai C, Chen Y, Hu L, Du J, Gong F, Dai J, et al. ZP1 mutations are associated with empty follicle syndrome: evidence for the existence of an intact oocyte and a zona pellucida in follicles up to the early antral stage. A case report. Hum Reprod. 2019;34(11):2201-7.
31. Hasegawa A, Tanaka H, Shibahara H. Infertility and Immunocontraception based on zona pellucida. Reprod Med Biol. 2013;13(1):1-9.

CHAPTER

63

Role of Aneuploidy Screening in Preimplantation Embryos

Jwal Banker, Manish Banker, Parul Arora

INTRODUCTION

Aneuploidy is the presence of abnormal number of chromosomes, either extra or missing, in the cell nucleus. It occurs due to failure of separation of the paired chromosomes during cell division (nondisjunction).[1] It is seen commonly in human oocytes and embryos. It is believed that most embryos with aneuploidy either fail to implant, undergo developmental arrest, or miscarry. Such chromosomal defects compromise the viability of embryos and explain the low success rates of in vitro fertilization (IVF) and the low fecundity in natural conceptions. Therefore, to obtain a healthy live birth in IVF, it is important that the embryos transferred are chromosomally normal.

Traditionally, the most competent embryos used in IVF have been evaluated and selected for transfer using morphology-based grading as the primary technique. Recent advances in technologies in the fields of genomics, transcriptomics, proteomics, metabolomics, and time-lapse imaging have assisted in embryo selection. Evaluation of chromosome copy number and transfer of only euploid embryos, also known as aneuploidy screening or testing, is now gradually becoming the preferred modality to screen and select the embryos.

Aneuploidy screening or preimplantation genetic screening (PGS) has been advocated for use in conjunction with IVF. It involves identification and transfer of only euploid embryos where parents are chromosomally normal to improve the likelihood for a successful pregnancy. Preimplantation genetic diagnosis (PGD) on the other hand involves looking for a specific mutation or an unbalanced chromosomal component in the embryo for which the parents are carriers. Both the terms PGS and PGD are now replaced by the term PGT (preimplantation genetic testing) as advocated by the International Committee for Monitoring Assisted Reproductive Technologies (ICMART) glossary 2017.[2] PGT is defined as a test performed to analyze the DNA from oocytes (polar bodies) or embryos (cleavage stage or blastocyst) for aneuploidies (PGT-A), single gene disorders (PGT-M), and chromosomal structural rearrangements (PGT-SR).

ORIGIN OF ANEUPLOIDY

Aneuploidy in preimplantation embryos (whether IVF or conceived naturally) can primarily arise during three developmental stages:

1. The premeiotic divisions during gametogenesis
2. The meiotic division of gametogenesis
3. The early mitotic divisions during embryogenesis stage.

Understanding the mechanisms behind the defects in segregation of chromosomes at these stages gives insight into the role of PGT when applied in clinical practice.

Abnormal separation of chromosomes in oogenic meiosis-I and meiosis-II is the most common cause of aneuploidy in human preimplantation embryos. More than 20% of oocytes from patients with an average age under 35 years have been reported to be aneuploid in cytogenetic studies on oocytes and first polar bodies (PB1) from assisted conception cycles.[3,4] This percentage of aneuploidy increases significantly with age, to >65% of oocytes in advanced maternal age of >40 years, and 80% in the age group of 43 years and older.[5,6]

In contrast to oocytes, incidence of aneuploidy in sperms is only around 4–14%.[7,8]

As compared to meiotic, mitotic nondisjunction during embryogenesis yields two or more distinct cell lines resulting in both normal and abnormal cells in the same embryo, called as mosaic embryos. The proportions of these normal and aneuploid cells in such an embryo may vary, depending on the point at which the failed separation of chromosomes has occurred.

PROPOSED INDICATIONS FOR PGT-A

By definition, PGT-A (as compared to PGT-M) is performed in patients having no known chromosomal anomaly, mutation, or other genetic abnormalities. As such, there are no specific indications for PGT-A. It should be considered in patients in whom the risk of having an aneuploid embryo is considered to be higher, such as:

- Advanced maternal age >35 years
- Patients with a history of recurrent early pregnancy loss
- Recurrent implantation failures
- Previous trisomic pregnancy
- Severe male factor infertility.

COUNSELING

Proper counseling is very critical because IVF patients planned for PGT-A do not have any inherent specific identifiable genetic abnormality, and PGT-A is recommended in order to detect aneuploidies so that the chances of pregnancy may be increased. The American Society for Reproductive Medicine (ASRM) Practice Committee guidelines[9] recommended certain key points that must be included at a minimum in the counseling before PGT **(Box 1)**.

TECHNIQUES AND LIMITATIONS

Biopsy for PGT is a two-step micromanipulation process that involves zona penetration and removal of one or more cells for chromosome analysis. The penetration or breaching of zona pellucida can be performed by different methods such as mechanical pipette-induced breakage, controlled acid tyrode treatment to dissolve part of zona, or by laser assistance. Various animals and humans have reported that zona breaching by the laser has no detrimental effects on embryo development, provided it is used appropriately.[10,11] Specialized micromanipulation pipettes are used to separate and remove the required cells from the embryo. Although PGT can be performed at any developmental stage starting from mature oocyte stage (metaphase II) to the blastocyst stage, generally this period has been divided into three discrete stages for clinical use: (1) Polar body (oocyte and/or zygote), (2) cleavage stage (day 3 embryo), and (3) blastocyst (day 5 or 6 embryo). Since each of these three stages is biologically different, PGT performed in each stage has different diagnostic relevance as well as limitations, both in terms of information gained and the risk to the viability of the embryo.

BOX 1: Key points that must be included in the counseling before preimplantation genetic testing (PGT).

- The risks associated with IVF
- The option of choosing not to proceed with IVF and PGT
- The risks associated with embryo biopsy and extended culture
- The possibility of a false-positive result that may lead to the discard of a normal embryo
- The possibility of a false-negative result that may lead to the transfer of an abnormal embryo
- The possibility that testing may yield inconclusive results
- The possibility that no embryos may be transferred if all appear abnormal
- Options relating to prenatal diagnostic testing and their associated risks:
  - Chorionic villus sampling
  - Amniocentesis
  - Ultrasonography with or without additional blood tests
  - No prenatal testing
- The nature and quality of the available evidence with regard to live-birth rates after IVF with PGT
- The disposition of embryos not transferred (e.g., discard, cryopreservation, research, or donation) as and when appropriate

(IVF: in vitro fertilization)
Source: ASRM Practice Committee guidelines[9]

Polar Body Biopsy

Through biopsy and analysis of the first and second polar body (PB1 and PB2), an indirect interpretation of the chromosome of the corresponding oocyte can be obtained. This helps in detecting aneuploidy of maternal origin in the embryos.[12] Removal of the polar bodies from a human oocyte does not have any deleterious effect on the development of the embryo, as these bodies have no role to play in fertilization or further embryonic growth.[13] There are two strategies for PB biopsy: (1) Biopsy of only PB1 and (2) combined biopsy of PB1 and PB2. However, isolated biopsy of PB1 has limited applicability as only metaphase-I errors can be detected in this, not including the chromatid segregation errors. Handyside et al.[14] have reported that biopsy of only PB1 can miss almost 30% of aneuploidy of maternal origin.

The other strategy of biopsy and analysis of both polar bodies can result in better detection of maternal-origin aneuploidy. This can be laborious and requires skill due to multiple micromanipulations steps which may be required—intracytoplasmic sperm injection (ICSI), PB1, PB2, and blastomere biopsy (in case of noninformative or ambiguous PB result). To minimize the multiple manipulations of sequential PB biopsy, there is a possibility of biopsying both PBs on the day of fertilization. However, there is a chance that PB1 may degenerate by that time, resulting in diagnostic failure. Another important limitation of polar body biopsy technique (either single or both) is that no information can be obtained on aneuploidies arising from paternal origin or postfertilization in the embryo.

Cleavage Stage Embryo Biopsy

Till some time back, cleavage stage embryo biopsy was the most common type of embryo biopsy performed worldwide. In a typical cleavage stage embryo biopsy, one or two blastomeres are taken from six to eight cell embryos. This is performed on day 3 following fertilization. Although the detection of aneuploidies of maternal and paternal origin as well as postzygotic origin is possible, it is not always possible to distinguish between these. The major shortcoming of cleavage stage biopsy results from the presence of the phenomenon of chromosomal mosaicism in the embryo, as discussed earlier. Mosaicism can result in both false positive

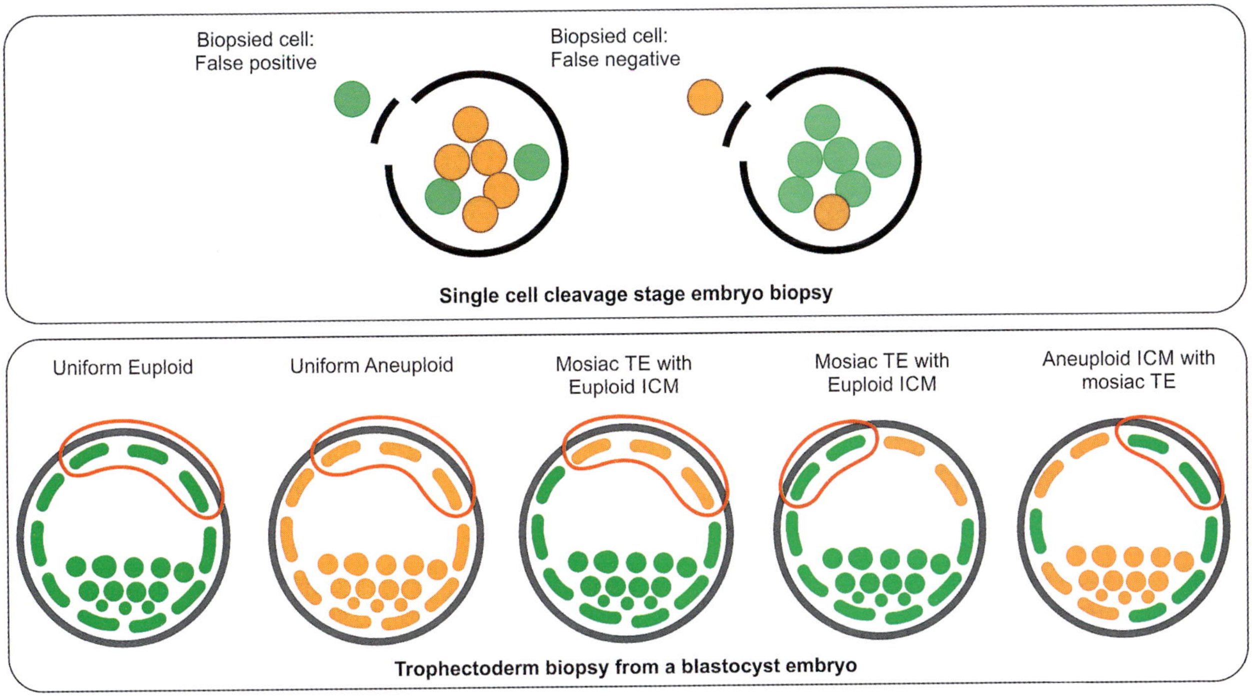

Fig. 1: Possible misdiagnosis following preimplantation genetic testing (PGT) biopsy. (ICM: inner cell mass; TE: trophectoderm;)

and false negative results in a single cell or even two- cell biopsy **(Fig. 1)**. Further, a study by Liu et al.[15] has shown that the potential for the embryo to continue to develop and implant can be adversely affected by cleavage stage biopsy, and this deleterious effect is directly proportional to the size of the sample removed from the embryo. The cleavage stage biopsy strategy has now become less popular because of these two reasons.

Blastocyst Stage Biopsy

This is the most preferred stage for embryo biopsy, and it involves the biopsying of 6–10 trophectoderm (TE) cells from a day 5 or day 6 blastocyst. Just like cleavage stage, TE biopsy can detect aneuploidy occurring at gametogenesis stage as well as embryogenesis stage. Compared to other biopsy stages, it is highly reliable as it involves the retrieval of up to 10 cells without causing any damage to the inner cell mass (ICM) which gives rise to the fetus. The conventional method for TE biopsy involves the partial zona dissection using laser, followed by a period of culture to allow blastocyst growth. This causes herniation of cells through this laser-induced artificial breach. These cells herniating through the breach (approximately 6–10 cells) are then easily biopsied by excision or aspiration using specialized micromanipulation tools with or without the aid of a laser shot. Analysis of multiple cells decreases the chances of missing potential mosaicism and eliminates the extreme sensitivity of single cell diagnosis. The concern of nonreflection of genetic composition of ICM[16] was negated by Johnson et al.[17] suggesting 100% concordance between TE and ICM genetic makeup with exception of structural abnormalities. A major benefit of blastocyst biopsy, compatibility of embryo to grow to the blastocyst stage, is also one of its main limiting factors, as not all good quality day 3 embryos will grow to blastocyst stage. If very few blastocysts are available, biopsy cannot be used for selection purposes. Moreover, another issue faced with blastocyst biopsy is that of time constraint while awaiting the diagnosis. This leads to the need for cryopreservation of biopsied blastocysts. Hence, the subsequent effects of cryopreservation as well as thawing on the embryo viability also become an issue for concern. However, such concerns have been taken care of by improved culture methods, improved outcomes of cryopreservation and thawing, and methods of rapid molecular analysis, thus making blastocyst biopsy the preferred option.[18]

The advantages and disadvantages of biopsy for PGT at different stages are compared in **Table 1**.

DIFFERENT METHODS FOR CHROMOSOMAL ANALYSIS

Once the oocyte or embryo is biopsied and material is available for analysis, a predefined screening protocol should be used. A cytogenetic technique with very high sensitivity and specificity is required for PGT, as it involves analysis of one or only a few cells to define the karyotype and identify chromosomal abnormalities. The testing process should also be fast enough so that fresh embryo transfer (ET) can be carried out if so desired. The classic karyotyping methods cannot be used for testing as it is

TABLE 1: Advantages and disadvantages of different biopsy techniques for preimplantation genetic screening.

Technique	Detail	Advantages	Disadvantages
PB biopsy	• Earliest stage at which cells can be obtained for genetic testing • Based on assumption that the chromosomal make-up of PBs reflects that of the oocyte[20]	• Provides maximum time for genetic analysis in case of fresh embryo transfer • Least invasive, as PBs do not make a physical contribution to the embryo[20] and hence, no effect on fertilization rates or further embryo development[21]	• Detects aneuploidies originating only from maternal origin which in fact accounts for only 66% of embryonic aneuploidies,[22] leaving one-third of aneuploidies undetected • Not very cost-effective and labor intensive as two PBs are sampled per oocyte, and not all of them will develop into embryos
Blastomere biopsy	• Biopsied on day 3 postinsemination at the 6- to 10-cell stage • Removal of blastomeres is facilitated by incubation in Ca^{2+}/Mg^{2+}-free medium, which disrupts cellular junctions[23]	As sample is taken from embryo itself, it allows aneuploidies of both maternal and paternal origin to be detected	• Requires removal of a significant proportion of the embryo's cells, which may adversely impact embryo developmental viability and implantation rates[24] • Normal reported embryos can be mosaic and mosaicism is seen up to 29% of preimplantation embryos at cleavage stage[25,26]
Blastocyst biopsy	• Hole drilled in the zona pellucida on day 3, then cultured to blastocyst stage (days 5–6) • Some trophectoderm cells herniate through the hole in the zona pellucida which are removed, leaving the inner cell mass intact	• Randomized controlled trial evidence of no adverse impact on embryo implantation potential[27] • Allows more cells to be taken for • analysis • Greater efficiency as many cleavage stage embryos do not grow till blastocyst[28]	• The results of biopsy may not come same day, mostly necessitating vitrification of embryos and transfer in subsequent cycle[24,25] • Trophectoderm biopsy may not be • representative of the inner cell mass[18] • Mosaicism is still an issue[19]

(PB: polar body)

difficult to achieve adequate metaphase spreads with very limited number of cells.[29]

Fluorescent In Situ Hybridization

The first technique used for PGT in 1992 was fluorescent in situ hybridization (FISH) for sex selection to prevent the X-linked recessive disorders.[30] This molecular cytogenetic tool is highly sensitive and comparatively inexpensive, and it assists in determining the number of chromosome copies in the cell (ploidy) as well as structural abnormalities in metaphase chromosomes and interphase nuclei.[31] The process involves fixation of the cells to be analyzed to a glass slide followed by visual assessment after hybridization with fluorescent DNA probes specific for each chromosome. Earlier, only 2 sets with 5 chromosomes (typically for chromosomes 13, 16, 18, 21, 22 or chromosomes 13, 18, 21, X, and Y) were used in a test. Later, 12 chromosomes could be analyzed (X, Y, 2, 4, 13, 15, 16, 18, 19, 20, 21, and 22) at the cleavage stage. This allowed detection of almost 91% of blastocyst stage embryos with chromosomal abnormalities.

However, in past two decades, multiple randomized controlled trials (RCTs) have found that FISH-based PGT did not improve clinical outcomes, including live birth rates (LBRs).[32-34] This could be due to the limited number of chromosomes that can be analyzed in FISH[35] or the early stage of embryogenesis at which the biopsy is performed. Further, because of the very limited number of cells that are assessed, mosaicism may also be responsible for this.[36] There are also some technical disadvantages of FISH. For example, the signals can overlap (so that two different signals are visualized as one, or three signals as two). The signal can also "split" depending on the current cell cycle stage of the cell being analyzed, thus making a single signal visualized as two different signals.[37]

This has led to more usage of microarray-based tests using the whole genome amplification (WGA) technology.

Whole Genome Amplification

The advent of WGA technology has significantly improved the efficacy for molecular karyotyping for the complete set of chromosomes. All 23 pairs of chromosomes can be analyzed simultaneously and with greater accuracy by microarray-based tests using this technology, resulting in a lower rate of misdiagnosis.[38]

The process involves transfer of the cell(s) to a microfuge tube and cell lysis followed by genome amplification. The genome amplification can be performed either by polymerase chain reaction (PCR) or multiple displacement amplification (MDA), which can yield >20 µg of DNA from a single cell. This DNA is then used for WGA studies

TABLE 2: Technical aspects of different genetic tests used in PGT.

aCGH	• Whole-genome amplification (WGA) of DNA from the biopsied cell(s)[51] • Followed by fluorescent labeling, denaturation, and hybridization to an array platform containing thousands of DNA probes specific to each of the human chromosomes • Then subjected to fluorescent intensity scanning for each probe on the array • By comparison of these intensities with that of control sample, copy number of each chromosome in the biopsied cell is determined[52,53]
qPCR	• Preamplification of DNA from the biopsied cell/s • Followed by a high-order multiplex PCR reaction that amplifies several loci from each chromosome • Real-time qPCR quantifies each product, allowing a comparison across the genome[43]
SNP arrays	• WGA of DNA from the biopsied cell/s • Followed by fragmentation and hybridization to SNP array platform containing probes for >500,000 different SNP sites across the genome • Followed by extension and staining step • SNP sites of A/T nucleotides are labeled with a red fluorochrome, and G/C nucleotides are labeled with a green fluorochrome • With intensity measurement of red-to-green fluorescence at each SNP site on the array, it is possible to simultaneously genotype >500,000 SNPs in each sample
NGS	• WGA of DNA from the biopsied cell/s • Followed by fragmentation and tagging with a specific barcode • Barcoded DNA fragments mixed together and sequenced in parallel • Specialized computer software segregates the results according to biopsy sample by reading the tracking barcodes • Followed by comparison of each fragment against a reference human genome • Trisomy or monosomy is identified based on a corresponding increase or decrease in the number of aligned sequences

(aCGH: array comparative genomic hybridization; NGS: next-generation sequencing; PGT: preimplantation genetic testing; qPCR: quantitative polymerase chain reaction; SNP: single nucleotide polymorphism)

to establish copy number of each chromosome with high accuracy.

The following are the different techniques utilizing genome amplification that are used for PGT **(Table 2)**.

Comparative Genomic Hybridization

This method was originally developed to carry out molecular karyotyping of tumor cells.[39,40] It has now been successfully used for the analysis of PGT samples.[41] The sample DNA is first amplified and then this amplified DNA and a normal reference sample are labeled separately with different fluorescent dyes. The material is then cohybridized to an array of several thousand probes printed on a glass slide, corresponding to known regions of the genome. Quantitative image analysis is used for fluorescent intensity scanning for each of these probes, and by comparing these fluorescent intensities between the sample and the control, gain or loss of the known regions is identified.[41] Since probes from all chromosomes are included, the copy number of all chromosomes can be determined simultaneously.[42] aCGH (array-comparative genomic hybridization) is rapid (24 hours) and has an error rate of <2%.[42]

This technique has some minor technical limitations. Since it shows only the deviations from the most frequent level of the combined fluorescence signal, as a result, haploid, polyploid, and normal (diploid) embryos will appear similar and chromosomal ploidy cannot be assessed. Further, the source of the chromosomal abnormality cannot be determined. For example, meiotic errors cannot be distinguished from postzygotic errors. Despite these limitations, aCGH has established itself as the "gold standard" for PGT, and most laboratories are now using aCGH in place of FISH-based approaches.

Quantitative Polymerase Chain Reaction

Quantitative polymerase chain reaction (qPCR) has traditionally been used for PGT-M (rather than PGT), as it is very effective in detection of known single gene defects. In recent years, the technique has been adapted for use in PGT.[43] The technique utilizes a high-order real-time multiplex PCR reaction to amplify multiple loci from each chromosome along with quantification. Genome-wide comparison can be made and it can give results in just 4 hours.[43]

Single Nucleotide Polymorphism Arrays

This is another commonly used technique for PGT-A. Single nucleotide polymorphism is a variation in a single nucleotide at a specific position in the genome, occurring at an appreciable frequency within a population. They represent the most frequent form of genomic variation. Over 6 million SNPs have been found in the human genome till date.[44] SNP microarrays are used in PGT to detect the specific alleles present in the sample cells at up to 500,000 SNP loci. Quantification of these alleles and assessment of heterozygosity enables diagnosis of aneuploidy in the cells. SNP arrays can also detect uniparental isodisomy.[45,46]

Next-generation Sequencing

The most advanced and recent technique used for PGT-A is next-generation sequencing (NGS) **(Fig. 2)**. DNA from the biopsied cell/s is amplified using WGA, fragmented, and then each fragment is tagged with a specific barcode. These small, barcoded DNA fragments (even from several samples) are mixed and sequenced parallelly. Specialized computer software is then used to read these barcoded fragments from each sample and align them against a reference human genome. Trisomy or monosomy can then be identified on the basis of increase or decrease in the number of sequences aligned against that chromosome.

The role of NGS in PGT was assessed by Yin et al.,[47] who compared SNP arrays with NGS in 38 blastocyst biopsy samples. They concluded that NGS could be used in PGT to detect chromosomal abnormality with a potentially higher accuracy and in a cost-effective manner. There have been many other retrospective[48] and prospective trials[49,50] that show that NGS for PGT is a highly accurate and cost-effective technology.

The advantages and disadvantages of these different PGT techniques are summarized in **Table 3**.

Noninvasive Preimplantation Genetic Testing

All the past and current methods of aneuploidy employ sampling of the genetic material from the oocytes/ trophectoderm and require micromanipulation techniques which are invasive and not entirely without risk. In addition, they need skilled embryologists and specialized laser equipment. The discovery of DNA within the blastocele fluid of the blastocyst and in the spent culture medium (SCM) during embryo development has promoted the development of the noninvasive methods of PGT.

- *Blastocentesis:* This procedure involves aspiration the blastocele fluid with an ICI pipette by piercing through the trophectoderm, leaving the embryo in a collapsed state.[51] Loss of the fluid from blastocoel is not detrimental to the embryo, which re-expands. However, the low quantity and poor quality of DNA extracted and

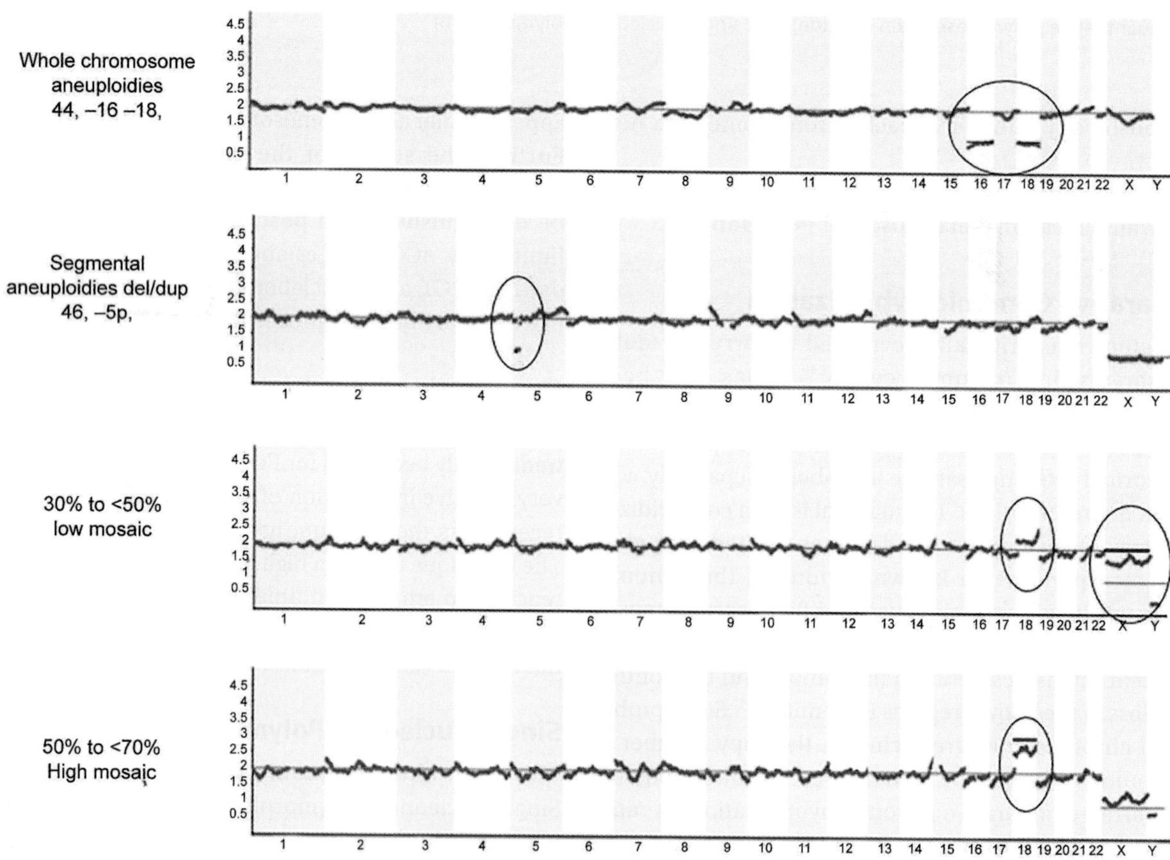

Fig. 2: Examples of next-generation sequencing (NGS) reporting. The top graph shows whole chromosome aneuploidy with deletion of chromosomes 16 and 18. Second graph shows segmental deletion at short arm of chromosome 5. Third and fourth graphs show low and high mosaic patterns.
(*Courtesy*: Igenomix SL, Spain.)

TABLE 3: Advantages and disadvantages of different PGT techniques.

	aCGH	*SNP array*	*qPCR*	*NGS*
Advantages	Widespread clinical application	Can detect the widest range of chromosomal abnormalities	Results are ready within very short time period	Increased resolution[49] Improved detection of mosaicism[49]
Disadvantages	Limited detection of mosaics	Relatively expensive	Due to assessment of small number of loci of each chromosome, it gives significantly low resolution[43]	Expensive initial set-up

(aCGH: array comparative genomic hybridization; NGS: next-generation sequencing; PGT: preimplantation genetic testing; qPCR: quantitative polymerase chain reaction; SNP: single nucleotide polymorphism)

difficulties in amplification have not made it a popular choice for genetic analysis [51]

- *Spent culture medium:* The embryo has been found to release various metabolites such as interleukins, proteins, micro RNAs along with DNA in the culture medium during its growth which may be used for genetic analysis. Studies have shown that the amount of genetic material in the SCM increases during embryo growth and has an embryonic origin.[52] The potential of the SCM analysis for PGT-A screening has incited a huge interest due to its noninvasiveness, but is having difficulty in gaining popularity due to technical complexity and low concordance with traditional trophectoderm biopsy.

Initial studies achieved a fair degree of ploidy agreement by performing cytogenetic and molecular analysis on the spent cultures and blastocele fluid. However, the ploidy agreement efficiency is restricted by the low quality and quantity of DNA, technical limitations, maternal contamination, and embryonic mosaicism. However, future research and long-term data may validate noninvasive PGT as a less expensive technique requiring less skills for micromanipulation and lower risk to embryos. Such methods may even allow genetic analysis of embryos which are often considered unsuitable for biopsy and are discarded without biopsy.

RESULTS OF ANEUPLOIDY SCREENING IN VARIOUS PATIENT GROUPS

For Advanced Maternal Age

Fertility decreases with increasing maternal age. Data derived from IVF centers in the United States show that LBRs decline with age (41.4% in women <35 years of age, 31.6% in women between 35 and 37 years of age, 22.3% between 38 and 40 years of age, 11.7% between 41 and 42 years, 3.8% for those older than 42 years). Along with it, there is increase in aneuploidy rates as well as spontaneous miscarriage rates.[53] The miscarriage rates increase in IVF from 12.6% in those younger than 35 years to 34.8% in women older than 42 years.[54,55]

This decrease in the LBRs and increase in spontaneous miscarriage rates is, to a large extent, because of the increase in aneuploidy with age. This is supported by data from Society for Assisted Reproductive Technology (SART) registry,[56] in which, the LBR (49.3%) did not vary with the age of the recipients in the group of patients who underwent fresh transfers using eggs obtained from healthy, young donors.

Thus, theoretically, by ensuring euploidy in the transferred embryos, PGT-A should result in better pregnancy rates and LBRs. However, the results for PGT-A in advanced maternal age reported in the literature have been mixed.

The initial results of PGT-A were discouraging. In a meta-analysis performed by Mastenbroek et al.,[57] in 2011, five out of the nine RCTs, which had studied the outcomes of PGT in advanced maternal age, concluded that PGT significantly decreased the LBR after IVF in this group. The main drawback of this systematic review was that FISH had been used in all the studies, which can study only 9 out of 24 chromosomes, and all but one trials used cleavage stage biopsy wherein only 1–2 cells can be biopsied, which may not be representative of the whole embryo. Moreover, later on Scott et al., in 2013,[27] demonstrated that cleavage stage biopsy may itself be harmful to embryo leading to lower pregnancy rates. Many technical improvements have been done in PGT since then, including utilization of comprehensive chromosomal screening (CCS) and doing TE biopsy at blastocyst stage (day 5/6).

Another more recent meta-analysis was performed by Lee et al., in 2015,[58] including 13 observational studies. In this, among the subgroup of studies which included a control group of embryos selected based on morphology, improved implantation rates were consistently found in the PGT arm.[18,53,59] Another RCT noted higher delivery rates after first transfer by selecting embryos after PGT-A, with lesser mean number of ETs required per live birth (1.8 vs. 3.7) as well as less time to pregnancy (7.7 vs. 14.9 weeks) and a lower miscarriage rate.[60]

The STAR trial by Munne et al. studied the benefit of PGT-A (n = 661) versus morphology (n = 331) for selection of embryo in frozen-thawed ET in women aged 25–40 years. 661 women (33.7 ± 3.6 years) were randomized to PGT-A (n = 330) or morphology alone (n = 331). The ongoing pregnancy rate (OPR) was similar in both the groups with no significant difference per ET [50% (137/274) vs. 46% (143/313)] or per intention to treat (ITT) [41.8% (138/330) vs. 43.5% (144/331)]. Post-hoc analysis of women between

35 and 40 years showed a significant increase in OPR per ET (51 vs. 37%) but not per ITT. They concluded that PGT-A did not improve overall pregnancy outcomes in all women, analyzed per ET or per ITT. However, a significant increment in OPR per ET was noted with the use of PGT-A in the subgroup of women aged 35–40 years who had two or more biopsiable embryos, but this was not significant when analyzed by ITT.[61] Pagliardini et al. reinterpretated that data from the STAR trial and attributed incorrect diagnosis and/or biopsy-related embryo damage might underlie reduction from 82.2 to 50.0% of the LBR for competent embryos, thus reiterating the fact that PGT-A may be associated with some embryo wastage.[62]

Thus, at present, the available evidence suggests that PGT-A for aneuploidy may increase the pregnancy rate per ET, thereby reducing the time to pregnancy in advanced age, although the cumulative pregnancy rates per oocyte retrieval may not increase.

For Recurrent Pregnancy Loss

Recurrent pregnancy loss (RPL) is classically defined as loss of three or more pregnancies under 500 g (or before 20 weeks of gestation). The most common reason for RPL is aneuploid embryos.[63,64] This has also been supported by a higher rate of aneuploidy in PGT of embryos from women with RPL, independent of the maternal age.[65,66] Hence, PGT has been proposed as a solution for RPL, as it can decrease the risk of another aneuploid pregnancy.

There are no randomized studies in the literature assessing the clinical utility or efficacy of PGT in RPL. In a prospective study,[67] assessing the role of PGT in women with RPL (69 cycles in 49 patients), a high proportion of embryos were found to be aneuploid in women younger than 37 years (43.85%) as well as in women 37 years and older (66.95%). However, in their study, PGT did not improve the OPRs per cycle in younger women (26%) as compared to those generally achieved in the general IVF population. In the older group also, PGT did not improve the already poor outcomes (2.9% OPR per cycle).

Murugappan et al.[68] compared PGT-A versus expectant management in a retrospective analysis of 300 patients. In this study, 112 patients underwent PGT-A and 188 were enrolled as control in expected management group. Between PGT and expectant management, clinical pregnancy rates (44 vs. 51%), LBRs (32 vs. 34%), and clinical miscarriage rates (20 vs. 24%) were similar. However, the cycles in which PGT was planned but cancelled had a significantly higher clinical miscarriage rate (50 vs. 14%) and lower LBR (15 vs. 36%) as compared to cycles in which PGT was performed, with similar maternal ages.

Musters et al.[69] reviewed the literature on efficacy of PGT in comparison with natural conception in women with unexplained recurrent miscarriages. The authors could not find any randomized or nonrandomized studies directly comparing PGT with natural conception for patients with recurrent miscarriage. The review of 12 observational studies suggested that PGT lowers the incidence of miscarriage; however, due to lower pregnancy rates after PGT, the overall live births decrease. On the other hand, Sato et al. prospectively studied patients undergoing IVF who had RPL, with at least one case of aneuploidy ascertained through point-of-care (POC) testing and in patients who had repeated implantation failures (RIFs, at least three failed transfers).[70] They noted no difference in the LBR per patient with or without PGT-A in the RPL group and no difference in the clinical miscarriage rates per clinical pregnancy. However, they did note improvement in LBR per ET and reduced biochemical pregnancy loss per pregnancy in the RPL group.

Bhatt et al. in 2021 studied the SART data for IVF–ICSI between 2010 and 2016 and assessed the utility of PGT-A in couples with RPL. In women with RPL, the adjusted odds ratio (OR) comparing IVF with PGT-A versus without for live birth outcome was 1.31 [for age >35 years; 95% confidence interval (CI) 1.12, 1.52], 1.45 (ages 35–37 years), 1.89 (38–40 years), and 3.80 (>42 years). The ORs for spontaneous abortion were 0.95 (<35 years), 0.85 (35–37 years), 0.81 (38–40 years), and 0.58 (>42 years). They concluded that PGT-A was associated with an improvement in LBR and clinical pregnancy rate with the largest difference in women >42 years.[71]

To summarize, the available evidence currently is equivocal regarding the role of PGT in patients with recurrent pregnancy loss, and more robust evidence is needed from properly designed RCTs.

For Repeated Implantation Failure

Repeated implantation failure is defined as failure of pregnancy after three or more IVF cycles, or after transfer of 10 morphologically good embryos. Although there is still no ideal management strategy for these couples, selective elimination of aneuploidy embryos via PGT has been offered as a treatment option worldwide.

Previously, many observational studies were unable to find significant improvement in pregnancy outcomes in these patients.[72-74] A RCT by Blockeel et al. failed to show any significant benefit of PGT in RIF patients.[75] Recently, Rubio et al.[32] conducted an RCT including 91 patients (43 in PGT group and 49 control group) and reported slightly higher LBRs in PGT (47.9%) as compared to control groups (27.9%), although the difference could not achieve statistical significance. Recent studies by Sato et al.[70] and Mantravadi et al.[76] have found no benefit of PGT-A in improving the LBRs in couples with RIF; another study by Tong et al.[77] noted no significant differences in pregnancy rates (43.5 vs. 64.7%), clinical pregnancy rates (39.1 vs. 48.0%), implantation rates (39.1 vs. 51.0%), and miscarriage rates (4.3 vs. 7.8%) per ET between RIF women stratified by age (<38 and >38 years) and concluded that maternal age does not affect the implantation potential of euploid blastocysts. Thus, the evidence so far has shown equivocal results for PGT in patients with RIF.

For Severe Male Infertility

Chromosomal abnormalities are reported in ejaculated or testicular sperms in 10–15% of azoospermic men and 5% of oligospermic men, as compared to <1% of men with semen of normal quality. A microdeletion in the Y chromosome may also be present in another 15% of infertile men having azoospermia or severe oligospermia.[78] Such high prevalence of abnormal karyotypes is expected to increase the risk of aneuploidy in the embryo, and this forms the theoretical basis for doing PGT in such patients. Initial studies focused on gene-specific testing for cystic fibrosis transmembrane conductance regulator gene mutation in cases of congenital bilateral absence of the vas deferens, Klinefelter syndrome, Y chromosome microdeletion, and known autosomal translocations and did not study PGT-A alone. Recent evidence from Asoglu et al. (2020) who studied PGT-A in cases with severe male factor undergoing IVF and noted LBRs of 55.6% in PGT-A group versus 51.1% in non-PGT-A (OR 1.19; 95% CI 0.62–1.80; p = 0.8) with similar IR and CPR. They noted that advanced maternal age was the only factor independently associated with live birth (OR 0.46; 95% CI 0.22–0.96; p = 0.04).[79]

CONCERNS WITH PREIMPLANTATION GENETIC TESTING

Testing for aneuploidy, though seems very safe and logical, is not without concerns. An important concern in PGT is chromosomal mosaicism, as discussed earlier. It results from mitotic errors occurring after fertilization. Cells obtained in TE biopsy may not represent the whole embryo, the unbiopsied TE cells, or the ICM.[80] Second, different techniques used for comprehensive screening of embryos have different sensitivity and specificity of detecting mosaicism.[81] Third and most important issue is how this mosaicism is clinically relevant, as there are mouse and now even human studies suggesting that aneuploid embryos do implant and can result in a healthy live birth.[82-84] Preimplantation Genetic Diagnosis International Society (PGDIS) is perhaps the only society which has stated its position on the use of PGT. After taking into consideration the abovementioned facts, this society has recently issued revised guidelines on PGT, including how it should be performed, how the laboratory reports should be issued, and how the clinicians should interpret these reports.[85] These guidelines are reprinted in **Boxes 2 to 5**.

BOX 2: Preimplantation Genetic Diagnosis International Society recommendations for preimplantation genetic testing (PGT) laboratories.

- For reliable detection of mosaicism, ideally five cells should be biopsied, with as little cell damage as possible. If the biopsy is facilitated using a laser, the identified contact points should be minimal and preferably at cell junctions. Overly aggressive use of the laser may result in cell damage and partial destruction of cellular DNA
- Only a validated next-generation sequencing (NGS) platform that can quantitatively measure copy number should be used for measurement of mosaicism in the biopsy sample. Ideally, a NGS methodology that can accurately and reproducibly measure 20% mosaicism in a known sample
- For reporting embryo results, the suggested cutoff point for definition of mosaicism is >20%, so lower levels should be treated as normal (euploid), >80% abnormal (aneuploid), and the remaining ones between 20 and 80% mosaic (euploid-aneuploid mosaics)

BOX 3: Preimplantation Genetic Diagnosis International Society recommendations for the clinicians.

- Patients should continue to be advised that any genetic test based on sampling one or small number of cells biopsied from preimplantation embryos cannot be 100% accurate for a combination of technical and biological factors, including chromosome mosaicism
- The patient information and consent forms for aneuploidy testing (if used) should be modified to include the possibility of mosaic aneuploid results and any potential risks in the event of transfer and implantation. This needs to be explained to patients by the clinician recommending the aneuploidy testing
- Transfer of blastocysts with a normal euploid result should always be prioritized over those with mosaic aneuploidy results
- In the event of considering the transfer of a blastocyst with only mosaic aneuploidies, the following options should be discussed with the patient:
  - A further cycle of in vitro fertilization with aneuploidy testing to increase the chance of identifying a normal euploid blastocyst for transfer
  - Transfer of a blastocyst with mosaic aneuploidies for low-risk chromosomes only, after appropriate genetic counseling if available
  - Appropriate monitoring and prenatal diagnosis of any resulting pregnancy, preferably by early amniocentesis (>14 weeks' gestation)

PREIMPLANTATION GENETIC TESTING AS UNIVERSAL SCREENING

The whole treatment of IVF is aimed at providing a singleton healthy live baby to the couple. To achieve this goal, most clinics transfer multiple embryos in order to increase the chances of a successful pregnancy in one cycle. However, transfer of multiple embryos has resulted in an increase in the incidence of multiple birth pregnancies which has its own medical and financial implications. Since the most important reason for implantation failure as well as miscarriage in IVF is embryonic aneuploidy (which increases significantly with advanced maternal age), PGT has been suggested in all IVF cycles to select a single embryo which has the maximum implantation potential.

BOX 4: Preimplantation Genetic Diagnosis International Society guidelines to prioritize mosaic embryos for transfer.

Based on our current knowledge of the reproductive outcomes of fetal and placental mosaicism from prenatal diagnosis, the following can be used as a guide by the clinician (or a genetic counselor if available) when a mosaic embryo is being considered for transfer:

- Embryos showing mosaic euploid/monosomy are preferable to euploid/trisomy, given that monosomic embryos (excepting 45, X) are not viable
- If a decision is made to transfer mosaic embryos trisomic for a single chromosome, one can prioritize selection based on the level of mosaicism and the specific chromosome involved. The preferable transfer category consists of mosaic embryos trisomic for chromosomes 1, 3, 4, 5, 6, 8, 9, 10, 11, 12, 17, 19, 20, 22, X, and Y. None of these chromosomes involve the adverse characteristics enumerated below:
  - Embryos mosaic for trisomies that are associated with potential for uniparental disomy (14 and 15) are of lesser priority
- Embryos mosaic for trisomies that are associated with intrauterine growth retardation (chromosomes 2, 7, and 16) are of lesser priority
- Embryos mosaic for trisomies capable of live born viability (chromosomes 13, 18, and 21) are of lowest priority, for obvious reasons

BOX 5: Key points for counselling regarding mosaic PGT-A results [American Society for Reproductive Medicine (ASRM), 2020].[86]

- Clinicians should understand the prevalence of mosaic PGT-A results issued by their reference laboratory
- Clinics should have a policy in place regarding the reporting and the management of mosaic PGT-A results. The policy should be known to staff and shared with patients before PGT-A testing
- Transfer of embryos deemed euploid should be prioritized before considering the transfer of embryos with mosaic results.
- If no embryos deemed euploid are available for transfer, patients should be offered, with due consideration of their clinical situation, the option of another IVF cycle, with or without PGT-A
- Patients considering the transfer of embryos with mosaic results should consult with a clinical genetics specialist, such as a board-certified genetic counselor, who has specific knowledge of perinatal and pediatric outcomes associated with chromosomal mosaicism
- Patient counseling should include a discussion of the various possible explanations for mosaic PGT-A results and potential outcomes
- A decision regarding the transfer of an embryo with mosaic result is optimally made with ample time for careful consideration of the risks, benefits, and alternatives associated with this option
- The limited outcomes reported after transfer of an embryo with mosaic results seem to be reassuring; however, current data are limited and should be interpreted with caution:
  - Lower implantation rates and higher miscarriage rates have been reported after the transfer of embryos with mosaic results compared with embryos deemed euploid; these outcomes may be due in part to biases in the patient populations studied
  - A small number of apparently healthy live births have been reported in the literature after the transfer of embryos with mosaic results
- In the prenatal and pediatric populations, cytogenetic mosaicism involving nearly every chromosome in monosomic and trisomic form has been reported in association with congenital anomalies, fetal growth restriction (also known as intrauterine growth restriction), intellectual disabilities, and/or long-term health problems. When an embryo with mosaic results successfully implants, the chance for the occurrence of such an adverse outcome is currently unknown. Nonetheless, until further data are available, patient should be counseled on these risks
- The following parameters for risk stratification of embryo with mosaic results have been proposed:
  - By percentage of mosaicism
  - By specific chromosome(s) involved
  - By monosomy versus trisomy
  - Whether full chromosome versus partial chromosome is affected
  - By the number of chromosomes involved (single vs. double vs. complex aneuploidies)
- However, no evidence-based classification system currently exists for prioritizing embryos based on these parameters. It remains to be determined whether prenatal or postnatal mosaicism data can be applied to predict outcomes for preimplantation embryos identified as mosaic
- Prenatal genetic counseling is strongly recommended for any pregnancy resulting from the transfer of embryos with mosaic results and should include a discussion of the risks, benefits, and limitations of chorionic villus sampling (CVS) and amniocentesis
- If prenatal diagnostic testing is performed, additional analyses beyond routine karyotyping should be considered depending on the specific PGT-A result. At the discretion of the ordering provider, these may include:
  - Chromosomal microarray, if a partial chromosome aneuploidy is involved
  - Uniparental disomy studies (UPD), depending on the chromosome involved
  - Additional cell counts, in an effort to identify lower level mosaicism
- Postnatal evaluation by peripheral blood karyotype and/or microarray should be considered, particularly if prenatal diagnostic testing is declined. Referral to a pediatric specialist in genetics is recommended in the event of an abnormal physical or developmental phenotype
- Large-scale outcome studies are needed to improve data available for patient counseling. Providers are encouraged to track and publish prenatal, perinatal, and pediatric outcomes following the transfer of embryo(s) with mosaic PGT-A results

A retrospective study[87] of 235 cycles of ICSI with PGT by using aCGH in Indian population, with different indications for PGT, has shown consistent implantation rates (33.3–42.9%) and pregnancy rates per transfer (31.8–54.9%) after transferring euploid embryos irrespective of indication for performing PGT and age of women.

An RCT in 2013 compared the pregnancy outcomes after transferring single euploid embryo versus two untested blastocysts.[88] The OPRs per patient after the first transfer remained similar between the two groups (60.7 vs. 65.1%), while the risk of multiple gestations was significantly reduced from 53.4% in two untested blastocysts transfer group to 0% after PGT and single euploid blastocyst transfer. The Blastocyst Euploid Selective Transfer (BEST) Trial by the same group of authors in 2015 comparing euploid elective single embryo transfer (eSET) and untested two-embryo transfer[89] found that the delivery rates were similar (69 vs. 72%) in the fresh cycle and up to one frozen transfer, with a huge and significant reduction in the incidence of multiple birth pregnancies (1.6 vs. 47%). The incidences of preterm delivery and low birthweight were also significantly lower after euploid eSET. The babies born following untested two-ET had higher chances of neonatal intensive care unit (NICU) admission and spent more than five times as many days in the NICU (479 vs. 93 days) as compared to those born after eSET.

A meta-analysis done in 2015 by Dahdouh et al.,[90] in which three RCTs with good prognosis patients were included, also concluded that PGT improved embryo selection and increased clinical and sustained implantation rates, particularly in women with normal ovarian reserve. However, few studies have concluded that the cumulative pregnancy rates per aspiration do not change with embryo selection with PGT.[91,92] Moreover, there are no studies on the cost-effectiveness of embryo selection with PGT as compared to transferring untested embryos because the intangible costs of failed implantation and spontaneous losses, variable treatment costs as well as costs due to multiple pregnancies are difficult to quantify.

After a comprehensive review, the ASRM published a practice guideline in 2018 which states "there is insufficient evidence to recommend the routine use of PGT-A for all infertile women."[88] The recent Cochrane database (2020) also concludes that "There is insufficient good-quality evidence of a difference in cumulative LBR, LBR after the first ET, or miscarriage rate between IVF with and IVF without PGT-A as currently performed."[93]

LEGAL ASPECTS AND REGULATIONS WITH PREIMPLANTATION GENETIC TESTING

While technological advancements enable new treatment modalities to patients leading to better outcomes and efficient results, legislation often lags and novel technology is often disputed. Consequently, PGT is subject to considerable regulation with variation in between countries internationally. While Western Europe has some restrictions and regulations on the use of PGT limiting use of PGT-M/SR to cases of serious hereditary disease, other countries, such as France, have a case-to-case approval by a multidisciplinary committee. In countries like the UK, specifications are in force for the conditions under which PGT can be performed and every new disease has to be approved by the Human Fertilization and Embryology Authority (HFEA). The situation in USA is quite different as no regulation exists on the application of PGT and IVF is commercially driven. These variations in legislation between countries promote reproductive tourism, that is, couples or individuals seeking treatment which is not permitted or accessible in their home country.

In India, The Assisted Reproductive Technology (Regulation) Act, 2021, has defined in Section 25 (1) "Pre-implantation genetic diagnosis" means the genetic diagnosis when one or both genetic parents has a known genetic abnormality and testing is performed on an embryo to determine if it also carries a genetic abnormality; and (2) "Preimplantation genetic testing" means a technique used to identify genetic defects in embryos created through IVF before pregnancy. It states that "Pre-implantation Genetic testing shall be used to screen the human embryo for known, pre-existing, heritable or genetic diseases only."[94]

The donation of an embryo after preimplantation genetic testing to an approved research laboratory for research purposes can be done only: (1) With the approval of the commissioning couple or woman; and (b) when the embryo suffers from pre-existing, heritable, life-threatening, or genetic diseases. In the Gazette dated June 7, 2020, the assisted reproductive technology (ART) rules have allowed PGT-A when medically indicated and have mandated clinics to ensure that no PGT shall be done for sex selection for nonmedical reasons or selection of particular traits due to personal preferences of the prospective parents or to alter or with a view to alter the genetic constitution of an embryo.

KEY POINTS

- Available evidence suggests that PGT can help in increasing both clinical and OPRs.
- The newer techniques of TE biopsy with analysis by array-based methods or better by NGS have allowed the testing of all chromosomes and hence have improved the PGT results considerably.
- By selecting the euploid embryo, PGT may decrease time to pregnancy and miscarriage rates but only in selected population which is not yet defined but can include women with advanced age.
- The cost-effectiveness of PGT needs to be evaluated before its widespread use in clinical practice.
- PGT may help in reducing the multiple gestation rate by transferring a single euploid embryo as opposed to multiple embryos.
- The concern regarding transfer of mosaic embryos needs more evidence and needs proper counseling based on the best new evidence.

- Newer technique such as the noninvasive PGT appears promising, but robust data is lacking for recommending its use in routine practice.
- One must keep updated on the latest guidelines by the regional authorities before implementing PGT in practice.
- PGT is a valuable procedure, but for the time being, it is not suitable for every patient and not for every IVF practice.

REFERENCES

1. Hassold T, Hunt P. To err (meiotically) is human: the genesis of human aneuploidy. Nat Rev Genet. 2001;2(4):280-91.
2. Zegers-Hochschild F, Adamson GD, Dyer S, Racowsky C, de Mouzon J, Sokol R, et al. The international glossary on infertility and fertility care, 2017. Fertil Steril. 2017;108(3):393-406.
3. Selva J, Martin-Pont B, Hugues JN, Rince P, Fillion C, Herve F, et al. Cytogenetic study of human oocytes uncleaved after invitro fertilization. Hum Reprod. 1991;6(5):709-13.
4. Fragouli E, Wells D, Thornhill A, Serhal P, Faed MJ, Harper JC, et al. Comparative genomic hybridization analysis of human oocytes and polar bodies. Hum Reprod. 2006;21(9):2319-28.
5. Kuliev A, Cieslak J, Verlinsky Y. Frequency and distribution of chromosome abnormalities in human oocytes. Cytogenet Genome Res. 2005;111(3-4):193-8.
6. Gutiérrez-Mateo C, Benet J, Wells D, Colls P, Bermúdez MG, Sánchez-García JF, et al. Aneuploidy study of human oocytes first polar body comparative genomic hybridization and metaphase II fluorescence in situ hybridization analysis. Hum Reprod. 2004;19(12):2859-68.
7. Martin RH, Ko E, Rademaker A. Distribution of aneuploidy in human gametes: comparison between human sperm and oocytes. Am J Med Genet. 1991;39(3):321-31.
8. Shi Q, Martin RH. Aneuploidy in human spermatozoa: FISH analysis in men with constitutional chromosomal abnormalities, and in infertile men. Reproduction. 2001;121(5): 655-66.
9. Practice Committee of Society for Assisted Reproductive Technology, Practice Committee of American Society for Reproductive Medicine. Preimplantation genetic testing: a Practice Committee opinion. Fertil Steril. 2008;90(5 Suppl):S136-43.
10. Park S, Kim EY, Yoon SH, Chung KS, Lim JH. Enhanced hatching rate of bovine IVM/IVF/IVC blastocysts using a 1.48-micron diode laser beam. J Assist Reprod Genet. 1999;16(2):97-101.
11. Han TS, Sagoskin AW, Graham JR, Tucker MJ, Liebermann J. Laser-assisted human embryo biopsy on the third day of development for preimplantation genetic diagnosis: two successful case reports. Fertil Steril. 2003;80(2):453-5.
12. Verlinsky Y, Cieslak J, Freidine M, Ivakhnenko V, Wolf G, Kovalinskaya L, et al. Polar body diagnosis of common aneuploidies by FISH. J Assist Reprod Genet. 1996;13(2):157-62.
13. Gianaroli L. Preimplantation genetic diagnosis: polar body and embryo biopsy. Hum Reprod. 2000;15 (Suppl 4):69-75.
14. Handyside AH, Montag M, Magli MC, Repping S, Harper J, Schmutzler A, et al. Multiple meiotic errors caused by predivision of chromatids in women of advanced maternal age undergoing in vitro fertilisation. Eur J Hum Genet. 2012;20(7):742-7.
15. Liu J, Van den Abbeel E, Van Steirteghem A. The invitro and in-vivo developmental potential of frozen and non- frozen biopsied 8-cell mouse embryos. Hum Reprod. 1993;8(9):1481-6.
16. Kalousek DK, Vekemans M. Confined placental mosaicism. J Med Genet. 1996;33(7):529-33.
17. Johnson DS, Cinnioglu C, Ross R, Filby A, Gemelos G, Hill M, et al. Comprehensive analysis of karyotypic mosaicism between trophectoderm and inner cell mass. Mol Hum Reprod. 2010;16(12):944-9.
18. Schoolcraft WB, Fragouli E, Stevens J, Munne S, Katz-Jaffe MG, Wells D. Clinical application of comprehensive chromosomal screening at the blastocyst stage. Fertil Steril. 2010;94(5):1700-6.
19. Fasouliotis SJ, Schenker JG. Preimplantation genetic diagnosis principles and ethics. Hum Reprod. 1998;13(8):2238-45.
20. De Vos A, Van Steirteghem A. Aspects of biopsy procedures prior to preimplantation genetic diagnosis. Prenat Diagn. 2001;21(9):767-80.
21. Verlinsky Y, Rechitsky S, Evsikov S, White M, Cieslak J, Lifchez A, et al. Preconception and preimplantation diagnosis for cystic fibrosis. Prenat Diagn. 1992;12(2):103-10.
22. Treff NR, Su J, Tao X, Frattarelli JL, Miller KA, Scott RT, et al. Characterization of the source of human embryonic aneuploidy using microarray-based 24 chromosome preimplantation genetic diagnosis (mPGD) and aneuploid chromosome fingerprinting. Fertil Steril. 2008;90:S37.
23. Dumoulin JC, Bras M, Coonen E, Dreesen J, Geraedts JP, Evers JL. Effect of Ca^{2+}/ Mg^{2+}-free medium on the biopsy procedure for preimplantation genetic diagnosis and further development of human embryos. Hum Reprod. 1998;13(10):2880-3.
24. Schoolcraft WB, Katz-Jaffe MG. Comprehensive chromosome screening of trophectoderm with vitrification facilitates elective single-embryo transfer for infertile women with advanced maternal age. Fertil Steril. 2013;100(3):615-9.
25. Scott KL, Hong KH, Scott RT Jr. Selecting the optimal time to perform biopsy for preimplantation genetic testing. Fertil Steril. 2013;100(3):608-14.
26. Munné S, Weier HU, Grifo J, Cohen J. Chromosome mosaicism in human embryos. Biol Reprod. 1994;51(3):373-9.
27. Scott RT, Upham KM, Forman EJ, Hong KH, Scott KL, Taylor D, et al. Blastocyst biopsy with comprehensive chromosome screening and fresh embryo transfer significantly increases in vitro fertilization implantation and delivery rates: a randomized controlled trial. Fertil Steril. 2013;100(3):697-703.
28. Harton GL, Munné S, Surrey M, Grifo J, Kaplan B, McCulloh DH, et al. Diminished effect of maternal age on implantation after preimplantation genetic diagnosis with array comparative genomic hybridization. Fertil Steril. 2013;100(6):1695-703.
29. Angell RR, Templeton AA, Aitken RJ. Chromosome studies in human in vitro fertilization. Hum Genet. 1986;72(4):333-9.
30. Griffin DK, Wilton LJ, Handyside AH, Winston RM, Delhanty JD. Dual fluorescent in situ hybridisation for simultaneous detection of X and Y chromosome-specific probes for the sexing of human preimplantation embryonic nuclei. Hum Genet. 1992;89(1):18-22.
31. Coonen E, Dumoulin JC, Dreesen JC, Bras M, Evers JL, Geraedts JP. Clinical application of FISH for sex determination of embryos in preimplantation diagnosis of X-linked diseases. J Assist Reprod Genet. 1996;13(2):133-6.

32. Rubio C, Bellver J, Rodrigo L, Bosch E, Mercader A, Vidal C, et al. Preimplantation genetic screening using fluorescence in situ hybridization in patients with repetitive implantation failure and advanced maternal age: two randomized trials. Fertil Steril. 2013;99(5):1400-7.
33. Gleicher N, Kushnir A, Barad DH. Preimplantation genetic screening (PGS) still in search of a clinical application: a systematic review. Reprod Biol Endocrinol. 2014;12:22.
34. Staessen C, Platteau P, Van Assche E, Michiels A, Tournaye H, Camus M, et al. Comparison of blastocyst transfer with or without preimplantation genetic diagnosis for aneuploidy screening in couples with advanced maternal age: a prospective randomized controlled trial. Hum Reprod. 2004;19(12):2849-58.
35. Wilton L, Voullaire L, Sargeant P, Williamson R, McBain J. Preimplantation aneuploidy screening using comparative genomic hybridization or fluorescence in situ hybridization of embryos from patients with recurrent implantation failure. Fertil Steril. 2003;80(4):860-8.
36. Fritz MA. Perspectives on the efficacy and indications for preimplantation genetic screening: where are we now? Hum Reprod. 2008;23(12):2617-21.
37. Munné S, Howles CM, Wells D. The role of preimplantation genetic diagnosis in diagnosing embryo aneuploidy. Curr Opin Obstet Gynecol. 2009;21(5):442-9.
38. Wells D, Alfarawati S, Fragouli E. Use of comprehensive chromosomal screening for embryo assessment: microarrays and CGH. Mol Hum Reprod. 2008;14(12):703-10.
39. Kallioniemi A, Kallioniemi OP, Sudar D, Rutovitz D, Gray JW, Waldman F, et al. Comparative genomic hybridization for molecular cytogenetic analysis of solid tumors. Science. 1992;258(5083):818-22.
40. Kallioniemi OP, Kallioniemi A, Sudar D, Rutovitz D, Gray JW, Waldman F, et al. Comparative genomic hybridization: a rapid new method for detecting and mapping DNA amplification in tumors. Semin Cancer Biol. 1993;4(1):41-6.
41. Voullaire L, Slater H, Williamson R, Wilton L. Chromosome analysis of blastomeres from human embryos by using comparative genomic hybridization. Hum Genet. 2000;106(2):210-7.
42. Gutiérrez-Mateo C, Colls P, Sánchez-García J, Escudero T, Prates R, Ketterson K, et al. Validation of microarray comparative genomic hybridization for comprehensive chromosome analysis of embryos. Fertil Steril. 2011;95(3):953-8.
43. Treff NR, Tao X, Ferry KM, Su J, Taylor D, Scott RT Jr. Development and validation of an accurate quantitative real-time polymerase chain reaction-based assay for human blastocyst comprehensive chromosomal aneuploidy screening. Fertil Steril. 2012;97(4):819-24.
44. Javed R, Mukesh. Current research status, databases and application of single nucleotide polymorphism. Pak J Biol Sci. 2010;13(13):657-63.
45. Northrop LE, Treff NR, Levy B, Scott RT Jr. SNP microarray-based 24 chromosome aneuploidy screening demonstrates that cleavage-stage FISH poorly predicts aneuploidy in embryos that develop to morphologically normal blastocysts. Mol Hum Reprod. 2010;16(8):590-600.
46. Brezina PR, Benner A, Rechitsky S, Kuliev A, Pomerantseva E, Pauling D, et al. Single-gene testing combined with single nucleotide polymorphism microarray preimplantation genetic diagnosis for aneuploidy: a novel approach in optimizing pregnancy outcome. Fertil Steril. 2011;95(5):1786.e5-8.
47. Yin X, Tan K, Vajta G, Jiang H, Tan Y, Zhang C, et al. Massively parallel sequencing for chromosomal abnormality testing in trophectoderm cells of human blastocysts. Biol Reprod. 2013;88(3):69.
48. Fiorentino F, Bono S, Biricik A, Nuccitelli A, Cotroneo E, Cottone G, et al. Application of next- generation sequencing technology for comprehensive aneuploidy screening of blastocysts in clinical preimplantation genetic screening cycles. Hum Reprod. 2014;29(12):2802-13.
49. Fiorentino F, Biricik A, Bono S, Spizzichino L, Cotroneo E, Cottone G, et al. Development and validation of a next-generation sequencing-based protocol for 24-chromosome aneuploidy screening of embryos. Fertil Steril. 2014; 101(5):1375-82.
50. Yang Z, Lin J, Zhang J, Fong WI, Li P, Zhao R, et al. Randomized comparison of next-generation sequencing and array comparative genomic hybridization for preimplantation genetic screening: a pilot study. BMC Med Genomics. 2015;8:30.
51. Magli MC, Pomante A, Cafueri G, Valerio M, Crippa A, Ferraretti AP, et al. Preimplantation genetic testing: polar bodies, blastomeres, trophectoderm cells, or blastocoelic fluid? Fertil Steril. 2016;105(3):676-683.e5
52. Hammond ER, Shelling AN, Cree LM. Nuclear and mitochondrial DNA in blastocoele fluid and embryo culture medium: evidence and potential clinical use. Hum Reprod. 2016;31(8):1653-61.
53. Keltz MD, Vega M, Sirota I, Lederman M, Moshier EL, Gonzales E, et al. Preimplantation genetic screening (PGS) with Comparative genomic hybridization (CGH) following day 3 single cell blastomere biopsy markedly improves IVF outcomes while lowering multiple pregnancies and miscarriages. J Assist Reprod Genet. 2013;30(10):1333-9.
54. American College of Obstetricians and Gynecologists Committee on Gynecologic Practice, Practice Committee of the American Society for Reproductive Medicine. Female age-related fertility decline. Committee Opinion No. 589. Obstet Gynecol. 2014;123(3):719-21.
55. Sunderam S, Kissin DM, Zhang Y, Jewett A, Hsiao YH, Liu A, et al. Assisted reproductive technology surveillance — United States, 2017. MMWR Surveill Summ. 2020;69(No. SS-9):1–20.
56. Society for Assisted Reproductive Technology. SART National Summary Report- Preliminary CSR for 2019 [online]. Available from: www.https://www.sartcorsonline.com/rptCSR_PublicMultYear.aspx. [Last accessed November 2022].
57. Mastenbroek S, Twisk M, van der Veen F, Repping S. Preimplantation genetic screening: a systematic review and meta-analysis of RCTs. Hum Reprod Update. 2011; 17(4):454-66.
58. Lee E, Illingworth P, Wilton L, Chambers GM. The clinical effective- ness of preimplantation genetic diagnosis for aneuploidy in all 24 chromosomes (PGD-A): systematic review. Hum Reprod. 2015;30(2):473-83.
59. Fishel S, Craig A, Lynch C, Dowell K. Assessment of 19,803 paired chromosomes and clinical outcome from first 150 cycles using array CGH of the first polar body for embryo selection and transfer. J Fertiliz In Vitro. 2011;1:101.

60. Rubio C, Bellver J, Rodrigo L, Castillón G, Guillén A, Vidal C, et al. In vitro fertilization with preimplantation genetic diagnosis for aneuploidies in advanced maternal age: a randomized, controlled study. Fertil Steril. 2017;107(5): 1122-9.
61. Munné S, Kaplan B, Frattarelli JL, Child T, Nakhuda G, Shamma FN, et al. Preimplantation genetic testing for aneuploidy versus morphology as selection criteria for single frozen-thawed embryo transfer in good-prognosis patients: a multicenter randomized clinical trial. Fertil Steril. 2019;112(6):1071-1079.e7.
62. Pagliardini L, Viganò P, Alteri A, Corti L, Somigliana E, Papaleo E. Shooting STAR: reinterpreting the data from the 'Single Embryo TrAnsfeR of Euploid Embryo' randomized clinical trial. Reprod Biomed Online. 2020;40(4):475-8.
63. Simpson JL. Genes, chromosomes, and reproductive failure. Fertil Steril. 1980;33(2):107-16.
64. Eiben B, Bartels I, Bähr-Porsch S, Borgmann S, Gatz G, Gellert G, et al. Cytogenetic analysis of 750 spontaneous abortions with the direct-preparation method of chorionic villi and its implications for studying genetic causes of pregnancy wastage. Am J Hum Genet. 1990;47(4):656-63.
65. Rubio C, Simón C, Vidal F, Rodrigo L, Pehlivan T, Remohí J, et al. Chromosomal abnormalities and embryo development in recurrent miscarriage couples. Hum Reprod. 2003;18(1):182-8.
66. Kahraman S, Benkhalifa M, Donmez E, Biricik A, Sertyel S, Findikli N, et al. The results of aneuploidy screening in 276 couples undergoing assisted reproductive techniques. Prenat Diagn. 2004;24(4):307-11.
67. Platteau P, Staessen C, Michiels A, Van Steirteghem A, Liebaers I, Devroey P. Preimplantation genetic diagnosis for aneuploidy screening in patients with unexplained recurrent miscarriages. Fertil Steril. 2005;83(2):393-7; quiz 525-6.
68. Murugappan G, Shahine LK, Perfetto CO, Hickok LR, Lathi RB. Intent to treat analysis of in vitro fertilization and preimplantation genetic screening versus expectant management in patients with recurrent pregnancy loss. Hum Reprod. 2016;31(8): 1668-74.
69. Musters AM, Repping S, Korevaar JC, Mastenbroek S, Limpens J, van der Veen F, et al. Pregnancy outcome after preimplantation genetic screening or natural conception in couples with unexplained recurrent miscarriage: a systematic review of the best available evidence. Fertil Steril. 2011;95(6):2153-7, 2157.e1-3.
70. Sato T, Sugiura-Ogasawara M, Ozawa F, Yamamoto T, Kato T, Kurahashi H, et al. Preimplantation genetic testing for aneuploidy: a comparison of live birth rates in patients with recurrent pregnancy loss due to embryonic aneuploidy or recurrent implantation failure. Hum Reprod. 2019;34(12):2340-8.
71. Bhatt SJ, Marchetto NM, Roy J, Morelli SS, McGovern PG. Pregnancy outcomes following in vitro fertilization frozen embryo transfer (IVF-FET) with or without preimplantation genetic testing for aneuploidy (PGT-A) in women with recurrent pregnancy loss (RPL): a SART-CORS study. Hum Reprod. 2021;36(8):2339-44.
72. Gianaroli L, Magli MC, Ferraretti AP, Munné S. Preimplantation diagnosis for aneuploidies in patients undergoing in vitro fertilization with a poor prognosis: identification of the categories for which it should be proposed. Fertil Steril. 1999;72(5):837-44.
73. Pehlivan T, Rubio C, Rodrigo L, Romero J, Remohi J, Simón C, et al. Impact of preimplantation genetic diagnosis on IVF outcome in implantation failure patients. Reprod Biomed Online. 2003;6(2):232-7.
74. Munné S, Sandalinas M, Escudero T, Velilla E, Walmsley R, Sadowy S, et al. Improved implantation after preimplantation genetic diagnosis of aneuploidy. Reprod Biomed Online. 2003;7(1):91-7.
75. Blockeel C, Schutyser V, De Vos A, Verpoest W, De Vos M, Staessen C, et al. Prospectively randomized controlled trial of PGS in IVF/ICSI patients with poor implantation. Reprod Biomed Online. 2008;17(6): 848-54.
76. Mantravadi K, Debnath S, Relekar S, Relekar N PGT-A doesn't seem to benefit recurrent implantation failure couples to optimize live births. Fertil Steril. 2020;114(3):E436.
77. Tong J, Niu Y, Wan A, Zhang T. Next-generation sequencing (NGS)-based preimplantation genetic testing for aneuploidy (PGT-A) of trophectoderm biopsy for recurrent implantation failure (RIF) patients: a RETROSPECTIVE STUDY. Reprod Sci. 2021;28(7):1923-9.
78. Schlegel PN, Sigman M, Collura B, De Jonge CJ, Eisenberg ML, Lamb DJ, et al. Diagnosis and treatment of infertility in men: AUA/ASRM Guideline Part I. J Urol. 2021;205(1):36-43.
79. Asoglu MR, Celik C, Serefoglu EC, Findikli N, Bahceci M. Preimplantation genetic testing for aneuploidy in severe male factor infertility. Reprod Biomed Online. 2020;41(4):595-603.
80. Vera-Rodriguez M, Rubio C. Assessing the true incidence of mosaicism in preimplantation embryos. Fertil Steril. 2017;107(5):1107-12.
81. Harton GL, Cinnioglu C, Fiorentino F. Current experience concerning mosaic embryos diagnosed during preimplantation genetic screening. Fertil Steril. 2017;107(5): 1113-9.
82. Gleicher N, Vidali A, Braverman J, Kushnir VA, Barad DH, Hudson C, et al. Accuracy of preimplantation genetic screening (PGS) is compromised by degree of mosaicism of human embryos. Reprod Biol Endocrinol. 2016;14(1):54.
83. Bolton H, Graham SJL, Van der Aa N, Kumar P, Theunis K, Fernandez Gallardo E, et al. Mouse model of chromosome mosaicism reveals lineage-specific depletion of aneuploid cells and normal developmental potential. Nat Commun. 2016;7:11165.
84. Greco E, Minasi MG, Fiorentino F. Healthy babies after intrauterine transfer of mosaic aneuploid blastocysts. N Engl J Med. 2015;373(21):2089-90.
85. PGDIS position statement on chromosome mosaicism and preimplantation aneuploidy testing at the blastocyst stage. PGDIS Newsletter 2016. [online] Available from: http://www.pgdis. org/docs/newsletter_071816.html. [Last accessed November 2022].
86. Practice Committees of the American Society for Reproductive Medicine and the Society for Assisted Reproductive Technology. Electronic address: ASRM@asrm.org; Practice Committees of the American Society for Reproductive Medicine and the Society for Assisted Reproductive Technology. The use of preimplantation genetic testing for aneuploidy (PGT-A): a committee opinion. Fertil Steril. 2018;109(3):429-36.

87. Kotdawala A, Patel D, Herrero J, Khajuria R, Mahajan N, Banker M. Aneuploidy screening by array comparative genomic hybridization improves success rates of in vitro fertilization: A multicenter Indian study. J Hum Reprod Sci. 2016;9(4):223-9.
88. Forman EJ, Hong KH, Ferry KM, Tao X, Taylor D, Levy B, et al. In vitro fertilization with single euploid blastocyst transfer: a randomized con- trolled trial. Fertil Steril. 2013;100(1): 100-7.e1.
89. Forman EJ, Hong KH, Franasiak JM, Scott RT Jr. Obstetrical and neonatal outcomes from the BEST Trial: single embryo transfer with aneuploidy screening improves outcomes after in vitro fertilization without compromising delivery rates. Am J Obstet Gynecol. 2014;210(2):157.e1-6.
90. Dahdouh EM, Balayla J, García-Velasco JA. Comprehensive chromosome screening improves embryo selection: a meta-analysis. Fertil Steril. 2015;104(6):1503-12.
91. Ubaldi FM, Capalbo A, Colamaria S, Ferrero S, Maggiulli R, Vajta G, et al. Reduction of multiple pregnancies in the advanced maternal age population after implementation of an elective single embryo transfer policy coupled with enhanced embryo selection: pre- and post-intervention study. Hum Reprod. 2015;30(9):2097-106.
92. Kang HJ, Melnick AP, Stewart JD, Xu K, Rosenwaks Z. Preimplantation genetic screening: who benefits? Fertil Steril. 2016;106(3):597-602.
93. Cornelisse S, Zagers M, Kostova E, Fleischer K, van Wely M, Mastenbroek S. Preimplantation genetic testing for aneuploidies (abnormal number of chromosomes) in in vitro fertilisation. Cochrane Database Syst Rev. 2020;9(9):CD005291.
94. The Gazette of India. The Assisted Reproductive Technology (Regulation) Act, 2021. [online] Available from: https://egazette.nic.in/WriteReadData/2021/232025.pdf. [Last accessed November 2022].

CHAPTER 64

Preimplantation Genetic Testing of Embryos

Rohit Gutgutia, Santosh Kumar Jena

INTRODUCTION

Preimplantation genetic testing can be defined as a test performed on the oocytes or the embryo to know any genetic abnormality or to know human leukocyte antigen (HLA) typing. This has replaced the previous terminologies, PGS (preimplantation genetic screening), and PGD (preimplantation genetic diagnosis).[1] PGT includes PGT-A (preimplantation genetic testing for aneuploidy), PGT-M (preimplantation genetic testing for monogenic disorders or single gene disorders), and PGT-SR (preimplantation genetic testing for structural chromosomal rearrangements). It essentially involves two steps, embryo biopsy or polar body biopsy (obtaining cells from the developing embryo or the oocyte) and genetic analysis of the cells by using different genetic platforms. PGT has evolved a lot in the last two decades, from being an experimental procedure during the 90s to a well-established procedure today. Shifting from day 3 (cleavage stage embryo biopsy) to day 5/6 (blastocyst) biopsy, from targeted genetic analysis to genome-wide analysis (all the 46 chromosomes and almost all single gene disorders) and robust vitrification program are few of the attributes to the present form of PGT (sometimes called PGT 2.0).

PREIMPLANTATION GENETIC TESTING FOR ANEUPLOIDY

Every human cell contains 46 chromosomes (22 pair of autosomes and sex chromosomes XY or XX). Aneuploidy can be defined as an extra or a missing chromosome. This can be detected in contemporary genetic testing by copy number variation. It is one of the most common causes of both early miscarriage and implantation failure. Few recent studies suggest that in an assisted reproductive technology (ART) cycle, >40% of all blastocysts across all age groups are aneuploid[2] and an unexpectedly high aneuploidy rate (>30%) even in oocyte donation cycles (donor age <36 years) as well.[3] Almost 90–99% of aneuploidy can be attributed to oocytes and the rest 1–10% due to sperm. Meiosis-I errors (nondisjunction giving rise to trisomy and early separation of sister chromatid giving rise to monosomy) during oogenesis result in aneuploidy. Meiosis-I errors and thus aneuploidy have a strong correlation with maternal age. Relation between age and aneuploidy can be very well-appreciated from one of the recent studies, which suggests when maternal age is between 22 and 28 years, percentage of euploid embryos ranges from 60 to 75% in contrast to just 10% embryos being euploid at 45 years.[4,5] To avoid such a negative outcome which has both financial and psychological impact, genetic testing of the preimplantation embryos and transferring only euploid embryos seems a noble step, although universal aneuploidy testing is severely criticized in recent times as evidence suggests it does not increase the cumulative live birth rate.[6] Advanced maternal age, recurrent miscarriage, recurrent implantation failure, and severe male factor infertility are the recommended indications for aneuploidy testing. Few recent studies suggest the role of aneuploidy testing in younger patients having good number of embryos to enhance the process of selection of embryo thus to reduce time to pregnancy (TTP) and encourage elective single embryo transfer (eSET), but in many countries, the local regulations do not allow aneuploidy testing for such indication.

A typical PGT cycle involves the following steps: (1) Pre-PGT work-up and counseling, (2) in vitro fertilization (IVF) cycle (3) embryo culture, (4) embryo biopsy (cleavage stage embryo or blastocyst), (5) genetic analysis and interpretation of results, (6) embryo transfer, and postpregnancy follow-up.

PRE-PREIMPLANTATION GENETIC TESTING FOR ANEUPLOIDY WORKUP AND COUNSELING

All patients undergoing PGT-A should ideally have a karyotyping done specifically so, if it is being done for recurrent miscarriage, implantation failure and severe male factor, as there is a high chance of structural chromosomal rearrangement in the above mentioned categories.

Counseling is the most important step in any PGT cycle. Patients should be counseled by a certified genetic counselor and all possible risks and outcomes of the test must be discussed beforehand including chances of having no embryo for transfer.

IN VITRO FERTILIZATION CYCLE

A conventional ovarian stimulation protocol (mild ovarian stimulation not preferred) is followed. Preferred method of fertilization should be intracytoplasmic sperm injection (ICSI) to avoid genetic contamination by granulosa cells and sperms [granulosa cell removal during oocyte-cumulus cell complex (OCC) denudation and use of single spermatozoa]. Embryos should ideally be cultured single again to avoid genetic contamination.

EMBRYO BIOPSY AND TUBING

Skill and experience of the embryologist performing biopsy is one of the most important factors for a successful PGT cycle, specifically as there is hardly any formal teaching and skill assessment methods in the field. In the Indian scenario, it is one of the limiting factors even in tier-I cities.

Day 3 versus Day 5 Biopsy

Few years back, the majority of embryo biopsies were performed on cleavage stage embryo (day 3), whereas presently blastocyst biopsy (day 5/6 or sometimes even on day 7) is the most favored one. Better embryo culture conditions (more confidence in growing embryos to blastocyst stage) and a robust vitrification program (nearly 100% post thaw survival rate) are primarily the factors of this recent shift from cleavage stage biopsy to blastocyst biopsy.

Advantages of blastocyst biopsy are as follows:

- More genetic material (removal of 5–10 cells from trophoectoderm) is obtained for analysis, which overcomes the problem of insufficient genetic material, frequently encountered on a day 3 embryo biopsy (removal of one or two cells).
- Percentage of cells removed from the embryo is lesser in a blastocyst (5–10 cells out of 64–128 cells) in comparison to cleavage stage embryo biopsy (1–2 cells out of 8 cells).
- It only removes cells from trophoectoderm and leaves the inner cell mass (ICM) undisturbed.
- As blastocyst is a more advanced stage in embryo selection method, so doing unnecessary biopsy of a day 3 embryo is avoided, which anyway won't survive till day 5/6.
- Chances of mosaicism are less in a blastocyst compared to cleavage stage embryos. Also, chances of errors (in mosaicism detection) are lower when more cells are analyzed.

Method of obtaining biopsy involves creating an opening in the zona (zona drilling) by either chemical or using noncontact LASER (commonly practiced method presently). This is followed by aspirating cells using embryo biopsy pipette and removing the cells from the trophoectoderm interface either by using LASER shots to favor detachment from embryo or gentle mechanical (flickering) movement. Blastocyst biopsy is only possible where there is a clear differentiation between the ICM and trophoectoderm. Throughout the biopsy procedure, the ICM should be positioned between 7 and 11 o'clock position[7] and biopsy site at 3 o'clock position to avoid any unintended injury to ICM. Each embryo should be individually tracked throughout the procedure of biopsy.

Tubing is an equally important step in embryo biopsy method. It involves transferring the genetic material with very minimal media into a container provided by the genetic laboratory. Sometimes there is a risk of losing the genetic material in the process of washing and transferring it to the tubes though it is extremely rare in experienced hands. Also, there is a chance of contamination by exogenous genetic material. Then the tubes containing cells can be transferred to the genetic laboratory for analysis following the service providers' recommendation or it can also be stored specially in cases where embryo pooling and PGT-A is planned, where collectively genetic materials from embryos obtained from different stimulation cycles are sent together. After biopsy, the embryos can be vitrified using a separate cryopreservation device for each embryo.

GENETIC ANALYSIS

The very first step in the genetic analysis is amplification of the genetic material. Multiple amplification cycles are run to obtain enough genetic material for analysis of all 24 chromosomes. The amplification can be of whole-genome amplification or even a targeted amplification, where a target area is amplified for studying specific regions. Targeted amplification increases the depth of genetic analysis in the region of interest at the cost of breadth of analysis. Postamplification the genetic analysis is carried out by using methods such as CGH (comparative genomic hybridization), array CGH, SNP (single nucleotide polymorphism), or a NGS (next-generation sequencing) based platform to detect the copy number variations. Among all, NGS-based platforms are widely followed and more popular nowadays.[8] FISH (fluorescent in situ hybridization) which was practiced in the initial days of genetic testing is almost completely replaced by these newer methods which can provide a comprehensive analysis of all 24 chromosomes with much accuracy and at the same time, less time-consuming.

COMPARATIVE GENOMIC HYBRIDIZATION

After amplification, the targeted DNA is labeled with green fluorescent dye, the same is repeated for a known reference sample (normal chromosome), which is labeled with red fluorescent dye. Both test and reference DNA after hybridization are added to a normal metaphasic spread. The color signal is read by a computer imaging system. Any deviation of color intensity from the 1:1 ratio indicates the copy number variation of the target chromosome.

ARRAY COMPARATIVE GENOMIC HYBRIDIZATION

Principle of the test remains the same, except in place of metaphasic chromosomes microarray-based solid support is used. This eliminates the use of metaphasic spread which is nonuniform and prone for errors and thus favors automation and rapid analysis.

SINGLE NUCLEOTIDE POLYMORPHISM MICROARRAYS

Single nucleotide polymorphism represents the variations at a single base position. SNP array contains probes of thousands of unique nucleotide sequences that are distributed across the length of chromosomes. Known nucleotide sequence is used as a probe and the tested DNA is hybridized with the known sequence and the fluorescent signal is analyzed both qualitatively and quantitatively. Its advantage being single gene disorders also can be diagnosed at the same time during aneuploidy testing.

NEXT-GENERATION SEQUENCING

Postamplification the product is fragmented to produce millions of short segments of DNA. These numerous short pieces are simultaneously sequenced in parallel. This greatly reduces the cost of sequencing as multiple samples can be run in one go. The depth of analysis is typically lower in a conventional NGS method (sometimes called "low pass" or "shallow" sequencing). This "low-depth analysis" is still considered adequate for numeric chromosomal analysis[9] (aneuploidy) but the information obtained regarding individual genes is negligible although targeted sequencing is also an option for studying monogenic disorders, where a deeper sequencing is essential. There are various commercially available platforms to run NGS.

INTERPRETATION OF RESULT

Results of a PGT-A testing are no longer just a binary division. We now have situations of mosaic embryo and segmental aneuploidy apart from usual euploid and aneuploid embryos. All these need special attention as these situations demand special counseling sessions and management challenges. Although genetic testing methodology has undergone a reform in the last two decades, the lack of standardization is still a major challenge. Aneuploidy can affect a single chromosome or even multiple chromosomes called complex aneuploidy. Aneuploid embryos are not suitable for transfer.

Complex Aneuploidy

When the aneuploidy involves two or more chromosomes in the same embryo. Complex aneuploidies are incompatible with life.

MOSAIC EMBRYOS

Mosaicism is the presence of two different cell lines with different chromosomal configurations (in context of PGT-A, co-presence of both euploid and aneuploid cells) in the same embryo. It is mostly a mitotic error that results from mal-segregation of sister chromatids during the cell division. Chances of mosaicism reduce as the embryo grows. In one of the studies where embryos found to be mosaic on day 5/6 biopsy were cultured till day 12 and rebiopsy is done on day 12. Surprisingly, only 20% of those embryos, previously diagnosed as mosaic, retain mosaicism and the rest corrected.[10] This phenomenon of autocorrection of mosaicism is a well-acknowledged fact now. Autocorrection mainly depends on the fraction of cells that have been affected by mosaicism. Chances of correction are lower if the mitotic event happens early in cell division (closer to zygote stage) as more fraction of cells are affected downstream, whereas if it affects remote from zygote stage, mosaicism fragment is less and chance of autocorrection is higher. Contrary to the meiotic errors (maternal age-related aneuploidy risk), mitotic errors are not age-related and there is a uniform baseline risk throughout the reproductive years.[11] Many laboratories report mosaicism according to the percentage of mosaic cells and categorized it into different categories such as low mosaic (20–30%), medium mosaic (30–50%), high mosaic (50–70%), and aneuploid (>70% mosaic fraction).[12]

MANAGEMENT OF MOSAIC EMBRYOS

Many recent reports have been published from various groups regarding the transfer of mosaic embryos and its outcome. All these evidences indicate that mosaic embryo can result in viable pregnancy, although the chances of implantation failure and miscarriage are higher compared to euploid embryos.[13] Mosaic embryos, specifically low mosaic ones, can be considered for transfer in the absence of euploid embryos. Before proceeding with transfer of mosaic embryos, patients must be counseled thoroughly regarding the need of invasive prenatal testing such as amniocentesis or chorionic villus sampling as the data regarding the outcome of mosaic embryos is still limited.

SEGMENTAL ANEUPLOIDY

Segmental aneuploidy, also called partial aneuploidy, affects subchromosomal area and it results due to regional loss or gain of a segment of a chromosome. Presently used PGT-A testing platforms can diagnose segmental aneuploidy in a chromosome if the segment is of 10–20 Mb or above. Many a times segmental aneuploidy of trophoectoderm biopsy does not properly represent the changes in ICM. Although presently there is no clarity regarding the management of segmental aneuploidy but very few studies suggest rebiopsy of trophoectoderm as an option. According to one such study, chances of ICM carrying the same segmental aneuploidy are just 21% if both biopsies are discordant, whereas this figure goes as high as 84% if both biopsies are concordant.[14]

LIMITATIONS OF PREIMPLANTATION GENETIC TESTING FOR ANEUPLOIDY TESTING

Current PGT-A testing has 1–2% chance of error, giving either false positive result (reported as aneuploidy when actually the embryo is euploid) or false negative result (reported as euploid when embryo is aneuploid). This is mainly due to mosaicism and the fact that trophoectoderm cells may not always be a true representation of the ICM, though there is a high concordance rate, documented from various studies. Routine prenatal screening and testing methodology should be followed in all patients undergoing PGT.

There can be other genetic or nongenetic causes of birth defects. PGT-A can detect it only if it results from chromosomal copy number variations. For example, single gene disorders can never be diagnosed in a PGT-A testing.

Preimplantation genetic testing for aneuploidy can only detect aneuploidy (either gain or loss of chromosomal copy number from euploid). It cannot detect situations involving alteration in an entire set of chromosome as in haploid (absence of a set of all 23 chromosomes) or triploid (presence of one extra set of all 23 chromosomes).

It cannot detect uniparental disomy (UPD), where both the sets of chromosomes come from a single parent only.

ADVERSE EFFECTS OF BIOPSY

One of the criticisms of doing an embryo biopsy is damage to the embryo and reduction in implantation potential due to the biopsy procedure itself although it is extremely rare in experienced hands but there can be situations of technical difficulty during biopsy procedure (sometimes due to poor embryo quality itself) resulting in damage to the embryo.

DIFFICULT SITUATIONS IN PREIMPLANTATION GENETIC TESTING

Insufficient Genetic Material

It is one of the situations which needs to be counseled with the patient properly specifically in situations of unavailability of euploid embryos. Many times it is due to compromised embryo quality itself. Rebiopsy of the embryo can be considered as an option along with transfer of the embryo without genetic analysis (benefits of PGT-A are lost).

No Transferable Embryos

This is a commonly encountered situation and needs proper counseling prior to starting the IVF cycle itself.

We have a balanced opinion about PGT-A, after analyzing our unit's PGT-A data from the last 2 years. Analysis of PGT-A result of 289 blastocysts (exclusive blastocyst biopsy) from 66 patients showed euploid rate of 40% and an implantation rate of 56.6% after the transfer of the resulting euploid embryos with maximum chance of implantation in subcategory of patient who had previous miscarriage due to aneuploid pregnancy. Success rate of euploid embryo transfer is fairly similar across all age groups. Noninformative results were obtained in 2.7% of the biopsied embryo. 11 patients (out of total 66) did not have any euploid embryo for transfer, either due to all embryos being aneuploid/mosaic or noninformative result. One such patient (out of 11) has an ongoing pregnancy that resulted from transfer of a rebiopsy-confirmed euploid embryo that had no DNA detected in the first biopsy attempt.

PREIMPLANTATION GENETIC TESTING FOR MONOGENIC DISORDERS OR SINGLE GENE DISORDERS

It is now possible to diagnose all kinds of single gene disorders using the trophectoderm biopsy and subsequent genetic analysis.

Most of the steps of PGT-M, except for the step of pre-PGT work-up and the genetic analysis, are similar to a PGT-A cycle and already discussed in this chapter.

INDICATION OF PREIMPLANTATION GENETIC TESTING FOR MONOGENIC DISORDERS OR SINGLE GENE DISORDERS

There is an extensive list of 1,380 single gene disorders approved by HFEA (Human Fertilisation and Embryology Authority), UK, which can be tested using PGT-M technique. Autosomal dominant disorders are the most common indication of PGT-M (64%), followed by autosomal recessive (21%) and X-linked disorders (15%), respectively. Ten common indications in decreasing order of prevalence (as per ESHRE PGT Consortium data)[15] are mentioned in **Table 1**.

In Indian scenario, as per our own experience, hematologic conditions are the most common indication for PGT-M followed by musculoskeletal and other indications such as cystic fibrosis and BRCA-1 mutation detection.

PRE-PREIMPLANTATION GENETIC TESTING WORK-UP

Fundamental basis of the pre-PGT-M work-up is identifying haplotype (group of alleles that are inherited together along with the gene of interest). First it is assessed whether a specific

TABLE 1: Commonest indication in decreasing order of prevalence.	
Huntington disease	9%
Cystic fibrosis	4.6%
Neurofibromatosis type 1	4.3%
Myotonic dystrophy type 1	4.3%
Breast ovarian cancer, familial susceptibility to, 1	4.3%
Beta-thalassemia	
Fragile X syndrome	
Breast ovarian cancer, familial susceptibility to, 2	
Marfan syndrome	
Muscular dystrophy, Duchenne type	

pattern is noted in affected members of the family that can be differentiated from nonaffected members. If a specific pattern can be identified, it is called high risk haplotype, then the embryo is tested for presence of the same, i.e., "the indirect method of testing." If a specific pattern cannot be identified because of either de novo mutation or absence of family members for pre-PGT work-up, then a direct method is followed to detect new mutations using different genetic markers.

First step in PGT-M work-up is a pedigree analysis by an expert geneticist to find out the inheritance in the family and the need of collecting blood samples from relevant family members apart from the couple.

After haplotype differentiation (high risk and low risk) test strategy is decided in the pre-PGT work-up itself and validation is checked.

GENETIC ANALYSIS IN CASE OF PREIMPLANTATION GENETIC TESTING FOR MONOGENIC DISORDERS OR SINGLE GENE DISORDERS

Genetic analysis that is most commonly followed in contemporary PGT-M analysis involves whole-genome amplification followed by downstream analysis either using SNP array or NGS-based methods to detect the presence of gene of interest in the embryo.

PREIMPLANTATION GENETIC TESTING FOR STRUCTURAL CHROMOSOMAL REARRANGEMENTS

Structural rearrangement is the most common indication for performing PGT-SR accounting 64% of all PGT-SR cases followed by Robertsonian translocation (22% of cases). Chromosomal inversion and deletion account for small fraction of cases of PGT-SR.[15]

Most unbalanced structural rearrangements can be diagnosed using modern-day NGS platforms for PGT-A detection, provided it is above the threshold level of detection, i.e., 10–20 Mb.

Balanced structural rearrangements, chromosomal inversion, and unbalanced translocation below the threshold level need different genetic analysis methods. In these categories of cases, there is still a role of the conventional FISH assay.

In pre-PGT-SR work-up, the karyotyping of the couple along with the exact structural change should be shared with the genetic laboratory to plan the testing strategy and validation of the same.

Analysis of single cell is preferred in few scenarios of genetic testing by the FISH method. So the genetic laboratory may suggest to do preferably a cleavage stage biopsy than a blastocyst biopsy (trophoectoderm cells are difficult to separate individually due to cohesive nature of trophoectoderm cells) in these scenarios.

HUMAN LEUKOCYTE ANTIGEN TYPING

Human leukocyte antigen typing of the embryo can also be done along with PGT-M keeping all the ethical concerns (creating a life for the purpose of helping the affected child) in mind and if permitted by local regulations.

MITOCHONDRIAL DNA QUANTIFICATION IN PREIMPLANTATION GENETIC TESTING

The basic principle behind this is mitochondrial DNA does not divide in a cell till blastocyst stage. So in slow growing embryos, the mitochondrial DNA content per cell is higher compared to a fast growing embryo. Few studies suggest the impaired implantation potential of embryo beyond certain level of mitochondrial DNA in embryos, though its application in routine practice is questionable. All euploid embryos should be considered for transfer but given situation to choose among euploid ones, embryo with lesser mitochondrial DNA score should be preferred as it has a better implantation potential.

NONINVASIVE PREIMPLANTATION GENETIC TESTING

Over the years, the genetic analysis of embryos has become very comprehensive to cover all 24 chromosomes and practically all single gene disorders. With more and more clients opting for PGT, even the cost of genetic analysis is reduced to a great extent and is no longer a limiting factor. Presently, biopsy procedure is one of the limiting steps considering the requirement of highly skilled personnel and hi-tech equipment. Added to that, invasive PGT cannot be performed in embryos having poor morphology.

BASIS OF NONINVASIVE PREIMPLANTATION GENETIC TESTING

It is based on the principle of detection of cell-free DNA in the spent culture medium (SCM) or blastocyst cavity (blastocele). This DNA can be extracted, amplified, and downstream genetic analysis can be performed to detect aneuploidy.

LIMITATION OF NONINVASIVE PREIMPLANTATION GENETIC TESTING

Amplification failure is one of the major concerns as the DNA content is very minimal.

Contamination from other genetic material (maternal cells contamination, cell-free DNA in some of media preparation, and from laboratory personnel) is the other major issue.

Cell-free DNA may not be a correct representation of the embryo and thought to be the byproduct cell repair mechanism. During autocorrection of the embryo, the defective cells undergo apoptosis and it is released into the culture media and blastocele fluid. So rather it may erroneously have false positive results when the embryo had already undergone correction after extruding the defective cells.

CURRENT STATUS OF NONINVASIVE PREIMPLANTATION GENETIC TESTING

Noninvasive PGT is now implemented in many IVF centers as one of the options of genetic testing though results from various studies about its concordance with the invasive PGT are contradictory.

One of the recent multicenter prospective studies conducted on 1,301 embryos showed a concordance rate of trophoectoderm biopsy with cell-free DNA assay of 78.2%, ranging from 72.5 to 86.3% among different centers. Concordance rate exceeded 86% when all the defined laboratory parameters were followed to minimize contamination. In a subgroup of 81 blastocysts, where ICM biopsy was also done, the comparison of the ICM with the embryonic cell-free DNA and the trophectoderm biopsies had shown similar concordance rates, 84.4% and 87.5%, respectively,[16] though many other small studies have contradictory findings. At this point in time, we still need more evidence before completely relying on a noninvasive method of testing.

FUTURE PERSPECTIVE

Considering the invasive nature of PGT and its limitations, a truly noninvasive PGT retaining its concordance rate with the invasive one will be a revolution in genetic testing of embryos. Many other markers such as microRNA (short noncoding RNA fragments) and EV (extracellular vesicles: nanoparticles of cellular metabolism byproducts made up of lipid bilayer which can readily cross cell membrane) are also studied by various researchers, which may be possible in future.

REFERENCES

1. Zegers-Hochschild F, Adamson GD, Dyer S, Racowsky C, de Mouzon J, Sokol R, et al. The international glossary on infertility and fertility care 2017. Hum Reprod. 2017;32(9):1786-801.
2. Franasiak JM, Forman EJ, Hong KH, Werner MD, Upham KM, Treff NR, et al. Aneuploidy across individual chromosomes at the embryonic level in trophectoderm biopsies: changes with patient age and chromosome structure. J Assist Reprod Genet. 2014;31(11):1501-9.
3. Munné S, Alikani M, Ribustello L, Colls P, Martinez-Ortiz PA, McCulloh DH, et al. Euploidy rates in donor egg cycles significantly differ between fertility centers. Hum Reprod. 2017;32(4):743-9.
4. Demko ZP, Simon AL, McCoy RC, Petrov DA, Rabinowitz M. Effects of maternal age on euploidy rates in a large cohort of embryos analyzed with 24-chromosome single-nucleotide polymorphism-based preimplantation genetic screening. Fertil Steril. 2016;105(5):1307-13.
5. Franasiak JM, Forman EJ, Hong KH, Werner MD, Upham KM, Treff NR, et al. The nature of aneuploidy with increasing age of the female partner: a review of 15,169 consecutive trophectoderm biopsies evaluated with comprehensive chromosomal screening. Fertil Steril. 2014;101(3):656-63.
6. Munné S, Kaplan B, Frattarelli JL, Child T, Nakhuda G, Shamma FN, et al. Preimplantation genetic testing for aneuploidy versus morphology as selection criteria for single frozen-thawed embryo transfer in good-prognosis patients: a multicenter randomized clinical trial. Fertil Steril. 2019;112(6):1071-9.
7. ESHRE PGT Consortium and SIG-Embryology Biopsy Working Group; Kokkali G, Coticchio G, Bronet F, Celebi C, Cimadomo D, et al. ESHRE PGT Consortium and SIG Embryology good practice recommendations for polar body and embryo biopsy for preimplantation genetic testing. Hum Reprod Open. 2020;2020(3):hoaa020.
8. Fiorentino F, Biricik A, Bono S, Spizzichino L, Cotroneo E, Cottone G, et al. Development and validation of a next-generation sequencing-based protocol for 24-chromosome aneuploidy screening of embryos. Fertil Steril. 2014;101(5):1375-82.
9. Deleye L, Dheedene A, De Coninck D, Sante T, Christodoulou C, Heindryckx B, et al. Shallow whole genome sequencing is well suited for the detection of chromosomal aberrations in human blastocysts. Fertil Steril. 2015;104(5):1276-85.
10. Popovic M, Dhaenens L, Taelman J, Dheedene A, Bialecka M, De Sutter P, et al. Extended in vitro culture of human embryos demonstrates the complex nature of diagnosing chromosomal mosaicism from a single trophectoderm biopsy. Hum Reprod. 2019;34:758-69.
11. McCoy RC, Demko ZP, Ryan A, Banjevic M, Hill M, Sigurjonsson S, et al. Evidence of selection against complex mitotic-origin aneuploidy during preimplantation development. PLoS Genet. 2015;11:e1005601.
12. Capalbo A, Poli M, Rienzi L, Girardi L, Patassini C, Fabiani M, et al. Mosaic human preimplantation embryos and their developmental potential in a prospective, non-selection clinical trial. Am J Hum Genet. 2021;108(12):2238-47.

13. Munné S, Spinella F, Grifo J, Zhang J, Beltran MP, Fragouli E, et al. Clinical outcomes after the transfer of blastocysts characterized as mosaic by high resolution next generation sequencing-further insights. Eur J Med Genet. 2020;63(2):103741.
14. Girardi L, Serdarogullari M, Patassini C, Poli M, Fabiani M, Caroselli S, et al. Incidence, origin, and predictive model for the detection and clinical management of segmental aneuploidies in human embryos. Am J Hum Genet. 2020; 106(4):525-34.
15. van Montfoort A, Carvalho F, Coonen E, Kokkali G, Moutou C, Rubio C, et al. ESHRE PGT Consortium data collection XIX-XX: PGT analyses from 2016 to 2017. Hum Reprod Open. 2021;2021(3):hoab024.
16. Rubio C, Navarro-Sánchez L, García-Pascual CM, Ocali O, Cimadomo D, Venier W, et al. Multicenter prospective study of concordance between embryonic cell-free DNA and trophectoderm biopsies from 1301 human blastocysts. Am J Obstet Gynecol. 2020;223(5):751.e1-13.

CHAPTER 65

Epigenetics and Assisted Reproductive Technology

Mandeep Kaur, Ajitabh Shukla

INTRODUCTION

There is growing evidence that epigenetics, an erstwhile obscure branch of medicine, may be increasingly more relevant in human reproduction than previously realized. Environmental and dietary influences may surreptitiously creep into the germ line, only to reflect in future generations in the form of intractable genetic diseases.

Assisted reproductive technology (ART) contributes to 1–2% of the total live births in developed countries.[1] ART has helped achieve pregnancies for millions of couples, grappling with infertility due to various physiological and anatomical obstacles. In view of the steadily rising interest and the immense possibilities in this field, it is imperative on the part of the reproductive specialist to be aware of the emerging evidence and be able to discuss them in an informed and responsible manner with the patients, as permitted by the current data.

This chapter aims at providing an insight into the basics of epigenetics, imprinting disorders, and the latest evidence of the impact of ART procedures on genetic imprinting. Comprehending the depths of the biochemistry involved in imprinting is rather arduous, so the authors have tried to lean more toward the clinical relevance of the same in this chapter.

EPIGENETICS

Waddington in 1942 introduced the term epigenetics.[2] It is the study of the changes in organisms caused by the modification of gene expression rather than the alteration of the genetic code. Epigenetics was later formally defined as "the study of mitotically and meiotically heritable changes in gene function that cannot be explained by changes in deoxyribonucleic acid (DNA) sequences."[3] This modification of the gene expression is heritable and can be influenced by environmental factors.[4] It may well be due to differences in chromosome packaging.[5]

Gene expression is influenced by changes in the chromatin structure **(Flowchart 1)**. Broadly stating, the genes are inactivated when the chromatin is condensed and expressed when the chromatin is open.

Methylation is the most well-studied epigenetic modification. DNA methylation is the addition of a methyl group to the DNA, which results in changed or altered gene expression, and is essential for embryonic development, genomic stability, gene silencing, and oncogenesis. Methylation usually occurs in the CpG site of the DNA ("p" in CpG stands for the phosphate group in the dinucleotide). This site is present in the promoter regions of the gene, which, according to the methylation status, activates or silences the gene.[6] Specific CpG methylation patterns are established in early development and are passed on during the process of DNA replication by DNA-methyltransferase-1 (DNMT-1).[7] Dietary deficiencies may result in low levels of folate, selenium, and methionine and this could lead to changes in DNA methylation, and as a result, clinical consequences, such as neural tube defects, cancers, and atherosclerosis.[8]

Histones are core proteins around which DNA is wound. The details of nucleosome structure are explained in **Flowchart 2**. Histone modifications can lead to

Flowchart 1: Epigenetic modifications.

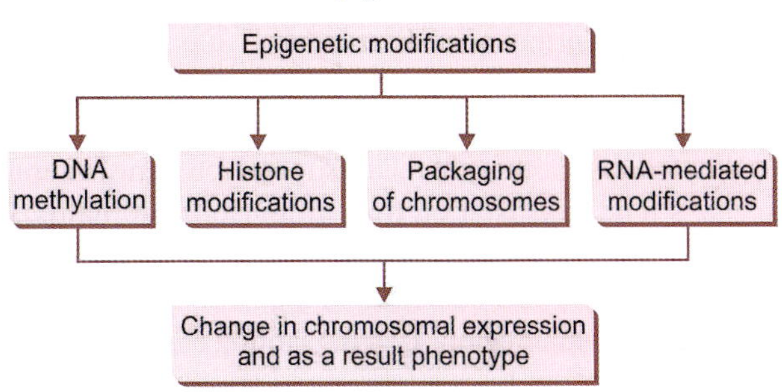

(DNA: deoxyribonucleic acid; RNA: ribonucleic acid)

Flowchart 2: Nucleosome.

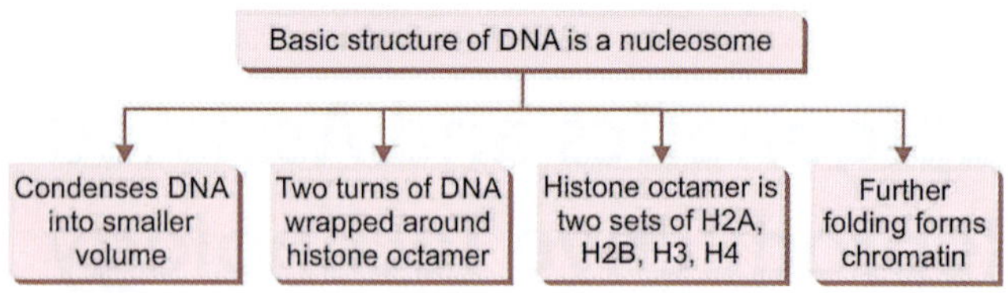

(DNA: deoxyribonucleic acid)

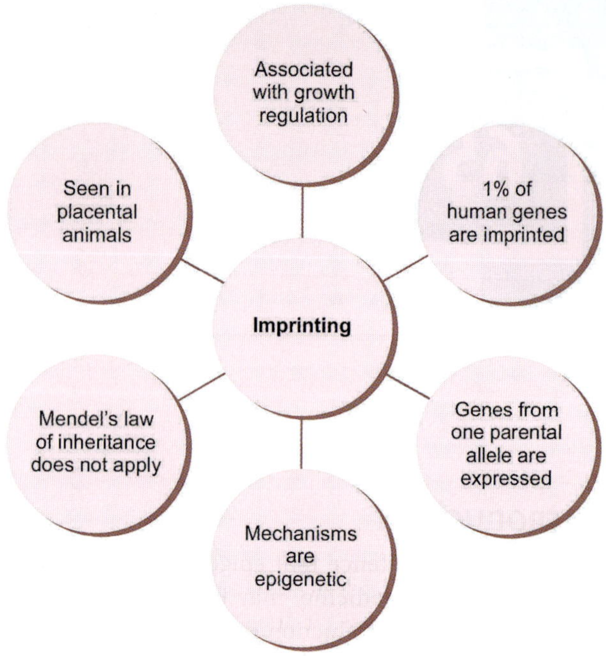

Fig. 1: Imprinting.

changes in gene expression (suppression or activation) depending upon the change in the amino acid sequence.[9]

GENOMIC IMPRINTING

According to Mendel's law of inheritance, genes from both parents play an equally important role in the process of development. However, genomic imprinting is an exception to this—it is a modification of the genome, selectively allowing *genes from only one parental allele to be expressed.* The underlying mechanism is mostly epigenetic, which implies a condition in which the DNA sequence is not changed, but the alleles are chosen to be expressed in a sex-specific manner.

We inherit two copies of all autosomal genes, and essentially almost all of them are expressed equally from maternally and paternally inherited alleles. However, some of the mammalian genes are expressed preferentially from either the paternal or the maternal alleles. The alleles are *stamped* by the epigenetic influences, which then continues throughout the pre and peri-implantation phases. This partial "favoritism" of some alleles is imprinting. Genomic imprinting, in other words, is the parental battle of the sexes to regulate the distribution of maternal resources to the offspring.[10] 1% of human genes are associated with imprinting.[11] Imprinting syndromes are the set of conditions that result from a disturbance in the expression of the genes that are known to be imprinted. Many of these genes are associated with the regulation of prenatal and postnatal growth.[12]

"Paternal disomy" appears to lead to retarded embryonic tissue but well-developed extraembryonic (placental) tissue development. "Maternal disomy," on the other hand, appears to be associated with poorly developed extraembryonic tissue with relatively normal or small embryos.[13] It is interesting to note that imprinting disorders are seen mainly in placental animals (summary in **Fig. 1**).

Clustering is another characteristic of imprinting, wherein the genes tend to cluster on the chromosome domains. In humans, these are seen on chromosomes 6, 7, 11, 14, 15, and 20. Clustering allows a coordinated regulation of genes in a given chromosomal region. Two imprinting clusters are well known: One on the human chromosome 11p15, which is associated with the *Beckwith-Wiedemann syndrome* (BWS), and another on 15q11-q13, related to the pathogenesis of the *Angelman syndrome* (AS) or the Prader-Willi syndrome (PWS). These clusters are regulated by imprinting centers (IC). Microdeletions in the ICs can affect the imprinting status of the genes even kilobases away.[14] The *insulin growth factor-2* (*IGF2/H19*), IC for example, coregulates *IGF2* and *H19*, and both these genes are located in the same imprinted domain, about 90 kb apart.[15]

HUMAN PHENOTYPES ASSOCIATED WITH IMPRINTED GENES

These include:
- BWS (11p15)
- PWS (15q11-q13)
- AS (15q11-q13)
- Silver-Russell syndrome (SRS) (11p15/7p11-p13)
- Transient neonatal diabetes mellitus (6q24)
- McCune-Albright syndrome (20q13)
- Familial nonchromaffin paraganglioma (11q13)
- Maternal and paternal UPD14 syndromes (14).

These are the known human phenotypes associated with imprinting genes (chromosome numbers in brackets).[16]

EPIGENETICS IN FETAL ORIGIN OF ADULT DISEASE

Mammalian phenotype can also be changed by the influence of nutrition on the epigenetic gene regulatory mechanisms. This forms the basis for the *"fetal origin of adult disease."* Epigenetic alterations associated with starvation of the mother in fetal life have an effect on adulthood, and thus have been known to be contributing to late-onset disorders, such as cardiovascular diseases and diabetes.[17]

BOX 1: Drawbacks of the studies showing a positive association between assisted reproductive technology and imprinting disorders.

- Small-sample size
- No correction for maternal age or diagnosis of infertility
- Statistical assumptions

TABLE 1: Mechanism of imprinting.

Event	*Timing*
Erasure	When germ cells enter the gonad
Acquisition	During oocyte and sperm maturation
Maintenance	After fertilization

In 2009, Katari et al. reported that there is a difference in some gene expression patterns between the babies who conceived naturally compared to the babies who conceived by means of in vitro fertilization (IVF). These changes were inherited by the future generations and were under epigenetic control. This mechanism could potentially place the children conceived by means of IVF at risk of certain diseases such as diabetes and obesity later in life.[18]

WHEN DID THE CONCERN START?

There is a general consensus that ART slightly increases the risk of congenital malformations in fetuses (3–4 vs. 2–3%). However, its association with epigenetic disorders is still debatable.[19]

In 2002, Cox et al. reported the association of AS with intracytoplasmic sperm injection (ICSI).[20] In 2003, the British[21] and French[22] medical registry data reported a higher incidence of BWS or the human overgrowth syndrome in ART conceptions. SRS[23] and retinoblastoma[24] were also reported to be higher in ART conceptions. It was also reported that the stimulation of the ovaries with gonadotropins causes differences in gene expression and methylation changes in the oocytes recovered from stimulated ovaries.[25]

Consequently, it was realized that these studies had a myriad of technical deficiencies. **Box 1** simplifies the drawbacks of these studies.[26] This led to a fallaciously exaggerated relative risk.

However, ensuing better-designed studies, and notably a systematic review and meta-analysis, also suggested an association of imprinting disorders with ART.[27]

WHAT IS THE MOST CRUCIAL PERIOD FOR IMPRINTING?

Germ cell development and early embryogenesis are the crucial times for erasure of the parental imprints, acquisition of the new imprints, and their maintenance during the process of embryogenesis. So, the concern with ART is valid as all these processes occur in artificial conditions, in comparison to the "in vivo" environment of spontaneous conceptions **(Table 1)**:

1. *Erasure:* When the germ cells enter the gonad, complete erasure of parental imprint occurs. Complete erasure of the entire genome of the parental imprints in the primordial germ cells occurs to serve the following three purposes:
   a. Totipotency of the gametes is restored.
   b. There is establishment of epigenetic equivalency before the establishment of new imprints during the process of gametogenesis.
   c. Any acquired epigenetic marks present in the adult somatic cells are removed.[28]
2. *Acquisition:* During the process of gametogenesis, primary imprints are established, and this occurs via the action of DNA methyltransferase enzymes.[29] The methylation programming of the sperms is complete by birth, whereas the methylation programming of the oocyte begins at puberty and is complete at the time of ovulation.
3. *Maintenance:* These primary parental imprints, established at the time of gametogenesis, are maintained during embryonic development and persist into adulthood. This maintenance occurs despite the second wave of erasure, which occurs just after fertilization. In order to ensure correct differentiation into the embryonic and extraembryonic cell lineages, methylation of the genome occurs at the blastocyst stage.

POTENTIAL RISKS IN ASSISTED REPRODUCTIVE TECHNOLOGY

Infertility, in itself, is a potential risk factor for imprinting. The additional effects of IVF, per se, further confound the issue. All the IVF-related manipulations take place almost exactly at the period when the epigenetic mechanisms too are active in the germ cells. The effect of the environment on the embryo is greater in the early stages of development. The epigenetic foci too are remodeled principally during the gametogenesis and early embryogenesis, so there is a legitimate concern with ART, wherein there is artificial manipulation of the gamete, potentially leading to increased susceptibility of the genome to epigenetic modulations.

We can divide the effects of ART on imprinting into the following categories as described here.

Male Gamete

Use of immature spermatids, surgically obtained germ cells, frozen–thawed gametes, and ICSI involving micromanipulation of both the gametes (postulations in **Box 2**) are the processes in ART where there is an apprehension of the increased susceptibility of acquisition of imprinting disorders. However, technically postulating, it is unlikely that ART involving the use of male gametes in the form of either surgically obtained immature sperms or elongated

BOX 2: How is intracytoplasmic sperm injection responsible for imprinting postulations?

- Disruption of the cytoskeleton of oocyte
- Leakage of cytoplasm
- Bypassing natural barrier/natural selection
- Paternal age/subfertility/genetic disorders
- Removal of cumulus
- Abnormal oocyte activation

sperms would interfere with the acquisition of imprinting disorders, as both erasure and the acquisition of new imprints appear to be completed by the spermatid phase of spermatogenesis. But this needs to be veritably proven with more studies.

Female Gamete

In vitro maturation, downregulation, superovulation, culturing and micromanipulation of mature oocytes, and freezing-thawing injuries are the concerns with the female gametes. Ovulation induction has been suggested to be one of the reasons for methylation errors, but it is still not clear whether ovulation induction is the root cause in itself or it is attributable to the backdrop of advanced age and underlying infertility.

Embryo Culture

Embryo culture, especially prolonged culture, manipulation, and cryopreservation, are the procedures that are thought to be related to imprinting. Preimplantation genetic screening (PGS), in fact, involves direct and invasive manipulation of the embryos. The temperature, pH, oxygen concentration, etc., in the culture media all are potential threats to the epigenetic modulation of the embryo.

The first concern of overgrowth due to culture media was the "large offspring syndrome" in cattle, characterized by high birth weight, organ overgrowth, and respiratory distress. This happened particularly when embryos were cultured with serum.[30] Weight is important as it is a marker of the growth and a harbinger of the future metabolic and cardiovascular diseases. The jury is still out on this, though with one study reporting a significant difference in the weight of the babies born after in vitro culture of embryos[31] and another refuting the same.[32] A study compiled 11 studies on media comparisons and found that while six studies showed differences, five did not. They made a note of the possibility of incomplete revelation of the culture conditions in at least some of these studies.[33] These concerns thus still await to be addressed, though it has been suggested recently that the presence of essential amino acids in culture on the first 3 days of embryo development reduces the chance of imprinting errors.[34] One impressive study reported a multitude of effects of culture media, including that on the metabolic cycles, of mouse embryos.[35]

The authors feel that in the backdrop of the above, there should, in fact, be a general shift toward disclosure of the contents, in which embryos are cultured, rather than veiling it behind a shroud of secrecy.

Ovarian Stimulation

Superovulation and pharmacological ovarian stimulation are unnatural procedures, leading to unnatural and accelerated growth of the follicles. It also leads to the atypical selection of multiple dominant follicles, bypassing the natural growth restriction mechanisms, thus potentially predisposing the eggs/embryos to epigenetic influences. A study has, in fact, incriminated ovarian stimulation with epigenetic changes at multiple loci.[36]

SPECIFIC IMPRINTING DISORDERS

- Beckwith-Wiedemann syndrome is reported to have an incidence of 1 in 14,500 live births.[37] It is a rare disorder characterized by a fetus which is large for gestational age. The placenta is large and thickened and the pregnancy may also be associated with polyhydramnios. Other characteristics include:
    - Macrosomia (newborn significantly larger than average)
    - Macroglossia (medical term for unusually large tongue)
    - Visceromegaly (enlargement of organs inside the abdomen)
    - Embryonal tumors (Wilms' tumor, hepatoblastoma, neuroblastoma, and rhabdomyosarcoma)
    - Omphalocele (a hernia in which the abdominal organs protrude in the umbilical cord)
    - Neonatal hypoglycemia
    - Ear creases or pits
    - Adrenocortical cytomegaly (presence of bizarre-looking eosinophilic cells in the adrenals)
    - Renal abnormalities.[38]

  Monochorionic twinning is also reported to be higher in BWS.[39] The disorder occurs due to *"paternal disomy and maternal deletion of chromosome 11p15.5."* Both BWS and SRS are related to chromosome 11p15.5. SRS is a condition characterized by severe intrauterine growth retardation, poor neonatal growth, and abnormalities in the craniofacial features, such as a broad forehead and a triangular face, also accompanied by asymmetry of the body and a variety of minor malformations.[40] Hypomethylation of *H19* at chromosome 11p15.5 (40%) occurs frequently in SRS.[41]

  Maternal UPD of chromosome 7 is also known to be associated in a few cases.
- "AS and PWS" are two distinct syndromes that map to the imprinting cluster on chromosome 15q11 to q13.[42]

Each syndrome is associated with mental retardation and other problems in growth, behavior, and sexual development.[43]

- Paternal deletion and maternal disomy of 15q11 to q13 lead to PWS.
- Maternal deletion and paternal disomy of 15q11 to q13 lead to AS.

Prader–Willi syndrome presents with developmental delay, endocrinological defects, and neural tube malformations. AS presents with developmental delay, intellectual disability, and speech, movement, and sleep disorders. Excessive laughter is a typical feature of AS.[44]

- Retinoblastoma is a malignant tumor of the retina which occurs during childhood and the incidence in the general population is 1:17,000.[45] It has been reported to be higher by a relative risk of 4.9–7.2 in IVF conceptions. The association between this tumor and imprinting has been suggested because hypermethylation of the *RB1* promoter has been linked to it.[46]

GLOBAL IMPRINTING DISORDERS

Embryos that completely lack one parental genome too can have global imprinting changes. Ovarian "teratomas" have been known to occur by spontaneous oocyte activation in situ with complete absence of paternal genome.[47] Complete hydatidiform mole is well known to form by the absence of maternal genome in the embryo and exhibits excessive development of placental tissue with the risk of choriocarcinoma formation.[48] Origin of pre-eclampsia too has recently been associated with the imprinting effects on certain trophoblastic cells.[49]

WHAT IS THE EVIDENCE OF ASSOCIATION?

- The only disease with a definite association with ART is BWS with a relative risk of 5.2. Considering the population prevalence of 1:13,700, it implies that 1 in every 2,700 children born out of ART would be affected by BWS. However, it is still not clear whether this association is due to the underlying (background) high-risk factors or because of the procedure-related effects. It is important to note that routine screening for imprinting disorders is not recommended as the absolute risk is <1%.[50]
- Another disease suspected to be associated is AS. The total number of reported cases is less, but still, there is a suggestion of positive correlation with ART.
- No significant positive correlation has yet been established between the twin syndromes of SRS and PWS with ART as the incidence of these maladies is very low. Other imprinting disorders, including transient neonatal diabetes mellitus and maternal hypomethylation syndrome, have been reported, but their relationship with ART is very low or nonexistent.[51]
- After correction for infertility, the incidence of retinoblastoma has not been found to increase. However, the conclusion is that rather than the direct effect of ART on imprinting diseases, the increased risk is linked with the parental causes of infertility. However, the possible relationship will hopefully be revealed in further larger studies. Caution, as well as avoidance of undue consternations, is worthwhile at this stage.[52]
- ICSI does not cause an increased incidence of epigenetic diseases compared with a regular IVF.[53] One fact that has already been highlighted in this chapter, but needs further stressing, is that the risks of ART on imprinting disorders cannot easily be evaluated because patients who undergo ART are different from the general population in their genetics and demography. They have lower fertility rates, increased abortion rates, and are usually of advanced age. For example, sperms of men with severe semenopathies have been linked to DNA methylation defects.[54] All these factors are independently associated with fetal and neonatal abnormalities. All these confounding factors make it difficult to evaluate and estimate the direct risk of ART, per se. At present, the data obtained in humans are inconclusive and controversial. Some studies do suggest an association between ART and imprinting disorders, but this could be a "tip of the iceberg" phenomenon.[55]

However, it is noteworthy that 90–100% of the children of BWS born after ART had imprinting defects, compared to 40–50% of the naturally born children with BWS, who had genetic (not epigenetic) defects. Similarly, in reported cases of AS, 71% of the children born after ART had imprinting defects, compared to 5% of the naturally conceived ones.[56]

PREVENTION

- Elucidating the exact trigger points for imprinting disorders during ART may allow protocols to be modified, therefore minimizing the risks.
- As mentioned earlier, the presence of essential amino acids in culture on the first 3 days of embryo development may safeguard against the risk of imprinting errors.
- Strict control of the embryology laboratory environment.

However, prevention can be efficacious only once epigenetic mechanisms are clearly understood.

IMPRINTING AND ASSISTED REPRODUCTIVE TECHNOLOGY: FUTURE CONSIDERATIONS

There are certain unanswered questions in this field:

- Whether embryo culture to the blastocyst stage is linked with a higher risk of imprinting disorders
- Role of superovulation and hormone stimulation in methylation defects.

- Whether cryopreservation of gametes and embryos leads to a higher risk.
- Whether it is the underlying infertility or the ART procedure that needs to be implicated in the causation of these disorders.

More studies are still needed to answer these questions. However, as detailed earlier, there are certain methodological issues, such as lack of control and very low prevalence of these disorders, which make this a difficult task. Only a large study can be reasonably expected to resolve this conundrum. But, such a survey would require an extensive international collaboration.[26]

OTHER EPIGENETIC ISSUES

In addition to the above-mentioned imprinting disorders, some neurodevelopmental disorders are also known to be associated with imprinting. Some examples include bipolar affective disorder, autism/intellectual disabilities, epilepsy, schizophrenia, Tourette syndrome, Turner syndrome, and late-onset Alzheimer's disease.[57]

Spontaneous abortions also have been proposed to occur in ART conceptions due to aberrations in the methylation levels on the imprinted loci. This possibility is yet to be conclusively proven.[58] Oxidative stress affects gametes and the developmental capability of embryos. Environmental endocrine disruptors can increase oxidative stress and methylation errors. ART may exacerbate these defects in methylation and epigenesis. Cardiovascular abnormalities are most widely prevalent among this class of epigenetic disorders as shown in a meta-analysis.[59]

The placenta is a specialized organ that supports fetal development and growth. Placental changes can have major effects on the fetus as well as on its adaptive mechanism. IVF or ICSI-derived pregnancies are known to have increased frequency of placenta-related complications, for example, an increased incidence of hypertensive disorders of pregnancy, third-trimester vaginal bleeding, placenta previa, and abruption.[60] Whether the imprinting errors lead to a change in placental function and maternal physiology, leading to long-term consequences, needs further evaluation. Choux et al. have shown the existence of alterations in the DNA methylation patterns in placentas derived from ART pregnancies.[61]

CONCLUSION

With growing popularity of ART/IVF procedures worldwide, the significance of epigenetics cannot be disregarded anymore. Genomic imprinting, clustering etc. are the concepts all clinicians should be versed with. Moreover, awareness of these disorders would lead to more accurate reporting. This is expected to lead to better understanding of the pathogenesis of these disorders, ultimately resulting in prevention strategies.

KEY POINTS

- Epigenetics is the study of the changes in organisms caused by a selective modification of gene expression, rather than alteration of the genetic code.
- Genomic imprinting is a genome modification, allowing genes from only one parental allele to be expressed.
- The effect of the environment on the embryo is greater in the early stages of development compared to later stages and so there is a concern with ART.
- Gamete maturation and postfertilization are the most important times when methylation changes occur.
- Studies suggesting a positive association between imprinting disorders and ART are marred by the small sample sizes, lack of correction for maternal age, or parental infertility diagnoses.
- It has been suggested that the presence of essential amino acids in culture on the first 3 days of embryo development reduces the chance of imprinting errors.
- Patients undergoing ART have lower fertility rates, increased abortion rates, and are usually of higher age groups; all of these are independently associated with fetal and neonatal abnormalities.
- The only disease with a definite association with ART is BWS with a relative risk of 5.2.
- More studies are required to elucidate the effect of the composition of the culture media on birth weight.
- There is upcoming evidence indicating an association between ART and long-term sequelae, such as cardiovascular disorders.
- Routine screening for imprinting disorders is not recommended as the absolute risk is <1%.

REFERENCES

1. Hiura H, Okae H, Miyauchi N, Sato F, Sato A, Van De Pette M, et al. Characterization of DNA methylation errors in patients with imprinting disorders conceived by assisted reproduction technologies. Hum Reprod. 2012;27:2541-8.
2. Waddington CH. The epigenotype. Endeavour. 1942;1:18-20.
3. Russo VEA, Martienssen RA, Riggs AD. Epigenetic Mechanisms of Gene Regulation. Monograph 32. Plainview, NY: Cold Spring Harbor Laboratory Press; 1996.
4. Jablonka E, Raz G. Transgenerational epigenetic inheritance: prevalence, mechanisms, and implications for the study of heredity and evolution. Q Rev Biol. 2009;84:131-76.
5. Margueron R, Reinberg D. Chromatin structure and the inheritance of epigenetic information. Nat Rev Genet. 2010;11:285-96.
6. Saxonov S, Berg P, Brutlag DL. A genome-wide analysis of CpG dinucleotides in the human genome distinguishes two distinct classes of promoters. Proc Natl Acad Sci USA. 2006;103:1412-7.
7. Jones PA. The DNA methylation paradox. Trends Genet. 1999;15:34.
8. Friso S, Choi SW. Gene-nutrient interactions and DNA methylation. J Nutr. 2002;132:2382S-7S.

9. Margueron R, Trojer P, Reinberg D. The key to development: interpreting the histone code. Curr Opin Genet Dev. 2005;15:163-76.
10. Moore T, Haig D. Genomic imprinting in mammalian development: a parental tug-of-war. Trends Genet. 1991;7:45-9.
11. Luedi PP, Dietrich FS, Weidman JR, Bosko JM, Jirtle RL, Hartemink AJ. Computational and experimental identification of novel human imprinted genes. Genome Res. 2007;17:1723-30.
12. Cutfield WS, Hofman PL, Mitchell M, Morison IM. Could epigenetics play a role in the developmental origins of health and disease? Pediatr Res. 2007;61(5 Pt. 2):68R-75R.
13. Lucifero D, Chaillet JR, Trasler JM. Potential significance of genomic imprinting defects for reproduction and assisted reproductive technology. Hum Reprod Update. 2004;10(1):3-18.
14. Spahn L, Barlow DP. An ICE pattern crystallizes. Nat Genet. 2003;35:11-2.
15. Gabory A, Jammes H, Dandolo L. The H19 locus: role of an imprinted non-coding RNA in growth and development. Bioessays. 2010;32:473-80.
16. Morison IM, Ramsay JP, Spencer HG. A census of mammalian imprinting. Trends Genet. 2005;21:457-65.
17. Mathers JC. Early nutrition: impact on epigenetics. Forum Nutr. 2007;60:42-8.
18. Katari S, Turan N, Bibikova M, Erinle O, Chalian R, Foster M, et al. DNA methylation and gene expression differences in children conceived in vitro or in vivo. Hum Mol Genet. 2009;18:3769-78.
19. Qin J, Sheng X, Wang H, Liang D, Tan H, Xia J. Assisted reproductive technology and risk of congenital malformations: a meta-analysis based on cohort studies. Arch Gynecol Obstet. 2015;292:777-98.
20. Cox GF, Bürger J, Lip V, Mau UA, Sperling K, Wu BL, et al. Intracytoplasmic sperm injection may increase the risk of imprinting defects. Am J Hum Genet. 2002;71:162-4.
21. Maher ER, Brueton LA, Bowdin SC, Luharia A, Cooper W, Cole TR, et al. Beckwith–Wiedemann syndrome and assisted reproduction technology (ART). J Med Genet. 2003;40(1):62-4.
22. Gicquel C, Gaston V, Mandelbaum J, Siffroi JP, Flahault A, Le Bouc Y. In vitro fertilization may increase the risk of Beckwith–Wiedemann syndrome related to the abnormal imprinting of the KCN1OT gene. Am J Hum Genet. 2003;72(5):1338-41.
23. Douzgou S, Mingarelli R, Tarani L, De Crescenzo A, Riccio A. Silver–Russell syndrome following in vitro fertilization. Pediatr Dev Pathol. 2008;11(4):329-31.
24. Moll AC, Imhof SM, Cruysberg JRM, Schouten-van Meeteren AYN, Boers M, van Leeuwen FE. Incidence of retinoblastoma in children born after in-vitro fertilisation. Lancet. 2003;361: 309-10.
25. Sato A, Otsu E, Negishi H, Utsunomiya T, Arima T. Aberrant DNA methylation of imprinted loci in superovulated oocytes. Hum Reprod. 2007;22:26-35.
26. Gosden R, Trasler J, Lucifero D, Faddy M. Rare congenital disorders, imprinted genes, and assisted reproductive technology. Lancet. 2003;361:1975-7.
27. Lazaraviciute G, Kauser M, Bhattacharya S, Haggarty P, Bhattacharya S. A systematic review and meta-analysis of DNA methylation levels and imprinting disorders in children conceived by IVF/ICSI compared with children conceived spontaneously. Hum Reprod Update. 2014;20:840-52.
28. Morgan H, Santos F, Green K, Dean W, Reik W. Epigenetic reprogramming in mammals. Hum Mol Genet. 2005;14: R47-58.
29. Allegrucci C, Thurston A, Lucas E, Young L. Epigenetics and the germline. Reproduction. 2005;129:137-49.
30. Young LE, Fernandez K, McEvoy TG, Butterwith SC, Gutierrez CG, Carolan C, et al. Epigenetic change in IGF2R is associated with fetal overgrowth after sheep embryo culture. Nat Genet. 2001;27:153-4.
31. Dumoulin JC, Land JA, Van Montfoort AP, Nelissen EC, Coonen E, Derhaag JG, et al. Effect of in vitro culture of human embryos on birthweight of newborns. Hum Reprod. 2010;25:605-12.
32. Lin S, Li M, Lian Y, Chen L, Liu P. No effect of embryo culture media on birthweight and length of newborns. Hum Reprod. 2013;28:1762-7.
33. Zandstra H, Van Montfoort APA, Dumoulin JCM. Does the type of culture medium used influence birthweight of children born after IVF? Hum Reprod. 2015;30:530-42.
34. Summers MC, Biggers JD. Chemically defined media and the culture of mammalian preimplantation embryos: historical perspective and current issues. Hum Reprod Update. 2003; 9:557-82.
35. Schwarzer C, Esteves TC, Araúzo-Bravo MJ, Le Gac S, Nordhoff V, Schlatt S, et al. ART culture conditions change the probability of mouse embryo gestation through defined cellular and molecular responses. Hum Reprod. 2012;27: 2627-40.
36. Khoueiry R, Ibala-Rhomdane S, Méry L, Blachére T, Guérin JF, Lornage J, et al. Dynamic CpG methylation of the KCNQ1OT1 gene during maturation of human oocytes. J Med Genet. 2008;45:583-8.
37. Sutcliffe A. Intracytoplasmic sperm injection and other aspects of new reproductive technologies. Arch Dis Child. 2000;83:98-101.
38. Choufani S, Shuman C, Weksberg R. Beckwith–Wiedemann syndrome. Am J Med Genet C Semin Med Genet. 2010;154C:343-54.
39. Weksberg R, Shuman C, Caluseriu O, Smith AC, Fei YL, Nishikawa J, et al. Discordant KCNQ1OT1 imprinting in sets of monozygotic twins discordant for Beckwith–Wiedemann syndrome. Hum Mol Genet. 2002;11:1317-25.
40. Saal HM. Russell–Silver syndrome. GeneReviews at GeneTests: Medical Genetics Information Resource (database online). Seattle: University of Washington; 2007.
41. Netchine I, Rossignol S, Dufourg MN, Azzi S, Rousseau A, Perin L, et al. 11p15 imprinting center region 1 loss of methylation is a common and specific cause of typical Russell–Silver syndrome: clinical scoring system and epigenetic–phenotypic correlations. J Clin Endocrinol Metab. 2007;92:3148-54.
42. Buiting K. Prader–Willi syndrome and Angelman syndrome. Am J Med Genet C Semen Med Genet. 2010;154C:365-76.
43. Nicholls RD, Saitoh S, Horsthemke B. Imprinting in Prader–Willi and Angelman syndromes. Trends Genet. 1998;14:194-200.
44. Williams CA, Driscoll DJ. Angelman syndrome. GeneReviews at GeneTests: Medical Genetics Information Resource (database online). Seattle: University of Washington; 2007.

45. Moll AC, Imhof SM, Schouten-van Meeteren AY, van Leeuwen FE. In-vitro fertilisation and retinoblastoma. Lancet. 2003;361(9366):1392.
46. Zeschnigk M, Böhringer S, Price EA, Onadim Z, Masshöfer L, Lohmann DR. A novel real-time PCR assay for quantitative analysis of methylated alleles (QAMA): analysis of the retinoblastoma locus. Nucleic Acids Res. 2004;32:e125.
47. Kuno N, Kadomatsu K, Nakamura M, Miwa-Fukuchi T, Hirabayashi N, Ishizuka T. Mature ovarian cystic teratoma with a highly differentiated homunculus: a case report. Birth Defects Res A Clin Mol Teratol. 2004;70(1):40-6.
48. Devriendt K. Hydatidiform mole and triploidy: the role of genomic imprinting in placental development. Hum Reprod Update. 2005;11:137-42.
49. van Dijk M, Mulders J, Poutsma A, Könst AA, Lachmeijer AM, Dekker GA, et al. Maternal segregation of the Dutch preeclampsia locus at 10q22 with a new member of the winged helix gene family. Nat Genet. 2005;37:514-9.
50. Bowdin S, Allen C, Kirby G, Brueton L, Afnan M, Barratt C, et al. A survey of assisted reproductive technology births and imprinting disorders. Hum Reprod. 2007;22:3237-40.
51. Amor DJ, Halliday J. A review of known imprinting syndromes and their association with assisted reproduction technologies. Hum Reprod. 2008;23:2826-34.
52. Doornbos ME, Maas SM, McDonnell J, Vermeiden JP, Hennekam RC. Infertility, assisted reproduction technologies and imprinting disturbances: a Dutch study. Hum Reprod. 2007;22:2476-80.
53. Santos F, Hyslop L, Stojkovic P, Leary C, Murdoch A, Reik W, et al. Evaluation of epigenetic marks in human embryos derived from IVF and ICSI. Hum Reprod. 2010;25:2387-95.
54. Marques CJ, Costa P, Vaz B, Carvalho F, Fernandes S, Barros A, et al. Abnormal methylation of imprinted genes in human sperm is associated with oligozoospermia. Mol Hum Reprod. 2008;14:67-74.
55. Maher ER, Afnan M, Barratt CL. Epigenetic risks related to assisted reproductive technologies: epigenetics, imprinting, ART and icebergs? Hum Reprod. 2003;18:2508-11.
56. Manipalviratn S, DeCherney A, Segars J. Imprinting disorders and assisted reproductive technology. Fertil Steril. 2009;91:305-15.
57. Isles AR, Wilkinson LS. Imprinted genes, cognition and behaviour. Trends Cogn Sci. 2000;4:309-18.
58. Zheng HY, Tang Y, Niu J, Li P, Ye DS, Chen X, et al. Aberrant DNA methylation of imprinted loci in human spontaneous abortions after assisted reproduction techniques and natural conception. Hum Reprod. 2013;28(1):265-73.
59. Guo XY, Liu XM, Jin L, Wang TT, Ullah K, Sheng JZ, et al. Cardiovascular and metabolic profiles of offspring conceived by assisted reproductive technologies: a systematic review and meta-analysis. Fertil Steril. 2017;107:622-31.e5.
60. Pandey S, Shetty A, Hamilton M, Bhattacharya S, Maheshwari A. Obstetric and perinatal outcomes in singleton pregnancies resulting from IVF/ICSI: a systematic review and meta-analysis. Hum Reprod Update. 2012;18:485-503.
61. Choux C, Binquet C, Carmignac V, Bruno C, Chapusot C, Barberet J, et al. The epigenetic control of transposable elements and imprinted genes in newborns is affected by the mode of conception: ART versus spontaneous conception without underlying infertility. Hum Reprod. 2018;33:331-40.

SECTION

9 Complications in ART

CHAPTER 66

Ovarian Hyperstimulation Syndrome

Surbhi Gupta, Divyashree PS

INTRODUCTION

Ovarian hyperstimulation syndrome (OHSS) is an iatrogenic complication of ovulation induction and ovarian stimulation for assisted reproductive technology (ART) and is characterized by cystic enlargement of the ovaries and rapid fluid shifts from the intravascular compartment to the third space. It is the most feared complication, potentially life threatening in its severe form, resulting in hospitalization in 1.9% cases,[1] and human chorionic gonadotropin (hCG), either exogenous or endogenous, is the triggering factor of the syndrome. The incidence of clinically significant OHSS is 2–3%; however, milder forms of OHSS develop in about 20–30% of in vitro fertilization (IVF) patients.[2] The mortality risk is estimated to be 1 in 450,000–500,000 cases.[3] It is second only to multiple gestations as the most common complication of ART. Young women, who wish to get pregnant, may face a potentially life-threatening condition. Therefore, every effort should be made to achieve an OHSS-free clinic.

CLASSIFICATION

Classification Schemes by Disease Severity

Over the past 25 years, several classification systems have evolved for categorizing OHSS so as to formulate uniform guidelines for prevention and treatment. Six major severity-based classifications, which have developed over a period of time, are as follows **(Table 1)**:

1. Rabau et al. (1967)—first classification combined both clinical and laboratory findings.
2. Scheneker and Weinstein (1978)—modified the classification and included three categories of mild, moderate, and severe as well as six grades of severity.
3. Golan et al. (1989)—made further changes including four major modifications to the earlier system: (1) Urinary assays of hormones were not taken into account, (2) the diagnosis of ovarian enlargement and the detection of ascites were ultrasound-based, (3) nausea, vomiting and diarrhea, and abdominal distension were classified into mild OHSS and not moderate (grade 2) OHSS, and (4) the detection of ascites on ultrasonography-classified OHSS to be moderate (grade 3).
4. Navot et al. (1992)—further contributed to the classification, based on clinical criteria and by reviewing and comparing the risk factors and previous treatment strategies. Mild OHSS was not included since it lacked clinical significance.
5. Rizk and Aboulghar (1999)—include specific laboratory values, and the major areas of the classification rely on qualitative clinical findings.
6. Royal College of Obstetricians and Gynaecologists (RCOG) Classification (2016)

Classification by Disease Onset

Ovarian hyperstimulation syndrome can be early or late based on the source of hCG **(Table 2)**.

ETIOLOGY AND PATHOPHYSIOLOGY

Ovarian hyperstimulation syndrome manifests systemically as a result of vasoactive mediators being released from hyperstimulated ovaries causing extravasation of protein-rich fluid into the third space. This leads to intravascular hypovolemia causing hypoalbuminemia, hemoconcentration, electrolyte imbalance, decreased renal perfusion and oliguria, ascites, and pleural/pericardial effusions, which may precipitate significant morbidity and mortality from thrombosis, renal, liver, and respiratory failure. Ovarian enlargement is also a risk factor for torsion and cyst rupture. Hemoconcentration can lead to complications such as hypercoagulability and reduction in organ perfusion **(Flowchart 1)**.

The exact etiology for the pathogenesis of OHSS is still unknown, but the syndrome is known to be dependent on hCG. The ovaries which are primed with gonadotropins and are subsequently exposed to hCG lead to pathophysiology of increased vascular permeability.[7]

TABLE 1: Classification of ovarian hyperstimulation syndrome (OHSS).[4]

Study	*Mild*	*Moderate*	*Severe*	
Rabau et al. (1967)	*Grade 1:* Estrogen >150 mg and pregnanediol >10 mg/24 h *Grade 2:* Grade 1 + enlarged ovaries and possibly palpable cysts. Grades 1 and 2 were not included under the title of mild OHSS	*Grade 3:* Grade 2 + confirmed palpable cysts and distended abdomen *Grade 4:* Grade 3 + vomiting and possibly diarrhea	*Grade 5:* Grade 4 + ascites and possibly hydrothorax	*Grade 6:* Grade 5 + changes in blood volume, viscosity, and coagulation time
Scheneker and Weinstein (1978)	*Grade 1:* Estrogen >150 mg/24 h and pregnanediol >10 mg/24 h *Grade 2:* Grade 1 + enlarged ovaries, sometimes small cysts	*Grade 3:* Grade 2 + abdominal distension *Grade 4:* Grade 3 + nausea, vomiting, and/or diarrhea	*Grade 5:* Grade 4 + large ovarian cysts, ascites, and/or hydrothorax	*Grade 6:* Marked hemoconcentration + increased blood viscosity and possibly coagulation abnormalities
Golan et al. (1989)	*Grade 1:* Abdominal distension and discomfort *Grade 2:* Grade 1 + nausea, vomiting and/ or diarrhea, enlarged ovaries 5–12 cm	*Grade 3:* Grade 2 + ultrasound evidence of ascites	*Grade 4:* Grade 3 + clinical evidence of ascites and/or hydrothorax and breathing difficulties	*Grade 5:* Grade 4 + hemoconcentration, increased blood viscosity, coagulation abnormality, and diminished renal perfusion
Navot et al. (1992)			*Severe OHSS:* Variable enlarged ovary; massive ascites ± hydrothorax; Hct >45%; WBC >15,000; oliguria; creatinine 1.0–1.5; creatinine clearance >50 mL/min; liver dysfunction; anasarca	*Critical OHSS:* Variable enlarged ovary; tense ascites 6 hydrothorax; Hct >55%; WBC >25,000; oliguria; creatinine >1.6; creatinine clearance <50 mL/min; renal failure; thromboembolic phenomena; ARDS
Rizk and Aboulghar (1999)		Discomfort, pain, nausea, distension, ultrasonic evidence of ascites and enlarged ovaries, normal hematological and biological profiles	*Grade A:* Dyspnea, oliguria, nausea, vomiting, diarrhea, abdominal pain, clinical evidence of ascites, marked distension of abdomen or hydrothorax, US showing large ovaries and marked ascites, normal biochemical profile *Grade B:* Grade A + massive tension ascites, markedly enlarged ovaries, severe dyspnea and marked oliguria, increased hematocrit, elevated serum creatinine, and liver dysfunction *Grade C:* Complications as respiratory distress syndrome, renal shutdown, or venous thrombosis	
RCOG Green-top Guidelines (2016)	Abdominal bloating, mild abdominal pain, ovarian size usually <8 cm^2	Moderate abdominal pain, nausea, vomiting, ultrasound evidence of ascites, ovarian size usually 8–12 cm^2	Clinical ascites (±hydrothorax), oliguria (<300 mL/day or <30 mL/h), hematocrit >0.45, hyponatremia (sodium <135 mmol/L), hypo-osmolality (osmolality <282 mOsm/kg), hyperkalemia (potassium >5 mmol/L), hypoproteinemia (serum albumin <35 g/L), ovarian size usually >12 cm^2	Tense ascites or large hydrothorax, hematocrit >0.55, white cell count >25,000/mL, oliguria/ anuria, thromboembolism, acute respiratory distress syndrome

(ARDS: acute respiratory distress syndrome; Hct: hematocrit; US: ultrasound; WBC: white blood cells)

Any molecule with an important role in pathophysiology of OHSS should fulfill the following prerequisites:[8]

- Its expression should be increased by hCG and should be higher in cases of OHSS.
- It should have a clear and strong effect on vascular permeability.
- Inhibition of such effect should ameliorate the clinical manifestations of OHSS.

TABLE 2: Classification on the basis of disease onset.[2,5,6]

	Early OHSS	*Late OHSS*
hCG	Exogenous	Endogenous
Time of onset	3–7 days after hCG trigger	>10 days after hCG trigger
Occurrence	Occurs in a stimulated cycle	Occurs in setting of a pregnancy
Associated with	Higher peak E2 levels, greater gonadotropin doses	Singleton or multiple pregnancy

(E2: estradiol; hCG: human chorionic gonadotropin; OHSS: ovarian hyperstimulation syndrome)

Flowchart 1: Pathophysiology of ovarian hyperstimulation syndrome (OHSS).

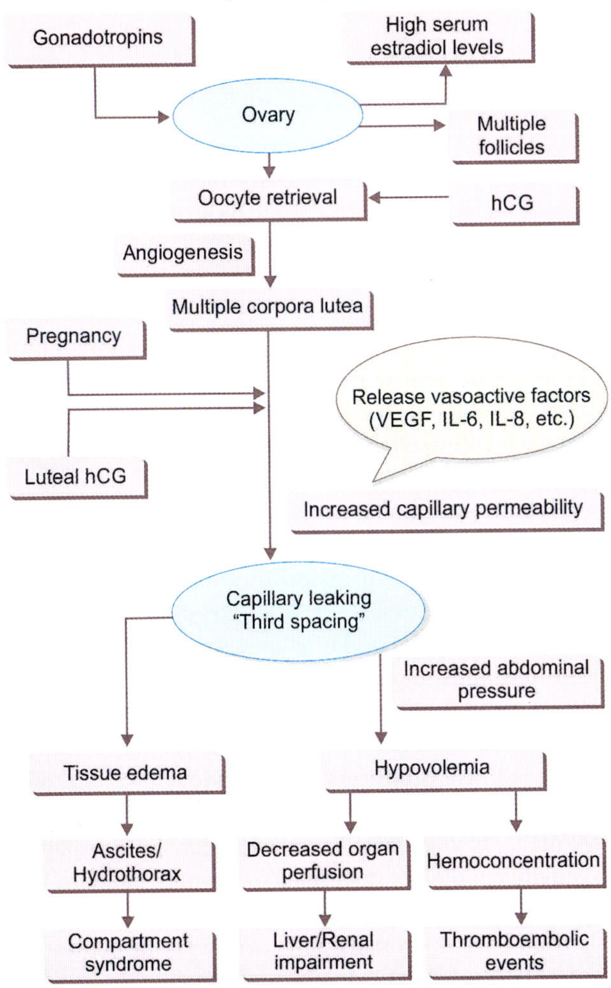

(hCG: human chorionic gonadotropin; IL: interleukin; VEGF: vascular endothelial growth factor)

Vascular endothelial growth factor (VEGF) has been found to be crucial for the development of OHSS, fulfilling all the aforementioned prerequisites. Cytokines and growth factors have been implicated in the inflammatory process associated with follicular maturation, ovulation, corpus luteum function, and embryo implantation. Renin-angiotensin-aldosterone system, prostaglandins, inhibin, endothelin-1, tumor necrosis factor α, and inflammatory mediators have all been implicated in the etiopathogenesis of OHSS.[9]

Factors implicated in the past in the pathogenesis of OHSS:[10]

- *Histamine and OHSS*: It was demonstrated that OHSS could be blocked in rabbits by the administration of antihistamine preparations.[11] It also caused a more rapid regression of the hyperstimulated ovaries. But later, no difference was demonstrated in histamine levels between rabbits in whom OHSS was induced and controls. Also, using two different H1 receptor blockers, the role of serotonin was not found in the pathogenesis of OHSS. The role of chlorpheniramine maleate, an H-1 receptor blocker, was also studied in OHSS.[12] This effectively blocked the ascites formation but did not prevent the ovarian enlargement and augmentation of the intraovarian prostaglandin F content.
- *Estrogen (E2) and OHSS:* Serum E2 has also been implicated in the pathogenesis of OHSS, but the exact role is still not clear. Although it is a known risk factor for OHSS, it is neither necessary nor sufficient for the development of the disease. High E2 levels are found in OHSS patients;[13] but no matter how high E2 levels may be, OHSS does not occur unless hCG is administered.[14] Also, OHSS can occur in patients with low E2 levels due to desmolase gene mutation[15] and those with hypogonadotropic hypogonadism.[16] Also, in experimental animals, OHSS was not prevented by extraperitonealization of ovaries.[17] E2 does not have a direct effect on vascular permeability[18] and high E2 is a mere marker of granulosa-lutein cell activity. Thus, increased capillary permeability in OHSS is caused by excess concentrations of the immediate metabolites secreted by the ovary after gonadotropin-hCG stimulation and not high E2 levels per se.
- *Prostaglandins and OHSS*: Experiments have been performed to determine whether prostaglandins are involved actively in the development of OHSS. Excessive E2 produced by the large number of developing follicles may lead to increased production of prostaglandins, which in turn may be responsible for the increased capillary permeability observed in OHSS. Indomethacin, a prostaglandin inhibitor, has not shown to improve ascites in cases of OHSS,[19] nor it has shown to improve the pathological process in the patients with severe OHSS.[20] Thus, the role of prostaglandins in triggering OHSS has not been proven.

The lead players currently implicated in the pathogenesis of OHSS are as follows:

- *hCG*: Human chorionic gonadotropin has a pivotal role in the development of OHSS, and this is based on the observation that OHSS rarely occurs when hCG is withheld as an ovulatory trigger during controlled ovarian stimulation (COS).[14] hCG has been used as a luteinizing hormone (LH) surrogate from the inception of COS. Its prolonged half-life and avid affinity to LH/hCG receptor results in prolonged ovarian stimulation and changes in periovarian vasculature in the postovulatory period. It also exerts follicle stimulation hormone (FSH)-like action in stimulating the ovaries.

In patients undergoing ART, hCG, apart from its role in ovulation triggering, adversely affects OHSS in a number of ways:

- hCG supplementation during the luteal phase makes OHSS worse.
- Pregnancy and, therefore, rising levels of hCG make OHSS much worse.
- Multiple-gestation pregnancy produces even higher levels of hCG, which is associated with more severe OHSS. Those cases, which constitute an early form followed by pregnancy, are serious and long lasting.[21]

Human chorionic gonadotropin is also implicated in the development of some cases of spontaneous OHSS, an extremely rare, noniatrogenic condition, unrelated to exogenous hormones and is usually seen to complicate both singleton and multiple pregnancy. Spontaneous OHSS is a rare but important differential diagnosis for abdominal distension in early pregnancy.[22,23]

High levels of glycoprotein hormones such as β-hCG, thyroid stimulating hormone (TSH), LH, and FSH with/without FSH receptor (FSHR) mutation are seen as the trigger for most cases of spontaneous OHSS.[24] These hormones are believed to release unknown mediators and vasoactive substances such as histamine, serotonin, prostaglandins, interleukins (ILs), E2, prolactin, the ovarian renin-angiotensin system (RAS), and VEGF leading to increased vascular permeability, extravascular fluid accumulation, hemoconcentration, deep vein thrombosis, and other complications observed in OHSS.

De Leener et al. classified spontaneous OHSS into four types **(Table 3)**. In both type I and type II, development of OHSS is hCG mediated. Mutations in FSHR may cause increased sensitivity to hCG. Type III is associated with hypothyroidism and type IV is caused by ectopic FSH-secreting neuroendocrine tumors.

TABLE 3: Modified De Leener's classification of spontaneous ovarian hyperstimulation syndrome.

Modified De Leener's classification	*Primary abnormality*	*Underlying trigger*
I	Mutated FSHR	Pregnancy
II	Elevated β-hCG	• Multiple pregnancies • Gestational trophoblastic disease (GTD) • β-hCG-secreting tumor
III	Elevated TSH	Hypothyroidism
IV	Elevated FSH/LH	• FSH/LH-secreting pituitary adenomas • Ectopic FSH-secreting tumors

(FSHR: follicle-stimulating hormone receptor; FSH: follicle stimulation hormone; hCG: human chorionic gonadotropin; LH: luteinizing hormone; TSH: thyroid-stimulating hormone)

- *VEGF:* Vascular endothelial growth factor is the key player in the pathophysiology of OHSS.

  In humans, there are five VEGF messenger ribonucleic acid (mRNAs), encoding $VEGF_{121}$, $VEGF_{145}$, $VEGF_{165}$, $VEGF_{189}$, and $VEGF_{206}$.[25] The isoforms $VEGF_{121}$ and $VEGF_{165}$, also known as VEGF A, are normal products of the ovary.[26] Two specific endothelial cell receptors for VEGF belonging to tyrosine kinase receptor family are known: VEGF receptor-1 (VEGFR-1) and VEGFR-2.[27] VEGFR-1 is also produced as a soluble receptor (sVEGFR-1) which modulates the bioactivity of VEGF.[28-30] These receptors are present not only in the endothelium but also in the ovarian follicles.[31] The binding of VEGF to VEGF-2 receptor determines the phosphorylation of intracellular domains and is critical for downstream signaling **(Figs. 1A and B)**, which is responsible for endothelial reorganization, membrane ruffling, and chemotactic contraction.[27] Expression of VEGF mRNA has been shown to be induced by hCG in a dose- and time-dependent fashion.

  Vascular endothelial growth factor has a very strong angiogenic effect in the ovary. hCG administration increases VEGF expression in granulosa-lutein cells, especially in patients at risk for OHSS. It has also been demonstrated that endothelium contains hCG receptors and responds to gonadotropin stimulation by releasing VEGF and increasing the amount of VEGF-2 receptor in the cell surface, recommending the role of endothelial cells as VEGF producers in the pathogenesis of OHSS.[32] Not only the ovarian vessels, but other endothelial cells of the body might also be the target for VEGF, explaining general circulatory disturbances in some patients.[33] The principal pathophysiologic events of typical OHSS are attributed to the gonads, and the ovary is the main source of VEGF and other cytokines responsible for increased capillary permeability and ascites.[34]

- *RAS*
  - *Local ovarian RAS*

    The RAS of the ovary also plays a causative role in the pathogenesis of OHSS and functions independently of the renal RAS **(Flowchart 2)**. It leads to the conversion of the avascular preovulatory follicle into a richly vascularized corpus luteum.

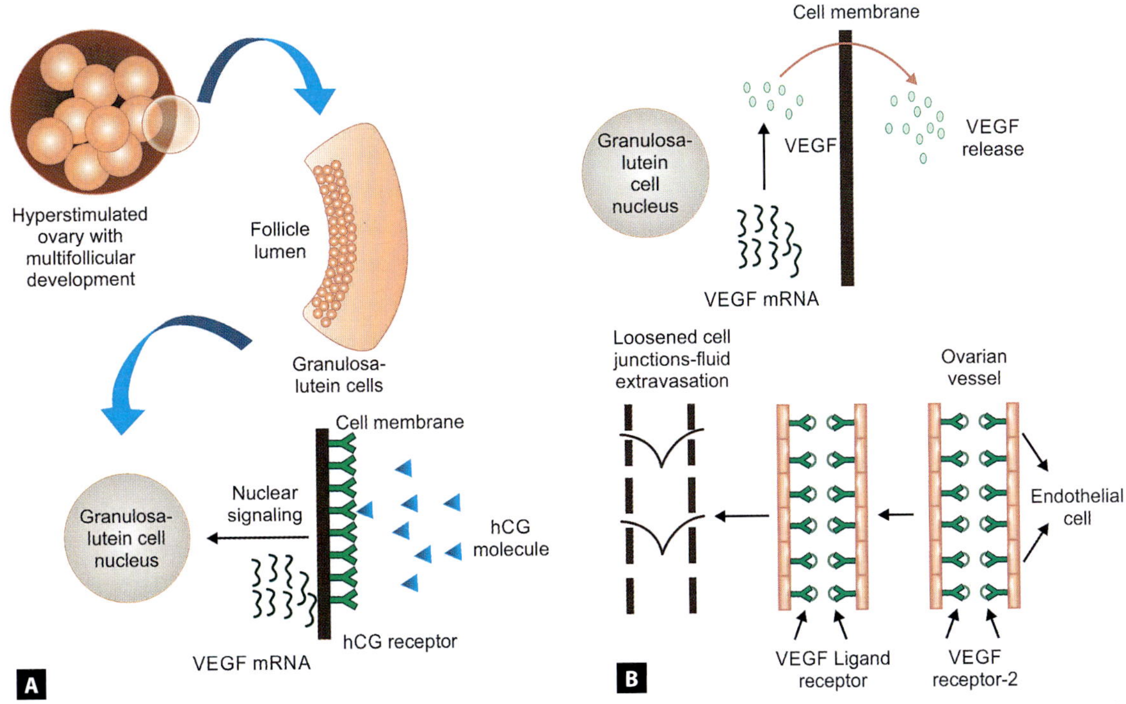

Figs. 1A and B: The pathogenesis of ovarian hyperstimulation syndrome (OHSS). (A) Human chorionic gonadotropin (hCG) stimulates a high number of granulosa-lutein cells leading to the increased production of vascular endothelial growth factor (VEGF) messenger ribonucleic acid (mRNA) (A); (B) VEGF receptor-2 (VEGFR-2) mRNA production in the granulosa-lutein and endothelial cells is also increased in response to hCG. High amounts of VEGF are produced and released from the granulosa-lutein cells and bind to VEGFR-2 on the endothelial cell membranes. Downstream signaling augments vascular permeability.

Flowchart 2: Suggested role of angiotensin–renin system and prostaglandins in the pathogenesis of ovarian hyperstimulation syndrome.

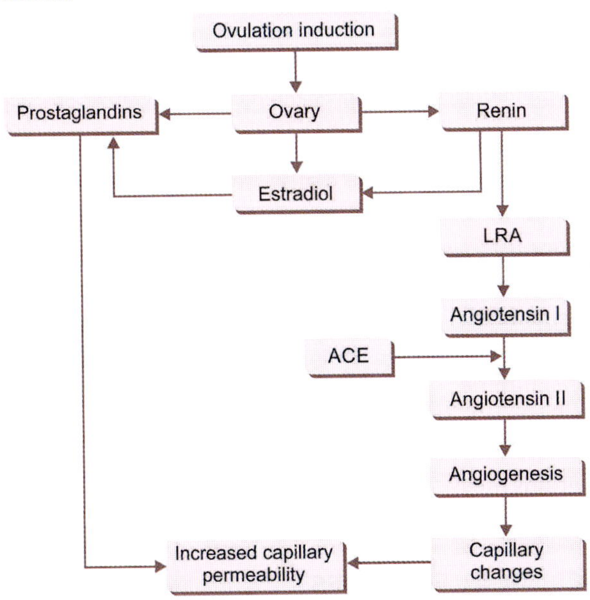

(ACE: angiotensin converting enzyme; LRA: luteal phase renin activity)

Ovarian follicles contain rennin in an inactive form, prorenin, which is activated at mid cycle, causing conversion of angiotensinogen to angiotensin I which in turn is converted to angiotensin II by the angiotensin-converting enzyme (ACE). Angiotensin II promotes angiogenesis, increased vascular permeability, and stimulates release of prostaglandins. hCG is a strong stimulant of RAS activity as high renin activity is observed in the follicular fluid and plasma of women with OHSS. Thus, ovarian RAS, in the same way as VEGF, brings about new vessel formation and increased capillary permeability leading to ovarian enlargement and extracellular fluid sequestration, characteristic of OHSS.[35] Overstimulation of the RAS cascade along with increasing VGEF levels can synergistically potentiate OHSS.

- *Systemic RAS*

  In the development of OHSS, another pathway thought to be is the arterial dilatation. This leads to underfilling of the arterial vascular component, arterial hypotension, and a compensatory increase in heart rate and cardiac output (CO).[36,37] If circulatory dysfunction occurs only as a result of extravascular fluid shift, then there will be a reduction in CO and increase in peripheral vascular resistance and atrial natriuretic peptide. On the contrary, there is an increase in CO and atrial natriuretic and a marked reduction in peripheral vascular resistance. This increase in CO is thought to be due to the activation of neurohormonal vasoconstrictor pathways including RAS.

Flowchart 3: Suggested role of cytokines and other factors in ovarian hyperstimulation syndrome.

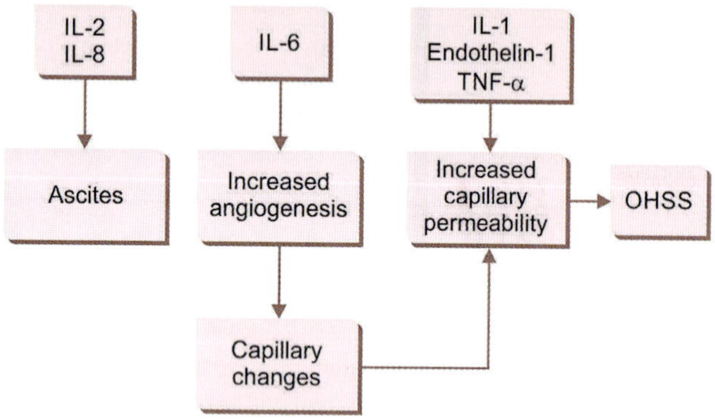

(IL: interleukin; OHSS: ovarian hyperstimulation syndrome; TNF: tumor necrosis factor)

- *Immune factors*: The immune system and the reproductive system have been found to be linked through cytokines and their receptors which in turn lead to the local and systemic effects of immune response.[38,39] Proinflammatory cytokines: IL-1β, IL-2, IL-6, IL-8, endothelin-1, and tumor necrosis factor α have been implicated to mediate the acute phase response, which leads to capillary leakage and the third space loss in OHSS **(Flowchart 3)**. Elevated serum levels of these cytokines have been found in OHSS.

RISK FACTORS FOR OVARIAN HYPERSTIMULATION SYNDROME

Identifying at-risk patients is critical in prevention of OHSS as it assists the clinician in making changes in the ovarian stimulation protocols or taking other preventive measures. Risk factors can be primary or secondary **(Table 4)**.

TABLE 4: Risk factors for ovarian hyperstimulation syndrome (OHSS).

Risk factor	***Increased risk***
Primary risk factors (patient related)	
Young age	<33 years predicts OHSS[38]
High-basal AMH	>3.36 ng/mL independently predicts OHSS[38]
High AFC	>14 may predict hyperresponse[38]
Previous OHSS	Moderate or severe cases especially those with hospitalization
PCOS/isolated PCOS characteristics	≥24 antral follicles in both ovaries combined[40]
BMI	Lower BMI predicts OHSS[41-43]
Race	Black race predicts OHSS[43]
Secondary risk factors (ovarian response related)	
Number of follicles on the day of hCG	>14 follicles of 11 mm^2; >11 follicles of 10 mm[38]
High and rapidly rising E2 levels and high number of follicles	E2 5,000 ng/mL and/or ≥18 follicles predictive of severe OHSS[39]
VEGF levels	Not applicable
Elevated inhibin-B levels	Elevated levels on day 5 of gonadotropin stimulation, at oocyte retrieval, and 3 days before oocyte retrieval appear to correlate with development of OHSS
hCG administration for LPS	Not applicable
Pregnancy (increase in endogenous hCG)	Not applicable

(AFC: antral follicle count; AMH: anti-müllerian hormone; BMI: body mass index; E2: estradiol; hCG: human chorionic gonadotropin; LPS: luteal phase support; OHHS: ovarian hyperstimulation syndrome; PCOS: polycystic ovarian syndrome)

Primary risk factors are patient-related and confer an increased risk of OHSS to the patients. They include young age, low body mass index (BMI), previous history of OHSS, polycystic ovary syndrome (PCOS), high basal anti-müllerian hormone (AMH), and antral follicle count (AFC). AMH is expressed in granulosa cells from preantral and small antral follicles and is a measure of ovarian reserve. It predicts ovarian response independent of age and PCOS.[45] AMH ≥ 3.36 ng/mL has a sensitivity of 90.5% and specificity of 81.3% in predicting OHSS.[44] Another primary risk factor is high AFC, that is, ≥12 follicles of 2–8 mm in each ovary, typically located in the periphery of the ovary, "necklace sign" or "string of pearls" appearance predicts OHSS with a sensitivity of 82% and specificity of 89%.[46] Only one study has evaluated black race as a predictor of OHSS, utilizing data from the Society for Assisted Reproductive Technology (SART) database.[43] Activating mutations in the *FSHR* gene have also shown to confer a higher response to FSH and, therefore, FSHR genotype may predispose women to OHSS.[47]

Secondary risk factors are related to ovarian response and become apparent during ovarian stimulation when patients with no predisposing factors develop an excessive response. The number of follicles on the day of trigger, E2 levels, number of oocytes retrieved, serum inhibin-B, and VEGF levels predict the risk of OHSS. But none of these has shown to independently predict the risk of OHSS. The data regarding measuring inhibin B levels and VEGF levels for the prediction of OHSS is still conflicting.

CLINICAL FEATURES

The clinical manifestations of OHSS are a cascade of pathophysiologic events resulting from increased vascular permeability. Symptoms of OHSS may begin as early as 24 hours after hCG administration and increase in severity over the next 7–10 days due to endogenous hCG rise resulting from early pregnancy.

- *Abdominal pain, nausea, and vomiting:* Ovarian hyperstimulation syndrome is marked by massive bilateral cystic ovarian enlargement. The ovaries show remarkable stromal edema, interspersed with multiple hemorrhagic follicular and theca-lutein cysts, areas of cortical necrosis, and neovascularization. This enlargement of the ovaries causes abdominal pain, nausea, and vomiting.
- *Third space fluid collection*: There is a generalized increase of vascular permeability, which results in decreased colloid oncotic pressure.[48] This causes fluid shift from intravascular to extravascular or "third" space resulting in ascites, pleural and pericardial effusion, and dependent edema. Dyspnea results due to mechanical impingement of diaphragm as a result of ascites. There can be rapid shift of fluid in the peritoneal cavity leading to ascites, increased intra-abdominal pressure (>20–25 mm Hg), and organ dysfunction. This is known as abdominal compartment syndrome (ACS). It is a triad consisting of:[49]
  - Respiratory compromise as a result of elevation of the diaphragm, thus affecting respiration resulting in dyspnea and pleural effusion[50]
  - Decreased venous return due to increased pressure compressing the inferior vena cava (IVC) and thus impeding blood return to heart
  - Intestinal obstruction because of compression of viscera, which can lead to decreased appetite and then nausea/vomiting[51-53]
- *Hypotension and hypovolemia*: The fluid shift into the third space depletes the intravascular volume, thus causing hypovolemia. Cardiac preload falls due to hypovolemia as well as compression of IVC due to increased intra-abdominal pressure leading to decreased CO. There is arterial vasodilatation leading to decreased peripheral resistance which in turn leads to decreased renal perfusion.[36,37]
- *Renal manifestations*: Decreased renal perfusion leads to increased proximal tubular reabsorption of salt and water and thus decreased sodium urinary excretion and oliguria.

  There is also impairment of sodium-hydrogen/potassium exchange in the distal tubule, leading to hyperkalemic acidosis.

  Decreased renal perfusion also decreases the glomerular filtration rate, which can result in oliguria or anuria and acute renal failure.
- *Hypercoagulable state and thromboembolic episodes*: A combination of hemoconcentration, high levels of ovarian steroids, and changes in liver perfusion and, thus, decreased hepatic protein synthesis and depletion of antithrombotic factors[54] results in a hypercoagulable state. Thromboses are mostly venous (67–75%) involving the upper limbs and neck and then arterial (25–33%), which are mainly cerebrovascular events usually occurring concurrently with the onset of OHSS.

TABLE 5: Classification of ovarian hyperstimulation syndrome (OHSS) symptoms.[52]

OHSS stage	Clinical feature	Laboratory feature
Mild	• Abdominal distension or discomfort • Mild nausea or vomiting • Mild dyspnea • Enlarged ovaries	No important alterations
Moderate	• Mild features • Ultrasonographic evidence of ascites	• Hemoconcentration (Hct >41%) • Elevated WBC (>15,000)
Severe	• Mild and moderate features • Clinical evidence of ascites • Hydrothorax • Severe dyspnea • Oliguria or anuria • Intractable nausea or vomiting	• Severe hemoconcentration (Hct >55%) • WBC >25,000/mL • CrCl <50 mL/min • Cr >1.6 mg/dL • Na^+ <135 mEq/L • K^+ >5 mEq/L • Elevated liver enzymes
Critical	• Low blood or central venous pressure • Pleural effusion • Rapid weight gain (>1 kg in 24 h) • Syncope • Severe abdominal pain • Venous thrombosis • Anuria or acute renal failure • Arrhythmia • Thromboembolism • Pericardial effusion • Massive hydrothorax • Arterial thrombosis • Adult respiratory distress syndrome • Sepsis	Worsening of findings

(Cr: creatinine; CrCl: creatinine clearance; Hct: hematocrit; K^+: potassium; Na^+: sodium; ; WBC: white blood cell)

OHSS is classified into mild, moderate, severe, and critical based on symptoms and laboratory features **(Table 5)**.

Humaidan et al. proposed a more objective classification system[55] incorporating vaginal ultrasound and laboratory parameters **(Table 6)**.

PREVENTION

Preventive strategies[56] for OHSS include

- Identifying "at risk" women and thus classifying the risk factors as primary or secondary **(Table 7)**

TABLE 6: Proposed new clinical grading system for ovarian hyperstimulation syndrome.

	Mild	Moderate	Severe
Objective criteria:			
Fluid in Douglas pouch	+	+	+
Fluid around uterus (major pelvis)		+	+
Fluid around intestinal loops			+
Hematocrit >45%		+*	+
White blood cells >15,000/mm^3		±*	+
Low urine output <600 mL/24 h		±*	+
Creatinine >1.5 mg/dL		±*	±
Elevated transaminases		±*	±
Clotting disorder			±‡
Pleural effusion			±‡
Subjective criteria:			
Abdominal distension	+	+	+
Pelvic discomfort	+	+	+
Breathing disorder	±†	±†	+
Acute pain	±†	±†	±†
Nausea or vomiting	±	±	±
Ovarian enlargement	+	+	+
Pregnancy occurrence	±	±	+

*If two of these present, consider hospitalization.
†If present, consider hospitalization.
‡If present, consider intensive care.

- Risk stratification into high, normal, or low risk and thus following preventive strategies. Prevention is either primary or secondary.
  Primary prevention: It involves classifying a person on the basis of their risk factors and then accordingly individualizing treatment regimens.
  Secondary prevention: It focuses on methods used in patients who have displayed an excessive response to ovarian stimulation during a cycle and aims to prevent progression to OHSS.

Primary Prevention

- *Reducing exposure to gonadotropins*: Gonadotropins have the capacity to enhance follicular recruitment and serum E2 concentrations, thus increasing the risk for OHSS. The exposure to gonadotropins can be minimized by reducing both dose and duration of administration of gonadotropins. The concept of individualized controlled ovarian stimulation (iCOS) should be followed for ovarian stimulation in patients at risk for OHSS.[57]
  Polycystic ovary syndrome is one of the major risk factors for the development of OHSS and, thus, this subgroup of women should be targeted for monofollicular ovulation. Thus, the protocols which stimulate the ovaries without exceeding FSH threshold and facilitate the development of a single dominant follicle are employed. Hence, either a chronic low-dose step-up or a step-down protocol regimen is favored. It is associated with a lower risk of OHSS and cycle cancellation and favors monofollicular development.[58,59] The duration of gonadotropin exposure can be reduced by mild stimulation protocols which delay the administration of FSH till the mid or late follicular phase.[55,60] In addition to reducing the risk of OHSS, mild stimulation protocols are also cost-effective as compared to standard agonist or antagonist protocols.
  In a Cochrane review published in 2018, it was highlighted that lower doses of FSH seemed to reduce the overall incidence of moderate and severe OHSS.[57]
- *Use of follitropin delta (follitropin δ)*: Follitropin δ is a new recombinant FSH derived from the cell line of human fetal retinal origin. The sialic acid of this FSH molecule is higher as compared to α and β subunits. It has a longer elimination half-life (30 vs. 24 hours) and induces a higher ovarian response when administered at equal doses of biological activity.
  The individualized dose for follitropin δ was determined on the basis of body weight and serum AMH levels. In Phase III ESTHER (Evidence-based Stimulation Trial With Human rFSH in Europe and Rest of World) trial,[61] its noninferiority to follitropin α was established. Also, the use of follitropin δ leads to decreased risk of moderate/severe OHSS as well as OHSS preventive interventions.[61,62]
- *Avoiding adjunct gonadotropin-releasing hormone agonist (GnRHa) utilization*: GnRH agonist protocol is employed to downregulate the endogenous pituitary secretion of LH to prevent premature luteinization. GnRHa plays a paradoxical role by causing profound ovarian suppression. The FSH rise in the late luteal phase is prevented. This process ends up in requiring increased doses of gonadotropins, more follicles attaining maturity with consequent rise in serum estradiol values and hence increased risk of OHSS.[55] It is also hypothesized that pituitary downregulation interferes with natural cohort selection and prevents smaller atretic follicles from becoming atretic.[63]
  Moreover, GnRHa cannot be utilized to trigger final oocyte maturation.
  It also adds to the cost of treatment without an increase in pregnancy rate. A Cochrane review by Nugent et al. demonstrated an increased risk of hyperstimulation with the use of GnRHa [odds ratio (OR) 3.15; 95% confidence interval (CI) 1.48–6.70].[64]
- *GnRH antagonist protocol*: GnRH antagonists are associated with a decreased risk of OHSS. The mechanism is thought to be related to reduction in circulating estradiol levels with GnRH antagonists.[65]

TABLE 7: Preventive measures for ovarian hyperstimulation syndrome (OHSS).

Preventive measures	***Rationale***	***Level of evidence***
Primary prevention		
Reducing gonadotropin exposure(both dose and duration)	Increased gonadotropins enhance both follicular recruitment and serum E2 concentrations with increased risk of OHSS	Grade A
Use of follitropin delta	Newer FSH with a long half-life and higher response with decreased incidence of OHSS	Grade B
Avoiding adjunct GnRH agonist (GnRHa) utilization	Pituitary downregulation prevents FSH rise in the luteofollicular transition; so, no atresia of follicles; hence cohort of follicles recruited for stimulation is more. More gonadotropin requirement, more E2 levels	Grade A
GnRH antagonist protocol	More physiological follicular selection, recruitment of smaller number of follicles, less gonadotropin requirement, less E2, and hence reduced risk of OHSS	Grade A
Avoidance of hCG for luteal phase support	• hCG increases the risk for OHSS • Progesterone significantly reduces the risk of OHSS without affecting pregnancy rates	Grade B
Insulin sensitizing agents (metformin)	By improving hyperinsulinemia and intraovarian hyperandrogenism, reduces number of nonperiovulatory follicles and hence estradiol secretion	Grade A
Secondary prevention		
Alternative agents for triggering ovulation [GnRha or recombinant LH (rLH)]	• GnRHa triggers cause massive luteolysis and thus less E2 levels in luteal phase • hCG itself is a risk factor for OHSS	Grade A
Reduced dose of hCG for triggering ovulation	Appears to decrease the risk of severe OHSS	Grade C
Cryopreservation of all embryos	Avoids endogenous hCG rise in fresh transfer cycles which can exacerbate late onset OHSS	Grade B
Cycle cancellation	Cycle cancellation and withholding hCG is definitive method for preventing OHSS	Grade C
Coasting	Withholding gonadotropins and delaying hCG reduces the risk of OHSS. Also alters the capacity of granulosa cells to produce VEGF	Grade C
Dopamine agonists	Prevents phosphorylation of VEGF receptor-2 and thus reduces the release of vasoactive angiogenic agents	Grade A
Calcium infusion	Inhibition of cAMP dependent renin secretion leading to decreased angiotensin-II production and thus VEGF synthesis	Grade B
Aspirin	Inhibits platelet activation thus inhibiting release of substances that can potentiate OHSS	Grade A
Glucocorticoids	Inhibitory effect on VEGF gene expression	Grade C
Colloid (albumin and hydroxyethyl starch) infusion	Increases plasma oncotic pressure and counteracting the permeability effect of angiotensin II	Grade C
Aromatase inhibitors	Inhibits aromatase enzyme and prevents excessive synthesis of estrogen	Grade C
Follicular aspiration		Grade C
Experimental		
In vitro maturation (IVM)	Aspiration of immature oocytes helps in preventing OHSS	
VEGF antagonists	Blocks action of VEGF	
Kisspeptin trigger for oocyte maturation	Stimulates GnRH release and in turn FSH and LH release	
Vasopressin V1a receptor antagonist	Inhibits vasopressin-induced VEGF secretion	

(cAMP: cyclic adenosine monophosphate; E2: estradiol; FSH: follicle-stimulating hormone; GnRH: gonadotropin-releasing hormone; hCG: human chorionic gonadotropin; LH: luteinizing hormone; VEGF: vascular endothelial growth factor)

The action of GnRH antagonists mimics the normal physiology in selection of follicles as a smaller number of follicles are recruited, thus requiring less dose of gonadotropins and decreased risk of OHSS. Also, they constitute a more rational way of inhibiting premature LH surge as compared to GnRHa. The differential action of GnRH antagonists at both pituitary and ovarian receptors is also thought to be responsible for reduced risk of OHSS.[55]

A Cochrane review compiled 29 randomized controlled trials (RCTs) and demonstrated statistically significant lower incidence of OHSS in the GnRH antagonist group (OR –0.43, 95% CI 0.33–0.57) as compared to GnRHa group with no difference in live birth rates.[66]

The advantages of using GnRH antagonists are lack of flare effect, absence of menopausal symptoms, no refractory period, reduced risk of ovarian cyst formation, shorter treatment cycle, and reduced gonadotropin dose requirement. Most importantly, because of lack of desensitization, GnRHa can be employed to trigger ovulation. It is mandatory to give full progesterone (P) support during luteal phase while using GnRHa to trigger ovulation.

- *Avoiding hCG for luteal phase support (LPS)*: The supraphysiological levels of E2 and progesterone due to COS result in low endogenous LH levels and, thus, defective luteal phase and impaired endometrial receptivity. Hence, LPS is crucial to improve these parameters.[67-69] hCG has been used for LPS, but it also increases the risk for OHSS. Use of P halves the risk of OHSS without affecting pregnancy rates.[70]

  As an alternative to P, GnRHa as repeated intranasal administration can be used for LPS, but more studies are required to support this.[71] It is recommended that in high-risk cases, LPS should be given in the form of P and not hCG.
- *Insulin sensitizing agents (metformin):* Metformin is an insulin-sensitizing agent widely used in PCOS patients. The concept of "androgen priming" states that androgens increase the ovarian response to gonadotropin stimulation. By improving intraovarian hyperandrogenism, metformin affects the ovarian response by reducing the number of nonperiovulatory follicles and hence estradiol secretion. Metformin is also hypothesized to inhibit the secretion of vasoactive molecules such as VEGF and thereby modulating vascular permeability and preventing OHSS.[72] A recent meta-analysis analyzing 12 studies and 1,516 participants showed that the use of metformin significantly reduced the risk of OHSS in PCOS patients.[73]

  In a recent Cochrane review based upon eight RCTs with 798 women, it was noted that there was a decreased risk of OHSS with metformin use (OR 0.29, 95% CI 0.18–0.49).[74]

Secondary Prevention

- *Alternative agents for triggering ovulation*: Utilizing exogenous hCG to mimic endogenous preovulatory LH surge and trigger ovulation has been in use for decades. However, due to its longer half-life, hCG results in prolonged luteotropic effect. This results in stimulation of LH receptors on multiple post-retrieval corpora lutea and raised E2 and P levels throughout the luteal phase and thus increasing the risk of OHSS. Therefore, alternative agents for triggering final oocyte maturation have been investigated so as to prevent OHSS.
  - *GnRHa trigger*: GnRHa, when administered as a bolus, results in a flare of gonadotropins (LH and FSH) released by the pituitary, mimicking the natural mid-cycle surge and triggering final oocyte maturation.[55] Moreover, it produces a more moderated and shorter gonadotropin surge in contrast to hCG, thus virtually eliminating the risk of OHSS.[75-77] However, it causes a profound luteal phase insufficiency due to massive luteolysis and hence, LPS in the form of E2 and P is required in patients receiving GnRHa trigger.

    A Cochrane review published in 2014 found that GnRHa as compared to hCG triggers results in lower incidence of OHSS in fresh autologous as well as donor-recipient cycles. It was also associated with lower live birth rate in fresh autologous cycles.[78]

    Although GnRHa is said to virtually eliminate the risk of OHSS, there have been case reports demonstrating OHSS even with OHSS trigger.[79-81] This was attributed to massive luteinization of the follicles after exaggerated stimulation and OHSS occurred independently of the ovulation triggering agent. Also, it cannot be used as a trigger in GnRHa cycles where the risk of OHSS is higher as compared to antagonist cycles.
  - *Recombinant LH (rLH)*: Recombinant LH closely mimics natural LH surge and a single peak of rLH is sufficient to induce final oocyte maturation. One preliminary comparison of rLH and recombinant hCG (rhCG) has demonstrated a lower incidence of moderate to severe OHSS with a single dose of rLH.[82] However, because of poor cost–benefit ratio, its use as a trigger is limited in routine clinical practice.
- *Reducing dose of hCG for triggering ovulation*: Human chorionic gonadotrophin is a known risk factor for OHSS; thus, different doses of hCG for triggering ovulation have been assessed. There has been no difference in the clinical outcome between 5,000 and 10,000 IU of hCG.[83,84] Low-dose hCG does not eliminate the risk of OHSS in high-risk patients. However, further studies are required before very low doses of hCG can be recommended.
- *Cryopreservation of all embryos*: During cryopreservation, COS and oocyte retrieval are performed, followed by

cryopreservation of all the embryos and their subsequent transfer in nonstimulated cycles. This prevents endogenous hCG rise in fresh-transfer cycles, which can exacerbate late-onset OHSS.

The routine use of elective cryopreservation has not been validated because, with routine culture of embryos to blastocyst stage, the degree of OHSS can be accurately assessed prior to embryo transfer as blastocyst transfer takes place on the 7th day after hCG and in the absence of moderate degree OHSS, fresh transfer can be safely done.[85,86] Cryopreservation also increases the cost of the treatment.

Another concern which was previously associated with cryopreservation was lower pregnancy rates owing to slow freezing methods; however, with the advent of vitrification, pregnancy rates with cryopreserved embryos exceed fresh embryo transfer.[87-90]

A Cochrane review analyzed two RCTs and concluded that there was insufficient evidence to recommend routine cryopreservation.[86]

A recent meta-analysis by Roque et al. supports the use of elective FET in hyper-responders as it increases live birth rate and significantly decreases the risk of moderate and severe OHSS.[91] Also, the evidence supports the use of GnRHa trigger followed by cryopreservation for "OHSS-free clinic" which is discussed subsequently.[92]

- *Cycle cancellation*: Withholding hCG and cycle cancellation guarantees prevention of early OHSS.[93] However, natural LH surge resulting in ovulation and natural conception may still occur in some cases, with a possibility of late OHSS.

  Although cycle cancellation is effective in preventing OHSS, it is not recommended because of the financial burden and psychological distress it causes to the patient.[55,94]
- *Coasting*: It is a preventive strategy of withholding gonadotropins at the end of COS for up to 4 days when a certain E2 concentration and/or a critical number of follicles are reached. hCG trigger is subsequently delayed until E2 levels significantly decrease or plateau.[94] Initial studies showed that coasting is associated with a lower risk of OHSS without compromising the pregnancy rate.[95,96] However, a Cochrane review in 2017 analyzed 8 RCTs and 702 women and concluded that there was insufficient evidence to suggest that coasting reduced moderate and severe OHSS. Also, there was no evidence to suggest that coasting was more beneficial than other interventions.[97] As a routine, coasting is not recommended for the prevention of OHSS.
- *Dopamine agonists*: As discussed previously, the pathophysiology of OHSS is mainly attributed to an increased vascular permeability of ovarian and peritoneal capillaries caused by ovarian hypersecretion of VEGF. Cabergoline is a dopamine receptor-2 agonist and inhibits the phosphorylation of VEGFR-2.[98] This results in reduction of VEGF production and subsequently decreased risk of OHSS.

  It has also been demonstrated that tyrosine hydroxylase enzyme, rate-limiting enzyme for dopamine synthesis, was downregulated in overstimulated ovaries.[99] High VEGF expression and activity in OHSS were associated with reduced dopamine production. Hence, it was postulated that dopamine could be used as an anti-angiogenic factor in ovary.[100] Also, with cabergoline, there was a dopaminergic control of LH release and thus a better clinical control of ovarian response and consequently reduced risk of OHSS.[101] Cabergoline in low doses does not produce any anti-angiogenic activity; states of high-level VEGFR-2-dependent vascular activity such as corpus luteum physiology or pregnancy development are not affected.[8,102-104]

  A daily administration of 0.5 mg/day for 8 days starting from the day of hCG administration has shown to reduce the incidence of moderate OHSS by 50%.[105] A Cochrane review in 2016 by Tang H et al., including 16 RCTs and 2,091 women, concluded that dopamine agonists reduce the incidence of moderate and severe OHSS in high-risk women and do not affect the pregnancy outcome in fresh embryo transfer cycles.[106]

  Therefore, use of cabergoline in a dose of 0.5 mg/day for 8 days commencing on the day of hCG trigger is recommended.
- *Calcium infusion*: As discussed previously, the ovarian renin–angiotensin system is involved in the etiopathogenesis of OHSS. Calcium infusion inhibits cyclic adenosine monophosphate (cAMP) synthesis and cAMP-dependent renin secretion from juxtaglomerular cells in the kidneys.[107,108] Decreased renin secretion leads to decreased angiotensin II production and consequently decreased angiotensin II-mediated stimulation of VEGF synthesis.[65] Intravenous infusion of 10 mL of 10% calcium gluconate in 200 mL normal saline on the day of oocyte retrieval and 3 days thereafter decreases the risk of mild and severe OHSS.[109,110] This preventive strategy has a potential benefit but further studies are required for routine recommendation.
- *Aspirin*: Increased VEGF levels lead to increased platelet activation, which causes release of substances such as histamine, serotonin, platelet-derived growth factor, or lysophosphatidic acid, further potentiating the physiologic cascade of OHSS. Aspirin is associated with reduced incidence of OHSS with no effect on pregnancy outcome and is routinely recommended.[65,111]
- *Glucocorticoids*: Glucocorticoids and their synthetic derivatives have an inhibitory effect on *VEGF* gene expression in vascular smooth muscle cells.[112]

By inhibiting vasodilatation and preventing increase in vascular permeability, they ameliorate the inflammatory response and prevent edema formation, thus helping in treating early signs of developing OHSS.[55,113] One randomized trial has demonstrated a beneficial role of corticosteroids in conjunction with aspirin in preventing OHSS; the treatment begins on the day of starting COS.[114] However, there is insufficient evidence to recommend the use of glucocorticoids in preventing OHSS.[115,116]

- *Colloids (albumin and hydroxyethyl starch)*: As third spacing and intravascular volume depletion due to increased capillary leakage are hallmarks of OHSS, use of intravenous infusion of colloidal agents (albumin and hydroxyethyl starch) for prevention of OHSS has been investigated.[117-119] Albumin has a low molecular weight and an average half-life of 20 days. It increases plasma oncotic pressure, counteracting the permeability effect of angiotensin II and thus attenuates the effects of hypovolemia, hemoconcentration, and ascites. It also binds to vasoactive substances such as VEGF and factors related to RAS.

  In a Cochrane review analyzing nine RCTs, albumin infusion administered on the day of oocyte retrieval reduce rates of moderate and severe OHSS in high risk women, but at the same time it is associated with reduced pregnancy rates.[120] The data on hydroxyethyl starch is limited. Moreover, as albumin is a blood-derived product, it leads to allergic reactions and transmission of viruses and prions. The benefits of colloidal agents still remain unclear and further studies are required to recommend their use as preventive strategies.
- *Aromatase inhibitors*: The aromatase enzyme catalyzes the rate-limiting step in E2 synthesis. Aromatase inhibitors, therefore, help to reduce excessive E2 and reduces the risk of OHSS. The antiestrogenic effects of these agents are promising, but further studies are required for their routine use in prevention of OHSS in a clinical setting.[55,121]
- *Follicular aspiration*: It means aspiration of granulosa cells from one ovary 10–12 hours post hCG injection or at the time of oocyte retrieval as a means of inducing intraovarian bleeding and limiting the production of OHSS mediators while allowing continued contralateral ovarian development.[122]

  There is insufficient data to prove its role in preventing OHSS. Moreover, it leads to increased cost, discomfort, and invasive procedures requiring anesthesia. Hence, this approach is not recommended.
- *Miscellaneous treatments*: There is insufficient data to make recommendations regarding the use of luteal antagonist administration, intramuscular P, or ketoconazole to reduce the risk of OHSS.[65]

EXPERIMENTAL METHODS

- *In vitro maturation (IVM)*: In patients having high risk of OHSS, IVM helps in OHSS prevention.[55] It is the process of aspirating antral follicles of unstimulated or minimally stimulated ovaries and thus retrieving immature oocytes. Although the clinical outcome has improved in the recent years,[123] it is not widely used. It is still in the experimental stages and further trials are needed to use it in clinical practice.
- *VEGF antagonists*: A compound SU4516 blocks the intracellular phosphorylation of VEGFR-2 and acts as a VEGF antagonist and helps in preventing OHSS.[35] Similarly, FMS-like tyrosine kinase, which binds to VEGF and decreases its concentration, is available for endothelial cells.[124] However, it has side effects such as thromboembolism, severe vomiting, and teratogenicity; hence, it has not been used in clinical practice.
- *Kisspeptin trigger for oocyte maturation*: A group of peptides in the hypothalamus encoded by *KISS1* gene plays an important role in the reproductive pathway. Through a G protein-coupled receptor, it increases the secretion of GnRH and in turn FSH and LH. Kisspeptin-54, 54-amino acid peptide trigger, acts as a trigger for final oocyte maturation without causing OHSS or affecting implantation rates. It can also be utilized to control LH pulsatility and, thereby, secretion of sex hormones. It is still in the experimental stages and holds a high potential in prevention of OHSS.[125,126]
- *Vasopressin V1a receptor antagonist*: Relcovaptan is a vasopressin V1a receptor antagonist and blocks vasopressin-induced VEGF secretion. It alters vasoconstriction and proliferation of vascular smooth muscles.[56] During experiments, it has been found that relcovaptan decreases the number of corpora lutea, and the increase in the weight of ovaries is also less. However, further studies are required before it is brought into clinical practice.[127]

Thus, we have seen that there are many methods to prevent OHSS. The following flowchart is an example of how we can use the above-mentioned measures for the prevention and treatment of OHSS **(Flowchart 4)**.

Hence, in the present day, we should aim to achieve an "OHSS fee clinic," a concept given by Paul Devroey,[128] by incorporating a segmentation approach for IVF treatment **(Flowchart 5)**.

MANAGEMENT

The management depends on the severity of OHSS and guides the clinician on whether it should be done on an outpatient basis or admission is required. The initial assessment[129] of the patient with suspected OHSS is done on the following basis:

Flowchart 4: Prevention and treatment of ovarian hyperstimulation syndrome (OHSS).

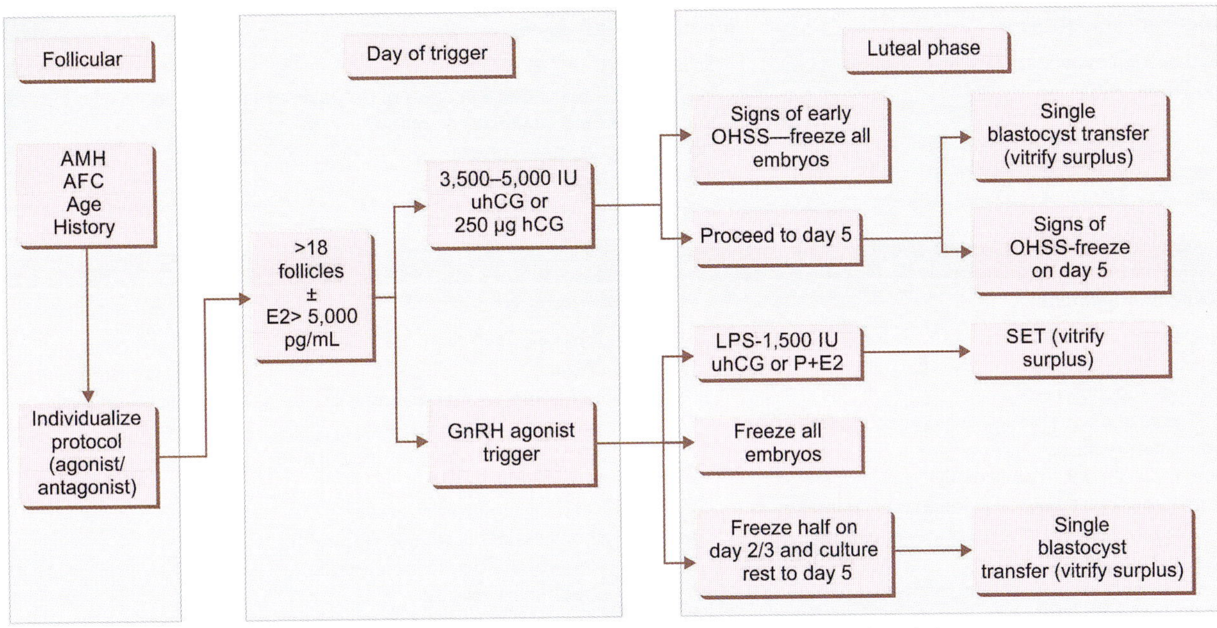

(AMH: anti-müllerian hormone; AFC: antral follicle count; E2: estradiol; LPS: luteal phase support; SET: single embryo transfer; uhCG: urinary human chorionic gonadotropin)

Flowchart 5: Segmentation approach for obtaining ovarian hyperstimulation syndrome-free clinic.

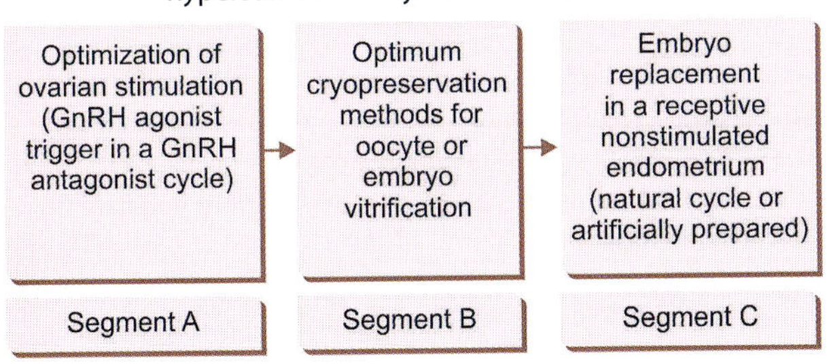

(GnRH: gonadotropin-releasing hormone)

- *History:*
  - Presence of high-risk factors for OHSS
  - Time of onset of symptoms from the time of trigger
  - Trigger used (hCG or GnRHa)
  - Number and size of follicles on the day of trigger
  - E2 levels
  - Fresh embryo transfer done or not
  - Presentation of the patient: Abdominal pain, discomfort, nausea, vomiting, difficulty in breathing, decreased urine output, swelling in legs or vulva, or any other co-morbidities.
- *Examination:*
  - General examination:
    - Assess for dehydration
    - Weight
    - Heart rate
    - Blood pressure
    - Respiratory rate
    - Saturation
  - Abdominal examination: Girth, ascites, any palpable mass, guarding, rigidity
  - Respiratory examination: Signs of pulmonary edema or pleural effusion
- *Investigations:*
  - Complete blood count
  - Hematocrit
  - Liver function tests
  - Renal function tests
  - Electrolytes (sodium and potassium)
  - Coagulation profile
  - Serum E2 (if required)
  - Ultrasound (ovarian size, ascites, pleural effusion; Doppler in cases of suspected torsion).

Other tests which might be indicated in critical cases are:
- C-reactive protein (CRP)
- Arterial blood gases
- D-dimers
- Electrocardiogram (ECG)/echocardiogram
- Chest X-ray.

Based on this, the severity and hence management of OHSS are decided **(Table 8)**.

Outpatient Management

Patients who are managed on an outpatient basis **(Table 9)** should be counseled in detail about symptoms such as abdominal pain, bloating, breathing difficulty, and decreased urinary output. The seriousness of the condition should be explained to the patients. Strict instructions should be given to take oral fluids abundantly as it is more

TABLE 8: Indications for outpatient and inpatient management.

Outpatient management	*Inpatient management*
• Mild ovarian hyperstimulation syndrome (OHSS) • Moderate OHSS	• Severe or critical OHSS • Worsening signs of OHSS in cases of outpatient management • Inadequate fluid intake due to nausea • Nonsatisfactory pain control • Noncompliance of the patient

TABLE 9: Management of ovarian hyperstimulation syndrome on an inpatient basis.

Medical management	*Paracentesis*	*Surgical management*
• Daily assessment of body weight, abdominal girth, input–output, full blood count, hematocrit, electrolytes, creatinine, and liver function tests • Analgesia and antiemetics (avoid nonsteroidal anti-inflammatory drugs) • Fluid replacement (mainly orally) • Intravenous crystalloids if inadequate oral intake • Intravenous colloids in cases of persistent hemoconcentration or oliguria • Diuretics only in cases of tense ascites with oliguria despite adequate hemodilution • Anticoagulants (low-molecular-weight heparin)	• Tense ascites • Oliguria • Increasing serum creatinine or falling creatinine clearance • Hemoconcentration nonresponsive to medical treatment • Need for symptomatic relief • Shortness of breath and respiratory compromise due to increased intra-abdominal pressure	• Adnexal torsion • Ovarian rupture • Ectopic pregnancy • Hemorrhage

BOX 1: Management on an outpatient basis.

Outpatient management:
- Counsel about symptoms
- Avoid intense exercises, sexual intercourse
- Fluid intake guided by thirst
- Weight, abdominal girth measurement
- Input–output chart
- *Analgesics:* Paracetamol or opioids; avoid nonsteroidal anti-inflammatory drugs
- Monitor every 2–3 days till symptoms resolve or onset of menses

physiological. Oral fluids, especially isotonic electrolyte solutions and sports drinks, help in optimum rehydration. Patients should be instructed to keep a diary of their daily weight, abdominal girth, urine output, fluid intake, and symptoms including abdominal discomfort, shortness of breath, and gastrointestinal complaints **(Box 1)**. They should report to the hospital immediately if any of the symptoms worsen. Nonsteroidal anti-inflammatory agents (NSAIDs) can be toxic to the kidney and hence should be avoided. Instructions should be given to avoid intense physical exercises and sexual intercourse so as to prevent injury/torsion of hyperstimulated ovaries. Women managed on an outpatient basis should be reviewed urgently if they develop signs and symptoms of worsening OHSS. If the signs do not worsen, patients can be reviewed every 2–3 days till resolution of symptoms or until menstrual bleeding ensues. OHSS is usually a self-limiting condition; however, it can worsen in case pregnancy occurs. Women with moderate OHSS should be evaluated for predisposing risk factors for thrombosis and prescribed either anti-embolism stockings or low-molecular-weight heparin (LMWH).

BOX 2: Parameters to indicate worsening of ovarian hyperstimulation syndrome.

Clinical findings:
- Weight gain: ≥2 lbs (0.91 kg)/day for 2 days
- Heart rate: >100 beats/min
- Respiratory rate: >20 breaths/min at rest
- Oliguria: <0.5 mL/kg/h for >6 hours or a 24-hour negative fluid balance of 500 mL
- Ascites:
  - Grade 1: Visible only on ultrasound
  - Grade 2: Detectable with flank bulging or shifting dullness
  - Grade 3: Marked distension

Laboratory findings:
- Hematocrit: >45%
- Liver function tests: >2 times normal range
- Electrolytes:
  - Sodium: <132 mEq/L
  - Potassium: >5 mEq/L
- Renal function:
  - Serum creatinine increases to ≥0.3 mg/dL or increases to ≥150% above initial baseline levels

The deterioration of the following parameters **(Box 2)** indicates the worsening of OHSS,[130] and inpatient management may be indicated:

Baseline laboratory investigations should be repeated if severity of OHSS is thought to be worsening. Hematocrit is a useful guide to the degree of intravascular volume depletion.

Inpatient Management

Women admitted with OHSS should be assessed at least once daily. Assessment should be done more frequently for those with critical OHSS and with complications.

Severe and critical OHSS should be managed on an inpatient basis and may also require admission to the intensive care unit. It is usually managed medically, but surgical intervention in the form of paracentesis, laparoscopy, or laparotomy **(Table 9)** might be required. A multidisciplinary approach should be used for the management of critical OHSS.

Strict monitoring of inpatients should be done. Body weight, abdominal girth, input-output, complete blood count with hematocrit, electrolytes, and liver and renal function tests should be monitored on a daily basis. CRP also helps in monitoring severity.[131] As OHSS resolves, diuresis ensues along with reduction in hematocrit, abdominal girth, and body weight.[65,132] Supportive treatment should be given in the form of analgesics and antiemetics for the relief of pain and nausea. NSAIDs should be avoided because of their toxic effects on the kidneys. Intravenous fluid therapy forms an important part of treatment when oral fluid intake is inadequate or if the patient is unable to take it orally because of severe nausea. Isotonic crystalloids should be given though they might not restore the balance because of increased capillary permeability and massive protein loss. Intravenous colloids are given if there is markedly decreased urine output or persistent hemoconcentration.

If oliguria persists despite adequate fluid replacement and drainage of ascites, diuretics can be used but with caution. Intravenous furosemide is given in a dose of 10–20 mg when adequate fluid replacement has been done, but still the urine output is markedly decreased.

Ovarian hyperstimulation syndrome is a hypercoagulable state, and anticoagulation therapy should be instituted prophylactically in the form of LMWH. The dose and duration of LMWH are given depending on the patient's risk factors.

Tense ascites with oliguria, respiratory compromise, or deteriorating renal function require paracentesis. It is tapping of the ascetic fluid and should be done under ultrasound guidance using all aseptic precautions. It can be done transabdominally or transvaginally. Up to 4 L of fluid can be drained by gravity or by using negative pressure.[133] Paracentesis should not be done in the presence of hemoperitoneum or if the patient is not stable hemodynamically. Another novel technique under research for the management of severe OHSS is peritoneovenous shunting.[134]

The chances of ovarian torsion or rupture are increased in OHSS. Usually, laparoscopy is employed for untwisting of ovaries in case of torsion. Ectopic pregnancy should always be kept as a differential diagnosis in cases of severe pain and if fresh embryo transfer has been done.[135] Rarely, late-onset critical OHSS might require termination of pregnancy.[135] In addition to the usual symptoms and signs of venous thromboembolism (VTE), thromboembolism should be suspected in women with OHSS who present with unusual neurological symptoms, even if they appear several weeks after improvement of OHSS. Clinicians should be aware and the patients be informed that pregnancies complicated by OHSS might be at an increased risk of preterm delivery and preeclampsia.

CONCLUSION

Ovarian hyperstimulation syndrome is a threat to every patient undergoing ovulation induction. It is important to understand the pathophysiology of OHSS and take appropriate measures for its prevention. All efforts should be made to make ART clinics OHSS-free clinics and prevent the fatal complications of this iatrogenic condition.

KEY POINTS

- OHSS is a threat to every patient undergoing ovulation induction.
- It is life threatening in its severe form resulting in hospitalization in 1.9% cases.
- It has been classified in various ways but the most commonly being practiced is the RCOG classification classifying it into mild, moderate, severe, and critical. It is also classified on the basis of onset, whether early or late onset.
- It is important to understand the pathophysiology of OHSS and take appropriate measures for its prevention. The most important factors implicated in its pathogenesis are hCG, VEGF, renin–angiotensin system, and certain immune factors.
- The primary risk factors include young, thin women with high basal AMH and AFC, having PCOS with history of OHSS.
- Prevention should be at both primary and secondary levels. Primary prevention involves using iCOS and GnRH antagonist protocol and avoiding GnRHa trigger.
- The most important secondary preventive measure is segmentation of the cycle with cryopreservation of embryos.
- The clinical features of OHSS should be recognized as early as possible and appropriately managed.
- All efforts should be made to make ART clinics OHSS-free clinics and prevent the fatal complications of this iatrogenic condition.

REFERENCES

1. Mocanu E, Redmond ML, Hennelly B, Collins C, Harrison R. Odds of ovarian hyperstimulation syndrome (OHSS)—time for reassessment. Hum Fertil (Camb). 2007;10(3):175-81.

2. Papanikolaou EG, Pozzobon C, Kolibianakis EM, Camus M, Tournaye H, Fatemi HM, et al. Incidence and prediction of ovarian hyperstimulation syndrome in women undergoing gonadotropin-releasing hormone antagonist in vitro fertilization cycles. Fertil Steril. 2006;85:112-20.
3. Brinsden PR, Wada I, Tan SL, Balen A, Jacobs HS. Diagnosis, prevention and management of ovarian hyperstimulation syndrome. Br J Obstet Gynaecol. 1995;102:767-72.
4. Aboulghar MA, Mansour RT. Ovarian hyperstimulation syndrome: classifications and critical analysis of preventive measures. Human Reprod Update. 2003;9(3):275-89.
5. Lyons CA, Wheeler CA, Frishman GN, Hackett RJ, Seifer DB, Haning Jr RV. Early and late presentation of the ovarian hyperstimulation syndrome: two distinct entities with different risk factors. Hum Reprod. 1994;9:792-9.
6. Mathur RS, Akande VA, Keay SD, Hunt LP, Jenkins JM. Distinction between early and late ovarian hyperstimulation syndrome. Fertil Steril. 2000;73:901-7.
7. Vlahos NF, Gregoriou O. Prevention and management of ovarian hyperstimulation syndrome. Ann N Y Acad Sci. 2006;1092:247-64.
8. Soares SR, Gómez R, Simón C, García-Velasco JA, Pellicer A. Targeting the vascular endothelial growth factor system to prevent ovarian hyperstimulation syndrome. Hum Reprod Update. 2008;14(4):321-33.
9. Nastri CO, Ferriani RA, Rocha IA, Martins WP. Ovarian hyperstimulation syndrome: pathophysiology and prevention. J Assist Reprod Genet. 2010;27:121-8.
10. Elchalal U, Schenker JG. The pathophysiology of ovarian hyperstimulation syndrome—views and ideas. Human Reprod. 1997;12(6):1129-37.
11. Knox GE. Antihistamine blockade of the ovarian hyperstimulation syndrome. Am J Obstet Gynecol. 1974;118:992-4.
12. Pride J, Ho YI. The ovarian hyperstimulation syndrome. Semin Reprod Endocrinol. 1990;8:247-53.
13. Haning Jr RV, Austin CW, Carlson IH, Kuzma DL, Shapiro SS, Zweibel WJ. Plasma estradiol is superior to ultrasound and urinary estriol glucuronide as a predictor of ovarian hyperstimulation during induction of ovulation with menotropins. Fertil Steril. 1983;40:31-6.
14. Schenker JG. Prevention and treatment of ovarian hyperstimulation. Hum Reprod. 1993;8:653-9.
15. Pellicer A, Miró F, Sampaio M, Gómez E, Bonilla-Musoles FM. In vitro fertilization as a diagnostic and therapeutic tool in a patient with partial 17,20-desmolase deficiency. Fertil Steril. 1991;55:970-5.
16. Levy T, Orvieto R, Homburg R, Peleg D, Dekel A, Ben-Rafael Z. Severe ovarian hyperstimulation syndrome despite low plasma oestrogen concentrations in a hypogonadotrophic, hypogonadal patient. Hum Reprod. 1996;11:1177-9.
17. Yarali H, Fleige-Zahradka BG, Yuen BH, McComb PF. The ascites in the ovarian hyperstimulation syndrome does not originate from the ovary. Fertil Steril. 1993;59:657-61.
18. Delvigne A, Rozenberg S. Systematic review of data concerning etiopathology of ovarian hyperstimulation syndrome. Int J Fertil Womens Med. 2002;47:211-26.
19. Pride SM, Yuen BH, Moon YS, Leung PCS. Relationship of gonadotropin-releasing hormone, danazol, and prostaglandin blockade to ovarian enlargement and ascites formation of the ovarian hyperstimulation syndrome in the rabbit. Am J Obstet Gynecol. 1986;154:1155-60.
20. Borenstein R, Elhalah U, Lunenfeld B, Schwartz, ZS. Severe ovarian hyperstimulation syndrome: a reevaluated therapeutic approach. Fertil Steril. 1989;51:791-5.
21. Golan A, Ron-el R, Herman A, Soffer Y, Weinraub Z, Caspi E. Ovarian hyperstimulation syndrome: an update review. Obstet Gynecol Surv. 1989;44:430-40.
22. Chae HD, Park EJ, Kim SH, Kim CH, Kang BM, Chang YS. Ovarian hyperstimulation syndrome complicating a spontaneous singleton pregnancy: a case report. J Assist Reprod Genet. 2001;18(2):120-3.
23. Oztekin O, Soylu F, Tatli O. Spontaneous ovarian hyperstimulation syndrome in a normal singleton pregnancy. Taiwan J Obstet Gynecol. 2006;45(3):272-5.
24. Mittal K, Koticha R, Dey AK, Anandpara K, Agrawal R, Sarvothaman MP, et al. Radiological illustration of spontaneous ovarian hyperstimulation syndrome. Pol J Radiol. 2015;80:217-27.
25. Neufeld G, Cohen T, Gengrinovitch S, Poltorak Z. Vascular endothelial growth factor (VEGF) and its receptors. FASEB J. 1999;13:9-22.
26. Olson TA, Mohanraj D, Carson LF, Ramakrishnan S. Vascular permeability factor gene expression in normal and neoplastic human ovaries. Cancer Res. 1994;54:276-80.
27. Waltenberger J, Claesson-Welsh L, Siegbahn A, Shibuya M, Heldin CH. Different signal transduction properties of KDR and Flt1, two receptors for vascular endothelial growth factor. J Biol Chem. 1994;269:26988-95.
28. Kendall RL, Thomas KA. Inhibition of vascular endothelial cell growth factor activity by an endogenously encoded soluble receptor. Proc Natl Acad Sci U S A. 1993;90: 10705-9.
29. Kendall RL, Wang G, Thomas KA. Identification of a natural soluble form of the vascular endothelial growth factor receptor, flt-1, and its heterodimerization with KDR. Biochem Biophys Res Commun. 1996;226:324-8.
30. Roeckl W, Hecht D, Sztajer H, Waltenberger J, Yayon A, Weich HA. Differential binding characteristics and cellular inhibition by soluble VEGF receptors 1 and 2. Exp Cell Res. 1998;241:161-70.
31. Gómez R, Simón C, Remohí J, Pellicer A. Administration of moderate and high doses of gonadotropins to female rats increases ovarian vascular endothelial growth factor (VEGF) and VEGF receptor-2 expression that is associated to vascular hyperpermeability. Biol Reprod. 2003;68:2164-71.
32. Albert C, Garrido N, Mercader A, Rao CV, Remohí J, Simón C, et al. The role of endothelial cells in the pathogenesis of ovarian hyperstimulation syndrome. Mol Hum Reprod. 2002;8:409-18.
33. Manau D, Balasch J, Arroyo V, Jiménez W, Fábregues F, Casamitjana R, et al. Circulatory dysfunction in asymptomatic in vitro fertilization patients. Relationship with hyperestrogenemia and activity of endogenous vasodilators. J Clin Endocrinol Metab. 1998;83:1489-93.
34. Blumenfeld Z, Shabadash V, Shen-Or Z, Arnon R, Israeli E, Makler A. The origin of ascites in the ovarian hyperstimulation syndrome is mainly ovarian in humans. In: Program and Abstracts of the Annual Meeting of the Society for

Gynecological Investigation, San Diego, CA. J Soc Gynecol Invest. 1997;(Suppl. 4). Abstract 123.
35. Naredi N, Talwar P, Sandeep K. VEGF antagonist for the prevention of ovarian hyperstimulation syndrome: current status. Med J Armed Forces India. 2014;70(1):58-63.
36. Balasch J, Arroyo V, Fábregues F, Saló J, Jiménez W, Paré JC, et al. Neurohormonal and hemodynamic changes in severe cases of the ovarian hyperstimulation syndrome. Ann Intern Med. 194;121:27-33.
37. Balaśch J, Arroyo V, Carmona F, Llach J, Jiménez W, Paré JC, et al. Severe ovarian hyperstimulation syndrome: role of peripheral vasodilation. Fertil Steril. 1991;56(6):1077-83.
38. Adashi EY, Resnick CE, Packman JN, Hurwitz A, Payne DW. Cytokine-mediated regulation of ovarian function: tumor necrosis factor alpha inhibits gonadotropin-supported progesterone accumulation by differentiating and luteinized murine granulosa cells. Am J Obstet Gynecol. 1990;162: 889-96.
39. Dinarello CA. Interleukin-1 and its biologically related cytokines. Adv Immunol. 1989;44:153-205.
40. Aramwit P, Pruksananonda K, Kasettratat N, Jammeechai K. Risk factors for ovarian hyperstimulation syndrome in Thai patients using gonadotropins for in vitro fertilization. Am J Health Syst Pharm. 2008;65:1148-53.
41. The European Orgalutran Study Group, Borm G, Mannaerts B. Treatment with the gonadotrophin-releasing hormone antagonist ganirelix in women undergoing ovarian stimulation with recombinant follicle stimulating hormone is effective, safe and convenient: results of a controlled, randomized, multicentre trial. Hum Reprod. 2000;15:1490-8.
42. Danninger B, Brunner M, Obruca A, Feichtinger W. Prediction of ovarian hyperstimulation syndrome by ultrasound volumetric assessment [corrected] of baseline ovarian volume prior to stimulation. Hum Reprod. 1996;11:1597-9.
43. Luke B, Brown MB, Morbeck DE, Hudson SB, Coddington 3rd CC, Stern JE. Factors associated with ovarian hyperstimulation syndrome (OHSS) and its effect on assisted reproductive technology (ART) treatment and outcome. Fertil Steril. 2010;94:1399-404.
44. Lee TH, Liu CH, Huang CC, Wu YL, Shih YT, Ho HN, et al. Serum anti-müllerian hormone and estradiol levels as predictors of ovarian hyperstimulation syndrome in assisted reproduction technology cycles. Hum Reprod. 2008;23:160-7.
45. Nardo LG, Gelbaya TA, Wilkinson H, Roberts SA, Yates A, Pemberton P, et al. Circulating basal anti-müllerian hormone levels as predictor of ovarian response in women undergoing ovarian stimulation for in vitro fertilization. Fertil Steril. 2009;92:1586-93.
46. Kwee J, Elting ME, Schats R, McDonnell J, Lambalk CB. Ovarian volume and antral follicle count for the prediction of low and hyper responders with in vitro fertilization. Reprod Biol Endocrinol. 2007;5:9.
47. Rizk B. Symposium: update on prediction and management of OHSS. Genetics of ovarian hyperstimulation syndrome. Reprod Biomed Online. 2009;19:14-27.
48. Tollan A, Holst N, Forsdahl F, Fadnes H, Oian P, Maltau JM. Transcapillary fluid dynamics during ovarian stimulation for in vitro fertilization. Am J Obstet Gynecol. 1990;162:554-8.
49. Grossman LC, Michalakis KG, Browne H, Payson MD, Segars JH. The pathophysiology of ovarian hyperstimulation syndrome: an unrecognized compartment syndrome. Fertil Steril. 2010;94:1392-8.
50. Abramov Y, Elchalal U, Schenker JG. Pulmonary manifestations of severe ovarian hyperstimulation syndrome: a multicenter study. Fertil Steril. 1999;71(4):645-51.
51. Hecker A, Hecker B, Hecker M, Riedel JG, Weigand MA, Padberg W. Acute abdominal compartment syndrome: current diagnostic and therapeutic options. Langenbecks Arch Surg. 2016;401:15-24.
52. Chopra SS, Wolf S, Rohde V, Freimann FB. Pressure measurement techniques for abdominal hypertension: conclusions from an experimental model. Crit Care Res Pract. 2015;2015:278139.
53. De Waele JJ, De Laet I, Malbrain ML. Understanding abdominal compartment syndrome. Intensive Care Med. 2016;42:1068-70.
54. Fábregues F, Balasch J, Ginès P, Manau D, Jiménez W, Arroyo V, et al. Ascites and liver test abnormalities during severe ovarian hyperstimulation syndrome. Am J Gastroenterol. 1999;94:994-9.
55. Humaidan P, Quartarolo J, Papanikolaou EG. Preventing ovarian hyperstimulation syndrome: guidance for the clinician. Fertil Steril. 2010;94:389-400.
56. Smith V, Osianlis T, Vollenhoven B. Prevention of ovarian hyperstimulation syndrome: a review. Obstet Gynecol Int. 2015;2015:514159.
57. Lensen SF, Wilkinson J, Leijdekkers JA, La Marca A, Mol BJ, Marjoribanks J, et al. Individualised gonadotropin dose selection using markers of ovarian reserve for women undergoing in vitro fertilisation plus intracytoplasmic sperm injection (IVF/ICSI). Cochrane Database Syst Rev. 2018;2:CD012693.
58. Christin-Maitre S, Hugues JN, Recombinant FSH Study Group. A comparative randomized multicentric study comparing the step-up versus step-down protocol in polycystic ovary syndrome. Human Reprod. 2003;18(8):1626-31.
59. Homburg R, Levy T, Ben-Rafael Z. A comparative prospective study of conventional regimen with chronic low-dose administration of follicle-stimulating hormone for anovulation associated with polycystic ovary syndrome. Fertil Steril. 1995;63(4):729-33.
60. Mahajan N. Should mild stimulation be the order of the day? J Hum Reprod Sci. 2013;6(4):220-6.
61. Andersen AN, Nelson SM, Fauser BC, García-Velasco JA, Klein BM, Arce JC, et al. Individualized versus conventional ovarian stimulation for in vitro fertilization: a mutlicenter, randomized, controlled, assessor-blinded, phase 3 noninferiority trial. Fertil Steril. 2017;107(2):387-96.
62. Fernández-Sánchez M, Visnova H, Yuzpe A, Klein BM, Mannaerts B, Arce JC, et al. Individualization of the starting dose of follitropin delta reduces the overall OHSS risk and/or the need for additional preventive interventions: cumulative data over three stimulation cycles. Reprod Biomed Online. 2018;38:528-37.
63. Jayaprakasan K, Hopkisson JF, Campbell BK, Clewes J, Johnson IR, Raine-Fenning NJ. Quantification of the effect of pituitary down-regulation on 3D ultrasound predictors of ovarian response. Hum Reprod. 2008;23:1538-44.
64. Nugent D, Vandekerckhove P, Hughes E, Arnot M, Lilford R. Gonadotrophin therapy for ovulation induction in subfertility

associated with polycystic ovary syndrome. Cochrane Database Syst Rev. 2000;(4):CD000410.
65. Practice Committee of the American Society for Reproductive Medicine. Prevention and treatment of moderate and severe ovarian hyperstimulation syndrome: a guideline. Fertil Steril. 2016;106:1634-47.
66. Al-Inany HG, Youssef MA, Aboulghar M, Broekmans F, Sterrenburg M, Smit J, et al. Gonadotrophin-releasing hormone antagonists for assisted reproductive technology. Cochrane Database Syst Rev. 2011:CD001750.
67. Pritts EA, Atwood AK. Luteal phase support in infertility treatment: a meta-analysis of the randomized trials. Human Reprod. 2002;17(9):2287-99.
68. Fatemi HM, Kolibianakis EM, Camus M, Tournaye H, Donoso P, Papanikolaou E, et al. Addition of estradiol to progesterone for luteal supplementation in patients stimulated with GnRH antagonist/rFSH for IVF: a randomized controlled trial. Human Reprod. 2006;21(10):2628-32.
69. Young SL. Oestrogen and progesterone action on endometrium: a translational approach to understanding endometrial receptivity. Reprod Biomed Online. 2013;27(5):497-505.
70. van der Linden M, Buckingham K, Farquhar C, Kremer JA, Metwally M. Luteal phase support for assisted reproduction cycles. Cochrane Database Syst Rev. 2011;10:CD009154.
71. Pirard C, Donnez J, Loumaye E. GnRH agonist as novel luteal support: results of a randomized, parallel group, feasibility study using intranasal administration of buserelin. Human Reprod. 2005;20:1798-804.
72. Elia EM, Quintana R, Carrere C, Bazzano MV, Rey-Valzacchi G, Paz DA, et al. Metformin decreases the incidence of ovarian hyperstimulation syndrome: an experimental study. J Ovarian Res. 2013;6(1):62.
73. Huang X, Wang P, Tal R, Lv F, Li Y, Zhang X. A systematic review and meta-analysis of metformin among patients with polycystic ovary syndrome undergoing assisted reproductive technology procedures. Int J Gynaecol Obstet. 2015;131:111-6.
74. Tso LO, Costello MF, Albuquerque LE, Andriolo RB, Macedo CR. Metformin treatment before and during IVF or ICSI in women with polycystic ovary syndrome. Cochrane Database Syst Rev. 2020;12:CD006105.
75. Emperaire JC, Ruffie A. Triggering ovulation with endogenous luteinizing hormone may prevent the ovarian hyperstimulation syndrome. Human Reprod. 1991;6(4):506-10.
76. Itskovitz J, Boldes R, Levron J, Erlik Y, Kahana L, Brandes JM. Induction of preovulatory luteinizing hormone surge and prevention of ovarian hyperstimulation syndrome by gonadotropin-releasing hormone agonist. Fertil Steril. 1991;56(2):213-20.
77. Kol S, Humaidan P. GnRH agonist triggering: recent developments. Reprod Biomed Online. 2013;26(3):226-30.
78. Youssef MA, Van der Veen F, Al-Inany HG, Mochtar MH, Griesinger G, Nagi Mohesen M, et al. Gonadotropin-releasing hormone agonist versus HCG for oocyte triggering in antagonist-assisted reproductive technology. Cochrane Database Syst Rev. 2014:CD008046.
79. Van der Meer S, Gerris J, Joostens M, Tas B. Triggering of ovulation using a gonadotrophin-releasing hormone agonist does not prevent ovarian hyperstimulation syndrome. Hum Reprod. 1993;8:1628-31.
80. Kol S, Lewit N, Itskovitz-Eldor J. Ovarian hyperstimulation: effects of GnRH analogues. Ovarian hyperstimulation syndrome after using gonadotrophin-releasing hormone analogue as a trigger of ovulation: causes and implications. Hum Reprod. 1996;11:1143-4.
81. Casper RF. Ovarian hyperstimulation: effects of GnRH analogues. Does triggering ovulation with gonadotrophin-releasing hormone analogue prevent severe ovarian hyperstimulation syndrome? Hum Reprod. 1996;11:1144-6.
82. European Recombinant LH Study Group. Human recombinant luteinizing hormone is as effective as, but safer than, urinary human chorionic gonadotropin in inducing final follicular maturation and ovulation in in vitro fertilization procedures: results of a multicenter double-blind study. J Clin Endocrinol Metab. 2001;86:2607-18.
83. Schmidt DW, Maier DB, Nulsen JC, Benadiva CA. Reducing the dose of human chorionic gonadotropin in high responders does not affect the outcomes of in vitro fertilization. Fertil Steril. 2004;82:841-6.
84. Kolibianakis EM, Papanikolaou EG, Tournaye H, Camus M, Van Steirteghem AC, Devroey P. Triggering final oocyte maturation using different doses of human chorionic gonadotropin: a randomized pilot study in patients with polycystic ovary syndrome treated with gonadotropin-releasing hormone antagonists and recombinant follicle-stimulating hormone. Fertil Steril. 2007;88:1382-8.
85. Navot D, Bergh PA, Laufer N. Ovarian hyperstimulation syndrome in novel reproductive technologies: prevention and treatment. Fertil Steril. 1992;58:249-61.
86. D'Angelo A, Amso N. Embryo freezing for preventing ovarian hyperstimulation syndrome. Cochrane Database Syst Rev. 2007;(3):CD002806.
87. Herrero L, Martínez M, Garcia-Velasco JA. Current status of human oocyte and embryo cryopreservation. Curr Opin Obstet Gynecol. 2011;23(4):245-50.
88. Dolmans MM, Marotta ML, Pirard C, Donnez J, Donnez O. Ovarian tissue cryopreservation followed by controlled ovarian stimulation and pick-up of mature oocytes does not impair the number or quality of retrieved oocytes. J Ovarian Res. 2014;7:80.
89. Roque M. Freeze-all policy: is it time for that? J Assist Reprod Genet. 2015;32(2):171-6.
90. Roque M, Lattes K, Serra S, Solà I, Geber S, Carreras R, et al. Fresh embryo transfer versus frozen embryo transfer in in vitro fertilization cycles: a systematic review and meta-analysis. Fertil Steril. 2013;99(1):156-62.
91. Roque M, Haahr T, Geber S, Esteves SC, Humaidan P. Fresh versus elective frozen embryo transfer in IVF/ICSI cycles: a systematic review and meta-analysis of reproductive outcomes. Hum Reprod Update. 2019;25(1):2-14.
92. Devroey P, Adriaensen P. OHSS free clinic. Facts Views Vis Obgyn. 2011;3(1):43-5.
93. Schenker JG, Weinstein D. Ovarian hyperstimulation syndrome: a current survey. Fertil Steril. 1978;30:255-68.
94. Mathur RS, Tan BK. British fertility society policy and practice committee: prevention of ovarian hyperstimulation syndrome. Hum Fertil (Camb). 2014;17(4):257-68.

95. Al-Shawaf T, Zosmer A, Hussain S, Tozer A, Panay N, Wilson C, et al. Prevention of severe ovarian hyperstimulation syndrome in IVF with or without ICSI and embryo transfer: a modified 'coasting' strategy based on ultrasound for identification of high-risk patients. Hum Reprod. 2001;16:24-30.
96. Dhont M, Van der Straeten F, De Sutter P. Prevention of severe ovarian hyperstimulation by coasting. Fertil Steril. 1998;70:847-50.
97. D'Angelo A, Amso NN, Hassan R. Coasting (withholding gonadotrophins) for preventing ovarian hyperstimulation syndrome. Cochrane Database Syst Rev. 2017;5(5): CD002811.
98. Ata B, Seyhan A, Orhaner S, Urman B. High dose cabergoline in management of ovarian hyperstimulation syndrome. Fertil Steril. 2009;92:1168.e1-e4.
99. Gomez R, Gonzalez M, Simón C, Remohí J, Pellicer A. Tyroxine hydroxylase (TH) downregulation in hyperstimulated ovaries reveals the dopamine agonist bromocriptine (Br2) as an effective and specific method to block increased vascular permeability (VP) in OHSS. Fertil Steril. 2003;80:43-4.
100. Busso CE, Garcia-Velasco J, Gomez R, Alvarez C, Simón C, Pellicer A. Symposium: update on prediction and management of OHSS. Prevention of OHSS—dopamine agonists. Reprod Biomed Online. 2009;19(1):43-51.
101. Papaleo E, Doldi N, De Santis L, Marelli G, Marsiglio E, Rofena S, et al. Cabergoline influences ovarian stimulation in hyperprolactinaemic patients with polycystic ovary syndrome. Hum Reprod. 2001;16:2263-6.
102. Zimmermann RC, Hartman T, Bohlen P, Sauer MV, Kitajewski J. Preovulatory treatment of mice with anti-VEGF receptor 2 antibody inhibits angiogenesis in corpora lutea. Microvasc Res. 2001;62:15-25.
103. Pauli SA, Tang H, Wang J, Bohlen P, Posser R, Hartman T, et al. The vascular endothelial growth factor (VEGF)/VEGF receptor 2 pathway is critical for blood vessel survival in corpora lutea of pregnancy in the rodent. Endocrinology 2005;146:1301-11.
104. Mornex R, Orgiazzi J, Hugues B, Gagnaire JC, Claustrat B. Normal pregnancies after treatment of hyperprolactinemia with bromoergocryptine, despite suspected pituitary tumors. J Clin Endocrinol Metab. 1978;47:290-5.
105. Alvarez C, Martí-Bonmatí L, Novella-Maestre E, Sanz R, Gómez R, Fernández-Sánchez M, et al. Dopamine agonist cabergoline reduces hemoconcentration and ascites in hyperstimulated women undergoing assisted reproduction. J Clin Endocrinol Metab. 2007;92:2931-7.
106. Tang H, Mourad S, Zhai SD, Hart RJ. Dopamine agonists for preventing ovarian hyperstimulation syndrome. Cochrane Database Syst Rev. 2016;11(11):CD008605.
107. Ortiz-Capisano MC, Ortiz PA, Harding P, Garvin JL, Beierwaltes WH. Decreased intracellular calcium stimulates renin release via calcium-inhibitable adenylyl cyclase. Hypertension. 2007;49:162-9.
108. Beierwaltes WH. The role of calcium in the regulation of renin secretion. Am J Physiol Renal Physiol. 2010;298:F1-11.
109. Yakovenko SA, Sivozhelezov VS, Zorina IV, Dmitrieva NV, Apryshko VP, Voznesenskaya JV. Prevention of OHSS by intravenous calcium. Hum Reprod. 2009;24(Suppl. 1):i61.
110. Gurgan T, Demirol A, Guven S, Benkhalifa M, Girgin B, Li TC. Intravenous calcium infusion as a novel preventive therapy of ovarian hyperstimulation syndrome for patients with polycystic ovarian syndrome. Fertil Steril. 2011;96:53-7.
111. Várnagy A, Bódis J, Mánfai Z, Wilhelm F, Busznyák C, Koppán M. Low-dose aspirin therapy to prevent ovarian hyperstimulation syndrome. Fertil Steril. 2010;93:2281-4.
112. Nauck M, Karakiulakis G, Perruchoud AP, Papkonstantinou E, Roth M. Corticosteroids inhibit the expression of the vascular endothelial growth factor gene in human vascular smooth muscle cells. Eur J Pharmacol. 1998;341:309-15.
113. Perretti M, Ahluwalia A. The microcirculation and inflammation: site of action for glucocorticoids. Microcirculation. 2000;7:147-61.
114. Revelli A, Dolfin E, Gennarelli G, Lantieri T, Massobrio M, Holte JG, et al. Low-dose acetylsalicylic acid plus prednisolone as an adjuvant treatment in IVF: a prospective, randomized study. Fertil Steril. 2008;90:1685-91.
115. Lainas T, Petsas G, Stavropoulou G, Alexopoulou E, Iliadis G, Minaretzis D. Administration of methylprednisolone to prevent severe ovarian hyperstimulation syndrome in patients undergoing in vitro fertilization. Fertil Steril. 2002;78:529-33.
116. Tan SL, Balen A, el Hussein E, Campbell S, Jacobs HS. The administration of glucocorticoids for the prevention of ovarian hyperstimulation syndrome in in vitro fertilization: a prospective randomized study. Fertil Steril. 1992;58: 378-83.
117. Shalev E, Giladi Y, Matilsky M, Ben-Ami M. Decreased incidence of severe ovarian hyperstimulation syndrome in high risk in-vitro fertilization patients receiving intravenous albumin: a prospective study. Hum Reprod. 1995;10:1373-6.
118. Isik AZ, Gokmen O, Zeyneloglu HB, Kara S, Keles G, Gulekli B. Intravenous albumin prevents moderate-severe ovarian hyperstimulation in in-vitro fertilization patients: a prospective, randomized and controlled study. Eur J Obstet Gynecol Reprod Biol. 1996;70:179-83.
119. Gokmen O, Ugur M, Ekin M, Keles G, Turan C, Oral H. Intravenous albumin versus hydroxyethyl starch for the prevention of ovarian hyperstimulation in an *in-vitro* fertilization programme: A prospective randomized placebo controlled study. Eur J Obstet Gynecol Reprod Biol. 2001;96:187-92.
120. Youssef MA, Mourad S. Volume expanders for the prevention of ovarian hyperstimulation syndrome. Cochrane Database Syst Rev. 2016;2016(8):CD001302.
121. Santen RJ. Inhibition of aromatase: insights from recent studies. Steroids. 2003;68:559-67.
122. Gonen Y, Powell WA, Casper RF. Effect of follicular aspiration on hormonal parameters in patients undergoing ovarian stimulation. Hum Reprod. 1991;6:356-8.
123. Suikkari AM. In-vitro maturation: its role in fertility treatment. Curr Opin Obstet Gynecol. 2008;20:242-8.
124. McElhinney B, Ardill J, Caldwell C, McClure N. Preventing ovarian hyperstimulation syndrome by inhibiting the effects of vascular endothelial growth factor. J Reprod Med. 2003;48:243-6.
125. Skorupskaite K, George JT, Anderson RA. The kisspeptin-GnRH pathway in human reproductive health and disease. Hum Reprod Update. 2014;20:485-500.
126. Abbara A, Jayasena CN, Christopoulos G, Narayanaswamy S, Izzi-Engbeaya C, Nijher GM, et al. Efficacy of kisspeptin-54 to trigger oocyte maturation in women at high risk of

ovarian hyperstimulation syndrome (OHSS) during in vitro fertilization (IVF) therapy. J Clin Endocrinol Metab. 2015;100:3322-31.

127. Cenksoy C, Cenksoy PO, Erdem O, Sancak B, Gursoy. A potential novel strategy, inhibition of vasopressin-induced VEGF secretion by relcovaptan, for decreasing the incidence of ovarian hyperstimulation syndrome in the hyperstimulated rat model. Eur J Obstet Gynecol Reprod Biol. 2014;174(1): 86-90.
128. Devroey P, Polyzos NP, Blockeel C. An OHSS-Free Clinic by segmentation of IVF treatment. Hum Reprod. 2011;26(10):2593-7.
129. Royal College of Obstetricians and Gynaecologists. (2016). The management of ovarian hyperstimulation syndrome (Greentop Guideline No. 5). [online] Available from: https://www.rcog.org.uk/guidance/browse-all-guidance/green-top-guidelines/the-management-of-ovarian-hyperstimulation-syndrome-green-top-guideline-no-5/ [Last accessed November, 2022].
130. Humaidan P, Nelson SM, Devroey P, Coddington CC, Schwartz LB, Gordon K, et al. Ovarian hyperstimulation syndrome: review and new classification criteria for reporting in clinical trials. Hum Reprod. 2016;31(9):1997-2004.
131. Nowicka MA, Fritz-Rdzanek A, Grzybowski W, Walecka I, Niemiec KT, Jakimiuk AJ. C-reactive protein as the indicator of severity in ovarian hyperstimulation syndrome. Gynecol Endocrinol. 2010;26:399-403.
132. Fábregues F, Balasch J, Manau D, Jiménez W, Arroyo V, Creus M, et al. Haematocrit, leukocyte and platelet counts and the severity of the ovarian hyperstimulation syndrome. Hum Reprod. 1998;13:2406-10.
133. Thaler I, Yoffe M, Kaftory JK, Brandes JM. Treatment of ovarian hyperstimulation syndrome: the physiologic basis for a modified approach. Fertil Steril. 1981;36:110-3.
134. Koike T, Araki S, Minakami H, Ogawa S, Sayama M, Shibahara H, et al. Clinical efficacy of peritoneovenous shunting for the treatment of severe ovarian hyperstimulation syndrome. Hum Reprod. 2000;15:113-7.
135. Gorkemli H, Camus M, Clasen K. Adnexal torsion after gonadotrophin ovulation induction for IVF or ICSI and its conservative treatment. Arch Gynecol Obstet. 2002; 267:4-6.

CHAPTER

67 Ectopic Pregnancy

Rishma Dhillon Pai, Hrishikesh Pai, Nidhi Shah Gandhi, Navina Singh

INTRODUCTION

For pregnancy to occur, the egg has to enter the fallopian tube, where it survives for 24 hours. If it gets fertilized with a sperm, the embryo stays in the fallopian tube for 3 days or 4 days before it reaches the uterus. There it attaches to the endometrium and continues to grow until a baby is born.

DEFINITION

An ectopic pregnancy (EP) occurs when the embryo is implanted anywhere other than the cavity of the uterus. It could get implanted within the fallopian tube, ovary, abdomen, etc.

HETEROTOPIC PREGNANCY

A heterotopic pregnancy is a combination of two pregnancies occurring simultaneously at two different implantation sites. The most frequent combination is an intrauterine and an extrauterine pregnancy. The most common extrauterine site is the fallopian tube (90%); however, an EP can also be seen in the cervix, ovary, abdomen, or even a previous cesarean scar.

HISTORY OF ECTOPIC PREGNANCY

Abulcasis was the first to describe an EP as early as the 10th century AD. The first known surgical procedure for EP was performed in France in 1714. In the late 19th century, Robert Lawson Tait, a British surgeon performed laparotomy and salpingectomy for ruptured tubal EP. The first ever in vitro fertilization (IVF) conception was also known to be an EP.

INCIDENCE

Among the general population, EP is known to occur in 19/1,000 pregnancies. The incidence is higher—4% in women undergoing assisted reproductive techniques for conception.

Ectopic pregnancy is considered the number one cause for maternal deaths during the first trimester of pregnancy, accounting for approximately 10% of the total deaths.[1]

COMMON SITES FOR ECTOPIC PREGNANCY

Approximately 93–97% of all ectopic pregnancies occur within the fallopian tube.[2] The other lesser frequently involved sites include the ovary, cervix, abdomen, and a previous cesarean scar **(Table 1)**.

RISK FACTORS

The blastocyst travels along the fallopian tube as a result of smooth muscle contractions and ciliary beating.[3]

Any condition that interferes with this tubal transport mechanism or damages the tubes may predispose to EP.[4-6]

Abnormality of the tubes can occur as a result of any of the following:

- Pelvic inflammatory disease (PID)
- History of a previous EP
- Infertility ≥2 years
- Pelvic/abdominal surgery resulting in adhesions and interference with the normal anatomical structure
- Endometriosis
- Sexually transmitted infections such as *Chlamydia* and gonorrhea
- Previously failed tubal surgery such as tubal sterilization or a tubal ligation reversal procedure.

Relative risk (RR) factors **(Flowchart 1)** include the following:

- Cigarette smoking increases the risk by twofold.
- Increased maternal age.

TABLE 1: Common sites for ectopic pregnancy.

Site	%
Fallopian tubes	93%
Ampulla	70%
Isthmus	12%
Fimbria	11%
Ovarian	3.2%
Cornual/interstitial	2.4%
Abdominal	1.3%
Cervical	<1%

Flowchart 1: Risk factors for an ectopic pregnancy.

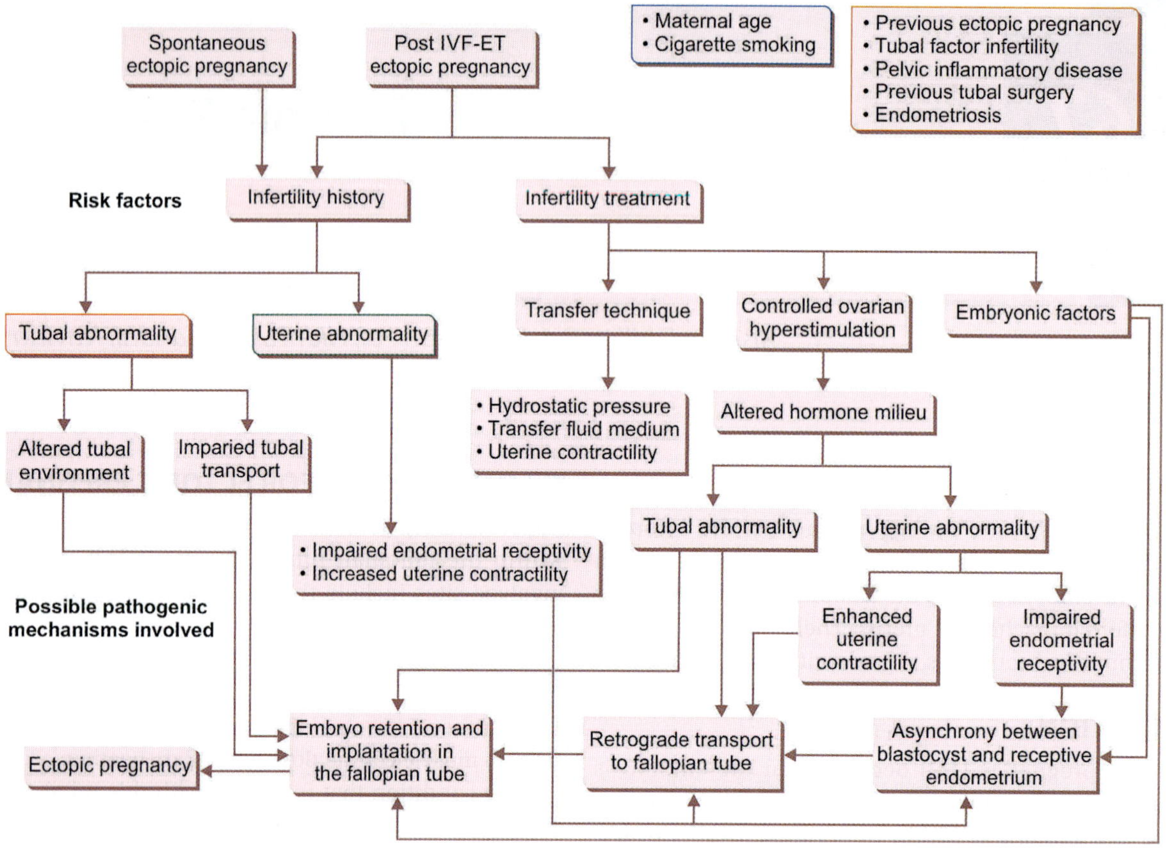

(ET: embryo transfer; IVF: in vitro fertilization)

- Multiple sexual partners probably due to increased risk of exposure to sexually transmitted diseases (STDs).
- Intrauterine exposure to diethylstilbestrol increases the risk by twofold.
- Pregnancy with an intrauterine device (IUD) in situ.
- IVF/assisted reproductive technology (ART) increases the risk by twofold.

CLINICAL FEATURES

Ectopic pregnancy can manifest differently in different individuals. Patients may be symptom-free or may present with more than or equal to one of the following symptoms:

- *Amenorrhea*—generally of 5–6 weeks
- *Abnormal vaginal bleeding:* Any bleeding that manifests at times other than your normal menstrual period is called abnormal vaginal bleeding. It could be either scanty in the form of spotting or heavy with passage of clots/tissues.
- *Lower abdominal pain:* It may be unilateral/bilateral. The pain may arise acutely as a sudden sharp ache or it may occur gradually over several days. The pain generally does not respond to painkillers and is not relieved on rest.
- *Shoulder pain if it is a ruptured tubal pregnancy.* Accumulated blood within the peritoneal cavity irritates the diaphragm and causes shoulder ache.
- *Weakness, lightheadedness, or syncope* because of sudden, excessive blood loss from a ruptured EP.

Currently, we seldom come across such advanced cases with vast majority of women presenting with either low-grade pain or vaginal spotting, and fortunately, they are promptly identified using highly sensitive and specific methods available.

DIAGNOSIS

History

When a woman of the reproductive age presents with the classical triad of amenorrhea, abnormal vaginal bleeding, and abdominal pain, one should think "ectopic."

Hence, the clinician should carefully evaluate the period of amenorrhea/gestational age, the onset, and severity of the symptoms.

The clinician must try to look for any possible risk factors for an EP.

Note: The woman may be unaware of her pregnancy. Hence, any fertile woman presenting with pelvic pain or abnormal vaginal bleeding should undergo a pregnancy test as part of the initial evaluation.

Physical and Pelvic Examination

On General Examination

Look for pulse rate and volume, blood pressure, pallor, and peritoneal signs, such as guarding, rigidity, and rebound tenderness which indicate the possibility of hemoperitoneum.

On Pelvic Examination

Per speculum examination: This is done to visualize the cervix and look for positive signs of pregnancy. Rule out a local cause for the abnormal bleeding.

Bleeding arising from the cervical os with visualization of the gestational products in the vagina will confirm the diagnosis of spontaneous abortion and rule out an EP.

Per vaginal examination: This is done to assess the uterine size, feel for an adnexal mass and look for cervical motion tenderness.

Urine Pregnancy Test

This test is done to confirm the pregnancy.

Biochemical Investigations

β-human Chorionic Gonadotropin

β-human chorionic gonadotropin (β-hCG) is secreted by the syncytiotrophoblast and becomes detectable in maternal serum as early as 8–10 days postovulation in normal conception cycles.

Modern assays for the β-subunit of hCG are highly sensitive and specific, with detection limits below 5 IU/L.

Serial β-hCG levels: Serum β-hCG concentrations rise predictably, at an exponential pace, during the early weeks of normal intrauterine pregnancy. After 7 weeks, the titer doubles every 3.5 days and the β-hCG levels peak between 50,000 and 100,000 IU/L at 8–10 weeks of gestation.[2]

Compared to the pattern observed in women with viable intrauterine pregnancies, serum β-hCG levels increase at a slower rate in most of the women with an ectopic or nonviable intrauterine pregnancy.

β-hCG discriminatory level: It is the value (1,500 IU/L) beyond which an intrauterine pregnancy should be visualized on transvaginal ultrasonography. Failure to do so is highly suggestive of an EP.

Combined use of history, clinical symptoms, and early first quantitative hCG drawn approximately 15 days after oocyte retrieval is an effective means to predict EP after IVF.[7]

There is a misconception that EP is unlikely in cases with serum β-hCG levels >1,000 IU/L.

Meta-analysis indicates that an isolated titer of serum β-hCG cannot predict an EP.[8]

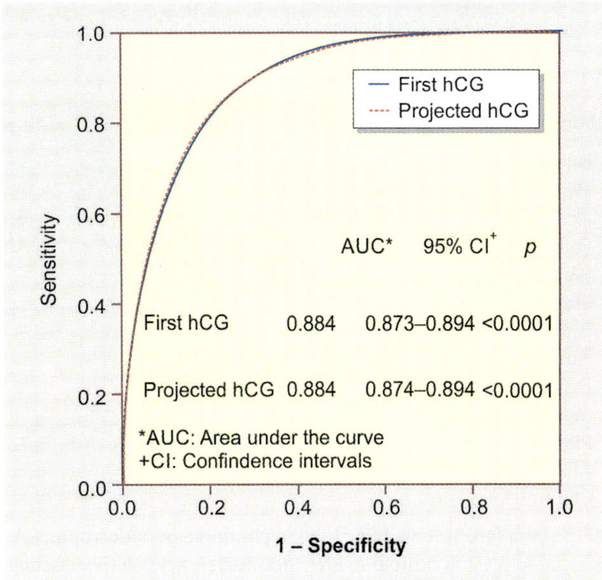

Fig. 1: Receiver operating characteristic (ROC) curves of first and projected human chorionic gonadotropin (hCG) levels to predict ectopic pregnancy.

Serum β-hCG levels are used in the management of an EP.

The key prognostic indicator for successful conservative management of ultrasound-visualized tubal ectopic pregnancies is initial serum β-hCG levels.

The receiver operating characteristic (ROC) curves of first and projected hCG levels to predict EP have been shown in **Figure 1**.

Serum Progesterone Levels

Serum progesterone levels are not useful (grade C evidence) in predicting ectopic pregnancies.

Different biomarkers for determination of tubal EP are enlisted in **Table 2**.

Blood Group and Rhesus Typing

Blood grouping with rhesus (Rh) typing should be done on all women with suspected EP. As per the Royal College of Obstetricians and Gynecologists (RCOG) guidelines 2016, anti-D prophylaxis should be offered to all RhD-negative women with the following:

- Has undergone surgical removal
- Has recurrent, heavy bleeding
- Has pain in lower abdomen to protect them against the development of Rh alloimmunization.

Imaging Techniques

Transvaginal sonography is the primary diagnostic tool in patients suspected of having an EP. It is superior to the abdominal route because of its close proximity to the adnexa allowing direct visualization of an ectopic mass.[9]

TABLE 2: Biomarkers of tubal ectopic pregnancy.

Related to embryo			*Related to implantation milieu*	
Abnormal trophoblast function	***Abnormal corpus luteal function***	***Angiogenesis***	***Normal uterine implantation***	***Abnormal tubal implantation***
• β-hCG • Hyperglycosylated hCG • Activin • Follistatin • PAPP-A • Pregnancy specific β-glycoprotein-1 • Human placental lactogen • Disintegrin and metalloproteinase-12 • Placental micro-RNA • AFP • Cell-free fetal DNA	• Progesterone • Estradiol • Inhibin A • Relaxin and rennin	• VEGF • Placental-like growth factor • Angiopoietins	• Leukemia inhibitory factor • Glycodelin • Mucin-1 • Adrenomedullin • Activin B	• Markers of compromised tubal musculature—creatine kinase, smooth muscle heavy chain myosin, and myoglobin • Markers of inflammation and peritoneal irritation—cytokines, CA-125, and antibodies to C1q

(AFP: alpha-fetoprotein; hCG: human chorionic gonadotropin; CA: cancer antigen; DNA: deoxyribonucleic acid; PAPP-A: pregnancy-associated plasma protein A; RNA: ribonucleic acid; VEGF: vascular endothelial growth factor)

By 5.5–6 gestational weeks, an intrauterine pregnancy is generally seen in the form of a gestational sac with a yolk sac ± fetal pole ± cardiac activity.[10] Visualizing these structures inside the uterine cavity effectively rules out an EP since we know that only about 1 in every 4,000 spontaneous conceptions results in a heterotopic pregnancy.[11]

The "intradecidual sac sign" is a useful feature in identifying an early intrauterine pregnancy as early as 25 days of gestation. As per this sign, the site of implantation is seen as a collection of fluid or as an echogenic area in an excessively thickened decidua on one side of the uterine cavity.

The "double decidual sac sign" is another useful finding to confirm an early intrauterine pregnancy. It involves the decidua parietalis and the decidua capsularis and is seen as two concentric rings surrounding an anechoic gestational sac.

A tiny collection of anechoic fluid in the cul-de-sac is seen in both intrauterine and EP.

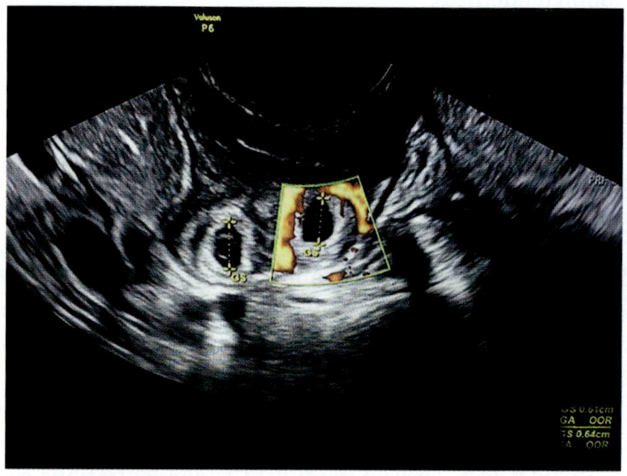

Fig. 2: Ring of fire appearance of tubal ectopic pregnancy in color Doppler view.

TUBAL PREGNANCY

A transvaginal sonography showing an adnexal mass that moves separately from the ovary along with an empty uterine cavity is highly suggestive of an EP with a sensitivity of 87–99% and a specificity of 94–99%.

The initial sonographic findings may be as follows:

- 50–60% of patients present with a nonhomogeneous/noncystic adnexal mass.
- 20–40% of patients present with an empty gestational sac.
- 15–20% of patients show an extrauterine gestational sac + yolk sac ± fetal pole ± cardiac activity.
- 10% of patients may present with a "pseudosac"—blood collected within the uterine cavity and may be erroneously diagnosed as having a small intrauterine gestational sac.
- 28–56% of patients present with free fluid in the pelvis secondary to tubal rupture with leakage from the fimbrial end of the fallopian tube.

The color and pulsed Doppler sonography can improve the diagnostic accuracy as follows:

- The blood flow in the arteries of the fallopian tube harboring the EP is 20–40% greater than that seen in the contralateral tube.
- Similarly, the adnexa will show numerous tiny vessels with increased velocity and low impedance signals. This is known as ring of fire appearance as depicted in **Figure 2**.
- Visualizing the ipsilateral corpus luteum blood flow is an important diagnostic feature of tubal pregnancy.[12]

Note: Some pregnancies are too early to be visualized on initial scans and are termed "pregnancy of unknown location (PUL)."

NONTUBAL ECTOPIC PREGNANCY

Cervical Pregnancy

Cervical pregnancy is rare and seen in <1% of all ectopic pregnancies.

Rubin's ultrasonographic criteria for the diagnosis of cervical pregnancy include:

1. The presence of cervical glands opposite to the site of attachment of the placenta.
2. The placenta and the cervix should be intimately attached with each other.
3. The placenta should be implanted below the level of peritoneal reflection on the uterine surfaces.
4. The uterine cavity should be devoid of any fetal elements.

Other ultrasonography features consist of:

- An empty uterus.
- Presence of a barrel-shaped cervix.
- A gestational sac presents below the level of the internal os of the cervix.
- Absent "sliding sign." When the gestational sac slides over the endocervical canal on applying pressure on the cervix, the diagnosis goes in favor of an ongoing miscarriage rather than a cervical pregnancy.
- Doppler studies to analyze the blood flow around gestational sac.

In the 20th century, Paalman and McElin proposed additional *clinical criteria* for the diagnosis of cervical pregnancy. They believed that one should think of an EP in cases of:

- Painless uterine bleeding following a period of amenorrhea.
- A soft and enlarged cervix equal to or bigger than the size of a uterine fundus.
- Endocervical confinement and attachment of the gestational products.
- A closed internal cervical os with a partially open external cervical os.

CESAREAN SCAR PREGNANCY

Cesarean scar pregnancy is defined as the implantation of the products of conception in a myometrial defect seen at the level of a previous uterine incision.

It is seen in 1 in 2,000 pregnancies and can present in the form of a potentially ongoing viable pregnancy or as a miscarriage within the scar.

However, its true prevalence is much higher than estimated as some cases are misdiagnosed as cervical pregnancies or end as miscarriages and thus go unreported.

There are two types of cesarean scar pregnancies. In the first type, the products of conception grow into the uterine cavity and can reach a viable age. However, the implantation site may bleed heavily. In the second type, the pregnancy grows toward the serosal surface. This can result in an early uterine rupture with massive hemorrhage.[13]

A transvaginal sonography along with a transabdominal approach is the first choice of diagnosis. Magnetic resonance imaging (MRI) may be helpful in equivocal cases.

Jurkovic's diagnostic criteria on transvaginal ultrasound include:

- An empty uterus and endocervical canal
- Gestational sac lies anteriorly at the level of the internal os
- The presence of a thin layer/absence of myometrium between the gestational sac and the bladder
- Evidence of placental/trophoblastic circulation on color and pulsed Doppler.

There is no role in measuring serum β-hCG level in diagnosing a cesarean scar pregnancy.

INTERSTITIAL PREGNANCY

In interstitial pregnancy, the products of conception implant within the interstitial part of the fallopian tube. It occurs in 1–6.3% of all ectopic pregnancies and has an increased risk of rupture resulting in hemorrhagic shock and maternal death. This is due to the high vascularity seen in this area.

The following *ultrasonographic criteria* may be used for the diagnosis of interstitial pregnancy:

- An empty uterus
- The gestational sac is located laterally within the intramural portion of the tube and is surrounded by <5 mm of myometrial thickness in all imaging planes.
- The presence of the "interstitial line sign"—it is a thin echogenic line that extends from the uterine cavity echo in the center to the periphery of the interstitial sac.

Three-dimensional (3D) ultrasonography can be used to differentiate a pregnancy implanted into the lateral angles of the uterus from an interstitial pregnancy. In a 3D coronal view, we can see the connection between the endometrial cavity and the interstitial part of the tube. These findings can be corroborated with those of an MRI.

On MRI, the cornu lies medial to the gestational sac, which is surrounded by myometrium. The diagnosis is confirmed by visualizing an intact endomyometrial junction between the uterine cavity and the gestational sac.

Two β-hCG levels, 48 hours apart, are useful in the decision of management.

CORNUAL PREGNANCY

Cornual pregnancy is an extremely rare type seen in 1/76,000 pregnancies.

The *ultrasonographic criteria* for the diagnosis of a cornual pregnancy are as follows:

- A single interstitial portion of the fallopian tube is seen within the uterine body.
- The visualization of a gestational sac surrounded on all sides by the myometrium and seen separated from the uterus.
- Doppler studies show that the gestational sac is joined to the unicornuate uterus by a vascular pedicle.

Serial serum β-hCG levels are useful for further management.

OVARIAN PREGNANCY

Ovarian pregnancy is seen in 3% of patients presenting with an ectopic.

Spiegelberg's ultrasonographic criteria for its diagnosis are as follows:

- The gestational sac is seen and lies within the ovary.
- The ovarian ligament connects the gestational sac to the uterus.
- Histopathologic evidence of ovarian tissue from the products retrieved
- The ovary along with the gestational sac is seen separate from the ipsilateral tube.
  Note: A corpus luteum and an ovarian pregnancy can be mistaken for each other and should always be differentiated.
- Color Doppler will confirm the presence of a fetal heartbeat within the ovary.

Negative sliding organ sign—the pregnancy cannot be felt separately from the ovary on deep palpation.

Any complex adnexal mass with free fluid in the pelvis—suspect a ruptured ovarian pregnancy.

Diagnosis is generally confirmed at surgery and made histologically as ovarian pregnancies are difficult to differentiate from hemorrhagic corpus luteal cysts, germ-cell tumors, and other ovarian pathologies.

Serial serum β-hCG levels are used for further management.

ABDOMINAL PREGNANCY

Abdominal pregnancy is the implantation of the products of conception in the peritoneal cavity, excluding the tubes, ovaries, or intraligamentary structures.

Implantation may occur anywhere within the omentum, pelvic sidewalls, broad ligament, pouch of Douglas, liver, spleen, bowel, diaphragm, and uterine serosa.

It is a rare obstetric complication seen in 1/10,000 pregnancies with a high maternal and perinatal mortality.

There are two types of abdominal pregnancies:

1. The primary type where the pregnancy is implanted in the peritoneal cavity from the beginning
2. The secondary type is more common. Here, the pregnancy continues its development within the abdominal cavity after expulsion from its primary organ of implantation.

Studdiford criteria for the diagnosis of primary peritoneal pregnancies are as follows:

- Both the fallopian tubes and ovaries are normal with no history of a recent/past pregnancy.
- The absence of a uteroperitoneal fistula.
- Visualization of a pregnancy attached exclusively to the peritoneal surface with elimination of a secondary implantation following a primary implantation elsewhere.

Another classification important from the point of view of management is early peritoneal pregnancy when the products of conception are ≤20 weeks and an advanced abdominal pregnancy for ≥20 weeks.

The *ultrasonographic criteria* by Gerli et al.[14] for diagnosing an early abdominal pregnancy are:

- An empty uterine cavity.
- The absence of a complex adnexal mass and a dilated fallopian tube.
- The presence of a gestational sac surrounded by bowel loops but separated by peritoneum.
- A wide range of mobility that occurs as a result of pressure with a probe toward the pouch of Douglas similar to that of a fluctuating sac.

Diagnosis is at laparoscopy performed for persistently raised serum β-hCG levels.

Advanced abdominal pregnancies account for 1 in 25,000 pregnancies. It is a life-threatening condition with risk of massive hemorrhage leading to shock and very poor fetal outcome.

Prompt management with preoperative arterial embolization along with methotrexate (MTX) administration will minimize the volume of blood lost during surgery and aid in the maximal removal of placental tissue.

Magnetic resonance imaging is useful in confirming the diagnosis and identifying the sites of placental attachment.

HETEROTOPIC PREGNANCY

The incidence of heterotopic pregnancy is increased substantially due to increasing use of exogenous gonadotropins and artificial reproductive techniques. It is seen in 1/3,900 pregnancies.

Heterotopic pregnancies are often missed initially because both the serum β-hCG and ultrasonography can be misleading.

The clinician should suspect a heterotopic pregnancy when a patient complains of persistent pelvic pain along with an intrauterine pregnancy and when a woman presents with persistent high levels of serum β-hCG following a miscarriage or a medical termination of pregnancy **(Flowchart 2)**.

Flowchart 2: Representing initial diagnostic intervention.

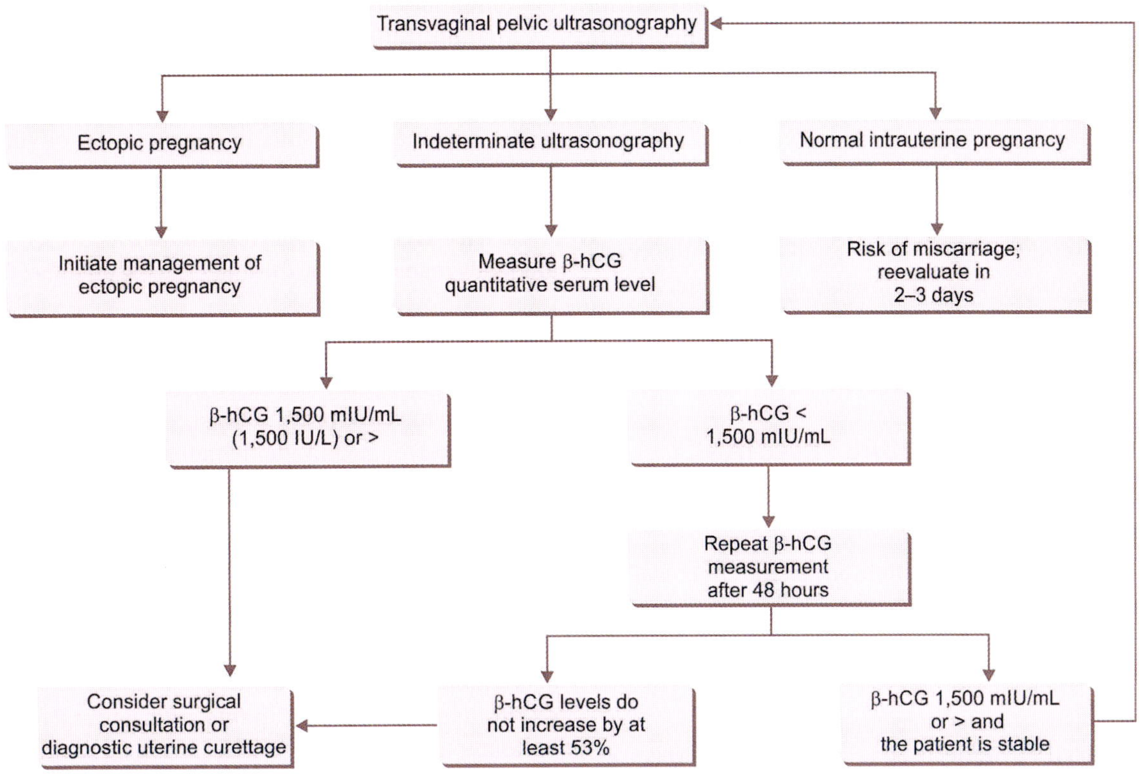

(hCG: human chorionic gonadotropin)

An ultrasound showing a coexisting intrauterine and extrauterine pregnancy confirms the diagnosis.

Differential diagnosis with partial or complete mole should be made.

LAPAROSCOPY

The pregnancy should be located within 7–10 days with the help of blood tests and ultrasonographies provided there is no major risk to the patient.

A diagnostic laparoscopy should be considered if there is uncertainty in the diagnosis.

However, in a woman with a previous history of an ectopic or in the presence of other high-risk factors, a diagnostic laparoscopy may be considered earlier. During laparoscopy, tubal ectopic is seen as dilated bluish discoloration with hemoperitoneum as shown in **Figure 3**.

Earlier, laparoscopy was the gold standard for the diagnosis of an EP, but as high as 3–4.5% of cases of false-negative laparoscopies were reported when they were performed too early.

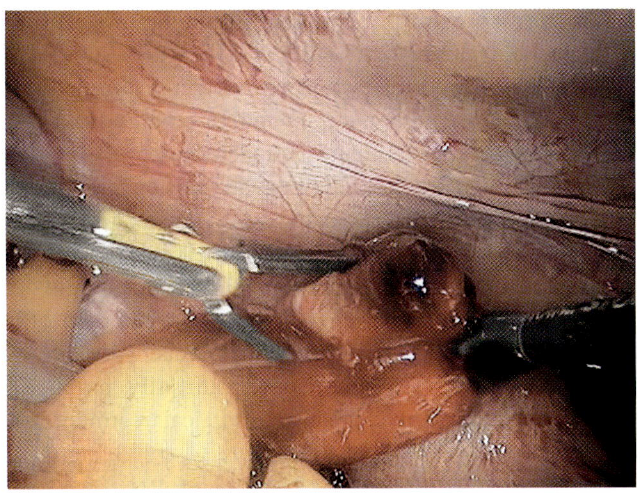

Fig. 3: Tubal ectopic pregnancy during laparoscopy.

PRIMORDIAL AND PRIMARY PREVENTION OF ECTOPIC PREGNANCY DURING IN VITRO FERTILIZATION

The lowest risk of EP is associated with a single blastocyst transfer in a frozen embryo transfer cycle. This approach leads to better perinatal outcomes and overall increase in pregnancy and birth outcomes.[15]

Approximately 2–5% of all clinical pregnancies following an IVF-embryo transfer are ectopic in nature.

Following IVF, tubal pregnancies occur as a result of:

- Injecting the transfer medium directly into the fallopian tubes
- Reflux expulsion of the embryos into the tubes secondary to uterine contractions

The junctional activity of the uterine musculature, especially that of stratum subvasculare, decreases with increasing time interval from oocyte retrieval. Thus, there is a lower risk of EP with day 3 transfer as opposed to day 2 transfer secondary to reduced uterine contractions toward the luteal phase.[16]

The incidence of EP is lower following blastocyst transfer as opposed to cleavage stage transfer due to the following:
- Reduced retrograde uterine contractions from the cervix to the fundus on day 7 following an hCG injection as compared to the first 4 days.
- A bigger diameter and integrin expression resulting in the resting stage of the blastocyst.

MANAGEMENT OF TUBAL PREGNANCY (FLOWCHARTS 3 TO 5)

Expectant Management

Expectant management is defined as watchful waiting or close monitoring of the clinical symptoms, the serum β-hCG levels, and transvaginal sonographies instead of any immediate intervention.

Indications of expectant management:
- Low (1,500 IU/L) or decreasing serum β-hCG levels
- Clinically and hemodynamically stable women
- Patient has minimal pain.
- An ultrasonography showing a small, unruptured, nonviable (absent heartbeat) EP.

When opting for expectant management, the patient should be counseled about the need for continuous, close monitoring and the possibility of tubal rupture.

Serial β-hCG levels, initially every 48 hours until the blood levels begin to drop and then weekly thereafter, should be checked until the levels become normal (<5 IU/L).

Immediate termination of expectant management—if the patient complains of increasing abdominal pain or if there is an increase in the serum β-hCG levels.

Approximately 25% of women initially managed expectantly go on to need medical or surgical treatment.

Medical Management

Before the 1980s, the management of EP was only surgical. Evolving knowledge and experience with MTX has revolutionized the treatment of ectopic pregnancies.

The advantages of medical management over surgical management are:
- It eliminates the morbidity arising out of anesthesia and surgery.
- Comparatively, there is lesser tubal damage.
- It is more cost-effective.

Methotrexate is a folate antagonist that causes acute deficiency of a folate coenzyme, tetrahydrofolate, essential for the synthesis of ribonucleic acid (RNA) and deoxyribonucleic acid (DNA) in rapidly multiplying cells.

Methotrexate is structurally similar to norethindrone with five times higher affinity for the progesterone receptors.

It competitively binds to the progesterone receptors in the decidua and results in degeneration of villi tissue, atrophy, and necrosis of decidual tissue, eventually leading to embryo death.[19, 20]

It selectively kills the cytotrophoblasts, which are then gradually reabsorbed by the body leaving an intact fallopian tube.

As per the National Institute for Health and Care Excellence (NICE) guidelines, MTX should be the first-line management if the following criteria are fulfilled:
- A hemodynamically stable patient with no evidence of rupture
- A serum β-hCG level between 1,500 and 5,000 IU/L
- Minimal pain
- No visible intrauterine pregnancy on sonography
- Ultrasound showing absent fetal cardiac activity
- An adnexal mass <3.5 cm size
- Hemoperitoneum <100 mL
- Women should be capable and willing for regular follow-ups.

The mean resolution time is 32 days following a single dose and 58 days following repeated doses of MTX.

Mechanism of Action

Methotrexate acts as an antifolic acid.

Dosage

Single-dose regimen: Administer a single dose of MTX intramuscularly, 1.0 mg/kg or 50 mg/m^2 on day 1 and follow it with serum β-hCG level measurements on days 4 and 7. If the serum β-hCG level drops by >15%, then repeat β-hCG levels every week until it reaches the normal range (<5 IU/L).

If the level does not drop by 15%, then a repeat ultrasonography should be done to rule out the presence of an ectopic fetal heartbeat and significant hemoperitoneum.

A second dose of intramuscular MTX 50 mg/m^2 can be given in such cases.

The success rate of a single dose of MTX ranges from 65 to 95%, with 3–27% of women requiring a second dose.[21]

Multiple-dose regimen: MTX 1.0 mg/kg intramuscularly on 0, 2, 4, and 6 days alternated with folinic acid 0.1 mg/kg orally on days 1, 3, 5, and 7.

If the serum β-hCG level drops by >15% on 2nd day, measure β-hCG levels weekly until it reaches <5 IU/L.

If the level does not reduce by 15%, repeat intramuscular MTX 1 mg/kg on day 2 and leucovorin (folinic acid) 0.1 mg/kg orally on day 3.

Flowchart 3: Algorithm for the management of a suspected ectopic pregnancy.[1,17,18]

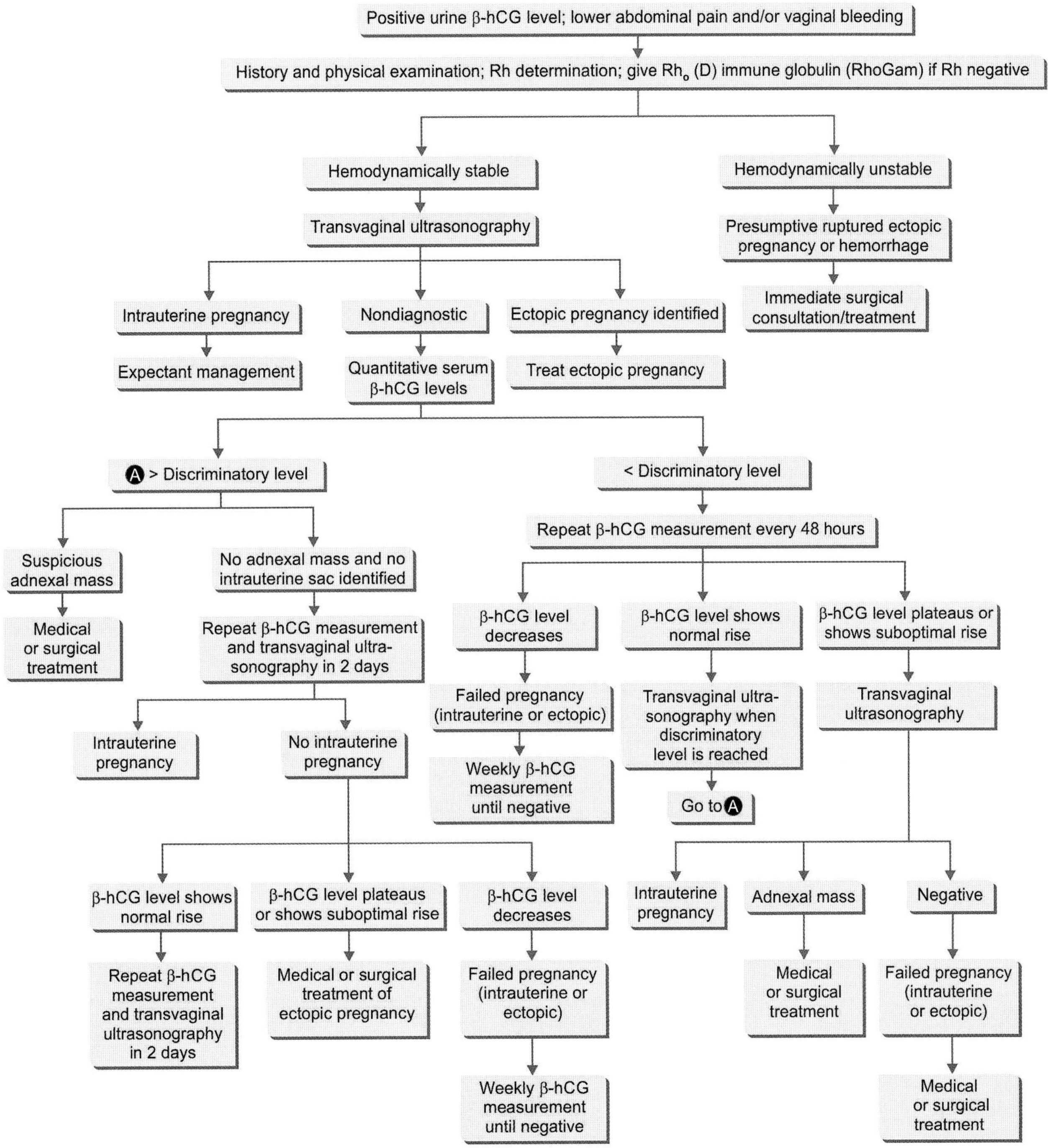

Advise patient of ectopic pregnancy risks and precautions

(hCG: human chorionic gonadotropin; Rh: rhesus)

Women presenting with pain following MTX administration should be thoroughly evaluated before assuming the treatment has failed and rushing into surgical intervention.

Regardless of the regimen selected pretreatment evaluation consisting of complete blood count, kidney, and liver function tests, and blood grouping with Rh factor typing should be done in all patients on day 1 prior to MTX administration.

Adverse Effects

- Side effects of MTX are relatively common but usually minor and transient; their prevalence is somewhat

Flowchart 4: Management of ectopic tubal pregnancy.

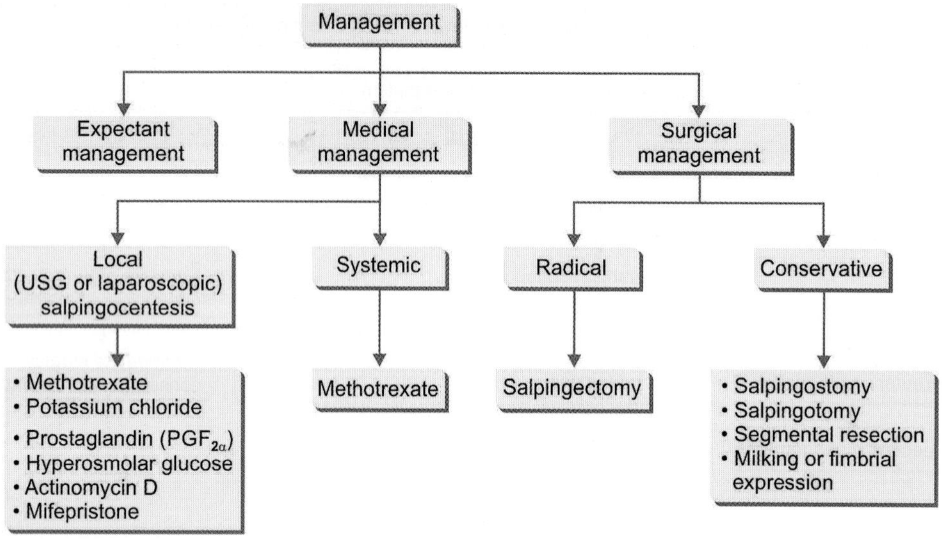

(USG: ultrasonography)

Flowchart 5: Management according to the size of adnexal mass.

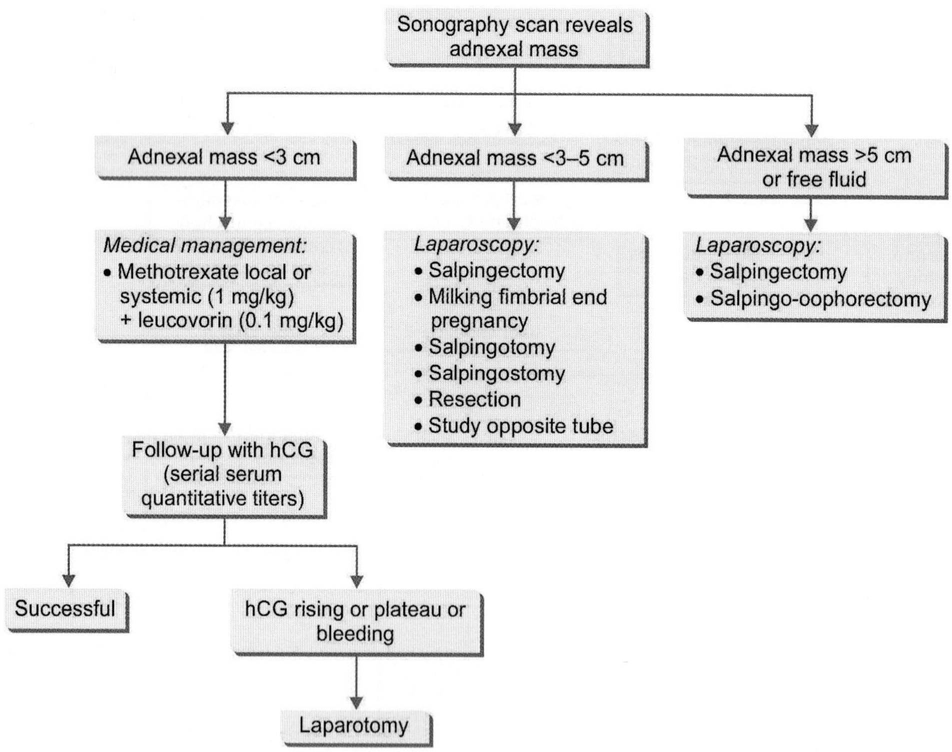

(hCG: human chorionic gonadotrophin)

higher with multidose regimen as compared to single-dose therapy.

- Gastrointestinal effects such as gastric pain, nausea, vomiting, and stomatitis are the most common side effects seen with MTX.
- Other rare adverse effects include bone marrow depression with severe neutropenia, elevated liver enzymes, reversible alopecia, dermatitis, and pneumonitis.[22]

Contraindications to Methotrexate Treatment

- Hemodynamically unstable patient
- Presence of an intrauterine pregnancy
- Breastfeeding
- Noncompliance for follow-up
- Known sensitivity to MTX
- Chronic liver disease

- Preexisting blood dyscrasia such as severe anemia, leukopenia, and thrombocytopenia
- Active pulmonary disease
- Immunodeficiency conditions
- Active peptic ulcer disease
- Renal dysfunction.

Lower abdominal pain is usually seen 3–7 days after the initiation of treatment. This pain occurs due to dilatation of the fallopian tubes secondary to tubal abortion or hematoma formation.[23] Generally, the pain is mild and lasts for 4–12 hours in a hemodynamically stable patient. Immediate surgery should be considered for tubal rupture as indicated by hemodynamic instability, dropping hemoglobin levels, or visualization on ultrasonography.[1]

In a meta-analysis conducted of 15 studies including 1,573 women diagnosed with EP and managed nonsurgically, there was no significant difference in the success rate of treatment; however, single-dose MTX was associated with fewer side effects than two-dose/multiple-dose regimen.[24,25]

Surgical Treatment

If the serum β-hCG level is high (>5,000 IU/L), the EP is larger than 4 cm or there has been significant internal bleeding, and if the patient is hemodynamically unstable, surgery becomes the first choice of management.

Surgery is also indicated in cases of failed expectant or medical management.

Surgery can be performed laparoscopically or by conventional laparotomy. Laparotomy is generally reserved for hemodynamically unstable patients with a ruptured ectopic and massive hemoperitoneum or in patients with poor visualization of the pelvis at the time of laparoscopy.[26] The type of procedure will be salpingectomy or salpingostomy based upon the damage to the affected tube and the condition of the contralateral tube.

Salpingectomy (removal of the affected tube) is the procedure of choice if the contralateral tube is normal, especially if the affected tube looks unhealthy or is adherent.

Salpingostomy is the removal of an EP by making a small cut on the tube while leaving the tube in situ. It is the surgery of choice in women with:

- History of a previous EP
- Damaged/unhealthy contralateral tube
- Previous history of an abdominal surgery
- A previous PID
- Preservation of fertility.

There is a minimum chance of persistent ectopic pregnancy (PEP) in these patients. Hence, they should be informed and counseled regarding the same and they should be closely followed up with serum β-hCG levels. In case the PEP is not resolved, these patients may need systemic MTX or salpingectomy.

As per the NICE guidelines, serum β-hCG levels should be repeated after a week following salpingotomy and then weekly until normal levels are reached.

In a randomized controlled trial on 446 women—after 2 years of trying for natural conception, 60.7% after salpingotomy and 56.2% after salpingectomy, persistent trophoblast occurred more frequently in the salpingotomy group [14 (7%) vs. 1 (<1%); RR 15.0, 95% confidence interval (CI) 2.0–113.4].

Repeat EP occurred in 18 (8%) women in the salpingotomy group and 12 (5%) in the salpingectomy group (RR 1.6, 95% CI 0.8–3.3).

It was concluded that in women with a tubal EP and a healthy contralateral tube, salpingotomy does not significantly improve fertility prospects compared with salpingectomy.[27]

Higher rates of subsequent intrauterine pregnancy have been found if salpingotomy is done versus salpingectomy in women with a history of fertility-reducing factors.

Becker et al. found a subsequent intrauterine pregnancy rate of 75% with salpingotomy and 40% with salpingectomy in such women. However, subsequent intrauterine pregnancy rates were >90% in both groups in women without fertility-reducing factors.[28]

A 2007 Cochrane review found no difference in the success rates, tubal patency, and subsequent fertility rates between laparoscopic salpingostomy and medical treatment with intramuscular MTX.[29]

Laparoscopic Surgical Approach is Preferred than Conventional Open Approach

The advantages of laparoscopy over laparotomy are:

- A shorter operative time
- Lower intraoperative blood loss
- A shorter hospital stay
- Lower cost
- Lesser quantity of analgesia is required.
- Lower rate of adhesion formation.

No differences have been noted in subsequent successful pregnancy outcomes.

MANAGEMENT OF NONTUBAL ECTOPIC PREGNANCY

Interstitial Pregnancy

Management depends upon the clinical presentation, the presence of fetal cardiac activity, and serum β-hCG levels.

Medical management with MTX or surgical management by laparoscopic cornual resection or salpingotomy are effective options.

Cornual Pregnancy

Treatment involves open/laparoscopic excision of the fibrous band that attaches the rudimentary horn to the unicornuate uterus with removal of the rudimentary horn.

Laparoscopic technique is safe, but the possibility of associated urinary tract anomalies should be kept in mind.

Cervical Pregnancy

If cervical pregnancy is diagnosed early, medical treatment with MTX is recommended, either administered directly into the gestational sac under ultrasound guidance or systemically by intramuscular injection. Local administration is more effective.

The disadvantage of medical treatment is that the trophoblast remains in situ, causing hemorrhage. Thus, simultaneous suction evacuation or uterine artery embolization is preferred.

In late cases, hysterectomy may be needed.

Cesarean Scar Pregnancy

Wedge resection and repair of the implantation site by laparotomy or laparoscopy is often needed along with medical management with MTX.[12]

Ovarian Pregnancy

Definitive surgical treatment in the form of minimal access surgery is preferred if laparoscopy is required to make the diagnosis of ovarian EP.

The gestational products can be removed either by enucleation or by wedge resection. This should be carried out bluntly to avoid damage to the surrounding ovarian tissue. Electrocautery can be used to achieve hemostasis.

Intramuscular MTX is recommended when the surgery is high risk or postoperatively in patients with residual trophoblastic disease or with persistently raised β-hCG levels.

Oophorectomy is done in case of a coexisting pathology or when there is excessive bleeding from the ovary.

Heterotopic Pregnancy

Utmost care of the intrauterine pregnancy should be taken in the management of a heterotopic pregnancy.

Methotrexate to be given only in case of a nonviable intrauterine pregnancy or if the woman wishes to discontinue the pregnancy, in which case the Regulations of the Abortion Act will apply.

Local injection of potassium chloride or hyperosmolar glucose with aspiration of the sac contents is an option for clinically stable women.

Laparoscopic surgical removal of the EP is the method of choice for hemodynamically unstable women and may also be an option for hemodynamically stable women.

Expectant management is an option in heterotopic pregnancies, where the ultrasound findings are of a nonviable pregnancy.

POST-TREATMENT

After medical treatment with MTX, it is important to wait for at least 3 months after the treatment has finished before getting pregnant again.

Methods of Contraception

- Combined oral contraceptive pill
- Contraceptive vaginal ring/patch
- Progestogen-only pill (POP)
- Barrier methods—condoms
- Natural methods of family planning.

LONG-TERM FERTILITY PROSPECTS FOLLOWING AN ECTOPIC PREGNANCY (ROYAL COLLEGE OF OBSTETRICIANS AND GYNAECOLOGISTS, 2016)

There is no difference in the fecundity rates, tubal patency, and risk of future tubal EP with the different types of management methods in the absence of any cause for subfertility or history of tubal pathology.

Women with a history of subfertility should be managed expectantly and medically to improve the reproductive outcomes as compared to radical surgical management.

Methotrexate with either single- or double-dose protocol has no effect on the ovarian reserve.

For nontubal ectopic pregnancies, uterine artery embolization with systemic MTX can be tried. Live births have been reported after that.

COUNSELING AND PSYCHOLOGICAL SUPPORT

Women should be educated about the advantages and disadvantages of each and every approach. Along with the recommendations of the treating clinician, she should make an appropriate decision.

The psychological impact of early pregnancy loss may seriously affect a large number of women and their families. She should be encouraged to talk with support groups such as the Ectopic Pregnancy Trust or utilize the local bereavement counseling services.

Further plans of management should be explained to the patient properly.

KEY POINTS

- Women should be made aware that the recurrence rate in a woman with a history of one EP is 10%. Hence, an early sonography at 6 weeks of gestation is recommended to confirm an intrauterine pregnancy.
- Along with a history of tubal infertility and PID, the embryo transfer technique is significant for late cases of EP.

- A high level of suspicion along with an early measurement of serum β-hCG and transvaginal sonography as early as the 5th gestational week can identify an early EP. These women should be closely monitored with repeated ultrasound and serum β-hCG levels until a definitive diagnosis is reached.
- Treatment must be customized according to the clinical condition of the patient and her future fertility requirements.
- In heterotopic pregnancy, a viable intrauterine pregnancy can be preserved with removal of extrauterine pregnancy with laparoscopic surgical management.

REFERENCES

1. Seeber BE, Barnhart KT. Suspected ectopic pregnancy. Obstet Gynecol. 2006;107(2 Pt. 1):399-413.
2. Speroff L, Glass RH, Kase NG. Clinical Gynecological Endocrinology and Infertility, 6th edition. Lippincott Williams and Wilkins; 1999. p. 1149ff.
3. Shaw JL, Oliver E, Lee KF, Entrican G, Jabbour HN, Critchley HO, et al. Cotinine exposure increases fallopian tube PROKR1 expression via nicotinic AChRalpha-7: a potential mechanism explaining the link between smoking and tubal ectopic pregnancy. Am J Pathol. 2010;177(5):2509-15.
4. Ankum WM, Mol BW, Van der Veen F, Bossuyt PM. Risk factors for ectopic pregnancy: a meta-analysis. Fertil Steril. 1996;65(6):1093-9.
5. Mol BW, Ankum WM, Bossuyt PM, Van der Veen F. Contraception and the risk of ectopic pregnancy: a meta-analysis. Contraception. 1995;52(6):337-41.
6. Bouyer J, Coste J, Shojaei T, Pouly JL, Fernandez H, Gerbaud L, et al. Risk factors for ectopic pregnancy: a comprehensive analysis based on a large case-control, population-based study in France. Am J Epidemiol. 2003;157(3):185-94.
7. Cookingham LM, Duran EH, Goossen RP, Shah DK, Sparks A, Van Voorhis BJ. First hCG level as a predictor of ectopic pregnancy after in vitro fertilization. Fertil Steril. 2014;101(2):e25.
8. van Mello NM, Mol F, Opmeer BC, Ankum WM, Barnhart K, Coomarasamy A, et al. Diagnostic value of serum hCG on the outcome of pregnancy of unknown location: a systematic review and meta-analysis. Hum Reprod Update. 2012;18:603-17.
9. Kirk E, Bourne T. Diagnosis of ectopic pregnancy with ultrasound. Best Pract Res Clin Obstet Gynaecol. 2009;23(4):501-8.
10. Levine D. Ectopic pregnancy. Radiology. 2007;245(2):385-97.
11. Ory SJ. New options for diagnosis and treatment of ectopic pregnancy. JAMA. 1992;267(4):534-7.
12. Honemeyer U, Alkatout I, Kupesic-Plavsic S, Pour-Mirza A, Kurjak A. The value of color and power Doppler in the diagnosis of ectopic pregnancy. Donald School J Ultrasound Obstet Gynecol. 2013;7(4):429-39.
13. Vial Y, Petignat P, Hohlfeld P. Pregnancy in a cesarean scar. Ultrasound Obstet Gynecol. 2000;16:592-3.
14. Gerli S, Rossetti D, Baiocchi G, Clerici G, Unfer V, Di Renzo GC. Early ultrasonographic diagnosis and laparoscopic treatment of abdominal pregnancy. Eur J Obstet Gynecol Reprod Biol. 2004;113:103-5.
15. Li Z, Sullivan EA, Chapman M, Farquhar C, Wang YA. Risk of ectopic pregnancy lowest with transfer of single frozen blastocyst. Hum Reprod. 2015;30(9):2048-54.
16. Milki AA, Jun SH. Ectopic pregnancy rates with day 3 versus day 5 embryo transfer: a retrospective analysis. BMC Pregnancy Childbirth. 2003;3:7.
17. Lozeau AM, Potter B. Diagnosis and management of ectopic pregnancy. Am Fam Physician. 2005;72(9):1707-14.
18. Tulandi T. (2009). Ectopic pregnancy: clinical manifestations and diagnosis. [online] Available from: http://www.uptodate.com/contents/clinical-manifestations-diagnosis-and-management-of-ectopic-pregnancy. [Last accessed March, 2018].
19. Gazvani MR, Baruah DN, Alfirevic Z, Emery SJ. Mifepristone in combination with methotrexate for the medical treatment of tubal pregnancy: a randomized, controlled trial. Hum Reprod. 1998;13:1987-90.
20. Li ZH, Quan S. Mifepristone combined with methotrexate for conservative treatment of tubal ectopic pregnancy. Di Yi Jun Yi Da Xue Xue Bao. 2004;24:829-31.
21. Kirk E, Condous G, Bourne T. The non-surgical management of ectopic pregnancy. Ultrasound Obstet Gynecol. 2006;27:91-100.
22. American College of Obstetricians and Gynecologists. ACOG practice bulletin No. 94: medical management of ectopic pregnancy. Obstet Gynecol. 2008;111(6):1479-85.
23. Lipscomb GH, Puckett KJ, Bran D, Ling FW. Management of separation pain after single-dose methotrexate therapy for ectopic pregnancy. Obstet Gynecol. 1999;93(4):590-3.
24. Xiao C, Shi Q, Cheng Q, Xu J. Non-surgical management of tubal ectopic pregnancy: a systematic review and meta-analysis. Medicine. 2021;100(50):e27851.
25. Lin Q, Lin N, Wang G, Zheng X, Hua R. Fallopian tube pregnancy following methotrexate treatment. Ann Transl Med. 2021;9(2):146.
26. Barnhart KT. Clinical practice. Ectopic pregnancy. N Engl J Med. 2009;361(4):379-87.
27. Mol F, van Mello NM, Strandell A, Strandell K, Jurkovic D, Ross J, et al. Salpingotomy versus salpingectomy in women with tubal pregnancy (ESEP study): an open-label, multicentre, randomised controlled trial. Lancet. 2014;383:1483-9.
28. Becker S, Solomayer E, Hornung R, Kurek R, Banys M, Aydeniz B, et al. Optimal treatment for patients with ectopic pregnancies and a history of fertility-reducing factors. Arch Gynecol Obstet. 2011;283:41-5.
29. Hajenius PJ, Mol F, Mol BW, Bossuyt PM, Ankum WM, van der Veen F. Interventions for tubal ectopic pregnancy. Cochrane Database Syst Rev. 2007;2007(1):CD000324.

CHAPTER 68

Multiple-order Births

Veronica Irene Yuel

INTRODUCTION

After Louise Brown was born in 1975, assisted reproductive technique (ART) has reached great heights. Also, there has been a proportionate rise in the number of infertile couples, hence, leading to a rise in the number of couples opting for fertility treatment much earlier. A rise in fertility treatment has in turn shown its impact on the number of multiple-order pregnancies referred to as twins, triplets, and a higher number of fetuses (quadruplets, quintuplets, etc.).

Multifetal pregnancies have a higher risk of maternal and neonatal morbidities and mortality.[1] This is because these pregnancies have higher chances of preterm deliveries leading to low-birth-weight babies and, thus, the associated morbidities due to prematurity.

INCIDENCE

Owing to the increase in the number of multiple births, its incidence has also risen.[2] On an average, multiple pregnancies constitute about 3 in 100 births and the incidence is constantly rising. The incidence of multiple-order births is significantly different in different regions and countries. Smits et al. in their study have reported a twining rate of <9/1,000 births in India.[3] The National Center for Health Statistics has reported a twin birth rate of up to 70%. It is now 32.6/1,000 live births. Differences in twining rates in various geographical distributions can be attributed to differences occurring in the frequencies of dizygotic twinning. However, the frequency of monozygotic twins remains constant worldwide at about 4/1,000 births.

Higher order births are much less in incidence. Naturally occurring triplets happen in about 1 in 10,000 pregnancies[4] and quadruplets in about 1 in 700,000 pregnancies.[5]

Quintuplets (five babies), sextuplets (six babies), septuplets (seven fetuses), and octuplets (eight fetuses) have also been reported though their incidence is extremely rare.

ETIOLOGY

The exact etiology of multiple gestations remains unknown. Several factors have been associated in causing this rise in higher order births. These causes are enumerated in the following text.

Maternal Age

A higher incidence of multiple-order births has been seen in women of advanced age. In developed nations, the average reproductive age at which women plan their childbirth has gone up on the scale to around and above 30 years.[6] This could be attributed to more women attending fertility clinics and seeking treatments as many of them are delaying childbearing in the present era. Also, higher age, as an independent variable, is associated with multiple pregnancies.[7]

Parity

It has been shown that multiparous ladies have higher chances of developing multiple-order pregnancies when compared to nulliparous ones[8] as an independent factor.

Geographical Distribution

The rates of multiple gestation pregnancies vary in different geographical distributions. The authors have mentioned earlier in the chapter that the incidence of multiple-order births differs among countries; Australia and USA seem to be following a similar pattern compared to the UK. The lowest twinning rates have been found in Japan, Singapore, and Hong Kong though these, in turn, have also increased from 0.05% in 1972 to 0.09% in 2001.[8] The highest rates of dizygotic twinning have been reported in Nigeria and Zimbabwe and the least in Asian countries,[9] whereas the rate of monozygous twins remains constant.

Socioeconomic Strata

Multiple-order birth has been found to be more prevalent among the high socioeconomic strata. This can be directly related to those women who delay childbearing due to their careers and thus seek fertility treatments for conception at a higher age, though fertility treatment is an independent factor affecting the incidence of multifetal gestation.

Genetic Predisposition

Studies have shown that multiple pregnancies run in families which are passed down from both maternal and paternal sides.[9]

Use of Fertility Drugs

Over the years, there has been a tremendous rise in couples seeking fertility treatments. This may be due to an increase in awareness about fertility, an increase in the educational status of the couple, and better and affordable services offered by the fertility clinics. A rise in the liberal use of ovulogens and gonadotropins is the most important factor associated with multifetal pregnancy.[10] In fact, the use of these drugs is more commonly associated with multiple births than in vitro fertilization (IVF) techniques.

Assisted Reproductive Techniques

Assisted reproductive technique procedures such as intrauterine insemination (IUI) and IVF are commonly associated with multiple births. There has been a direct relationship between multifetal pregnancies and the number of embryos transferred[10] during the IVF procedures.

Maternal Weight (Body Mass Index) and Height

A positive association of body mass index (BMI) with multiple pregnancies has been reported in the observation by Basso et al., who referred to the Danish National Birth Registry, which reported a statistically significant correlation of women who had a BMI ≥30 kg/m^2 with a higher rate of naturally conceived twins. Further, they also observed that women whose BMI was <20 kg/m^2 had a lower rate of naturally conceived twins even after correcting for maternal age and parity. They further observed that women who were tall were more likely to give birth to twins.[11]

Miscellaneous

Maternal smoking, a seasonal variation where the length of the day and food supply is affected, and usage of drugs such as oral contraceptives and folic acid are some factors mentioned in the literature; however, more definite evidence is needed to support these causes. An increase in the frequency of coitus has also been reported to be an independent factor behind the increase in twinning rate, although this needs to be supported with more research.

PATHOPHYSIOLOGY

Zygosity is determined at the time when splitting occurs after fertilization. Monozygous twins occur when a fertilized ovum splits within 48 hours leading to the formation of amnion and chorion separately. Thus, there are two separate placentae, which may be fused off separately. Nearly 30% of all monozygous twins are dichorionic diamniotic **(Figs. 1A and B)**.

When the splitting occurs after 72 hours till 8 days, monochorionic diamniotic twins are formed, which comprise around 70% of the twins **(Figs. 2A and B)**.

Monochorionic monoamniotic **(Figs. 3A and B)** twins develop when splitting happens between 9 and 12 days. These twins are rare, comprising only 1% of the monozygous twins. These twins have a higher incidence of complication rates, especially cord accidents, twin-to-twin transfusion, etc.

Splitting of fertilized ovum beyond 12 days leads to only partial splitting resulting in the development of conjoined twins.

Higher order pregnancies, such as triplets and quadruplets, i.e., dizygotic and trizygotic births, occur when two or three or multiple separate ova fuse with sperms separately and therefore will have separate amnion, chorion, and placentae. The placentae in dizygotic twins are fused,

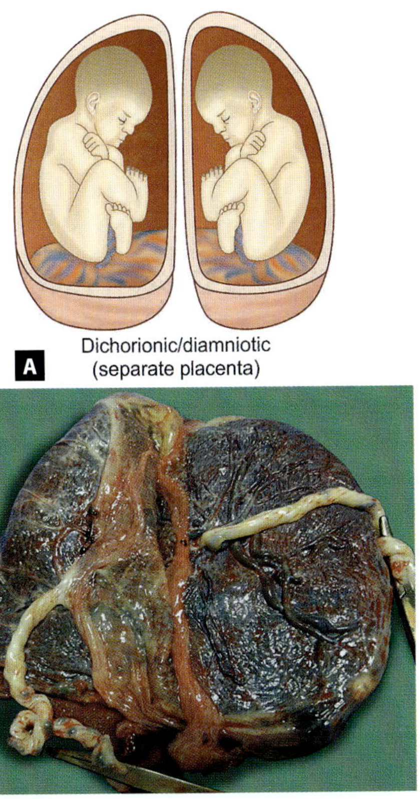

Figs. 1A and B: Dichorionic/diamniotic twin/placenta.
Source: (A) https://eatinfor3.wordpress.com/tag/monozygotic/; (B) Author's own image.

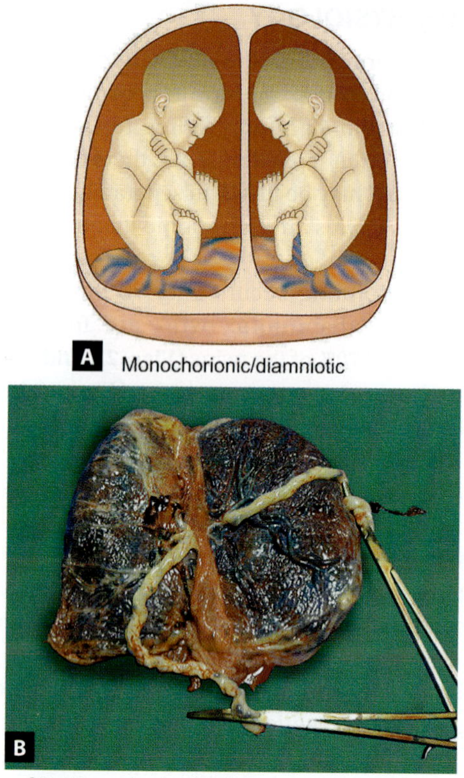

Figs. 2A and B: Monochorionic/diamniotic twin/placenta.
Source: (A) https://eatinfor3.wordpress.com/tag/monozygotic/; (B) Author's own image.

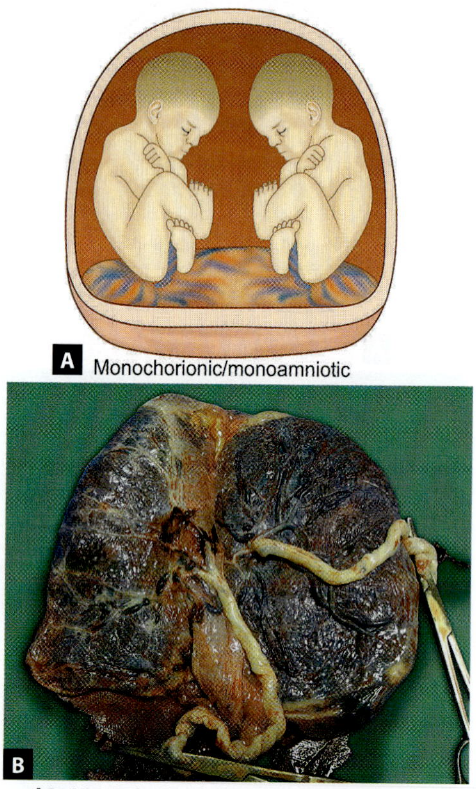

Figs. 3A and B: Monochorionic/monoamniotic twin/placenta
Source: (A) https://eatinfor3.wordpress.com/tag/monozygotic/; (B) Author's own image.

if the area of implantation is close by, but, at birth, they are easily separable.

Pregnancy with triplets occurs when fertilization, then splitting, and later development of ovum and sperm occur at separate levels. Triplet pregnancies may be, therefore, monozygotic, dizygotic, or trizygotic. Trizygotic triplets are formed when three different sperms fertilize with three different ova. Dizygotic triplets develop when one set of monozygotic co-triplets and another co-triplet develop from a different zygote. Rarely, two consecutive zygotic splittings with a vanished fetus can also give rise to monozygotic triplets. Zygosity in quadruplets and higher order multiples varies.

The examination of the placentae after birth is an important feature in all higher order births, as it helps in identifying the chorionicity and zygosity: however, it may not always be helpful.[12]

PATHOGENESIS

Ultrasonographic evaluation of the placenta to determine chorionicity during the early gestational period and later following the birth of babies helps us in determining the type of multifetal gestation.

Monozygotic twins develop when the splitting of a fertilized ovum occurs within 48 hours of conception producing chorions and amnions separately. These twins have separate placentae and can be separated, forming the dichorionic-diamniotic placenta, or fused forming the monochorionic-diamniotic placenta. When this splitting of the zygote occurs between 3 and 8 days after fertilization, it leads to the formation of monochorionic/diamniotic placentation. Further, if the splitting happens between 9 and 12 days of fertilization, monochorionic/monoamniotic placentation occurs. Splitting beyond 12 days after fertilization leads only to partial split, which further leads to the formation of conjoined twins.

Higher order pregnancies, such as triplets and quadruplets, i.e., dizygotic and trizygotic births, occur when two or three or multiple separate ova fuse with sperms separately and therefore will have separate amnion, chorion, and placentae.

The pathogenesis of multiple births has been shown in **Table 1 and Figure 4**.

CLINICAL FEATURES

In the current times, most women are already aware of their diagnosis and they visit the doctor with the diagnosis (based on history) and a variety of symptoms.

History

The history of the patient may reveal about the lady carrying multifetal pregnancy. Women who are not aware may give a history of using ovulation-inducing drugs. Along with this, all the other symptoms of pregnancy may be exaggerated in presentation. Patients will give a history of hyperemesis, excessive weight gain, excessive fetal movements, etc. A family history of twins or triplets may be there.

Symptoms

Excessive weight gain, dehydration—if the patient has hyperemesis, and all other symptoms of pregnancy may be exaggerated. On examination, the uterine height will be more than the period of gestation, striae gravidarum and chloasma may be severely increased, multiple fetal parts will be felt on palpation, and multiple fetal heart sounds will be heard on auscultation. Along with this, there may be other systemic features. Many a times, multifetal pregnancies are associated with high blood pressure recordings, i.e., pregnancy-induced hypertension (PIH), and thus, may be comorbidly associated with all the other features of PIH.

TABLE 1: Pathogenesis of twins.

Dividing membrane	*Type of placenta*	*Type of twin*
None	Monochorionic monoamniotic	Monozygotic
Amnion	Monochorionic diamniotic	Monozygotic
Amnion + Chorion	Dichorionic diamniotic	Monozygotic or dizygotic
No common membrane	Dichorionic diamniotic	Dizygotic

Conjoined Twins

Twins that are joined at various levels of the body parts, i.e., fused at various levels, are called conjoined twins. Conjoined twins have a very rare incidence, ranging from 1 in 50,000 to 1 in 100,000.[10] "Pagus" means "fusion" and therefore conjoined twins are named depending on the level of fusion. The varieties of conjoined twins are depicted in **Figure 5**.

Discordant Twins

When there is a difference in the weights of the twins, they are called discordant twins. It is defined as a discrepancy of ≥10% difference in the weights of the twins. This occurs in around 16% of all the twins, where the discordancy is around 20%.[13] This commonly occurs due to hyperperfusion of one sac, while the other is hypoperfused. A variety of associated maternal comorbidities, fetal abnormalities, and placental causes seems to be causing the discordancy, but the exact cause remains unknown.

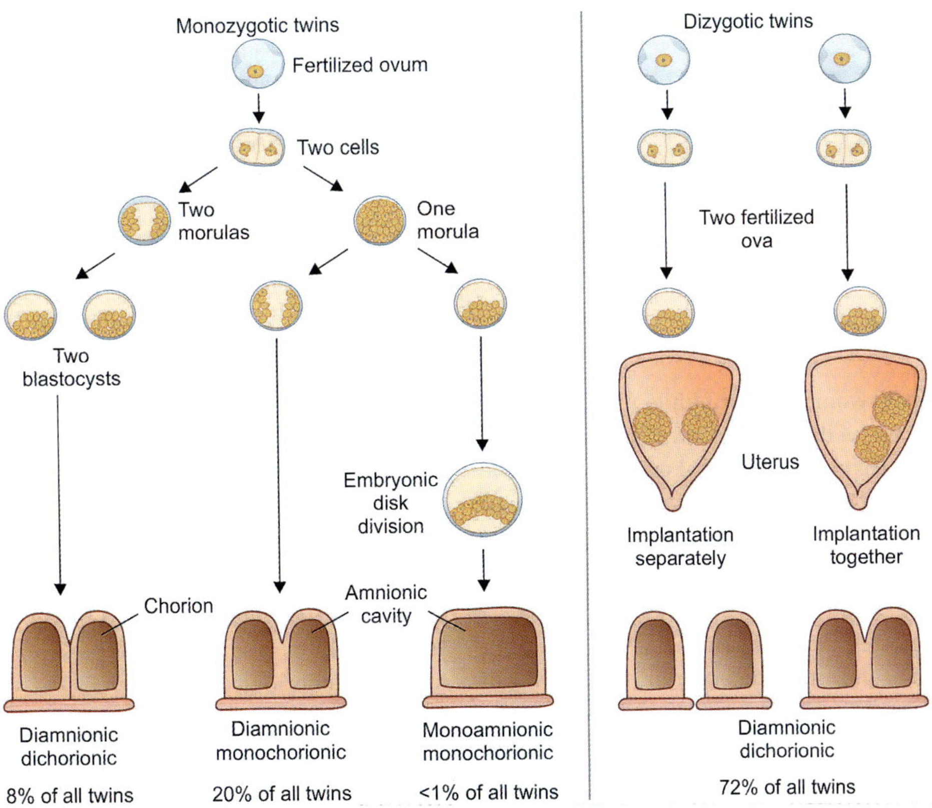

Fig. 4: Pathogenesis of twins.
Source: Pathologyoutlines.com. (2017). Placenta: Placental findings in specific newborn/fetal or maternal conditions. [online] Available from: http://www.pathologyoutlines.com/topic/placentatwins.html. [Accessed March, 2018].

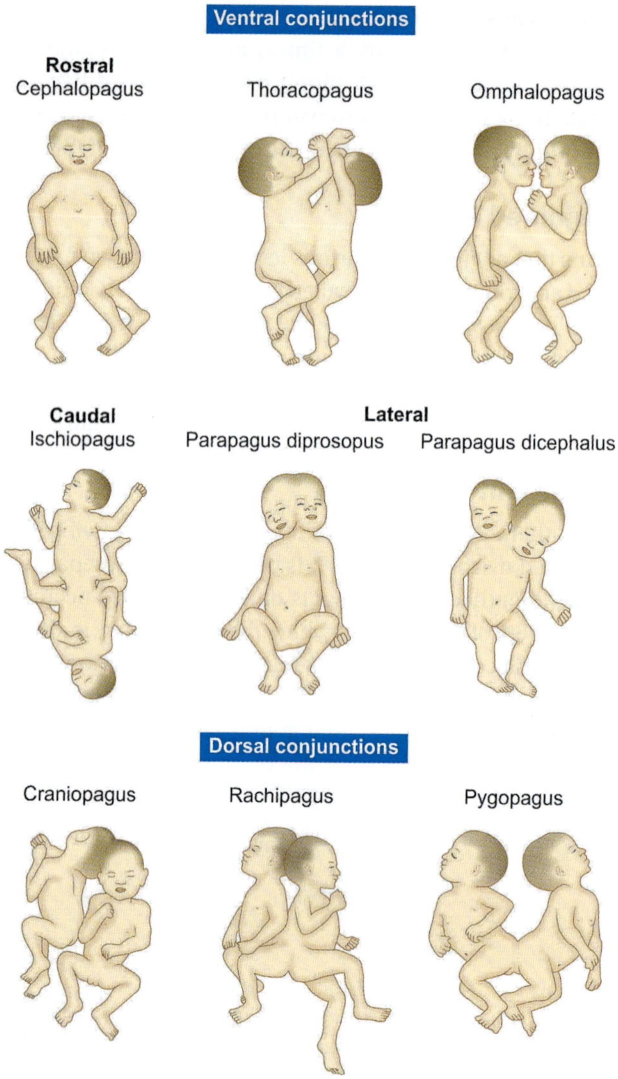

Fig. 5: Various types of conjoined twins.
Source: Twins. [online] Available from: https://smithlhhsb122.wikispaces.com/Bhumika+P. [Accessed March, 2018].

DIAGNOSIS

Diagnosing a pregnant woman with multiple-order gestation should be on the basis of history, clinical examination, and imaging modalities. History and clinical examination have already been discussed earlier in this chapter. Imaging and other diagnostic studies include the following.

Placental Examination

Since time immemorial, examination of the placenta after delivery has been a useful tool in determining the zygosity of multiple pregnancies.[14] Earlier, it was believed that a single placenta meant monozygous twins, while two separate placentae were dizygotic. However, this was found to be quite incorrect because if the eggs implant close together, the placentae can become fused and take on the appearance of one placenta, and in such a case twins will then be wrongly diagnosed as monozygotic. Therefore, more important than the placenta itself is an examination of the membranes. Amnion is the inner membrane and chorion is the outer membrane. If the amnion is common between the two fetuses, it always means monozygotic twins, but this is very rare. Two amnions and one chorion also mean monozygotic twins (monochorionic diamniotic). If there are two amnions and two chorions, the twin type can be either mono- or dizygotic (dichorionic diamniotic).

Dizygotic twins will have separate placentae; however, sometimes they may be fused, leading to a confusion, but this placenta is very easily separable into two separate placentae.

Clinical Features

Dizygotic twins are known to be genetically similar with nearly 50% similarity in the genetic constitution, an observation similar to that in the nontwin sibling. They are also known as "fraternal twins." Among these twins, half of the twins are of the same sex and half of different sex, but each fetus has its own placenta, which is continuous with the chorion.

Monozygotic twins, also known as "identical" twins, develop when an ovum is fertilized by a sperm and during the first 2 weeks after conception; this embryo then splits into two, forming two identical babies of almost the same sex and genetic constitution. One third of the monozygotic twins have separate placentae, while the other two thirds have a single placenta though they have their own amnion, umbilical cord, and placental mass.

Imaging Modality

Ultrasonography is the test to confirm multiple-order pregnancies. It is also to be carried out for antenatal surveillance of these pregnancies. Chorionicity of twin fetuses is detected on ultrasonography by 10–14 weeks of gestation at the earliest by visually inspecting the intervening membrane of the fetuses. Demonstration of "T-sign" at the intertwin membrane-placental junction suggests monochorionic-diamniotic twins (this is the junction between the intertwin membrane and the external rim forming a right angle), whereas dichorionic twins present with a "lambda (λ) sign" (that is the chorion forms a wedge-shaped protrusion into the intertwin space, creating a rather curved junction). This "lambda sign" is also known as the "twin peak sign" **(Fig. 6)**. In the ultrasound assessment at 16–20 weeks of pregnancy, the presence of "lambda sign" suggests dichorionicity; however, if this sign is not found at this gestation, it does not exclude the diagnosis.[15]

Ultrasonography is also a diagnostic tool to assess multiple pregnancies in those who develop complications such as twin-to-twin transfusion syndrome, growth discordancy, conjoined twins, malpresentations, intrauterine demise of one twin, and abnormal Dopplers.[16]

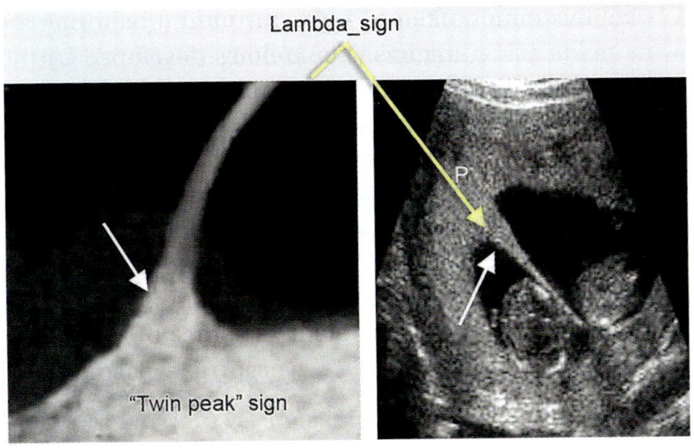

Fig. 6: Ultrasonographic feature of dichorionic-diamniotic placentae. *Source:* Twins for Undergraduate. (2014). Lambda Sign (Slide 21). [online] Available from: https://www.slideshare. net/MBHRY/ twins-for-undergraduate-32772937. [Accessed March, 2018]. Twins Clinical Management. (2012). Twin Peak Sign. [online] Available from: https://image.slidesharecdn.com/ twinsclinicalmanagement2012-120605164954-phpapp01/95/ twins-clinical-management-2012-15-728. jpg?cb=1338915097. [Accessed March, 2018].

Magnetic Resonance Imaging

Magnetic resonance imaging (MRI) is another modality in diagnosing multiple pregnancies, especially conjoined twins. Diagnostic features in conjoined twins include a bifid fetal pole, absence of separating membranes between fetuses, unseparated fetuses and their parts, number of blood vessels in the umbilical cord exceeds three, fetal heads and bodies positioned in the same plane, unusual extension of the fetal spines, unusual proximity of fetal extremities, and fetal positions.[17]

COMPLICATIONS

Multiple-order gestations are known to have both fetal and maternal risks.[18] Mortality in both cases is currently less due to better medical facilities.

Maternal Complications

Higher order pregnancies lead to a higher incidence of maternal complications such as preeclampsia, anemia, labor difficulties, postpartum hemorrhage, failed lactation, and, last but not the least, psychological disturbances in a woman.[19] In 2005, Flanders, from Belgium, reported the perinatal outcome in 26,656 ART pregnancies in the study conducted at Study Center for Perinatal Epidemiology (SPE);[20] preterm delivery was the most common: 95.9% of triplet pregnancies (mean gestation of 32.7 weeks) and 53.8% among twins (mean gestation of 35.6 weeks). Early preterm delivery (<32 weeks) and very-low-birth-weight infants (<1,500 g) were almost three times more among triplets compared with twins after assisted reproduction. Thus, it was clearly observed that as the number of fetuses increased, the duration of gestation reduced to a mean of 3 weeks per additional fetus. A comparable figure was also reported by Martin et al.[4] Twin-to-twin transfusion[21] and conjoined twins[22] are separate complications associated with multiple pregnancies. Many studies evaluated psychosocial risks such as quality of life, depression, and social stigma prevailing in families who underwent ART treatment, resulting in multiple birth children. They found a greater incidence of parenting stress and decreased parenting satisfaction when compared with families who conceived twins spontaneously.[21] Thus, these studies suggested that the infertility treatment experienced by these couples makes them more vulnerable to psychosocial stress.

Neonatal Complications

Prematurity is the most common morbidity associated with multiple pregnancies leading to low-birth-weight babies. Intrauterine growth restriction (IUGR) also leads to low-birth-weight babies. Various studies have reported that the average birth weight of these babies range between 1.1 and 2.5 kg.[5,23] All these factors independently lead to higher chances of neonatal morbidity and intensive care unit admission, birth asphyxia, neonatal metabolic complications such as hypoglycemia and hypocalcemia, respiratory distress, and eventually mortality.[5,23] It should be mentioned here that the higher the number of fetuses, the more the severity of morbidity and, thus, mortality.

In monozygotic pregnancies with single chorion and amnion (monochorionic-monoamniotic), both fetuses have one large amniotic sac. These twins not only possess all the risks of monochorionic-diamniotic twins, but they also have the risk of fetal and umbilical cord entanglement which have a reported fetal mortality rate of up to 60%.[24]

TREATMENT

Prophylactic Management

Strategies aimed at reducing multifetal gestation and thus reduce the morbidity and mortality in multiple-order births. These include the following:

Elective Single Embryo Transfer

Currently, elective single embryo transfer (eSET) has been advocated to be adopted as a standardized practice in those ART cycles where the chance of resulting in a live birth is high.[25] However, considering the live birth rates may be reduced with single embryo transfer; therefore, a careful selection of patients is advocated who would benefit from eSET and result in a live birth. Also, strategies to improve culture conditions, embryo grading, and selecting the most viable and competent embryo need to be developed.[26]

Excess Oocyte Aspiration and Vitrification

In patients undergoing ART and ovarian stimulation, a direct correlation between the number of follicles and multiple pregnancy rates has been observed. Studies have shown that cycles in which three or four follicles result in no substantial gain in the overall pregnancy rate, but there occurs an increase in multiple fetuses, thus increasing the multiple pregnancy rate.[27] A low-dose or minimal-stimulation protocol can therefore be advocated for such women to prevent multifollicular development and thus reduce the multiple pregnancies after ovarian stimulation.[28] The use of excess oocyte retrieval and vitrification technique may further improve the cost-effectiveness in stimulated IUI cycles by reducing multiple pregnancy rates and increasing the overall chances of pregnancy by cryopreserving the excess embryos. This technique, however, should not become a substitute for carefully monitored ovulation induction (OI). This modality of treatment has been widely studied, reporting excellent outcomes for oocyte cryopreservation.[29]

Fetal Reduction

Fetal reduction in multifetal pregnancies has been advocated to reduce them to twin pregnancies in order to improve perinatal outcomes.[30] This also decreases the early miscarriage rates, antenatal complications, preterm births, cesarean deliveries, low birth weight, and neonatal mortality. Outcomes from multifetal reduction to twins have been found to be comparable to those obtained from twin pregnancies conceived either spontaneously or through assisted reproductive technologies.[31]

Others

Cycle cancellation, coasting in ovarian stimulation, aspiration of follicles before human chorionic gonadotropin (hCG) administration, and switching to IVF in an IUI cycle are some of the other strategies advocated that help in the reduction of multiple pregnancies.[32-34]

Definite Management

Treatment of multiple-order births is directed toward its type. Monochorionic-monoamniotic twins carry maximum risk during the antenatal period; hence, they need extra attention and care.

Antenatal

Pregnancies complicated with multiple fetuses are high-risk pregnancies; therefore, these women should have regular and frequent antenatal checkups. Initially, monthly checkups are up to 24 weeks and then every fortnight. These pregnancies are at an increased risk of preterm deliveries, PIH, anemia, and antepartum hemorrhage (abruptio placentae) warranting close monitoring. Antepartum surveillance with nuchal translucency (NT) scan, level II anomaly scan, and time-to-time obstetric Doppler studies is indicated at 10–12, 18–20, and >28 weeks onward, respectively.[2]

The recommendations[16] for ultrasound monitoring for twins made according to the guidelines developed by the Canadian Task Force on Preventive Health Care are as follows:

- All patients who are suspected to have a twin pregnancy on first-trimester physical examination or who are at risk (e.g., pregnancies resulting from ART) should have a first-trimester ultrasound performed (II-2A).
- Every attempt should be made to determine and report amnionicity and chorionicity when a twin pregnancy is identified (II-2A).
- Although the accuracy in confirmation of gestational age at the first and second trimesters is comparable, dating should be done with first-trimester ultrasound (II-2A).
- Beyond the first trimester, a combination of parameters rather than a single parameter should be used to confirm gestational age (II-2C).
- When twin pregnancy is the result of IVF, accurate determination of gestational age should be made from the date of embryo transfer (II-1A).
- There is insufficient evidence to make a recommendation of which fetus (when discordant for size) to use to date a twin pregnancy. However, to avoid missing a situation of early IUGR in one twin, most experts agree that the clinician may consider dating pregnancy using the larger fetus (III-C).
- In twin pregnancies, aneuploidy screening using NT measurements should be offered (II-2B).
- Detailed ultrasound examination to screen for fetal anomalies should be offered, preferably between 18 and 22 weeks' gestation, in all twin pregnancies (II-2B).
- When ultrasound is used to screen for preterm birth in a twin gestation, endovaginal ultrasound measurement of the cervical length should be performed (II-2A).
- Increased fetal surveillance should be considered when there is either growth restriction diagnosed in one twin or growth discordancy (II-2A).
- Umbilical artery Doppler should not be routinely offered in uncomplicated twin pregnancies (I-E).
- For defining oligohydramnios and polyhydramnios, the radiologist should use the deepest vertical pocket in either sac—oligohydramnios when <2 cm and polyhydramnios when >8 cm (II-2B).

Folic acid, hematinics, calcium, and other dietary supplements should be prescribed. Immunization schedule is to be followed as in any other pregnancy.

If the twins are conjoined, it should be clearly decided whether they would be viable after birth following a corrective surgery. Such twins should be allowed to continue and electively terminated at 36 weeks by cesarean section. This should be in a tertiary care unit with a neonatal intensive care unit (NICU) backup. However, if the twins are not viable, termination should be offered like any other pregnancy within legal limits.

Discordant twins and twin-to-twin transfusions are to be managed as "high risk" on similar lines with closed surveillance.

Intrapartum

Management depends on the number of fetuses. Pregnancies with more than two fetuses should be delivered by cesarean section. Twins where both the fetuses are either cephalic or first twin cephalic and second breech can have vaginal births with close intrapartum monitoring. Malpresentations are to be planned for the cesarean section.

Postpartum

Multifetal pregnancies have an increased risk of postpartum hemorrhage; hence, they should be encouraged to deliver in a well-equipped facility, preferably under a tertiary care unit. Failed lactation and postpartum blues are also associated with a higher frequency than singleton pregnancies.

Neonatal Care

Most outcomes from multifetal pregnancies if born after 34 weeks require only routine pediatric care; though some may require specialized care, NICU admissions, and regular close follow-up. The American College of Obstetricians and Gynecologists has postulated guidelines for the evaluation and management of such newborns, which include the following:[2]

- *Neonatal:* A complete blood count (CBC) for evaluating anemia and polycythemia
- *Neonatal arterial blood gas and cord blood gas:* To evaluate for respiratory distress, hypoxia, acidosis, and perinatal depression
- *Metabolic panel:* Fluid status and electrolyte levels should be evaluated and metabolic status should be determined, including through screening for hypoglycemia and hypocalcemia
- *Bilirubin level:* This is obtained to screen for increased risk of hyperbilirubinemia associated with prematurity and polycythemia.

CONCLUSION

A significant rise in multiple-order births has been there because of a rise in women taking fertility drugs and assisted reproduction. Twin pregnancies are more common than triplets and quadruplets; though higher-order births are rare, nevertheless they have also been reported. Zygosity of twins is dependent on the timing of splitting after fertilization and is diagnosed with a placental examination at birth, ultrasonography, and features of the twins after birth. Preterm delivery is the most common complication associated with multifetal gestation. Other comorbidities may be PIH, anemia, twin-to-twin transfusion, growth discordancy, etc. Prematurity leading to the birth of low-birth-weight babies is the most common neonatal morbidity and is thus associated with neonatal complications. All possible efforts should be made to reduce the occurrence of multifetal pregnancies; some strategies in this direction include eSET, excess oocyte aspiration and vitrification, coasting, cycle cancellation, converting IUI cycle to IVF, and multifetal reduction. All these pregnancies should be monitored with regular antenatal surveillance. Delivery should be in a well-equipped hospital because there are higher chances of operative intervention and babies requiring NICU care.

Multiple-order births are frequent as more couples are seeking fertility treatments. These are high-risk pregnancies and are often complicated with PIH, anemia, abruption, and the most common being preterm deliveries. Prematurity leads to the birth of low-birth-weight babies and higher associated morbidity and mortality. Ultrasonography is the simplest, easiest, and noninvasive test used for diagnosis and also antenatal surveillance though MRI may be better in select cases. Regular antenatal monitoring, nutritional supplements, immunization, and delivery in tertiary care unit are recommended.

KEY POINTS

- Multiple-order births have increased as more couples are opting for infertility treatments.
- Zygosity depends on the timing of splitting after fertilization.
- The most common order of multiple gestations is twin pregnancy—monochorionic-diamniotic being the most common, though triplets and higher-order births also occur.
- Preterm delivery is common, which leads to prematurity, and low-birth-weight babies and hence leading to increased neonatal morbidity and mortality.
- Recommended guidelines that lower the chances of multiple pregnancies during assisted reproductive technique (ART) procedures should be followed.
- Recommended guidelines should be followed for fetal surveillance and maternal treatment.
- Delivery should be planned in a tertiary care unit with neonatal intensive care.

REFERENCES

1. Blickstein I, Shinwell ES. Obstetric management of multiple gestation and birth. In: Martin RJ, Fanaroff AA, Walsh MC (Eds). Fanaroff and Martin's Neonatal-Perinatal Medicine: Diseases of the Fetus and Infant, 9th edition. Philadelphia, PA: Saunders/Elsevier; 2011. p. 343.
2. ACOG practice bulletin no. 144: multifetal gestations: twin, triplet and higher-order multifetal pregnancies. Obstet Gynecol. 2014;123(5):1118-32.
3. Smits J, Monden C. Twinning across the developing world. PLoS One. 2011;6(9):e25239.

4. Martin JA, Hamilton BE, Ventura SJ, Osterman MJ, Wilson EC, Mathews TJ. Births: final data for 2010. Natl Vital Stat Rep. 2012;61(1):1-72.
5. Singh L, Trivedi K. Study of maternal and fetal outcome in twin pregnancy. Int J Reprod Contracept Obstet Gynecol. 2017;6(6):2272-8.
6. Jacobsson B, Ladfors L, Milsom I. Advanced maternal age and adverse perinatal outcome. Obstet Gynecol. 2004;104(4):727-33.
7. Tough SC, Greene C, Svenson L, Claro A, Belik J. Maternal age and its relationship to multiple birth, low birth weight and preterm delivery in in vitro fertilization (IVF) pregnancies. Pediatr Res. 1999;45:257.
8. Imaizumi Y. Demographic trends in Japan and Asia. In: Blickstein I, Keith L, Keith D (Eds). Multiple Pregnancy, 2nd edition. London and New York: Taylor and Francis Group; 2005. pp. 33-8.
9. Hoekstra C, Zhao ZZ, Lambalk CB, Willemsen G, Martin NG, Boomsma DI, et al. Dizygotic twinning. Hum Reprod Update. 2008;14(1):37-47.
10. Kulkarni AD, Jamieson DJ, Jones Jr HW, Kissin DM, Gallo MF, Macaluso M, et al. Fertility treatments and multiple births in the United States. New Engl J Med. 2013;369:2218-25.
11. Basso O, Nohr EA, Christensen K, Olsen J. Risk of twinning as a function of maternal height and body mass index. JAMA. 2004;291(13):1564-6.
12. Qiu X, Lee SK, Tan K, Piedboeuf B, Canning R, Canadian Neonatal Network. Comparison of singleton and multiple-birth outcomes of infants born at or before 32 weeks of gestation. Obstet Gynecol. 2008;111(2 Pt 1):365-71.
13. Miller J, Chauhan SP, Abuhamad AZ. Discordant twins: diagnosis, evaluation and management. Am J Obstet Gynecol. 2012;206(1):10-20.
14. Potter EL. Twin zygosity and placental form in relation to the outcome of pregnancy: Adair Award address. Am J Obstet Gynecol. 1963;87(5):566-77.
15. Sepulveda W, Sebire NJ, Hughes K, Kalogeropoulos A, Nicolaides KH. Evolution of the lambda or twin-chorionic peak sign in dichorionic twin pregnancies. Obstet Gynecol. 1997;89(3):439-41.
16. Morin L, Lim K, Diagnostic Imaging Committee; Special Contributor; Genetics Committee; Maternal Fetal Medicine Committee. Ultrasound in twin pregnancies. J Obstet Gynaecol Can. 2011;33(6):643-56.
17. Çetin O, Kurdoğlu Z, Çim N, Yildizhan R, Sahin G, Kurdoglu M. Early prenatal diagnosis of conjoined twins: case series. Int J Womens Health Reprod Sci. 2015;3(3):168-70.
18. Norwitz ER, Edusa V, Park JS. Maternal physiology and complications of multiple pregnancy. Semin Perinatol. 2005;29(5):338-48.
19. Ellison MA, Hotamisligil S, Lee H, Rich-Edwards JW, Pang SC, Hall JE. Psychosocial risks associated with multiple births resulting from assisted reproduction. Fertil Steril. 2005;83:1422-8.
20. Ombelet W, De Sutter P, Van der Elst J, Martens G. Multiple gestation and infertility treatment: registration, reflection and reaction—the Belgian project. Hum Reprod Update. 2005;11:3-14.
21. Ortibus E, Lopriore E, Deprest J, Vandenbussche FP, Walther FJ, Diemert A, et al. The pregnancy and long-term neurodevelopmental outcome of monochorionic diamniotic twin gestations: a multicenter prospective cohort study from the first trimester onward. Am J Obstet Gynecol. 2009;200(5):494.e1-8.
22. de Silva RS, Amaradivakara PW. Antenatal diagnosis and management of conjoined twins: a case report. Sri Lanka J Obstet Gynaecol. 2015;37(2):24-6.
23. Irene YV, Kaur V. An analytical study of pregnancy outcome in multifetal gestation. J Obstet Gynecol India. 2007;57(6): 509-12.
24. Paek B, Shields LE. Twin-to-twin transfusion syndrome: diagnosis and treatment. Curr Women Health Rev. 2005;1:43-7.
25. Söderström-Anttila V, Vilska S. Five years of single embryo transfer with anonymous and non-anonymous oocyte donation. Reprod Biomed Online. 2007;15:428-33.
26. Gardner DK, Sakkas D. Assessment of embryo viability: the ability to select a single embryo for transfer—a review. Placenta. 2003;24(Suppl. B):S5-12.
27. Van Rumste MM, Custers IM, van der Veen F, van Wely M, Evers JL, Mol BW. The influence of the number of follicles on pregnancy rates in intrauterine insemination with ovarian stimulation: a meta-analysis. Hum Reprod Update. 2008;14:563-70.
28. Dickey RP, Taylor SN, Lu PY, Sartor BM, Rye PH, Pyrzak R. Effect of diagnosis, age, sperm quality, and number of preovulatory follicles on the outcome of multiple cycles of clomiphene citrate-intrauterine insemination. Fertil Steril. 2002;78:1088-95.
29. Antinori M, Licata E, Dani G, Cerusico F, Versaci C, Antinori S. Cryotop vitrification of human oocytes results in high survival rate and healthy deliveries. Reprod Biomed Online. 2007;14:72-9.
30. Ombelet W, Camus M, de Catte L. Relative contribution of ovarian stimulation versus in vitro fertilization and intracytoplasmic sperm injection to multifetal pregnancies requiring reduction to twins. Fertil Steril. 2007;88:997-9.
31. Dodd J, Crowther C. Multifetal pregnancy reduction of triplet and higher-order multiple pregnancies to twins. Fertil Steril. 2004;81:1420-2.
32. Urman B, Pride SM, Yuen BH. Management of overstimulated gonadotropin cycles with a controlled drift period. Hum Reprod. 1992;7:213-7.
33. Albano C, Platteau P, Nogueira D, Cortvrindt R, Smitz J, Devroey P. Avoidance of multiple pregnancies after ovulation induction by supernumerary preovulatory follicular reduction. Fertil Steril. 2001;76:820-2.
34. Haydardedeoglu B, Bagis T, Simsek E, Cok T, Hacivelioglu SO, Erkanli S. The impact of rescue in vitro fertilization converted from high-response gonadotropin intrauterine insemination cycles in terms of implantation and pregnancy rates as compared with matched controls. Fertil Steril. 2009;92:137-42.

SECTION 10

Third Party Reproduction

Figs 2A and B: [illegible]
Source: (A) https://[illegible]
(B) Author's own image.

The history of the patient may reveal about the lady carrying multifetal pregnancy. Women who are not aware may give a

CHAPTER 69

Oocyte and Sperm Donation

Jaideep Malhotra, Ashwini Mohandas, Narendra Malhotra, Neharika Malhotra

INTRODUCTION

If we conceive society as a cultural concept in which the people's behaviors are representative of the types of relationships they have with each other, then it necessitates evaluating the cultural aspect of each event for investigating its social dimension. Therefore, in order to have an accurate understanding of fertility and infertility as a social phenomenon and for evaluating its social dimensions, a careful review of the event's cultural background is required

Human response to new developments regarding birth, death, marriage, and divorce is largely shaped by religious beliefs.

The possibility of conceiving through assisted reproductive technologies (ARTs), more specifically from a third-party, has provoked different reactions in different cultures, which have received and interpreted them to befit their own reproductive norms and practices. As Unnithan-Kumar points out "[Reproductive] technologies in themselves do not bring about social transformation but it is in how they are made socially meaningful that their power lies."

Third party reproduction is a form of assisted reproduction in which woman agrees to bear child on behalf of and relinquish the child to and individual or couple who intend to rear the child. Introducing a stranger's gamete to conceive has the potential of disrupting the biological continuity and, inevitably, leads to a redefinition of what is "biological" and what is "social" as far as family and kinship are concerned. When assisted reproduction was introduced into medical practice in the last quarter of the 20th century, it was fiercely attacked by some religious groups and highly welcomed by others. Today, assisted reproduction is accepted in nearly all its forms.

Unlike the recent advances in assisted reproduction, the concept of third-party reproduction is not new and has been in vogue since the mythological era **(Figs. 1 and 2)**.

With the advent of ART and gamete freezing, anonymous gamete donation has become feasible/possible. It involves use of sperms (sperm donation) or eggs (oocyte donation) or uterus (surrogacy) from persons other than the commissioning couple involved. This was limited initially to sperm donation till egg donation came into the picture

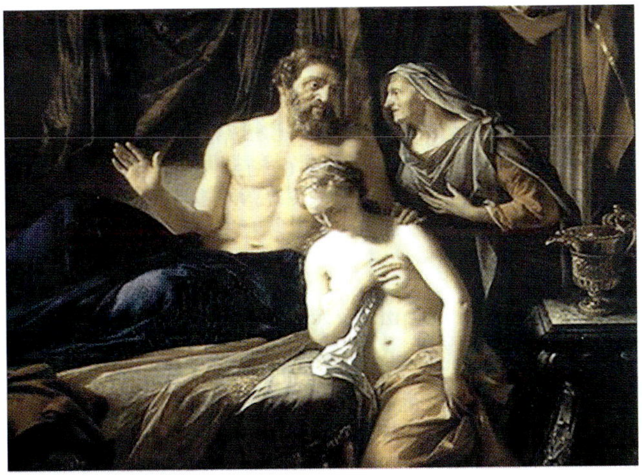

Fig.1: Abraham with Sarah and Hagar.

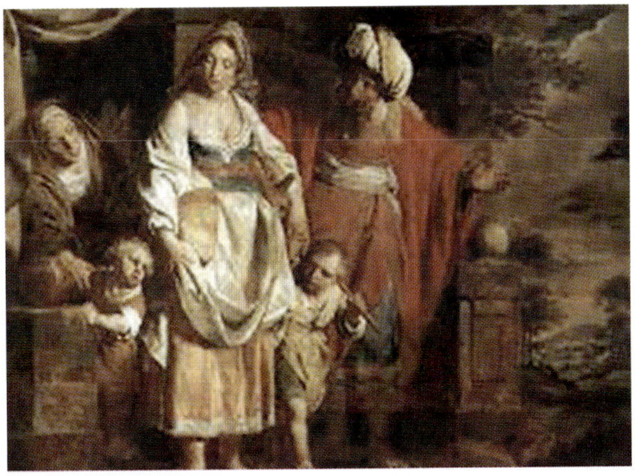

Fig. 2: Sarah exiles Hagar and her child.

with the development of techniques for oocyte harvesting. Trounson et al. reported the first pregnancy using donor eggs in 1983. The first conception was reported after transplanting an unhatched embryo flushed out from the donor by uterine lavage using a special device into the recipient uterus. Over the past 20 years, the number of births from gamete donation has increased exponentially from 30,000–60,000 in the United States.[1]

This chapter reviews the need, clinical effectiveness, and implications of oocyte donation and sperm donation.

OOCYTE DONATION

In vitro fertilization with the use of donor oocytes (IVF-OD) has become an integral part of infertility treatment today. The procedure is used to achieve pregnancy in women with premature and age-related ovarian failure, poor ovarian reserve (due to disease or advanced age), Turner's syndrome, recurrent implantation failure due to poor oocyte quality, and recurrent abortions.[1,2] Couples also opt to use donated oocytes to avoid transmission of severe genetic diseases.[3]

Results achieved in recipients surpass those attained with use of autologous oocyte IVF[4-6] in good prognosis patients, resulting in an exponential rise in the procedure. In the USA, the annual number of donor oocyte cycles increased from 10,801–18,306 between 2000–2010,[7] whilst the European IVF Monitoring (EIM) consortium for the European Society of Human Reproduction and Embryology (ESHRE)[4] reported 7,171 IVF-OD cycles in 2006 and 33,605 cycles in 2012. Indeed, couples will travel outside their country if local laws forbid oocyte donation. The procedure is so popular that oocyte banks[8] have been established to allow for sharing of oocytes from a donor, reduced waiting times involved in sourcing and screening donors, and circumventing donor-recipient synchronization. Cross-border reproductive care too is gaining attention, as ART practices and obstetric care may differ between countries.[9]

The donor-recipient model has provided an insight into various aspects of ART, such as the importance of oocyte age in implantation,[11] endometrial receptivity,[12,] and the contribution of male factors to IVF failure.[13] Perhaps the most thought-provoking realization is the knowledge that the reproductive system can function perfectly in the absence of a genetic connection.[2]

Indications for Oocyte Donation

Premature Ovarian Insufficiency

Premature ovarian insufficiency (POI) is defined as cessation of menstrual cycle, increased serum follicle-stimulating hormone (FSH) levels, and decreased serum estradiol levels in women before the age 40 years.[14] POI concerns about 1% of women and is characterized by severely diminished fertility.

BOX 1: Causes of premature ovarian failure.

- Gonadal dysgenesis
- Turner syndrome
- Perrault syndrome
- 46, XX gonadal dysgenesis/46, XY gonadal dysgenesis
- Genetic associations
- Familial ovarian failure
- Galactosemia
- Enzyme defects—P450c17
- FRAXA premutation
- Blepharophimosis, ptosis, and epicanthus inversus syndrome (also called BPES)
- Small X chromosome defects
- FSH receptor mutations/LH receptor mutations

Autoimmune:

- Autoimmune polyendocrinopathy syndrome 1
- Autoimmune polyendocrinopathy-candidiasis-ectodermal dystrophy/autoimmune Polyendocrinopathy syndrome 2
- Association with various autoimmune diseases
- Isolated autoimmune ovarian failure
- Iatrogenic chemotherapy
- Radiotherapy
- Pelvic surgery
- Environmental toxins
- Idiopathic

(FRAXA: fragile X; FSH: follicle-stimulating hormone; LH: luteinizing hormone).

The etiopathogenesis of this disorder is related to a multifactoral background **(Box 1)**. A major part is regarded as idiopathic, although it is suspected to be genetically determined.[4,5] Autoimmunological causes are involved in the pathogenesis of 4–30% of POI cases.[14] The presence of antiovarian autoantibodies (AOAs), lymphocytic oophoritis, and associated autoimmune disorders are key evidence of autoimmunological background.

Over the past decades, many genes have emerged as POI candidates, but only a minority has been proven causative by functional validation.

These include genes involved in primordial germ cell migration and proliferation (NANOS3), in cell death (PGRMC1 and FMR1), oocyte specific transcription factors (FIGLA and NOBOX genes).[2]

The increasing number of POI cases is also related to iatrogenic background (use of radiotherapy, chemotherapy, and pelvic surgery in patients treated due to oncological diseases).

Turner Syndrome

One of the most common chromosomal abnormalities is Turner syndrome (TS), its incidence being 1 in 2,000 live born female infants. These women have an absent or partial loss of one X chromosome leading to severe and often irreversible POF, presenting prior to menarche. Though sporadic spontaneous pregnancies are reported among women with

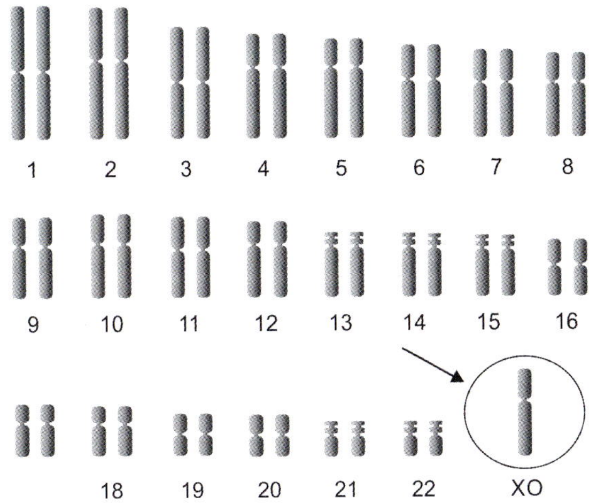

Fig. 3: Turner syndrome.

TS these can be associated with a high risk of miscarriage and an increased risk of trisomy 21 in the offspring **(Fig. 3)**.[3]

Turner syndrome patients are also candidates for in vitro fertilization with oocyte donation. However, it is well known that in these patients a high rate of cardiovascular anomalies is observed. There have been studies associated with early implantation failure after oocyte donation in these women possibly due to an inherent endometrial abnormality.[3] Therefore, according to the American Society of Reproductive Medicine (ASRM), women with TS before attempting to become pregnant should undergo medical and cardiovascular control[13]; this can decrease the high rate of cardiovascular mortality during pregnancy.

In a retrospective study, conducted in 10 of the 27 French oocyte donation centers between 2012–2016, on all the patients presenting with TS included in an oocyte donation program, the pregnancy rates were 53%. Pregnancies were complicated by gravid arterial hypertension in 28.2% of cases, preeclampsia in 10.3% of cases, and gestational diabetes in 7.7% of cases.[15]

Diminished Ovarian Reserve

Women with greatly reduced ovarian reserve as determined by ovarian reserve markers [anti-Müllerian hormone (AMH) <0.5 ng/mL, FSH >15 IU/L] or previous poor response to stimulation or advanced age can opt for oocyte donation after proper counseling.

Women with diminished ovarian reserve can be categorized and treated accordingly as per the POSEIDON criteria. The POSEIDON stratification helps to not only guide clinicians regarding clinical management of the patient, but also to be a counseling tool to help set patient expectations prior to initiation of ovarian stimulation. Various clinics can have different cutoffs of age and ovarian reserve tests above which ovarian stimulation is deferred.

In such patients IVF with oocyte donation has seen benefits.

Repeated Implantation Failure Due to Poor Quality Oocytes

In patients with repeated implantation failure (RIF), oocyte donation has been suggested as an alternative especially if oocyte quality is implicated and offers an option with acceptable pregnancy rates although sometimes couples with unexplained RIF are also treated using this method.

Genetic Disorders

In women not willing or affording for preimplantation genetic diagnosis, egg donation is an acceptable alternative for the prevention of heritable genetic disorders such as single gene defects or balanced translocations with good success rates.

LEGALITIES PERTAINING OOCYTE DONATION AS PER ASSISTED REPRODUCTIVE TECHNOLOGY (REGULATION) ACT, 2021

In 2021, the Parliament passed the Assisted Reproductive Technology (Regulation) Act, 2021 (hereinafter referred to as "ART Act") which received the assent of the President on 18.12.2021 and came into force on 25.01.2022 vide the notification in the Gazette of India No. CG-DL-E-21012022-232818.

The aim of the ART Act is regulation and supervision of the ART Banks, prevention of misuse, and safe and ethical practices of ART Services for addressing the issue of reproductive help where ART is required for becoming a parent or for freezing gametes, embryos, embryonic tissues for further use due to infertility, decease or social or medical concerns and regulation and supervision of research and development.

The Commissioning Couple

An infertile married couple who approaches an ART Clinic or an ART Bank for obtaining the services authorized by such clinics or banks for the purpose of bearing a child is referred to as a commissioning couple.

Regulatory Authority

The *"National Assisted Reproductive Technology and Surrogacy Board"* constituted under Section 15(1) of the Surrogacy (Regulation) Act, 2021 is the National Board that regulates ART in India and exercises and discharges various functions.

The *"State Assisted Reproductive Technology and Surrogacy Board"* constituted under Section 24(1) of the Surrogacy Act, 2021 acts as the State Board for the purposes of the ART Act and has the responsibility to follow the policies and plans laid by the National ART Board for ART Clinics and

Banks in the State. Further, the ART Board is responsible to follow the policies and plans made by the National Board and take into account its recognition, and policies and regulating and coordinating enforcement and implementation of such policies and guidelines for assisted reproduction.

The Registry

The Central Government under Section 9 of the ART Act has established a registry called the *National Assisted Reproductive Technology and Surrogacy Registry,* which consists of scientific and other technical information pertaining to surrogacy.

- It acts as a central database in the country through which the details of all the clinics and banks of the country including the nature and types of services provided by them, the outcome of the services, and other relevant information obtained on regular basis.
- It assists the National Board in its functioning by providing the data generated from the central database of the Registry.
- The data generated from the National Registry are utilized by the National Board for making policies, and guidelines and to help in identifying new research areas and conducting research in the area of assisted reproduction and other related fields in the country.

Appropriate Authority

The Central and State Governments appoint Appropriate ART and Surrogacy Authorities for each Union Territories and state.

The appropriate authority under Section 13 of the ART Act discharges the following functions:

- To grant, suspend or cancel the registration of a clinic or bank.
- To enforce the standards to be fulfilled by the clinic or bank.
- To investigate complaints relating to the breach of the provisions of this Act and take appropriate legal actions regarding misuse of ART by any person and also to initiate independent investigations in such matters.
- To recommend to the National Board and State Boards the modifications required in the rules, in accordance with changes in technology or social conditions.
- To take action after investigation of complaints received by it against the ART clinics or banks or discharge any other function as may be prescribed by the Central Government.

IMPORTANT POINTS REGARDING OOCYTE DONATION IN THE ART ACT

- A bank shall not supply the sperm or oocyte of a single donor to more than one commissioning couple.
- The donor eggs should be obtained from women between 23–35 years of age.
- An oocyte donor shall be an ever-married woman having at least one live child of her own with a minimum age of 3 years and should donate oocytes only once in her life.
- All unused oocytes shall be preserved by the banks for use on the same recipient or given for research to an organization registered under this Act after seeking written consent from the commissioning couple.
- Assisted reproductive technology clinics should ensure the eligibility of both recipients and the donors by medically testing them for sexually transmitted diseases (STDs) and other communicable diseases, which can be harmful to anyone.
- They should elicit all relevant information for donor selection.
- Sperm or egg donation by any person known or related to the recipients should not be permitted.
- Full confidentiality should be maintained regarding the identity of the couple/woman/donor. Disclosure of information regarding the donor by any staff is a punishable offence under ART Bill regulations.
- Recipient is entitled to know about physical characteristics of donor, her ethnicity, educational background, and relevant medical history and family background.
- Counseling regarding implications and chances of success should be done and written consent forms to be signed.
- Couple and donor should be made aware of the rights of the children born using third-party reproduction.
- No clinic can advertise for oocyte, semen donors, and surrogates apart from registered ART banks.
- It is essential that detailed records should be maintained in the laboratory of all aspects of gamete donation such as the number of oocytes retrieved from donor, quality of oocytes, number of recipients, details of recipients, and pregnancy outcome.
- Records should be maintained up to 10 years and then transferred to centralized registry. Immediate transfer of all records to central data base has to be done in case of closure of ART bank or clinic before 10 years.
- It is a gross violation to treat any woman with gametes or embryos of different origins during a treatment cycle or mix semen of two individuals for any ART procedure.
- If multiple pregnancies occur, it is responsibility of the respective clinic to inform patient immediately of its medical implications and fetal reduction may be thought of after appropriate counseling.
- Preimplantation genetic diagnosis should not be used to screen embryos except in couples who are known carriers of inheritable genetic disorders.
- Embryos can be cryopreserved for a maximum period of 5 years with appropriate consent. Consent should also

include information whether the couple wants to donate these embryos for research or discard them at the end of this tenure and manner of their use in case of death of one partner.

- According to the ART Bill 2020, insurance cover should be provided to the oocyte donor by the commissioning couple from any registered insurance company .
- The child born through ART shall be deemed to be a biological child of the commissioning couple and the said child shall be entitled to all the rights and privileges available to a natural child only from the commissioning couple under any law for the time being in force.
- A donor shall relinquish all parental rights over the child or children which may be born from his or her gamete.
- Under Section 26 of the ART Act, no ART clinic can offer to provide a couple or woman the child of a predetermined sex and the same is also subject to the provisions of the Pre-complication and Pre-natal Diagnostic Techniques (Prohibition of Sex Selection) Act, 1994.
- It is also prohibited for anyone to do any act at any stage to determine the sex of the child to be born during the process of the ART, support, or yield fractions enriched in sperm of x or y variation.
- It is also prohibited for any person to knowingly provide, prescribe, or administer anything that can ensure or increase the probability that an embryo shall be of a particular sex or that can identify the sex of an in-vitro embryo, except to diagnose, prevent or treat the sex-linked disorder or disease.

EVALUATION

Recipient

- Thorough evaluation of the recipient (complete history, general and local examination) should be performed to rule out any abnormalities which can affect pregnancy outcome.
- Endocrinological investigations that affect the fertility potential and subsequent pregnancy prognosis such as thyroid function test, serum prolactin, fasting glucose, etc., should be done.
- Serological screening for human immunodeficiency virus (HIV) 1 and 2, hepatitis B by hepatitis surface antigen or hepatitis core antibody (IgG and IgM), hepatitis C by hepatitis C antibody, syphilis by venereal disease research laboratory is mandatory and investigations for other reproductive tract infections such as chlamydia, and tuberculosis should be done if deemed necessary.
- A good two-dimensional (2D) ultrasonography (USG) to rule out the presence of any uterine or ovarian pathology such as fibroids, polyps, hydrosalpinx, ovarian cyst, uterine anomalies should be performed and confirmed by three-dimensional (3D) USG. Mock endometrial preparation cycle should be a part of the protocol with enrolment in the program only once an adequate response is observed.
- Uterus can be evaluated for any abnormality by sonohysterography, 3D scans, or any another suitable procedure. Hysteroscopy is indicated in case of suspicion of any abnormality.
- Endometrial biopsy for histopathological examination, TUBERCULOSIS-PCR (Polymerase chain reaction), and culture may be done if previous history of TB or RIF or persistently thin endometrium with visible lesions or adhesions on hysteroscopy.
- Screening for concurrent medical conditions such as hypertension, cardiac diseases, Pap smear, and mammography should be done, especially if the woman is >40 years old.
- The risks related to pregnancy increases as women approach their 50s hence additional testing such as screening for diabetes and ECG to assess heart health as well as a clearance by a high-risk obstetrician.
- Rubella and varicella titer scan be done, and non-immune recipients should be immunized (not mandatory).
- Genetic tests should be prescribed depending on the history, ethnic background, and current recommendations.[8]
- Special tests such as karyotype and autoimmune screening in women with POI and cardiac evaluation in known case of Turner syndrome.
- Psychological screening of the couple is recommended.

Recipient Partner

- Thorough evaluation of the recipient partner (complete history, general, and local examination) should be performed to rule out any abnormalities, which can affect pregnancy outcome.
- It is essential that a detailed evaluation of semen sample has been done and appropriate therapy initiated. In case of any abnormality, semen analysis should be repeated 1–3 months later[9].
- Serological screening of the partner for hepatitis B, hepatitis C, and HIV should be done.
- Endocrinological investigations as appropriate should be carried out in oligospermic and azoospermic men.
- It is advised to have at least two frozen samples of the partner as a backup for the day of donor pickup in case, he is not able to supply a fresh sample.

Donor Selection and Evaluation

- Screening of gamete donors has to be done by an independently registered ART bank. A thorough medical history, physical examination, lab evaluation, and screening for hereditary disorders should be carried out.

BOX 2: Checklist of investigations for the donor.

- Complete blood count
- ABO and Rh
- Peripheral smear
- Random blood sugar
- Blood urea or serum creatinine
- SGPT
- Routine urine examination
- HBsAg status
- Hepatitis C status
- HIV status
- VDRL for syphilis
- Hemoglobin A2 (for thalassemia) status
- Anti-Müllerian hormone (AMH)—optional

(ABO: A,B,O blood group; HBsAg: hepatitis B surface antigen; HIV: human immunodeficiency virus; Rh: Rhesus factor; SGPT: serum glutamic pyruvic transaminase; VDRL: venereal disease research laboratory).

- Donors should be screened for STDs or any other communicable diseases liable to endanger the health of the recipient.
- Donor should undergo appropriate genetic evaluation based on history, in accordance with ethnic background and current guidelines. Though ART bill does not specify any genetic tests for oocyte donors' other societies such as ASRM recommend genetic screening. Implementation of expanded carrier screening (ECS), in a recent study has resulted in 63% risk reduction in adverse outcomes observed in oocyte donation program from a potential adverse event rate of 4.2% to an actual 1.55% incidence of adverse outcomes.[11]
- According to the Human Fertilisation and Embryology Authority (HFEA) 2009 guidelines (revised in October 2017), if there is history of poor-quality gamete formation with oocytes from a particular donor or any history of serious physical, psychological or medical harm to the resulting progeny then that donor should not be accepted again.[12]
- Women with high-risk sexual behavior, close contact with hepatitis B (HepB) or hepatitis C (HepC) infected persons, history of treatment for STDs in last 12 months, recent blood transfusion, and transplant recipients should not be accepted as donors.
- Oocyte donors should have a good screening transvaginal sonography to rule out any pelvic pathology and to assess the ovarian reserve using the astral follicle count.[13]
- Checklist of blood investigations for the donor is described in **Box 2**.

COUNSELING

Recipient Couple

Assisted reproductive technology bill stresses the need to counsel the commissioning couple regarding the implications and chances of success of all ART procedures including cost, side effects, risks especially that of multiple births, limitations of donor screening, to help them make an informed decision. The decision to opt for oocyte donation itself can be taxing for the couple as there can be fear of unknown genetic material.

TABLE 1: Various consent forms under Indian Council of Medical Research.

FORM - K	Consent form for the donor of oocytes
FORM - L	Consent form for the donor of sperm
FORM - M	Information on semen donor
FORM - M1	Information on oocytes donor
FORM - R	Contract between the assisted reproductive technology bank and the semen donor
FORM - R1	Contract between the assisted reproductive technology bank and the oocyte donor

In a systematic review of 144 couples choosing oocyte donation, given a choice, about two-thirds opted for known donors and one-thirds only opted for anonymous donors. Counseling the couple regarding the laws related to third party reproduction and reassurance of confidentiality is very important.[16] Couple should be reassured that the process of gamete donation shall be kept confidential in accordance with the National ART Bill and identity of the donor can be disclosed only in unexceptional circumstances by a court order.

Donors

Professional counseling of the donor should be a part of the clinic's protocol. It should include assessment of the mental wellbeing and understanding regarding details of the procedure, need for regular visits, and possible complications due to ovarian stimulation such as nausea, headaches, abdominal bloating, and rarely ovarian hyperstimulation. Furthermore, donors should understand that they will, before going any right to future offspring, need to be fully capable and free from any kind of coercion in giving informed consent.

Consent of an oocyte donor should be obtained in local language or in presence of an interpreter if necessary and can be withdrawn at any time before embryos are created. Consent of the spouse of oocyte donor must also be obtained if there **(Table 1)**.

Offspring of Gamete Donation

Controversy exists regarding the disclosure of the facts of conception via gamete donation and identity of donor to the children born via this method. As per the ACT, a child born through ART will be deemed to be a biological child of the commissioning couple, and the said child will be entitled to all the rights and privileges available to a natural child only from the commissioning couple, under any law for the time being in force. A donor relinquishes all parental rights to offspring born by gamete donation. Various ethical committees and human right organizations are encouraging ART programs and ART banks to conduct gamete donation in ways that promote interests of offspring in learning the facts of their conception while respecting the privacy interests of donors and recipient parents.[17]

According to Indian Council of Medical Research (ICMR), a child >18 years or legal guardian of a minor can ask for information about the donor except for identification if necessary for the child's welfare. The identity of a donor can be divulged only if there is a life-threatening medical emergency. ASRM recommends that provisions to be made in such a way that, if consented by the donor, the identity can be revealed by the ART bank at the request of the offspring.[18]

SEX-SELECTIVE ASSISTED REPRODUCTIVE TECHNOLOGY PRACTICE

Any clinic must not issue, publish, distribute, or communicate any advertisement in any manner including the internet, regarding facilities of sex-selective ART. Doing so is a punishable offense.

Anyone who is found guilty of sex-selective ART practice will be punishable with imprisonment for a term, which is not <5 years but may extend to 10 years or with a fine, which shall not be <10 lakh rupees but may extend to 25 lakh rupees.

STIMULATION PROTOCOLS IN OOCYTE DONOR IN VITRO FERTILIZATION CYCLE

There has been a steady shift toward the use of gonadotropin hormone-releasing hormone (GnRH) antagonist protocol for stimulation of oocyte donors from the earlier cycles when agonist protocols were preferred. Antagonist cycles in donors offer the advantage of ease, fewer injections, lower cost, and most importantly lower incidence of hyper stimulation without compromising the oocyte or embryo quality.

A Cochrane review also suggested similar clinical outcomes using either GnRH agonist or antagonist cycles in donor oocyte cycles, providing clinicians' reassurance for using either option without compromising results.[19]

Gonadotropin hormone-releasing hormone antagonist protocols also allow the use of GnRH agonist trigger further reducing the risk of ovarian hyperstimulation syndrome (OHSS). Several prospective and randomized studies have found that GnRH agonist trigger does not negatively impact oocyte quality, embryo quality or recipient pregnancy rates while reducing the risk of OHSS when compared to human chorionic gonadotropin (HCG) trigger.

A recent meta-analysis by Guan et al. published in 2021, also did not find any difference between agonist and antagonist protocols or with the use of progesterone primed ovarian stimulation protocols.[16]

Random-start ovarian stimulation protocols have emerged allowing treatment to begin at any day of the menstrual cycle. Concomitantly, in what is called progestin primed oocyte stimulation (PPOS), the use of progestins seem similarly as effective as GnRH antagonists in preventing LH surge as suggested in a recently published study by Farfan et al.[18]

ENDOMETRIAL PREPARATION OF RECIPIENT

The key challenges to a successful oocyte donation program are endometrial preparation of the recipient and embryo-endometrial synchronization. Endometrial preparation is a key factor for successful ART outcomes, particularly in oocyte donation (OD) cycles.

In case of anovulatory recipients, either a fresh transfer can be planned by synchronizing the recipient with the donor or freezing the embryos and plan for frozen embryo transfer (FET). The easiest way to synchronize and plan for a fresh embryo transfer is by downregulating the recipient. The benefit of a fresh cycle transfer is that patient can avoid the cost of freeze-thaw cycle. The downside of a fresh cycle is the task of synchronizing the cycle of a recipient with that of a donor, which is not needed in FET cycles.

- Methods of synchronizing recipient cycle with that of donor is to give a GnRH depot to the recipient on D21-D22 of the pre-transfer cycle. Hormone replacement therapy (HRT) can be started after 2 weeks of depot after confirming for downregulation using a serum estradiol and serum progesterone level, (E2 <60 pg/mL; P4 <0.5 ng/mL) or clinically by USG measurement of endometrial thickness <5 mm. Donor stimulation should be started 3–4 days after initiating HRT in the recipient. The aim is to prime the endometrium with estrogen for at least minimum 10 days before oocyte retrieval of the donor.[20]
- Oral contraceptive pills can also be started from the 2nd day of pre-transfer cycle in recipient and withdrawn 7 days before the expected menses of the donor. The recipient usually starts bleeding from the 7th day after stopping the pills.
- In woman with complete cessation of cycles due to premature ovarian failure, it is advised to give at least one cycle of trial HRT to assess the endometrial response and prime the uterus as well. In these women use of GnRH agonists for downregulation is not required.
- Hormone replacement cycles involve sequential administration of estrogen followed by progesterone. Estrogen preparations with either (oral estradiol 4–8 mg or transdermal 0.2–0.4 mg) are usually initiated 3–4 days before stimulation in donor. There is no difference in the use of constant or increasing dosages of estrogen for endometrial preparation as well as route of administration.[21] Progesterone is started for the recipient from the day of oocyte retrieval if the endometrium is at least 7 mm thick.

- In FET cycles, embryo transfer is planned on the 4th day of progesterone for a day 3 transfer and similarly on the 6th day for a blastocyst embryo. Recent prospective study carried out in donor oocyte recipients found that serum P levels <9.2 ng/mL on the day of ET were associated with poor outcomes in patients on vaginal P. In case of ovulatory patients, transfer can be planned in a natural cycle such that blastocysts are replaced 5 days after an LH surge is detected. Similarly in a cycle using cryopreserved oocytes, they can be thawed 1 day post LH surge with subsequent transfer of day 3/5 embryos.

Several meta-analyses have demonstrated equal efficacy of different protocols of endometrial preparation in maximizing the endometrial receptivity. However natural cycle transfers have less flexibility and increased chance of cancellation. Large RCT showed that pregnancy rates in natural transfers are higher if vaginal (400 mg) progesterone is initiated after embryo transfer compared to no progesterone.[22]

FACTORS PREDICTING SUCCESS OF A DONOR PROGRAM

Recipient Related Factors

Maternal Age

The age of the recipient seems to be the most important factor predicting a successful outcome. In a prospective study of 270 cycles, woman <40 years had significantly higher implantation rate and ongoing pregnancies as compared to those >40 years (22.1% vs. 11.5%; 36.8% vs. 23.6% p = 0.001). The importance of age was emphasized by another retrospective cohort study of 27,959 fresh donor oocyte transfer cycles from the Society for Assisted Reproduction Technology (SART) registry which concluded that donor oocyte recipients have stable rates of pregnancy outcomes before age 45 years, after which there is a small but steady and significant decline. This is indicative probably of uterine senescence leading to decreased fertility potential, despite younger oocytes.[23]

Paternal Age

There are conflicting reports in literature regarding the effect of paternal age on the pregnancy rates of donor oocyte cycles. A systemic review and meta-analysis including 12,538 oocyte-donation cases concluded that the available evidence did not suggest an association between advanced paternal age and adverse reproductive outcome in donor oocyte cycles, although the quality of evidence was suboptimal.[24]

Endometrial Thickness

The evidence regarding impact of endometrial thickness on oocyte donation cycles is conflicting. Whereas a recently published retrospective analysis of 4,070 cycles reported that endometrial thickness ≥5 mm is a reasonable parameter for determining success in oocyte donation cycles.[25] The best reproductive outcomes tend to be achieved if the endometrium is >8–9 mm. There is no consensus in literature regarding the impact of trilaminar hypoechogenic pattern of endometrium on reproductive outcomes.[26] Another 2022 study revealed that ENT change after 6 days of progesterone administration, whether increased or decreased, does not have any significant effect on LBR and clinical pregnancy rates (CPR) in fresh OD recipients.[27]

Recipient Diagnosis

The cause of infertility in the recipient did not seem to affect the reproductive outcome of the donor cycle.[25,26]

High Body Mass Index

It is not an independent predictor of live birth in recipient cycles. Large meta-analysis comparing pregnancy outcomes amongst obese and non-obese recipients of egg donation cycles did not find any difference in implantation, clinical pregnancy, and live birth or miscarriage rates.[28] This was contrary to cohort and cross-sectional studies showing a poorer reproductive outcome of obese women using their own oocytes. This might imply that high body mass index (BMI) might have a significant negative impact on the quality of the oocyte rather than endometrial receptivity which is overcome in an obese recipient by using an oocyte donor.[28] Interestingly though, study by Cardozo et al. found increased donor BMI to be associated with decreased pregnancy and live birth rates.[29] In a most recent September 2022 study conducted over 5 years aimed to determine if overweight and obese oocyte recipients had similar pregnancy outcomes compared with healthy weight controls after the transfer of a single euploid frozen–thawed embryo transfer (FET).[30] The results of the study showed that BMI alone does not adversely alter endometrial receptivity and is not the cause of poor IVF outcomes in patients with increased BMI. These deleterious IVF outcomes might be the result of diminished oocyte and/or embryo quality or other factors that have not yet been elucidated.

Blastocyst Transfer

Advances in the culture systems and improved blastocyst cryopreservation programs have played a major role in improving the success rates of oocyte donation cycles. Various prospective randomized and retrospective series have shown superior results per transfer in blastocyst cycles compared to cleavage day 3 embryo cycles. Thus, recipients of oocyte donation cycles can opt for blastocyst transfer as an effective method for increasing pregnancy rates and reducing multiple pregnancies.[31]

This has led to a recommendation in 2013 from the American Society for Reproductive Medicine stating that in the case of young oocyte donors, only a single blastocyst-stage (eSET) or no more than two cleavage-stage embryos may be transferred. However there has been poor compliance with these guidelines and a retrospective analysis of 13,939 cycles found only 18% to be complaint. A study conducted in March 2022 stated that among fresh donor oocyte transfers, only (55%) underwent eSET. Non-adherence with transfer guidelines was associated with dramatically increased multiple pregnancies, preterm births, and low birth weights.[32]

Fresh versus Frozen Embryo Transfer

Frozen embryo transfer (ET) with vitrification has been associated with improved pregnancy rates, but also increased rates of large for gestational age infants.[38] Donor oocyte recipients represent an attractive biological model to attempt to isolate the impact of embryo cryopreservation on IVF outcomes, yet there is a paucity of studies in this population. Recent retrospective cohort study of the SART data from 2014–17 analyzing 33,893 cycles also found that that in cycles using fresh donor oocytes, live birth rates were statistically significantly higher following fresh embryo transfer compared with cryopreserved-thawed embryo transfer, even when PGT-A was performed.[33] However, this study is limited by the potential for selection and confounding bias.

Recent study in 2022 suggested that there was no significant difference between the fresh ET and FET groups in terms of mean birth weight. However, artificial endometrial preparation was associated with a higher birth weight when compared with a transfer in a natural cycle. No other statistically significant differences were found in the remaining neonatal and maternal outcomes studies between the fresh ET and FET groups.

On the contrary another 2022 study in October stated that vitrified donor oocytes were associated with improved pregnancy outcomes compared with fresh donor oocytes in patients undergoing single embryo transfer.[34]

Preimplantation Genetic Testing

Although a study of US data from the Society for Assisted Reproductive Technology Clinic Outcome Reporting System from 2005–2013, found the adjusted odds of live birth to be reduced by 35% in donor recipient cycles, this could be as they included cleavage stage PGT-A, which is no longer in clinical practice.[35] A retrospective analysis of 398 donor frozen ET (FET) cycles comparing blastocyst embryos that either underwent trophectoderm biopsy PGT-A using array comparative genomic hybridization or next-generation sequencing (NGS) versus unbiopsied and untested embryos demonstrated higher live birth rate for PGT-A embryos.[39]

TABLE 2: Correlation between number of retrieved oocytes with live birth rates.

Oocyte source and day of transfer	*No. of retrieved oocytes*	*Overall live birth rate in %*
Donor, day 2–3 (n = 14,744)	1–5	15.1
	6–10	23.6
	11–15	27.5
	16–25	33.5
	>26	46.3
p value for trend	<.0001	

On the contrary, a most recent 2021 cohort study stated that preimplantation genetic testing for aneuploidies does not increase success rates in fresh oocyte donation cycles.[36,37]

Donor Factors

Age

Age of the donor seems to be the only factor influencing the outcome in egg donation cycles. Study was conducted by Wang et al. to compare the pregnancy and live delivery rates in oocyte recipients of various age groups as well as different donor age groups. Donor age was found to have the most significant effect with the highest live birthrate observed in cycles with donors aged 30–34 years (25.0%), followed by 24.1% in donors aged <30 years and lowest rates in cycles with donors aged >40 years. A recent population-based cohort study also found donor age to be critical to cumulative birth rates in recipients, irrespective of recipient age.[40]

Although previous reproductive outcome of donor has been shown to have a positive effect on reproductive outcome in egg donation cycles, there is no evidence suggesting a significant difference.

Number of Mature Oocytes (MII) Retrieved

A retrospective cohort study in Massachusetts of 237 fresh donor oocyte ET cycles, the greatest probability of live birth was observed in cycles with more oocytes retrieved (>10), more mature oocytes, and an increased number of cleavage stage embryos.[41]

An analysis of Society for Assisted Reproductive Technology data has revealed a positive correlation between number of retrieved oocytes with live birth rates and embryos available for cryopreservation even after adjusting for age and previous births **(Table 2)**.

REPRODUCTIVE AND OBSTETRIC OUTCOMES

Pregnancy and Implantation Rates

The European IVF Monitoring (EIM) consortium report of 2014 on reproductive outcome with use of donor oocytes, reported a PR of 50.4% per fresh embryo transfer, and 48.7% using frozen oocytes.[42] In comparison, use of autologous oocytes resulted in a CPR of 29.9% per aspiration, 35.8% per transfer, and 27 .6 % with FET, and an overall multiple PR of 17.9%. The rate of twin pregnancy was also significantly higher in women with IVF-oocyte donation compared to IVF and spontaneous pregnancy (39.4% vs. 15.0% with IVF and 2.5% with spontaneous, $p<0.001$).[43]

A recent study of 40,485 IVF cycles using donor oocytes reported to the Society for Assisted Reproductive Technology registry in 2016–2018 was published. There was decline in LBR with increasing age and BMI of the recipients. They observed an increase in LBR with >16 oocytes retrieval as well as with blastocyst transfer versus a cleavage transfer.[44]

Maternal Outcomes

Most studies have demonstrated good obstetric outcomes for recipients of egg donation cycles except for an increase in hypertensive disorders and cesarean section rates.[45]

A total of 217 OD and 363 control singleton pregnancies were compared for percentage of hypertensive disorders of pregnancy for OD versus controls.[46] The results of this large, comparative, matched cohort study detected a tripling of the pregnancy induced hypertension (PIH) risk for young women with OD pregnancies that was confirmed by multivariate analyses. In addition, they demonstrated an increase in the severity of PIH among OD recipients, as evidenced by higher rates of preeclampsia and even eclampsia compared with controls.[47] The underlying cause for this increase in hypertensive disorder is believed to be placental dysfunction. It is postulated that the trophoblastic human leukocyte antigen-C in donated oocytes is less recognizable to the maternal immune system, leading to an altered functionality of the uterine natural killer cells and consequently an altered maternal blood supply to the placenta.

Studies have also found an increased occurrence of first-trimester bleeding, gestational diabetes,[39] placental abnormalities,[40] intrauterine growth restriction (IUGR), preterm delivery,[40,41] prolonged maternal hospitalization after delivery, and increased prevalence of cesarean section in oocyte donation recipients.[48]

Neonatal Outcomes

Neonatal complications include an increased risk of prematurity, extreme prematurity, small for gestational age (SGA), low birth weight (LBW), and very LBW (VLBW). The perinatal outcomes between pregnancies with donor and autologous eggs have been found to be similar in a meta-analysis of 23 studies by Adams et al.[49] Subsequently Kamath et al. analyzed large HFEA data and found the adjusted odds ratio to be significantly higher for preterm birth and LBW after oocyte donation.[50]

On Donor

Women who donate their oocytes to others are exposed to physical and psychological burdens they would not otherwise face. There is some risk of unintentional pregnancy because hormonal contraceptives must be discontinued for donation to occur. Donors also are exposed to risks of morbidity and a remote risk of mortality from controlled ovarian stimulation and oocyte retrieval. Young women may be prone to dismiss the potential psychological consequences of donation, particularly those that could arise if they later experience infertility problems themselves. In addition, they may underestimate the psychological and legal consequences of their agreement to forgo parental rights and future contact with children born to oocyte recipients.

There is still not much evidence and many unanswered questions regarding the long-term medical and psychological effects of egg donation on donors.

Short-term risks of egg donation include OHSS (0.38%), intra-abdominal bleeding, infection, ovarian torsion, and short-term subfertility (5–10%). Serious complications seem to be rare (<1%).[51,52] Few studies have examined the long-term medical effects of egg donation, such as fertility, cancer, and other potential health risks.

OOCYTE BANKING

The first pregnancy using cryopreserved oocyte was reported in 1986 and in India in 2009. Advances in cryopreservation techniques especially vitrification led to the ASRM revoking the experimental tag for oocyte cryopreservation in 2012.[53]

In the first reported experience with the establishment of a commercial donor egg bank in 2007, Akin et al. recruited donors according to ASRM guidelines for gamete and embryo donation. Studies have shown comparable ongoing pregnancy rates in oocyte donor IVF cycles utilizing either cryobanked oocytes or fresh oocyte donation **(Figs. 4A and B)**. Owing to the advances in vitrification, comparable survival rates, and reproductive outcomes, there has been shift in trend with more couples opting for oocyte banking.

Potential Benefits of Commercial Egg Banks

Commercial egg banks offer multiple potential benefits over conventional donor oocyte programs. Benefits of oocyte cryopreservation include simplified IVF logistics since coordinating donor and recipient cycles is no longer necessary, reduced costs, and a faster flow as donors can be selected from a bank and used relatively quickly.[54] According to the ASRM guideline, recipients can be counseled that cryopreserved donor oocytes are a reasonable option with no significant difference in per transfer pregnancy rates compared to fresh donor oocytes.[55] In addition, the ability to routinely implement a quarantine period for infectious

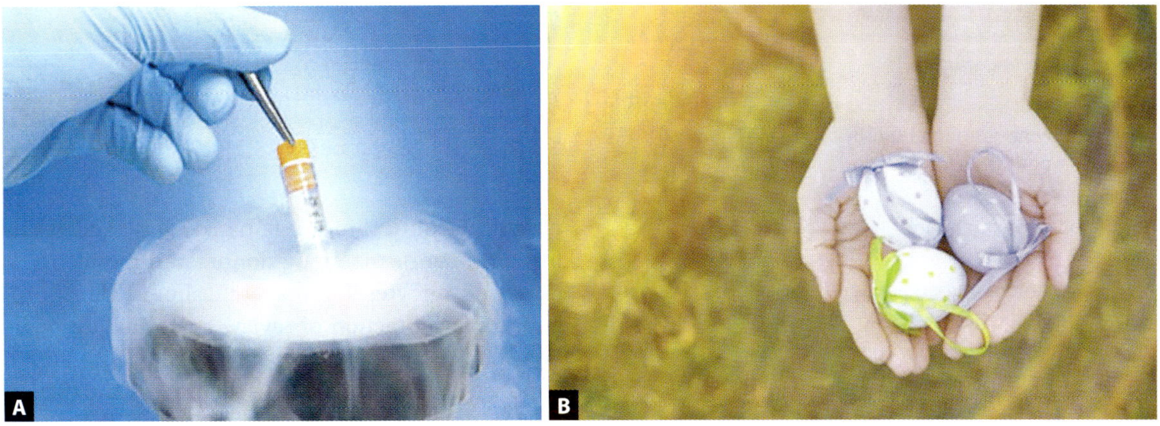

Figs. 4A and B: Oocyte banking.

disease testing, analogous to the practice in sperm banking, increases patient safety. Furthermore, an increasingly global network of commercial egg banks will permit a larger pool of ethnically diverse donors for selection.

Apart from the cost-effectiveness, the waiting time for a donor is also significantly lesser when an oocyte bank comes into picture. This also ensures reduction in wastage of gametes. Donor oocyte vitrification has become more commercialized in recent years with the development of multiple egg bank programs.[56] As per the ART ACT in India, it states that oocytes collected from "donors" shall be stored for 10 years.

OOCYTE SHARING

The system of oocyte sharing is that in which an indigent infertile couple that needs to raise resources for ART agrees to donate oocytes to an affluent infertile couple wherein the wife can carry a pregnancy through but cannot produce her own oocyte, for IVF with the sperm of the male partner of the affluent couple, for a monitory compensation that would take care of the expenses of an ART procedure on the indigent couple.[58] This concept has generated considerable interest, especially in countries where commercial egg donation is not allowed or there is paucity of egg donors.[57]A successful cycle needs careful assessment of the donor by antral follicle count, AMH, age, and cause of infertility.[59] If the number of eggs recovered is lower or of poor quality, both donor and recipient's cycles may be compromised with neither having sufficient good quality embryos to transfer and/or cryopreserve, necessitating a fresh IVF cycle with its inherent costs.

Oocyte vitrification and banking have changed the concept of oocyte sharing from one that involved sharing of oocytes between two sub fertile couples to one where the eggs of a commercial donor are shared. A second scenario is where the number of oocytes obtained from a single donor is shared between two recipients and the cost of the cycle is shared between the recipients. In vitro fertilization patients in these sharing arrangements generally donate up to half the oocytes retrieved in a single cycle to another patient, in return for a 50–60% reduction in the total costs of the IVF cycle. Oocyte-sharing programs reportedly exist in a number of other countries, including the United Kingdom, Israel, Denmark, Australia, Spain, and Greece.

Donors in oocyte-sharing programs also may be required to undergo the additional medical and psychological screening required of oocyte donors. They also may experience extra psychological burdens. A donor who remains childless may feel added distress based on her knowledge that another couple may become the parents of a child genetically related to her. The major advantage of oocyte sharing is drop in financial burden. However, as per the new rules in the ART ACT in India, a bank shall not supply the sperm or oocyte of a single donor to more than one commissioning couple.

OOCYTE DONOR PROGRAMS FOR STEM CELL RESEARCH

The IVF procedures may also be used to create blastocysts for non-reproductive purposes. Blastocysts may be created for fundamental research to study basic biological mechanisms of early embryo development. Human embryonic stem cells (ESCs) typically derived from human blastocysts have been used to develop specific human ESC lines, thus enabling the study of specific diseases[55]

REMUNERATION

In recognition of the significant time, inconvenience, and discomfort associated with oocyte donation, two types of remuneration are common. One is monetary compensation to women who undergo COS and oocyte retrieval for the sole purpose of providing donor oocytes. Another form of financial compensation involves an arrangement known as oocyte sharing as described formerly in this chapter.

The legal status and cost or compensation models of egg donation vary significantly from one country to another **(Table 3)**.

TABLE 3: Legal implications of donor cycle.

Legal status of oocyte donation[44]	*Country*
Totally legal	Italy, Germany, Austria
Legal only if anonymous and gratuitous. Without any compensation for the egg donor	France
Legal only if non-anonymous and gratuitous	Canada
Legal only if anonymous, but egg donors may be compensated	Spain, Czech Republic, South Africa, India
Legal only if non-anonymous, but egg donors may be compensated	UK
Legal whether or not it is anonymous, and egg donors may be compensated	USA

Compensation for egg donors is another ethical gray area with much debate regarding adequate compensation amount which should at least be generous enough for undergoing the necessary medical procedures rather than according to number of eggs. The regulations of the respective country influence the reproductive process in the sense that, in countries that prohibit compensation there is an extreme dearth of young women willing to go through this procedure. There is an increase in medical tourism to countries where the process is legal and anonymous. Half the donor cycles in Europe occur in Spain as egg donation is illegal in a number of European countries including Germany, Austria, and Italy.[60] Similarly many Canadians travel to the US for ART procedures due to lenient laws. A law enacted in California in 2019 likewise requires women who provide human oocytes for research to be compensated for their time, discomfort, and inconvenience in the same manner as other research subjects, removing a previous prohibition of compensation of research donors.

Additionally, in most countries where it is legal and compensated, the law places a cap on the compensation and that cap tends to be in the vicinity of $1,000–$2,000 in western countries while maybe a meager 25,000–30,000 rupees in India. Higher compensation may be offered in some clinics according to favorable physical attributes, educational qualifications, or previous good outcomes in recipients.

In India, as per ART ACT 2021, clause 3.9.2. banks will be encouraged to obtain (for example, through appropriate advertisement) and maintain information on possible oocyte donors. The oocyte donor may be compensated suitably (e.g., financially) by the bank when the oocyte is donated.

DISCLOSURE AND COUNSELING

Prospective donors should be fully informed about the potential medical and psychological risks of undergoing oocyte retrieval for reproduction or research. This ethical obligation to ensure the informed consent of prospective donors attaches to any party or program seeking the services of an oocyte donor, including providers assisting intended parents, fertility clinics, egg banks, and agencies involved in recruiting or matching donors and recipients. Women donating oocytes for research should be afforded the additional protection of review by an institutional review board or other required oversight body with authority for approval of the informed consent process and documents.

BOX 3: Advantages of donor regulations.

- Protection of intended couple rights
- Protection of donor rights
- Avoiding physical and psychological exploitation of donors
- Increase in medical tourism

The potential negative health and psychological effects of oocyte donation should be openly acknowledged **(Box 3)**. Prospective donors should understand the measures they must take to avoid unwanted pregnancy during a stimulation cycle. They also should understand that they could later develop desires to establish contact with their genetically related children, desires that may be difficult to satisfy because of legal or other barriers. Alternatively, donors should be apprised that remaining anonymous to the recipient(s) or resulting offspring may not be possible because of increasingly sophisticated genetic tracing and social-media technologies.

ETHICAL CONCERNS REGARDING OOCYTE DONATION

Both monetary compensation and oocyte sharing create the possibility of undue inducement and exploitation in the oocyte donation process. Women may agree to provide oocytes in response to financial need. High payments could lead some prospective donors to conceal medical information relevant to their own health or that of their biologic offspring. Patients undergoing IVF who cannot afford the procedure may, because of the intensity of their desire to have children, consent to share oocytes without careful consideration of risks and burdens. With both types of compensation, there is a possibility that women will discount the physical and emotional risks of oocyte donation out of eagerness to address their financial situations or their infertility problems. Financial compensation also could be challenged on grounds that it conflicts with the prevailing belief that gametes should not become products bought and sold in the marketplace.

OFFENSES AND THEIR IMPLICATIONS

Any registered medical practitioner is bound to perform certain duties, and under any circumstances, the person must not:

- Abandon, disown or exploit (or cause to be abandoned, disowned, or exploited) the child born through ART.
- Sell human embryos or gametes or run an agency, a racket, or an organization for selling, purchasing, or trading in human embryos or gametes.

- Import, or help in getting imported the human embryos or human gametes.
- Exploit the commissioning couple, woman, or gamete donor in any form.
- Transfer a human embryo into a male person or an animal.
- Sell any human embryo or gamete for the purpose of research.
- Use any intermediates to obtain gamete donors or purchase gamete, donors.

The ART Act has made the abovementioned acts punishable under the law. Anyone found guilty of the commission of any of these acts is punishable with a fine which is not <5 lakh rupees but may extend to 10 lakh rupees for the first contravention; and for subsequent contravention, will be punishable with imprisonment for a term which is not <3 years but may extend to 8 years and with fine which is not <10 lakh rupees but can extend to 20 lakh rupees.

Courts can only take cognizance of an offense punishable under the ART Act if a complaint is made to it by the National Board or the State Board, or by an officer authorized by it.

No court inferior to that of a Metropolitan Magistrate or a Judicial Magistrate of the first class can try any offense punishable under the ART Act. Further, all offenses under this Act are cognizable and bailable.

In addition, it is pertinent to add that where an offense under the ART Act has been committed by any clinic or bank, the executive head of such clinic or bank will be deemed to be guilty of an offense and will be liable to be proceeded against and punished accordingly, unless he/she proves that the offense was committed without their knowledge or that he/she exercised all due diligence to prevent the commission of such offense.

SPERM DONATION

Indications

Donor semen insemination is mainly used for couples where the male partner is suffering from azoospermia or severe oligoasthenoteratozoospermia **(Box 4)**.

The rules, duties, and regulations regarding sperm banking have been discussed earlier.

BOX 4: Common indications for artificial insemination with donor sperm.

- Non-obstructive azoospermia with failure to retrieve testicular sperms
- Severe oligozoospermia with financial restrictions
- Hereditary genetic defect in male partner not willing for PGD
- The couple has Rh incompatibility
- Anejaculation or retrograde ejaculation not willing for sophisticated ART such as ICSI
- Failed fertilization on ICSI

(ART: assisted reproductive technology; ICSI: intracytoplasmic sperm injection; PGD: preimplantation genetic diagnosis).

Quarantine of Semen Samples

One of the important reasons for freezing semen from donors is that any donor semen has to be quarantined for 6 months. Donors whose semen is frozen for future use are required to report to the ART bank 6 months after donation to be checked for HIV infection or disease status. This helps in avoiding donors who are infected of with venereal diseases, hepatitis B or C, or HIV. The safety of using frozen sperm has been abundantly proven, both by experimental work and the actual results in humans. The only drawback of sperm freezing is the likelihood of an approximately 20% loss in motility after thawing which is an acceptable bargain compared with the risk of acquiring infections.[60,61]

Sperm Donor Screening

The investigation described in **Box 5** should be performed on the intended donor.

Apart from this, the basic information that has to be obtained is listed in **Box 6**.

BOX 5: Investigations for sperm donor.

- Complete blood picture, blood group, and Rh status:
  - Hemoglobin
  - Total RBC count
  - Total WBC count
  - Differential WBC count
  - Platelet count
  - Peripheral smear
- Random blood sugar
- Blood urea or Serum creatinine
- SGPT
- Routine urine examination
- HBsAg status
- Hepatitis C status
- HIV1 status with date of the tests done
- Hemoglobin A2 (for thalassemia) status
- HIV PCR2 (positive or negative)

(HIV PCR2: human immunodeficiency virus polymerase chain reaction 2; SGPT: serum glutamic pyruvic transaminase).

BOX 6. Information to be obtained from the donor.

- Identification number (Donor ID)
- Age or date of birth
- Marital status
- Education: a. Donor b. Spouse
- Occupation: a. Donor b. Spouse
- Monthly income
- Religion
- Obstetric history of wife: a. Number of deliveries b. Number of abortions c. Other points of note
- History of use of contraceptives
- Medical history
- Family history from the medical point of view
- History of any abnormality in a child of the donor
- History of blood transfusion
- History of substance abuse

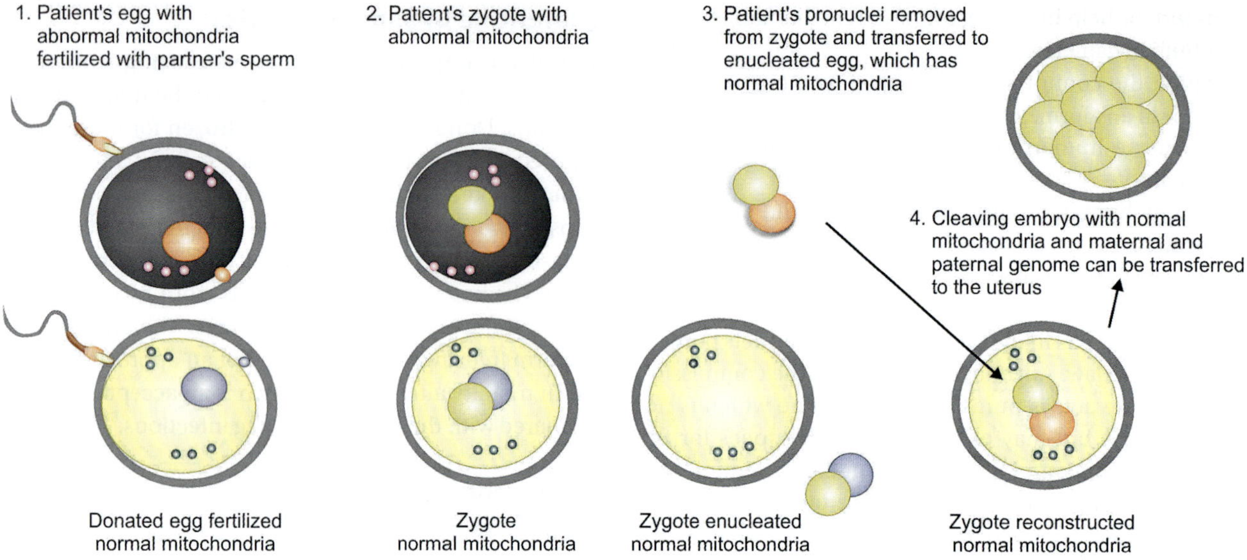

Fig. 5: Use of assisted reproductive technology to prevent inheritable mitochondrial disease.

The consent for the husband is mandatory to perform a donor insemination.

Consent for semen freezing should also include clauses such as ownership of semen sample in case of the death of the donor. If there is non-payment of fees, ART bank would have the right to destroy the semen sample or donate it for research in case due charges are not paid or if there are no bona fide claimants in case of death of the donor.

Posthumous Artificial Insemination Husband through Sperm Bank

Since according to Indian Evidence Act, 1872, a child born within 280 days after dissolution of marriage (by death or divorce) is a legitimate child; the same can be extrapolated in context of ART using cryopreserved semen to bear a child after death of the husband. Thus, a child born via posthumous autoimmune hepatitis through sperm banking is considered legitimate.

THREE-PARENT ASSISTED REPRODUCTIVE TECHNOLOGY

Mitochondrial diseases arise due to mutations in either mitochondrial DNA or in nuclear genes involved in mitochondrial function. The morbidity of such diseases is severe because they affect critical organs such as brain, heart, muscle, and central nervous system and are non-curative. Novel ART techniques to prevent inheritable mitochondrial disease include transfer of genetic material between oocytes and embryos.

Either replacement of the nucleus from the pronuclear stage zygote of an affected woman to a healthy enucleated zygote; in the second technique, the metaphase II spindle from the unfertilized oocyte of an affected woman is transferred to an enucleated donor oocyte.[61] These technologies have been found encouraging in animal models but need more robust human data before implementation. Offspring resulting from such fertilized ova containing ooplasm (including mitochondria) from a donor ovum now have three genetic parents. In such cases, ooplasm donor must be thoroughly screened and give consent **(Fig. 5)**.

KEY POINTS

- Third-party reproduction is an essential part of ART helping infertile couples to achieve the dream of parenthood.
- Meticulous evaluation of the recipients and donors coupled with adequate counseling helps in the smooth running of a donor program.

REFERENCES

1. HuffPost. (2015). 30k–60k US sperm and egg donor births per year. [online] Available from https://www.huffpost.com/entry/a-call-to-to-stop-using-t_b_8126736 [Last accessed December, 2022].
2. Swapp GH, Johnston AW, Watt JL, Couzin DA, Stephen GS. A fertile woman with non-mosaic Turner's syndrome. Case report and review of the literature. Br J Obstet Gynaecol. 1989;96:876-80.
3. Yaron Y, Ochshorn Y, Amit A, Yovel I, Kogosowki A, Lessing JB. Patients with Turner's syndrome may have an inherent endometrial abnormality affecting receptivity in oocyte donation. Fertil Steril.1996;65(6):1249-52.
4. Mercadal BA, Imbert R, Demeestere I, Englert Y, Delbaere A. Pregnancy outcome after oocyte donation in patients with Turner's syndrome and partial Xmonosomy. Hum Reprod. 2011;26(8);2061-8.
5. Hagman A, Loft A, Wennerholm UB, Pinborg A, Bergh C, Aittomäki K, et al. Obstetric and neonatal outcome after oocyte donation in 106 women with Turner syndrome: a Nordic cohort study. Hum Reprod. 2013; 28(6):1598-609.
6. Lok Sabha. (2021). The Assisted Reproductive Technology (Regulation) Bill, 2021. [online] Available from

http://164.100.47.4/BillsTexts/LSBillTexts/Passed Loksabha/97-C_2020_LS_Eng.pdf [Last accessed December, 2022].
7. Burton G, Abdalla HI, Kirkland A, Studd JW. The role of oocyte donation in women who are unsuccessful with in-vitro fertilization treatment. Hum Reprod. 1992;7:1103-5.
8. Jurkovic D, Geipel A, Gruboeck K, Jauniaux E, Natucci M, Campbell S. Three-dimensional ultrasound for the assessment of uterine anatomy and detection of congenital anomalies: a comparison with hysterosalpingography and two-dimensional sonography. Ultrasound Obstet Gynecol. 1995;5:233-7.
9. Clua Obradó E, Palacios-Verdú G, Sumarroca M, Martínez F, Polyzos N, O-144 Adverse pregnancy and neonatal outcomes in an oocyte donation program. Expanded Carrier Screening can substantially decrease the risk of recessive conditions, Hum Reprod. 2022;37(Suppl 1):deac105.044.
10. Cohen MA, Lindheim SR, Sauer MV. Donor age is paramount to success in oocyte donation. Hum Reprod.1999;14:2755-8.
11. Practice Committee of the American Society for Reproductive Medicine and the Practice Committee of the Society for Assisted Reproductive Technology. Recommendations for gamete and embryo donation: a committee opinion. Fertil Steril. 2013;99(1):47-62.e1.
12. ACOG committee opinion. Genetic screening of gamete donors. Number 192, October 1997. Committee on Genetics. American College of Obstetricians and Gynecologists. Int J Gynaecol Obstet.1998;60:190-2.
13. Męczekalski B, Maciejewska-Jeske M, Podfigurna A. Reproduction in premature ovarian insufficiency patients - from latest studies to therapeutic approach. Prz Menopauzalny. 2018;17(3):117-9.
14. Andre H, Pimentel C, Veau S, Domin-Bernhard M, Letur-Konirsch H, Priou G, et al. Pregnancies and obstetrical prognosis after oocyte donation in Turner syndrome: a multicentric study. Eur J Obstet Gynecol Reprod Biol. 2019;238:73-7.
15. Alyasin A, Mehdinejadiani S, Ghasemi M. GnRH agonist trigger versus hCG trigger in GnRH antagonist in IVF/ICSI cycles: a review article. Int J Reprod Biomed. 2016; 14(9):557-566
16. Guan S, Feng Y, Huang Y, Huang J. Progestin-Primed Ovarian Stimulation Protocol for Patients in Assisted Reproductive Technology: A Meta-Analysis of Randomized Controlled Trials. Front Endocrinol (Lausanne). 2021;12:702558.
17. Ethics Committee of the American Society for Reproductive Medicine. Informing offspring of their conception by gamete donation. Fertil Steril. 2004;81(3).
18. Farfan JC, Guerrero J, García AB. Outcomes Following Random Start Plus Progestin Primed Ovarian Stimulation In An Oocyte Donation Program. Fertil Steril. 2022;118.4:e315.
19. Sagi-Dain L, Sagi S, Dirnfeld M. Effect of paternal age on reproductive outcomes in oocyte donation model: a systematic review. Fertil Steril. 2015;104:857-65.
20. Yeh JS. Pregnancy outcomes decline in recipients over age 44: an analysis of 27,959 fresh donor oocyte in vitro fertilization cycles from the Society for Assisted Reproductive Technology. Fertil Steril. 2014;101:1331-6.
21. Ameratunga D, Weston G, Osianlis T, Catt J, Vollenhoven B. In vitro fertilization (IVF) with donor eggs in post-menopausal women: are there differences in pregnancy outcomes in women with premature ovarian failure (POF) compared with women with physiological age-related menopause? Assist Reprod Genet. 2009;26:511-4.
22. Gupta P, Banker M, Patel P, Joshi B. A study of recipient related predictors of success in oocyte donation program. J Hum Reprod Sci. 2012;5(3):252-7.
23. Dviri M, Madjunkova S, Koziarz A, Madjunkov M, Mashiach J, Nekolaichuk E, et al. Is there an association between paternal age and aneuploidy? Evidence from young donor oocyte-derived embryos: a systematic review and individual patient data meta-analysis. Hum Reprod Update. 2021;27(3):486-500.
24. Jungheim ES, Schon SB, Schulte MB, DeUgarte DA, Fowler SA, Tuuli MG. IVF outcomes in obese donor oocyte recipients: a systematic review and meta-analysis. Hum Reprod. 2013;28:2720-7.
25. Arce H, Velilla E, López-Teijón M. Association between endometrial thickness in oocyte donation cycles and pregnancy success rates. Reprod Fertil Dev. 2015. doi: 10.1071/RD14459. Epub ahead of print. PMID: 25707405.
26. Gursu T, Goksever Celik H, Eraslan A, Angun B, Ozaltin S, Yeh J, et al. Impact of endometrial thickness change in response to progesterone on live birth rates embryo transfers with fresh oocyte donation cycles. J Obstet Gynecol. 2022;1-8.
27. Rittenberg V, Seshadri S, Sunkara SK, Sobaleva S, Oteng-Ntim E, El-Toukhy T. Effect of body mass index on IVF treatment outcome: an updated systematic review and meta-analysis. Reprod Biomed Online. 2011;23:421-39.
28. Cardozo ER, Karmon AE, Gold J, Petrozza JC, Styer AK. Reproductive outcomes in oocyte donation cycles are associated with donor BMI. Hum Reprod. 2016;31(2):385-92.
29. Moreta LE, Hanley W, Lee JA, Copperman AB, Stein D. Elevated Body Mass Index in Donor Oocyte Recipients Does Not Affect Implantation of Euploid Embryos. J Womens Health (Larchmt). 2022;31(9):1364-8.
30. Brady PC. Serum progesterone concentration on day of embryo transfer in donor oocyte cycles. J Assist Reprod Genet. 2014;31:569-75.
31. Gingold JA, Fazzari M, Gerber R, Kappy M, Goodman M, Lieman H, et al. Adherence to embryo transfer guidelines in favorable-prognosis patients aged less than 35 years using autologous oocytes and in recipients using donor oocytes: a Society for Assisted Reproductive Technology Clinic Outcome Reporting System study. Fertil Steril. 2022;117(3):548-59.
32. Noyes N. Factors useful in predicting the success of oocyte donation: a 3-year retrospective analysis. Fertil Steril.2001;76.
33. Glatthorn HN, Klimczak AM, Herlihy N, Margolis CK, Roberts LM, Reig A, et al. Vitrified Donor Oocytes Are Associated With Improved Pregnancy Outcomes Compared With Fresh Donor Oocytes In Patients Undergoing Single Frozen Embryo Transfer. Fertil Steril. 2022;118(4):e380.
34. Schoolcraft WB, Gardner DK. Blastocyst culture and transfer increases the efficiency of oocyte donation. Fertil Steril. 2000;74:482-6.
35. Van der Auwera I, Debrock S, Spienssens C, Afschrift H, Bakelants E, Meuleman C, et al. A prospective randomized study: day 2 versus day 5 embryo transfer. Hum Reprod. 2002;17:1507-12.
36. Martello CL, Kulmann MIR, Donatti LM, Bos-Mikich A, Frantz N. Preimplantation genetic testing for aneuploidies does not increase success rates in fresh oocyte donation cycles: a paired cohort study. J Assist Reprod Genet. 2021;38(11):2909-14.
37. Check JH, Choe JK, Nazari A, Fox F, Swenson K. Fresh embryo transfer is more effective than frozen for donor oocyte recipients but not for donors. Hum Reprod. 2001;16(7):1403-8.

38. Coates A, Bankowski BJ, Kung A, Griffin DK, Munne S. Differences in pregnancy outcomes in donor egg frozen embryo transfer (FET) cycles following preimplantation genetic screening (PGS): a single center retrospective study. J Assist Reprod Genet. 2017;34:71-8.
39. Wang YA, Farquhar C, Sullivan EA. Donor age is a major determinant of success of oocyte donation/recipient programme. Hum Reprod. 2012;27(1):118-25.
40. Baker VL. Association of number of retrieved oocytes with live birth rate and birth weight: an analysis of 231,815 cycles of in vitro fertilization. Fertil Steril. 2015;103:931-8.
41. Letur H. Hypertensive pathologies and egg donation pregnancies: results of a large comparative cohort study. Fertil Steril. 2016;106:284-90.
42. Sheffer-Mimouni G, Mashiach S, Dor J, Levran D, Seidman DS. Factors influencing the obstetric and perinatal outcome after oocyte donation. Hum Reprod. 2002;17(10):2636-40.
43. Williams RS, Ellis DD, Wilkinson EA, Kramer JM, Datta S, Guzick DS. Factors affecting live birth rates in donor oocytes from commercial egg banks vs. program egg donors: an analysis of 40,485 cycles from the Society for Assisted Reproductive Technology registry in 2016–2018. Fertil Steril. 2022;117(2):339-48.
44. Malchau SS. Perinatal outcomes in 375 children born after oocyte donation: a Danish national cohort study. Fertil Steril. 2013;99:1637-43.
45. Davies MJ. Reproductive technologies and the risk of birth defects. N Engl J Med. 2012;366:1803-13.
46. Bodri D. Risk and complications associated with egg donation. In: Sauer MV, (Ed). Principles of oocyte and embryo donation. New York: Springer; 2013:205-19.
47. Rodriguez-Wallberg KA, Berger AS, Fagerberg A, Olofsson JI, Scherman-Pukk C, Lindqvist PG, et al. Increased incidence of obstetric and perinatal complications in pregnancies achieved using donor oocytes and single embryo transfer in young and healthy women. A prospective hospital-based matched cohort study. Gynecol Endocrinol. 2019;35(4):314-319.
48. Stoop D, Vercammen L, Polyzos NP, de Vos M, Nekkebroeck J, Devroey P. Effect of ovarian stimulation and oocyte retrieval on reproductive outcome in oocyte donors. Fertil Steril. 2012;97:1328-30.
49. Woodriff M, Sauer MV, Klitzman R. Advocating for longitudinal follow-up of the health and welfare of egg donors. Fertil Steril. 2014; 102(3):662-6.
50. Bukulmez O. Repetitive oocyte donation does not decrease serum anti-Müllerian hormone levels. Fertil Steril. 2010; 94:905-12.
51. Domingues TS, Aquino AP, Barros B, Mazetto R, Nicolielo M, Kimati CM, et al. Oocyte survival rate highly affect the outcomes of an oocyte bank for an egg donation program. Fertil Steril. 104(3):e225.
52. Li L, Fischer E, Castaneda D, Conaghan J, Ryan I. Frozen thawed donor oocytes have equivalent embryo developmental competency compared to fresh donor oocytes – a single center experience from pacific fertility egg bank (PFEB). Fertility and Sterility. 2017;107(3):e30-1.
53. Glujovsky D. A shared egg donor program: which is the minimum number of oocytes to be allocated? J Assist Reprod Genet. 2011;28:263-7.
54. Carson SA. Proposed oocyte donation guidelines for stem cell research. Fertil Steril. 2010;94:2503-6.
55. Fox News. (2012). Fertility treatment bans in Europe draw criticism. 04-13.
56. Kovacs P. Seeking IVF Abroad: Medical Tourism for Infertile Couples. Medscape. 2010;06:24.
57. Check JH, Wilson C, Jamison T, Choe JK, Cohen R. The sharing of eggs by infertile women who are trying to conceive themselves with an egg recipient for financial advantages does not jeopardize the donor's chance of conceiving. Clin Exp Obstet Gynecol. 2012;39(4):432-3.
58. Kunt C, Ozaksit G, Keskin Kurt R, Cakir Gungor AN, Kanat-Pektas M, Kilic S, et al. Anti-Müllerian hormone is a better marker than inhibin B, follicle stimulating hormone, estradiol, or antral follicle count in predicting the outcome of in vitro fertilization. Arch Gynecol Obstet. 2011;283:1415-21.
59. Hughes EG, Dejean D. Cross-border fertility services in North America: a survey of Canadian and American providers. Fertil Steril. 2010;94(1):e16-9.
60. Nazari H, Ahmadi E, Hosseini Fahraji H, Afzali A, Davoodian N. Cryopreservation and its effects on motility and gene expression patterns and fertilizing potential of bovine epididymal sperm. Vet Med Sci. 2020;7(1):127–35.
61. Amato P, Tachibana M, Sparman M, Mitalipov S. Three-parent in vitro fertilization: gene replacement for the prevention of inherited mitochondrial diseases. Fertil Steril. 2014;101(1):31-5.

ANNEXURE

FORM-L

Consent Form for the Donor of Sperm.

I, Mr. .... consent to donate my sperm to couples/individuals who are unable to have a child by other means. I have had a full discussion with Dr............................. .... (Name and address of the clinician) on ...., I have been counseled by.............. .... (Name and address of independent counselor) on I understand that there will be no direct or indirect contact between the recipient, and me, and my personal identity will not be disclosed to the recipient or to the child born through the use of my gamete. I understand that I shall have no rights whatsoever on the resulting offspring and vice versa. (If applicable) My wife has agreed to the donation of my sperm. (Strike off if not applicable.) Endorsement by the ART bank I/we have personally explained to................. ....the details and implications of his signing this consent/ approval form and made sure to the extent humanly possible that he understands these details and implications.

Signed: ....

Name and address of the donor ....

Name and signature of the Doctor

Name, address, and signature of the witness from the ART bank

Name and address of the ART bank

Dated:

CHAPTER 70

Surrogacy in Assisted Reproductive Technology

Nayana H Patel, Yuvraj D Jadeja, Harsha K Bhadarka, Niket H Patel, Molina N Patel, Harmi Thakkar

WHAT IS SURROGACY?

The word "surrogate" is rooted in Latin "Subrogare" (to substitute), which means "appointed to act in the place of." It means a substitute, especially a person deputizing for another in a specific role. As per draft ART Bill, 2014, "Surrogacy" means an arrangement in which a woman agrees to a pregnancy, achieved through assisted reproductive technology (ART), in which neither of the gametes belongs to her or her husband, with the intention to carry it and hand over the child to the commissioning couple for whom she is acting as a surrogate.[1] It is important to be noted that the definition from the European Society for Human Reproduction and Embryology (ESHRE)[2] does not state the sexuality of the intended parents.

HISTORY

The first surrogacy arrangement is believed to have happened about 2,000 years before the birth of Christ and was mentioned in the Old Testament of the Bible. Sarah and Abraham were unable to conceive and Sarah hired her maid Hagar to carry a child for her husband. Subsequently, Hagar gave birth to a son, Ishmael, for Sarah and Abraham. The concept of surrogacy is also rooted in Hindu mythology, as despite of taking birth from the womb of Rohini, Balraam was regarded as the son of mother Devaki and the elder brother of Lord Krishna.

TYPES OF SURROGACY

Surrogacy is of two types—*traditional* and *gestational*.

Traditional (also called genetic or partial) surrogacy is the result of artificial insemination of the surrogate mother with the intended father's sperm, making her a genetic parent along with the intended father.

Gestational [in vitro fertilization (IVF)/host/full] surrogacy is defined as an arrangement in which an embryo from the intended parents, or from a donated oocyte or sperm, is transferred to the surrogate's uterus. In gestational surrogacy, the gestational carrier has no genetic connection to the child.

Surrogacy may be *commercial (compensated)* or *altruistic*, depending upon whether the surrogate receives monetary benefits for her pregnancy. In commercial surrogacy, the surrogate is reimbursed for medical costs and paid for her gestational services. With altruistic surrogacy, the surrogate who could be a friend or acquaintance or relative may be reimbursed for medical costs directly related to the pregnancy and for loss of income due to the pregnancy.

To be a surrogate mother could be a life-changing choice that can be tremendously rewarding, but with challenges. Surrogate requires commitment for a year or more as she has to undergo medical and psychological evaluations, procedures, and challenges related to pregnancy with a baby that is not her own. Surrogacy not only gives surrogate the unique opportunity to give an incredible and selfless gift to another person or couple but also provides her with financial benefits and can create lasting, meaningful relationships between her and the family she helped in creating.

WHO NEEDS SURROGACY? THE INDICATIONS

- *Congenital or acquired absence of a functioning uterus:* Congenital absence of the uterus such as Mayer-Rokitansky-Küster-Hauser (MRKH) syndrome is relatively rare with an incidence of 1 per 4,000–5,000 newborn girls.[3,4]
- *Hysterectomy for various reasons:* Obstetric complications during delivery or medical diseases, such as cervical cancer, could also be a cause for hysterectomy and lead to uterine infertility in spite of healthy ovaries.
- Significant *structural abnormalities* and the presence of *multiple fibroids*
- *Severe adenomyosis*
- *Persistently thin endometrium due to endometrial tuberculosis (TB)*
- *Asherman's syndrome*

- *Repeated miscarriages* and repeated *unexplained IVF failures* despite good-quality embryo
- Repeated IVF failure due to nonreceptive uterus
- Heart and renal diseases and other *medical conditions*, which might be life threatening for a woman during pregnancy, are also considered indications for surrogacy only if her life expectancy is reasonable to take care of a child after birth.
- Biological inability to conceive or bear a child, which applies to same-sex male couples or single men, also approaches surrogacy.
- **Figure 1** depicts indications that required treatment by gestational surrogacy; these data were acquired from one private IVF setup in India.

STEPS INVOLVED IN THE SURROGACY PROCESS

The steps involved in the surrogacy process are:

1. Patient selection
2. Source of the surrogate (ART bank)
3. Selection and screening of the prospective surrogate

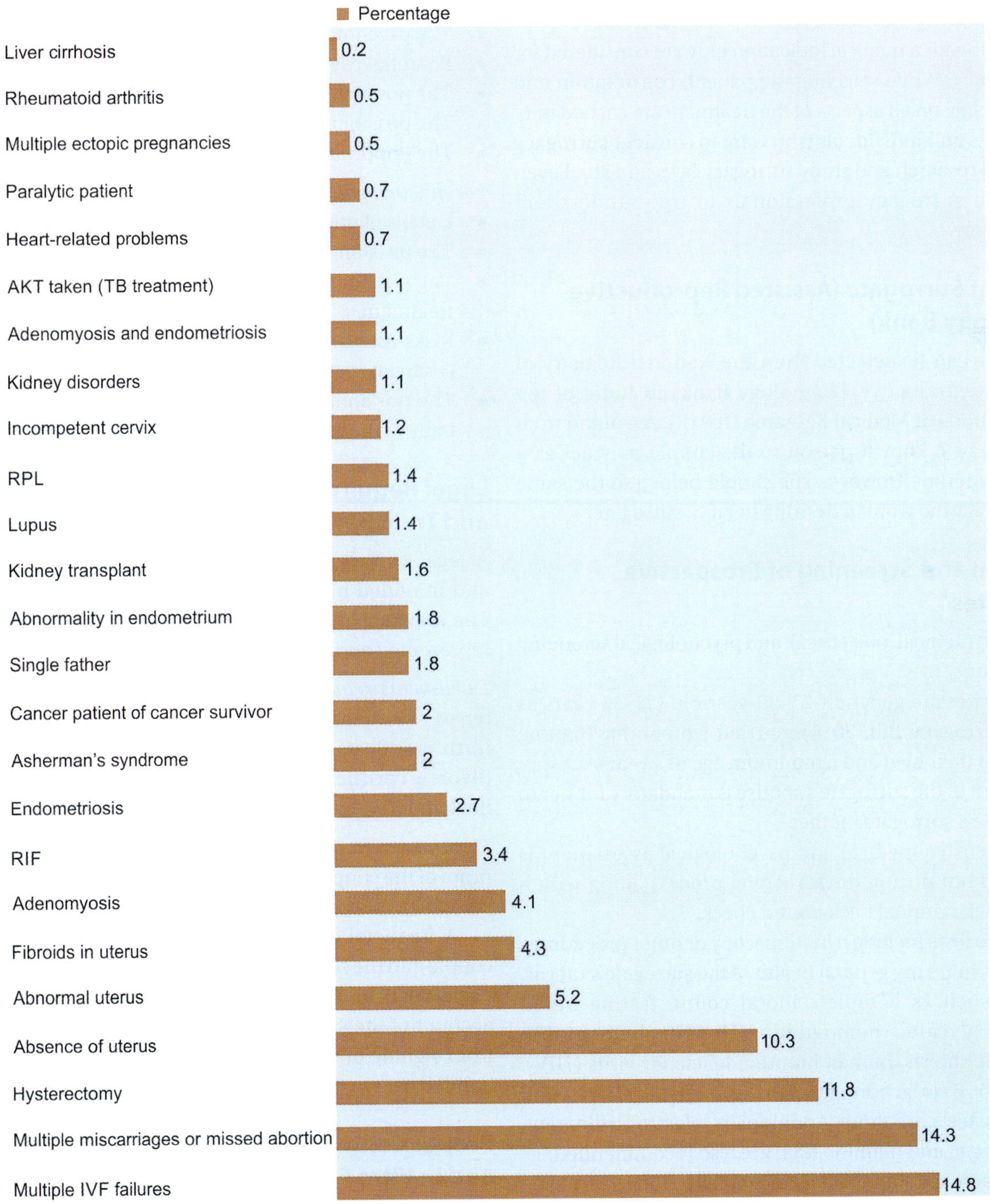

Fig. 1: Indications for surrogacy.
(AKT: assisted reproductive technology; IVF: in vitro fertilization; RIF: repeated implantation failure; RPL: recurrent pregnancy loss; TB: tuberculosis)

4. Intensive counseling—the key factor
5. Legal requirements, financial contracts, and transparency of arrangement
6. Proper controlled ovarian stimulation and IVF technique
7. Preparing the surrogate
8. Synchronizing the cycles of the surrogate and the genetic mother
9. Window period for embryo transfer
10. Obstetrics care of the surrogate.

Selection of Patient

- Patients with a medical indication only are considered for surrogacy. While selecting the patient, consultation and counseling on all aspects of the treatment are carried out.
- Couples and individuals who want to consider surrogacy should research and study surrogacy laws and shall even consult surrogacy professionals to truly understand surrogacy.

Source of Surrogate (Assisted Reproductive Technology Bank)

Surrogates can be selected from the National Registry of Assisted Reproductive Technology Banks in India of the Indian Council of Medical Research (ICMR). A woman from the family or a known person to the couple may act as a surrogate mother. However, she should belong to the same generation as the woman desiring her as a surrogate.

Selection and Screening of Prospective Surrogates[4]

A thorough medical, obstetrical, and psychological screening is mandatory.

- Surrogates are generally 21–35-year-old (25–35 years as per Surrogacy Bill, 2016) married women having one child of their own and a minimum age of 3 years.
- Consent of the surrogate's spouse is mandatory for her to become a surrogate mother.
- An extensive medical and psychological assessment is carried out during the screening process along with a thorough criminal background check.
- Routine tests include a hysteroscopy or other procedures to determine the general health of the surrogate's uterus.
- Tests such as complete blood count, fasting blood sugar, glycated hemoglobin (HbA1c), hemoglobin electrophoresis, human immunodeficiency virus (HIV), hepatitis B surface antigen (HBsAg), hepatitis C virus, and genetic tests are done. Additionally, electrocardiogram, Pap smear, and mammogram are also recommended.
- Pelvic and abdominal ultrasonography is done to evaluate the capability of her uterus to carry a pregnancy to term.
- Medical fitness from a physician.

Intensive Counseling

In-depth counseling of all the parties engaged in surrogacy arrangements is very crucial. They must have trust among themselves, and they must be confident and comfortable with their decisions. Many concerns must be discussed with both the genetic couple and the proposed surrogate, including:

For the genetic couple:

- Consideration of alternative treatment options
- The need for a detailed counseling
- The practical difficulty and cost of treatment of gestational surrogacy
- The psychological risks of surrogacy
- Potential psychological risk to the child
- The possibility of multiple pregnancies
- The possibility of the birth of an abnormal child
- The importance of obtaining legal advice.

For the surrogate:

- Details of undergoing treatment by IVF surrogacy
- The possibility of multiple pregnancies
- The possibility of family and friends being against such treatment
- Risks associated with pregnancy and the possibility of cesarean section
- The possibility of a sense of bereavement while giving baby to the genetic parents.

Legal Requirements, Financial Contracts, and Transparency of Arrangement

A legal contract is drafted and signed by the surrogate and intended parents once they decide to move forward. The attorney of each party ensures that legal interests are represented and protected for everyone.

Documents required from the surrogate: Identity proof in terms of Aadhaar card, voter ID, school leaving certificate, birth certificate for age verification, marriage certificate, divorce certificate if divorced, and death certificate of husband if widow.

Documents required from the couple or single parent: Identity proof of the couple, address proof (Aadhaar card, voter ID, or passport), and marriage certificate.

A financial contract is signed between the intended couple and the surrogate mother as per the ICMR guidelines. As per ART Guideline 2014, funds are transferred to the bank account of the surrogate mother at different stages starting from signing of the agreement till the child/children is/are handed over to the commissioning parents.

Proper Controlled Ovarian Stimulation and In Vitro Fertilization Technique

If women requesting treatment by gestational surrogacy are perfectly normal with regard to their ovarian function, the management of their IVF treatment cycle is straightforward. Ovarian follicular stimulation, monitoring, and oocyte recovery methods are practiced as previously described.[5] Sperm used in surrogacy cases should be treated in the same way as donor sperm and must be frozen and quarantined for 6 months before use.[6]

With the ovarian stimulation, the job of the infertility specialist doctor is to:

- Select a proper medication protocol and dosing regimen
- Monitor the patient's stimulation progress so that medication doses can be adjusted properly
- Trigger with human chorionic gonadotropin or gonadotropin-releasing hormone agonist at the ideal time.

Preparing the Surrogate

- Start estrogen from D2 or D3 of the recipient's cycle after confirming a thin endometrium (<5 mm) on the scan. The dose of estrogen can vary from 4 to 6 mg/day as per individual preference.
- Follow-up on the 10th day for the scan to see for the growth of the endometrium, a minimum of 8 mm (triple line), is ideal before starting progesterone.
- 5 or 3 days of progesterone is required either intramuscularly (50 mg/100 mg a day) or intravaginally (400 mg/day) before transfer.
- 5 days progesterone for a blastocyst transfer and 3 days for a cleavage-stage transfer
- Various protocols have been suggested; the other popular protocol for surrogate preparation is the leuprolide protocol due to its feasibility and flexibility in adjustment of transfer date with cycle control.
- Here suppression with leuprolide is done along with the previously mentioned endometrial preparation method.
- Either starting from day 21 of the previous cycle agonist injection for downregulation or stopping it at one-fourth dose on their own till the day of progesterone.
- Luteal phase support has to be decided accordingly.

Synchronizing the Cycles of the Surrogate and the Genetic Mother

- The surrogate embryo transfer could be fresh or frozen transfer and is subject to the availability of the gestational carrier. With the advent of excellent vitrification techniques, surrogacy cycles have become less difficult for the ART clinic with good embryology laboratory and freezing facility.
- For a fresh surrogate transfer, the surrogate's and the intended mother's cycle may be synchronized with oral contraceptive (OC) pills or progesterone pills or the surrogate may be put on agonist injection for flexibility of transfer dates.
- The surrogate is started on estrogen tablets from the third day of her cycle for around 10 days before her endometrium is assessed. On reaching a minimum of 8 mm, she is then put on progesterone supplementation for 3 or 5 days before a planned cleavage or blastocyst transfer.

Obstetrics Care of the Surrogate

Once a pregnancy is confirmed in the gestational carrier depending on the facility of the ART clinic, she stays either in the surrogate house or at her home. The concept of surrogate house has recently caught a lot of attention for various reasons. The idea of *surrogate house* was developed from the wish of many surrogates to be provided a shelter during the pregnancy as many of them wish to hide the practice from relatives and friends due to the stigma that prevails in rural areas owing to of awareness of the scientific procedures behind surrogacy. A surrogate house is a place where a surrogate stays for her entire antenatal period till the date of delivery and all her medical and personal requirements are taken care of. The obstetrics care of a surrogate is extensive due to the preciousness of the pregnancy. In the surrogate house, surrogates stay under the supervision of 24-hour nursing staff along with dieticians, physiotherapists, counselors, and gynecologists for their medical care. Surrogates get complete rest and healthy, nutritionally complete meals which turn out to be beneficial for their health during pregnancy. As they stay under one roof, they get a lot of emotional, moral, and psychological support from each other. Also, they are allowed to meet their family and kids and be in constant touch with their families via phone. They can go to their place as and when they want; also, young kids of surrogates are allowed to stay with them at surrogate houses during weekends and school holidays. It is voluntary for surrogates to stay in the surrogate house. Any surrogate who wishes to stay at her home can always do so.

In the surrogate house, she has obstetric assessment every 20 days till the date of delivery: Obstetric scans at 6–8 and 11–13 weeks; anomaly scan at 20–22 weeks (anomaly scan 3D–4D); and growth scan at 28 and 34–36 weeks. Any additional scan is subject to the obstetric needs.

The intended couple is sent regular mail regarding the surrogate's pregnancy in the form of her weight gain, vitals, fetal growth, and antenatal investigation reports and scans. Post delivery, the surrogate is kept under observation for a minimum of 15 days before discharge.

Inducing Lactation in Genetic Mother

The genetic mother is excluded from breastfeeding if she suffers from any malignancy or disease which has the risk of transmission to the infant via breastfeeding.

- "Active" birth control pill each day and 10 mg domperidone 4 times per day for 1 week are started in the intended mother, 6 months before the baby is due. Then the dosage is increased to 20 mg 4 times per day.
- Six weeks before the baby is due, birth control pills are discontinued while continuing domperidone. During

this course, generally mothers experience vaginal bleeding which is normal. Mothers shall be examined for potential pregnancy if she does not experience withdrawal bleeding.

- One month before the baby is due, the mother should pump the milk at least once during the night. Serum prolactin levels reach to peak between 1 and 5 AM.
- After the birth of the baby, the mother should continue the domperidone dosage of 20 mg 4 times per day until she achieves a substantial milk supply. The domperidone shall be decreased slowly once the milk supply is well established.

RISKS ASSOCIATED WITH SURROGACY

The major risks associated with surrogacy are obstetric complications and multiple-order pregnancy, which is most common. Recently, a lot of recommendations have been made by the Association of Reproductive Managers and ESHRE committees for single-embryo transfer, yet only 15–20% of the clinics follow single-embryo transfer norms. But it is an improvement from the previous years and more and more clinics are accepting this policy. Pregnancy, birth, and the postpartum period include complications such as preeclampsia and eclampsia, urinary tract infections, stress incontinence, gestational diabetes, and rare complications such as amniotic fluid embolism and the possibility of postpartum hemorrhage (PPH), but these risks are associated with pregnancy in general and not specific to surrogacy.

Apart from physical risk, surrogacy may be the reason for emotional trauma, surrogate mothers face emotional problems after having to relinquish the child. However, a study by Jadva et al.[7] indicates that although some women experience emotional problems in handing over the baby, these feelings appeared to lessen during the weeks following the birth.

VARIOUS ASPECTS AND CONCERNS INVOLVED IN SURROGACY

- *Ethical aspects:* Surrogacy has raised a large ethical debate in the past. The prime ethical concerns raised in the whole system of surrogacy are regarding exploitation and commodification as women are paid to be pregnant and deliver babies. The commodification arrangement raises the argument of whether women are being given control over their body or being exploited for their individual body parts.[8,9] The other major argument against womb commodification is that it allows the rich to take advantage of the willingness of a poor woman to perform any job as long as she is able to earn a wage.[7] A woman may choose to commodify her womb for money because she is faced with no other possible options for employment.
- *Religious aspects and issues:* Various religions around the world take different stances with regard to surrogacy practice and ART in general. Paragraph 2376 of the Catechism of the Catholic Church states that "Techniques that entail the dissociation of husband and wife, by the intrusion of a person other than the couple (donation of sperm or ovum, surrogate uterus), are gravely immoral." Islam also has a similar approach regarding their Chastity. Jewish religious establishments have now accepted surrogacy only if it is full gestational surrogacy with both intended parents' gametes included and fertilization done via IVF.[10,11] The religious stands for surrogacy are all with regard to traditional surrogacy, as that was the only way during ancient time, but with the advent of IVF and gestational surrogacy, the relevance of these beliefs is being questioned.
- *Psychological impact of surrogacy:* Despite the increasing success rates, surrogacy poses a new complexity on psychological aspects and again requires a multidisciplinary approach. Surrogacy brings to light a cobweb of possible relationships which could sometimes be emotionally taxing. The main element in the success of surrogacy lies in exploring and deeply understanding its psychological arm and the key to it is the quality of relationship between the intended parents and gestational carrier. Unlike the donor egg programs in which the intended parent does not share a relationship with the donor and know only nonidentifying information about her, intended parents working with a gestational surrogate typically share a personal relationship with her that will last throughout the pregnancy and often beyond. Studies have convincingly shown that children through third-party reproduction do well psychologically and developmentally and do not appear to be adversely affected by the lack of a genetic or gestational link to the intended parents.[12,13]

Identity and rights of the child: A child born through ART shall be presumed to be the legitimate child of the couple and shall have legal rights of parental support, inheritance, and all other privileges as of a child born to a couple through natural intercourse. Upon reaching the age of 18 years, the child can ask for any information relating to the donor or surrogate. However, the personal identification of the donor or surrogate may be released only in cases of life-threatening medical conditions which require physical testing or samples of the donor or parents or surrogate. Children born through the use of donor gametes shall not have any right whatsoever to know the identity (name, address, parentage, etc.) of their genetic parent(s).

SURROGACY LEGISLATION: THE INTERNATIONAL SCENARIO

- Surrogacy is not allowed in Austria, Bulgaria, Denmark, Finland, France, Germany, Italy, Malta, Norway, Portugal,

Spain, Sweden, Japan, and Saudi Arabia.[14] However, altruistic surrogacy is allowed in Belgium, Greece, the Netherlands, UK, Australia, Canada, New Zealand, and in many states of USA.

- Poland and the Czech Republic currently have no laws regulating surrogacy.[15,16] Commercial surrogacy is legal in Georgia, Israel, Ukraine, Russia, and California.
- In China, the Ministry of Health banned surrogacy in 2001. However, illegal surrogacy "black market" is still flourishing in China. Anxious about such a situation, strict legislation has been suggested by the political parties.[3] Surrogacy was previously illegal in Bulgaria, but as the procedure is still practiced illegally, the government decided to sanction it. Instead of using the term surrogate, though, Bulgaria calls it the "substitute mother."[17]

SURROGACY IN INDIA AND GUIDELINES FOR SURROGACY

Commercial surrogacy has been legalized in India since 2002. Till the implementation of ART Bill 2015, when surrogacy was allowed for foreigners, overseas citizens of India (OCI), persons of Indian origins (PIOs), and others, India was emerging as a leader in international surrogacy and as a destination in surrogacy-related fertility tourism because of good medical skills, infrastructure, transparency of procedure, favorable guidelines, and relatively low cost. Here, surrogacy was found to be a symbiotic arrangement as infertile couple gets a baby which completes their family and the needy surrogate gets compensation which helps for the betterment of her entire family. Indian surrogates see surrogacy as "Hope for a better future." The common motives for which women in India practice surrogacy vary individually, but most women become surrogates as they want monetary compensation for the education of their children, construction of their houses, start-up of small business, treatment of family members, payment of loans, or other as demonstrated in **Figure 2** (data from a private IVF setup in India).

However, one after the other regulations from the regulatory authority of India is pushing surrogacy practice almost to a ban. The proposed ART Bill 2015 bans foreign nationals from commencing surrogacy in India while an overnight notification in November 2015 restricted OCIs and PIOs as well. The effect of such an approach of government toward surrogacy practice has evidently affected the industry negatively and a reduction in the number of surrogate babies born was noted in private clinics. **Figure 3** depicts data from one private IVF setup to justify this impact. Furthermore, August 24, 2016, has to be considered a Black Day for surrogacy in India, as the Surrogacy (Regulation) Bill 2016 received the cabinet approval. The bill bans the commercial form of surrogacy, allowing only altruistic arrangement with many other constraints on this practice.

Assisted Reproductive Technology Regulation Bill, 2021[18]

- Registration of the ART clinic or ART bank is a must.
- Registration is to be made to the National Registry.

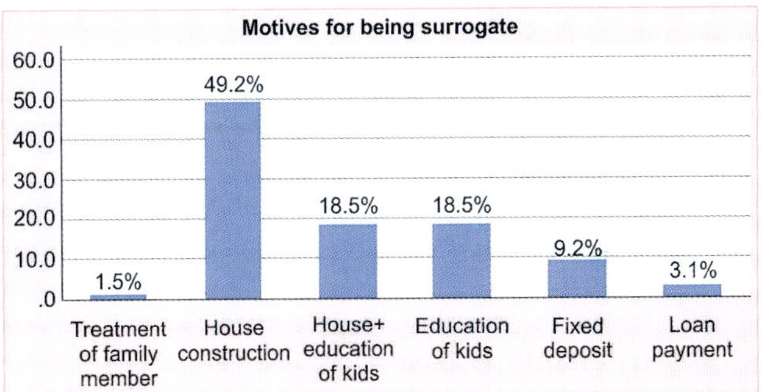

Fig. 2: Motives of surrogate mothers for practicing surrogacy.

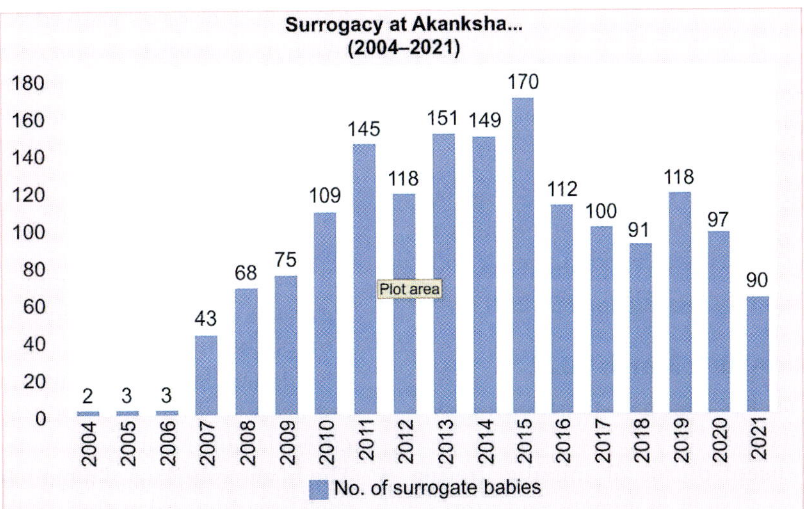

Fig. 3: Yearly frequency of birth of surrogate babies at a private in vitro fertilization (IVF) clinic in India.

- After 60 days of establishment, a clinic or a bank must register itself.
- The registration, if granted, may be renewed for a further period of 5 years by the appropriate authority.
- A national board is to be established for the regulation and to advise the central government.
- A State-Assisted Reproductive Technology and Surrogacy Board (SART and SB) is to be constituted.
- SART and SB will have the responsibility to follow the policies and plans laid by the national board.
- Clinics shall apply the ART services to a woman above the age of 21 years and below the age of 55 years and to a man above the age of 21 years and below the age of 55 years.
- Every clinics and every bank should maintain a grievance cell in respect of matters relating to the clinics/banks.
- No cryopreservation of any human embryo or gamete.
- Clinics to retrieve oocytes as specified by the regulations
- Clinics to not implant/place more than three embryos in the uterus of a woman during the treatment cycle.
- Preimplantation genetic diagnosis (PGD) shall only be used to screen the human embryo for known, preexisting, heritable, or genetic diseases only.
- Regarding donor gametes.
- The banks shall obtain semen from males between 21 and 55 years of age.
- The banks shall obtain oocytes from females between 23 and 35 years of age.
- The sperm or oocytes should not be supplied to more than one commissioning couple.
- An oocyte donor shall donate only once in her lifetime, and not more than seven oocytes shall be retrieved from the oocyte donor.
- All unused oocytes shall be preserved by the banks for use on the same recipient.
- The gamete of a donor or embryo shall be stored for a period of not more than 10 years.
- The use of any human gamete and embryos or their transfer to any country outside India for research is strictly prohibited.
- Harsh fines for offences.
- Sex Selective Assisted Reproductive Technology and Offences and Penalties; whoever contravenes shall be punishable with imprisonment for a term for 5 years but may extend up to 10 years or with fine not less than 10 lakh rupees but may extend up to 20 lakh rupees or both.

(For more details please refer ART Regulation Bill, 2021).

Surrogacy (Regulation) Bill, March 2022[18]

- Medical indications necessitating gestational surrogacy
- Surrogacy can be opted if:
    - A woman has absent uterus or missing uterus or abnormal uterus (such as hypoplastic uterus, intrauterine adhesions, thin endometrium, small unicornuate uterus, T-shaped uterus) or if the uterus is surgically removed due to any medical conditions such as gynecological cancers
    - Intended parents/women have repeatedly failed to conceive after multiple IVF/intracytoplasmic sperm injection (ICSI) attempts (recurrent implantation failure)
    - Multiple pregnancy losses resulting from an unexplained medical reason. Unexplained graft rejection due to exaggerated immune response.
    - Any illness that makes it impossible for a woman to carry a pregnancy to viability or a pregnancy that is life threatening
- The intending couple is in possession of a certificate of essentiality issued by the appropriate authority, after satisfying itself, for the reasons to be recorded in writing.
- The intending couple needs a certificate of proven infertility from a District Medical Board.
- The intending couple have not had any surviving child biologically or through adoption or through surrogacy. Provided if the child is mentally challenged or suffers from life-threatening disorder or fatal illness with no permanent cure and approved by the appropriate authority with due medical certificate from a district medical board.
- Intending couple married and between the age of 23 and 50 years in case of females and 26 and 55 years in case of males.
- Surrogacy is to be done only for altruistic purposes and not for commercial purpose.
- The surrogate should be between 25 and 35 years of age, married, and having a child of her own.
- A woman shall act as a surrogate for *only one successful live birth* in her life.
- Surrogate shall be medically tested for HIV or acquired immunodeficiency syndrome (AIDS) and all other communicable diseases and conditions such as cardiovascular disease and thyroid problem.
- She must not have received a blood transfusion or a blood product in the *last 6 months.*
- *No surrogate* shall undergo *only 1 embryo transfer more than three times* for the same couple.
- A surrogate shall *relinquish all parental rights over the child* or children.
- The couple and the surrogate shall enter into a surrogacy agreement or contract.
- All medical expenses, including insurance of the surrogate, should be given by the commissioning couple.
- Complications that arise during pregnancy (i.e., gestational diabetes, chronic hypertension, etc.), which are likely to continue for the rest of her life, shall be covered under insurance.
- The birth certificate of a baby born through surrogacy shall bear the name of the couple who commissioned the surrogacy, as parents.

- Surrogacy shall be allowed for foreigners but permissible to OCIs, PIOs, nonresident Indians (NRIs), and a foreigner married to an Indian citizen.
- The surrogate mother needs an eligibility certificate issued by the appropriate authority.
- *Registration of surrogacy clinics:* Every certificate of registration shall be valid for a period of 3 years and shall be renewed.
- There shall be established a Registry to be called the National Assisted Reproductive Technology and Surrogacy Registry for the purposes of registration of surrogacy clinics under this act.
- Any intending couple or any person who seeks the aid of any surrogacy clinic, laboratory, or a registered medical practitioner, gynecologist, pediatrician, human embryologist, or any other person for commercial surrogacy or for conducting surrogacy procedures for commercial purposes shall be punishable with imprisonment for a term which shall not be <5 years and with a fine which may extend to 5 lakh rupees for the first offence and for any subsequent offense with imprisonment which may extend to 10 years and with fine which may extend to 10 lakh rupees.
- *ICMR portal for surrogacy bill was open for public opinion till April 2, 2022. [For more details, please refer Surrogacy (Regulation) Bill, March 2022].*

CONCLUSION

In conclusion, surrogacy is a hope for the couples who are facing serious fertility issues which cannot be treated directly. Banning the surrogacy is not a solution for unethical practices rather appropriate regulations can be formulated and implemented to handle the misconduct on surrogates.

KEY POINTS

- Surrogacy is an important method of ART wherein a woman carries a pregnancy for another couple.
- A numbers of couples around the world require surrogacy services for various reasons.
- Since legislation in 2002 till the Surrogacy (Regulation) Bill, 2021, surrogacy in India has traveled a long path.
- Although this arrangement seems to be beneficial for all parties concerned, there are multifarious social, ethical, and legal issues associated with it, which have made this practice unpopular in many parts of the world.
- In recent times, where the need for surrogacy is increasing day by day, delicate issues associated with this practice are ought to be addressed properly. Efforts shall be taken to spread awareness about surrogacy in society to make this arrangement more open and acceptable.
- Formulation of laws, appropriately designed to protect the rights of surrogate mothers, intended parents, and children, can make this practice an approachable and gratifying experience for all the parties involved.
- Banning surrogacy will only give rise to underground arrangements. To solve this issue, national and international frameworks must be set up.
- Proper regulation, ethical practice, and commitment from all the stakeholders can help to solve the associated issues and put an end to all the controversies.

REFERENCES

1. Ministry of Health and Family Welfare, Government of India; New Delhi: Indian Council of Medical Research. Draft Assisted Reproductive Technology (Regulation) Bill. 2014.
2. Shenfield F, Pennings G, Cohen J, Devroey G, de Wert G, Tarlatzis B, et al. ESHRE task force on ethics and law 10: surrogacy. Hum Reprod. 2005;20:2705-7.
3. Lindenman E, Shepard MK, Pescovitz OH. Mullerian agenesis: an update. Obstet Gynecol. 1997;90:307-12.
4. Aittomaki K, Eroila H, Kajanoja P. A population-based study of the incidence of Mullerian aplasia in Finland. Fertil Steril. 2001;76:624-5.
5. Wikland M, Enk L, Hamberger L. Transvesical and transvaginal approaches for the aspiration of follicles by the use of ultrasound. Ann N Y Acad Sci. 1985;442;683-9.
6. Brinsden PR. Surrogacy. In: Brinsden PR (Ed). Textbook of In Vitro Fertilization and Assisted Reproduction. London: Taylor & Francis; 2005. pp. 393-404.
7. Jadva V, Murray C, Lycett E, MacCallum F, Golombok S. Surrogacy: the experiences of surrogate mothers. Hum Reprod. 2003;18(10):2196-204.
8. Kimbrell A. The Human Body Shop: The Engineering and Marketing of Life. New York: HarperSanFrancisco; 1993. p. 101.
9. Honjo S, Arai S, Kaneko H, Ujiie T, Murase S, Sechiyama H, et al. Antenatal depression and maternal-fetal attachment. Psychopathology. 2003;36:304-11.
10. MacCallum F, Lycett E, Murray C, Jadva V, Golombok S. Surrogacy: the experience of commissioning couples. Hum Reprod. 2003;18(6):1334-42.
11. Inhorn MC, Patrizio P. Rethinking reproductive "tourism" as reproductive "exile". Fertil Steril. 2009;92(3):904-6.
12. Golombok S, Blake L, Casey P, Roman G, Jadva V. Children born through reproductive donation: a longitudinal study of psychological adjustment. J Child Psychol Psychiatry. 2013;54(6):653-60.
13. Golombok S, Murray C, Jadva V, Lycett E, MacCallum F, Rust J. Non-genetic and non-gestational parenthood: consequences for parent-child relationships and the psychological well-being of mothers, fathers and children at age 3. Hum Reprod. 2006;21(7):1918-24.
14. Brunet L, Carruthers J, Davaki K, King D, Marzo C, Maccandless J. A comparative study on the regime of surrogacy in EU member states. LSE Research Online, 2013.
15. Deomampo D. Defining parents, making citizens: nationality and citizenship in transnational surrogacy. Med Anthropol. 2015;34:210-25.
16. Aramesh K. Iran's experience with surrogate motherhood: an Islamic view and ethical concerns. J Med Ethics. 2009;35:320-2.
17. Pennings G. Reply: reproductive exile versus reproductive tourism. Hum Reprod. 2005;20:3571-2.
18. ART Bill and Surrogacy Regulation Bill. Government of India 2022.

CHAPTER 71

Assisted Reproductive Technology Guidelines

(Brig.) RK Sharma

INTRODUCTION

Infertility, though not life-threatening, causes intense mental agony and trauma that can only be best described by infertile couples themselves. There are no detailed figures of the extent of infertility prevalent in India, but a multinational study carried out by the World Health Organization (WHO)[1] that included India places the incidence of infertility between 10 and 15%. Out of a population of 1,000 million Indians, an estimated 25% (250 million individuals) may be conservatively estimated to be attempting parenthood at any given time; by extrapolating the WHO estimate, approximately 13–19 million couples are likely to be infertile in the country at any given time.

Prevention and appropriate treatment of infertility has been included in the International Conference on Population and Development (ICPD) Program of Action; it follows that alleviation of infertility should be included as a component of the primary healthcare system. Most types of infertility, such as reproductive tract infections (RTIs) and genital tuberculosis, are preventable and amenable to treatment. About 8% of infertile couples, however, need serious medical intervention involving the use of advanced assisted reproductive technology (ART) procedures, such as in vitro fertilization (IVF) or intracytoplasmic sperm injection (ICSI). Such advanced treatment is expensive and not easily affordable to the majority of Indians. Further, the successful practice of ART requires considerable technical expertise and expensive infrastructure. Moreover, the success rate of any ART procedure is below 30% under the best of circumstances. Infertility, especially in our country, also has far-reaching societal implications. Today, infertility is the most common medical problem in 30–40 years age group of couples in India, and ART was valued at $793.27 million in 2020 and is projected to reach $3,721.99 million by 2030, registering a compound annual growth rate (CAGR) of 16.45% from 2021 to 2030. 20,000 ART clinics across the country are providing IVF and intrauterine insemination (IUI) services. However, a fraction of these clinics have applied for registration.[2]

Therefore, with the rapidly increasing use of ART in our country, it has become imperative to ensure their safety and safeguard against their possible misuse.[3]

Scientific societies around the world, such as the American Society for Reproductive Medicine (ASRM), European Society of Human Reproduction and Embryology (ESHRE), and International Federation of Fertility Societies (IFFS), have drawn up guidelines for the safe and ethical practice of ART. The European Union and the governments of several countries such as Australia, the United Kingdom, and the United States of America have taken steps to accredit and supervise the performance of infertility clinics.

The United States notably has few federal or state regulations pertaining to the ART industry. This is in contrast to other developed nations, which provide more extensive regulations on the use of ART, and, in many cases, restrict its use for certain ends, such as reproductive cloning. While some of these regulations may not be ideal, there are steps taken to ensure the health and safety of women utilizing ART and the children resulting from these technologies as well as the ethical use of ART by all participants.[4]

Australia regulates ART at both the federal and the state levels, with the states providing the most regulation. The key federal law is the Prohibition of Human Cloning for Reproduction and the Regulation of Human Embryo Research Amendment Act, 2006. This law prohibits reproductive cloning and allows states to either permit or prohibit research cloning. Research cloning is permitted in Victoria, New South Wales, Tasmania, Queensland, South Australia, and the Australian Capital Territory. Additionally, this law prohibits germline modification and the commercial trading of human eggs, sperm, or embryos. The National Health and Medical Research Council publishes ethical guidelines on the use of ART in clinical practice and research. These general guidelines must be followed for ART centers to be accredited by the reproductive technology accreditation committee. These guidelines encourage limiting the number of embryos created to those needed during the course of treatment, strict recording of the outcomes of ART, and the prohibition of nonmedical sex selection and commercial surrogacy. Noncommercial or altruistic surrogacy is permitted by some Australian states.[5]

In 2008, after extensive consultations held at both the Indian Council of Medical Research (ICMR) and other national institutions, with scientists, medical practitioners, lawyers, social scientists, and activists, the ICMR developed a draft for ART (Regulation) Bill which was meant to ensure that ART clinics in India are accredited, regulated, and supervised to assure the patients as well as the public that our ART clinics offer services that are at par with those available anywhere in the world and sent it to the Ministry of Health and Family Welfare, which was then revised by the Ministry of Law and Justice as ART (Regulation) Bill, 2013. In 2016, the ART (Regulation) Bill, 2016, came before the Cabinet for consideration. The ART (Regulation) Bill proposed to establish national board, state boards, and national registry of ART in India for accreditation and supervision of ART clinics and ART banks, ensuring that services provided by these are ethical and that the medical, social, and legal rights of all the concerned are protected with maximum benefit to all the stakeholders within a recognized framework of ethics and good medical practices.[6]

The Assisted Reproductive Technology (Regulation) Bill, 2020 was introduced in Lok Sabha on September 14, 2020. On March 19, 2021, Standing Committee Report was formed. On December 1, 2021, it was passed in Lok Sabha, and by December 08, 2021, it was passed by the Rajya Sabha. The Bill seeks to provide for the regulation of ART services in the country.

ART CLINIC AND BANK: MINIMAL PHYSICAL REQUIREMENTS

A well-designed ART clinic of level 1 or level 2[7] should have a nonsterile and a strictly sterile area. Some of the spaces could be used for more than one purpose as long as such a step does not compromise the quality of service. However, the space provision for the sterile area cannot be combined with those for the nonsterile area and vice versa. For level 1B infertility care units,[8] a strictly sterile area will not be required. The space requirement, however, will include a reception area, a waiting room for the patients, and a consulting room for the gynecologist.

The minimum equipment in ART clinics and banks are:[9]

- *ART level 1 clinics:*
    - Microscope
    - Centrifuge
    - Refrigerator
- *ART level 2 clinics:*
    - Microscope
    - Incubator (minimum two in number)
    - Laminar airflow
    - Sperm counting chambers
    - Centrifuge
    - Refrigerator
    - Equipment for cryopreservation
    - Ovum aspiration pump
    - Ultrasonography (USG) machine with transvaginal probe and needle guard
    - Test tube warmer
    - Anesthesia resuscitation trolley
- *ART banks:*
    - Centrifuge machine
    - Incubator
    - Microscope
    - Laminar airflow.

Semen Collection Room

The semen collection room must be a well-appointed room with privacy and an appropriate environment; it should be located in a secluded area close to the laboratory. Such a facility must be available in-house rather than making the patient collect the sample and bring it to the laboratory for analysis as, in the latter case, semen quality and identity are likely to be compromised. Procedures for collection of semen as described in the WHO Semen Analysis Manual must be followed with special reference to the type of container used; these containers must be sterile, maintained at body temperature, and nontoxic. This room must have a washbasin with availability of soap and clean towels. The room must also have a toilet and must not be used for any other purpose.[10]

Semen Processing Laboratory

There must be a separate room with a laminar airflow for semen processing, preferably close to the semen collection room. This laboratory must also have facilities for microscopic examination of postcoital test smears. Good laboratory practice (GLP) guidelines as defined internationally must be followed. Care must be taken for the safe disposal of biological waste and other materials (syringes, glass slides, etc.). Laboratory workers should be immunized against hepatitis B and tetanus.

Sterile Area

The sterile area shall house the operation theater, a room for intrauterine transfer of sperm or embryos, and an adjoining embryology laboratory. Entry to the sterile area must be strictly controlled by an anteroom for changing footwear, area for changing into sterile garments, and a scrub station. The sterile area must be air-conditioned where fresh air filtered through an approved and appropriate filter system is circulated at an ambient temperature (22–25°C).

Operation Theater

The operation theater must be well equipped with facilities for carrying out transvaginal ovum pickup. It must be equipped for emergency resuscitative procedures.

Embryology Laboratory Complex

The embryology laboratory must have facilities for the control of temperature and humidity and must have filtered air with an appropriate number of air exchanges per hour. Walls and floors must be composed of materials that can be easily washed and disinfected; the use of carpeting must be strictly avoided. The embryology laboratory must have the following:

- Laminar flow bench with a thermostatically controlled heating plate
- Stereo zoom microscope
- Routine high-powered binocular light microscope
- "High-resolution" inverted microscope with phase contrast or Hoffman optics, preferably with facilities for video recording
- Micromanipulator (if ICSI is done)
- CO_2 incubator, preferably with a backup
- Hot air oven
- Laboratory centrifuge
- Equipment for freezing embryos in a programmed manner
- Liquid nitrogen cans
- Refrigerator.

Appropriate steps need to be taken for the correct identification of gametes and embryos to avoid mix-ups. All material from the operation room, culture dishes and plastic wares, must bear the name of the patient. In the incubator, identified oocytes and sperm should be kept together on the same tray and double-checked. Pipettes used should be disposed of immediately after use. The embryology laboratory must have a daily logbook in which all the day's activities are recorded, including the performance of the equipment.

Maintenance of the Laboratories

Each laboratory should be maintained by writing standard operating manuals for the different procedures carried out in the laboratory. It should be ensured that there is no "mix-up" of gametes or embryos. The patient's name should be clearly labeled on all the tubes, dishes, and pipettes containing the gametes and embryos. All pipettes should be immediately discarded after use. Laminar flow hoods, laboratory tables, incubators, and other areas where sterility is required must be periodically checked for microbial contamination using standard techniques, and a record of such checks must be kept. A logbook should be maintained which records the temperature, carbon dioxide content and humidity of the incubators, and the manometer readings of the laminar airflow. All instruments must be calibrated periodically (at least once every year) and a record of such calibration maintained.

Power Supply Backup

There should not be any interruption in power supply to the incubator and to other essential services in the clinic. Given the power supply situation in India, it is, therefore, imperative that a power backup in the form of uninterruptible power supply systems and/or a captive power generation system is available in infertility clinics offering ART services.

ART: CLINICS AND BANKS CLASSIFICATIONS AS PER THE ASSISTED REPRODUCTIVE TECHNOLOGY (REGULATION) BILL, 2021[11]

There shall be two levels of clinics, namely:

- Level 1 ART clinics, where only IUI procedure is carried out as part of treatment
- Level 2 ART clinics, where the procedures, or as the case may be, and techniques that attempt to obtain a pregnancy shall be carried out by any or all of the following, namely:
    - Surgical retrieval of gametes
    - Handling the oocyte outside the human body
    - Using sperms for fertilization of oocytes
    - Transfer of the embryo into the reproductive system of a woman
    - Carryout storage of gametes or embryos or perform any kind of procedure or technique involving gametes or embryos.

Assisted reproductive technology banks shall:

- Be responsible for screening, collection and registration of the semen donor, and cryopreservation of sperms
- Perform screening and registration of oocyte donor
- Operate as semen banks or oocyte banks or both
- Maintain the records or data of all the donors and shall regularly update the National Registry as provided in sections 23, 27, and 28 of the Act.
- Perform screening and registration of surrogate.

ART TEAM: ESSENTIAL QUALIFICATIONS AS PER THE ASSISTED REPRODUCTIVE TECHNOLOGY (REGULATION) BILL, 2021[12]

- *ART level 1 clinic:* Minimum one gynecologist
  Qualification: The gynecologist shall be a medical postgraduate in Gynecology and Obstetrics.
- *Staffing of ART level 2 clinic:* ART clinic level 2 shall have a minimum of one gynecologist, one anesthetist, one embryologist, and one counselor. The additional staff at

the level of director and andrologist may be employed by the ART level 2 clinics.

- Qualification of staff in ART level 2 clinics shall be as follows:
  - *Gynecologist:* The gynecologist will be a medical postgraduate in Gynecology and Obstetrics and should have a record of performing 50 ovum pickup procedures under the supervision of a trained ART specialist with at least 3 years of working experience in an ART clinic under supervision. (In the case of gynecologists practicing ART or IVF and are working in ART clinics before the commencement of this Act, a postgraduate degree in Gynecology and Obstetrics with at least 3 years' experience and record of 50 ovum pickup procedures shall be acceptable.)
    Or
    A medical postgraduate in Gynecology and Obstetrics with super specialist Doctorate of Medicine or fellowship in reproductive medicine with experience of not <3 years of working in an ART clinic.
  - *Andrologist:* The andrologist in a clinic or a bank will be a MCh or DNB in Urology with special training in diagnosing and treating male infertility.
  - *Embryologist:* From the date of commencement of these rules, clinics will hire embryologists only with the following qualifications and experience, namely: Postgraduate in Clinical Embryology (graduated with full-time program with minimum four semesters) from a recognized university with additional 3 years of human ART laboratory experience in handling human gametes and embryos
    Or
    PhD holder or one with full-time PhD project shall be related to Clinical Embryology or ART or fertility from a recognized university with an additional 1 year of human ART laboratory experience in handling human gametes and embryos
    Or
    Medical graduate (MBBS) or veterinary graduate (BVSc) with a postgraduate degree in Clinical Embryology (full-time program) from a recognized university with additional 2 years of ART laboratory experience in handling human gametes and embryos
    Or
    Postgraduate in Life Sciences or Biotechnology with a minimum of 1 year of on-site, full-time clinical embryology certified training in addition to 4 years of experience in handling human gametes and embryos in a registered ART level 2 clinic.
    Note: As a one-time measure, all embryologists working in ART or IVF clinics before the commencement of these rules, with the below-mentioned qualifications and experience, may be allowed to continue as an embryologist. However, after the commencement of these rules, all clinics will hire embryologists with any of the above-mentioned qualifications and experience as criteria: Graduate in Life Sciences or Biotechnology or Reproductive Biology/Veterinary Science with at least 5 years of working experience in a registered ART or IVF clinic, who have performed at least 500 IVF laboratory procedures (including ICSI and at least 100 cycles of cryopreservation of embryos)
  - *Counselor:* A person who is a graduate in Psychology or Clinical Psychology or Nursing or Life Sciences
  - *Anesthetist:* Anesthetist will be a medical postgraduate in Anesthesia.
  - *Director:* The director shall have a postgraduate degree in Medical or Life Sciences or Management Sciences.
- *ART bank:* The ART bank shall have a minimum of one registered medical practitioner trained in the handling, preparation, and storage of semen samples.

ARTIFICIAL INSEMINATION WITH DONOR SEMEN

The indications for artificial insemination with donor semen (AID) are:

- When there is nonobstructive azoospermia
- When the husband has a hereditary genetic defect
- When the couples have Rh incompatibility

The main advantage of AID is that it enables a couple to achieve pregnancy even though the husband is not the biological father. However, the possible transmission of diseases from the donor to the future child and the risk of consanguinity constitute some drawbacks that must be brought to the notice of the patients. It is necessary to get the informed consent of both the partners after they are counseled about the possible psychological conflict they may face later in their life with the knowledge that one of them is not the biological parent of their child. AID is an ethically acceptable procedure, provided there is a medical indication and psychological confirmation for its use. Also, the normal conditions of anonymity and screening of the donor must be met, and only frozen sperm samples that have passed appropriate quarantining for infectious diseases, such as human immunodeficiency virus (HIV), hepatitis B and C, and syphilis, should be used.

OOCYTE DONATION OR EMBRYO DONATION

Oocyte donation (OD) would necessitate using the husband's semen for fertilization and transferring the resultant embryo to the infertile female partner. Embryo donation (ED) would obviate the necessity of using the husband's semen. The choice of oocytes and embryos for OD or ED would depend entirely on the circumstances prevalent at the time the infertile couple comes for treatment and the access of the infertility clinic to frozen oocytes or embryos.

Indications for Oocyte or Embryo Donation

- Gonadal dysgenesis
- Premature ovarian failure
- Iatrogenic (due to ovarian surgery or radiation, or chemical castration) ovarian failure
- Women who have resistant ovary syndrome or who are poor responders to ovulation induction
- Women who are carriers of recessive autosomal disorders
- Women who have attained menopause

Donors should be healthy (as determined by medical and psychological examination, screening for sexually transmitted diseases, and absence of HIV antibodies) women in the age group of 18–35 years. Oocytes may be obtained for donation, mostly by surgical intervention from women participating in an IVF program or those undergoing elective sterilization or surgery. The recipient should be a healthy woman (determined by medical and psychological examination) having normal genitalia (as determined by physical examination) and uterine cavity (as determined by hysterosalpingography). In case of OD, the semen characteristics of the husband must be determined to see if they are in conformity with those associated with normal fertility. The blood group of the donor should be noted; the donor should also be tested for antibodies to rubella, HIV, hepatitis, *Cytomegalovirus*, gonorrhea, syphilis, *Chlamydia*, *Mycoplasma*, and trichomonas. Ovum or ED can be carried out in menopausal women with no surviving child and desiring to have a child. The endometrium of menopausal women has the ability to respond to sex hormones and provide a receptive environment for the implantation of an embryo. Various protocols are now available to prepare the endometrium of the recipient for OD or ED with estrogens and progestogens until the placenta takes over the function of maintaining the gestation.

Meanwhile, the expansion and proliferation of ART has been facilitated by economic globalization wherein reproductive tissues such as sperm, ova, and uteri are traded like any other commodity to make profit, and India emerged as the surrogacy outsourcing capital of the world.

Due to the proliferation of surrogacy and India becoming a center for medical tourism, some interesting and difficult cases of surrogacy-related legal issues, especially involving foreigners, surrogacy became the most "contentious" issue in the country. It was felt by the government that "there is a need to regulate surrogacy for the time being and that is why it was decided to separate it from the earlier proposed ART Bill so as to get going."

This resulted in the Surrogacy (Regulation) Bill, 2016, by the Health Ministry that proposed to legalize altruistic, domestic surrogacy. The Bill seeks to control exploitation of the surrogate child and mother for unethical purposes.

The Cabinet approved certain amendments in the Surrogacy (Regulation) Bill, 2016, on March 21, 2018. Commercial surrogacy is prohibited, whereas altruistic surrogacy is allowed for the benefit of "needy and infertile" married Indian couples. The Cabinet proposed the formation of a National Surrogacy Board.[13]

KEY HIGHLIGHTS OF THE ASSISTED REPRODUCTIVE TECHNOLOGY (REGULATION) BILL, 2021

- *Registration:* An application for registration shall be made by the ART clinics or any such health facility which are carrying out procedures related to the ART to the appropriate authority in Form-1 and by the ART banks in Form-2. Every application for registration shall be accompanied with a fee of:[14]
  - ₹ 50,000 for level 1 ART clinic
  - ₹ 200,000 for level 2 ART clinic
  - ₹ 50,000 for ART bank
- Under the Bill, every ART clinic and bank must be registered under the National Registry of Banks and Clinics of India, which will act as a central database for all facilities providing ART services in India.
- *Regulation of ART clinics and banks*: The Bill provides that every ART clinic and bank must be registered under the National Registry of Banks and Clinics of India. The National Registry will be established under the Bill and will act as a central database with details of all ART clinics and banks in the country. State governments will appoint registration authorities for facilitating the registration process. Clinics and banks will be registered only if they adhere to certain standards (specialized manpower, physical infrastructure, and diagnostic facilities). The registration will be valid for 5 years and can be renewed for a further 5 years. Registration may be canceled or suspended if the entity contravenes the provisions of the Bill.
- *National and State Boards*: The Bill provides that the National and State Boards for Surrogacy, constituted under the Surrogacy (Regulation) Bill, 2019, will act as the National and State Boards, respectively, for the regulation of ART services. Key powers and functions of the National Board include (1) advising the central government on ART-related policy matters, (2) reviewing

and monitoring the implementation of the Bill, (3) formulating code of conduct and standards for ART clinics and banks, and (4) overseeing various bodies to be constituted under the Bill. The State Boards will coordinate enforcement of the policies and guidelines for ART as per the recommendations, policies, and regulations of the National Board.

- *Conditions for gamete donation and supply*: Screening of gamete donors, collection and storage of semen, and provision of oocyte donor can only be done by a registered ART bank. A bank can obtain semen from males between 21 and 55 years of age and oocytes from females between 23 and 35 years of age. An oocyte donor should be an ever-married woman having at least one alive child of her own (minimum 3 years of age). The woman can donate oocyte only once in her life and will be minimally stimulated. A bank cannot supply gamete of a single donor to more than one commissioning couple (couple seeking services).
- *Conditions for offering ART services*: ART procedures can only be carried out with the written informed consent of both the party seeking ART services and the donor. The party seeking ART services will be required to provide insurance coverage in favor of the oocyte donor (for any loss, damage, or death of the donor). A clinic is prohibited from offering to provide a child of pre-determined sex.
- *Rights of a child born through ART*: A child born through ART will be deemed to be a biological child of the commissioning couple and will be entitled to the rights and privileges available to a natural child of the commissioning couple. A donor will not have any parental rights over the child.
- *Offenses and penalties*: Offenses under the Bill include (1) Abandoning or exploiting children born through ART; (2) selling, purchasing, trading, or importing human embryos or gametes; (3) using intermediates to obtain donors; (4) exploiting commissioning couple, woman, or the gamete donor in any form; and (5) transferring the human embryo into a male or an animal. These offenses will be punishable with a fine between 5 and 10 lakh rupees for the first contravention. For subsequent contraventions, these offenses will be punishable with imprisonment for a term between 8 and 12 years and a fine between 10 and 20 lakh rupees.
- Any clinic or bank advertising or offering sex-selective ART will be punishable with imprisonment between 5 and 10 years, or a fine between 10 and 25 lakh rupees, or both.
- No court will take cognizance of offenses under the Bill, except on a complaint made by the National or State Board or any officer authorized by the Boards.

OTHER DUTIES OF ASSISTED REPRODUCTIVE TECHNOLOGY CLINIC[15]

- The ART clinic shall ensure that all unused gametes or embryos shall be preserved by the ART clinic for use on the same recipient and shall not be used for any other couple.
- Allow cryopreservation of oocytes, sperms for onco-fertility patients undergoing treatment and for other such conditions, for duration longer than 10 years with the permission from the National Board.
- Ensure the controlled ovarian stimulation of woman in order to prevent ovarian hyperstimulation.
- Ensure that preimplantation genetic testing shall be used to screen the human embryos for known preexisting heritable or genetic diseases and when medically indicated.
- Ensure that no preimplantation genetic testing shall be done for sex selection for nonmedical reasons or selection of particular traits due to personal preferences of the prospective parents or to alter or with a view to alter the genetic constitution of an embryo.
- Maintain consent form to be signed by the couple or woman as specified in Form 6, IUI with husband's semen or sperm as specified in Form 7, IUI with donor semen as specified in Form 8, freezing of embryos as specified in Form 9, freezing gametes as specified in Form 10, freezing of gametes sperm or oocytes and parental consent as specified in Form 11, oocyte retrieval as specified in Form 12, and oocyte donor as specified in Form 13.

NEED FOR ASSISTED REPRODUCTIVE TECHNOLOGY (REGULATION) BILL, 2021[16]

- *To standardize protocols:*
  - There are so many such ART clinics that have been running without regulation and there are implications on the health of those who undertake the procedure.
  - If there is no regulation, unethical practices will increase.
- *To protect women and children:* The oocyte (a cell in an ovary) donor needs to be supported by an insurance cover. Multiple embryo implantation needs to be regulated and children born through ART need to be protected.

CONCERN FOR ASSISTED REPRODUCTIVE TECHNOLOGY (REGULATION) BILL, 2021[16]

- *Discrimination in accessibility:* The Bill allows for a married heterosexual couple and a woman above the age of marriage to use ARTs and excludes single men, cohabiting heterosexual couples and lesbian, gay, bisexual, transgender, or queer (LGBTQ+) individuals and couples from accessing ARTs.

- *Duplicity:*
  - Both Surrogacy and ART Bills will set up multiple bodies for registration which will result in duplication or worse, lack of regulation.
  - For example, a surrogacy clinic is not required to report surrogacy to the National Registry.
- *Violates Article 14:*
  - The bill violates Article 14 of India's constitution and is also silent on the rights of children.
  - According to Article 14, equality before law and equal protection of law to any person within India cannot be denied.
- *Cost of the services:* The cost of the procedure should be effectively monitored so that even the poor can avail of its services which may not be possible in third-party reproduction.

EVOLUTION IN SURROGACY LAW—LEGAL INSIGHTS[17]

- *Assisted Reproductive Technology Bill, 2013:* The ART Bill, 2013 was pending for quite a while, which did not allow commercial surrogacy that involves exchange of money for anything other than paying for medical expenses for the mother and the child. The Bill also prohibited couples already having one child, foreigners or overseas citizens of India (OCI), holders as well as live-in-partners, single people, homosexuals, and widows for opting surrogacy.
- *Surrogacy (Regulation) Bill, 2016 and 2019:* In 2016, a Surrogacy (Regulation) Bill was introduced and passed in Lok Sabha, the lower house of the Indian parliament, proposing to permit only Indian heterosexual couples married for at least 5 years with infertility problems to access altruistic or unpaid surrogacy and thereby banning commercial surrogacy. The 2016 Bill lapsed owing to the adjournment of the parliament session. The bill was reintroduced and passed by the Lok Sabha in 2019.
- *Surrogacy (Regulation) Act, 2021:*
  - This Act explains surrogacy as a practice in which if a couple is incapable of producing a child of their own due to infertility or any disease is eligible for the surrogacy process with certain guidelines. It is permitted only for altruistic purposes or for couples who suffer from proven infertility or disease.
  - Altruistic surrogacy includes no money-related pay to the surrogate other than the clinical costs and protection inclusion during the pregnancy. In vitro treatment (IVF) is the most widely recognized and powerful sort of ART. The ART Regulation 2021 gives a framework to the execution of the law on surrogacy by setting up of the National Assisted Reproductive Technology and Surrogacy Board.
  - In order to improve the facilities provided in surrogacy clinics, the Ministry of Health and Family Welfare came up with Surrogacy (Regulation) Rules, 2022, on June 21, 2022, under the ministry of Mansukh Mandaviya, which elaborates the requirement of number of persons employed and the qualifications that they must possess. In addition to that, it also provides for the form and manner in which the registration will take place and the procedure to pay the fees for the surrogacy clinic **(Table 1)**.

TYPES OF SURROGACY

- *Altruistic surrogacy:* It involves no monetary compensation to the surrogate mother other than the medical expenses and insurance coverage during the pregnancy.
- *Commercial surrogacy:* It includes surrogacy or its related procedures undertaken for a monetary benefit or reward (in cash or kind) exceeding the basic medical expenses and insurance coverage.

TABLE 1: Difference between Surrogacy Act and Assisted Reproductive Technology (ART) Act.[20]

Surrogacy Act	*ART Act*
Relates to surrogacy, an infertility treatment, where a third person, a woman, is the surrogate mother	Treatments can be availed by the commissioning couple themselves and it is not always necessary that a third person is involved
Surrogacy is allowed for only Indian married couples	ART procedures are open to married couples, live-in partners, single women, and also foreigners
It prohibits the commissioning of surrogacy in India by foreigners or OCI or PIO cardholders, but NRIs holding Indian citizenship can avail of surrogacy	Foreigners can visit India under medical tourism to avail ART services
There will be a National Surrogacy Board that will be involved in policy making, and act as a supervisory body, and State Boards that will act as executive bodies	The ART Act provides for a National Board, with the powers vested in a civil court under the Code of Civil Procedure
About 1,000 clinics are practicing surrogacy in India according to the Health Ministry	ART practicing clinics are likely >20,000

(NRI: nonresident Indian; OCI: overseas citizens of India; PIO: persons of Indian origin)

ELIGIBILITY CRITERIA FOR COUPLES INTENDING SURROGACY[18]

- Couple is having a proven infertility condition, either male or female suffering from infertility.
- Couple should have Indian citizenship.
- Couple should be married for at least 5 years.
- Age of wife should be between 23 and 50 years old and husband's age between 26 and 55 years old.
- They do not have any surviving child (biological, adopted, or surrogate)—this would not include a child who is mentally or physically challenged or suffers from a life-threatening disorder or fatal illness.
- Not for commercial purposes
- Not for producing children for sale, prostitution, or other forms of exploitation
- For any condition or disease specified through regulations
- Insurance coverage for 16 months covering postpartum delivery complications for the surrogate.

If all the above criteria are met, then only a couple will be issued a certificate of essentiality and a certificate of eligibility by the appropriate authority to make them eligible for the altruistic surrogacy process.

ELIGIBILITY CRITERIA FOR A SURROGATE MOTHER[18]

- A close relative of the intending couple
- Age has to be between 25 and 35 years old
- A married woman
- Already having a child of her own
- Permitted to be a surrogate mother only once in her life
- Possess a certificate of medical and psychological fitness for surrogacy.
- The surrogate mother is not allowed to give her own eggs for surrogacy.
- The surrogate mother should not have any history of miscarriage or complications during her previous pregnancy and childbirth.

ABORTION DURING SURROGATE PREGNANCY

- An abortion of the surrogate child requires the written consent of the surrogate mother and the authorization of the appropriate authority with compliance to the Medical Termination of Pregnancy Act, 1971.
- The surrogate mother has an option to withdraw from surrogacy before the embryo implantation.

OFFENSES AND PENALTIES RELATED TO SURROGACY IN INDIA[19]

In order to stop the exploitation of surrogate mothers and children, some penalties have been established by the Indian government.

- The penalty for such offenses is imprisonment up to 10 years and a fine of up to 10 lakh rupees.
- Undertaking or advertising commercial surrogacy
- Exploiting the surrogate mother
- Abandoning, exploiting, or disowning a surrogate child
- Selling or importing human embryos or gametes for surrogacy.

CIRCUMSTANCES FOR OPTING SURROGACY[17]

- When a woman has no uterus or missing uterus or abnormal uterus or the uterus is surgically removed due to any disease
- Failed to conceive even after multiple IVF or ICSI attempts
- In case of multiple pregnancy losses and the medical reason is unexplained
- If pregnancy is impossible due to some illness.

ANALYSIS OF KEY POINTS OF SURROGACY (REGULATION) RULES, 2022[17]

- Central government, by issuing a notification, declared the eligibility criteria and number of persons required at a registered surrogacy clinic. Further, the details for the minimum equipment required at such clinics are also specifically mentioned.
- The composition of such clinics as per the notification is that any such clinics shall have at least one gynecologist, anesthetist, embryologist, and counselor and the clinic may employ additional staff by the ART level 2 clinics.
- Gynecologist at surrogacy clinics shall be a medical postgraduate in Gynecology and Obstetrics and should have record of performing 50 ovum pickup procedures and at least 3 years of working experience in an ART clinic under supervision of a trained ART specialist.
- ART is defined as "assisted reproductive technology" with its grammatical variations and cognate expressions, means all techniques that attempt to obtain a pregnancy by handling the sperm or the oocyte outside the human body and transferring the gamete or the embryo into the reproductive system of a woman." Henceforth, it is very essential for a gynecologist to have expertise in this technology.
- Form 1 in the notification specifies the application to receive a certificate of recommendation from the board.
- To safeguard the rights of the surrogate mother, the provision for insurance coverage has been introduced, which mandates the intending couple or woman to purchase a health insurance for the surrogate mother for 36 months.
- An affidavit before a Metropolitan Magistrate or a Judicial Magistrate of the first class shall be signed by the woman

or couple with the intention of giving guarantee under section 2 of the Surrogacy (Regulation) Act, 2021.
- The maximum number of attempts of the surrogacy procedure shall not be more than three times.
- The surrogate mother shall give her free consent as per the specifications provided in the form.
- It has been decided that the gynecologist shall implant only one embryo, with an exception of three embryos in special cases.
- In case where a surrogate mother wants to abort the child, the abortion process is to be followed as per the Medical Termination of Pregnancy Act, 1971.

INFERTILITY—A TABOO

Assisted reproductive technology and surrogacy procedures have emerged essentially due to increasing infertility in the society. The current Bill defines infertility as the inability to conceive after 5 years, whereas the previous draft bills defined it as the inability to conceive after 1 year.

The Committee has compared this definition of infertility with that given by the WHO and suggested that "since conception has many interplay functions, a 5-year time bar would add to the misery of already distressed intending couples. The 5-year waiting period is therefore arbitrary, discriminatory, and without any definable logic. The Committee, therefore, recommends that the definition of infertility should be made commensurate with the definition given by WHO. The words "five years" in clause 2(p) and 4 (iii)(c) II, be, therefore, replaced with "one year" and consequential changes be made in other relevant clauses of the Bill."[21]

This suggestion by the Committee is based on the basic fundamental right to reproduction and the right to privacy.

How and when individuals wish to reproduce is their own personal discretion. The government can impose limitations and set criteria; however, the same should be rational and not arbitrary.

Other Suggestions

The Committee made several other laudable suggestions, some of which take root from the previous ART bills and some of which are based on reasonable analysis of the current social-medical scenario. It suggested that "compensated surrogacy" should be allowed and that single parents and live-in partners should be allowed to commission surrogacy.

The Committee also recommended that there should be a provision of breast milk banks for the surrogate child, and a tripartite surrogacy agreement should be entered between the parties instead of separate agreements to make the process easier.

Thus, a Bill to regulate surrogacy is found to have elements far removed from ground realities and certain provisions would need to be recast for it to serve its intended purpose. The committee, which has raised several issues with the Bill, has "strongly" recommended that the ART Bill be brought forth before it.

"The committee failed to comprehend the reasons behind bringing a fresh bill specifically on surrogacy, when a detailed, comprehensive and all-encompassing bill on ART services had already been drafted by the department," the committee stated.

At the same time, it observed that surrogacy could not be a way out for women living in poverty and should not be allowed as a profession—it supported the provision that restricts a woman from becoming a surrogate more than once.

The Bill aims to control exploitation and safeguard interests of poor women who become surrogates for money, but the potential for exploitation is linked to lack of regulatory oversight and legal protection to these women, according to the report.

Despite this, the Bill, in opinion of many ART experts, fails to address various issues, including transparency and fair practices.

One of the major issues is that of lack of screening guidelines of couples based on their socioeconomic background, criminal records in the past, their health, age, and family information check before they are permitted to commission surrogacy. In the absence of such screening guidelines, the surrogate child's interests suffer considerable risk from being put under the guardianship of those who lack credibility or even be detrimental to the child's security.

Although the Bill prohibits and penalizes abandonment, rejection of the surrogate by couple postbirth, it defines "abandoned child" by defining grounds of abandonment as "physical or mental defect or infirmity, or being more than one in number," excluding "sex of the child" among the same. In this aspect, the Bill does not address the plight of such surrogate child found nongenetically connected with either of the parents post birth due to mishaps arising out of switching or swapping of donated frozen gametes of couples in clinics, laboratories, or sperm banks. The Bill is unclear if such a surrogate child is allowed to be abandoned, rejected, or left in adoption home or orphanage.

Among the biggest misses of the Bill is sex-selective surrogacy or family balancing surrogacy done to have child of a predetermined sex, in which the earlier ART Bill prohibited and penalized the same by adding relevant provisions of Prenatal Diagnostic Techniques (Regulation and Prevention of Misuse) Act, 1994, in ART.[22] Among other offenses and punishments, the Bill does not talk about "trafficking or sale, abduction of surrogate child" in the guise of either altruistic or commercial surrogacy arrangement in any form under the same.

Apart from the above-mentioned aspects, there are various other aspects in relation to the rights of the surrogate mother and the child. The Bill lacks in clarity and transparency required to protect these rights sufficiently in case legal issues arise.

Health experts believe that dealing in surrogacy in isolation and in separation with other important issues such as ART clinics, gamete donation, sperm donation, and IVF practices (which had been earlier the part of the broad ART Bill) will serve no purpose. Earlier, the ART Bill had surrogacy as one of the parts of the Bill and should be taken as such, with more clarification and provisions for surrogacy as it evolves, like other areas of ART. ART, such as all other advances in medical profession, is ever evolving and any legislation or bill will have to be revised as such from time to time, depending on the scientific advancements and societal changes.

ASSISTED REPRODUCTIVE TECHNOLOGY BANK

Facilities for cryopreservation are an essential component of an ART clinic as they are to be used under a variety of conditions.

Freezing Semen

Men who are likely to suffer from psychological stress at the time of ovum pick-up or those who cannot be present at the time of ovum pick-up are recommended to have their semen frozen for use at the appropriate time. One of the important reasons for freezing semen from donors is that any donor semen has to be quarantined for 6 months. The safety of using frozen sperm has been abundantly proven by both experimental work and the actual results in humans. Matters of concern are the donor's health and the necessity to avoid donors who are infected with venereal diseases, hepatitis B or C, or HIV. One of the drawbacks of sperm freezing is an approximate 20% loss in motility after thawing. Donors whose semen is frozen for future use are required to report to the semen bank 6 months after donation to be checked for HIV, hepatitis B or C virus infection, or disease status.[23]

Freezing Embryos

Embryos are routinely cryopreserved to enable storage of supernumerary embryos, as up to a maximum of only three embryos is allowed for transfer to avoid the risk of multiple pregnancies. Embryo freezing is a widespread routine procedure to increase cumulative pregnancy rates. Human embryos can be successfully cryopreserved at any stage from zygote to blastocyst, using 1,2-propanediol (PrOH) or dimethyl sulfoxide (DMSO) for zygotes and cleaved embryos and glycerol for blastocysts. Straws or ampoules used for freezing embryos should be carefully and permanently labeled for identification purpose. Patients should be fully informed before the treatment cycle on the procedure of cryopreservation, the risks and, particularly, what is to be done with their embryos if they do not use them. They should sign a consent form concerning the agreement for embryo freezing as well as for the future use of the embryos.[24] When a serum supplementation is used in the preparation of freezing and thawing solutions, one must carefully avoid any risk of viral transmission to the embryo through the serum.

Oocyte Cryopreservation

This procedure has been successfully used in cases where a large number of immature oocytes have been retrieved during ovum pickup. The oocyte can be thawed at a later date, matured in vitro, and used for OD or similar procedures either on the person from whom the oocytes were retrieved or on other prospective recipients. However, the success rates in terms of fertilization, pregnancy, and live births with the use of cryopreserved oocytes are not very encouraging. ART clinics are the only source of embryonic stem cells. Spare embryos are either frozen or returned to the infertile couple for replacement during a later cycle, or donated to another infertile couple, or discarded after 5 years using a suitable protocol.[25] The stand taken by the foreign governments on embryo research might promote commercial exploitation (selling of embryos) of developing countries that do not have appropriate national guidelines. Therefore, sale or transfer of human embryos or any part thereof, or of gametes in any form, directly or indirectly to any party outside the country, must be prohibited. Within the country, such embryos or gametes could be made available to bona fide researchers only as a gift, with both parties having no commercial transaction, interest, or intent.

CONCLUSION

As India is one of the significant center points of these practices, the Act is surely a positive development, but there are few aspects on which the laws on surrogacy stand contradictory. According to Article 21, "Right to Life" is a fundamental aspect and right to reproduction has been embraced under it. The right for women to have children and the right to bring a pregnancy to term are all included in their reproductive rights. Therefore, it is clearly a violation of Articles 21 and 14 to limit surrogacy while denying reproductive options.

However, it is very crucial to maintain certain standards in the professions where risk to life of a person is involved; with the same motive, the Central Government issued the guidelines to establish quality surrogacy clinics and explained the prerequisites that the surrogacy clinics shall comply with before providing the services. In addition to that, certain guidelines are also provided for an intending couple or woman who is opting for surrogacy. With these measures, a protective process for a surrogate mother is created.

Since the enactment of new rules and regulations, there have been many debates on the shortcomings of the present bill. There are likely to be some changes to make it more patient friendly. Hence as of today, this is not the last word. Regulated ART and surrogacy will not only be beneficial for the patients but also for the doctors. More deliberations and changes will make this cost effective. Till then, many patients will approach the courts for redressal and the Judiciary will be flooded with such issues.

REFERENCES

1. Rowe PJ, Vikhlyaeva EM. Diagnosis and Treatment of Infertility. Toronto: Hans Huber Publishers; 1988. pp. 15-39.
2. Allied Market Research. (2022). India in-vitro fertilization (IVF) services market. [online] Available from https://www.alliedmarketresearch.com/india-ivf-services-market. [Last accessed October, 2022].
3. ICMR/NAMS. Guidelines for ART Clinics in India, 2016.
4. Kristen R. Global Bioethics Public Policy Reproductive Ethics. 2009;16:4.
5. National Health and Medical Research Council. Ethical Guidelines on the use of ART. Australia: NHMRC; 2006.
6. Ministry of Law and Justice. Assisted Reproductive Technology (Regulation) Bill 2013 and Bill 2016, India.
7. ICMR/NAMS. Guidelines for ART Clinics in India. 2016 [Sections 2.5.3 and 2.5.4].
8. ICMR/NAMS. Guidelines for ART Clinics in India. 2016 [Section 2.5.2].
9. The Constitution of India DHR. The Assisted Reproductive Technology (Regulation) Act, 2021, PART II—SEC. 3(i) Notification June 07, 2022 Part 2.
10. ICMR/NAMS. Guidelines for ART Clinics in India. 2016 [Section 1.3.1.8, 1.3.1.9 and 1.3.1.10].
11. The Constitution of India DHR. The Assisted Reproductive Technology (Regulation) Act, 2021, PART II—SEC. 3(i) Notification June 07, 2022, S. No. 3.
12. The Constitution of India DHR. The Assisted Reproductive Technology (Regulation) Act, 2021, PART II—SEC. 3(i) Notification June 07, 2022, Schedule 1, Part 1.
13. Ayushman Bharat-National Health Protection Mission (AB-NHPM), India. 2018.
14. The Constitution of India DHR. The Assisted Reproductive Technology (Regulation) Act, 2021, PART II—SEC. 3(i) Notification June 07, 2022, S. No. 7.
15. The Constitution of India DHR. The Assisted Reproductive Technology (Regulation) Act, 2021, PART II—SEC. 3(i) Notification June 07, 2022, S. No. 13.
16. Drishti IAS. (2021). Assisted Reproductive Technology (Regulation) Bill, 2021. [online] Available from https://www.drishtiias.com/daily-updates/daily-news-analysis/assisted-reproductive-technology-regulation-bill-2021. [Last accessed October, 2022].
17. Lawrbit. (2022). Analytical study on Surrogacy (Regulation) Rules, 2022. [online] Available from https://www.lawrbit.com/article/analytical-study-on-surrogacy-regulation-rules-2022/Lawrbit. [Last accessed October, 2022].
18. The Constitution of India DHR. The Surrogacy (Regulation) Act, 2021, PART II—SEC. 1, Dec 25, 2021, Chapter 3, S. No. 4.
19. The Constitution of India DHR. The Surrogacy (Regulation) Act, 2021, PART II—SEC. 1, Dec 25, 2021, Chapter 7, S. No. 38.
20. ClearIAS. (2022). Assisted reproductive technology. [online] Available from https://www.clearias.com/assisted-reproductive-technology/. [Last accessed October, 2022].
21. World Health Organization. WHO infertility definition. Clause 2(p) and 4 (iii) (c) II.
22. Government of India. Prenatal Diagnostic Techniques (Regulation and Prevention of Misuse) Act in ART, 1994.
23. ICMR/NAMS. Guidelines for ART Clinics, India. 2016:1.6.8.1.
24. ICMR/NAMS. Guidelines for ART Clinics, India. 2016:1.6.8.2 [Section 3.11].
25. ICMR/NAMS. Guidelines for ART Clinics, India. 2016:1.6.8.3 [Section 3.11].

CHAPTER 72

Adoption

Himanshu Singhal, Anubhuti Patel

INTRODUCTION

Having children has always been important since time immemorial, and the continuity of the family unit has been of major significance in every culture. Infertility affects millions of people of reproductive age worldwide—and has an impact on their families and communities. Estimates suggest that between 48 million couples and 186 million individuals live with infertility globally as per the World Health Organization report in 2020.

Childlessness in India is estimated at around 2.5% (5.5% for the 30–49 year age group and 5.2% for the 45–49 year age group). In absolute terms, it is around 4.9 million, and if secondary infertility is also added, then it increases to 17.9 million.[1]

Due to advancement in fertility treatment, more babies are being born using techniques ranging from minimally invasive medications to assisted conception techniques such as intrauterine insemination (IUI) to in vitro fertilization (IVF).

In vitro fertilization, which is often pursued as the last option, is one of the most complex treatments in infertility with success rates up to 30% which decrease further as women get older.[2]

Dropout rate reaches up to 65% after three cycles of IVF in countries offering free/subsidized cycles[2-4] versus one cycle in self-funded treatment. Various reasons for discontinuation of treatment were found to be financial burden in majority of self-funded cycles, while prognosis being another major factor affecting a patient's decision of continuing the treatment (25% dropout due to poor prognosis). Other reasons for dropout were psychological in 26%, social in 15% (such as marital problems), and physical burden in 6% [ovarian hyperstimulation syndrome (OHSS), infection, and pain due to injections], while it was not related to the cause of infertility.[2,5-7]

Infertile couples undergoing IVF may experience significant psychosocial stress, problems in the marital relationship, divorce, difficulties in sexual adjustment, blame for the infertility, lower self-esteem, loss of hope, and social isolation following the unsuccessful completion of treatment.[3,8-19]

Little is known about their final probability of having a child. 10% of them may conceive spontaneously.[9,20] Another recent study reported live birth rate up to 24% after spontaneous conception in couples who remained childless after treatment.[21] A follow-up study reported women being less satisfied with their lives who remained childless compared with those who were parenting a biological or an adopted child.[12]

After unsuccessful treatment or not achieving parenthood, couples may pass through different stages of grief including denial of them not having children biologically, and then the final stage of acceptance comes when they begin to see adoption as a solution to become parents. Parenthood after discontinuation of IVF in majority (46%) is due to adoption.[22]

Adoption is not a new concept. Its roots may be traced to ancient India. Indian mythology is full of stories about what couples have done in the past to overcome their problem of infertility. One such example of adoption was when Rishi Kanva adopts and raises an abandoned child that he finds in the forest who grows up to be Shakuntala who, when rejected by her husband, Dushyanta, raises her son, Bharata, on her own. The son becomes such a great king that the land he rules comes to be known as "Bharata-varsha," now known as "India."

"The bond that links your true family is not one of blood, but of respect and joy in each other's life."

DEFINITION

Adoption is a social, emotional, and legal process that provides a new family for a child when the birth family is unable or unwilling to parent.[23] It is the creation of a parent–child relationship by judicial order between two parties who usually are unrelated. This relationship is brought about only after a determination that the child is an orphan or has been abandoned, or that the parents' parental rights have been terminated by court order.[24]

Modern systems of adoption, arising in the 20th century, tend to be governed by comprehensive statutes and regulations.

TYPES OF ADOPTION

Open Adoption

This kind of adoption is open, which means that the adoptive parents and the birth parents keep in touch with each other through letters, emails, phone calls, and may even visit each other, and the birth mother can meet the child.

Advantages

- There is substantial medical information available to the adopted child, which is very important to assess some genetic disorders and other medical purposes.
- The adoptee has an extended family and more people who love and support him.
- The adoptee has access to his ancestry and lineage.

Disadvantages

- There may be a difference in expectations from adoptive or birth parents.
- The boundary issues may occur, where both the parties may struggle with drawing the line.
- The morals and values of both the families may not match, and this may cause confusion.

Semiopen Adoption

This is a kind of adoption that does not involve direct contact between the birth parents and the adoptive parents. However, the mother may keep receiving letters or photographs from the adoptive parents or through the adoption agency she is registered with. This may continue until the child reaches the legal age. At any given point of time, semi-adoption may get converted into an open or closed adoption.

Advantages

- Adoptive parents have access to the medical records and other information of the birth parents.
- This kind of adoption helps you maintain your privacy.
- Birthing parents have the information on how their child is taken care of.
- Adoptees may contact the birthing parents in future.

Disadvantages

- Both parties have to rely on the mediator agency.
- A semiopen adoption may become closed adoption in case the adoption agency goes out of business or stops functioning.
- The communication may stop if either of the party loses contact with the agency.

Closed Adoption

As the name suggests, this kind of adoption involves absolutely no contact between the adoptive parents and the birth parents.

Advantages

- The adoptee will not feel torn between two families.
- There is a sense of closure for both the sets of parents.
- The adoptee will have a close-knit family.
- There will not be any intrusion from the birth parents.

Disadvantages

- The child on knowing that he is adopted may become obsessed with finding birth parents in case of a closed adoption.
- There may be limited medical information available.
- The adoptee may face an identity crisis.

Intra-family Adoption/Relative Adoption

This is a kind of adoption that happens within the family.

Advantages

- The child stays within the biological family.
- The adoptive parents are in full control of taking various important decisions concerning the child.
- The adopted child in most cases gets to keep his original name.

Disadvantages

- The change in relation to the adoptive parents may confuse the child (in case the child is old enough).
- The time to contact and visitation is usually decided by the adoptive parents.

Domestic Adoption

Domestic adoption refers to adoption that happens within the country.

Advantages

- This type of adoption is less expensive as compared to international adoption.
- It also involves lesser paperwork in contrast to international adoption.
- Couples who intend on adopting a newborn baby may adopt him easily.
- The information of the birth parents may be accessible to the adoptive parents.

- You may keep in contact with the birth parents, or the contact may vary as per the requirements of both the parties.
- It does not require any international travel.

Disadvantages

- There may not be enough information on the medical history of the birth parents.
- The rules are very strict, and the eligibility criteria of adoptive parents are very strict.
- Adoptive parents may have to choose from a limited number of children.
- The mother may refuse the adoption, which may amount to termination of adoption.

International Adoption

It involves adopting a child from outside the country or in other words giving a child to the couple (adoptive parents) who are not a native of that country.

Advantages

- International adoption may usually happen with orphaned children, and thus birth parents may not be involved.
- There are a wide variety of children to choose from in terms of sex, race, health, and age.
- There is no interference of birth parents.
- Once the home approval is received, it increases the chances of adoption tremendously.

Disadvantages

- This type of adoption is expensive as the adoptive parents are required to travel to foreign lands.
- There are chances of fraud and scams in international adoption.
- As the adoption procedure may take a while, it may not be feasible to adopt a newborn baby.
- If the child is a bit older, he may take considerable time to adjust to a new setting, new country, and new ways of life.

RULES AND REGULATIONS OF ADOPTION IN INDIA

In India, only agencies recognized by the government can deal with adoption placement. Direct placement by hospitals or maternity homes is not permitted.

Central Adoption Resource Authority

The Central Adoption Resource Authority (CARA) is a statutory body of the Ministry of Women and Child Development, Government of India, and functions as the nodal body, which regulates and monitors in-country and inter-country adoption (in accordance with the provisions of the Hague Convention on Inter-country Adoption, 1993, ratified by Government of India in 2003) of Indian orphan, abandoned, or surrendered children through recognized adoption agencies. In 2018, CARA allowed individuals in a live-in relationship to adopt children from and within India. (For details, we can visit www.cara.nic.in.)

Stakeholders in the adoption process

- *CARA:* It ensures smooth functioning of the adoption process from time to time and issues adoption guidelines laying down procedures.
- *State Adoption Resource Agency (SARA):* It acts as a nodal body within the state to promote and monitor adoption and noninstitutional care in coordination with CARA.
- *Specialized Adoption Agency (SAA):* SAA is recognized by the state government under subsection 4 of section 41 of the Act for the purpose of placing children in adoption.
- *Authorized Foreign Adoption Agency (AFAA):* AFAA is recognized as a foreign social or child welfare agency that is authorized by CARA on the recommendation of the concerned central authority or government department of that country for coordinating all matters relating to the adoption of an Indian child by a citizen of that country.
- *District Child Protection Unit (DCPU):* It means a unit set up by the state government at the district level under section 61A of the Act. It identifies orphan, abandoned, and surrendered children in the district and gets them declared legally free for adoption by the Child Welfare Committee.

Adoption Regulations, 2017

Fundamental Principles Governing Adoption

During the adoption process:

- Child's best interest is of paramount consideration.
- Preference is given to Indian citizens in their own sociocultural environment.
- All the adoptions are registered on CARA and confidentiality is maintained.

Child Eligible for Adoption

- Any orphan, abandoned, or surrendered child declared legally free for adoption by the Child Welfare Committee.
- Child of a relative defined under subsection (52) of section 2 of the Act.
- Child or children of spouse from an earlier marriage, surrendered by the biological parent(s) for adoption by the stepparent.

Eligibility Criteria for Prospective Adoptive Parents

- They shall be physically, mentally, and emotionally stable and financially capable with no life-threatening medical condition.

TABLE 1: Age of adoptive parents to apply for children of different age groups.

Age of the child	*Maximum composite age of prospective adoptive parents (couple)*	*Maximum age of single prospective adoptive parent*
Up to 4 years	90 years	45 years
Above 4 and up to 8 years	100 years	50 years
Above 8 and up to 18 years	110 years	55 years

- Any prospective adoptive parent, irrespective of his marital status and whether or not he has his own biological son or daughter, can adopt a child, but should fulfill the following:
  - Consent of both the spouses is needed in case of a married couple, and they should be in a stable marital relationship for at least 2 years.
  - Single female is eligible to adopt a child of any gender.
  - Single male cannot adopt a girl child.
- The age of adoptive parents shall be counted for deciding the eligibility to apply for children of different age groups as shown in **Table 1**.
- The minimum age difference between the child and either of the prospective adoptive parents shall not be <25 years. The age for eligibility will be as on the date of registration of the prospective adoptive parents.
- Age criteria are not applicable for relative or step-children adoption.
- Couple with three or more children shall not be considered for adoption except in case of special need children and in case of relative adoption and adoption by step-parent.

Procedure Relating to Orphan or Abandoned Children

- Abandoned or orphaned child is first presented to the Child Welfare Committee (within 24 hours) who holds the sole authority to declare the child free for adoption.
- Child's details and the photograph are entered online within 3 days of receiving, and the same can be advertised in a national newspaper to trace biological parents/legal guardians.
- Abandoned or orphan child is free for adoption in 2 or 4 months, in case of child up to 2 or above 2 years, respectively.
- In case biological parents want to relinquish a child, they have to execute a document in favor of adoption agency, witnessed by the authority of hospital and relative. After a waiting period of 2 months given to biological parents to reconsider the decision, the child is free for adoption.

Availability of Child for Adoption

Adoption to resident or nonresident Indian is allowed once the child is legally free for adoption by the Child Welfare Committee.

Intercountry adoption is allowed after:

- 60 days if child is <5 years of age
- 30 days if child is >5 years of age or sibling
- 15 days in the presence of physical or mental illness.

Adoption Procedure for Resident Indians

Such couples have to go to a registered agency licensed by both the state government and CARA.

- *Registration:* Filling online application form, uploading the relevant documents regarding their health, financial status, etc., following which they get a registration number.
- *Home study report:* Within 30 days from the date of submission of requisite documents and remain valid for 3 years.
- Once their adoption is approved, the suitable child is shown, and if accepted placement is legalized.
- *Follow-up of the progress of adopted child:* 6 monthly for 2 years
- In case of an adjustment problem, required counseling is arranged.

Adoption Procedure for Nonresident Indians, Overseas Citizen of India, and Foreign Prospective Adoptive Parents

- Nonresident Indian prospective adoptive parents shall be treated at par with Indians living in India in terms of priority for adoption.
- Nonresident Indian, overseas citizen of India, or foreign prospective adoptive parents, living in a country which is a signatory to the Hague Adoption Convention and wishing to adopt an Indian child, can approach the AFAA or the Central Authority concerned.
- In case there is no AFAA or Central Authority in their country, then the government department or Indian diplomatic mission in that country can be approached.
- After ascertaining their eligibility, a home study report is completed.
- The child can be taken in preadoption foster care for a temporary period within India after issuance of "no objection certificate" by the authority while the court order is pending (Schedule VIII).
- Final custody of the child is received from the specialized adoption agency once the passport and visa are issued to the child after issue of adoption order from the competent court.
- *Follow-up of progress:* On a quarterly basis during first year and on a 6-monthly basis in the second year.

Adoption by Lesbian, Gay, Bisexual, and Transgender

It may be a joint adoption by both partners which is legalized in 26 countries, five countries legalize step-child adoption among lesbian, gay, bisexual, and transgender (LGBT), or it can be adoption by a single LGBT.

CARA does not allow adoption to the same-sex foreigner couples, but many LGBT in India have adopted as single parent. In such cases, their partner does not have any legal rights over the child.

Adoption of Children with Special Needs

- The adoption process for children with special needs to be completed as expeditiously as possible.
- Children with special needs shall be available for adoption by resident Indians and nonresident Indians from the date they are declared legally free for adoption by the Child Welfare Committee.
- These children are available for adoption by overseas citizen of India or foreign adoptive parents, after 15 days from the date they are declared legally free for adoption.
- Adoptive parents are made aware of the exact medical condition.

Procedure for Adoption of a Child from a Foreign Country by Indian Citizens

Necessary formalities for the adoption of a child from a foreign country by Indian citizens shall initially be completed in that country as per their law and procedure.

PEDIATRICIAN'S ROLE

A pediatrician plays a major role in guiding families through the medical aspect of adoption (helping them interpret the information provided to them, risks inherent to international adoption, information on a child's growth and development, ordering essential blood and stool tests, reviewing the immunization, and providing a schedule) as well as helps in improving the health and well-being of children in foster care.

After adoption, a pediatrician helps parents deal with challenges in rearing the adopted child and helps the child in dealing with differences and losses associated with the adoption process.

POSTADOPTION FAMILY CONCERNS

Child Concerns

Children's interest in adoption varies throughout the developmental stages of childhood and adolescence. Parents can facilitate this developmental process by being knowledgeable and supportive and by continuing to retell their child his or her adoption story, thus assisting this natural grieving process.

Infancy and Early Childhood

During this period, a child attaches to and bonds with the primary caregiver. The child must understand that places and people exist outside of his or her immediate environment. Telling a child his or her adoption story at this early age may help parents to become comfortable with the language of adoption and the child's birth story.[25]

School-aged Child

Operational thinking and logical planning start at this age. They realize that most other children live with at least one biological relative[26] and may see themselves as being different from other children, feel abandoned, angry or face withdrawal, and self-image problems. A parent's patience and understanding are crucial at this point of an adopted child's life. School personnel education about the natural grieving issues need to be discussed.[27,28]

Adolescent

Adolescents are in a phase to establish an identity while actively seeking independence and separation from family. Adopted adolescents' search for information about themselves is very normal, and parents should not see this as a threat. Instead, parents' willingness to accept their child's dual heritage of biology and environment will help their child to accept that reality.[27,28]

All adopted children grieve the loss of identity, their biological family, their heritage, and culture at some point in their lives when they learn that they were adopted and may have feelings of depression, anger, anxiety, numbness, or fear.[29] An adopted child wants to learn more about their biological family members and why were they left by their birth parents for adoption. Their grief is real and should not be denied or avoided. Support from knowledgeable healthcare providers is invaluable in helping adoptive parents and their child.

Child Abuse

Child abuse has been estimated to occur in 1% of adoptive families. An Ankeny couple who adopted nine children with disabilities from foster care has been charged for physical abuse. Recently, an Indian-American couple was booked for the death of their adopted daughter. Stringent rules for adoption and follow-up by the regulatory body may help in reducing the same.

Family Concerns

Adoptive parenthood, such as other types of parenthood, can bring tremendous joy and a sizable amount of stress. Some challenges are same that all families—biological and adoptive—face; however, other potential stressors are unique to adoption. Most adoptive children settle in with their new families, and research shows that the great majority of adoptive parents are satisfied with their decision to adopt.[30] Adoptive parents may worry that they do not "feel" like parents, even after the adoption is complete; a small percentage will have a feeling of "let down" or sadness much like postpartum depression.[31,32]

Number of things can be done to help adjust to the new identity:

- Connect with parents who have completed a similar adoption.
- Establish family traditions or rituals, e.g., bedtime reading or family movie night.
- Create a family story beginning with your own story from childhood through the decision to adopt.
- Connect with your child's birth culture.
- Prepare to respond to outsiders (relatives, friends, or strangers) about the adoption.
- Find support services tailored for adoptive families such as respite care, support groups, counselors or therapists, and educational advocates to help parents of children with special needs.

Most adopted children and families adjust well and lead healthy, productive lives. Disruption rates are higher among children adopted at the older ages and their histories of multiple placements prior to adoption.

KEY POINTS

- Adoption has given and continues to give people the opportunity to lead fulfilling, meaningful lives alongside their children, and in turn provides children opportunities in life once thought unachievable.
- Adoption is a lifelong commitment, and adoption-related issues may arise at any point in the parents' or their child's lifetime.
- A willingness to learn about the issues and seek support if necessary can help to ensure that parents and children experience happy and healthy family lives.

REFERENCES

1. Shivaraya M, Halemani B. Infertility: psycho-social consequence of infertility on women in India. Indian J Soc Dev. 2007;7:309-16.
2. Olivius C, Friden B, Borg G, Bergh C. Why do couples discontinue in vitro fertilization treatment? A cohort study. Fertil Steril. 2004;81:258-61.
3. Land JA, Courtar DA, Evers JL. Patient dropout in an assisted reproductive technology program: implications for pregnancy rates. Fertil Steril. 1997;68:278-81.
4. Olivius K, Friden B, Lundin K, Bergh C. Cumulative probability of live birth after three in vitro fertilization/intracytoplasmic sperm injection cycles. Fertil Steril. 2002;77:505-10.
5. Sharma V, Allgar V, Rajkhowa M. Factors influencing the cumulative conception rate and discontinuation of in vitro fertilization treatment for infertility. Fertil Steril. 2002;78:40-6.
6. Domar AD. Impact of psychological factors on dropout rates in insured infertility patients. Fertil Steril. 2004;81:271-3.
7. Walschaerts M, Bujan L, Parinaud J, Mieusset R, Thonneau P. Treatment discontinuation in couples consulting for male infertility after failing to conceive. Fertil Steril. 2013;99:1319-23.
8. Filetto JN, Makuch MY. Long-term follow-up of women and men after unsuccessful IVF. Reprod Biomed Online. 2005;11(4):458-63.
9. Baram D, Tourtelot E, Muechler E, Huang KE. Psychosocial adjustment following unsuccessful in vitro fertilization. J Psychosom Obstet Gynaecol. 1988;9:181-90.
10. Newton CR, Hearn MT, Yuzpe AA, Houle M. Motives for parenthood and response to failed in vitro fertilization: implications for counseling. J Assist Reprod Genet. 1992;9:24-31.
11. Newton CR, Hearn MT, Yuzpe AA. Psychological assessment and follow-up after in vitro fertilization: assessing the impact of failure. Fertil Steril. 1990;54:879-86.
12. Leiblum SR, Aviv A, Hamer R. Life after infertility treatment: a long-term investigation of marital and sexual function. Hum Reprod. 1998;13:3569-74.
13. Verhaak CM, Smeenk JM, Eugster A, van Minnen A, Kremer JA, Kraaimaat FW. Stress and marital satisfaction among women before and after their first cycle of in vitro fertilization and intracytoplasmic sperm injection. Fertil Steril. 2001;76:525-31.
14. Hjelmstedt A, Widström AM, Wramsby H, Collins A. Emotional adaptation following successful in vitro fertilization. Fertil Steril. 2004;81:1254-64.
15. Callan VJ, Hennessey JF. Emotional aspects and support in in vitro fertilization and embryo transfer programs. J In Vitro Fert Embryo Transf. 1988;5:290-5.
16. Hynes GJ, Callan VJ, Terry DJ, Gallois C. The psychological well-being of infertile women after a failed IVF attempt: the effects of coping. Br J Med Psychol. 1992;65:269-78.
17. Boivin J, Takefman JE, Tulandi T, Brender W. Reactions to infertility based on extent of treatment failure. Fertil Steril.1995;63:801-7.
18. Mahlstedt P, Macduff S, Bernstein J. Emotional factors and the in vitro fertilization and embryo transfer process. J In Vitro Fert Embryo Transf. 1987;4:232-6.
19. Dyer SJ, Abrahams N, Hoffman M, van der Spuy ZM. 'Men leave me as I cannot have children': women's experiences with involuntary childlessness. Hum Reprod. 2002;17:1663-8.
20. Bryson CA, Sykes DH, Traub AI. In vitro fertilization: a long-term follow-up after treatment failure. Hum Fertil (Camb). 2000;3:214-20.
21. Troude P, Bailly E, Guibert J, Bouyer J, de la Rochebrochard E, DAIFI Group. Spontaneous pregnancies among couples previously treated by in vitro fertilization. Fertil Steril. 2012;98:63-8.
22. de La Rochebrochard E, Quelen C, Peikrishvili R, Guibert J, Bouyer J. Long-term outcome of parenthood project during in vitro fertilization and after discontinuation of unsuccessful in vitro fertilization. Fertil Steril. 2009;92:149-56.
23. Kliegman RM. Adoption. Nelson Textbook of Pediatrics, 19th edition. Philadelphia, PA: Saunders Elsevier; 2012.
24. Garner BA. Black's Law Dictionary, 9th edition. Eagen, MN: Westlaw; 2009.

25. Canadian Paediatric Society (CPS). Understanding adoption: a developmental approach. Paediatr Child Health. 2001;6(5):281-3.
26. Melina L. Talking to children about being adopted: when to start, what to say, what to expect. Adopted Child. 2000;19:1-4.
27. Okun BF. Understanding Diverse Families: What Practitioners Need to Know. New York: Guilford Press; 1996. p. 376.
28. Derdeyn A, Graves CL. Clinical vicissitudes of adoption. Child Adolesc Psychiatr Clin N Am. 1998;7:373-88.
29. Brodzinsky DM, Schechter MD, Henig RM. Being Adopted: The Lifelong Search for Self. New York: Doubleday; 1992.
30. Vandivere S, Malm K, Radel L. Adoption USA: A Chartbook Based on the 2007 National Survey of Adoptive Parents. Washington, DC: The U.S Department of Health and Human Services, Office of the Assistant Secretary for Planning and Evaluation; 2009.
31. Foli KJ. Depression in adoptive parents: a model of understanding through grounded theory. West J Nurs Res. 2010;32(3):379-400.
32. Senecky Y, Agassi H, Inbar D, Horesh N, Diamond G, Bergman YS, et al. Post-adoption depression among adoptive mothers. J Affect Disord. 2009;115(1-2):62-8.

CHAPTER 73

LGBTQ and Fertility

Utpala Sen, Gautam Khastgir

INTRODUCTION

Lesbian, gay, bisexual, or transgender (LGBT) people are a group referred to as the LGBT community and forms a minority section of the society. Not all people consider themselves part of the LGBT community. Homosexual women are known as lesbians, which depicts their sexual identity and sexual behavior regardless of their sexual orientation. Similarly, a homosexual man is referred to as a gay individual. A transgender man is defined as a person who was assigned female at birth but identifies and expresses her gender as male and vice versa. The equality and nondiscrimination guarantee provided by international human right laws applies to all people regardless of sex, sexual orientation, and gender identity or other status. All human beings have the right to express themselves and their identities without fear of violence or retribution. The human rights of this community have been coming into sharper focus around the world, with wider acceptance and legal protection in recent years.

Gender variance is when a person's sex assigned at birth is inappropriate to what they identify themselves to be. These people desire a permanent transition to the sex or gender with which they identify by seeking medical help in the form of hormone therapy with or without sex reassignment surgery (SRS). In 1923, Hirschfeld in Germany first introduced the term trans-sexualismus, which was later translated by Cauldwell into English as transsexualism and transsexual.[1,2] Historically, transsexual people encompassed heterosexual, gay, lesbian, or bisexual. In 1965, John Oliven, for the first time introduced the term "transgender." By early 1990s, transsexual had become a subset of the umbrella term "transgender," which is now more common. The scenario has further altered with evolution of the term "gender dysphoria" in 2013, which has been described as the distress of persons who sense a mismatch between their gender identity with their sex assigned at birth.[3] All transgenders are not gender dysphoric as gender dysphoria is a diagnosis only for those who seek medical treatment, excluding those who have sexual identity disorders without gender concerns.

Those with gender dysphoria have a strong desire to modify her or his appearance and express themselves by doing surgical procedures, taking medicines, and using attire consistent with their gender identity. Transgender persons are subjected to social harassment, discrimination, and abandonment by family or friends, in addition to poor access to healthcare.[4] This psychological suffering leads to psychiatric problems such as self-harming behavior, depressive symptoms, and suicidal ideas. These problems can be lowered by gender-affirming treatment.[5]

The number of LGBT people having babies is unknown in most countries due to lack of published data. In the year 2019, data from Human Fertilization and Embryology Authority (HFEA) and birth registration in the United Kingdom identified that lesbian couples are one of the fastest growing client groups within maternity services seeking fertility treatment. The UK gender clinics have risen proportionally more for transgender men who wish to be parents. Pregnant transgender men may also be a growing population with maternity services.[6]

Over the decades, there has been a distinct paradigm shift in terms of the social existence of LGBT groups globally. A multidisciplinary tailor-made team approach is required to help them with professional assistance to fulfill their reproductive desire. This would help them to enjoy sexual relationship and skills which would strengthen their relationship. Different forms of infertility treatment involving assisted reproductive technology (ART) have been offered to these individuals or couples toward achieving pregnancy and childbirth.

The live birth rate in this group has increased by 15–20% for the past decade. Surrogacy has also shown a similar increase with respect to live birth rate. However, it is unknown what proportion of parents are heterosexual. This uncertainty exists because fertility clinic statistics assume a female partner and report statistics as "male partner, female partner, no partner, or surrogacy." No figures are available for transgender people becoming pregnant or impregnating their partners.[7]

Universal access to reproductive health is one of the goals of the Millennium Declaration 2000 and the World Summit 2005 of the United Nations.[8] According to the guidelines of the Ethics Committee for the American Society of Reproductive Medicine (ASRM), Endocrine Society, and World Professional Association for Transgender Health, fertility preservation should be discussed before any hormonal treatment or gender-affirming surgery.

The United Nations Human Rights Committee has advocated that it is unlawful to make any discrimination of people, based on their gender and sexual orientation. In 2021, The Ethics Committee of ASRM suggested that fertility programs should be same for single individuals, unmarried couples and LGBT group, and cisgender heterosexual married couples as well.[9] The European Society of Human Reproduction and Embryology (ESHRE) Task Force on Ethics and Law have suggested avoiding the use of double standard in terms of assisted reproductive therapy effect of ART on any of the persons involved, including the future child as well as the surrogate mother or the applicants themselves. All these concerns have to be considered on the basis of available scientific evidence, especially for single women, gay, lesbians, and transgenders.[10]

It is beyond the scope of this chapter to discuss the controversies with regard to the fertility issues of this particular group of people and related legislation. Nevertheless, the authors aim to provide an insight to the readers regarding the global scenario of the fertility options of LGBT groups, including various guidelines and related legislations **(Table 1)**. The changing situation in the Indian subcontinent will also be discussed.

TABLE 1: Fertility options for LGBT community.

Transgender men	Multiple options	• Oocyte cryopreservation • Ovarian tissue cryopreservation • Embryo cryopreservation
Transgender women	Limited options	• Sperm freezing • Testicular tissue cryopreservation
Lesbian	Range of options	• IUI with donor sperm • IVF with donor sperm • Co-IVF with donor sperm
Gay	Limited options	• Ovum donation with surrogacy • Embryo donation with surrogacy

(IUI: intrauterine insemination; IVF: in vitro fertilization; ; LGBT: lesbian, gay, bisexual, or transgender)

TRANSGENDER PEOPLE

Lesbians, gays, and bisexuals are equally concerned about their sexuality, but the problems of transsexuals and transgenders are completely different. Transsexual people often seek medical or surgical consultation, with an intent to satisfy their sexual needs. On the other hand, not all transgender people pursue medical treatment, though they believe that their gender behavior and culture assigned to their sex is not conforming to their gender identity described by the society. Transgender men are biologically born female but wish to be identified as male and vice versa. Fertility potential and options for transgender men and transgender women are distinctly different. A retrospective study in Sweden has reported that 69.5% of trans men and 82% of trans women wished to have parenthood. However, the desire to preserve fertility prior to hormonal or surgical treatment was higher in trans women than trans men.[11]

The process of transition from biological sex to the desired gender starts from early adolescence. Sex reassignment treatment generally starts at a younger age when reproductive desires are not clearly defined. The fertility potential of transgender people may be impaired by gender-affirming hormonal treatment (GAHT) and also suppressed by SRS. Hormonal and surgical treatment may have a devastating effect on the possibility of having a family for these people. GAHT is the most common treatment opted by transgender people to modify secondary sexual characteristics of their desired sex. All medical treatments related to sex reassignment of transgender and intersex people are named as sex reassignment therapy (SRT). A diagnosis of gender identity disorder is the prerequisite to obtain SRT. A multidisciplinary team comprising healthcare professionals, counselors, psychotherapists, and social support groups is required to provide tailor-made treatment to these people according to their wishes. For gender dysphoric children, pubertal suppression with gonadotropin-releasing hormone (GnRH) agonist at puberty can be offered to avoid the development of undesired secondary sexual characteristics.[12]

Fertility preservation should ideally be offered prior to initiation of any hormonal or surgical treatment. In 2021, a French case series has reported that 96% of transgender women who had not started treatment benefitted from sperm cryopreservation compared to 50% who were on GAHT treatment.[13] Therefore, fertility preservation options should be discussed with all transgender people before GAHT or SRS.

The guidelines published by the World Professional Association for Transgender Health are intended to ensure that the clients are adequately informed, having sound psychological health to have realistic expectations. All treatment should be done under supervision of physician and psychiatrist as unsupervised discontinuation of medicine or even change of dose may lead to physical and psychological health risk.[14]

Gender-affirming hormone therapy facilitates breast growth of thin trans-females, but reduction of breast size in trans-males with such treatment is often suboptimal. Similarly, prompt facial hair growth can be seen on trans men, while regression of hair growth is very rare in trans women. Distribution of body fat and muscle and cessation of menstruation can be achieved by GAHT in trans men. Hormones used for GAHT are testosterone, estrogen, and antiandrogen. Testosterone is used to enhance vocal cord and skin thickness in trans men.

Sex reassignment surgery is done to change the physical appearance and genital anatomy according to their gender identity. Mastectomy along with male chest reconstruction, phalloplasty for trans men, and breast augmentation with vaginoplasty for trans women are common surgeries done in this subset of patients.

For transgender men, the fertility preservation options are oocyte cryopreservation, ovarian tissue cryopreservation, and embryo cryopreservation.[15] Slow freezing cryopreservation of ovarian tissue is the standard method, but vitrification has shown good results in recent years for people who are assigned female at birth. However, in January 2022, Borrás et al. in their study have shown that both cryopreservation techniques are accurate to maintain the number of follicles as well as stromal tissue.[16] Embryo cryopreservation involves fertilization of transgender men oocyte with a donor or partner sperm. They also have the opportunity to preserve their fertility without consenting to a male partner at the time of cryopreservation. However, their future option for fertilizing the egg with another partner or donor would not exist after SRS.[17]

Ovarian tissue cryopreservation is an upcoming experimental method in this group and may be performed during SRS; however, there are limited centers where this option is offered to transgender men. In some centers, it is considered at prepubertal age when ovarian stimulation is not possible. A single case report in 2021 has showed that cryopreservation of mature oocyte is possible for transgender men who are on continuous long-term testosterone therapy.[18]

In 2021, Martin et al. have used letrozole to maintain lower level of estradiol in adolescent transgender men for ovarian stimulation. They reported that low estradiol minimizes pubertal development and possibly prevents gender dysphoria symptoms.[19]

Prolonged use of testosterone in transgender men may lead to follicular atresia, hyperplasia of stroma, and polycystic ovarian look on ultrasonography.[20,21] In 2017, De Roo et al. in their study reported that long-term use of testosterone for 1 year did not induce any significant change in ovarian morphology. In these patients, presence of a large number of primordial follicles ensures potential for in vitro maturation of cumulus–oocyte complexes.[22]

Feigerlová et al. in 2019 reported that 61% of transgender men had testosterone treatment before pregnancy and 88% used the oocytes from their own ovaries. Majority of them became pregnant spontaneously within 4 months, 7% requested fertility drugs, and only 12% required ART [intrauterine insemination (IUI), in vitro fertilization (IVF), and gamete intrafallopian transfer].[23]

There is paucity of evidence with regard to fertility potential for transgender women. The potential for fertility preservation procedures in this group have been questioned though sperm cryopreservation may be an option for them. Experimental techniques including spermatogonium stem cells and testicular tissue preservation are currently under research in prepubertal individuals. There are no reports of such procedures in clinical practice till date. Long-term effects of estrogen and antiestrogen formulations on testicular morphology and function are still not clear. Impaired steroidogenesis and involution of Leydig cells are observed following treatment with combination of estrogen and antiestrogen drugs. A multicenter study on different treatment regimens (antiestrogen with different doses of estrogen, estrogen only, or combination of spironolactone and estrogen) reported unaltered spermatogenesis in 24% of orchidectomy specimens. They also reported that spermatogenic suppression is reversible.[24] Satisfactory recovery of spermatogenesis was observed in 3–4 months after treatment cessation.[25]

LESBIANS

Lesbian single women who wish to have family can opt for IUI with donor sperm if the fallopian tubes are patent with good ovarian reserve (anti-Müllerian hormone and antral follicle count). For older women, IUI may not be the best option. IVF is the option for those lesbian couples where both the partners want to get physically involved in the treatment. Here, one partner may choose to donate egg and the other partner will carry the pregnancy. The partner donating the egg would be stimulated with hormones and have her eggs fertilized with donor sperm and then transferred into the other partner's uterus. This is called co-IVF or reciprocal IVF. They also have the option to donate eggs and the same partner has the embryos transferred. The sperm used for fertilization can be taken from a friend, known donor, or anonymous donor through a sperm bank.

GAY COUPLES

With an increasing number of gay couples willing to have biological parenthood, there is a rise in the demand for IVF. To accomplish this, gay couples need access to fertility clinics, where facility for egg donation and surrogacy is available. Occasionally, insemination may be carried out with sperms equally shared by both partners. The embryos are transferred into the uterus of the surrogate. The other option for this group is embryo donation, which means that there is no biological involvement of both the partners. Both sperm and egg are collected from the donors and the embryos are put into the surrogate's uterus. Most of the agencies who are providing the service have a customized treatment plan along with legal support, which help the couple to go through the journey smoothly.

SCENARIO IN INDIA

LGBT rights in India have been attracting more social and administrative attention over the past decade, with increasing tolerance and social acceptance. Nevertheless, discrimination still exists, especially in the rural areas where these people face rejection from their family and the society at large. The concept of gender is generally beyond the understanding of common people, who often consider the terms "gender" and "sex" to be synonymous.[19] According to the human rights campaign, gender is defined as the innermost concept of self as male, female, absence of both, or neither depending on how individuals perceive themselves and what they call themselves. There are many genders outside of just men or women that people can identify with. It can be the same as what was assigned at birth or may be entirely different.[26]

Historically, exclusion of LGBT community from the rest of the society was legalized by section 377 of the Indian penal code in 1860. It took one and a half century to change this law when the Supreme Court of India decriminalized all consensual sex among adults including homosexual sex in 2009 and subsequently in 2018.[27] In a landmark ruling by the Supreme Court of India in 2014, transgender has been recognized as a legal third gender. Transgender people now have constitutional rights to change their legal gender and to register themselves under a third gender following a reassignment surgery.[28] Legislations with regard to same-sex marriage are also emerging. The first marriage in lesbian community was officially recognized by the Gurgaon High Court in 2017.[29] In April 2022, private member's bill was introduced to legalize same-sex marriage under the Special Marriage Act, 1954.[30]

Despite the emerging Indian legislations and strong political movements in favor of LGBT rights, a large section of Indian citizens is yet to come out of the social stigma and generally disapprove such changing practice in the society. In addition, the LGBT community often face violence and discrimination in employment, education, and healthcare services. In 2014, Badgett has reported that 41% of Indians do not want their neighbor to be homosexual and 64% believe that homosexuality is not justified.[31] A public opinion poll in 2019 showed that 25% of Indians were still objecting to same-sex relationship.[32]

In India, when single parents and live-in couples with children are facing burdensome battle, the discrimination against lesbian, gay, bisexual, transgender, or queer (LGBTQ) parents is not even a part of public conversation. The right to parenthood for people of this group is not recognized or accommodated by law or even by society. Most laws and rights that fall in the domain of family law in India including adoption, surrogacy, guardianship, and assisted reproductive therapy are all tied to marriage. Adoption regulation in India, published officially by Central Adoption Resource Authority in 2017 for couple who have been married for at least 2 years, states that a single woman can adopt a child of any gender while a single man is eligible only to adopt a male child and there is no mention about live-in couples, same-sex couples, and transgender individuals. Until April 2022, when LGBT people could not get married legally, they were forced to find all sorts of other ways such as adopting in one partner's name instead of together. Currently, there is no law that unequivocally stops or supports adoption by LGBTQ people in India, and it needs to be more clarified as now the marriage is legal in this group.

The recent ART bill, 2021, strictly says that married heterosexual couple and a woman above the age of marriage can opt for ART treatment. However, single men, cohabiting heterosexual couples, and LGBT individuals and couples have been excluded. The surrogacy bill in 2022 is also far from clear in terms of the legal rights of LGBT individuals who seek treatment for childbirth and parenthood.

SUPPORT GROUPS

In the continued struggle for this particular community throughout the world to get their choice and rights accepted legally and socially, various support groups have had substantial contributions.

LGBT Mummies

The purpose of this organization is to support LGBT women and people globally on the path to motherhood or parenthood. They passionately campaign for LGBT family through their recommendation, training and conversation with government, National Health Service (NHS), corporate and charitable organization to improve support for LGBT families in healthcare, law, and society. They provide guidance on the different family creation pathways through their social media and support groups and also provide access to their global community to meet like-minded families. Their mission is to acquire true equality and equity for LGBT families to that of their heterosexual counterparts.

TwoDads (UK)

This organization commenced operation in 2004 by two male partners who are now dads to three children. They have their own networks of clinics, surrogacy agencies, family lawyers, surrogacy experts, egg banks, counselors, and regulators.

Pride

LGBT pride is a social group who promotes the dignity and equality of this group of people across the world. Pride supports LGBT-themed organizations and foundations by lending its name.

CONCLUSION

LGBT community is a component of human civilization, which has emerged over past centuries. However, this particular community has been underrepresented in the area of human rights throughout the world. Though there has been a significant revolution with regard to legal and social acceptance of this particular group of the global community, very little has been done so far regarding their fertility options being legalized. In some parts of the world, partnership rights or marriage have been extended to same-sex couples. Advocates of same-sex marriage believe that a range of benefits are denied to unmarried live-in partners. This includes immigration, health care, inheritance and property rights, and other family obligations and protections.

In summary, there has been a distinct paradigm shift in terms of the social existence and enhanced human rights of this group of people globally. New legislations and novel fertility management protocols are evolving which would pave the way forward for this community to fulfill their dream to have a child.

KEY POINTS

- LGBT community forms a minor section of the society.
- This section of people are subjected to social harassment, discrimination, and abandonment by family or friends.
- LGBTQ subjects face challenges while looking for options to have offspring.
- Fertility options for these people are limited but evolving.
- Tailormade medical treatment reinforced by social and administrative support is crucial.

REFERENCES

1. Hirschfeld M. Die intersexuelle Konstitution. Jahrbuch für sexuelle Zwischenstufen; 1923.
2. Cauldwell DO. Psychopathia Trassexualis. London: Routledge; 1949. p. 16.
3. Diagnostic and Statistical Manual of Mental Disorders, 5th edition. USA: American Psychiatric Association; 2013.
4. James SE, Herman JL, Rankin S, Keisling M, Mottet L, Anafi M. The Report of the 2015 U.S. Transgender Survey. Washington, DC: National Center for Transgender Equality; 2016.
5. Michel A, Mormont C, Legros JJ. A psycho-endocrinological overview of transsexualism. Eur J Endocrinol. 2001;145;365-76.
6. von Doussa H, Power J, Riggs D. Imagining parenthood: the possibilities and experiences of parenthood among transgender people. Cult Health Sex. 2015;17(9):1119-31.
7. Darwin Z, Greenfield M. Mothers and others: the invisibility of LGBTQ people in reproductive and infant psychology. J Reprod Infant Psychol. 2019;37:341-3.
8. United Nations Millenium Declaration 2000. A/55/305-S/2000/809; Official Records of the Security Council, Fifty-fifth Year, Supplement for July, August and September 2000, document S/2000/809
9. Ethics Committee of the American Society for Reproductive Medicine. Access to fertility treatment irrespective of marital status, sexual orientation, or gender identity: an ethics committee opinion. Fertil Steril. 2021;116(2):326-30.
10. De Wert G, Dondorp W, Shenfield F, Barri P, Devroey P, Diedrich K, et al. ESHRE task force on ethics and law 23: medically assisted reproduction in singles, lesbians, gay couples and transsexual people. Hum Reprod. 2014;29(9):1859-65.
11. Mattelin E, Strandell A, Bryman I. Fertility preservation and fertility treatment in transgender adolescents and adults in a Swedish region, 2013–2018. Hum Reprod Open. 2022;2022(2):hoac008.
12. Hagen CP, Sørensen K, Anderson RA, Juul A. Serum levels of antimüllerian hormone in early maturing girls before, during, and after suppression with GnRH agonist. Fertil Steril. 2012;98:1326-30.
13. Sermondade N, Benaloun E, Berthaut I, Moreau E, Prades M, Béranger A, et al. Reproductive functions and fertility preservations in transgender women: a French case series. Reprod Biomed Online. 2021;43(2):339-45.
14. Deutsch MB, Feldman JL. Updated recommendations from the world professional association for transgender health standards of care. Am Fam Physician. 2013;87(2):89-93
15. De Roo C, Tilleman K, T'Sjoen G, De Sutter P. Fertility options in transgender people. Int Rev Psychiatry. 2016;28(1):112-9.
16. Borrás A, Manau D, Fabregues F, Peralta S, Calafell JM, Casals G, et al. Comparison between slow freezing and vitrification of ovarian tissue cryopreservation in assigned female at birth transgender people receiving testosterone therapy: data on histological and variability parameters. J Assist Reprod Genet. 2022;39:527-41.
17. Mattawanon N, Spencer JB, Schirmer 3rd DA, Tangpricha V. Fertility preservation options in the transgender people: a review. Rev Endocr Metab Disord. 2018;19(3):231-42.
18. Gale J, Magee B, Forsyth-Greig A, Visram H, Jackson A. Oocyte cryopreservation in a transgender man on long-term testosterone therapy: a case report. F S Rep. 2021;2(2):249-51.
19. Martin CE, Lewis C, Omurtag K. Successful oocyte cryopreservation using letrozole as an adjunct to stimulation in a transgender adolescent after GnRH agonist suppression. Fertil Steril. 2021;116(2):522-7.
20. Miller N, Bédard YC, Cooter NB, Shaul DL. Histological changes in the genital tract in transsexual women following androgen therapy. Histopathology. 1986;10:661-9.
21. Caanen MR, Schouten NE, Kuijper EAM, van Rijswijk J, van den Berg MH, van Dulmen-den Broeder E, et al. Effects of long-term exogenous testosterone administration on ovarian

morphology, determined by transvaginal (3D) ultrasound in female-to-male transsexuals. Hum Reprod. 2017;32; 1457-64.

22. De Roo C, Lierman S, Tilleman K, Peynshaert K, Braeckmans K, Caanen M, et al. Ovarian tissue cryopreservation in female-to-male transgender people: insights into ovarian histology and physiology after prolonged androgen treatment. Reprod Biomed Online. 2017;34:557-66.
23. Feigerlová E, Pascal V, Ganne-Devonec MO, Klein M, Gerci B. Fertility desires and reproductive needs of transgender people: challenges and considerations for clinical practice. Clin Endocrinol (Oxf). 2019;91(1):10-21.
24. Schneider F, Newhaus N, Wistuba J, Zitzmann M, Heß J, Mahler D, et al. Testicular functions and clinical characterization of patients with gender dysphoria (GD) undergoing sex reassignment surgery (SRS). J Sex Med. 2015;12:2190-200.
25. Adeleye AJ, Reid G, Kao CN, Mok-Lin E, Smith JF. Semen parameters among transgender women with a history of hormonal treatment. Urology. 2019;124:136-41.
26. Adams C. The difference between sexual orientation and gender identity. CBC News; 2017.
27. Johar NS, Ors. V. Union of India Thr. Secretory, Ministry of Law and Justice, W. P. (crl no. 762 2016. Supreme Court of India). [online] Available from https://indiankanoon.org/doc/119980704/ [Last accessed November, 2022].
28. Global Human Rights Defense. [online] Available from https://ghrd.org/ [Last accessed November, 2022].
29. In a first, Gurgaon court recognize. http://timesofindia.indiatimes.com/articleshow/9401421.cms?utm_source=contentofinterest&utm_medium=text&utm_campaign=cppst
30. NCP's Supriya Sule brings bill to legalize same-sex marriage. The Indian Express. 2022. [online] Available from https://indianexpress.com/article/india/ncps-supriya-sule-brings-bill-to-legalise-same-sex-marriage-7848768/ [Last accessed November, 2022].
31. Badgett MVL. (2014). The Economic Cost of Stigma and the Exclusion of LGBT People: A Case Study of India. Washington, DC: World Bank. [online] Available from https://openknowledge.worldbank.org/handle/10986/21515. [Last accessed November, 2022].
32. Centre for the Study of Developing Societies. (2019). Politics and society between elections. Regional political democracy. 2-Social Identity. https://www.lokniti.org/media/upload_files/politics-and-society-between-elections-2019-report.pdf. [Last accessed November, 2022]. pp. 88-92.

CHAPTER 74

Transgender Population and Fertility

HK Nagaraj, Arjun N

INTRODUCTION

Gender dysphoria is a term used to define the psychological distress experienced by transgender people because of the incongruence between the birth assigned sex and one's gender identity. However, transgender is a term used to denote a person whose birth assigned sex differs from their gender identity.

As per the 2011 census, India's transgender population is around 4.88 lakh. In Karnataka, the total population of transgenders is about 20,266, with a literacy rate of 58.82%. This population has lesser access to jobs, education or community/family support and hence these people are subject to inequality in their social and economic status.

There has been an increased demand for gender affirmation surgery and specialized care to meet the expanding needs for this specific population, but only a small portion of them undergo both chest and genital surgeries. This indicates that the needs of the patient may be varied may it be surgical or otherwise.

GENDER AFFIRMATION SURGERY

In gender dysphoria, gender affirmation surgery is often the last and most considered step in the process of treatment as compared to the other modalities.

It includes a large selection of procedures which can be broadly classified into male-to-female (MTF) or female-to-male (FTM). The most common procedures opted for are given in **Tables 1 and 2**.

TABLE 1: Common surgical procedures for male-to-female (MTF).

Surgical procedures for MTF	*Process*
Chest surgery	Breast augmentation
Genital surgery	Penectomy, orchidectomy, vaginoplasty
Others	Facial feminization surgery, esthetic procedures, hair reconstruction, liposuction/lipofilling, thyroid cartilage reduction

TABLE 2: Common surgical procedures for female-to-male (FTM).

Surgical procedures for FTM	*Process*
Chest surgery	Bilateral mastectomy
Genital surgery	Hysterectomy, salpingo-oophorectomy, metoidioplasty, phalloplasty, vaginectomy, scrotoplasty, insertion of prosthesis
Others	Facial reconstruction, pectoral implants, esthetic procedures

Criteria for Gender Affirmation Surgery

At our institute we follow certain criteria that the patients have to fulfill before they are deemed to be considered for surgery. Any patient who comes for sex reassignment procedures would be referred to the department of psychiatry for diagnosis, counseling and confirmation of gender dysphoria. After the patient has undergone the requisite counseling, letters of recommendation are requested from the mental healthcare professionals for the surgical procedure considered.

Among others, a recommendation letter from one mental health professional is required for chest surgery and letters from two mental health professionals is required for genital surgery.

Hormone therapy is a prerequisite for surgery in the case of genital surgery for a minimum continuous period of 12 months, however not so in the case of chest surgery as per the *WPATH guidelines.*

The two major goals of hormonal therapy are:

1. To reduce endogenous sex hormone levels to reduce the secondary sex characteristics of the individual's designated gender, and

TABLE 3: Hormone regimes for transgender females [male-to-female (MTF)].

Antiandrogens
• GnRH agonists – leuprolide depot – 3.75 mg subcutaneously monthly or 11.25 mg subcutaneously 3 monthly • If the patient cannot afford GnRH agonists then, the following can be given • Spironolactone 100–200 mg/day (up to 300 mg) • Cyproterone acetate 25–50 mg/day
Estrogen
• *Oral estradiol:* – Estradiol valerate 2–6 mg/day, initially low doses are started, then increased every 2–3 months • *Transdermal estrogen:* – Estradiol patch 0.025–0.2 mg/d (new patch placed every 3–5 d) • *Parenteral:* – Estradiol valerate or cypionate - 5–30 mg IM every 2 weeks - 2–10 mg IM every 2 weeks

BOX 1: Hormonal therapy for transgender males [female-to-male (FTM)].

Testosterone:
- *Parenteral testosterone (IM or subcutaneous)*
- Testosterone enanthate or cypionate 100–200 mg every 2 weeks or 250 mg every 3–4 weeks
- Testosterone undecanoate 1,000 mg every 12 weeks

Transdermal testosterone:
- Testosterone gel 1% w/v 5 g: 50–100 mg/d
- Testosterone transdermal patch: 2.5–7.5 mg/d

2. To replace endogenous sex hormone levels consistent with the individual's gender identity by using hormone replacement therapy of the identified gender

The hormone replacement therapy routinely used at our institute is given in **Table 3 and Box 1**.

Additionally, we also get an affidavit done with relevant declarations through the legal process prior to surgery. Below we will discuss a few procedures involved in gender affirmation surgery.

Surgical Procedures in Male-to-Female

This includes breast augmentation, orchidectomy, feminizing urethroplasty, vaginoplasty, etc. **(Table 1)**.

Vaginoplasty includes creation of a neovagina of adequate depth and width which can be done in various techniques. An average depth of around 12–15 cm is achievable by using the penile skin technique. The procedure involves bilateral orchidectomy and creation of the neo-vaginal canal initially. The neovaginal canal is made in a space in-between the urethra along with the bladder superiorly and the rectum inferiorly. The penis is separated into its component parts, after which based on the type of the vaginoplasty, the procedure is taken forward. The skin of the penis is used to cover the neovaginal canal when doing a penile skin inversion vaginoplasty, the urethra is shortened and feminizing urethroplasty is done and the neovascular bundle along with a part of the glans is used to create the neoclitoris.

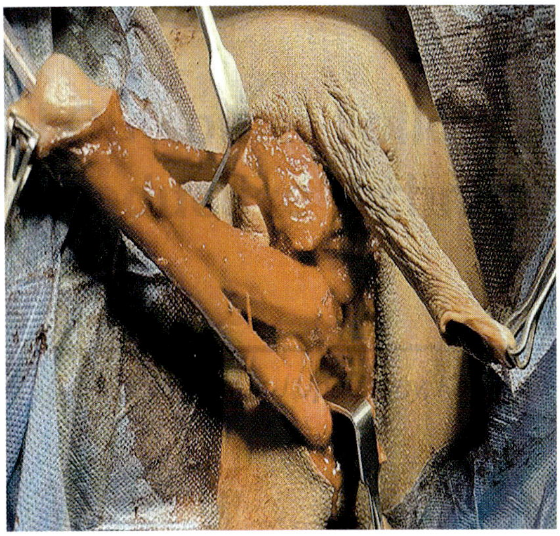

Fig. 1: Components separated showing the penile skin, urethra, corpora cavernosal bundles and neurovascular bundle with glans penis. Retractor showing the neovaginal canal.

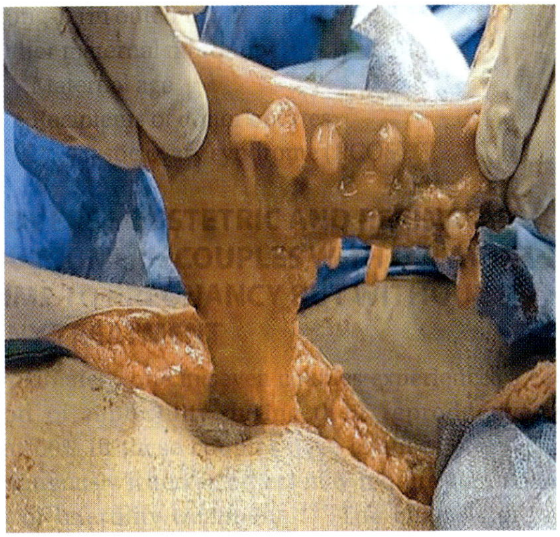

Fig. 2: Colon segment used for vaginoplasty.

Vaginoplasty can be done in various methods including the penile skin inversion vaginoplasty as described. Others include using pedicled intestinal segments such as sigmoid colon, ileum, etc. Also we can include a peritoneal or skin flap and partial or full thickness skin grafts for the same among others **(Fig. 2)**.

Reconstruction is done using the available tissue along with the scrotal skin. Postoperatively patients are given vaginal dilators for up to 6 months for regular dilatation of the neo vaginal canal based on the procedure they have undergone **(Figs. 1 to 4)**.

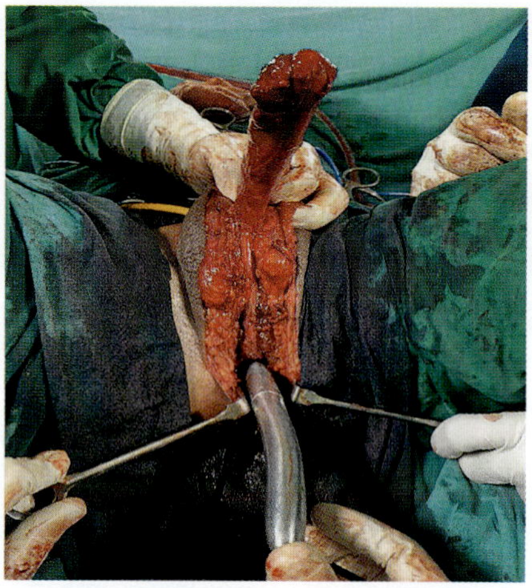

Fig. 3: Neovaginal canal created.

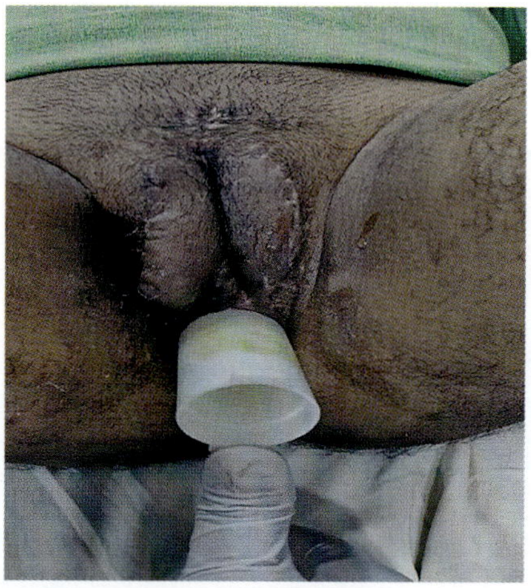

Fig. 4: Vaginal dilators.

Majority of the Indian patients do not opt for a vaginoplasty but only removal of the male genitalia with a feminizing urethroplasty or a zero depth vaginoplasty.

Other Procedures

The other common procedures include breast augmentation which is done either by using breast implants or by fat augmentation, facial feminization surgery, aesthetic procedures, hair reconstruction, liposuction/lipofilling, thyroid cartilage reduction, etc.

Surgical Procedures in FTM

This includes bilateral mastectomy, hysterectomy, salpingo-oophorectomy, metoidioplasty, phalloplasty, etc., as discussed in **Table 2**.

Bilateral Mastectomy (Chest Surgery)

This includes removal of breast tissue bilaterally usually via a periareolar incision, inframammary incision, double incision, transaxillary being some of the methods used.

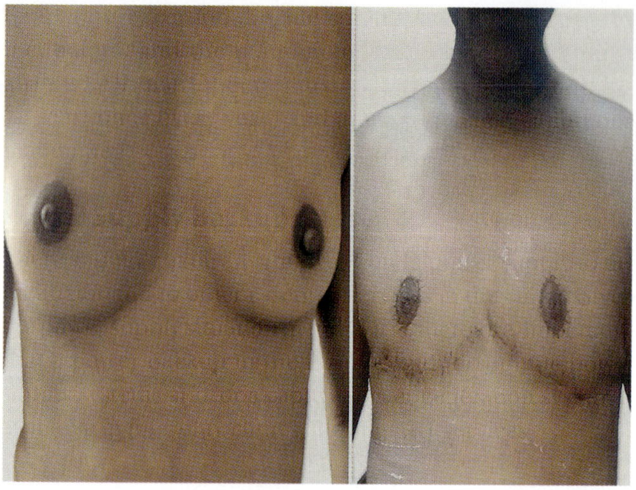

Fig. 5: Bilateral mastectomy.

The procedure used is dependent on the size of the breast and is evaluated preoperatively and the patient is counseled accordingly **(Fig. 5)**.

Metoidioplasty and Phalloplasty

Metoidioplasty is a one stage procedure for the creation of a microphallus. The patient is required to undergo a minimum of 1 year of hormone replacement therapy prior to the procedure. This ensures an adequate growth of the genital tissues which can be used for reconstruction required for metoidioplasty. Metoidioplasty of an adequate length ensures that the patient can micturate in the standing position. However, it is not adequate for the purpose of intercourse. This can be done with phalloplasty.

Phalloplasty is one of the most challenging procedures in gender affirmation surgery. It involves creation of a neophallus using a well vascularized flap. It can be combined with other procedures such as reconstruction of the urethra, closure of the vaginal canal, creation of scrotum, implants, etc., in a single stage or a two stage procedure.

Various flaps are used for the purpose of phalloplasty including radial artery forearm free flap, anterolateral thigh flap, latissimus dorsi flap, abdominal flap, etc., based on the patient requirements and body habitus. The length of the neo phallus depends on the flap taken.

Below we have described the procedure of a radial artery forearm free flap phalloplasty in brief. The flap was marked as shown. The radial artery and cephalic vein were identified and divided. Centrally, the neourethra was planned as shown and tubularized. This would be connected later on with the native urethra along with tissue obtained from the vagina and labial skin to gain adequate length of the urethra for anastomosis. The flap is wrapped around the neo urethra to form the neophallus. The corona is fashioned on the neo phallus. The neophallus is brought to the recipient site and the neourethra is anastomosed to the native reconstructed urethra over a Foleys catheter. The arterial and venous

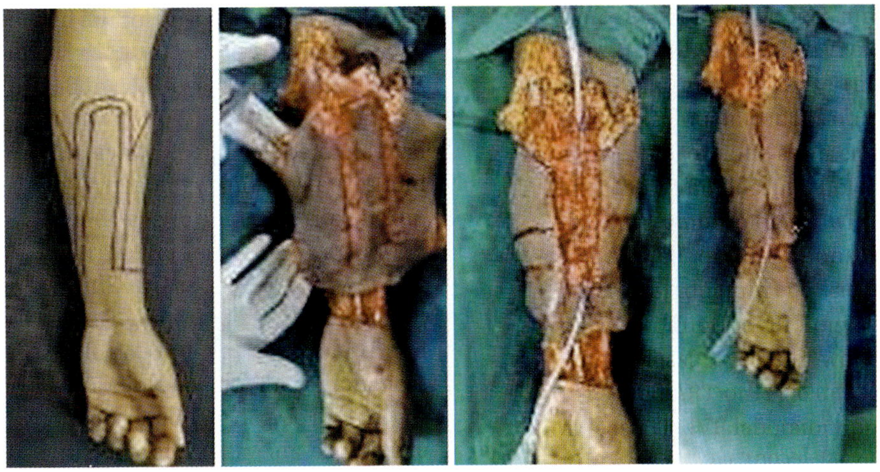

Fig. 6: Radial artery free flap marked, raised and tubularized.

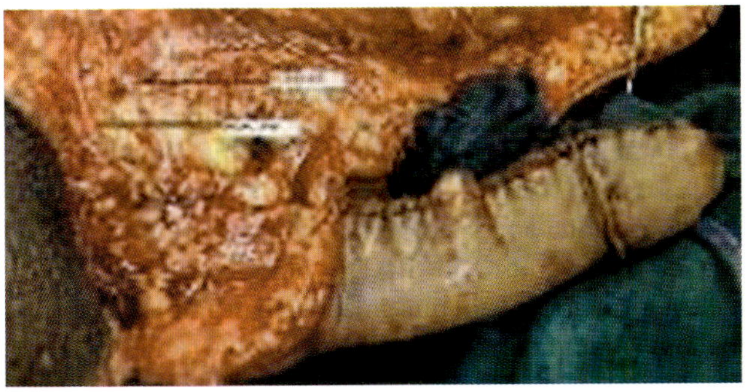

Fig. 7: Flap after anastomosis.

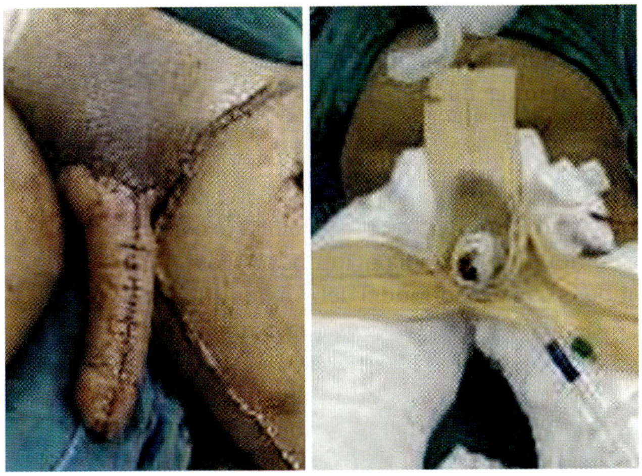

Fig. 8: Created neophallus and dressing.

anastomoses are done. We use a saphenofemoral AV loop, which is made to facilitate the arterial and venous anastomosis. The left ilioinguinal nerve was coapted with the lateral antebrachial cutaneous nerve. The flap inset is completed and the vagina is closed. The donor forearm site is covered with a skin graft. We usually plan for placement of penile and scrotal implants at a second stage **(Figs. 6 to 8)**.

Other Procedures

The other commonly done procedures include hysterectomy with or without bilateral salpingo-oophorectomy which may be done by the open abdominal, vaginal, laparoscopic or robotic method. The other procedures include supplemental or esthetic procedures, facial reconstructive procedures, etc.

COMPLICATIONS OF GENDER AFFIRMATION SURGERY

The purpose of gender affirmation surgery though done regularly comes with a set of complications that the patient has to be counseled and aware of. Depending on the type of surgery the complications may vary. In chest surgeries, the most commonly encountered complications are that of wound infection, necrosis of the nipple areola complex in mastectomy, complications of the breast implants including infection of the implant and capsular fibrosis are seen. In both, scarring may be a significant feature with keloid formation at the incision site in a few.

In genital surgeries, the more serious complications include neovaginal canal stenosis **(Fig. 9)**, rectal or bladder fistulas with the neovaginal canal, urethral stenosis in the case of vaginoplasty. As with phalloplasty, urethral strictures, necrosis of the neophallus and urethrocutaneous fistulas are the more morbid complications usually requiring a second procedure for correction. The above are just a few of the complications encountered during gender affirmation surgery **(Fig. 10)**.

The most common problem in the present scenario arises with patients who undergo these procedures in the hands of surgeons or others who are not trained to do these procedures, those who do not follow guidelines for the same or procedures done at low volume centers. In many cases, there is no diagnosis of gender dysphoria or the patient has not undergone hormone replacement therapy. This leads to a significant morbidity to the patient in terms of a bad

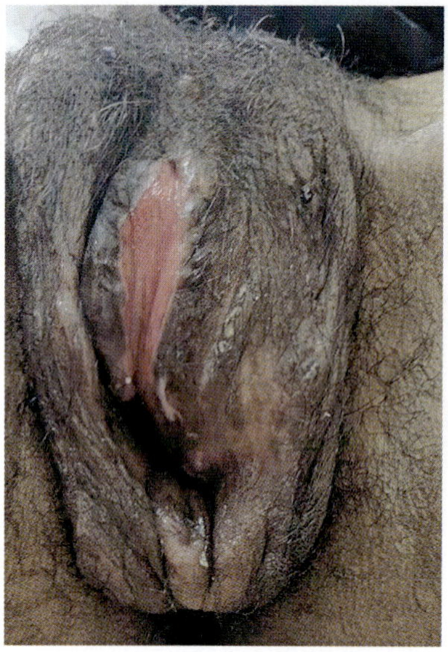

Fig 9: Stenosis of neovaginal canal.

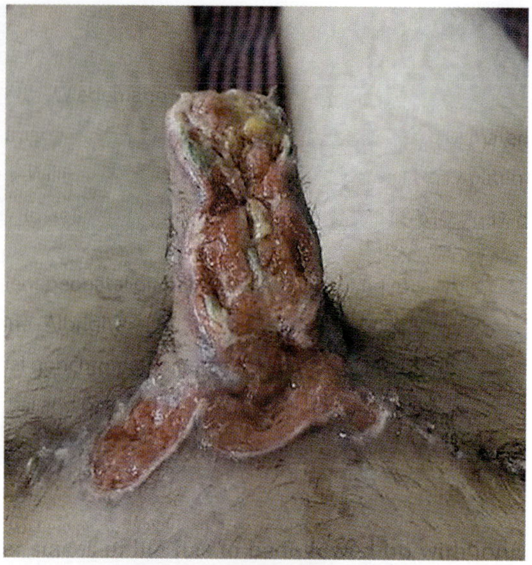

Fig. 10: Necrosis of neophallus.

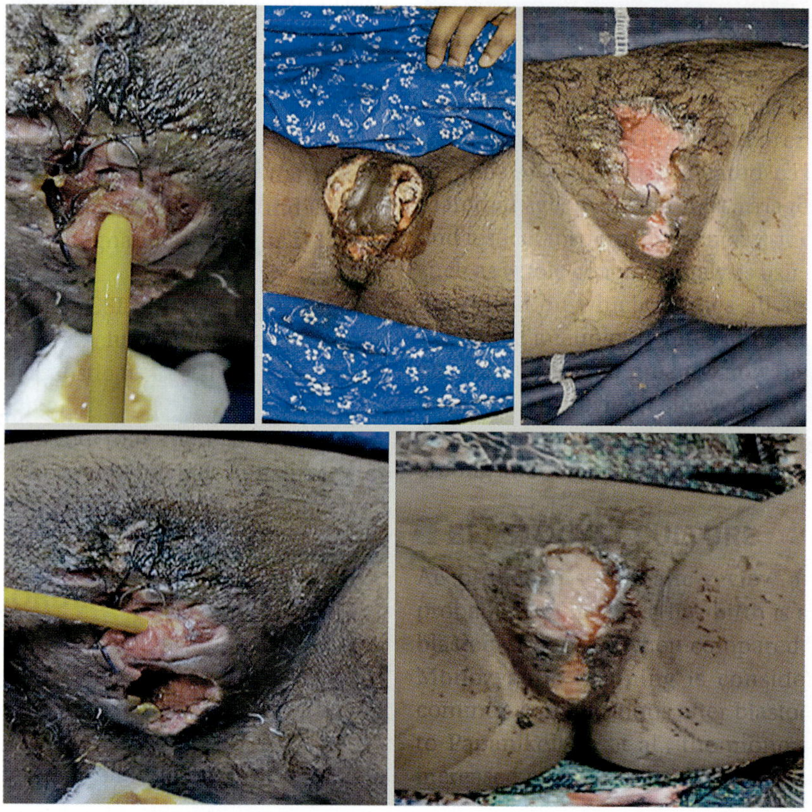

Fig. 11: Complications of surgery with urethral injury.

reconstructive procedure or long-term implications to the patient for the same. This leads to added procedures, health risks and an additional financial burden to these patients. Most commonly encountered are shown in the images **(Fig. 11)**.

Urethral stenosis is a very commonly seen complication of urethroplasty in gender affirmation surgery. The patients usually realize the thinning of urinary stream with recurrent urinary infections and some patients tend toward home-made solutions for the purpose of urethral dilatation with the use of thin metal rods/wires, clove, hair accessories, etc. The treatment of the same includes urethral dilatation as a temporary procedure or meatoplasty as a permanent measure. An adequate spatulation of the urethra during

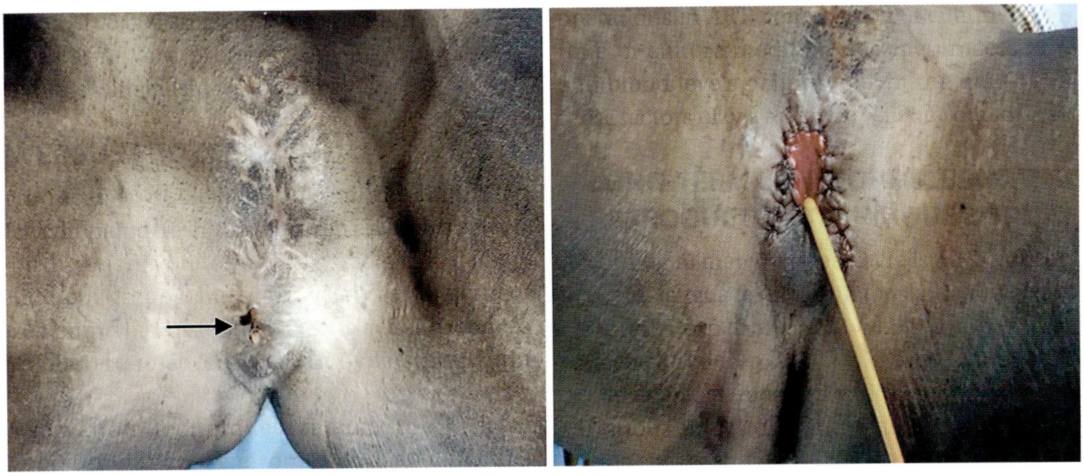

Fig. 12: Urethral stenosis with clove inserted by patient for dilatation.

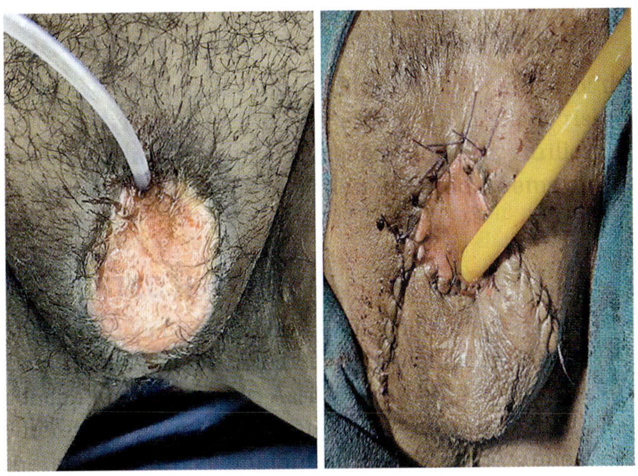

Fig. 13: Urethral injury with stenosis.

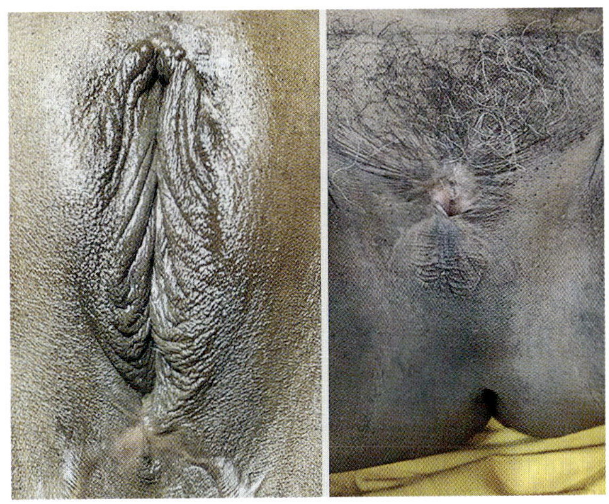

Fig. 14: Urethral stenosis postsurgery.

reconstruction with adequate skin flap cover are a few techniques utilized to prevent this complication. The other complications include infection and necrosis of the surgical flaps which require debridement and secondary reconstruction in certain cases **(Figs. 12 to 14)**.

There are incidents in certain patients living within transgender communities wherein they are made to under genital mutilation procedures using knives or other sharp instruments which require an additional reconstructive procedure either in the short- or long-term periods as shown in **Figure 13**.

FERTILITY PRESERVATION

After a patient undergoes orchidectomy or oophorectomy for gender affirmation, fertility is a concern as it causes irreversible effects in the patient. Hence the fertility preservation should be discussed with the patient before they undergo any treatment for the same. The methods of fertility preservation in transgender patients have been discussed here.

Fertility Preservation in MTF Transgender Patients

Hormonal interventions for transgender people down-regulate the HPG axis and the estrogen therapy causes reduced testosterone and in turn reduced sperm count and motility and surgical orchidectomy would be irreversible. Methods for fertility preservation in MTF include sperm cryopreservation. Cryopreservation of testicular tissue for intracytoplasmic sperm injection is an experimental option but feasible in azoospermic men. The collection is ideally done before hormone therapy is started as studies have shown azoospermia in around 75% of men who have been started on hormone therapy after 6 months of use.

Fertility Preservation in FTM Transgender Patients

Embryo and oocyte cryopreservation are first-line methods in postpubertal women. Metaphase II oocyte cryopreservation is the preferred option. Oocyte cryopreservation, embryo cryopreservation and ovarian tissue cryopreservation are the three methods for fertility preservation in FTM transgender patients of which ovarian tissue cryopreservation is in an experimental stage. Oocyte cryopreservation includes a controlled ovarian hyperstimulation but the patient will need to stop hormone therapy for the same. Embryo cryopreservation is similar to oocyte cryopreservation, but once mature oocytes are retrieved, they are inseminated on the same day to create embryos and then vitrified for future use.

There is a need for further studies in this area with the focus on transgender population. With breakthrough examples such as uterine transplantation in the field of reproductive medicine which has been proven to be successful in a controlled setting, there is a need for detailed discussion with the patient regarding fertility preservation prior to the commencement of any therapy for gender dysphoria.

CONCLUSION

Gender dysphoria and gender affirmation surgery involves multiple considerations which may be different for each individual. It is necessary to be aware of the options available and the protocols to be followed so that proper guidance can be given in this aspect.

KEY NOTES

- There is an increasing awareness for gender dysphoria with an increasing population of transgender patients requiring specialized treatment.
- Gender affirmation surgery is always followed by the diagnosis of gender dysphoria with relevant counseling and hormone treatment when necessary.
- The main modality of fertility preservation in MTF is sperm cryopreservation.
- Fertility preservation in FTM mainly includes oocyte cryopreservation, embryo cryopreservation and ovarian tissue cryopreservation.

SUGGESTED READING

1. American Psychiatric Association. Diagnostic and Statistical Manual of Mental Disorders, 5th edition (DSM-5). Washington, DC: American Psychiatric Association; 2013.
2. An Interim National Guideline—Good Practices for Sex Reassignment Surgeries (SRS) for Male-to-Female Transgender People in India, could be accessed, that is prepared by UNAIDS India-constituted Working Group in 2011. New Delhi: Ministry of Social Justice and Empowerment; 2011.
3. Gupta R, Murarka A. Treating transsexuals in India: History, prerequisites for surgery and legal issues. IJPS. 2009;42(2): 226-33.
4. Hembree WC, Cohen-Kettenis PT, Gooren L, Hannema SE, Meyer WJ, Murad MH, et al. Endocrine Treatment of Gender-Dysphoric/Gender-Incongruent Persons: An Endocrine Society Clinical Practice Guideline. J Clin Endocrinol Metab. 2017;102(11):3869-903. Erratum in: J Clin Endocrinol Metab. 2018;103(2):699. Erratum in: J Clin Endocrinol Metab. 2018; 103(7):2758-9.
5. Hovatta O. Cryopreservation of testicular tissue. Mol Cell Endocrinol. 2000;169(1-2):113-5.
6. Jagadeesh N. Third Sex and Gender Equity. J Clin Biomed Sci. 2015;5(4):141-2.
7. Johannesson L, Järvholm S. Uterus transplantation: current progress and future prospects. Int J Womens Health. 2016; 8:43-51.
8. Kumbar L, Bobba R, Arjun N, Kalra P. Demographic data of transgender population from a tertiary care centre in south India. Med J DY Patil Vidyapeeth. 2022:21.
9. Li JS, Crane CN, Santucci RA. Vaginoplasty tips and tricks. Int Braz J Urol. 2021;47(2):263-73.
10. Majumder A, Chatterjee S, Maji D, Roychaudhuri S, Ghosh S, Selvan C, et al. (2020). IDEA Group Consensus Statement on Medical Management of Adult Gender Incongruent Individuals Seeking Gender Reaffirmation as Female. Indian J Endocrinol Metab. 2020;24(2):128-35.
11. Martinez F. Update on fertility preservation from the Barcelona International Society for Fertility Preservation-ESHRE-ASRM 2015 expert meeting: indications, results and future perspectives. Hum Reprod. 2017;32(9):1802-11.
12. Mattawanon N, Spencer JB, Schirmer DA 3rd, Tangpricha V. Fertility preservation options in transgender people: A review. Rev Endocr Metab Disord. 2018;19(3):231-42.
13. Mittra A. Educational inequality in India: A review paper for transgender population. Int J Trend Sci Res Dev. 2017;2:1578-84.
14. Schneider F, Kliesch S, Schlatt S, Neuhaus N. Andrology of male-to-female transsexuals: influence of cross-sex hormone therapy on testicular function. Andrology. 2017;5(5):873-80.
15. Taliat G, Kumar KM, Nagaraj A. Phalloplasty - Sensate radial forearm free flap for creation of neourethra and neophallus in gender affirmation surgery: a case report. J Surg Med. 2021;5(12):1224-6.
16. World Health Organization Task Force on Methods for the Regulation of Male Fertility. Contraceptive efficacy of testosterone-induced azoospermia and oligozoospermia in normal men. Fertil Steril. 1996;65(4):821-9.
17. WPATH. Standard of care - version 8. Minneapolis: World Professional Association for Transgender Health; 2020.
18. Zhao LC. Gender affirming surgery. Urol Clin North Am. 2019;46(4):1.

SECTION 11

Outcome Following Assisted Reproductive Technique

CHAPTER 75

Maternal and Fetal Outcomes Following Assisted Reproductive Technique

Navya V, Amit J Upadhyay, Kamini A Rao

INTRODUCTION

Infertility is defined as an inability to conceive after 1 year of attempting pregnancy.[1] Infertility itself acts as an independent predictor of adverse pregnancy and perinatal outcomes.[2-4] Assisted reproductive techniques (ARTs) contribute to 1.4–7% of total pregnancies.[5] ART helps couples suffering from primary or secondary infertility.[6] But nowadays, it has been extended to help patients undergoing gonadotoxic treatments for fertility preservation,[7] to help same-sex couples, single women, and men to conceive and have their biological children,[8] and to facilitate the services of surrogate gestational carriers. The global incidence of multiple pregnancies is on the rise due to ART and advancing maternal age.[9,10]

The ART involves any procedure which includes handling of human gametes outside a body such as in vitro fertilization (IVF), intracytoplasmic sperm injection (ICSI), cryopreservation, donor gamete usage, assisted zona hatching (AZH), preimplantation genetic screening (PGS), and intrauterine insemination (IUI).[11] In the initial days, success of ART was a primary concern now with an exponentially escalating number of children born through ART poses multiple challenges on maternal as well as fetal outcomes.

POSSIBLE CAUSES OF ADVERSE OUTCOMES AT VARIOUS LEVELS

- Specific IVF-related outcomes **(Table 1)**[11]
- Perinatal risks
  - Multiple gestations
  - Preterm birth
  - Low birth weight and small for gestation age (SGA)
  - Congenital anomalies
  - Perinatal mortality
- Long-term outcomes of children
- Other maternal morbidity
  - Maternal age
  - Recipients of donor oocytes
  - Polycystic ovary syndrome (PCOS).

ADVERSE OBSTETRIC AND PERINATAL OUTCOME IN COUPLES WITH DELAY IN TIME TO PREGNANCY BUT WITHOUT ANY TREATMENT

Approximately, one in seven couples experiences a certain period of subfertility during their reproductive life.[12] About 50% of these couples have chances of conceiving spontaneously whereas others may require some or other form of infertility treatment.[13-15] The chances of having high obstetric and perinatal adverse outcomes are more in subfertile population when compared to women who are fertile.[16,17] There are evidences showing the increased risk of obstetric complications and interventions in women with subfertility, which are independent of age, parity, and fertility treatment. The risk of preterm delivery and low birth weight is high among ART-born babies.[18] In comparison with women in the general population,

TABLE 1: Specific in vitro fertilization-related outcomes.[11]

At gamete level	*At embryo level*	*At embryo transfer level*	*At endometrial level*
• Maternal and paternal age • Environment • Genetics • Male factor • Ovarian stimulation • In vitro maturation	• Culture systems • Assisted hatching • Blastomere biopsy	• Number of embryos transferred • Day of transfer • Quality • Cryopreservation • Imprinting disorders • PGD/PGS	• Endometrial receptivity • Placentation • Maternal health • Uterine environment • Gestation order

(PGD: preimplantation genetic diagnosis; PGS: preimplantation genetic screening)

there is a twofold increased risk of preeclampsia, placental abruption, cesarean section and vacuum extraction, and a fivefold increased risk of placenta previa in spontaneous singleton pregnancies in women with a history of infertility.[18]

MULTIPLE PREGNANCY AND ADVERSE OBSTETRICAL AND PERINATAL OUTCOMES

Multiple pregnancy is the most debatable issue associated with ART. Multifetal gestations are considered as high-risk pregnancies with higher perinatal morbidity and mortality rate. The prime determinant of pregnancy and its long-term sequelae depends on whether the pregnancy is a singleton or multiple gestation, irrespective of whether it is a natural or assisted conception.[19,20]

Worldwide, there is a drastic increase in the multiple-order births associated with advancing maternal age due to increased focus on career orientation and seeking fertility treatment.[21,22] Following ovulation induction with drugs and controlled ovarian hyperstimulation, multiple gestation rates range between 5 and 40%.[23] The 2011 published rate of multiple pregnancies as a result of IVF reported by the Canadian Assisted Reproductive Technologies Register (CARTR) in Canada is approximately 30%.[24]

The risk of adverse outcomes increases with high-order gestation and even worsens with monozygous gestation as it poses two- to threefold increased risk when compared to natural conceptions although the incidence of monozygotic twins, even after IVF, remains very low.[25]

Approximately, monozygotic twinning (meaning having a monochorionic placentation) accounts for 0.4% of live births among pregnancies which are conceived spontaneously when compared to 0.9–2% of IVF pregnancies.[25-27] The percentage of monozygotic twinning is almost 6% after transferring day 5 blastocyst in IVF pregnancies when compared to day 3 cleavage embryo transfer which accounts for 2%.[28]

One of the recent systematic reviews in 2009 compared the live birth rate of elective double embryo transfer (DET) with that of elective single, triple, or quadruple embryo transfer. The review concluded that a single cycle of elective single embryo transfer (eSET) resulted in a lower live birth rate than DET, but that the cumulative live birth rate in a fresh eSET cycle followed by a frozen eSET was not significantly different from a single DET cycle.[29]

A meta-analysis by Grady et al. in 2012 compared perinatal outcomes between DET and eSET pregnancies. eSET is associated with decreased risks of preterm births and low birth weight compared with DET but poses a high risk when compared to singleton pregnancies conceived spontaneously. They found a randomized controlled trial (RCT)-based relative risk of 0.37 (0.25–0.55) for preterm birth <37 weeks and an RCT-based relative risk of 0.25 (0.15–0.45) for birth weight <2,500 g in the eSET group.[30]

As evidence in the literature shows, there may be a sevenfold increase in mortality among twins and 20-fold increase in mortality among triplets when compared to singletons.[31-33] The risks of perinatal mortality, growth restriction, cerebral palsy, and congenital anomalies are also increased in multiple-order gestation than in singletons, not only in monochorionic twins but also in dichorionic twins.[22,34,35]

Multiple-order gestation involves higher perinatal complications including fetal anomalies, fetal demise, intrauterine growth restriction, prematurity, polyhydramnios, and oligohydramnios.[36]

Some rare complications such as twin oligohydramnios-polyhydramnios sequence (TOPS), twin-to-twin transfusion syndrome (TTTS), acardiac twins, conjoined twins, co-twin demise, and heterotopic pregnancies, which affect both maternal and perinatal outcomes negatively, are seen with multiple gestations.[37]

Nowadays, adopting eSET in assisted reproductive technologies demonstrates a rapid downfall in unnecessary complications to mother such as preeclampsia and cerebral palsy for fetus.[38]

PRETERM DELIVERY

Various meta-analyses in the literature showed that singleton pregnancies born through assisted reproductive technologies after single-embryo transfer or multiple-embryo transfer are 1.8–2.1 times more prone to the risk of preterm delivery when compared to pregnancies which are conceived spontaneously.[39-42]

De Neubourg et al. study compared single-embryo transfer versus spontaneous singletons, which found a 10% risk of preterm delivery in the single-embryo transfer group compared to a 6.8% risk among spontaneously conceived singletons.[43]

Hayashi et al. concluded that infertility itself is a risk factor of preterm delivery and also there is no significant difference in the risk of prematurity between various methods of infertility treatment groups such as ovulation induction, IUI, and IVF. He also derived a conclusion that prematurity risk is more in the infertility-treated singleton groups in comparison to singletons born in fertile groups.[44]

According to Adam et al. study, the production of high levels of steroid hormones and other protein peptides resulting after ovarian stimulation during IVF also increases the risk of prematurity, hence performing an embryo transfer in artificially prepared luteal cycles after cryopreservation of embryos was shown beneficial. Along with ovarian steroid hormones, maternal serum relaxin, which is produced from the corpus luteum also known to be increased after controlled superovulation, which is associated with an increased risk of preterm delivery in singleton.[45]

In view of Maheshwari et al., there is a lower risk of preterm deliveries in singleton pregnancies conceived with frozen embryo transfer when compared to fresh embryo transfer cycles. In this study, following frozen thawed transfer, singleton pregnancies were 16% less likely to deliver before 37 weeks in comparison to those pregnancies following fresh IVF cycles.[46]

Therefore, it is well documented that ART singleton pregnancies have a little increased risk of preterm compared to singleton from spontaneous conceptions. Preterm birth after ART is considered as a syndrome with multifactorial etiology.

LOW BIRTH WEIGHT

In the literature, all systematic reviews showed that IVF pregnancies are associated with low birth weight babies.[40,42,47-49] Sazonova et al. performed logistic regression analysis between 2002 and 2006 on 8,941 singleton pregnancies, and four major outcomes were investigated such as very preterm birth, SGA, placenta previa, and placental abruption. Maternal factors such as age, parity, body mass index (BMI), smoking, and years of infertility and other variables such as number of oocytes retrieved, number of embryo culture days, number of transferred and cryopreserved embryos, and "vanishing twin" were studied and it was concluded that primiparity, smoking, BMI, and the vanishing twin phenomenon increased the risk of preterm birth and that maternal age, smoking, BMI, and duration of infertility increased the risk of low birth weight.[50]

Various studies compared fresh versus cryopreserved embryos, which showed that frozen embryo transfers result in higher birth weights and decrease the chances of low birth weight infants in addition to preterm births.[51-54] A systematic review analyzed that the risk of low birth weight can be unchanged or improved with frozen embryo transfers whereas the risk of preterm births is either unchanged or decreased.[55]

An interesting study of 292 singletons examined serum estradiol levels during IVF cycles adjusted for patient's age, BMI, parity, number of embryos transferred, day of transfer, and gonadotropin dose, and high serum estradiol levels (>3,450 pg/mL or >90th percentile) were associated with preeclampsia [odds ratio (OR) 4.8; 95% confidence interval (CI) = 1.6–14.8] and SGA (OR 9.4; 95% CI = 3.2–27.5).[56]

The most recent data from a cohort of 25,777 births documents a significant difference in birth weight of 90.9 g in singletons conceived in frozen versus fresh transfer cycles.[57] The Society for Assisted Reproductive Technology (SART) report comparing 60,037 standard IVF cycles with 10,176 donor egg cycles and 1,180 gestational carrier cycles found an adjusted odds ratio (aOR) of 1.21 (95% CI = 1.13–1.30) for birth weight <2,500 g and 1.28 (95% CI = 1.10–1.49) for birth weight <1,500 g when comparing donor egg with autologous egg IVF cycles.[58]

PERINATAL MORTALITY

A prospective follow-up study of 20,166 singleton pregnancies at Denmark compared the risk of stillbirths between fertile women, subfertile women (time to natural conception >12 months), and women pregnant after fertility treatment (IVF and non-IVF ART).[59] Women who conceived with IVF had a statistically significant fourfold increased risk of stillbirth as compared with fertile women. However, this is in contrast to the findings from three studies of perinatal mortality in singletons conceived naturally following a prolonged time to conception, which found a two- to three-fold increased risk of perinatal death compared with singletons naturally conceived without a prolonged time to conception.[60-62]

OTHER OBSTETRICAL OUTCOMES

A prospective cohort study that included 1,000 ART pregnancies when compared to 2,593 spontaneously conceived pregnancies, where all women were screened for first-trimester screening, showed that false-positive rates in ART groups were significantly higher when compared with the control population which is 9 versus 6%.[63]

Other adverse outcomes of ART conceptions include the placentation abnormalities, which indirectly lead to low birth weight babies, preeclampsia, abnormal placentation, placenta accreta, antepartum hemorrhage (APH), and postpartum hemorrhage. One of the retrospective studies showed that the association of placenta accreta and IVF pregnancies, which showed higher chances of developing the same in IVF pregnancies, may be related to the altered endometrial environment, repeated curettages, advanced maternal age, and multiparity.[64]

A large retrospective cohort study between 1990 and 2004 in Australia compared the occurrence of placental conditions such as placenta previa, placental abruption, APH, and primary postpartum hemorrhage in women, 6,730 IVF/ICSI cycles versus 24,619 general population, 2,167 non-ART population, and 779 gamete intrafallopian transfer (GIFT). Logistic regressions and exploratory analysis showed that obstetric hemorrhages are common in IVF, ICSI, and GIFT cycles which can be attributed to the defective endometrial environment around implantation due to fresh embryo transfers in controlled stimulated cycles, endometriosis, and hormone treatments.[65]

Postpartum depression is another outcome, which is significantly increased in a group of pregnancies conceived with ART, showed by a systematic review. Small study samples and a lack of psychiatric history lead to further research in this area.[66]

The procedures such as induction of labor, operative deliveries, cesarean sections, perinatal complications, neonatal deaths, and neonatal intensive care unit (NICU) admissions tend to be more associated with the ART conceptions, which can be explained with the occurrence of maternal complications such as APH and preeclampsia.[67]

CONGENITAL ANOMALIES

Among 3–5% of total congenital anomalies are associated with ART pregnancies which contribute to 30–40% more in comparison with natural conceptions. Common anomalies include gastrointestinal, cardiovascular and musculoskeletal, cardiac septal defects, etc.[47,68,69]

According to one retrospective cohort study in IVF/ICSI cycles, the prevalence of cardiac septal defects is around 1.1% more when compared to spontaneously conceived infants, which was around 0.4% which can be attributed to an increased BMI of >30 kg/m^2.[70]

Meta-analysis showed that there is no difference in occurrence of congenital anomalies between IVF and IVF/ICSI pregnancies.[71]

CHROMOSOMAL DISORDERS

Compared to ART pregnancies as a whole, the rate of occurrence of chromosomal anomalies is around 0.2% in spontaneously conceived pregnancies, and in IVF/ICSI cycles, it is around 1%.[72]

Women conceived with ICSI are at a higher risk of chromosomal aberrations, including sex chromosomal abnormalities; hence, diagnostic testing should be offered after appropriate counseling.

Various studies observed that there are no major significant differences between nuchal translucencies among ART pregnancies and spontaneously conceived pregnancies.[73]

IMPRINTING DISORDERS

Nowadays, with increasing technology, industrialization, career orientation, advanced maternal age, and availability of ART techniques everywhere, the percentage of babies born through ART was around 1.7–4%.

Imprinting is a process of modification of complete deoxyribonucleic acid (DNA) structure by methylation or histone that occurs over a period of time by which that gene becomes nontranscriptable but with no alteration in actual DNA coding sequence **(Table 2)**.[74-76]

Most probable mechanisms include the composition of media, culture conditions, gas phase in incubators, oil overlay, superovulation, hypomethylation of maternal and paternal genes, underlying conditions of infertility, etc.[77]

Due to reduced imprinting gene activity leading to dysregulation in tumor suppression causing malignancies in later stages of life has to be followed up with long-term follow-up studies.[76]

TABLE 2: Human phenotypes identified and associated with imprinted genes.[76]

Beckwith–Wiedemann	11p15
Angelman	15q11-q12 maternal
Prader–Willi	15q11-q12 paternal
Silver–Russell	7p11-p13, 7q31-qter, 11p15
Transient neonatal diabetes mellitus	6q24
McCune–Albright	20q13
Familial nonchromaffin paraganglioma	11q13
Maternal and paternal uniparental disomy	2, 14, 16
Turner	X

PREIMPLANTATION GENETIC SCREENING

Preimplantation genetic screening is a procedure where an adequate number of blastomeres are taken for biopsy to study the whole genome. The role of most recent advances, which include PGS/PGD (preimplantation genetic diagnosis) usage in indicated cases such as increased maternal age, recurrent miscarriage, repeated IVF failures, and testicular sperm extraction using the latest technologies such as whole genomic analysis using comparative genomic hybridization which studies all sets of chromosomes to detect the aneuploidy rates to be done in large samples of population, are required to know the long-term effects. One of the recent reviews showed that there is no significant difference found in birth weights and major anomalies among infants born after PGS.[78]

BLASTOCYST CULTURE

According to systematic review and meta-analysis, the probability of having a live birth is almost 40% higher with blastocyst transfer when compared to cleavage transfers.[79] Monozygotic twinning is considered to be one of the common complications after blastocyst transfer. According to Papanikolaou et al., the monozygotic twinning is not increased after a single blastocyst transfer when compared with a single cleavage transfer.[80-82] Some other authors concluded that there is an increased risk of monozygotic twinning after blastocyst transfer.[83] However, the reason might be related to the usage of various culture media during ART. In the near future, to avoid complications, eSET will be an effective option.

However, blastocyst transfer ensures good embryo selection and also encourages single embryo transfer. Two systematic reviews and meta-analyses on perinatal outcomes after blastocyst versus cleavage embryo transfers which included >100,000 singletons born with fresh cycles found that preterm, very preterm, and SGA babies are comparatively less with blastocyst transfer.[80-82]

FRESH VERSUS FROZEN

According to recently published randomized controlled studies which compared fresh versus frozen embryo transfer; the mean birth weight, preterm birth, and birth defects were same in both groups, but while safety is concerned, elective frozen embryo transfer (eFET) significantly reduces the risk of moderate-to-severe ovarian hyperstimulation syndrome.[80-82]

Cryopreservation techniques reduce the risk of ovarian hyperstimulation syndrome, and an effective synchronization between the embryo and endometrium is possible, thus reducing the incidence of prematurity.

VITRIFICATION VERSUS SLOW FREEZING

There were no significant negative effects of either of the cryopreservation techniques except for a slight risk of preterm deliveries with vitrification. However, vitrification or ultrarapid cryopreservation method seems to be reassuring.[80-82]

ASSISTED HATCHING

Sometimes, because of the inability of blastocyst to escape from its thick shell called zona, implantation failure and conception may result. Assisted hatching is a procedure where an aperture is created in zona which facilitates the embryo to get implanted. This method appears to increase the clinical pregnancy rate whereas the live birth rates and take-home baby rates are yet to be proven. Long-term sequences are yet to be studied in larger study groups.[84,85]

IN VITRO MATURATION

In vitro maturation (IVM) is a process where immature oocytes are collected and cultured in vitro to change them to metaphase II oocytes, and then ICSI is conducted. This procedure has a promising role in fertility preservation, patients with PCOS, etc. As the number of babies born through IVM worldwide are less, their long-term their long-term sequences are yet to be reported. As such, there are no major significant neurological disturbances noted in children born with IVM in the study reported by Söderström-Anttila et al.[86-88]

Intracytoplasmic Sperm Injection versus In Vitro Fertilization

Some researchers strongly believe that ART complications are due to many manipulation factors such as using ovulation induction drugs, addition of many nonphysiological operations in ART, composition of culture medium, storage time in culture medium, freezing process of the embryo, and blood levels of hormones at the time of implantation; these factors play a role in pregnancy outcomes.[87,88]

LONG-TERM CONSEQUENCES IN ASSISTED REPRODUCTIVE TECHNIQUE BORN CHILDREN

According to many studies, there is no significant difference between language, neuromotor skills, and cognition among children born from ART when compared to naturally conceived children.[89]

Ceelen et al. reported various cardiometabolic diseases, variations in systolic and diastolic blood pressures, and fasting sugars among children born through ART.[90]

Therefore further studies are mandatory which include adolescents and adults born through ART studying various metabolic disorders, cardiovascular disorders, obesity, etc.

OTHER MATERNAL FACTORS WHICH INFLUENCE THE OUTCOME

In this modern era, with the increase in the average age of marriage and conception increases, maternal and perinatal complications have increased too. Complications which may be related to infertility, miscarriages, APH, postpartum hemorrhage, operative deliveries, pregnancy-induced hypertension, and gestational diabetes may increase. As comorbidities improve along with age, pre-IVF counseling and screening should be offered in routine for couples opting for ART.

Polycystic ovary syndrome being one of the main causes of infertility poses a long-term risk for diabetes, cardiovascular disorders, obesity, neonatal complications including preterm births, low birth weight babies, increased perinatal mortality, operative deliveries, cerebral palsy, etc. Hence, this mandates a very well-explained thorough preconceptional counseling for women who are associated with PCOS and emphasis is to be imposed on lifestyle changes and weight management.[91]

With increasing usage of donor, oocyte programs among women with increased maternal age, and premature ovarian failures, an increased risk of maternal and perinatal complications is seen; however studies has to be done to show the longterm sequelae of children born after ART.[92]

Barker's hypothesis showed that baby's nourishment before birth and during infancy manifests in patterns of fetal and infant growth and may program the various risk factors such as raised blood pressure and glucose intolerance which are the key role players of coronary heart diseases **(Fig. 1)**.[93,94]

Preexisting maternal medical conditions were present in 15.1% of women, with a consistent increase from 9.7% in women <31 years old to 27.8% in women >40 years.

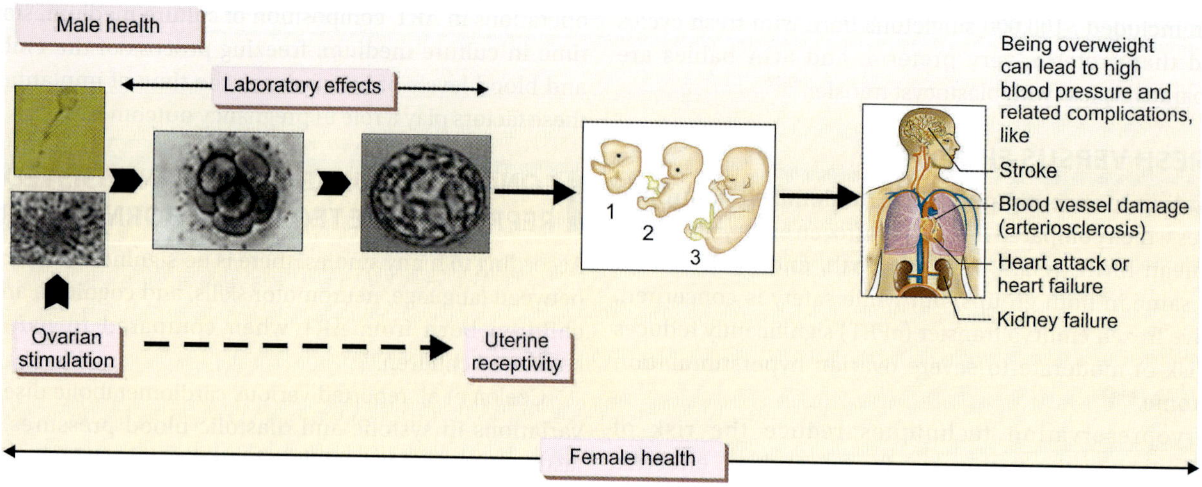

Fig. 1: Barker's hypothesis.[93,94]

INTRACYTOPLASMIC SPERM INJECTION WITH EJACULATED VERSUS NONEJACULATED SPERM

The evidence shows that there is no major difference in the rate of birth defects in children conceived with ICSI using non-ejaculated sperm compared with ICSI using ejaculated sperm.[95]

Genetic counseling plays a pivotal role in those individuals who have oligozoospermia, azoospermia, aspermia, etc.

KEY POINTS

- As ART is always evolving because of its dynamic and ever-changing nature, there will be newer developments at each and every step.
- ART poses a clear high risk of adverse perinatal and maternal outcomes; proper counseling about IVF, the risks involved in it, and assessment of risk during the antenatal period with an apt time of referral are very important.
- Constantly ongoing studies on larger populations are always required, and continuous fine-tuning of the technologies and its application become mandatory.
- Continuous supervision after ART is needed to ensure safety and quality, especially when new techniques are introduced.
- In conclusion, women who undergo ART may have an increased risk of obstetric and perinatal outcomes due to multiple pregnancies; hence, eSETs are strongly recommended.

REFERENCES

1. Lobo R, Mishell DR, Davajan V. Mishell's Textbook of Infertility, Contraception, and Reproductive Endocrinology. Philadelphia: Mosby Elsevier; 1997.
2. Joffe M, Li Z. Association of time to pregnancy and the outcome of pregnancy. Fertil Steril. 1994;62(1):71-5.
3. Sutcliffe AG, Ludwig M. Outcome of assisted reproduction. Lancet. 2007;370:351-9.
4. Reddy UM, Wapner RJ, Rebar RW, Tasca RJ. Infertility, assisted reproductive technology, and adverse pregnancy outcomes: executive summary of a National Institute of Child Health and Human Development workshop. Obstet Gynecol. 2007;109(4):967-77.
5. Talaulikar VS, Arulkumaran S. Reproductive outcomes after assisted conception. Obstet Gynecol Surv. 2012;67(9): 566-83.
6. European Society of Human Reproduction and Embryology. ART fact sheet. [online] Available from https://www.eshre.eu/Press-Room/Resources.aspx. [Last accessed March, 2018].
7. Rodriguez-Wallberg KA, Oktay K. Fertility preservation medicine: options for young adults and children with cancer. J Pediatr Hematol Oncol. 2010;32(5):390-6.
8. Buckett W. Infertility treatment for non-traditional families. Canada Infertility Awareness Association; 2011.
9. Surrogacy in Canada online. (2011). Information, referral and support. [online] Available from http://www.surrogacy.ca. [Last accessed March, 2018].
10. van de Mheen L, Everwijn SM, Knapen MFC, Oepkes D, Engels M, Manten GT, et al. The effectiveness of multifetal pregnancy reduction in trichorionic triplet gestation. Am J Obstet Gynecol. 2014;211(5):536.e1-6.
11. Pregnancy outcomes after assisted human reproduction principal authors Nanette Okun MD. Sony Sierra MD. Genetics committee. Special contributors DOI: https://doi.org/10.1016/S1701-2163(15)30685-X.SOGC clinical practice guidelines/volume 36, Issue 1, P64-83, January 01,2014.
12. Templeton A, Ashok P, Bhattacharya S, Gazuani R, Hamilton M, S M. Management of Infertility for the MRCOG and Beyond, 1st edition. London: RCOG Press; 2000.
13. Jones HW Jr, Toner JP. The infertile couple. N Engl J Med. 1993;329:1710-5.
14. Reubinoff BE, Samueloff A, Ben-Haim M, Friedler S, Schenker JG, Lewin A. Is the obstetric outcome of in vitro fertilized singleton gestations different from natural ones? A controlled study. Fertil Steril. 1997;67(6):1077-83.

15. Li TC, MacLeod I, Singhal V, Duncan SL. The obstetric and neonatal outcome of pregnancy in women with a previous history of infertility: a prospective study. Br J Obstet Gynaecol. 1991;98(11):1087-92.
16. Isaksson R, Tiitinen A. Obstetric outcome in patients with unexplained infertility: comparison of treatment-related and spontaneous pregnancies. Acta Obstet Gynecol Scand. 1998;77(8):849-53.
17. Pandian Z, Bhattacharya S, Templeton A. Review of unexplained infertility and obstetric outcome: a 10 year review. Hum Reprod. 2001;16(12):2593-7.
18. Thomson F, Shanbhag S, Templeton A, Bhattacharya S. Obstetric outcome in women with subfertility. BJOG. 2005; 112(5):632-7.
19. British Fertility Society. In vitro fertilisation: perinatal risks and early childhood outcomes. Scientific impact paper no. 8. London: Royal College of Obstetricians and Gynaecologists; 2012.
20. Okun N, Sierra S, Genetics Committee. Pregnancy outcomes after assisted human reproduction. J Obstet Gynaecol Can. 2014;36(1):64-83.
21. Blondel B, Kaminski M. Trends in the occurrence, determinants, and consequences of multiple births. Semin Perinatol. 2002;26(4):239-49.
22. Liu S, Allen A, Fraser W. Preterm birth rate. Ottawa: Minister of Public Works and Government Services; 2008. pp. 123-6.
23. Fauser BC, Devroey P, Macklon NS. Multiple birth resulting from ovarian stimulation for subfertility treatment. Lancet. 2005;365(9473):1807-16.
24. Gunby J, Bissonnette F, Librach C, Cowan L, IVF Directors Group of the Canadian Fertility and Andrology Society. Assisted reproductive technologies (ART) in Canada: 2007 results from the Canadian ART Register. Fertil Steril. 2011;95(2):542-7.e1-10.
25. Vitthala S, Gelbaya TA, Brison DR, Fitzgerald CT, Nardo LG. The risk of monozygotic twins after assisted reproductive technology: a systematic review and meta-analysis. Human Reprod Update. 2009;15:45-55.
26. Blickstein I. Estimation of iatrogenic monozygotic twinning rate following assisted reproduction: pitfalls and caveats. Am J Obstet Gynecol. 2005;192(2):365-8.
27. Vela G, Luna M, Barritt J, Sandler B, Copperman AB. Monozygotic pregnancies conceived by in vitro fertilization: understanding their prognosis. Fertil Steril. 2011;95(2): 606-10.
28. Milki AA, Jun SH, Hinckley MD, Behr B, Giudice LC, Westphal LM. Incidence of monozygotic twinning with blastocyst transfer compared to cleavage-stage transfer. Fertil Steril. 2003;79(3):503-6.
29. Pandian Z, Bhattacharya S, Ozturk O, Serour G, Templeton A. Number of embryos for transfer following in-vitro fertilisation or intra-cytoplasmic sperm injection. Cochrane Database Syst Rev. 2013;(7):CD003416.
30. Grady R, Alavi N, Vale R, Khandwala M, McDonald SD. Elective single embryo transfer and perinatal outcomes: a systematic review and meta-analysis. Fertil Steril. 2012; 97(2):324-31.
31. Beral V, Doyle P, Tan SL, Mason BA, Campbell S. Outcome of pregnancies resulting from assisted conception. Br Med Bull. 1990;46:753-68.
32. Doyle P. The outcome of multiple pregnancy. Hum Reprod. 1996;11(Suppl 4):110-7.
33. Schieve LA, Meikle SF, Ferre C, Peterson HB, Jeng G, Wilcox LS. Low and very low birth weight in infants conceived with use of assisted reproductive technology. N Engl J Med. 2002;7(346):731-7.
34. Alexander GR, Slay Wingate M, Salihu H, Kirby RS. Fetal and neonatal mortality risks of multiple births. Obstet Gynecol Clin North Am. 2005;32(1):1-16.
35. Pharoah PO. Risk of cerebral palsy in multiple pregnancies. Clin Perinatol. 2006;33(2):301-13.
36. Divon MY, Weiner Z. Ultrasound in twin pregnancy. Semin Perinatol. 1995;19(5):404-12.
37. Allaf MB, Campbell WA, Vintzileos AM, Haeri S, Javadian P, Shamshirsaz AA, et al. Does early second-trimester sonography predict adverse perinatal outcomes in monochorionic diamniotic twin pregnancies? J Ultrasound Med. 2014;33(9):1573-8.
38. Finnström O, Källén B, Lindam A, Nilsson E, Nygren KG, Olausson PO. Maternal and child outcome after in vitro fertilization—a review of 25 years of population-based data from Sweden. Acta Obstet Gynecol Scand. 2011;90(5): 494-500.
39. Helmerhorst FM, Perquin DA, Donker D, Keirse MJ. Perinatal outcome of singletons and twins after assisted conception: a systematic review of controlled studies. BMJ. 2004;328(7434):261.
40. Jackson RA, Gibson KA, Wu YW, Croughan MS. Perinatal outcomes in singletons following in vitro fertilization: a meta-analysis. Obstet Gynecol. 2004;103(3):551-63.
41. McGovern PG, Llorens AJ, Skurnick JH, Weiss G, Goldsmith LT. Increased risk of preterm birth in singleton pregnancies resulting from in vitro fertilization-embryo transfer or gamete intrafallopian transfer: a meta-analysis. Fertil Steril. 2004;82(6):1514-20.
42. McDonald SD, Han Z, Mulla S, Murphy KE, Beyene J, Ohlsson A, et al. Preterm birth and low birth weight among in vitro fertilization singletons: a systematic review and meta-analyses. Eur J Obstet Gynecol Reprod Biol. 2009;146(2): 138-48.
43. De Neubourg D, Gerris J, Mangelschots K, Van Royen E, Vercruyssen M, Steylemans A, et al. The obstetrical and neonatal outcome of babies born after single-embryo transfer in IVF/ICSI compares favourably to spontaneously conceived babies. Hum Reprod. 2006;21(4):1041-6.
44. Hayashi M, Nakai A, Satoh S, Matsuda Y. Adverse obstetric and perinatal outcomes of singleton pregnancies may be related to maternal factors associated with infertility rather than the type of assisted reproductive technology procedure used. Fertil Steril. 2012;98(4):922-8.
45. Fechner AJ, Brown KR, Onwubalili N, Jindal SK, Weiss G, Goldsmith LT, et al. Effect of single embryo transfer on the risk of preterm birth associated with in vitro fertilization. J Assist Reprod Genet. 2015;32(2):221-4.
46. Maheshwari A, Pandey S, Shetty A, Hamilton M, Bhattacharya S. Obstetric and perinatal outcomes in singleton pregnancies resulting from the transfer of frozen thawed versus fresh embryos generated through in vitro fertilization treatment: a systematic review and meta-analysis. Fertil Steril. 2012; 98(2):368-77.e1-9.

47. McDonald S, Murphy K, Beyene J, Ohlsson A. Perinatal outcomes of in vitro fertilization twins: a systematic review and meta-analyses. Am J Obstet Gynecol. 2005;193(1):141-52.
48. Skiadas CC, Missmer SA, Benson CB, Acker D, Racowsky C. Spontaneous reduction before 12 weeks' gestation and selective reduction similarly extend time to delivery in in vitro fertilization of trichorionic-triamniotic triplets. Fertil Steril. 2011;95:596-9.
49. Klemetti R, Sevón T, Gissler M, Hemminki E. Health of children born as a result of in vitro fertilization. Pediatrics. 2006;118(5):1819-27.
50. Sazonova A, Källen K, Thurin-Kjellberg A, Wennerholm UB, Bergh C. Factors affecting obstetric outcome of singletons born after IVF. Hum Reprod. 2011;26(10):2878-86.
51. Belva F, Henriet S, Van den Abbeel E, Camus M, Devroey P, Van der Elst J, et al. Neonatal outcome of 937 children born after transfer of cryopreserved embryos obtained by ICSI and IVF and comparison with outcome data of fresh ICSI and IVF cycles. Hum Reprod. 2008;23(10):2227-38.
52. Pinborg A, Loft A, Aaris Henningsen AK, Rasmussen S, Andersen AN. Infant outcome of 957 singletons born after frozen embryo replacement: the Danish National Cohort Study 1995–2006. Fertil Steril. 2010;94(4):1320-7.
53. Pelkonen S, Koivunen R, Gissler M, Nuojua-Huttunen S, Suikkari AM, Hydén-Granskog C, et al. Perinatal outcome of children born after frozen and fresh embryo transfer: the Finnish cohort study 1995–2006. Hum Reprod. 2010;25(4):914-23.
54. Shih W, Rushford DD, Bourne H, Garrett C, McBain JC, Healy DL, et al. Factors affecting low birthweight after assisted reproduction technology: difference between transfer of fresh and cryopreserved embryos suggests an adverse effect of oocyte collection. Hum Reprod. 2008;23(17):1644-53.
55. Wennerholm UB, Söderström-Anttila V, Bergh C, Aittomäki K, Hazekamp J, Nygren KG, et al. Children born after cryopreservation of embryos or oocytes: a systematic review of outcome data. Hum Reprod. 2009;24(9):2158-72.
56. Imudia AN, Awonuga AO, Doyle JO, Kaimal AJ, Wright DL, Toth TL, et al. Peak serum estradiol level during controlled ovarian hyperstimulation is associated with increased risk of small for gestational age and preeclampsia in singleton pregnancies after in vitro fertilization. Fertil Steril. 2012;97(6):1374-9.
57. Nakashima A, Araki R, Tani H, Ishihara O, Kuwahara A, Irahara M, et al. Implications of assisted reproductive technologies on term singleton birth weight: an analysis of 25,777 children in the national assisted reproduction registry of Japan. Fertil Steril. 2013;99(2):450-5.
58. Gibbons WE, Cedars M, Ness RB, Society for Assisted Reproductive Technologies Writing Group. Toward understanding obstetrical outcome in advanced assisted reproduction: varying sperm, oocyte, and uterine source and diagnosis. Fertil Steril. 2011;95(5):1645-9.
59. Wisborg K, Ingerslev HJ, Henriksen TB. IVF and stillbirth: a prospective follow-up study. Hum Reprod. 2010;25(5):1312-6.
60. Jaques AM, Amor DJ, Baker HW, Healy DL, Ukoumunne OC, Breheny S, et al. Adverse obstetric and perinatal outcomes in subfertile women conceiving without assisted reproductive technologies. Fertil Steril. 2010;94(7):2674-9.
61. Draper ES, Kurinczuk JJ, Abrams KR, Clarke M. Assessment of separate contributions to perinatal mortality of infertility history and treatment: a case-control analysis. Lancet. 1999;353(9166):1746-9.
62. Basso O, Olsen J. Subfecundity and neonatal mortality: longitudinal study within the Danish national birth cohort. BMJ. 2005;330:393-4.
63. Gjerris AC, Loft A, Pinborg A, Tabor A, Christiansen M. First-trimester screening in pregnancies conceived by assisted reproductive technology: significance of gestational dating by oocyte retrieval or sonographic measurement of crown–rump length. Ultrasound Obstet Gynecol. 2008;32(5):612-7.
64. Esh-Broder E, Ariel I, Abas-Bashir N, Bdolah Y, Celnikier DH. Placenta accreta is associated with IVF pregnancies: a retrospective chart review. BJOG. 2011;118(9):1084-9.
65. Healy DL, Breheny S, Halliday J, Jaques A, Rushford D, Garrett C, et al. Prevalence and risk factors for obstetric haemorrhage in 6730 singleton births after assisted reproductive technology in Victoria Australia. Hum Reprod. 2010;25(1):265-74.
66. Ross LE, McQueen K, Vigod S, Dennis CL. Risk for postpartum depression associated with assisted reproductive technologies and multiple births: a systematic review. Hum Reprod Update. 2011;17(1):96-106.
67. Bell J, Campbell DM, Graham WJ, Penney GC, Ryan M, Hall MH. Do obstetric complications explain high caesarean section rates among women over 30? A retrospective analysis. BMJ. 2001;322:894-5.
68. Rimm AA, Katayama AC, Diaz M, Katayama KP. A meta-analysis of controlled studies comparing major malformation rates in IVF and ICSI infants with naturally conceived children. J Assist Reprod Genet. 2004;21(12):437-43.
69. Hansen M, Bower C, Milne E, de Klerk N, Kurinczuk JJ. Assisted reproductive technologies and the risk of birth defects—a systematic review. Hum Reprod. 2005;20(2):328-38.
70. Wen SW, Leader A, White RR, Léveillé MC, Wilkie V, Zhou J, et al. A comprehensive assessment of outcomes in pregnancies conceived by in vitro fertilization/intracytoplasmic sperm injection. Eur J Obstet Gynecol Reprod Biol. 2010;150(2):160-5.
71. Chen T, McDonald A, Shadbolt B, Talaulikar D. Precision of histological bone marrow staging in follicular lymphoma and diffuse large B-cell lymphoma. Clin Invest Med. 2012;35(6):E358-64.
72. Wennerholm UB, Bergh C, Hamberger L, Lundin K, Nilsson L, Wikland M, et al. Incidence of congenital malformations in children born after ICSI. Hum Reprod. 2000;15(4):944-8.
73. Shulman A, Maymon R. Mid-gestation Down syndrome screening test and pregnancy outcome among unstimulated assisted-conception pregnancies. Prenat Diagn. 2003;23(8):625-8.
74. Ishida M, Moore GE. The role of imprinted genes in humans. Mol Aspects Med. 2013;34(4):826-40.
75. Iliadou AN, Janson PC, Cnattingius S. Epigenetics and assisted reproductive technology. J Intern Med. 2011;270:414-20.
76. Lim DH, Maher ER. Genomic imprinting syndromes and cancer. Adv Genet. 2010;70:145-75.

77. Jenkins J, Daya S, Kremer J, Balasch J, Barratt C, Cooke I, Lawford-Davies J, De Sutter P, Suikari AM, Neulen J, Nygren K. European Classification of Infertility Taskforce (ECIT) response to Habbema et al., 'Towards less confusing terminology in reproductive medicine: a proposal'. Hum Reprod. 2004;19(12):2687-8. DOI:10.1093/humrep/deh499. Epub 2004 Aug 27. PMID: 15333591.
78. Liebaers I, Desmyttere S, Verpoest W, De Rycke M, Staessen C, Sermon K, et al. Report on a consecutive series of 581 children born after blastomere biopsy for preimplantation genetic diagnosis. Hum Reprod. 2010;25(1):275-82.
79. Papanikolaou EG, Kolibianakis EM, Tournaye H, Venetis CA, Fatemi H, Tarlatzis B, et al. Live birth rates after transfer of equal number of blastocysts or cleavage-stage embryos in IVF. A systematic review and meta-analysis. Hum Reprod. 2008;23(1):91-9.
80. Papanikolaou EG, Fatemi H, Venetis C, Donoso P, Kolibianakis E, Tournaye H, et al. Monozygotic twinning is not increased after single blastocyst transfer compared with single cleavage-stage embryo transfer. Fertil Steril. 2010; 93(2):592-7.
81. Wennerholm UB, Bergh C. Perinatal outcome in children born after assisted reproductive technologies. Ups J Med Sci. 2020;125:158-66.
82. Banica AM, Popescu SD, Vladareanu S. Obstetric and perinatal complications associated with assisted reproductive techniques—review. Maedica (Bucur). 2021;16(3):493-8.
83. Kawachiya S, Bodri D, Shimada N, Kato K, Takehara Y, Kato O. Blastocyst culture is associated with an elevated incidence of monozygotic twinning after single embryo transfer. Fertil Steril. 2011;95(6):2140-2.
84. Das S, Blake D, Farquhar C, Seif MM. Assisted hatching on assisted conception (IVF and ICSI). Cochrane Database Syst Rev. 2009;(2):CD001894.
85. Martins WP, Rocha IA, Ferriani RA, Nastri CO. Assisted hatching of human embryos: a systematic review and meta-analysis of randomized controlled trials. Hum Reprod Update. 2011;17(4):438-53.
86. Shu-Chi M, Jiann-Loung H, Yu-Hung L, Tseng-Chen S, Ming-I L, Tsu-Fuh Y. Growth and development of children conceived by in-vitro maturation of human oocytes. Early Hum Dev. 2006;82(10):677-82.
87. Söderström-Anttila V, Salokorpi T, Pihlaja M, Serenius-Sirve S, Suikkari AM. Obstetric and perinatal outcome and preliminary results of development of children born after in vitro maturation of oocytes. Hum Reprod. 2006;21(6): 1508-13.
88. Tai W, Hu L, Wen J. Maternal and neonatal outcomes after assisted reproductive technology: a retrospective cohort study in China. Front Med (Lausanne). 2022;9:837762.
89. Middelburg KJ, Heineman MJ, Bos AF, Hadders-Algra M. Neuromotor, cognitive, language and behavioural outcome in children born following IVF or ICSI—a systematic review. Hum Reprod Update. 2008;14(3):219-31.
90. Ceelen M, van Weissenbruch MM, Vermeiden JP, van Leeuwen FE, Delemarre-van de Waal HA. Cardiometabolic differences in children born after in vitro fertilization: follow-up study. J Clin Endocrinol Metab. 2008;93:1682-8.
91. Boomsma CM, Eijkemans MJ, Hughes EG, Visser GH, Fauser BC, Macklon NS. A meta-analysis of pregnancy outcomes in women with polycystic ovary syndrome. Hum Reprod Update. 2006;12(6):673-83.
92. Wiggins DA, Main E. Outcomes of pregnancies achieved by donor egg in vitro fertilization—a comparison with standard in vitro fertilization pregnancies. Am J Obstet Gynecol. 2005;192(6):2002-6.
93. Wadhwa PD, Buss C, Entringer S, Swanson JM. Developmental origins of health and disease: brief history of the approach and current focus on epigenetic mechanisms. Semin Reprod Med. 2009;27(5):358-68.
94. Chinea E, Hernandez J, Sanabria V, Gonzelez L, Martin-casanas F, Palumbo A. Maternal and perinatal outcomes in assisted reproductive technology (ART) singleton and twin pregnancies stratified by increasing maternal age. Fertil Steril. 2007;88(1):S112-3.
95. Holte TO, Hofmann B, Lie RT, Norderhaug IN, Romundstad P, Sæterdal I, et al. Male infertility: intracytoplasmic sperm injection (ICSI) using surgically retrieved sperm from the testis or the epididymis. NIPH Systematic Reviews: Executive Summaries. Oslo, Norway; 2007.

CHAPTER 76

Early Pregnancy Scan

Srividhya GK

INTRODUCTION

The availability of the modern ultrasound technology has increased the understanding of early pregnancy development and antenatal management. The high-frequency transvaginal probe improves the image quality in such a way that detailed imaging of the embryonic morphology has become possible. Early human embryo changes its anatomical appearance rapidly with uniform development and continuous growth. Hence, first trimester defines the most critical period of human development.[1]

The duration of first trimester is from conception up to 12 weeks of gestation. The accurate method to calculate the duration of pregnancy is by knowing the date of conception. As most women are not aware of the date of conception, the last menstrual period (LMP) date is noted to calculate the gestational age (GA) and expected date of delivery (EDD). The embryological age of the gestation is calculated from the conception date and is usually 2 weeks less than the menstrual age.[2]

Ultrasonography is used in the first trimester for the pregnancy confirmation, its location, molar pregnancy, first-trimester vaginal bleeding, or pain in the abdomen, to determine the GA, to assess multiple gestations and its chorionicity, to assess fetal viability, as an adjunct to invasive procedures such as chorionic villus sampling (CVS) and fetal reduction, and to evaluate adnexal masses or uterine abnormalities. The diagnostic ultrasound is considered safe during all trimesters of pregnancy and has no harmful bioeffects demonstrated. However, a fundamental principle for the safe usage of ultrasound is to use the lowest power output and the shortest scan time for acquiring the required diagnostic information. This is called ALARA principle (i.e., as low as reasonably achievable). The serum beta-human chorionic gonadotropin (β-hCG) levels and ultrasonography make the diagnosis of pregnancy more specific and help in identifying women with abnormal or high-risk pregnancies.[3] Furthermore, with the introduction of three-dimensional and four-dimensional ultrasound, the fetal embryological developments are still more accurately documented.[3]

It is important to understand normal development and to appreciate the rapid and critical sequential changes that are occurring and thus helps us to identify normal and abnormal sonographic findings in early pregnancy.

NORMAL SONOEMBRYOLOGY

Sonoembryology is defined as the description of the normal embryonic anatomical relations as visualized by ultrasound. To make the diagnosis of an anomaly, the knowledge of the normal embryonic development is needed. The GA is subclassified into distinct gestational periods. The first 2 weeks of prenatal development are referred to as the *preembryonic stage*. The conceptus phase is from 3 to 5 weeks, embryonic phase is from 6 to 10 weeks, and fetal phase is from 10 weeks onward.

First 3 Weeks of Development

The duration of pregnancy from the LMP is an average of 280 days to delivery. This period consists of:

- *Ovulation and oocyte migration:* The oocytes fertilize in the tube within 24 hours of ovulation.
- Fertilization and zygote migration
- *Implantation:* It is the process of attachment and invasion of the endometrium by the blastocyst (conceptus). Implantation occurs about 9 days after ovulation, ranging between 6 and 12 days. hCG produced by the trophoblasts enters the maternal circulation approximately 2 weeks postconception.

On ultrasound, a gestational sac develops after implantation.

- *Gastrulation:* The inner cell mass forms and it consists of two layers—an upper epiblast and a lower hypoblast. Gastrulation converts this bilaminar disk into three layers: (1) Upper ectoderm, (2) middle mesoderm, and (3) lower endoderm **(Fig. 1)**.

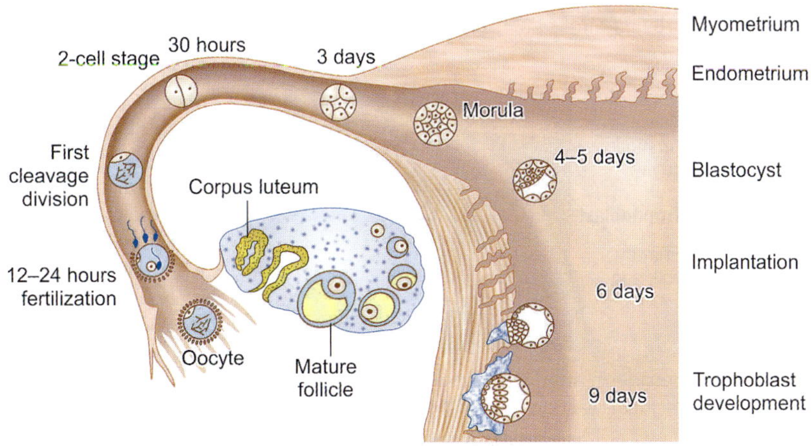

Fig. 1: Sequence of ovulation, fertilization, and early development of the embryo.
Source: Moore KL, Persaud TVN, Torchia MG. The Developing Human: Clinically Oriented Embryology, 9th edition. Philadelphia: WB Saunders; 2011.

FIRST-TRIMESTER ULTRASOUND: NORMAL LANDMARKS

The chronologic developmental features of the embryo or fetus are well defined in an orderly manner like the visualization of gestational sac, then the yolk sac, and then the embryo with heartbeat at a given number of days from the onset of the LMP. These features help us in identifying the structural defects as early as the first 12 weeks of pregnancy. These can be identified during the first-trimester scan, thus differentiating the pregnancy into a normal and at-risk pregnancy **(Table 1)**.

Gestational Sac

Gestational sac is seen as a round, fluid-filled area with echogenic rim. The central fluid is the chorionic cavity, and the echogenic rim is due to the chorionic decidual complex. The growth rate of the sac is 1 mm/day. The sac is usually round in shape initially and later becomes oval. The gestational sac measurements are taken as the mean sac diameter (MSD). The measurements from three orthogonal planes [anterior-posterior (AP), transverse, and longitudinal] are averaged. The calipers are placed at the inner margin of the sac for measuring the MSD **(Figs. 10A to C)**. It is measured in all pregnancies <10 weeks of gestation. The GA can be calculated by using MSD when the pregnancy is <6 weeks of gestation or until the crown-rump length (CRL) is seen. There is a percentile graph available for the gestational sac at different GA.[4,5]

The sac must be distinguished from other cystic areas seen in the cavity, such as nabothian cyst in the upper cervix, decidual cyst, decidual cast, or pseudogestational sac (hypoechoic cystic area in the cavity without echogenic rim due to fluid). The sac may become irregular in shape due to fibroid uterus, focal myometrial contraction, large subchorionic hemorrhage (SCH), and distended bladder.[3]

The lowest β-hCG level by which a normal intrauterine sac is possibly visible is called *threshold level*. The level of β-hCG above which a gestational sac should be visualized is called *discriminatory level*. Nyberg et al. described the discriminatory level as 1,000 mlU/mL for a transvaginal scan (TVS).[5]

Yolk Sac

During early pregnancy, the yolk has nutritive, metabolic, endocrine, immunological, and hematopoietic functions. It is a well-defined echogenic rim with anechoic center and is round in shape. It identifies the true gestation sac. The yolk sac is seen by TVS by 5–6 weeks of GA and when the sac diameter is 8 mm. The yolk sac normally grows 0.1 mm/day to a maximum of 5 mm (*see* **Figs. 10A to C**).[3]

Embryo

The embryo is initially seen as an echogenic line next to the yolk sac by 5 weeks. It is measured from crown to rump and termed "crown-rump length" (CRL)," the most precise method for assessing the GA in the first trimester. The fetal pole should always be seen when the sac is around 25 mm.

An amniotic sac separates the embryo from the extraembryonic celom (chorionic cavity), and the obliteration of the celomic cavity happens by 14–16 weeks. There is a proportional growth of the chorionic cavity, amniotic cavity, and CRL in normal gestation till about 10 weeks of gestation. Later, the fetal urine production disproportionately enlarges the amniotic cavity, and hence obliteration of chorionic cavity. The percentile chart for the CRL and GA is available in the literature and has to be used to assess the fetal growth.

Embryonic morphology is featureless till about 7–8 weeks. At approximately 8 weeks of gestation, the cranial portion is well defined and thus differentiated from the body. The rhombencephalon (which develops into hindbrain) is an important structure seen at >7 weeks of gestation. It is seen

<table>
<tr><th colspan="2">TABLE 1: Embryonic developmental landmarks and sonoembryology.</th></tr>
<tr><th>Sonoembryology</th><th>Embryonic developmental landmarks</th></tr>
<tr><td>
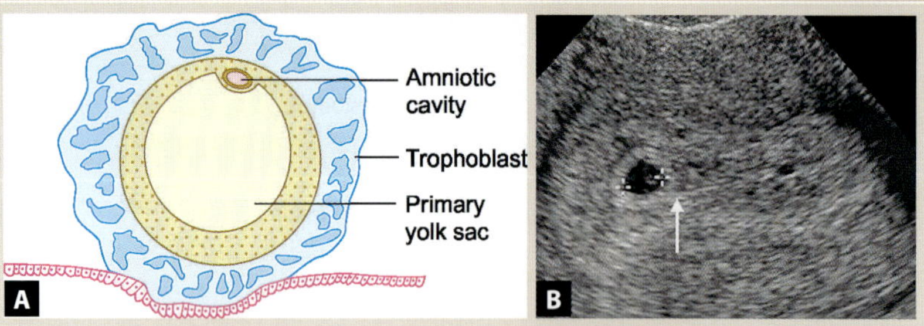

Figs. 2A and B: (A) Formation of the mesoderm after implantation; (B) On ultrasound, small gestational sac with good choriodecidual reaction seen within the endometrium.
</td><td>
Menstrual age—4th week (Figs. 2A and B):
<ul>
<li>The first feature on ultrasound is the presence of a decidualized endometrium with vascular corpus luteum</li>
<li>A small regular and spherical sac seen in the mid-to-upper uterine cavity. (approximately 2–5 mm in size)</li>
<li>The threshold value for the gestational sac to be seen on TVS is when the beta-human chorionic gonadotropin values are 1,000 mUI or above</li>
</ul>
</td></tr>
<tr><td>
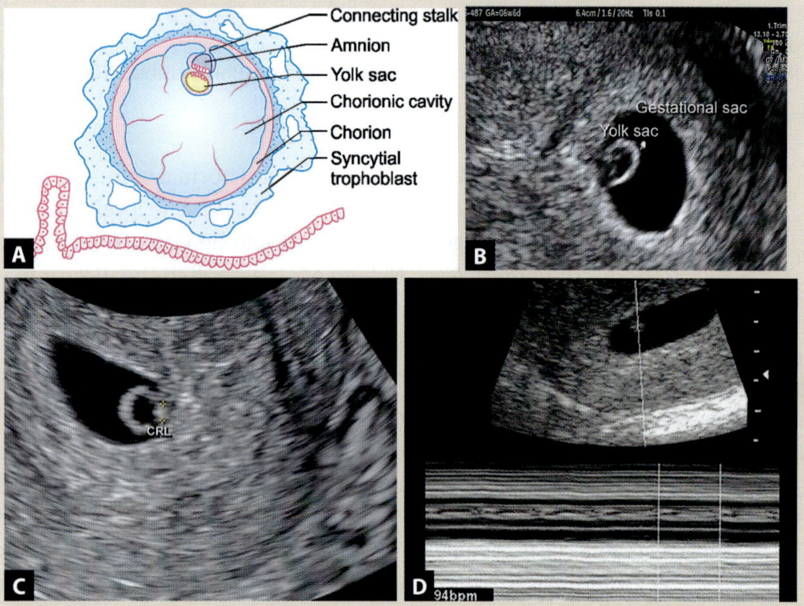

Figs. 3A to D: (A) The mesodermal migration around endodermal pouch creates yolk sac; (B to D) On ultrasound, gestational sac appears regular with echogenic trophoblastic rim and a small yolk sac is seen within.
</td><td>
Menstrual age—5th week (Figs. 3A to D):
<ul>
<li>MSD is around 7–10 mm in size</li>
<li>Yolk sac (YS) is visible</li>
<li>The embryo appears as a thickened linear structure adjacent to the yolk sac ("=" sign) and measured as crown–rump length (CRL). The embryo appears more echogenic when the size is around 2 mm
<ul><li>Cardiac activity can be seen within the embryo on real-time imaging</li></ul></li>
</ul>
</td></tr>
<tr><td>
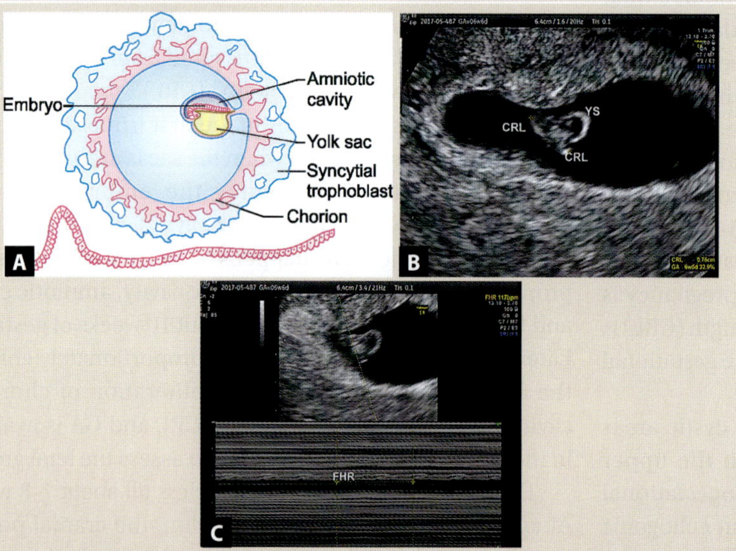

Figs. 4A to C: (A) The embryonic disk bulges into the amniotic cavity at the head fold; (B) On ultrasound, fetal pole is well visualized and measured as CRL. Fetal pole and yolk sac appear floating in the chorionic cavity; (C) FHR increases with gestational age.
</td><td>
Menstrual age—6th week (Figs. 4A to C):
<ul>
<li>The fetal pole can be easily identified and it measures around 2–4 mm in length</li>
<li>Cardiac activity when measured at this gestation is around 90–120 BPM</li>
<li>The fetal pole and YS appear floating in the chorion cavity</li>
<li>The fetal pole needs be seen when the MSD is of 18 mm (on TVS) and 25 mm (on TAS)</li>
<li>The fetal pole is measured as crown–rump length (CRL)</li>
<li>The embryo grows at the rate of around 1 mm/day</li>
</ul>
</td></tr>
</table>

Contd...

Contd...

Sonoembryology	***Embryonic developmental landmarks***

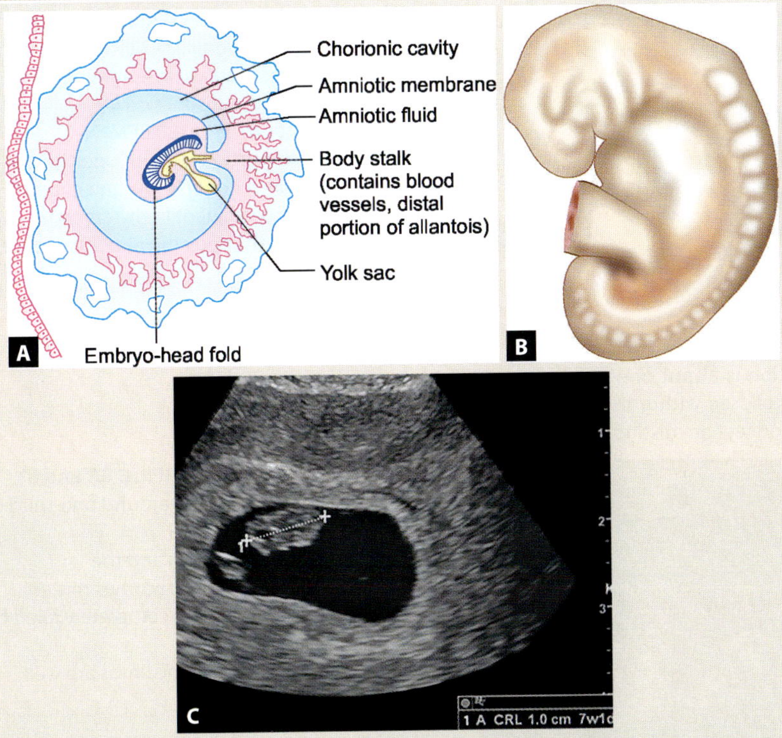

Figs. 5A to C: (A) The developing embryo and extraembryonic membrane bulge into the uterine cavity. The folded embryo moves away from the placenta and umbilical stalk develops; (B) Embryo is "C" shaped due to lateral and craniocaudal folds; (C) On ultrasound, fetal pole moves away from the yolk sac.

Menstrual age—7th week **(Figs. 5A to C)**:
- The CRL increases up to around 16 mm, with yolk sac reaching the maximum diameter of 5 mm
- CRL moves further away from the yolk sac. CRL appears as a "C"-shaped structure due to lateral and craniocaudal fold of the embryo
- The rhombencephalon (brain development) is a cystic space seen at the cranial end of the embryo
  - Spine seen as parallel echogenic line
  - The amniotic cavity is seen as a distinct entity from the chorionic cavity. The short cord is seen

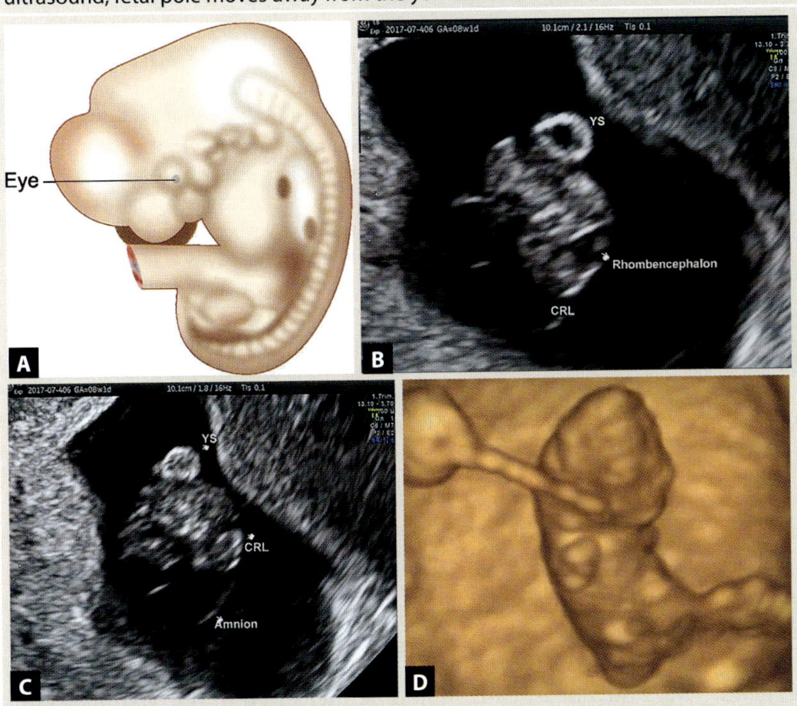

Figs. 6A to D: (A) The cranial end of the embryo appears large. Facial features are now apparent and small limb buds seen; (B) On ultrasound, the diamond-shaped cystic area (rhombencephalon) at the cranial end is more obvious now; (C) Amniotic cavity expands and amnion is seen clearly; (D) 3D picture of the embryo showing small limb buds and the umbilical cord.

Menstrual age—8th week **(Figs. 6A to D)**:
- The extremities (limb buds) are seen as round in shape close to the body
- CRL is around 17–23 mm by 8 weeks
- Midgut hernia is an echogenic protruding solid mass (the bowels loops) seen at the base of the umbilical cord, adjacent to the anterior abdominal wall. The size is usually small (<7 mm) and returns into the abdominal cavity by the 11th week
- The head end is large. The facial features can be identified but clearly visible at later gestational age
- The amniotic cavity enlarges and the umbilical cord lengthens
- Occasionally, small body movements can be seen
- The placental site can be identified

Contd...

Contd...

Sonoembryology	**Embryonic developmental landmarks**
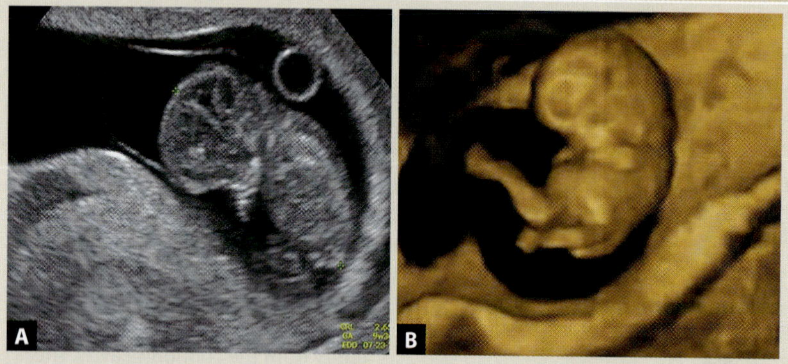 **Figs. 7A and B:** On ultrasound, (A) Cephalic portion is about one-third of the body. Fetus is seen within the amniotic cavity and the yolk sac within the chorionic cavity; (B) The limb buds increase in length and the hand and feet are distinct now.	*Menstrual age—9th week* **(Figs. 7A and B)**: • CRL measures around 23–32 mm • The limb buds increase in length and the hand and feet are distinct now • FHR increases to 170–180 BPM • The cephalic portion is about one-third of the body. The echogenic falx and choroid plexuses are prominent in the cranium • Distinct frequent body movements are seen
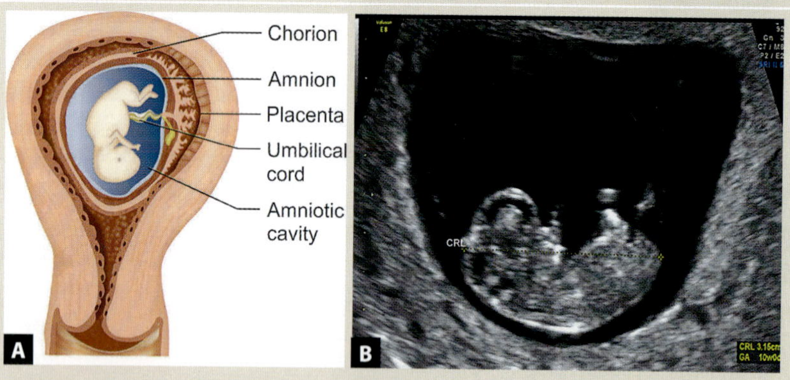 **Figs. 8A and B:** (A) Amniotic cavity rapidly expands and fills the uterine cavity. Fetus is connected to the placenta by cord; (B) On ultrasound, CRL is measured in sagittal section.	*Menstrual age—10th week* **(Figs. 8A and B)**: • The fetus grows and fills around one-third of the sac space • CRL is around 32–41 mm and the craniocaudal curvature becomes more • The lateral ventricles are completely filled by choroid plexus • The three segments of the limbs are well defined
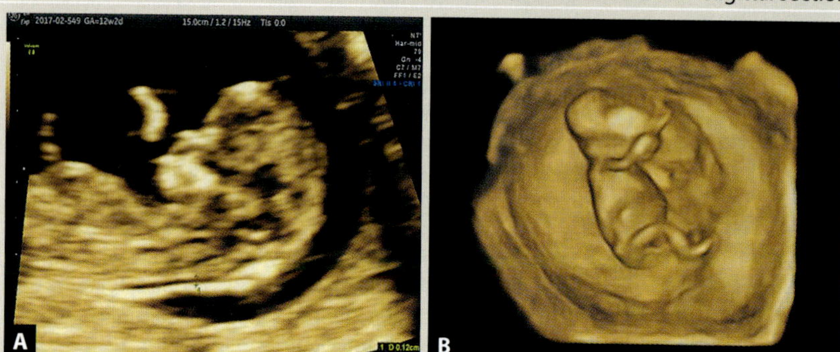 **Figs. 9A and B:** (A) Ultrasound image of the fetus in mid-sagittal section with magnification of head and thorax portion and measurement of the NT; (B) 3D image of the fetus.	*Menstrual age—11–13 + 6 weeks* **(Figs. 9A and B)**: • The CRL is >42 mm at around 11 weeks and reaches to about 76 mm by 13 weeks • Detailed anatomical survey is done, the cerebral, cardiovascular systems, digestive and urinary tracts. Stomach, bladder, and the kidneys are visible. The hernia returns into the abdominal cavity • NT scan is done when the CRL is around 45–84 mm • The important aneuploidy markers are nuchal translucency (NT) and nasal bone. The normalcy of the Doppler flow across tricuspid valve and ductus venosus needs to be established • Fusion of the two decidual layers happens by the end of first trimester (parietal and capsular) and nonfusion of which is abnormal

(FHR: fetal heart rate; MSD: mean sac diameter; TAS: transabdominal scan; TVS: transvaginal scan)

as a cystic space (diamond shaped) within the head. The limb buds are prominently seen. The body movements are seen as early as 8–9 weeks of gestation.[5]

The CRL is the measurement of the maximum length of an embryo **(Figs. 10A to C)**. Prior to 7 weeks of gestation, the mean of three CRLs should be obtained. Later, as the GA advances, CRL should be measured in the sagittal section and as a straight line. The magnification should be such that the sac and the embryo occupy most of the width of screen. The endpoints should be clearly made out. Beyond 10 weeks as the fetal curvature increases, the fetus should be measured in neutral position.

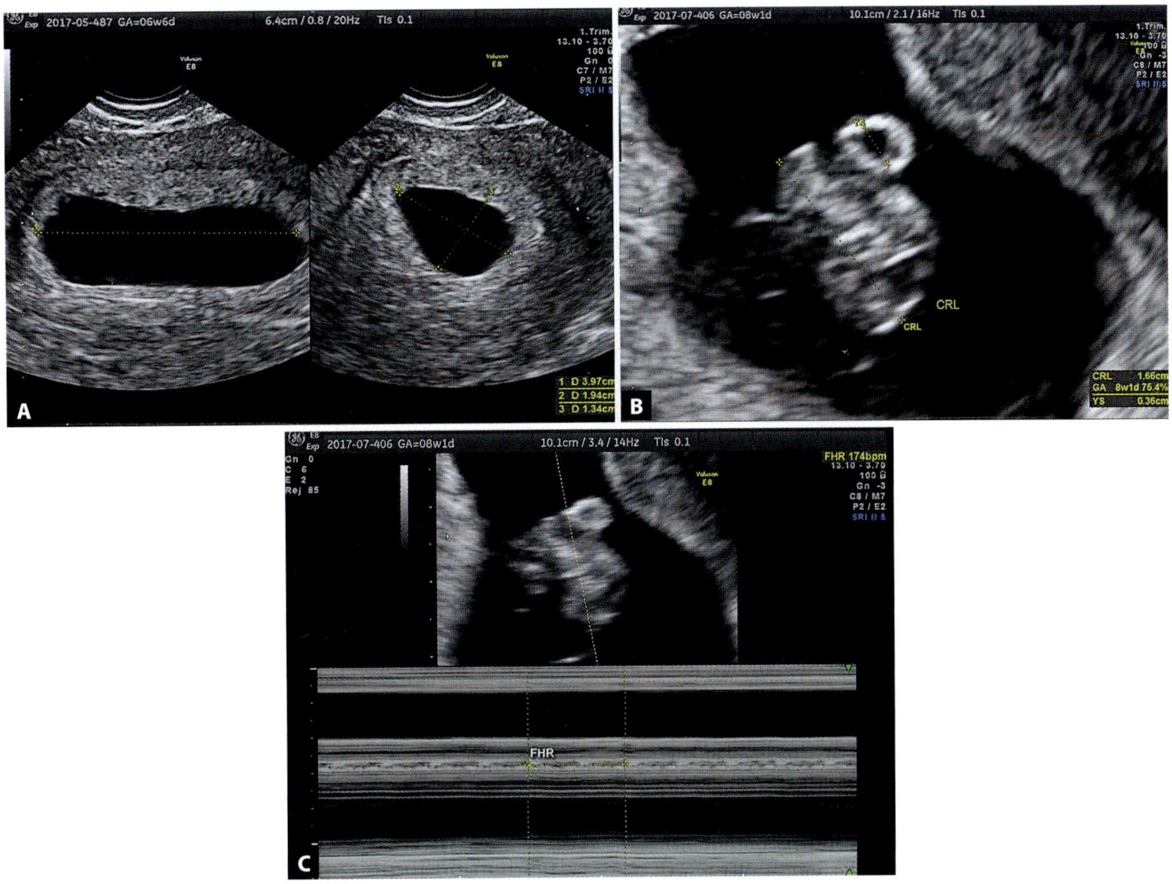

Figs. 10A to C: (A) Measurement of gestational sac; (B) Yolk sac and crown–rump length (CRL); (C) Fetal heart rate (FHR) in M mode.

Cardiac Activity

Cardiac pulsation is seen at around 5–6 weeks of gestation. The cardiac activity is always seen by CRL of 7 mm and larger and thus enables in diagnosis of early pregnancy loss. During the first trimester, fetal heart rate is always recorded by M-mode and it varies with GA.

The heart rate increases over the first 6–8 weeks of gestation. The lower limit of normal is 100 BPM at around 6 weeks of gestation and reaches to 120 BPM at 6–7 weeks of gestation. The heart rate reaches to 170–180 BPM by 8–9 weeks of gestation.[5]

Assessment of Gestational Age

Accurate dating is a very essential part of the first-trimester scan and helps in proper follow-up of the pregnancies. It is one of the main indications of ultrasound in the first trimester. Ultrasound CRL measurement determines GA, and it is based on the assumption that the size of the embryo is consistent with its age. Biological variation in the size of the embryo is less during the first trimester compared to later gestations.[6,7]

Dating of the pregnancy can be done by two different methods. The age calculated from the conception date is referred to as conception/fertilization age. The GA calculated from the LMP is referred to as "menstrual age," which is commonly used. Only in case of in vitro fertilization (IVF)-assisted reproduction pregnancies, the day of conception is determined reliably. Else, the true GA is established accurately by ultrasound. All the guidelines recommend that the early pregnancy ultrasound should be advised to all pregnant women to determine the GA.

The CRL up to 84 mm size is the most precise in dating the pregnancy or determining the GA, and the difference is usually ±5–7 days in 95% of cases. The period for CRL assessment for assigning the GA is between 7 and 13 + 6 weeks by either a transabdominal or transvaginal sonography.[8] After that, head circumference is used to calculate GA as it is more precise than biparietal diameter (BPD). The American College of Obstetricians and Gynecologists (ACOG) committee's expert opinion is that when the CRL is at least 10 mm (i.e., by 7 weeks), the reliability and measurability are best. Nomograms are available for the singleton and are also applicable in multiple pregnancy.[6]

Dates are reassigned when:

- In case of spontaneous conception and assisted reproductive technologies (ART) except for IVF:
  Expected delivery date (EDD) should be changed to correspond with the ultrasound age when:

    - *11–14 weeks period of gestation:* When CRL and the menstrual age differ by >7 days.
    - *7–10 weeks period of gestation:* When CRL and the menstrual age have a discrepancy of >5 days.
- If the patient does not know her LMP, EDD is assigned as per the ultrasound examination, and the earliest CRL measurement is the most reliable.
- In case of an ART–IVF pregnancy, the conception date should be used to assign the EDD. For example, in an IVF pregnancy, the delivery date is assigned by the embryo age and the date of transfer, i.e., when the embryo is transferred on for the day-5/fifth day after fertilization, the EDD is 261 days from the embryo transfer (ET) date. Likewise, for a day-3 embryo/third day after fertilization, EDD is 263 days from the ET date.[7]

Assessment of GA in twin pregnancy: The CRL of both the fetuses is measured. The larger CRL is used for assigning or confirming the GA. Differences of >1 week between the fetuses in the first trimester should be noted. These fetuses need to be monitored with serial ultrasound scans. The discrepancy is often due to constitutional differences, but however, the early onset fetal growth restriction (FGR), structural, and/or karyotype abnormality need to be excluded.

MULTIPLE PREGNANCY

The incidence of multiple pregnancy is increasing, mainly due to widespread use of assisted reproduction techniques. Ultrasound examination in the first trimester tells us about the number of fetuses and the chorionicity of pregnancy. It is important to determine the type of twining.

The fertilized egg is termed "the zygote." If there is ovulation and fertilization of two eggs, it results in dizygotic twin, and in case of a single oocyte, it leads to monozygotic twin. All dizygotic twins have two placentas and hence have two chorionic sacs and two amniotic sacs. They are called "diamniotic dichorionic" twins. The *monozygotic twin* divide at different stages of development, resulting in three types of monozygotic twins:

- *Dichorionic diamniotic (DCDA twin):* They will have two placentas (chorion) and two amniotic cavities (when the embryo splits within the first 48 hours). They are similar to dizygotic twins but will be of the same sex and constitute around one-third of monozygotic twins.
- *Monochorionic diamniotic (MCDA twin):* There is one placenta (chorion) and two separate amniotic cavities (when the embryo splits after 72 hours but within 8 days). Majority of the monozygotic twins are MCDA (around two-third).
- *Monochorionic monoamniotic (MCMA):* They have one placenta and one amniotic cavity (when the embryo splits between 9 and 12 days). It constitutes <1% of monozygotic twins.

All dizygotic twins are dichorionic and not all monozygotic twins are monochorionic. Dizygotic twins can be either of same sex or of different sex, but all monozygotic twins are of same sex.

Ultrasound Assessment of Multiple Pregnancy

Multiple gestation can be seen as singleton during early scans (from 4 to 5 weeks). All twin pregnancies seen in the early GA might not result in twin live birth. The twin conception rate is usually high, but unfortunately, the early single embryo or fetal loss is approximately around 30% in the first trimester.

The visualization of two different gestational sacs on ultrasound before 6 weeks of gestation confirms the diagnosis of dichorionicity; however, it could be either dizygotic or monozygotic. The number of sacs is not used as a predictor of the number of future embryos as the sac might contain more than one embryo. Many a time, an empty sac in twin gestation regresses spontaneously, and it is known as "vanishing twin" phenomenon (20% of multiple pregnancies).

Presence of two or more embryos in a sac by 6–7 weeks of gestation confirms the diagnosis of monochorionic multiple pregnancy. But however, the amnionicity is established only by 8–9 weeks of gestation as the amount of amniotic fluid increases, thus facilitating the visualization of amniotic membrane by ultrasound **(Table 2)**.

Ultrasound Labeling of Twins

On ultrasound, each fetus or fetuses has to be identified correctly to ensure proper fetal assessment throughout the pregnancy. The position of the sac in relation to the cervix remains almost constant throughout the gestation and hence is used for labeling of the multiple pregnancies.

The fetus in the sac closer to the cervix is identified as twin/fetus 1 or A and the twin in the sac further from the cervix as fetus/twin 2 or B. In case of multiple pregnancy (multiple order), further labeling goes anticlockwise from fetus one, two, and so forth. This notation should be strictly applied from the very beginning of pregnancy **(Figs. 12A to C)**.

Establishing Chorionicity and Amnionicity

Ultrasound between 10 and 14 weeks of gestation is the ideal time for multiple pregnancy as dichorionic (DCDA) or monochorionic (MCDA/MCMA) twin pairs.

DCDA twin: The presence of two placentas in the later gestation is diagnostic of a dichorionic twin pregnancy. However, the presence of a single placenta on ultrasound can indicate either a dichorionic pregnancy with adjacent implantation of the two placentas or a monochorionic pregnancy with a single placenta. It is important to establish

TABLE 2: Ultrasound diagnosis of type of twin pregnancy.

Gestational age (weeks)	*Dichorionic diamniotic*	*Monochorionic diamniotic*	*Monochorionic monoamniotic*
5	Two separate sacs **(Fig. 11A)** 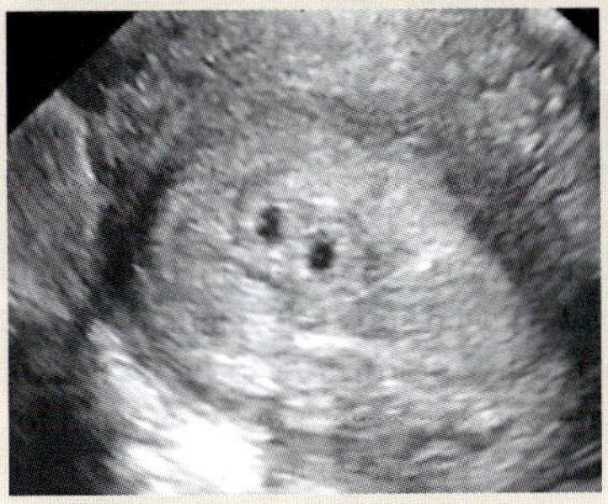 **Fig. 11A:** Two separate sacs.	Single sac **(Fig. 11B)** 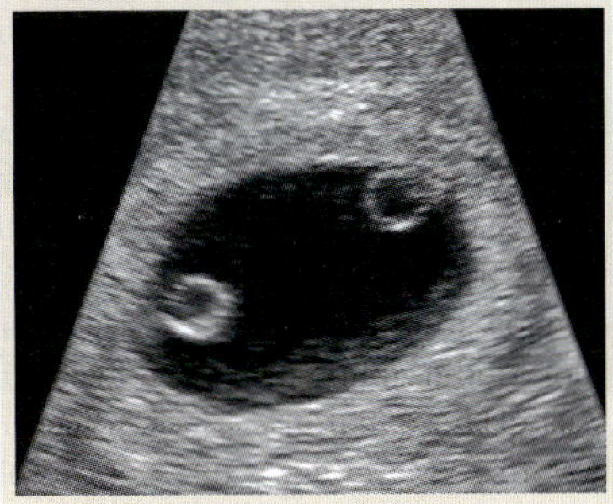 **Fig. 11B:** Single sac with two yolk sacs.	Single sac **(Fig. 11C)** 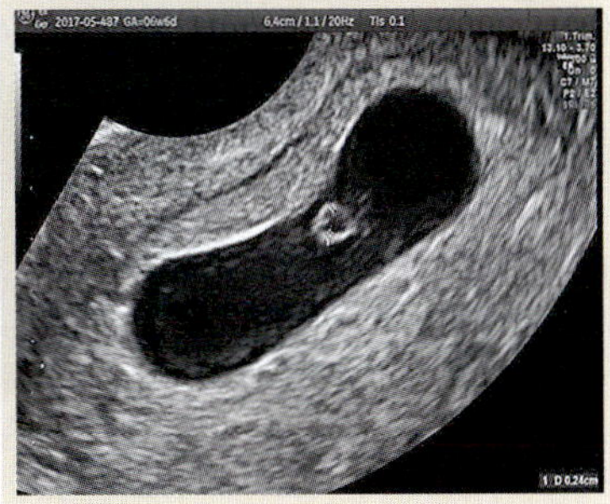 **Fig. 11C:** Single sac with one yolk sac.
6	Two sacs with embryo in each **(Fig. 11D)** 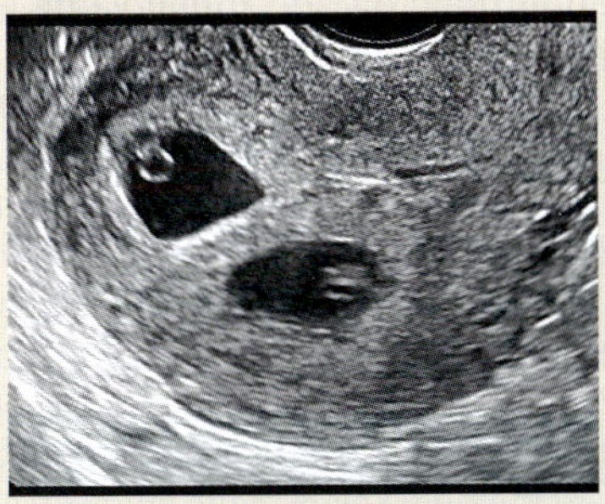 **Fig. 11D:** Two sacs with embryo in each.	Single sac with two embryos **(Fig. 11E)** 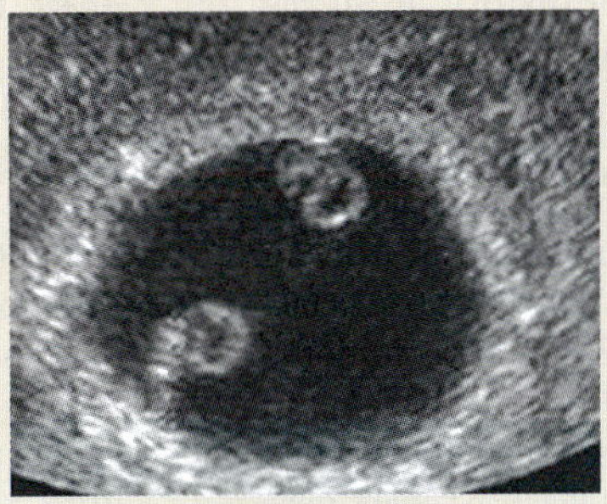 **Fig. 11E:** Single sac with two yolk sacs and two embryos.	Single sac with two embryos **(Fig. 11F)** 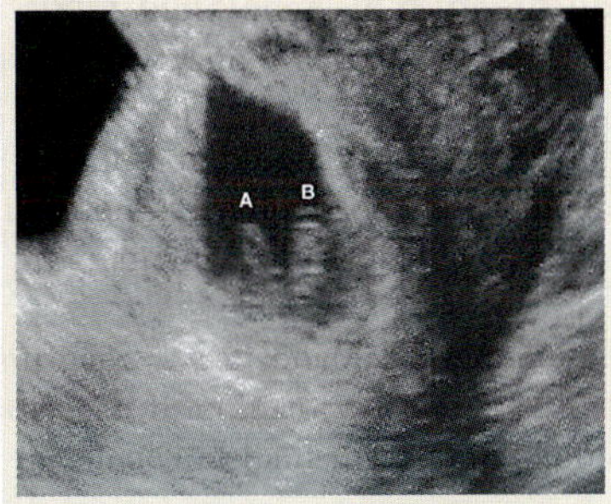 **Fig. 11F:** Single sac with one yolk sac and two embryos.
9	Two sacs with embryo and amniotic cavity in each **(Fig. 11G)** 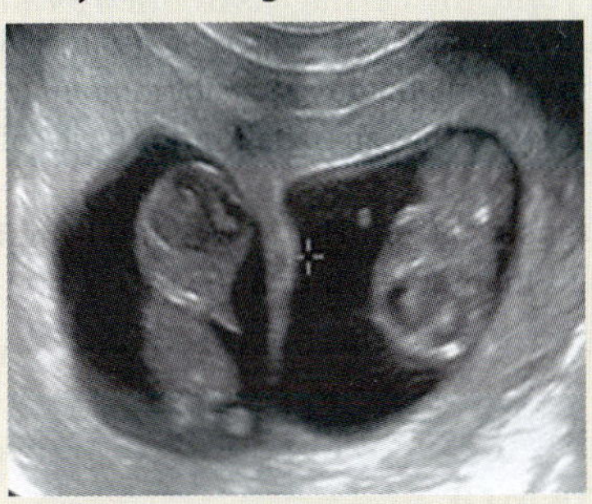 **Fig. 11G:** Two sacs with embryo and amniotic cavity in each.	Single sac with two embryos in two amniotic sacs **(Fig. 11H)** 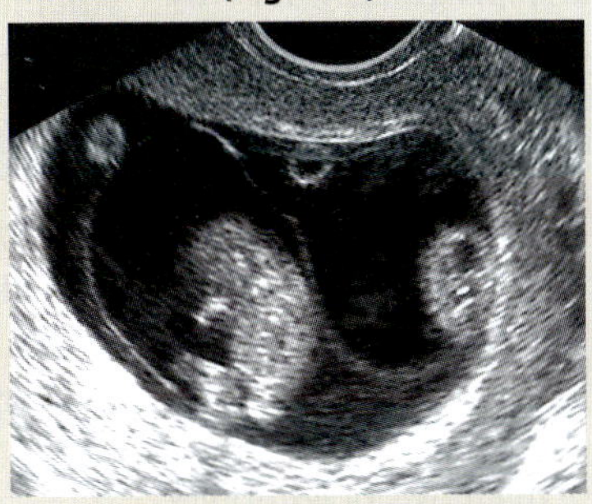 **Fig. 11H:** Single sac with two embryos in two amniotic sacs.	Single sac with two embryos in single amniotic sac **(Fig. 11I)** 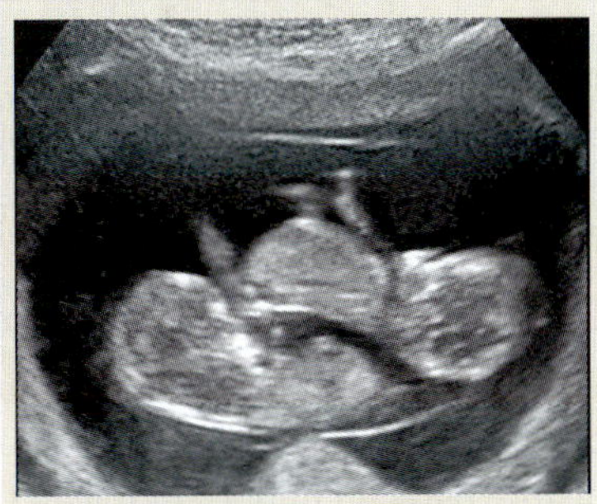 **Fig. 11I:** Single sac with two embryos in single amniotic sac.

the chorionicity correctly for further antenatal management, as monochorionic pregnancy is associated with more complications than dichorionic pregnancy. The dichorionic placenta will demonstrate *the "twin peak" sign* or *"lambda" sign* **(Figs. 12A to C)**. It comprises the two amniotic and two chorionic membranes separated slightly at the insertion site by a tongue of placental tissue.

MCDA twin: A monochorionic placenta will demonstrate the *"T sign"* when the two amniotic membranes insert into the shared placenta **(Figs. 12A to C)**.

MCMA twin: If there is no dividing membrane seen between the fetuses, MCMA twins have to be suspected. The confirmation is always to be made in the late first trimester or early second trimester.

FIRST-TRIMESTER COMPLICATIONS

The fetal demise, empty sac, and disproportionate fetal growth can be a feature of abnormal development in early pregnancy. The vaginal bleeding and pain in the abdomen are symptoms of early pregnancy loss but could also be seen

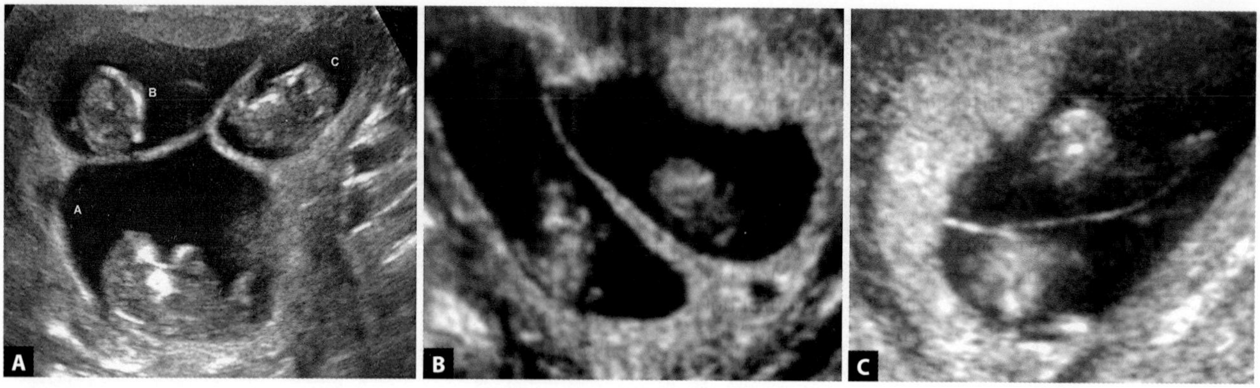

Figs. 12A to C: (A) Labeling of fetuses in multiple pregnancy; (B) Twin peak sign in dichorionic diamniotic (DCDA) twin; (C) T-sign in monochorionic diamniotic (MCDA) twin.

in normal gestation. The ultrasound helps in identifying the first-trimester complications and thus to prognosticate the pregnancy. A detailed medical history, examination, sonography, and serum β-hCG help in making a more specific diagnosis.

Approximately 40% of early pregnancies can result in early pregnancy loss. The causes of miscarriages could be due to unknown causes, chromosomal defects, viral infections, uterine malformation, maternal endocrine problems, autoimmune antibodies—immunologic factors, and maternal systemic disease. As the pregnancy advances, the risk of miscarriage decreases.[3]

Early Pregnancy Loss

The criteria for diagnosing an early pregnancy loss by ultrasound were reported in the early 1990s, immediately after vaginal sonography was widely available. Based on the ultrasound findings, the miscarriages are labeled as threatened, missed, incomplete, and complete.

Complete and Incomplete Miscarriage

The experience of the operator is important in the diagnosis of complete and incomplete miscarriage. The clinical history plays an important role in the diagnosis of complete or incomplete miscarriage. Ultrasound should always be combined with clinical and biochemical assessment. When the endometrium is thin, regular, and comparable to that of early proliferative phase on ultrasound, probability of complete miscarriage is high.

The ultrasound diagnosis of incomplete miscarriage is difficult. The diagnostic criteria of endometrial thickness vary between 5 and 15 mm. Using fixed cutoff values are difficult as blood clots cannot be always differentiated from retained conception products within the cavity at the time of miscarriage. Therefore, subjective assessment is preferred over quantitative assessment. The retained conception products appear as a well-defined hyperechoic area within the cavity as opposed to blood clots which are more irregular. Clots are seen sliding within the cavity when pressure is applied by the transvaginal probe. However, the Doppler examination may not add much value to the diagnosis of incomplete miscarriage.[9]

Threatened Miscarriage

Threatened miscarriage is associated with vaginal bleeding with or without abdominal cramps, and ultrasound gives valuable information about the prognosis and the treatment options. The cervical os is closed. It occurs in about 20% of the recognized pregnancies. The subchorionic hematoma does not always predict poor outcomes **(Figs. 13A to C)**.[9]

Anembryonic Miscarriage

Anembryonic miscarriage is defined as an empty gestational sac, previously known as blighted ovum **(Figs. 13A to C)**.

Missed Miscarriage

Missed miscarriage is defined as embryonic demise or early fetal death in utero. Absence of cardiac activity in the embryo or fetus on ultrasound aids in the diagnosis of missed miscarriage. The cardiac activity either does not develop (up to CRL of 7 mm) or appears and then later disappears **(Figs. 13A to C)**.

According to the previous studies, the diagnostic criteria to confirm early pregnancy loss were either a CRL of 5 mm without a cardiac activity or an empty sac with a diameter of 16 mm.[10-12] In the recent time, two large prospective studies challenged these cutoffs.[13,14] In one of the studies, when the CRL cutoff of 5 mm was used for diagnosis of early pregnancy loss, the false-positive rate was 8.3% and for CRL cutoff of 7 mm, a false-positive rate was decreased with high specificity.[13] Similarly, the authors said that when the MSD cutoff of 16 mm was used for early pregnancy loss, the false-positive rate was 4.4%. An MSD cutoff of 25 mm (without an embryo and with or without a yolk sac) was used to achieve 100% specificity for the early pregnancy loss. However, the authors also concluded that if the sac remained

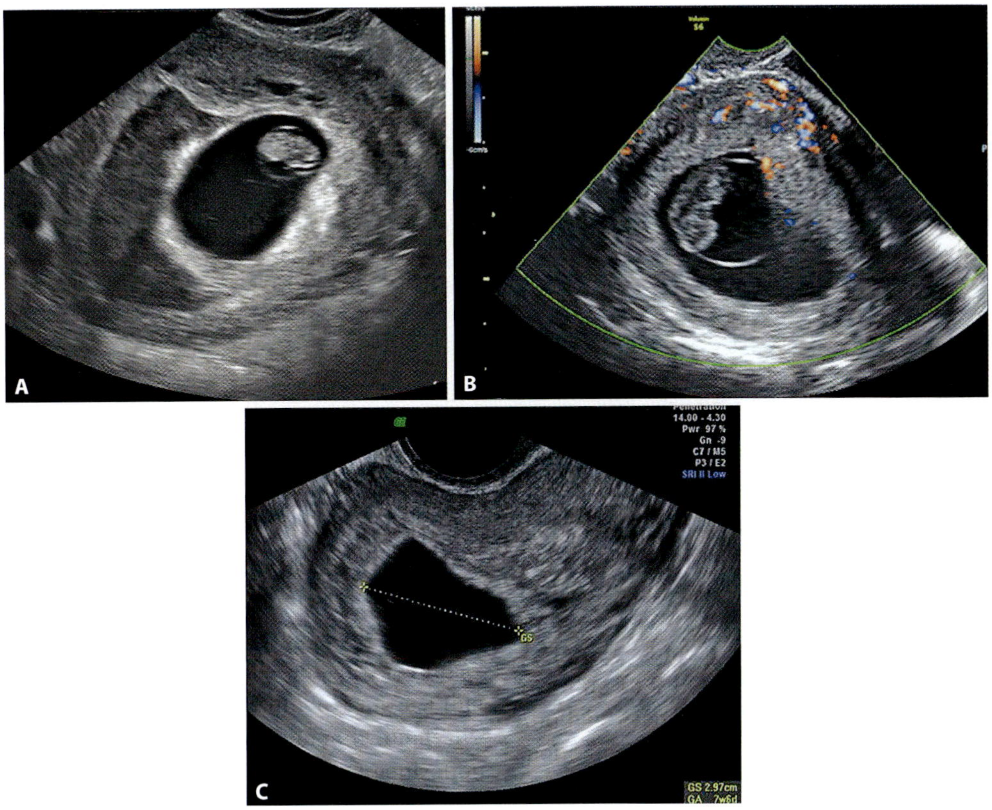

Figs. 13A to C: (A) Threatened miscarriage; (B) Absent cardiac activity suggestive of missed miscarriage; (C) Empty gestational sac suggestive of anembryonic miscarriage.

empty after reassessment in 7 days, then it was labeled as pregnancy loss.[14]

Based on these studies, the Society of Radiologists in Ultrasound Multispecialty Panel on Early First Trimester Diagnosis of Miscarriage created guidelines which are more conservative than the previous guidelines and has a strict cutoff for the diagnosis of early pregnancy loss.[15]

Individualizing these guidelines according to the patient circumstances is very important. According to the ACOG committee opinion, few criteria are considered suggestive of early pregnancy loss but not diagnostic, and these are listed in **Table 3**. Examples of slow fetal heart rate at 7–8 weeks of gestation are associated with early pregnancy loss. When these findings are present, it warrants repeat ultrasound in 7–10 days.[15]

Pregnancy of Unknown Location

When there is no sign of intrauterine or extrauterine pregnancy on transvaginal ultrasound, in spite of the pregnancy test being positive, it is defined as pregnancy of unknown location (PUL). It is a transient situation and not a final diagnosis. At this stage, the differential diagnoses are early intrauterine pregnancy (IUP), ectopic pregnancy, and complete miscarriage. Serial ultrasound evaluation and also serum hCG are necessary for the follow-up, especially for localization of pregnancy. In women with an hCG result below the discriminatory level, it may be too early to visualize the gestational sac. In a multiple pregnancy, serum β-hCG levels are high at the early gestation when compared with those in a singleton pregnancy. The possibility of ectopic pregnancy is high when there is no intrauterine sac and β-hCG is above the discriminatory level, particularly if the level is >3,000 IU/L. The Doppler finding of focal low-resistance arterial trophoblastic flow may not be useful as it can have adverse effect on the IUP.

There is a small intrauterine collection seen in PUL, which could be a decidual cyst or localized intrauterine fluid. When a patient with PUL is hemodynamically stable, it is less harmful to wait. It is recommended that serum β-hCG levels and endovaginal scan need to be repeated after 7–10 days.[4] The combination of ultrasound findings and quantitative β-hCG levels help in the diagnosis of normal IUP, nonviable IUP, and ectopic pregnancy.

ECTOPIC PREGNANCY (FIGS. 14A TO C)

Implantation of the embryo outside the uterine cavity is defined as an ectopic pregnancy. Majority of the ectopic pregnancies are tubal (93%). The rate of ectopic pregnancy is 11/1,000 pregnancies, with a maternal mortality of 0.2/1,000 estimated ectopic pregnancies.[16] Clinically, a patient

TABLE 3: Society of Radiologists in Ultrasound Guidelines for Transvaginal Ultrasonographic Diagnosis of Early Pregnancy Loss*—ACOG, Committee Opinion Number 700, May 2017.

Findings diagnostic of early pregnancy loss†	*Findings suggestive, but not diagnostic, of early pregnancy loss‡*
Crown–rump length of 7 mm or greater and no heartbeat	Crown–rump length of <7 mm and no heartbeat
Mean sac diameter of 25 mm or greater and no embryo	Mean sac diameter of 16–24 mm and no embryo
Absence of embryo with heartbeat 2 weeks or more after a scan that showed a gestational sac without a yolk sac	Absence of embryo with heartbeat 7–13 days after an ultrasound scan that showed a gestational sac without a yolk sac
Absence of embryo with heartbeat 11 days or more after a scan that showed a gestational sac with a yolk sac	Absence of embryo with heartbeat 7–10 days after an ultrasound scan that showed a gestational sac with a yolk sac
	Absence of embryo for 6 weeks or longer after last menstrual period
	Empty amnion (amnion seen adjacent to yolk sac, with no visible embryo)
	Enlarged yolk sac (>7 mm)
	Small gestational sac in relation to the size of the embryo (<5 mm difference between mean sac diameter and crown-rump length)

*Criteria are from the Society of Radiologists in Ultrasound Multispecialty Consensus Conference on early first-trimester diagnosis of miscarriage and exclusion of a viable intrauterine pregnancy, October 2012.

†These are the radiologic criteria only and do not replace clinical judgment.

‡When there are findings suspicious for early pregnancy loss, follow-up ultrasonography at 7–10 days to assess the pregnancy for viability is generally appropriate.

Source: Doubilet PM, Benson CB, Bourne T, Blaivas M, Society of Radiologists in Ultrasound Multispecialty Panel on Early First Trimester Diagnosis of Miscarriage and Exclusion of a Viable Intrauterine Pregnancy, Barnhart KT, et al. Diagnostic criteria for nonviable pregnancy early in the first trimester. N Engl J Med. 2013;369:1443-51.

may present with abdominal pain with or without vaginal bleeding.[9]

Usually, the finding of pregnancy test being positive and on ultrasound, no IUP suggests ectopic pregnancy. On TVS, majority of the ectopic pregnancies can be visualized at the initial ultrasound scan; however, index suspicion should be high. A sac-like structure within the uterus, known as pseudosac, is seen in around 10–29% of ectopic pregnancies and should not be mistaken for an early gestational sac. In longitudinal section, the gestational sac is round, and pseudosac is elongated in appearance. Absence of good choriodecidual reaction and vascularity on Doppler helps in differentiating pseudosac from gestational sac.[16]

In about 78% of the cases, ectopics are on the same side as the corpus luteum, and few times it is difficult to differentiate corpus from the ectopic. The "sliding sign" helps to distinguish a corpus luteum from an ectopic pregnancy. In this technique, a gentle pressure is applied with the tip of the transvaginal probe to observe whether the mass moves separately from the ovary. In addition to the adnexal mass, presence of internal hemorrhage which is indicative of tubal abortion or a ruptured ectopic has to be noted. On ultrasound, hemorrhage is seen as hyperechoic fluid in the pouch of Douglas **(Table 4)**.

Differential diagnosis of an ectopic (false positive diagnosis) is static bowel loop, hydrosalpinx, adhesions, or an endometrioma. Direct visualization of the adnexal ectopic mass facilitates the diagnosis and helps to decide the best management option. The ultrasound appearance of ectopic pregnancies varies and the diagnosis depends on the quality of the equipment and the experience of the sonographers.

Interstitial pregnancy is defined as implantation in the interstitial portion of the fallopian tube. On ultrasound, gestational sac or the mass is seen in the upper lateral aspect of the uterus and outside the uterine cavity, surrounded with a thin myometrial mantle. A *cervical pregnancy* occurs when the conceptus is implanted in the cervical canal. The ultrasound diagnostic criteria for the diagnosis of cervical ectopic are no evidence of an intrauterine gestational sac,

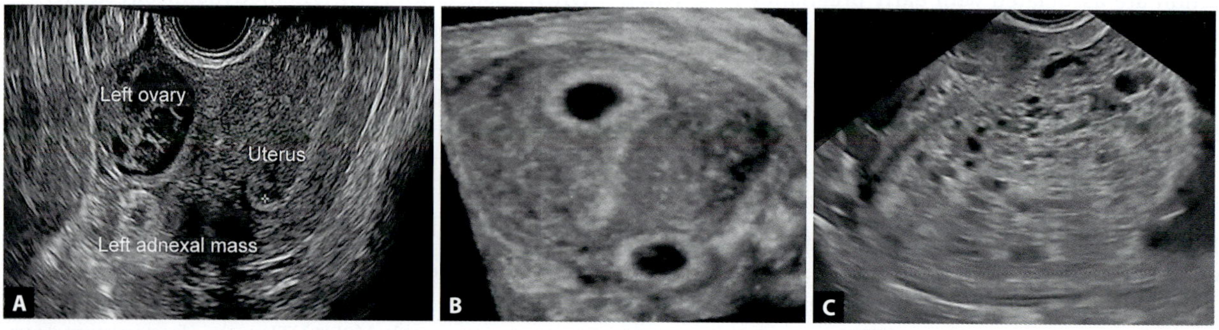

Figs. 14A to C: (A) Transvaginal scan showing an adnexal mass adjacent to left ovary—left-sided ectopic pregnancy; (B) 3D rendered image of heterotrophic pregnancy shows presence of intrauterine and extrauterine gestational sac; (C) Transvaginal scan image showing homogeneous distribution of cystic areas within the uterine cavity. Suggestive of complete molar pregnancy.

TABLE 4: Ultrasound (transvaginal scan) findings of tubal ectopic pregnancy.

Intrauterine	*Adnexal findings*
• Empty uterus with or without increased endometrial thickness • Fluid collection within the uterine cavity (i.e., pseudosac, must be differentiated from an intrauterine sac, which is identified by the presence of an eccentrically located hypoechoic structure with a double decidual sign in the endometrium) • Concurrent intrauterine pregnancy	• Adnexal mass, moving separate to the ovary (sometimes called the "sliding sign"): – Comprising a gestational sac with a yolk sac or fetal pole (with or without fetal heartbeat) or an empty gestational sac (described as a "tubal ring" or "bagel sign") – A complex, inhomogeneous adnexal mass moving separate to the ovary • Moderate or large amount of free fluid collection is seen in the peritoneal cavity or pouch of Douglas, suggestive of hemoperitoneum

Source: Ectopic pregnancy and miscarriage: diagnosis and initial management (update) (NG126) April 2019.[17]

ballooning of the cervical canal (hourglass uterine shape), the presence of a gestation sac within the cervical canal, and internal os is closed. Ovarian ectopic can be diagnosed on scan when the gestation sac is seen within the ovary or when sac cannot be separated from the ovary. It is essential that the corpus luteum is identified separately from the gestational sac to avoid misinterpreting the corpus luteum as an ovarian pregnancy.

HETEROTOPIC PREGNANCY (FIGS. 14A TO C)

When there is an intrauterine gestational sac along with an ectopic pregnancy, it is termed "heterotopic pregnancy." The incidence of heterotopic pregnancy is high in women undergoing assisted reproductive treatment, and in the general population it is about 1:6,000. The diagnosis of a normal IUP thus cannot rule out a concomitant ectopic pregnancy. A careful and thorough examination has to be made to exclude the presence of heterotopic pregnancy in a symptomatic patient and a high index of suspicion is necessary for the diagnosis.

MOLAR PREGNANCY

The generalized swelling of the chorionic villous and diffuse trophoblastic hyperplasia in the absence of embryonic or fetal tissue are the features of complete molar pregnancy. The ultrasound appearance of molar pregnancy is described as "snowstorm appearance," i.e., homogenous distribution of cystic areas within the uterus. The gestational sac or fetal pole is not separately seen **(Fig. 14C)**. Serum hCG will be high in these women, usually >2.5 multiples of median (MoM), and will continue to increase as the pregnancy advances.

Partial hydatidiform moles are characterized by focal swelling of the villous tissue and focal trophoblastic hyperplasia in the presence of embryonic or fetal tissue. The sonolucent areas seen within the placenta might represent either a partial mole or a twin pregnancy with one conceptus normal and the other complete mole. In partial moles, the molar structures are dispersed inside the placental mass. With triploid partial moles, major fetal abnormalities or severe intrauterine growth restriction are most commonly present.

RISK FACTORS FOR EARLY PREGNANCY FAILURE (FIGS. 15A TO C)

- *GA:* An inverse relationship exists between GA and an adverse outcome.
- *SCH:* Intrauterine collections of blood are found in many women with first-trimester threatened miscarriage as well as some asymptomatic patients. Bleeding in the early pregnancy period occurs in about 5–25% of all pregnancies. During very early pregnancy, bleeding could be implantation bleed. Later, it is likely due to venous bleeding associated with separation or abruption of the placental margin or marginal sinus. The blood dissects along paths of least resistance and ultimately can be located in a variety of positions relative to the developing sac and placenta. The echogenicity of the blood depends on its age and the amount of associated clot. *Subchorionic hematoma is defined as hypoechoic or anechoic areas between the chorionic membrane and the myometrium adjacent to gestational sac.*[18-21]

  The SCH can be quantified by measuring the volume of the hematoma. The volumes can be estimated by measuring the anteroposterior, longitudinal, and transverse diameters and multiplying these values by 0.523 (the ellipsoid formula). However, the *size of the hematoma can be assessed relative to the gestational sac because this method is simple and well-established.*
  - *Small:* When SCH encircles less than one-third of the gestational sac.
  - *Moderate:* When SCH encircles around one-third to half of the gestational sac.
  - *Large:* When SCH encircles around one-half to two-thirds or greater of the gestational sac.
- *Growth delay:*
  - *CRL:* A smaller-than-expected first-trimester CRL measurement reflects early growth restriction that persists throughout pregnancy and is associated with low birth weight, premature delivery, and an increased risk for miscarriage, approximately 25%. It is not surprising when a small sac is present; other adverse prognostic indicators such as embryonic

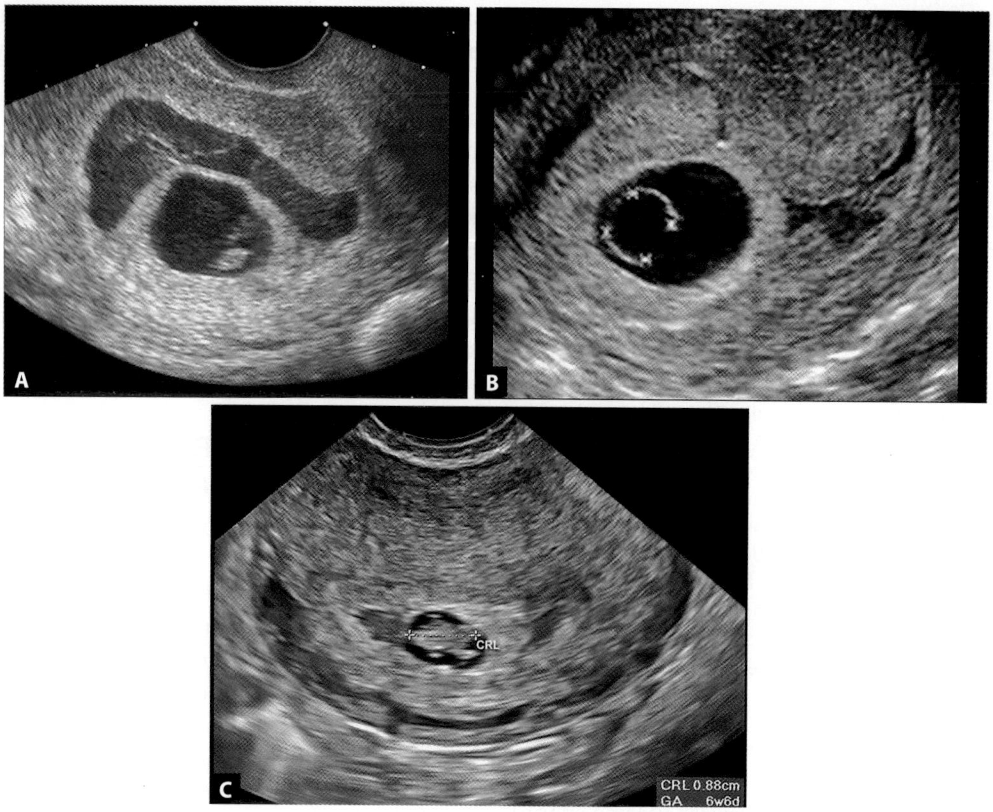

Figs. 15A to C: (A) Large subchorionic hemorrhage; (B) Large yolk sac; (C) Small gestational sac with small amniotic cavity. (CRL: crown–rump length; GA: gestational age)

bradycardia, maternal bleeding, or delay in embryonic growth may also be present.[22]

- *Yolk sac:* The size and characteristics of the yolk sac should be assessed in early pregnancy. An abnormal-appearing yolk sac is also associated with early pregnancy failure. Sporadic case reports suggest that yolk sacs that are abnormally shaped, calcified, echogenic, or double (vitelline duct cyst) are associated with either antecedent or subsequent embryonic demise. Despite an abnormal-appearing yolk sac, whenever cardiac activity is present, follow-up imaging is recommended because, in rare and exceptional cases, the pregnancy may continue to term.[22,23]
- *Cardiac activity:* When embryonic cardiac activity is first detected between 5 and 6 weeks' GA, the rate is relatively slow. The mean heart rate increases to approximately 140 BPM by 9 weeks' GA. Bradycardia is defined as <90 BPM after 6 weeks of gestation. There is a 25% risk of fetal demise by the end of the first trimester.

  Analysis of first-trimester bradycardia also confirms an association with structural and chromosome abnormalities, especially trisomy 18 and triploidy. In contrast, other chromosome defects, including trisomy 21, and especially trisomy 13 and Turner syndrome, have all been associated with first-trimester tachycardia (determined at 10–14 weeks of GA).[23-28]
- *Maternal factors:* These factors that may increase the risk of spontaneous miscarriage include age, smoking, structural uterine abnormalities, and a history of miscarriages.

Adnexa

The anatomical area adjacent to the uterus is called adnexa, and it contains the fallopian tube, ovary, associated vessels, ligaments, and connective tissue. The incidence of adnexal masses in pregnancy is around 1 in 81 to 1 in 8,000 pregnancies. Usually, the diagnosis is incidental. The adnexal mass is commonly complicated by torsion, rupture, or bleeding/infection. Ultrasound allows stratification of risk in women with adnexal mass during pregnancy without compromising maternal or fetal safety. The adnexal mass in pregnancy is classified as simple, complex, solid-benign, and solid-malignant. Functional cyst and corpus luteum account for 13–17% of all cystic adnexal masses in pregnancy. Other adnexal masses seen in pregnancy are benign masses (dermoid cyst, serous cystadenoma, mucinous cystadenoma), ovarian malignancy (approximately 1–8% of adnexal masses in pregnancy), endometrioma, hydrosalpinx, and leiomyoma. Complications such as torsion of the ovary have no definitive ultrasound features. The ovary may appear congested, edematous, and markedly enlarged ovary. However, Doppler may show the absence of blood flow in case of torsion, though this is not universal as torsion may be complete or intermittent. Both transabdominal scan and TVS should be used together as complementary techniques. However, the detailed morphological assessment of the mass is better with TVS, especially in early pregnancy. The color Doppler imaging significantly improves the ability to distinguish benign from malignant masses.[29]

KEY POINTS

- The TVS and the quantitative β-hCG levels are the great tools available for the diagnosis of normal and abnormal early pregnancy.
- The Society of Radiologists in Ultrasound 2012 consensus panel of radiologists, obstetricians, and emergency medicine physicians has established new terminology and a new set of discriminatory criteria for the diagnosis of the abnormal early pregnancy and would improve patient care and reduce the risk of inadvertent harm to potentially normal pregnancies.
- The aim of these guidelines is to protect the mother and baby by providing accurate and correct interpretations of the ultrasound findings. Therefore, sonologists should have a knowledge of the progression of normal early pregnancy ultrasound features and abnormal first-trimester ultrasound findings.
- The importance of using the accepted terminology in reporting helps the referring physicians to understand the findings and treat the patients safely.

REFERENCES

1. Kurjak A, Chervenak CFA. Donald School Textbook of Ultrasound in Obstetrics and Gynecology. Boca Raton, Florida, United States: CRC Press; 2004.
2. Callen PW. Ultrasonography in Obstetrics and Gynecology, 5th edition. The University of Michigan: Saunders; 2008.
3. Yigiter AB. Early normal and abnormal pregnancy. Donald School J Ultrasound Obstet Gynecol. 2011;5(4):385-404.
4. Rodgers SK, Chang C, DeBardeleben JT, Horrow MM. Normal and abnormal US findings in early first-trimester pregnancy: review of the society of radiologists in ultrasound 2012 consensus panel recommendations. Radiographics. 2015;35(7):2135-48.
5. Bickhaus J, Perry E, Schust DJ. Re-examining sonographic cut-off values for diagnosing early pregnancy loss. Gynecol Obstet (Sunnyvale). 2013;3(1):141.
6. Salomon LJ, Alfirevic Z, Bilardo CM, Chalouhi GE, Ghi T, Kagan KO, et al. ISUOG practice guidelines: performance of first-trimester fetal ultrasound scan. Ultrasound Obstet Gynecol. 2013;41:102-13.
7. ACOG, Committee Opinion Number 700, May 2017. Committee on Obstetric Practice, American Institute of Ultrasound in Medicine, Society for Maternal-Fetal Medicine. [online] Available from https://www.acog.org/clinical/clinical-guidance/committee-opinion/articles/2017/05/methods-for-estimating-the-due-date [Last accessed November, 2022].
8. SOGC Clinical Practice Guidelines. Determination of gestational age by ultrasound. J Obstet Gynaecol Can. 2014;36(2):171-81.
9. Chudleigh T, Thilaganathan B. Obstetric Ultrasound: How, Why and When, 3rd edition. London: Churchill Livingstone; 2004.
10. ACOG. (2015). Early pregnancy loss. ACOG Practice Bulletin. [online] Available from https://www.acog.org/clinical/clinical-guidance/practice-bulletin/articles/2018/11/early-pregnancy-loss [Last accessed November, 2022].
11. Brown DL, Emerson DS, Felker RE, Cartier MS, Smith WC. Diagnosis of early embryonic demise by endovaginal sonography. J Ultrasound Med. 1990;9:631-6.
12. Pennell RG, Needleman L, Pajak T, Baltarowich O, Vilaro M, Goldberg BB, et al. Prospective comparison of vaginal and abdominal sonography in normal early pregnancy. J Ultrasound Med. 1991;10:63-7.
13. Abdallah Y, Daemen A, Kirk E, Pexsters A, Naji O, Stalder C, et al. Limitations of current definitions of miscarriage using mean gestational sac diameter and crown-rump length measurements: a multicenter observational study. Ultrasound Obstet Gynecol. 2011;38:497-502.
14. Abdallah Y, Daemen A, Guha S, Syed S, Naji O, Pexsters A, et al. Gestational sac and embryonic growth are not useful as criteria to define miscarriage: a multicenter observational study. Ultrasound Obstet Gynecol. 2011;38:503-9.
15. Doubilet PM, Benson CB, Bourne T, Blaivas M, Society of Radiologists in Ultrasound Multispecialty Panel on Early First Trimester Diagnosis of Miscarriage and Exclusion of a Viable Intrauterine Pregnancy, Barnhart KT, et al. Diagnostic criteria for nonviable pregnancy early in the first trimester. N Engl J Med. 2013;369:1443-51.
16. National Collaborating Centre for Women's and Children's Health (UK). Ectopic pregnancy and miscarriage: Diagnosis and initial management in early pregnancy of ectopic pregnancy and miscarriage. NICE clinical guideline 154. 2012.
17. Ectopic pregnancy and miscarriage: diagnosis and initial management (update) (NG126) April 2019.
18. Institute of Obstetricians and Gynaecologists, Royal College of Physicians of Ireland. Ultrasound diagnosis of early pregnancy miscarriage. Clinical practice guideline. Guideline No. 1. 2010.
19. Kolte AM, Bernardi LA, Christiansen OB, Quenby S, Farquharson RG, Goddijn M, et al. Terminology for pregnancy loss prior to viability: a consensus statement from the ESHRE early pregnancy special interest group. Hum Reprod. 2015;30(3):495-8.
20. Leite J, Ross P, Rossi AC, Jeanty P. Prognosis of very large first-trimester hematomas. J Ultrasound Med. 2006;25(11):1441-5.
21. Falco P, Milano V, Pilu G, David C, Grisolia G, Rizzo N, et al. Sonography of pregnancies with first-trimester bleeding and a viable embryo: a study of prognostic indicators by logistic regression analysis. Ultrasound Obstet Gynecol. 1996;7:165.

22. Harris RD, Vincent LM, Askin FB. Yolk sac calcification: a sonographic finding associated with intrauterine embryonic demise in the first trimester. Radiology. 1988;166:109-10.
23. Barzilai M, Lyons EA, Levi CS, Lindsay DJ. Vitelline duct cyst or double yolk sac. J Ultrasound Med. 1989;8:523.
24. Merchiers EH, Dhont M, De Sutter PA, Beghin CJ, Vandekerckhove DA. Predictive value of early embryonic cardiac activity for pregnancy outcome. Am J Obstet Gynecol. 1991;165:11.
25. Doubilet PM, Benson CB. Outcome of first-trimester pregnancies with slow embryonic heart rate at 6-7 weeks gestation and normal heart rate by 8 weeks at US. Radiology. 2005;236:643.
26. Vaccaro H, Arnor F, Leyton M, Sepulveda W. Arrhythmia in early pregnancy: a predictor of first-trimester pregnancy loss. Ultrasound Obstet Gynecol. 1998;12:248.
27. Wong SF, Chau KT, Ho LC. Fetal bradycardia in the first trimester: an unusual presentation of atrial extrasystoles. Prenat Diagn. 2002;22:976.
28. Moore KL, Persaud TVN. The Developing Human: Clinically Oriented Embryology, 7th edition. Philadelphia: WB Saunders; 2003.
29. Yakasai IA, Bappa LA. Diagnosis and management of adnexal masses in pregnancy. J Surg Tech Case Rep. 2012;4(2): 79-85.

CHAPTER 77

Recurrent Pregnancy Loss: From Diagnostic Dilemmas to Clinical Decisions

Smitha AP, Sushma Baxi, Sushma Madhuprakash

DEFINING PREGNANCY LOSS AND RECURRENT PREGNANCY LOSS

Recurrent pregnancy loss (RPL) is a rising concern today. Most of the clinicians face ambiguity as to defining RPL. With more and more couples facing infertility, may be it is time to redefine RPL.

The term "miscarriage" is applied to many complications of early pregnancy, and it is important to be clear on terminology. A pregnancy loss that occurs after a positive urinary human chorionic gonadotropin (hCG) or a raised serum beta-hCG but before ultrasound or histological verification is defined as a "biochemical loss" [the European Society of Human Reproduction and Embryology (ESHRE) 2005]. In general, these occur before 6 weeks of gestation. The term clinical miscarriage is used when ultrasound examination or histological evidence has confirmed that an intrauterine pregnancy has existed. Ectopic, biochemical, and molar pregnancies are thus not included. Clinical miscarriages may be subdivided into early clinical pregnancy losses (before gestational week 12) and late clinical pregnancy losses (gestational weeks 12–21).

The new sonographic diagnostic criteria for early pregnancy loss [the American College of Obstetricians and Gynecologists (ACOG)] are shown in **Table 1**.

TABLE 1: New sonographic diagnostic criteria for early pregnancy loss.

Absent embryonic cardiac activity	*Gestational sac diameter*	*Empty gestational sac with no yolk sac/fetal pole on a repeat scan >1 week*
• CRL cut off 5–5.3 mm • False positive reduced from 8.3 to 0%	• 21 mm without embryo • False positive reduced from 4.4 to 0%	Always associated with pregnancy loss

Prompt reevaluation of both clinical and sonological parameters is warranted within a week where there is evidence of a subchorionic hematoma or a slow fetal heart of <100 beats per minute (bpm).

There is no consensus on the number of pregnancy losses needed to fulfill the criteria for recurrent miscarriage (RM), but ESHRE guidelines define RM as three or more consecutive pregnancy losses before 22 weeks of gestation.

In primary RPL, a woman has multiple losses with no previous viable pregnancies, whereas, in secondary RPL, it occurs in a woman who had a pregnancy beyond 20 gestational weeks. In tertiary RPL, multiple pregnancy losses occur between normal pregnancies **(Fig. 1)**.

Recurrent pregnancy loss has been redefined as two or more clinical pregnancy losses, which are not necessarily consecutive [American Society for Reproductive Medicine (ASRM) 2012].

TIP OF THE ICEBERG

Recurrent pregnancy loss encompasses a wide spectrum from nonviable intrauterine pregnancy for early pregnancy loss to midtrimester abortions and more complex late intrauterine devices (IUDs). The workup and evaluation for each of these presentations vary with specific treatment directed at the primary pathology.

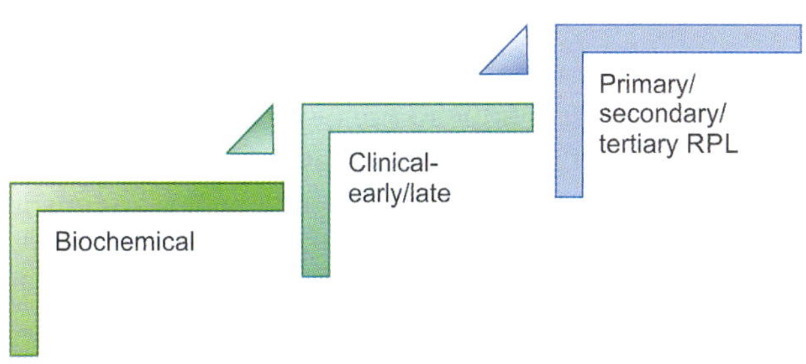

Fig. 1: Spectrum of pregnancy loss.
(RPL: recurrent pregnancy loss)

TABLE 2: Etiological features of recurrent pregnancy loss.

Uterine factors	• *Anatomic defects congenital:* Septate, bicornuate, unicornuate, arcuate, didelphic • *Acquired:* Intrauterine adhesions, myoma, endometrial polyps • *Chronic endometritis*
Thrombophilias	• *Inherited:* Factor V Leiden (FVL), prothrombin gene (PT G20210A) mutation, protein C and protein S deficiency (PSD), antithrombin III (ATIII) deficiency, and methylenetetrahydrofolate reductase (MTHFR) mutation • *APS:* Lupus anticoagulant, anticardiolipin antibody, and anti-β2 glycoprotein I
Endocrine factors	Hyperprolactinemia, hypothyroidism, PCOS, uncontrolled diabetes
Environmental and psychological factors	High BMI, smoking, high caffeine consumption >300 mg/day, excess alcohol intake, and cocaine
Genetic factors	Embryonic aneuploidy, balanced translocations (reciprocal/Robertsonian)
Unexplained	

(APS: antiphospholipid syndrome; BMI: body mass index; PCOS: polycystic ovarian syndrome)

TABLE 3: Etiological features: Diagnostic tests and treatment options.

Etiology	*Diagnostic tests*	*Treatment options*
Uterine factor	3D USG, HSG, hysteroscopy, MRI	Myomectomy, hysteroscopic removal of polyp, septum, adhesion
APS	aCL, anti-β2 glycoprotein, lupus anticoagulant	Heparin, aspirin
Endocrine abnormality	TSH, prolactin, FBS/HbA1c	Appropriate therapy
Genetic	Karyotype of POC parental karyotype	PGD for balanced translocation

(aCL: anticardiolipin; APS: antiphospholipid syndrome; FBS: fasting blood sugar; HbA1c: glycated hemoglobin; HSG: hysterosalpingography; MRI: magnetic resonance imaging; PGD: preimplantation genetic diagnosis; POC: products of conception; TSH: thyroid-stimulating hormone; USG: ultrasonography)

The turmoil a couple go through facing RPL is beyond description, and it is futile to run a whole plethora of tests on them and add to their agony. Targeted tests to identify the primary pathology and specific treatment plans ensure optimal outcomes. In more than half of couples facing RPL, there is no discernible cause, and tender loving care (TLC) plays a crucial role as proven time and again in achieving clinical end points, at times probably the only evidence-based treatment in such couples **(Tables 2 and 3)**.

Flowchart 1: Immunological milieu in recurrent pregnancy loss.

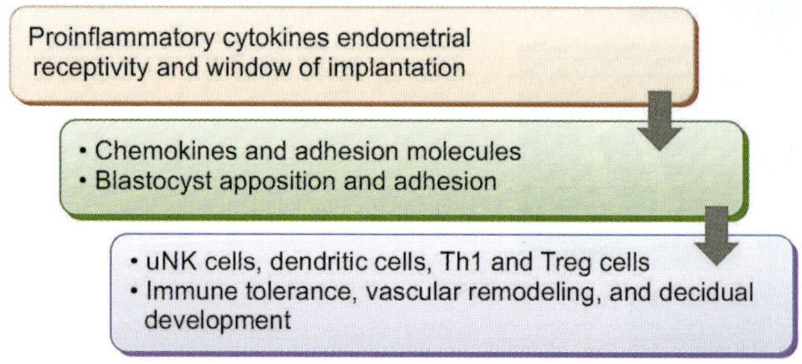

(Treg: regulatory T; Th1: T helper 1; uNK: uterine natural killer)

IMMUNOLOGICAL MILIEU IN RECURRENT PREGNANCY LOSS

Disproving the historical statement that pregnancy is a state of immunological suppression with inhibition of T helper 1 (Th1)-mediated cytotoxic responses. The newer theory defines that pregnancy encompasses a state of altered immunological milieu with pro- and anti-inflammatory phases during specific stages in pregnancy. A complex network of receptors and cytokines orchestrate an intricate communication between the fetus and the maternal immune cells, which ultimately results in a successful pregnancy **(Flowchart 1)**.

NATURAL KILLER CELLS: FRIEND OR FOE?

Maternal–fetal interface is a site of intense immunological activity. The natural killer (NK) cells present here are not a threat to pregnancy but are recruited and harnessed by the trophoblast favorably for promoting trophoblast invasion and vascular remodeling. Reduced decidual NK (dNK) cells mark limited trophoblast invasion, a hallmark of fetal growth restriction **(Fig. 2)**.

Decidual NK cells communicate with the invading extravillous trophoblast (EVT). Paternal human leukocyte antigen (HLA)-C is the major histocompatibility complex (MHC) class I molecule that is expressed by the EVT, which binds to killer immunoglobulin-like receptor (KIR) on NK cells. This triggers the release of angiogenic growth factors, thereby promoting trophoblastic invasion and spiral artery remodeling.

Extravillous trophoblast-mediated expression of Fas ligand (FasL) causes apoptosis of Fas-bearing activated $CD3^+$ T cells and endothelial cells (ECs), thereby protecting against the maternal immune system. Failure of any of these mechanisms predisposes to preeclampsia **(Figs. 3A and B)**.

Regulatory T Cells

Regulatory T (Treg) cells play an important role by recognizing self and nonself antigens. They help in recognizing fetal tissue and are responsible for maternal

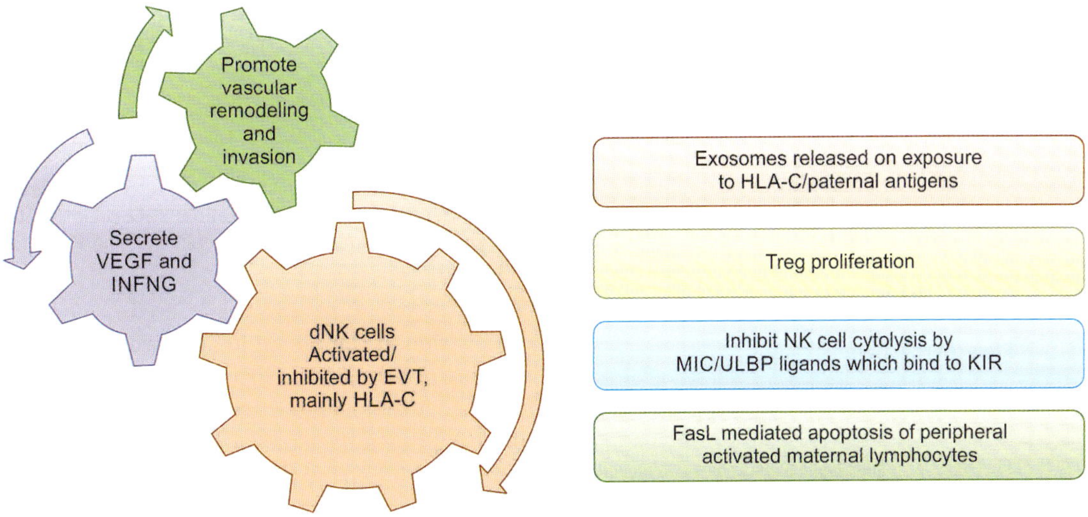

Fig. 2: Features of natural killer (NK) cells as well as decidual NK (dNK) cells.
(EVT: extravillous trophoblast; FasL: Fas ligand; HLA: human leukocyte antigen; INFNG: interferon gamma; KIR: killer immunoglobulin-like receptor; MIC: MHC class I related chain; Treg: regulatory T; ULBP: UL16-binding proteins; VEGF: vascular endothelial growth factor)

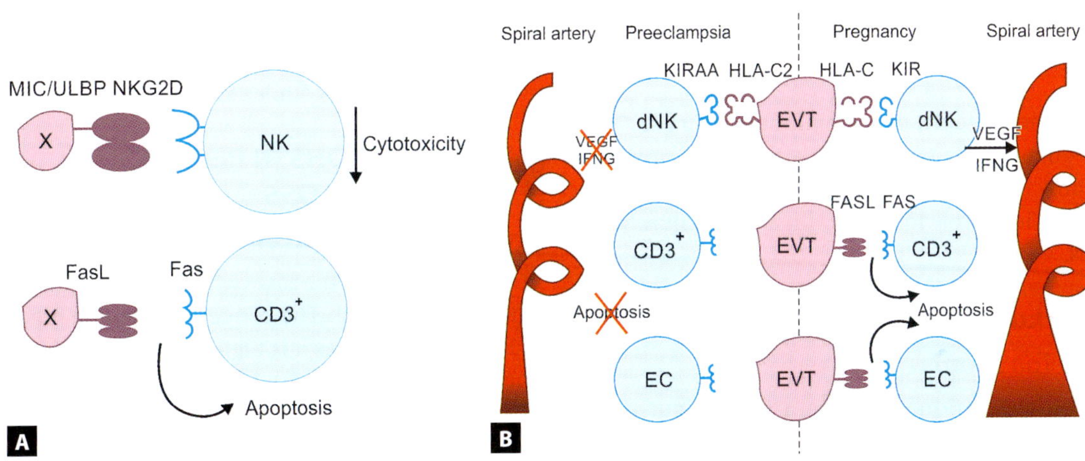

Figs. 3A and B: (A) Maternal periphery; (B) Extravillous trophoblast-mediated expression of Fas ligand (FasL).
(dNK: decidual natural killer; EC: endothelial cells; EVT: extravillous trophoblast; HLA: human leukocyte antigen; INFNG: Interferon gamma; KIR: killer immunoglobulin-like receptor; KIRAA: combination of two KIR A haplotypes; MIC: MHC-I class-related chain; NK: natural killer; NKG2D: natural-killer group 2, member of CD94/NKG2 family an activating receptor; ULBP: UL16-binding proteins; VEGF: vascular endothelial growth factor)

immune tolerance. They secrete transforming growth factor (TGF)-β and interleukin (IL)-10 and mediate both Th1 and Th2 responses. Granulocyte colony-stimulating factor (G-CSF) may reduce the incidence of miscarriage by promoting the proliferation of these Tregs by recognizing HLA-C on extravillous cytotrophoblasts.

In autoimmune diseases, there is evidence of Treg dysfunction. Overexpression of Th1 with low levels of Tregs has been found in RPL and primary infertility.

Angiogenesis and trophoblast invasions are immunologically active processes; rather than passively "escaping" maternal recognition, the fetus actively harnesses the maternal immune surveillance system to facilitate its survival and growth.

PLASTICITY OF REGULATORY T AND T HELPER 17 CELLS (FIG. 4)

Genetic Factors (Flowchart 2)

More than half of early pregnancy losses are the consequence of chromosomal abnormalities. These can arise de novo as commonly encountered or can be of parental origin.

Accounting for 2–4% of cases of RPL, balanced translocations are the most common parental causes and account for more than double than those seen in the general population.

Unbalanced translocations are found in more than a third of miscarried embryos. Most couples with balanced translocations have healthy live births.

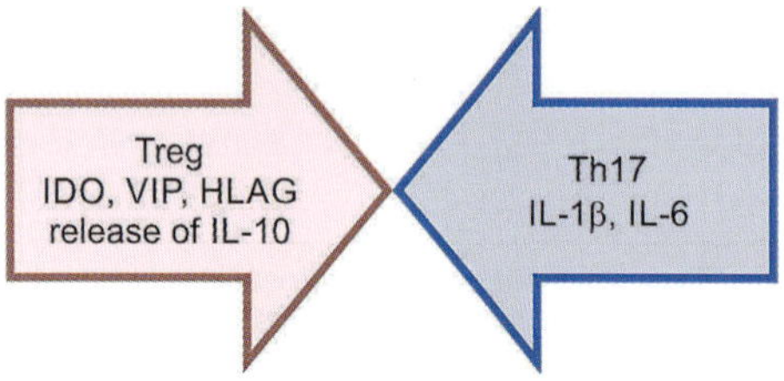

Fig. 4: Plasticity of regulatory T (Treg) and T helper 17 (Th17) cells. (HLAG: human leukocyte antigen-G; IDO: indoleamine-2,3-dioxygenase; IL: interleukin; VIP: vasoactive intestinal peptide)

Flowchart 2: Genetic causes.

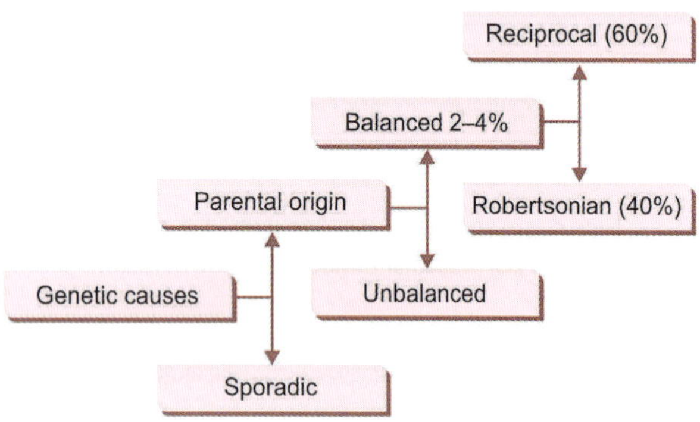

Embryonic aneuploidy, most commonly seen (60–70%) in early pregnancy loss <10 weeks, is generally numeric, namely trisomy (60%), monosomy X (20%), and polyploidy (20%). They are less likely to occur with a higher number of miscarriages.

Genetic Workup (Flowchart 3)

How Soon is Too Soon?

Selective RPL evaluation could be a tool to cut down expenses involved in evaluating a couple which is done if second miscarriage is euploid and <10 weeks.

Based on this concept, genetic evaluation of couples with RPL can be done, thereby enabling early diagnosis and targeted treatment and minimizing the valuable time for these couples.

Preimplantation genetic screening (PGS) is offered to couples with RPL for global assessment of the embryo, unlike the more specific preimplantation genetic diagnosis (PGD) where more specific genetic abnormalities are looked at. PGS use is yet controversial in couples with RPL.

Among the other modalities, comparative genomic hybridization (CGH) is gaining popularity in present day as it can be used even when conventional cytogenetic analysis and cell culture fails or when maternal contamination is present or in tissues preserved in formalin or embedded in paraffin. However, it has its own limitations as in balanced structural chromosome rearrangements cannot be identified, and flow cytometry is required to detect polyploidy. Array CGH (aCGH) testing of products of conception (POCs) do not need live cells, cell culture, or

Flowchart 3: Genetic workup.

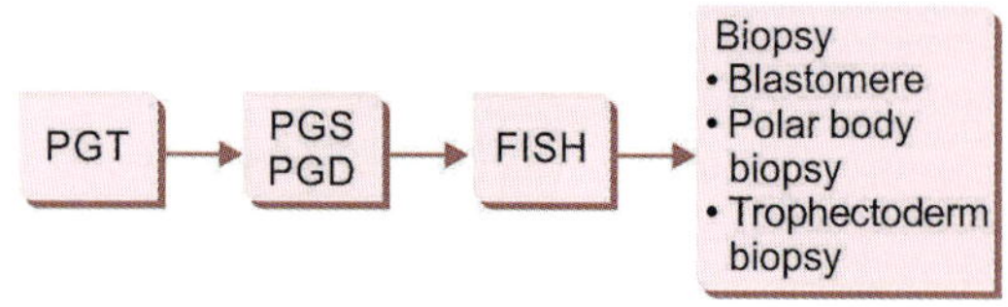

(FISH: fluorescent in situ hybridization; PGD: preimplantation genetic diagnosis; PGS: preimplantation genetic screening; PGT: preimplantation genetic testing)

cell division. It is more rapid and flexible. Single nucleotide polymorphism (SNP) chromosomal microarray analysis can detect the overall distribution of microdeletions and microduplications across a genome. SNP arrays can also be used with CGH to detect aneuploidies and single-gene disorders through linkage analysis.

Next-generation sequencing (NGS) for preimplantation embryo assessment may provide information to such intricacies whose clinical relevance is questionable. With the dawn of "omics," deploying noninvasive technologies for PGS, such as transcriptomics, epigenomics, metabolomics, and mitochondrial function tests, may prove to be a promising future for couples facing RPL.

INTERVENTIONS IN RECURRENT PREGNANCY LOSS

Unexplained Recurrent Pregnancy Loss

In more than half of the cases with RPL, there is no underlying pathology detected. The concept of genetic predisposition to RPL is emerging as it is higher in siblings of patients with unexplained RPL (URPL). Most commonly associated with RPL are the IL genes, especially IL-1β, IL-6, IL-10, and IL-18. More studies on establishing HLA haplotypes in couples with URPL are required. Immune dysregulation has long been postulated with various immune modulatory therapies such as the use of synthetic corticosteroids and more recently hydroxychloroquine sulfate (HCQS).

Hydroxychloroquine Sulfate

Hydroxychloroquine sulfate is a lysosomotropic amine and interferes with lysosomal acidification, which in turn inhibits proteolysis, chemotaxis, phagocytosis, and antigen presentation. As a result, cells are not able to proceed with endocytosis, exosome release, and phagolysosomal fusion in an orderly manner. It could probably prove to be the "wonder drug" in URPL by its various methods of action as enumerated in **Figure 5**.

Aspirin or/and Low-molecular-weight Heparin

Aspirin

Aspirin has been used widely in the prevention of preeclampsia and in RPL secondary to antiphospholipid

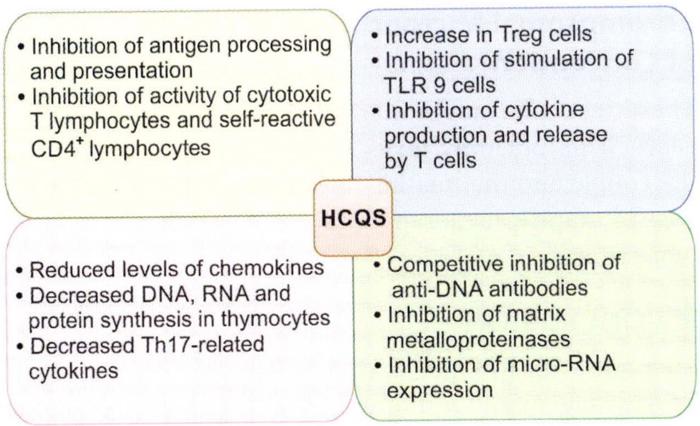

Fig. 5: Various methods of action of hydroxychloroquine sulfate (HCQS).
(DNA: deoxyribonucleic acid; RNA: ribonucleic acid; Th17: T helper 17; TLR: toll-like receptors; Treg: regulatory T)

Flowchart 4: Method of action of aspirin.

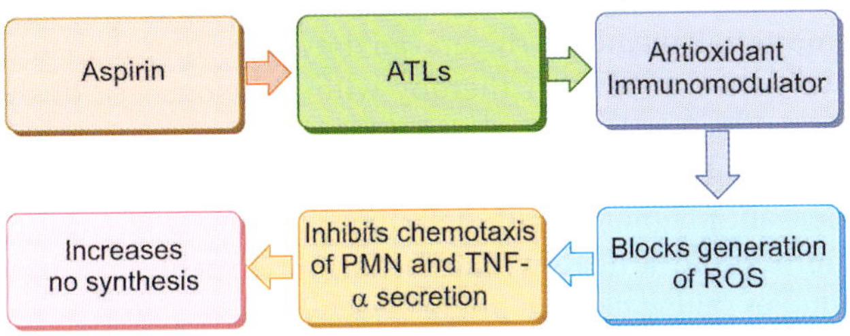

(ATLs: aspirin-triggered lipoxins; PMN: polymorphonuclear; ROS: reactive oxygen species; TNF: tumor necrosis factor)

syndrome (APS). The mechanism is not a mere reduction of prostaglandins/thromboxanes but the production of aspirin-triggered lipoxins (ATLs) **(Flowchart 4)**.

Low-molecular-weight Heparin

Though low-molecular-weight heparin (LMWH) use is rampant in clinical practice, unfortunately, its benefits have not been reflected in randomized controlled trials (RCTs). LMWH might regulate in vitro trophoblast invasiveness and placental production of matrix metalloproteinases (MMPs) and tissue inhibitors of metalloproteinases (TIMPs). Heparin significantly enhanced both pro-MMPs and the active forms, and increased the invasiveness of EVT. The increase in trophoblast invasion by heparin is probably due to a specific protein playing a role in placental invasion. Treatment with LMWH and low-dose aspirin in high-risk patients with low pregnancy-associated plasma protein-A (PAPP-A) has shown improvement in overall clinical outcomes as well.

Synthetic Corticosteroids

Synthetic corticosteroids have been the gold standard in the treatment of RPL because of their known immuno-suppressive effect. Prednisolone effectively reduces the number of uterine NK cells in women with RPL and is most widely used in this patient population. Though some studies showed an improvement in live birth rate (LBR) when prednisolone was combined with aspirin or LMWH, their safety in the first trimester is of concern albeit its effect on increasing risk of maternal hypertension, diabetes, and prematurity. What makes the scenario complex is the presence of multiple confounding factors, thereby masking each individual component from being assessed for the efficacy of this drug. Their use should be limited in women with proven immunological backgrounds for RPL.

Intravenous Immunoglobulin

Intravenous immunoglobulin (IVIg) has long been used in women with URPL despite several trials failing to show any positive impact. A recent meta-analysis of 11 randomized trials in women with URPL showed no difference in LBR between IVIg and placebo. IVIg is, therefore, not recommended for women with URPL.

TUMOR NECROSIS FACTOR-ALPHA ANTAGONISTS

Tumor necrosis factor-alpha (TNF-α) is involved in fetal loss via thrombotic and inflammatory factors. TNF-α antagonists, such as adalimumab, have been used for URPL. Improved LBRs were found when a combination of adalimumab and IVIg was added to anticoagulants compared to anti-coagulants alone in a retrospective analysis of 75 patients. Further studies are required for supporting their use in RPL.

Intralipids

Intralipids have immune modulatory properties and act by inhibiting NK cell activity.

Granulocyte Colony-stimulating Factor

Granulocyte colony-stimulating factor is a cytokine that stimulates neutrophilic granulocyte proliferation and differentiation and is produced by decidual cells. G-CSF administration significantly increased LBR in women with URPL compared to placebo (82.8 vs. 48.5%, $p = 0.006$) without major side effects in one trial. However, G-CSF use in clinical practice warrants evidence from larger trials.

Sperm Deoxyribonucleic Acid Fragmentation and Unexplained Recurrent Pregnancy Loss

Sperm DNA fragmentation (SDF) is commonly tested using terminal deoxynucleotidyl transferase dUTP nick end labeling (TUNEL) assay, the sperm chromatin dispersion test, and the sperm chromatin structure assay. A meta-analysis of 16 cohort studies involving 2,969 couples found a significant increase in miscarriage in patients with high SDF. Sperm DNA fragmentation testing should be offered to couples with otherwise unexplained RPL. Besides advanced paternal age, many environmental factors, such as cigarette smoking, obesity, exogenous heat, and exposure to toxins, have been associated with increased SDF. Testing for SDF could aid in bringing necessary lifestyle modifications.

Progesterone Supplementation for Unexplained Recurrent Pregnancy Loss

Progesterone supplementation has been proposed as a treatment for URPL and has proven beneficial. What makes the situation complex is the numerous preparations, routes, doses, and duration of therapy. A meta-analysis of 10 RCTs, including 1,586 women with URPL, found a significantly lower risk of RM [RR: 0.72, 95% confidence interval (CI): 0.53–0.97] and a higher chance of live birth (RR: 1.07, 95% CI: 1.02–1.15) following supplementation with progesterone. However, natural and micronized progesterone had no impact, whereas the use of synthetic progestogens made the difference. In a more recent observational cohort study, vaginal micronized progesterone started 3 days after the urinary luteinizing hormone (LH) surge resulting in improved pregnancy rates in women with URPL.

Overall, progesterone administration seems to be beneficial for women with URPL. But to answer our questions on the ideal progestogen, its dose and route of administration, further studies are required.

RECENT ADVANCES

Chronic Endometritis

Chronic endometritis has been seen in 7–58% of women with RPL. However, prevalence is largely influenced by the method of detection. Antibiotics have been found to be effective in treating endometritis with an apparent improvement in the live birth rate.[1] More studies are required to validate these evidences in clinical practice.

Endometrial Decidualization

Endometrium acts as a checkpoint for embryo quality with decidualization for normal embryos and rapid demise of endometrium with abnormal embryos. Abnormal endometrial decidualization leads to an excessively permissive endometrium to implantation of embryo and not sustenance.[2]

Chromosomal Microarray on Products of Conception

These tests offer more clarity on the etiology in 90% of cases. This not only gives answers to the questions of the couple and the treating doctor but also minimizes the cost of empirical therapy and the emotional turmoil of uncertainty.[3]

CONCLUSION

A couple with RPL needs evaluation with the right tools and management with appropriate interventions. These interventions could be as minimal as TLC and as complex as involving genetic workup with PGS or use of therapeutic agents altering immunologic mechanisms of RPL. Although more than half of these patients conceive on their own in due course of time, these interventions are required to minimize time lag and ensure successful outcomes. Over vigorous workup draining the couple financially, on a superseded emotional turmoil, triggers anxiety and apprehension. Avoidance of blanket therapy with judicious use of the available parameters and evidence-based approach is warranted. Optimization of complex clinical situations into pleasant pregnancy with definitive end points of "healthy mother and a healthy baby" become a reality for these couples sailing through troubled waters.

STRONG PRACTICE RECOMMENDATIONS IN RECURRENT PREGNANCY LOSS

- Optimal BMI: Neither obesity/underweight is recommended.
- aCGH is recommended.
- Thyroid screening and anti-thyroid peroxidase (TPO) antibody testing are recommended.
- Assessment of uterine anatomy is mandatory.

REFERENCES

1. Cicinelli E, Matteo M, Trojano G, Mitola PC, Tinelli R, Vitagliano A, et al. Chronic endometritis in patients with unexplained infertility: prevalence and effects of antibiotic treatment on spontaneous conception. Am J Reprod Immunol. 2018;79(1).
2. Lucas ES, Vrljicak P, Muter J, Diniz-da-Costa MM, Brighton PJ, Kong CS, et al. Recurrent pregnancy loss is associated with a pro-senescent decidual response during the peri-implantation window. Commun Biol. 2020;3:37.
3. Khalife D, Ghazeeri G, Kutteh W. Review of current guidelines for recurrent pregnancy loss: new strategies for optimal evaluation of women who may be superfertile. Semin Perinatol. 2019;43(2):105-15.

SECTION

12 Recent Advances

CHAPTER 78

Bioengineered Human Endometrium In Vitro

Satish Patki, Ujjwala Patki, Shweta Patki

INTRODUCTION

Since the birth of the first test tube baby in 1978, many technological advances have taken place in the field of assisted reproductive technology (ART). In spite of these advances, the implantation rate in all the ART procedures is 25–30%.[1] The problem of failure of implantation is due to the difficulties in getting the process of synchronization between the competent embryo and the receptive endometrium.[2] It is now proved that in 65% cases of the failure of implantation, the cause is the nonreceptive endometrium, while in 35% cases, the poor embryo is the cause. The research in the field of creating a good-quality embryo "in vitro" is evolving rapidly by the use of different culture media, advanced incubators, and monitoring systems such as embryo scopes and metabolomics. However, the research in the field of endometrial assessment is not progressing with a similar pace. Animal studies cannot mimic the human "in vivo" conditions. In mice, natural killer (NK) cells are not present in the nonpregnant endometrium, decidualization occurs only after implantation, and during pregnancy, there is minimal trophoblastic invasion.[3] To understand the cellular and molecular events in the human endometrium, especially during the process of implantation, the procedure of getting the endometrial tissue by biopsy itself is invasive and cannot be performed repeatedly. The procedure of endometrial biopsy cannot be performed during the conception cycle. Hence, most of the data on endometrial receptivity are based on noninvasive procedures such as assessing endometrial thickness and blood flow by vaginal sonography. However, their positive predictive value is limited.[4,5] Doing repeated endometrial biopsies in the preembryo transfer cycle and assessment of the endometrial gene expression by the procedures of endometrial receptor array (ERA) tests are expensive and also have limitations.

Thus, there is a need for a process to develop a bioengineered human endometrium in a Petri dish for the following reasons:

- Such bioengineered endometrium will be at hand any time and can obviously avoid the traumatic procedures of repeated endometrial biopsies, especially to study the sequential changes in the endometrium during the window of implantation (WOI).
- It will avoid animal model studies, which are scientifically never matching the human physiological processes.
- Such bioengineered endometrium will be useful to study the effects of hormones or drugs at a cellular level.
- It will be easier to study the morphological and molecular status of the bioengineered endometrium available in Petri dish.
- The bioengineered endometrium will be helpful as a model for implantation research.
- Finally, the embryos cultured on this autologous bioengineered endometrium will be sensitized for the process of implantation, before they are actually transferred to the uterus. This will definitely increase the implantation rates of the procedures of ART following their transfer.

INDICATIONS OF THE CULTURE OF ENDOMETRIUM

The indications for endometrium culture are as follows:

- As a research tool for the evaluation of the process of implantation
- It is more useful in the management of the patients with previous implantation failure with a high index of suspicion of inadequate endometrial receptivity.

Tissue Culture Protocol for the Development of Bioengineered Endometrium in Culture Dish

The entire procedure has to be performed in a class 10,000 tissue culture laboratory, well equipped with air management by air handling unit (AHU). The cells handling should be performed in a laminar flow with class 100 atmosphere. All the disposable ware should be made up of tissue culture grade polypropylene of BD Falcon make, and the culture media used should be from Sigma-Aldrich. The patients undergoing in vitro fertilization (IVF) procedures are posted for diagnostic hysteroscopy and endometrial scratch during the cycle prior to IVF cycle in the proliferative phase. After the hysteroscopy, the endometrial samples are obtained by sharp curettage. Even in a situation where hysteroscopy is not planned, blind endometrial biopsy from the uterine fundus is adequate. The endometrial bits should be placed in a beaker containing phosphate buffered saline (PBS).

CONTRAINDICATIONS

The procedure is contraindicated in patients with genital tuberculosis, Asherman's syndrome, where the amount of endometrium obtained for culture is usually inadequate. Similarly, patients with pelvic inflammatory disease and large hydrosalpinges are also not good candidates as their endometrium may be contaminated and hence difficult to culture.

THREE-DIMENSIONAL CULTURE SYSTEM

Human endometrium is a layered tissue with basically three components **(Fig. 1)**:

1. The surface epithelium which invaginates down to form the glands.
2. The stroma underneath the epithelium actually keeps the glands intact and supports the vessels.
3. The coiled vessels running in the stroma between the glands.

It is relatively easy to culture the stromal cells in vitro but to culture and propagate the epithelium, glands, and vessels are extremely difficult and need a three-dimensional (3D) culture system. Scientists have made attempts to culture both glandular epithelial and stromal cells in the canine endometrial model[6] and rabbit endometrial model.[7]

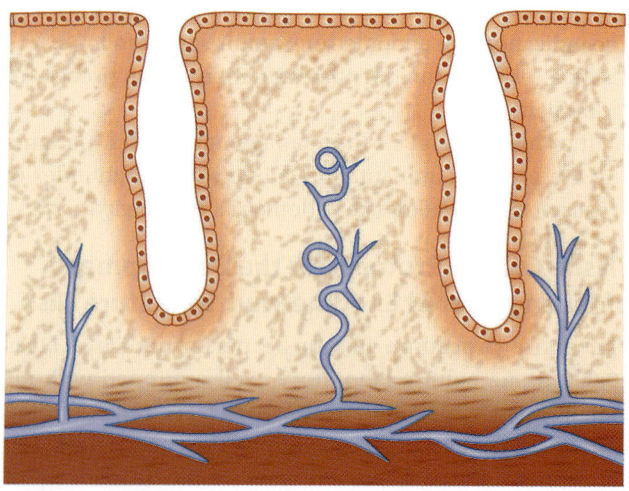

Fig. 1: Histology of human endometrium.

The culture model of human endometrium and cell sheet engineering has been tried.[8,9]

Preparation of Three-dimensional Culture System

Matrigel (BD) is used as an extracellular matrix platform to culture all three components of the human endometrium. A total of 300 μL of red Matrigel is added to each well of four-well dishes, and the dish is kept in the carbon dioxide incubator for 30 minutes to solidify the gel. Such 3D culture system has the following advantages:

- It is helpful for detailed morphological studies of all three components of endometrium under phase contrast and scanning electron microscopy.
- It helps for gene and protein expression studies at each cellular component.
- It helps for the differentiation of each component with suitable sequential hormonal stimulation of estradiol followed by progesterone.
- It is easy to study the response of each endometrial component to the type of stimulus.

Preparation of the Component Cells for Seeding and Subsequent Culture

The endometrial bits are initially washed several times with PBS to remove the red blood cells. These bits are taken in a Petri dish and are minced with number 20 surgical blade and forceps. The endometrial glands can be isolated by mechanical dissection under a stereo zoom microscope **(Figs. 2A and B)**. The fine paste of the tissue is made which is then transformed into a 10 mL conical tube. 0.5 mL trypsin is added to the cell paste for 3 minutes, and vigorous mixing of cells in the enzyme is done at room temperature. To prevent the overaction of trypsin and to avoid overdigestion of the stromal cells, 1 mL of filtered human serum (patient's own) is added after 3 minutes. The human serum neutralizes the action of trypsin. The tube is then centrifuged at 2,000 RPM for 20 minutes to wash the trypsin and get the cell pellet. After centrifugation, the supernatant is removed, and 5 mL of mixture of Dulbecco's Modified Eagles Medium (DMEM) and Ham F-12 is added to the cell pellet. This cell pellet is seeded on Matrigel floor prepared in a four-well dish **(Fig. 3)**.

The dish is kept in a carbon dioxide incubator at 37°C at 5% CO_2 atmosphere. The medium is replenished every 48 hours. The stromal cells predominate in the culture plate because they form the 85% component of endometrium and look like circular, spherical cells at 0 hour **(Fig. 4)** while epithelial cells look like smaller and brighter circular cells at 0 hour **(Fig. 5)**. After 48 hours, the stromal cells start attaching the floor of the dish and look like fibroblast **(Fig. 6)** while the epithelial cells show cobblestone appearance and glandular differentiation **(Fig. 7)**.

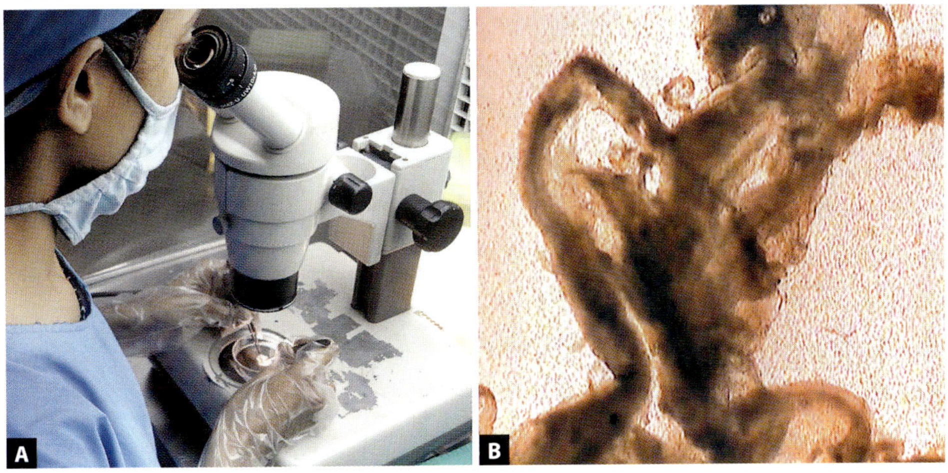

Figs. 2A and B: Endometrial glands isolation under stereo microscope.

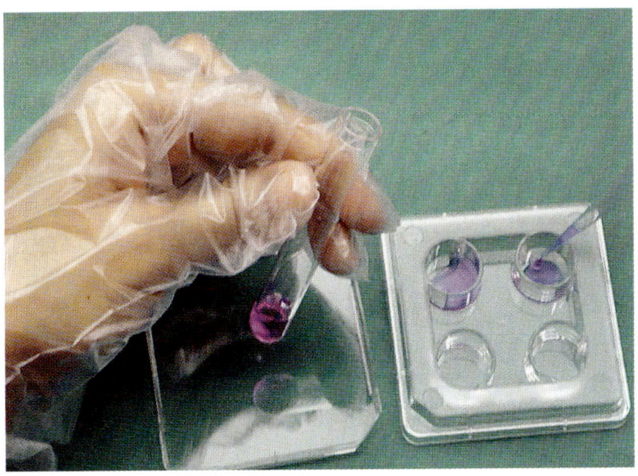

Fig. 3: Seeding of the cell pellet.

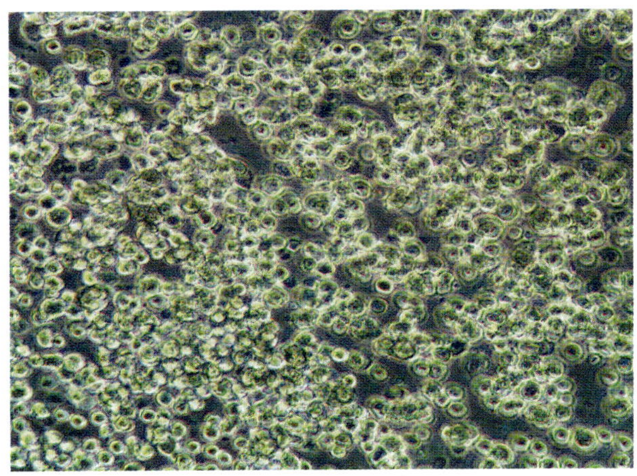

Fig. 5: Epithelial cells at 0 hour.

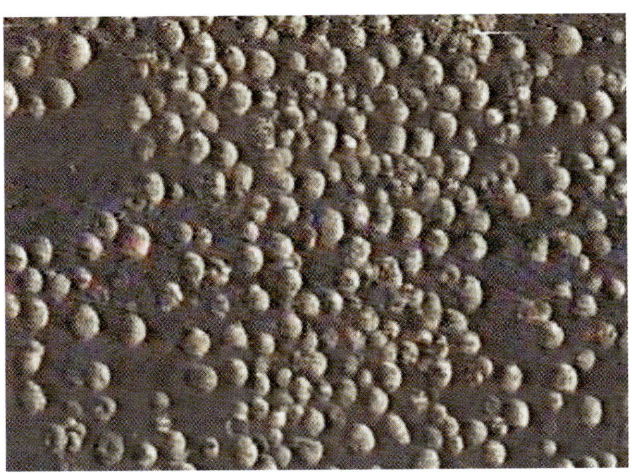

Fig. 4: Stromal cells at 0 hour.

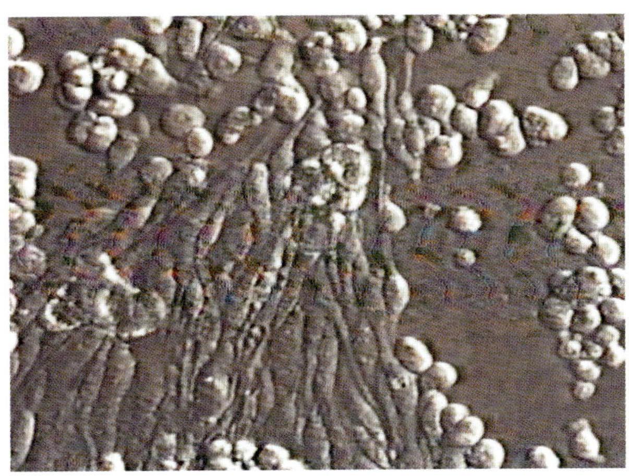

Fig. 6: Stromal cells after 48 hours.

Stimulation of the Bioengineered Endometrium with Sequential Hormonal Therapy

About 48–72 hours after the primary 3D culture of all the three endometrial components, the culture medium is supplemented with 17β-estradiol dissolved in DMEM. The epithelium, glands, and the stromal cells start rapidly proliferating under the stimulation of estradiol. The change of medium is done every 48 hours, and the supernatant containing floating dead cells is removed. Usually, by the

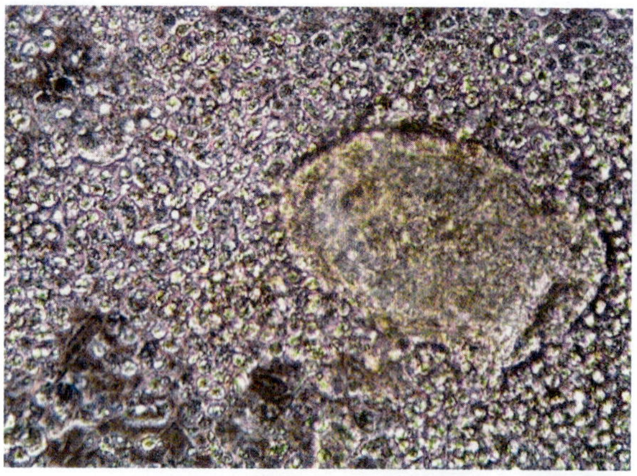

Fig. 7: Epithelial cells after 48 hours.

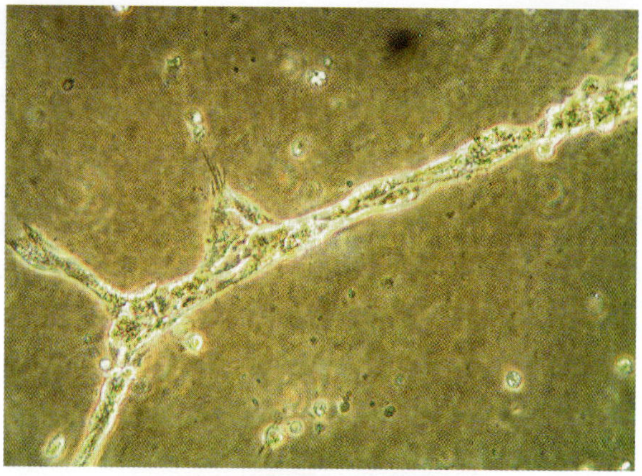

Fig. 9: Vessel formation.

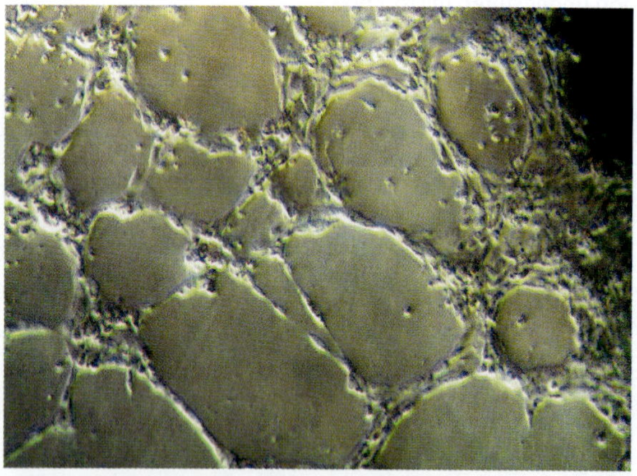

Fig. 8: Ring formation test—angiogenesis.

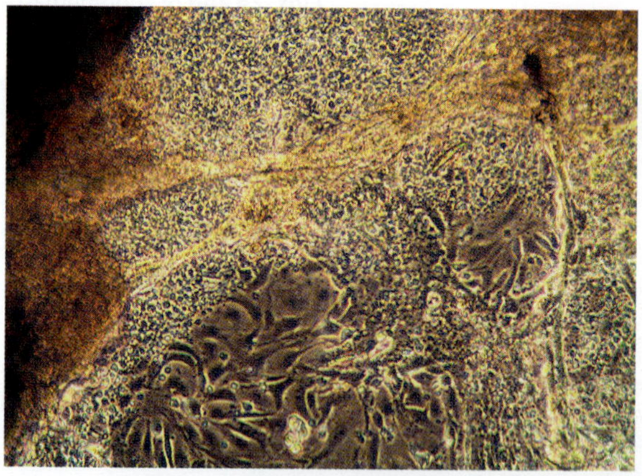

Fig. 10: Fully developed endometrium.

fourth or fifth day of estradiol supplementation, each well is fully confluent with the layered endometrium. In order to induce the process of angiogenesis, vascular endothelial growth factor (VEGF) is added to the medium in a very small quantity. Usually within 24 hours, the new vessels are seen developing from epithelial and endothelial cells which form ring-like structures **(Figs. 8 and 9)**. The aqueous progesterone is then additionally supplemented to the culture medium from day 5 of culture. This will bring about the early secretory stage.

COMPLICATIONS

As such, the procedure of culture does not have any complications. However, sometimes the contamination in the culture system can prevent cell proliferation, and on some occasions, may spoil the entire culture with the resultant degeneration of all the cells.

STUDY OF WINDOW OF IMPLANTATION ON BIOENGINEERED ENDOMETRIUM

The endometrium which is normally nonreceptive for the embryo becomes receptive for a very small period of 3–4 days, after the appearance of progesterone on the endometrium, which is adequately primed with estradiol.[10] During this period, all three components of the endometrium support the process of implantation of blastocyst through mediation by immune cells, cytokines, growth factors, and adhesion molecules.[11-13]

The bioengineered endometrium demonstrates all the sequential morphological changes during WOI. The epithelial proliferation, glandular enlargement with early secretions, stromal proliferation, and angiogenesis are the endometrial changes during WOI. All changes can be very well appreciated through a phase-contrast microscope in the bioengineered endometrium in the culture dish **(Fig. 10)**.

The most notable change in the epithelium is the appearance of "pinopode" which is believed to be involved in embryo opposition and attachment.[14,15] The pinopodes cover not only the entire surface but also cover and go deep down in the lumen of the glands also. When the culture dish of bioengineered endometrium is subjected to the scanning electron microscopy, the pinopodes can be clearly identified on the surface as well as inside the glands **(Figs. 11 and 12)**. Pinopodes are considered as a marker of endometrial receptivity.[16] The newly formed vessels can also be clearly seen under an electron microscope with their endothelial lining **(Fig. 13)**.

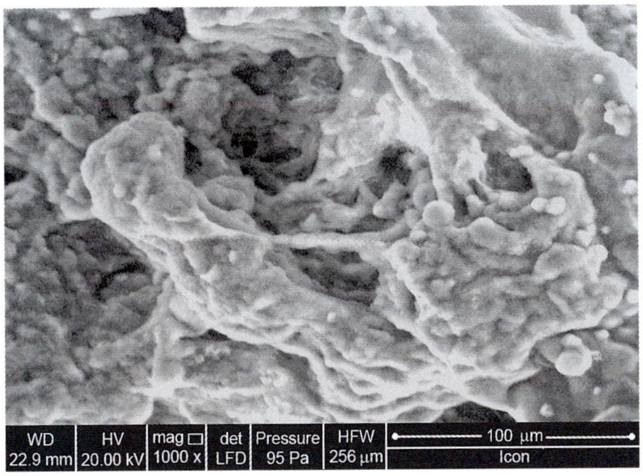

Fig. 11: Pinopodes on surface of endometrium.

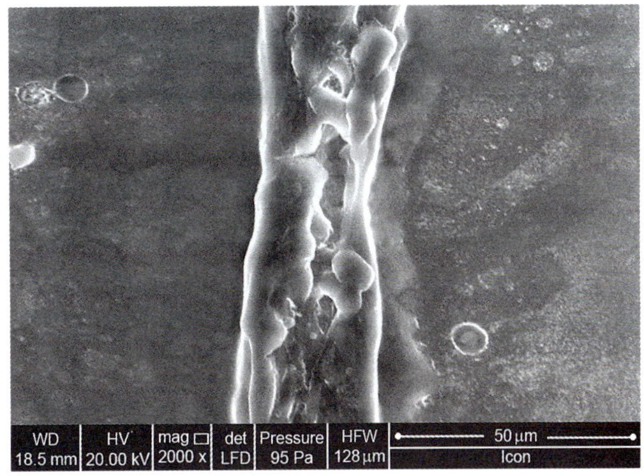

Fig. 13: New vessel observed under scanning electron microscope.

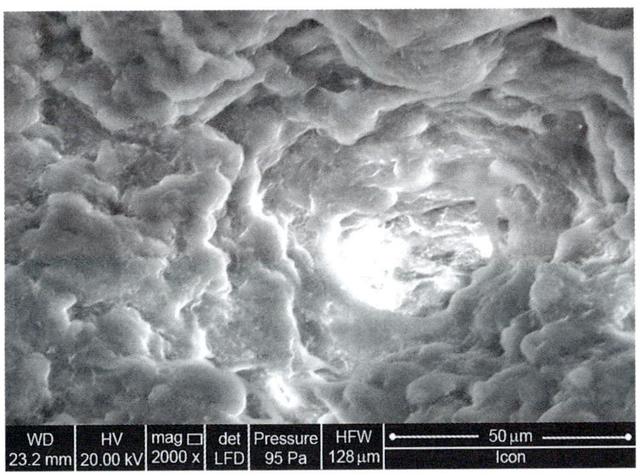

Fig. 12: Pinopodes over the glands.

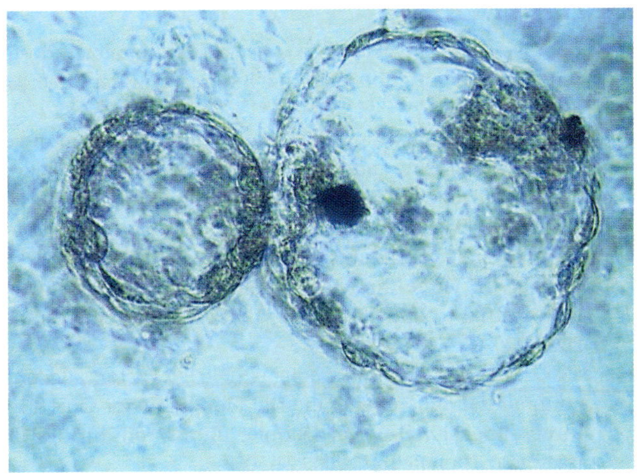

Fig. 14: In vitro hatching blastocyst on bioengineered endometrium.

Some of the genes in the endometrium are upregulated while some are downregulated making a "gene signature" during WOI.[13] Such molecular studies can be done on the cells obtained from the bioengineered endometrium.

"In vitro" Sensitization of Embryo Prior to Embryo Transfer

The embryo resulting from the procedures of ART can be cultured on such bioengineered endometrium. It is better to culture the embryo of a stage of morula as it mimics in vivo process. It is not physiological to coculture the 8-16-cell-stage embryo. Interestingly, sometimes even hatching of the blastocyst can be observed in the culture dish **(Fig. 14)**. Such sensitized embryos can then be transferred to the uterus which will have a high chance of implantation. Future research in this field can further throw light on these events.

Thus, the bioengineered endometrium is in fact a "mini uterus" in Petri dish, which can be used to study the morphological as well as molecular studies beneficial for the research not only in the field of reproduction but also in the fields of various endometrial pathologies such as hyperplasia or malignancies.

LIMITATIONS OF THE PRESENT STUDY AND FUTURE RESEARCH

The present research is the morphological evaluation of the bioengineered endometrium in culture dish, using phase contrast and scanning electron microscopy. The future research should be the molecular evaluation of the bioengineered endometrium by doing gene studies of the cultured cells. The marker studies throwing light on the various endometrial components will further widen the horizon of the research.

CONCLUSION

Bio engineered Endometrium gives opportunity to study the various components of endometrium, specially during the window of implantation. Histological, electron microscopy and molecular studies can be performed without repeated invasive procedures of endometrial biopsy. It can be tried to sensitize the blastocysts before embryo transfer.

KEY POINTS

- Culture of the endometrial components, i.e., epithelium glands, stroma, and vessels, is possible with 3D culture techniques.
- Such bioengineered endometrium can be used as a research tool for the study of the implantation process.
- Sequential stimulation of such bioengineered endometrium with estradiol and progesterone can mimic the events which occur "in vivo" during WOI.
- The embryos can be cocultured on such bioengineered endometrium for better development "in vitro" followed by high chances of implantation after transfer.

REFERENCES

1. Boomsma CM, Macklon NS. What can the clinician do to improve implantation? Reprod Biomed Online. 2006;13: 845-55.
2. Nardo LG, Li TC, Edwards RG. Introduction: human embryo implantation failure and recurrent miscarriages: basic science and clinical practice. Reprod Biomed Online. 2006;13(1):11-2.
3. Carson DD, Bagchi I, Dey SK, Enders AC, Fazleabas AT, Lessey BA, et al. Embryo implantation. Dev Biol. 2000;223:217-37.
4. Alcázar JL. Three-dimensional ultrasound assessment of endometrial receptivity: a review. Reprod Biol Endocrinol. 2006;4:56.
5. Ng EH, Chan CC, Tang OS, Yeung WS, Ho PC. Factors affecting endometrial and subendometrial blood flow measured by three-dimensional power Doppler ultrasound during IVF treatment. Hum Reprod. 2006;21:1062-9.
6. Bartel C, Tichy A, Schoenkypl S, Aurich C, Walter I. Effects of steroid hormones on differentiated glandular epithelial and stromal cells in a three dimensional cell culture model of the canine endometrium. BMC Vet Res. 2013;9:86.
7. Wang HB, Lü SH, Lin QX, Feng LX, Li DX, Duan CM, et al. Reconstruction of endometrium in vitro via rabbit uterine endometrial cells expanded by sex steroid. Fertil Steril. 2010; 93(7):2385-95.
8. Bläuer M, Heinonen PK, Martikainen PM, Tomás E, Ylikomi T. A novel organotypic culture model for normal human endometrium: regulation of epithelial cell proliferation by estradiol and medroxyprogesterone acetate. Hum Reprod. 2005;20:864-71.
9. Takagi S, Shimizu T, Kuramoto G, Ishitani K, Matsui H, Yamato M, et al. Reconstruction of functional endometrium-like tissue in vitro and in vivo using cell sheet engineering. Biochem Biophys Res Commun. 2014;446(1):335-40.
10. Navot D, Scott RT, Droesch K, Veeck LL, Liu HC, Rosenwaks Z. The window of embryo transfer and the efficiency of human conception in vitro. Fertil Steril. 1991;55(1):114-8.
11. Kämmerer U, von Wolff M, Markert UR. Immunology of human endometrium. Immunobiology. 2004;209:569-74.
12. Giudice LC. Implantation and endometrial function. In: Fauser BC (Ed). Reproductive Medicine: Molecular, Cellular and Genetic Fundamentals. New York: Parthenon Publishing; 2002. pp. 439-65.
13. Dimitriadis E, White CA, Jones RL, Salamonsen LA. Cytokines, chemokines and growth factors in endometrium related to implantation. Hum Reprod Update. 2005;11:613-30.
14. Anderson TL, Olson GE, Hoffman LH. Stage-specific alterations in the apical membrane glycoproteins of endometrial epithelial cells related to implantation in rabbits. Biol Reprod. 1986;34:701-20.
15. Bentin-Ley U. Relevance of endometrial pinopodes for human blastocyst implantation. Hum Reprod. 2000;15:67-73.
16. Qiong Z, Jie H, Yonggang W, Bin X, Jing Z, Yanping L. Clinical validation of pinopode as a marker of endometrial receptivity: a randomized controlled trial. Fertil Steril. 2017;108(3):513-7.e2.

CHAPTER 79

Recent Trends in Assisted Reproductive Technique

Arya Rajendran, Baiju Pookilath

INTRODUCTION

Ever since the birth of Louise Brown in 1978, with every passing decade, there have been spectacular advances in assisted reproductive technique (ART) that have revolutionized and revamped its practice. The introduction of transvaginal scans, transvaginal oocyte retrieval, intracytoplasmic sperm injection (ICSI), preimplantation genetic screening (PGS)/ preimplantation genetic diagnosis (PGD), and time-lapse imaging are to name a few.

The current worldwide trends causing a paradigm shift include **(Flowchart 1)**:

- ART during COVID-19 pandemic
- ART and COVID-19 vaccination
- Routine blastocyst transfer instead of cleavage stage embryo transfer
- Replacement of fresh embryo transfer with embryo cryopreservation and subsequent transfer in a frozen-thawed cycle
- PGS for all
- Single embryo transfer
- Stimulation protocols—minimal stimulation protocols and progestin-primed ovarian stimulation (PPOS).

Flowchart 1: Approach to recent trends in assisted reproductive technique (ART).

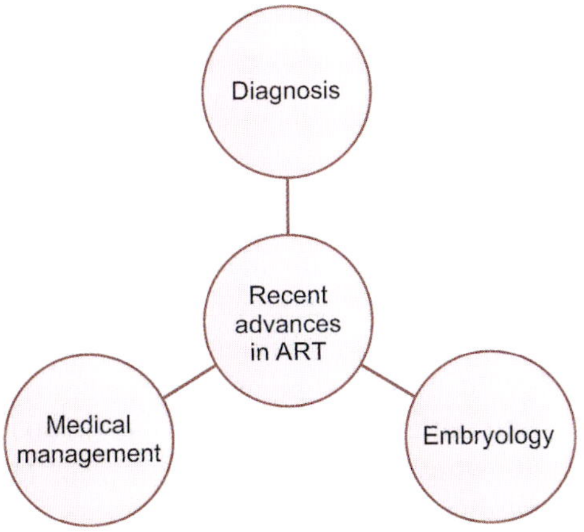

ASSISTED REPRODUCTIVE TECHNIQUE DURING COVID-19 PANDEMIC

Advent of novel severe acute respiratory syndrome coronavirus 2 (SARS-CoV-2) (COVID-19) as a global pandemic has changed the way humans live worldwide due to the widespread devastation caused due to death, morbidity, and economic collapse. With the first wave of COVID-19, European Society of Human Reproduction and Embryology (ESHRE) and American Society for Reproductive Medicine (ASRM) issued advice to stop all ART procedures as the risks outweighed the benefit of continuing treatment. With the pandemic well into the second year of rampage, the world has learned to adapt to the new normal and restart routine activities.

Indian Council of Medical Research (ICMR) has brought forth the following steps to be part of restarting ART clinical practice:

- *Patient information and counseling:*
  - Research on impact of COVID-19 on ART and pregnancy is still evolving.
  - Evidence so far does not indicate increased risk of congenital malformations or adverse pregnancy outcomes in association with COVID-19 disease.
  - All patients need to be educated regarding the methods of spread of COVID-19, importance of social distancing, and use of personal protection equipment—masks and hand sanitization.
  - Patients should be educated that treatment will be discontinued in case they get infected with COVID-19.
- *Consent to start treatment:*
  - Patients should be counseled regarding the risks and benefits involved in starting ART treatment during the pandemic. This decision should be individualized considering the age and severity of underlying conditions of the couple. They should be given the choice whether to start or postpone treatment to a future date; however, the virus is

likely to remain in transmission in the community for an extended period of time. After thorough discussion, the patient's choice to start treatment should be documented using the consent form given below.
- Patients with high-risk health conditions such as diabetes, cardiovascular illness, and respiratory conditions should have their present status evaluated by a specialist and fitness should be issued prior to start of ART.

- *Patient and ART clinic staff risk assessment triage:*
  - *Recommendations for patients, donors, and surrogates:*
    - ICMR risk assessment triage questionnaire must be self-answered by the patient before each visit to the clinic.
    - Following triage, patients suspected to be infected should undergo reverse transcription-polymerase chain reaction (RT-PCR) testing for COVID-19.
    - Those who have recovered from COVID-19 should be assessed by a physician and fitness to start ART should be obtained.
    - Patient and partner, all potential oocyte/sperm donors, and gestational surrogates must undergo COVID-19 RT-PCR test prior to start of treatment. Once ovarian stimulation is started, they are advised to self-isolate themselves until oocyte retrieval to prevent getting infected during the course of ovarian stimulation.
    - RT-PCR testing must be repeated on the day of human chorionic gonadotropin (hCG)-trigger and if found positive at any point during the ovarian stimulation, cycle must be canceled.
  - *Recommendations for staff working at ART clinics:*
    - ICMR risk assessment triage questionnaire must be self-answered every day.
    - Staff suspected of infection during triage must get RT-PCR testing done and self-quarantine if positive. Further, contact tracing and testing must be performed.
    - Staff should be divided into mini-teams with minimal interaction between different teams and work, so that if one gets infected, the spread can be contained.
    - Work at home must be encouraged whenever possible.
    - Reduce physical contact with patients with physical barriers and use personal protection equipment.
    - Organize virtual meetings instead of conventional ones.
- *Modification of ART clinic layout and services:*
  - Physical modifications should be brought about at the ART clinics to enable social distancing—such as separation of furniture and putting up physical barriers.
  - Thermal scanning at entrance to ART clinic
  - Scheduling outpatient (OP) visits to prevent overcrowding at the center.
  - Restrictions on number of bystanders attending the clinic along with the couple undergoing treatment, so as to prevent overcrowding.
  - Use of Arogya Setu application must be made mandatory for all staff and patients attending the clinic.
  - Friendly relationship must be maintained with a nearby ART clinic, so that in the event of breakout of COVID-19 infection at the clinic, patients can be diverted for emergency care.
- *Planning treatment specific to individual:*
  - *OP visits:*
    - Each patient's treatment plan must be individualized and properly planned so as to reduce number of visits to the center to minimum and judiciously reduce number of scan visits/blood tests.
    - Encourage home collection of semen samples with proper instructions to carry out the same.
    - Use of telemedicine to reduce the number of outpatient department (OPD) visits.
  - *OP and ART procedures:*
    - Questionnaire-based triage is adequate for attending OP, scan visits, blood tests, semen analysis, sonosalpingography (SSG), and hysterosalpingography (HSG).
    - RT-PCR testing must be undergone prior to office hysteroscopy (under paracervical block or regional analgesia).
    - Laparoscopy procedures must be categorized into emergent and elective, and planned accordingly. RT-PCR testing is mandatory prior to the procedure.
    - General anesthesia should be avoided due to risk of aerosol exposure to anesthesiologist. Regional analgesia is preferred.
    - Bipolar energy source must be preferred in comparison to ultrasonic instruments during laparoscopy to reduce transmission of virus through fumes.
  - *Embryology laboratory:*
    - Separate instruments (keyboards, pens, microscope eyepiece) should be used, as far as possible, to prevent transmission among embryologists.
    - Separate cryo-containers and closed system of vitrification must be used for embryos obtained from patients who are detected COVID-positive following oocyte retrieval and prior to embryo freezing.

- Careful disposal of follicular fluid and semen as evidence is incomplete as to whether transmission of virus is possible via these body fluids.
- *Mental health of healthcare workers and patients:*
    - Patients and health workers are at increased risk of anxiety related to treatment delays, risk of exposure to disease at the clinic, unanticipated interruptions in treatment due to infection or lockdown, etc.
    - Adequate counseling of patients regarding treatment steps and infection-preventing strategies at the ART clinic can help in mitigating undue stress to patients.
    - Prompt referral to psychological counseling sessions[1] (which can be accessed via telemedicine as well).

ASSISTED REPRODUCTIVE TECHNIQUE AND COVID-19 VACCINATION

Different types of vaccines [inactivated, messenger ribonucleic acid (mRNA), and protein subunit] are available presently in the armamentarium against COVID-19 infection during this pandemic. Information regarding the safety of vaccination against COVID-19 during pregnancy and preconceptional period is still in the emerging phase. Presently, vaccination is approved during preconceptional period, pregnancy, and lactation.

Who all should get vaccinated?

- All pregnant women are advised to get vaccinated, irrespective of the period of gestation as severity of COVID-19 disease is found to be higher during pregnancy.
- In preconceptional period, vaccination should be offered to patients at high risk of exposure to the disease (e.g., healthcare workers) or who have high-risk health conditions (diabetes, respiratory, or cardiovascular illnesses).
- Patients should not be refused ART services due to their unvaccinated status.
- *How long should couples wait to start ART treatment following vaccination?*
- ESHRE recommends completion of vaccination prior to start of ART procedures and to wait at least for a few days after vaccination, before starting ART procedures in order to provide time for immune reaction to settle down.
- In the event of allergic reaction to vaccination, ART procedures should not commence until the reaction settles down completely and physician has assessed the candidate as fit to resume treatment.
- ESHRE recommends monitoring of ART outcome in vaccinated and nonvaccinated patients to further the research on impact of vaccination on ART outcome, if any.
- Presently, there is no recommendation on the choice of which vaccine to be taken during preconceptional period.[2]

NEWER DIAGNOSTIC MODALITIES IN ASSISTED REPRODUCTIVE TECHNIQUE

Recent Trends in Ultrasonography in Reproductive Medicine

Doppler and 3D

These are the epochal recent advances in ultrasonography (USG) in reproductive medicine. Doppler studies allow evaluation of direction and magnitude of blood flow. Three-dimensional (3D) USG can provide multiplanar images, volume rendering, and surface rendering. Apart from USG, 3D dynamic magnetic resonance hysterosalpingography (dMR-HSG) and multislice computed tomography (CT) HSG are advances in tubal patency evaluation with more clarity on myometrium as well.[3,4]

Uterus

- *Endometrial blood flow:* Uterine artery resistance index (RI), pulsatility index (PI), and subendometrial RI and PI measurements as well as Applebaum's classification of endometrial blood flow have become common practice now for endometrial tracking prior to embryo transfer.
- *Myomas:* 3D USG has been seen to have diagnostic sensitivity as high as that of hysteroscopy in identifying submucosal and myometrial components of myomas, information that is critical for deciding between hysteroscopic and laparoscopic route of excision. Magnetic resonance-guided ultrasound energy has been used for thermoablation of myomas with two instances of pregnancies being achieved post-treatment.[5,6]
- *Adenomyosis:* On USG, adenomyosis appears as asymmetrical thickening of uterine walls or poorly defined heterogenous areas.
- *Müllerian anomalies:* 3D USG is a diagnostic modality of choice in detecting Müllerian anomalies.

Ovaries

- *Antral follicle count (AFC):* Sonography-based automated volume count (SonoAVC) is a volumetric analysis of follicles in ovary and is useful for careful estimation of AFC, especially in a polycystic ovarian morphology (PCOM) ovary. Receiver operating curve (ROC) analysis in a meta-analysis has shown superiority of AFC in prediction of in vitro fertilization (IVF) cycle outcome over serum follicle-stimulating hormone (FSH).[7]
- *Stromal ovarian blood flow* has lower impedance in PCOM ovaries, reflecting with lower RI and PI. These are

responsible for greater delivery of gonadotropins to such ovaries during stimulation.

- *3D evaluation of cysts* can give better delineation of cyst characteristics, especially with regard to septations, contents, etc., and to differentiate benign from malignant features.
- Measurement of *ovarian perifollicular blood flow* characteristics can be used to follow-up follicles during stimulation.

Fallopian Tubes

Three-dimensional USG is highly useful in assessment of hydrosalpinges that present as retort-shaped hypoechoic area between uterus and ovaries. Assessment of tubes to rule out hydrosalpinges is essential in pre-IVF workup since patients with hydrosalpinges have up to 50% lower implantation and pregnancy rates.

Self-operated Endovaginal Telemonitoring (SONAURA) System

This system consists of a vaginal probe connected by a USB (universal serial bus) to a small tablet. A specific website application to which the recorded data are immediately uploaded allows the operator to perform follicular and endometrial two-dimensional (2D) measurements using the video recorded by the patient. Self-operated endovaginal telemonitoring (SOET) increases patient and partner participation, decreases stress, and saves time and cost. The minor variations in folliculometry have not shown to alter treatment decisions.[8]

Smartphone USG

The transducer probe can be attached by USB cable to smartphone. After downloading the application for the scan settings, this combination of devices can be used as a portable scanning machine. Philips and MobiUS SP1 are popular brands of smartphone USG probes.

Fertiloscopy

Fertiloscopy is the performance of laparoscopy through the vagina using saline solution instead of CO_2 as working medium. It holds potential use in the evaluation of unexplained infertility as an alternative to diagnostic laparoscopy **(Fig. 1)**.

Advantages of Fertiloscopy over Laparoscopy

- Safer since neither Trendelenburg position nor CO_2 insufflation is needed.
- Evaluation of genital tract in its anatomical position
- Minimally invasive.

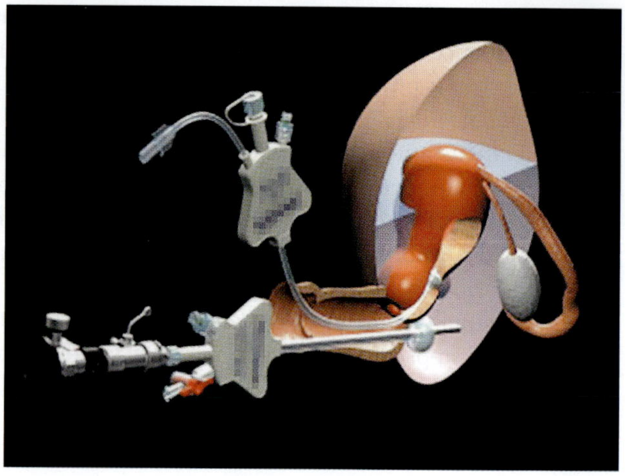

Fig. 1: Fertiloscopy.

Technique

- Careful vaginal examination is the first step to rule out contraindications for fertiloscopy such as fixed retroverted uterus [where there will be no space for penetration into pouch of Douglas (POD)] and nodules in rectovaginal septum (indicative of posterior endometriosis with close proximity to rectum and possible adherence to rectal wall).
- *Anesthesia:* (1) Local anesthesia with anesthetic swab for 10 minutes followed by a paracervical block with lignocaine; (2) Short general anesthesia is an alternative as in ovum pickup.
- *Hydropelviscopy:* Veress needle is introduced into POD 1 cm below cervix. 100–200 mL of saline should be introduced followed by removal of Veress and introduction of fertiloscope. Optic will be introduced through the scope (preferably 30° scope). Careful examination of genital structures will be carried out.
- *Hysteroscopy* is performed in collaboration to rule out intrauterine disease.

Fertiloscopy versus Laparoscopy

Fertiloscopy versus Laparoscopy (FLY) study was a multicenter randomized prospective study in which fertiloscopy and laparoscopy were performed in same patient by two surgeons randomized for the procedure. The video recording of the procedures was reviewed by two independent reviewers. Sensitivity, specificity, and concordance of both studies were evaluated. FLY study concluded that fertiloscopy should replace laparoscopy in infertile women with no obvious pathology.[9]

Endometrial Receptivity Array

Implantation of embryo requires a complex cross-talk between embryo and endometrium, which involves over

236 genes expression. The transcriptomic signature of the window of receptivity or window of implantation (WOI) of the endometrium can be identified by advances in microarray technology. Endometrial receptivity array (ERA) is a molecular diagnostic tool developed on this premise. Among women with recurrent implantation failure (RIF), use of ERA has shown that WOI is displaced in at least a quarter of them. Detecting the WOI in a woman and performing embryo transfer on a specific day is called "personalized embryo transfer (PET)" and has improved pregnancy rates making women with RIF achieve ongoing pregnancy rates at par with women without RIF (52%).[10]

How to Perform Endometrial Receptivity Array?

Endometrial receptivity array has been developed and patented by Igenomix. Endometrial biopsy is performed on luteinizing hormone (LH)+7 days (natural cycle) or on P+5 days [in hormone replacement treatment (HRT) cycle]. After obtaining a sample of endometrial tissue using a Pipelle brush, it is transferred to the vial of fixative provided with ERA kit. The sample should occupy one third of the vial. The sample is shaken well for approximately 40 seconds and then stored at 4°C for 4 hours for the cryofixation to happen. The fixed sample is then sent to the designated laboratory. The ERA test is performed with next-generation sequencing (NGS) technology. The ERA test has proven highly sensitive and accurate in detecting gene expression profiles associated with receptivity. If the report of ERA comes as "receptive", the embryo transfer should be planned on the same day of menstrual cycle as when ERA was performed. If it comes as "nonreceptive", then ERA test must be repeated on a subsequent cycle according to the predicted date given by the first test. Once the second test confirms receptive status, embryo transfer must be performed on the revised day of cycle.

Mahajan reported that 27.5% of women with RIF showed a displaced WOI. Pregnancy rates, ongoing pregnancy rates, and implantation rates improved after PET in the RIF group and became similar to non-RIF IVF cycles. Similar improvement was seen in above results for the subgroup of women with persistently thin endometrium as well.[11]

A recent prospective study assessed patients by ERA test at their first presentation for fertility treatment. They were excluded if they had RIF, recurrent pregnancy loss, stage 3–4 endometriosis, and abnormal uterine cavity or fibroids. After completion of the study, patients returned to routine clinical care as deemed appropriate by their provider. Infertility treatments and pregnancy outcomes were assessed 2 years after ERA testing. Patients who had a nonreceptive ERA were compared to those who had a receptive ERA on initial testing. The study concluded that nonreceptive ERA group had similar live birth rates as the receptive ERA group; however, majority of nonreceptive group women conceived in ovulatory cycles whereas majority of receptive group women conceived in embryo transfer cycles. Hence, a nonreceptive ERA in an HRT cycle does not seem to have prognostic value in naturally ovulating women.[12]

DNA Fragmentation Index

Sperm DNA fragmentation index (DFI) denotes the degree of damage to the genetic integrity of sperm DNA. Higher DFI rates are associated with subfertility and IVF failure. A routine semen analysis comments only on sperm concentration, motility, and morphology. Specialized tests are required to assess sperm DNA fragmentation.

Sperm Chromatin Structure Assay

Sperm chromatin structure assay (SCSA) test has been tried and tested over many years. It is technically less challenging than other tests and can be performed in minutes. It is a fluorescence cell sorter test and measures susceptibility of sperm DNA to damage after exposure to acid or heat. It measures single-stranded fragments and has high sensitivity. It simultaneously detects both DFI and the presence of immature sperm nuclei with abnormal proteins and altered protamine/histone ratios.

It has only two steps: (1) Treat the raw semen dilution with pH 1.2 buffer for 30 seconds; and (2) stain the spermatozoa with acridine orange, a dye that reveals broken DNA strands as red fluorescence and unbroken DNA strands as green fluorescence.[13]

A DFI of 30% is a widely accepted clinical threshold for significant DNA damage.

TUNEL Assay

It detects free ends of DNA by adding fluorescent stained nucleotides [labeling of the 3′-ends of single- and double-strand breaks with biotinylated deoxyuridine triphosphate (dUTP)], enabling single- and double-stranded DNA damage, either by fluorescent microscopy or by flow cytometry. The test has been further modified by adding a viability stain, thereby measuring the damage level in live sperms alone.

Sperm Chromatin Dispersion Test (Halo Test)

Halo test is "kit" form, convenient for testing for DNA without DNA damage, contrary to other tests that look for damaged sperms. It estimates the level of DNA fragmentation indirectly by quantification of the amount of nuclear dispersion or halo after sperm lysis and acid denaturation to remove excess nuclear proteins.

Comet Test

Comet test quantifies the amount of DNA damage per sperm by means of a single-cell gel electrophoretic assay. Applicable to both single- and double-stranded damage detection.

Within an agarose gel, the sperm membranes are lysed and the DNA is decondensed in a high-concentration salt solution. Disulfide bridges are broken down and then the spermatozoon is placed in an electrophoretic field where strands of charged broken DNA stream towards the cathode. As the mass of DNA fragments stream out from the "head" of unbroken DNA they resemble a "comet tail," hence the name of the assay.[14]

Higher DFI has been associated with poorer IVF outcomes (impaired fertilization and disrupted preimplantation embryo development[5]) and higher miscarriage rates[15,16] as well as birth defects in offsprings and even childhood cancers. The major limitation of testing for sperm DNA damage is that the assay renders the tested sperm unsuitable for clinical purpose. Intracytoplasmic morphologically selected sperm injection (IMSI) and hyaluronic acid selection of sperm for ICSI [physiological ICSI (PICSI)] are noninvasive methods for testing sperm DNA integrity that enable the use of normal sperms for ART.

Follicle-stimulating Hormone Receptor Polymorphism

Follicle-stimulating Hormone Receptor

The FSH and the LH are glycoprotein hormones secreted from anterior pituitary. They are heterodimers with alpha subunit being common to FSH, LH, hCG, and thyroid-stimulating hormone. Beta subunit is specific for each hormone with receptor binding specificity. FSH receptors are G protein-coupled receptors present on the plasma membrane of granulosa cells and Sertoli cells. FSH receptor gene is 192 kb in size and has 10 exons and 9 introns. Among the 10 exons, the first 9 code for N-terminal of extracellular domain of FSH receptor. The 10th exon is large and codes for C-terminal of extracellular domain, transmembrane domain as well as intracellular domain of FSH receptor.[17] The transmembrane domain has seven alpha helices and inner domain is coupled to G protein that initiates the series of events that culminate in the biological function of the receptor. FSH gene and receptor gene activity are absolutely essential for female fertility whereas in males, some degree of spermatogenesis is possible even with abnormal FSH genes.[18]

The FSH receptor gene is highly polymorphic. Single nucleotide polymorphisms (SNPs) at positions 29, 307, and 680 are extensively studied. Loss-of-function mutations in FSH receptor have been found in women with ovarian dysgenesis and primary and secondary amenorrhea. Gain-of-function mutations have been found in women with ovarian hyperstimulation syndrome (OHSS).

Single Nucleotide Polymorphisms of Follicle-stimulating Hormone Receptor Gene

There are eight SNPs in coding region and >1,300 SNPs in noncoding region of FSH receptor gene. Out of the eight SNPs in coding region, six are asymptomatic. The two polymorphisms at position p Thr^{307}Ala (rs6165) and p Asn^{680}Ser (rs 6166) are most extensively investigated.

Ser^{680} allele is clinically important in prediction of ovarian response to gonadotropin stimulation. Women with Ser/Ser and Asn/Ser genotype showed significantly higher FSH dose for ovarian stimulation when compared with Asn/Asn genotype. Peak estradiol levels, number of follicles, and oocytes were similar in all three.[19]

Women with Ala^{307}Ala genotype are significantly associated with lower dose of exogenous FSH and higher estradiol levels. 85% of women with Ala-Ala genotype developed OHSS.[20]

Asn^{680} allele is associated with a lower risk for polycystic ovary syndrome (PCOS) and Ala^{307}-Ser^{680} genotype has increased risk of developing PCOS. In a study among women with PCOS, Ser/Ser genotype at 608 showed resistance to clomiphene citrate (CC) and favorable response to exogenous FSH.[21] Asn/Thr genotype at position 307 showed higher response to FSH stimulation than both homozygous states.[22]

Homozygous Ala^{307}/Ser^{680} has been shown to be associated with higher risk of occurrence and recurrence of ovarian cancer.[23]

Alternately spliced variants of FSH receptor gene are also encountered. Alternately spliced exon 9 has been observed in normal testicular tissue.[24] Deletion of exons 6 and 9 has been seen in infertile men.[25] Among women, deletion of exon 9 has been associated with poor response and deletion of exon 6 is associated with a high response.[26]

RECENT TRENDS IN MEDICAL MANAGEMENT IN ASSISTED REPRODUCTIVE TECHNIQUE

Corifollitropin Alfa/Delta/Epsilon

Corifollitropin Alfa

Corifollitropin alfa (Elonva®) is the first hybrid FSH molecule and has sustained follicle-stimulating activity.

The beta subunit of this molecule contains the carboxy-terminal peptide of human chorionic gonadotropin. This imparts a longer half-life (approximately 69 hours), which is two times higher and slower absorption (fourfold higher time to peak serum levels) when compared with recombinant FSH (rFSH).

Pharmacodynamic properties of corifollitropin alfa are identical to rFSH as it interacts only with the FSH receptor. Corifollitropin alfa is able to sustain multiple follicular growth for a week, with a similar ovarian response and safety profile as rFSH. A single injection of corifollitropin alfa can replace seven daily injections of rFSH during the first week of ovarian stimulation in gonadotropin-releasing hormone (GnRH) antagonist protocols.

Therefore, corifollitropin alfa presents a simplified treatment protocol and reduces the burden of multiple daily injections.[27]

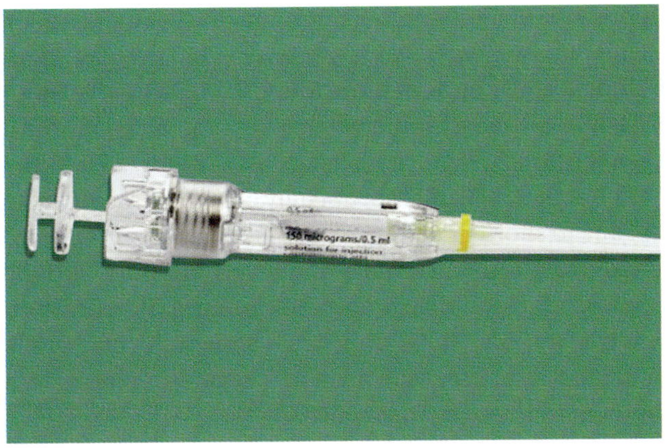

Fig. 2: Corifollitropin alfa.

Corifollitropin alfa is given as a single subcutaneous injection on menstrual day 2/3 (stimulation day 1). A GnRH antagonist can be added on stimulation day 5, depending on follicular response, to prevent a premature LH surge. Daily rFSH doses should be instituted from stimulation day 8 as required.

The optimal dose is 100 μg (<60 kg, <36 years) and 150 μg (>60 kg or >36 years) **(Fig. 2)**.[28]

Meta-analysis has shown that corifollitropin alpha is as effective as rFSH in terms of live birth rate, ongoing pregnancy rate, and clinical pregnancy rate. There is an increased number of eggs retrieved after corifollitropin; hence, a careful patient selection to screen out hyperresponders is mandatory to prevent OHSS.[29]

Corifollitropin Delta

Corifollitropin delta is the first rFSH product that has been developed from human cell line, namely PER.C6. It is unique in that dosing is optimized based on patient's body mass index (BMI) and anti-Müllerian hormone levels. Both alpha and delta have the same amino acid sequence but vary in their glycosylation and subsequently in the pharmacodynamics in humans. Steelman–Pohley bioassay done on Chinese hamster ovarian cells revealed similar pharmacodynamic curves; whereas in humans, the pharmacodynamics are different for the two. Corifollitropin delta has slower serum clearance and hence greater exposure and higher pharmacodynamic response.[30]

Corifollitropin Epsilon

Also a human cell line derived rFSH, at similar doses epsilon, has been shown to have a greater effect on follicular growth, not only on diameters but also on the follicular numbers.[75] IU corifollitropin epsilon given daily produces comparable response as that of 150 IU of rFSH (Gonal-f) and 150 IU of epsilon given on alternate days produces a greater response than 150 IU of rFSH given daily. There is a similar increase in estradiol and inhibin B levels produced while on epsilon than on rFSH or on corifollitropin delta. The drug is currently in clinical trial.[31]

Synthetic Kisspeptins

The neuropeptide kisspeptin and its receptor Kiss1R modulate the reproductive timeline of mammals by triggering puberty onset and promoting ovulation by stimulation of GnRH secretion. Kisspeptin interacts with other neuropeptides like dynorphin and neurokinin B to influence the GnRH release. Loss of kisspeptin signaling causes hypogonadotropic hypogonadism.

Kisspeptin was initially discovered as a factor that inhibits metastasis in melanoma cell lines.[32] Kisspeptin comprises a group of peptides encoded by the *Kiss1* gene. These peptides are derived from the common precursor—prepro-kisspeptin. The most abundant kisspeptin in humans is kisspeptin-54.[33]

Kisspeptin receptor belongs to rhodopsin family of G protein-coupled receptors.[33]

The short half-life of kisspeptin has been overcome by modifications that reduce proteolytic degradation and renal clearance. These modifications have increased the potency of the drug.

Different Roles of Kisspeptin

- *Regulation of gonadal steroid feedback to hypothalamus:* Kisspeptin plays a key role in mediating the positive feedback effect of estrogen via estrogen receptor alpha at the hypothalamus, which in turn causes the LH surge and ovulation. Kisspeptin gene expression is under epigenetic modulation.[34]
- *Direct action on gonads:*
  - Kisspeptin and its receptor genes are expressed in ovary and testes as well. Reduced kisspeptin gene expression in ovaries has been associated with premature ovarian failure in mice.
  - Neurotrophin signaling via NTRK2 receptor which is essential for oocyte maturation following LH surge is dependent upon kisspeptin signaling, as evident in knockout mice.[35]
  - In testes, kisspeptin potentiates the release of testosterone on hCG administration via a peripheral pathway.[36]
  - Kisspeptin and its receptor expression in spermatozoa mediate a biphasic rise in intracellular calcium release and increase sperm motility and in capacitation.[37]
- *Pregnancy and implantation:*
  - Syncytiotrophoblastic cells have the highest level of peripheral kisspeptin expression in the body. The levels increase with gestation and are more in gestational trophoblastic disease. Kisspeptin plays a role in trophoblastic cell invasion.[38]
  - Kisspeptin levels are lower in pregnancy associated with type 1 diabetes mellitus (T1DM), gestational

diabetes mellitus (GDM), hypertension, placental dysfunction, and recurrent miscarriage.[39]

- *Regulation of nutrition and fertility:* Kisspeptin plays an intermediary role between leptin and GnRH neurons. Leptin is a peptide hormone secreted by adipocytes. GnRH neurons do not have leptin receptors. Kisspeptin neurons have leptin receptors. Kisspeptin expression increases after exogenous leptin administration.[40] Deficiency of leptin results in delayed puberty and hypogonadotropic hypogonadism.

Applications of Synthetic Kisspeptins

- Manipulation of kisspeptin signaling can be made use in disorders related to decreased GnRH signaling as in hypogonadotropic hypogonadism and where the hormones need to be suppressed as in hormone-sensitive cancers.
- Kisspeptin administration in males has shown to increase plasma gonadotropin and testosterone levels.[41]
- A single bolus of kisspeptin-10 induces an immediate LH pulse, irrespective of when the previous endogenous LH pulse was, and the amplitude is higher than normal LH pulse. The next endogenous LH pulse is delayed by the normal interpulse interval; hence, it is suggestive that kisspeptin administrations reset the GnRH pulse generator.[42]
- In women with hypothalamic amenorrhea, twice daily administration of kisspeptin resulted in desensitization whereas twice weekly administration retained the response in healthy women.[43]
- Kisspeptin neurons express prolactin receptors. High prolactin levels suppress kisspeptin expression and thereby prevent the LH surge. This provides the application of synthetic kisspeptin in treatment of anovulation due to hyperprolactinemia, which is not amenable to usual medications.[44]
- Jayasena et al. investigated the effect of varying doses of kisspeptin in GnRH antagonist protocol IVF stimulation to bring about triggering of oocyte maturation. Egg maturation was achieved at 36 hours after kisspeptin administration and the mean number of mature eggs increased with increase in kisspeptin dosage. Since this involves stimulation of endogenous gonadotropin release to bring about egg maturation, the risk of OHSS is minimized.[45]

Elagolix—The Oral Gonadotropin-releasing Hormone Antagonist

Elagolix is a highly potent, short-duration, nonpeptide, orally active, competitive GnRH antagonist. Due to the entirely revised properties, it is called "second-generation GnRH antagonists." It causes rapid and dose-dependent suppression of pituitary gonadotropins, the peak effect being reached in 4–6 hours. The target dose is 150 mg/day. Phase II clinical trials have demonstrated benefit in alleviation of dysmenorrhea, chronic pelvic pain, and dyspareunia of endometriosis.

The actions of GnRH are not fully blocked throughout the day, due to shorter half-life than regular antagonists. Hence, gonadotropin and sex hormone levels are only partially suppressed. Upon discontinuation of drug, its effects are rapidly reversible. These provide an easier tolerance profile upon long-term use, especially with regard to menopausal symptoms and bone mineral density.[46]

Uterine Transplantation

The first pelvic organ transplant was that of fallopian tube, tried in animal models to develop treatment for tubal infertility. With advent of IVF, tubes were bypassed and importance came on to uterine transplantation for curing uterine factor infertility. First uterine transplantation was performed in Saudi Arabia in 2002 but it ended in graft rejection and hysterectomy at 3 months posttransplantation. Second attempt was in Turkey and resulted in pregnancies that ended in miscarriages. Successful pregnancy posttransplant came later as Baby Vincent on October 14, 2014 in Gothenburg, Sweden, among a cohort of nine patients who underwent the procedure. In her, the first menstruation happened 43 days after transplantation.

Indications

- Uterine malformations: Most common being agenesis and hypoplasia
- Posthysterectomy for neoplasms, postpartum hemorrhage, etc.
- Asherman's syndrome

Assessment of Donor Eligibility

- Proved parity with no history or evidence of any uterine disease
- To be screened for genital infections and Pap smear
- History of risk factors for infection
- Malignancy in the past 5 years
- Presence of any comorbidities
- Serology, infectious, and malignant screening
- Human leukocyte antigen (HLA) typing
- ABO and Rh typing.

Tissue Typing

The tissue typing laboratory carries out three tasks:

1. To determine the HLA type of blood for both donor and recipient by PCR.
2. Lymphocyte cross-matching to exclude circulating antibodies in recipient against HLA expressed by donor.

3. HLA antibody screening and specificity in recipient before and after transplant to guide immunosuppressive therapy.

Donor Surgery

Donor can be living or deceased. Deceased subjects were opened by midline infraumbilical incision. Uterus is heparinized and perfused with saline solution before harvesting. Use of living donors was pioneered by Mats Brännström of Sweden. Infraumbilical midline incision is used to give adequate exposure. Uterus is dissected and supportive ligaments delineated. Bilateral salpingectomy is performed. With careful dissection, uterine artery and veins should be separated from the uterus. A 10–15 mm of vaginal cuff is needed for reanastomosis. After surgical isolation, uterus is flushed bilaterally through the arterial ends with cold histidine-tryptophan-ketoglutarate solution.

The human myometrial tissue is resistant to cold ischemia for a period of 6 hours if a protective buffer is used.[47]

Recipient Surgery

Both donor and recipient surgery must be synchronized to reduce ischemia time. Internal and external iliac vessels are dissected and anastomosed to donor vessels. Vagina will be sutured and subsequent fixation of transplanted uterus is performed. Fixation of uterus to the ligaments and suturing the bladder peritoneum on the uterine graft on top of the recipient's bladder provide extra structural support. Living donor uterus requires more extensive vascular anastomosis than dead donor organ.[47]

Immunosuppression is maintained till birth of child by cesarean section and discontinued with hysterectomy soon after. The Swedish group has subjects who were maintained on immunosuppression following first childbirth for uterine preservation for a subsequent gestation.

Monitoring for Immunological Rejection

Monitoring for immunological rejection is by:
- *Ultrasound:* Endometrium and the uterus
- *Doppler:* Blood flow in the uterine arteries
- Visual inspection of cervix
- Cervical cultures
- Cervical biopsies.

Birth of healthy babies from the Swedish study has opened up hope for the subgroup of women with severe uterine factor infertility.[48] Deceased donor organ transplant has lesser success rates than living donor, probably due to preexisting conditions such as vasoactive drug use, elevated serum inflammatory markers, duration of ischemia, and type of solution used for preservation. There is a need for improvement in technology for preservation of organ in deceased donor for better posttransplant results.

Ethical Issues

Uterine transplantation is fraught with ethical issues because of following reasons—not a lifesaving organ transplant, day-to-day physiological functioning is not compromised in its absence, alternatives such as surrogacy and adoption are available, temporary in nature—removed after one or two children, and possibility of failure of IVF.

Montreal Criteria for the Ethical Feasibility of Uterine Transplantation[49]

The recipient:
- Is a genetic female of reproductive age with no medical contraindications to transplantation.
- Has documented congenital or acquired uterine factor infertility, which has failed all current gold standard and conservative therapy.
- (1) has a personal or legal contraindication to surrogacy and adoption measures, or (2) seeks the uterus transplantation (Utx) solely as a measure to experience gestation, with an understanding of the limitations provided by the Utx in this respect.
- Has not had her decision to undergo Utx deemed as irrational by expert psychological evaluation.
- Does not exhibit frank unsuitability for motherhood, and
- Is responsible enough to consent, informed enough to make a responsible decision, and not under coercion.

The donor:
- Is a female of reproductive age with no medical contraindications to donation.
- (1) has repeatedly attested to her conclusion of parity, or (2) has signed an advanced directive for postmortem organ donation.
- Has no history of uterine damage or disease, and
- Is responsible enough to consent, informed enough to make a responsible decision, and not under coercion.

The healthcare team:
- Is part of an institution that meets Moore's third criteria as it pertains to institutional stability.
- Has provided adequate informed consent to both parties regarding risks, potential sequelae, and chances of success and failure.
- Has no conflict of interest independently or with either party, and
- Has the duty to preserve anonymity if donor or recipient does not explicitly waive this right.

First ICMR-approved uterine transplantation program in India is currently underway at our center, in collaboration with Mats Brännström (Sweden).

Bioengineered Uterus

Absolute uterine factor infertility (AUFI) is caused by congenital [absent uterus as in Mayer-Rokitansky-Küster-Hauser

(MRKH) syndrome, uterine malformations] or acquired uterine conditions (severe intrauterine adhesions, following hysterectomy) that preclude the possibility of pregnancy. Brännström of the Stockholm group pioneered uterine transplantation as a cure to AUFI. Among the nine women who underwent uterine transplantation, the indication was MRKH for eight of them and posthysterectomy for early-stage cervical cancer for one candidate. Among the nine, seven candidates had graft survival at 1-year postsurgery and were able to go ahead with embryo transfers and so far, five live births have been achieved of the lot.[47]

But uterine transplantation comes with its accompaniment of perils. A 10-hour long surgery for the recipient, long-term immunosuppressant use, and risks and health effects of tissue rejection reaction are to name a few. Long-term effects of immunosuppression include chronic conditions as well such as diabetes, hypertension, and accelerated arteriosclerosis.[50] Also there is a mismatch between demand and supply of matched donors to recipients. This has led to development of bioengineered uterus.

Bioengineering of organs is based on using a synthetic or biologically derived scaffold to provide structural support for pluripotent cell proliferation and differentiation.[51] A biological scaffold is produced by decellularization of an organ. Decellularization is the process of removal of immunologically active cells from a normal organ, leaving behind a framework of extracellular matrix.[52] Decellularization is carried out by exposure to detergents or to physical forces (freeze-thaw or pressure) or enzymatic activity. Embryonic and mesenchymal stem cells are the most used cell source for repopulation.[53] The vascular conduits in biological tissue-derived scaffolds are used to cannulate and connect to perfusion bioreactors during recellularization.[54] For whole uterus construction, larger scaffolds and vascular conduits will be necessary and is still in the stage of experimentation at level of rat uterus. Encouraging results have been obtained for strategies for partial uterine reconstruction with tissue-engineered uterine patch for use to cover partial uterine defects such as following resection of placental tumors, myomectomy, etc.[55]

Ectogenesis

- Artificial uterus (or artificial womb) is a hypothetical device that would allow for extracorporeal pregnancy or extrauterine fetal incubation by growing embryo or fetus outside of body of an organism that would normally internally carry the embryo or fetus to term.
- Extreme prematurity is the leading cause of neonatal morbidity and mortality. In particular, respiration is affected by bronchopulmonary dysplasia, which is the arrest in lung development secondary to premature transition from liquid to gas ventilation. There is circulatory failure as well due to imbalance between preload and afterload in artificial support circuits. Thirdly, there is a high chance for sepsis due to exposure to open fluid incubators. Lambs at 100–115 days of gestation are biologically equivalent to 22–24 weeks of premature human infant. An experimental team has successfully maintained preterm lambs in this artificial womb circuit and opens avenues of possibility in treatment of preterm human babies.
- Ectogenesis aims to overcome these three main obstacles by a system with following three components:
    1. *Pumpless arteriovenous circuit:* Blood flow is driven by the fetal heart and oxygenated by a low-resistance oxygenator.
    2. *Closed fluid environment with continuous fluid exchange:* A biobag, closed system, single-use design was used. Watertight ports were included for cannula access, suction, and temperature probes.
    3. Umbilical vascular access

A major concern in this artificial setup was anticoagulation, which has the risk of intracranial hemorrhage in preterm infants. Artificial womb has low effective surface area and hence the dose of anticoagulant is low and comparable to that used in extracorporeal membrane oxygenation **(Fig. 3)**.

Lambs grown in this external womb had no structural or ischemic defects. Myelination of nerves was also comparable to term offsprings. The target population for this therapy is 23–25 weeks extreme preterms.[56]

INVO Procedure (In Vivo Fertilization/ Vaginal Incubation)

Intravaginal culture of oocytes (INVO) procedure is an ART that makes use of a specially designed vaginal incubation device for oocyte fertilization and early embryogenesis **(Fig. 4)**. INVOcell™ intravaginal culture system has three parts:

1. *INVOcell culture device:* It consists of an inner vessel surrounded by an outer rigid shell. The inner vessel holds culture medium, eggs and sperm, or ICSI fertilized embryos. The inner vessel is placed into the outer rigid shell, which provides additional resistance to contamination. Made of polystyrene and silicone ring and medical grade synthetic rubber, all of which are nonembryotoxic.
2. *INVOcell retention device:* Helps in retention of the culture device within the vagina during the incubation period of 72 hours.
3. *INVOcell holding block:* For temperature maintenance during loading and collection procedures.

The sperm concentration is limited to 30,000/mL and not more than seven eggs are placed in the culture device. At the end of 72-hour incubation period, the device is collected and the contents are examined for viable embryos. Since its Food and Drug Administration (FDA) approval in November 2015, several hundred babies have been born in the United States by this technique.

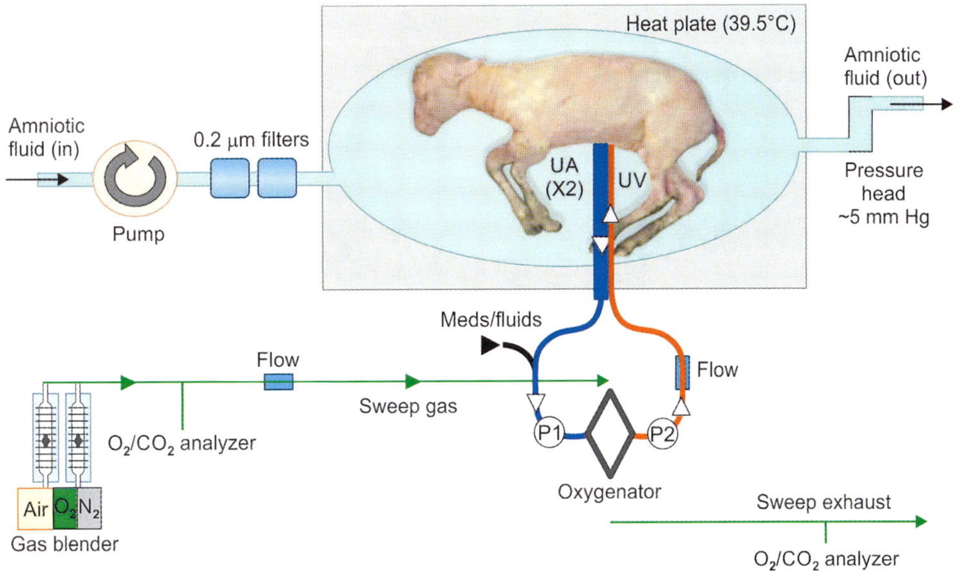

Fig. 3: Ectogenesis.

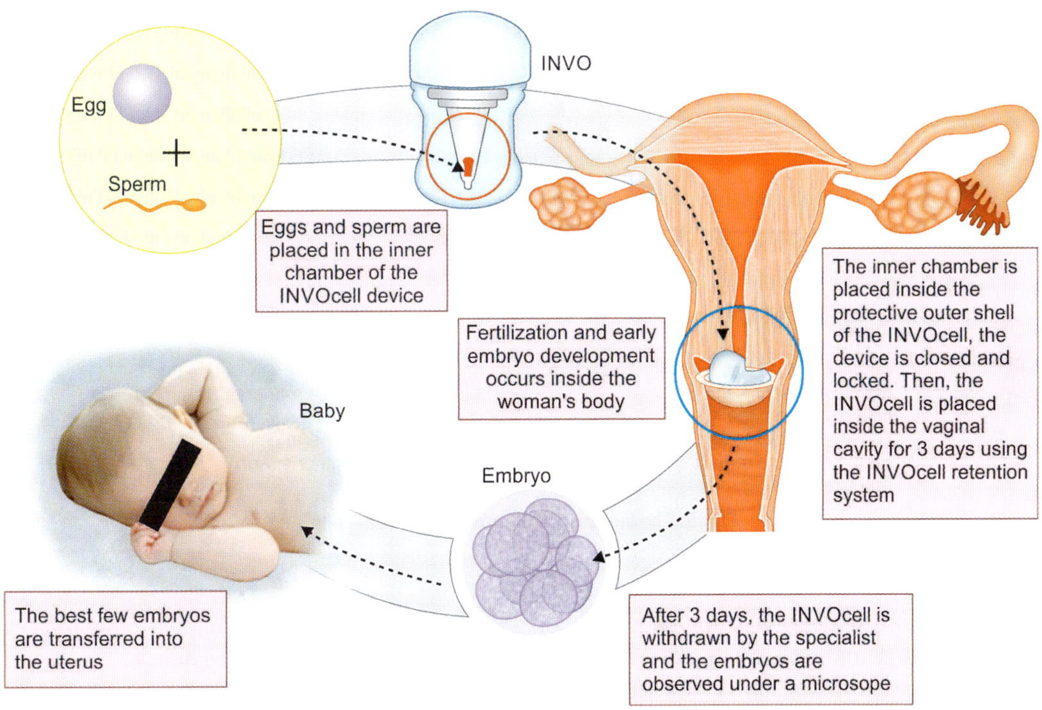

Fig. 4: In vivo procedure.

Benefits

Benefits of this procedure are:

- Greater patient involvement is a source of comfort to the couple
- Natural and stable culture environment
- Rules out the possibility of wrong embryo transfer
- Reduction in cost of IVF procedure.[57]

Embryonic Stem Cells

Embryonic stem cells are derived from cells of inner cell mass, which are removed and cultured under appropriate conditions. These cells have the ability to proliferate and develop into any cell type in the body **(Fig. 5)**.

Even though mouse embryonic stem cells were reported as early as 1981, the first reports of human embryonic stem

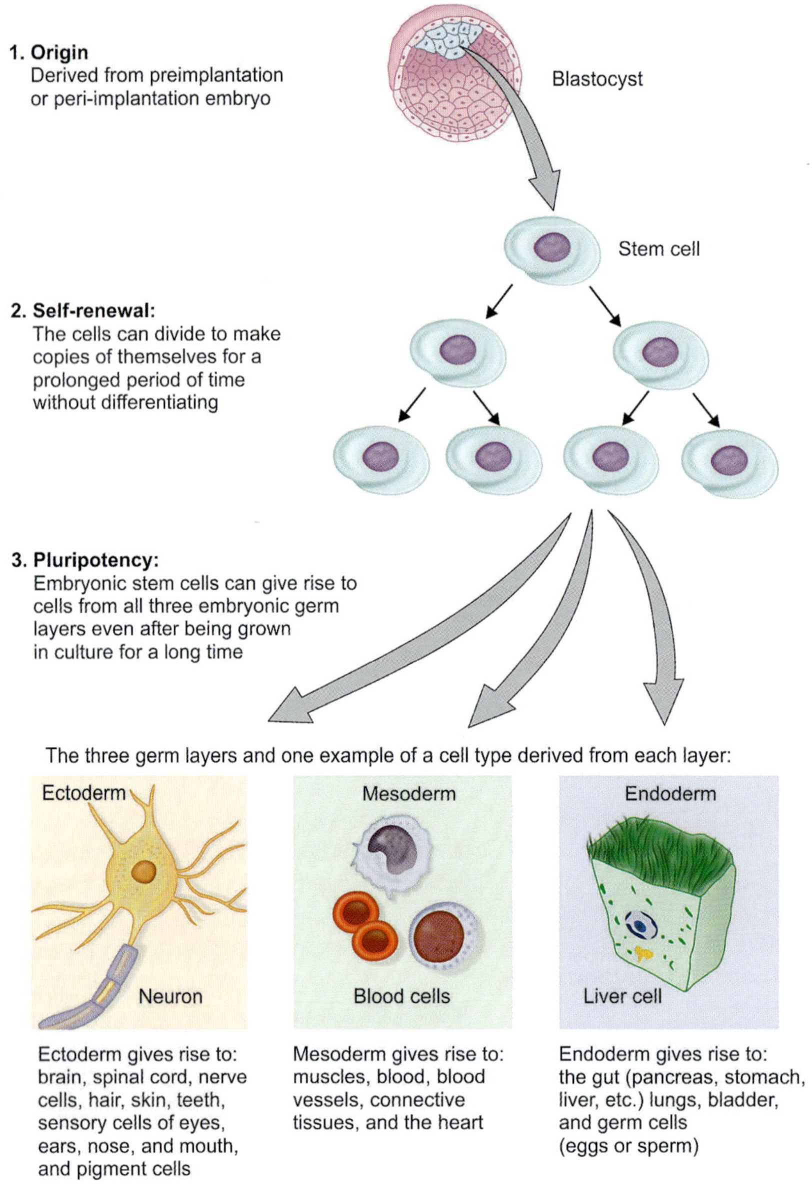

Fig. 5: Characteristics of embryonic stem cells.

cells came only in 1998.[58] The delay was due to scarcity of human embryos as a source for these cell lines. With advent of IVF, spare embryos became possible, which were no longer required by the commissioning couple. These became the source for extracting inner cell mass cells.

There are challenges in the culture of human stem cells:

- The cloning efficiency of human stem cells is low when compared to mouse cells.
- Initially, mouse fibroblasts were used for coculture of human embryonic stem cells. This provides a chance for introduction of pathogens as well as introduction of mouse cell strain impurities. Newer culture systems are being developed to avoid the use of mouse fibroblasts for coculture.[59]
- Another challenge is the possibility of accumulation of genetic and epigenetic changes over a period of stem cell culture.[60] The behavior of imprinted genes is also a matter of intrigue.[61]

Applications

- *Therapeutic drug research:* Access to unique stem cell lines can provide a platform for drug testing. This can prevent toxic drugs from reaching the level of clinical trials and harming participants.
- *Transplantation medicine:* Stem cells can provide a source for specific cells for substitution in diseased states, such as the use of insulin-producing cells in diabetes or dopaminergic neurons in Parkinson's disease.

- Human embryonic stem cells derived from samples taken for PGD can provide in vitro models to study the effect of these mutations on cell proliferation and differentiation and hence lead to a better understanding of the pathophysiology of these diseases.[62]

In Vitro Gametogenesis

The creation of human gametes in vitro [in vitro gametogenesis (IVG)] is an area of interest, related to embryonic stem cell research. IVG has been successfully completed in mice and has resulted in live birth.[63] Gametes were derived from embryonic stem cells obtained from inner cell mass of mice blastocyst. Similarly, gametes have been derived from human embryonic stem cells as well. Even primordial sperm cells have been formed from female human embryonic stem cells.[64] Even more outstanding achievement has been the creation of embryonic stem cell-like cells, which are pluripotent in nature, by the process of dedifferentiation of somatic cells and subsequent differentiation into spermatogenic cells and egg-like cells.[65]

Applications of In Vitro Gametogenesis

- To obtain gametes for IVF in patients with paucity of normal gametes such as poor ovarian reserve (POR), postmenopausal, and azoospermia. This obviates the need for gamete donors and allows them the possibility of their own genetic progeny.
- *Solo-IVG:* The concept of a single individual becoming a parent. Stem cells derived from epidermal cells can be used to create gamete of the opposite gender. This gamete and the normal self-gamete are fertilized to obtain an embryo.[66] There are greater technical challenges and genetic errors in this procedure because the entire genome is derived from a single individual.[67]
- Same-sex couple—can have their own child by using stem cell-derived gamete of one spouse and naturally derived gamete of the second spouse.
- *For PGD:* Greater number of embryos available can benefit PGD to select a disease-free embryo in individuals with multiple genetic defects.[68]
- *Multiplex parenting:* When four people want to have a genetic child together, embryos are formed from each couple respectively by conventional IVF, the inner cell mass is extracted from the embryos and cultured to differentiate into gametes. The fusion of these gametes will give rise to a second-generation embryo with 25% genetic contribution from each of the four individuals.[66]

Mitochondrial Replacement Therapy

Mitochondrial DNA constitutes <0.1% of total DNA content of a cell. Yet, defects in mitochondrial genes can lead to several debilitating diseases such as Duchenne muscular dystrophy, ragged-red fiber disease—mitochondrial myopathies, and Leber's hereditary optic neuropathy. The inheritance of mitochondrial defects will vary depending on the number of defective DNA copies per cell, ranging from asymptomatic to life-threatening.[69] At the time of fertilization and formation of zygote, the entire cytoplasm is derived from the mother and consequently, mitochondria are exclusively maternally inherited.[70]

Mitochondrial replacement therapy (MRT) aims at avoiding inheritance of defective mitochondrial genes in women with known mitochondrial disorders. There are two ways to achieve MRT:

1. *Maternal spindle transfer:* An oocyte sourced from a healthy donor is enucleated and the nucleus isolated from the genetic mother (who has the mitochondrial disease) is transferred into the enucleated donor oocyte. This is followed by ICSI and fertilization. The embryo is followed up for development for 5 days. The embryos are checked for mitochondrial heteroplasmy by quantitative PCR to confirm the absence of mitochondrial disease.[71]
2. *Pronuclear transfer:* One donor oocyte and a self-oocyte are sourced from the donor and the intended parent, respectively. Both the oocytes are fertilized with the male parent's sperm. Once fertilization is at the two-pronuclei stage, the female pronucleus derived from the genetic mother is isolated. The female pronucleus derived from the egg donor is removed. The genetic mother-derived female pronucleus is inserted into the donor-derived embryo, whose female pronucleus has been removed.[72]

Ethical Concerns

- Concerns that alterations in germ cells may produce heritable changes have been quenched by the explanation that mitochondrial DNA constitutes <0.1% of total DNA content and also that external characteristics of humans are not coded by these genes.
- *Designer babies:* Since MRT aims at removal of disease-causing mitochondrial genes and not at enhancing normal embryos, it does not come under the purview of "designer babies".
- There is a concern that there is a possibility of interaction between mitochondrial DNA derived from the donor and nuclear DNA derived from the genetic mother. The ramifications of such an interaction are yet unknown.
- Safer options such as egg donation, PGD, and prenatal screening for fetal diseases have been proposed. Egg donation takes away the mother's right to have her own genetic child. Whereas PGD and prenatal testing are neither well-established nor are they totally accurate, with regard to mitochondrial diseases.
- Widespread use of MRT might fuel the need for more donor oocytes and possibly can lead to exploitation of egg donors.[73]

Mitochondrial Replacement Therapy Today

The United States FDA has not approved of human clinical trials to establish the efficacy of MRT as a clinical modality. However, MRT-derived embryos and stem cell lines have been cultured in research setting in New York.[71] In the UK, HFE (Human Fertilisation and Embryology) Act has been amended in October 2015 to allow the use of MRT.

Gene Editing

Gene editing is a biotechnological advancement that enables us to produce permanent and heritable changes in genome. Earlier, advances in this regard were thwarted by poor targeting efficiency of techniques. This has been recently overcome by obtaining double-strand breaks adjacent to integration sites.[74] This has led to the development of sequence-specific nucleases (SSNs) such as CRISPR (clustered regularly interspaced short palindromic repeats).

The CRISPR/Cas9 are endonucleases that can cleave DNA and store short sequences in the genome. These can be expressed as RNA molecules that search for complementary DNA sequences and can produce double-strand breaks at specific sites.[75]

Applications

- *Preimplantation embryos:* The endonuclease is injected into the zygote and embryos are screened for selection of embryos with correct genome.[76]
  A challenge in this selection process is brought about by mosaic nature of corrected embryos that precludes the use of PGD as a selection tool.
- *Germ cells:* Errors can be corrected in sperm cell or oocytes to prevent their transmission to embryo. Spermatogonial cells are technically easier target than oocytes.
- *Pluripotent cells:* Corrected pluripotent stem cells can be differentiated into sperm or oocyte and can be used for ART.[76]

Uses

- *Correction of mutations* is responsible for monogenic disorders such as cystic fibrosis and sickle cell disease. Affected genomes as well as carrier state can be prevented henceforth. Robertsonian translocations such as trisomy 21 can also be edited and restored to normalcy.[77]
- *Enhancement of phenotype:* Traits such as poor eyesight, short stature can be attempted, to be resolved using this technology. Even though, the polygenic nature and influence of environment are facts that make the likelihood of such a possibility dimmer.

Newer Strategies in Management of Thin Endometrium

Persistent thin endometrium is a frequently encountered problem in ART. Endometrial thickness of 7 mm is commonly accepted as the lower limit to define thin endometrium, even though pregnancies have been reported with endometrium as low as 5 mm.[78] Estrogen supplementation, low-dose aspirin, vitamin E, sildenafil, pentoxifylline, and acupuncture are the various modalities in practice to tackle thin endometrium. Newer strategies have been envisaged for thin endometrium but are associated with controversial evidence as to their benefits.

Human Chorionic Gonadotropin Injections

Endometrial cells express hCG receptors and produce hCG during the secretory phase. hCG has local paracrine and immune-modulating effects that enhance endometrial receptivity.

On the eighth day of estradiol administration, hCG 150 IU subcutaneous injections were started for 7 days and endometrial thickness was monitored in a study. There was >10% increase in endometrial thickness in 52.9% of patients and >20% increase in 35.3%. Forty-one percent had live birth. This study showed improvement in both endometrial thickness and clinical outcome.[79] However, at higher doses, the benefits are lost.[80]

Granulocyte Colony-stimulating Factor

Granulocyte colony-stimulating factor (GCSF) is a glycoprotein that has proliferative and decidualizing influence on endometrium. GCSF supplementation on endometrial cell cultures showed that GCSF modulates gene pathways involved in endometrial vascularity and remodeling.[81] But a well-powered randomized controlled trial (RCT) in this regard has showed no difference in either endometrial thickness or in clinical pregnancy rates.[82]

Platelet-rich Plasma

Platelet-rich plasma (PRP) is a source of vascular endothelial growth factor, platelet-derived growth factor, epidermal growth factor, and transforming growth factor. Combined, these enhance the cellular migration and proliferation as well as laying down of extracellular matrix in the endometrium.[83] Marked improvement has been noted in endometrial thickness with the use of intrauterine PRP instillation.[84]

Since it is an autologous product, there is limited risk of infection and autoimmunity.

Preparation of Platelet-rich Plasma

About 15 mL of venous blood of patient is collected in a syringe with 5 mL of acid citrate dextrose (ACD)—an anticoagulant solution. This is centrifuged at 200 g for 10 minutes. There is formation of three layers in the tube—topmost is plasma, buffy coat in middle, and red cells in bottom. The upper two layers are removed into a second tube and recentrifuged at 500 g for 10 minutes. The pellet obtained at the bottom of this tube is resuspended with 0.5 mL of supernatant. This 0.5 mL solution contains platelets at a concentration 4–5 times that of blood. This is loaded into an intrauterine catheter and instilled into the uterus on the 10th day of cycle and can be repeated on the day of the start of progesterone.[83]

Gonadotropin-releasing Hormone Analogs

Qublan et al. conducted an RCT that administered 0.1 mg triptorelin subcutaneous injections on the day of ovum pickup, the day of embryo transfer, and one dose 3 days later. The control arm was given conventional luteal support. Significant improvement in pregnancy rates was noted.[85] But further studies have not come up in this regard to support this use.

Stem Cell Therapy

Stem cells can be sourced from bone marrow or from embryonic stem cells and instilled in uterus where they can differentiate into epithelial and stromal cell lines within the endometrium. Among patients who have received bone marrow transplantation, 1–10% of them have been documented to have donor-derived cells in their endometrium.[86] Nagori et al. have reported a case of live birth following instillation of autologous bone marrow stem cells extracted from iliac crest in a patient with Asherman's syndrome.[87]

Role of Endometrial Receptivity Array in Thin Endometrium

A thin endometrium is not always a nonreceptive one. ERA can be used to assess the displacement of WOI, and PET can aid in overcoming the change in WOI. A study performed on women with endometrium ≤6 mm found ERA to be nonreceptive in 23% and receptive in 77%.[11]

NEWER TRENDS IN CONTROLLED OVARIAN STIMULATION

Minimal Stimulation Protocols

The concept of minimal stimulation protocols was envisaged by Edwards et al. in 1996 as a means to provide ovarian stimulation with minimal treatment risks and to be more patient friendly.[88]

Endocrine Basis for Minimal Stimulation

In a normal ovarian cycle, the increased estrogen output by granulosa cells of the dominant follicle will cause negative feedback effect on pituitary secretion of FSH. Thus, the lower FSH blood levels become inadequate to sustain the growth of smaller preantral and antral follicles, leading to their atresia.

Controlled ovarian stimulation (COS) is based on exogenous gonadotropin supplementation, which lengthens the FSH window wherein more antral follicles continue to grow and become multiple dominant follicles.

Studies have shown that even mild interference in the FSH reduction in midfollicular phase is enough to sustain the growth of more dominant follicles.[89] This is the crux of minimal stimulation protocol wherein a normal intercycle rise of FSH is utilized to initiate follicular recruitment and smaller gonadotropin doses in combination with oral ovulogens are used to lengthen the FSH window.

Oral Ovulogens Combined with Gonadotropins

Use of CC in early follicular phase and further supplemented with gonadotropins produces synergistic beneficial effects and remove the adverse effects of CC on endometrium.

Aromatase inhibitors, by inhibiting conversion of androgens to estrogens in granulosa cells, increase intraovarian androgen milieu and help in recruitment of more antral follicles, possibly reducing the dose of gonadotropins require subsequently.[90]

Benefits of Minimal Stimulation[91]

- Less duration of treatment
- Lesser dose and expenditure of gonadotropins
- Lesser risk of hyperstimulation
- Less incidence of multiple pregnancies
- Improved embryo quality since high dose gonadotropin stimulation and supraphysiological E2 levels affect chromosomal segregation and impair embryo quality.
- Better endometrial receptivity due to absence of high E2 level mediated endometrial advancement and embryo-endometrial asynchrony.
- Cumulative live birth in a year is same as that of conventional stimulation
- Proven to have less psychological burden on couples receiving treatment, in comparison to conventional protocols.

Demerits of Minimal Stimulation

- Fewer embryos for transfer produced per oocyte retrieval cycle
- Higher cycle cancellation rates due to mono or bifollicular responses when gonadotropins are started on day 5 of the cycle.
- If more cycles are required to bring about a live birth, a greater number of oocyte retrievals will be necessary, which is the most invasive step in IVF. This can contribute to anxiety and emotional stress.

Role of Growth Hormone in Poor Responders

Growth hormone (GH) is a peptide hormone secreted by lactotrophic cells of anterior pituitary gland and exerts its action through insulin-like growth factor-1 (IGF-1) generated in the liver. IGF-1 receptors are present on oocytes, granulosa cells, and theca cells. IGF-1 facilitates the action of FSH during follicular growth. Use of GH during COS has been shown to increase the receptor density of GH, LH, FSH, and bone morphogenic protein (BMP-1B). Use of GH in COS has crossed 25 years; however, its role is still debatable and newer evidence is emerging.

Use of GH in COS has shown to reduce the duration of COS, reduce the total dose of gonadotropins used, increase the peak estradiol level, and increase the number of oocytes retrieved and embryos generated. However, there is no improvement in live birth rate. It is unclear as to whether the absence of benefit in live birth rate is absolute or whether the studies are underpowered to discern the benefit.

Australian multicenter study, "LIGHT" trial, randomized women with previous poor response to IVF stimulation to those who received 12 IU of GH from the start of stimulation and those who received gonadotropin alone. About 98.5% of women in intervention arm achieved an oocyte retrieval as compared to 78% in placebo group, and the number of oocytes retrieved was greater by 1 in the study arm. However, there was no difference in the number of women who reached embryo transfer neither in the quality of embryos formed.

It is put forth that use of GH may benefit a subgroup of poor responders who have poor oocyte/embryo quality, the so-called suboptimal responder. Recent evidence is also emerging on usefulness of GH in women with refractory thin endometrium. Both of these concepts warrant further validation.[92,93]

Long Antagonist Protocol

A novel protocol using a single-dose long-acting GnRH antagonist injection, degarelix, on day 24 of menstrual cycle preceding the COS cycle was introduced as a proof of concept study by Papanicolao et al. in 2018. No LH rise was noted in any of the 10 oocyte donors on whom the study was conducted. The same oocyte donors underwent a conventional antagonist protocol stimulation 6 months later and served as their own control arm. There was no significant difference in ART outcome parameters including oocytes retrieved, embryo output, and clinical pregnancy rates. The advantage of this protocol is that it issues greater flexibility to the programming of IVF cycles as COS can be started as late as 10 days into the follicular phase of menstrual cycle. Secondly, agonist triggering is possible, avoiding the perils of OHSS.

Degarelix is available in the Indian market, being used in the treatment of carcinoma prostate.[94]

Double Stimulation Protocols

Double stimulation protocols involve COS during follicular and luteal phase of same menstrual cycle. This is based on the fact that follicular recruitment occurs in multiple waves spread across the menstrual cycle. Performing consecutive stimulations and oocyte retrievals within the same menstrual cycle aids in reducing time to collect more oocytes, which is useful among women with rapidly declining ovarian reserve such as age >40 years and also in oncofertility.

Different protocols have evolved with double stimulation as its crux.

Shanghai protocol uses letrozole/CC and human menopausal gonadotropin (hMG) for COS in follicular phase, GnRH antagonist for prevention of LH surge, and GnRH agonist for triggering of oocyte maturation. DuoStim protocol (Ubaldi et al.) uses rFSH and hMG for COS and after 5 days of oocyte retrieval, second COS is started. According to Ubaldi et al., the number of euploid embryos increased from 41.9% (among oocytes obtained from follicular phase stimulation alone) to 69.8% (among oocytes pooled from both follicular and luteal phase stimulation). This increase in the number of euploid embryos is of paramount importance in the subgroup of women with poor ovarian reserve. This was further substantiated by a case series done in 2020 by Vaiarelli et al. Obtaining euploid blastocyst increased from 14% to 31% with luteal stimulation and cumulative live birth rate increased from 7% to 15%. Reducing the duration of time needed to create more embryos reduces the emotional burden on couple undergoing treatment and reduces the treatment dropout rate.[95,96]

ADVANCES IN EMBRYOLOGY LABORATORY TECHNIQUES

Newer Sperm Selection Techniques

Intracytoplasmic Morphologically Selected Sperm Injection/Physiological Intracytoplasmic Sperm Injection

Intracytoplasmic morphologically selected sperm injection involves the injection of sperm into oocyte after the selection of sperm with good morphology under a magnification of 6,300.

Intracytoplasmic sperm injection, performed under a magnification of 200–400, excludes spermatozoa with major morphological defects. Whereas IMSI can look for subtle nuclear defects. MSOME (Motile Sperm Organelle Morphology Examination) criteria for normal nucleus include smooth, symmetrical, and oval nucleus with homogenous chromatin material with not more than one vacuole occupying <4% of nucleus.[97]

Use of IMSI to rule out subtle nuclear defects has a definite role in improving pregnancy outcome.[98] The fertilization rate with IMSI is significantly greater than that with ICSI, especially among oligoasthenospermic males.[99] Blastocyst conversion rate is also higher post-IMSI.[100]

Physiological ICSI identifies and uses mature hyaluronan-binding sperm for injection into oocyte.

Immaturity of sperm is known to cause aneuploidies.[101] Live birth rates with PICSI are higher than in ICSI,[102] especially in male factor infertility. Some studies have also documented improved embryo quality and implantation rates with PICSI.[103]

Electrophoretic Sperm Separation

Electrophoretic sperm separation is a membrane-based electrophoretic separation that can separate sperms with maturity and least DNA damage. It works on the premise that sperm cells with least DNA damage and more maturity will carry a greater negative charge. This allows their separation from leukocytes and immature germ cells.[104] Spermatozoa are highly susceptible to oxidative stress due to the high content of unsaturated fatty acids. Leukocytes generate reactive oxygen species that create oxidative stress. Hence the separation of sperms from leukocytes is imperative.[105] Negative charge on mature spermatozoa is acquired by sialic acid residues on CD52 molecules on sperm surface.

CD52 molecules are acquired during epididymal transit and reflect on the maturity of sperms.[106]

Electrophoretic sperm separation works with a cassette that has two separate chambers of 400 μL each, separated by a filter and sealed by polyacrylamide gel, which allows permeation of buffer. Semen is put into one cabin, 75 mA of current is applied, and a filtered sperm suspension is obtained in adjacent cabin.[104]

Magnetic-assisted Cell Sorting

Magnetic-assisted cell sorting (MACS) is an efficient way to identify and separate functional sperms. Apoptotic sperms show loss of membrane integrity and phosphatidyl serine is exposed. Annexin V conjugated with magnetic microspheres and exposed to a magnetic field can segregate the apoptotic sperms from the nonapoptotic sperms.[107]

By removal of apoptotic sperms, there is improvement in embryo quality and pregnancy rates but there is no difference in the miscarriage rates. Density gradient centrifugation combined with MACS is a preferred method for sperm selection.[108]

Polscope and Rescue Intracytoplasmic Sperm Injection

Oocyte morphology has always been a focus of interest, primarily to choose the best oocytes for IVF or ICSI with the probability of development of good quality embryos. Assessment of cumulus, zona, and cytoplasm for granulation, vacuoles, and polar body configuration has been a widespread practice.

With the advent of orientation-independent polarizing microscope "polscope," meiotic spindle examination of living and unstained oocytes has become a reality.

When two orthogonally polarized light rays pass through an orderly arrangement of filamentous structures such as the microtubules constituting the meiotic spindle, the light rays get slowed down or retarded. The retardance is in direct proportion to the density of the structure that they pass through. This is the principle underlying the phenomenon of birefringence.[109]

In this manner, meiotic spindle of oocytes can be assessed as part of morphological assessment of oocytes. Disorganized meiotic spindles result in segregation errors and aneuploid embryos.[110] Meiotic spindle can be damaged by temperature fluctuations and also inadvertently by the ICSI procedure itself.[111] To prevent damage to spindle, ICSI needle is always positioned at 90° to polar body.

Mature (MII) oocytes with a single meiotic spindle show the highest fertilization rates.[112]

Clinical Application: Rescue Intracytoplasmic Sperm Injection

Intracytoplasmic sperm injection performed on day 1 of unfertilized matures oocytes (at 18–21 hours postoocyte retrieval) is called as rescue ICSI. Examination of meiotic spindle helps in selection of oocytes for ICSI. By seeing a single meiotic spindle and single polar body, it can be confirmed that there has been no fertilization so far and hence prevent three pronuclei (3PN) state following ICSI of such an oocyte. Presence of MII oocytes with two spindles indicates sperm penetration of oocyte followed by oocyte activation failure. Such oocytes are ineligible for rescue ICSI. Rescue ICSI can yield good quality embryos and often need cryopreservation of embryos to achieve better embryo-endometrial synchrony. This can come as a big relief to patients who were otherwise destined for total fertilization failure and cycle cancellation.[113]

Assisted Oocyte Activation

Total fertilization failure happens in 2–3% of ICSI cases. Oocyte activation following fertilization is mediated by a biphasic rise of intracellular calcium.

Step 1—Trigger: The trigger originates from the oocyte cortex, following interaction of oocyte membrane with sperm.

Step 2—Oscillator: Around 30 minutes following trigger, there are sustained short-duration and high-amplitude pulses of calcium release. A soluble factor from sperm is postulated to bring about the oscillator.[114]

Total fertilization failure ensues when the calcium release fails or is suboptimal. This might be due to inherent defects in sperm (severe teratospermia and globozoospermia) or in oocyte. To discriminate between sperm and oocyte defect, heterologous ICSI with mouse oocyte is performed [mouse oocyte activation test (MOAT)]. If fertilized also, developmental defects such as cleavage arrest are seen with suboptimal calcium rise.

In ICSI, the injection process by itself triggers calcium rise. In failed fertilization, use of calcium ionophores is known to restore the calcium release and aid in fertilization in majority of cases. Assisted oocyte activation (AOA) is brought about by exposure to $CaCl_2$ followed by calcium ionophores.

Other less effective means of AOA are use of electrical pulses, mechanical, and vigorous cytoplasmic aspiration.[115]

Globozoospermia

Globozoospermia is a rare form of teratospermia that accounts for 0.1% of male infertility. It is characterized by absent acrosome and rounded nucleus in majority of sperms. It causes fertilization failure due to inability of sperm to bind to zona pellucida in the absence of an acrosome reaction. Even with ICSI, fertilization rates are poor due to absence of oocyte activation factor, phospholipase C zeta. Calcium ionophore activation is especially useful in these patients to bring about successful fertilization.[116]

Elongated Spermatid Injection

In patients with nonobstructive azoospermia, surgically retrieved spermatids (haploid in nature) can be used for ICSI. Round spermatids have lesser fertilization rate compared to elongated spermatids. Due to absence of phospholipase C zeta, calcium ionophores are required to bring about oocyte activation when elongated spermatids are used for ICSI.[117]

Time-lapse Monitoring of Embryos

- Time-lapse monitoring (TLM) of embryos is the most significant advancement in ART of this decade. It enables the continuous monitoring of embryos, to observe the cleavage pattern, morphological changes, and growth dynamics without having to take the embryos out of their ideal culture conditions.
- Built-in digital inverted microscope within the incubator takes photographs at distinct time intervals and the data are automatically compiled into a video sequence by software.
- Presently available TLM technologies are Primo Vision (Vitrolife), EmbryoScope (FertiliTech), and Eeva (Early Embryonic Viability Assessment, Auxogyn).
- Embryos whose cleavage times occupy the two middle quartiles have the maximum implantation potential. Also, adherence to time pattern of development showed greater correlation with euploidy. Thus, the best embryo of the lot can be selectively transferred, aiding in the practice of single embryo transfer.[118]

CONCLUSION

- The major change that has come in the world of ART recently is the advent of COVID-19 pandemic that necessitated changes in functioning of ART centers. The change encompasses modifications in patient counselling, treatment recommendations for couples, donors and surrogates, recommendations for staff working at ART centers, modifications in ART center layout and functionality.
- Vaccination against Covid-19 has been made mandatory at a national level.
- Newer diagnostic modalities in ART include Self operated endovaginal telemonitoring, Smartphone USG, Fertiloscopy, Endometrial receptivity array (ERA), Sperm DNA fragmentation index (DFI).
- Recent trends in ART medicines include newer gonadotropin preparations such as Corifolitropin Alpha/delta/epsilon, synthetic kisspeptins. Uterine transplantation has emerged as a ground-breaking treatment modality in absolute uterine factor infertility with its arrival in India. Bio-engineered uterus, ectogenesis, in-vitro vaginal incubation of embryos, embryonic stem cell technology, in-vitro gametogenesis, mitochondrial replacement therapy, gene editing are some of the cutting edge research happening in the field of ART.
- Thin endometrium has always been a tough and enigmatic challenge for clinicians of ART. Newer strategies in the arsenal against thin endometrium include intrauterine HCG, intrauterine platelet rich plasma infusion (PRP), intrauterine granulocyte colony stimulating factor (gCSF) and stem cell therapy.
- Newer trend in ovarian stimulation protocols is Minimal stimulation IVF,use of growth hormone as adjuvant in ovarian stimulation, long antagonist protocol and double stimulation protocols.
- Advances in embryology lab procedures include newer sperm selection techniques such as IMSI/PICSI/Electrophoretic sperm sorting/Magnetic assisted cell sorting.
- Newer embryology lab techniques include rescue ICSI, assisted oocyte activation and Polscope and Time-Lapse imaging (Embryoscope).

REFERENCES

1. ICMR. (2020). Guidelines for recommending ART services during COVID-19 pandemic. [online] Available from: https://www.icmr.gov.in/pdf/covid/techdoc/Guidelines_ART_during_COVID19_revised.pdf [Last accessed November, 2022].
2. ESHRE. (2021). COVID-19 vaccination and assisted reproduction. [online] Available from: https://www.eshre.eu/Europe/Position-statements/COVID19 [Last accessed November, 2022].
3. Carrascosa M, Baronio M, Capuñay C, López EM, Sueldo C, Papier S. Clinical use of 64-row multislice computed

tomography hysterosalpingography in the evaluation of female factor infertility. Fertil Steril. 2008;90:1953-8.
4. Baronio JM, Carrascosa P, Ulla M, Papier S, Borghi M, Sueldo C. Virtual hysterosalpingography: a novel painless technique for the study of the female reproductive tract in infertile patients. Fertil Steril. 2006;86:S51.
5. Rabinovici J, Inbar Y, Eylon SC, Schiff E, Hananel A, Freundlich D. Pregnancy and live birth after focused ultrasound surgery for symptomatic focal adenomyosis: a case report. Hum Reprod. 2006;21:1255-9.
6. Hanstede MF, Tempany CM, Stewart EA. Focused ultrasound surgery of intramural leiomyomas may facilitate fertility: a case report. Fertil Steril. 2007;88:497.e5-7.
7. Hendriks DJ, Mol BWJ, Bancsi LFJMM, Te Velde ER, Broekmans FJM. Antral follicle count in the prediction of poor ovarian response and pregnancy after in vitro fertilization: a meta-analysis and comparison with basal follicle-stimulating hormone level. Fertil Steril. 2005;83:291-301.
8. Pereira I, von Horn K, Depenbusch M, Schultze-Mosgau A, Griesinger G. Self-operated endovaginal telemonitoring: a prospective, clinical validation study. Fertil Steril. 2016;106(2):306-10.e1.
9. Watrelot A, Nisolle M, Chelli H, Hocke C, Rongières C, Racinet C, et al. Is laparoscopy still the gold standard in infertility assessment? A comparison of fertiloscopy versus laparoscopy in infertility. Results of an international multicenter prospective trial: the 'FLY' (Fertiloscopy-LaparoscopY) study. Hum Reprod. 2003;18(4):834-9.
10. Ruiz-Alonso M, Blesa D, Diaz-Gimeno P, Gómez E, Fernández-Sánchez M, Carranza F, et al. The endometrial receptivity array for diagnosis and personalized embryo transfer as a treatment for patients with repeated implantation failure. Fertil Steril. 2013;100:818-24.
11. Mahajan N. Endometrial receptivity array: clinical application. J Hum Reprod Sci. 2015;8(3):121-9.
12. Churchill S, Comstock I, Lathi R. Pregnancy outcomes after endometrial receptivity array in an infertile population. Fertil Steril. 2017;108(3):E360.
13. Darzynkiewicz Z, Traganos F, Sharpless T, Melamed MR. Thermal denaturation of DNA in situ as studied by acridine orange staining and automated cytofluorometry. Exp Cell Res. 1975;90:411-28.
14. Simon L, Lutton D, McManus J, Lewis SEM. Sperm DNA damage measured by the alkaline Comet assay as an independent predictor of male infertility and in vitro fertilization success. Fertil Steril. 2011;95:652-7.
15. Simon L, Proutski I, Stevenson M, Jennings D, McManus J, Lutton D, et al. Sperm DNA damage has a negative association with live-birth rates after IVF. Reprod Biomed Online. 2013;26:68-78.
16. Robinson L, Gallos ID, Conner SJ, Rajkhowa M, Miller D, Lewis S, et al. The effect of sperm DNA fragmentation on miscarriage rates: a systematic review and meta-analysis. Hum Reprod. 2012;27(10):2908-17.
17. Gromoll J, Dankbar B, Gudermann T. Characterization of the 5' flanking region of the human follicle-stimulating hormone receptor gene. Mol Cell Endocrinol. 1994;102:93-102.
18. Tapanainen JS, Aittomaki K, Min J, Vaskivuo T, Huhtaniemi IT. Men homozygous for an inactivating mutation of the follicle-stimulating hormone (FSH) receptor gene present variable suppression of spermatogenesis and fertility. Nat Genet. 1997;15:205-6.
19. Perez Mayorga M, Gromoll J, Behre HM, Gassner C, Nieschlag E, Simoni M.. Ovarian response to follicle-stimulating hormone (FSH) stimulation depends on the FSH receptor genotype. J Clin Endocrinol Metab. 2000;85:3365-9.
20. Achrekar SK, Modi DN, Desai SK, Mangoli VS, Mangoli RV, Mahale SD. Follicle-stimulating hormone receptor polymorphism (Thr307Aa) is associated with variable ovarian response and ovarian hyperstimulation syndrome in Indian women. Fertil Steril. 2007;91:432-9.
21. Overbeek A, Kujiper EA, Hendriks ML, Blankenstein MA, Ketel IJG, Twisk JWR, et al. Clomiphene citrate resistance in relation to follicle-stimulating hormone receptor Ser680Ser-polymorphism in polycystic ovary syndrome. Hum Reprod. 2009;24:2007-13.
22. Dolfin E, Guani B, Lussiana C, Mari C, Restagno G, Revelli A. FSH-receptor Ala307Thr polymorphism is associated to polycystic ovary syndrome and to a higher responsiveness to exogenous FSH in Italian women. J Assist Reprod Genet. 2011;28:925-30.
23. Ludwig AH, Murawska M, Panek G, Timorek A, Kupryjanczyk J. Androgen, progesterone, and FSH receptor polymorphisms in ovarian cancer risk and outcome. Endocr Relat Cancer. 2009;16:1005-16.
24. Gromoll J, Gudermann T, Nieschlag E. Molecular cloning of a truncated isoform of the human follicle stimulating hormone receptor. Biochem Biophys Res Commun. 1992;188:1077-83.
25. Song GJ, Park YS, Lee YS, Lee CC, Kang IS. Alternatively spliced variants of the follicle-stimulating hormone receptor gene in the testis of infertile men. Fertil Steril. 2002;77:499-504.
26. Gerasimova T, Thanasoula MN, Zattas D, Seli E, Sakkas D, Lalioti MD. Identification and in vitro characterization of follicle stimulating hormone (FSH) receptor variants associated with abnormal ovarian response to FSH. J Clin Endocrinol Metab. 2010;95:529-36.
27. Ledger WL, Fauser BC, Devroey P, Zandvliet AS, Mannaerts BMJL. Corifollitropin alpha doses based on body weight: clinical overview of drug exposure and ovarian response. Reprod Biomed Online. 2011;23:150-9.
28. de Greef R, Zandvliet AS, de Haan AF, Ijzerman-Boon PC, Marintcheva-Petrova M, Mannaerts BMJL. Dose selection of corifollitropin alpha by modeling and stimulation in controlled ovarian stimulation. Clin Pharmacol Ther. 2010;88:79-87.
29. Fensore S, Di Marzio M, Tiboni GM. Corifollitropin alpha compared to daily FSH in controlled ovarian stimulation for in vitro fertilization: a meta-analysis. J Ovarian Res. 2015;8:33.
30. Koechling W, Plaksin D, Croston GE, Jeppesen JV, Macklon KT, Andersen CY. Comparative pharmacology of a new recombinant FSH expressed by a human cell line. Endocr Connect. 2017;6:297-305.
31. Abd-Elaziz, Duijkers I, Stockl L, Dietrich B, Klipping C, Eckert K, et al. A new fully human recombinant FSH (follitropin epsilon): two phase I randomized placebo and comparator-controlled pharmacokinetic and pharmacodynamic trials. Hum Reprod. 2017;32(8):1639-47.
32. Lee JH, Miele ME, Hicks DJ, Phillips KK, Trent JM, Weissman BE, et al. KiSS-1, a novel human malignant melanoma metastasis-suppressor gene. J Natl Cancer Inst. 1996;88:1731-7.

33. Kotani M, Detheux M, Communi D, Communi D, Vanderwinden JM, Le Poul E, et al. The metastasis suppressor gene KiSS-1 encodes kisspeptins, the natural ligands of the orphan G protein-coupled receptor GPR54. J Biol Chem. 2001;276:34631-6.
34. Wintermantel TM, Campbell RE, Porteous R, Bock D, Gröne HJ, Todman MG, et al. Definition of estrogen receptor pathway critical for estrogen positive feedback to gonadotropin-releasing hormone neurons and fertility. Neuron. 2006;52: 271-80.
35. Gaytan F, Garcio-Galiano D, Dorfman MD, Manfredi-Lozano M, Castellano JM, Dissen GA, et al. Kisspeptin receptor haplo-insufficiency causes premature ovarian failure despite preserved gonadotropin secretion. Endocrinology. 2014; 155:3088-97.
36. Irfan S, Ehmcke J, Wahab F, Shahab M, Schlatt S. Intratesticular action of kisspeptin in rhesus monkey (*Macaca mulatta*). Andrologia. 2014;46:610-7.
37. Pinto FM, Cejudo-Roman A, Ravina CJ, Fernández-Sánchez M, Martín-Lozano D, Illanes M, et al. Characterization of kisspeptin system in human spermatozoa. Int J Androl. 2012;35:63-73.
38. Roseweir AK, Katz AA, Millar RP. Kisspeptin-10 inhibits cell migration in vitro via a receptor-GSK3 beta-FAK feedback loop in HTR8SSVneo cells. Placenta. 2012;33:408-15.
39. Cetkovic A, Miljic D, Ljubic A, Patterson M, Ghatei M, Stamenković J, et al. Plasma kisspeptin levels in pregnancies with diabetes and hypertensive disease as a potential marker of placental dysfunction and adverse perinatal outcome. Endocr Res. 2012;37:78-88.
40. Smith JT, Acohido BV, Clifton DK, Steiner RA. KiSS-1 neurons are direct targets for leptin in the ob/ob mouse. J Neuroendocrinol. 2006;18:298-303.
41. Dhillo WS, Chaudhri OB, Patterson M, Thompson EL, Murphy KG, Badman MK, et al. Kisspeptin-54 stimulates the hypothalamic-pituitary gonadal axis in human males. J Clin Endocrinol Metab. 2005;90:6609-15.
42. Chan YM, Butler JP, Pinnell NE, Pralong FP, Crowley Jr WF, Ren C, et al. Kisspeptin resets the hyptothalamic GnRH clock in men. J Clin Endocrinol Metab. 2011;96:E908-15.
43. Jayasena CN, Nijher GM, Chaudhri OB, Murphy KG, Ranger A, Lim A, et al. Subcutaneous injection of kisspeptin-54 acutely stimulates gonadotropin secretion in women with hypothalamic amenorrhea, but chronic administration causes tachyphylaxis. J Clin Endocrinol Metab. 2009;94:4315-23.
44. Araujo-Lopes R, Crampton JR, Aquino NS, Miranda RM, Kokay IC, Reis AM, et al. Prolactin regulates kisspeptin neurons in the arcuate nucleus to suppress LH secretion in female rats. Endocrinology. 2014;155:1010-20.
45. Jayasena CN, Abbara A, Alexander N, Nijher GMK, Christopoulos G, Narayanaswamy S, et al. Kisspeptin-54 triggers egg maturation in women undergoing in vitro fertilization. J Clin Invest. 2014;124:3667-77.
46. Ezzati M, Carr BR. Elagolix, a novel, orally bioavailable GnRH antagonist under investigation for the treatment of endometriosis-related pain. Womens Health (Lond). 2015; 11(1):19-28.
47. Brännström M, Johannesson L, Bokstrom H, Kvarnström N, Mölne J, Dahm-Kähler P, et al. Live birth after uterus transplantation. Lancet. 2015;385(9968):607-16.
48. Ejzenberg D, Mendes LRBC, Haddad LBP, Baracat EC, D'Albuquerque LAC, Andraus W. Uterine transplantation: a systematic review. Clinics (Sao Paulo). 2016;71(11):679-83.
49. Lefkowitz A, Edwards M, Balayla J. The Montreal criteria for the ethical feasibility of uterine transplantation. Transpl Int. 2012;25(4):439-47.
50. Azimzadeh AM, Lees JR, Ding Y, Bromberg JS. Immunobiology of transplantation: impact on targets for large and small molecules. Clin Pharmacol Ther. 2011;90:229-42.
51. Peloso A, Dhal A, Zambon JP, Li P, Orlando G, Atala A, et al. Current achievements and future perspectives in whole-organ bioengineering. Stem Cell Res Ther. 2015;6:107.
52. Badylak SF, Taylor D, Uygun K. Whole-organ tissue engineering: decellularization and recellularization of three-dimensional matrix scaffolds. Annu Rev Biomed Eng. 2011;13:27-53.
53. Scarritt ME, Pashos NC, Bunnell BA. A review of cellularization strategies for tissue engineering of whole organs. Front Bioeng Biotechnol. 2015;3:43.
54. Song JJ, Guyette J, Gilpin S, Gonzalez G, Vacanti JP, Ott HC. Regeneration and experimental orthotopic transplantation of a bioengineered kidney. Nat Med. 2013;19:646-51.
55. Raya-Rivera AM, Esquiliano D, Fierro-Pastrana R, López-Bayghen E, Valencia P, Ordorica-Flores R, et al. Tissue-engineered autologous vaginal organs in patients: a pilot cohort study. Lancet. 2014;384:329-36.
56. Partridge EA, Davey MG, Hornick MA, McGovern PE, Mejaddam AY, Vrecenak JD, et al. An extra-uterine system to physiologically support the extreme preterm lamb. Nat Comm. 2017;8:15112.
57. INVO Bioscience. Frequently asked questions. [online] Available from: https://invobioscience.com/about-us/faq/. [Last accessed March, 2018].
58. Thomson JA, Itskovitz-Eldor J, Shapiro SS, Waknitz MA, Swiergiel JJ, Marshall VS, et al. Embryonic stem cell lines derived from human blastocysts. Science. 1998;282:1145-7.
59. Amit M, Margulets V, Segev H, Shariki K, Laevsky I, Coleman R, et al. Human feeder layers for human embryonic stem cells. Biol Reprod. 2003;68:2150-6.
60. Draper JS, Smith K, Gokhale P, Moore HD, Maltby E, Johnson J, et al. Recurrent gain of chromosomes 17q and 12 in cultured human embryonic stem cells. Nat Biotechnol. 2004;22: 53-4.
61. Mann MR, Lee SS, Doherty AS, Verona RI, Nolen LD, Schultz RM, et al. Selective loss of imprinting in the placenta following preimplantation development in culture. Development. 2004;131:3727-35.
62. Zakrzewski W, Dobrzyński M, Szymonowicz M, Rybak Z. Stem cells: past, present, and future. Stem Cell Res Ther. 2019;10:68. https://doi.org/10.1186/s13287-019-1165-5.
63. Newson A, Smajdor A. Artificial gametes: new paths to parenthood? J Med Ethics. 2005;31:184-6.
64. Nayernia K, Lee JH, Lako M, Armstrong L, Herbert M, Li M, et al. In vitro derivation of human sperms from embryonic stem cells. Stem Cells Dev. 2009.
65. Easley CA, Phillips BT, McGuire MM, Barringer JM, HannaValli H, Hermann BP, et al. Direct differentiation of human pluripotent stem cell into haploid spermatogenic cells. Cell Rep. 2012;2(3):440-6.
66. Palacios-Gonzales C, Harris J, Testa G. Multiple parenting: IVG and the generations to come. J Med Ethics. 2014;40:752-8.

67. Xue Y, Chen Y, Ayub Q, Huang N, Ball EV, Mort M, et al. Deleterious- and disease-allele prevalence in healthy individuals: insights from current predictions, mutation databases, and population-scale resequencing. Am J Hum Genet. 2012;91(6):1022-32.
68. Bourne H, Douglas T, Savulescu J, Huang N, Ball EV, Mort M, et al. Procreative beneficence and in vitro gametogenesis. Monash Bioethics Rev. 2012;30(2):29-48.
69. Taylor RW, Turnbull DM. Mitochondrial DNA mutations in human disease. Nat Rev Genet. 2005;6(5):389-402.
70. Schwartz MK, Vissing J. Paternal inheritance of mitochondrial DNA. N Engl J Med. 2002;347:576-80.
71. Fischer C, Prosser R, Engelstad K, Lobo R, Sauer MV, Egli D. Toward clinical use of mitochondrial replacement therapy. Fertil Steril. 2017;108:E155.
72. Castro RJ. Mitochondrial replacement therapy: the US and UK regulatory landscapes. J Law Biosci. 2016;3(3):726-35.
73. Appleby JB. The ethical challenges of the clinical introduction of mitochondrial replacement techniques. Med Health Care Philos. 2015;18:501-14.
74. Donoho G, Jasin M, Berg P. Analysis of gene targeting and intrachromosomal homologous recombination stimulated by genomic double-strand breaks in mouse embryonic stem cells. Mol Cell Biol. 1998;18:4070-8.
75. Mojica FJM, Díez-Villaseñor C, García-Martínez J, Soria E. Intervening sequences of regularly spaced prokaryotic repeats derive from foreign genetic elements. J Mol Evol. 2005;60: 174-82.
76. Vassenna R, Heindryckx B, Peco R, Pennings G, Raya A, Sermon K, et al. Genome engineering through CRISPR/Cas9 technology in the human germline and pluripotent stem cells. Hum Reprod Update. 2016;22(4):411-9.
77. Carroll JM, Quaid KA, Stone K, Jones R, Schubert F, Griffith CB. Two is better than one: a case of homozygous myotonic dystrophy type 1. Am J Med Genet A. 2013;161A:1763-7.
78. Cai QF, Wan F, Huang R, Zhang HW. Factors predicting the cumulative outcome of IVF/ICSI treatment: a multivariable analysis of 2450 patients. Hum Reprod. 2011;26:2352-540.
79. Papanikolaou EG, Kyrou D, Zervakakou G, Paggou E, Humaidan P. Follicular hCG endometrium priming for IVF patients experiencing resisting thin endometrium. A proof of concept study. J Assist Reprod Genet. 2013;30:1341-5.
80. Prapas N, Tavaniotou A, Panagiotidis Y, Prapa S, Kasapi E, Goudakou M, et al. Low-dose human chorionic gonadotropin during the proliferative phase may adversely affect endometrial receptivity in oocyte recipients. Gynecol Endocrinol. 2009;25:53-9.
81. Rahmati M, Petitbarat M, Dubanchet S, Bensussan A, Chaouat G, Ledee N. Granulocyte-colony stimulating factor related pathways tested on an endometrial ex-vivo model. PLoS One. 2014;9:e102286.
82. Barad DH, Yu Y, Kushnir VA, Shohat-Tal A, Lazzaroni E, Lee HJ, et al. A randomized clinical trial of endometrial perfusion with granulocyte colony-stimulating factor in in vitro fertilization cycles: impact on endometrial thickness and clinical pregnancy rates. Fertil Steril. 2014;101:710-5.
83. Lee JW, Kwon H, Kim TK, Cho YK, Choi KY, Chung HY, et al. Platelet-rich plasma: quantitative assessment of growth factor levels and comparative analysis of activated and inactivated groups. Arch Plast Surg. 2013;40:530-5.
84. Chang Y, Li J, Chen Y, Wei L, Yang X, Shi Y, et al. Autologous platelet-rich plasma promotes endometrial growth and improves pregnancy outcome during in vitro fertilization. Int J Clin Exp Med. 2015;8(1):1286-90.
85. Qublan H, Amarin Z, Al-Qudah M, Diab F, Nawasreh M, Malkawi S, et al. Luteal phase support with GnRH-a improves implantation and pregnancy rates in IVF cycles with endometrium of <7mm on day of egg retrieval. Hum Fertil (Camb). 2008;11:43-7.
86. Gargette CE, Ye L. Endometrial reconstruction from stem cells. Fertil Steril. 2012;98:11-20.
87. Nagori CB, Panchal SY, Patel H. Endometrial regeneration using autologous adult stem cells followed by conception by in vitro fertilization in a patient of severe Asherman's syndrome. J Hum Reprod Sci. 2011;4:43-8.
88. Edwards RG, Lobo R, Bouchard P. Time to revolutionize ovarian stimulation. Hum Reprod. 1996;11:917-9.
89. Schipper I, Hop WC, Fauser BC. The follicle-stimulating hormone (FSH) threshold/window concept examined by different interventions with exogenous FSH during the follicular phase of the normal menstrual cycle: duration, rather than magnitude of FSH increase affects follicle development. J Clin Endocrinol Metab. 1998;83:1292-8.
90. Mitwally MFM, Casper RF. Aromatase inhibition reduces gonadotropin dose required for controlled ovarian stimulation in women with unexplained infertility. Hum Reprod. 2003;18:1588-97.
91. Verberg MFG, Macklon NS, Nargund G, Frydman R, Devroey P, Broekmans FJ, et al. Mild ovarian stimulation for IVF. Hum Reprod Update. 2009;15(1):13-29.
92. Hart RJ. Use of growth hormone in IVF of treatment of women with poor ovarian reserve. Front Endocrinol (Lausanne). 2019;10:500.
93. Norman RJ, Alvino H, Hull LM, Mol BW, Hart RJ, Kelly TL, et al. Human growth hormone for poor responders: a randomized placebo-controlled trial provides no evidence for improved live birth rate. Reprod Biomed Online. 2019;38:908-15.
94. Papanikolaou E, Timotheou E, Tatsi P, Chartomatsidou T, Najdecki R. Long antagonist protocol; luteal administration of a single dose of degarelix (long-acting GnRH-antagonist) for controlled ovarian stimulation. A new protocol for IVF. Fertil Steril. 2018;110:E336-7.
95. Ubaldi FM, Capalbo A, Vaiarelli A, Cimadomo D, Colamaria S, Alviggi C, et al. Follicular versus luteal phase ovarian stimulation during the same menstrual cycle (DuoStim) in a reduced ovarian reserve population results in a similar euploid blastocyst formation rate: new insight in ovarian reserve exploitation. Fertil Steril. 2016;105:1488-95.e1.
96. Vaiarelli A, Cimadomo D, Conforti A, Schimberni M, Giuliani M, D'Alessandro P, et al. Luteal phase stimulation after conventional stimulation in the same ovarian cycle might improve the management of poor responder patients fulfilling the Bologna criteria: a case series. Fertil Steril. 2020;113:121-30.
97. Berkovitz A, Eltes F, Ellenbogen A, Peer S, Feldberg D, Bartoov B, et al. Does the presence of nuclear vacuoles in human sperm selected for ICSI affect pregnancy outcome? Hum Reprod. 2006;21:1787-90.
98. Tasaka A, Doshida M, Sato Y, Kyoya T, Nakajo Y, Kyono K, et al. Outcome of IMSI (intracytoplasmic morphologically selected sperm injection) in patients with repeated ICSI failures. Fertil Steril. 2009;92(3);S76.

99. Figueira RCS, Setti A, Braga D, Pasqualotto F, Iaconelli Jr A, Borges Jr E, et al. Intracytoplasmic morphologically morphologically-selected sperm injection (IMSI) benefits on severe male factor profiled according to the 2010 WHO reference values. Fertil Steril. 2010;94(4):S14.
100. Zukin VD, OO Barash. Effectiveness of ART treatment using ICSI and IMSI in sibling oocyte study. Fertil Steril. 2008;90:S12.
101. Sauerbrun-Cutler MT, Ozensoy S, Vega M, Keltz M. Does PICSI offer an advantage over ICSI in ART for patients with male factor. Fertil Steril. 2013;100:S516.
102. Alegre L, Garrido N, Munoz M, de los Santos M, Remohi Gimenez J, Meseguer M. Sperm selection with hyaluronic acid (PICSI) improves LBR in IVF treatments. Fertil Steril. 2017;108:E130.
103. Alegre L, Garrido N, Romero J, Palma AE, Remohi Gimenez J, Meseguer M. Embryo quality is improved by PICSI sperm selection. A randomized controlled trial. Fertil Steril. 2016;106:E307.
104. Ainsworth C, Nixon B, Aitken RJ. Development of a novel electrophoretic system for the isolation of human spermatozoa. Hum Reprod. 2005;20:2261-70.
105. Aitken RJ, Buckingham DW, Brindle J, Gomez E, Baker HW, Irvine DS. Analysis of sperm movement in relation to oxidative stress created by leucocytes in washed sperm preparations and seminal plasma. Hum Reprod. 1995;10:2061-71.
106. Kirchhoff C, Schröter S. New insights into the origin, structure and role of CD52: a major component of the mammalian sperm glycocalyx. Cells Tissues Organs. 2001;168:93-104.
107. Gil M, Sar-Shalom V, Carreras R, Carreras R, Checa MA. Sperm selection using magnetic activated cell sorting (MACS) in assisted reproduction: a systematic review and meta-analysis. J Assist Reprod Genet. 2013;30:479-85.
108. Bochev I, Gavrilov P, Kyurkchiev S, Shterev A. 27th Annual Meeting of the European Society on Human Reproduction and Embryology (ESHRE). Sperm motility improvement after magnetic-activated cell sorting in men with astheno/oligo-asthenozoospermia. Hum Reprod. 2011;26:i133.
109. Sato H, Ellis GW, Inoué S. Microtubular origin of meiotic spindle from birefringence. Demonstration of the applicability of Wiener's equation. J Cell Biol. 1975;67:501-17.
110. Eichenlaub-Ritter U, Shen Y, Tinneberg HR. Manipulation of the oocyte: possible damage to the spindle apparatus. Reprod Biomed Online. 2002;5:117-24.
111. Sun XF, Wang WH, Keefe DL. Overheating is detrimental to meiotic spindles within in vitro matured human oocytes. Zygote. 2004;12:65-70.
112. Korkmaz C, Baykal B, Ceyhan ST, Mutlu Ercan C, Muslu Bal E, Seferbay S, et al. Long term analysis of polscope data from Gülhane Military Medical Faculty ART Center. Reprod Biomed Online. 2014;28:S20-21.
113. Moon JH, Henderson S, Gaqrcia-Cerrudo E, Mahfoudh A, Reinblatt S, Son WY. Successful live birth after transfer of blastocyst and frozen blastocyst from rescue ICSI with application of polarized light microscopy for spindle examination on unfertilized eggs. J Ovarian Res. 2015;8:22.
114. Tesarik J, Mendoza C, Greco E. The activity (with calcium oscillator?) responsible for human oocyte activation after injection with round spermatids is associated with spermatic nuclei. Fertil Steril. 2000;74:1245-7.
115. Heindryckx B, Van der Elst J, De Sutter P, Dhont M. Treatment option for sperm- or oocyte-related fertilization failure: assisted oocyte activation following diagnostic heterologous ICSI. Hum Reprod. 2005;2(8):2237-41.
116. Grasa P, Coward K, Young C, Parrington J. The pattern of localization of the putative oocyte activation factor, phospholipase Czeta, in uncapacitated, capacitated, and ionophore-treated human spermatozoa. Hum Reprod. 2008;23(11):2513-22.
117. Vanderzwalmen P, Lejeune B, Nijs M, Segal-Bertin G, Vandamme B, Schoysman R. Fertilization of an oocyte microinseminated with a spermatid in an in-vitro fertilization programme. Hum Reprod. 1995;10:502-3.
118. Kovacs P. Embryo selection: the role of time-lapse monitoring. Reprod Biol Endocrinol. 2014;12:124.

CHAPTER 80

Uterine Transplantation: Research, Techniques, and Results

Mats Brännström, Jana EJ Pittman

INTRODUCTION

Prior to the successful evolvement of uterus transplantation (UTx), as a treatment option for women with absolute uterine factor infertility (AUFI), these women were considered unconditionally infertile. Women with AUFI have either a congenital/surgical uterine absence or a uterine abnormality (anatomic/functional) that impedes embryo implantation or further pregnancy.[1] It is estimated that the prevalence of AUFI is around 20,000 women of fertile age, in a total population of 100 million.[2] Gestational surrogacy can provide genetic and, after adoption from the gestational carrier, also legal motherhood. However, in most countries, gestational surrogacy is either prohibited or highly restricted due to ethical, religious, and/or legal reasons. For a woman with AUFI who desire motherhood, UTx allows the ability to be both a gestational and genetic mother.

A uterine allograft is unique from all other organ transplants. It is a type of vascularized composite allograft (VCA) transplantation, like the hand and face. However, the donor can be either a live donor (LD) or a deceased donor (DD), in the case of UTx, but for other VCAs, only the DD alternative is available. Furthermore, the uterus graft is an ephemeral organ, as the allograft will be removed when the woman has achieved the desired number of children or after a specified time to reduce the risk of side effects associated with immunosuppression (IS). Unlike other solid organ transplants, the blood flow of the graft will be shared by mother and fetus. While surgical success (SS) of a UTx procedure can be determined soon after transplantation by the three findings of normal blood flow, cervical biopsies with no signs of necrosis, and menstruations, the determination of overall success is prolonged until a live birth occurs. Consequently, it will typically take at least 1.5 years after the Utx procedure until it can be concluded that the transplantation was successful.

The world's first human UTx case was an LD UTx case performed in Saudi Arabia in 2000, but this pioneering surgical procedure was not successful and ended in removal of a necrotic graft 99 days after transplantation.[3] This first case of human UTx sheds light on the issue that animal-based research is needed before a possible reintroduction in humans and stimulated several centers around the world to start research activities within the field. The evolution of UTx, from basic animal studies toward clinical application, has then followed both Moore criteria[4] and IDEAL recommendations[5] for the introduction of major surgical innovations.

ANIMAL RESEARCH IN UTERUS TRANSPLANTATION

Animal UTx research, performed during the last two decades, has paved the way for clinical UTx trials. The research has involved all classical experimental animals and followed a well-established sequential approach in each animal species, testing and improving multiple factors of importance for the development of a safe and effective UTx procedure for human use. The central aspects of surgery and fertility outcomes in the important UTx models are discussed below.

Surgery in Animal Models

Surgery of UTx has to be accustomed to the size of the vasculature and the opportunity to accomplish vascular connections. In the rodent models (mouse, rat), DD UTx models were developed since central parts of the vascular tree (aorta, caval vein, common iliac vessels) had to be harvested alongside the uterine graft, in order to gain large enough vessels to undertake the vascular anastomoses. The mouse UTx model was with the uterine graft transplanted into a heterotopic position in the upper abdomen, with end-to-side caval–caval and aortic–aortic vascular anastomoses.[6] In the rat, with considerably larger sizes of blood vessels and uterus, a model was developed to place the uterus orthotopically and perform end-to-side anastomoses between the common iliacs of the graft and the recipient.[7]

The sheep has been the most commonly used large-domestic species in animal UTx research. This model was originally explored as an autologous UTx model with anastomoses of the anterior branch of the internal iliac artery and the complete utero-ovarian vein of the graft end-to-side to the external iliac vessels.[8] To allow for fertility studies in this autologous model, with the inclusion of undisturbed blood flow to the utero-tubal-ovarian unit, surgery was later modified to also include the ovarian artery, which, by a patch, was anastomosed to the aorta.[9] In an allogeneic LD ovine UTx model, end-to-end anastomosis of the uterine vessels was performed, but this model necessitated simultaneous hysterectomy surgery in the recipient, in order to have pedicles of uterine vessels of the recipient to carry out the anastomoses of the uterine vessels.[10] The latter model was tested as an LD UTx concept, with the uterus switched within pairs of sheep. The DD sheep UTx model involves anastomosis with a caval-aortal macrovascular patch technique.[11]

Uterus transplantation models have also been developed in nonhuman primate species. The importance of that is the near-human anatomy and physiology of these species. The initial nonhuman primate UTx model was the autologous baboon model with surgery involving a side-to-side fusion of the internal iliac arteries and the ovarian veins of the graft on the back table and then unilateral end-to-side anastomosis to the external iliac vessels.[12] By adapting minor modifications, the functionality, in terms of menstruation, increased threefold in this auto-UTx model.[13] In the LD allogeneic baboon model,[14] vessel anastomosis was end-to-side to the external iliac vessels as described above. The baboon DD UTx model, to carry out allogeneic UTx, utilized a macrovascular aortic-caval patch technique which was anastomosed on the subrenal aorta and vena cava of the recipient.[15] The cynomolgus macaque is the nonhuman primate species which has been most widely used in UTx research. The anatomy of this species is similar to the baboon and the human, but since the body size is only around a third of the baboon, surgery is more challenging. Initially, an autologous UTx model was developed in the cynomolgus macaque, with the uterus retrieved together with bilateral uterine arteries and the deep uterine veins and anastomoses on the external iliacs.[16] The dissection of deep uterine veins was complex, and the technique was modified to use the ovarian veins as outflow vessels, resulting in a considerably shorter surgical time.[17] Furthermore, surgery of DD UTx was performed in the cynomolgus macaque and in this allogeneic setting, a comparison was made with models including retrievals of either the common iliacs or parts of the aorta/vena cava.[18] Anastomoses were performed on the corresponding vessels.

Fertility in Animal Models

Fertility is the important endpoint of UTx, and thus it is essential to evaluate this component in UTx, which may be autologous, syngeneic, or allogeneic transplantation. In the animal models that have been explored, the autologous and syngeneic models have initially been tested for fertility and those experiments, in nonrejection settings, have then been followed by allogeneic transplantation models. Allogeneic transplantations would need IS treatment to prevent rejection. Several UTx-specific factors may affect the fertility potential such as changed uterine position, denervation, altered blood flow and outlet, and naturally negative side effects of IS.

The first demonstration of pregnancy in a UTx model was in a syngeneic transplantation model between inbred mice, with no need for IS, since the donor and recipients had full histocompatibility.[19] In this initial study, with the uterus in a heterotopic position and the cervix positioned intra-abdominally, only occasional early pregnancies were seen after transmyometrial embryo transfer (ET). The reason for a low pregnancy rate was most likely damaging effects on the endometrium, secondary to accumulation of cervical mucus within the uterine cavity.[19] The mouse UTx model was then modified with a cervical cutaneous stroma, which allowed proper drainage of mucus.[6] In that syngeneic model, the pregnancy rate per uterus was equal in the transplanted uteri as compared to the native control uteri and also in comparison to the uteri of nontransplanted animals with sham operations.[6] The pregnancies went to term. Weights of offspring and growth trajectory up to adulthood were normal. No studies on fertility after allogeneic UTx in the mouse have been performed.

In the rat UTx model, fertility was first tested in a syngeneic setting between inbred rats, with no need for IS.[20] In this syngeneic model, the pregnancy rate and the number of pups per pregnancy were similar in transplanted animals as in sham-operated control animals. Furthermore, the growth trajectory of offspring was similar in offspring from the UTx group and the control group. Fertility after allogeneic UTx was first reported in a rat model, with discordances between two major histocompatibility sites.[21] Tacrolimus IS was given via mini-osmotic pumps. The pregnancy rates, assed around pregnancy date 13, were comparable in the UTx group and in the control group.[21] In a follow-up study, with another allogeneic combination of rats and tacrolimus as IS, the pregnancies went to term.[22] The pregnancy rate was somewhat lower in the UTx group as compared to the two sham-operated control groups. However, birth weights of UTx offspring and growth trajectory of the pups until postnatal week 16 were unaffected in comparison to controls.[22]

The first large-animal UTx model to be tested for fertility was the sheep, and initial experiments were performed in an autologous UTx model. This autologous UTx model was with uterine-tubal-ovarian transplantation and end-to-side vascular anastomoses of the uterine artery, utero-ovarian vein, and ovarian artery, including an aortic patch, to the external iliacs.[9] The reason for transplanting the uterine-tubal-ovarian en bloc was to allow for natural mating and conception. Conception occurred spontaneously and offspring of normal sizes were delivered by cesarean section, around 2 weeks before term.[9] The allogeneic sheep UTx model involved surgery, where the uteri were switched between two animals and with cyclosporine as IS.[23] After ET in five ewes, pregnancies were seen in three animals. A live birth occurred via cesarean section at day 138 of pregnancy. This was the first birth after allogeneic UTx in a large animal.[23]

Concerning fertility in UTx models of nonhuman primates, experiments have only been conducted in the cynomolgus macaque. In the first study on fertility after auto-UTx, two animals underwent UTx with unilateral preservation of the oviduct and the ovary and anastomoses between the uterine arteries and the external iliac arteries bilaterally, with venous outflows of deep uterine vein and ovarian vein ipsilaterally.[24] Menstruation resumed spontaneously and pregnancy occurred post three menstruations and after spontaneous mating. Prematurely, around 3 weeks before expected delivery, a cesarean section was performed due to bleeding and partial placental abruption. A live offspring was delivered but with fetal respiratory distress.[24] No attempts were done to secure further survival of the fetus. This birth, which was reported already in 2012, was very important for the field of UTx and the coming human clinical trials (see below), since it was a proof-of-concept of live birth after UTx in a primate. The same Japanese team published in 2020[25] the first live birth in a nonhuman primate species after allogeneic UTx. Although this was a great accomplishment, the importance for the UTx field was less than the live birth after auto-UTx in macaque from 2012,[24] since human UTx had already been proven successful, with five live births reported already in the interval from 2014 to 2016 within the first human UTx trial,[26,27] as further discussed in a section below. Allogeneic UTx was performed between major histocompatibility complex (MHC)-defined cynomolgus macaques, which were haploidentical, thus providing a semi-allogenic transplantation setting.[25] Anastomoses were end-to-side aortal-aortal and caval-caval at an infrarenal site, with transplantations carried out in six animals. The IS was induction with both antithymocyte globulin and rituximab and then triple maintenance IS. Although donor-specific antibodies, posttransplantation lymphoproliferative disease, and two spontaneous abortions after ET occurred in one specific animal, this animal became successfully pregnant around 2 years after UTx. A cesarean section was performed at full-term and the offspring was healthy. This birth represents the first and the only birth after UTx in an allogeneic nonhuman primate model.

SURGICAL TECHNIQUES IN HUMAN UTERUS TRANSPLANTATION

A number of clinical UTx trials have been initiated, involving either LD UTx procedures or DD UTx procedures and in some comparative trials, inclusion of both LD UTx and DD UTx. This first section provides an overview of the different surgical techniques in LDs, DDs, and recipients, where it has been an evolution from classical laparotomy, toward the introduction of minimal invasive surgery (MIS). The results of the trials are summarized in sections further below.

Laparotomic Uterus Procurement in Live Donor

The classical approach of organ retrieval in LD UTx is by laparotomy. The technique has been described in detail[26] and a briefer description is given below. The laparotomic uterus retrieval in LD UTx starts with a subumbilical, midline abdominal incision. To ensure long ligaments on the graft, for later fixation in the recipient, the round ligaments are divided laterally and tagged. Subsequently, using monopolar diathermy, a large bladder flap, nearly to the bladder dome, is dissected. This peritoneal sheet is created to cover the vesicouterine fossa and for fixation in the recipient, by suturing the sheet on top of the bladder at transplantation. The surgery then moves toward the pelvic sidewalls. The initial focus is to isolate and dissect the ureters. Complete ureterolysis, from around 2 cm below the iliac crossing until the inlet into the bladder, should be performed, which also includes dissection of the ureteric tunnel. At dissection of the ureteric tunnel, care must be taken not to cause any injury to the uterine artery, passing over the ureter, and handle the thinned-wall deep uterine veins, which often ride under the ureter, in a delicate fashion. Several venous plexuses are firmly attached to the ureters and must be gently dissected off the ureter. The surgery should advance equally on both sides. Once the ureters are free, the focus moves to the arterial supply of the graft. In most cases, only one major arterial segment remains with the graft on each side and that segment is mostly made up of the complete major trunk of the anterior portion of the internal iliac artery. All other branches from the anterior iliac artery are ligated and transected, and these distinct branches include the iliolumbar artery and pudendal artery. Importantly, to ensure uncompromised blood flow to the gluteal muscles, the gluteal artery, which commonly is the first major posterior branch of the internal iliac artery, should be preserved in the donor. Subsequently, venous dissection begins, which is challenging and time-consuming. Venous anatomy differs substantially between each donor, and there may be one or two large deep uterine veins bilaterally and they will reach the internal iliac veins on the pelvic side wall just above the pelvic floor. The venous vascular pedicles should include segments of the internal iliac veins, which ensure wider vessel diameters for anastomoses in the recipient and thereby decrease the risk of venous thrombosis over the anastomosis line. The dissection approach of the distal part of the deep uterine veins is preferably from the pelvic sidewalls toward the graft. Lastly, the rectovaginal space is opened to separate the upper, posterior parts of the vagina from the rectum, and the remaining ligaments, including the sacrouterine ligaments, are divided. The small vaginal arteries are also divided in the paravaginal tissue and the vagina is then transected by scissors and bipolar diathermy. To ensure an uncomplicated vaginal–vaginal end-to-end anastomosis during recipient surgery, at least 20 mm of a vaginal rim should be included in the graft. The large vessels are then clamped and divided, starting with the internal iliac arteries and then the veins. The graft, with long vascular pedicles, is then taken to the back table for chilling and flushing.

Robotic-assisted Uterus Procurement in Live Donor

The robotic donor surgery approach has become more widely used in LD hysterectomy. The methodology has recently been described in detail and with illustrative material.[28] A brief description of donor hysterectomy by robotics is given below. It is recommended that two experienced robotic surgeons, preferably one gynecologist and one transplantation surgeon, should work in collaboration in dual consoles by a four-arm setup. The robotic instruments which are recommended include Maryland bipolar forceps, monopolar curved scissors, a large needle driver, a clip applier for medium and large clips, ProGrasp forceps, and a vessel sealer. In most cases, additional laparoscopic ports are also used to enable a laparoscopic surgeon to assist to apply clips on vessels and for retraction of tissue. Before docking, the donor is placed in a steep Trendelenburg (up to 28°) position and then 45° side-docking, toward the hip of the donor, is performed to provide access to the vaginal route for alternate uterine positioning during surgery. This is performed by an assisting surgeon, using a hand-held, atraumatic vaginal probe, which does not cause any damage to the cervical canal. Initially, the surgery involves isolating the large bladder peritoneal flap for subsequent fixation in the recipient, followed by divisions of the round ligaments. Differing from laparotomy, it is recommended to concentrate dissection on one side of the graft at a time and to continue on one side until the ureter and the vessels are fully dissected. The unilateral dissection will start with the identification and gross dissection of the uterine arteries, anterior portions of internal iliac arteries, and umbilical arteries. Subsequently to this, complex ureteric isolation is performed, requiring delicate dissection in the ureteric tunnel and also separating the ureter from its attachments, caudally of the crossing of the uterine artery. Bipolar diathermy and scissors should be used with dissection at a fair distance from the ureter, in order to avoid thermal ureteric injury. There exist venous irregularities and uterine veins and their branches are well hidden within the tissue. A ureteric stent may aid in the dissection and fluorescent dye could help to identify the vessels that are hidden in the tissue. Once the ureter is fully isolated, the surgery focuses on the dissection of the internal iliac vein in the region of the inlet of the deep uterine vein(s). Following full mobilization of the ureter, the finer dissection of the uterine artery should be performed, with prolongation to include the anterior portion of the internal iliac artery. All branches of the internal iliac artery are dissected and transected after securing blood flow. Hemoclips, with a securing suture, or titanium clips are placed on either side of the transections, depending on the size of the vessels. Then the deep uterine vein is dissected free from the paravaginal tissue, so it is fully mobilized until the inlet into the deep uterine vein. All steps are then repeated on the contralateral side. On completion of both pelvic sidewalls, dissection of proximal parts of the utero-ovarian vein from the corner of the uterus up until the ovarian branch of the utero-ovarian vein is performed to secure additional venous outflow. The pouch of Douglas is then dissected, with separation of the rectum from the posterior vagina and including division of the sacrouterine ligaments. By alternate use of bipolar diathermy and scissors, the vagina is transected, leaving a cuff on the graft of around 2 cm for attachment to the recipient vaginal tissue. Finally, as with the laparotomy, the six vascular pedicles are clamped (often with a laparoscopic staple instrument) and transected. The graft is then placed in a sterile laparoscopic specimen bag and extracted through the vagina. The vaginal cuff is closed by a V-lock suture and the large vessels are secured. All instruments and ports are then extracted and the port sites on the skin are sutured accordingly.

Uterus Procurement in Deceased Donor

For obvious reasons, only laparotomic uterus procurement for the DD is performed. The recovery of the uterus graft from a DD is often part of a multiorgan donor retrieval process. The donor hysterectomy in DD has been described in detail[29] and is briefly outlined below. A large midline incision is usually performed from the xiphisternum to the pubic symphysis and for greater access to the pelvis, the incision can include bilateral inguinal extensions. The ureters are ligated, transected, and tagged (to mark the uterine artery location). Following this, the round ligaments are also ligated, transected, and tagged. The bladder flap is then extensively dissected, taking care not to damage the uterine veins which may curve upward close to the lateral aspects of the bladder. At the level of the distal common iliac vessels, the internal iliac artery and vein dissections begin, taking the vessels caudally. The gluteal, obturator, and inferior rectal branches of the internal iliac artery are all ligated. After vessel dissection, the rectovaginal space is opened, and good lengths of the uterosacral ligaments are preserved for use as fixation points in the recipient. The external iliac arteries should be exposed for catheterization to enable separate flushing of the uterus, while the other organs are flushed through the aorta. After procurement of thoracic and abdominal organs, with the uterus being flushed and cooled during this procedure via the femoral artery catheters, uterus procurement can begin. The vagina is transected, and the internal iliac vessels are clamped and ligated before removing the graft to the back table.

Uterus Transplantation by Laparotomy

Recipient surgery is typically done by laparotomy. In laparotomic transplantation into the recipient,[26] a subumbilical midline incision is performed and the external iliac vessels are dissected with veins and arteries separated. In patients with the Mayer–Rokitansky–Küster–Hauser (MRKH) syndrome, further dissection of the pelvic sidewall structures, including the round ligament, may be required due to presence of rudimentary uterine-tissue buds, typically positioned between the round ligament and the external iliac vein. In the MRKH patient, which so far has been the typical UTx patient, the vaginal vault is prepared, often with the use of a vaginal probe which is pushed in the direction of the umbilicus. This is necessary to expose the vaginal vault, which typically is hidden under a midline, uterine rudiment as well as the overfolding bladder. The midline rudiment is cleaved down to the fascia, which is overlaying the vault and the rectum is then separated from the posterior of the vagina. An area of the vaginal vault of about 50 mm longitudinally and 40 mm transversely should be freed from the bladder and rectum for subsequent vaginal–vaginal anastomosis. The chilled graft is then positioned inside the pelvis, and end-to-side vascular anastomoses are performed between the internal iliac segments of the graft and the external iliacs of the recipient, starting with the vein and then moving onto the artery on one side at a time. The vagina is then opened by monopolar diathermy in the midline and the vaginal vault of the recipient is secured to the vaginal rim of the graft by end-to-end fashion. Uterine fixation is then performed to the round ligaments, cleaved midline rudiments, and sacrouterine ligaments. Noteworthy, in patients post subtotal hysterectomy, the cervical stump should be removed or in women who have a normal-sized but nonfunctional uterus, such as a patient with Asherman's syndrome, a total hysterectomy will need to be performed as part of the preparatory surgery of the recipient. In both these cases, it is important that the vagina is closed temporarily to avoid transcending infection.

Uterus Transplantation by Robotic-assisted Laparoscopy

Fully robotic-assisted transplantation of the uterus in the recipient was introduced by the Swedish team in 2021. For this robotic implantation procedure, a similar setup is used as per the donor hysterectomy (four-arm robot, dual consoles, similar instruments, two robotic surgeons, and a laparoscopist). Additionally, one extra assisting surgeon is required to maneuver the vaginal probe during vault preparation. The surgical procedure starts with the preparation of the recipient vessels for the anastomosis. The surgery is then directed toward the vaginal vault, where anatomical variations exist depending on the cause for uterine infertility, as outlined in the paragraph above. The rectum and bladder are then gently separated from the vagina and the chilled graft is brought into the abdomen through a small supraumbilical midline incision, which is covered by a GelPort. One significant difference in the robotic transplantation, as compared to the laparotomic implantation of the uterus, is the recommendation for only two venous and two arterial end-to-side anastomoses in robotics, since anastomosis surgery will be prolonged in the robot and rewarming ischemia should not be extended. Anastomoses are by two continuous sutures on each anastomosis using Gore-Tex, CV-6. On each side, the deeper-positioned vein is the first site for anastomosis. End-to-end vaginal anastomosis is then performed by V-lock sutures after a sagittal opening of the vaginal has been accomplished. Fixation is by suturing the end of the round ligaments to the remnants of the round ligament, and the bladder flap is sutured to the top of the recipient bladder rather than via several ligamentous fixation points as in laparotomic implantation.

RESULTS OF THE ONLY COMPLETED HUMAN UTERUS TRANSPLANTATION TRIAL

The first registered UTx clinical trial was initiated in Sweden in 2012, including nine LD UTx procedures, with recipient age range of 27–38 years.[26] This is so far the only trial with completed reproduction,[27] after hysterectomies of the grafts[30]) within the time frame of up to 6.5 years after UTx. One recipient had acquired AUFI after a radical hysterectomy for cervical cancer and the remaining eight had MRKH syndrome. This is a congenital syndrome, with uterine and upper vaginal aplasia in a female with normal karyotype and normal secondary sex characteristics.[31] The LDs were either genetically related (mother, sister, maternal aunt) or close family friend (mother-in-law, friend). The donors were 37–62 years old and five of the nine donors were postmenopausal.[26] Comprehensive medical and psychological investigations were completed in all recipients, partners, and donors.[26,32] Uterus recovery by laparotomy was lengthy and had durations of 10.5–13 hours.[26] The deep uterine veins and uterine arteries on the graft were procured with segments of the internal iliac arteries and in a few procedures, portions of the utero-ovarian veins, between the uterus and ovary, were harvested. Pre- and postoperative outcomes of LDs were favorable, but with one case of a ureteric-vaginal fistula which necessitated ureteric reimplantation surgery repaired 3 months postuterus donation.[26] All donors were in good psychological and medical health at follow-up 1 year after surgery.[33] The duration of recipient surgery was 4–5 hours, including dissection of the external iliacs and preparation of the vaginal vault. SS, defined as a viable graft 1 month after transplant, was evident in seven out of nine grafts.[26] Graft failures because of immediate vascular thrombosis in one case and hypoperfusion with secondary infection occurred in two cases within the first months.[26,30] The psychosocial health of the recipient and their partners were in general fine during the first posttransplantation year, although initial worries concerning rejection were seen during this time frame.[34] Single ETs were to be performed from around 12 months after UTx in the seven patients with successful UTx procedures. Further follow-up of psychological health of donors during years two and three showed that they were relatively stable regarding health-related quality of life, mood, and marital relationship, but slight negative deviations existed in some patients, with possible associations with older age and continued nonpregnancy results from their donations.[35] Concerning the psychological health of recipients and their partners during the interval from 1 year after transplantation to 3 years after transplantation, it was evident that graft failure and failure to achieve parenthood pose psychological strains on couples during this time period after transplantation.[36]

The world's first human live birth after UTx was reported from the Swedish trial in September 2014, when a boy was born in gestational week 31+6, after a pregnancy that was complicated by preeclampsia.[37] The Swedish trial, with surgeries in 2012–2013, is the first UTx trial to present full data of reproductive and obstetrical outcomes.[27] The complete dataset is from the seven women with surgically successful graft after UTx and with initiated ETs from 12 months after transplantation. Six of the seven women had in total nine live births, with three women giving birth twice. Five out of nine live births were after the transfer of day 5 (D5) embryos and the same number of live births were from in vitro fertilization (IVF) treatments after UTx. One patient, a woman who never achieved a live birth, underwent 16 ETs, which resulted in six miscarriages, some as late as gestational week 15. The overall clinical pregnancy rate (CPR) per ET was 32.6% and the live birth rate (LBR) per ET was 19.6% in the seven women undergoing ETs. The total LBR is lower than in a usual IVF population, with possible explanations being that one out of seven women had a very high number of implantation failures or miscarriages and that as many as 76% ETs were with day 2 (D2) embryos. A subgroup analysis of ETs of D2 and D5 embryos showed that LBRs per ET were 8.6% for D2 and 45.4% for D5 in the seven women undergoing ET and 12.5% for D2 and 83.3% for D5 in the six women who gave birth. The cumulative LBR for the seven women with viable grafts was 85.7%.[27] The nine children were all delivered by cesarean section and deliveries were either per protocol (n = 5; range 35+0 to 38+0) or due to obstetric complication (n = 4; range 31+6 to 35+3). The obstetric complications which caused acute delivery were preeclampsia in three women and intrahepatic cholestasis of pregnancy in one woman. The weight deviations [median (range)] were –1% (–13 to +23%) and Apgar scores (1 and 5 minutes) were 9 (3–9) and 10 (8–10). Four of nine neonates developed mild respiratory distress syndrome and they were all born in the interval 31+6 to 35+0. The growth trajectories and health follow-up for the first 2 years were normal for all children. Longer follow-up studies of UTx children have not yet been published.

RESULTS OF UNCOMPLETED STUDIES AND SINGLE CASES OF UTERUS TRANSPLANTATION

There exist a number of UTx studies that have been initiated worldwide, with some presenting interim results of as many as 20 procedures and some that have only published results of single cases. The number of published UTx studies/cases, where information of SS can be extracted, is so far 67 procedures **(Table 1)**. SS is defined as a graft with uncompromised blood flow during the initial months after UTx and with resumed menstruations, as signs of functionality. Two menstruations should be seen so, typically, it will be at least 2–4 months after UTx until success or no success can be decided. Concerning reproductive and obstetrical outcomes, it is not meaningful to look at these parameters until a study is completed, by graft removal, in all patients of the study cohort. Thus, interim results concerning reproduction and obstetrics are not further discussed in the section below, which focus on reported cases, SS, and postoperative complications in LDs and recipients.

One case report warrants special attention and this is the first published live birth after DD donor UTx, with the birth taking place in Brazil in late 2017.[38] A 32-year-old woman with MRKH received a uterus from a 45-year-old DD, with brain death due to subarachnoid bleeding. Pregnancy occurred at the second single ET, which was 7 months post-UTx. The pregnancy was uneventful and delivery was by cesarean section in gestational week 35+3. The neonate was healthy. The uterus was removed in the same surgical procedure as the delivery.

As shown in **Table 1**, LD UTx procedures have involved donor hysterectomy by laparotomy (n = 33), robotic-assisted laparoscopy (n = 17), and traditional laparoscopy

TABLE 1: Summary of published (n = 67) cases of uterus transplantation (UTx). Data on surgical success (SS), rate of major (≥Clavien–Dindo class 3) postoperative live donor complications (DC), and rate of major (≥Clavien–Dindo class 3) surgery-related postoperative complications in recipients with successful grafts (RC).

Type of UTx	*Country*	*UTx year(s)*	*n*	*RC*	*SS*	*DC*
DD	Turkey	2011	1	0/1	1/1	–
DD	Czech Republic	2016–2018	5	2/3	3/5	–
DD	USA	2016–2018	6	1/4	4/6	–
DD	Brazil	2016	1	0/1	1/1	–
LD laparotomy	Saudi Arabia	2000	1	0/1	1/1	0/1
LD laparotomy	Sweden	2012–2013	9	0/7	7/9	0/9
LD laparotomy	Germany	2016–2019	4	0/4	4/4	0/4
LD laparotomy	Czech Republic	2016–2018	5	1/4	4/5	2/5
LD laparotomy	USA	2016–2019	13	1/8	8/13	2/13
LD laparotomy	Lebanon	2018	1	0/1	1/1	0/1
LD robotics	China	2015	1	0/1	1/1	0/1
LD robotics	Sweden	2017–2019	8	0/6	6/8	1/8
LD robotics	USA	2016–2019	5	0/5	5/5	2/5
LD robotics	France	2019	1	0/1	1/1	1/1
LD robotics	Spain	2020	1	0/1	1/1	0/1
LD robotics	Brazil	2021	1	0/1	1/1	0/1
LD laparoscopy	India	2018–2019	4	0/4	4/4	0/4
Summary		2000–2021	67	5/53	53/67	8/54

(DD: deceased donor; LD: live donor)

(n = 4). Thirteen DD UTx procedures have been reported **(Table 1)**. The 31 LD UTx procedures by laparotomy have been reported from trials/cases in Saudi Arabia,[3] Sweden,[26] Germany,[39] Czech Republic,[40] Lebanon,[41] and USA.[42] The 17 LD UTx procedures by robotic-assisted laparoscopy have been reported from trials/cases in China,[43] Sweden,[28,44] USA,[42] Spain,[45] France,[46] and Brazil.[47] The four LD UTx procedures by traditional laparoscopy have been reported from one trial in India.[48,49] The 13 DD UTx procedures have been performed in Turkey,[50] Czech Republic,[40] USA,[42,51-53] and Brazil.[38]

Table 1 summarizes SS, defined as a graft with uncompromised blood flow during the initial 3–4 months after UTx and with resumed menstruations. **Table 1** also provides information on the rate of major surgery-related postoperative complications in LDs and recipients. The distinction of a major postoperative complication is based on the Clavien–Dindo (CD) score system,[54] where we have chosen to classify complications higher than CD 2 as major **(Table 1)**. Grade 3 includes complications requiring radiological, endoscopic, or surgical intervention. Grade 4 includes complications involving single-organ dysfunction or multiorgan dysfunction.

Concerning SS, the overall success rate was 79%, which has to be considered acceptable in this new type of transplantation, which involves complex surgery both in the LD and the recipient. There are too few cases published yet to determine if the SS is higher in any type of Utx, and it has to be taken into consideration that there is a learning curve in this type of surgery. Major postsurgical complications in recipients occurred in 9% of the surgically successful procedures. The complications were mostly related to occurrence of vaginal stenosis over the anastomosis line between the vaginal vault of the recipient and the vaginal rim of the graft. This complication was seen in recipients of both LD UTx and DD UTx procedures. Vaginal stenosis is corrected by dilatation or vaginal surgery, or a combination of these.

Rejection episodes occur in a majority of the UTx procedures and they are commonly subclinical and diagnosed on histology of cervical biopsies.[55] The rejection episodes are reversed by corticosteroid treatment or by an increased dose of maintenance IS.

The rate of major postoperative complications in LDs was 15% and they were distributed equally between procedures by laparotomy and robotics. A majority of these postoperative complications in LDs have been related to the ureters, with ureteric laceration, ureteric-vaginal fistula, and hydronephrosis reported.

TABLE 2: Reported pregnancies with live births (n = 35) after uterus transplantation.

	Week of live birth	*Pregnancy complication*	*Indication for delivery*	*Apgar (1/5 minutes)*	*Neonatal complication*
LD laparotomy (Sweden)	31+6	PE	PE	9/10	RDS
	34+4	ICP	ICP	9/10	RDS
	35+0	–	Per protocol	8/8	RDS
	37+0	–	Per protocol	9/10	–
	34+4	PE, ICP, PPROM	PE	3/7	RDS
	35+3	PE	PE	9/10	–
	35+6	–	Per protocol	9/9	–
	37+1	–	Per protocol	9/10	–
	38+0	–	Per protocol	9/10	–
LD laparotomy (USA)	33+1	SCH	Low renal function	8/9	RDS
	36+6	–	Per protocol	9/9	–
	38+0	–	Per protocol	9/9	–
	35+6	GD	Per protocol	8/8	RDS
	30+6	–	PTL	7/8	RDS
	37+2	–	Per protocol	8/8	–
	37+0	PP	Per protocol	8/9	–
	36+6	PE	PE	8/9	–
LD laparotomy (Germany)	35+1	–	PPROM	9/10	RDS
	36+3	–	GH	8/8	–
LD laparotomy (Czech Republic)	35+3	GD	Per protocol	9/10	–
	36+2	PH	Per protocol	10/10	–
LD laparotomy (Lebanon)	35+2	–	PTL	9/10	–
LD robotics (China)	33+6	SCH	PTL	10/10	–
LD robotics (Sweden)	36+1	–	Per protocol	9/10	RDS
LD robotics (USA)	37+0	GH, PH	Per protocol	4/8	RDS
	32+4	PP	PTL	7/8	RDS
	35+6	–	PTL	8/8	–
DD (Brazil)	35+3	PN	Per protocol	9/10	–
DD (USA)	34+1	PA, IRF	Unknown	8/9	–
	37+6	GH	Per protocol	9/9	–
	34+6	SCH	Unknown	7/8	–
	34+2	GD, GH, PPROM	Unknown	8/9	–
	37+1	–	Unknown	8/9	–
DD (Czech Republic)	34+6	GD	Per protocol	7/9	–
DD (Turkey)	28+0	IUGR, PE	PPROM, PE, IUGR	7/8	RDS

(DD: deceased donor; GD: gestational diabetes; GH: gestational hypertension; ICP: intrahepatic cholestasis of pregnancy; IRF: impaired renal function; IUGR: intrauterine growth restriction; LD: live donor; PA: placenta accreta; PH: polyhydramnion; PN: pyelonephritis; PP: placenta previa; RDS: respiratory distress syndrome; SCH: subchorionic hematoma)

LIVE BIRTHS AFTER UTERUS TRANSPLANTATION

Up until today 35 live births after UTx have been published **(Table 2)**. The great majority (27/35) of the live births have been after LD UTx and most of the births have occurred in Europe[27] and USA.[56] There is a wide variation in gestational length of the births, ranging from gestational week 28+0 until 38+0. As shown in **Table 2**, maternal pregnancy complications and respiratory distress syndrome of the neonate were common events. It is predicted that this rate will decrease in the future since per protocol delivery has been adjusted from 35 weeks until 37–38 weeks in many centers.

CONCLUSION

Uterus transplantation is the first and only treatment for the hundreds of thousands of women around the world with AUFI. The UTx procedure is still in the phases for development and evaluation and should therefore be considered as an experimental procedure within the field of infertility treatments.

REFERENCES

1. Hur C, Rehmer J, Flyckt R, Falcone T. Uterine factor infertility: a clinical review. Clin Obstet Gynecol. 2019;62(2):257-70.
2. Sieunarine K, Zakaria F, Boyle D, Corless DJ, Noakes DE, Iain Lindsay I, et al. Possibilities for fertility restoration: a new surgical technique. Int Surg. 2005;90(5):249-56.
3. Fageeh W, Raffa H, Jabbad H, Marzouki A. Transplantation of the human uterus. Int J Gynaecol Obstet. 2002;76(3):245-51.
4. Moore FD. Ethical problems special to surgery: surgical teaching, surgical innovation, and the surgeon in managed care. Arch Surg. 2000;135(1):14-6.
5. McCulloch P, Altman DG, Campell WB, Flum DR, Glasziou P, JC Marshall, et al. No surgical innovation without evaluation: the IDEAL recommendations. Lancet. 2009;374(9695):1105-12.
6. El-Akouri RR, Kurlberg G, Brännström M. Successful uterine transplantation in the mouse: pregnancy and postnatal development of offspring. Hum Reprod. 2003;18(10):2018-23.
7. Wranning CA, Akhi SN, Kurlberg G, Brännström M. Uterus transplantation in the rat: model development, surgical learning and morphological evaluation of healing. Acta Obstet Gynecol Scand. 2008;87(11):1239-47.
8. Dahm-Kähler P, Wranning C, Lundmark C, Enskog A, Mölne J, Marcickiewicz J, et al. Transplantation of the uterus in sheep: methodology and early reperfusion events. J Obstet Gynaecol Res. 2008;34(5):784-93.
9. Wranning CA, Marcickiewicz J, Enskog A, Dahm-Kähler P, Hanafy A, Brännström M. Fertility after autologous ovine uterine-tubal-ovarian transplantation by vascular anastomosis to the external iliac vessels. Hum Reprod. 2010;25(8): 1973-79.
10. Ramirez ER, Ramirez DK, Pillari VT, Vasquez H, Ramirez HA. Modified uterine transplant procedure in the sheep model. J Minim Invasive Gynecol. 2008;15(3):311-14.
11. Gauthier T, Bertin F, Fourcade L, Maubon A, Saint Marcoux F, Piver P, et al. Uterine allotransplantation in ewes using an aortocava patch. Hum Reprod. 2011;26(11):3028-36.
12. Enskog A, Johannesson L, Chai DC, Dahm-Kähler P, Marcickiewicz J, Nyachieo A, et al. Uterus transplantation in the baboon: methodology and long-term function after auto-transplantation. Hum Reprod. 2010;25(8):1980-87.
13. Johannesson L, Enskog A, Dahm-Kähler P, Hanafy A, Chai DC, Mwenda JM, et al. Uterus transplantation in a non-human primate: long-term follow-up after autologous transplantation. Hum Reprod. 2012;27(6):1640-48.
14. Johannesson L, Enskog A, Dahm-Kähler P, Diaz-Garcia C, Hanafy A, Dahm-Kähler P, et al. Preclinical report on allogeneic uterus transplantation in non-human primates. Hum Reprod. 2013;28(1):189-98.
15. Tryphonopoulos P, Tzakis AG, Tekin A, Johannesson L, Rivas K, Morales PR, et al. Allogeneic uterus transplantation in baboons: surgical technique and challenges to long-term graft survival. Transplantation. 2014; 98(5):e51-56.
16. Kisu I, Mihara M, Banno K, Hara H, Yamamoto T, Araki J, et al. A new surgical technique of uterine auto-transplantation in cynomolgus monkey: preliminary report about two cases. Arch Gynecol Obstet. 2012;285(1):129-37.
17. Mihara M, Kisu I, Hara H, Iida T, Yamamoto T, Araki J, et al. Uterus autotransplantation in cynomolgus macaques: intraoperative evaluation of uterine blood flow using indocyanine green. Hum Reprod. 2011;26(11):3019-27.
18. Obara H, Kisu I, Kato Y, Yamada Y, Matsubara K, Emoto K, et al. Surgical technique for allogeneic uterus transplantation in macaques. Sci Rep. 2016;6:35989.
19. El-Akouri RR, Kurlberg G, Dindelegan G, Mölne J, Wallin A, Brännström M. Heterotopic uterine transplantation by vascular anastomosis in the mouse. J Endocrinol. 2002;174(2): 157-66.
20. Wranning CA, Akhi SN, Diaz-Garcia C, Brännström M. Pregnancy after syngeneic uterus transplantation and spontaneous mating in the rat. Hum Reprod. 2011;26(3): 553-58.
21. Díaz-García C, Akhi SN, Wallin A, Pellicer A, Brännström M. First report on fertility after allogeneic uterus transplantation. Acta Obstet Gynecol Scand. 2010;89(11):1491-94.
22. Díaz-García, C, Johannesson L, Shao R, Bilig H, Brännström M. Pregnancy after allogeneic uterus transplantation in the rat: perinatal outcome and growth trajectory. Fertil Steril. 2014; 102(6):1545-52.
23. Ramirez ER, Ramirez Nessetti DK, Nessetti MB, Khatamee M, Wolfson MR, Shaffer TH, et al. Pregnancy and outcome of uterine allotransplantation and assisted reproduction in sheep. J Minim Invasive Gynecol. 2011;18(2):238-45.
24. Mihara M, Kisu I, Hara H, Iida T, Araki J, Shim T, et al. Uterine autotransplantation in cynomolgus macaques: the first case of pregnancy and delivery. Hum Reprod. 2012;27(8):2332-40.
25. Kisu I, Kato Y, Masugi Y, Ishigaki H, Yamada Y, Matsubara K, et al. First successful delivery after uterus transplantation in MHC-defined cynomolgus macaques. J Clin Med. 2020; 9(11):3694.
26. Brännström M, Johannesson L, Dahm-Kähler P, Enskog A, Mölne J, Kvarnström N, et al. First clinical uterus transplantation trial: a six-month report. Fertil Steril. 2014;101(5): 1228-36.
27. Brännström M, Dahm-Kähler P, Kvarnström N, Enskog A, Olofsson JI, Olausson M, et al. Reproductive, obstetrical and long-term health outcome after uterus transplantation: results of the first clinical trial. Fertil Steril. 2022; 118(3):576-85.
28. Brännström M, Kvarnström N, Groth K, Akouri R, Wiman L, Enskog A, et al. Evolution of surgical steps in robotics-assisted donor surgery for uterus transplantation: results of the eight cases in the Swedish trial. Fertil Steril. 2020;114(5): 1097-107.
29. D'Amico G, Quintini C, Eghtesad B, Hashimoto K, Ricci S, Flyckt R, et al. Uterus recovery from deceased donor: simple technique securing safety of vital organs and uterus graft. J Am Coll Surg. 2021;232(3):e1-6.
30. Karlsson CC, Dahm-Kähler P, Kvarnström N, Mölne J, Broecker V, Brännström M, et al. Hysterectomy after uterus transplantation and detailed analyses of graft failures. Acta Obstet Gynecol Scand. 2022;101(3):355-63.

31. Krogh Herlin M, Petersen MB, Brännström M. Mayer-Rokitansky-Küster-Hauser (MRKH) syndrome: a comprehensive update. Orphanet J Rare Dis. 2020;15(1):214.
32. Järvholm S, Johannesson L, Brännström M. Psychological aspects in pre-transplantation assessments of patients prior to entering the first uterus transplantation trial. Acta Obstet Gynecol Scand. 2015;94(10):1035-38.
33. Kvarnström N, Järvholm S, Johannesson L, Dahm-Kähler P, Olausson M, Brännström M. Live donors of the initial observational study of uterus transplantation-psychological and medical follow-up until 1 year after surgery in the 9 cases. Transplantation. 2017;101(3):664-70.
34. Järvholm S, Johannesson L, Clarke A, Brännström M. Uterus transplantation trial: psychological evaluation of recipients and partners during the post-transplantation year. Fertil Steril. 2015;104(4):1010-15.
35. Järvholm S, Kvarnström N, Dahm-Kähler P, Brännström M. Donors' health-related quality-of-life and psychosocial outcomes 3 years after uterus donation for transplantation. Hum Reprod. 2019;34(7):1270-77.
36. Järvholm S, Dahm-Kähler P, Kvarnström N, Brännström M. Psychosocial outcomes of uterine transplant recipients and partners up to 3 years after transplantation: results from the Swedish trial. Fertil Steril. 2020;114(2):407-15.
37. Brännström M, Johannesson L, Bokström H, Kvarnström N, Mölne J, Dahm-Kähler P, et al. Livebirth after uterus transplantation. Lancet. 2015;385(9968):607-16.
38. Ejzenberg D, Andraus W, Baratelli Carelli Mendes LR, Ducatti L, Song A, Tanigawa R,, et al. Livebirth after uterus transplantation from a deceased donor in a recipient with uterine infertility. Lancet. 2019;392(10165):2697-704.
39. Brucker SY, Strowitzki T, Taran FA, Rall K, Schöller D, Hoopmann M, et al. Living-donor uterus transplantation: pre-, intra-, and postoperative parameters relevant to surgical success, pregnancy and obstetrics with live births. J Clin Med. 2020;9(8):2485.
40. Fronek J, Kristek J, Chlupac J, Janousek L, Olausson M. Human uterus transplantation from living and deceased donors: the interim results of the first 10 cases of the Czech trial. J Clin Med. 2021;10(4):586.
41. Akouri R, Maalouf G, Abboud J, Nakad T, Bedran F, Hajj P, et al. First live birth after uterus transplantation in the Middle East. MEFS J. 2020;25:30-7.
42. Testa G, McKenna G, Bayer J, Wall A, Fernandez H, Martinez E, et al. The evolution of transplantation from saving lives to fertility treatment: DUETS (Dallas UtErus Transplant Study). Ann Surg. 2020;272(3):411-17.
43. Wei L, Xue T, Tao KS, Zhang G, Zhao G-Y, Yu S-Q, et al. Modified human uterus transplantation using ovarian veins for venous drainage: the first report of surgically successful robotic-assisted uterus procurement and follow-up for 12 months. Fertil Steril. 2017;108(2):346-56.
44. Brännström M, Dahm-Kähler P, Ekberg J, Akouri R, Groth K, Enskog A, et al. Outcome of recipient surgery and 6-month follow-up of the Swedish live donor robotic uterus transplantation trial. J Clin Med. 2020;9(8):2338.
45. Carmona F, Rius M, Díaz-Feijoo B, Musquera M, Tort J, Alcaraz A. Uterine transplantation. First viable case in southern Europe. Med Clin (Barc). 2021;26;156(6):297-300.
46. Ayoubi JM, Carbonnel M, Kvarnström N, Revaux A, Poulain M, Vanlieferinghen S, et al. Case report: post-partum SARS-CoV-2 infection after the first French uterus transplantation. Front Surg. 2022;9:854225.
47. Vieira MA, Souza C, Nobrega L, Reis R, Andrade C, Schmidt R, et al. Uterine transplantation with robot-assisted uterus retrieval from living donor: first case in Brazil. Minim Invasive Gynecol. 2021;28(11):1817.
48. Puntambekar S, Telang M, Kulkarni P, Puntambekar S, Jadhav S, Panse M, et al. Laparoscopic-assisted uterus retrieval from live organ donors of uterine transplant: our experience of two patients. J Minim Invasive Gynecol. 2018;25(4):622-31.
49. Puntambekar S, Puntambekar S, Telang M, Kulkarni P, Date S, Panse M, et al. Novel anastomotic technique for uterine transplant using utero-ovarian veins for venous drainage and internal iliac arteries for perfusion in two laparoscopically harvested uteri. J Minim Invasive Gynecol. 2019;26(4):628-35.
50. Ozkan O, Ozkan O, Dogan NU, Bahceci M, Mendilcioglu I, Boynukalin K, et al. Birth of a healthy baby 9 years after a surgically successful deceased donor uterus transplant. Ann Surg. 2022;275(5):825-32.
51. Flyckt RL, Farrell RM, Perni UC, Tzakis AG, Falcone T. Deceased donor uterine transplantation: innovation and adaption. Obstet Gynecol. 2016;128(4):837-42.
52. Flyckt R, Falcone T, Quintini C, Perni U, Eghtesad B, Richards EG, et al. First birth from a deceased donor uterus in the United States: from severe graft rejection to successful cesarean delivery. Am J Obstet Gynecol. 2020;223(2):143-51.
53. Richards EG, Farrell RM, Ricci S, Perni U, Quintini C, Tzakis A, et al. Uterus transplantation: state of the art in 2021. J Assist Reprod Genet. 2021;38(9):2251-59.
54. Dindo D, Demartines N, Clavien PA. Classification of surgical complications: a new proposal with evaluation in a cohort of 6336 patients and results of a survey. Ann Surg. 2004;240(2):205-13.
55. Mölne J, Broecker V, Ekberg J, Nilsson O, Dahm-Kähler P, Brännström M. Monitoring of human uterus transplantation with cervical biopsies: a provisional scoring system for rejection. Am J Transplant. 2017;17(6);1628-36.
56. Johannesson L, Testa G, Putman JM, McKenna GJ, Koon EC, York JR, et al. Twelve live births after uterus transplantation in the Dallas Uterus Transplant Study. Obstet Gynecol. 2021; 137(2):241-49.

CHAPTER 81

Ovarian Transplant

Pravin Mhatre, Jyoti Mhatre

HISTORY OF OVARIAN TRANSPLANT

Man has always been fascinated with the idea of longevity and eternity. However, the main desire was youth forever. This eternal youth desire leads to the idea of gonadal transplantation. Browsing through the history, there are many examples in the world literature. Almost all religions are replicated with such stories. The famous example of king Yayāti taking the youth from his son Pururava is well known in Hindu mythology **(Fig. 1A)**.

Not only mythological events but well-documented events in Christian literature also exist. Emperor Caligula used to have decoction prepared with testicular extracts to achieve eternal youth, while Pope Pius II used what was described as a fountain of youth **(Fig. 1B)**, where he drank the juice prepared from semen and blood of young boys.

The story of a famous Chinese general in the 18th century is very fascinating. He was a *eunuch* and carried his castrated gonads around his waist and believed to draw energy for all his great achievements from them **(Figs. 2A and B)**. He was the most powerful general and had traveled half the world in his naval fleet.

Although the discovery of hormones and their role in imparting the youth made these practices unworthy, the continuation of such treatment in the modern era is extremely shocking. The famous examples of Sophia Lauren and Charlie Chaplin using these modalities to achieve eternal youth are well documented.

Charles-Édouard Brown-Séquard, well known for his work in physiology, neurology, and anatomy, declared the use of such treatment on himself and in achieving the youth **(Figs. 3A to G)**. This work was presented at a world conference held in Paris. His famous quote was

"Everything I have done badly due to advancing age, I am able to perform most admirably today".

The most surprising fact is that such clinics are running even today and boasting of their elite *clientele* **(Figs. 3A to G)**.

Christiaan Barnard, noted for his first heart transplant after 1980, started such a clinic in Switzerland and is still operating, having done 65,000 treatments till 1990.

The gonadal or testicular transplant was carried out in a big way in USA. These were more testicular implants than transplants. Frank Lydston from Chicago first reported these testicular implants in 1916 to achieve rejuvenation. In 1919, the largest series of more than 1,000 patients were carried out unethically in San Quentin prison. Surprisingly, these experiments were continued unofficially till 1960. Brinkley from Kansas performed 16,000 such cases of testicular

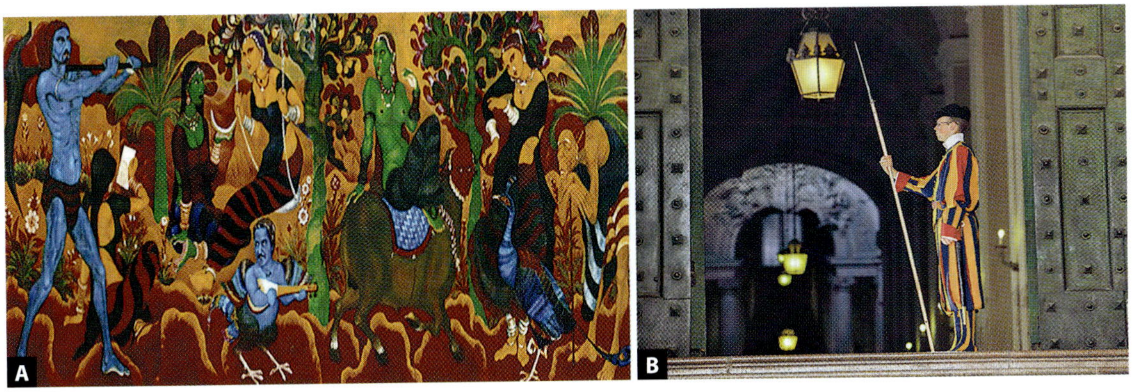

Figs. 1A and B: (A) King Yayāti and Pururava; (B) Pope Pius II and the Fountain of Youth.

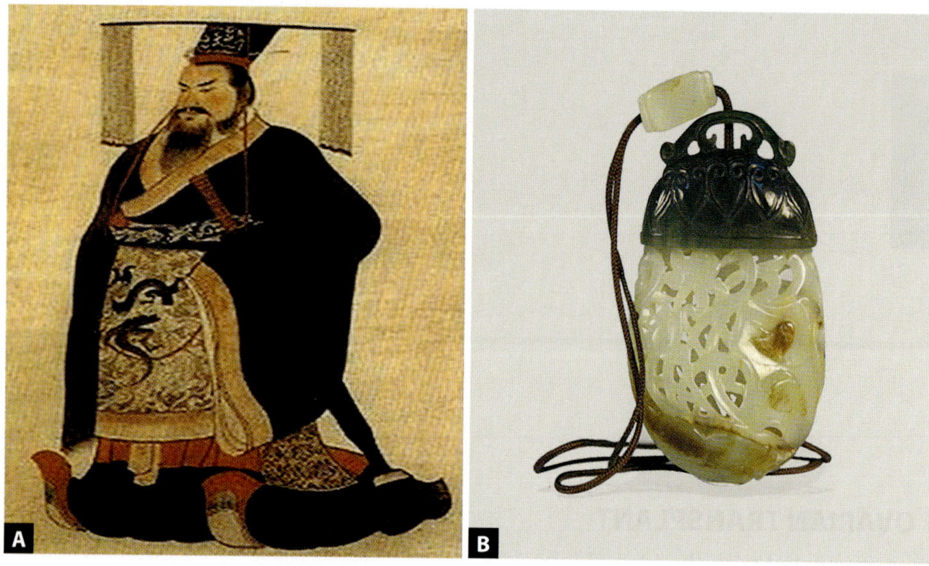

Figs. 2A and B: (A) 18th century Chinese general; (B) Preserved gonads.

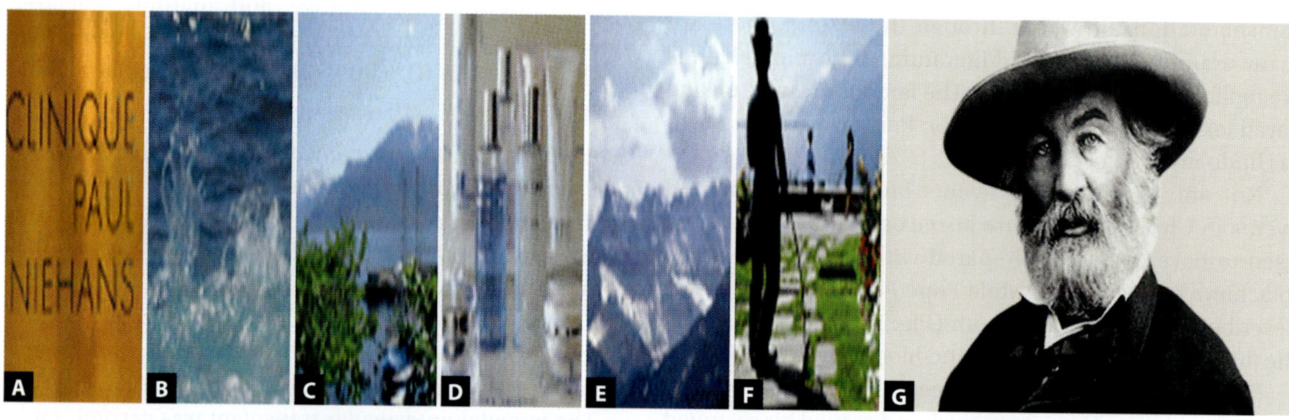

Figs. 3A to G: (A to F) Clinique Paul Niehans; (G) Charles-Édouard Brown-Séquard.

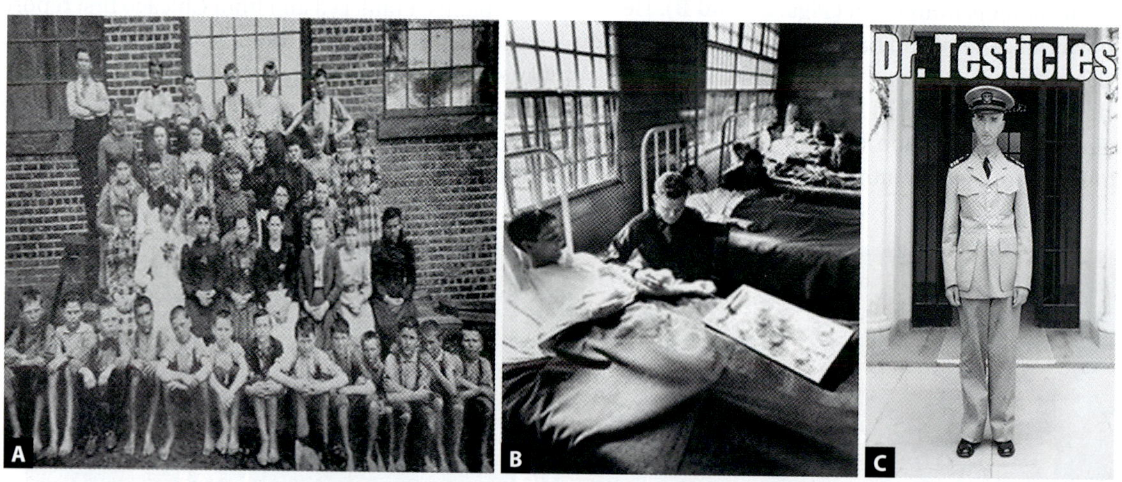

Figs. 4A to C: San Quentin prison and testicular implants.

implants in 1930 alone **(Figs. 4 and 5)**. With the increasing demand resulting in dwindling supply, some researchers started to use monkey or goat glands for rejuvenation.

The real scientific transplantation began in India 600 years before Christ, and the sage Sushruta is credited for the first nose transplant. Sushruta is credited to be the

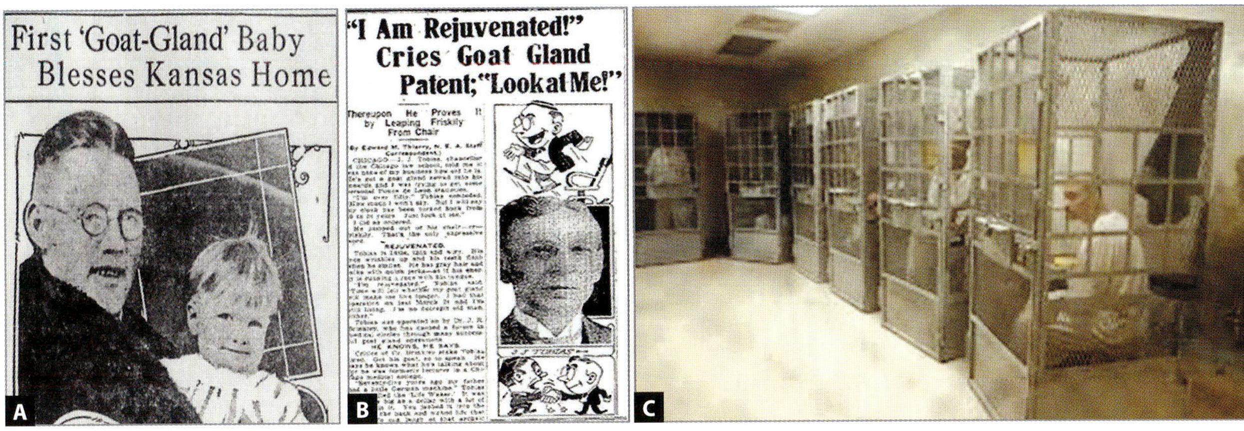

Figs. 5A to C: Frank Lydston and testicular implants.

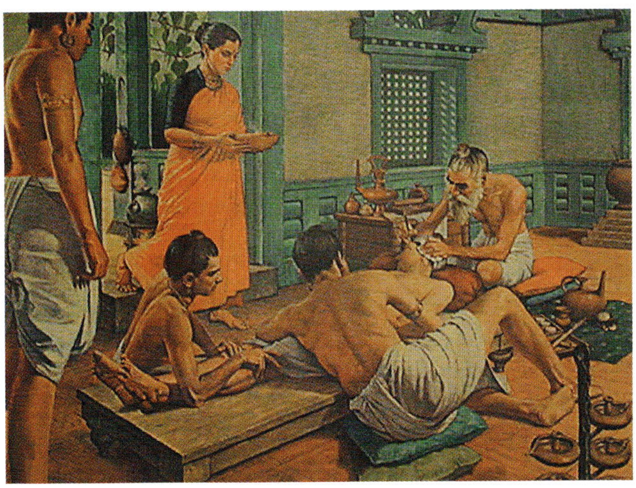

Fig. 6: Sushruta 600 BC.

father of transplantation **(Fig. 6)**. However, Alexis Carrel in 1900 developed the technique of vascular anastomosis leading to a revolution in organ transplant and hence should be called the father of modern transplant history **(Fig. 7)**. He was the first surgeon to receive the noble prize although he was barred from medical practice. His contribution opened a plethora of organ transplants till 1930, but the lack of knowledge of immunology resulted in failures and was followed with a period of lull till 1950.

The work of Medawar on understanding immunology gave an impetus to organ transplantation, resulting in true success. The first successful renal transplant was performed in 1954, paving a wave of organ transplants. The actual credit goes to Yu Yu Voronoy from Russia, who performed the first renal transplant in 1933 and a successful one in 1950 from a cadaveric donor **(Fig. 8)**. The authorities who were dissatisfied asked him to repeat the procedure and gave him a person who was dead for 8 days, thus resulting in failure, and denounced his experiment, which is a classical case of rivalry and jealousy.

Many workers have worked scientifically on ovarian transplant.

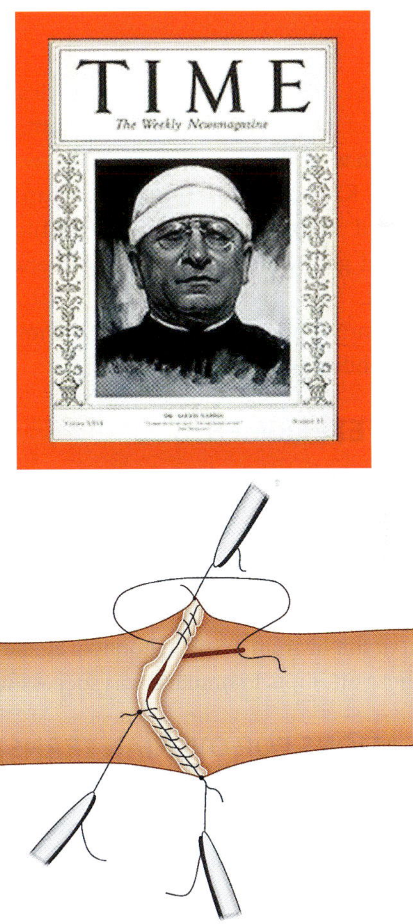

Fig. 7: Alexis Carrel and technique of vascular anastomosis.

ANIMAL EXPERIMENTS

Foa in 1900 showed that neonatal ovarian tissue in rabbits survives against the adult one in ovarian homografts.

Harris and Eakin in 1949 showed that ovarian homografts in rats survived better only after removing the recipient ovaries. They showed that the recipient oophorectomy improved success by reducing the lymphatic response.

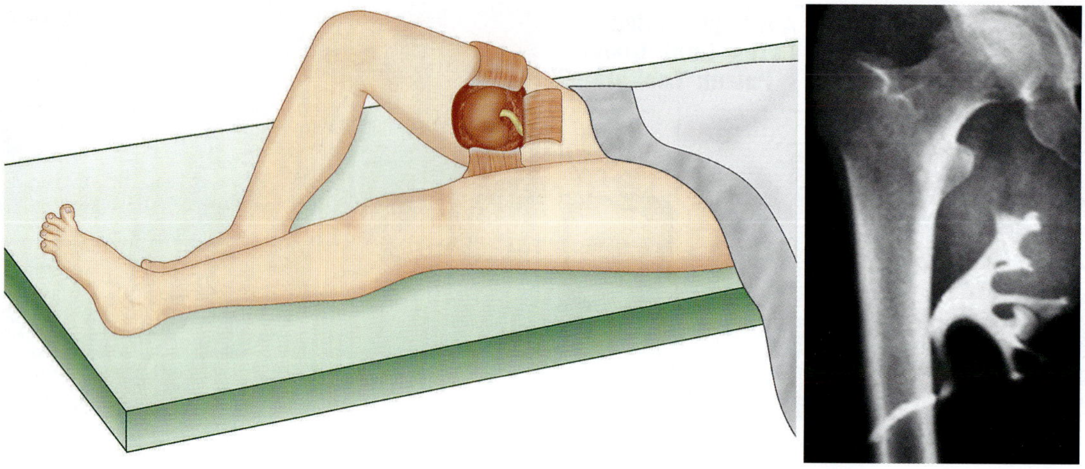

Fig. 8: Yu Yu Voronoy from Russia who performed the first renal transplant.

Deanesly in 1956 described the histological appearance and function of long-term subcutaneous homografts in rats, some of which were frozen prior to grafting.

In 1955, Krohn noted that homotransplantations in mice had improved results by using cortisone. Estrogen and gonadotropins were also beneficial in the improvement.

Hicken and Krohn were the first to show the role of histocompatibility genes.

HUMAN EXPERIMENTS

Sturgis and Castellanos in 1958 demonstrated the survival of human ovarian homograft in the Millipore chamber of six patients of Turner syndrome.

Desaire transplanted the ovary in spleen in the patient having generalized cancer and was castrated. Holmer transplanted the ovarian tissue in gonadal agenetic patients. None of these attempts in humans was successful.

INDICATIONS FOR OVARIAN TRANSPLANT

Theoretically, there are many indications for ovarian transplant; however, ethical considerations are more important in the decision-making. Unlike other solid organ transplants where they are more of lifesaving, ovarian transplant is for improving the quality of life. The indications are as follows:

- Dysgenetic gonads—as in Turner syndrome—is the most important indication
- Ovarian agenesis
- Bilateral oophorectomy or post onco- or radiotherapy
- Fertility restoration
- Treatment of menopause.

Whatever may be the indication, it must be a long-term therapeutic and not a one-time procedural gain as to achieve pregnancy.

PROBLEMS ASSOCIATED WITH OVARIAN TRANSPLANT

- It is vital to understand that ovarian transplant, unlike other solid organ transplant, is not lifesaving but only improves the quality of life.
- The second major issue is that as of today, ovarian transplant is from a live donor only. The cadaveric ovarian transplant is not possible as the primordial follicles are extremely susceptible to oxygen concentration and are lost almost immediately following death. The safety time zone between the time of death and organ retrieval is practically absent. The ovarian function of hormone production is maintained for a long time, even in low oxygen concentration. The follicles are extremely susceptible to low oxygen, and there is a significant loss of primordial follicles due to hypoxia **(Table 1)**.
- Cryopreservation of ovarian grafts and tissue is now standardized and has a fair success rate; however, the entire ovarian cryopreservation is not yet successful.
- One of the major problems is immunological rejection. On the scale of immunogenicity, tissues such as cornea, cartilage, and cardiac muscles are at the bottom due to the paucity of cell nucleus, and there is great evidence to believe that the ovary also has less immunogenicity. It was believed for a long time that the ovary is privileged for transplant; however, our experience in human ovarian transplantation paints a different picture. It has been found that the ovary has one dominant system of transplantation antigen and probably 30 or more so-called weaker systems. An incompatible dominant system results into a marked graft rejection within 8–10 days, while when the weaker systems are involved, rejection occurs after a considerable length of time. Thus, it was found that the ovaries are resistant to graft rejection across minor histocompatibility barriers and are highly resistant to homograft reactivity.

TABLE 1: Oxygen uptake of endocrine tissues.

Tissue	*QO_2 (μM/g tissue/h)*
Liver	35
Adrenal	26
Thyroid	17
Placenta	11
Ovary	9
Parathyroid	7

- Special position on transplantability scale: Less human leukocyte antigen (HLA) antigens.
- Master organ in terms of cell potential so more acceptability.
- O_2 requirements for growth and function are less.
- Ability to be fragmented and transplanted and take new blood supply is good.
- Endocrine function of the transplanted ovary is achieved easily. Blood supply and nutrition are of greater importance for ovulation.
- Ovary transplanted from immature to a functional environment develops more rapidly than it would ordinarily be expected to do so (Foa 1900).

The *immunological rejection* can be prevented by three different ways:

1. *Central inhibition:* This is achieved by thymectomy and splenectomy in which the aim is to reduce the lymphoid tissue. The other way is general or selective radiation. None of these methods are practicable.
2. *Efferent inhibition:* The most important part of immunosuppression is brought about by pharmacological therapy. Two types of drugs mainly used are steroids and cytotoxic drugs. The basic drug is prednisolone and the most important cytotoxic drugs are azathioprine and cyclosporine. The second principle of immunosuppression is the removal of or destruction of circulating immunized lymphocytes. This can be achieved by prolonged irradiation of extracorporeally shunted blood. Recently, antilymphocytic globulins have also been introduced for the similar effect.
3. *Local inhibition:* The third principle of immunosuppression is to protect the allograft from immunological attack. This can be achieved by local infusion of steroids into the allograft artery.

The most important problem is ovarian vasculature. The orthotopic placement of the ovary poses the real challenge in achieving the transplant. Various attempts were done in graft placement in heterotopic sites.

OVARIAN VASCULATURE

The ovary has a low metabolic activity as compared to other vital organs; however, it receives the arterial blood supply directly from the heart at substantial high pressure. To circumvent this discrepancy in anatomical supply and the physiological need, the ovarian vasculature undergoes unique changes **(Fig. 9)**.

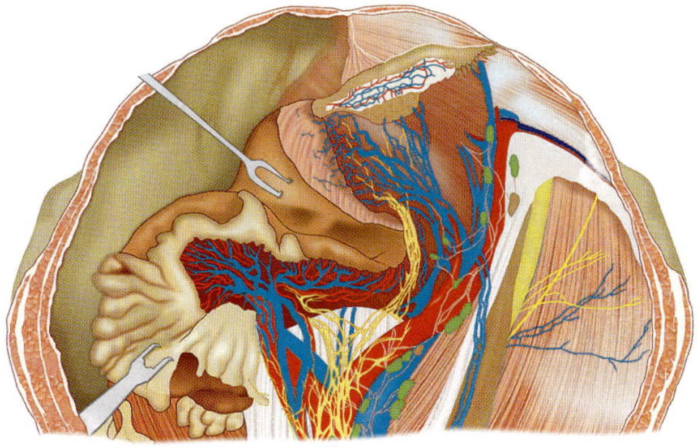

Fig. 9: Pelvic vasculature.

The ovarian artery after arising from the aorta runs a straight course and before it enters the ovary, it has distinct convolutions. There are three sets of convolutions in the ovarian artery course—upper, middle, and lower **(Figs. 10A to C)**. With the help of these anatomic convolutions, the ovary achieves reduction in the arterial force to match its physiological needs.

This is an extremely unique anatomical arrangement probably not seen in any other organ.

Ovary being a pelvic organ also has its unique nature of venous drainage system. As the ovarian veins drain directly into the vena cava, a high-flow drainage system, it requires to change its anatomical structure. The ovarian vein no more remains a single large drainage system but gets replaced by a multitude of small drainage vessels forming a confluence. These ovarian vessels form a mesh around the ovarian artery.

By far these unique anatomical changes occurring in the ovarian vasculature pose the greatest challenge in the ovarian transplant and form a major stumbling block in achieving its success **(Figs. 11 and 12)**.

The larger vessel diameter for anastomosis and the availability of a large single drainage vein are the hallmarks of success in the solid organ transplant.

SITE OF OVARIAN TRANSPLANTATION

Orthotopic Transplant

To achieve both the reproductive and the hormonal function, it is paramount to transplant the ovary in its orthotopic site. Although the most ideal, the following factors affected its success:

- Unique vasculature
- Difficult anatomical position
- Nonavailability of matching vessels in the pelvis
- Need of its proximity to the fallopian tube for fertility.

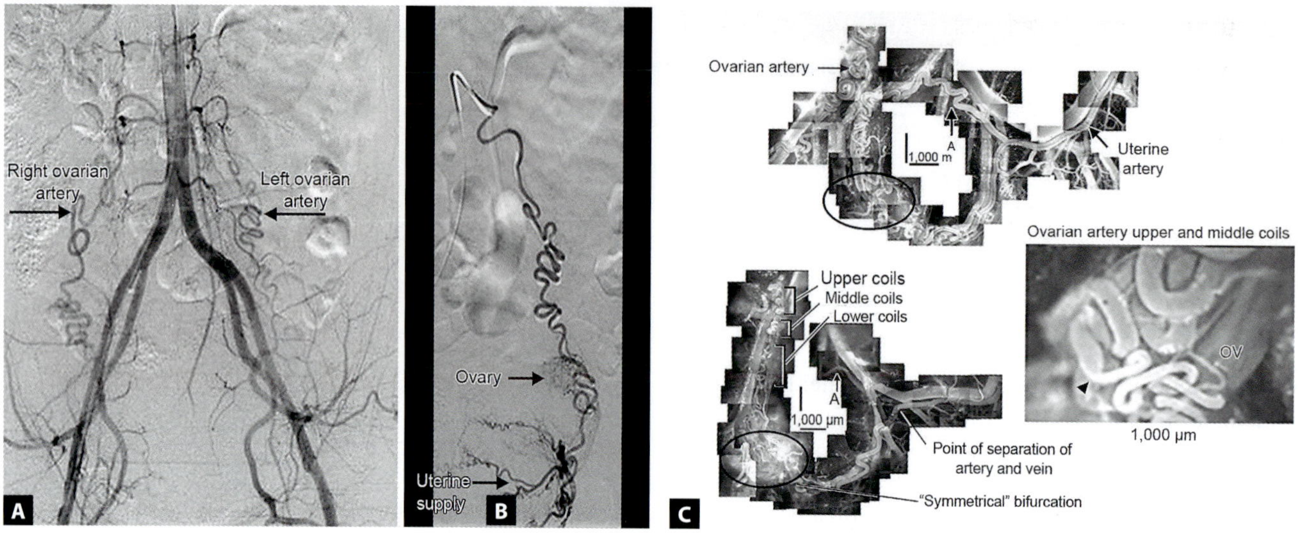

Figs. 10A to C: Ovarian artery and its convolutions.

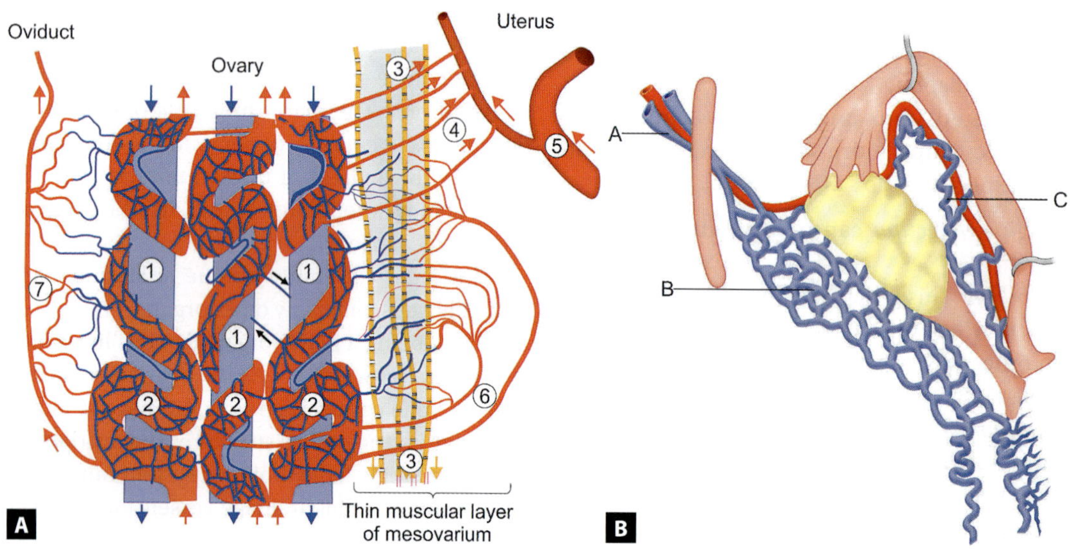

Figs. 11A and B: Ovarian vasculature. (A) Relation of ovarian vasculature with oviduct and uterus; (B) Mesoovarian vasculature; (C) Tubo ovarian vasculature. (1) Ovarian vein; (2) Ovarian artery; (3) Lymphatics; (4) Utero-ovarian connections; (5) Uterine artery; (6) Arteriovenous shunts.

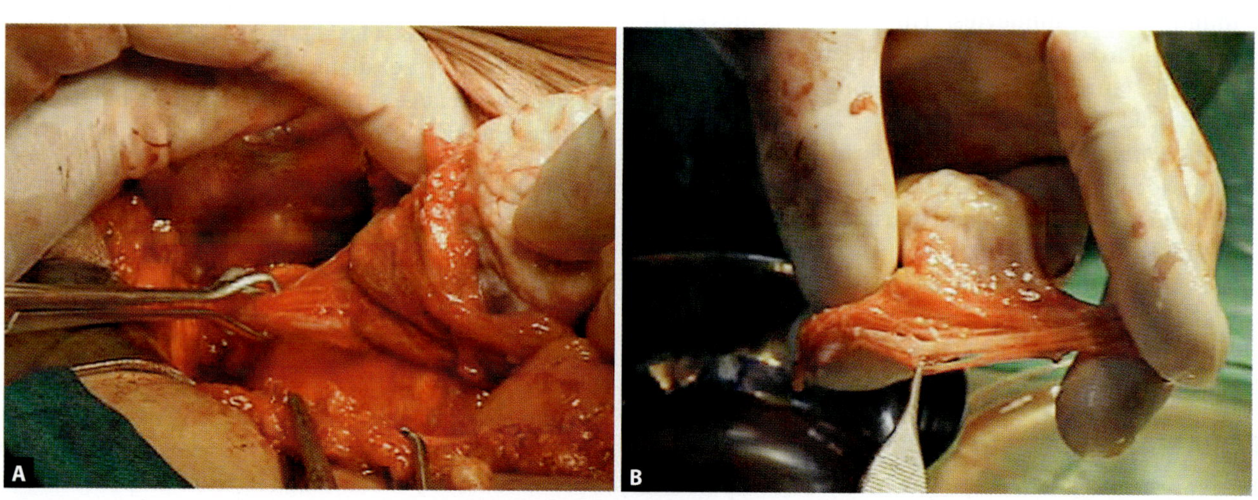

Figs. 12A and B: Ovarian vasculature.

Subcutaneous or Intramuscular Ovarian Grafts

Many workers have shown the subcutaneous survival of the ovarian tissue in both animals and humans. However, the graft did survive for a short time span. These ovarian tissues underwent neoangiogenesis and developed their blood supply from the surrounding tissues but eventually underwent atrophy.

Anterior Chamber of the Eye

This is an extremely common site for the transplant of endocrine tissues in the animals as it allows direct visualization of the graft. Over a period of time, the graft undergoes vascularization in the eye chamber and the rejection of the ovarian graft occurs. Interesting work from Woodruff needs a special mention. The thyroid tissue when transplanted initially in the eye chamber and later placed in the subcutaneous tissue survives. This probably shows the principle of adaptation.

Uterine Fundus and Uterine Cornu

Robert Tuttle Morris did a pioneering work when he implanted the ovaries in the uterine fundus. The Estes operation is well known where ovaries are stitched to the cornu of the uterus. This operation was devised for the irreversible tubal pathology rather than ovarian transplant.

The Spleen

The spleen has been a popular site of ovarian transplant in the animals and early human transplants. The rich vascularity of the spleen was a major factor of consideration in the survival of the graft.

THE SOLUTIONS

- The main problem for ovarian transplant is the unique nature of ovarian vessels. In an effort to maintain the arterial coiling, we dissected the ovarian vessels at a high level. This was done by extraperitoneal dissection of the infundibulopelvic ligament. The ovarian artery was taken much above the pelvic brim maintaining the arterial coils. This dissection at a higher point also allowed selecting a large diameter vein for anastomosis.
- Nonavailability of matching size vessel is the second major issue in ovarian transplantation. This problem was the main stumbling block in achieving success.

After many cadaveric dissections, the solution was identified.

- *Arterial anastomosis:* The ovarian artery has a diameter of 1–1.5 mm. The various arteries available for the anastomoses are native ovarian artery, uterine artery, internal iliac artery, and inferior epigastric artery. The native ovarian vessels usually are not developed or have undergone atrophy. The uterine vessel (4–5 mm) is too large and cannot be used due to its disproportionate size. The internal iliac artery is also too large (10 mm). The only matching diameter is of the inferior epigastric artery. The inferior epigastric artery is in the anterior abdominal wall and after dissecting, it is brought into the extraperitoneal space to be anastomosed to the donor ovarian artery.
- *Venous anastomosis:* As discussed before, the ovarian vein is not a single large vein but a confluence and a mesh. There are no matching size veins in the pelvis. The native ovarian veins are practically atrophied; the uterine veins are also a confluence of veins not suitable for anastomosis. The only large vein available is the external iliac vein. After a lot of deliberation and many cadaver dissections, it was decided to use the external iliac vein. The greatest problem is that the external iliac vein has a high flow velocity unsuitable for the low drainage of ovarian venous flow. However, with no other better choice available, the external iliac vein drainage was used. The postoperative findings of the transplanted ovary showed a dramatic adaptation of the venous flow pattern over a period of time, showing a change from high to low drainage system (unpublished data).

Venous flow after 1 month and 6 months posttransplant **(Figs. 13A and B)**: The greatest breakthrough was the selection of the appropriate vessels for anastomosis and the technique of using the extraperitoneal dissection for the surgery. These two factors were most important for the success of achieving the first successful orthotopic, vascular, and whole ovarian transplant by the author in March 2002.

- Unlike other solid organ transplants, ovarian vasculature cannot be studied prior to transplant. Therefore, the exact nature of this vasculature remains an enigma and prior planning is not possible. The decision-making happens only on table, keeping the surprise element. Contrary to this, renal, hepatic, cardiac, pulmonary, or small bowel vasculature can be documented prior to surgery and the surgeon is well prepared for the same.
- Although there are many factors against the success of the ovarian transplant, an important factor favors its success. What makes ovarian transplant different? It is the process of vasculogenesis and angiogenesis. The ovary is the only organ having vasculogenesis and angiogenesis as a normal physiological event. Its ability to be fragmented and transplanted and take new blood supply is good; hence, ovarian grafting succeeds even in the absence of vascular anastomosis.
- Ovarian follicles and corpora lutea have been shown to contain and produce angiogenic factors.
- These angiogenic factors appear to be heparin-binding and belong to the fibroblast growth factor (FGF) and vascular endothelial growth factor (VEGF) families of

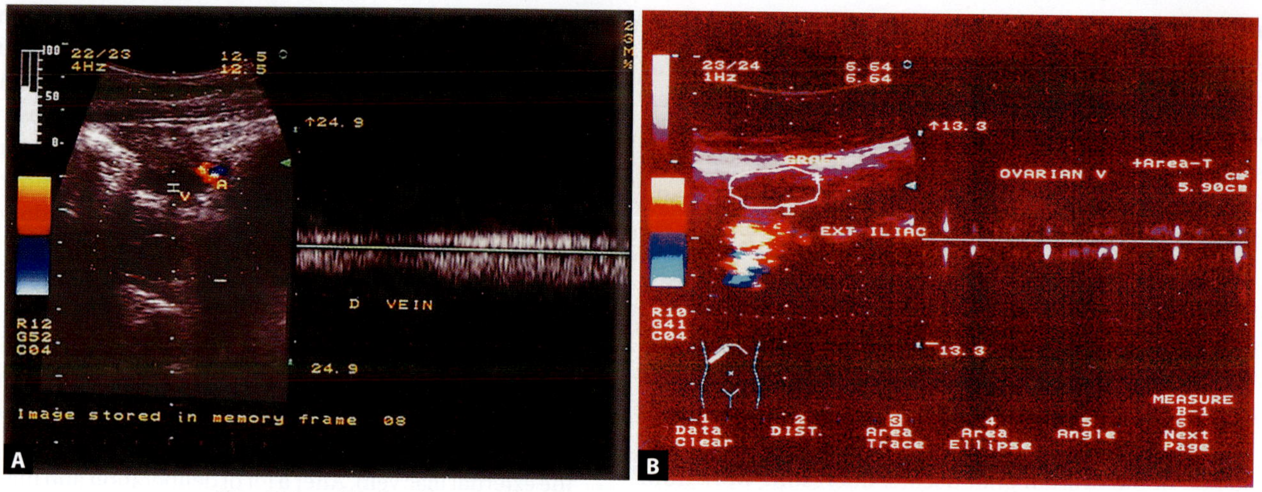

Figs. 13A and B: Ovarian vein Doppler blood flow 1 month and 6 months post operation.

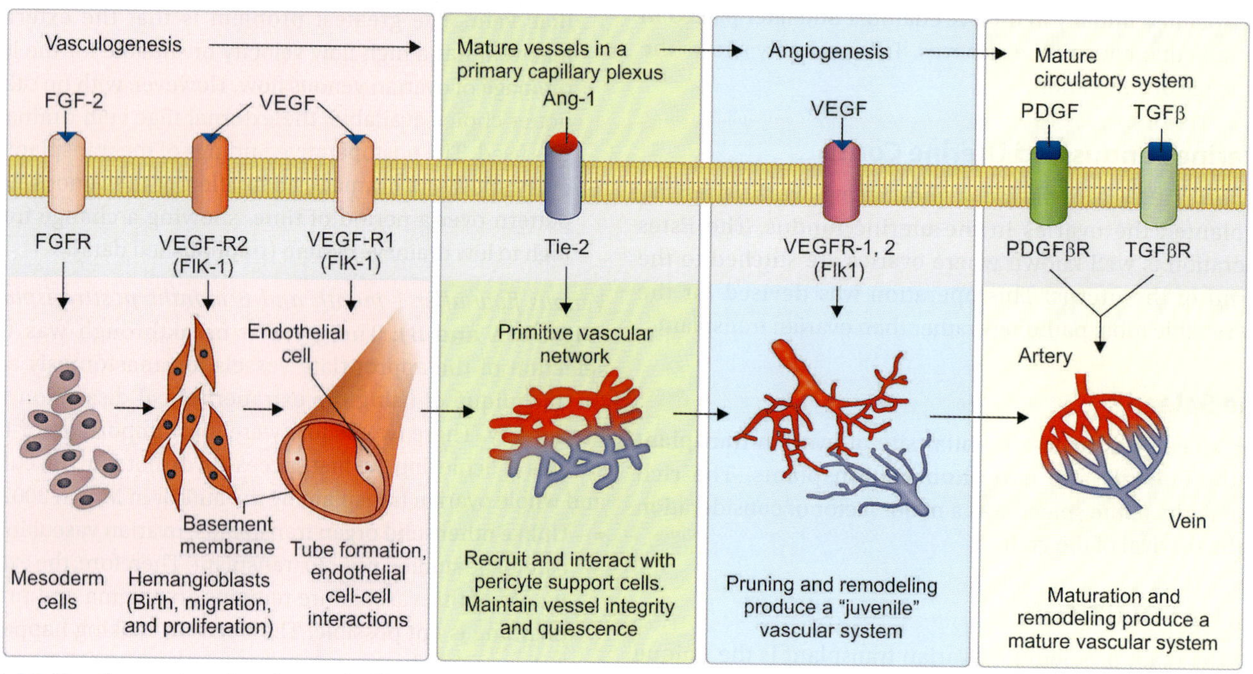

Fig. 14: Vasculogenesis and angiogenesis. (Ang-1: angiopoietin-1; FGF-2: fibroblast growth factor 2; FGFR: fibroblast growth factor receptor; PDGF: platelet-derived growth factor; PDGFβR: platelet-derived growth factor beta receptor; TGFβ: transforming growth factor beta; TGFβR: transforming growth factor beta receptor; VEGF: vascular endothelial growth factor; VEGF-R1: vascular endothelial growth factor-receptor 1; VEGF-R2: vascular endothelial growth factor-receptor 2)

proteins. In addition, factors regulating gap junctional communication may play a critical role in coordinating the interactions between luteal vascular and nonvascular tissues.

- Further elucidation of the specific physiological roles of these factors in follicular and luteal growth, development, and function will ultimately lead to improved methods for regulating fertility in mammals. Immune cells are active players in luteal angiogenesis.
  - Neutrophils stimulate the formation of luteal endothelial cells and capillary-like structures.
  - Macrophages play a crucial role in maintaining vascular integrity.
  - Bone marrow-derived vascular progenitor cells and macrophages contribute to neovascularization during corpus luteum (CL) formation.
  - The role of macrophages is potentially the most important since these cells can be differentiated into the "tissue remodeling" M2 phenotype by the luteal microenvironment. M2 macrophages then produce various proangiogenic factors including VEGFA, VEGFC, and FGF2 to promote angiogenesis.
- The vasculogenesis and angiogenesis are two separate entities, and one must understand the difference between them **(Fig. 14)**.

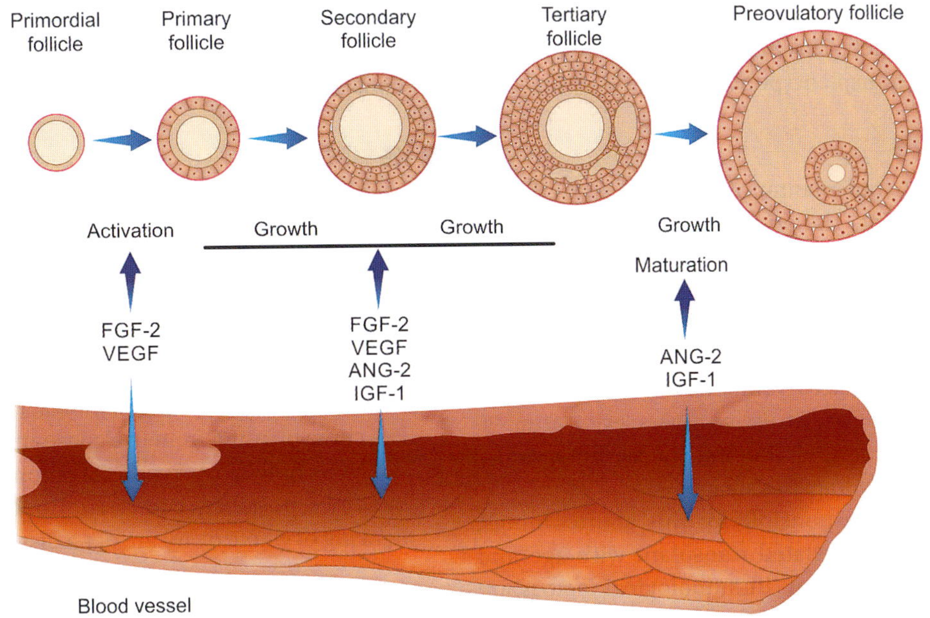

Fig. 15: Angiogenesis factors. (ANG-2: angiopoietin-2; FGF-2: fibroblast growth factor 2; IGF-1: insulin-like growth factor 1; VEGF: vascular endothelial growth factor)

The vasculogenesis has a primary role in the early development of gonads and in the formation of ovarian development. However, in testicular development, angiogenesis plays an important role. Angiogenesis has a role in the follicular development and in formation of CL. The factors governing these are different.

- In a transplanted ovary, the donor ovary has its own set of vasculogenesis factors, while the angiogenetic factors come from the recipient **(Fig. 15)**. This may be an important cause of ovarian rejection. This remains still an ill-understood topic.

JOURNEY TO THE FIRST TRANSPLANT[1-3]

The author achieved the first ever successful ovarian transplant on March 29, 2002. This was a whole ovary, vascular, and orthotopic transplant achieved from a live-related donor to her sister. The success story was long spanned over a period of 20 years of research spanning from conceiving the idea to a fruitful culmination.

- *Animal experiments:* These were carried out with the help of the National Institute for Research in Reproductive Health (NIRRH). These experiments were done primarily on rats to find about the subcutaneous grating of ovarian tissues and their fate over a period of time interval.
  The dog sterilization units from the municipal corporation were chosen to learn the testicular vasculature and the anastomosis techniques. Similar exercises were done on animals from the abattoir.
- *Cadaver dissections:* Permission was obtained to perform the cadaveric dissection to understand the ovarian and pelvic vasculature. It is extremely important to understand that the pelvic vasculature not only differs from individual to individual but also from right to left side. More than 20 cadaveric dissections were carried out for understanding the vasculature. The experience during extraperitoneal dissections of oncological surgical procedures was also helpful.
- *Immunology:* The immunological matching was based on the knowledge from other solid organ transplants. It was decided to do the matching by both major and minor HLA systems as well as to do lymphocytic crossmatch.
- *Renal transplant:* Observer ship—I was fortunate to be an observer in many renal transplant units to understand the entire process—surgical, medical, and social aspects of the transplants.
- *Microvascular surgery:* It is extremely important to have sound knowledge of vascular surgery and it challenges both intra- and postoperative and the management of the complications.

GOVERNMENT PERMISSION

- As per the transplant law, I first obtained the necessary skills for becoming a gynecological transplant surgeon.
- A transplant center was formed as per the law and was certified.
- Necessary permission was obtained from the transplant coordinating committee for conducting the first ovarian transplant.
- On March 29, 2002, an ovarian transplant was performed on a 17-year-old recipient suffering from Turner's syndrome. The donor was her 26-year-old sister, with two living children. The donor and recipient were immunologically

matched by major and minor HLA matching and lymphocytic crossmatch. This happened to be the first successful ovarian transplant (published data).

CONCLUSION

- The history of transplantation actually started with gonadal transplant. The primary goal being achieving immortality with permanent youth by gonadal transplant. This is evident by many mythological stories, as well as recent past experiments conducted almost till 1990.
- The other solid organ transplants flourished exponentially over the last 60 years, however the ovarian transplant has not grown in numbers even after 20 years since we described the first successful vascular orthotopic whole ovarian transplant.
- Many factors are responsible for this shortcomings, namely it being live related transplant with age and fertility bar for the donor. Immunological factors are responsible for failure to ovulatory function. The recent studies have indicated incompetence in vasculogenic and angiogenesis factors which comes from recipient and donor respectively.
- The heart and liver donations can never come from live donors but the ovarian donation such as the renal ones can come plentiful from live consenting donors.
- As the technique of cryopreservation of the entire ovary becomes possible, cadaveric donation and ovarian banking of whole ovary are not a distant dream.

KEY POINTS

- The ovary, unlike kidney, liver, or heart, is not a vital organ required for life sustenance and therefore not lifesaving in true sense of words, but it definitely improves the quality of life and is life producing for the recipient.
- The heart and liver donations can never come from live donors but the ovarian donation such as the renal ones can come plentiful from live consenting donors.
- As the technique of cryopreservation of the entire ovary becomes possible, cadaveric donation and ovarian banking of whole ovary are not a distant dream.

REFERENCES

1. The first orthotopic ovarian transplant in Turner's syndrome. Int J Gynaecol Obstet. 2003;83(Suppl. 3).
2. The first orthotropic ovarian transplant in Turner's syndrome. Int Pediatr. 2003;18:4.
3. Mhatre P, Mhatre J. Orthotopic ovarian transplant—review and three surgical techniques. Pediatr Transplant. 2006; 10(7):782-7.

CHAPTER

82 Novel Ways of Creating Vagina

Pravin Mhatre, Jyoti Mhatre

INTRODUCTION

Almost 200 years have passed since Peter Muller described the Müllerian ducts. However, we are still groping in the dark to understand the nuances. The development of the Müllerian duct is one of the most ill-understood topics in gynecology and remains an enigma. Surprisingly, it is impossible to find the total absence or aplasia of the Müllerian structure, but it always presents as a partial absence or hypoplasia. Its correlation with anti-Müllerian hormone (AMH) is still unclear.

DEVELOPMENT OF MÜLLERIAN DUCT

- The Müllerian duct appears close to the region of primitive gonads at about the 7th week of pregnancy.
- The caudal tip of this Müllerian duct is comprised of a solid band of cells, which continues to grow from cephalic end to caudal end.
- As they grow caudally after some distance, they turn medially across the mesonephric duct and lie in close proximity to each other.
- Partial fusion occurs in the Müllerian duct and they continue to grow caudally.
- The lower end of the fused Müllerian ducts projects into the urogenital sinus as a Müllerian tubercle.
- The upper part of Müllerian duct develops into the fallopian tubes, the fused part into the uterus, and the upper three-fourths of the vagina. While the lower one-fourth develops from sinovaginal bulbs. The hymen is developed from the junction of sinovaginal bulbs and the urogenital sinus.
- The uterus develops by the end of 3rd month. During the 5th month of intrauterine life, the septum disappears and a single uterus results. The muscle wall also starts developing, and a circular muscle layer is identified by the 5th month. The longitudinal muscle layer develops during 7th month of pregnancy.
- In summary, Müllerian ducts appear at 6 weeks of gestation:
  - By 10 weeks, they fuse to form the uterus.
  - By 22 weeks, the lining is formed.
  - By 32 weeks, it become an adult uterus ready to bleed, as witnessed by witch menstruation.

The fusion of the two Müllerian ducts with subsequent canalization and hypertrophy leads to the development of the adult female genital tract. The total absence of Müllerian development will lead to aplasia, while the partial development, which is a common occurrence, leads to tubal and partial uterine development and complete absence of upper three-fourths of vagina. It is commonly observed that absence of Müllerian tubercle in urogenital sinus leads to absence of lower one-fourth of vagina. In some rare cases, the lower one-fourth of the vagina may develop in absence of Müllerian counterpart. Failure of canalization in the sinovaginal bulb may lead to an imperforate hymen to complete the absence of lower one-fourth of the vagina.

CLINICAL PRESENTATION

- In most of the cases of upper vaginal absence, the uterus is usually duplicated, hypoplastic, or rudimentary. The ovaries are normal but are placed on lateral pelvic wall along with the uterus. Classically, this is described as the "Mayer-Rokitansky-Küster-Hauser" (MRKH) syndrome. Probably, it has autosomal recessive genetic transmission. These patients have normal secondary sexual development.
- The other presentation is rather rare in the form of lower one-fourth of vaginal atresia with normal Müllerian counterpart. These girls may present early in age as cases of hydrocolpos or hydrometrocolpos, where there is a collection of watery fluid in the vagina and uterus, causing distention and an abdominal mass. These girls, at the time of puberty, develop hematocolpos or hematometrocolpos, causing acute distention

and abdominal mass. Very often, but not always these girls may be operated upon with a wrong diagnosis of duplication cyst or ovarian tumor.

- Another common presentation is in the form of testicular feminization syndrome or androgen insensitivity syndrome, where the patient is 46, XY but phenotypic female having a short, blind lower one-fourth of vagina and absent pubic and axillary hair.
- The classical clinical presentation of imperforate hymen is cryptomenorrhea, cyclical abdominal pain from pubertal age to the development of hematocolpos, hematometra, etc.

  All these types of presentations are as a result of developmental errors; the etiology remains unexplained. Contrary to this, the group of patients with intersexuality also presents with absent vaginal or fusion defects, where the etiological factors are known.

  As a dictum, when the vagina is absent, the uterus is absent too. However, there are many minor differences noted and must be given importance while planning the treatment. Suffice to say, there cannot be a single method of vaginoplasty for all the conditions, but the patient needs to be catered to according to their individual merits.
- Almost all the Müllerian malformations must be suspected of having concomitant urinary developmental defects unless proved otherwise. As a result, all the patients must be subjected to ultrasound sonography (USG), intravenous pyelography, and in some selective cases, magnetic resonance imaging (MRI).
- It is commonly associated with single kidney, horseshoe-shape kidney, and pelvic kidney. Ureteric developmental defects in the form of duplication and absence are also found.
- Laparoscopy, till recently, was considered as an unnecessary investigation. However, according to the authors' study, it forms a very important diagnostic tool, not only to assess the defect in detail but also confirms the utricle and gonadal size and position, rules out or details the pelvic kidney. The size of utricles can help in deciding future uterine implantation.

USE OF PERITONEUM IN NEOVAGINAL LINING

Many surgical techniques such as use of colon, intestine, and skin have been described for the creation of neovagina; however, none of them are successful in developing a normal vagina (**Figs. 1A to C**). Almost all of them are surgically challenging, multistage involving gross technique and resulting in cosmetic disfigurement.

The use of peritoneum in vaginoplasty was first described in Russian literature. This method was popularized by Davydov (**Figs. 2A and B**). The peritoneal use procedure was done by the open laparotomy method. Semm first described the creation of neovagina using a laparoscope. He used dura mater cerebri grafts (Semm 1983). His procedure was time-consuming, required extra instrumentation, and was associated with complications. The more recently reported technique describes laparoscopic application to modify the original Davydov procedure.

Dr Mhatre's Modifications

The author has described three different techniques of peritoneal vaginoplasty:

1. Use of thin peritoneal graft
2. Use of thick peritoneal graft with substratum
3. Combined use of peritoneum with amnion grafts in cases of MRKH syndrome along with pelvic kidney, where retrieval of peritoneum is difficult and is associated with complications.

Apart from routine preoperative work-up, a diagnostic laparoscopy was performed to determine mobilization and feasibility of creating anterior and posterior flaps for peritoneal pull through and to see the size and position of the utricles on lateral pelvic walls to determine the possibility of uterine implantation in the neovagina.

PROCEDURE (FIGS. 3 TO 6)

- The neovaginal space is created by making a horizontal incision below the urethral orifice, taking care not to damage the urethra. The further dissection is carried out by blunt dissection, creating an adequate length.
- With the help of operative laparoscope, anterior and posterior thin peritoneal flaps are created.
- The attachment of these peritoneal flaps to the parent peritoneum is maintained.
- In some cases, thick peritoneal flaps along with substratum were obtained. Care must be exercised to achieve hemostasis in cases of thick peritoneal grafts. Hemostasis may be achieved with the use of bipolar cautery or the use of harmonics.
- These peritoneal flaps are brought down in the neovaginal space and sutured to the introital mucosal edges.
- The vault is closed either vaginally or laparoscopically maintaining adequate vaginal length.
- The peritoneal flaps are kept in continuation with the parent site through the attachment, thus ensuring continuation of blood supply.
- In select cases, the utricles were implanted either as a single or after unification to the neovagina as a separate second stage procedure.
- In patients who underwent peritoneal pull-through surgery, vaginal mold was not required. The peritoneal lining prevents vaginal shrinkage and adhesions.
- During follow-up, the neovaginal space can be dilated gradually to maintain the desired length till sexual activity

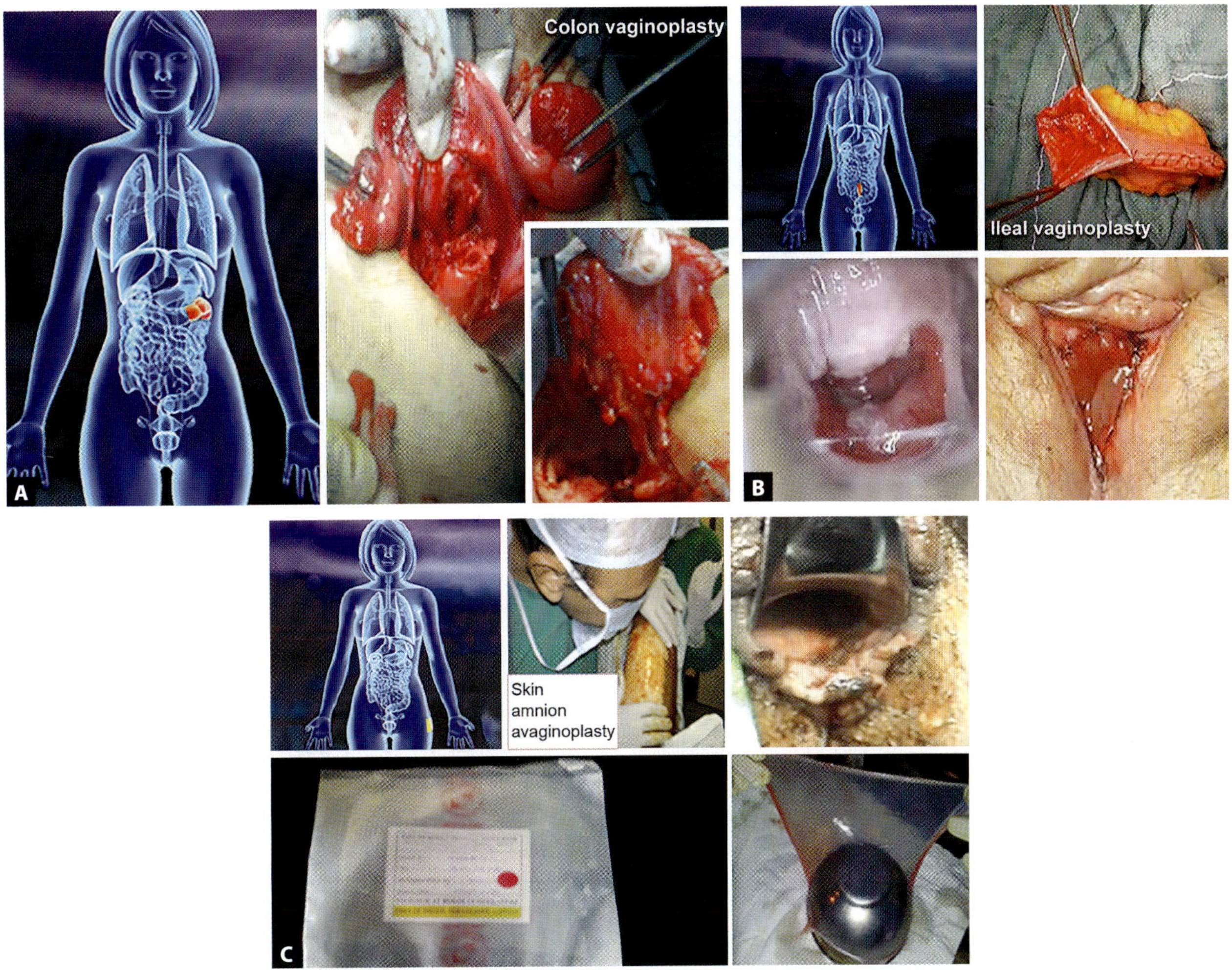

Figs. 1A to C: Surgical techniques for creation of neovagina with the use of (A) Colon; (B) Ileum; and (C) Skin.

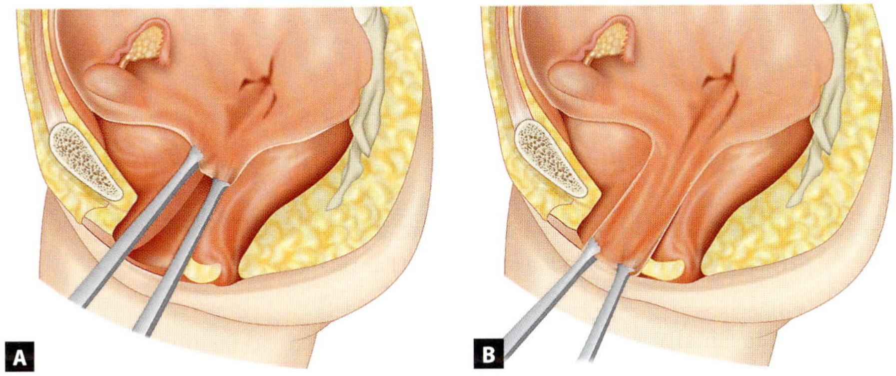

Figs. 2A and B: Application of laparoscopy for the creation of neovagina.

is resumed. Dilatation using glass dilator increases the length and diameter of neovagina and also changes the axis to one which is ideal for intercourse. The neovagina is in correct anatomical axis. The pelvic peritoneum lining the neovagina is responsive to estrogen. It is imperative to remember that the vascular anatomy differs drastically from patient-to-patient and even in the same patient from either side. It is very important to identify uterine artery and vesical arterial disposition during the dissection.

- These patients with Müllerian agenesis have different anatomical presentations, and many of them have associated renal anomalies making this dissection

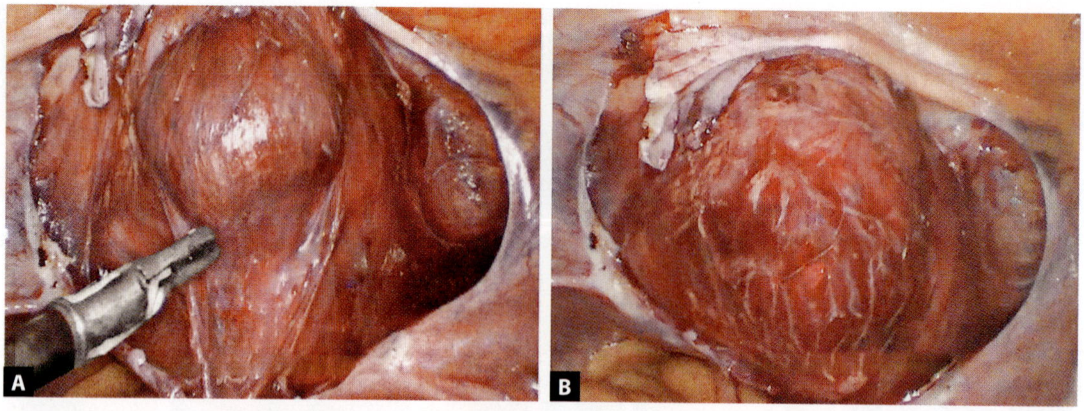

Figs. 3A and B: Dissection of anterior and posterior peritoneal flaps.

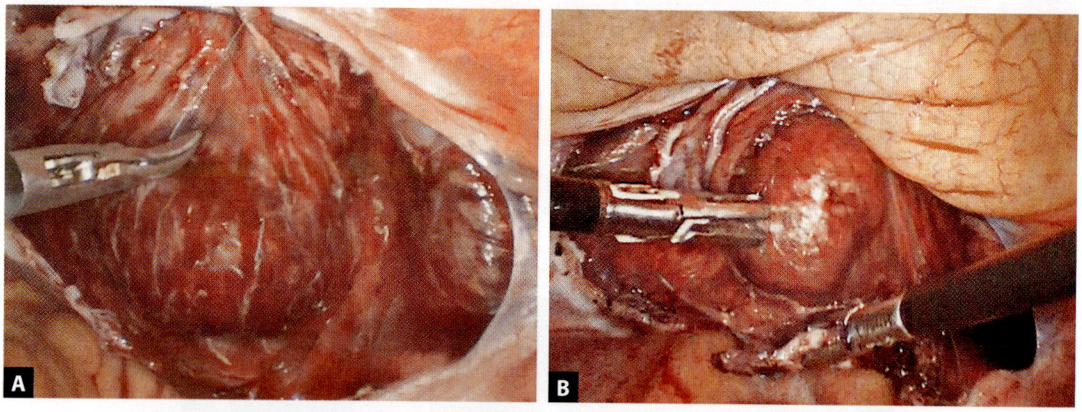

Figs. 4A and B: Dissection of bladder and rectum, and opening of vault of neovagina.

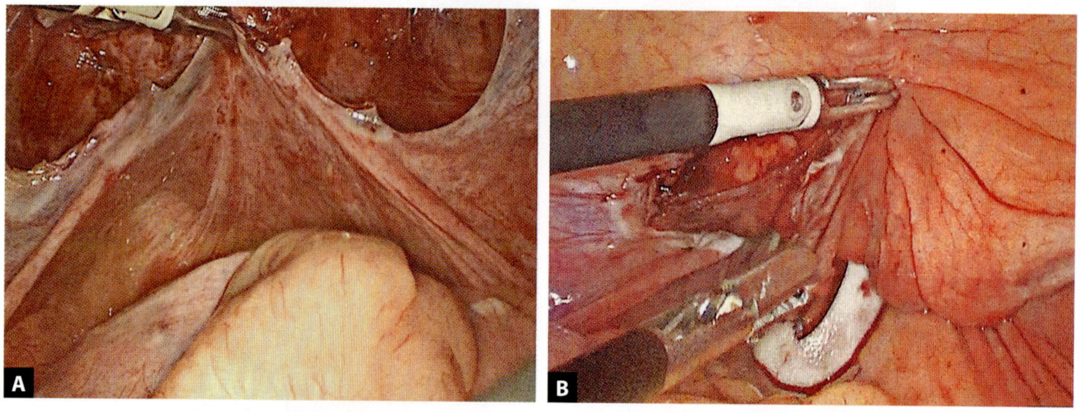

Figs. 5A and B: Mobilization of peritoneal flaps in the neovaginal space.

surgically challenging. Classically single kidney, malrotated kidney, pelvic kidney, and anomalies of ureter such as double ureter pose great surgical challenges **(Fig. 7)**.

- Modification of the peritoneal flaps may be done depending on the availability of free peritoneum. In number of cases, posteriorly the rectum is in close apposition and for fear of rectal damage; it is advisable not to take a posterior peritoneal graft. In such an event, both the flaps may be designed from the anterolateral pelvic peritoneum.
- In such cases, fashioning of peritoneal grafts may be difficult and may be combined with freeze-dried or fresh amnion grafts.

RESEARCH HYPOTHESIS

The ability of the peritoneum to undergo metaplasia is a well-documented fact. It can transform itself into a variety of tissues such as endometrium, cartilage, intestinal epithelium, etc. This knowledge has helped us to understand the genesis of endometriosis and a variety of ovarian neoplasms.

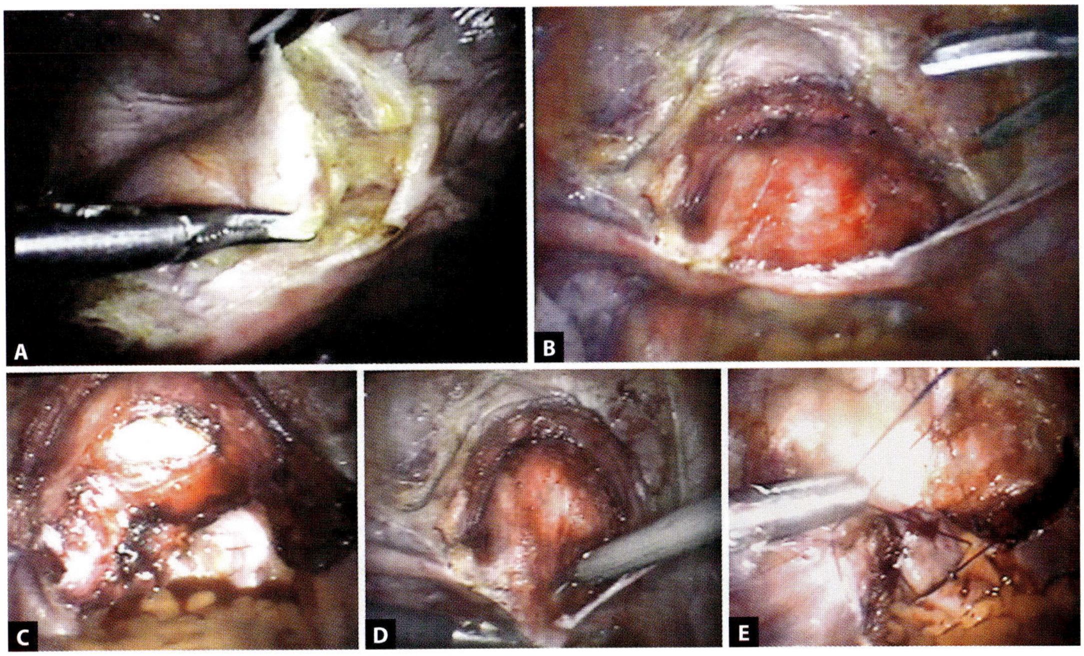

Figs. 6A to E: Technique of using thick peritoneal grafts.

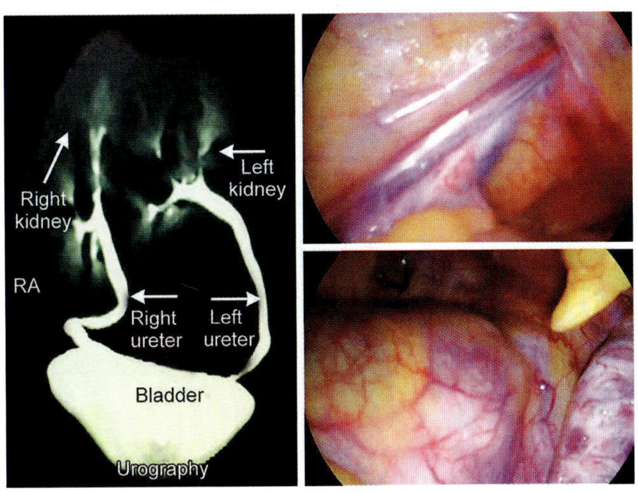

Fig. 7: Single pelvic kidney, fused pelvic kidney with two ureters, and single kidney with double ureter.

The peritoneum and the Müllerian ducts have the same parentage. Both develop from celomic epithelium. The Müllerian ducts develop as invagination of the celomic epithelium finally leading to fusion and canalization. This knowledge prompted us to carry out research in peritoneal vaginoplasty, to find out how the peritoneal metaplastic conversion occurs in the vaginal epithelium.

The peritoneum, when displaced in the vaginal space, undergoes metaplastic stimulation. The nature of the stimulus is still unknown; however, we wish to put forward some hypothetical considerations.

- Anatomically when exposed to the exterior environment, the metaplastic stimulus starts to play its role.
- The dilatation and the friction by the glass dilator provide a mechanical stimulus responsible for the metaplastic conversion.

  The peritoneal metaplasia is not from simple multiplication of low-cuboidal epithelium but a complex phenomenon passing through activation followed by suppression of mesothelial progenitor cells.

  The research was directed toward documenting exactly the stages of these metaplastic conversions. This was achieved by studying the neovaginal biopsies done at regular interval documenting the histological events. These changes were documented at three levels:
  1. Epithelial changes
  2. Stromal changes
  3. Neoangiogenesis.
- All the biopsies performed of the neovagina showed stratified squamous epithelium. The keratinization occurred after 3–5 months of surgery. Serial transformation was demonstrated by biopsies taken at weekly intervals **(Figs. 8 and 9)**.

Day 7 of Neovagina

Day 7 of neovagina shows single layer epithelium with loose adventitial layer below it. Vaginoscopy of neovagina at day 7 showed pink-color lining with healthy look **(Fig. 10)**.

Day 14 of Neovagina

Day 14 of neovagina shows polymorph and mononuclear infiltrate along with vascular endothelium. Adventitial layer is dense as compared to day 7. The vaginoscopy shows pale neovaginal mucosa **(Fig. 11)**.

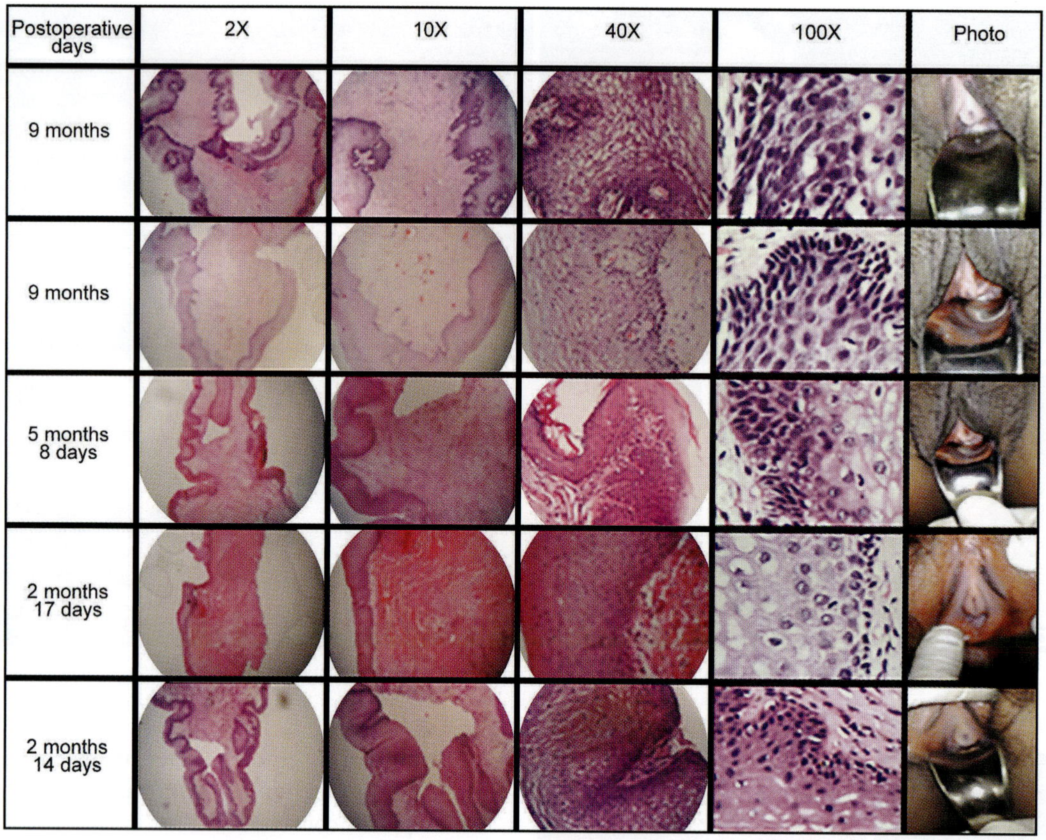

Fig. 8: Vaginal biopsies and vaginoscopic pictures of neovagina.

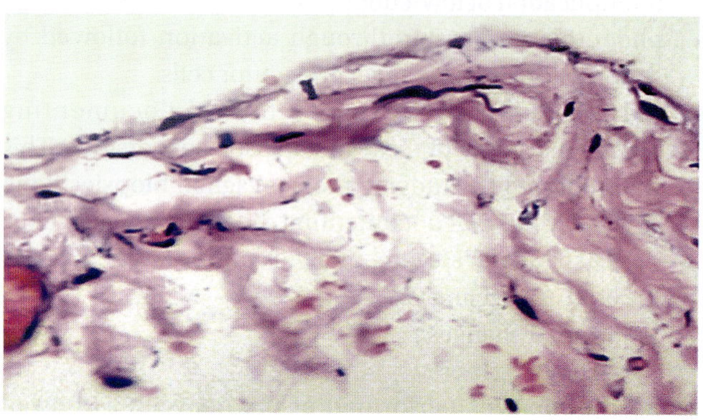

Fig. 9: Normal peritoneal epithelium and loose adventitial layer.

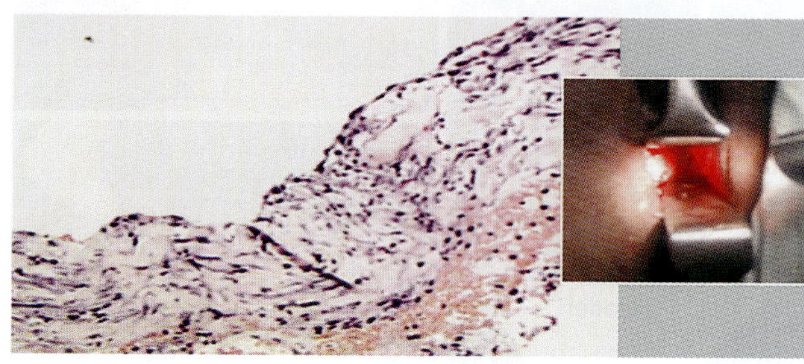

Fig. 10: Day 7 of neovagina with single layer epithelium and loose adventitial layer.

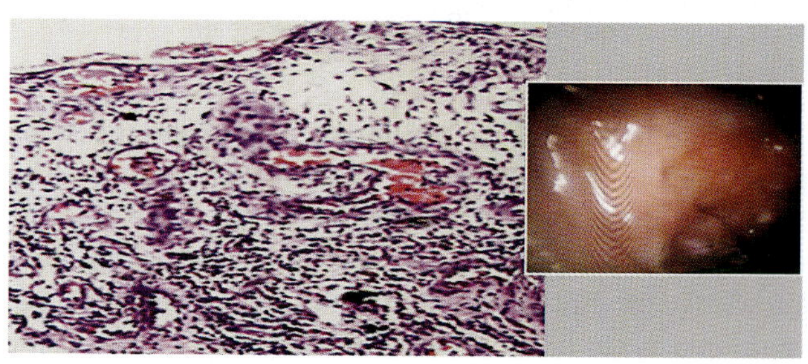

Fig. 11: Day 14 of neovagina with—multilayer, polymorph, and mononuclear infiltrate with vascular endothelium and dense adventitial layer.

Day 21 of Neovagina

Day 21 of neovagina shows increased polymorph and mononuclear infiltrate with angiogenesis. Adventitial layer is dense and compact as compared to day 14. The vaginoscopy shows metaplastic white areas with normal looking pink posterior wall **(Fig. 12)**.

Day 28 of Neovagina

Day 28 of neovagina shows increased polymorph and mononuclear infiltrate with well-organized capillaries and edematous adventitial layer. Vaginoscopy shows white lesions on the vaginal wall representing metaplastic activity **(Fig. 13)**.

Having confirmed this histological conversion, the research was directed toward identification of specific progenitor cell in the peritoneum responsible for this metaplasia.[1]

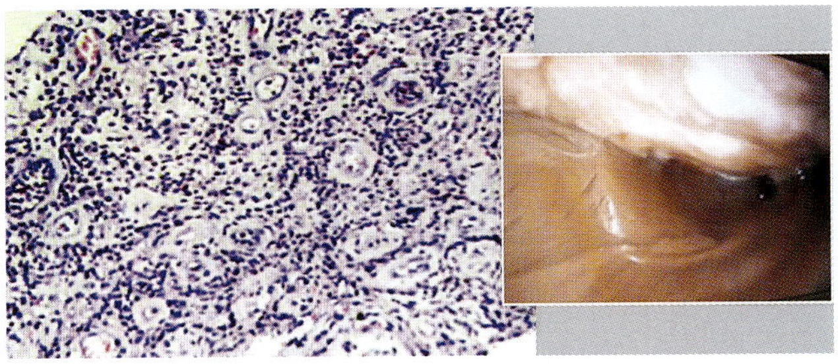

Fig. 12: Day 21 of neovagina with—increased polymorph and mononuclear infiltrate with angiogenesis and dense adventitial layer.

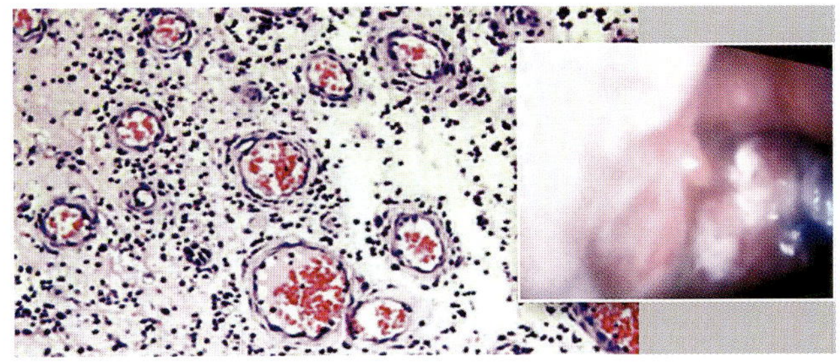

Fig. 13: Day 28 of neovagina with—increased polymorph and mononuclear infiltrate with well-organized capillaries and edematous adventitial layer.

IMMUNOHISTOCHEMISTRY

Neovagina sections of 5 mm thickness were deparaffinized and rehydrated using descending grades of methanol. Endogenous peroxidase activity was quenched by incubating the sections in 0.3% hydrogen peroxide for 30 minutes. This was followed by microwave treatment of the sections for 10 minutes in an antigen unmasking solution (Vector Laboratories, Burlingame, CA, USA). Sections were blocked with 2% goat serum (for the section to be incubated with polyclonal antibodies against all antigens) in phosphate-buffered solution for 1 hour at room temperature. Sections were then incubated with the respective primary antibodies for 16 hours at 4–8°C. The negative control sections were incubated with rabbit or mouse immunoglobulin G in place of primary antibodies. This was followed by incubations of the sections with fluorescent-labeled secondary antibodies raised in goat (Vector Laboratories, Burlingame, CA, USA) for 1 hour at 37°C. Sections were then counterstained with hematoxylin and gradually dehydrated, cleared in xylene, and mounted. The staining intensities for immunoreactive antigens were determined using confocal microscope (Zeiss, Germany). At least 10 areas from each section were randomly selected for measuring the integrated optical density (IOD). The IOD values of the respective negative control (without primary antibody) were subtracted from the IOD values for the sections stained with primary antibody.

Immunohistochemistry tests (IHC) were performed on peritoneal biopsy samples and the presence of progenitor cells was demonstrated by octamer-binding transcription factor 4 (OCT4) and SRY-Box 2 (SOX2) as markers. Immunostaining with stem cell marker OCT4 is seen in the nucleus in green; whereas 4',6-diamidino-2-phenylindole (DAPI) fluorescent stain is used as nuclear stain in blue. The immunostained images have been overlaid with the differential interference contrast image (DIC is the bright field contrast image of the unstained sample) to show the localization of OCT4. Immunostaining with stem cell marker SOX2 is seen in the nucleus as green, whereas DAPI is used as nuclear stain in blue. The immunostained images have been overlaid with the DIC image to show the localization of SOX2.

Peritoneal biopsies were taken and subjected for identification of the progenitor cell using SOX2 and OCT4 IHC markers **(Fig. 14)**.

Day 7 of Neovagina

Immunostaining with stem cell marker SOX2 is seen in the nucleus as green. The expression is scattered in the tissue and in some areas it is seen in parallel distribution **(Figs. 15A and B)**.

Day 14 of Neovagina

The expression of OCT4 is scattered in the tissue. The expression of SOX2 is increased as compared to day 7. The expression is seen in two distribution patterns—(1) tubular and (2) circular **(Figs. 16A and B)**.

Day 21 of Neovagina

Comparing with day 14, OCT4 expression is reduced on day 21, and the SOX2 expression is increased with wide distribution **(Figs. 17A and B)**.

Day 28 of Neovagina

Expression of OCT4 and SOX2 is very low in the day 28 vaginal biopsy.

In seven cases, we were able to connect the utricles to the neovagina and achieve menstrual function. **Figure 18** shows the left utricle almost of normal size, uterus having normal blood flow pattern, and a right rudimentary utricle. Pregnancy was attempted in this patient but failed. However, in three patients, we achieved the pregnancy using surrogacy, thus making this vaginoplasty a fertility-enhancing procedure **(Figs. 19 to 22)**.[2]

Having confirmed the histological metaplastic conversion and identifying the progenitor cell responsible, the research was continued toward evaluation of the neovagina on various anatomical, physiological, and functional parameters.

- The anatomical parameters were histology, cell cytology, and neoangiogenesis.

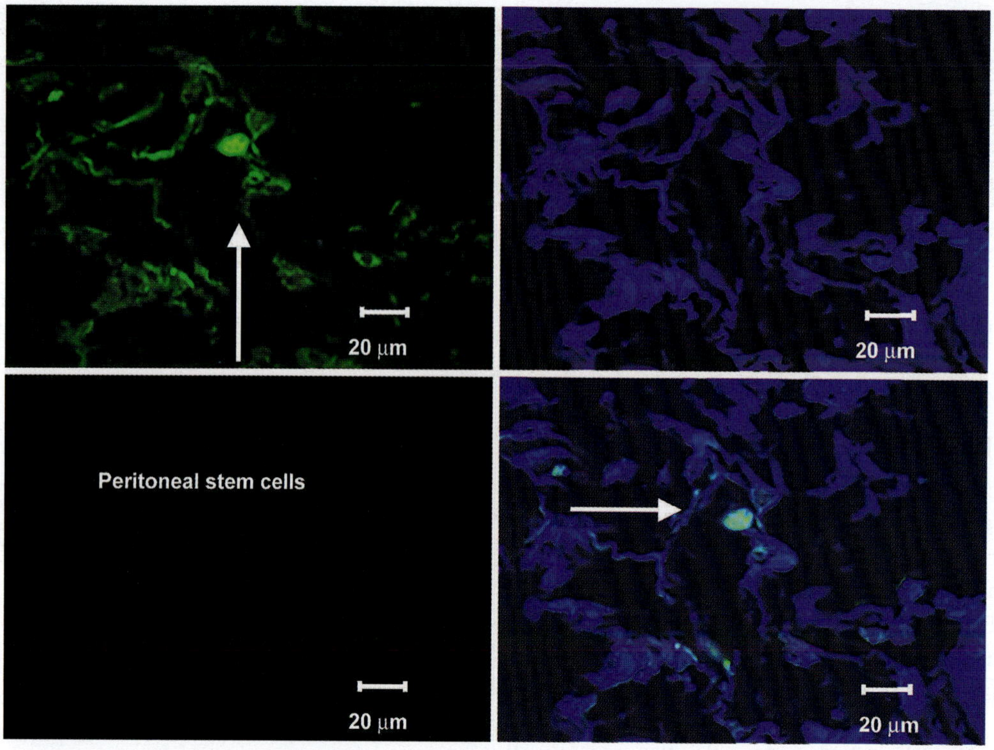

Fig. 14: Identification of peritoneal stem cells using SRY-Box 2 (SOX2) and octamer-binding transcription factor 4 (OCT4) immunohistochemistry markers.

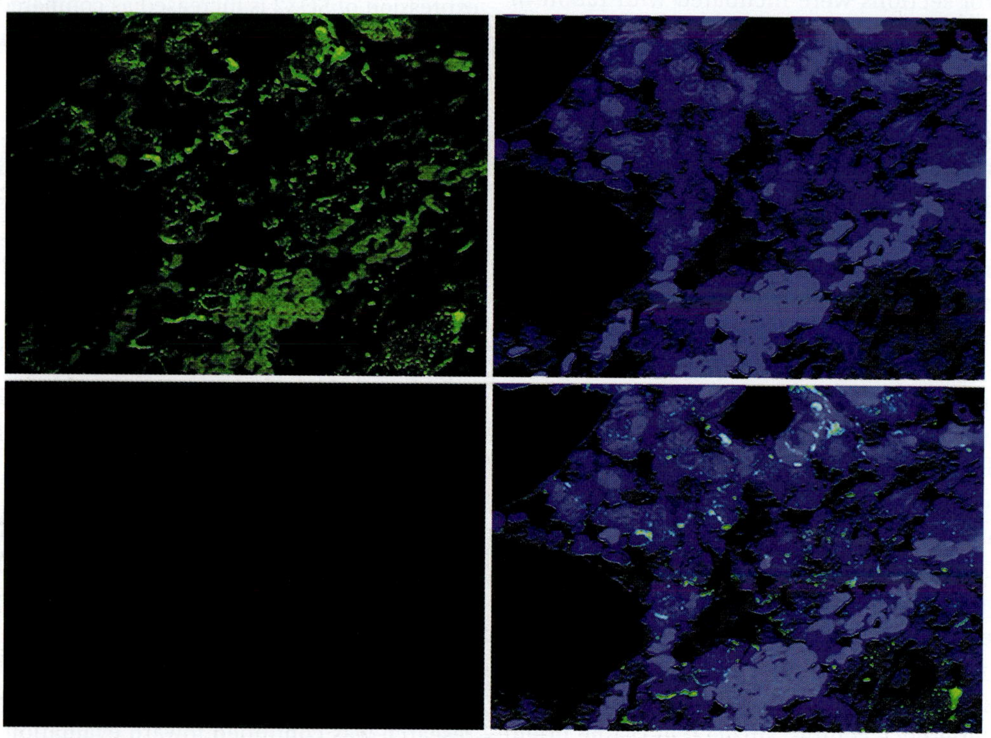

Fig. 15A

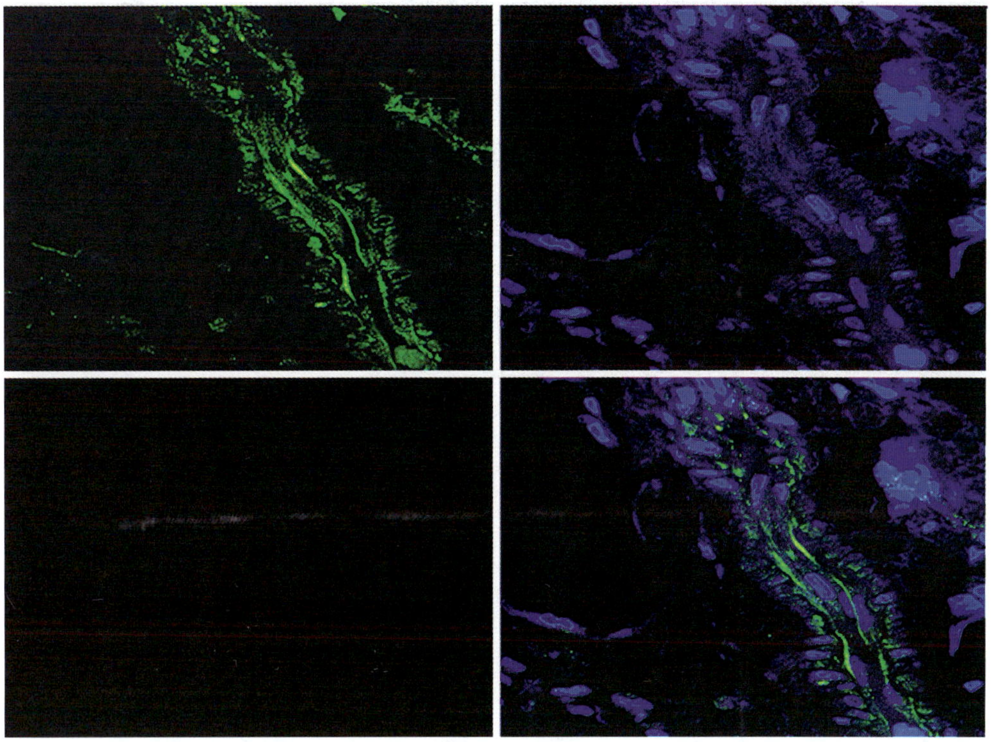

Fig. 15B

Figs. 15A and B: Day 7 neovagina SRY-Box 2 (SOX2) and octamer-binding transcription factor 4 (OCT4) staining of progenitor cells.

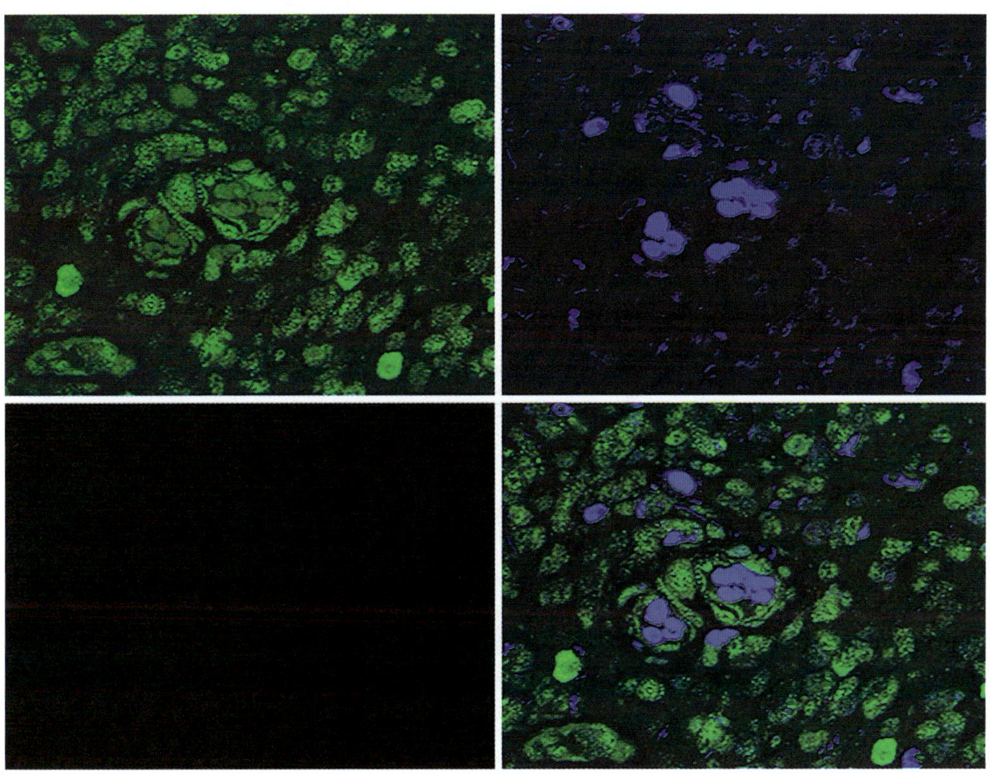

Fig. 16A

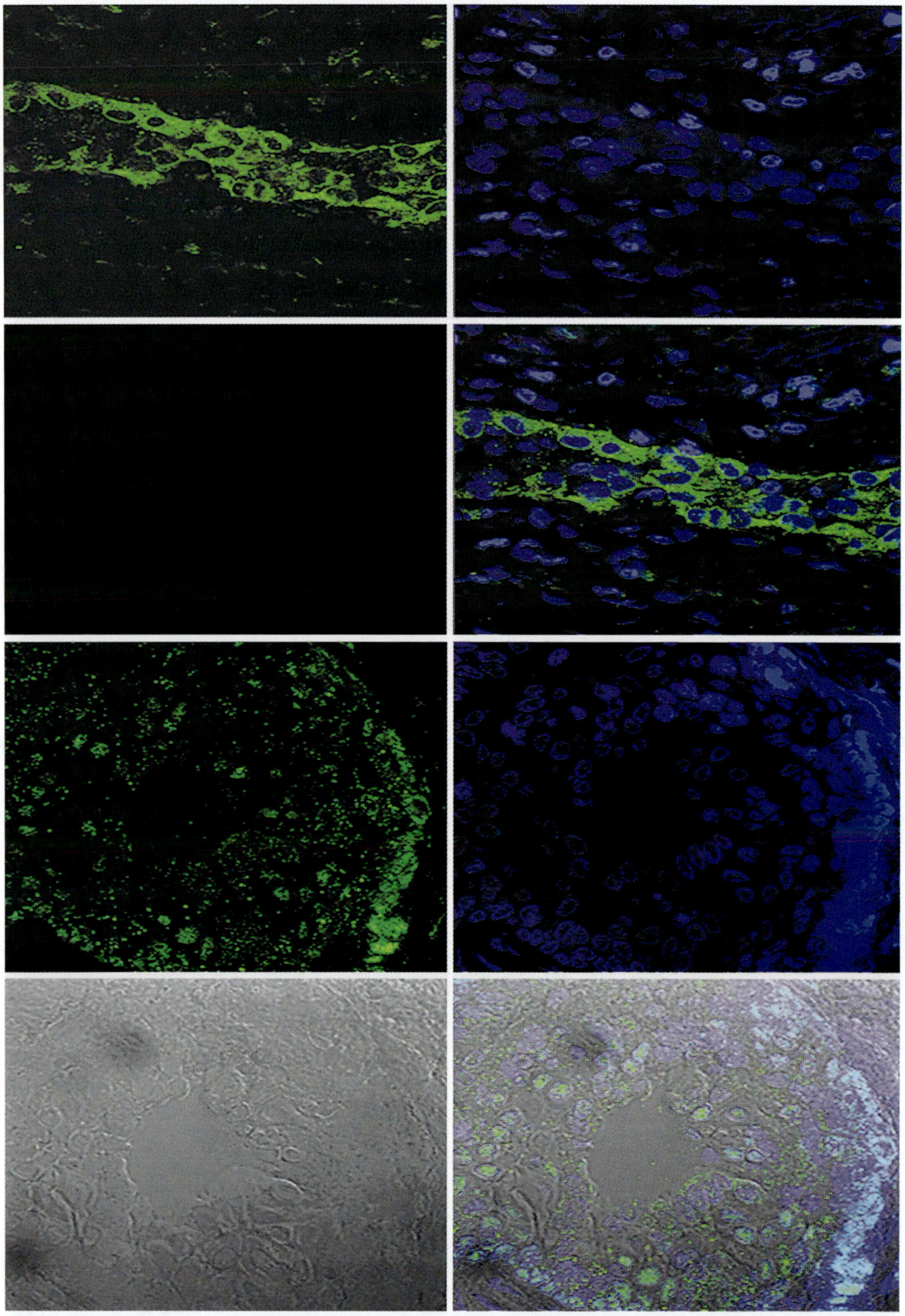

Fig. 16B

Figs. 16A and B: Day 14 of neovagina octamer-binding transcription factor 4 (OCT4) and SRY-Box 2 (SOX2) staining of progenitor cells.

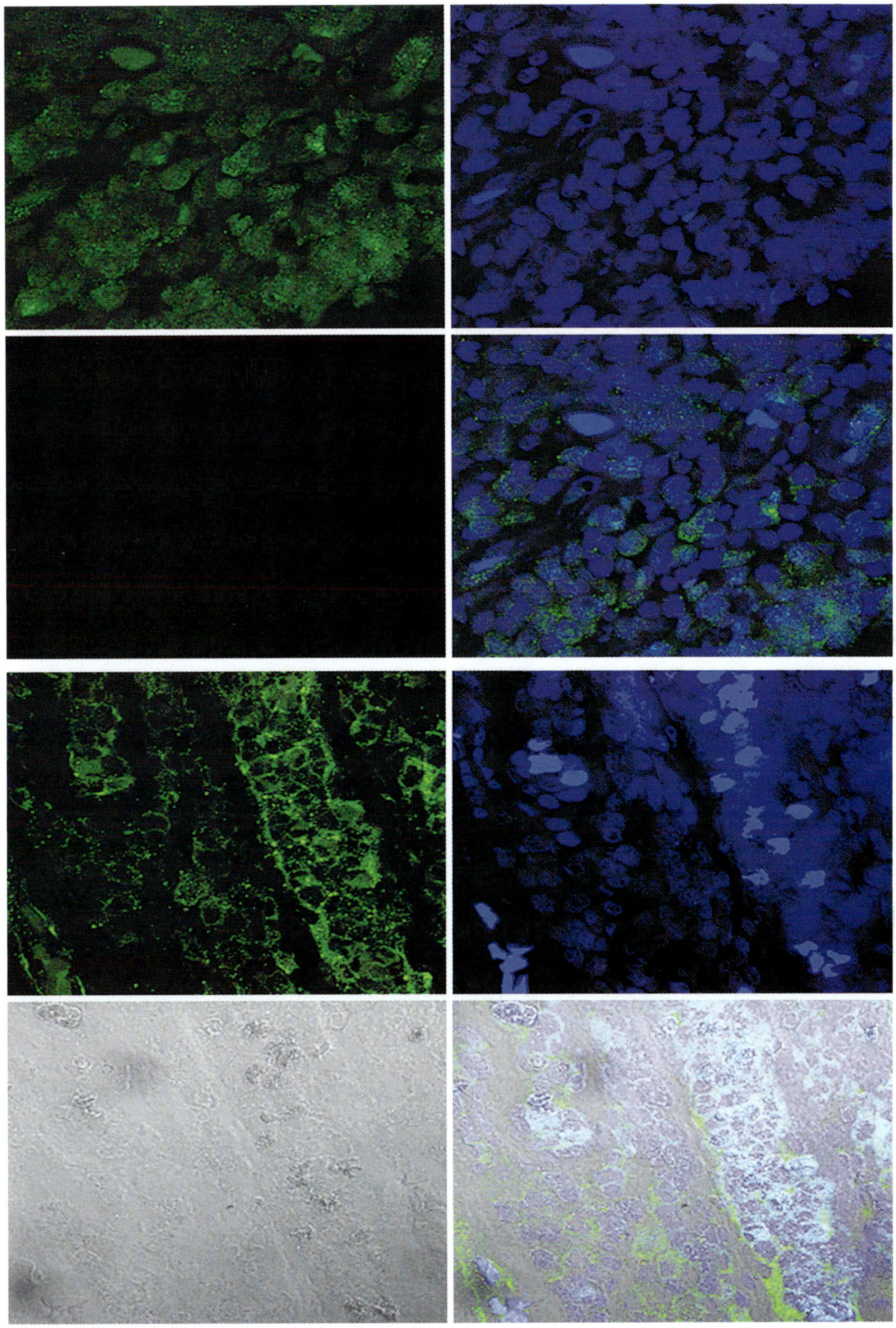

Fig. 17A

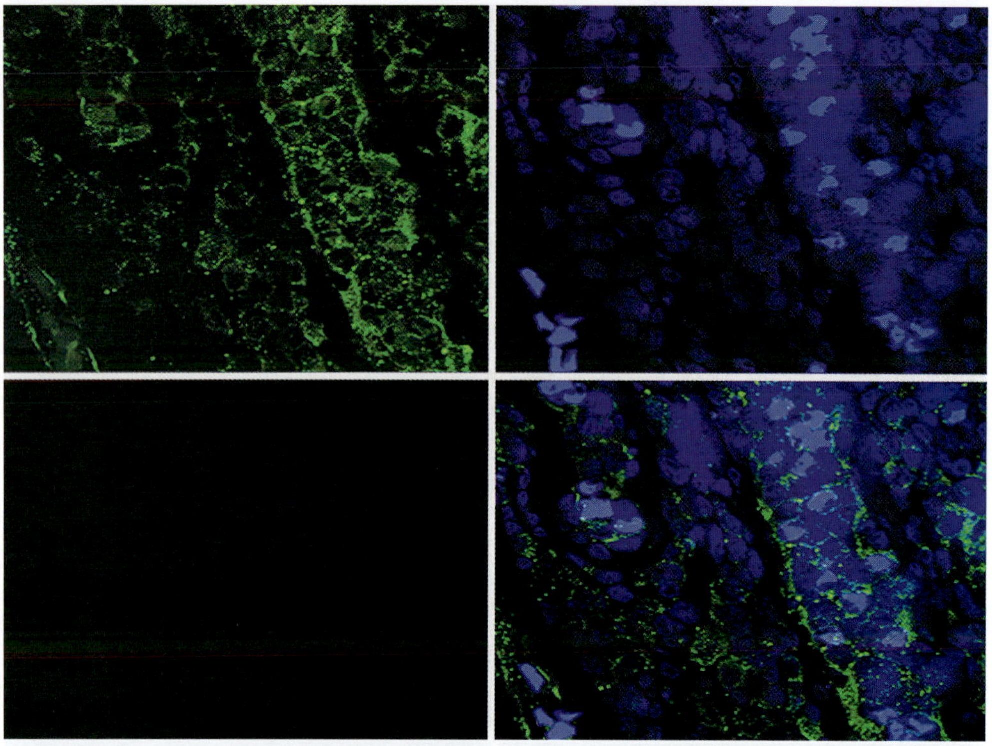

Fig. 17B

Figs. 17A and B: Day 21 of neovagina octamer-binding transcription factor 4 (OCT4) and SRY-Box 2 (SOX2) staining of progenitor cells.

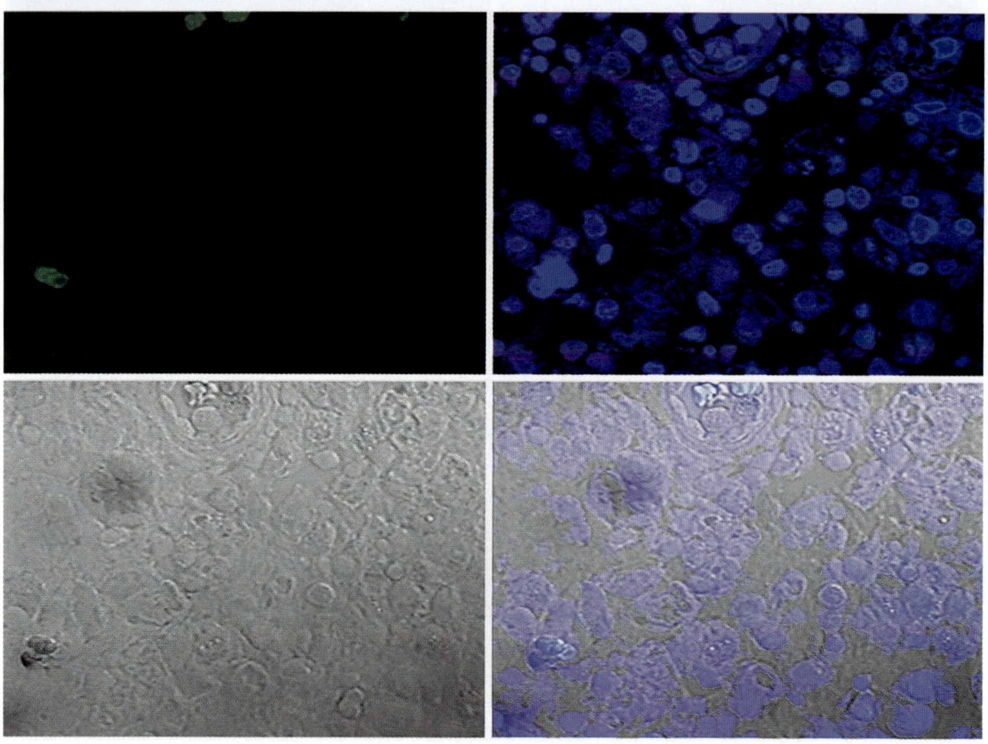

Fig. 18A

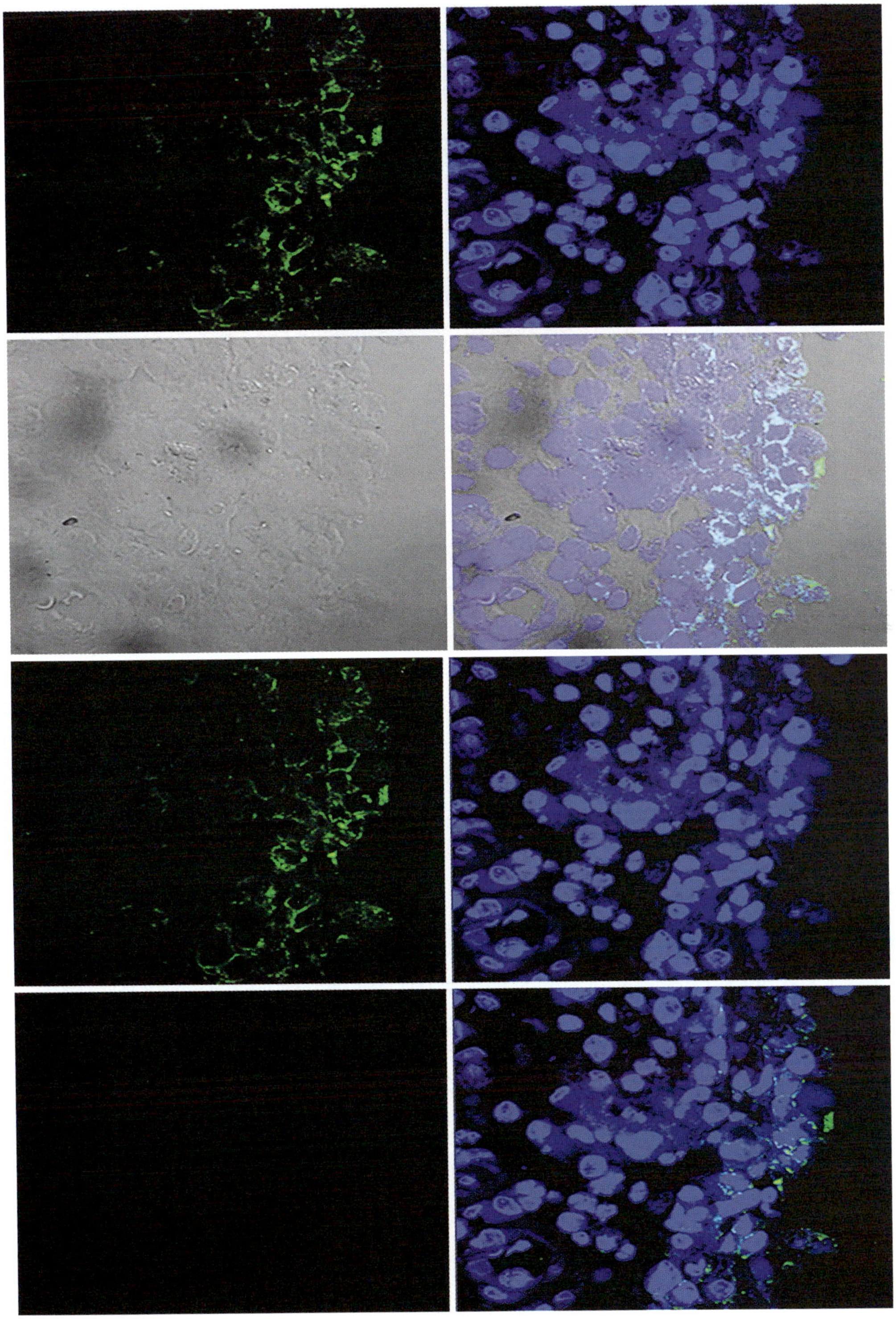

Fig. 18B

Figs. 18A and B: Day 28 neovagina octamer-binding transcription factor 4 (OCT4) and SRY-Box 2 (SOX2) staining of progenitor cells.

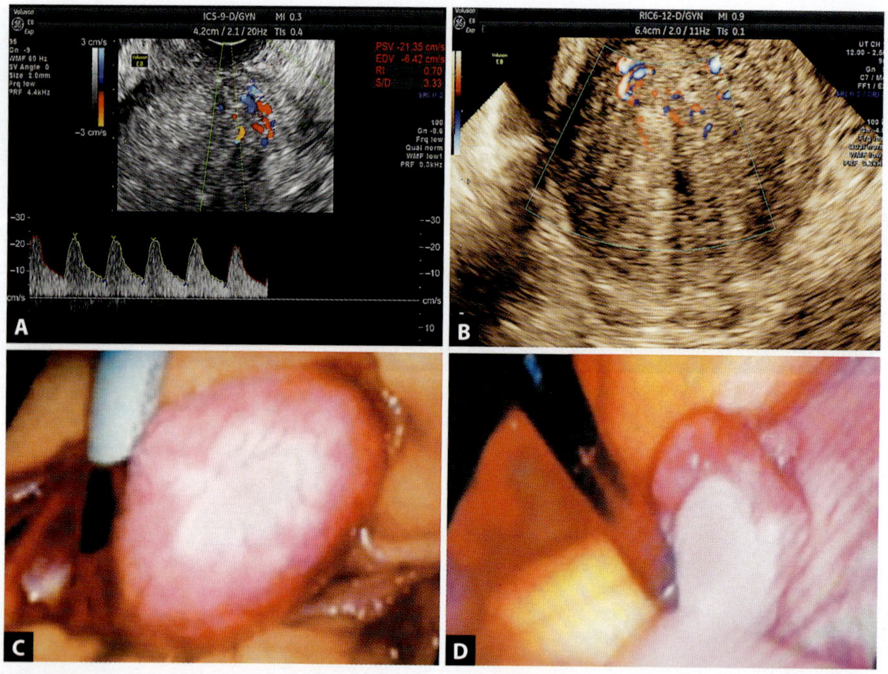

Figs. 19A to D: Normal size left utricle with normal blood flow pattern and right rudimentary utricle.

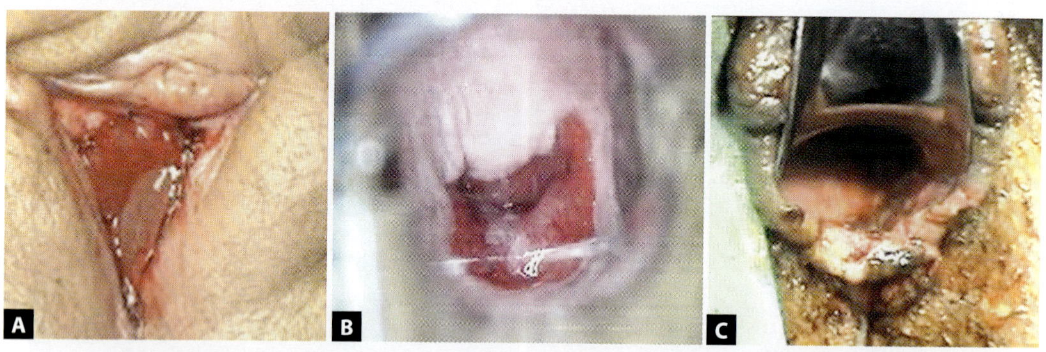

Figs. 20A to C: Vaginoplasty pictures by using (A) Colon; (B) Small intestine; and (C) Skin.

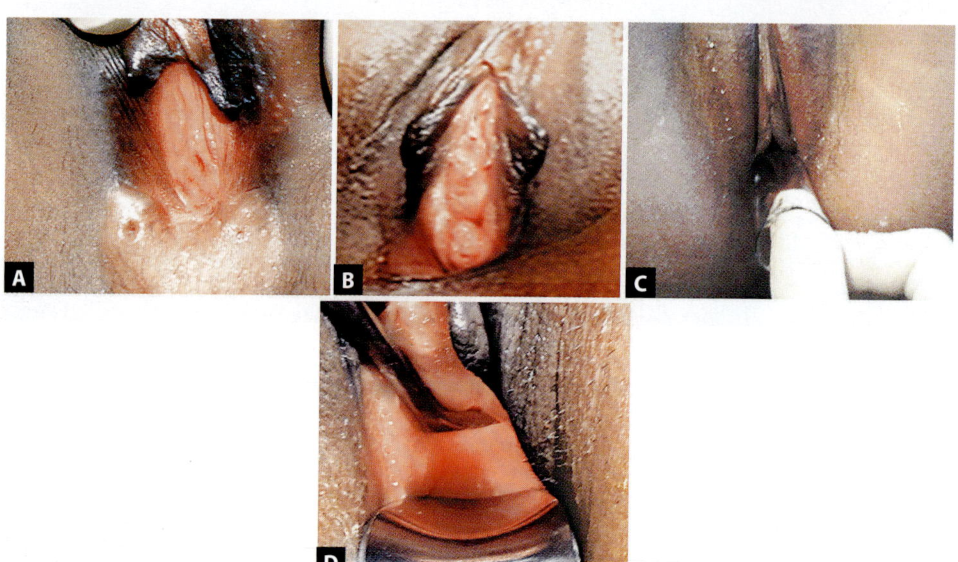

Figs. 21A to D: Pre- and postoperative pictures of dilatation and speculum examination showing near normal look of neovagina.

- The physiological parameters were pH, Doppler blood flow, and USG.
- The functional parameter was applying sexual satisfaction score.

The neovagina was comparable with the normal on all these parameters including the sexual satisfaction score. However, we found a stark difference in the three-dimensional USG studies in the neovagina (**Figs. 23A and B**).

The normal vaginal cavity is a potentially closed space due to the presence of abundant elastic tissue, while the neovagina remains an open space due to lack of elastic tissue (**Figs. 24A and B**). It was observed that the neovagina remains open in the upper half while it mimics normal vaginal contour in the lower half. This is achieved by the contraction of pelvic floor muscles (**Figs. 25A and B**). This fact has led us to routinely teach pelvic floor muscles exercises to all our patients undergoing the vaginoplasty.

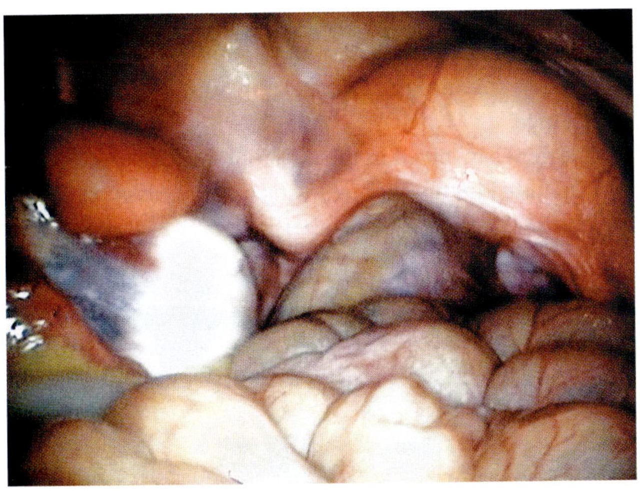

Fig. 22: Second look laparoscopic picture 1 year postsurgery, showing virgin pelvis with no telltale signs of surgery.

These observations and the lacunas due to lack of the elastic tissue prompted for the further research.

The problem was addressed by three different ways:

1. With the idea that a thick peritoneal graft could probably give a good substratum, six cases were subjected to this modified procedure. However, it was noticed that the end results are the same. The disadvantage was increased operating time and comparatively increased blood loss.
2. After using the pelvic floor exercises, a significant difference was noticed in the anatomical contour of the neovagina.
3. Efforts are on developing auto stem cell culture. These mesothelial stem cells will be used for the development of elastic tissue in the neovagina.

Finally, we have undertaken a pilot study to identify the genes responsible for the Müllerian hypoplasia to offer a genetic solution to this devastating problem.

ROLE OF STEMNESS MARKERS AND TRANSLATIONAL GENES IN CREATING NEOVAGINA

Peter Muller described the Müllerian duct in 1730, almost 300 years ago; however, the genetic information regarding its normal and anomalous development is still ill understood.

Regression of Müllerian duct is an important event in sex differentiation and main genes in formation of reproductive tract in mice are as follows:

- *Pax 2:* Null mice show lack of kidneys, ureters and genital tract.
- *Emx2:* Null mice show lack of kidneys, ureters, gonads and genital tract.
- *Lim1:* Female null mice lack Müllerian duct.

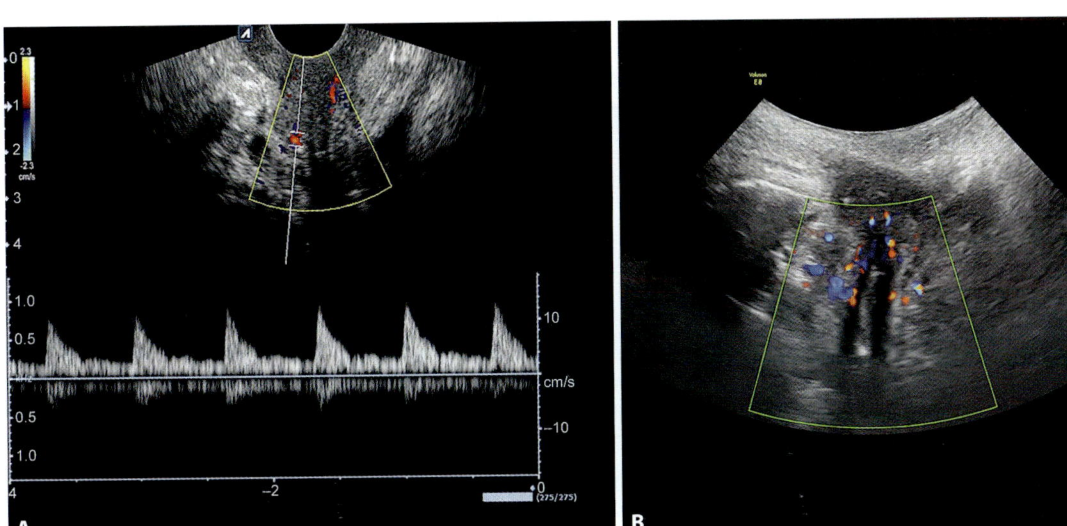

Figs. 23A and B: Functional evaluation of neovagina: (A) 3D USG; (B) Doppler angiogenesis.

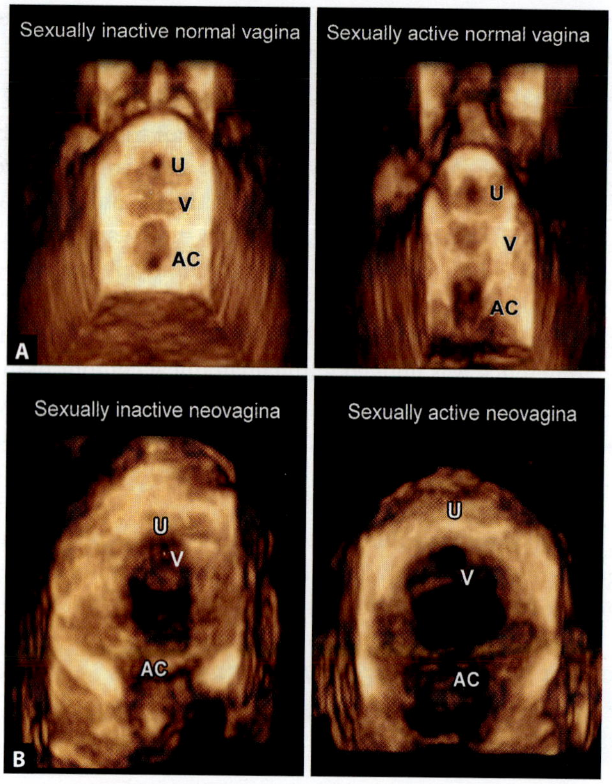

Figs. 24A and B: Comparison of normal vagina and neovagina.

- *WNT4:* It is essential for development of Müllerian duct. Both male and female null mice lack Müllerian duct. It is expressed in the mesonephros at E day 10 and also seen in mesenchyme of indifferent gonads at E day 11 and stays in female gonads and surrounding mesenchyme of Müllerian duct.
- *WNT7A:* This also plays an important role and is expressed in Müllerian epithelium at E day 12.5 and continues through life.
- *WNT5A:* This is expressed in high amount in uterus and has helps the differentiation process of reproductive tract in first 2 weeks of postnatal life.
- *HOXA 10 and 11:* Associated with correct anterior and posterior patterning of reproductive tract.
- Summarizing, *WNT4* initiates the ductal formation and morphogenesis of ductal derivatives, which are regulated by *WNT7*.

Previously, it was assumed that MRKH syndrome has sporadic genetic etiology, but familial cases have been reported in the literature suggesting autosomal dominant inheritance.

The genes involved in the development of the Müllerian tract include Lim homeobox 1 (*Lim1*), wingless-type MMTV integration site family, member 4 (*WNT4*),[3] Paired box 2

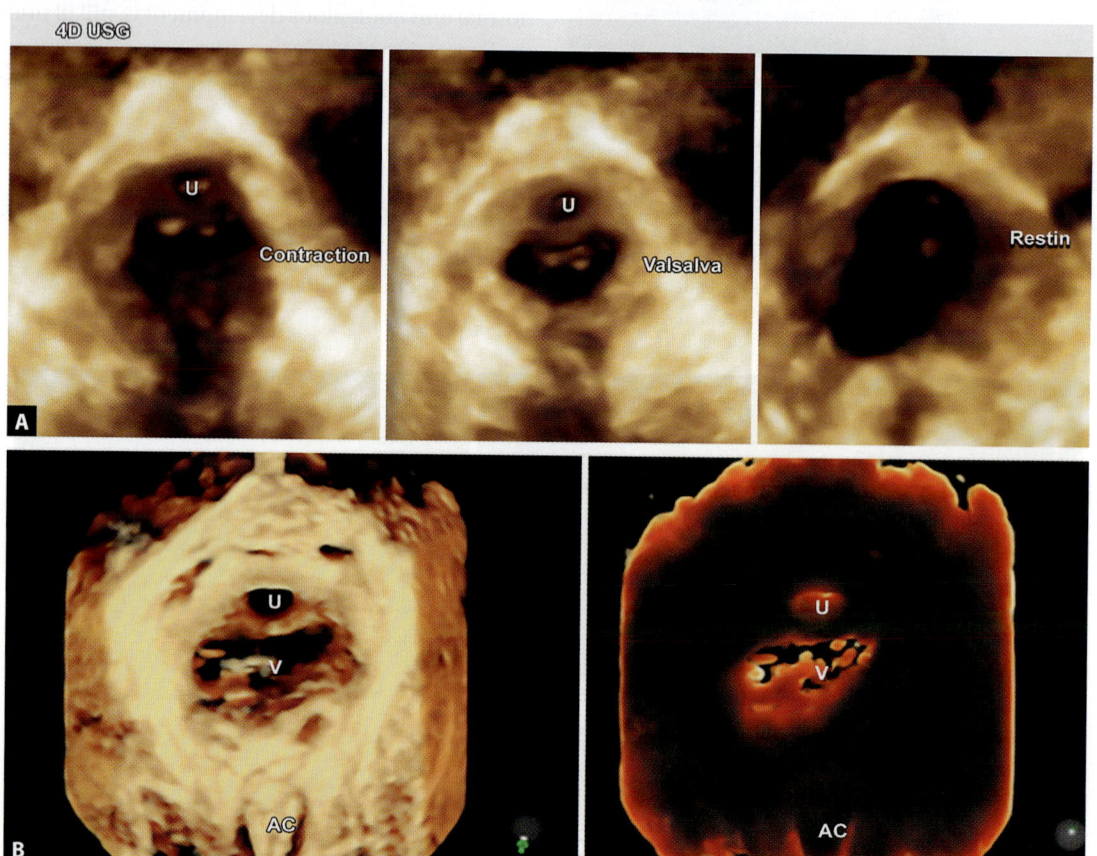

Figs. 25A and B: Contraction of pelvic floor muscles.

(*Pax2*), Empty spiracles homeobox 2 (*Emx2*), POU domain-containing transcription factor 2 (*Tcf2*), large homolog 1 (*Dlgh1*), dachshund homolog 1 and 2 (*Dach1 and Dach2*), *Hoxa13, Wnt5a, Wnt7a*, Catenin (cadherin-associated protein), beta 1 (*Ctnnb1*) and forkhead box A2 (*Foxa2*).

Three types of MRKH syndrome have been described in the literature. The first being pure MRKH syndrome, the second being associated with renal, somatic, and cardiac anomalies and the third type is in association with hyperandrogenism. No mutations in AMH or activating mutation of its associated receptor, *WT1, PBX1, PAX2, Hoxa10, Hoxa11*, a cofactor of HOX genes, have been linked to MRKH syndrome.

The third type of MRKH syndrome, which is associated with hyper-androgenism and renal malformations, is implicated to have WNT4 mutation. WNT4 mutation confirms that this signaling molecule is involved in Müllerian development and androgen repression in the ovary, WNT4, HNF1B, and LHX1 have been studied in genetic analysis of MRKH syndrome. A study using whole genome expression was done to identify the etiology of MRKH syndrome and it suggested that increased expression of estrogen receptors 1 (ESR1), Wilms Tumor 1 (WT1), and GATA-binding protein 4 (GATA4) might lead to abnormal development of the female reproductive tract. Ectopic expression of certain *HOXA* genes may also be implicated. There were three microdeletions at 16p11.2, 17q12, and 22q11.2 that were found in syndromic Müllerian aplasia case population was compared to the control population. Ledig et al. found recurrent deletions affecting TBX6, HNF1β, and LHX1 in their cohort of MRKH patients. Duplication in the *SHOX* gene has recently been identified in two daughters with MRKH type I; miRNAs may have an important role in the development and function of the female reproductive tract.

The literature remains inconclusive on genetic etiology of MRKH syndrome. Having identified the progenitor cell an attempt is made to identify the specific translational stemness markers and the activation of specific genomes in the neovagina. In the previous study presence of stemness markers was shown by staining technique using IHC. This was not specific with the DNA material hence RNA latter was prepared from the neovaginal tissue and specific cDNA was obtained. The serial expression and concentration of translational stemness markers (NANOG, OCT4, and SOX2) were identified by using the conventional PCR. The activation of various genes (*HOXA9, HOXA10A, HOXA11, HOX13, WNT4, WNT5A*, and *WNT7A*) and their concentration was identified in neovaginal tissue.

Our current research has shown the following findings:

- The study shows peritoneal metaplastic conversion to normal vagina by laparoscopic peritoneal vaginoplasty. The translational stemness markers (NANOG, OCT4, and SOX2) and expression of the specific genes (*WNT4, WNT5A*, and *WNT7A*) responsible for the neovaginal formation were identified.
- The translational stemness markers (NANOG, OCT4, and SOX2) appearance and concentration at different stages of conversion were demonstrated. The neovagina has shown upregulation of these translational stemness markers. The expression of developmental genes namely *HOXA9, HOXA10A, HOXA11, HOX13* were found to be lesser than the control samples as expected. The expressions of WNT4, WNT5A, and WNT7A were found to be increased compared to the control.
- The study confirms the normal vaginal development by peritoneal metaplasia. This technique should replace current treatment of absent vagina.
- *Research implications:* Furthering this research, manipulating and activating these genes by genetic engineering may lead to treatment of developmental defects of Müllerian duct and developing the rudimentary uterus to normal size, obviating the need of transplant. To the best of our knowledge, this study is the first to show the metaplastic conversion peritoneum to normal vagina, identifying the progenitor cell, expression of translational stemness markers and upregulation of specific genes **(Fig. 26)**.

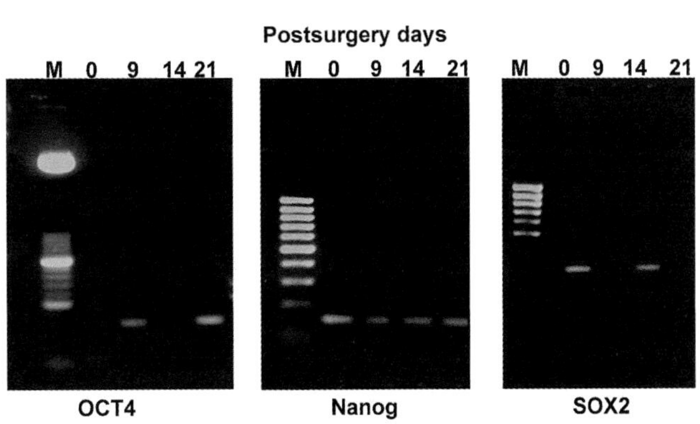

Fig. 26: Stemness markers in cDNA-OCT4-Nanog-SOX2.

The expression of candidate genes (viz., *HOXA9, HOXA10A, HOXA11, HOX13, WNT4, WNT5A, and WNT7A*)

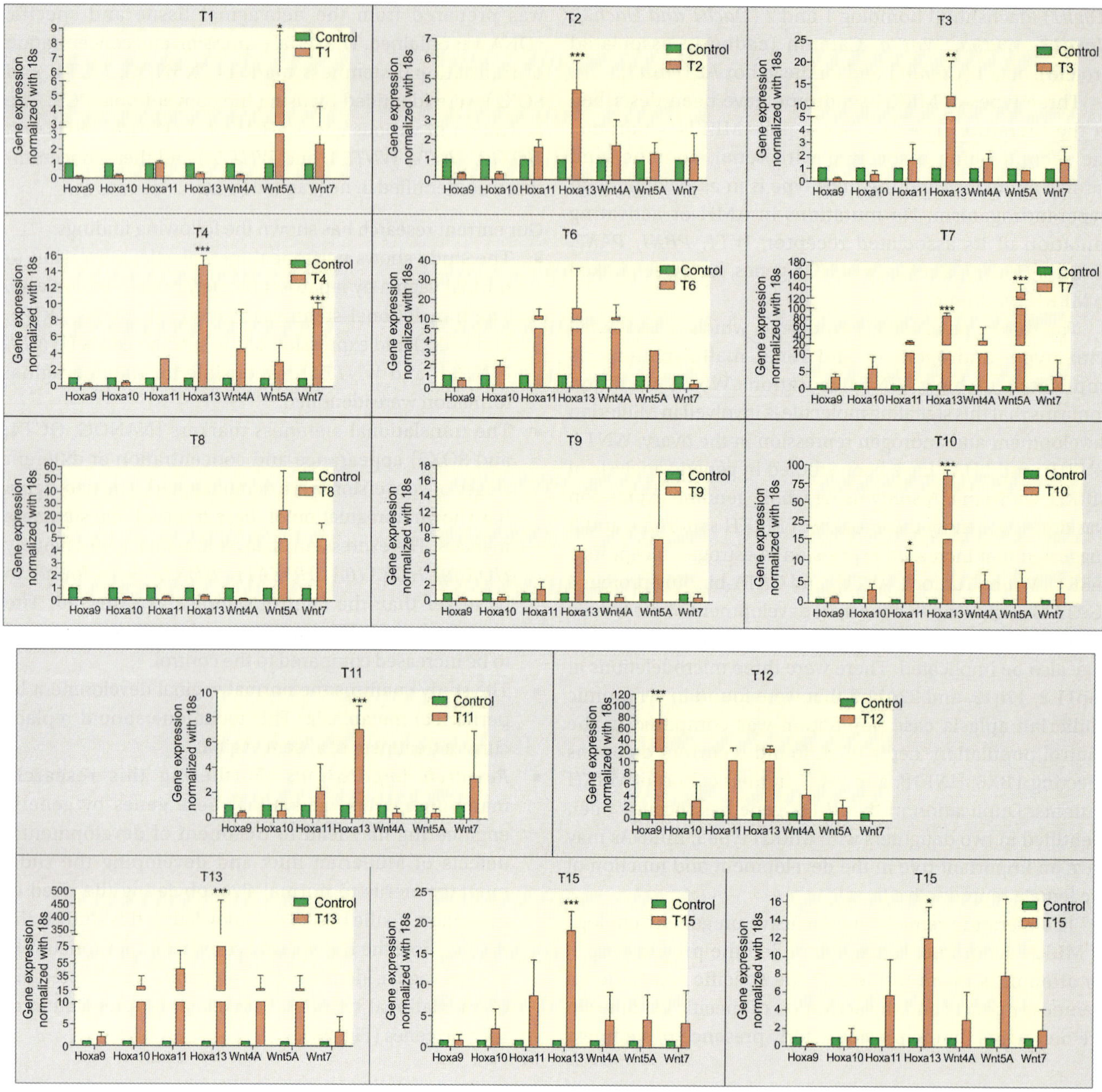

REFERENCES

1. Mhatre PN, Narkhede HR, Pawar PA, Mhatre PJ, Kumar DD. Role of progenitor cell producing normal vagina by metaplasia in laparoscopic peritoneal vaginoplasty. J Hum Reprod Sci. 2016;9(4):215-22.
2. Mhatre P, Mhatre J, Sahu R. New laparoscopic peritoneal pull-through vaginoplasty technique. J Hum Reprod Sci. 2014;7(3):181-6.
3. Mhatre P, Dighe V, Das DK, Pawar A. Novel technique of vaginoplasty developing normal vagina, role of stemness markers and translational genes. J Hum Reprod Sci. 2020;13(4):303-9.

CHAPTER 83

Genitoplasty

Prashant Puranik

INTRODUCTION

Genitoplasty refers to reparative surgery of genital organs (genito refers to genitals and plasty refers to molding or formation of specified part of body). Female genitoplasty can involve vulva, clitoris, labia, vagina, or a combination of above structures. It can be broadly classified into reconstructive and aesthetic.

Aim of surgical procedures in reconstructive genitoplasty is to reconstruct genital structures in anomalies occurring due to congenital or acquired (traumatic or oncological or dermatological disease) deformities. One of the common congenital genital anomalies encountered in gynecological services is vaginal agenesis.

Recent advances in artificial reproduction techniques have led to noninvasive methods of harvesting of ovum or insemination by vaginal approach. Patients with developmental anomalies or congenital absence of vagina can pose a technical difficulty for the same. This chapter focuses on congenital absence of vagina and its management.

EMBRYONAL BASIS

Vaginal agenesis occurs due to Müllerian dysgenesis, the most common form of it is Mayer–Rokitansky–Küster-Hauser (MRKH) syndrome. In MRKH syndrome, intermediate mesoderm is affected. Intermediate mesoderm provides blastema of cervicothoracic somites and pronephric ducts. Intermediate mesoderm anomalies can lead to coexistence of skeletal and urinary system anomalies. Pronephric ducts differentiate to mesonephric ducts. Mesonephric ducts differentiate to Wolffian ducts and Müllerian ducts. Müllerian duct affection in MRKH leads to incomplete differentiation. This is supported by the presence of Müllerian structures.[1] Cervix and vagina initially form a solid unit embryologically, vaginal agenesis occurs due to lack of cavitation, and cell death needed to form vagina.[2]

ETIOLOGY OF VAGINAL AGENESIS AND CLINICAL PRESENTATION

Mayer–Rokitansky–Küster–Hauser Syndrome

Mayer–Rokitansky–Küster–Hauser syndrome is the most common cause of vaginal agenesis. It is the second most common cause of primary amenorrhea. The most common being gonadal dysgenesis. Other names for MRKH syndrome are Müllerian aplasia, genital renal ear syndrome, or congenital absence of the uterus and vagina. The incidence ranges from 1 in 4,000 to 10,000.[3]

Genetics

Normal female morphology and endocrine status have increased the interest for study of genetic anomalies of MRKH. A wide range of malformations in closely associated organ systems suggest developmental field defect.[4] *WT1*, *PAX2*, *HOXA* cluster genes, and *PBX1* genes are involved in related organogenesis during early embryogenesis.[5,6] Deletion or duplication sequences point to the involvement of *LIM* homeobox 1 (*LHX1*), *HNF1* homeobox B (*HNF1B*), and *T-Box 6* (TBX6). *LHFX1* and *HNF1B* are located on 17q12 chromosome. Haploinsufficiency of *HNF1B* leads to *LHX1* downregulation leading to uterine hypoplasia.[7-9]

WISP2, *HOXA5*, *HOXA9*, *CDH5*, *MFAP5*, and *PEG10* genes are involved in development of female genital tract. Epigenetic abnormalities of *WISP2*, *HOXA5*, *HOXA9*, *GATA4*, and *WT1* have a key role in MRKH syndrome. These epigenetic changes could be due to environmental and stochastic factors. Epigenetic abnormality is further substantiated by development of MRKH syndrome in only one of the monozygotic twins. Chromosomal translocations are a rare cause of MRKH syndrome. Single-gene mutations and epigenetic changes are postulated to be the cause but definitive etiology is still not determined. Hence, prenatal diagnosis and genetic counseling are not useful.

Anti-Müllerian hormone (AMH) plays an important role in pathogenesis by disrupting the formation of Müllerian structures. Activating mutation of AMH gene or its receptor leads to MRKH syndrome. Estrogen regulates the level of AMH expression. Increased levels of estrogen lead to activation of AMH promoters. *WT1* and *GATA4* genes are involved in regulation of AMH. Endocrine-disrupting agents or high maternal hormonal levels lead to ectopic expression of *HOXA* genes leading to MRKH syndrome.[10-13]

Renal anomalies and skeletal anomalies occur in mothers and relatives of MRKH patients.[14,15] Hence, vaginal agenesis can be a manifestation of a variably expressing genetic abnormality. Incomplete penetrance and variable expression of an autosomal dominant gene or small chromosomal imbalances which are undetectable in standard karyotypes are suggested modes of inheritance. The majority of cases are sporadic,[16] but familial cases are also described.[17]

Mayer-Rokitansky-Küster-Hauser based on the extent of anomaly is categorized into two types. Type I/typical or Rokitansky sequence has only isolated uterovaginal agenesis. Type II/atypical has additionally, other systemic anomalies. Type II is known as *MURCS* association. It is an abbreviation for *MU*llerian duct aplasia, *R*enal dysplasia and *C*ervical *S*omite anomalies. Types 1 and 2 account for 44 and 56%, respectively.

- Urinary system anomalies occur in 40% cases.
  They can be unilateral renal agenesis, ectopic or horseshoe kidneys and pelviureteric junction obstruction.
- Skeletal anomalies occur in 30–40% cases. Vertebral anomalies are the most common.
  They can be Klippel-Feil anomaly, fused vertebrae, cervical scoliosis, or rib abnormalities.
- Auditory defects occur in 10–25% cases.
- Other rare associations are cardiac anomalies and hand anomalies such as syndactyly (fused fingers) and polydactyly (multiple fingers).

Clinical Presentation

The most common presenting symptoms are amenorrhea, inability to intercourse, and dyspareunia. Typically, medical evaluation is sought for the absence of menstruation at the age of 14–16 years. The classical presentation is primary amenorrhea in a normal female phenotype. Secondary sexual characteristics are normal except for absence of menarche. The MRKH syndrome is associated with developmental absence of the uterus and upper two thirds of vagina leading to amenorrhea. 8–10% have functioning uterus with variable development of cervix. This results in concealed menstruation and hematometra. This can present as a large, painful abdominal mass.

Clinical examination reveals well-developed secondary sexual characteristics (pubic hair and breast development are Tanner stage 5) and external genitalia **(Figs. 1A and B)** with primary amenorrhea. The vagina is reduced to a dimple (2–7 cm). There are no signs of hyperandrogenism. Inspection of genitalia at the time of birth can diagnose the condition.[3]

DIFFERENTIAL DIAGNOSIS

Differential diagnosis of MRKH syndrome includes patients presenting with primary amenorrhea and normal secondary sexual characteristics. The differential diagnoses are isolated vaginal atresia, WNT4 syndrome, and androgen insensitivity **(Table 1)**.

Transverse vaginal septum and imperforate hymen are not included. Patients with these latter conditions have normal cervix and uterus, both of which are palpable on rectal examination.[3]

Complete Androgen Insensitivity Syndrome/ Testicular Feminization Syndrome

It is the second most common cause of vaginal agenesis. It is a male pseudohermaphrodite disorder. Incidence is 1/13,000 to 40,000 live births. Androgen insensitivity syndrome is an X-linked recessive disorder with a female phenotype and 46XY karyotype. Mutation in the androgen receptor gene renders receptors insensitive to testosterone and results in female phenotype.

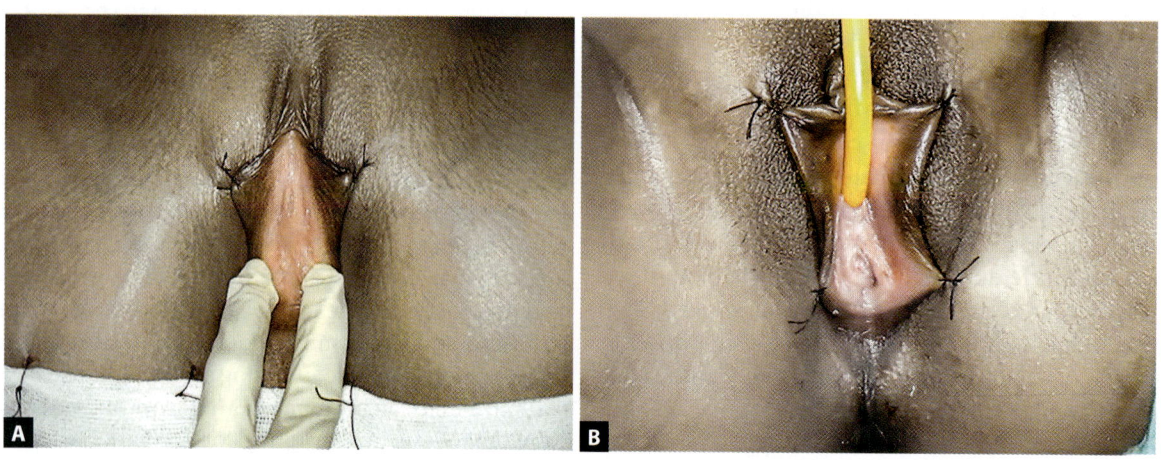

Figs. 1A and B: Vaginal agenesis with normal external genitalia—vaginal dimple in normal position.

TABLE 1: Differential diagnosis of Mayer–Rokitansky–Küster–Hauser syndrome.

	MRKH syndrome	Isolated vaginal atresia	WNT4 syndrome	Complete androgen insensitivity syndrome
Upper vagina	Absent	Variable	Absent	Absent
Uterus	Absent	Present	Absent	Absent
Gonads	Ovary	Ovary	Masculinized testis	Testis
Breast development	Normal	Normal	Normal	Normal
Pubic hair development	Normal	Normal	Normal	Sparse
Hyperandrogenism features	No	No	Yes	No
Karyotype	46XX	46XX	46XX	46XY

Clinical manifestations are normal female breast and external genitalia development with a blind vagina. Müllerian duct structures are absent with abdominal or inguinal testes. Partial androgen insensitivity presents as micropenis with or without hypospadias with gynecomastia.[18]

Isolated Vaginal Atresia

Clinical presentation is pelvic pain with cryptomenorrhea on physical examination. Vaginal atresia can be syndromic as in Winter syndrome (renal, genital, and middle ear defects)[19] or McKusick–Kaufman syndrome (hydrometrocolpos, digital anomalies such as postaxial polydactyly and cardiac malformation). In McKusick–Kaufman syndrome, pathology lies in *MKKS* gene mutations on chromosome 20p12.[20] Vaginal atresia is also a component of Bardet–Biedl syndrome and Fraser syndrome.

Müllerian aplasia of MRKH syndrome leads to irreversible sterility. Surgical correction of isolated vaginal atresia with a normal uterus can lead to pregnancy.

WNT4 Syndrome

This is characterized by XX karyotype with absence of Müllerian structures, hyperandrogenism, and renal dysplasia. Normal female phenotypes with features of hyperandrogenism are pointers to WNT4 syndrome.[21]

DIAGNOSTIC METHODS

Universal principles in the management of congenital malformations should be followed. Congenital malformations can have associated disorders of other organ systems, which also need to be investigated. Complete investigation (genetic and endocrine) with accurate diagnosis is crucial. MRKH is a diagnosis of exclusion and merits thorough evaluation.

Workup would include karyotype, hormonal study, and ultrasound of the abdomen. A pelvic magnetic resonance imaging (MRI) is needed in difficult cases.

Biological Status

The karyotype in MRKH syndrome is 46XX without major genetic abnormality. The karyotype in androgen insensitivity syndrome is 46XY.

Hormonal Studies

These are the indicators of ovarian function. In MRKH syndrome, hormonal studies (follicle-stimulating hormone, luteinizing hormone, and 17-β estradiol) are normal. Androgen levels (plasma level of testosterone, delta-4-androstenedione, 17-hydroxyprogesterone, and dehydroepiandrosterone) are also normal.[22]

Transabdominal Ultrasonography

Transabdominal ultrasonography is the first investigation to evaluate Müllerian structures. Transvaginal, transperineal, or even transrectal ultrasonography can also be performed. It is a simple, noninvasive test. It is characterized by the absence of the Müllerian structures between the bladder anteriorly and rectum posteriorly.

Mayer–Rokitansky–Küster–Hauser type I syndrome has normal fallopian tubes with rudimentary horns. Rudimentary horns are linked with peritoneal fold.[23] MRKH type 2 is characterized by symmetric or asymmetric uterine hypoplasia, accompanied by hypoplasia or aplasia of one or both the fallopian tubes with aplasia of one of the two horns or by a size difference between the two horn rudiments.[24] A quadrangular retrovesical structure, noncavitated vestigial lamina can give a pseudo appearance of hypoplastic or juvenile uterus.[25] Urinary system malformations can be evaluated systemically.

Magnetic Resonance Imaging

Magnetic resonance imaging is a noninvasive technique with higher sensitivity and specificity than ultrasonography. It is the gold standard for evaluation of Müllerian agenesis. It is indicated in an inconclusive ultrasonographic study. It provides an accurate evaluation of Müllerian structures and other pelvic organs. Nonvisualization of ovaries, uterus, or Müllerian rudiments in ultrasound is not confirmatory of their absence. MRI provides an accurate evaluation of uterine aplasia with clear visualization of the rudimentary horns and ovaries. Uterine aplasia is best visualized on sagittal views and vaginal aplasia on transverse section images.[26-28] MRI can simultaneously evaluate for renal and skeletal anomalies.

Laparoscopy

This is an invasive technique requiring anesthesia. It is indicated in cases of diagnostic uncertainty after ultrasonography and/or MRI. Laparoscopy is preferred in cases needing additional interventions. It defines the precise anatomical location and abnormalities of the uterus, tubal remnants, the vestigial lamina, and the ovaries. It can also be used as a therapeutic modality to drain hematometra, excise symptomatic remnants of the Müllerian system, or achieve uterine–vaginal anastomosis with a well-developed uterus.

A systemic evaluation must be done to identify associated malformations. Asymptomatic nature of renal and skeletal abnormalities necessitates at least a screening transabdominal ultrasonography and spine radiography. Intravenous pyelogram may be needed to diagnose urinary system anomalies. Suspected hearing impairment or cardiac anomaly necessitates screening with an audiogram or echography and specialist consultation. In familial cases, investigation of the patient's relatives may be recommended for renal and skeletal malformations.[3]

PSYCHOLOGICAL ASPECTS OF MÜLLERIAN APLASIA

Evaluation of the psychological status of MRKH patients is important. Müllerian agenesis deprives the woman, both coitus and childbearing, thus doubting her femininity. Vaginal agenesis can have significant consequences on self-image and sexual identity, as well as serious social problems considering engagement and marriage. This leads to negative impact on her psychological, sexual, and social well-being. Psychological harm sustained during early adolescent years can lead to difficulty in sustaining relationships. They are also at risk of long-term sexual dysfunction and face difficulties to integrate with society.

Psychological difficulties of adolescence are more complex, making assessment difficult in comparison with children or adults. Intellectual development in adolescence varies widely. There is a complete discrepancy between physical maturity and intellectual maturity. Physical maturity can be attained by the age of 15 or 16 years, but intellectual maturity cannot be reached until the age of 18–20 years. This discordance poses problems in evaluation. This necessitates specially trained psychological counselors.[29]

Physician's lack of appreciation of the difficulties and inability to communicate affect patients negatively.[30] Degree of emotional reactions to the diagnosis and treatment is influenced by age and relationship with her parents and partner. Doubts about gender, inability to fulfill female roles, lead to depression. Infertility is more difficult to accept than coital inability. Prolonged counseling with positive reinforcement is vital and input from psychological services improves the outcome.[31] Group programs can be useful.

Psychological input into the preparation of patients is essential. It helps them to adapt to their abnormality, prepare for neovaginal creation techniques, and address the infertility component. They can achieve good sexual function after treatment and build a genetically related family utilizing in vitro fertilization (IVF) with a gestational carrier.[32-35] Creation of a neovagina helps restore self-confidence. This has been proven in quality-of-life studies.[36] As a general rule, it is useful to counsel patients that after the creation of neovagina, it is possible to have normal sexual activity and build healthy sexual relationships.[37]

Treatment of patients with vaginal aplasia requires psychological support, adequate information to the fulfillment of the complexities of female sexual response, together with the creation of a neovagina to give the patient the prospect of a normal sexual life.

MANAGEMENT

Neovaginal creation can be done by either nonsurgical or surgical techniques. Motivation of the patient and individual needs can be considered to decide the best treatment option for a patient. There is no ideal method of reconstruction, substantiated by multiple treatment options. Treatment consists of creating a neovagina. This must be offered to patients, when they are emotionally mature and preferably starting sexual activity **(Table 2)**.

An ideal neovagina must be satisfying in appearance, function, and sensation. Reconstruction should recreate neovagina in a normal position with normal dimensions directed posterior-superiorly. It should be sensate, at least at introitus level. The technique should be simple, reliable, one staged with minimal morbidity **(Fig. 2)**.[38]

TABLE 2: Procedures to create neovagina.

Nonsurgical creation of neovagina	• Frank method • Ingram method
Surgical creation—traction method	Vecchietti operation: • Laparotomy • Laparoscopic
Surgically created neovaginal lined with or without grafts	• Split-thickness skin graft • Full-thickness skin graft • Amnion • Peritoneum • Buccal mucosa • Absorbable adhesion barriers • Tissue expansion
Neovagina lined with flaps	• Pudendal flap • Gracilis myocutaneous flap • Rectus abdominis flap • Scapular free flap
Vulvovaginoplasty	William's operation
Bowel vaginoplasty	• Sigmoid colon • Ileum • Cecum

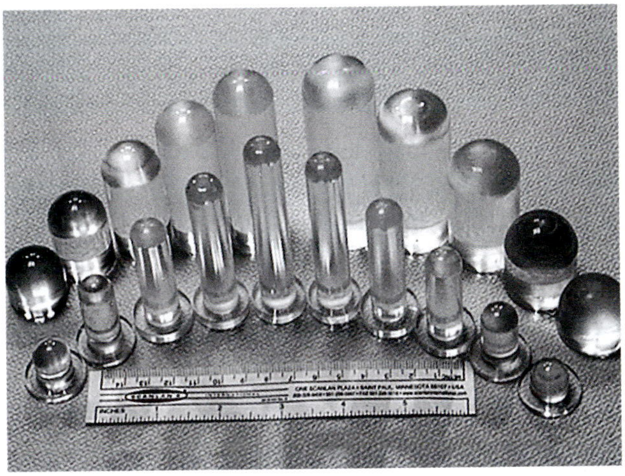

Fig. 2: Acrylic dilators of increasing size.
Source: Lee MH. Non-surgical treatment of vaginal agenesis using a simplified version of Ingram's method. Yonsei Med J. 2006;47(6):892-5.

NONSURGICAL CREATION OF A NEOVAGINA

Nonsurgical approach is recommended as a first-line therapy. It is noninvasive and complications are rare. These methods can be applied in incomplete vaginal agenesis, when the vaginal dimple is deep (2–4 cm).

Frank Dilator Method

This is the most commonly used nonsurgical method. It is a form of tissue expansion. The technique involves dilatation of the vaginal dimple with progressively increasing dimensions of vaginal dilators or mold with active participation of the patient **(Figs. 3A to C)**. Dilators are placed on the vaginal dimple for at least 20 minutes a day. 6 months is a typical time to attain functional depth and width of neovagina. Regular follow-ups are recommended to evaluate patient motivation and skills in using the dilator.

The dilators come in a number of formats, made of different materials. Well-motivated, well-supported patients achieve good results. In a compliant and well-motivated patient, satisfactory length of the vagina for intercourse can be achieved in 75–85% of cases.[39]

Ingram Method

This variation of Frank's method uses a bicycle stool.[40] Ingram introduced a bicycle seat stool, where the patient could sit and use her trunk weight to hold in place the vaginal dilators and create pressure over the vaginal dimple **(Figs. 3A to C)**. The whole process requires 6 weeks to several months using dilators of increasing size, with a success rate varying from 78% to 92%.[41,42]

The advantages of nonsurgical treatment are outpatient treatment, patient control, cost-effectiveness, minimal morbidity, and complications. If the patient is not able to complete treatment or achieve adequate dimensions, surgical intervention is an option. Patient's familiarity with vaginal mold can also help in postoperative period. Disadvantages include the length of time required to achieve a functional vagina, discomfort, risk of urethritis, cystitis, fistula, and vaginal prolapse.

Common difficulties experienced by patients are cramping, pain, fatigue, lack of comfort, unpleasantness, privacy issues, and lack of time to dilate daily. These lead to poor compliance with higher failure rates, unless patients are persistent and well motivated.[39,43]

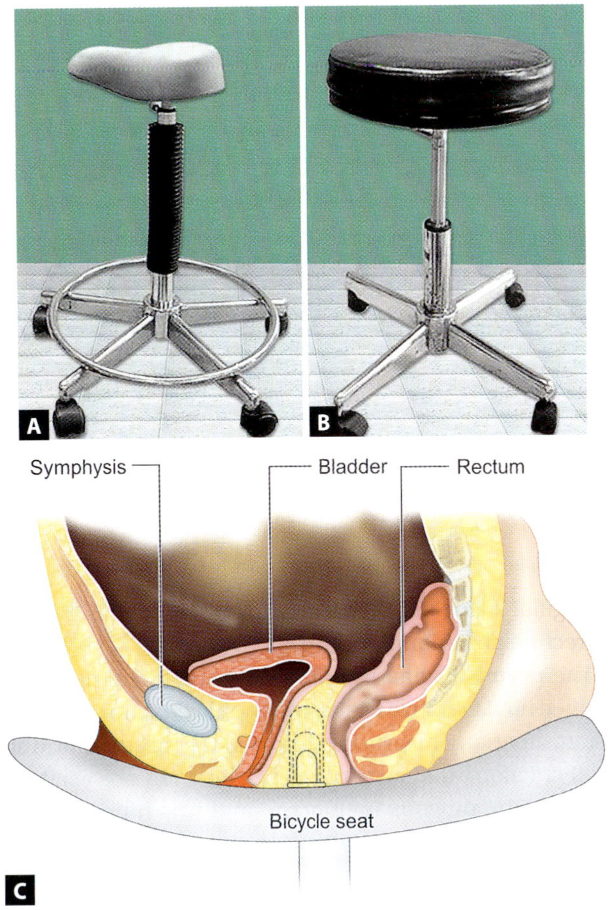

Figs. 3A to C: Bicycle seat stool or ordinary stool can be used to hold acrylic dilators.
Source: https://www.qrcodematrix.com/ingram-bicycle-seat-stool.

SURGICAL CREATION OF A NEOVAGINA

Vaginal reconstruction for vaginal agenesis is a challenging procedure. Failed nonsurgical methods or refusal of nonsurgical treatment is an indication for surgical treatment. Surgery should be done on a mature and motivated patient, ideally starting active sexual life. There is no consensus on the best modality of surgical creation of neovagina. The approach is often based on the surgeon's experience.

Preoperative bowel preparation should be done. Surgical creation of neovagina can be performed in spinal or general anesthesia. Surgery has two components. First is creation of

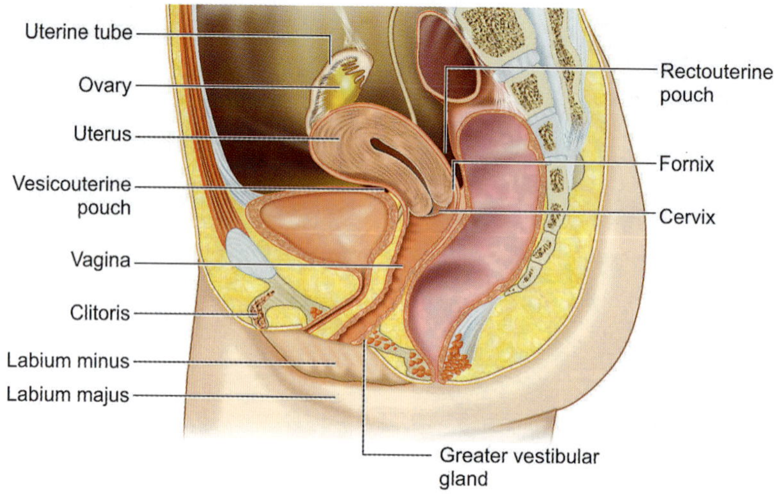

Fig. 4: Anatomical relations of vagina.

neovaginal space between urethra and bladder anteriorly and rectum posteriorly **(Fig. 4)**.

The normal vagina is a fibromuscular tube lined with stratified nonkeratinized squamous epithelium. It is inclined posterosuperiorly measuring 7.5 cm along the anterior wall and 9 cm along the posterior wall. There are no secretory glands in the mucous membrane and it is lubricated by mucus derived from cervical glands.

The second component is the lining of this neovaginal cavity with skin or mucous membrane, to maintain neovaginal dimensions and prevent contracture. Surgical creation of the neovaginal cavity is universal for all techniques. The source of the vaginal lining can be diverse. The lining can be a nonvascularized graft or vascularized flap.

Creation of Neovaginal Cavity

Transverse or Y incision is made at the apex of the vaginal dimple and blunt dissection is done between the urethra and bladder anteriorly and the rectum posteriorly. Dissection is done in cephalon-posterior direction. Neovaginal cavity must reach the peritoneum to prevent excessive contracture postoperatively. Depth of dissection should be in the range of 10–14 cm. The risk of injury to the rectum, urethra, or bladder and fistula formation ranges between 0% and 7.6%. Urinary catheter anteriorly and assistant's gloved finger in the rectum posteriorly help to prevent injury to the bladder and rectum. Trendelenburg position during neovaginal cavity creation displaces the bowel from the pelvis and helps prevent bowel injury **(Figs. 5A and B)**.[44]

Abbe–McIndoe Procedure

Abbe–McIndoe operation is an easy and commonly used technique. Neovaginal space is lined with a partial-thickness skin graft. Skin graft is spread over a stent, placing dermal side outward for lining the cavity **(Figs. 6A to D)**.

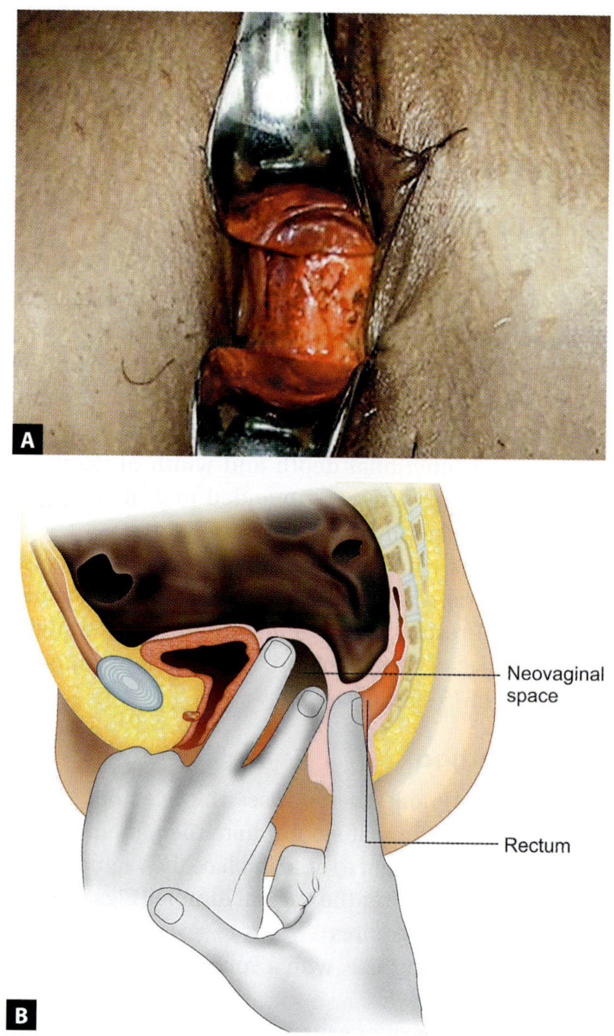

Figs. 5A and B: Neovaginal cavity creation between urethra, bladder, and rectum.

Source: For Figure 5B—Gebhart JB, Breech LL, Hurst BS, Rock JA. Congenital Vaginal Abnormalities. [online] Available from https://clinicalgate.com/congenital-vaginal-abnormalities/ [Last accessed November, 2022].

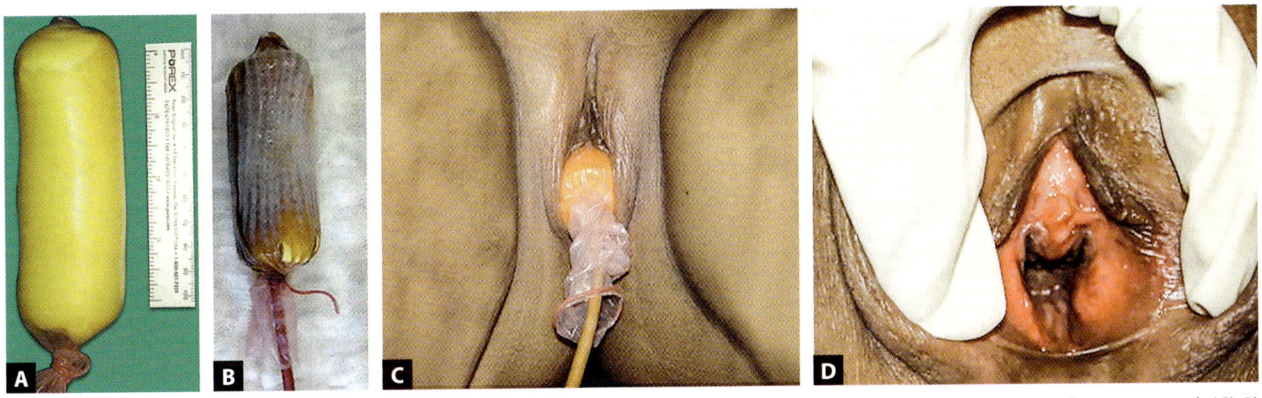

Figs. 6A to D: Abbe–McIndoe procedure: (A) Vaginal mold; (B) Skin graft placed over vaginal mold with dermal side facing upward; (C) Skin graft with vaginal mold in the neovaginal cavity; and (D) Postoperative result.
Courtesy: Dr Vinita Puri, Professor and Head, Department of Plastic and Reconstructive Surgery, Seth GS Medical College, Mumbai, Maharashtra.

Two to three sheets of skin graft are needed to achieve the required dimensions. The skin grafts can be harvested from the gluteal region or thigh. Postoperative vaginal dilatation is pivotal for good outcomes **(Figs. 6A to D)**.

Graft take can be unpredictable and mold has to be used continuously for 3 months, at least during nighttimes. Vaginal stents or conformers or molds are used for up to 3–6 months. 3–4 months after surgery, once the skin graft matures, intercourse should be encouraged. If the patient has intercourse two to three times per week, conformer elimination can be considered, else night stenting should be continued. Intercourse acts as an effective obturator.

Historically candle wax, carved balsa wood, gauze packing, syringe casing, dental wax, and hard plastic conformers have been used as vaginal stents. Mold consistency can be soft, semirigid, or rigid. Soft molds have a lower incidence of fistula formation due to reduced pressure and lesser risk of avascular necrosis. An alternative is the use of the inflatable soft stent with reduced risk of hematoma and fistula formation without affecting healing.

All other methods of reconstruction are compared with the traditional Abbe–McIndoe procedure. Skin graft donor-site morbidity, graft contracture, and dryness are the disadvantages of Abbe–McIndoe procedure. Shrinkage of neovagina, especially in the upper third, can lead to partial or total vaginal obliteration. Preferably, patients should use dilated postoperatively for 6 months to 1 year, even with regular sexual activity. Lubrication is required before intercourse.

Modifications of this procedure have been devised to reduce donor morbidity. Absence of external scars (skin graft donor scars) is the main advantage of these modifications. It could be spontaneous epithelialization or the use of different materials such as peritoneum,[45] buccal mucosa, amnion,[46] labia minora grafting, or synthetic materials.[47,48] The use of freeze-dried amnion has been described by Ashworth. Donors should be screened for human immunodeficiency virus and other infectious diseases.[49]

Fasciocutaneous Flaps

Neurovascular pudendal thigh flap or Singapore flap of Wee and Joseph, modified Singapore flap of Karl Podratz and Woods and lotus petal flaps in vulvovaginal reconstruction of Niranjan have been used for vaginal reconstruction. These are inferiorly based axial pattern flaps.

Vascular supply is from posterior labial arteries. Innervation of flaps from posterior labial branch of pudendal nerve and perineal branch of posterior cutaneous nerve thigh provides sensation. Flaps are harvested from the thigh crease lateral to hair-bearing area. Flaps of dimension 9 × 4 cm to 15 × 6 cm are raised on either side. Posterior margin of flap is at the posterior fourchette. Flaps are tunneled under labia majora or after the division at the level of fourchette. Flaps are tubed for neovaginal creation **(Figs. 7A to F)**.

These flaps do not require long-term dilatation of neovagina through mold **(Figs. 7A to F)**.[50]

Skin flaps have the advantage of full-thickness vascularized skin, which resists shrinkage. These flaps are highly vascularized, thin, pliable, and reliable. These flaps are sensate, at least at introitus. The disadvantage of this technique is hair growth in the created vagina, which can result in dyspareunia and discharge. Laser epilation or harvesting flap from nonhearing portion can be done.

Vulvovaginoplasty Procedure

Williams vulvovaginoplasty creates vagina using the labia majora and minora. "U"-shaped flap from nonhair-bearing skin within the labia majora is used to create a new vagina. In O'Brien's vulvovaginoplasty, vulval tissue is used. This flap divides all the neurovascular input coming from the internal pudendal system.[38,51]

Labial tissue transfers distort the external appearance of the genitalia with the conspicuous scar. Abnormal angle may result in dyspareunia in the long term. Neovagina is of smaller diameter; hence, regular use of dilator is advised to increase the dimensions of the cavity.

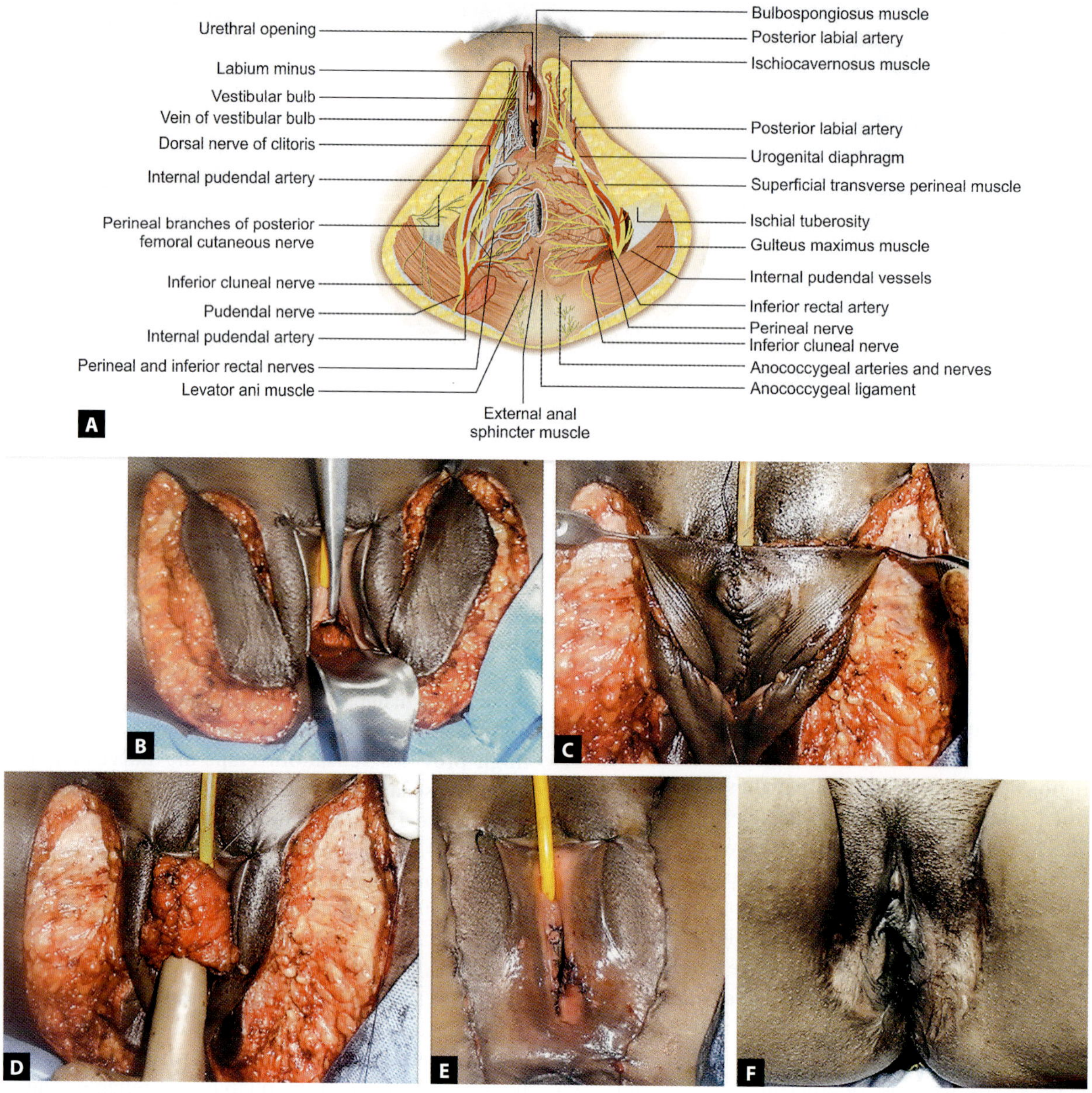

Figs. 7A to F: (A) Neurovascular pudendal thigh flap; (B) Neural and vascular basis of pudendal thigh flap; (C) Raised bilateral pudendal thigh flap; (D) Formation of tubed neovagina; (E) Tubed neovagina; and (F) Postoperative result: 4 months postoperative result.

Vecchietti Procedure

The Vecchietti operation combines both surgical and nonsurgical techniques. This is similar to nonsurgical dilatation without relying on the patient. Neovagina is created by a traction device placed over the anterior abdominal wall, which exerts traction over the vaginal skin. It can be performed through the open technique or a less invasive laparoscopic approach.

The technique involves placing plastic olive over the vaginal dimple. Sutures anchored to plastic olive pass through rectovesical space and preperitoneally to the anterior abdominal wall skin. These sutures are attached to the traction device. Traction on the suture stretches the vaginal skin through the olive and creates vagina **(Figs. 8A to E)**.

Dilatation is done daily or on alternative days. Vaginal length of 10–12 cm is created over 7–9 days. Vaginal dilators should be used after creation of neovagina to prevent shrinkage **(Figs. 8A to E)**.[52-54]

Main disadvantage is the pain due to the traction device and prolonged hospitalization. Prolonged hospitalization is needed for managing pain. This technique is difficult to perform after failed surgeries.

Intestinal Transfers

Intestinal transfers are generally reserved for more difficult cases where simple vaginoplasties have failed with postsurgical scarring. Previously scarred area is excised and

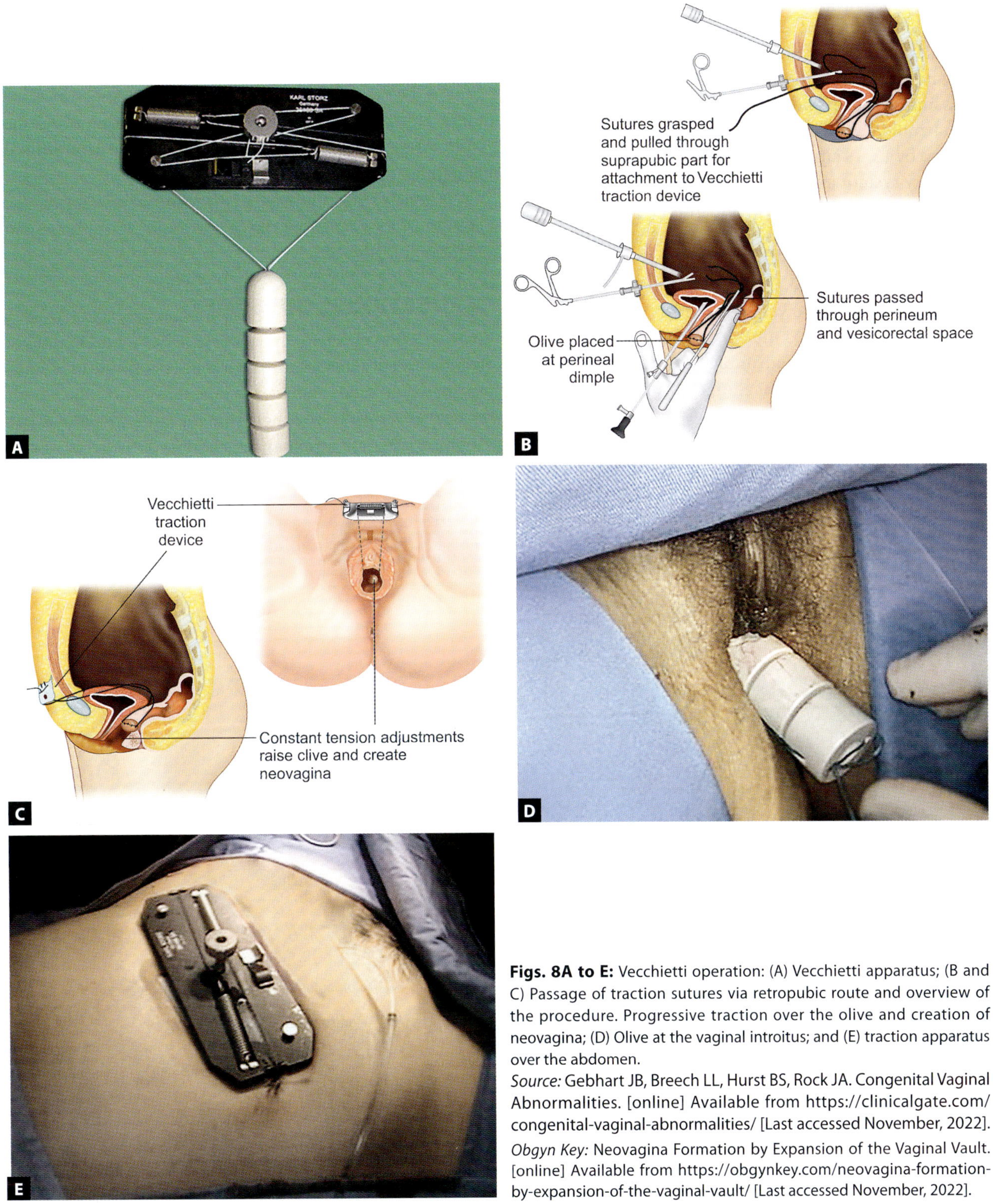

Figs. 8A to E: Vecchietti operation: (A) Vecchietti apparatus; (B and C) Passage of traction sutures via retropubic route and overview of the procedure. Progressive traction over the olive and creation of neovagina; (D) Olive at the vaginal introitus; and (E) traction apparatus over the abdomen.

Source: Gebhart JB, Breech LL, Hurst BS, Rock JA. Congenital Vaginal Abnormalities. [online] Available from https://clinicalgate.com/congenital-vaginal-abnormalities/ [Last accessed November, 2022].

Obgyn Key: Neovagina Formation by Expansion of the Vaginal Vault. [online] Available from https://obgynkey.com/neovagina-formation-by-expansion-of-the-vaginal-vault/ [Last accessed November, 2022].

neovaginal cavity is created; neovagina is resurfaced with a loop of bowel. Sigmoid colon is the best segment to use.[29]

Surgery involves mobilizing a segment of intestine with its feeding blood supply into the surgically created neovaginal cavity. It can be performed as pedicled transfer or free tissue transfer. In pedicled transfer, a segment of intestine with its intact blood supply is transposed into the neovaginal cavity. In free tissue transfer, blood supply needs to be re-established by anastomosing intestinal blood vessels to the perineal blood vessel.

Baldwin's ileal procedure utilizes the ileal segment of intestine. Constant caliber of the ileum with good lubrication is the advantage. Traumatization of mucosa during intercourse, with bleeding and chronic secretion of mucus, makes it a less popular procedure.

In sigmoidal vaginoplasty or Ruge procedure, neovagina is created by 12–18 cm segment of sigmoid[55] **(Figs. 9A to C)**.

Urinary system anomalies in MRKH syndrome such as single kidney or left pelvic kidney impair this procedure. Restoration of coital function may require prolonged care and support **(Figs. 9A to C)**.[56]

Intestinal transfers require laparotomy or laparoscopy. Anastomotic leaks of bowel anastomosis, adhesive bowel obstruction, and copious mucous secretion which can be foul smelling are the disadvantages. Bowel necrosis and fistula are potential complications. Hiroi et al.[57] recently reported a mucinous adenocarcinoma arising in a neovagina using the sigmoid colon.

Postoperative Care

Postoperative care would involve complete immobilization for 5–7 days. Low-fiber diet and constipation are advised for 3–5 days. Local hygiene is crucial due to the proximity to anus. First dressing of skin graft is usually done at 5–7 days. Manual support of mold is advised during straining and coughing.

Potential problems are shortening of vagina, fecal contamination, postoperative immobilization, bowel, and bladder injuries.

FUNCTIONAL OUTCOMES

Partner's perception of the neovagina has found that there is a high level of satisfaction and has not been able to identify it as a newly created vagina.[58,59] Sexual satisfaction and length of neovagina are not correlated from the patient's perspective.[31] Highest subjective sexual satisfaction of 97.8% in sexually

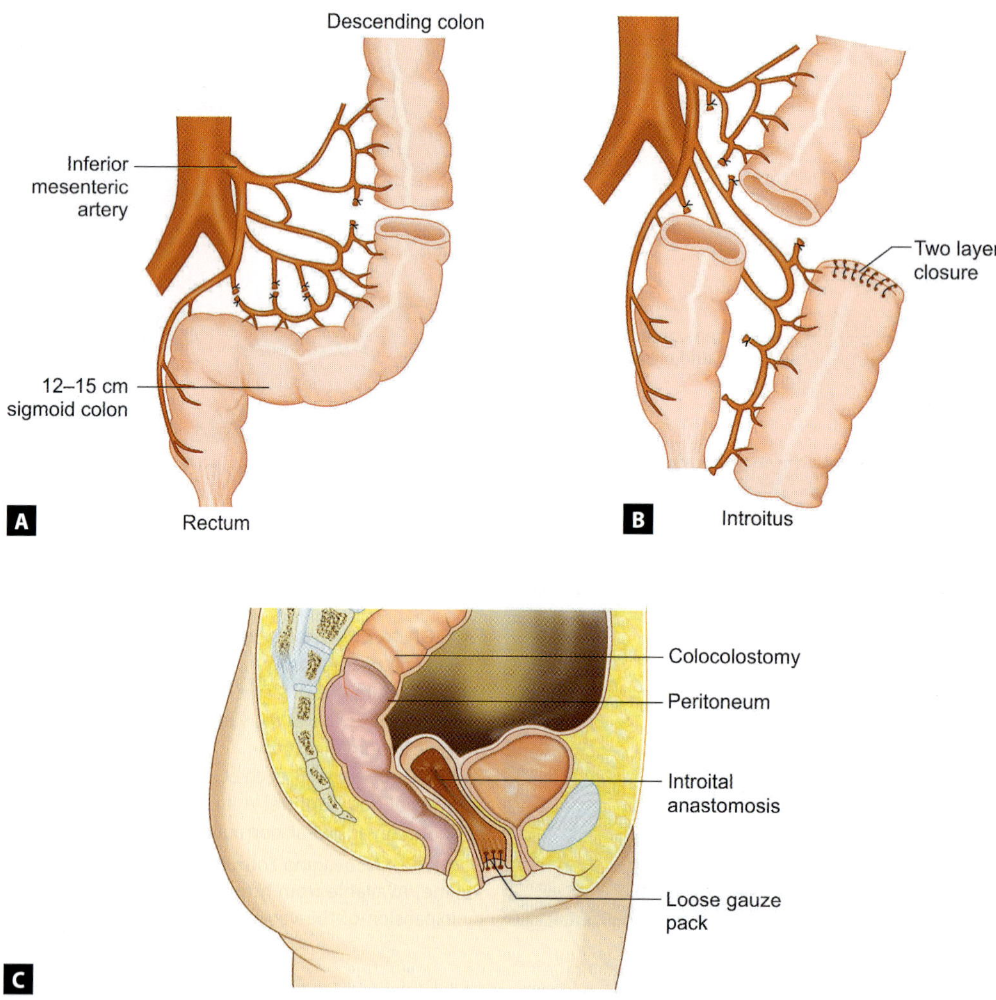

Figs. 9A to C: Sigmoid vaginoplasty. (A) Isolation of 12–15 cm of sigmoid mucosa; (B) Sigmoid colon is placed in neovaginal position and anchored to vulvar mucosa; (C) Colocolostomy is completed and peritoneum is closed above transposed bowel. Neovagina between rectum and bladder.

Source: Nowier A, Esmat M, Hamza RT. Surgical and functional outcomes of sigmoid vaginoplasty among patients with variants of disorders of sex development. Int Braz J Urol. 2012;38(3):380-6; discussions 387-8.

active is found in flap reconstruction cases. Overall, assessing the results and treatment success of various techniques in relation to patient satisfaction is difficult.[60]

MANAGEMENT OF INFERTILITY

Most difficult aspect in MRKH is infertility. MRKH syndrome causes uterine factor infertility, due to absence of anatomical or functional uterus. However, there are rare reports of conception after neovagina reconstruction and establishing continuity with developed uterus. Adoption or utilization of gestational surrogacy is an option to attain a biological child.[61]

Ovaries, due to different embryonic origin, are normal and respond to ovarian hyperstimulation to obtain oocytes.[31-35] Ovarian hyperstimulation for harvest of ovum can be started with random start protocols, since there is no need to collaborate embryo transfer and endometrial lining, similar to oncological patients.[62]

The response to ovarian hyperstimulation is measured by number of oocytes harvested and fertilization rate. The quality of embryos in MRKH syndrome is slightly lower than average. Pregnancy rates are also below the average for infertile patients. Additionally, pelvic anatomy in MRKH patients favors oocyte retrieval via transabdominal route than the transvaginal approach.[34]

Gestational surrogacy in MRKH syndrome is an attractive alternative, even though the reported number of pregnancies after IVF is small. Children of patients born to MRKH mothers have been normal, but due to relative uncertainty of the etiology of MRKH, children born after such procedures should be evaluated. In a series of 162 IVF cycles in MRKH syndrome patients, 34 children were born. MRKH transmission risk is difficult to evaluate as the genetic basis is unclear. However, no congenital abnormalities were found in these offspring ruling out dominant fashion of inheritance.[63] Similarly, Beski et al. have reported similar outcome figures and no congenital abnormalities.[64] Goldfarb et al. in their surrogacy program also had equally encouraging results.[65] Infertility treatment options through IVF can be utilized as part of the long-term care of these patients. Clinicians can therefore consider IVF surrogacy as an option for MRKH patients, who wish to attempt pregnancy. However, counseling of patients about risk should be done till a definitive level of evidence is reached. Gestational surrogacy is currently banned in many countries. Uterine transplant is an emerging treatment for uterine factor infertility.

Uterine transplant is a complex procedure with ethical, moral, cultural, legal, and social concerns. In comparison with other transplants, it risks four parties—donor, recipient, partner of recipient, and the possible future child. Pregnancies are planned after onset and regularization of menstrual cycles following uterine transplantation. During pregnancies, regular monitoring of immunosuppressive drug levels is preferred. Evaluation for rejection, fetal growth, uterine and cord vessel blood flow, and regular cardiotocography are advised.[61]

Uterine transplant for MRKH syndrome was first performed in 2011.[66] First clinical series involving nine patients, from living donor, was performed in Sweden between 2012 and 2013. Seven of them had MRKH syndrome. Live birth after uterine transplantation was first reported in 2014, showing uterine factor infertility is now treatable.[67]

FUTURE SCOPE

Tissue engineering of skin can provide full-thickness skin grafts without donor-site scar morbidity. Modification of McIndoe procedure using autologous in vitro cultured vaginal tissue as a graft for neovaginal creation has been reported.[68] This technique can produce similar vaginal lining tissue without any donor-site scarring.

Organ engineering is advancing rapidly, though in its infancy. Significant efforts are being made to bioengineer the uterus. Organ engineering requires creation of matrix, recellularization of matrix followed by transplant into the recipient. Matrix for organ regeneration can be from synthetic matrix or decellularized donated uterus. Recellularization of the uterine matrix is done by recipients' own stem cells or somatic cells. This bioengineered uterus after transplant would theoretically function as a transplanted uterus without donor morbidity and immunosuppression, as in uterine transplantation. Several scaffolds have been promising. Major limitation is the efficiency of recellularization in vitro and in vivo.[61,69] Successful tissue-engineered uterus supporting pregnancy has been reported in rats. Studies on engineering various components of human uterus on sterile model or animal scaffold are underway.[70-74]

Molecular genetics may identify gene sequences responsible for etiology of MRKH syndrome. This knowledge may help guide treatment and development.

CONCLUSION

- Most common cause of vaginal agenesis is MRKH syndrome.
- Vaginal agenesis can be associated with skeletal and urinary anomalies.
- Evaluation and management of psychological difficulties is crucial.
- Nonsurgical management should be preferred initial treatment.
- Surgery consists of creating neovaginal cavity and lining the cavity.
- Lining can be achieved with skin or mucosal graft, flap, labial tissue or intestinal segment.
- Newer advances in artificial reproduction techniques like oocyte retrieval, gestational surrogacy, uterine transplant give hope of attaining genetic child.

REFERENCES

1. Karam KS, Salti I, Hajj SN. Congenital absence of the uterus. Clinicopathologic and endocrine findings. Obstet Gynecol. 1977;50:531-5.
2. Counseller VS. Congenital absence of the vagina. JAMA. 1948;136:861.
3. Morcel K, Camborieux L, Guerrier D. Mayer-Rokitansky-Küster-Hauser (MRKH) syndrome. Orphanet J Rare Dis. 2007;2:13.
4. Duncan PA, Shapiro LR, Stangel JJ, Klein RM, Addonizio JC. The MURCS association: Mullerian duct aplasia, renal aplasia, and cervicothoracic somite dysplasia. J Pediatr. 1979;95:399-402.
5. Guerrier D, Mouchel T, Pasquier L, Pellerin I. The Mayer-Rokitansky-Küster-Hauser syndrome (congenital absence of uterus and vagina)—phenotypic manifestations and genetic approaches. J Negat Results Biomed. 2006;5:1.
6. Burel A, Mouchel T, Odent S, Tiker F, Knebelmann B, Pellerin I, et al. Role of HOXA7 to HOXA13 and PBX1 genes in various forms of MRKH syndrome (congenital absence of uterus and vagina). J Negat Results Biomed. 2006;5:4.
7. Kobayashi A, Shawlot W, Kania A, Behringer RR. Requirement of Lim1 for female reproductive tract development. Development. 2004;131:539-49.
8. Ledig S, Brucker S, Barresi G, Schomburg J, Rall K, Wieacker P. Frame shift mutation of LHX1 is associated with Mayer-Rokitansky-Küster-Hauser (MRKH) syndrome. Hum Reprod. 2012;27:2872-5.
9. Coffinier C, Barra J, Babinet C, Yaniv M. Expression of the vHNF1/HNF1beta homeoprotein gene during mouse organogenesis. Mech Dev. 1999;89:211-3.
10. Rall K, Barresi G, Walter M, Poths S, Haebig K, Schaeferhoff K, et al. A combination of transcriptome and methylation analyses reveals embryologically-relevant candidate genes in MRKH patients. Orphanet J Rare Dis. 2011;6:32.
11. Miyamoto Y, Taniguchi H, Hamel F, Silverside DW, Viger RS. A GATA4/WT1 cooperation regulates transcription of genes required for mammalian sex determination and differentiation. BMC Mol Biol. 2008;9:44.
12. Aubin J, Lemieux M, Tremblay M, Behringer RR, Jeannotte L. Transcriptional interferences at the Hoxa4/Hoxa5 locus: importance of correct Hoxa5 expression for the proper specification of the axial skeleton. Dev Dyn. 1998;212:141-56.
13. Watanabe K, Kobayashi Y, Banno K, Matoba Y, Kunitomi H, Nakamura K, et al. Recent advances in the molecular mechanisms of Mayer-Rokitansky-Küster-Hauser syndrome. Biomed Rep. 2017;7(2):123-7.
14. van Lingen BL, Reindollar RH, Davis AJ, Gray MR. Further evidence that the WT1 gene does not have a role in the development of the derivatives of the mullerian duct. Am J Obstet Gynecol. 1998;179:597-603.
15. van Lingen BL, Reindollar RH, Davis AJ, Gray MR. Molecular genetic analysis of the PAX2 gene in patients with congenital absence of the uterus and vagina. Fertil Steril. 1998;70:S402.
16. Carson SA, Simpson JL, Malinak LR, Elias S, Gerbie AB, Buttram Jr VC, et al. Heritable aspects of uterine anomalies. II. Genetic analysis of Mullerian aplasia. Fertil Steril. 1983; 40:86-90.
17. Tiker F, Yildirim SV, Barutcu O, Bağiş T. Familial mullerian agenesis. Turk J Pediatr. 2000;42:322-4.
18. Sultan C, Lumbroso S, Paris F, Jeandel C, Terouanne B, Belon C, et al. Disorders of androgen action. Semin Reprod Med. 2002;20:217-28.
19. King LA, Sanchez-Ramos L, Talledo OE, Reindollar RH. Syndrome of genital, renal, and middle ear anomalies: a third family and report of a pregnancy. Obstet Gynecol. 1987;69:491-3.
20. Slavotinek AM, Searby C, Al-Gazali L, Hennekam RCM, Schrander-Stumpel C, Orcana-Losa M, et al. Mutation analysis of the MKKS gene in McKusick-Kaufman syndrome and selected Bardet-Biedl syndrome patients. Hum Genet. 2002;110:561-7.
21. Biason-Lauber A, Konrad D, Navratil F, Schoenle EJ. A WNT4 mutation associated with Mullerian-duct regression and virilisation in a 46,XX woman. N Engl J Med. 2004;351:792-8.
22. Fraser IS, Baird DT, Hobson BM, Michie EA, Hunter W. Cyclical ovarian function in women with congenital absence of the uterus and vagina. J Clin Endocrinol Metab. 1973;36:634-7.
23. Jones KL. Rokitansky sequence. In: Smith DW, Jones KL (Eds). Smith's Recognizable Patterns of Human Malformations, 4th edition. Philadelphia, PA: Saunders WB; 1988. pp. 570-1.
24. Strubbe EH, Willemsen WN, Lemmens JA, Thijn CJ, Rolland R. Mayer-Rokitansky-Küster-Hauser syndrome: distinction between two forms based on excretory urographic, sonographic, and laparoscopic findings. Am J Roentgenol. 1993;160:331-4.
25. Paniel J, Haddad B, el Medjadji M, Vincent Y. Value of ultrasonography in utero-vaginal aplasia. J Gynecol Obstet Biol Reprod (Paris). 1996;25:128-30.
26. Maubon A, Ferru JM, Courtieu C, Mares P, Rouanet JP. Gynecological malformations. Classification and contribution of different imaging methods. J Radiol. 1996;77:465-75.
27. Carrington BM, Hricak H, Nuruddin RN, Secaf E, Laros Jr RK, Hill EC. Mullerian duct anomalies: MR imaging evaluation. Radiology. 1990;176:715-20.
28. Troiano RN, McCarthy SM. Mullerian duct anomalies: imaging and clinical issues. Radiology. 2004;233:19-34.
29. Edmonds DK. Congenital malformations of the genital tract and their management. Best Pract Res Clin Obstet Gynaecol. 2003;17(1):19-40.
30. Kaplan EH. Congenital absence of the vagina. Psychoanal Q. 1970;39:52-70.
31. Poland ML, Evans TN. Psychologic aspects of vaginal agenesis. J Reprod Med. 1985;30:340-4.
32. Raziel A, Friedler S, Gidoni Y, Ben Ami I, Strassburger D, Ron-El R. In vitro fertilization surrogacy in rare coexisting Mayer-Rokitansky-Küster-Hauser syndrome and triple X karyotype. Fertil Steril. 2011;95(5):1788.e11-3.
33. Raziel A, Friedler S, Gidoni Y, Ben Ami I, Strassburger D, Ron-El R. Surrogate in vitro fertilization outcome in typical and atypical forms of Mayer-Rokitansky-Küster-Hauser syndrome. Hum Reprod. 2012;27(1):126-30.
34. Londra L, Chuong FS, Kolp L. Mayer-Rokitansky-Küster-Hauser syndrome: a review. Int J Womens Health. 2015;7:865-70.
35. Brinsden PR. Gestational surrogacy. Hum Reprod Update. 2003;9(5):483-91.
36. Bean EJ, Mazur T, Robinson AD. Mayer-Rokitansky-Küster-Hauser syndrome: sexuality, psychological effects, and quality of life. J Pediatr Adolesc Gynecol. 2009;22(6):339-46.
37. Committee on Adolescent Health Care Committee opinion: no. 562: mullerian agenesis: diagnosis, management, and treatment. Obstet Gynecol. 2013;121(5):1134-7.

38. Purushothaman V. Horse shoe flap vaginoplasty—a new technique of vaginal reconstruction with labia minora flaps for primary vaginal agenesis. Br J Plast Surg. 2005;58(7):934-9.
39. Callens N, De Cuypere G, De Sutter P, Monstrey S, Weyers S, Hoebeke P, et al. An update on surgical and non-surgical treatments for vaginal hypoplasia. Hum Reprod Update. 2014;20(5):775-801.
40. Ingram JM. The bicycle seat stool in the treatment of vaginal agenesis and stenosis: a preliminary report. Am J Obstet Gynecol. 1981;140:867-73.
41. Rock JA, Reeves LA, Retto H, Baramki TA, Zacur HA, Jones Jr HW. Success following vaginal creation for Müllerian agenesis. Fertil Steril. 1983;39:809-13.
42. Roberts CP, Haber MJ, Rock JA. Vaginal creation for mullerian agenesis. Am J Obstet Gynecol. 2001;185:1349-52; discussion 1352-3.
43. Willemsen WN, Kluivers KB. Long-term results of vaginal construction with the use of Frank dilation and a peritoneal graft (Davydov procedure) in patients with Mayer-Rokitansky-Küster syndrome. Fertil Steril. 2015;103(1):220-227.e1.
44. Hojsgaard A, Villadsen I. McIndoe procedure for congenital vaginal agenesis: complications and results. Brit J Plast Surg. 1995;48:97-102.
45. Davydov SN. Colpopoeisis from the peritoneum of the uterorectal space. Akush Ginekol (Mosk). 1969;45:55-7.
46. Dhall K. Amnion graft for treatment of congenital absence of the vagina. Br J Obstet Gynaecol. 1984;91:279-82.
47. Jackson ND, Rosenblatt PL. Use of Interceed absorbable adhesion barrier for vaginoplasty. Obstet Gynecol. 1994;84: 1048-50.
48. Motoyama S, Laoag-Fernandez JB, Mochizuki S, Yamabe S, Maruo T. Vaginoplasty with Interceed absorbable adhesion barrier for complete squamous epithelialization in vaginal agenesis. Am J Obstet Gynecol. 2003;188:1260-4.
49. Ashworth MF, Morton KE, Dewhurst J, Lilford RJ, Bates RG. Vaginoplasty using amnion. Obstet Gynecol. 1986;67: 443-6.
50. Mostafa W. Pudendal thigh flap in vaginal agenesis. Egypt J Plast Reconstr Surg. 2012;36(1):99-108.
51. O'Brien B, Mellow MC, MacIsaac IA, Maher PJ, Barbaro C. Treatment of vaginal agenesis with a new vulvovaginoplasty. Plast Reconstr Surg. 1990;85(6):942-8.
52. Borruto F. Mayer-Rokitansky-Küster syndrome: Vecchietti's personal series. Clin Exp Obstet Gynecol. 1992;19(4):273-4.
53. Borruto F, Chasen ST, Chervenak FA, Fedele L. The Vecchietti procedure for surgical treatment of vaginal agenesis: comparison of laparoscopy and laparotomy. Int J Gynaecol Obstet. 1999;64:153-8.
54. Borruto F, Camoglio FS, Zampieri N, Fedele L. The laparoscopic Vecchietti technique for vaginal agenesis. Int J Gynaecol Obstet. 2007;98(1):15-19.
55. Freundt I, Toolenaar TA, Huikeshoven FJ, Drogendijk AC, Jeekel H. A modified technique to create a neovagina with an isolated segment of sigmoid colon. Surg Gynecol Obstet. 1992;174:11-6.
56. Louis-Sylvestre C, Haddad B, Paniel BJ. Creation of a sigmoid neovagina: technique and results in 16 cases. Eur J Obstet Gynecol Reprod Biol. 1997;75:225-9.
57. Hiroi H, Yasugi T, Matsumoto K, Fujii T, Watanabe T, Yoshikawa H, et al. Mucinous adenocarcinoma arising in a neovagina using the sigmoid colon thirty years after operation: a case report. J Surg Oncol. 2001;77:61-4.
58. Weijenborg PT, Ter Kuile MM. The effect of a group programme on women with the Mayer-Rokitansky-Küster-Hauser syndrome. BJOG. 2000;107(3):365-8.
59. Sanfilippo JS. Mayer-Rokitansky-Küster-Hauser (MRKH) syndrome: it's more than the anatomy. J Pediatr Adolesc Gynecol. 2009;22(6):337-8.
60. McQuillan SK, Grover SR. Systematic review of sexual function and satisfaction following the management of vaginal agenesis. Int Urogynecol J. 2014;25(10):1313-20.
61. Johannesson L, Järvholm S. Uterus transplantation: current progress and future prospects. Int J Womens Health. 2016;8:43-51.
62. Cakmak H, Rosen MP. Random-start ovarian stimulation in patients with cancer. Curr Opin Obstet Gynecol. 2015;27(3): 215-21.
63. Petrozza JC, Gray MR, Davis AJ, Reindollar RH. Congenital absence of the uterus and vagina is not commonly transmitted as a dominant genetic trait: outcomes of surrogate pregnancies. Fertil Steril. 1997;67:387-9.
64. Beski S, Gorgy A, Venkat G, Craft IL, Edmonds K. Gestational surrogacy: a feasible option for patients with Rokitansky syndrome. Hum Reprod. 2000;15:2326-8.
65. Goldfarb JM, Austin C, Peskin B, Lisbona H, Desai N, de Mola JR. Fifteen years experience with an in vitro fertilization surrogate gestational pregnancy programme. Hum Reprod. 2000;15:1075-8.
66. Ozkan O, Akar ME, Erdogan O, Ozkan O, Hadimioglu N. Uterus transplantation from a deceased donor. Fertil Steril. 2013;100(6):e41.
67. Brannstrom M, Johannesson L, Bokstrom H, Kvarnström N, Mölne J, Dahm-Kähler P, et al. Livebirth after uterus transplantation. Lancet. 2015;385(9968):607-16.
68. Benedetti Panici P, Maffucci D, Ceccarelli S, Vescarelli E, Perniola G, Muzii L, et al. Autologous in vitro cultured vaginal tissue for vaginoplasty in women with Mayer-Rokitansky-Küster-Hauser syndrome: anatomic and functional results. J Minim Invasive Gynecol. 2015;22(2):205-11.
69. Hellström M, Bandstein S, Brännström M. Uterine tissue engineering and the future of uterus transplantation. Ann Biomed Eng. 2017;45(7):1718-30.
70. Campbell GR, Turnbull G, Xiang L, Haines M, Armstrong S, Rolfe BE, et al. The peritoneal cavity as a bioreactor for tissue engineering visceral organs: bladder, uterus and vas deferens. J Tissue Eng Regen Med. 2008;2:50-60.
71. Ding L, Li X, Sun H, Su J, Lin N, Peault B, et al. Transplantation of bone marrow mesenchymal stem cells on collagen scaffolds for the functional regeneration of injured rat uterus. Biomaterials. 2014;35:4888-900.
72. Hellström M, El-Akouri RR, Sihlbom C, Olsson BM, Lengqvist J, Bäckdahl H, et al. Towards the development of a bioengineered uterus: comparison of different protocols for rat uterus decellularization. Acta Biomater. 2014;10:5034-42.
73. Hellström M, Moreno-Moya JM, Bandstein S, Bom E, Akouri RR, Miyazaki K, et al. Bioengineered uterine tissue supports pregnancy in a rat model. Fertil Steril. 2016;106(2):487-96.e1.
74. Hiraoka T, Hirota Y, Saito-Fujita T, Matsuo M, Egashira M, Matsumoto L, et al. STAT3 accelerates uterine epithelial regeneration in a mouse model of decellularized uterine matrix transplantation. JCI Insight. 2016;1(8):e87591.

CHAPTER 84

Endometrial Rejuvenation

Satish Patki, Shweta Patki, Surhud S Patki, Aditi M Kunte

INTRODUCTION

Human endometrium is one of the highly regenerative tissues of the body with its regenerative potential comparable to that of the bone marrow, hematopoietic tissue, and epidermis. It is a dynamic tissue, undergoing more than 400 menstrual cycles of regeneration following shedding during a woman's reproductive life.[1,2]

Primarily the increasing levels of the hormone estrogen is the main stimulus behind the rapid proliferation of the endometrium during a span of 8–10 days. The upper two-thirds of the endometrium is called stratum functionalis, which contains glands supported by the stroma and is supplied by the spiral arteries. The lower one-third is the basal layer and contains the lowermost branching portions of the glands and dense stroma with radial arteries at their origin. The basalis layer does not take part in the event of menstruation. However, the process of endometrial regeneration after menstruation is initiated from the basalis layer, which contains mesenchymal stem cells (MSCs) possessing a high potential of differentiation and multiplication under the influence of estrogen produced by the leading follicle.

ROLE OF ENDOMETRIUM IN THE PROCESS OF IMPLANTATION

After the procedure of "embryo transfer (ET)", the successful implantation is dependent on the quality of the endometrium and the quality of the embryo, the concept of "soil and seed". In about 65% cases of the failure of implantation, faulty endometrium is the responsible factor, while in 35% cases, the faulty embryo is the reason.

The quality of the endometrium during ET cycle is best assessed by transvaginal sonography. The parameters studied by vaginosonography are endometrial thickness, endometrial pattern, endometrial volume, and endometrial and subendometrial blood flow.[3,4]

In several studies, the minimum endometrial thickness during the ET was reported to be 7 mm.[5,6] It has been observed that if the endometrial thickness is <7 mm, a successful pregnancy is unlikely. The mechanism explaining the correlation between thin endometrium and inverse in vitro fertilization (IVF) outcome is not yet clear. It has been speculated that in patients with thin endometrium, the oxygen concentration in the basalis layer is higher, which might be detrimental for embryo implantation.[7]

It has been observed that the endometrial thickness <7 mm has a negative predictive value for IVF outcomes[8-10] and clinical pregnancy as well as live birth rates are significantly higher when the endometrial thickness is >9 mm.[11]

Endometrial patterns observed on vaginosonography are classified as:

- Pattern A: "Triple layer", characterized by a central hyperechogenic line representing the empty uterine cavity and hyperechogenic endometrium on either side.
- Pattern B: Isoechoic endometrium with poorly defined outer walls and central echogenic line.
- Pattern C: Homogeneous hyperechoic endometrium.

A triple-line endometrial pattern on the day of progesterone administration in a frozen embryo transfer (FET) cycle is associated with higher pregnancy rates versus a homogenous and hyperechogenic endometrial pattern.[12]

The color Doppler study of the endometrial and periendometrial areas also throws the light on the endometrial receptivity. These areas are divided into four zones:

1. Zone 1: A 2-mm thick area surrounding the hyperechoic outer layer of the endometrium
2. Zone 2: The hyperechoic outer layer of the endometrium
3. Zone 3: The hypoechoic inner layer of the endometrium
4. Zone 4: The endometrial cavity

Chien et al.[13] have shown that the pregnancy rates are significantly higher in the patients with multifocal vascularity in zone 3. Maugey-Laulom et al.[14] have demonstrated that absent endometrial vascularization was associated with a significantly lower pregnancy rate. It has been postulated that a good endometrial vascularity can lead to better placentation resulting in a higher chance of live births following an ET.[15]

CAUSES AND PATHOPHYSIOLOGY OF THIN ENDOMETRIUM

Thin endometrium is caused by diminished normal endometrial growth. Certain temporary causes like administration of antiestrogenic drugs like clomiphene citrate can cause thin endometrium. In such cases, the superficial layer of functionalis of the endometrium is affected due to suppression of the endometrial components of epithelium, glands, stroma, and vasculature. Impaired epithelial cell proliferation and delayed glandular maturation are often found in endometrial biopsies from the patients treated with clomiphene.[16] The number as well as diameter of the glands are also observed to be lower in such patients.[17] Reducing the dosage of clomiphene, administration of clomiphene in the early part of the menstrual cycle, and addition of estrogens or gonadotropins can help such patients by improving the thickness of their endometrium. In some cases, the treatment with clomiphene citrate needs to be abandoned.

The real problem which is more serious and difficult to treat arises when there is a destruction of the basalis layer of the endometrium. Iatrogenic thin endometrium due to destruction of the basalis layer is caused by surgical procedures such as repeated curettage, polypectomy, laparoscopic and hysteroscopic myomectomies, hysteroscopic septal resection, and lateral wall metroplasty.

Acute infections such as pelvic inflammatory diseases or chronic infections such as genital tuberculosis often result in the destruction of endometrial basalis. In genital tuberculosis, fallopian tubes are affected in 95% cases, while the endometrium and the ovaries are affected in 60 and 20% cases, respectively. The disease starts in the ampullary portion of the fallopian tube. Tubercular endometritis in the initial stage is often focal and pathological changes such as ulceration and caseous necrosis occur later. In advanced stages, intrauterine adhesions result in shrunken uterine cavity. The classical findings of genital tuberculosis on hysterosalpingography are lead pipe, coiled and blocked tubes, smaller and irregular uterine cavity, and intravasation of the dye into the uterine vessels.

Asherman's syndrome, due to the surgical trauma to the endometrium of the pregnant uterus, is often a cause of thin endometrium in patients with secondary infertility. Over enthusiastic curettage during evacuation of the pregnant uterus or repeated events of medical termination of pregnancy by suction and evacuation often leads to intrauterine adhesions. Sometimes, post cesarean section, intrauterine adhesions develop. Such patients often have scanty menses, dysmenorrhea, and sometimes secondary amenorrhea.

Thin endometrium with reduced blood flow, as seen on sonography, is often associated with a partially damaged basalis layer. The glands, radial arteries, and especially the stroma are damaged, with a low potential of regeneration in response to estrogens. Rejuvenation of the endometrium in these patients is a real challenge.

PRINCIPLES OF ENDOMETRIAL REJUVENATION

Since a thin endometrium is a multifactorial condition, its management should be cause related with the aim of increasing endometrial receptivity and ultimately facilitating the process of implantation. Angiogenesis plays a key role in the process of endometrial regeneration, which is regulated by a vascular endothelial growth factor (VEGF), expressed in the stroma of the endometrium.[18] The principle of endometrial rejuvenation is to increase the angiogenesis in the endometrium by using various drugs, cell therapies, and growth factors. The aim is to facilitate endometrial regeneration using medical treatment with or without surgical procedures such as hysteroscopic adhesiolysis, to restore anatomy.

There are various methods of endometrial rejuvenation which can be tried either individually or can be combined, depending upon the cause and severity of the thin endometrium **(Table 1)**. They can be broadly classified as:

- Use of drugs, hormones, and growth factors
- Use of cell-based therapies
- New technologies such as use of extracellular vesicles (EVs).

The endometrial rejuvenation is a challenging job for the infertility specialist and every case has to be individualized for selecting the modality of treatment.

METHODS OF ENDOMETRIAL REJUVENATION

Drugs, Hormones, and Growth Factors

Estrogen

Endometrium is a hormone-dependent tissue. Continuous administration of estrogen is the foundation of endometrial rejuvenation. Estrogen supports the endometrial proliferation by causing contraction of the spiral arteries and decreasing the oxygen tension in the functional layer.[19,20] Estradiol valerate or hemihydrate can be started with the dosage of 4 mg/day and can be stepped up to the dose of 12 mg/day till the endometrium reaches a thickness of 7 mm or above when progesterone can be added and FET can be performed on day 3 or day 5 depending on the stage of the embryo. The duration of the therapy to achieve the desired endometrial thickness can vary from 15 days to 1 month. The estrogen administration should be continued following ET though the dose can be stepped down to 6 mg/day and should

TABLE 1: Methods of endometrial rejuvenation and mechanism of action.

No.	Method	Mode of administration	Mechanism
1.	Estrogens	Oral	• Contraction of spiral arteries, reduction in oxygen tension in functionalis layer leading to proliferation • Priming of progesterone receptors
2.	hCG	• IM/SC injection • Intrauterine instillation	• Upregulation of endometrial VEGF and MMP-9 • Increasing angiogenesis
3.	Aspirin	Oral	Increasing endometrial blood flow
4.	GCSF	• SC injection • Intrauterine instillation	• Mobilization of stem cells from bone marrow • Tissue remodeling and angiogenesis • Autocrine and paracrine role
5.	PRP	• Intrauterine instillation • Subendometrial injection through hysteroscopy • Subendometrial injection using vaginosonography	Secretion of VEGF, EGF, IGF-1, and tissue healing promoting molecules such as fibrinectin and vitronectin
6.	Autologous stem cell from bone marrow/adipose tissue/endometrium	• Intrauterine perfusion • Subendometrial injection through hysteroscopy • Subendometrial injection using vaginosonography • Intra-arterial (uterine circulation) • Tissue engineering	• Angiogenesis • Secretion of growth factors • Tissue regeneration
7.	Extracellular vesicles (EVS) from endometrial stem cells	Subendometrial injection	• Serve as biological cargos of proteins, Lipids, RNAs, and DNAs • Regenerative
8.	Extracellular vesicles (EVs) released from cultured blastocysts	During embryo transfer procedure	• Cell to cell cross talk between blastocysts and endometrium • Endometrial microrejuvenation

(DNA: deoxyribonucleic acid; EGF: epidermal growth factor; GCSF: granulocyte colony-stimulating factor; hCG: human chorionic gonadotropin; IGF-1: insulin-like growth factor 1; IM: intramuscular; MMP-9: matrix metallopeptidase 9; PRP: platelet-rich plasma; RNA: ribonucleic acid; SC: subcutaneous; VEGF: vascular endothelial growth factor)

be further continued after confirmation of pregnancy till 8 weeks when the placentation begins. Additional advantage of estrogen supplementation is that it helps in priming of the progesterone receptors (PR). Transdermal estrogen can be added to oral estrogen.

Human Chorionic Gonadotropin

Human chorionic gonadotropin (hCG) plays a local paracrine role in the process of endometrial differentiation by stimulating different cytokines and growth factors.[21,22] Various protocols of hCG administrations are suggested by different researchers. Davar et al. recommend daily intramuscular administration of 150 IU of hCG for 7 days after initial 8–10 days of daily 8 mg oral estradiol valerate. It helps to improve the endometrial thickness and vascularity.[23] The latest studies report that intrauterine injection of 0.04 mL of recombinant hCG just before ET significantly improves pregnancy rates. It is suggested that hCG exerts multiple direct local effects on the endometrium. hCG provokes significant upregulation of endometrial VEGF and matrix metalloproteinase (MMP)-9 leading to angiogenesis.

Aspirin

The effect of low-dose aspirin on the endometrial thickness is still debated in literature. Some studies have reported the positive impact of low-dose aspirin (150 mg) on the endometrial thickness, pattern, and endometrial blood flow.[24] Hsieh et al. have demonstrated a higher percentage of trilaminar endometrium in a group of patients receiving low-dose aspirin therapy than the nonaspirin group.[25]

Sildenafil Citrate

Sildenafil citrate prevents the breakdown of cyclic guanosine monophosphate (cGMP) and increases the effect of nitric oxide on vascular smooth muscles. In combination with estrogen, sildenafil citrate administration causes an improvement in uterine blood flow and proliferation of uterine epithelium.[26] It also elevates VEGF levels leading to increased radial artery resistance index and endometrial thickness.

In FET cycles, sildenafil can be administered in a dose of 25 mg by vaginal route from the first day of progesterone administration till the day of ET.

Granulocyte Colony-stimulating Factor

Granulocyte colony-stimulating factor (GCSF) is one of the cytokine family members including colony-stimulating factors. It stimulates the mobilization of stem cells from the bone marrow into the systemic circulation and further helps in their differentiation. GCSF plays an important role in tissue remodeling and angiogenesis, which are essential for endometrial growth. GCSF also stimulates various endogenous endocrine mechanisms such as the secretion of endogenous cytokines which act through autocrine as well as paracrine routes.

Granulocyte colony-stimulating factor can be administered by subcutaneous injectable route or direct intrauterine route. During pickup cycles if the endometrium is observed to be thin, 300 μg of GCSF is instilled in the uterine cavity by using an ET catheter on the day of oocyte retrieval if fresh ET is planned. For FET cycles, on day 12–14th of estrogen therapy if the endometrium is thin, then 300 μg of GCSF can be instilled in the uterine cavity and endometrial thickness and vascularity is assessed after 48 hours. The instillation can be repeated if the endometrium still is thin. The progesterone is started after desired endometrial thickness and vascularity, and ET can be done on day 3 or day 5 as per the stage of embryos.

Granulocyte colony-stimulating factor can also be given by subcutaneous route in a dose of 300 μg if the endometrial thickness is observed to be less on the 12th day of estrogen therapy. The same dose can be repeated 48 hours after the first dose if the endometrium is still thin. Once the optimum endometrium is observed, injection progesterone can be started and ET is done subsequently.

Cell-based Therapies for Endometrial Rejuvenation

- Use of autologous platelet-rich plasma (PRP)
- Stem cells therapy for endometrial rejuvenation
- Endometrial micro-rejuvenation by EVs—newer technology under research.

Use of Autologous Platelet-rich Plasma

Platelets are cytoplasmic fragments of megakaryocytes. They are formed in the bone marrow. They contain >30 bioactive proteins which have a role in the process of hemostasis and tissue healing.

Platelets actively secrete seven fundamental protein growth factors, namely VEGF, epidermal growth factor (EGF), fibroblast growth factor (FGF), insulin-like growth factor 1 (IGF-1), platelet-derived growth factor (PDGF), transforming growth factor (TGF), and connective tissue growth factor (CTGF). In addition to these growth factors, platelets secrete important cell adhesion and tissue healing, promoting molecules such as fibrin, fibronectin, and vitronectin.

Activation of the platelets causes the granules present in the platelets to fuse to their cell membranes, leading to active secretion of the proteins and growth factors. The active secretion of the proteins begins within 10 minutes and >90% of the growth factors are secreted within 1 hour.[27,28] The process of regeneration is initiated within 24 hours and continues for 2 months. There are various studies mentioning the minimal requirement of platelet count in the final preparation of PRP. Marx proposed that platelet count of 10 lakhs/mL in 5 mL of PRP is a working definition of PRP for the process of angiogenesis and regeneration.[28]

Types of PRP preparations: The classification of types of PRP is done by Ehrenfest et al.[29] depending on their cell content and fibrin architecture. The important types for clinical use are as follows:

- Pure platelet-rich plasma (P-PRP) or leukocyte poor PRP: These are the preparations without leukocytes.
- Leukocyte-rich PRP (L-PRP): These are preparations with leukocytes.

Protocol for PRP preparation: PRP is prepared by two step or differential centrifugation. The steps are as follows:

1. Collect 30 cc venous blood, which will yield 3–5 cc of PRP. The blood is collected in four different tubes containing anticoagulant acid citrate dextrose A (ACD-A), with the ratio of blood to ACD-A to be 9:1. Follow strict aseptic precautions at each step.
2. Do not chill the blood at any time before or during platelet separation.
3. Blood is centrifuged immediately at 1200 RPM (soft spin) for 12 minutes.
4. After the first spin, the blood separates into three layers: The upper layer that contains mostly platelets and white blood cell (WBC), an intermediate thin layer called buffy coat which is rich in WBCs, and bottom layer that consists mostly of red blood cells (RBCs).
5. For the production of P-PRP, the upper layer and superficial buffy coat are transferred to an empty sterile tube. For the production of leukocyte-rich PRP (L-PRP), the entire layer of buffy coat and few RBCs are transferred to an empty sterile tube, along with the upper layer.
6. Centrifuge the tube containing P-PRP at 3300 RPM (hard spin) for 7 minutes.
7. The platelet pellets are formed at the bottom.
8. The upper two-thirds platelet-poor plasma (PPP) is removed, and the lower one-third platelet-rich plasma is used for therapy.
9. Homogenize platelet pellet by thoroughly mixing with plasma before collecting in the syringe for therapy.

Modes and timing of administration of PRP for endometrial rejuvenation: PRP can be administered by two routes:

1. Intrauterine perfusion of PRP (IU-PRP)
2. Subendometrial multiple injections of PRP during one cycle prior to FET cycle by two techniques (SE-PRP):
    a. Hysteroscopic subendometrial multiple PRP injections *or*
    b. Transvaginal sonographically guided multiple subendometrial PRP injections.

Intrauterine perfusion of PRP (2015): Chang et al. were the first study who reported a pilot study of intrauterine perfusion of PRP in five patients with thin endometrium who had poor response to standard therapies.[30] In this study, all five patients had successful pregnancies. Four women had babies while one aborted.

In the latest study by the same group in 2019, intrauterine perfusion of 0.5–1 mL PRP was performed on the 10th day of the FET cycle in the cases when the endometrial thickness was <7 mm. The procedure was repeated on the day when progesterone was started prior to the procedure of ET. The clinical pregnancy rate in the PRP group was 44.12% as compared to 20% in no PRP group. The clinical pregnancy rate in patients with normal endometrium (10 mm and above) in their study was 50–55%.

Whenever the intrauterine PRP infusion is considered for endometrial rejuvenation, it is given during the FET cycle. It is suggested that the growth factors in PRP stimulate the mitogenesis and proliferation of the endometrial cells and MSCs in the endometrium and then activate endocrine—paracrine pathways to promote the implantation process. Platelets also activate peripheral blood mononuclear cells (MNCs), which release an anti-inflammatory cytokine interleukin-10 (IL-10), which in turn accelerates tissue regeneration.[31]

Hysteroscopic subendometrial PRP injection: This procedure is done one cycle prior to the FET cycle. In this procedure, autologous PRP is injected in the subendometrial area at multiple sites using an ovum pick single lumen needle of 22G size. About 0.5–1 mL PRP is injected per site in about five sites. Latest study by Shawki has shown significant improvement in endometrial thickness in a series of 51 patients,[32] where hysteroscopic subendometrial PRP injection was given **(Figs. 1 and 2)**.

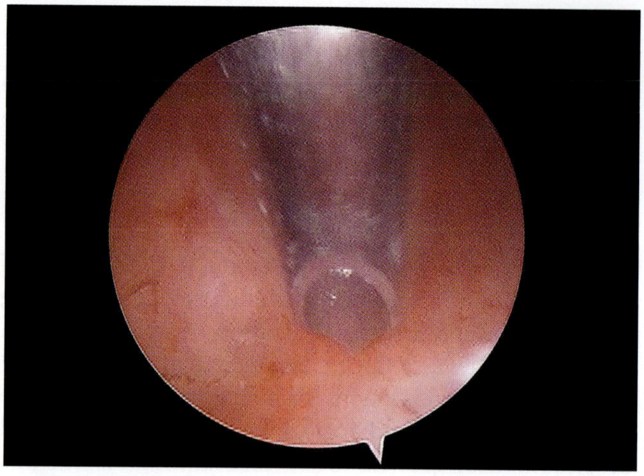

Fig. 1: Hysteroscopic subendometrial injection of platelet-rich plasma (PRP). Needle in the uterine cavity.

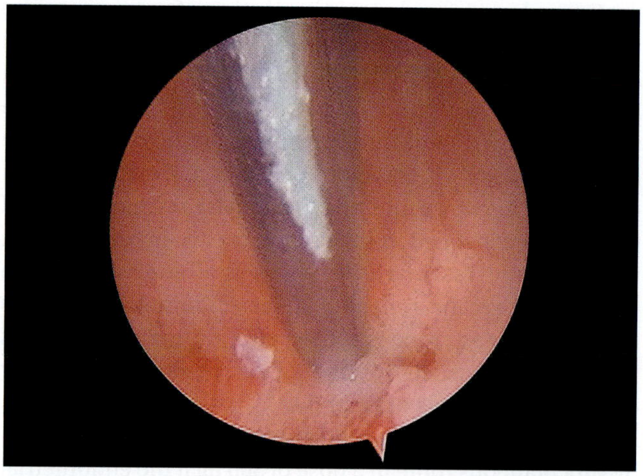

Fig. 2: Hysteroscopic subendometrial injection of platelet-rich plasma (PRP). Needle penetrating endometrial layer.

Transvaginal sonography guided subendometrial PRP injection: This procedure is done during the proliferative phase of the menstrual cycle prior to the FET cycle. Autologous PRP is injected under vaginal ultrasound guidance into subendometrial regional multiple sites using a 35-cm 17G single lumen needle. In a latest study, Cakiroglu et al. have shown that subendometrial PRP injections under vaginosonography guidance have resulted in significant improvement in endometrial thickness and higher clinical pregnancy rate (28% vs. 7% in non-PRP group).[33]

A recent study by Noushin et al. has shown that PRP treatment definitely improves endometrial thickness as well as clinical pregnancy rates. However, the study has concluded that SE-PRP does not offer any advantage over less invasive intrauterine PRP (IU-PPP) treatment.[34]

Adjuncts to PRP treatment: The drugs which stimulate angiogenesis can be combined with PRP treatment. Noushin et al. have recommended subcutaneous administration of 300 µg of GCSF for three successive days from the day of the procedure (SE-PRP or IU-PRP) to boost WBCs and growth factors production.

Our own experience of adding 300 µg of GCSF and 2,000 IU of hCG to the PRP preparation itself for SE-PRP procedures have shown significant improvement in the endometrial thickness, endometrial pattern, and vascularity in the subsequent cycle of actual FET.

Stem Cells Therapy for Endometrial Rejuvenation

Adult stem cells are pluripotent cells with self-renewal and differentiation potentials. It has been documented that adult stem cells are responsible for cyclical regeneration of the endometrium. The adult stem cells reside in the basalis layer and are even present in the atrophic endometrium of postmenopausal women.

Mesenchymal stem cell is the most important type of stem cell, which is present in the basalis layer of the endometrium. Apart from these tissue residential MSCs, another significant source of endometrial stem cells is bone marrow. There is a trafficking of the stem cells from the bone marrow to the endometrium, which is estrogen dependent.[35]

There are two types of stem cells released from the bone marrow to the endometrium. One is bone marrow MSCs, which along with endometrial MSCs mainly contribute to the regeneration of the stroma, glands, and epithelium. The other important stem cell which is released from the bone marrow is endothelial progenitor cell (EPC), which contributes to the formation of new blood vessels (angiogenesis) in the endometrium.[36]

Apart from the endometrium and bone marrow, MSCs can be harvested from adipose tissue, Wharton's jelly of umbilical cord, amniotic fluid, and menstrual blood.

Mesenchymal stem cells as well as other adult stem cells are used for endometrial rejuvenation inpatients having thin endometrium. There are various mechanisms which are postulated to promote the regenerative effects of stem cell therapy.

Mesenchymal stem cells can secrete several growth factors such as VEGF, hepatocyte growth factor (HGF), and TGF. They also exert anti-inflammatory effects. MSCs are immunomodulatory and regulate the functions and proliferation of T cells balancing the activity of T helper cell type 2 (Th2) and T helper cell type 1 (Th1).

The most common source of MSCs and EPCs used for endometrial rejuvenation is autologous bone marrow.

Methodology of preparation of autologous bone marrow derived stem cells:

- *Invasive method:* Bone marrow aspiration is done under all aseptic precautions from the posterior superior iliac spine under general anesthesia using a J (Jamshidi) needle (13G) and 20 mL. Syringe, prewashed with heparin. Around 150–200 mL bone marrow is aspirated. From this aspirate, around 15 mL bone marrow derived stem cells are separated by optical sensor technology. We have isolated the MNCs, which predominantly contain stem cells by Ficoll centrifugation and buffy coat method. Stem cell counting in the final product can be done by using a flow cytometer or hemocytometer. Usually, the stem cell count varies from 5 to 15 million cells/mL of the final product.
- *Noninvasive method:* In this method, stem cells from the bone marrow are mobilized to the peripheral circulation by administration of injection GCSF (10 MU/kg/day on day-4, -3, -2, and -1). 5 days after injection, isolation of MNCs is performed by apheresis through peripheral venous access using a cell separator. Minimum 50 million CD133+ (EPCs) are required.

Modes of administration of stem cells for endometrial rejuvenation:

- Intrauterine perfusion
- Subendometrial injection of stem cells at multiple sites under hysteroscopy or transvaginosonography guidance
- Intra-arterial injection of stem cells in the catheterization laboratory into uterine or spiral arteries
- Tissues engineering and endometrial reconstruction using collagen scaffolds.

Zhao et al. demonstrated that intrauterine perfusion with bone marrow derived stem cells in rat models resulted in increased endometrial thickness. They also have documented the upregulation of vimentin and cytokeratin which are marker proteins of the endometrial cells.[37]

Stem cells can also be injected at multiple sites in subendometrial areas through hysteroscopy. Wang et al. have shown that the bone marrow derived stem cells repair the damaged endometrium through upregulation of estrogen receptors (ER) and PR expression.[38]

Santamaria et al. have shown that intra-arterial injection of CD133+ bone marrow derived cells in patients with Asherman's syndrome led to increase in the endometrial thickness as well as vascularity.[39] In this study, the femoral artery was approached and the uterine artery was catheterized till the most distal spiral arterioles, where the isolated CD133+ cells were injected. Patients in this study showed significant improvement in the duration as well as intensity of their menstrual flow. Achievement of pregnancy was observed in three patients out of the total series of sixteen patients. Post-therapy hysteroscopic evaluation of remaining patients after 3 months revealed good uterine cavity and vascularized thick endometrium.

Some studies have avoided using bone marrow derived stem cells. They have used MSCs from other sources, such as endometrium or adipose tissue.

Sudoma et al. have used adipose tissue derived stem cells (ASCs) because they could not get adequate endometrium for isolating MSCs in the cases of Asherman's syndrome.[40] In this study adipose tissue was derived by aspiration from the patient's anterior abdominal wall. The cells were cultured "in vitro" for four passages till pure stem cells were finally isolated. These cells were injected in the subendometrial area at multiple sites under vaginosonography guidance using a 17G needle which is used for oocyte retrieval **(Figs. 3 and 4)**.

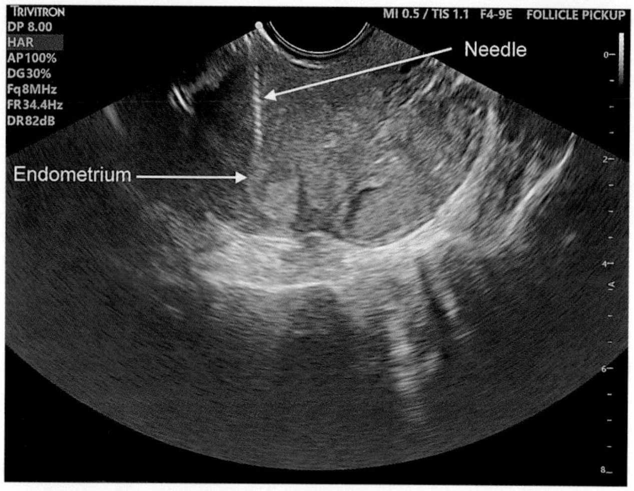

Fig. 3: Vaginosonography-guided injection of cells. Needle in the subendometrial zone.

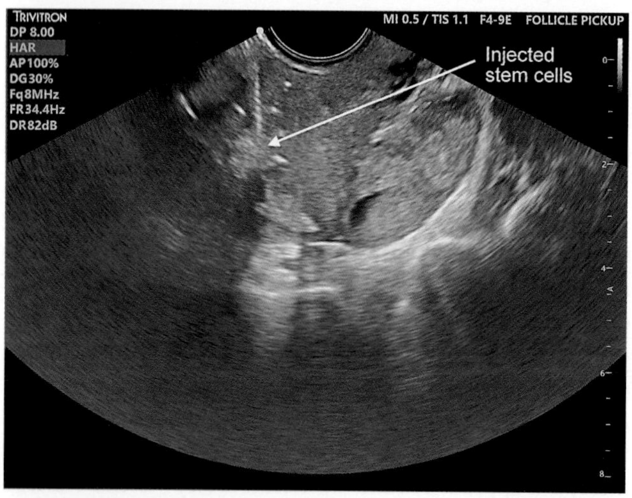

Fig. 4: Vaginosonography-guided injection of stem cells. Needle in subendometrial zone and echogenic areas of stem cells infiltration with vascularity.

There are studies in the literature where umbilical cord-derived stem cells and amniotic tissue-derived stem cells are used for endometrial rejuvenation.

In order to utilize MSCs after transplantation, the tissue engineering techniques such as use of scaffolds or gels loaded with stem cells are under consideration and development.

The collagen scaffolds have a three-dimensional structure which can guide the stem cells to grow rapidly. These scaffolds have good histocompatibility with no inflammation or immune rejection at the endometrial site.

Adjuncts to stem cell therapy for endometrial rejuvenation: Estrogen is an important hormone to promote the mobilization of stem cells from the bone marrow to the endometrium. It also stimulates the proliferation of MSCs in the basalis layer of the endometrium. Hence, cyclical administration of estradiol valerate in the dose of 4–6 mg followed by the addition of progesterone in the last 8 days are necessary for 1 month prior and 2–3 months after stem cell therapy.

Endometrial Micro-rejuvenation by EVs—Newer Technology Under Research

Extracellular vesicles are lipid bilayer enclosed nanoparticles released mainly by stem cells. They are spherical structures with a diameter of 30–80 nm. They serve as biological cargos of proteins, lipids, ribonucleic acids (RNAs), and deoxyribonucleic acids (DNAs). They promote angiogenesis.[41] They have immunomodulatory properties and reduce oxidative stress at cellular levels. EVs are active paracrine components with a high potential for repairing damaged tissues.

They play an important role in intercellular communication by autocrine and paracrine signaling. These signaling molecules stay within the membranes of EVs and hence are protected from degradation by enzymes. They play an important role in the cell-to-cell cross talk of many physiological processes.

Many studies have isolated EVs from cultured endometrial MSCs.[42] The surface markers of EVs, CD9, and CD63 are detected in the supernatants of cultured endometrial stem cells. Recently, it has been documented that the regenerative benefits of stem cell therapy are not due to the stem cells themselves. It is the regenerative mechanism mediated through the EVs secreted by the stem cells. The conditioned culture medium from the endometrial stem cells can be used for endometrial rejuvenation by administering it in various subendometrial regions under hysteroscopy guidance.

The role of EVs in implantation and endometrial micro-rejuvenation: The process of implantation involves a cross talk between the blastocyst and the endometrium. A recent study has demonstrated the important role of EVs secreted by the endometrial stem cells from the maternal side and those secreted by the inner cell mass of the blastocyst in the process of implantation.

The endometrial stromal and glandular cells secrete EVs during the window of implantation. Similarly, the cells, especially from the inner cell mass of the blastocyst also secrete EVs.[43] The EVs secreted from the inner cell mass are also detected in the blastocoel fluid. They play an important role in the development of embryos. The EVs which come out of the blastocyst are playing an important role in the process of immunomodulation and induction of endometrial angiogenesis, which is a prerequisite for the process of implantation.[44]

The time lapse imaging of the process of fertilization from the day of intracytoplasmic sperm injection (ICSI) of an oocyte to the stage of formation of a fully expanded blastocyst on day 5 at our center has shown a rapid expulsion of the cellular matter from the blastocyst during the period

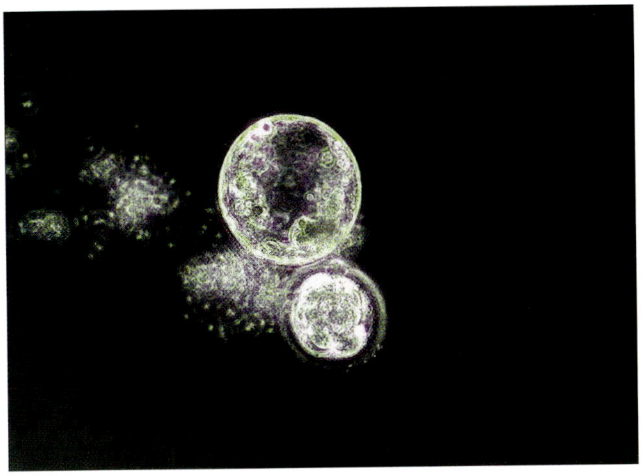

Fig. 5: Microphotograph of expelled cellular matter from blastocyst. Microphotograph showing expulsion of cellular matter from the fully expanded blastocyst. The other embryo is arrested at a stage of morula.

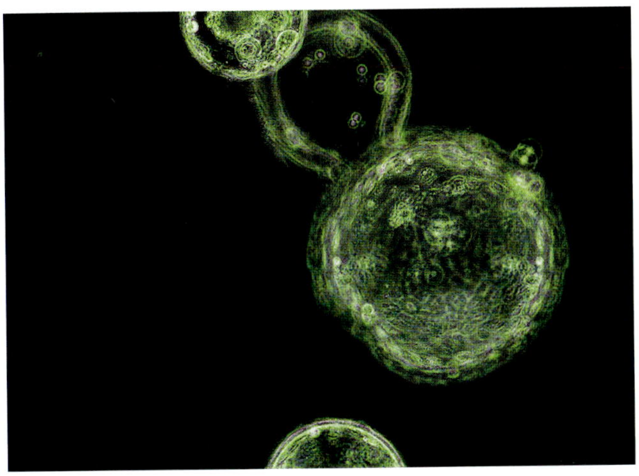

Fig. 6: Hatched blastocyst with expulsion of cellular matter.

of last 2 days of the 5 days culture (microphotograph) **(Figs. 5 and 6)**.

Giacomini in his study has also documented that the conditioned media of the IVF embryos from the period of day 3–5 of the culture contain a significant amount of EVs.[45] He has confirmed their presence by scanning electron microscopy (SEM) and by demonstrating EVs markers CD63 and CD9.

It is thus suggested that the embryos "in vitro", communicate with each other through EVs. This concept favors the culture of the IVF embryos in groups to promote the growth of each other through the mechanism of cell-to-cell cross talk rather than doing the culture of a solitary embryo per droplet of the culture medium.

The conditioned culture medium of the endometrial MSCs rich in EVs, when added to the culture medium in which the embryos are cultured, has been shown to significantly enhance the total number of the embryonic cells and grade of the blastocyst.[43]

It is hypothesized that if the blastocyst transfer is done along with its own autologous conditioned culture medium supplemented with autologous conditioned medium of endometrial MSCs, it should improve the implantation and clinical pregnancy rates of IVF procedures. The EVs thus transferred can bring about endometrial micro-rejuvenation leading to firm implantation and invasion which may reduce the complications such as pregnancy losses and conditions such as pregnancy-induced hypertension (PIH), leading ultimately to higher "take-home baby rates". Further research in this direction is needed on this concept of micro-rejuvenation of receptive endometrium with EVs.

CONCLUSION

- Management of a patient with thin endometrium is really a challenge to Assisted Reproductive Technology (ART) specialists. The implantation rates as well as clinical pregnancy rates are very poor when the endometrium is <7 mm with poor vasculature.
- Genital tuberculosis is the important cause among infective etiological factors of thin endometrium.
- Iatrogenic thin endometrium is due to over enthusiastic curettage of gravid uterus, endoscopic surgeries such as polypectomy, myomectomy and septal resection, and post cesarean intrauterine adhesions.
- Endometrial rejuvenation can be done by medical treatment with or without hysteroscopic adhesiolysis for anatomical correction.
- Estrogens, sildenafil, or GCSF can be used as a first-line treatment in mild cases.
- Autologous PRP, bone marrow stem cells can be administered by various routes for endometrial rejuvenation.
- EVs secreted by endometrial MSCs and blastocysts can be considered for endometrial regeneration.
- EVs in the blastocyst culture medium can be considered for endometrial micro-rejuvenation during ET.
- There is no definitely proven method for endometrial rejuvenation and the subject needs a lot of research.

REFERENCES

1. Jabbour HN, Kelly RW, Fraser HM, Critchley HO. Endocrine regulation of menstruation. Endocr Rev. 2006;27:17-46.
2. Gargett CE. Uterine stem cells: what is the evidence? Hum Reprod Update. 2007;13:87-101.
3. Basir GS, O WS, So WW, Ng EH, Ho PC. Evaluation of cycle-to-cycle variation of endometrial responsiveness using transvaginal sonography in women undergoing assisted reproduction. Ultrasound Obstet Gynecol. 2002;19:484-9.
4. Wang L, Qiao J, Li R, Zhen X, Liu Z. Role of endometrial blood flow assessment with color Doppler energy in predicting pregnancy outcome of IVF-ET cycles. Reprod Biol Endocrinol. 2010;8:122.

5. El-Toukhy T, Coomarasamy A, Khairy M, Sunkara K, Seed P, Khalaf Y, et al. The relationship between endometrial thickness and outcome of medicated frozen embryo replacement cycles. Fertil Steril. 2008;89:832-9.
6. Richter KS, Bugge KR, Bromer JG, Levy MJ. Relationship between endometrial thickness and embryo implantation, based on 1,294 cycles of in vitro fertilization with transfer of two blastocyst-stage embryos. Fertil Steril. 2007;87:53-9.
7. Casper RF. It's time to pay attention to the endometrium. Fertil Steril. 2011;96:519-21.
8. Traub ML, Van Arsdale A, Pal L, Jindal S, Santoro N. Endometrial thickness, Caucasian ethnicity, and age predict clinical pregnancy following fresh blastocyst embryo transfer: a retrospective cohort. Reprod Biol Endocrinol. 2009;7:33.
9. Zhao J, Zhang Q, Li Y. The effect of endometrial thickness and pattern measured by ultrasonography on pregnancy outcomes during IVF-ET cycles. Reprod Biol Endocrinol. 2012;10:100.
10. Zhao J, Zhang Q, Wang Y, Li Y. Endometrial pattern, thickness and growth in predicting pregnancy outcome following 3319 IVF cycles. Reprod Biomed Online. 2014;29:291-8.
11. Kovacs P, Matyas S, Boda K, Kaali SG. The effect of endometrial thickness on IVF/ICSI outcome. Hum Reprod. 2003;18:2337-41.
12. Chen SL, Wu FR, Luo C, Chen X, Shi XY, Zheng HY, et al. Combined analysis of endometrial thickness and pattern in predicting outcome of in vitro fertilization and embryo transfer: a retrospective cohort study. Reprod Biol Endocrinol. 2010;8:30.
13. Chien LW, Au HK, Chen PL, Xiao J, Tzeng CR. Assessment of uterine receptivity by the endometrial-subendometrial blood flow distribution pattern in women undergoing in vitro fertilization-embryo transfer. Fertil Steril. 2002;78(2):245-51.
14. Maugey-Laulom B, Commenges-Ducos M, Jullien V, Papaxanthos-Roche A, Scotet V, Commenges D. Endometrial vascularity and ongoing pregnancy after IVF. Eur J Obstet Gynecol Reprod Biol. 2002;104(2):137-43.
15. Ng EH, Chan CC, Tang OS, Yeung WS, Ho PC. Endometrial and subendometrial vascularity is higher in pregnant patients with livebirth following ART than in those who suffer a miscarriage. Hum Reprod. 2007;22(4):1134-41.
16. Bonhoff AJ, Naether OG, Johannisson E. Effects of clomiphene citrate stimulation on endometrial structure in infertile women. Hum Reprod. 1996;11:844-9.
17. Sereepapong W, Suwajanakorn S, Triratanachat S, Sampatanukul P, Pruksananonda K, Boonkasemsanti W, et al. Effects of clomiphene citrate on the endometrium of regularly cycling women. Fertil Steril. 2000;73:287-91.
18. Hyder SM, Stancel GM. Regulation of VEGF in the reproductive tract by sex-steroid hormones. Histol Histopathol. 2000;15(1):325-34.
19. Bedaiwy MA, Abdelaleem MA, Hussein M, Mousa N, Brunengraber LN, Casper RF. Hormonal, follicular and endometrial dynamics in letrozole-treated versus natural cycles in patients undergoing controlled ovarian stimulation. Reprod Biol Endocrinol. 2011;9:83.
20. Young SL. Oestrogen and progesterone action on endometrium: a translational approach to understanding endometrial receptivity. Reprod Biomed Online. 2013;27(5): 497-505.
21. Licht P, Fluhr H, Neuwinger J, Wallwiener D, Wildt L. Is human chorionic gonadotropin directly involved in the regulation of human implantation? Mol Cell Endocrinol. 2007;269:85-92.
22. Eftekhar M, Rahmani E, Eftekar T. Effect of adding human chorionic gonadotropin to the endometrial preparation protocol in frozen embryo transfer cycles. Int J Fertil Steril. 2012;6:175-8.
23. Davar R, Miraj S, Mojtahedi MF. Effect of adding human chorionic gonadotropin to frozen thawed embryo transfer cycles with history of thin endometrium. Int J Reprod Biomed. 2016;14:53-6.
24. Kuo HC, Hsu CC, Wang ST, Huang KE. Aspirin improves uterine blood flow in the peri-implantation period. J Formos Med Assoc. 1997;96:253-7.
25. Hsieh YY, Tsai HD, Chang CC, Lo HY, Chen CL. Low-dose aspirin for infertile women with thin endometrium receiving intrauterine insemination: a prospective, randomized study. J Assist Reprod Genet. 2000;17:174-7.
26. Sher G, Fisch JD. Effect of vaginal sildenafil on the outcome of in vitro fertilization (IVF) after multiple IVF failures attributed to poor endometrial development. Fertil Steril. 2002;78:1073-6.
27. Raja VS, Naidu EM. Platelet-rich fibrin: evolution of a second-generation platelet concentrate. Indian J Dent Res. 2008;19:42-6.
28. Marx RE. Platelet-rich plasma (PRP): what is PRP and what is not PRP? Implant Dent. 2001;10:225-8.
29. Ehrenfest DM, Bielecki T, Mishra A, Borzini P, Inchingolo F, Sammartino G, et al. In search of a consensus terminology in the field of platelet concentrates for surgical use: platelet-rich plasma (PRP), platelet-rich fibrin (PRF), fibrin gel polymerization and leukocytes. Curr Pharm Biotechnol. 2012;13:1131-7.
30. Chang Y, Li J, Chen Y, Wei L, Yang X, Shi Y, et al. Autologous platelet-rich plasma promotes endometrial growth and improves pregnancy outcome during in vitro fertilization. Int J Clin Exp Med. 2015;8:1286-90.
31. Chang Y, Li J, Wei LN, Pang J, Chen J, Liang X. Autologous platelet-rich plasma infusion improves clinical pregnancy rate in frozen embryo transfer cycles for women with thin endometrium. Medicine (Baltimore). 2019;98:e14062.
32. Shawki YO. Hysteroscopic subendometrial PRP injection in cases of infertility. J Minim Invasive Gynecol. 2020;27:119.
33. Cakiroglu Y, Tohma YA, Yuceturk A, Karaosmanoglu O, Kopuk SY, Korun ZEU, et al. Effects of subendometrial autologous platelet rich plasma injection on endometrium and pregnancy rates in patients with unresponsive thin endometrium undergoing frozen-thawed embryo transfer. Fertil Steril. 2021;116(3):E103.
34. Noushin MA, Ashraf M, Thunga C, Singh S, Singh S, Basheer R, et al. A comparative evaluation of subendometrial and intrauterine platelet-rich plasma treatment for women with recurrent implantation failure. F S Sci. 2021;2(3):295-302.
35. Masuda H, Kalka C, Takahashi T, Yoshida M, Wada M, Kobori M, et al. Estrogen-mediated endothelial progenitor cell biology and kinetics for physiological postnatal vasculogenesis. Circ Res. 2007;101:598-606.
36. Mayani H, Alvarado-Moreno JA, Flores-Guzmán P. Biology of human hematopoietic stem and progenitor cells present in circulation. Arch Med Res. 2003;34:476-88.

37. Zhao J, Zhang Q, Wang Y, Li Y. Uterine infusion with bone marrow mesenchymal stem cells improves endometrium thickness in a rat model of thin endometrium. Reprod Sci. 2015;22(2):181-8.
38. Wang J, Ju B, Pan C, Gu Y, Zhang Y, Sun L, et al. Application of bone marrow-derived mesenchymal stem cells in the treatment of intrauterine adhesions in rats. Cell Physiol Biochem. 2016;39:1553-60.
39. Santamaria X, Cabanillas S, Cervelló I, Arbona C, Raga F, Ferro J, et al. Autologous call therapy with CD133+ bone marrow-derived stem cells for refractory Asherman's syndrome and endometrial atrophy: a pilot cohort study. Hum Reprod. 2016;31(5):1087-96.
40. Sudoma I, Pylyp L, Kremenska Y, Goncharova Y. Application of autologous adipose-derived stem cells for thin endometrium treatment in patients with failed ART programs. J Stem Cell Ther Transplant. 2019;3:001-8.
41. Saribas GS, Ozogul C, Tiryaki M, Pinarli FA, Kilic SH. Effects of uterus derived mesenchymal stem cell and their exosomes on Asherman's syndrome. Acta Histochem. 2020;122(1):151465.
42. Yáñez-Mó M, Siljander PR, Andreu Z, Zavec AB, Borràs FE, Buzas EI, et al. Biological properties of extracellular vesicles and their physiological functions. J Extracell Vesicles. 2015;4:27066.
43. Blázquez R, Sánchez-Margallo FM, Álvarez V, Matilla E, Hernández N, Marinaro F, et al. Murine embryos exposed to human endometrial MSCs-derived extracellular vesicles exhibit higher VEGF/PDGF AA release, increased blastomere count and hatching rates. PLoS One. 2018;13:e 0196080.
44. Desrochers LM, Bordeleau F, Reinhart-King CA, Cerione RA, Antonyak MA. Microvesicles provide a mechanism for intercellular communication by embryonic stem cells during embryo implantation. Nat Commun. 2016;7:11958.
45. Giacomini E, Vago R, Sanchez AM, Podini P, Zarovni N, Murdica V, et al. Secretome of in vitro cultured human embryos contains extracellular vesicles that are uptaken by the maternal side. Sci Rep. 2017;7:5210.

CHAPTER 85

Ovarian Rejuvenation

Manjunath C Swamy

INTRODUCTION

Due to various causative factors, Infertility is becoming one of the major global concerns. Among the various causes of infertility, premature ovarian insufficiency (POI) and premature ovarian failure (POF) is increasingly becoming common across the globe. Clinics across the globe are reporting more women with loss of oocytes. In India it is more so, maybe because of ethnic/racial differences compared to Caucasian women. Similarly, there are rising trends in infertile men presenting with low spermatogenesis problems or with azoospermia. In case of POI or POF, women can still ovulate and may result in natural pregnancy erratically. The chance of natural conception varies widely among these groups of patients. Generally, many studies have shown 4.5–5% of POI/POF women conceive naturally by erratic ovulation. But the majority of them require medical help.

The only well accepted proven treatment is IVF using donor eggs. Women who wish to have their own genetic material (oocytes) are often met with limited options. Stem cell therapy (cell-based therapy) is increasingly explored with some amount of progress in clinical settings.[1] Even though many studies have shown that less percentage of stem cell treated couples conceive naturally, their hormonal milieu has improved. This may avoid unnecessary low prognostic procedures like IVF in this group of patients.

WHAT ARE STEM CELLS?

Stem cells are specialized pluripotent (means not yet differentiated cells) cells which have capacity to develop into distinct specific cells based on the environmental stimuli, with the purpose to develop, repair or regenerate tissues and organs **(Fig. 1)**.

CLASSIFICATION

There are five types of stem cells which vary from less differentiated (but with more potency) stem cells to more differentiated (but with less potency) stem cells.

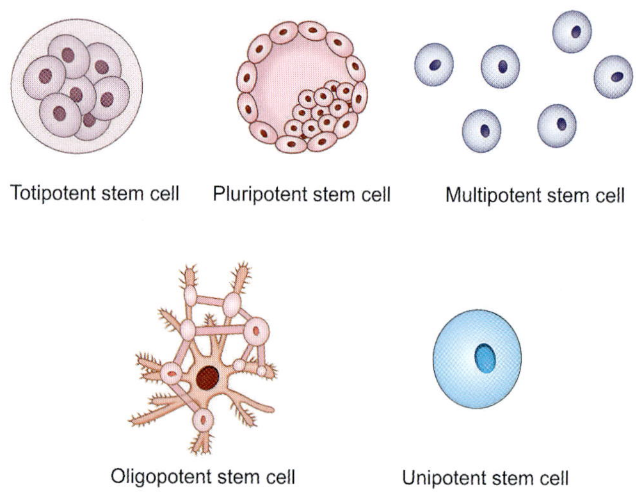

Fig. 1: Stem cell potency.

- Embryonic stem cells (ESCs)
- Induced pluripotent stem cells (iPSCs)
- Mesenchymal stem cells (MSCs)
- Hematopoietic stem cells (HSCs)
- Spermatogonial and oogonial stem cells (SSCs and OSC, respectively).

All these varieties of stem cells are used in different conditions of infertility with varying success **(Table 1)**.

One more way of classifying stem cells is based on potency:

- Pluripotent:
  - Embryonic stem cells (ESCs)
  - Induced pluripotent stem cells (iPSCs)
- Multipotent:
  - Mesenchymal stem cells (MSCs)
  - Hematopoietic stem cells (HSCs)
- Unipotent:
  - Spermatogonial stem cells (SSCs)
  - Oogonial stem cells (OSCs).

Embryonic Stem Cells

Induced pluripotent stem cells (iPSCs) and ESCs are derived from inner cell mass of the blastocyst. These cells

TABLE 1: Different type of fertility issues addressed with stem cells therapy.

		Female fertility issues (Fig. 2)	
	Conditions	***Stem cell types***	***Effects/Reference***
Endometrium	• Asherman's syndrome (Partial/complete) • Thin endometrium • Recurrent pregnancy loss • Recurrent implantation failure	• MenSCs (Menstrual-humans) • UCSCs (umbilical cord-humans) • ESCs (epithelial-mouse) • MSCs (mesenchymal)	• Endometrium↑[2] • LBR ↑[3,4]
Ovary	• PCOS • POF	• ADSc (adipose tissue) • AFSCs (amniotic fluid), BMSCs (bone marrow)	↑Follicles, ↑E2[5-8]
		Male fertility issues	
Testis	• Azoospermia	• UCSCs (Umbilical cord)	Spermatogenesis↑
	• Aspermia	• MSCs (mesenchymal)	Testicular tissue↑
	• Oligospermia	• iPSCs (induced pluripotent) • ADSc (adipose tissue)	Births↑ (only animal studies)[9,10]

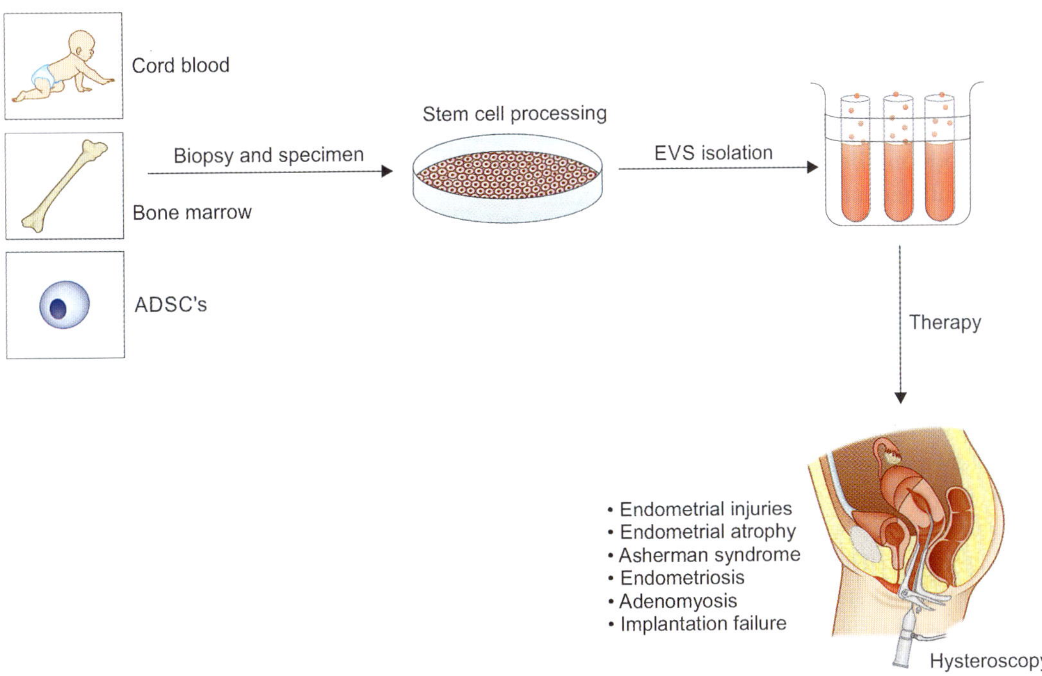

Fig. 2: A schematic representation various sources of stem cells and their application in disorders of female reproductive system.

are pluripotent which means apart from having self-renewal capacity they can differentiate into any cells of three germ layers (endoderm, mesoderm and ectoderm) and germ cells. Many studies have shown iPSCs can be achieved by reprogramming somatic cells. These cells have identical characteristics to ESCs but have advantage of no ethical involvement.[11]

Even though a lot of preclinical/clinical studies focusing on stem cells are underway for many other diseases, none of them are studying infertility management. The in vitro creation of "artificial gametes" from ESCs or iPSCs is still a long way to go in humans.

Mesenchymal Stem Cells

Mesenchymal stem cells are the ones which are widely used for treating infertility conditions. They are derived from mesoderm layers which can be obtained from various adult tissues such as bone marrow, adipose tissue, placenta, umbilical cord (Wharton's jelly) and blood **(Fig. 3)**.[12,13]

Great advantage of these MSCs is that they can be easily isolated from many adult tissues without any ethical issues. Many clinical trials have shown MSCs has potential application for various infertility conditions such as endometrial diseases, ovarian insufficiency and erectile dysfunction.[12,13]

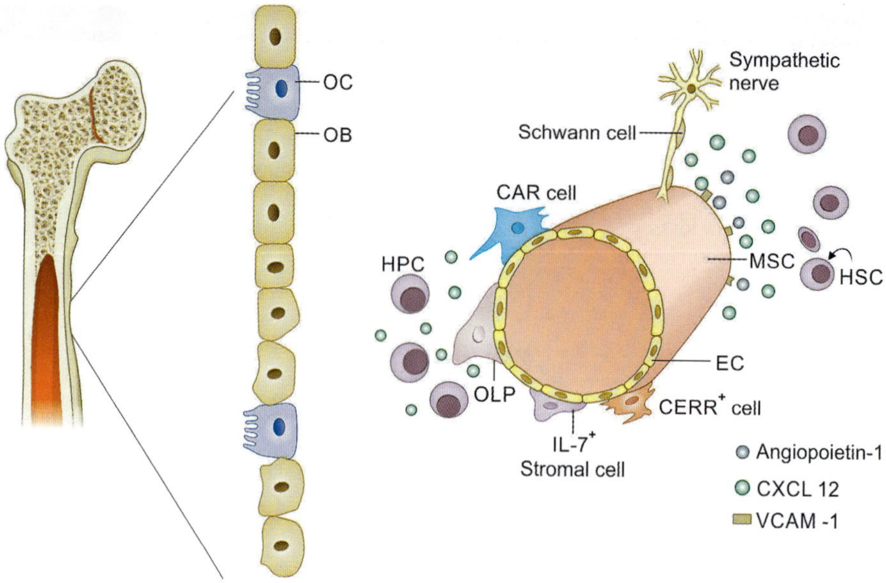

Fig. 3: Bone marrow derived mesenchymal stem cells (MSCs) in repair of injured tissues.

Hematopoietic Stem Cells

These are adult mesoderm - derived multipotent stem cells which can be differentiated into many types of blood cells. Particularly CD 133+ cells from bone marrow have high regenerative capacity. Clinical trials using these CD 133+ cells to treat endometrial disorders have shown promising results.

Spermatogonial and Oogonial Stem Cells

Spermatogonial sperm cells and OSCs are germline stem cells that are unipotent and can give rise to fully differentiated gametes (sperm and oocytes). Biggest drawback is the amount of SSCs and OSCs in testis and ovaries, respectively, is very low which impedes their maintenance and growth in vitro in comparison to other stem cells. Till today there are no human clinical trials using SSCs therapy.

Oogonial stem cells: Many commercial companies are studying the use of OSCs in infertility issues, there is presently no strong evidence of their presence, origin and function.[1]

STEM CELLS "NICHE"

The term "stem cell niche" was first proposed by Schofield in 1978. The self-renewal capacity of stem cells is believed due to the specific microenvironment provided by the neighboring cells of the stem cells. Stem cells niches or the specialized microenvironment in which the stem cells are located are complex structures which include different components.

Components of the Stem Cell "Niches"

- Cellular components (e.g., stem cells and differentiated cells)
- Secreted factors (e.g., chemokines, growth hormones and Wnt)
- Extracellular matrix (e.g., collagen fibers and fibronectin)
- Physical parameters (e.g., shear stress and tissue stiffness)
- Environmental signals (e.g., hypoxia and metabolism) and
- Bidirectional regulation of stem cells and their micro-environment.

In endometrium, these niches are found near rapidly growing spiral arteries which promote the renewal of the stem cells which promotes endometrial cyclical regeneration. In case of ovaries these niches help in the activation of remaining primordial follicles.

STEM CELL BASED THERAPY FOR FEMALE INFERTILITY

Most preclinical trials of stem cells for female infertility have used MSCs and HSCs with varying degree of expected results. Most of them have used autologous MSCs from bone marrow and adipose tissue. Few studies have used allogeneic umbilical cord MSCs for POF. Many studies have reported positive result[14-16] as:

- Improvement of overall ovarian function
- Increase in ovarian volume
- Resumption of menstrual cycle
- Endometrial improvement
- Increase in estradiol concentration
- Improved follicular development
- Increased number of antral follicles.

Premature Ovarian Insufficiency

It is defined as setting of amenorrhea or oligomenorrhea before the age of 40 (In Indian scenario we can take it as

35 years) increase in gonadotropins [follicle-stimulating hormone (FSH)], and decrease in estradiol (E2).[17] Even though older studies have shown that in general it is 2–4%, recently there is an increase in its prevalence. In the majority of POI, the cause is unexplained.

In clinical set up ovarian regeneration is attempted generally by injecting prepared autologous MSCs (mostly derived from bone marrow and adipose tissue) into the ovaries, mostly by laparoscopy and in few studies by transvaginal sonography guided procedure. Bone marrow aspiration is generally done at the iliac crest. The first child born after autologous BM-MSCs is by Edessy et al.[18] After this many clinical human studies have been conducted and many more are still in trials.

Proposed Mechanism of Ovarian Regeneration

Animal studies have shown that transplanted stem cells are not directly becoming oocytes.[19] These stem cells are differentiated into granulosa cells which in turn rescued or directed the oocyte maturation which were otherwise destined to apoptosis. These stem cells decreased apoptosis and pushed them into development. This process of improving ovarian function by MSCs transplantation is due to various molecular mechanisms (inhibition of autophagy of theca-interstitial cells via AMPK/mTOR signaling pathway;[20] activation of PI3K pathway[21] and ECM-development FAK/AKT signaling pathway; improved ovarian metabolome; paracrine activity by releasing different growth factor such as NGF, EGT, VEGT, etc.

The expected results are usually seen after 2–3 months. Many studies have shown that it is better to consider hormonal support after MSCs transplantation. HRT using a cyclical combination of estradiol plus dydrogesterone is considered in many studies.[1]

Proposed Mechanism of Endometrial Regeneration

Endometrium is a dynamic endocrine organ just like the ovary which plays an important role during embryo implantation. Dynamic dialog between endometrium and embryo will determine strong implantation. Adequate thickness (7–13 mm), morphology (triple-like pattern) and good functionality is crucial to achieve a successful pregnancy.[22]

The four components of human endometrium are the epithelium, stroma, vascular network and immune components. There are dynamic changes which continuously keep happening in these components throughout the menstrual cycle and during the implantation process. These four components will form two layers of endometrium, the stratum basalis and stratum functionalis.

Stratum basalis which usually would not shed during menstrual phase contains permanent somatic stem cell population, which is responsible for cyclical regeneration of the functionalis layer. So, this intrinsic capacity of endometrium to regenerate itself is due to the NICHE of stem cells population located in the stratum basalis. This set of cell population aptly called as NICHE of endometrium not only contains, endogenous endometrial stem cells but also bone marrow derived stem cells, extracellular component of stem cells and other structures, which may migrate to endometrium on stimulation such as endometrial injury.[23] Two main endometrial pathologies where stem cell therapy is explored are Asherman's syndrome and endometrial atrophy.

Asherman Syndrome

Asherman syndrome (AS) consists of the presence of intrauterine adhesions (IUAs) which occurs when normal endometrium is replaced by fibrotic tissue. Usual clinical presentations are scanty menstruation, infertility, recurrent miscarriage, abnormal placentation and pelvic pain.[24]

American fertility society (1988) AFS classification of AS includes three groups.

1. *Stage I (mild):* Few flimsy IUAs involving less than one-third of the cavity and normal to mild hypomenorrhea.
2. *Stage II (moderate):* Flimsy to dense IUAs involving one-third to two-thirds of the cavity and hypomenorrhea.
3. *Stage III (severe):* Dense IUAs involving more than two-thirds of the cavity and amenorrhea.[25]

Usually etiology of AS is, genital infections (Tuberculosis common in India), iatrogenic trauma such as D&C, miscarriage, post-partum curettage or hysteroscopic surgery. Other causes are induced uterine artery embolization, cesarean sections, IUD insertions, Mullerian duct malformation.

Endometrial Atrophy

Generally endometrial thickness (measured by TVS—maximum distance between echogenic interfaces at junction of endometrium and myometrium) varies from 7to 13 mm during implantation phase. Clinical consensus is that embryo implantation cannot be achieved if the thickness is below 6 mm[26] (though few cases have achieved pregnancy below this cut-off).

Endometrial atrophy (EA) is caused by decreased endometrial thickness also termed as thin or refractory endometrium. General incidence varies from 2.2 to 4.2% among patients undergoing IVF cycles. Most common causes of EA are inflammatory such as acute/chronic infections or iatrogenic causes such as excessive curettage or hysteroscopic surgeries - all leading to destruction of stratum basalis.

STEM CELL THERAPY FOR ENDOMETRIAL REGENERATION

The presence of bone marrow derived stem cells apart from endogenous endometrial stem cells hypothesize that we can induce BMDSC to accumulate in the endometrium or we can inject these cells directly into the endometrium by process of stem cells transplantation **(Fig. 4)**. This BMDSC hypothesis-postulated to use granulocyte-colony stimulating factor (G-CSF) which pushes stem cell and its progenitor from bone marrow into peripheral blood stream, which in turn gets accumulated in the endometrium. But G-CSF studies remain controversial. Many studies reported that this G-CSF does not significantly increase endometrial thickness. But a meta-analysis of 11 different studies[27] indicated that when G-CSF was used as intrauterine perfusion, it improved endometrial thickness and clinical pregnancy and implantation rate.

Stem cell transplantation for AS or EA involves bone marrow aspiration of 15–20 mL at anterior or posterior iliac crest and the preparation of stem cells using refrigerated centrifuge at 20–21°C. This stem cell mixed plasma is immediately injected into the uterine cavity at multiple sites using hysteroscopy. Injection of these stem cells has to be in the subendometrial zone **(Figs. 5 to 7)**. Similarly, in conditions of ovarian impairment such as POF, the prepared stem cell extract is injected laparoscopically into the bilateral rugosed ovaries. Various clinical studies have shown benefits of using these stem cells in the form of increased ET, increased endometrial functionality markers (ER2, Ki67), increase in pregnancy rate in ART, increased LBR, increased vascular density, and increased menstruation duration.

Many studies using BMDSCs have an effect of increase in ET but it was transient. They could see this maximum effect up to 3 months after injection and then it diminished after 6 months. Mechanism of these stem cells effectiveness could be due to the paracrine effect. Stem cells create an immunomodulatory change which drives the regenerative procedure such as proliferation and angiogenesis.[28]

Bioengineering Material Along with Stem Cell

Bioengineering materials are known to strengthen the cell's regenerative actions. Collagen scaffolds (three-dimensional porous biomaterials), polyglycerol sebacate (PGS) scaffolds, lactic-coglycolic acid scaffolds and hydrogels are being used. Ding et al. (2014) mixed BMMSCs and collagen scaffolds and transplanted the mix onto the basal endometrial layer of rats with an injured uterus,[29] and have shown increased endometrial functional markers.

Endometrial regeneration using other sources of stem cells have been attempted using umbilical cord mesenchymal stem cells (UCMSCs), menstrual blood stem cells, amniotic membrane, adipose tissue mesenchymal stem cells have been tried.

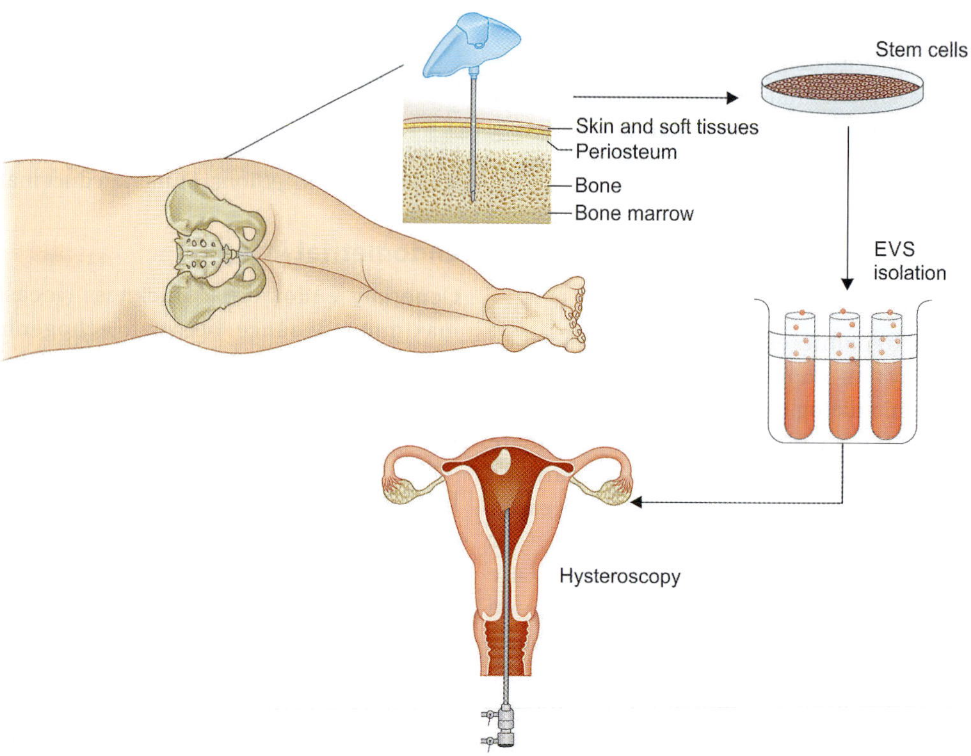

Fig. 4: Stem cell preparation from bone marrow and stem cell implantation.

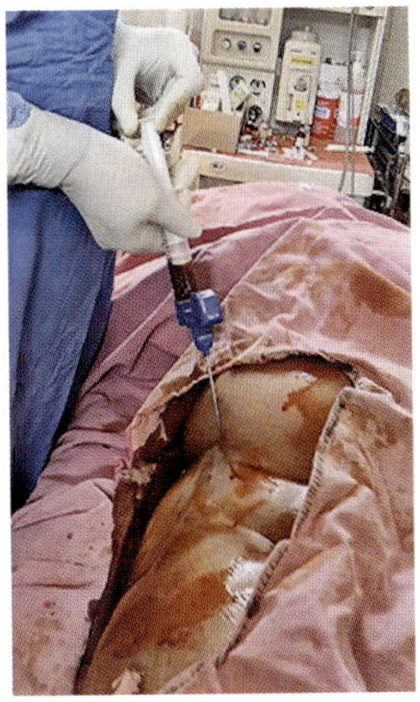

Fig. 5: Bone marrow aspiration.

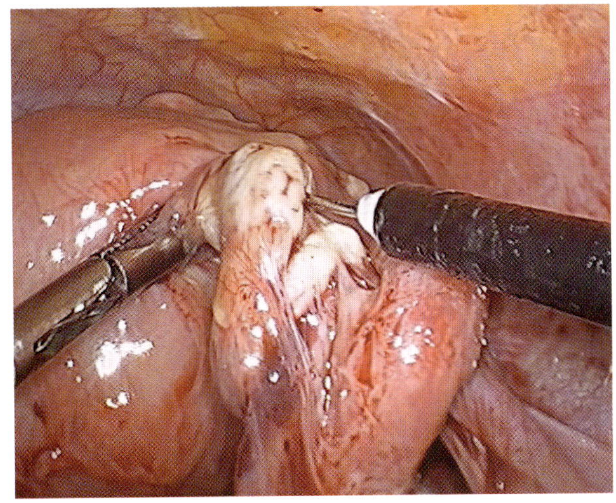

Fig. 7: Laparoscopic ovarian injection of stem cells.

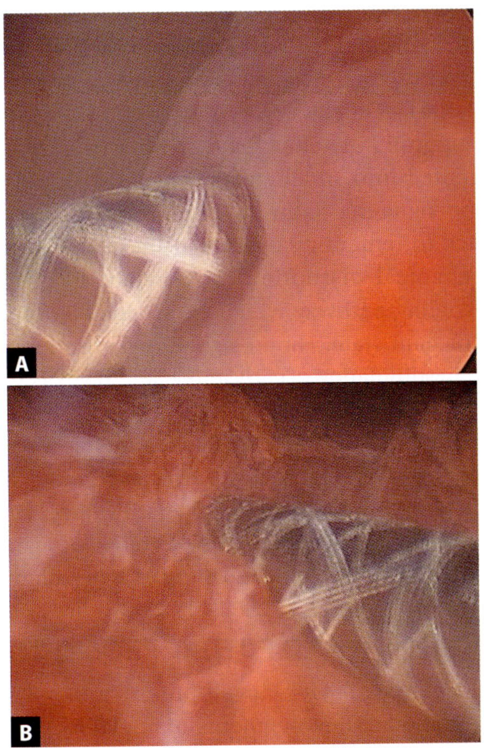

Figs. 6A and B: Hysteroscopic subendometrial stem cell injection.

DERIVATIVES OF STEM CELLS: EXPLORED FOR REGENERATING ENDOMETRIUM

In general, various studies using stem cells for regenerating endometrium highlighted that regeneration happens because of the stem cells paracrine hypothesis. This also means that the effect of this stem cell action is for shorter duration (low retention of the cells) and also there may be the theoretical risk of teratoma development.[30]

So, researchers are trying to develop therapeutic approaches using derivation of stem cells instead of using direct stem cells for regenerating the endometrium. Few things they are exploring include stem cells secretome, stem cell exosomes (extracellular vesicles paracrine factors) and specific molecules from cells (e.g., cell growth factors, cytokines). Granulocyte-colony stimulating factor is one such cell factor which promotes stem cells progenitors and increases regenerative capacity of endometrium which has been studied extensively in human clinical studies. Others include hepatocyte growth factor (HGF), transforming growth factor-beta (TGF-β), platelet derived growth factor (PDGF), and fibroblast growth factor (FGF). Many of these growth factors are presumably present in plasma rich protein (PRP). The use of PRP for generating endometrium has been studied with varied results.

Platelet Rich Plasma

It is a peripheral blood derived mixture of platelets and its growth factor (which has above average platelet concentration) which has potential to repair and regenerate tissues.[31] PRP mainly consists of α-granules inside the platelets which contain bioactive molecules (which are released after activation) such as cytokine, growth factors, (IGF-1, HCF, FGF) and other biologically active proteins which will actively take part in tissue repairs and regeneration. Prior use of G-CSF 2–3 days before taking peripheral blood for preparation of PRP may increase these regenerating factors.

Various clinical studies using PRP have been published. Most of these studies are smaller in number. Only two randomized clinical trials using PRP have been published. In RCT by Eftekhar M et al., PRP has been used for EA cases, which showed improvement in endometrial thickness, clinical pregnancy rate and implantation rate were observed.[32] In RCT by Javaheri A et al., PRP was used for AS patients. They reported no improvement in endometrial thickness or restoration of menstrual patterns.[33]

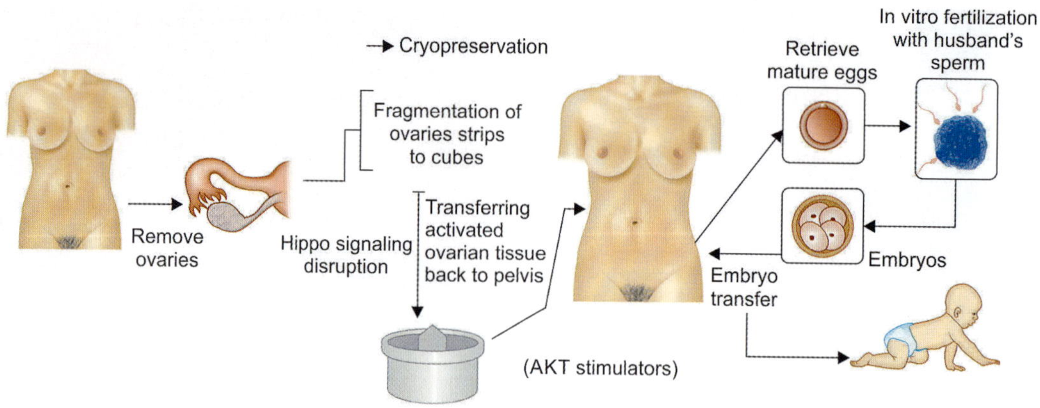

Fig. 8: In vitro activation of the ovary.

Paracrine Factors

Many paracrine factors have been explored along with stem cell therapy to make this regenerative treatment simpler. At present there are varied results in terms of effectiveness and safety. This relatively recent therapeutic approach needs further larger well designed studies. It is prudent to wait for a better understanding on regenerative capacity of these factors.

IN VITRO ACTIVATION OF OVARY

In order to develop mature oocytes, plenty of small primordial follicles (PFs) are constantly activated from the pool of PFs. In many cases as the doctrine of ovarian follicles progresses, the activation of dormant follicles eventually arrests or temporarily stops despite still having a reasonable amount of residual PFs. So, these women with limited numbers of growing follicles present with poor ovarian response and many fail to conceive on their own or on stimulation with ovulogens.

So, this can be addressed by activating their residual dormant PFs using a new method of infertility treatment called in vitro activation (IVA) and drug-free IVA. By doing so it stimulates early gonadotropin-independent stage follicles to grow which may benefit a few POI and POR-DOR patients.

Mechanism of In Vitro Activation

Exact mechanism of how dormant PFs activation happens is not clearly understood. Many intracellular signaling pathways have been described.[34] Three important pathways studied in activation of PFs are phosphatidyl inositol-3-kinase (PI3k-AKT), mammalian target of rapamycin (mTOR) signaling pathways[35] and Hippo signaling pathway.

What is IVA?

This is a procedure in which laparoscopy is used to remove one or both ovaries. Then cortex of the ovaries around 2 mm thickness is removed (since majority of PFs are located within 2 mm of cortex surface) and then immediately this cortical tissue is cut into small strips (1–2 mm thickness) **(Fig. 8)**. Then these cortical strips were cryopreserved for subsequent tissue culture with AKT activators and auto grafting (usually in the pouch created in mesosalpinx-using second laparoscopy). This method of IVA can be treated as conventional IVA or classical IVA.

In drug-free IVA, after removing the ovarian cortex it is fragmented into small cubes (1–2 mm) to just disturb the Hippo signaling pathway. Then immediately grafting them back to remaining ovaries or mesosalpinx pouch.[36] The mechanical disruption is sufficient to disturb the Hipposignaling pathway which is responsible for keeping PFs in dormant state. Hippo signaling disruption alone is sufficient in stimulation of early follicular growth. Few studies have shown clinical improvement with drug-free IVA,[37] but the number of cases is small. Extrapolating this mechanism, a group published the clinical outcome of the disruption of Hippo signaling pathway by ovarian biopsy/scratch in 80 patients with POI women. They were able to get follicle growth with FSH stimulation in almost 14% of patients.[38]

CONCLUSION AND FUTURE PROSPECTIVE

With >43 years of ART development and >8 million babies born so far, new segments of infertility population such as POI, POR, poor endometrium and disturbed spermatogenesis have been added to the infertility pool. These segments of the infertility population require newer therapeutic approaches. One such approach is in considering stem cells and its derivatives as an alternative approach to ART and or to improve the success of IVF outcomes in these couples. Clinical and preclinical studies have shown some light on how stem cell therapy can be of assistance in infertility management. But at present stem cell therapies are largely in the preclinical phase and several ethical issues need to be addressed. Since autologous stem cells are ethical, safe, and nonimmune, the clinical use of these autologous stem cells is more convenient and has great potential in the future.

REFERENCES

1. Varsena R, Eguizabal C, Heindry CKB, ESHRE Special Internet Group Stem Cell. Stem cells in reproductive medicine: ready for the patient? Human Reprod, 2015;30:2014-21.
2. Tan J, Li P, Wang Q, Li Y, Li X, Zhao D, et al. Autologous menstrual blood derived stromal cell transplantation for secure Asherman's syndrome. Human Reprod. 2016;31(12): 2723-9.
3. Cao Y, Sun H, Zhu H. Allogenic cell therapy using umbilical cord MSCs on collagen scaffolds for patients with recurrent uterine adhesions: a phase 1 clinical trial stem cell res ther 2018;9(1);192
4. Park SR, Kin SR, Park CH. Sonic hedgehog, a novel endogenous damage signal, activates multiple beneficial functions of human endometrial stem cells. Mol Ther. 2020;28(2):452-65.
5. Su J, Ding L, Cheng J. Transplantation of adipose-derived stem cell combined with collagen scaffolds restores ovarium functions in a rat model of POI. Hum Reprod. 2016;31(5):1075-86.
6. Xioo GY, Liu IH, Cheng CC. Amniotic fluid stem cells prevent follicular atresia and rescue fertility of mice with POF induced by chemotherapy . PLOS One. 2014;(9):106538.
7. Ghadami M, EL-Denordash E, Zhang D. Bone marrow transplantation restores follicular maturation and steroid hormone production in a mouse a model for POF. PLOS One. 2012;7(3):e32462.
8. While YAR, Woods DC, Talkar Y. Oocyte formation by mitotically active germ cells purified from ovaries of reproductive age women. Nat Med. 2012;18(3)413-76.
9. Calcici C, Buyruka B, Duruksu G. Recovery of fertility in azoospermia rats after injection of adipose-tissue derived mesenchymal stem cell: the sperm generation. Biomed Res Int. 2013;529589.
10. Mouka A, Izard V, Tachdjian G. Induced pluripotent stem cell generation from a man carrying a complex chromosomal rearrangement as a genetic model for Infertility studies. Sci Rep. 2017;7:39760.
11. Takahashi K, Tanabe K, Ohnuki M, Narita M, Ichisaka T, Tomoda K, et al. Induction of pluripotent stem cell from adult human fibroblasts by defined factors. Cell. 2007;131:872.
12. He M, von Schwarz ER. Stem cell therapy for erectile dysfunction: a review of clinical outcomes. Int J Impot Res. 2021;33(3):271-7.
13. Zhao Y, Chen S, Su P. Using MSCs to treat female infertility: An update on female reproductive disease. Stem cells Int. 2019;2019:9071720 .
14. Xie Y, Liu W, Liu S. The quality evaluation system establishment of MSCs for cell based therapy products. Stem cell Res Ther. 2020;11:176 .
15. Edessy M, Hosni H, Wafer Y. Stem cells transplantation in premature ovarian failure. World J Med Sci. 2014;10:12-6 .
16. Herraiz S, Buigues A, Díaz-García C, Romeu M, Martínez S, Gómez-Seguí I, et al. Fertility rescue and ovarian follicle growth promotion by bone marrow stem cell infusion. Fertile Steril. 2018;109:908-18.
17. De Vos M, Devroey D, Fausev BC. Primary ovarian insufficiency. Lancet. 2010;376:911-21.
18. Edessy M, Hosni HN, Shady Y, Waf Y, Bakr S, Kamel M. Autologous stem cells therapy, the first baby of idiopathic premature ovarian failure. Acta Media Int 2016;3:19-23.
19. Reig A, Mamillapall R, Coolodge A. Uterine cells improved ovarian function in a murine model of ovarian insufficiency. Reprod Sci 2019;26:1633-9 .
20. Lu X, Bao H, Cui L. hUMSC transplantation restores ovarian function in POI rats by inhibiting autophagy of theca-interstitial cells via the AMPK/m TOR signalling pathway. Stem Cell Res Ther 2020;11:268.
21. Cui L, Bao H, Liu Z. hUMSCs regulate the differentiation of ovarian stromal cells via TGF-β(1)/smad 3 signalling pathway to inhibit ovarian fibrosis to repair ovarian function in POI rats. Stem Cell Res Ther. 2020;11:386.
22. Cunnigham F, Leveno K. WilliamsObstetrics, 24th edition. New York: McGraw Hill Education; 2015.
23. Gargett CE, Masuda H. Adult stem cells in the endometrium. Mol Hum Reprod. 210;16:818-34.
24. Santamaria X, Mas A, Cervelló I, Taylor H, Simon C. Uterine stem cells: From basic research to advanced cell therapies. Hum Reprod update. 2018;24:673-93.
25. Smikle C, Yarrarapy S, Khetarpal S. Asherman syndrome. Treasure Island (FL): StatPearls Publishing; 2022.
26. Senturic LM, Erel CT. Thin endometrium in assisted reproductive technology. Curr Opin Obstet Gynaecol. 2008; 20:221-8.
27. Xie Y, Zhang T, Tian Z, Zhang J, Wang W, Zhang H, et al. Efficacy of intrauterine perfusion of G-CSF for infertile women with thin endometrium: a Systematic review and meta-analysis. Am J Reprod Immunol. 2017;78:1-10.
28. de Miguel-Gómez L, Ferrero H, López-Martínez S, Campo H, López-Pérez N, Faus A, et al. Stem cell paracrine actions in tissue regeneration and potential therapeutic effect in human endometrium: a retrospective study. BJOG. 2019;127:551-60.
29. Ding L, Li X, Sun H, Su J, Lin N, Péault B, et al. Transplantation of BMSCs on collagen scaffolds for the functional regeneration of injured rat uterus. Biomaterials. 2014;35:4888-900.
30. Musiał-Wysocka A, Kot M, Majka M. The pros and cons of mesenchymal stem cells-based therapies. Cell Transplant. 2019;28:801-12.
31. Alves R, Grimalt R. Clinical indications and treatment protocols with platelet rich plasma in dermatology. Barcelona: Ediciones Mayo; 2016.
32. Eftekhar M, Tabibnejad N, Alsadat A. The thin endometrium in assisted reproductive technology: an ongoing challenge. Middle East Fertile Soc J. 2018;23:1-7.
33. Javaheri A, Kianfar K, Pourmasumi S, Eftekhar M. Platelet-rich plasma is the management of Asherman's syndrome: an RCT. Int J reprod Biomed 2020;18:113-20.
34. Adhikari D, Liu K. Molecular mechanisms underlying the activation of mammalian primordial follicles. Endoc Res. 2009;30:438-64.
35. Tian T, Li X, Zhang J. mTOR signaling in the control of activation of PFs cell cycle. Int J Mol Sci. 2019;20(3):755.
36. Kawamura K, Ishizuka B. Drug free IVA of follicles for infertility treatment is POR patients with decreased ovarian reserve. RBM online. 2020;40:245-53.
37. Tanaka Y, Hsueh AJ. (2020) Surgical approaches of drug free IVA and laparoscopic ovarian incision to treat patients with ovarian infertility. Fertil Steril. 2020;114;1355-7.
38. Zhang X, Han T, Yan L. Resumption of ovarian function after ovarian biopsy/scratch in patients with POI. Reprod Sci. 2019;26:207-13.

SECTION 13

Miscellaneous

CHAPTER 86

Batch In Vitro Fertilization

Sandhya Krishnan

INTRODUCTION

Even with an increasing number of in vitro fertilization (IVF) centers, the demand for batch IVF still remains high due to the limited number of senior embryologists available and the better convenience of patients and clinicians. Here, the menstrual cycles of multiple women are programmed such that they can undergo all the processes, from stimulation until embryo transfer around the same time frame. There is sufficient evidence on scheduling cycles with steroids in gonadotropin-releasing hormone (GnRH)-agonist and antagonist protocols without compromising success.[1] This chapter will highlight the clinical concept of scheduling cycles in a "batch IVF" setup.[2]

Batch IVF is a planned process of recruiting a group of patients, such that the stimulation is started on the same day (±1–2 day window) and oocyte retrieval (OCR) falls on the same day (±1–2 day window).[3] The embryo transfer, if in a fresh cycle, falls on the same day (±1–2 day window), day 2, or day 3 following OCR. The aim is to facilitate OCR, intracytoplasmic sperm injection (ICSI), or IVF, and embryo transfer within a designated period when a visiting senior embryologist is available.

In full-fledged laboratories with an in-house senior embryologist, where two batches may be planned in the same month, so that time for laboratory maintenance is available and quality control could be implemented in a better way, all staff are better prepared and media utilization is done to the maximum.[4,5] It is cost-effective in terms of better utilization of media and gonadotropins, and benefits can be passed on to patients as well.

Batching has its advantages and disadvantages, but its necessity in some settings cannot be underestimated. Weekend-free scheduling of procedures without compromising results is important that is appreciated by all hospital staff.[6]

Standard guidelines to facilitate the smooth running of batch IVF are needed to ensure increased success without compromising results and patient care.

Patient selection is crucial for batch IVF for optimum results.

DIFFERENT SETTINGS WHERE BATCH IN VITRO FERTILIZATION IS DONE[1]

- A well-equipped laboratory with in-house senior embryologist and infertility consultant may choose to have IVF in batch in order to optimize the use of media consumables, drugs, incubator operation theater, anesthetist, ancillary staff, etc. Even though there is no time constraint in such laboratories, batching allows them time to recover and audit. Gonadotropins and media can be shared. In centers where other gynecological procedures are practiced, facilities can be streamlined, and a team can be geared up for batch and better-quality control guaranteed. The quality technician can be designated to come a week before the batch to check the laboratory air quality, pH, humidity and temperature, and incubator swab test for infection control.
- A setup with an in-house infertility specialist and visiting embryologist would do batching as per the availability of embryologist. Here also, optimum resource utilization is the advantage. Results can also be optimized if availability of embryologist in case needed is arranged, when a case or two do not get ready on expected batch dates.
- A setup run by a gynecologist with visiting fertility specialist and embryologist coming for a specified duration can do batching. Here, batching is done due to necessity and lack of full-time available specialists. The gynecologist recruits a batch, and stimulation is done as per remote instructions by a fertility specialist who may not be aware of the patient's clinical details. There is the risk of suboptimal stimulation or overstimulation, and results may be compromised. The advantages and disadvantages of batch IVF thus depend on the setting and organization of the batch. Strategies to identify ideal patients and refer or recruit patients with complex issues outside the batch are vital to the batch's success;

for example, poor responders, hyperresponders, and recurrent implantation failure are the groups who need individualized care and are not ideal for batch IVF.

PREPARATION FOR A BATCH IN VITRO FERTILIZATION

Clinical Aspects

- Number of couples to be recruited
- Pretreatment with the oral contraceptive pill (OCP)
- Previous month's depot preparation
- *Protocol*: Agonist versus antagonist
- *Stimulation*: Starting dose of gonadotropins
- Other protocols
- Monitoring
- Advantages
- Disadvantages
- Summary.

The number of couples to be recruited: This depends on:

- Days of availability of embryologist
- The capacity of the laboratory and the number of incubators available.
- Most recommend four patients per incubator, or if a benchtop is available, the numbers may be increased.
- The number of OCRs around five per day is ideal. Maximum is seven to eight OCR per day. The time required for embryo transfers should also be allotted.

The embryologist should be available on the day of OCR, taken as day 0, on day 1 to check fertilization and additional 2 days to plan day 2 or day 3 for embryo transfer. If complex procedures such as testicular sperm aspiration (TESA), MicroTESA, or blastocyst transfer are planned, additional staff and extra time must be allotted.

Pretreatment with OCP: For batch IVF, pretreatment with OCP is a must to facilitate cycle synchronization.

- It helps to avoid cyst formation.
- It prevents premature luteinizing hormone (LH) surge.[7]
- It maintains persistent reduced LH till trigger.
- Serum level of progesterone is decreased to levels incompatible with ovulation.[1,4]
- Sensitization of receptors to follicle-stimulating hormone (FSH).[1,8]

Disadvantages: The endometrial shedding or thinning effect may last until mid of the stimulation cycle.[8]

This may be beneficial in the antagonist cycle, where advanced endometrial maturation supposedly decreases implantation rates.[9] Pill pretreatment does not improve the number of oocytes obtained and may even have a negative effect on outcome.[10] However, studies have shown the effect as the number needed to treat (NNT) = 20 for 1 less number of live birth rate. The use of oral contraceptive pretreatment in antagonist IVF cycles showed a relatively small but statistically significant reduction of ongoing pregnancy when a pill-free interval of 2–5 days is used before starting gonadotropin stimulation. Based on the incidence of ongoing pregnancies in the randomized controlled trials included in this meta-analysis, the NNT to harm is 20 patients [95% confidence interval (CI): 10–100]. For example, for every 20 patients pretreated with oral contraceptives, one ongoing pregnancy will be missed.[11,12]

It may also increase the duration of stimulation and the dose of gonadotropins.[11,12] Profound LH suppression may increase miscarriage rate and reduce pregnancy rates and thus lead to poor oocyte quality in poor responders.[13,14]

The endometrial thinning effect may persist and reduce fresh cycle transfer success rates.[15]

Recent Cochrane on pill pretreatment in antagonist cycle:[16] Among women undergoing ovarian stimulation in antagonist protocols, combined oral contraceptive pill (COCP) pretreatment was associated with a lower rate of live birth or ongoing pregnancy than no pretreatment. There was insufficient evidence to determine whether live birth rates or ongoing pregnancy were influenced by pretreatment with progestogens or estrogens or by COCP pretreatment using other stimulation protocols. Findings on adverse events were inconclusive, except that progesterone pretreatment may reduce the risk of ovarian cysts in agonist cycles, and COCP in antagonist cycles may reduce the risk of pregnancy loss compared with no pretreatment in agonist cycles.[17-21]

The use of estradiol in the luteal phase of the previous cycle is another protocol with the advantage of synchronization of antral follicles and the disadvantage of missing the batch by 1–2 days if not careful.[22]

Previous month's depot preparation:[23] Administration of a single-dose depot of GnRH agonist preparation (leuprolide 3.75 mg) on day 21 of a prestimulated cycle was assessed in a Cochrane review.[24] The authors observed no evidence for differences between the long protocols using depot or daily GnRH agonist for IVF cycles. Nonetheless, depot GnRH agonist is associated with increased requirements for gonadotropins and a longer time for ovarian stimulation.[25,26] If these differences could be shown to decode into economic benefit, depot GnRH agonist would increase the overall costs of IVF treatment which is not in favor of this protocol.

Protocol—agonist versus antagonist: As a routine, the agonist-long protocol was always recommended for batch IVF as timing and synchronization are easier.[27,28]

However, with pretreatment with combined pills, the antagonist protocol is also used with equal efficacy and comparable success rates.[29]

The calendar also shows a typical agonist-long protocol cycle. However, the agonist-long protocol will be disadvantageous for some patients, especially poor responders, last-minute recruits to the batch, and hyperresponders.

The antagonist cycle can be considered where OCP is stopped 5 days before the stimulation date and irrespective of periods.[30]

When patients received the pill for only 12–16 days, and stimulation started after a wash-out period of at least 5 days, no differences could be found in live birth rates. Also, when cycles planned with OCP were compared with cycles pretreated with estrogens only, again, no differences could be found in live birth rates.[31]

Periods can also be induced using PGE1 200 µg 2 doses 12 hours apart or by coring (mechanical aspiration of the endometrium) for the patient's psychological satisfaction.[32]

Stimulation—starting dose of gonadotropin: Initial starting dose of gonadotropin should be individualized to get optimal response and prevention of hyperstimulation.

Consort algorithm: The daily FSH dose may be calculated based on age and two markers of ovarian reserve, namely antral follicle count (AFC) and anti-Müllerian hormone (AMH), with the last two variables being the most significant predictors.[33-35]

However, standard dosing with 150 IU FSH, with the option of increasing or decreasing the dosage as per response, is a standard protocol with triggering final oocyte maturation by a GnRH agonist with or without deferred embryo transfer.[36]

Individualized FSH dosing based on the AFC does not improve live birth rates or reduce costs. Ovarian reserve test-based treatment for the IVF/ICSI population as a whole should, therefore, not be pursued. Women scheduled for IVF/ICSI with a regular menstrual cycle are therefore recommended to a standard FSH starting dose of 150 IU/day.[37]

Ordering for gonadotropins: Once the initial starting dose is calculated for each patient, this is multiplied by 10 to get the amount of gonadotropin to be ordered. An extra 10% of the calculated dose is kept for backup in case of any additional requirement. The choice of gonadotropin depends on the center's experience and personal preference. A trained staff nurse should be available to check the stocks and administer injections to a patient. A separate refrigerator with an uninterrupted power supply is a must for gonadotropins to maintain the cold chain.[38]

Other protocol—microflare for poor responders:[1,38] The microflare protocol is designed to optimize ovarian response in women with a previous poor response to a routine protocol or who have low AMH and AFC. The term "microflare" is derived in two parts: "micro" refers to the use of a diluted dose of Lupron, micrograms instead of milligrams, and "flare" refers to the stimulatory or flare effect of Lupron when given this way—hence the term microflare. Starting on cycle day 3--two to three (sometimes up to four) weeks of OCPs, then start microdose Lupron (0.2 cc twice daily) 3 days after stopping OCPs, and then add gonadotropins 2 days after starting Lupron. The gonadotropin start day is the cycle start day or stimulation day 1 **(Table 1)**.

Dosage is also based on baseline FSH, AMH, body mass index, age, and AFC.

Additional LH may be added and is helpful in hypogonadotropic hypogonadism and poor responders.[39,40]

Monitoring: Aim for an optimum number of oocytes to avoid overburdening of resources. Most studies put the optimal number of retrieved oocytes between 10 and 15.[41,42]

Use standardized protocol for batches to avoid confusion among staff and easy counseling of patients. Optimal stimulation will avoid ovarian hyperstimulation syndrome (OHSS)[43]

TABLE 1: Microdose Lupron Flare protocol.

Sunday	*Monday*	*Tuesday*	*Wednesday*	*Thursday*	*Friday*	*Saturday*
Combined oral contraceptive pill (COCP) (continue for 2–3 weeks)						
	Baseline sonogram take last OCP			Diluted Lupron 0.02 cc 2 times each day until hCG		Stimulation medication (gonadotropins) Start to continue Lupron two times each
		E2	(Completion of the cycle may vary depending on individual patient's response)	Sono and E2		
	Sono and E2	Sono and E2 hCG (PM)		Oocyte retrieval time in (AM)		

(E2: estradiol; hCG: human chorionic gonadotropin; OCP: oral contraceptive pill) and provide better endometrial receptivity and endocrine environment.[44]

- Baseline ultrasound
- *Day 2:* Hormone levels to confirm downregulation (optional)
- *Day 2:* Scan to confirm downregulation
- *Day 6:* Scan and hormone level (optional) to confirm optimum dosage of gonadotropins and response to prevent OHSS or suboptimal stimulation.
- *Day 8:* Scan.

Day 10: Scan + hormones assay to check progesterone level (only if planning fresh transfer) on trigger day and decide regarding a fresh transfer.

- *Day 12:* OCR and IVF or ICSI by the embryologist
- *Day 13:* Fertilization check
- *Day 14:* Day 2 embryo check--day 2 embryo transfer or freeze can be done. The sample batch calendar for D2 transfer is given in **Table 2**.
- *Day 15:* Day 3 embryo transfer--day 3 embryo transfer or freeze can be done.
- The batch completes treatment for that particular cycle, and the embryologist leaves to join another center for another batch.

Advantages of the batch IVF compared to regular batch are given in **Table 3**.

Disadvantages of batch IVF compared to a regular cycle are given in **Table 4**.

Suggested checklist for optimum results in batch IVF:

- Detailed clinical and hormonal evaluation of each couple. Better to include prior cycle monitoring to have an idea of the patient's response to stimulation.

TABLE 2: Sample batch calendar for D2 transfer.

Sunday	Monday	Tuesday	Wednesday	Thursday	Friday	Saturday
		1	2	3	4 GnRH agonist depot (long protocol)	5
6	7	8	9	10	11 Stop OCP	12
13	14	15	16	17 S1 Start gonadotropin	18 S2	19 S3
20 S4	21 S5	22 S6 Start antagonist in antagonist cycle	23 S7	24 S8	25 S9	26 S10
27 S11 Trigger on S10 or S11	28	29 Oocyte retrieval Embryologist available	30 Embryologist available	31 Embryologist available: D2 embryo transfer		

(GnRH: gonadotropin-releasing hormone; OCP: oral contraceptive pill)

TABLE 3: Advantages of batch in vitro fertilization (IVF) compared to regular batch.

	Batch IVF	*Regular IVF*
Availability	It makes IVF available at peripheral centers at an affordable price	Only a few centers are available
Access	Access to more people	Less number of populations covered
Long-distance travel	Traveling distance can be avoided for IVF treatment	Long distance to be traveled for treatment which increases the cost
Quality control	Laboratory gets time to get ready and quality control possible, as enough time is available	Laboratory quality assessment incomplete as no gap time to follow the standard operations for quality assessment and appraisal
Maintenance of equipment	Tasks such as incubator cleaning, calibration, pH assessment, sperm survival test, and maintenance of instruments can be easily undertaken during free time. This is not feasible at centers with ongoing cycles throughout the month	Laboratory cleaning and instrument calibration compromised
Results	The cumulative pregnancy rate in batch IVF is the same as routine IVF if standards and protocols are followed	Success rates are almost the same as a batch for a normal responder

TABLE 4: Disadvantages of the batch in vitro fertilization (IVF) compared to a regular cycle.

	Batch IVF	*Regular IVF*
Flexibility	Lack of flexibility of cycle and days	Days flexible
Time frame	Rigid time frames to be followed	Time frame flexible
Patient response to stimulation	Some patients may not respond as expected, leading to cycle cancellation and unsatisfied patient	Oocyte retrieval date can be adjusted as per response
Protocol	The antagonist cycle may be difficult to control and synchronize. Last-minute cancellation would reduce the number of cases and lead to media wastage	The protocol can be individualized
Privacy	Patients would be well acquainted with each other. If the results are low, they can cause trouble in groups which would be difficult for the doctor to deal with	Privacy maintained for both patient and center
Mishap	If any technical mishap happens, it will affect the whole group	Mishap, if any, would include a few numbers of patients
Skills	Accountability and skills of visiting embryologists may not be assured always	Embryologist and reproductive medicine consultant are accountable and more responsible as they directly deal with the patient
Operator	Operator-induced mistakes are more common due to workload and time constraints	Operator-induced error is less common as the staff is more relaxed with routine work
Sample mixing	More risk of mixing of samples	Mixing of the sample can be avoided
Individualized treatment	Individualized treatment difficult	Individualized treatment possible
OCP pretreatment	OCP pretreatment may affect cycle outcome and increase gonadotropin dose required	Pretreatment not necessary
Minimum number of recruits	If a minimum number of patients are not recruited, the batch may turn as overexpensive	The number of patients does not affect treatment
Incubator overload	Incubator overload is a concern if more patients are recruited and center not prepared	Incubator load not compromised
Cycle cancellation	Cancellation and rescheduling will be expensive, demoralizing, and inconvenient for both patient and the center	The patient feels more confident as embryologists, and reproductive medicine specialists are always available
Embryo transfer	Usually must do D2 or D3 transfer, and blastocyst transfer is not feasible even if indicated. Advanced procedures such as PGD and PGS cannot be done due to short stay of embryologist	Blastocyst culture can always be considered. PGD/PGS feasible in indicated cases
Complex procedures	A complex procedure such as TESA challenging to be implemented	Complex procedures such as TESA, PESA, and microsurgical testicular sperm extraction (microTESE) can always be considered when needed
Freeze–thaw quality	Freezing and thawing compromised due to time constraints	Embryology procedures such as freezing and thawing can be done at ease with no time constraints[45]
Quality control	Quality control may not be up to the mark if the visiting embryologist is dependent upon junior staff to maintain laboratory equipment and incubator	A full-time single-center-focused embryologist would be able to focus more on quality control. They can supervise the juniors directly

(OCP: oral contraceptive pill; PESA: percutaneous epididymal sperm aspiration; PGD: preimplantation genetic diagnosis; PGS: preimplantation genetic screening; TESA: testicular sperm aspiration)

- Individualize dosage and protocol according to patient's age, weight, hormonal, and ultrasound parameters.
- The number of patients per batch is decided as per the center's capacity.
- Have a referral protocol for the patients who need individualized care and for patients where stimulation has started. But patients get ready early or late for the planned dates of OCR–ICSI-embryo transfer in batch IVF.
- Well-trained counselors for patients who need extra time for explanation of cycle cancellation and transfer to other centers.
- It is better to stick to the services of a senior embryologist throughout, ideally a person who has been involved in the setting up of the laboratory so that they are interested in laboratory management/logistics, statistics, and results.

- Ensure availability of additional backup embryologist and ancillary staff in case of emergency leave of designated staff. Ensure additional junior embryologist who can coordinate with senior embryologist regarding laboratory maintenance.
- Well-planned billing system to minimize losses to the patient as well as the center.
- Good counseling services for patient satisfaction and patient feedback.
- Use standardized protocol but also individualize as and when required.
- Regular auditing and implementing corrections
- Records, labels, and documents to be well maintained. Ensure photographic records of the embryology laboratory.
- Avoid overcrowding
- Assistant staff to ensure proper and up-to-date documentation.

PREPARATION FOR A BATCH IN VITRO FERTILIZATION: LABORATORY ASPECTS[2,3]

- Check stocks for disposables, consumables, equipment, and culture media.
- Check the laboratory stocks and keep an adequate supply at least 1 week before the batch.
- Disposables should be stored close to the laboratory, separate but near. This is to off-gas the volatile organic compounds (VOCs). The OCR needles such as single- and double-lumen needles, embryo transfer catheters, and stylets have a long shelf-life and can be stocked in more numbers.
- A laboratory maintenance technician can be hired from outside who does the quality check of equipment and air quality every month, a week before IVF. Also, check uninterruptible power supply (UPS) connections, and an extra pressure pump is always recommended.
- The amount of media needs to be calculated and made available 5 days before the beginning of the batch.
- Media to be kept in separate refrigerators close to the laboratory. All new media to be checked for sperm survival test. Daily, weekly, and monthly readings of humidity, pH, and temperature are to be recorded as routine.
- Temperature and CO_2 control of all incubators and all heated stages to be verified and adjusted.
- Embryo safe cleaning solutions such as Oosafe and Fertisafe to be used as well as embryo culture grade water for cleaning. Excess alcohol can have a harmful effect on embryo development.

Disposables Required Per Patient[38]

- Semen collection container: 1
- Sterile probe cover: 1
- OCR needle: 1
- Embryo transfer catheter with stylet: 1
- Handcare gloves: 5
- Powder-free latex gloves: 5
- Round bottom tube 14 mL: 20
- Round bottom tube 6 mL: 2
- Screening dish 3034: 10
- Serological pipette 10 mL: 2
- Serological pipette 5 mL: 2
- Pasteur pipette 5.0 in.: 3
- Falcon centrifuge tube 15 mL: 2
- BD 7575 pipette 3 mL: 10
- Denuding pipette 170 µm: 2
- Denuding pipette 140 µm: 2
- Diamond microtip: 2
- Disposable BD syringe 1.0 mL: 7
- ICSI dish: 1
- Holding pipette: 1
- Injection needle: 1
- Nunc 4-well dish: 4
- Nunc culture dish: 1
- Goblet: 1
- Cry lock: 3
- Aluminum cane: 1

Amount of Different Media Required Per Patient[38]

- Cleavage media: 2.5 mL
- Extended culture media: 1.5 mL
- Fertilization media: 5 mL
- Sperm rinse: 5 mL
- Flushing media-MOPS: 15 mL
- Hyaluronidase: 0.05 mL
- ICSI polyvinylpyrrolidone (PVP): 0.03 mL
- Double density gradient: 1.0 mL
- Paraffin oil: 12 mL
- Vitrification kit: 4 mL for nine patients
- Warming kit: 4 mL for eight patients.

Optimum Number of Incubators

Minimum two incubators: One incubator is used to store culture media, oil, dishes, and consumables to off-gas before use and the second one is to keep the oocytes after denudation.

Four to five cases can be done at a time with two incubators. So, one extra incubator is needed for every five cases.

If 15–20 cases are in a batch, four to five incubators are needed.

With a benchtop incubator, usually 10 numbers can be done at a time.

Shutting down the laboratory completely in-between batches is not a good practice. Regular inspection of equipment and laboratory cleaning, as well as the air handling unit, need to be monitored regularly in-between batches.[46-48] An external validation of the laboratory by a quality control expert, if available, would maintain the quality and success of IVF.

CONCLUSION

The outcome of batch IVF depends on laboratory settings, the consultant involved, the clinician, and the embryologist and their availability, planning, and staff. The whole team should be passionately concerned regarding implementing the batch.

KEY POINTS

- Batch IVF still remains in high demand due to the limited number of senior embryologists available and the better convenience of the patients and clinicians.
- Batch IVF is a planned process of recruiting a group of patients, such that the stimulation is started on the same day (±1–2 day window) and OCR falls on the same day (±1–2 day window).[3] The embryo transfer, if in a fresh cycle, falls on the same day (±1–2 day window), day 2, or day 3 following OCR.
- Patient selection is crucial for batch IVF for optimum results.
- Embryologist should be available on the day of OCR, taken as day 0, on day 1 to check fertilization and additional 2 days to plan day 2 or day 3 embryo transfer. If complex procedures such as TESA, MicroTESA, or blastocyst transfer are planned, additional staff and extra time must be allotted.
- Have a referral protocol for the patients who need individualized care and for patients where stimulation has started. But patients get ready early or late for the planned dates of OCR–ICSI-embryo transfer in batch IVF.
- Check the laboratory stocks and keep an adequate supply at least 1 week before the batch.
- Shutting down the laboratory completely in-between batches is not a good practice. Regular inspection of equipment and laboratory cleaning, as well as air handling unit, needs to be monitored regularly in-between batches. External validation of the laboratory by a quality control expert, if available, would maintain the quality and success of batch IVF.

REFERENCES

1. Chandrareddy A, Kutty BA, Pandey S. Batch in vitro fertilisation: practical considerations. In: Rao KA (Ed). Principles and Practice of Assisted Reproductive Technology, Vol. 1. New Delhi: Jaypee Brothers Medical Publishers; 2014. pp. 827-33.
2. Varghese AC, Das MC, Jayaprakashan K, Angras S. Batch IVF program. In: Varghese AC, Sjöblom Peter, Jayaprakasan K (Eds). A Practical Guide for Setting up an IVF Lab, Assessment of Embryo Culture Systems and Running the Unit, Vol. 1. New Delhi: Jaypee Brothers Medical Publishers (P) Ltd; 2014. pp. 181-92.
3. Gianaroli L, Plachot M, van Kooij R, Al-Hasani S, Dawson K, DeVos A, et al. ESHRE guidelines for good practice in IVF laboratories. Hum Reprod. 2000;15(10):2241-6.
4. Gaspard UJ, Romus MA, Gillain D, Duvivier J, Demey-Ponsart E, Franchimont P. Plasma hormone levels in women receiving new oral contraceptives containing ethinyl estradiol plus levonorgestrel or desogestrel. Contraception. 1983;27(6):577-90.
5. Gardner DK, Weissman A, Howles CM, Shoham Z (Eds). Textbook of Assisted Reproductive Techniques, 5th edition. Boca Raton: CRC Press; 2017.
6. Feichtinger M, Karlström PO, Olofsson JI, Rodriguez-Wallberg KA. Weekend-free scheduled IVF/ICSI procedures and single embryo transfer do not reduce live-birth rates in a general infertile population. Acta Obstet Gynecol Scand. 2017;96(12):1423-9.
7. Borini A, Dal Prato L, Bianchi L, Violini F, Cattoli M, Flamigni C. Effect of duration of estradiol replacement on the outcome of oocyte donation. J Assist Reprod Genet. 2001;18:185-90.
8. Pinkas H, Sapir O, Avrech OM, Ben-Haroush A, Ashkenzi J, Fisch B, et al. The effect of oral contraceptive pill for cycle scheduling prior to GnRH-antagonist protocol on IVF cycle parameters and pregnancy outcome. J Assist Reprod Genet. 2008;25(1):29-33.
9. Rombauts L, Healy D, Norman RJ, Orgalutran Scheduling Study Group. A comparative randomized trial to assess the impact of oral contraceptive pretreatment on follicular growth and hormone profiles in GnRH antagonist-treated patients. Hum Reprod. 2006:21(1):95-103.
10. Farquhar C, Rombauts L, Kremer JAM, Lethaby A, Ayeleke R. (2017). Pretreatments in in vitro fertilisation/intra-cytoplasmic sperm injection cycles. Cochrane. [online] Available from https://www.cochrane.org/CD006109/MENSTR_pretreatments-vitro-fertilisationintra-cytoplasmic-sperm-injection-cycles [Last accessed November, 2022].
11. Garcia-Velasco JA, Bermejo A, Ruiz F, Martinez-Salazar J, Requena A, Pellicer A. Cycle scheduling with oral contraceptive pills in the GnRH antagonist protocol vs the long protocol: a randomized, controlled trial. Fertil Steril. 2011;96:590-3.
12. Karande VC. Use of oral contraceptives in assisted reproductive cycles. IVF Lite. 2014;1:6-11.
13. Xiao B, von Hertzen H, Zhao H, Piaggio G. Menstrual induction with mifepristone and misoprostol. Contraception. 2003;68(6):489-94.
14. Badawy A, Wageah A, El Gharib M, Osman EE. Strategies for pituitary down-regulation to optimize IVF/ICSI outcome in poor ovarian responders. J Reprod Infertil. 2012;13(3):124-30.
15. Kovacs P, Matyas S, Boda K, Kaali SG. The effect of endometrial thickness on IVF/ICSI outcome. Hum Reprod. 2003;18(11):2337-41.
16. Garcia-Velasco JA, Fatemi HM. To pill or not to pill in GnRH antagonist cycles: that is the question! Reprod Biomed Online. 2015;30:39-42.
17. Bermejo A, Iglesias C, Ruiz-Alonso M, Blesa D, Simón C, Pellicer A, et al. The impact of using the combined oral contraceptive pill for cycle scheduling on gene expression related to endometrial receptivity. Hum Reprod. 2014;29:1271-8.
18. Griesinger G, Venetis CA, Marx T, Diedrich K, Tarlatzis BC, Kolibianakis EM. Oral contraceptive pill pretreatment in ovarian stimulation with GnRH antagonists for IVF:

a systematic review and meta-analysis. Fertil Steril. 2008;90:1055-63.
19. Griesinger G, Kolibianakis EM, Venetis C, Diedrich K, Tarlatzis B. Oral contraceptive pretreatment significantly reduces ongoing pregnancy likelihood in gonadotropin-releasing hormone antagonist cycles: an updated meta-analysis. Fertil Steril. 2010;94:2382-4.
20. Hauzman EE, Zapata A, Bermejo A, Iglesias C, Pellicer A, Garcia-Velasco JA. Cycle scheduling for in vitro fertilisation with oral contraceptive pills versus oral estradiol valerate: a randomised, controlled trial. Reprod Biol Endocrinol. 2013;28:96-9.
21. Venetis CA, Kolibianakis EM, Bosdou JK, Tarlatzis BC. Progesterone elevation and probability of pregnancy after IVF: a systematic review and meta-analysis of over 60000 cycles. Hum Reprod Update. 2013;19(5):433-57.
22. Fanchin R, Salomon L, Castelo-Branco A, Olivennes F, Frydman N, Frydman R. Luteal estradiol pre-treatment coordinates follicular growth during controlled ovarian hyperstimulation with GnRH antagonists. Hum Reprod. 2003;18(12):2698-703.
23. Jenkins JM, Anthony FW, Wood P, Rushen D, Masson GM, Thomas E. The development of functional ovarian cysts during pituitary down-regulation. Hum Reprod. 1993;8(10):1623-7.
24. Oyesanya OA, Teo SK, Quah E, Abdurazak N, Lee FY, Cheng WC. Pituitary down-regulation prior to in-vitro fertilisation and embryo transfer: a comparison between a single dose of Zoladex depot and multiple daily doses of Suprefact. Hum Reprod. 1995;10(5):1042-4.
25. La Marca A, Sunkara SK. Individualisation of controlled ovarian stimulation in IVF using ovarian reserve markers: from theory to practice. Hum Reprod Update. 2014;20(1):124-40.
26. Ulug U, Bahceci M, Erden HF, Shalev E, Ben-Shlomo I. The significance of coasting duration during ovarian stimulation for conception in ART cycles. Hum Reprod. 2002;17(2):310-3.
27. Barmat LI, Chantilis SJ, Hurst BS, Dickey RP. A randomised prospective trial comparing gonadotropin-releasing hormone (GnRH) antagonist/recombinant follicle-stimulating hormone (rFSH) versus GnRH-agonist/rFSH in women pretreated with oral contraceptives before in vitro fertilisation. Fertil Steril. 2005;83:321-30.
28. Al-Inany HG, Youssef MA, Aboulghar M, Broekmans F, Sterrenburg M, Smit J, et al. GnRH antagonists are safer than agonists: an update of a Cochrane review. Hum Reprod Update. 2011;17:435.
29. Viardot-Foucault V, Nadarajah S, Lye WK, Tan HH. GnRH antagonist pre-treatment: one centre's experience for IVF–ICSI cycle scheduling. Reprod Biomed Online. 2015;30:366-72.
30. Kolibianakis EM, Venetis CA, Kalogeropoulou L, Papanikolaou E, Tarlatzis BC. Fixed versus flexible gonadotropin-releasing hormone antagonist administration in in vitro fertilization: a randomised controlled trial. Fertil Steril. 2011;95(2):558-62.
31. Melado L, Fatemi HM. Individualised ovarian stimulation for normal and high responders. In: Fatemi HM, Lawrenz B (Eds). Individualized In-Vitro Fertilization: Delivering Precision Fertility Treatment. Cambridge: Cambridge University Press; 2021. pp. 1-13.
32. Duijkers IJ, Klipping C, Verhoeven CH, Dieben TO. Ovarian function with the contraceptive vaginal ring or an oral contraceptive: a randomised study. Hum Reprod. 2004;19:2668-73.
33. La Marca A, Grisendi V, Giulini S, Argento C, Tirelli A, Dondi G, et al. Individualization of the FSH starting dose in IVF/ICSI cycles using the antral follicle count. J Ovarian Res. 2013,6:11.
34. Olivennes F, Howles CM, Borini A, Germond M, Trew G, Wikland M, et al. Individualizing FSH dose for assisted reproduction using a novel algorithm: the CONSORT study. Reprod Biomed Online. 2009;18(2):195-204.
35. Olivennes F, Trew G, Borini A, Broekmans F, Arriagada P, Warne DW, et al. Randomized, controlled, open-label, non-inferiority study of the CONSORT algorithm for individualised dosing of follitropin alfa. Reprod Biomed Online. 2015;30(3):248-57.
36. Broekmans FJ. Individualization of FSH doses in assisted reproduction: facts and fiction. Front Endocrinol (Lausanne). 2019;10:181.
37. van Tilborg TC, Oudshoorn SC, Eijkemans MJC, Mochtar MH, van Golde RJT, Hoek A, et al. Individualized FSH dosing based on ovarian reserve testing in women starting IVF/ICSI: a multicentre trial and cost-effectiveness analysis. Hum Reprod. 2017;32(12):2485-95.
38. Ahemmed, BP, Varghese AC. Batch IVF program in ART: practical considerations. In: Fleming S, Varghese AC (Eds). Organisation and Management of IVF Units: A Practical Guide for the Clinician. New York: Springer; 2017. pp. 27-50.
39. Wong PC, Qiao J, Ho C, Ramaraju GA, Wiweko B, Takehara Y, et al. Current opinion on use of luteinising hormone supplementation in assisted reproduction therapy: an Asian perspective. Reprod Biomed Online. 2011;23:81-90.
40. Hill MJ, Levy G, Levens ED. Does exogenous LH in ovarian stimulation improve assisted reproduction success? An appraisal of the literature. Reprod Biomed Online. 2012;24(3):261-71.
41. Van der Gaast MH, Eijkemans MJ, van der Net JB, de Boer EJ, Burger CW, van Leeuwen FE, et al. Optimum number of oocytes for a successful first IVF treatment cycle. Reprod Biomed Online. 2006;13(4):476-80.
42. Kovacs P. (2015). The ideal number of oocytes for IVF. Medscape. [online] Available from: https://www.medscape.com/viewarticle/839982 [Last accessed November, 2015].
43. Yovich J, Stanger J, Hinchliffe P. Targeted gonadotrophin stimulation using the PIVET algorithm markedly reduces the risk of OHSS. Reprod Biomed Online. 2012;24(3):281-92.
44. Haouzi D, Bissonnette L, Gala A, Assou S, Entezami F, Perrochia H, et al. Endometrial receptivity profile in patients with premature progesterone elevation on the day of hCG administration. Biomed Res Int. 2014;2014:951937.
45. Orvieto R, Meltcer S, Volodarski M, Scharf S, Rabinson J, Zohav E, et al. Luteal phase support for patients undergoing frozen-thawed embryo transfer cycles—the required progesterone dose. Clin Exp Obstet Gynecol. 2007;34(1):25-6.
46. Lee W, Lingham E, Catt J, Catt S, Pangestu M. (2011). Changing old trends in IVF laboratory cleaning and disinfection. [online] Available from: www.gynemed.de. [Last accessed November, 2022].
47. Practice Committee of American Society for Reproductive Medicine; Practice Committee of Society for Assisted Reproductive Technology. Revised guidelines for human embryology and andrology laboratories. Fertil Steril. 2008;90(5):S45-59.
48. Higdon 3rd LH, Blackhurst DW, Boone WR. Incubator management in an assisted reproductive technology laboratory. Fertil Steril. 2008;89(3):703-10.

CHAPTER

87 Frozen Embryo Transfer

Hrishikesh Pai, Nandita Palshetkar, Rishma Dhillon Pai, Kinjal Shah, Rohan Palshetkar, Arnav Pai

INTRODUCTION

The field of assisted reproductive technology (ART) has witnessed innumerable developments in the last few decades after the benchmark set by the birth of Louise Brown in 1978 through in vitro fertilization (IVF).

The success in ART depends on multiple factors such as:

- Etiology of infertility and selection of patients
- Multiple follicular stimulations and optimization of stimulation protocols
- Improvements in the oocyte retrieval technique and getting an optimum number of fertilizable oocytes
- Introduction of intracytoplasmic sperm injection (ICSI)
- Proper embryological technique with high-quality embryos
- Dramatic improvements in culture conditions
- Move toward extended embryo culture and blastocyst transfer
- *Efficient cryopreservation program*
- Optimization of laboratory techniques
- Highly receptive endometrium
- Skilled atraumatic embryo transfer (ET)
- Adequate luteal support
- Competent antenatal management.

Cryopreservation means preserving cells and tissues in live condition at such low temperatures that all the cell metabolisms come to a standstill.

The first-ever pregnancy derived from a frozen human embryo was reported by Alan Trounson and Linda Mohr in 1983 (although the fetus aborted spontaneously at about 20 weeks of gestation). The first-term pregnancy derived from a frozen embryo was born in 1984.

Earlier, only the "second best" embryos were frozen after the morphologically best embryos were transferred in fresh cycles. But today with improved cryopreservation techniques, which reduce embryo cryodamage, the confidence in cryopreservation and frozen embryo transfer (FET) has substantially increased. Cohort banking is also becoming a routine after the use of gonadotropin-releasing hormone (GnRH) agonist "trigger" to prevent ovarian hyperstimulation syndrome (OHSS) in high responders. Other reasons for the increased use of FET include an overall reduction in the average number of embryos transferred each time, thus allowing surplus embryos to be cryopreserved. Also, the increased use of genetic screening increases the use of cryopreservation because embryos are often frozen while awaiting test results, and the transfer of confirmed euploid embryos may contribute to increasing FET success rates. Thus, the last decade has seen a tremendous uphill in the use of FET and the live births resulting thereof.

Why should one go for a FET?

The rationale of a FET:[1]

Controlled ovarian stimulation (COS) with exogenous gonadotropins

⇓

Promotes multifollicular development

⇓

Supraphysiological levels of estrogen and progesterone

⇓

Affects endometrial development and maturation

Two frequently observed features in the endometrium after COS are as follows:[2-4]

1. Advanced histology
2. Advanced downregulation of progesterone receptors.

Both are suggestive of an advanced receptive phase resulting in:

↓

↓Endometrial receptivity

↓

Embryo-endometrium asynchrony

↓

Implantation failure

Whether one should go for fresh or FET for a patient depends on several factors such as age, diagnosis, history, follicular stimulation protocol, trigger agent, embryo developmental pace, cryopreservation technique, and its outcome at the respective center.

Although the trends have been rapidly shifting toward cohort cryopreservation and FET on the basis of success rates, there is no standardized single choice for all patients at all centers, and therefore, individualized approach remains appropriate.

Today, ART has progressed to a point where we can offer high success rates to our patients. Our goal must therefore be to give a safe and healthy pregnancy rather than just a pregnancy which may be complicated. One must not take pride in giving multiple pregnancies, but on the contrary, decrease adverse perinatal outcomes by offering single-embryo transfer whenever possible.

Frozen embryo transfers may not be feasible or necessary for all patients, but this approach appears to be an efficient way to decrease morbidity in patients at high risk for adverse outcomes, especially those with high estradiol (E2) levels, early elevated progesterone levels, and those at high risk for OHSS.

INDICATIONS FOR A FROZEN EMBRYO TRANSFER

Frozen embryo transfer can be recommended in the following subset of patients:

- Surplus good-quality embryos
- Follicles >14 on the day of trigger (at high risk for OHSS)
- Fluid in the cavity
- Endometrial thickness is <7 mm or >14 mm
- Previous history of OHSS
- Previous failed fresh transfers
- Spotting on the day of ET
- Serum progesterone is >1.5 ng/mL in normoresponders[5]
- Difficult ET
- Applebaum score <14
- Preimplantation genetic testing
- Before cancer chemotherapy or radiotherapy for fertility preservation.

DIFFERENT METHODS FOR ENDOMETRIAL PREPARATION FOR FROZEN EMBRYO TRANSFER

Frozen Embryo Transfer Preparation Methods

Frozen embryo transfer preparation methods are shown in **Flowchart 1**.

Natural Cycle-frozen Embryo Transfer (Table 1)[12]

- Here, no medication is administered to the patient prior to ovulation.
- Replacement of embryos is done in a woman's natural ovulatory cycle with the help of endocrine and ultrasound monitoring.

Flowchart 1: Frozen embryo transfer preparation methods.

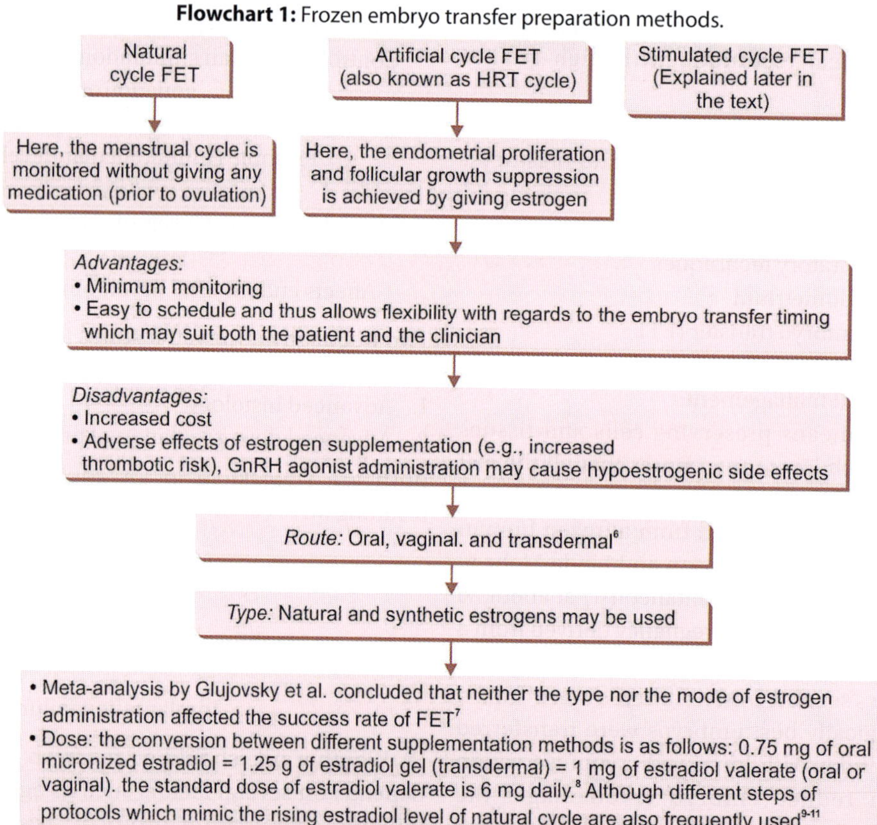

(FET: frozen embryo transfer; GnRH: gonadotropin-releasing hormone; HRT: hormone replacement therapy)

TABLE 1: Natural cycle-frozen embryo transfer (NC-FET).

True NC-FET	Modified NC-FET
• Here, ovulation is monitored by serial blood luteinizing hormone (LH) or till LH peak is observed, and/or ultrasound • Here, ovulation occurs spontaneously	• Here, triggering of ovulation is done by giving hCG once the dominant follicle is >16 mm

Advantage: Absence of estrogen supplementation

Disadvantages:

- Recommended only in women with regular ovulatory cycles. Cannot be used in women with irregular or anovulatory cycles as in polycystic ovary syndrome (PCOS)
- More frequent visits to the clinic. Only clinics which are functional 7 days a week must offer natural cycle-frozen embryo transfer (NC-FET) to their patients.
- Less cycle control and flexibility
- Higher cycle cancellation rate (up to 6%).[13]

The role of endocrine along with ultrasonography (USG) monitoring is controversial in both true and modified NC-FET. Difficulty arises in assigning an endocrine definition of luteinizing hormone (LH) surge. In clinical practice, many definitions are used including a value of 180% above the latest value of that patient and a continued rise after that[14] to a level of ≥10 IU/L.[15]

Studies comparing the above two types of NC-FET have not shown any significant difference in the clinical outcomes.[16] However, one large retrospective study[17] showed a significant difference in the clinical pregnancy rate (CPR), thus favoring true NC-FET [without luteal phase support (LPS)] compared to the modified NC-FET (with LPS).

But still, we do not have an answer to the best approach.

Is administration of progesterone required in NC-FET? Prevalence of luteal phase defect (LPD) in normo-ovulatory subfertile patients is around 8%.[18] Here, the serum progesterone level in the midluteal phase is <10 ng/mL.[19]

Overall, the time to initiate LPS in an NC-FET is not clear. Some advocate that starting progesterone soon after the LH surge or human chorionic gonadotropin (hCG) trigger may be too early, thus having a deleterious effect on the window of implantation (WOI). Thus, different protocols will be used in day-to-day practice till further data analysis is obtained.[20]

Stimulated Cycle Frozen Embryo Transfer

- Exogenous mild ovarian stimulation with clomiphene citrate (CC), aromatase inhibitors (AIs), gonadotropins, CC or AI + gonadotropins, and GnRH analogs with hCG trigger with/without LPS has been advocated to increase serum estrogen levels in turn enhancing the endometrial receptivity.
- Here, patients require increased monitoring, are relatively expensive, and do not have the advantages of flexibility with regard to the timing of embryo replacement. Only a few centers use this regimen.
- A recent systematic review[21] concluded that ovarian stimulation with gonadotropins or CC did not increase the live birth rate as compared to the NC.
- Until further research, no strong recommendation can be made for using stimulated cycle FET.

Hormone Replacement with/without Gonadotropin-releasing Hormone Against Downregulation

- In this regimen, the endometrium is prepared with estrogen. It is started on the first or the second of the cycle (which prevents follicular recruitment) in *high-dose fixed regimen* starting with 6 mg/day of E2 valerate or 1.8 mg conjugated equine estrogen (CEE) or 300 µg of transdermal estrogen patches which is given daily for 8–9 days, and then the woman is called for USG or *low variable dose step-up regimen* in which hormones are started with a lower dose and gradually stepped up as the cycle progresses. Tablet E2 valerate may be started at a lower dose of 2 mg once a day for 2 days followed by 2 mg twice a day for 2 days which again is stepped up to thrice a day for 2–3 days. Woman is recalled for endometrial monitoring after 8–9 days of medication for further dose titration. Some clinics also use E2 patches of 100 µg for 2 days followed by 200 µg for next 4 days again stepping up to 300 µg for next 2–3 days.
- Estrogen must be started on day 1 or day 2 of the cycle as starting estrogen after day 3 may cause an LH surge resulting in luteinization of the endometrium. This is especially important when the pituitary is not suppressed with a GnRH agonist.
- Duration of estrogen priming should be minimal of around 8 days and can be extended up to 40–60 days without affecting the cycle outcome.
- This protocol is beneficial for women with irregular cycles.
- Less frequent monitoring required and is more patient-friendly and cost-effective. Also, it allows better control and flexibility of transfer timing.

Downregulated Frozen Embryo Transfer

- This is the most popular method in which endometrial preparation is achieved with exogenous estrogens and progesterone after pituitary downregulation with a GnRH analog so as to prevent spontaneous ovulation.
- This regimen is recommended in women with endometriosis, PCOS, adenomyoma, and history of cycle cancellation in previous FET cycles due to premature luteinization and premature ovulation.

- The advantages include no endocrine monitoring, better patient convenience, and flexibility in scheduling transfer timing. The disadvantages include high cost, risk of hypoestrogenic side effects of the GnRH analog, and long preparation time.
- Ovarian downregulation is started in the previous cycle using daily injections/intranasal dose of GnRH agonist starting from day 21 of previous cycle or 7 days prior to expected menses. Some clinics prefer to use a depot dose 2–3 weeks prior to starting the endometrium preparation using estrogens.

In the hormone replacement, FET with/without prior downregulation, day of initiating progesterone administration corresponds to the day of ovum pick-up (OPU) or the day after OPU for the purpose of synchronization. In the case of day 2 or day 3 cryopreserved embryos, most retrospective studies have commenced progesterone 3 days prior to ET, while in the case of blastocyst transfer, high pregnancy rates have been reported replacing embryos after 5 days of progesterone. Vaginal (gel, suppositories) and intramuscular (IM) routes are common for giving progesterone.

The optimal means of endometrial preparation in frozen-thawed embryo transfer cycles?

A recent meta-analysis by Groenewoud et al.[22] did not find any significant difference in CPR, ongoing pregnancy rate, and live birth rate when comparing NC-FET versus modified NC-FET, NC versus artificial (hormone replacement) cycles, artificial cycles with and without GnRH agonist downregulation, and NC versus artificial cycles with GnRH agonist. Thus, it is not possible to differentiate any particular method of endometrial preparation in FET as being better than the other.

According to the Cochrane database 2008, a significantly higher live birth rate and favorable trends for other outcomes (CPR, endometrial thickness, and cycle cancellation rate) were observed in the GnRH agonist downregulated, hormone replacement FET group as against hormone replacement FET cycles alone.[23]

According to Cochrane Database 2010, which analyzed 22 randomized controlled trials (RCTs), when using GnRH agonist downregulation as against NC-FET, there was no significant advantage demonstrated. There was no evidence of any statistically significant benefit of one GnRH agonist compared to another.[7]

In a Cochrane review by Ghobara et al. in 2017[24] which analyzed 18 RCTs comparing different FET cycle regimens such as NC-FET versus hormone therapy (HT) FET, NC-FET versus HT plus GnRH agonist suppression, NC-FET versus modified NC-FET with hCG trigger, modified NC-FET versus HT FET, modified NC-FET versus HT plus GnRH agonist suppression, HT FET versus HT plus GnRH agonist suppression, and human menopausal gonadotropin (hMG) versus CC plus hMG-induced FET in 3,815 women did not find sufficient evidence to support the use of one cycle regimen in preference to another in subfertile women with regular ovulatory cycles.

IDEAL DURATION OF PROGESTERONE SUPPLEMENTATION BEFORE EMBRYO TRANSFER

In a prospective randomized trial by Van de Vijver et al.,[25] it was shown that when a cleavage stage day 3 embryo (vitrified-thawed) after overnight culture was transferred on the 3rd or on the 5th day of progesterone administration, the CPRs were similar. However, early pregnancy loss was significantly higher in the latter group. Thus, ET of a day 4 embryo (i.e., day 3 embryo warmed the day before, and thus, developed to a day 4 embryo at the time of transfer) on the 3rd day of progesterone administration appears to be almost deleterious.

The risk of early pregnancy loss is increased when progesterone is administered for a duration shorter than the age of the embryo. On the contrary, transferring a day 4 embryo on the 5th day of progesterone supplementation which might be too long, but there is no available evidence about the impact on success rates.[9]

An explanation to the above could be that 3 days of progesterone supplementation is not long enough to induce a sufficiently decidualized endometrium. Also, it could be hypothesized that a delayed embryo has a higher chance of still finding an open WOI and thus implanting but leading to an early pregnancy loss when progesterone was administered for 3 days before ET. Thus, the *optimal timing* has still not been established yet.[26]

It has been advised to commence progesterone from the theoretical day of oocyte retrieval in hormone replacement therapy (HRT), e.g., a day 3 embryo on the 4th day of progesterone written as P + 3, a day 5 embryo on the 6th day of progesterone written as P + 5, and to perform blastocyst transfer at hCG + 7 or LH + 6 in modified or true NC, respectively.[12]

A Cochrane database review by Glujovsky et al. concluded that starting progesterone at a time equivalent to the day of or the day after OPU results in a significantly increased pregnancy rate compared to starting progesterone a day before the day equivalent to oocyte retrieval.[7]

After a failed fresh transfer when can one go for a frozen embryo transfer?

In a retrospective cohort study by Santos-Ribeiro et al.[27] (i.e., <22 days of oocyte retrieval), FET performed immediately after fresh IVF cycles had CPR similar to those postponed to a later date (>22 days of oocyte retrieval). Therefore, postponing FETs may unnecessarily prolong time to pregnancy.

Thus, this above study proved that ovarian stimulation did not seem to have a carryover effect on CPR per FET, thus allowing patients to choose FET without delay or at their own convenience, thus reducing their frustration associated with the waiting period of IVF treatment.

In clinical practice, commonly followed is:

Previous cycle downregulation with single-dose GnRH agonist 3.6 mg goserelin acetate subcutaneous (SC)

Or

3.75 mg single-dose leuprolide acetate SC/IM (approximately 10 days prior to expected menses)

↓

Day 2 scan to confirm downregulation

ET <5 mm, E2 <50 pg/mL, absence of any ovarian cyst. To start estrogen 2–6 mg/day

↓

Optimum ET 9–12 mm triple line. Progesterone started depending on the embryonic status.

Limited need for endocrine monitoring in FET. Measurement of serum progesterone (highly controversial)—not usually measured.

TO BRIEFLY UNDERSTAND THE TECHNIQUE OF CRYOPRESERVATION

Cryoprotectant Agents

Both permeable and nonpermeable cryoprotectant agents (CPAs) are used usually in a mixture for freezing either by the slow freezing method or vitrification. They protect the cells from cryoinjuries, stabilize intracellular proteins, lower the intracellular water freezing point, and most importantly, they reduce or eliminate lethal intracellular ice formation. Examples of permeable CPAs are glycerol, ethylene glycol (EG), 1,2-propanediol (PrOH), dimethyl sulfoxide (DMSO), propylene glycol, acetamide, and raffinose. Examples of nonpermeable CPAs are sugars such as sucrose, trehalose and glucose, galactose, polymers such as polyvinylpyrrolidone, polyethylene glycol, ficoll, dextran, hydroxypropyl cellulose, polyvinyl alcohol, and proteins like egg yolk. The strategy to decrease the toxicity of one CPA is to use a mixture of two permeable CPAs. EG and DMSO combination is the most frequently used. EG is an almost indispensable component of all CPAs due to low toxicity, high permeability, and excellent prevention of ice crystal formation. Recently, sucrose has become a standard component in vitrification solutions (VS).

Techniques of Cryopreservation

There are two techniques of cryopreservation:

1. Slow freezing method
2. Vitrification method

Slow Freezing Method (Equilibrium Cooling)

This is a slow-rate freezing method. Here, extracellular ice formation drives cellular dehydration through an equilibrium process.

Embryos are exposed to 1–2 mol/L solutions of permeable and nonpermeable CPAs, and then loaded into straws, sealed and cooled rapidly to –6°C by placing the straws into a controlled-rate freezer. With this low concentration of CPAs, no spontaneous ice crystal formation occurs at this temperature. But ice nucleation is induced by "seeding," i.e., touching the straw with forceps that has previously been immersed into liquid nitrogen (LN_2), which is performed far away from the embryo and this ice grows stepwise toward the embryo. The controlled-rate freezer is adjusted to make a very slow cooling (usually 0.3°C/min to around –30°C) after which the straws are immersed into LN_2 for a final cooling and storage. The slow rate of this procedure permits solution exchange between the extracellular and intracellular fluids without any serious osmotic effects (this fact is reflected in the other method called vitrification).

Problems usually encountered with slow freezing are intracellular ice crystal formation, increased exposure to CPAs as it is a slow procedure, abnormal concentration of intracellular solutes due to excessive dehydration, and ice crystal formation during thawing. Also, the equipment is expensive.

Vitrification Method (Nonequilibrium Cooling)

It is a form of rapid cooling which utilizes very high concentrations of CPAs that solidify without forming ice crystals **(Fig. 1)**.

Procedure: The main purpose of this method is the complete elimination of ice crystal formation in the whole solution containing the oocytes and embryos. The reduction in the ice crystal formation rate can be achieved by either increasing the concentration of CPAs or by increasing the cooling and the warming rates. If the cooling rate is higher, then lower concentration of CPA is required and vice versa. Recent vitrification methods have focused on increasing the cooling and warming rates to decrease the potential osmotic and toxic damage caused by the high concentration of CPAs.

Vitrification process: It involves the use of two cryosolutions: (1) Equilibration solution (ES)—a HEPES

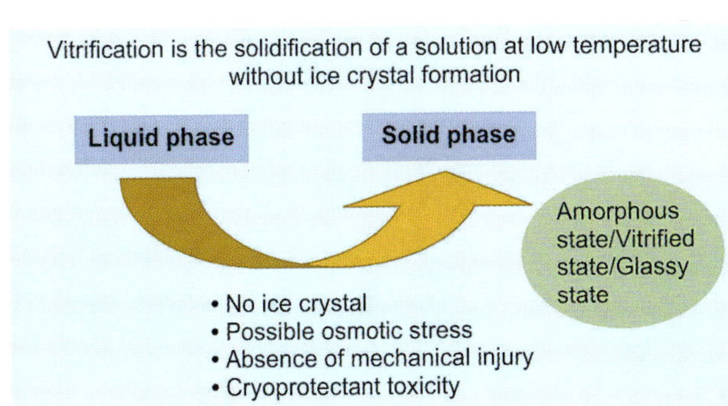

Fig. 1: Vitrification method.

[4-(2-hydroxyethyl)-1-piperazineethanesulfonic acid]-buffered medium containing 7.5% (v/v) of each DMSO and EG and 20% (v/v) of serum protein substitute and (2) VS—a HEPES-buffered medium, 15% (v/v) of each DMSO and EG and 20% (v/v) serum protein substitutes and 0.5 M sucrose. The oocytes/embryos/blastocysts are suspended initially in the ES (approximately 12 minutes for embryos and approximately 15 minutes for oocytes and blastocyst) **(Figs. 2 and 3)** and then washed serially in the VS for approximately 90 seconds. Then depending on the carrier used, it may be open-system freezing (carrier: CryoTop, CryoTech, CryoLock, and CryoLoop) or closed-system freezing (carrier: high security vitrification (HSV) straw and CryoTip).

Cryoinjuries may occur at all phases of the procedure. There is an increasing concern about possible disease transmission between the stored samples mediated by LN_2, even though there are no reported cases in literature involving embryos.

Embryos subjected to cryopreservation may undergo considerable damage during cooling and warming. Fortunately, these embryos have the ability to repair fully or partially this damage and thus continue with normal development.

The main difference between slow freezing and vitrification is that in vitrification, the oocyte/embryo and the surrounding solution solidify in an amorphous structure similar to glass but without ice crystal formation.

Various studies and the meta-analysis by Loutradi et al.[28] proved that vitrification was associated with higher post-thaw survival rate than slow freezing. Today, vitrification as a method to cryopreserve oocytes and embryos has achieved remarkable success due to its multiple advantages such as being rapid, simple, inexpensive, higher survival, and developmental rates.

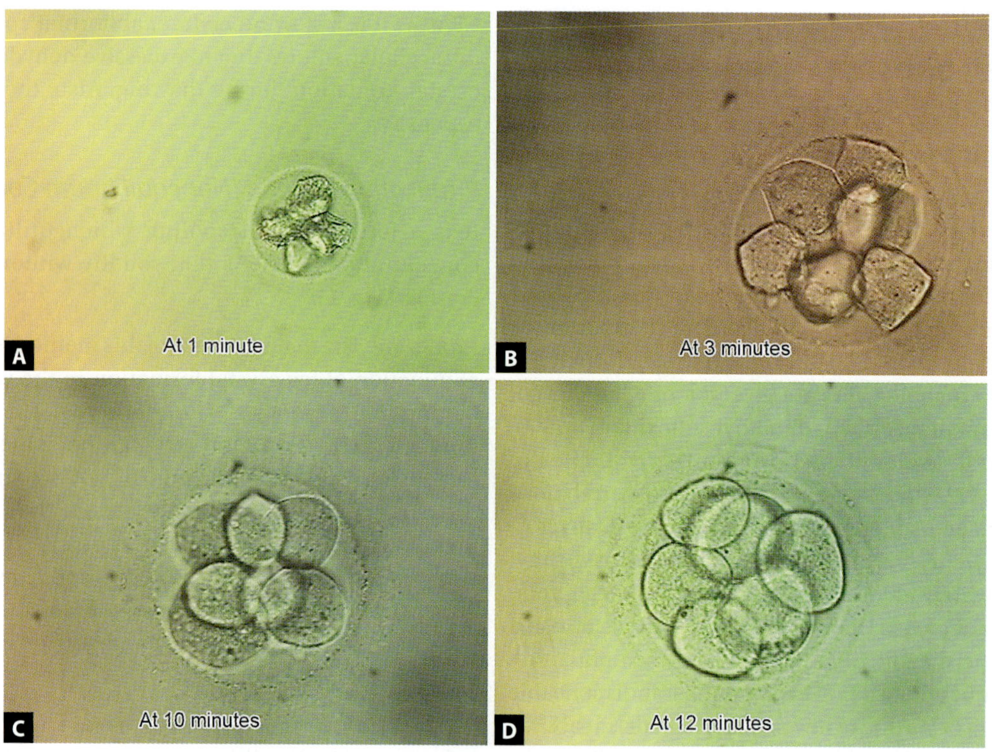

Figs. 2A to D: Vitrification of embryos showing initial shrinkage and recovery of embryos in equilibration solution (ES).

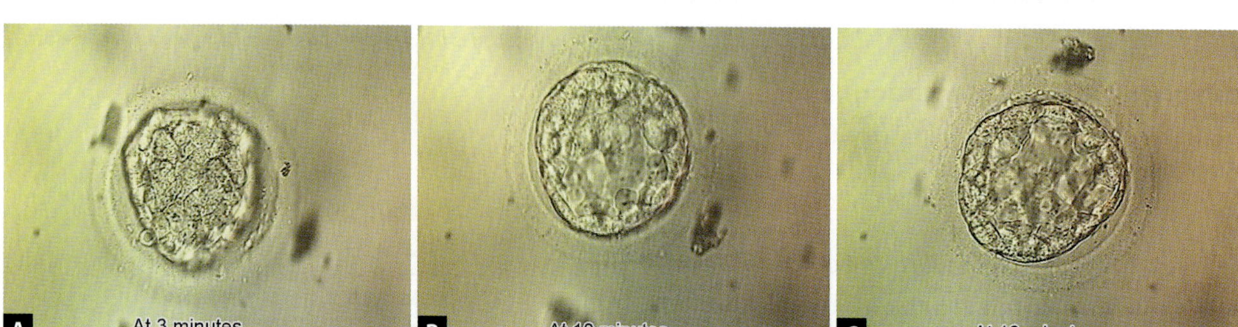

Figs. 3A to C: Vitrification of blastocyst showing initial shrinkage and recovery of blastocysts in equilibration solution (ES).

There are certain controversial areas with cryopreservation:
- Toxicity and long-term effects of the CPAs used
- Chances of viral transmission in open systems
- Higher miscarriage rate.

Potential sources of contamination include:
- Within the freezing apparatus
- During storage
- From LN_2.

European Union directive dictates that cooling and storage of embryos must be performed in a way that minimizes the risk of contamination. Basic recommendations [Human Fertilization and Embryology Authority (HFEA), 1998] for safe storage are:
- Patient screening for hepatitis B, hepatitis C, and human immunodeficiency virus (HIV)
- Careful hygiene throughout
- Double containment of storage straws
- Use of sealed ampoules.

Regarding the safety of vitrification, no currently available data indicate a higher incidence of malformation, which is reassuring but needs to be confirmed on a large scale. Theoretical risk of disease transmission with the open system is there which can be taken care of by the closed system.

There is no doubt that closed system should be preferred provided the outcome is comparable with open systems. Results achieved by using closed system for cleavage stage embryos and blastocysts are promising.[29,30] Studies have shown that open systems are more likely to produce superior results when oocytes are vitrified and to preserve the original physiological cell condition.[31,32]

FRESH VERSUS FROZEN EMBRYO TRANSFER

A randomized trial has shown that FET has been associated with a reduced risk of implantation failure when compared with fresh transfer. This randomized trial involved conventional slow freezing of entire cohorts of bipronuclear oocytes, with subsequent thaw of the entire cohorts, post-thaw extended culture to the blastocyst stage, and transfer of the two best blastocysts from each cohort. Post-thaw culture was used to ensure that transferred embryos were free of cryodamage, as demonstrated by their resumed development to morphologically acceptable blastocysts. Resumed development is a more rigorous indicator of post-thaw viability than immediate post-thaw survival assessment alone.[1]

Advantages of frozen-thawed ET:
- Separation of ET from the stress and rigors of ovarian stimulation
- Decrease in uterine stress, childhood, and adulthood diseases (Barker hypothesis)[33]
- Transferring embryos in a more physiologic rather than a hyperstimulated environment
- Ideal endometrial receptivity and high pregnancy rates
- An increase in cumulative pregnancy rate
- Lesser monitoring which ensures a better patient compliance
- Decreasing the risk of OHSS (OHSS-free clinic)
- Providing a more objective decision to transfer fewer embryos (or a single embryo)
- Possibility of genetic testing
- Decreasing perinatal and maternal morbidity benefits of FET
- In case of surplus embryos which are cryopreserved, it gives psychological support to the patient and clinician that FET can be done even though the fresh cycle has failed.

Disadvantages of frozen-thawed ET:
- Exposure to high concentration of chemicals
- Exposure to extreme temperature gradients
- Increased manipulation of the embryo
- Long-term studies on effects on pregnancy following vitrification not available
- Some studies have shown that FETs are 1.7 times more likely to result in *spontaneous abortions* than those following fresh ETs.[34]

Frozen embryo transfer with respect to maternal and fetal risks has been shown in **Table 2**.[35]

In a multicenter trial[36] involving randomly assigned 1,508 infertile women with PCOS who were undergoing their first IVF cycle underwent either fresh ET or embryo cryopreservation followed by FET. The primary outcome was a live birth after the first ET. They found FET resulted in a higher frequency of live birth after the first transfer than did fresh ET (49.3 vs. 42.0%), a lower frequency of pregnancy loss (22.0 vs. 32.7%), and of OHSS (1.3 vs. 7.1%), but a higher frequency of preeclampsia (4.4 vs. 1.4%). There were no significant differences between groups in rates of other pregnancy and neonatal complications. The study concluded that in subfertile women with PCOS, FET was associated with

TABLE 2: Comparison of the risks in frozen embryo transfer (FET).

Reduced risks in FET	*Increased risks with FET*
• Ovarian hyperstimulation syndrome (OHSS) • Low birth weight (LBW) (<2,500 g) • Small for gestational age (SGA) • Preterm birth (<37 weeks) • Preterm LBW • Antepartum hemorrhage • Placenta previa • Abruptio placenta • Perinatal mortality	• Placenta accreta • Macrosomia (>4,500 g) • Large for gestational age (LGA) • Increased C-section rate

a higher rate of live birth, a lower risk of OHSS, and a higher risk of preeclampsia after the first transfer than with the fresh ET.

In a meta-analysis of RCTs by Matheus Roque[37] comparing IVF outcomes between fresh and FETs showed that FET resulted in significantly increased clinical and ongoing pregnancy rates. The authors suggest that there is evidence that IVF outcomes may be improved by performing FET compared with fresh ET due to a better embryo-endometrium synchrony achieved with endometrium preparation cycles.

In a meta-analysis,[38] comparing obstetric and perinatal outcomes in singleton pregnancies after a frozen-thawed ET compared to a fresh ET, singleton pregnancies after FETs had better perinatal outcomes compared with those after fresh transfer. The relative risks (RRs) and 95% confidence interval (CI) of antepartum hemorrhage, preterm birth, small for gestational age, low birth weight, and perinatal mortality were lower in women who had FET. This meta-analysis suggested that pregnancies resulting from FET seemed to have better obstetric and perinatal outcomes.

Freeze All: The Debate Continues?

In a prospective cohort study by Matheus Roque,[39] which compared IVF outcomes between fresh ET and FET (the freeze all) where fresh ET was performed only in cases without progesterone elevation, the IVF outcomes were significantly better in the group using the freeze-all policy compared with the group using fresh ET. These results suggest that even in a select group of patients that underwent fresh ET (progesterone levels ≤1.5 ng/mL), endometrial receptivity may have been impaired by COS and outcomes may be improved by using a freeze-all policy.

In a Cochrane review by Wong et al.[40] where four randomized clinical trials were analyzed, there was no clear evidence of a difference in cumulative live birth rate between freeze-all strategy and the conventional IVF-ICSI strategy. The prevalence of OHSS was lower after the freeze-all strategy (1–3%) compared to the conventional IVF/ICSI strategy (7%). There was low-quality evidence to suggest that freeze-all strategy was associated with fewer miscarriages [odds ratio (OR) 0.67, 95% CI 0.52–0.86] and a higher rate of pregnancy complications (OR 1.44, 95% CI 1.08–1.92).

Although the major advantage of a freeze-all strategy is the potential for eliminating OHSS, several other factors also support a move toward this approach in ART. Enhanced cycle scheduling and improved organization of the IVF unit are elements that should not be overlooked. Taken together, these developments may lead to a new era in modern ART. Nevertheless, confirmation of the clinical benefits of a freeze-all strategy through well-designed clinical trials are mandatory prior to shifting our current ART practice.

A recent strengths, weaknesses, opportunities, and threats (SWOT) analysis with freeze all was summarized by Christophe Blockeel[41] in **Figure 4**.

For a successful freeze-all program, it would be mandatory to have the "best" laboratory and vitrification technique to implement freeze all on a routine basis. Although preclinical data suggest an inverse relationship between COS and endometrial receptivity, clinical data are controversial. Benefits of elective FET are likely limited to women with hyperovarian response. Clinical evidence is against elective FET for women with poor/suboptimal ovarian response. Current data regarding ART or obstetric outcome do not support a universal freeze-all strategy.[42]

Also, safety with regards to any long-term implications with FET, primarily due to its technique, is a concern which only will be proven with time.

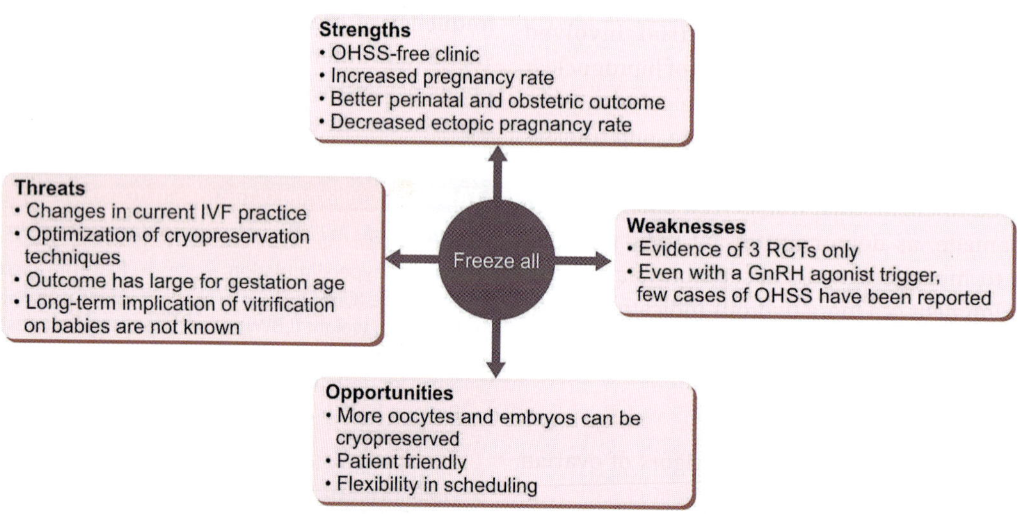

Fig. 4: Strengths, weaknesses, opportunities, and threats (SWOT) analysis. (GnRH: gonadotropin-releasing hormone; IVF: in vitro fertilization; OHSS: ovarian hyperstimulation syndrome; RCTs: randomized controlled trials)

CONCLUSION

- Years ago, cryopreservation techniques were relatively poor, and this balance leaned heavily toward fresh transfer. With the introduction of vitrification, cryopreservation techniques have significantly improved.[43] Vitrification/warming gives a significantly higher survival, fertilization, embryo cleavage and development, and CPRs.[28]
- As there began improvements in this technique, the balance now shifts more in favor of FET.
- Controlled ovarian hyperstimulation in ART cycles causes an asynchrony between the endometrium and the transferred embryos, which may lead to an implantation failure.
- In FETs, this synchrony can be achieved with natural/HRT. This improves the pregnancy rate.
- Increasing numbers of elective single-ETs are also resulting in more frozen embryos (blastocysts) available for subsequent FET cycles.
- In a subset of patients such as high anti-Müllerian hormone (AMH) or out-of-phase endometrium or for prevention of OHSS, FET gives a better pregnancy rate than fresh transfers.
- Time and, hopefully, high-quality research will establish if we are ready to eliminate the transfer of "fresh" embryos in IVF. However, the practice is already shifting.

KEY POINTS

- Natural cycles benefit from vaginal progesterone starting after ET. They are most appropriate for patients with regular ovulatory cycles who are able to comply with strict regimen of frequent urine and blood hormonal measurements.
- Modified natural FET cycles need USG monitoring and blood hormonal testing to decide the optimal time for hCG trigger. Luteal support with progesterone may not be given due to the luteotropic effect of hCG. Thus, progesterone support after ET is optional.
- Programed FET cycles are the most convenient because of limited monitoring requirements and flexibility of scheduling. However, they have not been shown to be superior to properly timed natural or modified natural FET protocols. There is no one single optimal form of progesterone from the available data. Patients' preference, convenience, and cost must be considered when choosing either vaginal or IM progesterone preparations. Alternative options for progesterone supplementation in FET cycles—SC and oral—should be evaluated with adequately powered RCTs.[44]

REFERENCES

1. Shapiro BS, Daneshmand ST, Garner FC, Aguirre M, Hudson C, Thomas S. Evidence of impaired endometrial receptivity after ovarian stimulation for in vitro fertilization: a prospective randomized trial comparing fresh and frozen-thawed embryo transfer in normal responders. Fertil Steril. 2011;96:344-8.
2. Nikas G, Develioglu OH, Toner JP, Jones Jr HW. Endometrial pinopodes indicate a shift in the window of receptivity in IVF cycles. Hum Reprod. 1999;14:787-92.
3. Develioglu OH, Hsiu JG, Nikas G, Toner JP, Oehninger S, Jones Jr HW. Endometrial estrogen and progesterone receptor and pinopode expression in stimulated cycles of oocyte donors. Fertil Steril. 1999;71:1040-7.
4. Mirkin S, Nikas G, Hsiu JG, Díaz J, Oehninger S. Gene expression profiles and structural/functional features of the peri-implantation endometrium in natural and gonadotropin-stimulated cycles. J Clin Endocrinol Metab. 2004;89:5742-52.
5. Griesinger G, Mannaerts B, Andersen CY, Witjes H, Kolibianakis EM, Gordon K. Progesterone elevation does not compromise pregnancy rates in high responders: a pooled analysis of in vitro fertilization patients treated with recombinant follicle-stimulating hormone/gonadotropin-releasing hormone antagonist in six trials. Fertil Steril. 2013;100:1622-8.
6. Scott Jr RT, Ross B, Anderson C, Archer DF. Pharmacokinetics of percutaneous estradiol: a crossover study using a gel and a transdermal system in comparison with oral micronized estradiol. Obstet Gynecol. 1991;77:758-64.
7. Glujovsky D, Pesce R, Fiszbajn G, Sueldo C, Hart RJ, Ciapponi A. Endometrial preparation for women undergoing embryo transfer with frozen embryos or embryos derived from donor oocytes. Cochrane Database Syst Rev. 2010;(1):CD006359.
8. Cobo A, de los Santos MJ, Castellò D, Gámiz P, Campos P, Remohí J. Outcomes of vitrified early cleavage-stage and blastocyst-stage embryos in a cryopreservation program: evaluation of 3,150 warming cycles. Fertil Steril. 2012;98:1138-46.e1.
9. Escribá MJ, Bellver J, Bosch E, Sánchez M, Pellicer A, Remohí J. Delaying the initiation of progesterone supplementation until the day of fertilization does not compromise cycle outcome in patients receiving donated oocytes: a randomized study. Fertil Steril. 2006;86:92-7.
10. Soares SR, Troncoso C, Bosch E, Serra V, Simón C, Remohí J, et al. Age and uterine receptiveness: predicting the outcome of oocyte donation cycles. J Clin Endocrinol Metab. 2005;90:4399-404.
11. Van de Vijver A, Polyzos NP, Van Landuyt L, De Vos M, Camus M, Stoop D, et al. Cryopreserved embryo transfer in an artificial cycle: is GnRH agonist down-regulation necessary? Reprod Biomed Online. 2014;29:588-94.
12. Mackens S, Santos-Ribeiro S, van de Vijver A, Racca A, Van Landuyt L, Tournaye H, et al. Frozen embryo transfer: a review on the optimal endometrial preparation and timing. Hum Reprod. 2017;32(11):2234-42.
13. Sathanandan M, Macnamee MC, Rainsbury P, Wick K, Brinsden P, Edwards RG. Replacement of frozen-thawed embryos in artificial and natural cycles: a prospective semi-randomized study. Hum Reprod. 1991;6:685-7.
14. Testart J, Frydman R, Feinstein MC, Thebault A, Roger M, Scholler R. Interpretation of plasma luteinizing hormone assay for the collection of mature oocytes from women: definition of a luteinizing hormone surge-initiating rise. Fertil Steril. 1981;36:50-4.

15. Groenewoud ER, Macklon NS, Cohlen BJ, ANTARCTICA Study Group. The effect of elevated progesterone levels before HCG triggering in modified natural cycle frozen-thawed embryo transfer cycles. Reprod Biomed Online. 2017;34:546-54.
16. Tomás C, Alsbjerg B, Martikainen H, Humaidan P. Pregnancy loss after frozen-embryo transfer—a comparison of three protocols. Fertil Steril. 2012;98:1165-9.
17. Montagut M, Santos-Ribeiro S, De Vos M, Polyzos NP, Drakopoulos P, Mackens S, et al. Frozen-thawed embryo transfers in natural cycles with spontaneous or induced ovulation: the search for the best protocol continues. Hum Reprod. 2016;31:2803-10.
18. Rosenberg SM, Luciano AA, Riddick DH. The luteal phase defect: the relative frequency of, and encouraging response to, treatment with vaginal progesterone. Fertil Steril. 1980;34:17-20.
19. Jordan J, Craig K, Clifton DK, Soules MR. Luteal phase defect: the sensitivity and specificity of diagnostic methods in common clinical use. Fertil Steril. 1994;62:54-62.
20. Weissman A, Horowitz E, Ravhon A, Steinfeld Z, Mutzafi R, Golan A, et al. Spontaneous ovulation versus HCG triggering for timing natural-cycle frozen-thawed embryo transfer: a randomized study. Reprod Biomed Online. 2011;23:484-9.
21. Yarali H, Polat M, Mumusoglu S, Yarali I, Bozdag G. Preparation of endometrium for frozen embryo replacement cycles: a systematic review and meta-analysis. J Assist Reprod Genet. 2016;33:1287-304.
22. Groenewoud ER, Cantineau AE, Kollen BJ, Macklon NS, Cohlen BJ. What is the optimal means of preparing the endometrium in frozen-thawed embryo transfer cycles? A systematic review and meta-analysis. Hum Reprod Update. 2013;19(5):458-70.
23. Ghobara T, Vandekerckhove P. Cycle regimens for frozen-thawed embryo transfer. Cochrane Database Syst Rev. 2008;(1):CD003414.
24. Ghobara T, Gelbaya TA, Ayeleke RO. Cycle regimens for frozen-thawed embryo transfer. Cochrane Database Syst Rev. 2017;7:CD003414.
25. Van de Vijver A, Polyzos NP, Van Landuyt L, Mackens S, Stoop D, Camus M, et al. What is the optimal duration of progesterone administration before transferring a vitrified-warmed cleavage stage embryo? A randomized controlled trial. Hum Reprod. 2016;31(5):1097-104.
26. Nawroth F, Ludwig M. What is the 'ideal' duration of progesterone supplementation before the transfer of cryopreserved-thawed embryos in estrogen/progesterone replacement protocols? Hum Reprod. 2005;20:1127-34.
27. Santos-Ribeiro S, Siffain J, Polyzos NP, van de Vijver A, van Landuyt L, Stoop D, et al. To delay or not to delay a frozen embryo transfer after a failed fresh embryo transfer attempt? Fertil Steril. 2016;105:1202-7.
28. Loutradi KE, Kolibianakis EM, Venetis CA, Papanikolaou EG, Pados G, Bontis I, et al. Cryopreservation of human embryos by vitrification or slow freezing: a systematic review and meta-analysis. Fertil Steril. 2008;90:186-93.
29. Van Landuyt L, Stoop D, Verheyen G, Verpoest W, Camus M, Van de Velde H, et al. Outcome of closed blastocyst vitrification in relation to blastocyst quality: evaluation of 759 warming cycles in a single-embryo transfer policy. Hum Reprod. 2011;26(3):527-34.
30. Vanderzwalmen P, Ectors F, Grobet L, Prapas Y, Panagiotidis Y, Vanderzwalmen S, et al. Aseptic vitrification of blastocysts from infertile patients, egg donors and after IVM. Reprod Biomed Online. 2009;19(5):700-7.
31. Bonetti A, Cervi M, Tomei F, Marchini M, Ortolani F, Manno M. Ultrastructural evaluation of human metaphase II oocytes after vitrification: closed versus open devices. Fertil Steril. 2011;95(3):928-35.
32. Papatheodorou A, Vanderzwalmen P, Panagiotidis Y, Prapas N, Zikopoulos K, Georgiou I, et al. Open versus closed oocyte vitrification system: a prospective randomized sibling-oocyte study. Reprod Biomed Online. 2013;26(6):595-602.
33. Shapiro BS, Daneshmand ST, Garner FC, Aguirre M, Thomas S. Gonadotropin-releasing hormone agonist combined with a reduced dose of human chorionic gonadotropin for final oocyte maturation in fresh autologous cycles of in vitro fertilization. Fertil Steril. 2008;90:231-3.
34. Zenzes MT, Bielecki R, Casper RF, Leibo SP. Effect of chilling to 0 degrees C on the morphology of meiotic spindles in human metaphase II oocytes. Fertil Steril. 2001;75:769-77.
35. Shapiro BS, Daneshmand ST, Garner FC, Aguirre M, Hudson C. Clinical rationale for cryopreservation of entire embryo cohorts in lieu of fresh transfer. Fertil Steril. 2014;102:3-9.
36. Chen ZJ, Shi Y, Sun Y, Zhang B, Liang X, Cao Y, et al. Fresh versus frozen embryos for infertility in the polycystic ovary syndrome. N Engl J Med. 2016;375(6):523-33.
37. Roque M, Lattes K, Serra S, Solà I, Geber S, Carreras R, et al. Fresh embryo transfer versus frozen embryo transfer in in-vitro fertilization cycles: a systematic review and meta-analysis. Fertil Steril. 2013;99:156-62.
38. Maheshwari A, Pandey S, Shetty A, Hamilton M, Bhattacharya S. Obstetric and perinatal outcomes in singleton pregnancies resulting from the transfer of frozen thawed versus fresh embryos generated through in vitro fertilization treatment: a systematic review and meta-analysis. Fertil Steril. 2012; 98(2):368-77.
39. Roque M, Valle M, Guimarães F, Sampaio M, Geber S. Freeze-all policy: fresh vs. frozen-thawed embryo transfer. Fertil Steril. 2015;103:1190-3.
40. Wong KM, van Wely M, Mol F, Repping S, Mastenbroek S. Fresh versus frozen embryo transfers in assisted reproduction. Cochrane Database Syst Rev. 2017;3:CD011184.
41. Blockeel C, Drakopoulos P, Santos-Ribeiro S, Polyzos NP, Tournaye H. A fresh look at the freeze-all protocol: a SWOT analysis. Hum Reprod. 2016;31(3):491-7.
42. Ata B, Seli E. A universal freeze all strategy: why it is not warranted. Curr Opin Obstet Gynecol. 2017;29:136-45.
43. Balaban B, Urman B, Ata B, Isiklar A, Larman MG, Hamilton R, et al. A randomized controlled study of human day 3 embryo cryopreservation by slow freezing or vitrification: vitrification is associated with higher survival, metabolism and blastocyst formation. Hum Reprod. 2008;23:1976-82.
44. Casper RF, Yanushpolsky EH. Optimal endometrial preparation for frozen embryo transfer cycles: window of implantation and progesterone support. Fertil Steril. 2016;105:867-72.

CHAPTER 88

Evidence-based Practice in Reproductive Medicine

Parimala Chinta, Mohan S Kamath, Korula George

INTRODUCTION

The use of assisted reproductive technology (ART) for the treatment of infertility has been increasing across the world. In view of the limited success following ART, newer treatments and interventions are being introduced in clinical practice at a very rapid pace. In many cases, the effectiveness of these treatments may not be clearly established at the time of introduction in the clinical setting.

In this chapter, we have examined the current evidence status for many of the controversial areas in the field of ART which are of importance in the daily clinical practice of ART.

CONTROVERSIAL AREAS IN PRACTICE

- Preimplantation genetic test (PGT)
- Time-lapse technology
- Screening hysteroscopy pre-in vitro fertilization (IVF)
- Luteal phase support in IVF
- Metformin before IVF
- Freeze-all strategy.

Preimplantation Genetic Testing

Background

One of the reasons for low live birth rate (LBR) post IVF is the transfer of chromosomally abnormal embryos. It is hypothesized that transfer of euploid embryos may increase the LBR.[1] PGT, formerly known as preimplantation genetic screening/preimplantation genetic diagnosis (PGS/PGD), involves an embryo biopsy and screening of embryo for chromosomal abnormalities.[2] This includes PGT for screening aneuploidy (PGT-A), PGT for monogenic or single-gene defects (PGT-M), and PGT for structural rearrangements of chromosomes (PGT-SR).[3] The suggested indications for PGT include women with advanced age, recurrent implantation failure (RIF), severe male infertility, and recurrent pregnancy loss (RPL) that are all likely to be associated with higher aneuploid embryos.[2,4,5]

Evidence

Initial PGT involved cleavage stage biopsy of one or two blastomeres and aneuploidy screening with fluorescence in situ hybridization (FISH). In a large multicenter, randomized, double-blinded trial, investigators included a total of 408 women of advanced age and compared three cycles of IVF with (n = 206) or without PGT (n = 202).[6] The main outcome, i.e., the ongoing pregnancy rate per woman, was significantly lower following PGT compared to the control group [25 vs. 37%; risk ratio (RR) 0.69; 95% confidence interval (CI) 0.51–0.93]. The live birth was significantly lower following PGT (25 vs. 35%; RR 0.68, 95% CI 0.50–0.92). Other trials also obtained lower pregnancy rates following PGT compared to the control group. The reason for lower pregnancy rates was mainly attributed to the limitations of FISH to screen all the chromosomal abnormalities and deleterious effect of blastomere biopsy on LBRs.[7] Hence, uptake of PGT with cleavage stage biopsy using FISH has reduced, and the search for more advanced aneuploidy screening method continued.

Technology for comprehensive chromosomal screening (CCS) was combined with trophectoderm biopsy at the blastocyst stage for PGT.[8,9] A platform for CCS includes array comparative genomic hybridization (aCGH), single nucleotide polymorphism microarrays, quantitative polymerase chain reaction (qPCR), and next-generation sequencing (NGS).[8-11] NGS results have been found to be comparable to aCGH for PGT.[11] NGS has advantages due to potential automation, which reduces human errors and results in higher consistent output.[11] In smaller randomized controlled trials (RCTs) involving women with good prognosis, PGT with CCS has been found to have significantly higher LBRs per cycle in comparison to IVF without PGT.[9,12,13] A systematic review included three RCTs with good prognosis women and found significantly higher ongoing pregnancy rates following CCS with PGT as compared to those women doing IVF without PGT.

The multiple pregnancy rates were significantly lower in PGT group compared to IVF without PGT, though the authors did not present the pooled results in this review.[2] In another systematic review that analyzed RCTs and cohort studies comparing IVF with a normal morphological screening versus PGT screening of embryos, four RCTs were included, but results for clinical pregnancy and ongoing pregnancy rates were available for only two trials. The pooled results showed that the clinical pregnancy (RR 1.26, 95% CI 0.83–1.93) and ongoing pregnancy (RR 1.31, 95% CI 0.64–2.66) rates did not reach a statistically significant difference.[14] The review did show significantly better outcomes following the pooling of results from cohort studies.

A recent multicenter RCT [STAR (Single Embryo TrAnsfeR of Euploid Embryo) trial] has evaluated the use of NGS-based PGT-A (n = 661) for selecting the embryos. The authors concluded that PGT-A showed no improvement in the overall ongoing pregnancy outcomes in women between 25 and 40 years as analyzed per embryo transfer (50% in the PGT-A group and 45.7% in the control group; $p = 0.32$) or per woman randomized (41.8 vs. 43.5%; $p = 0.65$).[15] However, in the subgroup of women of age 35–40 years, the ongoing pregnancy rates per embryo transfer were significantly higher (50.8 vs. 37.2%; $p = 0.035$), but when analyzed by intention-to-treat (ITT), there was no significant difference (41.1 vs. 35.7%; $p = 0.35$).[15]

A Cochrane update included 13 trials and evaluated the role of PGT-A in women undergoing ART for blastocyst biopsy. Evidence shows that it is uncertain if LBR after the first embryo transfer increases following PGT-A [n = 661, odds ratio (OR) 0.93, 95% CI 0.69–1.27, one RCT] and the quality of evidence is low. Similarly, whether PGT-A reduces miscarriage rate is also uncertain (n = 661, OR 0.89, 95% CI 0.52–1.54, one RCT) and the evidence quality is low.[16] In a multicenter randomized trial, women aged between 20 and 37 years with blastocysts screening done by NGS were divided into PGT-A group (n = 606) and conventional-IVF group (n = 606). The primary outcome was the cumulative LBR after three embryo transfers within a year post randomization. LBRs were 77.2% in the PGT-A group versus 81.8% in the conventional-IVF group [absolute difference (AD), –4.6; 95% CI, –9.2 to –0.0; $p < 0.001$]. Conventional IVF has shown to have a cumulative LBR similar to the rate following PGT-A among women with three or more high-quality blastocysts.[17]

Overall, the current evidence from large RCTs suggests lack of benefit of PGT-A compared to routine IVF in women. A paucity of high-quality trials comparing CCS with PGT to routine IVF in women with RIF, RPL, and severe male factor has been observed. There have been concerns raised on the widespread adoption of PGT technologies without clear benefits being shown.[18,19] Further, one group reported deliveries of healthy babies following the transfer of mosaic aneuploid blastocysts.[20] This finding raised questions on the practice of not transferring mosaic aneuploid embryos, which potentially influenced the outcomes following PGS.

Evidence Summary

- Earlier, PGT, which involved cleavage stage biopsy and FISH, was shown to have a significantly lower LBR in women with advanced age.
- PGT with newer CCS technologies along with trophectoderm biopsy has shown lack of benefit in good prognosis women as compared to routine IVF.
- Presently, there is a lack of trials comparing ART with and without newer PGT technologies in women with RIF, RPL, and severe male factor.

Practice Point

Currently, PGT can be offered only under the research setting after proper counseling in women with advanced age, RIF, RPL, and severe male factor.

Time-lapse Technology

Background

Time-lapse system (TLS) is a device with a technology that captures multiple images of embryo development at set time intervals. The integrated TLS has time-lapse camera and the incubator in one device. Images that are displayed can be assessed for morphology by the embryologist without taking the embryo out of the incubator. Some of these systems utilize software algorithms using morphokinetic parameters, which help in noninvasive way of embryo assessment and selection.

Evidence

A systematic review critically evaluated morphokinetic parameters as assessed by time-lapse microscopy (TLM) and clinical outcomes. The studies included in the review suggested that the implantation rate was higher among the embryos which cleaved early and those with timely duration of two-cell and three-cell stages, but no single parameter which could predict implantation potential was identified. The review concluded that no high-quality evidence is available to support routine use of TLM for embryo selection.[21]

A systematic review evaluating TLS versus single-point morphological assessment included five RCTs analyzing 1,637 women.[22] The pooled ongoing pregnancy rates (51 vs. 39.9%; $p < 0.0001$) and LBRs (44.2 vs. 31.3%; $p = 0.004$) were significantly higher following TLM as compared to conventional incubation, and the quality of evidence was moderate. However, three trials reported live birth as an outcome, and one of the trials was categorized at a high risk of bias.

A Cochrane systematic review compared the effectiveness of TLS with conventional morphology assessment of still images and conventional incubation and embryo assessment. The authors reported no significant differences in the LBR/ongoing pregnancy (OR 0.91; 95% CI 0.67–1.23, three RCTs) or the clinical pregnancy rates (OR 1.06, 95% CI 0.79–1.41, four RCTs) between the two methods of assessment and the evidence quality was low.[23] Comparing TLS utilizing embryo selection software versus conventional incubation of embryos and assessment in women undergoing ART, they found three RCTs involving 1,617 women. It is unclear whether there is any difference in LBR (OR 1.12; 95% CI 0.92–1.36) between TLS versus conventional embryo assessment. It was unclear, based on low-quality evidence, whether there is any difference in clinical pregnancy rates following TLS utilization of embryo selection software and conventional assessment (OR 0.95; 95% CI 0.78–1.16). The review concluded that there is lack of high-quality evidence to choose between conventional incubation systems versus TLS with or without the embryo selection software.[23]

Evidence Summary

- While TLS appears to be a promising tool for noninvasive methods of embryo selection, no single morphokinetic parameter is predictive of higher implantation potential.
- Low-quality evidence suggests higher clinical pregnancy rates following TLS versus conventional incubation.

Practice Points

- It is not clear if the suggested benefit of TLS is due to undisturbed culture condition or improved embryo selection.
- High-quality trials are needed to further validate the effectiveness of TLS and evaluate the cost-effectiveness before it can be adopted in routine clinical practice.

Pre-In Vitro Fertilization Screening Hysteroscopy

Background

Hysteroscopy is a commonly performed diagnostic procedure to evaluate the uterine cavity. It allows simultaneous detection and treatment of uterine cavity abnormalities during the same sitting and the procedure then being called an operative hysteroscopy. During the procedure, a telescope is introduced into the cervix and advanced into uterine cavity, and it can be usually carried out as an outpatient procedure.

Screening hysteroscopy is performed in asymptomatic woman without any abnormalities detected during routine pelvic imaging (e.g., transvaginal ultrasound). It is now being offered commonly before IVF as a screening procedure.[24]

Evidence

Initial randomized trials included women with at least previous two IVF failures, and significantly higher pregnancy rates were reported in women undergoing pre-IVF hysteroscopy versus no hysteroscopy.[25,26] A systematic review (n = 1,691) included two randomized and three nonrandomized trials to evaluate the role of outpatient hysteroscopy prior to IVF.[27] Most of the studies have included women with at least two previous IVF failures, and the pooled results (RR 1.75; 95% CI 1.51–2.03; $p < 0.00001$) suggested that pregnancy rates were significantly higher following hysteroscopy in relation to the control arm. Another systematic review evaluated the role of hysteroscopy in women undergoing their first IVF.[28] It included (n = 3,179) one randomized and five nonrandomized trials. The pooled results suggested a significantly increased clinical pregnancy rate (RR 1.44; 95% CI 1.08–1.92) per cycle with hysteroscopy followed by IVF, while the LBR per cycle did not show any significant difference (RR 1.30; 95% CI 1.00–1.67) after hysteroscopy. A high-quality, multicenter, randomized trial evaluated the role of screening hysteroscopy in women undergoing RIF (at least two unsuccessful IVF ending in embryo transfers) and included 350 and 352 women in hysteroscopy and control arm, respectively.[29] No significant difference was observed between LBR per woman randomized (29 vs. 29%; RR 1.00; 95% CI 0.79–1.25; p = 0.96). During the trial, 26% women had uterine abnormalities detected during hysteroscopy. Another similar multicenter randomized trial evaluated the role of pre-IVF hysteroscopy in women undergoing their first IVF and included 373 women in hysteroscopy and 377 in the control group.[30] The LBR per woman randomized was not significantly different (57 vs. 54%; RR 1.06; 0.93–1.20; p = 0.41) between the two groups. The live birth among women with treated uterine abnormalities as compared to those with untreated abnormalities was not significantly different as well (p = 0.69).

A recent Cochrane systematic review analyzed 10 trials with women who had a screening hysteroscopy (n = 1,836) and women who did not undergo hysteroscopy prior to ART (n = 1,914). Low-quality evidence suggests that screening hysteroscopy before ART may increase LBR (RR 1.26, 95% CI 1.11–1.43; six RCTs). However, analyzing the pooled results from high-quality trials showed no increase in LBR with the intervention (RR 0.99, 95% CI 0.82–1.18; two RCTs). Performing a screening hysteroscopy before ART may show an increase in the clinical pregnancy rate (RR 1.32, 95% CI 1.20–1.45; 10 RCTs), but the evidence quality is low.[31]

Evidence Summary

- While early studies show some beneficial effects with screening hysteroscopy before IVF in RIF, the recent systematic review reported uncertain evidence whether

performing routine screening hysteroscopy increases live birth, either for all women or for those women with two or more unsuccessful IVF cycles
- Current evidence does not support screening hysteroscopy before the first IVF.

Practice Points

Screening hysteroscopy may be considered in a selected group of women with RIF and suspected intracavitary pathology or previous history of difficult embryo transfer.

Luteal Support in In Vitro Fertilization

Background

Following controlled ovarian hyperstimulation (COH) during IVF, the steroid hormones, namely estrogen and progesterone, attain supraphysiological levels. These high levels of steroids lead to negative feedback on the hypothalamic–pituitary axis and consequently lower luteinizing hormone (LH), resulting in withdrawal of support to the corpus luteum and defective luteal phase.[32] This shortened and defective luteal phase, commonly known as premature luteolysis, can reduce pregnancy rates following IVF.

Since levels of progesterone are insufficient due to premature luteolysis, additional progesterone supplement is needed. Progesterone is given either alone or in combination with estrogen. Progesterone levels can be maintained indirectly by administering human chorionic gonadotrophin (hCG) or gonadotropin-releasing hormone (GnRH). Only progesterone is the most common form of luteal support and is usually given by vaginal, intramuscular (IM), or oral routes.

Evidence

The recent Cochrane update evaluated different luteal support protocols and routes of progesterone administration.[33] A single RCT result suggests no difference in LBR per woman randomized to IM versus oral route (OR 0.71, 95% CI 0.14–3.66), and the evidence was of very low quality. Similarly, very low-quality evidence from seven RCTs showed no difference in live birth per woman randomized for IM versus vaginal or rectal route (OR 1.37, 95% CI 0.94–1.99); and vaginal/rectal versus oral route (four RCTs, OR 1.19, 95% CI 0.83–1.69) subcutaneous (SC) versus vaginal gel route (two RCTs, OR 0.92, 95% CI 0.74–1.14) and the quality of evidence was low. The update concluded that no particular route of progesterone administration is superior.

A systematic review comparing oral progesterone (dydrogesterone) versus vaginal route progesterone included eight RCTs.[34] The ongoing pregnancy rates were not significantly different between both the groups (RR 1.04, 95% CI 0.92–1.18, seven RCTs, 3,134 women). Two out of three included studies reported on lower dissatisfaction rates following oral progesterone compared to vaginal option. Overall, the authors concluded that oral progesterone is as effective as vaginally administered progesterone.

A randomized trial compared the efficacy and safety of oral progesterone ($n = 520$) versus micronized progesterone ($n = 511$).[35] The ongoing pregnancy rates in oral (37.6%) and vaginal progesterone groups (33.1%) were similar. The authors concluded that since the oral route was more patient friendly, it may replace the vaginal route in clinical practice.

An open-label RCT, which included 800 women, evaluated SC progesterone versus vaginal progesterone.[36] The live birth (41.1 vs. 43.1%) and ongoing pregnancy rates (41.6 vs. 44.4%) were not significantly different in this non-inferiority trial. An individualized patient data meta-analysis compared the effectiveness of SC versus vaginal route and included 1,435 women. The ongoing pregnancy likelihood (OR 0.86, 95% CI 0.69–1.07) between both the groups did not reach statistical significance.[37]

Five RCTs with $n = 833$ women showed that hCG regimens alone or along with progesterone did not increase the live birth outcomes as compared to progesterone alone (OR 0.95, 95% CI 0.65–1.38).[33] The ovarian hyperstimulation syndrome (OHSS) rate was significantly lower with progesterone alone versus hCG regimens (five RCTs, 1,293 women, OR 0.46, 95% CI 0.30–0.71).

Progesterone alone versus combination of progesterone and GnRH agonist resulted in lower LBR (nine RCTs, $n = 2,861$, OR 0.62, 95% CI 0.48–0.81) though the quality of evidence was low.[33] There was no difference in LBR when progesterone alone was compared with progesterone with estrogen combination (OR 1.12, 95% CI 0.91–1.38, nine RCTs, 1,651 women). According to the recent European Society of Human Reproduction and Embryology (ESHRE) guideline on controlled stimulation during IVF, in cycles with hCG as trigger, a GnRH agonist bolus along with progesterone for luteal phase support can be used in a clinical trial context only.[38]

In case GnRH agonist is used as trigger instead of hCG, modified luteal support is advocated. In case a fresh transfer is planned, then small bolus of hCG (1,500 IU) is given post-oocyte retrieval, and intensive support of estradiol and progesterone is started.[39]

Use of aspirin during IVF as compared to placebo/no treatment did not show any increase in clinical pregnancy rate (RR 1.03, 95% CI 0.91–1.17, 10 RCTs, $n = 2,142$).[40] There is a lack of robust evidence favoring use of vasodilators such as sildenafil citrate or heparin as IVF adjuvants.[41] Addition of low-dose prednisolone to progesterone for luteal support has also not shown improved clinical pregnancy rates.[42]

Evidence Summary

- Among vaginal, oral, and IM administration of progesterone, no one route is superior to another for luteal support during IVF.
- Recent studies indicate similar efficacy for oral progesterone versus vaginal progesterone but with the advantage of being more patient friendly.
- Recent studies also indicate the effectiveness of SC progesterone as compared to vaginal progesterone.

Practice Points

- Since all the routes of progesterone administration are similar in efficacy, patient's preference and comfort is an important factor while choosing progesterone support during IVF.
- Vaginal micronized progesterone is most widely used, sometimes alone and other times in combination with IM route.
- Since oral progesterone has been shown to be equally efficacious as vaginal progesterone due to patient-friendly profile, the oral route may gain more widespread acceptance.
- The addition of hCG for luteal support increases OHSS risk and should be avoided in women at risk. The routine addition of hCG to progesterone needs to be avoided.
- The use of GnRH agonist in combination with progesterone for luteal support appears to be beneficial.
- There is no evidence of benefit by addition of adjuvants such as vasodilators (e.g., sildenafil), prednisolone, or heparin for luteal support during routine IVF.

Metformin before In Vitro Fertilization

Background

Metformin is commonly used as a drug of first choice for diabetes. It has got an anti-hyperglycemic effect mainly by inhibiting hepatic glucose production and increasing peripheral glucose uptake and utilization.[43]

It is commonly used in clomiphene-resistant women for ovulation induction and polycystic ovary syndrome (PCOS) women with impaired glucose.[44] Metformin is also used prior to starting IVF in PCOS women to increase pregnancy rates and reduce the risk of OHSS.[45]

Evidence

The efficacy of metformin prior to the long protocol in IVF was evaluated in a placebo-controlled double-blinded study.[46] The clinical pregnancy rates did not differ between the groups. However, spontaneous pregnancies were higher prior to starting IVF in the metformin group. Hence, when an ITT analysis was done, LBR was significantly increased with metformin (48.6 vs. 32%, p = 0.03). Another RCT evaluated metformin's role in reducing OHSS in PCOS group with GnRH antagonist protocol.[47] There was no significant reduction in moderate-severe OHSS rate in metformin group as compared to the placebo (16 vs. 12.2%, p = 0.66). However, the LBR was significantly reduced in the metformin group (27.6 vs. 51.6%, p = 0.02).

A systematic review observed the effectiveness of metformin in PCOS group (10 trials, n = 845) undergoing IVF and noted no significant difference in LBRs after metformin. There was a significant reduction in OHSS rates following metformin (OR 0.27, 95% CI 0.16–0.46) in relation to the control group.[48]

The updated Cochrane review included 13 RCTs and 1,132 women. The analysis was stratified based on the type of protocol, i.e., long agonist (six RCTs), antagonist and short protocol (one RCT), and included studies which reported live births. In the long protocol GnRH-agonist subgroup, an uncertain effect of metformin on LBR per woman was observed when compared with the control (RR 1.30, 95% CI 0.94–1.79; n = 651), and the quality of evidence was low. Only one trial used GnRH-antagonist protocol and reported LBR. The authors reported that metformin may reduce LBR in the antagonist protocol group versus control (RR 0.48, 95% CI 0.29–0.79; one RCT; n = 153). However, low-quality evidence also showed that metformin may lower the incidence of OHSS (RR 0.46, 95% CI 0.29–0.72; 11 RCTs; n = 1,091) in the long protocol GnRH-agonist ovarian stimulation protocol, but not in the antagonist ovarian stimulation protocol. There is uncertain evidence on miscarriage rate per woman in metformin versus placebo (RR 0.86, 95% CI 0.56–1.32; eight RCTs; 821 women). Intake of metformin increases the risk of side effects (RR 3.35, 95% CI 2.34–4.79; eight RCTs; 748 women).[45]

A recent systematic review and meta-analysis was done to investigate the association of metformin with pregnancy outcomes in PCOS women undergoing IVF. The risk of OHSS in women (n = 1,123, 12 RCTs) randomized to metformin was lower compared to control arm (OR, 0.43; 95% CI, 0.24–0.78), although this difference lost significance for women with a body mass index (BMI) of <26 kg/m^2 (OR, 0.67; 95% CI, 0.30–1.51). Among the 11 trials included, 10 trials used long agonist protocol and no significant difference was observed in clinical pregnancy rate (OR, 1.24; 95% CI, 0.82–1.86) or LBR (OR, 1.23; 95% CI, 0.74–2.04). However, in a post hoc analysis with a BMI of ≥26 kg/m^2, metformin treatment showed higher clinical pregnancy rates (OR, 1.71; 95% CI, 1.12–2.60).[49]

Evidence Summary

- Use of metformin pre-IVF in PCOS women does not increase LBRs.
- Metformin may reduce OHSS risk in PCOS women undergoing IVF on long agonist protocol.

- There is no clear evidence showing reduction of OHSS in PCOS women on GnRH antagonist protocol.
- Metformin may be associated with increased clinical pregnancy rates in PCOS women with higher BMI.

Practice Points

- Metformin can be started in 3 months pre-IVF in PCOS women who are planned for long agonist protocol.
- Benefits of metformin may not be substantial if PCOS women are on GnRH antagonist protocol which is a preferred option for women who are at OHSS risk.
- Metformin has gastrointestinal side effects, and long-term use may cause vitamin B12 deficiency.

Freeze-all Strategy

Background

The freeze-all strategy consists of cryopreserving all the embryos from an ART cycle and transferring them later in either a natural cycle or a hormone-primed replacement cycle, thus avoiding a fresh embryo transfer. This is mainly to avoid the deleterious effects of supraphysiological levels of hormones during COH, which may negatively impact endometrial receptivity and consequently embryo implantation.[50] The subtle rise in progesterone levels during COH may also lead to the advancement of endometrial receptivity, and consequent asynchrony may lower the implantation.[51] In women at high risk of OHSS, the freeze-all strategy along with antagonist protocol with an agonist trigger is considered an effective option to reduce OHSS risk.[52]

Due to the above stated reasons, the freeze-all embryos strategy has been incorporated into the routine clinical practice.

However, the long-term impact of freezing and cost implications are not yet clear.

Evidence

Earlier trials by Shapiro et al. evaluated the freeze-all strategy at the blastocyst stage in high responders and normoresponders in two separate trials.[53,54] In the trial involving high-responder women, a total of 122 women were randomized (62 in fresh and 60 in frozen).[51] The ongoing pregnancy rate per transfer between fresh versus frozen cycles did not show any significant difference (65.4 vs. 77.6%; $p = 0.19$). In the trial consisting of normoresponder women, a total of 53 fresh and 50 frozen cycles were analyzed.[54] The ongoing pregnancy rates were significantly lower in fresh compared to frozen (50.9 vs. 78%; $p = 0.007$). The authors suggested altered endometrial receptivity as the likely reason for lower pregnancy rates in the fresh cycles. In another RCT, fresh versus freeze-all strategy was compared involving day 3 stage embryos in PCOS women.[55] The trial involved a total of 1,508 women. The LBR after the first transfer was significantly higher following freeze-all versus fresh day 3 transfer (49.3 vs. 42%, $p = 0.004$), and pregnancy losses were significantly lower (22 vs. 32.7%, $p < 0.001$). While the OHSS rate was significantly lower after freeze-all strategy (1.3 vs. 7.1%, $p < 0.001$), the preeclampsia rate was significantly increased after freeze-all strategy (4.4 vs. 1.4%, $p = 0.009$).

The recent Cochrane review included 15 studies and a total of 4,712 women. The results show minimal or no difference in cumulative LBR (OR 1.08, 95% CI 0.95–1.22; eight RCTs) and cumulative pregnancy rates (OR 0.95, 95% CI 0.75–1.19; four RCTs, 1,245 women) between the freeze-all versus conventional ART strategy and the quality of evidence was moderate. Low-quality evidence suggests that women might develop less OHSS after the "freeze-all" strategy compared to the conventional strategy (OR 0.26, 95% CI 0.17–0.39; six RCTs, 4,478 women). There is uncertain evidence regarding the difference in miscarriage rate as the evidence is of very low quality (Peto OR 1.06, 95% CI 0.72–1.55; two RCTs, 986 women).[56]

A pragmatic two-arm parallel RCT (E-Freeze) included a total of 619 women between ages ≥18 and <42 years and evaluated the effectiveness of elective freezing versus fresh transfer.[57] The treatment outcomes following elective freeze compared to the fresh embryo transfer showed no significant difference in healthy baby rate (20.3 vs. 24.4%; RR, 95% CI: 0.84, 0.62–1.15); live birth (28.3 vs. 34.3%; RR, 99% CI: 0.83, 0.65–1.06); miscarriage rate (14.3 vs. 12.9%; RR, 99% CI: 1.09, 0.72–1.66), and OHSS rate (3.6 vs. 8.1%; RR, 99% CI: 0.44, 0.15–1.30). The participant adherence was lower, and the cost was higher in freeze-all group.

Summary

- The current evidence suggests that freeze-all strategy reduces OHSS risk in women at high risk compared to fresh transfer.
- The evidence is not clear regarding the benefit of freeze-all strategy on cumulative live birth compared to the conventional IVF strategy.
- There is some evidence which suggests that higher pregnancy complications following frozen transfer as compared to fresh transfers.

Practice Points

- For women at high risk of OHSS (e.g., PCOS), freeze-all strategy can be offered to reduce the risk.
- Since the present evidence is unclear with regard to the impact of freeze-all strategy on cumulative live birth, routine use of this strategy for all IVF cycles is not advised.
- Long-term effect of freezing on perinatal outcomes and cost implications has to be considered before wider use can be recommended.

CONCLUSION

The incorporation of newer interventions or adjuncts must be based on evolving evidence. Changes in the practice should be guided by the improvement in the pregnancy outcomes with patient safety and cost taken into consideration.

KEY POINTS

- PGT with newer CCS technologies along with trophectoderm biopsy has shown lack of benefit in good prognosis women as compared to routine IVF.
- TLS appears to be a promising tool for noninvasive methods of embryo selection, though no single morphokinetic parameter is predictive of higher implantation potential.
- Evidence shows lack of benefit with routine screening hysteroscopy before the first IVF.
- Among vaginal, oral, and intramuscular administration of progesterone, no one route is superior to another for luteal support during IVF, hence the choice can be decided according to patient comfort, compliance, and physician's discretion.
- Use of metformin pre-IVF does not increase the live births in PCOS women, but OHSS risk might be reduced in women with long agonist protocol.
- For women at high risk of OHSS, freeze all strategy can be offered.

REFERENCES

1. Wilton L. Preimplantation genetic diagnosis for aneuploidy screening in early human embryos: a review. Prenat Diagn. 2002;22(6):512-8.
2. Dahdouh EM, Balayla J, García-Velasco JA. Impact of blastocyst biopsy and comprehensive chromosome screening technology on preimplantation genetic screening: a systematic review of randomized controlled trials. Reprod Biomed Online. 2015;30(3):281-9.
3. Zegers-Hochschild F, Adamson GD, Dyer S, Racowsky C, de Mouzon J, Sokol R, et al. The international glossary on infertility and fertility Care. 2017. Fertil Steril. 2017;108(3):393-406.
4. Munné S, Alikani M, Tomkin G, Grifo J, Cohen J. Embryo morphology, developmental rates, and maternal age are correlated with chromosome abnormalities. Fertil Steril. 1995;64(2):382-91.
5. Rubio C, Bellver J, Rodrigo L, Bosch E, Mercader A, Vidal C, et al. Preimplantation genetic screening using fluorescence in situ hybridization in patients with repetitive implantation failure and advanced maternal age: two randomized trials. Fertil Steril. 2013;99(5):1400-7.
6. Mastenbroek S, Twisk M, van Echten-Arends J, Sikkema-Raddatz B, Korevaar JC, Verhoeve HR, et al. In vitro fertilization with preimplantation genetic screening. N Engl J Med. 2007;357(1):9-17.
7. Mastenbroek S, Twisk M, van der Veen F, Repping S. Preimplantation genetic screening: a systematic review and meta-analysis of RCTs. Hum Reprod Update. 2011; 17(4):454-66.
8. Wells D, Alfarawati S, Fragouli E. Use of comprehensive chromosomal screening for embryo assessment: microarrays and CGH. Mol Hum Reprod. 2008;14(12):703-10.
9. Scott RT, Upham KM, Forman EJ, Hong KH, Scott KL, Taylor D, et al. Blastocyst biopsy with comprehensive chromosome screening and fresh embryo transfer significantly increases in vitro fertilization implantation and delivery rates: a randomized controlled trial. Fertil Steril. 2013;100(3): 697-703.
10. Bisignano A, Wells D, Harton G, Munné S. PGD and aneuploidy screening for 24 chromosomes: advantages and disadvantages of competing platforms. Reprod Biomed Online. 2011;23(6):677-85.
11. Fiorentino F, Biricik A, Bono S, Spizzichino L, Cotroneo E, Cottone G, et al. Development and validation of a next-generation sequencing-based protocol for 24-chromosome aneuploidy screening of embryos. Fertil Steril. 2014;101(5): 1375-82.
12. Forman EJ, Hong KH, Ferry KM, Tao X, Taylor D, Levy B, et al. In vitro fertilization with single euploid blastocyst transfer: a randomized controlled trial. Fertil Steril. 2013;100(1):100-7.e1.
13. Yang Z, Liu J, Collins GS, Salem SA, Liu X, Lyle SS, et al. Selection of single blastocysts for fresh transfer via standard morphology assessment alone and with array CGH for good prognosis IVF patients: results from a randomized pilot study. Mol Cytogenet. 2012;5(1):24.
14. Chen M, Wei S, Hu J, Quan S. Can comprehensive chromosome screening technology improve IVF/ICSI outcomes? A meta-analysis. PLoS One. 2015;10(10):e0140779.
15. Munné S, Kaplan B, Frattarelli JL, Child T, Nakhuda G, Shamma FN, et al. Preimplantation genetic testing for aneuploidy versus morphology as selection criteria for single frozen-thawed embryo transfer in good-prognosis patients: a multicenter randomized clinical trial. Fertil Steril. 2019;112(6):1071-9.e7.
16. Cornelisse S, Zagers M, Kostova E, Fleischer K, van Wely M, Mastenbroek S. Preimplantation genetic testing for aneuploidies (abnormal number of chromosomes) in in vitro fertilisation. Cochrane Database Syst Rev. 2020;9(9):CD005291.
17. Yan J, Qin Y, Zhao H, Sun Y, Gong F, Li R, et al. Live birth with or without preimplantation genetic testing for aneuploidy. N Engl J Med. 2021;385(22):2047-58.
18. Gleicher N, Kushnir VA, Barad DH. Preimplantation genetic screening (PGS) still in search of a clinical application: a systematic review. Reprod Biol Endocrinol. 2014;12:22.
19. Mastenbroek S, Repping S. Preimplantation genetic screening: back to the future. Hum Reprod. 2014;29(9):1846-50.
20. Greco E, Minasi MG, Fiorentino F. Healthy babies after intrauterine transfer of mosaic aneuploid blastocysts. N Engl J Med. 2015;373(21):2089-90.
21. Kaser DJ, Racowsky C. Clinical outcomes following selection of human preimplantation embryos with time-lapse monitoring: a systematic review. Hum Reprod Update. 2014;20(5):617-31.
22. Pribenszky C, Nilselid A-M, Montag M. Time-lapse culture with morphokinetic embryo selection improves pregnancy

and live birth chances and reduces early pregnancy loss: a meta-analysis. Reprod Biomed Online. 2017;35(5):511-20.
23. Armstrong S, Bhide P, Jordan V, Pacey A, Marjoribanks J, Farquhar C. Time-lapse systems for embryo incubation and assessment in assisted reproduction. Cochrane Database of Syst Rev. 2019;5(5):CD011320.
24. Campo R, Meier R, Dhont N, Mestdagh G, Ombelet W. Implementation of hysteroscopy in an infertility clinic: The one-stop uterine diagnosis and treatment. Facts Views Vis Obgyn. 2014;6(4):235-9.
25. Rama Raju GA, Shashi Kumari G, Krishna KM, Prakash GJ, Madan K. Assessment of uterine cavity by hysteroscopy in assisted reproduction programme and its influence on pregnancy outcome. Arch Gynecol Obstet. 2006;274(3):160-4.
26. Demirol A, Gurgan T. Effect of treatment of intrauterine pathologies with office hysteroscopy in patients with recurrent IVF failure. Reprod Biomed Online. 2004;8(5):590-4.
27. El-Toukhy T, Sunkara SK, Coomarasamy A, Grace J, Khalaf Y. Outpatient hysteroscopy and subsequent IVF cycle outcome: a systematic review and meta-analysis. Reprod Biomed Online. 2008;16(5):712-9.
28. Pundir J, Pundir V, Omanwa K, Khalaf Y, El-Toukhy T. Hysteroscopy prior to the first IVF cycle: a systematic review and meta-analysis. Reprod Biomed Online. 2014;28(2):151-61.
29. El-Toukhy T, Campo R, Khalaf Y, Tabanelli C, Gianaroli L, Gordts SS, et al. Hysteroscopy in recurrent in-vitro fertilisation failure (TROPHY): a multicentre, randomised controlled trial. Lancet. 2016;387(10038):2614-21.
30. Smit JG, Kasius JC, Eijkemans MJ, Koks CAM, van Golde R, Nap AW, et al. Hysteroscopy before in-vitro fertilisation (inSIGHT): a multicentre, randomised controlled trial. Lancet. 2016;387(10038):2622-9.
31. Kamath MS, Bosteels J, D'Hooghe TM, Seshadri S, Weyers S, Mol BWJ, et al. Screening hysteroscopy in subfertile women and women undergoing assisted reproduction. Cochrane Database Syst Rev. 2019;4(4):CD012856.
32. Fatemi HM. The luteal phase after 3 decades of IVF: what do we know? Reprod Biomed Online. 2009;19(Suppl. 4):4331.
33. van der Linden M, Buckingham K, Farquhar C, Kremer JA, Metwally M. Luteal phase support for assisted reproduction cycles. Cochrane Database Syst Rev. 2015;(7):CD009154.
34. Barbosa MWP, Silva LR, Navarro PA, Ferriani RA, Nastri CO, Martins WP. Dydrogesterone vs progesterone for luteal-phase support: systematic review and meta-analysis of randomized controlled trials. Ultrasound Obstet Gynecol. 2016;48(2):161-70.
35. Tournaye H, Sukhikh GT, Kahler E, Griesinger G. A phase III randomized controlled trial comparing the efficacy, safety and tolerability of oral dydrogesterone versus micronized vaginal progesterone for luteal support in in vitro fertilization. Hum Reprod. 2017;32(5):1019-27.
36. Baker VL, Jones CA, Doody K, Foulk R, Yee B, Adamson GD, et al. A randomized, controlled trial comparing the efficacy and safety of aqueous subcutaneous progesterone with vaginal progesterone for luteal phase support of in vitro fertilization. Hum Reprod. 2014;29(10):2212-20.
37. Doblinger J, Cometti B, Trevisan S, Griesinger G. Subcutaneous progesterone is effective and safe for luteal phase support in IVF: an individual patient data meta-analysis of the phase III trials. PLoS One. 2016;11(3):e0151388.
38. The ESHRE Guideline Group on Ovarian Stimulation, Bosch E, Broer S, Griesinger G, Grynberg M, Humaidan P, et al. ESHRE guideline: ovarian stimulation for IVF/ICSI. Hum Reprod Open. 2020;2020(2):hoaa009.
39. Humaidan P, Kol S, Papanikolaou EG, Copenhagen GnRH Agonist Triggering Workshop Group. GnRH agonist for triggering of final oocyte maturation: time for a change of practice? Hum Reprod Update. 2011;17(4):510-24.
40. Siristatidis CS, Basios G, Pergialiotis V, Vogiatzi P. Aspirin for in vitro fertilisation. Cochrane Database Syst Rev. 2016;11:CD004832.
41. Nardo LG, El-Toukhy T, Stewart J, Balen AH, Potdar N. British Fertility Society Policy and Practice Committee: adjuvants in IVF: evidence for good clinical practice. Hum Fertil (Camb). 2015;18(1):2-15.
42. Ubaldi F, Rienzi L, Ferrero S, Anniballo R, Iacobelli M, Cobellis L, et al. Low dose prednisolone administration in routine ICSI patients does not improve pregnancy and implantation rates. Hum Reprod. 2002;17(6):1544-7.
43. Dunn CJ, Peters DH. Metformin. A review of its pharmacological properties and therapeutic use in non-insulin-dependent diabetes mellitus. Drugs. 1995;49(5):721-49.
44. George SS, George K, Irwin C, Job V, Selvakumar R, Jeyaseelan V, et al. Sequential treatment of metformin and clomiphene citrate in clomiphene-resistant women with polycystic ovary syndrome: a randomized, controlled trial. Hum Reprod. 2003;18(2):299-304.
45. Tso LO, Costello MF, Albuquerque LET, Andriolo RB, Macedo CR. Metformin treatment before and during IVF or ICSI in women with polycystic ovary syndrome. Cochrane Database Syst Rev. 2020;12(12):CD006105.
46. Kjøtrød SB, Carlsen SM, Rasmussen PE, Holst-Larsen T, Mellembakken J, Thurin-Kjellberg A, et al. Use of metformin before and during assisted reproductive technology in non-obese young infertile women with polycystic ovary syndrome: a prospective, randomized, double-blind, multi-centre study. Hum Reprod. 2011;26(8):2045-53.
47. Jacob SL, Brewer C, Tang T, Picton HM, Barth JH, Balen AH. A short course of metformin does not reduce OHSS in a GnRH antagonist cycle for women with PCOS undergoing IVF: a randomised placebo-controlled trial. Hum Reprod. 2016;31(12):2756-64.
48. Palomba S, Falbo A, La Sala GB. Effects of metformin in women with polycystic ovary syndrome treated with gonadotrophins for in vitro fertilisation and intracytoplasmic sperm injection cycles: a systematic review and meta-analysis of randomised controlled trials. BJOG. 2013;120(3):267-76.
49. Wu Y, Tu M, Huang Y, Liu Y, Zhang D. Association of metformin with pregnancy outcomes in women with polycystic ovarian syndrome undergoing in vitro fertilization: a systematic review and meta-analysis. JAMA Netw Open. 2020;3(8):e2011995.
50. Kolibianakis E, Bourgain C, Albano C, Osmanagaoglu K, Smitz J, Van Steirteghem A, et al. Effect of ovarian stimulation with recombinant follicle-stimulating hormone, gonadotropin releasing hormone antagonists, and human chorionic gonadotropin on endometrial maturation on the day of oocyte pick-up. Fertil Steril. 2002;78(5):1025-9.
51. Venetis CA, Kolibianakis EM, Bosdou JK, Lainas GT, Sfontouris IA, Tarlatzis BC, et al. Estimating the net effect of progesterone elevation on the day of hCG on live birth rates

after IVF: a cohort analysis of 3296 IVF cycles. Hum Reprod. 2015;30(3):684-91.

52. Griesinger G, Schultz L, Bauer T, Broessner A, Frambach T, Kissler S. Ovarian hyperstimulation syndrome prevention by gonadotropin-releasing hormone agonist triggering of final oocyte maturation in a gonadotropin-releasing hormone antagonist protocol in combination with a "freeze-all" strategy: a prospective multicentric study. Fertil Steril. 2011;95(6):2029-33.
53. Shapiro BS, Daneshmand ST, Garner FC, Aguirre M, Hudson C, Thomas S. Evidence of impaired endometrial receptivity after ovarian stimulation for in vitro fertilization: a prospective randomized trial comparing fresh and frozen-thawed embryo transfers in high responders. Fertil Steril. 2011;96(2):516-8.
54. Shapiro BS, Daneshmand ST, Garner FC, Aguirre M, Hudson C, Thomas S. Evidence of impaired endometrial receptivity after ovarian stimulation for in vitro fertilization: a prospective randomized trial comparing fresh and frozen-thawed embryo transfer in normal responders. Fertil Steril. 2011;96(2):344-8.
55. Chen Z-J, Shi Y, Sun Y, Zhang B, Liang X, Cao Y, et al. Fresh versus frozen embryos for infertility in the polycystic ovary syndrome. N Engl J Med. 2016;375(6):523-33.
56. Zaat T, Zagers M, Mol F, Goddijn M, van Wely M, Mastenbroek S. Fresh versus frozen embryo transfers in assisted reproduction. Cochrane Database Syst Rev. 2021;2(2):CD011184.
57. Maheshwari A, Bell JL, Bhide P, Brison D, Child T, Chong HY, et al. Elective freezing of embryos versus fresh embryo transfer in IVF: a multicentre randomized controlled trial in the UK (E-Freeze). Hum Reprod. 2022;37:476.

CHAPTER 89

Ethical, Legal, and Social Issues of Modern Assisted Reproductive Technology Practice

Petra De Sutter, Pankaj Talwar

INTRODUCTION

Infertility is still considered a social stigma for both men and women in India, damaging their mental, social, and physical experiences. While assisted reproductive technology (ART), including in vitro fertilization (IVF), has given hope to millions of couples suffering from infertility, it has also introduced countless ethical, legal, and social challenges. Surrogacy guidelines were laid out in 2002 by the Indian Council of Medical Research (ICMR). Further, "National Guidelines for Accreditation, Supervision and Regulation of ART Clinics in India" were described by ICMR in 2005, which prescribed the conditions that ART clinics need to comply with. No legislative backing was there for both the initiatives. In 2008, the ART Bill was first proposed, with the final version being brought out in 2017.[1-3]

ASSISTED REPRODUCTIVE TECHNOLOGY (REGULATION) RULES, 2022[4,5]

Assisted Reproductive Technology Clinics and Banks

There shall be two levels of clinics, namely:

- *Level 1 ART clinics,* where only intrauterine insemination (IUI) procedure is carried out as part of treatment.
- *Level 2 ART clinics,* where the procedures, or as the case may be, techniques, that attempt to obtain a pregnancy shall be carried out by any or all of the following, namely:
  - Surgical retrieval of gametes
  - Handling the oocyte outside the human body
  - Using sperms for fertilization of oocytes
  - Transfer of the embryo into the reproductive system of a woman
  - Carrying out storage of gametes or embryos or performing any kind of procedure or technique involving gametes or embryos.

ART banks shall:

- Be responsible for screening, collection and registration of the semen donor, and cryopreservation of sperms
- Perform screening and registration of oocyte donor
- Operate as semen banks or oocyte banks or both
- Maintain the records or data of all the donors and shall regularly update the National Registry.

Requirements and Qualifications of the Staff in the Assisted Reproductive Technology Clinics

- *ART level 1 clinic:* Minimum one gynecologist
- *Qualification:* The gynecologist shall be a medical postgraduate in Gynecology and Obstetrics.
- *ART level 2 clinic:* ART level 2 clinic shall have a minimum of one gynecologist, one anesthetist, one embryologist, and one counselor.

The additional staff at the level of director and andrologist may be employed by the ART level 2 clinics.

- *Qualification of staff in ART level 2 clinics* shall be as follows:
  - *Gynecologist:* The gynecologist will be a medical postgraduate in Gynecology and Obstetrics and should have a record of performing 50 ovum pickup procedures under the supervision of a trained ART specialist with at least 3 years of working experience in an ART clinic under supervision. (In the case of gynecologists practicing ART or IVF and are working in ART clinics before the commencement of this Act, a postgraduate degree in Gynecology and Obstetrics with at least 3 years' experience and record of 50 ovum pickup procedures shall be acceptable.)

    Or

    A medical postgraduate in Gynecology and Obstetrics with super specialist Doctorate of Medicine or fellowship in reproductive medicine with experience of not <3 years of working in an ART clinic.

- *Andrologist:* The andrologist in a clinic or a bank will be a MCh or DNB in Urology with special training in diagnosing and treating male infertility.
- *Embryologist:* From the date of commencement of these rules, clinics will hire embryologists only with the following qualifications and experience, namely: Postgraduate in Clinical Embryology (graduated with full-time program with minimum four semesters) from a recognized university with additional 3 years of human ART laboratory experience in handling human gametes and embryos

  Or

  PhD holder or doing full-time PhD project shall be related to clinical embryology or ART or fertility from a recognized university with an additional 1 year of human ART laboratory experience in handling human gametes and embryos

  Or

  Medical graduate (MBBS) or Veterinary graduate (BVSc) with a postgraduate degree in Clinical Embryology (full-time program) from a recognized university with additional 2 years of ART laboratory experience in handling human gametes and embryos

  Or

  Postgraduate in Life Sciences or Biotechnology with a minimum of 1 year of on-site, full-time clinical embryology certified training in addition to 4 years of experience in handling human gametes and embryos in a registered ART level 2 clinic.

  Note: As a one-time measure, all embryologists working in ART or IVF clinics before the commencement of these rules, with the below-mentioned qualifications and experience, may be allowed to continue as an embryologist. However, after the commencement of these rules, all clinics will hire embryologists with any of the above-mentioned qualifications and experience as criteria: Graduate in Life Sciences or Biotechnology or Reproductive Biology/Veterinary Science with at least 5 years of working experience in a registered ART or IVF clinic, who have performed at least 500 IVF laboratory procedures (including intracytoplasmic sperm injection and at least 100 cycles of cryopreservation of embryos).
- *Counselor:* A person who is a graduate in Psychology or Clinical Psychology or Nursing or Life Sciences
- *Anesthetist:* Anesthetist will be a medical postgraduate in Anesthesia
- *Director:* The director shall have a postgraduate degree in Medical or Life Sciences or Management Sciences

- *ART bank:* The ART bank shall have a minimum of one Registered Medical Practitioner trained in the handling, preparation, and storage of semen samples.

Minimum Equipment in Assisted Reproductive Technology Clinics and Banks

- *ART level 1 clinics:*
  - Microscope
  - Centrifuge
  - Refrigerator
- *ART level 2 clinics:*
  - Microscope
  - Incubator (minimum two in number)
  - Laminar airflow
  - Sperm counting chambers
  - Centrifuge
  - Refrigerator
  - Equipment for cryopreservation
  - Ovum aspiration pump
  - Ultrasonography (USG) machine with transvaginal probe and needle guard
  - Test tube warmer
  - Anesthesia resuscitation trolley
- *ART banks:*
  - Centrifuge machine
  - Incubator
  - Microscope
  - Laminar airflow.

Registration Fees

Every application for registration shall be accompanied with a fee of:

- ₹ 50,000 for level 1 ART clinic
- ₹ 200,000 for level 2 ART clinic
- ₹ 50,000 for ART bank

If an application for registration of any ART clinic or ART bank has been rejected by the appropriate authority, no fee shall be required to be paid on resubmission of the application by the applicant for the same clinic and the application fees once paid shall not be refunded.

Provided further that no fee shall be required to be paid by the establishments run by the institute under the control of the Government.

Donor Gametes

All donors, both male and female, must be recruited through a registered ART bank.

Age of Donor and Recipient

Age of the recipient: Female: 21–50 years, male: 21–55 years

Age of the donor: Female: 23–35 years, male: 21–55 years.

Sex and Marital Status of Recipient

The recipient can be married or a single woman.

A bank shall not supply the sperm or oocyte of a *single donor* to more than *one commissioning couple.*

An *oocyte donor* shall be an ever-married woman having at least one live child of her own with a minimum age of 3 years and can donate oocytes only once in her life; not more than seven oocytes shall be retrieved from the oocyte donor.

All *unused oocytes* shall be preserved by the banks for use on the same recipient, or given for research to an organization registered under this Act after seeking written consent from the commissioning couple.

The gamete of a donor or embryo shall be *stored for a period of not more than 10 years,* and at the end of this period, the embryo or gamete shall be allowed to perish or be donated to a research organization registered under this Act for research purposes with the consent of the commissioning couple or individual, in the manner as prescribed.

Medical Examination of Donor

The sperm or oocyte donor shall be tested for the following communicable diseases, namely:

- Human immunodeficiency virus (HIV), types 1 and 2
- Hepatitis B virus (HBV)
- Hepatitis C virus (HCV)
- *Treponema pallidum* (syphilis) through Venereal Disease Research Laboratory (VDRL).

Insurance Coverage/Guarantee for Oocyte Donor

- The intending couple or woman will purchase a general health insurance coverage in favor of oocyte donor for a period of 12 months from an insurance company or an agent recognized by the Insurance Regulatory and Development Authority established under the provisions of the Insurance Regulatory and Development Authority Act, 1999, for an amount which is sufficient enough to cover all expenses for all complications arising due to oocyte retrieval.
- The intending couple shall sign an affidavit to be sworn before a Metropolitan Magistrate or a Judicial Magistrate of the first class.

Retrieval of Number of Oocytes from Donor

The clinics should make efforts to retrieve not more than 7–15 oocytes from the donor during one cycle. All formed follicles may be retrieved; however, the clinics shall ensure the controlled ovarian stimulation of donor women in order to prevent ovarian hyperstimulation. It is preferred over a coasting strategy in patients at risk of ovarian hyperstimulation syndrome (OHSS).

Other Duties of Clinics

The ART clinic shall:

- Ensure that all unused gametes or embryos shall be preserved by the ART clinic for use on the same recipient and shall not be used for any other couple or as the case may be woman.
- Allow cryopreservation of oocytes and sperms for oncofertility patients undergoing treatment and for other such conditions, for duration longer than 10 years with the permission from the National Board.
- Ensure the controlled ovarian stimulation of woman in order to prevent ovarian hyperstimulation.
- Ensure that preimplantation genetic testing shall be used to screen the human embryos for known preexisting heritable or genetic diseases and when medically indicated.
- Ensure that no preimplantation genetic testing shall be done for sex selection for nonmedical reasons or selection of particular traits due to personal preferences of the prospective parents or to alter or with a view to alter the genetic constitution of an embryo.
- A woman is not treated with gametes or embryos derived from more than one man or woman during any one treatment cycle.
- A clinic shall never mix semen from two individuals for the procedures specified under this Act.
- The embryos shall not be split and used for twinning to increase the number of available embryos.
- The collection of gametes posthumously shall be done only if prior consent of the commissioning couple is available.
- Maintain the following consent forms, namely:
    - Consent form to be signed by the couple or woman as specified in Form 6
    - Consent for IUI with husband's semen or sperm as specified in Form 7
    - Consent for IUI with donor semen as specified in Form 8
    - Consent for freezing of embryos as specified in Form 9
    - Consent for freezing gametes as specified in Form 10
    - Consent for freezing of gametes, sperm, or oocytes and parental consent as specified in Form 11
    - Consent for oocyte retrieval as specified in Form 12
    - Consent from oocyte donor as specified in Form 13.

The ART banks shall maintain the following, namely:

- Record of use of donor gametes as specified in Forms 14, 14A, and 14B
- Consent form for the donor of sperm as specified in Form 15.

Grievance Redressal

Every clinic and every bank shall maintain a grievance cell in respect of matters relating to such clinics and banks and the manner of making a complaint before such grievance cell be as specified in Form 5.

Number of Embryos to be Transferred

The gynecologist may transfer preferably one, and not more than two embryos; in cases with explainable circumstances, three embryos can be placed in the uterus of a woman during the treatment cycle.

Donor Embryos

Both donor gametes are allowed but only recommended for the same recipient.

Sale, Transfer, or Use of Gametes

The sale, transfer, or use of gametes, zygotes, and embryos, or any part thereof, or information related thereto, directly or indirectly to any party within or outside India, shall be prohibited except in the case of transfer of own gametes and embryos for personal use with the permission of the National Board.

SURROGACY (REGULATION) RULES, 2022[4,6]

Age of the Recipient Couple

Female: 23–50 years, male: 26–55 years
Surrogate: 25–35 years.

Insurance Coverage

- The intending woman or couple shall purchase a general health insurance coverage in favor of the surrogate mother for a period of 36 months from an insurance company or an agent recognized by the Insurance Regulatory and Development Authority established under the provisions of the Insurance Regulatory and Development Authority Act (41 of 1999) for an amount which is sufficient enough to cover all expenses for all complications arising out of pregnancy and also covering postpartum delivery complications.
- The intending couple/woman shall sign an affidavit to be sworn before a Metropolitan Magistrate or a Judicial Magistrate of the first class.

Number of Attempts of Surrogacy Procedure

The number of attempts of any surrogacy procedure on the surrogate mother shall not be more than three times.

Consent of a Surrogate Mother

The consent of a surrogate mother shall be as specified in Form 2.

Number of Embryos to be Implanted in the Uterus of the Surrogate Mother

The gynecologist shall transfer one embryo in the uterus of a surrogate mother during a treatment cycle.

It is only in special circumstances that up to three embryos may be transferred.

Medical Indications Necessitating Gestational Surrogacy

A woman may opt for surrogacy if:

- She has no uterus or missing uterus or abnormal uterus (such as hypoplastic uterus or intrauterine adhesions or thin endometrium or small unicornuate uterus, T-shaped uterus) or if the uterus is surgically removed due to any medical conditions, such as gynecological cancer.
- Intended parent or woman who has repeatedly failed to conceive after multiple IVF or intracytoplasmic sperm injection attempts (recurrent implantation failure).
- Multiple pregnancy losses resulting from an unexplained medical reason and unexplained graft rejection due to exaggerated immune response.
- Any illness that makes it impossible for a woman to carry a pregnancy to viability or pregnancy that is life threatening.
- Single woman (widow/divorced).

Offenses and Penalties

The offenses shall be punishable with a fine which shall not be less than 5 lakh rupees but may extend to 10 lakh rupees for the first contravention and for subsequent contravention, or shall be punishable with imprisonment for a term which shall not be less than 8 years but may extend to 12 years, or with fine which shall not be less than 10 lakh rupees but may extend to 20 lakh rupees.

TIMELINE OF ASSISTED REPRODUCTIVE TECHNOLOGY AND SURROGACY RULES (2021–2022)

The *Assisted Reproductive Technology (Regulation) Bill, 2017* was enacted by the Parliament in the 71st year of the Republic of India to establish the national board, the state boards, and the national registry for the regulation and supervision of ART clinics and ART banks, for prevention of misuse, for the safe and ethical practice of ART services, and for matters connected therewith or incidental thereto. This Act may be called the Assisted Reproductive Technology (Regulation) Act, 2017. It extends to the whole of India. It shall come into force on such date as the Central Government may, by notification in the Official Gazette, appoint an "appointed day" meaning the date with effect from which the National Board is established under subsection (1) of section 3. The Assisted Reproductive Technology (Regulation) Act of Parliament received the assent of the President on *December 18, 2021*, and this Act may be called the *Assisted Reproductive Technology (Regulation) Act, 2021*. In *March 2022*, the Central Government hereby makes the rules which may be called the *Assisted Reproductive Technology (Regulation) Rules, 2022.* They shall come into force on the date of their publication in the Official Gazette.

The *Surrogacy (Regulation) Bill, 2016* was enacted by the Parliament in the 72nd year of the Republic of India to constitute National Assisted Reproductive Technology and Surrogacy Board, State Assisted Reproductive Technology and Surrogacy Boards, and appointment of appropriate authorities for regulation of the practice and process of surrogacy, and for matters connected therewith or incidental thereto. The Surrogacy (Regulation) Act of Parliament received the assent of the President on *December 25, 2021* and this Act may be called the *Surrogacy (Regulation) Act, 2021*. In *March 2022*, the Central Government hereby makes the rules which may be called the *Surrogacy (Regulation) Rules, 2022*. They shall come into force on the date of their publication in the Official Gazette.

April 21, 2022: The Central Government hereby notifies the establishment of the National Assisted Reproductive Technology and Surrogacy Registry under the Department of Health Research for the purposes of *the Assisted Reproductive Technology (Regulation) Act, 2021 and the Surrogacy (Regulation) Act, 2021*. The said National Registry shall be in operation with effect from April 22, 2022.

May 4, 2022: The Central Government hereby notifies that the appropriate authority in respect of each Union Territory (UT) for the purposes of the Assisted Reproductive Technology (Regulation) Act, 2021 and the Surrogacy (Regulation) Act, 2021 consists of the following functionaries of respective UT:

- An officer of or above the rank of the Joint Secretary of the Health and Family Welfare Department as Chairperson, ex officio
- An officer of or above the rank of the Joint Director of the Health and Family Welfare Department as Vice Chairperson, ex officio
- An officer of the Law Department of the UT concerned not below the rank of a Deputy Secretary as a member, ex officio.

May 4, 2022: The Central Government hereby notifies that *composition of National Assisted Reproductive Technology and Surrogacy Board* for the purposes of the Assisted Reproductive Technology (Regulation) Act, 2021 and the Surrogacy (Regulation) Act, 2021 is as follows:

- The Minister-in-Charge of the Ministry of Health and Family Welfare as Chairperson, ex officio
- The Secretary to the Government of India in charge of the Department of Health Research as Vice-Chairperson, ex officio
- Dr Kakoli Ghosh Dastidar and Dr Bharatiben Dhirubhai Shiyal, Members of Lok Sabha as Members, ex officio
- Dr Rakesh Gupta, Joint Secretary, Ministry of Women and Child Development, Government of India, and Dr NR Battu, Joint Secretary and Legislative Counsel, Legislative Department, Ministry of Law and Justice, Government of India as Members, ex officio.
- The Director General of Health Services of the Central Government as Member, ex officio.
- The Chairpersons of the State/UT Boards:
  - Andaman and Nicobar Island
  - Andhra Pradesh
  - West Bengal
  - Uttarakhand as Members, ex officio.
- The Joint Secretary, Department of Health Research, Ministry of Health and Family Welfare, in charge of Surrogacy Division as Member Secretary, ex officio.

May 4, 2022: The Central Government hereby notifies that the UT Board in respect of each UT without Legislature for the purposes of the Assisted Reproductive Technology (Regulation) Act, 2021 and the Surrogacy (Regulation) Act, 2021 consists of the following *functionaries of respective UT*:

- Lieutenant Governor/Administrator of UT as Chairperson, ex officio
- The Secretary-in-Charge of the Department of Health and Family Welfare as Vice-Chairperson, ex officio
- Secretaries or Commissioners-in-charge of the Departments of Women and Child Development, Social Welfare, Law and Justice and Home Affairs or their nominees as members, ex officio.
- Director General of Health and Family Welfare of the State Government as member, ex officio
- An officer not below the rank of Joint Secretary, in charge of Family Welfare as Member Secretary, ex officio.

May 13, 2022: Assisted Reproductive Technology (Regulation) Rules, 2022 and Surrogacy (Regulation) Rules, 2022 are yet to be notified for the purposes of the Assisted Reproductive Technology (Regulation) Act, 2021 and the Surrogacy (Regulation) Act, 2021.

June 7, 2022: The Central Government hereby makes the rules which may be called the Assisted Reproductive Technology (Regulation) Rules, 2022.

June 21, 2022: The Central Government hereby makes the following rules which may be called the Surrogacy (Regulation) Rules, 2022.

August 4, 2022: The Central Government hereby makes the following order to remove the said difficulties, namely:

- This Order may be called the Assisted Reproductive Technology (Regulation) and Surrogacy (Regulation) (Removal of Difficulties) Order, 2022.
- It shall come into force with effect from July 25, 2022. Accordingly, the ART clinics, ART banks, and surrogacy clinics, falling under the jurisdiction of the 17 states as indicated below, are allowed to conduct counseling or procedures pertaining to ART and surrogacy beyond July 24, 2022 and up to a maximum period of 3 months (i.e., up to October 24, 2022):
  - Assam

- Bihar
- Chhattisgarh
- Goa
- Gujarat
- Haryana
- Himachal Pradesh
- Jharkhand
- Karnataka
- Manipur
- Meghalaya
- Nagaland
- Rajasthan
- Sikkim
- Tripura
- Uttar Pradesh
- Uttarakhand.

August 4, 2022: The Central Government hereby notifies the *appointment of the following experts as members of the National Assisted Reproductive Technology and Surrogacy Board* for the purposes of the Assisted Reproductive Technology (Regulation), Act 2021 and the Surrogacy (Regulation) Act, 2021:

- Dr Nitiz Murdia, Embryologist
- Dr Shubha Phadke, Medical Geneticist
- Dr Neeta Singh, Gynecologist and Obstetrician
- Dr RG Patel, Gynecologist and Obstetrician
- Smt. N Lalitha, Social Scientist.

October 10, 2022: The Central Government hereby makes the following rules, further to amend the Assisted Reproductive Technology (Regulation) Rules, 2022, namely:

- These rules may be called the *Assisted Reproductive Technology (Regulation) Amendment Rules, 2022*
- They shall come into force on the date of their publication in the Official Gazette.
- In the Assisted Reproductive Technology (Regulation) Rules, 2022, sub-rule (ii) of Rule 12 shall be substituted as under: (ii) The intending couple/woman shall sign an affidavit to be sworn before a Metropolitan Magistrate or a Judicial Magistrate of First Class or an Executive Magistrate or a Notary Public giving guarantee as per the section 22 (4) (ii) of the Assisted Reproductive Technology (Regulation) Act, 2021.

October 10, 2022: The Central Government hereby makes the following rules, further to amend the Surrogacy (Regulation) Rules, 2022, namely:

- These rules may be called the *Surrogacy (Regulation) Amendment Rules, 2022.*
- They shall come into force on the date of their publication in Official Gazette.
- In the Surrogacy (Regulation) Rules, 2022, sub-rule (2) of Rule 5 shall be substituted as under: (2) The intending couple/woman shall sign an affidavit to be sworn before a Metropolitan Magistrate or a Judicial Magistrate of First Class or an Executive Magistrate or a Notary Public giving guarantee as per the clause (q) of subsection (1) of section 2 of the Surrogacy (Regulation) Act, 2021 (47 of 2021).

ETHICAL, LEGAL, AND SOCIAL ISSUES[7-9]

Donor Gametes

- All donors, both male and female, must be recruited through a registered ART bank, but there are no registered ART banks formed yet.
- A bank shall not supply the sperm or oocyte of a single donor to more than one commissioning couple; however, this will increase the cost of IVF cycle.
- The intending couple or woman will purchase a general health insurance coverage in favor of an oocyte donor for a period of 12 months from an insurance company, but no donor compensation is recommended.
- The intending couple shall sign an affidavit to be sworn before a Metropolitan Magistrate or a Judicial Magistrate of first class; however, anonymity is not maintained.
- Known donor or anonymous donor is not clearly mentioned in the rules.

Donor Embryos

Both donor gametes are allowed but only recommended for the same recipient; however, this will increase the cost of IVF cycle.

Assisted Reproductive Technology Banks

All donors, both male and female, must be recruited through a registered ART bank, but there are no registered ART banks formed yet.

Surrogacy

- Only gestational surrogacy is allowed in India.
- Single/divorced women can opt for surrogacy, but same-sex couples cannot apply for surrogacy.
- A woman can become a surrogate only once in her lifetime and only for one commissioning couple.

CONCLUSION

Assisted reproductive technology has resulted in a tectonic shift in the way physicians and the general population perceive infertility and ethics. ART is directly challenging the society to reevaluate the way in which human life, social justice and equality, and claims to genetic offspring are viewed. Furthermore, these issues will force legal systems to modify the existing laws to accommodate the unique challenges created by ART. Society has a responsibility to ensure that the advances achieved through ART are implemented in a socially responsible manner.

REFERENCES

1. Malhotra N, Shah D, Pai R, Pai HD, Bankar M. Assisted reproductive technology in India: a 3 year retrospective data analysis. J Hum Reprod Sci. 2013;6(4):235-40.
2. Farquhar C, Marjoribanks J. Assisted reproductive technology: an overview of Cochrane reviews. Cochrane Database Syst Rev. 2018;8(8):CD010537.
3. Brezina PR, Zhao Y. The ethical, legal, and social issues impacted by modern assisted reproductive technologies. Obstet Gynecol Int. 2012;2012:686253.
4. The Assisted Reproductive Technologies (Regulation) Rules—2010; 2017 Indian Council of Medical Research New Delhi; Ministry of Health and Family Welfare, Government of India, New Delhi.
5. The Gazette of India. Ministry of Health and Family welfare, Assisted Reproductive Technology (Regulation) Rules, 2022, New Delhi, 2022.
6. The Gazette of India. Ministry of Health and Family welfare, Surrogacy (Regulation) Rules, 2022, New Delhi, 2022.
7. Scott R. Legal issues in IVF. Clin Obstet Gynaecol. 1985;12(4):893-910.
8. Kar S, Shah D, Patil M. Upper age limit for assisted reproductive technologies: ethics opinion. J Hum Reprod Sci. 2018;11(2):89-90.
9. Asplund K. Use of in vitro fertilization—ethical issues. Ups J Med Sci. 2020;125(2):192-9.

CHAPTER 90

Quality Management in Assisted Reproductive Techniques Laboratory

Surbhi Gupta, Divyashree PS

INTRODUCTION

"Quality of the IVF laboratory is invisible when it is good but impossible to ignore when it is bad".

The practice of in vitro fertilization (IVF) has evolved into a well-established routine treatment of infertility since its inception 40 years ago. It involves the integration of individuals from various disciplines, such as embryology, ultrasonography, medicine and nursing, and requires them to work together in a safe and productive atmosphere to ensure that the service is being delivered in the best way.

A quality management system (QMS) is a process within an organization to ensure that the service is provided consistently and with as little variation as possible.[1]

Total quality management (TQM) is a management approach of an organization centered on quality, based on the participation of all its members and aiming at long-term success through customer satisfaction and benefits to all members of the organization and society. It is restricted not only to IVF laboratory but also to every function in the assisted conception unit.

The markers of good quality of an IVF laboratory are:
- Highest patient care in the form of caring for their gametes
- Highest success rate.

The requirements involve organization, management, personnel, equipment and materials, facilities/premises, documentation, records, and quality review and include the following:
- Defining the responsibilities of each personnel
- Having validated and written standard operating procedures (SOPs) including those for adverse events
- Ensuring full traceability for everything including cells, tissues, equipment, and records
- Confirming that quality assays are being performed as and when required
- Ensuring proper and periodic maintenance, service, and calibration of equipment
- Reviewing performance to ensure continuous and systematic improvement
- Providing risk assessment analysis for all laboratory activities
- Record maintenance and upgradation.

Hence, QMS consists of:
- Quality control (QC)
- Quality assurance (QA)
- Quality improvement.

Quality Control

Quality control is a process that includes all activities or operational techniques carried out in order to meet the quality requirements. The main goal of QC is to evaluate the effectiveness of various policies and procedures, identify and correct problems, ensure the accuracy and precision of procedures, and monitor the performance of the laboratory staff.[2]

It is product oriented and ensures that what you have done is what you expected.

Quality Assurance

Quality assurance is the sum total of all the activities required to establish the confidence that the product or the service is meeting the determined quality requirements. QA is more expansive and involves monitoring and control of the ongoing and overall quality in laboratory processes.[2]

It is process oriented and ensures that you are doing the right thing in the right way.

REFERENCES FOR QUALITY GUIDELINES

- Association of Clinical Embryologists 1996—Accreditation Standards and Guidelines for IVF laboratories
- ISO 15189/2012—Medical laboratories—particular requirements for quality and competence[1]
- European Society of Human Reproduction and Embryology (ESHRE) 2015—Guidelines for good practice in IVF laboratories[3]

- American Society for Reproductive Medicine (ASRM) 2008—Guidelines for human embryology and andrology laboratories.[4]

MODELS FOR QUALITY MANAGEMENT[2]

- Total quality management based on Deming's cycle or plan-do-check-act (PDCA) cycle
- European Foundation of Quality Management (EFQM) based on radar logic.

Total Quality Management

The concept of PDCA **(Fig. 1)** was given by W. Edwards Deming who is known as the father of modern QC. It is based on the principle that once a hypothesis is confirmed (or negated), executing the cycle will extend the knowledge further and repeating the PDCA cycle can bring its users closer to the goal, usually a perfect operation and output.

European Foundation of Quality Management

The EFQM model allows organizations to determine their current "level of excellence" and where they need to improve their efforts. It provides a set of performance improvement tools in order to achieve and sustain success. The model is regularly reviewed to incorporate new ideas, concepts, and learning. It is based on RADAR logic **(Fig. 2)**; continuous improvement cycle is used by EFQM.

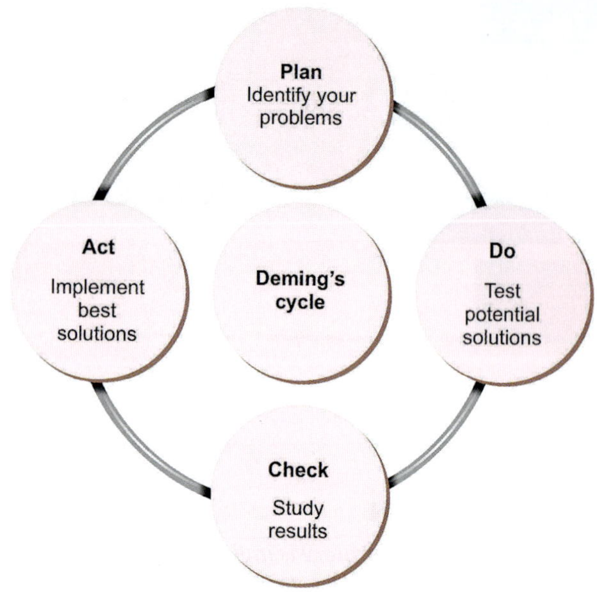

Fig. 1: Plan-do-check-act (PDCA) cycle.

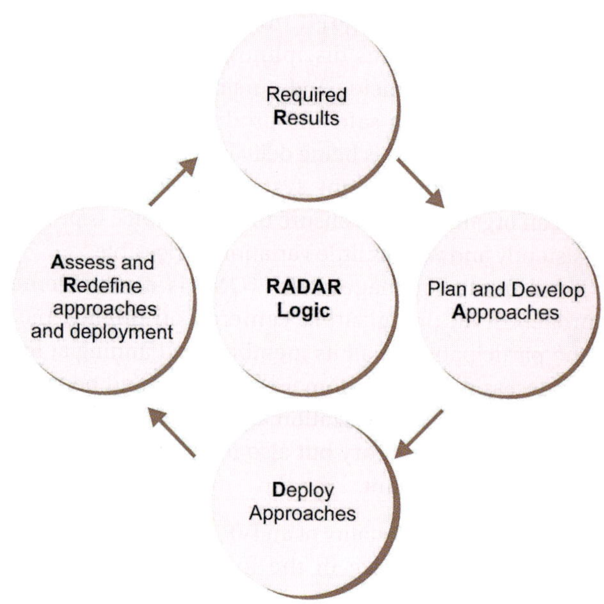

Fig. 2: European Foundation of Quality Management model using RADAR logic.

COMPONENTS OF QUALITY CONTROL PROGRAM

The components of QC program are depicted in **Flowchart 1**.

Laboratory Personnel

Laboratory personnel are one of the most important parts of an IVF laboratory and should be appropriately qualified, experienced, and responsible with the required expertise in the field of embryology and biological or medical sciences **(Table 1)**. The number of laboratory staff should reflect the number of cycles performed per year **(Table 2)**. There should be continuous upgradation for both new and senior embryologists by attending at least 12 hours of accredited continuing medical education (CME), conferences, and workshops annually.

Laboratory Safety and Equipment

Laboratory Design

- The IVF laboratory should be designed such a way as to minimize any damaging effects on gametes and embryos and to ensure good laboratory practice.[5]
- The laboratory should be in a low-traffic area, physically isolated from other laboratories, and in close proximity to the procedure room to ensure that oocyte or embryo viability is not compromised during transportation.
- The materials of the walls and floors should be easily washable and sterilizable. The materials used in laboratory construction, painting, flooring, and furniture should have minimized volatile organic compound (VOC) release and embryo toxicity. Low ceiling, granite wall, and vinyl floor are acceptable. Nontoxic, nonvaporizing paints such as epoxy paint should be used for floor, wall, and ceiling. There should be no carpeting.
- There should be optimal workflow over minimal distances while handling reproductive cells.

Flowchart 1: Components of quality control program.

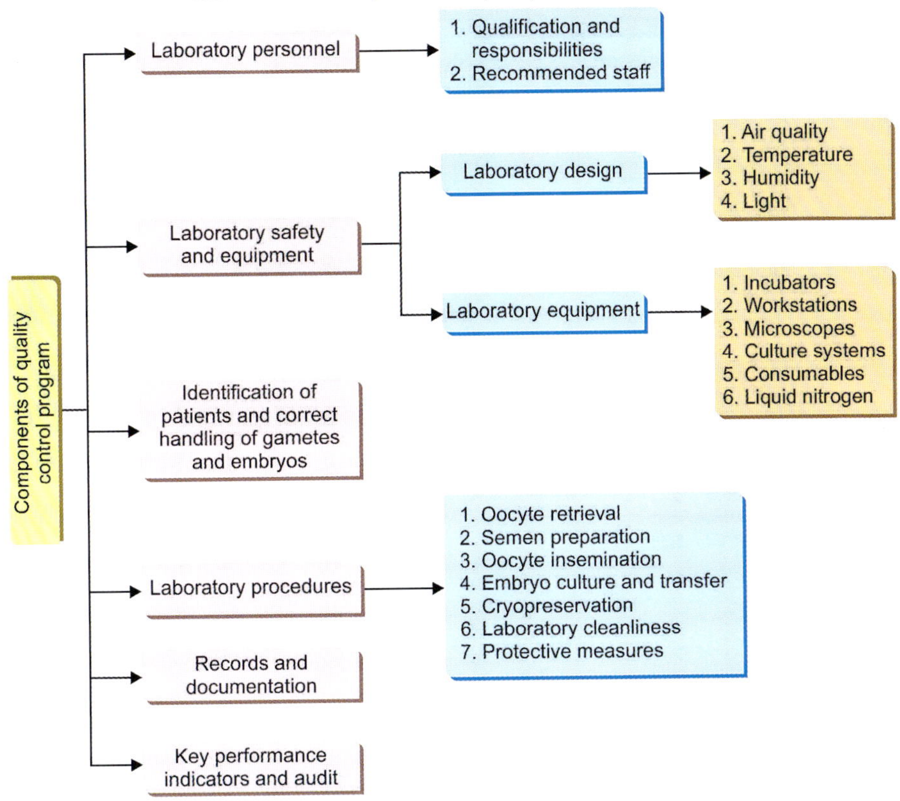

TABLE 1: Laboratory personnel and their responsibilities (ESHRE Guidelines 2015).

Position	*Qualification*	*Experience*	*Responsibilities*
Director	PhD/MD	2 years with minimum of 60 ART procedures	• To reach the highest standards in clinical IVF • Implementation of quality management system • Implementation of risk management and prevention policy • Ensuring sufficient staff members with appropriate skills • Management of staff training and continual scientific and biomedical education • Implementation and review of key performance indicators • Reporting of clinical data and adverse events • Approval of research projects
Supervisor	Master's/ Bachelor's	6 months with minimum of 60 ART procedures	• Efficient organization of daily work • Effective communication with laboratory staff and clinical colleagues • Continuous improvement wherever possible • Structured training of staff members and students
Technologist/ clinical embryologist	Master's/ Bachelor's	• Minimum of 30 ART procedures • 3 years experience as clinical embryologist • 6 years experience as senior clinical embryologist	• First-line of participation in daily clinical practice, communication, and organization • Execution of standard operating procedures • Contribution to laboratory clinical decisions • Training of staff members and students

(ART: assisted reproductive technique; IVF: in vitro fertilization)

- The laboratory access should be restricted only to laboratory personnel.
- There should be separate areas each for changing clothes, administrative work, cleaning and sterilization of materials, media preparation, and handwashing which should be outside the laboratory.

Air Quality

- Air quality monitoring consists of listing of particles and microorganisms, both in rest and in activity.
- Monitoring at rest **(Fig. 3)** ensures that the environment is ready for the forthcoming activity and aseptic process

TABLE 2: Recommended staff according to volume (ASRM guidelines 2008).

Number of laboratory cycles	Minimum number of embryologists
1–150	2
151–300	3
301–600	4
>600	1 additional embryologist per additional 200 cycles

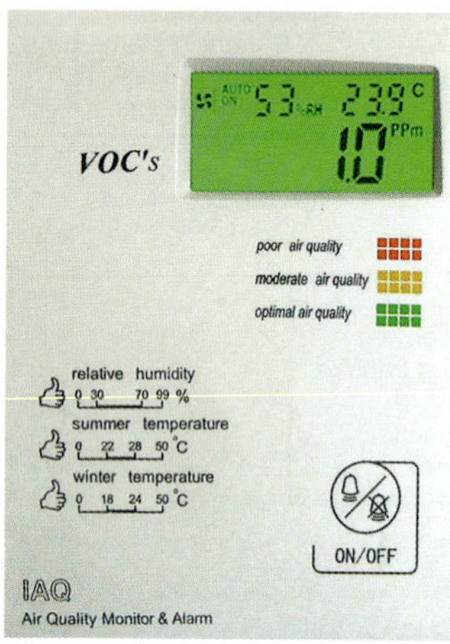

Fig. 3: Air quality monitor showing relative humidity (RH), temperature, and volatile organic compound (VOC) in the in vitro fertilization laboratory.

monitoring safeguards that the people, processes, and the environment remain under control during operation.

- Particulate matter (PM) and VOCs have effects on fertilization failure rate, delayed embryonic development, reduction in viability, implantation, and pregnancy rates.
- Positive pressure in the laboratory, high-efficiency particulate air (HEPA), filtration of laboratory air, filtration for VOCs, and the use of chemically active compounds are essential for high performance in IVF laboratories.

Air quality is divided into three parts: Air exchange, particle counts, and VOCs.

1. *Air exchange:*
   a. There should be an adequate number of air exchanges per hour in the laboratory so as to maintain positive pressure in the laboratory.
   b. It is calculated by dividing the cubic feet per minute of air exiting all the ducts by the total cubic feet of the room and multiplying by 60 minutes.
   c. Positive pressure air modules, such as Coda tower **(Fig. 4)**, within the laboratory are used to eliminate dust particles and microbes suspended in the laboratory air.
2. *Particle counts:*
   a. Bacteria and other contaminants attach themselves to particles and constitute the particle count.

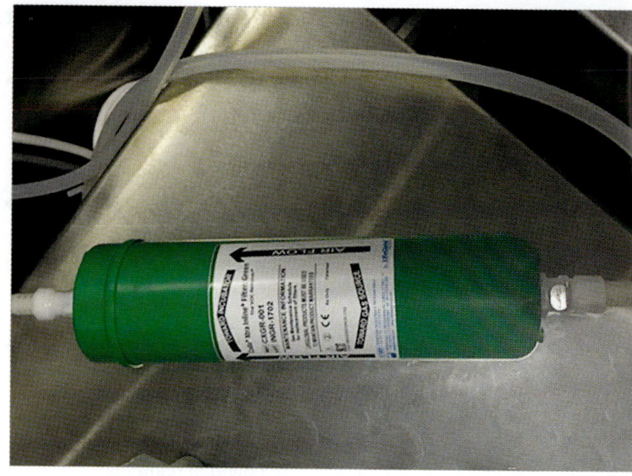

Fig. 4: Inline Coda filter.

   b. Individual and mean counts for different sizes (0.3, 0.5, and 5 μm) are measured.
   c. Decrease in particles equates to an increase in air quality and is done by adding HEPA or ultra-low penetration air (ULPA) filter to the heating, ventilation, and air conditioning (HVAC) systems.
   d. HEPA filter is 99.97% effective in removing particles with >0.3 m diameter. Laminar air flow equipped with HEPA filter is used for the manipulation of gametes.
   e. One study concluded that increased nitrogen dioxide (NO_2) is consistently associated with lower live birth rates. Fine $PM_{2.5}$ during embryo culture was associated with decreased conception rates, whereas no association was found with sulfur dioxide or large PM_{10}.[6]
3. *Volatile organic compounds:*
   a. VOCs are natural or synthetic chemicals that can vaporize under normal atmospheric conditions.
   b. HVAC systems can be equipped with filters embedded with charcoal and potassium permanganate to remove VOCs.
   c. Charcoal traps compounds such as benzene and formaldehyde, and potassium permanganate oxidizes alcohol and ketones.
   d. Oil overlays of culture media capture VOCs as they are oil soluble.
   e. Qualification is mostly done on a yearly basis and the maintenance schedule for service and replacement of filters is defined by particle count for HEPA filters and analysis of filter saturation for active carbon and chemical VOC filters.
   f. The records for filter replacement dates and batch numbers should be maintained.

Temperature

- The absolute value of ambient temperature in the clean room should not be >25°C.

- Elevated temperatures can increase the number of polar bodies formed and reduce oocyte and embryo competence, whereas lower temperatures can alter the cytoskeleton of oocyte, spindle fibers, and other organelles.
- Thus, for optimal laboratory performance, it is essential to keep ambient temperature constant and avoid fluctuations in the surface temperature of equipment (heated stages and incubators).
- The ambient temperature should be monitored and alarmed.

Relative Humidity

- Relative humidity (RH) is the amount of moisture in the air as compared to the maximum amount of moisture that the air will hold at the same temperature.
- The ideal RH of the clean room should be between 40 and 50%.
- RH >50% increases the risk of bacterial growth, whereas RH <35% promotes static electricity, personal discomfort, and irritation of mucous membranes and eyes.

Light

- The direct sunlight and the hard white fluorescent light, specifically the blue region (400–500 nm) of light, directly damage the gametes and the embryos. They can lead to impaired cell proliferation or alteration of DNA due to photooxidation.
- The use of green filters in microscopes is recommended.
- The use of plasticware also reduces light exposure because it absorbs almost all light waves <300 nm.
- The amount of light exposure can also be lowered simply by lowering light intensity in the room and on the microscope.

Laboratory Equipment

- The laboratory should be adequately and optimally equipped and the equipment must be easy to clean and disinfect (e.g., microscopes suitable for oocyte recovery, determination of fertilization, micromanipulators, devices to maintain temperature and pH of media, eggs, and embryos).
- Equipment should be appropriately validated and calibrated. Validation, calibration, maintenance, and repair must be documented and records should be retained.
- All critical equipment such as incubators and cryostorage units should be continuously monitored and must have alarm systems and an automatic emergency backup power system. There should be a minimum of two incubators.
- Gas cylinders should be located outside the laboratory **(Fig. 5)**. High-purity gas and inline HEPA and VOC filters **(Fig. 4)** are highly recommended.

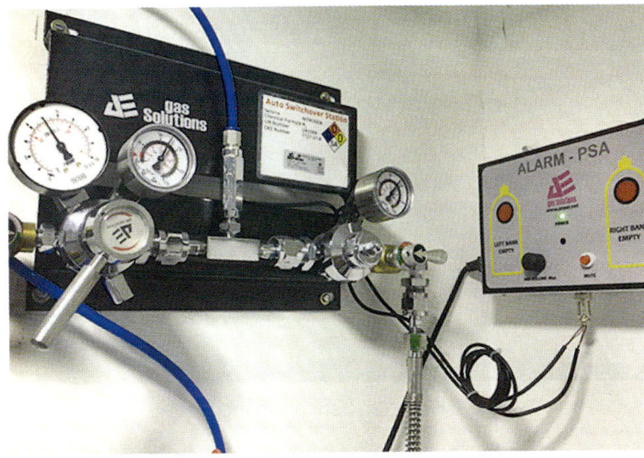

Fig. 5: Monitoring of CO_2 tank pressure with alarm system and autochange for gas cylinders.

TABLE 3: Types of incubators.

Box type	*Bench top*	*Others*
1. Water jacketed, 2. Air jacketed, e.g., Heracell incubator	1. Built in gas mixer: K-system 2. Premixed gases: 1. Minc 2. Planer BT 37 3. FIV-6	Mini incubator Portable incubator

- Heating devices to maintain the temperature of media and reproductive cells should be installed.
- Accepted ranges of use for all parameters should be determined and recorded.
- Malfunctioning equipment must be labeled as "out of use."
- For every equipment, an instruction manual should be available.
- All laboratory chemicals and reagents should be labeled including date of receiving, date of opening, and shelf life, wherever applicable.

Incubators: Incubators are the heart of the IVF laboratory. They are vital in providing a stable and appropriate culture environment for optimum embryo development and clinical outcome. The various types of incubators are ennumerated in **Table 3**.

Benchtop incubators **(Fig. 6)**

- They allow direct transfer of heat through the contact surfaces to the embryo culture dish.
- Rapidly equilibrate temperature and pH
- Heated chamber base plate and lid
- Compact size
- Digital record system for temperature and gas flow (24 hours)
- Time-stamped alarms
- Physiological culture environment is maintained by minimum premixed gas.

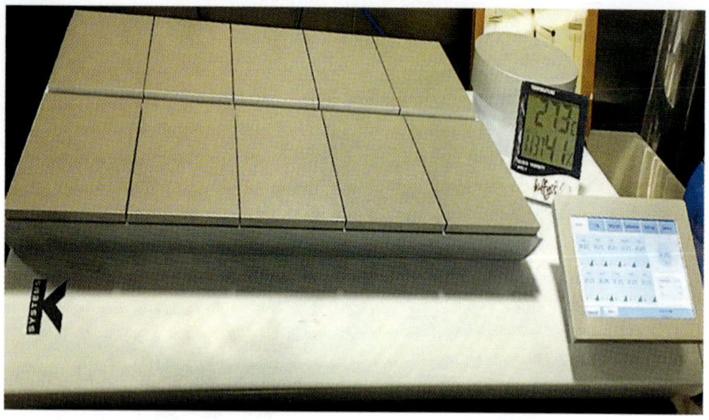

Fig. 6: K-system bench top incubator.

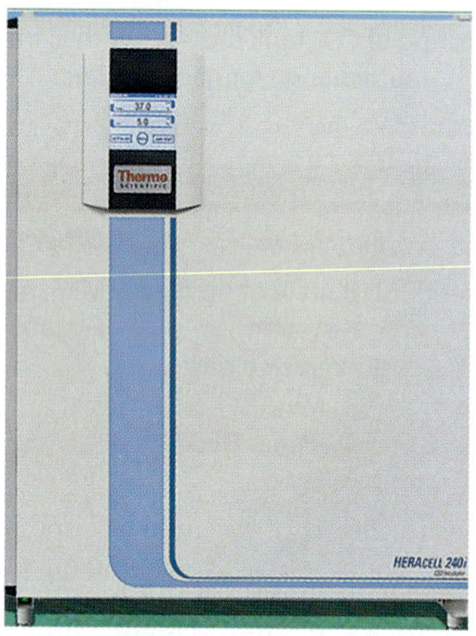

Fig. 7: Air jacketed (Heracell incubator).

The advantages of benchtop incubators are:
- Easy sterilization
- Less power consumption
- Cheaper to run than tri-gas big-box incubators
- Better embryo quality as compared to tri-gas big-box incubators as they can achieve low pO_2 culture easily.
- Less prone to fungal and bacterial contamination.

Most commonly used benchtop incubators are K-System G-185 and Minc. These are triple gas incubators with a built-in gas mixer. The concentrations of gases are 6% CO_2, 5% O_2, and 89% N_2.

Box incubators **(Figs. 7 and 8)**: Box incubators can be water jacketed or air jacketed **(Table 4)**.

The important environmental conditions that affect embryo culture are:
- Temperature
- Humidity
- Gas composition and pH
- Air quality.

Quality control of incubators[3]
- There should be a minimum of two incubators in any facility regardless of the type of incubator and the patient load and incubators must be connected to a 24-hour alarm system, monitoring all critical parameters.

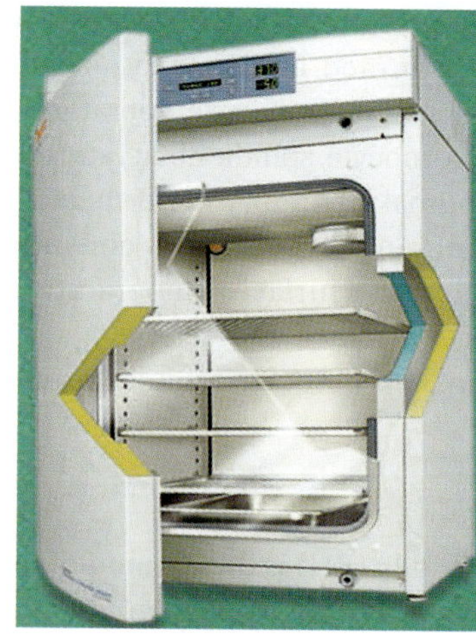

Fig. 8: Water jacketed incubator.

TABLE 4: Types of box incubators.

Water jacketed	*Air jacketed*
1. Retain heat longer in case of incubator opening or power failure	Warm up quickly but do not retain heat for longer periods
2. Heavy	Smaller size and light weight
3. Higher power consumption	Less power consumption
4. Preservation of chamber temperature is satisfactory	Preservation of chamber temperature is satisfactory
5. More chances of contamination and it may arise from the water jacket	Less chances of contamination
6. Decontamination cycles not possible	Decontamination cycles are possible
7. Maintenance is challenging	Maintenance is easy

- The temperature should be set at 37°C and should be monitored daily with an accurate and independent external thermometer.
- The humidity should be >90% (ideal 100%) inside the incubator.
- The pH should never exceed 7.4, even while evaluating embryos outside the incubator. The pH probe should always be calibrated with buffers and calibration should take place at the target temperature (37°C).
- Media pH is checked in each incubator for each new lot of media.
- Calibrated measuring devices should be used daily to monitor incubator temperature, CO_2 and O_2 concentrations, and RH levels. CO_2 settings should be determined based on pH measurements of culture media. Conventional incubators are equipped with infrared CO_2 sensors.
- All supply gases (CO_2, N_2, premix) to the incubators should pass through HEPA, activated carbon and permanganate

TABLE 5: Cleaning and disinfection of incubators.

Wipe/spray disinfection	*ContraCon decontamination*
Three stages: • Predisinfection: – Remove all samples – Pump the water off – Spray disinfectant (usually soft odorless soft solution to remove culture media and protein) • Cleaning: – Thoroughly remove dirt residues and wipe the surfaces clean using a clean cloth and plenty of clear water – Wipe accessories thoroughly dry • Final disinfection: – Spray disinfectant again (70% methanol to remove oil followed by distilled water) onto the work space, the shelf system, and the removed components and wipe them clean – Allow the disinfectant to react as specified by the manufacturer – Reinstall the shelf system The use of halogens such as bleach solution or betadine is contraindicated as they can persist for extended period and can potentially harm embryo cultures.	• Principle: – Takes approximately 25 hours – A hot and humid atmosphere at 90°C at 0% CO_2 with highly decontaminating effect is created in the work space • Procedure **(Figs. 9A and B):** – After cleaning, reinstall the shelf system components – Fill the floor pan with 350 mL processed water – Turn the device on – Activate and start the decontamination routine (90°C for 25 hours) – After the decontamination routine has been completed, remove the remaining water using a sterile cloth – Turn the device off or resume operation – Calibration is done using auto start at 5% CO_2 and 37°C for 9 hours and confirmed using sperm survival test.

filter. Monitor CO_2 supply cylinders regularly, and ensure that autochangers are functional **(Fig. 5)**.

- Water in the incubator pan (to maintain humidity) must be regularly changed before the new batch starts.
- Shelves should be changed every other week.
- Internal incubator filters, including VOC filters, are changed yearly.
- Coda filters are attached to medical-grade gas cylinders **(Fig. 4)**.
- A sperm survival test before every batch to ensure proper functioning of incubator or two-cell mouse embryo assay tests with 80% blastocyst rate are performed quarterly.
- Annual maintenance contract with the supplier for servicing must be regularly maintained.
- Incubators should not be opened frequently and widely. Consecutive opening and closing two to three times within 5 minutes can cause a significant fall in CO_2 concentration and temperature which will be detrimental for both the oocytes and embryos.
- Incubators must be regularly cleaned and decontaminated.

Cleaning of incubators: Regular cleaning and disinfection of CO_2 incubators should be performed once every 3–6 months. It can be done in two ways **(Table 5)**:

1. Wipe/spray disinfection
2. ContraCon decontamination.

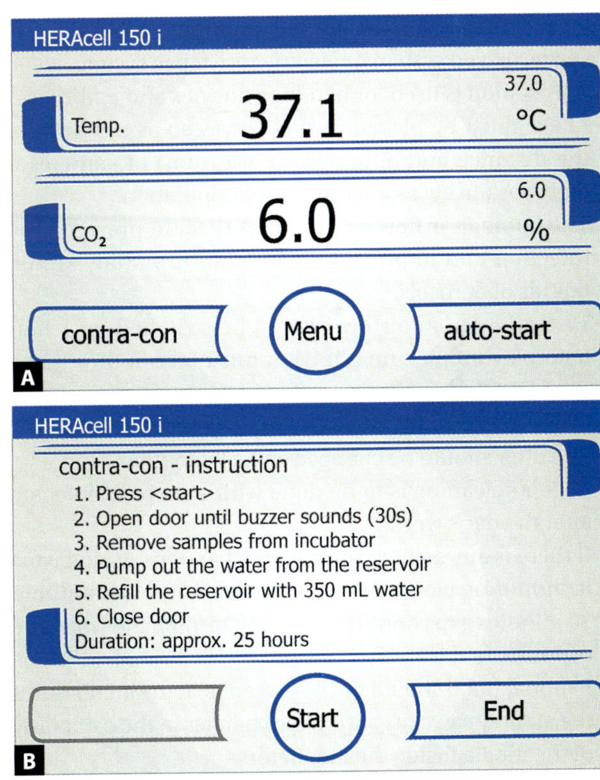

Figs. 9A and B: ContraCon™ decontamination of Heracell incubator.

In vitro fertilization workstations: The IVF workstations can be of three types:

1. *Open workstations:* Traditional flow cabinets and microscope stages
2. *Closed workstations:* To maintain the gas phase, controlling the CO_2 concentration, and improving the temperature control
3. *Time-lapse video systems:* Culture systems where the embryos can be manipulated without taking them outside the incubator.

Quality control of open (laminar airflow) workstations: The traditional workstation unit consists of a vertical laminar

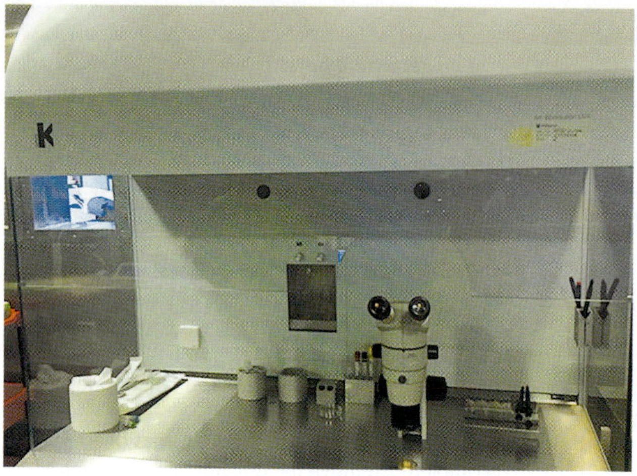

Fig 10: Laminar airflow workstation with stereomicroscope.

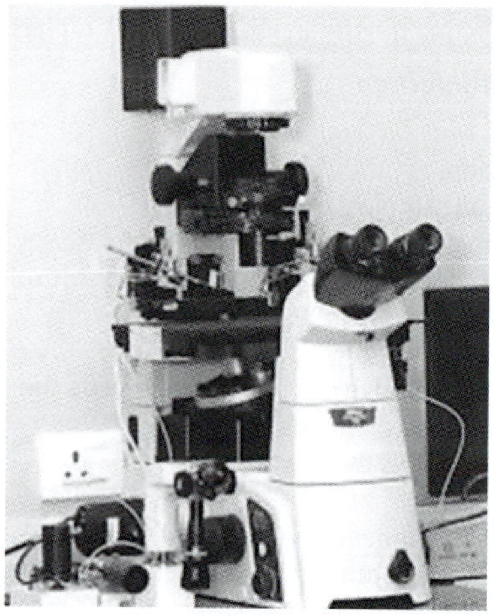

Fig. 11: Micromanipulator with inverted microscope.

flow cabinet **(Fig. 10)** together with a HEPA filter, a continuous heated surface with a stereomicroscope embedded, a working incubator inside or near the cabinet, and an inverted microscope on an antivibration table. Usually, under the heated surface are the aluminum blocks heated by a water-based system or electric resistance system.

- This station is used for handling oocytes and embryos.
- These must be placed in such a way so as to minimize the distance and optimize the transport of gametes or embryos during assessment or manipulation.
- The laminar airflow should be vertical to prevent cross infection and to protect the operator from any kind of liquids or aerosols.
- Vertical laminar airflow should be switched on 1 hour before ovum pick-up (OPU). It must be run throughout the day and switched off when the day's work is over.
- The filter should be changed every 6 months.
- Regular cleaning is to be done with surface disinfectant after the day's work.
- If there is any soiling/spillage that happens during work, it should be cleaned with 70% alcohol. A minimum of 30 minutes gap should be given, to resume the work after exposure to the alcohol.
- Laminar hood should not be placed near the incubator, as the air flow can cause dramatic changes in the osmolarity of the media inside the incubators.
- Regular servicing and cleaning of HEPA filter are a must.
- Ensure that the HEPA filter is working properly by testing the density of the PM in the air.

Quality control of closed workstations

- Closed workstations control temperature and pH and there is no need for HEPES buffer.
- There is a warm heated stage and a closed-circuit airflow which is also heated and sterile filtered (HEPA, VOC).
- Cleaning and decontamination are more complicated than laminar flow workstations.
- If methanol is used for cleaning, the workstation should be stopped and opened to prevent fumes from recirculating inside the workstation.

Microscopes: Microscopes used in an IVF laboratory are as follows:

- *Ordinary binocular microscope:* For evaluating semen parameters
- *Stereomicroscopes* **(Fig. 10)**: Workhorse of assisted reproductive technique (ART) laboratory. It is used when low magnification is needed, during cumulus isolation, washing and denuding, and embryo handling.
- *Inverted microscopes with micromanipulator* **(Fig. 11)**: Used for doing intracytoplasmic sperm injection (ICSI), and for oocyte and embryo assessment.

Quality control of microscopes

- Daily measurement of the temperature of the stage warmer should be done.
- Lack of clarity should be noted and rectified.
- Procedures for alignment of the optical path should be readily available.
- QC of image quality should be recorded and documented daily.
- Regular cleaning with surface disinfectant after each procedure must be followed.

Culture systems: The optimum environment of the culture systems is essential for the growth of embryos. The important conditions to control for providing an apt environment are:

- Temperature
- Culture media and pH
- Osmolality
- Oxygen tension
- Water quality
- Oil overlay
- Volume of culture media.

Temperature

- As discussed above, maintaining optimum temperature is very crucial for the gametes and the embryos.
- The human meiotic spindle is extremely sensitive to the variations in temperature and maintenance of temperature at 37°C is important for spindle integrity and thus normal fertilization and embryo development. The suboptimal temperatures should be avoided as the temperature effects are irreversible.[7-9]
- Temperature issues can occur during follicle puncture, on heated stages, in incubators and during embryo transfer.
- Temperature should be measured in culture dishes and in tubes with suitably calibrated probes. Thermistors with 0.1°C are widely available.

Culture media and pH

- The hydrogen ion concentration or pH is very important for embryo development. There is no ideal pH for culture media but is usually kept between 7.2 and 7.4.
- pH is dynamic and depends on association and dissociation of compounds in solution. It occurs in three phases in the laboratory: Equilibration, set point, and stabilization.
- Both extracellular pH (pHe) and intracellular pH (pHi) have to be regulated.

pH is extracellular (pHe) which is a balance between concentrations of CO_2 in the cell culture incubator and the amount of bicarbonate in the media. To regulate the set point of media pHe, CO_2 value is controlled on the incubator. This is an inverse relationship, pHe decreases as CO_2 concentration increases.[10]

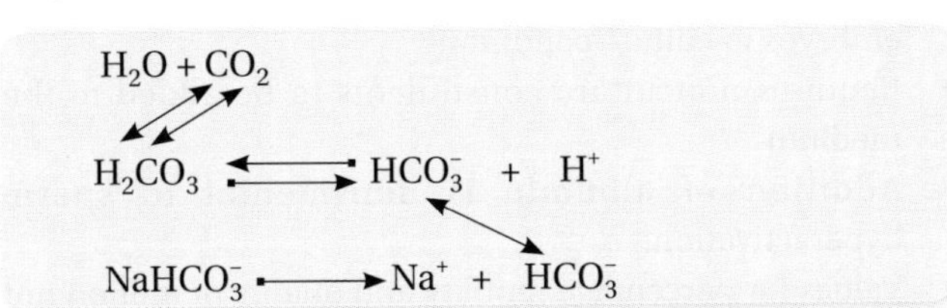

- Regulation of pHi is an important cellular function necessary to maintain intracellular homeostasis. Cells contain various mechanisms to regulate pHi. Short-term regulation of pHi is achieved by the physiochemical buffering capacity of the cytoplasm and proteins.
- Common regulatory systems to combat intracellular acidosis include the sodium-dependent HCO_3^-/Cl^- exchanger (HCE) and the Na^+/H^+ antiporter, which add and remove, respectively, bicarbonate and hydrogen ions from within the cell. To combat alkalosis, cells may contain the HCE.[7]
- The commonly used bicarbonate-buffered media added to culture media to regulate pH are N-(2-hydroxyethyl) piperazine-N′-(2-ethanesulfonic acid) (HEPES) or 3-(N-morpholino) propanesulfonic acid (MOPS). This is controlled by the amount of CO_2 dissolved in culture media which in turn is regulated by the partial pressure of CO_2 in incubator air.[11]
- The pH has a potential impact on the meiotic spindle. It affects embryo actin cytoskeletal elements and oocyte cytoskeleton responsible for positioning of the meiotic spindle. It affects both oocyte and embryo metabolism.[10]
- Presently, the culture media are built around 6% CO_2 instead of 5% CO_2. The 1% increase has been reported to increase blastocyst cell numbers and implantation rates.[8]
- On exposing the culture medium to ambient air, the pH starts rising immediately. However, if the lid is left on the culture dish after removing it from the incubator, the pH starts rising after 10 minutes; hence, lids should be left on the culture dishes during zygote and embryo scoring.
- For QC, the pH of each batch of culture medium after proper equilibration should be measured.
- A conventional pH meter with a glass electrode can be used (samples for measurement have to be removed from the incubator, measurements should be done at 37°C, and measurements have to be done in ambient air). Other methods are continuous pH recorders in incubators or the use of a point-of-care blood gas analyzer.

Osmolality

- The ideal osmolality is yet to be determined as it is dependent on cell stage and embryo quality but ranges from 255 to 298 mOsm/kg for the commercial media.[12]
- Osmolality measurement gives a sense of accuracy with which media was prepared and hence each laboratory should have a freezing point depression osmometer.
- It has been demonstrated that 3 mL of culture medium left out at room temperature for as little as 30 minutes causes osmolality to rise by 5%.[11]
- Each batch of culture media should be tested for osmolality before use.

Oxygen tension

- The two most commonly used O_2 levels are 5 and 20–21%.
- Oxygen is converted to superoxide radicals, which can be deleterious to cells.
- The O_2 level in the fallopian tube is 2–8%.[13-15]
- The best level for O_2 inside the incubator is shown to be 5%. Thus with less oxygen, there would be less chances of damage to gametes and embryos through free radicals.

Water quality

- Water is one of the most important ingredients in culture media.
- Water is purified with the use of carbon filtration and reverse osmosis and should be tested for bacterial endotoxins to ensure the levels <1.5 pg/mL.

Oil overlay

- Oil is often layered over culture media.
- The benefits include decreased media evaporation, heat loss, pH shift, and protection from outside contaminants. It can also extract harmful substances from the culture media.[16-18]
- However, it may contain contaminants that may affect embryo development.[19-22] To prevent this, before using, the media should be washed with various salt and protein solutions.[16,18,23-25]

Volume of the culture medium: The amount of culture medium used is based on three factors:

1. Type of culture vessel
2. Sperm density
3. Embryo culture (single or in groups).

As per one study, motile sperm concentration was more important for fertilization than the total number of sperms.[26] Another study reported that increased sperm concentration can reduce the pH because of sperm metabolism leading to increased CO_2 production.[27]

Group culture has been proven superior to single-embryo culture in terms of blastomere numbers and embryo quality.[28-34]

A smaller volume of culture medium should be used as it has been linked to increased fertilization rates[35-37] and better embryo quality.[29-31,38] This is because of the autocrine and paracrine factors produced by each embryo and thus the cross talk between them in a small volume of medium.[35,39]

Consumables: The various consumables in the IVF laboratory include oocyte retrieval needles, culture dishes, ICSI needles, transfer catheters, culture media, oil, pipettes, and other plastic wares. The QC of all the consumables is mandatory and should be provided by the manufacturer.

The various assays assess the ability to sustain sperm or achieve highly developed embryos. It is assumed that the optimal conditions for these assays mimic the conditions that are optimal for the maintenance of human gametes and culture of human embryos. But there is very little standardization of these assays in different laboratories. Bioassays must be capable of detecting any and all agents that are detrimental to gametes or embryos. At the same time, bioassays should be specific for agents that affect human embryos and not the nonhuman gametes used for testing. The assays commonly used are as follows:

- Hamster sperm motility assay
- Human sperm survival assay
- Mouse embryo assay (MEA)
- Limulus amoebocyte lysate (LAL) test.

Hamster sperm motility assay

Description

- *Hamster epididymis held in the medium*: Sperm allowed to swim through several lacerations
- *Test cultures*: Tyrode's solution modified by adding bovine serum albumin, lactate, and pyruvate[4]
- *Control cultures*: Prepared with a medium known to perform well in the assay previously
- *All media (testing and control)*: Added with polyvinyl alcohol, penicillamine, hypotaurine, and adrenergic agent (epinephrine or isoproterenol)
- *Sperm cultured* at a concentration of 1–2 mill/mL in 2 mL of medium, under oil, in an incubator at 37°C, 5% CO_2
- *Sperm examined* with a dissecting stereomicroscope after 4 hours (a time when sperm are expected to show maximal hyperactivation)
- *Motility score* calculated by multiplying percentage motility and quality of motility[4]
- *Assay relies upon* the timely appearance of hyperactivated sperm in high quantities, to achieve adequate scores.
- *Sperm motility scores compared* between test and control conditions using statistical comparisons of three or four replicates.

Sensitivity

Motility scores are affected by albumin. This assay's sensitivity is improved by using solutions without albumin.

Advantages

- Brief
- Requires only 4–6 hours for results
- Detect differences between media prepared with different water sources.

Disadvantages

- Requirement of hamsters
- Focuses only on hyperactivation (only one of the sperm function)
- May not represent the sensitivity of human sperm or embryos to culture conditions
- Requires nonculture constituents to be added to the medium
- Addition of albumin is detrimental to sperm hyperactivation.[4]
- Values for percentage motility and quality of motion not well defined: Need competent personnel.

Human sperm survival assay

Description

- Human sperm obtained from patient samples donated for research[40-46] or frozen sperm samples[47] are used.
- Sperm prepared for culture by separating from seminal plasma and cryoprotectants: By centrifugation of semen over density gradient media.
- *Control solution* which has previously supported the prolonged culture of sperms
- Sperm allotted to test solution and control solution in equal concentration
- Cultured for several minutes to days at constant room temperature (37°C)

- *Principle:* Sperm survival declines over time. Both test and control solutions are assessed at specific times.
- *Assessment of survival:* By determining percentage of motile sperms[41,47] or percentage of sperm with progressive motility.[40,43,44] (Vitality can also be assessed by using vitality stain exclusion or hypoosmotic swelling test, morphology, or mitochondrial function.)
- Statistical comparisons between sample replicates of the test group and control group done
- *Survival level:* Control solutions support motility of 70–85% of the initial motility. A defined survival level of 75% in the control is used as a threshold to measure.
- *If the sperm in the test solution is above the threshold value:* Test condition suitable for use in human gamete culture
- *Assay considered valid*: If control solution supports motility of 70–85% of initial motility after 48–96 hours

Sensitivity
- Duration of exposure and duration of culture improve sensitivity.
- Culture at 37°C improves sensitivity at shorter time intervals.
- Omission of protein/albumin from medium and decreasing concentration of sperm cultured have also shown to improve sensitivity.

Advantages
- Clinically applicable (uses human sperm)
- Ethical
- Detects conditions that are detrimental to human sperm survival, e.g., oil overlay, gloves, and probe covers which are not detected by other assays.

Disadvantages
- Sperm samples vary from male to male.
- Except survival, other functions of sperm in IVF (capacitation, hyperactivation, fertilization, oocyte activation) are not assessed.
- Qualitative scoring of motility is arbitrary and needs trained personnel.
- Sperm survival for 48 hours or more is not relevant in IVF (fertilization occurs within few hours of insemination).

Mouse embryo assay

Description
- *Mouse embryos:* Obtained by superovulation, mating and harvesting fresh embryos, or by thawing frozen embryos[44,45]
- *Culture of mouse embryos:* In test and culture media maintained at 37°C and 5% CO_2 in an incubator-like condition from early stages (one-cell or two-cell stage) to blastocyst stages
- Minimum of 69 mouse embryos in each (test group and control group)
- *Quantification:* Generally in the form of percentage of the embryos that achieve the advanced stage, and compared between test and control media
- If the percentage of embryos achieving the advanced stage is significantly lower in the test medium than in the control medium: Test conditions unsuitable for use in IVF laboratories.

Sensitivity

It is associated with
- *Strain of the mouse generating the gametes:* Inbred mice are less sensitive.
- *Starting stage of the embryos:* Embryos introduced as zygotes are more sensitive.
- *Stage that must be attained:* Reliance upon more advanced stages increases the sensitivity.

Advantages
- Tests the ability of embryos to undergo sustained development through the early stages and to result in embryos of a particular quality
- Conditions are quite similar to those used for culture of human embryos.
- Able to detect the presence or absence of pyruvate in the culture medium, the presence or absence of protein supplementation in the medium, and the quality of maternal serum used for supplementation.

Disadvantages
- May not be sensitive to the same array of culture conditions that may affect human embryo development
- Requires a lengthy duration of culture
- Not able to assess the ability of the conditions to support implantation, fetal growth, and delivery.

Limulus amoebocyte lysate test

Description
- Aqueous extract of blood cells (amoebocytes) from the horseshoe crab and limulus polyphemus
- LAL reacts with bacterial endotoxin or lipopolysaccharide (LPS), which is a membrane component of gram-negative bacteria.
- This reaction is the basis of the LAL test, which is used for the detection and quantification of bacterial endotoxins.

Advantages
- Simple and easy to perform
- Results obtained in a few hours
- Animals not used in testing.

Disadvantages
- High emphasis on the precise implementation of the test procedure
- Slight disturbances could influence the outcome of the test.[40]

Quality control of consumables

- There is no consensus on how these tests should be performed and different variables have an effect on their sensitivity.[48] Reagents, media, and consumables should be used prior to the expiry date.
- Sterile single-use disposables should be used.
- Appropriate refrigeration facilities for storage of media and reagents should be available and the maintenance of correct temperature during the shipment to the clinic must be verified.
- Documentation of QC is a must. The supply of commercial media should correspond with a delivered batch. A stock management system for media, oil, and consumables stating batch number, date of entry, shelf life, and date of expiry should be maintained **(Fig. 12)**.
- The protein source for medical use should be strictly defined. Use of blood-based media or blood-based media supplement (human fetal cord serum, maternal or donor serum, follicular fluid) is not allowed.
- Risk assessments should be done on all consumables.

Liquid nitrogen levels

- Liquid N_2 levels are measured using a measuring stick.
- The stick is lowered to the bottom of the tank and also allowed to cool for a few seconds. It is then taken out and shaken. Frost or condensation takes place when the measuring stick had contact with liquid N_2. The highest point of condensation value is recorded as the height of liquid nitrogen.
- The level should not be allowed to drop <5 inches as lower levels of liquid nitrogen could allow some of the product stored to thaw.
- Levels <2 inches are critical.

Electronic monitoring of liquid nitrogen

- Early alarm and alarm of sound and light for liquid N_2 level

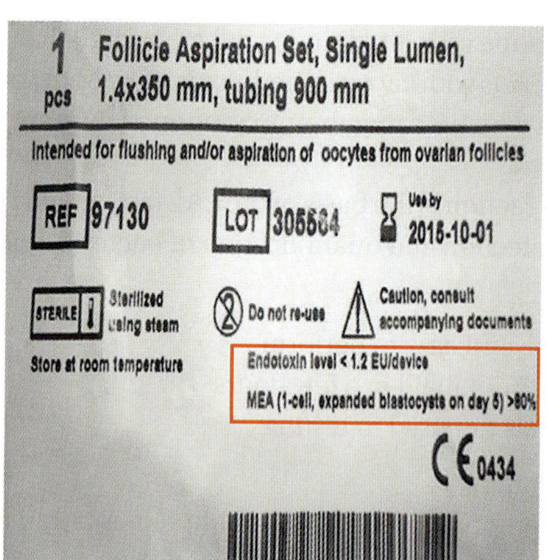

Fig. 12: Quality control of consumables (oocyte retrieval needle) on the cover.

- Temperature display, digital temperature adjustment, and calibration
- Threshold-crossing alarm signal should be set accurately.

Identification of Patients and Correct Handling of their Gametes and Embryos

- A proper and accurate system to correctly identify the patient and trace and locate their reproductive cells during each step is essential in ART treatment.
- Written SOPs **(Fig. 13)** should be made which should be followed strictly for correct identification and verification **(Figs. 14A to C)** of patients (or donors) and their tissues or cells.
- Proper documentation for products and materials coming into contact with them should be available all the time.

Laboratory Procedures

Semen Analysis

- Semen should be collected into sterile, plastic containers (tissue grade, sperm toxicity tested). Use of spermicidal condoms, creams, and lubricants must be avoided.
- The container must be properly labeled and correct identification **(Fig. 14A)** should be confirmed by the patient.
- Semen analysis and preparation should be commenced within 1 hour of collection as prolonged sperm exposure to seminal plasma is not recommended.
- Semen analysis should be performed according to World Health Organization (WHO) 2010 guidelines.
- Semen preparation is also advisable so as to suggest the most adequate insemination technique.
- Proper records should be maintained for each semen analysis.

Semen Preparation

- Before stating a treatment cycle, at least one diagnostic semen analysis should be performed according to WHO 2010 criteria. A frozen back-up sample should be kept if difficulty in semen collection is anticipated on the day of oocyte retrieval.
- Protocols for semen collection should be documented.
- Records should be maintained on the type of container used, time and place of collection, time interval between collection and analysis, use of medication in previous months, sample origin (ejaculate/epididymal/testicular, donor/partner, fresh/frozen), preparation method, and pre- and postpreparation sperm parameters.
- Sterile technique and universal precautions should be observed in all procedures.

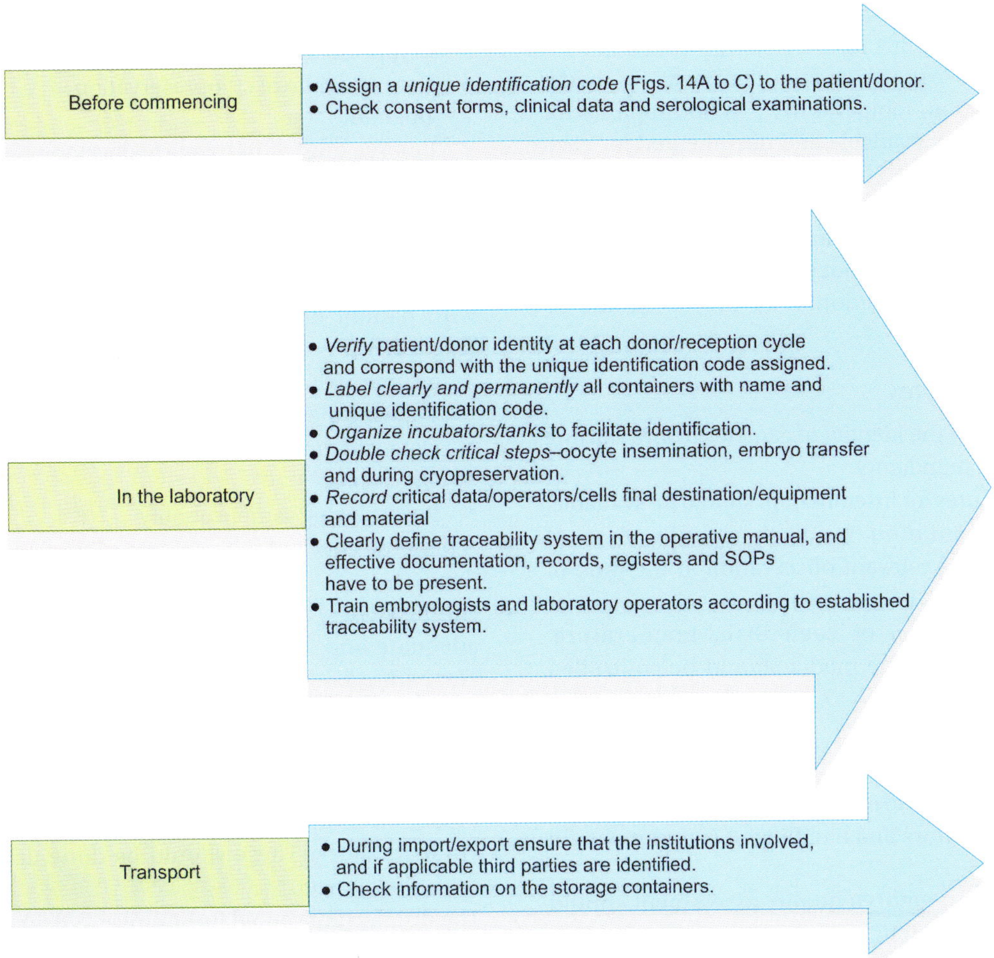

Fig. 13: Standard operating procedures for correctly identifying patients and handling their gametes. (SOP: standard operating procedures)

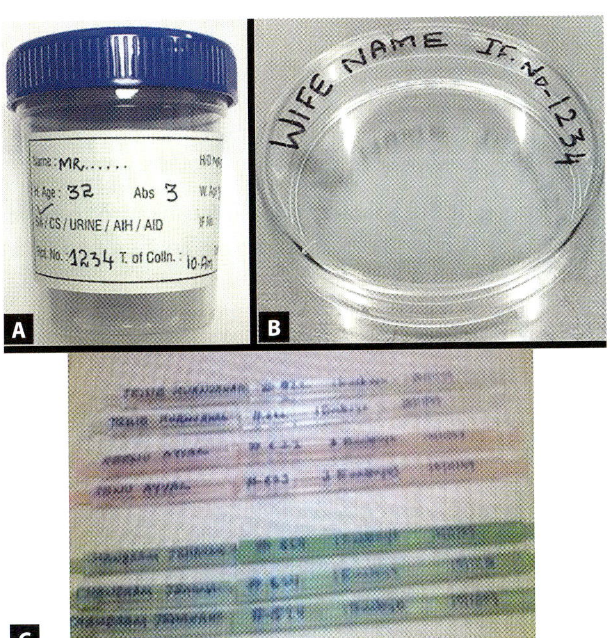

Figs. 14A to C: Verification of patient's identity.

- In cases of donor insemination, complete documentation including source and donor number should be done. Donors should be recruited only from the donor sperm banks which are accredited with the state.

Oocyte Retrieval

- An identity check before starting the procedure is mandatory.
- There should be efficient and quick handling and special attention to temperature and pH must be given. Appropriate equipment should be in place to maintain the temperature at 37°C. Flushing media, collection tubes, and dishes should be prewarmed. The egg retrieval room should be in close proximity to the laboratory and care must be taken to maintain temperature and pH during transportation.
- The time between oocyte retrieval and culture of washed oocytes should be kept at minimum and prolonged exposure of oocytes to follicular fluid is not recommended.

- Operator, timing of retrieval, and the number of collected oocytes must be documented.
- Written SOPs for egg search and identification, media used for aspiration, temperature, pH, and rapidity for evaluation must be available and documented for each procedure.
- Written protocols for description of stages of oocyte quality and maturity, magnification used, and remedies to be used for immature oocytes should be available. The morphological condition of all oocytes should be documented.

Insemination of Oocytes

- A double check of the identity of gametes before starting insemination is mandatory.
- Written procedures for insemination should be available.
- Proper documentation for each sample, time of insemination, and relevant observation at the time of insemination should be maintained.
- During insemination of each dish, temperature, humidity, and pH of the media should be controlled appropriately.

Embryo Culture and Transfer

- Appropriate measures to maintain adequate temperature and pH during culture and handling of embryos should be taken.
- Proper records on embryo quality assessment should be maintained which include the operator, date and time of assessment, and embryo morphological characteristics.
- A double identity check of the patient, the patient's file, and the culture dish(es) **(Fig. 14B)** are a must immediately before the transfer.
- For the transfer procedure, patient records should be maintained regarding:
    - Date and time of embryo transfer
    - Name of the operator
    - Name of the clinician performing the transfer
    - Number, developmental stage, and quality of embryos transferred
    - Type of catheter used
    - Fate of extra embryos and details about the procedure should be documented.

Cryopreservation

- A double check of the patient's identity is mandatory during the following steps:
    - Transfer of samples during labeled cryodish
    - Loading of labeled device **(Fig. 14C)**
    - Deposition in the cryobank
    - Removal from the cryobank
- At cryopreservation, proper documentation should be done on:
    - Device labeling
    - Cryopreservation method
    - Date and time of cryopreservation
    - Operator
    - Embryo quality and stage of development
    - Number of oocytes or embryos per device
    - Number of devices stored per patient
    - Location of stored samples (tank, canister)
- Cryodevices should be clearly and permanently labeled with patient details and unique identification code **(Fig. 14C)**.
- At the time of thawing, documentation should be done on
    - Thawing method
    - Date and time of thawing
    - Operator
    - Post-thawing sample quality
- A periodic check of the contents of cryobank should be done.
- During storage and handling of cryopreserved material, adequate and safe conditions should be maintained. Temperatures should never rise above –130°C. Liquid nitrogen levels should be checked and maintained.

In Vitro Fertilization Laboratory Cleanliness

- Proper cleaning and disinfection of the IVF laboratory are mandatory. These should be done daily after the day's work is over.
- The disinfectant should be nontoxic and odorless.
- Benzyl-alkyldimethyl chloride (Oosafe) or 70% alcohol (usually methanol) is used as disinfectant. Methanol is preferred over ethanol because of its lower vitality index and thus releasing lesser fumes in the laboratory environment.
- The use of halogens such as bleach solutions (chlorine) or betadine (iodine) is contraindicated because they are gamete and embryo toxic.

Protective Measures

The purpose of the protective measures is also to ensure personal safety and prevention of cross contamination and aseptic conditions for gametes and embryos:

- Use of nontoxic (nonpowdered) gloves and masks
- Use of vertical laminar-flow benches
- Use of mechanical pipetting devices
- Use of disposable materials: These must be discarded immediately after use in the proper waste containers. Potential infectious materials must be disposed of in a manner that protects laboratory workers and maintenance, service, and housekeeping staff from exposure to infectious materials in the course of their work.
- Needles and other sharps should be handled with extreme caution and discarded in special containers.

Special containers are used to discard used broken glassware and Pasteur pipettes.
- Use of cosmetics should be minimized and use of perfumes should be avoided.
- Vaccination of all personnel against hepatitis B
- Screening of all patients against infectious diseases
- Staff must be informed when a viral-positive patient has to be treated.

Laboratory Records and Documentation

Good documentation is an essential part of any QMS. The process and equipment validation and laboratory SOPs should be correctly and completely documented.

A document describing a method or process used in a laboratory is known as SOP. It should outline the competence demands on embryologists performing the process.

Records can be in the form of:
- *Paper records:*
  - Conventional method
  - Analysis not possible
- *Electronic records:*
  - Records in spreadsheets/database
  - Analysis possible immediately
  - Also ensures data backup.

It includes the following:
- Patients record in detail
- List of all instruments and their maintenance records
- Logbook of all disposable and culture media in the laboratory for day-to-day work, name of the suppliers, lot numbers, usage date, date of experiment
- Logbook record of all procedures done in the laboratory
- Records of grading the oocyte, embryo, and blastocyst and subsequent stages of development
- Log of laboratory incidents and milestones for future upgradation and modification
- Record of daily QC of equipment
- Record of all consent forms or legal papers regarding third-party reproduction
- Personnel records including educational credentials, continued education, and training
- Record of all publications and research programs essential for further progress of any ART center
- Records of license and registration
- Laboratory meeting minutes and documentation of the next objective

Advantages
- Available for review in future
- Helps in analysis later, when problems arise or improvements are desired
- Helps in determining corrective actions (QA) in future
- Helps to associate the maintained values with patient outcomes.

The records and documentation should be reviewed periodically by laboratory director or supervisory personnel:
- To confirm that the data were collected
- To confirm that corrective actions were taken when needed
- The corrective actions rectified the problem.

Key Performance Indicators

Performance indicators (PIs) are objective measures for evaluating critical healthcare domains (patient safety, effectiveness, equity, patient centeredness, timeliness, and efficiency). Key performance indicators (KPIs) are indicators deemed essential for evaluating the introduction of a technique or process, establishing minimum standards for proficiency, monitoring ongoing performance within a QMS for internal QC, external QA, benchmarking, and quality improvement. The best benchmarking for KPIs is done against an in-house-determined "gold standard." KPIs should be monitored for the whole laboratory **(Table 6)** and for each embryologist and doctor to maintain the principle of confidentiality and not ignoring the stress and decreased self-confidence it can lead to. The KPIs for ART laboratory have been proposed in Vienna Consensus.[49] The KPIs for cryopreservation have been proposed in alpha consensus.[50] These indicators typically assess cryosurvival being evaluated through return of apparently normal function or morphological development and implantation rate post embryo transfer. These are the most common indicators of cryosurvival for oocytes, zygotes, cleavage stage embryos, and blastocyst cryopreserved using either slow freezing or vitrification.

Audits

Clinical audit has been defined as a quality improvement process that seeks to improve patient care and outcomes through systematic review of care against explicit criteria and the implementation of change. Thus, an audit, be it of the IVF laboratory or the clinic, is an impartial and objective assessment. Done properly, it is a strong framework to objectively, dispassionately, and systematically improve patient care in an ongoing manner. It provides a unique opportunity to not only prove competence but also improve quality of care which will finally determine the success of the clinic. It is discussed in Chapter 91.

EMERGENCY PLAN IN IN VITRO FERTILIZATION LABORATORY

- Emergency planning aims to describe the actions to be taken for (in the order of importance):
  - Safety of personnel and patients
  - Protection of all fresh and cryopreserved human material

TABLE 6: Key performance indicators for the ART laboratory.[51]

Key performance indicator	*Calculation*	*Benchmark value (%)*
1. ICSI damage rate	$\frac{\text{No. of damaged or degenerated}}{\text{All oocytes injected}} \times 100$	≤5
2. ICSI normal fertilization rate	$\frac{\text{No. of oocytes with 2PN and 2PB}}{\text{No. of MII oocytes injected}} \times 100$	≥80
3. IVF normal fertilization rate	$\frac{\text{No. of oocytes with 2PN and 2PB}}{\text{No. of COCs inseminated}} \times 100$	≥75
4. Failed fertilization rate (IVF)	$\frac{\text{No. of cycles with no evidence of fertilization}}{\text{No. of stimulated IVF cycles}} \times 100$	<5
5. Cleavage rate	$\frac{\text{No. of cleaved embryos on day 2}}{\text{No. of 2PN/2PB oocytes on day 1}} \times 100$	≥99
6. D2 embryo development rate	$\frac{\text{No. of 4 – cell embryos on day 2}}{\text{No. of normally fertilized oocytes}^a} \times 100$	≥80
7. D3 embryo development rate	$\frac{\text{No. of eight cell embryos on day 3}}{\text{No. of normally fertilized oocytes}^a} \times 100$	≥70
8. Blastocyst development rate	$\frac{\text{No. of blastocysts day 5}}{\text{No. of normally fertilized oocytes}^a} \times 100$	≥60
9. Successful biopsy rate	$\frac{\text{No. of biopsies with DNA detected}}{\text{No. of biopsies performed}} \times 100$	≥95
10. Blastocyst cryosurvival rate	$\frac{\text{No. of blastocysts appearing intact}}{\text{No. of blastocyst warmed}} \times 100$	≥99
11. Implantation rate (cleavage stage)[b]	$\frac{\text{No. of sacs seen on ultrasound}}{\text{No. of embryos transferred}} \times 100$	≥35
12. Implantation rate (blastocyst stage)[b]	$\frac{\text{No. of sacs seen on ultrasound}}{\text{No. of blastocysts transferred}} \times 100$	≥60

[a]Defined as oocytes with 2PN and 2PB on Day 1

[b]Based on total no. of embryos transferred to all patients in the reference group, not just those for whom an implantation occurred (ART: assisted reproductive technique; ICSI: intracytoplasmic sperm injection; IVF: in vitro fertilization)

- Limitation of damage to equipment and medical records
- Communication measures in emergency situations should be clear for all personnel.
- Facilities:
  - Loss of electrical power should be compensated by generators or uninterrupted power supply (UPS) systems.
  - In case of failure of automatic supply lines of liquid N_2, tanks should be filled manually. A fully filled reserve tank should be kept as a backup.
- Equipment:
  - In case of power failure, critical equipment should be prioritized.
  - A backup of all critical equipment should be available which should be fully validated and ready for use.
  - Back-up cooled freezers and refrigerators should be available.
  - Cryopreservation vessels: It may be necessary to move tanks to another location.

TABLE 7: Checklist in in-vitro fertilization laboratory.[52-55]

Daily checklist	1. CO_2 incubator (temperature, CO_2, and humidity) 2. CO_2 cylinder (before and after procedure) 3. Temperature of Petri dish warmer 4. Temperature of heating stage, dry bath, and heating block 5. Bubbles in Teflon tubes of micromanipulator 6. Microscopes 7. Refrigerator 8. Media and consumable stocks 9. Overall cleaning 10. Daily disposable of waste materials is mandatory
Weekly checklist	1. Interiors of incubator—soiling and water level 2. Liquid nitrogen levels 3. pH meter check of the culture media 4. Circulating fan of the incubator
Monthly checklist	1. Stock of all disposables 2. Changing liquid paraffin of micromanipulator tubes 3. Checking uninterrupted power supply, alarm or call break system
Quarterly checklist	1. Servicing and calibration of incubator 2. Servicing of microscopes 3. Fumigation of laboratory
Half yearly checklist	1. Change of filter of laminar airflow 2. Change of filter of Coda tower
Annual checklist	1. Overall laboratory complex 2. Record keeping and maintenance

- Medical records to identify the ownership of human tissue should be kept on a secure Web server.
- Regular revision of the emergency plan is necessary.
- Third-party arrangements should be in place with another IVF laboratory for emergency transfer of gametes and embryos (fresh and cryopreserved).

CHECKLIST IN IN VITRO FERTILIZATION LABORATORY

A regular monitoring of laboratory on daily, weekly, monthly, quarterly, half yearly, or yearly basis is mandatory to ensure QC and optimum results **(Table 7)**.

BENEFITS AND DRAWBACKS OF QUALITY MANAGEMENT SYSTEM

Quality management is not a task that can be performed alongside regular work. It comes with its own advantages and disadvantages **(Table 8)**.

TABLE 8: Benefits and drawbacks of quality management system.

Benefits	***Drawbacks***
• *For patients:* Consistency, reproducibility, and highest quality of all diagnostic and therapeutic procedures • *For health insurance companies:* Highest quality care for their clients • *For IVF laboratory:* Trouble-shooting, maintenance of equipment and milieu, improved and standardized care • *For IVF clinic management:* – Optimization of working processes – Active risk management – Powerful mechanism for internal and external controls and decision making (saving costs) • Documented improvement of pregnancy rate	• Increased workload for management • Time consuming • Not always easy to motivate all the staff (increased competence, but also responsibility) • Expensive • Direct investments • Audits • Not easy to explain to patients

(IVF: in vitro fertilization)

CONCLUSION

Quality management is an ongoing process and is crucial for future follow up. At the beginning it appears to be endless, immense, time consuming, expensive, requiring lot of commitment, communication, cooperation and motivation, but once completed, it helps in standardization, reproducibility, traceability, transparency with increased efficiency and better results. It also helps in gaining trust and satisfaction of the patients. It is a never ending commitment and the only way by which we can promise safe and efficient IVF treatment for all patients.

KEY POINTS

- Quality management is an ongoing process and is crucial for future follow-up. At the beginning, it appears to be endless, immense, time consuming, expensive, requiring lot of commitment, communication, cooperation, and motivation but once completed, it helps in standardization, reproducibility, traceability, transparency with increased efficiency, and better results.
- It also helps in gaining trust and satisfaction of the patients.
- The QC should be at each level; laboratory personnel, equipment, consumables, procedures, record keeping and documentation, and also while doing audits.
- A proper plan including a backup plan and an emergency plan should always be ready.
- It is a never-ending commitment and the only way by which we can promise safe and efficient IVF treatment for all patients.

REFERENCES

1. Alper MM; International Standards Organization. Experience with ISO quality control in assisted reproductive technology. Fertil Steril. 2013;100:1503-8.
2. Kastrop PM. Quality management in the ART laboratory. Reprod Biomed Online. 2003;7(6):691-4.
3. Higdon HL 3rd, Blackhurst DW, Boone WR. Incubator management in an assisted reproductive technology laboratory. Fertil Steril. 2008;89(3):703-10.
4. Bavister BD, Andrews JC. A rapid sperm motility bioassay procedure for quality-control testing of water and culture media. J In Vitro Fert Embryo Transf. 1988;5:67-75.
5. Mortimer D, Cohen J, Mortimer ST, Fawzy M, McCulloh DH, Morbeck DE, et al. Cairo consensus on the IVF laboratory environment and air quality: report of an expert meeting. Reprod Biomed Online. 2018;36(6):658-74.
6. Legro RS, Sauer MV, Mottla GL, Richter KS, Li X, Dodson WC, et al. Effect of air quality on assisted human reproduction. Hum Reprod. 2010 May;25(5):1317-24.
7. Almeida PA, Bolton VY. The effect of temperature fluctuations on the cytoskeletal organization and chromosome constitution of the human oocyte. Zygote. 1995;3:357-65.
8. Pickering SJ, Braude PR, Johnson MH, Cant A, Currie J. Transient cooling to room temperature can cause irreversible disruption of the meiotic spindle in the human oocyte. Fertil Steril. 1990;54:102-8.
9. Wang WH, Meng L, Hackett RJ, Odenbourg R, Keefe DL. Limited recovery of meiotic spindles in living human oocytes after cooling-rewarming observed using polarized light microscopy. Hum Reprod. 2001;16:2374-8.
10. Swain JE. Optimizing the culture environment in the IVF laboratory: impact of pH and buffer capacity on gamete and embryo quality. Reprod Biomed Online. 2010 Jul;21(1):6-16.
11. Lane M, Mitchell M, Cashman KS, Feil D, Wakefi eld S, Zander-Fox DL. To QC or not to QC: the key to a consistent laboratory? Reprod Fertil Dev. 2008;20:23-32.
12. Swain JE, Pool TB. Culture media in IVF: Decisions for the laboratory. In: Zsolt PN, Alex CV, Ashok A (Eds). Practical Manual of In Vitro Fertilization: Advanced Methods and Novel Devices. New York, NY: Springer; 2012.
13. Mastroianni Jr L, Jones R. Oxygen tension within the rabbit fallopian tube. J Reprod Fertil. 1965;9:99-102.
14. Ross RN, Graves CN. O2 levels in the female rabbit reproductive tract. J Anim Sci. 1974;39:994.
15. Fischer B, Bavister BD. Oxygen tension in the oviduct and uterus of rhesus monkeys, hamsters and rabbits. J Reprod Fertil. 1993;99:673-9.
16. Miller KF, Goldberg JM, Collins RL. The result of an interlaboratory comparison of embryo culture media is dependent on culture method. J Assist Reprod Genet. 1993;(Suppl):226.
17. Shimada M, Kawano N, Terada T. Delay of nuclear maturation and reduction in developmental competence of pig oocytes after mineral oil overlay of in vitro maturation media. Reproduction. 2002;124:557-64.
18. Van den Abbeel E, Vitrier S, Lebrun F, Van Steirteghem A. Optimized mouse bioassays for the detection of embryology contaminants. Hum Reprod. 1999;14 (Suppl 1):114.
19. Boone WR, Shapiro SS. Quality control in the in vitro fertilization laboratory. Theriogenology. 1990;33:23-50.
20. Fleming TP, Pratt HPM, Braude PR. The use of mouse preimplantation embryos for quality control of culture reagents in human in vitro fertilization programs: a cautionary note. Fertil Steril. 1987;47:858-60.
21. Provo MB, Herr C. Washed paraffi n oil becomes toxic to mouse embryos upon exposure to sunlight. Theriogenology. 1998;49:21.
22. Otsuki J, Nagai Y, Chiba K. Peroxidation of mineral oil used in droplet culture is detrimental to fertilization and embryo development. Fertil Steril. 2007;88:741-3.
23. Bavister BD. A consistently successful procedure for in vitro fertilization of golden hamster eggs. Gamete Res. 1989;23:139-58.
24. Borque C, Pintado B, García P, Sánchez R. Effect of washing oil on in vitro development of mouse embryos. Theriogenology. 1996;45:206.
25. Li H, Zhang LX, Zhong Y, Zhu K, Zhang T, Wang MK. Effect of washing mineral oil on development of mouse embryos in vitro and in vivo after embryo transfer. Biol Reprod. 2006;(Suppl):133.
26. Dinnie H, Daniele A, Labrie S, Monte L, Grow D, Arny M. Microdrop insemination for optimal fertilization in an in vitro fertilization (IVF) program: a prospective study comparing sibling oocytes. Fertil Steril. 1995;64 (Suppl 1):S257.
27. Cunningham KJ, McCarthy CB, Russell JB. The pH change in a microdroplet system under oil with different numbers of sperm added for insemination. Fertil Steril. 1994;62 Suppl 1:S47.
28. Wiley LM, Yamami S, Van Muyden D. Effect of potassium concentration, type of protein supplement, and embryo density on mouse preimplantation development in vitro. Fertil Steril. 1986;45:111-9.
29. Paria BC, Dey SK. Preimplantation embryo development in vitro: cooperative interactions among embryos and role of growth factors. Proc Natl Acad Sci. 1990;87:4756-60.
30. Canesco RS, Sparks AET, Pearson RE, Gwazdauskas FC. Embryo density and medium volume effects on early murine embryo development. J Assist Reprod Genet. 1992;9: 454-7.
31. Lane M, Gardner DK. Effect of incubation volume and embryo density on the development and viability of mouse embryos in vitro. Hum Reprod. 1992;7:558-92.
32. Salahuddin S, Ookutsu S, Goto K, Nakanishi Y, Nagata Y. Effects of embryo density and co-culture of unfertilized oocytes on embryonic development of in-vitro fertilized mouse embryos. Hum Reprod. 1995;10:2382-5.
33. O'Neill C. Role of autocrine mediators in the regulation of embryo viability: lessons from animal models. J Assist Reprod Genet. 1998;15:460-5.
34. Gil MA, Abeydeera LR, Day BN, Vazquez JM, Roca J, Martinez EA. Effect of the volume of medium and number of oocytes during in vitro fertilization on embryo development in pigs. Theriogenology. 2003;60:767-76.
35. Ali J. Continuous ultra micro-drop (cUMD) culture yields higher pregnancy & implantation rates than either larger-drop culture or fresh-medium replacement. Clin Embryol. 2004;7(2):1-17.
36. Moinipanah R, Anderson R, Montgomery J, Steinberg J, Quinn P. Higher rates of fertilization in vitro of human oocytes using a smaller volume of medium for coincubation of gametes. Fertil Steril. 1994;62 Suppl 1:S228.

37. Goovaerts IGF, Leroy JLMR, Van Soom A, De Clercq JBP, Anries S, Bols PEJ. Effect of cumulus cell coculture and oxygen tension on the in vitro developmental competence of bovine zygotes cultured singly. Theriogenology. 2009;71: 729-38.
38. Wagner-Coughlin CM, Maravilla AE, Nikurs AR, Scoccia B, Scommegna A, Marut EL. Microdroplets under oil improves embryo quality even when an isolette is used. Fertil Steril. 1994;62 Suppl 1:S177.
39. Stokes PJ, Abeydeera LR, Leese HJ. Development of porcine embryo in vivo and in vitro: evidence for embryo 'cross talk' in vitro. Dev Biol. 2005;284:62-71.
40. Nijs M, Franssen K, Cox A, Wissmann D, Ruis H, Ombelet W. Reprotoxicity of intrauterine insemination and in vitro fertilization-embryo transfer disposables and products: a 4-year survey. Fertil Steril. 2009;92(2):527-35.
41. Hossain AM, Osuamkpe CO, Magamani M. Extended culture of human spermatozoa in the laboratory may have practical value in the assisted reproductive procedures. Fertil Steril. 2008;89:237-9.
42. Amaral A, Paiva C, Baptista M, Sousa AP, Ramalho-Santos J. Exogenous glucose improves long-standing human sperm motility, viability, and mitochondrial function. Fertil Steril. 2011;96(4):848-50.
43. Vargas J, Crausaz M, Senn A, Germond M. Sperm toxicity of "nonspermicidal" lubricant and ultrasound gels used in reproductive medicine. Fertil Steril. 2011;95:835-6.
44. Hughes PM, Morbeck DE, Hudson SB, Fredrickson JR, Walker DL, Coddington CC. Peroxides in mineral oil used for in vitro fertilization: defining limits of standard quality control assays. J Assist Reprod Genet. 2010;27(2-3):87-92.
45. Morbeck DE, Khan Z, Barnidge DR, Walker DL. Washing mineral oil reduces contaminants and embryotoxicity. Fertil Steril. 2010;94:2747-52.
46. Lierman S, DeSutter P, Dhont M, Van der Elst J. Doublequality control reveals high-level toxicity in gloves used for operator protection in assisted reproductive technology. Fertil Steril. 2007;88(Suppl 2):1266-72.
47. De Jonge CJ, Centola GM, Reed ML, Shabanowitz RB, Simon SD, Quinn P. Human sperm survival assay as a bioassay for the assisted reproductive technologies laboratory. J Androl. 2003;24(1):16-8.
48. Boone WR, Higdon HL, Johnson JE. Quality management issues in the assisted reproduction laboratory. J Reprod Stem Cell Biotechnol. 2010;1:30-107.
49. ESHRE Special Interest Group of Embryology and Alpha Scientists in Reproductive Medicine. Electronic address: coticchio.biogenesi@grupposandonato.it. The Vienna consensus: report of an expert meeting on the development of ART laboratory performance indicators. Reprod Biomed Online. 2017 Nov;35(5):494-510.
50. Alpha Scientists in Reproductive Medicine. The Alpha consensus meeting on cryopreservation key performance indicators and benchmarks: proceedings of an expert meeting. Reprod Biomed Online. 2012;25(2):146-67.
51. Nagy ZP, Varghese AC, Agarwal A. Practical Manual of In Vitro Fertilization: Advanced Methods and Novel Devices. New York: Springer; 2012.
52. ESHRE. (2015). Revised guidelines for good practice in IVF laboratories (2015). [online].
53. Practice Committee of American Society for Reproductive Medicine; Practice Committee of Society for Assisted Reproductive Technology. Revised guidelines for human embryology and andrology laboratories. Fertil Steril. 2008;90(5 Suppl):S45-59.
54. Blechová R, Pivodová D. Limulus amoebocyte lysate (lal) test—an alternative method for detection of bacterial endotoxins. Acta Vet Brno. 2001;70:291-6.
55. Gardner DK, Weissman A, Howles CM, Shoham Z. Textbook of Assisted Reproductive Techniques: Laboratory Perspectives. United Kingdom: Taylor and Francis Group; 2018.

CHAPTER 91

Auditing of Clinical Outcomes

Arati R Rao

INTRODUCTION

Clinical audit has been defined as a quality improvement process that seeks to improve patient care and outcomes through systematic review of care against explicit criteria and the implementation of change.

Aspects of the structures, processes, and outcomes of care are selected and systematically evaluated against explicit criteria. Where indicated, changes are implemented at individual, team, or service level and further monitoring is used to confirm improvement to healthcare delivery [National Institute for Health and Care Excellence (NICE) Guidelines, 2002].

The very first clinical audit was carried out by Miss Florence Nightingale during the Crimean War (1853–1855) where she meticulously demonstrated a significant reduction in mortality rates in the hospital wards by applying strict sanitary routines and standards of hygiene. Gradually, over the years conducting regular clinical audits has become quite the norm in many countries, but this unfortunately is not yet well accepted in India.

In fact, a study conducted by CMC Vellore in 2012 suggested that the root cause of noncompliance with audit was simply because it was not a priority in the busy schedules of practicing clinicians.[1] And, this was very likely due to a basic lack of understanding of the audit process.

BENEFITS OF AUDIT (BOX 1)

The benefits of a properly conducted audit are multifold—affecting not only the patients but also their caregivers (clinical staff) and the management too.

To the patient, regular audits will ensure quality, consistency, and efficacy of care.

To the staff, audits bring about significant professional development. They provide knowledge about newer developments in the field, current and established guidelines, and more importantly identifies the need for training. Data collection, an integral part of the audit, provides opportunities to publish.

BOX 1: Benefits of audit.

To the patient:
- Quality of care
- Consistency of care
- Effectiveness of care
- Patient satisfaction

To the staff:
- Professional development
- Awareness of current treatment guidelines and protocols
- Opportunities to publish
- Identifies training needs
- Improves clinical efficacy
- Improves communication

To the management:
- Strengthens self-regulation
- Improves cost effectiveness
- Reduces complaints and litigation
- Identifies the need for organizational change

All in all, *audits improve clinical effectiveness.*
They also help to improve communication—both interpersonal as well as intradepartmental.

To the management, audits will not only improve cost effectiveness, but will also reduce the risk of litigation and complaints. It also self-regulates and identifies the need for organizational change.

A properly conducted audit allows for an objective assessment of the quality of care with a focus on "how to improve". Transparency and accountability lead to high standards of care.

Who Should be Present at Audit Meetings?

Typically an audit meeting should have the primary caregivers—clinicians, nurses, andrologists, and embryologists—the persons who will implement the proposed changes; management representatives who will authorize any changes and whenever possible, the clinical audit team to regulate the entire process.

THE AUDIT CYCLE (FLOWCHART 1)

The audit cycle is a series of steps that are involved in a complete audit.

This cycle is closely interlinked with the reaudit cycle which is used to audit the changes that were suggested in the first audit—a sort of closing the loop process.

As is evident the audit is focused on quality of patient care. It is neither a research nor a process to collect and analyze data. Neither is it a criticism of clinical practices or technical competence **(Boxes 2 to 4)**.

SECTIONS TO BE AUDITED

Sections audited [International Organization for Standardization (ISO) 9001-2000]:

- Document control
- Record control
- Quality policy
- Quality objectives
- *Job description:* Responsibility and authority
- Provision of resources, infrastructure, and work environment
- *Human resources:* Competence, awareness, and training
- *Planning of product realization:* Process maps, documents, and records
- *Customer-related processes:* Consent, flow sheets, and communications
- Purchase
- *Service provision:* Procedures, validation, etc.
- Monitoring and measuring devices.

Flowchart 1: The audit cycle.

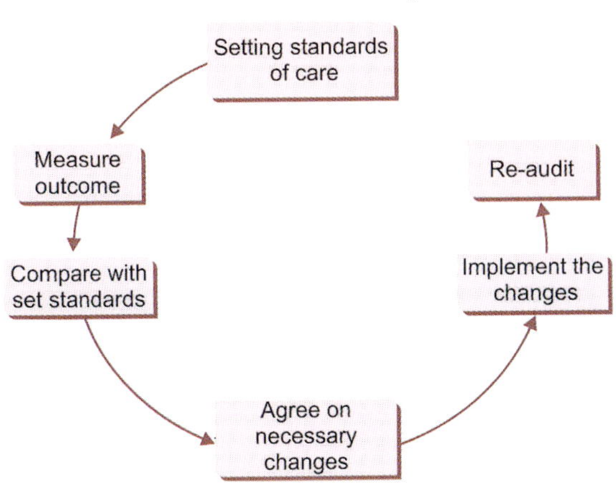

BOX 2: Differences between audit, research, and clinical service evaluation.[2]

- *Clinical audit:* Measures current practice against evidence-based clinical standards
- *Research:* Investigates the effects of new or existing treatment or technique on patients/carers
- *Service evaluation:* Evaluates the effectiveness or efficacy of current practice/services

An audit, be it of the in vitro fertilization (IVF) laboratory or the clinic is an impartial and objective assessment.

Done properly, it is a strong framework to objectively, dispassionately, and systematically improve patient care in an ongoing manner. It provides a unique opportunity to not only prove competence but to improve quality of care which will finally determine the success of the clinic.

SETTING STANDARDS

Audit is a process where actual practice is compared to established standards of good practice.

A standard is an explicit statement describing the area of care that is being measured.

The recommendations of standards are usually from international bodies such as the Royal College of Obstetricians and Gynaecologists (RCOG), American Society for Reproductive Medicine (ASRM), European Society of Human Reproduction and Embryology (ESHRE), etc.[3,4] Local consensus of expected practice norms may also be used.

BOX 3: Types of audit: horizontal, vertical and examination.

- *Horizontal audit:* Horizontal audit takes place within an organization and is often referred to as a "peer audit". This is used to evaluate the effectiveness of a process of one group as compared to another group within the same organization. An example of this type of audit is evaluation of pregnancy rates following frozen embryo transfer from two branches of the same clinic with the same quality management standards. A horizontal audit can be used to evaluate the shortcomings of a vertical audit
- *Vertical audit:* Vertical audits on the other hand dig deep. They focus on a single process or procedure. It may involve direct questioning of the operator, verification of related documents, and details of instrument calibration. This is easy to follow and can be used regularly. However, as it focuses on a single process, all aspects of the clinic may not be covered every time
- *Examination audit:* This is a type of vertical audit. It involves auditing of a procedure as it is being performed. It is used to ensure that the person has a good understanding of the procedure and adheres to the standard protocols set for this purpose. An example of this would be an audit of a clinician performing an embryo transfer

BOX 4: Types of audit: internal and external.

- *Internal audit:* Internal audits are conducted by the Internal Audit Committee composed of staff members/employees trained in the audit process. The management usually selects personnel who are familiar with the standards as well as the processes/activities performed. The audits may be conducted monthly or once in every 3 months (quarterly)
- *External audit:* External audits are conducted by outside organizations which are regulated by the International Organization for Standardization (ISO). Once a year (annual) along with a complete audit once in 3 years is recommended

In an IVF unit setting standards or benchmarking is used to compare services and results against the best in the field **(Box 5)**.

Obviously, the target of setting standards is to achieve 100% compliance with the set standards **(Boxes 6 and 7)**.[5]

SELECTING TOPICS FOR AUDIT

SMART forms the basis of selecting topics for an audit. Any area or process that is to be audited should basically fit the SMART criteria **(Box 8)**.

IN VITRO FERTILIZATION PROGRAM PERFORMANCE INDICATORS

For a patient, pregnancy and implantation rates are the most important indicators of a successfully run program. Cost and location of the clinic are also important.

While these indicators indicate the success of the IVF program as a whole, it must be remembered that standardizing performance indicators becomes difficult because of the multiple variables in this field. It is recommended that each program sets its own benchmarks for that particular function.

Listed here are the some examples of performance indicators **(Box 9)**.

It must be remembered that program performance indicators should be further classified based on the patient's age and the type of procedure used **(Boxes 10 to 14)**.

BOX 5: Types of benchmarking.

- *Internal:* Comparison between centers within a group. In an ideal world, each center within a group should have the same results anywhere in the world. This not only depends on the clinicians but on operational uniformity
- *Competitive:* Comparison with direct competitors
- *Functional:* Comparison with the best in the field. This will influence the stimulation protocols, drugs used, and technologies applied. For any of this to be successful, a strong internal quality management systems initiative is essential to maintain uniformity of practice

BOX 6: Classification of standards.

- *Structure:* What do you need?
- *Process:* What do you do?
- *Outcome of care:* What do you expect?

BOX 7: Tips for setting standards.

- Evidence-based
- Reflect current practice; not what was done 2 years ago
- It should be achievable and realistic
- It should have measurable parameters to allow for comparison

BOX 8: SMART criteria for selecting an audit topic.

S—specific
M—measurable
A—achievable
R—related
T—time bound

BOX 9: Program performance indicators.

- *Pregnancy rates:*
  - Biochemical [beta-human chorionic gonadotropin (hCG) positive]
  - Clinical (identification of the gestational sac)
  - Ongoing (fetal heart pulsations visualized by ultrasound at 7 weeks)
- *Implantation rates:*
  - Overall implantation rates = total number of gestational sacs seen on ultrasound/total number of embryos transferred
  - Multiple implantation = proportion of pregnancies with more than one gestational sac on ultrasound

BOX 10: Laboratory performance indicators.

- Oocyte grade/maturity
- IVF fertilization rates (proportion of inseminated oocytes that have 2 PN the day after insemination)
- ICSI fertilization rates (proportion of injected oocytes that have 2 PN the day after insemination)
- Poor or failed fertilization rated (proportion of cycles in which <25% of inseminated oocytes were fertilized)
- ICSI damage rates (proportion of oocytes that disintegrated during or just after the ICSI procedure)
- Zygote grade
- Cleavage rates (proportion of zygotes that have cleaved to become embryos)
- Embryo development rate (proportion of cleaved embryos that become four cells 2 days after insemination; proportion of cleaved embryos that become eight cells 3 days after insemination; proportion of cleaved embryos that become blastocysts 5 days after insemination)
- Embryo fragmentation rate (proportion of eight cell embryos with <5% fragmentation)
- Embryo grade (proportion of day 3 embryos with the highest grade)
- Embryo utilization rate (proportion of embryos that were either transferred or cryopreserved)
- Embryo cryosurvival rates (proportion of embryos that survived freezing and thawing cycle)

BOX 11: Efficiency indicators.

- Number of cases handled by individual operators
- Time lag between enquiry and response
- Proportion of patient records which are complete
- Number of phone calls answered
- Number of voicemails received
- Average time between conduction of a test and communication of results to clinician and patient

BOX 12: Best practice indicators.

- Incident reports
- Treatment complications
- Incidence of ovarian hyperstimulation syndrome (OHSS)
- Infection rates
- Number of positive and negative comments received

BOX 13: Laboratory indicators.

- Number of IVF and ICSI procedures done each month
- Utilization of consumables
- *Equipment efficacy:* For example, volume of liquid nitrogen required for top-up each month

(ICSI: intracytoplasmic sperm injection; IVF: in vitro fertilization)

BOX 14: Financial considerations.

- Revenue each month
- Comparison of fee structuring with other centers
- Number of referrals each month

The importance of identifying reference populations cannot be undermined. Stratification based on population demographics allows for more robust statistical data.

SETTING OBJECTIVES

An objective is a specific statement that clearly defines which aspects of quality are going to be measured in order to show that the purpose (aim) of the audit has been met.

It should be unambiguous so that there is no confusion about the focus and purpose of the audit.

While a center may have multiple objectives—this often may be difficult to handle for the audit team.

It will be better to divide the objectives into smaller and more manageable segments. As the proverb goes "one thing at a time and that done well".

It is always better to complete one audit, implement the changes, wait for them to work, and then move on to the next objective.

DATA COLLECTION

There are no specific definitions as to the sample sizes needed for clinical audits. This will depend on what is being audited and how easy it is to get the required information.

Random sampling is generally the best way to get a representation of the population being studied.

It is crucial that the sample is collected very carefully as inaccurate data can skew the audit results and give false results.

While clinical audits do not need ethical clearance, they are still bound by the data protection act and should be conducted within an ethical framework.

DATA ANALYSIS

The aim of data analysis is to convert data into useful information—in this case to see if the audit standards are complied with.

Details of statistical analysis are out of the scope of this chapter.

WRITING AN AUDIT REPORT[6]

An audit report outlines the measures taken to complete the audit.

Cover Sheet

It should include the audit title, date, name of lead auditor, and all the team members.

Introduction

It is a brief paragraph on the service being audited and the target group. It should also mention why the audit was undertaken and which standards were applied.

Aim

It is the purpose of the audit.

Standards

It is a list of the expected practice standards against which the audit will compare the current practice standards.

Methodology

It is the methods and tools used to collect data.

Size and Scope

This section documents—who was involved in conducting the audit, the target group, sample size, and the time frame when the audit was conducted.

Results/Findings

Results of the analyzed data should be presented in an easy-to-read graphical or tabular form.

Areas for change are identified along with any findings that may help in implementation of the changes.

Conclusion/Summary

It summarizes the findings of the audit along with evidence taken from within the results.

The report will indicate whether the set standards have been met—compliance or noncompliance when the standards have not been met. Noncompliance may be critical or noncritical.

Critical noncompliance is synonymous with a complete failure to adhere to the set standards. In other words, it is a system failure. On the other hand, a noncritical noncompliance is a failure to meet the set standards to a level where there will not be a total system failure.

Recommendations

Realistic changes are based on the audit findings.

The reaudit report should, in addition to the earlier, clearly state the changes that were proposed in the original

BOX 15: The action plan.

- Define what needs to change
- Define the actions necessary to bring about that change
- Establish a timeline for these actions to be carried out
- Identify person or persons responsible for these actions
- Indicate the evidence needed to show that these actions/ recommendations have been implemented

BOX 16: Simplified audit report.

- Observations
- Recommendations for improvement
- Timelines for implementation of change

audit and an assessment of the actions taken. A comparison of the findings of the current audit to the previous one must be documented.

RECOMMENDATIONS FOR CHANGE

Once the audit report has been accepted, the proposed changes must be discussed to fully understand why they are needed and how they will make a difference.

The proposed changes following a properly conducted audit constitute the action plan **(Box 15)**.

This should include clearly defined recommendations for change. Who should do it (named person) and by when (appropriate date and time) to give a realistic timeline for implementation.

Sample of audit information sheet	
Audit number	Date
Center name and address	
Department audited	
Lead auditor name:	Auditor 2 name
Supervisor name.	Signature
Section audited	

SCOPE OF THE AUDIT

Name the documents/processes audited. If only part of a process or document was completed—describe the same.

AUDIT REPORT

The final report should be simple, easy to read, and understand **(Box 16)**.

BOX 17: Traits of competent certification bodies.

- Accreditation to certify medical institutions
- Experience in certifying in vitro fertilization (IVF) clinics
- IVF specialists (clinicians and embryologists) on team
- Adequate time (at least 2 days) allotted to each center

Some organizations believe that by finding no non-conformances, i.e., a perfect audit indicates a clinic with an outstanding performance. However, this is more likely to indicate a poorly conducted audit as even the best clinics will always have scope for improvement.

Hence, the importance of finding suitable auditors/ certification bodies **(Box 17)**.

KEY POINTS

- An audit, be it of the IVF laboratory or the clinic is an impartial and objective assessment. Done properly it is a strong framework to objectively, dispassionately, and systematically improve patient care in an ongoing manner.
- It provides a unique opportunity to not only prove competence but to improve quality of care which will finally determine the success of the clinic.

REFERENCES

1. Chandy S, George O, Joseph L. Clinical Audit Program: A Feeder and a Model for the Nation. Vellore: Christian Medical College; 2012.
2. Daly M. (2008). Clinical Audit Criteria and Guidance Working Group. Accessed at https://www.lenus.ie/handle/10147/305196.
3. The European Society of Human Reproduction and Embryology (ESHRE). ESHRE Campus Symposium. London: ESHRE Symposium; 2010.
4. The International Organization for Standardization (ISO). (2018). All about ISO. [online] Available from: www.iso.org/about-us.html.
5. Mortimer D, Mortimer ST. Quality and risk management in the IVF laboratory. Cambridge: Cambridge University Press; 2005.
6. The National Institute for Health and Care Excellence (NICE). (2002). Principles for Best Practice in Clinical Audit. [online] Available from: www.nice.org.uk/media/default/About/what-we-do/Into-practice/principles-for-best-practice-in-clinical-audit.pdf.

CHAPTER 92

Periconceptional Challenges and Modifiable Risk Factors: Evidence to Practice

Revathi S Rajan

INTRODUCTION

Adverse outcomes due to dysfunctional placentation should be mapped from the time of implantation which is the essence of an "extended inverted pyramid" of prenatal care.[1]

This emphasizes the need to identify the possible risk factors that could complicate pregnancy especially in those undergoing "assisted reproduction" periconceptionally to optimize perinatal outcomes. Many of these women have no previous obstetric experience posing a challenge to the clinicians to decide risk modulation protocols that are conventionally based on previous obstetric outcomes.

Hence, it is quintessential to identify modifiable risk factors periconceptionally influencing conception and beyond.

BACKGROUND

Understanding of the complex interaction at the maternal fetal interface is crucial both in terms of challenges and adaptive mechanisms as any imbalance in these could lead to adverse pregnancy outcomes. This emphasizes the need for anticipating clinical stress prior to its onset based on the factors that help effective prediction; the true essence of risk modulation.

Here are listed various challenges and their implications encountered during the periconceptional period. Though their implications have not been fully understood; identifying modifiable risk factors prior to conception can contribute to better fertility and pregnancy outcomes.

OXIDATIVE STRESS

A disequilibrium between reactive oxygen species and processes of detoxification and restoration leads to oxidative stress. Evidence has shown that presence of inflammation without an adequate oxidizing environment may trigger complications including early pregnancy losses, preeclampsia and fetal growth restriction. Prediction of the same using biomarkers of oxidative stress is still not yet standardized. Hence, interventions to counter oxidative stress and its implications are still being researched.[2]

IMMUNE REGULATION IN PREGNANCY (FIG. 1)

The "placenta" which forms the maternal fetal interface is a complex unit that is composed of regulatory factors that could influence continuation of pregnancy.

As the pregnancy progresses, the regulatory mechanisms controlling these factors change and the process is almost clearly defined.

The trophoblasts primarily invade the uterus facilitating an active gas exchange including provision of nutrients and also simultaneously allow disposal of waste at the maternal-fetal interface.

The placenta allows for immune tolerance facilitating pregnancy progression. Any impairment of this results in a disease state-specific to pregnancy.

Maternal adaptive responses also occur allowing placental and fetal development. These include a shift of the immune response from T helper 1 (Th1) to Th2 profile which

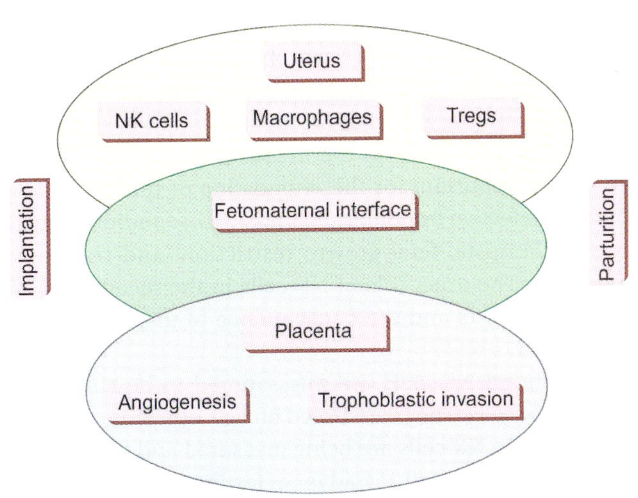

Fig. 1: Immune regulation pathway.
(NK: natural killer; Tregs: regulatory T cells)

is considered to be typical during pregnancy. The cluster of differentiation 4 (CD4) regulatory T cells (Tregs) which predominate in the latter half of the pregnancy modulate maternal immune responses directed toward the fetus and are triggered by paternal antigens.

The uterine natural killer (NK) cells ($CD56^{bright}$ and $CD16^{dim}$) have been recognized as the dominant cell type responsible for trophoblastic invasion.

"Implantation" is facilitated by the infiltration of the syncytiotrophoblasts into the endometrium and the differentiation of the trophectoderm into cytotrophoblasts for the embryo. The extravillous trophoblasts are those syncytiotrophoblasts in contact with the decidua and serve as an endocrine organ coordinating with maternal adaptive immune responses.

Fetus as an Allograft

"Pregnancy" is a complex regulatory mechanism involving both inflammatory and immunosuppressive responses leading to the acceptance of the fetal allograft. The immunoregulatory factors generated by the placenta help in establishing a state of immune tolerance and protects rejection of the developing fetus.

The trophoblastic invasion and angiogenesis are controlled by mechanisms involving both immune and vascular networks with maternal surveillance mechanisms in the fetus favoring progressive growth.

The trophoblasts are primarily important and crucial for the survival of the fetal allograft.

In a healthy pregnancy, these trophoblasts are resistant to "NK cells" and lymphocyte activated cells and define the fetoplacental interface. They also express NK cell type Fc-gamma receptor III (responsible for phagocytosis) and other immunosuppressive factors similar to transforming growth factor-beta (TGF-β).

Natural Killer Cells

Malfunction of the natural killer (NK) cells has been attributed to infertility and recurrent miscarriages.

Natural killer cells identified by CD56 predominantly inhabit the uterus especially at the implantation site. They are in close contact with the invading trophoblastic cells which are important for the remodeling of spiral arteries. There is defective trophoblastic invasion in conditions such as preeclampsia, fetal growth restriction, and recurrent abortions. The exact role of NK cells in the recognition of the trophoblasts and the consequence of this is yet to be established.

Peripheral NK cells are misassumed to be similar to uterine NK cells. They vary based on age, ethnicity, and sex. Though these NK cells are being measured and high values have been attributed for adverse fertility and pregnancy outcomes; they do not reflect the status or function of the uterine NK cells.

Hence therapies directed to suppress peripheral NK cells are not warranted. In fact, some of them have produced adverse effects to the mother and the fetus.[3]

Antinuclear Antibody Status

Antinuclear antibodies (ANA) are a group of antibodies that are directed against nuclear and nucleolar proteins of the biological cell. ANA is classically associated with systemic lupus erythematosus (SLE) but can be positive in other autoimmune disorders and some elderly individuals. Hence, clinical correlation with seropositivity is essential to make a working diagnosis.

Evidence has shown that ANA positivity could influence implantation. Implantation failures in in vitro fertilization (IVF)/intracytoplasmic sperm injection (ICSI) cycles; especially those in the first treatment cycle have shown a positive correlation with ANA positivity. However, this did not influence cumulative pregnancy rate without treatment. Hence, it was concluded that medications directed for the treatment of seropositive status would favor better implantation rates especially to those in the first treatment cycle.[4]

Antinuclear antibody positivity has also been shown to be associated with unexplained recurrent pregnancy loss (RPL) and also predicted unfavorable obstetric outcomes. Antinuclear antibody is to be measured by the immunofluorescence technique. Though enzyme-linked immunosorbent assay (ELISA) offers a high degree of sensitivity but has low specificity and hence could be used only as a screening test.

Structured and bigger studies are needed to prove the influence of ANA positivity on fertility and pregnancy.

Mapping Inflammatory Markers: Role in Immunomodulation

Methods to establish the diagnosis of NK cell malfunction and also those seronegative ANA category of patients with adverse fertility or pregnancy outcomes have still not been standardized. Any inflammatory trigger in the body can initiate hostile autoimmune responses unfavorable for conception. It is a challenge to make an accurate diagnosis of autoimmune conditions that could complicate fertility and pregnancy.

Measuring specific biochemical parameters reflective of the various organ systems of the body to map inflammatory responses could be an indirect method to measure hostile autoimmune responses.

Derangement of basic blood profiles such as complete blood count (CBC), metabolic profiles (abnormal levels of transaminases), acute phase reactants [C-reactive protein (CRP)], etc., could suggest a diffuse inflammatory process triggered by autoimmune etiology.

Parameters like elevated erythrocyte sedimentation rate (ESR) could be nonspecific but could reflect disease intensity.

Normalization of this parameter could be appreciated only after a while following the resolution of the inflammatory process.

Step-up immunological studies/serologies/flow cytometry/human leukocyte antigen (HLA) typing, etc., may also yield inconclusive results for making a diagnosis. Hence, basic and advanced testing (if suspicious of a defined autoimmune condition), together with clinical suspicion would add value in making a comprehensive clinical diagnosis.[5]

C-reactive Protein

It is an immune protein generated in the body and participates in defense against provoked antigens by opsonization and triggering the complement system.

Hence, if CRP in the blood is high, it could reflect an exaggerated inflammatory response triggered by a hostile autoimmune process.

A value of CRP <0.2 mg/dL is considered to be normal and any value more than 1 mg/dL could imply inflammation in the general population.

C-reactive protein levels during pregnancy:

- First trimester—not established. However, a value of >5 mg/dL has been known to be associated with low birth weight babies and neonatal complications.
- Second trimester—0.4–20.3 mg/dL
- Third trimester—0.4–8.1 mg/dL.[6]

Prednisolone and hydroxychloroquine are drugs [both classified as Food and Drug Administration (FDA) category C] that have been used extensively for immunomodulation during the periconceptional period and beyond. It is recommended for the clinician to explain with clarity the benefits of immunomodulation as against the probable risks before drug administration.

It is a challenge to make an accurate laboratory diagnosis of autoimmune disease which continues to remain so even in the periconceptional period. A battery of tests including basic laboratory investigations, metabolic panel, and acute phase reactants may add value apart from advanced immunological studies, serologies, and HLA typing.

The sensitivity for diagnosis and negative predictive values of ANA, which is one of the most common investigations that is performed in the general population, is low for autoimmune diseases. For specific rheumatic diseases, ANA yields a high negative predictive value of 97%, though the positive predictive value is 11%. However, the sensitivity and the specificity of ANA for the same are 42 and 85%, respectively.[7]

Application of clinical criteria and qualifying a particular disease state prior to testing significantly increases the sensitivity for diagnosis of autoimmune diseases.

Thyroid Peroxidase Antibody

Recent research has shown significant association between thyroid antibodies with infertility and recurrent miscarriage.

Effects on Fertility

High levels of thyroid peroxidase (TPO) antibody and high thyroid-stimulating hormone (TSH) have negative effect on IVF and embryo transfer in terms of embryo quality and abortion rates.

There has been an increased association of TPO antibody positivity with endometriosis as the latter is known to coexist with other autoimmune conditions. There has also been a similar association of polycystic ovarian syndrome (PCOS). This has been attributable to the increased estrogen to progesterone ratio usually seen in females with PCOS.

Effects on Pregnancy

Thyroid hormone is considered essential for normal placentation. Evidence has shown that preeclampsia, preterm delivery, and fetal growth restriction could be attributable to defective early placentation.[8] These effects are worsened in women with TPO positivity with thyroid dysfunction. A recent study has also shown that TPO-positive hypothyroid women are also more prone to midtrimester abortions compared to those who are hypothyroid and TPO-negative.

Another recent prospective study performed at a tertiary center for fertility and high-risk pregnancy in South India between August 2013 and September 2015 where outcomes of pregnancy in women with TPO positivity were mapped after appropriate dose adjustments of thyroxin concluded that there was a trend toward decrease in midtrimester abortions in these women. About 76.5% of these women were subclinically hypothyroid and hence emphasized the need for appropriate surveillance and management of this cohort to avert adverse obstetric consequences.

A positive TPO antibody test was diagnosed when the levels were equal to or >35 IU/mL. A TSH level of ≥2.5 mIU/L at booking in the first trimester was included under the category of subclinical hypothyroidism and was started on thyroxin supplements. Overt hypothyroid pregnant women who were already on thyroxin supplements were also included. Dose adjustments were made aggressively once in 4–6 weeks in the range of 1–2 µg/kg body weight. Trimester specific ranges to guide supplementation were followed as described in **Table 1**.

Adverse outcomes in pregnant women with thyroid peroxidase (TPO) positivity have been enumerated in **Table 2**.

In this study, pregnant women with TPO antibody levels of >600 IU/mL were significantly associated with gestational hypertension and fetal growth restriction.

Significant associations were found between pregnant women aged 30 years and older who were also TPO positive

TABLE 1: Trimester specific ranges to guide supplementation.

Trimester	Normal range of thyroid-stimulating hormone
First	0.1–2.5 mIU/mL
Second	0.2–3 mIU/mL
Third	0.3–3 mIU/mL

TABLE 2: Adverse outcomes in pregnant women with thyroid peroxidase (TPO) positivity.

Adverse outcomes	No. of patients (n = 115)	%
Gestational glucose intolerance/GDM	69	60
Hyperhomocysteinemia	50	43.5
Bad obstetric history/RPL	49	42.6
Threatened abortion	25	21.7
Gestational hypertension	17	14.8
Antinuclear antibody (ANA) positive status	17	14.8
Antiphospholipid antibody (APLA) positive status	14	12.2
Oligohydramnios	6	5.2
Second trimester abortion	6	5.2
Funneling of cervix	5	4.3
Premature rupture of membranes (PROM)	5	4.3
Missed abortion	5	4.3
Fetal growth restriction	4	3.5

(GDM: gestational diabetes mellitus; RPL: recurrent pregnancy loss)

with hyperhomocysteinemia, antiphospholipid antibody (APLA), bad obstetric history, and RPL.[9]

Adverse outcomes in pregnant women with thyroid peroxidase (TPO) positivity as per antibody levels have been enumerated in **Table 3**.

MICRONUTRIENTS AND METABOLIC FACTORS

Hyperhomocysteinemia

"Homocysteine" is a sulfur-containing amino acid synthesized in the body from an essential amino acid methionine. It is metabolized through two pathways: (1) remethylation and (2) transsulfuration. B_{12} and folic acid are essential for remethylation and B_6 is essential for transsulfuration **(Fig. 2)**.

Hyperhomocysteinemia is defined as levels ≥15 μmol/L.

Homocysteine levels decrease during pregnancy attributable to hemodilution, increased glomerular filtration along with increased utilization by the fetus apart from the hormonal changes during pregnancy.

Hyperhomocysteinemia in pregnancy is hence defined as any value >12 μmol/L.

It is more commonly due to combined deficiencies of B_6. B_{12} and folic acid in Southeast Asian countries unlike in the Caucasian population in whom genetic mutations in the enzymes involved in its metabolism are also common.[10]

The test is highly labile and needs standardization. A fasting ethylenediaminetetraacetic acid (EDTA) sample needs to be collected and centrifuged immediately. Values in early pregnancy are considered more reliable to predict adverse maternal and fetal outcomes.

TABLE 3: Adverse outcomes in pregnant women with thyroid peroxidase (TPO) positivity as per antibody levels.

Adverse outcomes	No. of patients (n = 115)	TPO-AB levels		p-value
		<600 (n = 100)	>600 (n = 15)	
Gestational glucose intolerance/GDM	69	61 (88.4%)	8 (11.6%)	0.572
Hyperhomocysteinemia	50	45 (90%)	5 (10%)	0.395
Bad obstetric history	49	45 (91.8%)	4 (8.2%)	0.181
Threatened abortion	25	23 (92%)	2 (8%)	0.518
Gestational hypertension	17	12 (70.6%)	5 (29.4%)	0.041
Antinuclear antibody (ANA) positive status	17	15 (88.2%)	2 (11.8%)	1.000
Antiphospholipid antibody (APLA) positive status	14	13 (92.9%)	1 (7.1%)	0.690
Oligohydramnios	6	4 (66.7%)	2 (33.3%)	0.175
Second trimester abortion	6	4 (66.7%)	2 (33.3%)	0.175
Cervical funneling	5	4 (80%)	1 (20%)	0.509
Premature rupture of membranes (PROM)	5	4 (80%)	1 (20%)	0.509
Missed abortion	5	5 (100%)	0 (0%)	1.000
Fetal growth restriction	4	2 (50%)	2 (50%)	0.082

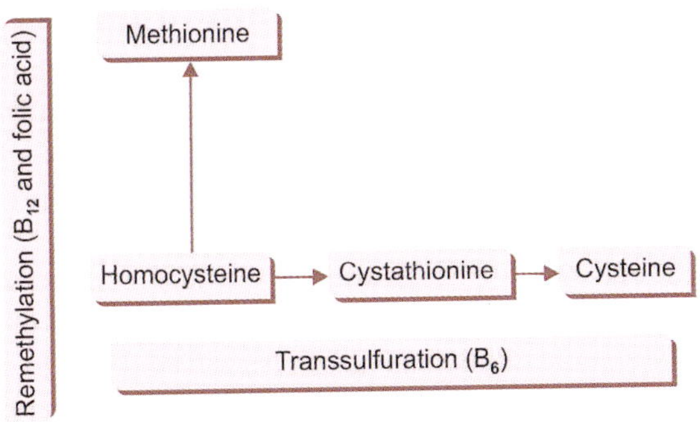

Fig. 2: Homocysteine metabolism.

Hyperhomocysteinemia could be attributable for adverse outcomes both during pregnancy and beyond. It has been established as independent causal factors for pregnancy complications. Suboptimal methylation could result in recurrent miscarriages, fetal structural defects, preeclampsia, fetal growth restriction/preterm labor, and intrauterine fetal demises. High levels of homocysteine could also adversely influence IVF outcomes. Attributable risks outside pregnancy include cardiovascular disease, vascular stroke, osteoporosis, and other neurodegenerative disorders.

Appropriate supplementation with B_6, B_{12}, and folic acid helps to control hyperhomocysteinemia in most of the Southeast Asian population where the cause of deficiency is nutritional.

A study conducted by Pratip Chakraborty et al., Kolkata in 2013, has depicted "hyperhomocysteinemia" as a significant risk factor in predicting pregnancy salvage rates in women with PCOS as obesity and insulin resistance controlled with other confounding factors. Anticoagulation with low-molecular-weight heparin and Ecosprin conferred an additional advantage in averting pregnancy wastage in those with the hyperhomocysteinemia phenotype.[11]

Hyperhomocysteinemia which is a consequence of altered micronutrients such as folic acid and B_{12} which could result in the generation of reactive oxygen species causing oxidative stress.

Another prospective study conducted at a tertiary center for fertility and high-risk pregnancy in South India that enrolled 442 pregnant women who were screened universally for a year (September 2012 to August 2013) reported a high prevalence of 28%, of which 37% of the women were primigravidae. The mean age of these women was 32 and the mean homocysteine level was 12.6 µmol/L. There was a strong positive correlation with ANA positivity and a trend toward a positive correlation with subclinical hypothyroidism (Pilot data).

Watchful surveillance for hyperhomocysteinemia and targeted value based supplementation would help avert adverse maternal and fetal outcomes and also contribute to a healthy adult life beyond pregnancy.

Flowchart 1: In utero fetal programming.

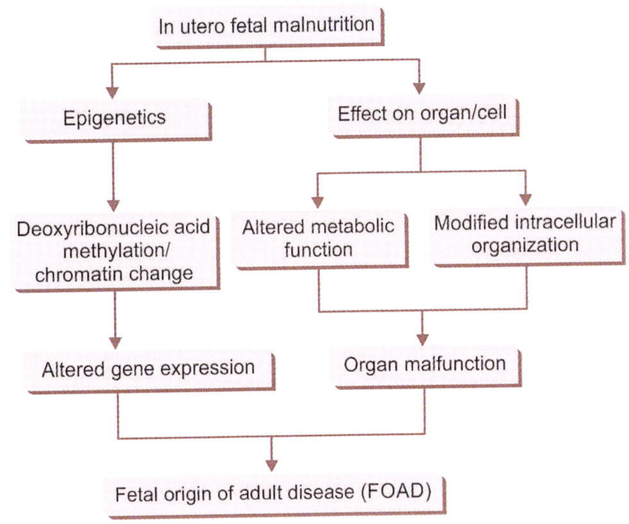

Hemoglobin A1c as a Predictor for Risk Modulation

Evidence has shown that there is a significant risk of congenital malformations for a hemoglobin A1c (HbA1c) value of >10.4%. However, the risk for adverse perinatal outcomes increases with an HbA1c of >6.9%.

Most studies recommend a pre pregnancy HbA1c levels of <7% in women with type 1 diabetes mellitus which further stresses the need for targeted preconceptional risk modulation.[12]

In Utero Fetal Programming (Flowchart 1)

"In utero fetal programming" is a novel concept that seems to have essential implications to Maternal Fetal Medicine translates to the fact that adverse intrauterine environment for the fetus can lead to irreversible change in the developing fetus contributing to "fetal origins of adult disease". Fetal overnutrition can predispose to permanent adverse changes in the genome overall influencing the metabolic homeostasis and neuroendocrine function, thus responsible for epigenetic changes resulting in changes in gene expression without any structural changes in the genome.[13]

Hence, effective surveillance for the risk factors complicating pregnancy adds value in delivering a mature fetus not only at birth but also ensures a healthy adulthood.

POST-IVF PREGNANCIES: SURVEILLANCE PATTERNS AND RATIONALE

Recent studies have established that the possible difference in perinatal outcomes between pregnancies due to assisted reproduction techniques (ARTs) and spontaneous conceptions cannot be attributed to ART per se suggesting that the inherent characteristics of the infertile population like high maternal age and low parity which could be a priori risk factors influencing poor perinatal outcomes.

Enumerating below a prospective matched case-control study comparing outcomes of IVF/ICSI pregnancies with non-IVF pregnancies **(Table 4)** between January 2009 and June 2010 under similar standards of maternal and fetal surveillance performed at a tertiary center for fertility and high-risk pregnancy in South India (Pilot data).

Majority of studies aimed at assessing ART outcomes have quoted a high incidence of preterm births and low birth weight babies. However, in this study, 35% of the IVF/ICSI group were born preterm as compared to 26.7% in the non-IVF/ICSI group. The mean pregnancy duration was 31.8 ± 10.31 weeks as compared to 32.92 ± 10.17 weeks in IVF/ICSI and non-IVF/ICSI pregnancies, respectively. As majority of the pregnancies have been delivered at or beyond 31 weeks, the incidence of low birth weight babies was 26.7% in the IVF/ICSI group as compared to 23.3% in the non-IVF/ICSI group. These rates were not statistically higher than the prevailing rates nationally during the time of the study. The increased rate of multiple pregnancies in both the groups could have contributed to increased incidence of preterm births in both the groups.

Though single embryo transfer has been advocated to check the rates of multiple pregnancies as a result of IVF/ICSI, iatrogenic multiple pregnancies will continue to occur provided strict guidelines for controlled ovarian stimulation are implemented even in ovulation induction-timed intercourse/intrauterine insemination (IUI) cycles.

To conclude, there were more elderly women and an increased number of plural pregnancies in the IVF/ICSI group as compared to the non-IVF/ICSI group. Hence, in vitro handling of gametes did not significantly affect perinatal outcomes which were probably influenced by the a priori maternal risk factors.

TABLE 4: Comparison of primary and secondary outcome variables between in vitro fertilization (IVF)/intracytoplasmic sperm injection (ICSI) and non-IVF/ICSI pregnancies.

Variable	*IVF/ICSI (n = 60)*	*Non-IVF/ICSI (n = 60)*	*p-value*
Age in years; mean ± standard deviation (SD)	31.02 ± 4.12	30.05 ± 3.45	0.166
Nullipara, No. (%)	56 (93.3%)	51 (85.0%)	0.239
P1, No. (%)	4 (6.7%)	8 (13.3%)	
P2, No. (%)	0	1 (1.7%)	
Singleton, No. (%)	43 (71.7%)	51 (85.0%)	0.121
Multiple pregnancy, No. (%)	17 (28.3%)	9 (15.0%)	
Duration of pregnancy (weeks)	31.80	32.92	0.551
• First trimester	8 (13.3%)	8 (13.3%)	1.000
• Second trimester	2 (3.3%)	5 (8.3%)	0.439
• Third trimester	0	1 (1.7%)	1.000
Preterm contractions, No. (%)	10 (16.7%)	5 (8.3%)	0.168
Gestational HTN/PE, No. (%)	10 (16.7%)	7 (11.7%)	0.432
Mode of delivery, No. (%)			
• Full-term vaginal delivery (FTVD)	2 (3.3%)	4 (6.7%)	0.679
• Lower segment cesarean section (LSCS)	46 (76.7%)	46 (76.7%)	1.000
• Blighted ovum	0	3 (5.0%)	0.244
• Missed abortion	7 (11.7%)	3 (5.0%)	0.322
• Spontaneous abortion	2 (3.3%)	4 (6.7%)	0.679
• Termination of pregnancy	3 (5.0%)	0	0.244
Fetal outcome, No. (%)			
• Intrauterine death (IUD)/neonatal death (NND)	4 (6.7%)	1 (1.7%)	0.364
Birth weight			
• Not known	1 (1.7%)	0	1.000
• <2.5 kg	16 (26.7%)	14 (23.3%)	0.833
• >2.5 kg	47 (78.3%)	48 (80.0%)	1.000
Preterm birth	21 (35.0%)	16 (26.7%)	0.323

Hence, appropriate/close maternal and fetal surveillance is important to optimize perinatal outcomes in IVF pregnancies. This was similar to the study conducted by De Sutter et al. (2005), where outcomes of IVF and non-IVF pregnancies were studied retrospectively **(Table 4)**.[14]

Larger studies need to be performed to aid better clinical extrapolation of the results.

ROLE OF ART/THIRD-PARTY REPRODUCTION AND PREIMPLANTATION GENETIC TESTING FOR ANEUPLOIDY IN CASES WITH RECURRENT PREGNANCY LOSS

Recent evidence does not support ART in cases with RPL without secondary infertility. Third-party reproduction for cases with RPL should be highly individualized based on the recurrence risk supported with a management strategy based on the latest evidence along with appropriate and relevant counseling. The use of preimplantation genetic testing for aneuploidy (PGT-A) has been supported by current and growing evidence in cases with RPL for idiopathic reasons.[15]

KEY POINTS

Evidence translated into practice:

- Surveillance for adverse outcomes as a consequence of dysfunctional placentation should be initiated during the peri-implantation phase—extended inverted pyramid of prenatal care shifting the focus too much earlier to clinical pregnancy.
- Predicting oxidative stress using biomarkers is still being researched which could pave the way to institute effective risk modulation strategies improving pregnancy outcomes.
- Several mechanisms influence immune tolerance at the maternal-fetal interface which involves effective angiogenesis and trophoblastic invasion. "Placenta" facilitates immune tolerance.
- Natural killer cell malformations have been attributed to infertility and RPL. However, peripheral NK cells do not reflect the status of uterine NK cells which are assumed to influence pregnancy outcomes. Hence therapies to suppress NK cells have shown no proven benefit.
- Isolated ANA positivity could influence fertility and pregnancy outcomes. However, its exact role and implications need to be researched with bigger studies.
- Thyroid peroxidase antibody positivity is known to be associated with adverse pregnancy outcomes. High levels of the antibody and high levels of TSH could have a negative effect on IVF. Dose-based adjustments of thyroxin with periodic surveillance could help avert adverse outcomes.
- Mapping inflammatory responses could be indirect but specific methods of measuring hostile autoimmunity in the body.
- Hyperhomocysteinemia could be attributed to adverse obstetric and fertility outcomes. Appropriate dietary supplementation of B_6, B_{12}, and folic acid could be beneficial especially when initiated periconceptionally.
- An HbA1c level of <7% preconceptionally is preferred for better outcomes in type 1 diabetes mellitus.
- Effective surveillance initiated periconceptionally for the identification of the probable risk factors that could complicate pregnancy helps to avert adverse irreversible changes in the genome aiding good in utero fetal programming.
- The perinatal outcomes of ART pregnancies do not differ significantly from non-ART pregnancies and effective surveillance for risk factors in ART pregnancies could result in better perinatal outcomes.
- Assisted reproductive technology can be recommended in cases with RPL only if there is associated secondary infertility. Third-party reproduction in RPL cases can only be suggested after judiciously weighing the recurrence risks. PGT-A can add value in idiopathic RPL.

REFERENCES

1. Ljubic A. Inverted pyramid of prenatal care – is it enough? Should it be – extended inverted pyramid of prenatal care? J Perinat Med. 2017;46(7):716-20.
2. Bak A, Roszkowski K. Oxidative stress in pregnant women. Arch Perinat Med. 2013;19(3):150-5.
3. Moffett A, Regan L, Braude P. Natural killer cells, miscarriage, and infertility. BMJ. 2004;329(7477):1283-5.
4. Kikuchi K, Shibahara H, Hirano Y, Kohno T, Hirashima C, Suzuki T, et al. Antinuclear antibody reduces the pregnancy rate in the first IVF-ET treatment cycle but not the cumulative pregnancy rate without specific medication. Am J Reprod Immunol. 2003;50(4):363-7.
5. Castro C, Gourley M. Diagnostic testing and interpretation of tests for autoimmunity. J Allergy Clin Immunol. 2010; 125(2 Suppl 2):S238-47.
6. Abbassi-Ghanavati M, Greer LG, Cunningham FG. Pregnancy and laboratory studies: a reference table for clinicians. Obstet Gynecol. 2009;114(6):1326-31.
7. Soto ME, Hernández-Becerril N, Perez-Chiney AC, et al. Pre dictive value of antinuclear antibodies in autoimmune diseases classified by clinical criteria: analytical study in a specialized health institute, one year follow-up. Results Immunol. 2013;5:13-22.
8. Saki F, Dabbaghmanesh MH, Ghaemi SZ, Forouhari S, Omrani GR, Bakhshayeshkaram M. Thyroid autoimmunity in pregnancy and its influences on maternal and fetal outcome in Iran (a prospective study). Endocr Res. 2015;40(3): 139-45.
9. Rajan RS, Malik P, Garg N, Avula S, Rao K. Outcomes of pregnancy in women with TPO positive status after

appropriate dose adjustments of thyroxin: a prospective cohort study. Int J Med Health Sci. 2016;10(3):114-7.
10. Herrmann W, Herrmann M, Obeid R. Hyperhomocysteinaemia: a critical review of old and new aspects. Curr Drug Metab. 2007;8(1):17-31.
11. Chakraborty P, Goswami SK, Rajani S, Sharma S, Kabir SN, Chakravarty B, et al. Recurrent pregnancy loss in polycystic ovary syndrome: role of hyperhomocysteinemia and insulin resistance. PLoS One. 2013;8(5):e64446.
12. Jensen DM, Korsholm L, Ovesen P, Beck-Nielsen H, Moelsted-Pedersen L, Westergaard JG, et al. Peri-conceptional A1c and risk of serious pregnancy outcome in 933 women with type 1 diabetes. Diabetes Care. 2009;32(6):1046-8.
13. Lehnen H, Zechner U, Haaf T. Epigenetics of gestational diabetes mellitus and offspring health: the time for action is in early stages of life. Mol Hum Reprod. 2013;19(7):415-22.
14. De Sutter P, Veldeman L, Kok P, Szymcza N, Van der Elst J, Dhont M. Comparison of outcome of pregnancy after intrauterine insemination (IUI) and IVF. Hum Reprod. 2005;20(6):1642-6.
15. Carp HJA. Recurrent Pregnancy Loss; Causes, Controversies and Treatment, 3rd edition. Florida: CRC Press; 2021. pp. 231-49.

CHAPTER

93 Emergencies in Infertility

Arunima Halder

INTRODUCTION

With the rise in infertility, more and more patients have been approaching infertility clinics for treatment. There has been rise in ovarian stimulation in the form of ovulation induction or controlled ovarian stimulation. With this has risen the increased chance of emergent complications during intrauterine insemination (IUI) or in vitro fertilization (IVF). Enlarged multicystic ovaries may release excess vascular endothelial growth factors (VEGFs) leading to extravasation of fluid to third space and ovarian hyperstimulation syndrome (OHSS) or may be too large and undergo torsion. Patients may present with vague pain and a high index of suspicion helps in early diagnosis of such a mishap in patients undergoing ovarian stimulation. Intra-abdominal and retroperitoneal bleed, which may occur during oocyte retrieval, though rare, is not unseen and may require immediate action. Extrauterine pregnancy is another complication, which is on the rise and may present with acute abdominal pain in case of rupture. In this chapter, we delve into these emergencies, which a reproductive medicine expert should always anticipate and be prepared for.

OVARIAN HYPERSTIMULATION SYNDROME

Ovarian hyperstimulation syndrome is the least common but most life-threatening iatrogenic complication of ovulation induction or controlled ovarian stimulation, which is characterized by ovarian enlargement, overproduction of ovarian hormones, and transudation of protein-rich fluid from vascular compartment to the extravascular compartment.

According to the Royal College of Obstetricians and Gynecologists (RCOG), OHSS should be considered as a possibility in any patient who is undergoing ovarian stimulation. However, the incidence of moderate-to-severe OHSS is around 3–8%.[1]

Classification of OHSS

Various authors have given various classifications of OHSS. RCOG 2016 in their Green-top guidelines has classified OHSS as described in **Table 1**.

Depending on the time of onset, OHSS can be classified into early- and late-onset OHSS.[2-4] Early-onset OHSS is milder, occurs within 3–7 days of human chorionic gonadotropin (hCG) trigger, and occurs in response to gonadotropin stimulation. On the other hand, late-onset OHSS, occurs around 10 days after the hCG trigger, is pregnancy related due to endogenous hCG of pregnancy, and is severe in nature.

Pathophysiology (Fig. 1)

Vascular endothelial growth factor is implicated as the key player in the genesis of OHSS and its action is propagated by hCG.[5-10] The renin-angiotensin system of the ovary as well as proinflammatory factors have also been shown to play a role in development of OHSS **(Table 2)**.

TABLE 1: Classification of ovarian hyperstimulation syndrome.

Mild	*Moderate*	*Severe*	*Critical*
• Bloating of the abdomen • Mild abdominal pain • Ovarian size <8 mL	• Moderate abdominal pain • Signs of ascites on ultrasonography • Nausea + Vomiting • Ovarian size 8–12 mL	• Clinical ascites with or without hydrothorax • Hyponatremia (<135 mmol/L) • Hyperkalemia (>5 mmol/L) • Oliguria (<30 mL/h or 300 mL/day) • Hematocrit >0.45 • Albumin <35 g/L • Hypo-osmolality <282 mOsm/kg • Ovarian size >12 mL	• Tense ascites • Hydrothorax • Hematocrit >0.55 • Oliguria/anuria • WBC count >25,000/mL • Thromboembolism • Acute respiratory distress syndrome

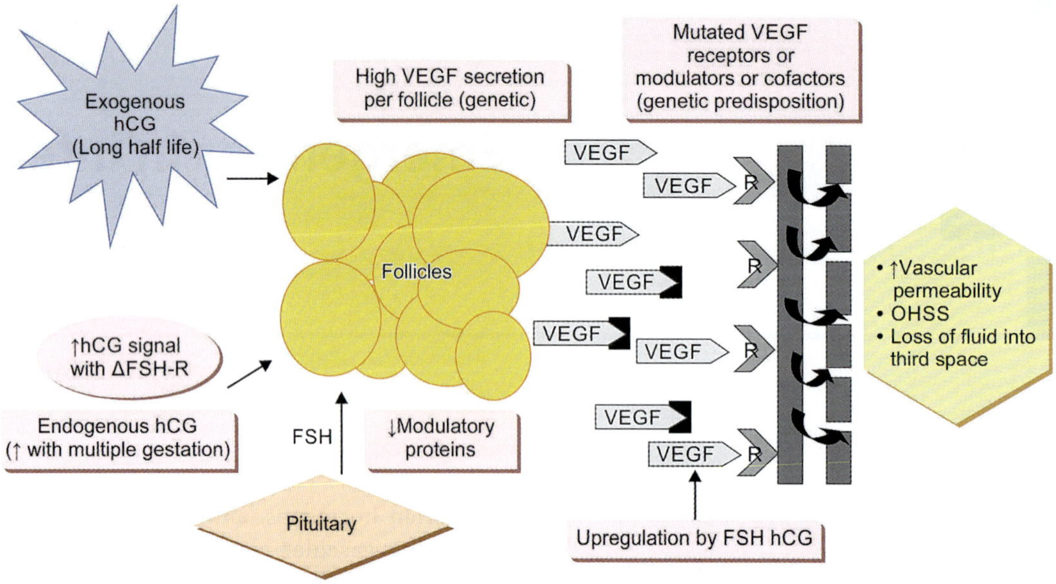

Fig. 1: Pathophysiology of ovarian hyperstimulation syndrome.
(hCG: human chorionic gonadotropin; VEGF: vascular endothelial growth factor; OHSS: ovarian hyperstimulation syndrome)

TABLE 2: Strategies for prevention of ovarian hyperstimulation syndrome.

Prevention	*Strategy*	*Advantage*	*Disadvantage*	*Evidence*
Primary	Chronic low dose step up protocol (decreasing the dose of gonadotropin)	• Decreasing the dose of gonadotropin • Decreases cost • Significantly decreases OHSS	Prolonged duration of stimulation	Orvieto et al.[11] with this protocol showed excellent safety profile
	GnRH antagonist protocol	• Significantly decreases • OHSS • Similar pregnancy rates as long protocol	Decreased flexibility of the protocol	Al Inany et al.[12] demonstrated that OHSS is decreased with GnRH antagonist protocol
	Metformin	• Reduces hyperinsulinemia and hyperandrogenism • Decreases number of follicles • Decreases OHSS		Tso et al.[13] suggested that metformin decreases the chance of OHSS (moderate quality evidence)
	Follitropin Delta	Provides statistically significant and clinically relevant decrease in incidence of OHSS without compromising live birth rates	May decrease the number of oocytes retrieved	Ishihara and Arce[14] (STORK group) suggested the use of Follitropin Delta for prevention of OHSS, which was reiterated by Yacoub et al., in his retrospective study.[15]
	Low Dose Aspirin	Well-known NSAID, inhibits the activity of COX1, preventing platelet aggregation thereby, preventing the pathological cascade of histamine, serotonin, PDGF, LPA thereby decreasing chance of OHSS	Minimal side effects	Guo et al., in their systematic review and network meta-analysis on the most appropriate pharmacological interventions for prevention of OHSS ranked low-dose aspirin as the Rank 1 choice of intervention. (Grade A evidence)[16]
Secondary	Agonist trigger	Elimination of OHSS	Luteolysis	Kol et al.,[17] suggested that GnRH-agonist is the key to prevention of OHSS. This was later supported by Cochrane meta-analysis by Youssef[18] in 2014 and Brown[19] in 2017. Several other studies have supported the same[20,21]
	Dopamine agonist	Reduces chance of moderate OHSS		Tang et al.,[22] proved in their Cochrane study that Cochrane decreases incidence of moderate OHSS

Contd...

Contd...

Prevention	*Strategy*	*Advantage*	*Disadvantage*	*Evidence*
Tertiary prevention	Freeze all strategy	Eliminates OHSS	Prolongs time to pregnancy	Blockeel et al.,[23] observed that one of the key strengths of freeze all protocol is prevention of OHSS
	Letrozole	Aromatase inhibitor decreases estrogen levels	Can be used only in oocyte donors and freeze all cases	Akman et al.,[24] found that letrozole reduces VEGF expression in OHSS and thus controls its occurrence
	Calcium gluconate	Decreases cAMP dependent rennin secretion decreasing VEGF synthesis	Monitoring required during calcium infusion	Naredi et al.,[25] demonstrated calcium gluconate to be extremely effective in prevention of OHSS
	Albumin/hetastarch	Borderline statistical decrease in OHSS	Heterogeneity of studies	Youssef et al.,[26] in their Cochrane analysis showed that plasma expanders were effective in prevention of moderate to severe OHSS
	Glucocorticoids	Affects VEGF gene expression	Insufficient evidence	Tan et al.,[27]; conflicting evidence available

(cAMP: cyclic adenosine monophosphate; GnRH: gonadotropin-releasing hormone; OHSS: ovarian hyperstimulation syndrome; VEGF: vascular endothelial growth factor)

TABLE 3: Evaluation of a patient with ovarian hyperstimulation syndrome (RCOG).

History	*Symptoms*	*Signs*	*Initial investigations*	*Subsequent tests*
• History of PCOS • Number of follicles at trigger • Drug used for trigger • Duration between trigger and onset of symptoms • Total number of oocytes retrieved • If embryo transfer was done or not	• Abdominal bloating or pain • Nausea and vomiting • Pedal edema • Vulval edema • Breathlessness • Reduced urine output • Other comorbidities like thrombosis	• Increase in weight • Tachycardia, tachypnea • Edema • Dehydration • Ascites, palpable abdominal mass • Peritonism • Signs of pleural effusion or pulmonary edema or pneumonia	• Complete blood count (CBC), Hematocrit (Hct), • Urea and electrolytes, osmolality, C-reactive protein (CRP), thrombophilia profile, liver function tests (LFT), ultrasound abdomen (USG) pelvis and thorax	• Electrocardiogram (ECG), chest X-ray, D-dimer • Arterial blood gas (ABG) • Ventilation perfusion scan

The concept of OHSS-free clinic was given by Devroey et al., where he emphasized the importance of segmentation of IVF.[28]

Evaluation of a Patient with OHSS

In the backdrop of ovarian stimulation, suspicion of OHSS should arise when a patient arrives with abdominal distension or pain. The symptoms for OHSS are vague and there are no particular investigations that pinpoint toward OHSS. Primary diagnosis of OHSS remains clinical.

RCOG[1] recommends the following evaluation in a patient with suspected OHSS **(Table 3)**.

Based on the initial assessment of the patient **(Table 3)**, and severity of OHSS **(Table 1)**, they can be treated as outpatient or inpatient.

Outpatient Treatment

Outpatient treatment can be offered to patients with mild or moderate OHSS and some patients with severe OHSS. All patients who are treated on an outpatient basis should comply with follow-up on a regular basis every 2–3 days.

- Verbal and written information should be given to the patient about their condition.
- Drink fluid as per thirst. Fluid intake should not be less than 1 L/day.
- Input output chart to be monitored. Urine output of less than 1,000 mL/day or a positive water deficit of more than 1,000 mL/day should imply immediate notification at the hospital.
- Low-molecular weight heparin (LMWH) should be given for thromboprophylaxis especially in cases of severe OHSS.
- Paracetamol or opioids for pain relief. Nonsteroidal anti-inflammatory drugs (NSAIDs) should be avoided as it can deteriorate renal function.
- Paracentesis, if required should be carried out trans-vaginally. Transabdominal paracentesis is preferred in a nonobese patient in whom large amount of ascitic fluid has to be drained (as it is feasible to put an indwelling catheter in this case).[1]

- Urgent reporting to hospital in case of worsening symptoms. Otherwise, a visit to the hospital every 2–3 days should be made.
- Hematocrit is a good tool to know the amount of hemoconcentration.

Need for Admission

- Inability to achieve adequate pain relief
- Inability to maintain required fluid intake due to nausea despite antiemetics
- Inability to follow-up routinely
- Worsening symptoms of OHSS despite outpatient interventions
- Critical OHSS.

Inpatient Treatment

Treatment of critical and severe OHSS should have a multidisciplinary approach and needs intensive care **(Figs. 2 and 3)**.

Several complications like thromboembolism **(Flowchart 1A)**, pleural effusion, adult respiratory distress syndrome (ARDS) **(Flowchart 1B)**, renal failure **(Flowchart 1C)**, and ascites **(Flowchart 1D)**, and should be looked out for and treated at the first suspicion.

Surgery in OHSS may be needed in cases of ovarian torsion, ovarian rupture, or ectopic pregnancy.

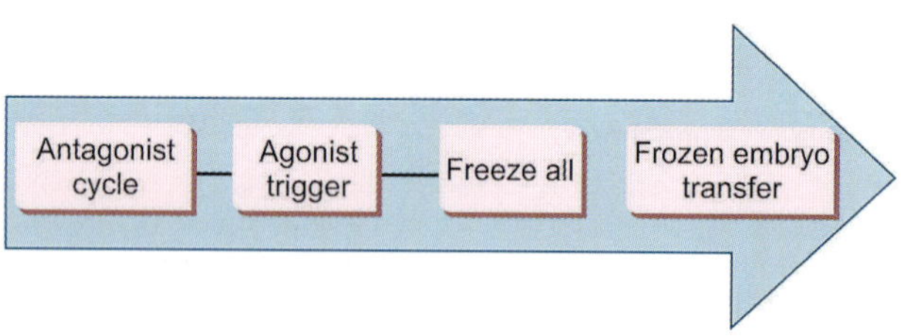

Fig. 2: Ovarian hyperstimulation syndrome-free clinic.

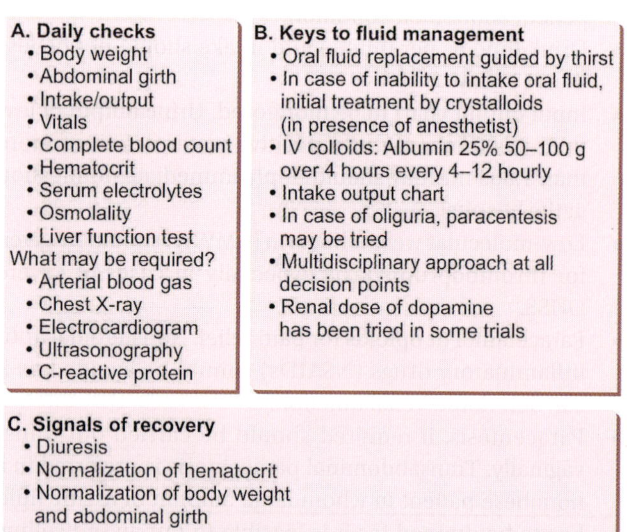

Fig. 3: Inpatient treatment.

ADNEXAL TORSION

Adnexal torsion may be defined as a complete or partial rotation of the ovarian pedicle along its own axis leading to an obstruction to the inflow and the outflow of blood eventually leading to ovarian ischemia and eventual demise, if left untreated.[29] In the general population, the incidence of ovarian torsion is around 2.7% and majority of these occur in the reproductive age group.[30] The incidence of ovarian torsion in women undergoing IVF–intracytoplasmic sperm injection (ICSI) is 0.08–0.13%,[31] the incidence may increase to 7.5% in case of OHSS.[32]

Adnexal torsion is a gynecological emergency needing immediate diagnosis and intervention. Diagnosing a case of adnexal torsion may not be easy and may involve high risk of suspicion.[33]

Anatomy of the Adnexa (Fig. 4)

The ovary lies in a hammock made by the infundibulopelvic ligament on one side and the utero-ovarian ligament on the other side. The infundibulopelvic ligament is a loose structure which connects the ovary to the lateral pelvic wall. It houses the ovarian artery and the vein. The utero-ovarian ligament is a fibromuscular band, which embodies the ovarian branches of the uterine vessels.[34]

Once the ovary gets twisted, there is an initial compression of the venous and lymphatic outflow. Since the arterial walls are muscular and less collapsible the arterial flow is maintained. Following this the ovary starts to become edematous. In due course, the diffuse ovarian stroma develops, increasing the intraovarian pressure, and stretching the ovarian capsule. This ultimately compresses the arteries leading to ischemia and necrosis.[35]

- *Normal ovary:* Torsion may occur in the normal ovary especially in young girls who are prepubertal because of the loose, mobile ovarian ligaments.[36,37] With the advent of puberty, the ligaments become shorter and sturdier decreasing the chance of ovarian torsion.[29]

  Torsion may also occur when one undergoes strenuous exercise with a stimulated ovary.[37,38] Littman et al.,[37] reported a case where a 38-year-old patient with secondary infertility had undergone gonadotropin stimulation with IUI, which had failed. Following this, in view of two cysts she had taken recess from treatment during which she resumed her normal activities. During an exercise session, she developed acute abdominal pain and was rushed to the emergency department. Hence, one must be careful to advise the patient to avoid any form of strenuous activity until the cysts following ovarian stimulation are resolved **(Table 4)**.
- *Ovarian cysts and tumors:* It has been seen that ovarian torsions are most often found with benign tumors as compared to malignant tumors.[29,39-42] The reason behind this discrepancy could be the fact that malignancies

Flowcharts 1A to D: Complications in inpatient treatment.

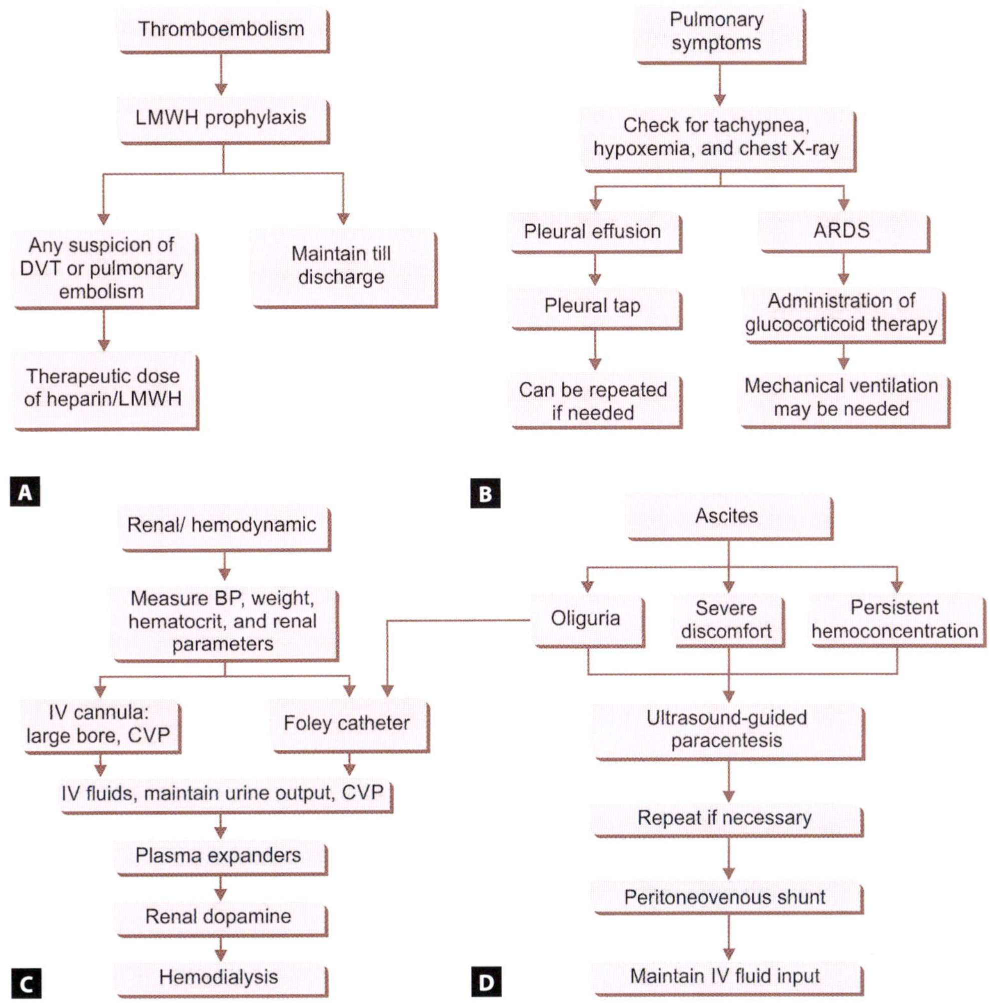

(ARDS: acute respiratory distress syndrome; CVP: central venous pressure; DVT: deep vein thrombosis; LMWH: low molecular weight heparin)

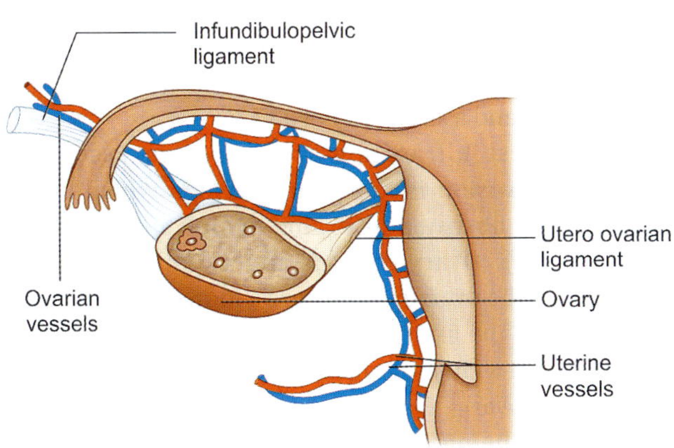

Fig. 4: Anatomy of adnexa.

are associated with adhesions, which decrease the incidence of the ovaries getting rotated around their axes. Of the benign tumors, benign cystic teratoma has been shown to be most commonly associated with ovarian torsion.[43,44]

TABLE 4: Predisposing factors to adnexal torsion.

Sl. No.	Predisposing factor	Probable reason
1.	Normal ovary	• Excessively mobile fallopian tubes and ovarian ligaments[33,34] • Long pelvic ligaments • Spasm of the tubes • Strenuous exercise[35] • Sudden changes in intra-abdominal pressure
2.	Ovarian tumors	• Benign ovarian tumors • Larger tumors >5 cm
3.	IVF	Larger ovaries due to multiple cysts
4.	Pregnancy	Physiological cysts
5.	Right side	Presence of sigmoid colon on the left side

- *In vitro fertilization:* According to Gelbaya et al.,[45] women who undergo assisted reproduction have 11-fold higher risk of ovarian torsion. Whether this is because of increase in size of ovaries or increase in ascitic fluid in the abdomen which increases the mobility of the ovaries is still unknown.[46]

- *Pregnancy:* There have been several reports of ovarian torsion during pregnancy.[47] This is more in cases where conception has occurred following ovarian stimulation. Ovarian torsion is most common in the first trimester with decreasing trends in the second and third trimester.[29]

Diagnosis of Adnexal Torsion

The clinical presentation of adnexal torsion may be non-specific **(Flowchart 2)**. It may present as an acute stabbing pain in the lower abdomen radiating to the groin. Sometimes, the patient may experience intermittent episodes of pain exhibiting an acute on chronic phenomenon.[48] Nausea and vomiting may be associated in 70–85% of cases. In undiagnosed cases, where necrosis of the ovary has set in, fever could also be a presenting symptom.[49] History of ovarian stimulation should be elicited. Pain may typically start following strenuous exertion[38] or straining at stools. Signs of abdominal tenderness, localized guarding, or rebound tenderness, tachycardia, and pyrexia may be noted. Cervical motion tenderness may be present.

Huchon et al.,[50] devised a predictive score for the preoperative diagnosis of adnexal torsion. According to this score, five criteria were included, which were given individual scores. Total score of less than 40 had a 3.7% risk of adnexal torsion, 40–60 had a 20% risk of adnexal torsion, and more than 60 had a 69% risk of adnexal torsion **(Table 5)**.

All said and done, a high index of suspicion is of utmost importance in diagnosing adnexal torsion especially in IVF patients.

Flowchart 2: Pathophysiology of adnexal torsion.

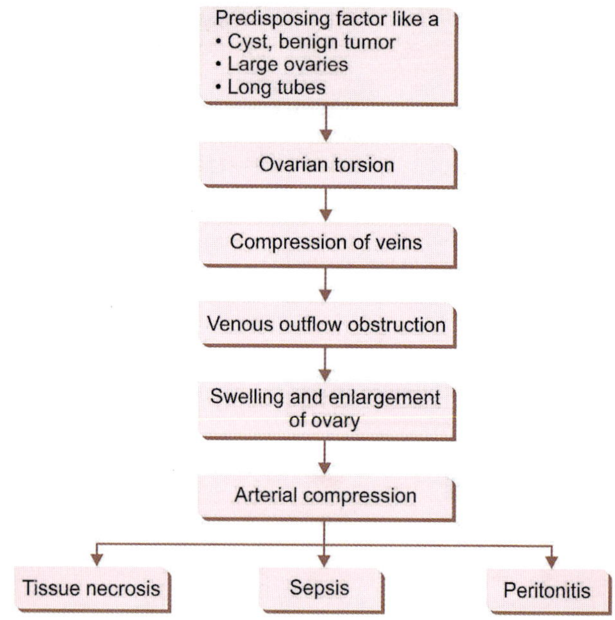

TABLE 5: Score for adnexal torsion.[50]

Sl. No.	*Parameter*	*Score*
1.	Spontaneous one-sided abdominal or lumbar pain	15
2.	Pain lasting <8 hours	20
3.	Vomiting	20
4.	Cyst >5 cm in the ovary on ultrasonography	25
5.	Absence of leukorrhea or metrorrhagia	25

Low risk: score <40, high risk : score >60

Laboratory Evaluation

No specific laboratory parameters have been seen to be associated with ovarian torsion. Torsion leads to ischemia followed by ischemia-reperfusion injury. This eventually leads to rise in acute phase proteins that seem to be elevated in this condition. Patient may present with leukocytosis and raised C-reactive protein.[51,52] According to Cohen et al., preoperative elevation of interleukin 6 and not TNF-alpha pointed to the diagnosis of ovarian torsion in a case of acute abdomen.[53] Aran et al., in their experimental study on rats demonstrated that a rise in ischemia-modified albumin was associated with ovarian torsion model and this could emerge as an early serum biomarker of ovarian torsion in humans.[54]

Imaging

Ultrasonography (Gray Scale)

When a woman in her reproductive age comes with an acute abdomen, the primary method of evaluation is an ultrasonography (USG). In a series by Graif et al.,[55] USG for adnexal torsion was found to have a positive predictive value of 87.5% and a specificity of 93%.

The earliest ultrasonographic feature associated with ovarian torsion is follicular ring sign which occurs when there is obstruction to the venous and lymphatic flow **(Fig. 5A)**. Ovary may be unilaterally enlarged.[56] Once twisted, the ovary may acquire a more central location almost close to the fundus of the uterus.[57] Ovarian size may be greater than 4 cm as compared to the normal appearing contralateral ovary. The stroma may appear hypoechoic with follicles being peripherally arranged **(Fig. 5B)**.[58] This may also be a feature in young women with polycystic ovary syndrome (PCOS) but in the setting of acute abdominal pain and associated clinical and sonographic findings, one must think of adnexal torsion. A cyst that may be present on the ovary may become hyperechoic due to hemorrhage.[58] Small follicles may be seen having a echogenic rim due to acoustic enhancement.[51] Hematosalpinx may be visible.[52]

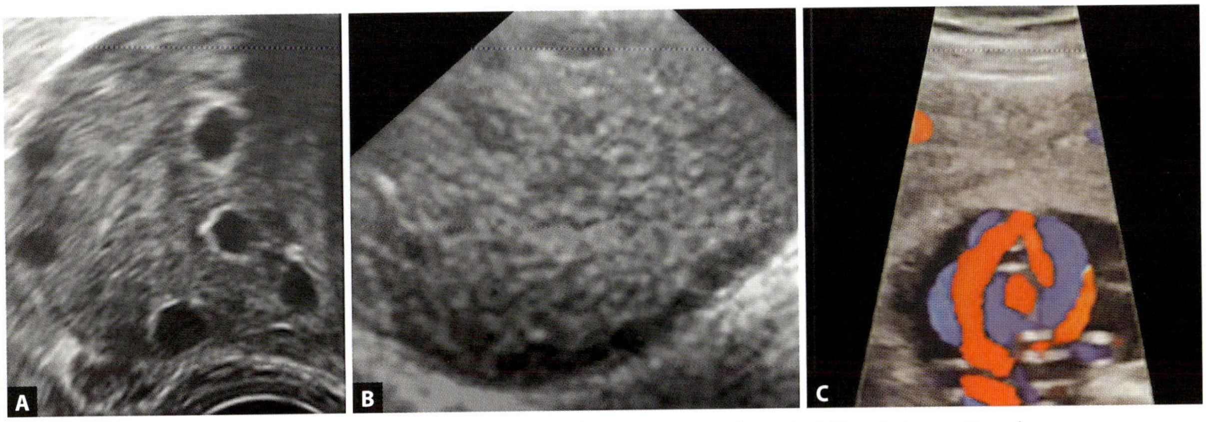

Figs. 5A to C: "Follicular ring sign", stromal edema on gray scale and whirlpool sign on Doppler.

TABLE 6: Summary of diagnosis of ovarian torsion.

Sl. No.	*Parameters*	*Findings*
1.	Symptoms	Sharp, stabbing pain radiating to the loin or thigh, vomiting, nausea, fever, history of strenuous exercise, or increased abdominal pressure
2.	Signs	Tachycardia, pyrexia, tenderness, and guarding of the affected side, rebound tenderness
3.	Gray scale ultrasound	• Unilateral ovarian enlargement • Hypoechoic stroma with peripherally arranged follicles • Hemorrhage within a cyst • Echogenic rim around follicles • Centrally located ovary • Twisted blood vessels at the pedicle • Free fluid in the pouch of Douglas
4.	Doppler	• Presence or absence of arterial blood flow depending on the progression of the disease • Whirlpool sign
5.	Serum markers	• Leukocytosis • C-reactive protein • Interleukin 6
6.	CT/MRI	• Ovary twisted to the contralateral side • Uterus deviated to the ipsilateral side • Thickened tubal walls • Fluid in pouch of Douglas

Free fluid may be visible, which may be hemorrhagic or nonhemorrhagic.[55] Twisted pedicle may be visible, which becomes enhanced on usage of color Doppler.[58]

On Doppler, blood flows may or may not be seen. The pathophysiology of ovarian torsion is a dynamic process. When only venous obstruction has occurred and the arterial blood flow is still maintained, ovarian blood flow may be visible. This however, does not rule out torsion.[53] The typical "whirlpool appearance" due to twisting of blood vessels may be seen **(Fig. 5C)**.[55]

Features on CT scan are mostly vague with the affected ovary rotated to the contralateral side. The uterus may appear shifted to the affected side. Ovary may also appear edematous with free fluid in the abdomen.[51,57,] On enhanced CT, the tubes may appear thickened.[57] MRI may not be of much help except in second and third trimesters where diagnosis by ultrasound is ambiguous **(Table 6)**.[58]

Management

Treatment for ovarian torsion is surgical. While deciding regarding the management, one should consider the progression of the condition, age of the patient, the desire for fertility, and presence of existing ovarian pathology **(Fig. 6 and Table 7)**. Traditionally, for such cases oophorectomy or salpingo-oophorectomy had been tried.[48]

However, recent studies emphasize the benefits of conservative surgery over radical surgery.[59-63] Despite the ovary appearing edematous and black, once detorted, it may still regain color and be viable. According to Chen et al.,[64] pain lasting for more than 48 hours may not correlate well with the successful outcome of the surgery. Recurrent torsion may implicate detorsion followed by oophoropexy.[65] If a leading point like a cyst has been identified it might be advisable to go ahead with cystectomy. This may however be risky as the tissues are friable.[53]

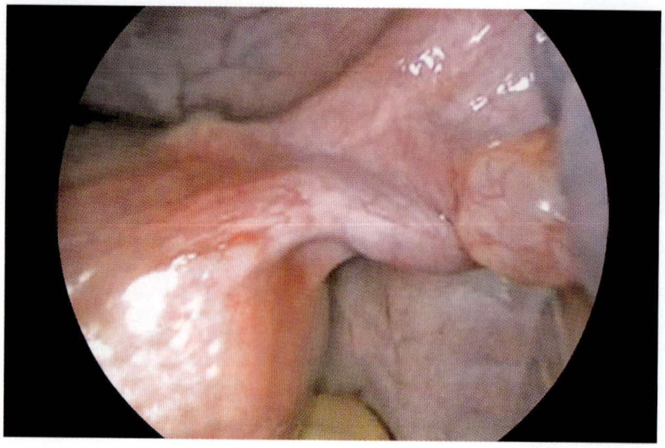

Fig. 6: Laparoscopic picture of ovarian torsion.

EMERGENCIES DURING OOCYTE RETRIEVAL

Bleeding

Vaginal bleeding during oocyte retrieval is common and occurs in up to 18% of the cases.[66] In most of the cases, this stops spontaneously. If it does not, pressure with sponge forceps or vaginal packing.

Intraperitoneal or retroperitoneal bleeding can occur with an incidence of around 1%.[67] Intraperitoneal bleed may be detected soon after the procedure. However, retroperitoneal bleed may have an indolent course.

Caution to be maintained, if such a bleed is suspected. Close monitoring of vitals should be done. Ultrasound may

TABLE 7: Management of ectopic pregnancy.

	Mode of treatment	***Indications***	***Regimen/method***	***Advantages***	***Disadvantages***	***Evidences***
Expectant	Close monitoring of BhCG	• Hemodynamically stable patient • Ectopic pregnancy detected on USG, falling BhCG level or initial level less than discriminatory zone	Close monitoring of clinical symptoms and BhCG until it reaches less than 15 IU/L	No side effects of methotrexate, no surgical or anesthesia related risks. No tubal damage as spontaneous regression occurs. Good fertility outcome	• Close monitoring required. • Risk of worsening leading to conversion to medical or surgical treatment	• *METEX trial*[91,92] by Mello et al., 60% of women with expectant management had an uneventful clinical course • *Cochrane 2007*[93] has not been able to adequately evaluate expectant management yet
Medical management	Single dose MTX	• Hemodynamically stable • Minimal or no symptoms • BhCG <5,000 IU/L • Size: <3.5 cm • No embryonic cardiac activity • Confirmed diagnosis of ectopic pregnancy • Compliance for follow-up	• $50 mg/m^2$ MTX given in D1 • BhCG on D4 and D7 • Expected drop in BhCG >15% • Follow-up till BhCG <5	Decreased side effects of MTX	Increased chance of requirement of a second dose of MTX	• *Cochrane 2007*:[93] Methotrexate was less effective than laparoscopic salpingotomy. However, RCOG 2016[90] suggests that methotrexate and laparoscopic surgery can be equally effective in tubal ectopic pregnancies • Elito et al.,[94] provided a score >5 entailed 97% success rate with single dose
	Two dose MTX		Two doses of MTX on D1 and D4 with no leucovorin rescue. Look for >15% fall in BhCG	• Lower number of days for BhCG to decrease as compared to single dose • Better balance between convenience and efficacy[95]		• *Barnhart et al.*:[95] Two dose regimen minimizes number of injections and decreases surveillance visits • *Song et al.*:[96] no overall difference in single and two dose. In subgroup with BhCG >5,000 two dose was better
	Multiple dose MTX		• MTX 1 mg/kg on D1, 3, 5, and 7 • Leucovorin rescue 0.1 mg/kg on D2, 4, 6, and 8 • A fall in BhCG >15% calls for stoppage of treatment and start of follow-up	Less chance of failure of treatment	Increased side effects of MTX like gastritis, stomatitis, leucopenia, hair fall	According to *ASRM: Practice committee guidelines 2013*,[97-99] multiple-dose regimen has a success rate significantly higher than single dose regimen

Contd...

Contd...

	Mode of treatment	Indications	Regimen/method	Advantages	Disadvantages	Evidences
Surgical management	Salpingotomy	• Only one patent tube Future pregnancy desired Patient hemodynamically stable • Contralateral abnormal tube • Unruptured ectopic of <5 cm	Longitudinal incision over the most bulged part with minimal usage of cautery followed by hydrodissection and removal of conceptus in to	Maintenance of fertility	Chance of persistent trophoblastic disease	• *ESEP trial:100* salpingotomy did not significantly improve fertility prospects as compared to salpingectomy. • *DEMETER trial:101* No significant difference in 2 years fertility for active ectopic pregnancy while comparing conservative versus radical surgery
	Salpingectomy	• Tube is severely damaged • Uncontrolled bleeding • Recurrent ectopic pregnancy in the same tube • Large tubal pregnancy of >5 cm • Woman has completed her family	Coagulation near the cornua followed by division and removal of the tube	Complete removal of trophoblastic tissue	Fertility not preserved. Theoretical chance of damage to ovarian blood supply	
Persistent trophoblastic disease	Single dose methotrexate		50 mg/m^2 single dose			Level 1: evidence. (RCOG)[90]

(MTX: methotrexate; BhCG: Beta-human chorionic gonadotropin)

not reveal a bleed especially in retroperitoneal bleed. Fall in hemoglobin is the best diagnostic tool.

Once diagnosed, urgent laparotomy with blood transfusion, if needed, should be done.[68]

Pelvic Infection[68]

There may be inadvertent insertion of cervicovaginal flora during oocyte pick-up (OPU) or accidental puncture of hydrosalpinx or endometriotic cyst. This can lead to pelvic infection. Pelvic inflammatory disease following OPU is rare. Patients may present with fever, offensive vaginal discharge, lower abdominal pain, or painful micturition.

Intravenous antibiotics are the treatment of choice in these cases.

EMERGENCY AFTER EMBRYO TRANSFER

Ectopic Pregnancy

Presence of a pregnancy other than within the uterine cavity is known as ectopic or extrauterine pregnancy. In the normal population, incidence of ectopic pregnancy is 1–3%.[69] Rise of assisted-reproductive technology (ART) has seen a corresponding rise in ectopic pregnancy and accounts for around 2–8.5% of all pregnancies, which may be even higher when tubal factor is the cause of ectopic.[70]

Various Sites of Ectopic Pregnancy

Sites of ectopic pregnancy have been described in **Figure 7**.

Pathophysiology[71]

The exact pathophysiology of ectopic pregnancy in IVF is not known. Various theories have been put forward **(Flowchart 3)**.

Risk Factors

Maternal age: Evidence is conflicting regarding the role of maternal age in the incidence of ectopic pregnancy. Patil et al.[72] and Rana et al.,[73] showed an increase in ectopic pregnancy with increasing maternal age. This could be because of genetically incompetent embryos or due age-related changes in the tubal physiology. However, studies by Malak et al.[74] and Li et al.[75] have not found an association between the two.

Tubal factor: Any factor that alters the tubal functionality can be implicated in causing ectopic pregnancy. The presence of pelvic inflammatory disease (PID), especially, Chlamydia trachomatis antibodies has been implicated in causing ectopic pregnancy.[75] Other causes associated could be, the presence of endometriosis, previous history of ectopic pregnancy, and previous tubal

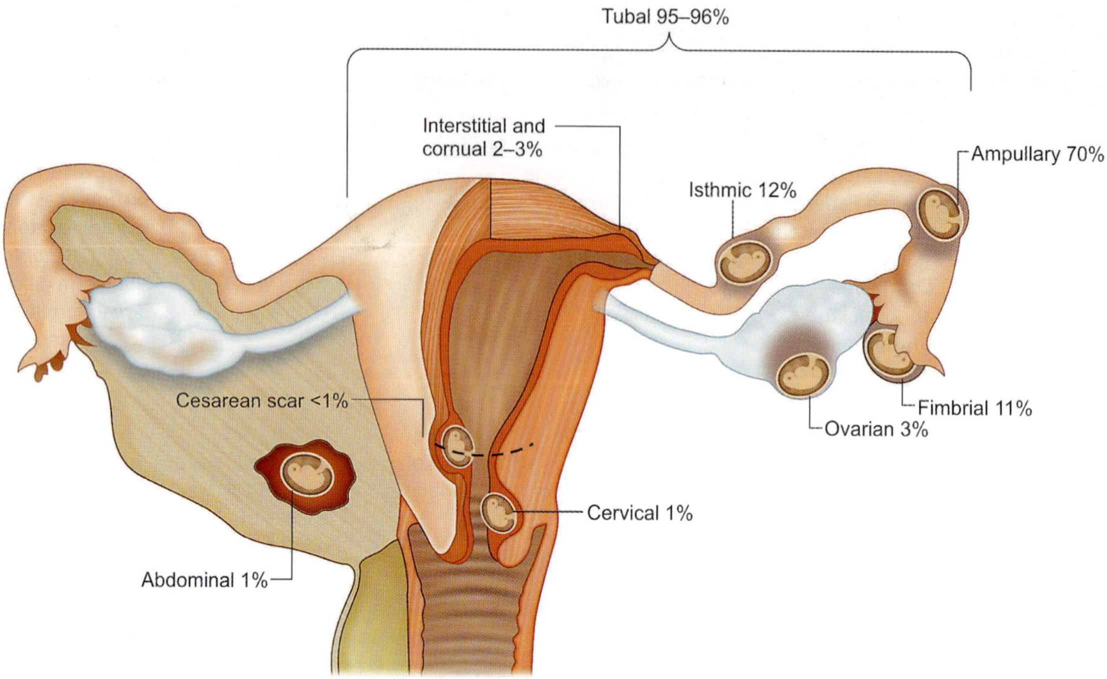

Fig. 7: Sites of ectopic pregnancy.

Flowchart 3: Pathophysiology of ectopic pregnancy in in vitro fertilization (IVF).

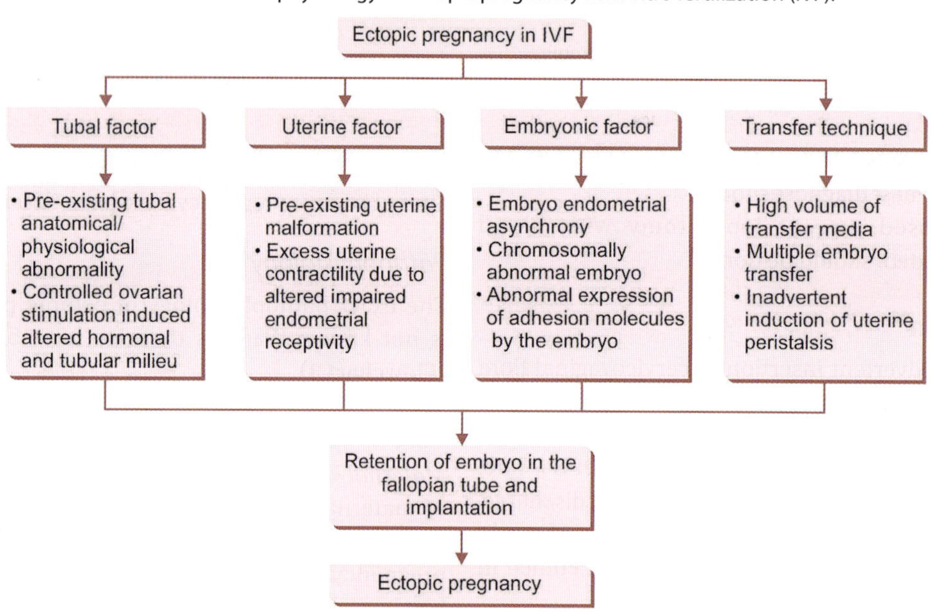

surgery. Cigarette smoking has been also associated with ectopic pregnancy especially because it decreases tubal and uterine motility.[76]

Uterine factors: Londra et al.,[77] suggested that there was an increase in incidence of ectopic pregnancy in fresh embryo transfer as compared to frozen embryo transfer. This could be because of the supraphysiological estrogen levels following ovarian stimulation rendering the uterus nonquiescent and nonreceptive. The same authors further went ahead to suggest that this risk was more with antagonist cycles as compared to agonist cycles.[78] Li et al.[79] corroborated the same by showing that there was significant reduction in ectopic pregnancy rates when frozen blastocyst was used for transfer. Effects of uterine abnormalities on ectopic pregnancy have not been adequately studied.[71,80]

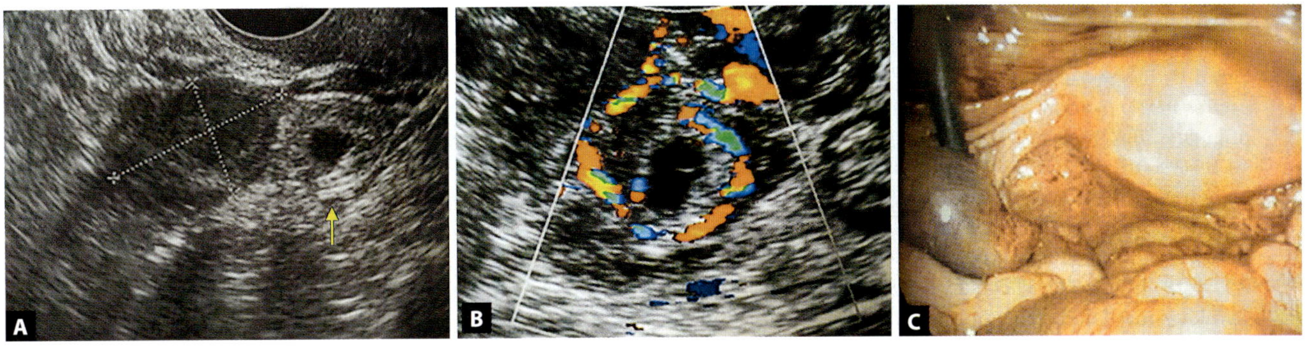

Figs. 8A to C: Diagnosis of ectopic pregnancy.

Embryonic Factors

Initially, it was theorized that assisted hatching may be associated with increased chance of ectopic pregnancy however in a recent study by Hageman et al.,[81] it was shown that assisted hatching neither improved pregnancy rates nor increased ectopic pregnancy rates. Tong et al.[82] demonstrated that there was a significant decrease in ectopic pregnancy rates with day 5 or day 6 embryo transfers. Job-Spira et al.,[83] suggested that chromosomal abnormalities increased ectopic pregnancy rates.

Transfer Techniques

Marcus et al., noted that patients with ectopic pregnancy were transferred larger volumes of culture media as compared to those with intrauterine pregnancy.[84] Knutzen et al.[85] also demonstrated that there was increased risk for tubal pregnancy to occur with larger volumes of culture media. Several authors have demonstrated that inadvertent touching of the uterine fundus caused onset of uterine peristalsis, which lead to ectopic pregnancy.[86-88] Also multiple embryo transfers were shown to be associated with ectopic pregnancy.[89]

Diagnosis of Ectopic Pregnancy

Beta-human chorionic gonadotropin (BhCG) alone does not have any role in diagnosing ectopic pregnancy.[90] It should be used along with ultrasound for the complete diagnosis of ectopic pregnancy. Serial quantitative BhCG measurements are better parameters in diagnosing ectopic pregnancy.[71] Transvaginal ultrasonography can effectively determine the presence of an intrauterine or ectopic sac at the level of a discriminatory zone of BhCG 2000 IU/L **(Fig. 8A)**. The features on ultrasonography may be presence of a pseudo sac without the presence of double decidual sign. An adnexal mass may be seen moving separately from the ovary. On Doppler, a ring of fire appearance **(Fig. 8B)** around the ectopic pregnancy may be seen with low-peak systolic velocity (PSV).[58] Ectopic pregnancy is usually ipsilateral to a corpus luteum cyst. The diagnosis of a heterotopic pregnancy remains elusive and one should be careful to look at the adnexa even after seeing a viable intrauterine pregnancy **(Fig. 8C)**.

KEY POINTS

- Assisted-reproductive technology is more or less a nonemergency field. However, emergencies may arise when least expected. One has to be vigilant to diagnose the pathological condition early.
- OHSS in its severe form needs a multidisciplinary and meticulous approach.
- Adnexal torsion on the other hand needs a high index of suspicion and needs urgent laparoscopy. Increased risk of ectopic pregnancy in COS has been attributed to the process of ovarian stimulation and embryo transfer and requires careful monitoring, medical or surgical treatment, and close follow-up. Overall, one has to be cautious of the complications that might be encountered during stimulation, retrieval, and post-transfer.

REFERENCES

1. Mathur RS, Drakeley AJ, Raine-Fenning NJ, Evbuomwan IO, Haitham H. The management of ovarian hyperstimulation syndrome. Green-top Guideline No. 5, RCOG Green Top Guideline. 2016.
2. Lyons CA, Wheeler CA, Frishman GN, Hackett RJ, Seifer DB, Haning RV Jr. Early and late presentation of the ovarian hyperstimulation syndrome: Two distinct entities with different risk factors. Hum Reprod. 1994;9:792-9.
3. Mathur RS, Akande VA, Keay SD, Hunt LP, Jenkins JM. Distinction between early and late ovarian hyperstimulation syndrome. Fertil Steril. 2000;73:901-7.
4. Papanikolaou EG, Pozzobon C, Kolibianakis EM, Camus M, Tournaye H, Fatemi HM, et al. Incidence and prediction of ovarian hyperstimulation syndrome in women undergoing gonadotropin releasing hormone antagonist in vitro fertilization cycles. Fertil Steril. 2006;85:112-20.
5. Golan A, Ron-el R, Herman A, Soffer Y, Weinraub Z, Caspi E. Ovarian hyperstimulation syndrome: an update review. Obstet Gynecol Surv. 1989;44:430-40.
6. Manau D, Balasch J, Arroyo V, Jiménez W, Fábregues F, Casamitjana R, et al. Circulatory dysfunction in asymptomatic in vitro fertilization patients. Relationship with

hyperestrogenemia and activity of endogenous vasodilators. J Clin Endocrinol Metab. 1998;83:1489-93.
7. Yarali H, Fleige-Zahradka BG, Yuen BH, McComb PF. The ascites in the ovarian hyperstimulation syndrome does not originate from the ovary. Fertil Steril. 1993;59(3):657-61. doi: 10.1016/s0015-0282(16)55815-4. PMID: 8458471.
8. Naredi N, Talwar P, Sandeep K. VEGF antagonist for the prevention of ovarian hyperstimulation syndrome: current status. Med J Armed Forces India. 2014;70(1):58-63.
9. Adashi E, Resnick C, Packman JN, Hurwitz A, Payne DW. Cytokine-mediated regulation of ovarian function: tumor necrosis factor alpha inhibits gonadotrophin-supported progesterone accumulation by differentiating and luteinized murine granulosa cells. Am J Obstet Gynecol. 1990;162:889-96.
10. Dinarello CA. Interleukin-1 and its related cytokines. Adv Immunol. 1989;44:153-205.
11. Orvieto R, Homburg R. Chronic ultra-low dose follicle-stimulating hormone regimen for patients with polycystic ovary syndrome: one click, one follicle, one pregnancy. Fertil Steril. 2009;91(4):1533-5.
12. Al-Inany HG, Youssef MA, Aboulghar M, Broekmans F, Sterrenburg M, Smit J, et al. GnRH antagonists are safer than agonists: an update of a Cochrane review. Hum Reprod Update. 2011;17(4):435.
13. Tso LO, Costello MF, Albuquerque LT, Andriolo RB, Freitas V. Metformin treatment before and during IVF or ICSI in women with polycystic ovary syndrome. Cochrane Database Syst Rev. 2014;(2):CD006105.
14. Ishihara O, Arce JC; Japanese Follitropin Delta Phase 3 Trial (STORK) Group. Individualized follitropin delta dosing reduces OHSS risk in Japanese IVF/ICSI patients: A randomized controlled trial. Reprod Biomed Online. 2021;42(5): 909-18.
15. Yacoub S, Cadesky K, Casper RF. Low risk of OHSS with follitropin delta use in women with different polycystic ovary syndrome phenotypes: a retrospective case series. J Ovarian Res. 2021;14:31.
16. Guo JL, Zhang DD, Zhao Y, Zhang D, Zhang XM, Zhou CQ, et al. Pharmacologic interventions in preventing ovarian hyperstimulation syndrome: A systematic review and network meta-analysis. Sci Rep. 2016;6:19093.
17. Kol S, Dor J. Prevention of OHSS: GnRH agonist versus hCG to trigger ovulation. Reprod BioMed Online. 2009;19(1):59-60.
18. Youssef MA, Van der Veen F, Al-Inany HG, Mochtar MH, Griesinger G, Nagi Mohesen M, et al. Gonadotropin-releasing hormone agonist versus HCG for oocyte triggering in antagonist-assisted reproductive technology. Cochrane Database Syst Rev. 2014;(10):CD008046.
19. Mourad S, Brown J, Farquhar C. Interventions for the prevention of OHSS in ART cycles: an overview of Cochrane reviews. Cochrane Database Syst Rev. 2017;(1):CD012103.
20. Krishna D, Dhoble S, Praneesh G, Rathore S, Upadhaya A, Rao K. Gonadotropin-releasing hormone agonist trigger is a better alternative than human chorionic gonadotropin in PCOS undergoing IVF cycles for an OHSS Free Clinic: a randomized control trial. J Hum Reprod Sci. 2016;9(3): 164-72.
21. Casper RF. Reducing the risk of OHSS by GnRH agonist triggering. J Clin Endocrinol Metab. 2015;100(12):4396-8.
22. Tang H, Mourad S, Zhai SD, Hart RJ. Dopamine agonists for preventing ovarian hyperstimulation syndrome. Cochrane Database Syst Rev. 2016;(11):CD008605.
23. Blockeel C, Drakopoulos P, Santos-Ribeiro S, Polyzos NP, Tournaye H. A fresh look at the freeze-all protocol: a SWOT analysis. Hum Reprod. 2016;31(3):491-7.
24. Akman L, Akdogan A, Erbas O, Aktug H, Sahin G, Tavmergen E. Effect of letrozole for prevention of ovarian hyperstimulation syndrome (OHSS) in a rat model. Fertil Steril. 2013;100(3):S258.
25. Naredi N, Karunakaran S. Calcium gluconate infusion is as effective as the vascular endothelial growth factor antagonist cabergoline for the prevention of ovarian hyperstimulation syndrome. J Hum Reprod Sci. 2013;6(4):248-52.
26. Youssef MA, Mourad S. Volume expanders for the prevention of ovarian hyperstimulation syndrome. Cochrane Database Syst Rev. 2016;(8):CD001302.
27. Tan SL, Balen A, el Hussein E, Campbell S, Jacobs HS. The administration of glucocorticoids for the prevention of ovarian hyperstimulation syndrome in in vitro fertilization: a prospective randomized study. Fertil Steril. 1992;58(2): 378-83.
28. Devroey P, Polyzos NP, Blockeel C. An OHSS-Free Clinic by segmentation of IVF treatment. Hum Reprod. 2011;26(10): 2593-7.
29. Huang Ci, Hong M-K, Ding D-C. A review of ovary torsion Ci Ji Yi Xue Za Zhi. 2017;29(3):143-7.
30. Hibbard LT. Adnexal torsion. Am J Obstet Gynecol. 1985; 152:456e61.
31. Roest J, Mous HV, Zeilmaker GH, Verhoeff A. The incidence of major clinical complications in a Dutch transport IVF programme. Hum Reprod Update. 1996;2(4):345-53.
32. Mashiach S, Bider D, Moran O, Goldenberg M, Ben-Rafael Z. Adnexal torsion of hyperstimulated ovaries in pregnancies after gonadotropin therapy. Fertil Steril. 1990;53(1):76-80.
33. Oelsner G, Shashar D. Adnexal torsion. Clin Obstet Gynecol. 2006;49:459-63.
34. Anne A, Dalley A. Grant's Atlas of Anatomy, 13th edition. Philadelphia: Lippincott Williams & Wilkins; 2012.
35. Chang HC, Bhatt S, Dogra VS. Pearls and pitfalls in diagnosis of ovarian torsion. Radiographics. 2008;28(5):1355-64.
36. Breech LL, Hillard PJ. Adnexal torsion in pediatric and adolescent girls. Curr Opin Obstet Gynecol. 2005;17(5):483-9.
37. Littman ED, Rydfors J, Milki AA. Exercise induced ovarian torsion in the cycle following gonadotrophin therapy: case report. Hum Reprod. 2003;18(8):1641-2.
38. Mordehai J, Mares AJ, Barki Y, Finaly R, Meizner I. Torsion of uterine adnexa in neonates and children: a report of 20 cases. J Pediatr Surg. 1991;26(10):1195-9.
39. Oltmann SC, Fischer A, Barber R, Huang R, Hicks B, Garcia N. Cannot exclude torsion--a 15-year review. J Pediatr Surg. 2009;44(6):1212-6.
40. White M, Stella J. Ovarian torsion: 10-year perspective. Emerg Med Australas. 2005;17(3):231-7.
41. Tsafrir Z, Azem F, Hasson J, Solomon E, Almog B, Nagar H, et al. Risk factors, symptoms, and treatment of ovarian torsion in children: the twelve-year experience of one center. J Minim Invasive Gynecol. 2012;19(1):29-33.

42. Rotoli JM. Abdominal pain in the post-menopausal female: Is ovarian torsion in the differential? J Emerg Med. 2017; 52(5):749-52.
43. Peterson WF, Prevost EC, Edmunds FT, Hundley JM Jr, Morris FK. Benign cystic teratomas of the ovary: a clinico-statistical study of 1,007 cases with a review of the literature. Am J Obstet Gynecol. 1955;70:368-82.
44. Kawahara Y, Fukuda T, Futagawa S, Sakamoto I, Takao M, Kinoshita Y, et al. Intravascular gas within an ovarian tumor: a CT sign of ovarian torsion. J Comput Assist Tomogr. 1996; 20(1):154-6.
45. Gelbaya TA. Short and long-term risks to women who conceive through in-vitro fertilisation. Hum Fertil. 2010;13: 19-27.
46. Zhu W, Li X, Chen X, Fu Z. Conservative management of adnexal torsion via transvaginal ultrasound guided ovarian cyst aspiration in patients with ovarian hyperstimulation. Fertil Steril. 2008;89:229e1-e3.
47. Tsai HC, Kuo TN, Chung MT, Lin MY, Kang CY, Tsai YC. Acute abdomen in early pregnancy due to ovarian torsion following successful in vitro fertilization treatment. Taiwan J Obstet Gynecol. 2015;54(4):438-41.
48. Dasgupta R, Renaud E, Goldin AB, Baird R, Cameron DB, Arnold MA, et al. Ovarian torsion in pediatric and adolescent patients: a systematic review. J Pediatr Surg. 2017;pii: S0022-3468.
49. Warner MA, Fleischer AC, Edell SL, Thieme GA, Bundy AL, Kurtz AB, et al. Uterine adnexal torsion: sonographic findings. Radiology. 1985;154(3):773-5.
50. Huchon C, Staraci S, Fauconnier A. Adnexal torsion: a predictive score for pre-operative diagnosis. Hum Reprod. 2010;25(9):2276-80.
51. Shadinger LL, Andreotti RF, Kurian RL. Preoperative sonographic and clinical characteristics as predictors of ovarian torsion. J Ultrasound Med. 2008;27:7-13.
52. Damigos E, Johns J, Ross J. An update on the diagnosis and management of ovarian torsion. Obstet Gynaecol. 2012;14:229-36.
53. Cohen SB, Wattiez A, Stockheim D, Seidman DS, Lidor AL, Mashiach S, et al. The accuracy of serum interleukin-6 and tumor necrosis factor as markers for ovarian torsion. Hum Reprod. 2001;16:2195-7.
54. Aran T, Guven S, Unsal MA, Alver A, Mentese A, Yulug E. Serum ischemia-modified albumin as a novel marker of ovarian torsion: an experimental study. Eur J Obstet Gynecol Reprod Biol. 2010;150(1):72-5.
55. Graif M, Itzchak Y. Sonographic evaluation of ovarian torsion in childhood and adolescence. Am J Roentgenol. 1988;150(3):647-9.
56. Albayram F, Hamper UM. Ovarian and adnexal torsion: spectrum of sonographic findings with pathologic correlation. J Ultrasound Med. 2001;20(10):1083-9.
57. Rha SE, Byun JY, Jung SE, et al. CT and MR imaging features of adnexal torsion. RadioGraphics. 2002;22(2):283-94.
58. Panchal S, Nagori C. Ultrasound in Infertility and Gynecology. Text and Atlas, 1st edition. New Delhi: Jaypee Brothers Medical Publishers (P) Ltd; 2015.
59. Descargues G, Tinlot-Mauger F, Gravier A, Lemoine JP, Marpeau L. Adnexal torsion: a report on 45 cases. Eur J Obstet Gynecol Reprod Biol. 2001;98:91-6.
60. Oelsner G, Bider D, Goldenberg M, Admon D, Mashiach S. Long-term follow-up of the twisted ischemic adnexal mass managed by detorsion. Fertil Steril. 1993;60:976-9.
61. Bayer AI, Wiskind AK. Adnexal torsion: can the adnexa be saved? Am J Obstet Gynecol. 1993;171:1506-10.
62. Ben-Rafael Z, Bider D, Mashiach S. Laparoscopic unwinding of twisted ischemic hemorrhagic adnexum after in-vitro fertilization. Fertil Steril. 1990;53:569-71.
63. Shalev E, Bustan M, Yarom I, Peleg D. Recovery of ovarian function after laparoscopic detorsion. Hum Reprod. 1995;10: 2965-6.
64. Chen M, Chang CD, Yang YS. Torsion of previously normal adnexa. Evaluation of the correlation between the pathological changes and the clinical characteristics. Acta Obstet Gynecol Scand. 2001;80:58-61.
65. Fuchs N, Smorgick N, Tovbin Y, Ben Ami I, Maymon R, Halperin R, et al. Oophoropexy to prevent adnexal torsion: how, when and for whom? J Minim Invasive Gynecol. 2010;17: 205-8.
66. Tureck RW, García CR, Blasco L, Mastroianni L. Perioperative complications arising after transvaginal oocyte retrieval. Obstet Gynecol. 1993;81(4):590-3.
67. Dicker D, Ashkenazi J, Feldberg D, Levy T, Dekel A, Ben-Rafael Z. Severe abdominal complications after transvaginal ultrasonographically guided retrieval of oocytes for in vitro fertilization and embryo transfer. Fertil Steril. 1993;59(6): 1313-31.
68. Gardner DK, Wiessman A, Howles C, Shoham Z. Textbook of Assisted Reproductive Techniques, Volume 2, 5th edition. US: CRC Press; 2018.
69. Jurkovic D, Wilkinson H. Diagnosis and management of ectopic pregnancy. BMJ. 2011;342:d3397.
70. Clayton HB, Schieve LA, Peterson HB, Jamieson DJ, Reynolds MA, Wright VC. Ectopic pregnancy risk with assisted reproductive technology procedures. Obstet Gynecol. 2006; 107:595-604.
71. Refaat B, Dalton E, Ledger WL. Ectopic pregnancy secondary to in vitro fertilisation-embryo transfer: pathogenic mechanisms and management strategies. Reprod Biol Endocrinol. 2015;13:30.
72. Patil M. Ectopic pregnancy after infertility treatment. J Hum Reprod Sci. 2012;5:154-65.
73. Rana P, Kazmi I, Singh R, Afzal M, Al-Abbasi FA, Aseeri A, et al. Ectopic pregnancy: a review. Arch Gynecol Obstet. 2013;288:747-57
74. Malak M, Tawfeeq T, Holzer H, Tulandi T. Risk factors for ectopic pregnancy after in vitro fertilization treatment. J Obstet Gynaecol Can. 2011;33:617-9.
75. Li C, Meng CX, Zhao WH, Lu HQ, Shi W, Zhang J. Risk factors for ectopic pregnancy in women with planned pregnancy: a case–control study. Eur J Obstet Gynecol Reprod Biol. 2014; 181:176-82.
76. Talbot P, Riveles K. Smoking and reproduction: the oviduct as a target of cigarette smoke. Reprod Biol Endocrinol. 2005;3:52.
77. Londra L, Moreau C, Strobino D, Garcia J, Zacur H, Zhao Y. Ectopic pregnancy after in vitro fertilization: differences between fresh and frozen-thawed cycles. Fertil Steril. 2015; 104(1):110-8.

78. Londra L, Moreau C, Strobino D, Bhasin A, Zhao Y. Is the type of gonadotropin-releasing hormone suppression protocol for ovarian hyperstimulation associated with ectopic pregnancy in fresh autologous cycles for in vitro fertilization? Fertil Steril. 2016;106(3):666-72.
79. Li Z, Sullivan EA, Chapman M, Farquhar C, Wang YA. Risk of ectopic pregnancy lowest with transfer of single frozen blastocyst. Hum Reprod. 2015;30(9):2048-54.
80. Galliano D, Bellver J, Diaz-Garcia C, Simón C, Pellicer A. et al. ART and uterine pathology: How relevant is the maternal side for implantation? Hum Reprod Update. 2015;21: 13-38.
81. Hagemann AR, Lanzendorf SE, Jungheim ES, Chang AS, Ratts VS, Odem RR. A prospective, randomized, double-blinded study of assisted hatching in women younger than 38 years undergoing in vitro fertilization. Fertil Steril. 2010;93: 586-91.
82. Du T, Chen H, Fu R, Chen Q, Wang Y, Mol BW, et al. Comparison of ectopic pregnancy risk among transfers of embryos vitrified on day 3, day 5, and day 6. Fertil Steril. 2017;108(1): 108-16.e1.
83. Job-Spira N, Coste J, Bouyer J, Tharaux-Deneux C, Fernandez H. Chromosomal abnormalities and ectopic pregnancy? New directions for aetiological research. Hum Reprod. 1996;11:239-42.
84. Marcus SF, Brinsden PR. Analysis of the incidence and risk factors associated with ectopic pregnancy following invitro fertilization and embryo transfer. Hum Reprod. 1995;10: 199-203.
85. Knutzen V, Stratton CJ, Sher G, McNamee PI, Huang TT, Soto-Albors C. Mock embryo transfer in early luteal phase, the cycle before in vitro fertilization and embryo transfer: a descriptive study. Fertil Steril. 1992;57:156-62.
86. Azem F, Yaron Y, Botchan A, Amit A, Yovel I, David MP, et al. Ectopic pregnancy after in vitro fertilization-embryo transfer (IVF-ET): the possible role of the ET technique. J Assist Reprod Genet. 1993;10: 302-4.
87. Nazari A, Askari HA, Check JH, O'Shaughnessy A. Embryo transfer technique as a cause of ectopic pregnancy in in vitro fertilization. Fertil Steril. 1993;60:919-21.
88. Keegan DA, Morelli SS, Noyes N, Flisser ED, Berkeley AS, Grifo JA. Low ectopic pregnancy rates after in vitro fertilization: do practice habits matter? Fertil Steril. 2007;88:734-6.
89. Pandian Z, Marjoribanks J, Ozturk O, Serour G, Bhattacharya S. Number of embryos for transfer following in vitro fertilization or intra-cytoplasmic sperm injection. Cochrane Database Syst Rev. 2013;7:CD003416.
90. Elson CJ, Salim R, Potdar N, Chetty M, Ross JA, Kirk EJ. Diagnosing and management of ectopic pregnancy. BJOG. 2016;123:e15-55.
91. van Mello NM, Mol F, Adriaanse AH, Boss EA, Dijkman AB, Doornbos JP, et al. The METEX study: Methotrexate versus expectant management in women with ectopic pregnancy: a randomised controlled trial. BMC Womens Health. 2008;8:10.
92. van Mello NM, Mol F, Verhoeve HR, van Wely M, Adriaanse AH, Boss EA,et al Methotrexate or expectant management in women with an ectopic pregnancy or pregnancy of unknown location and low serum hCG concentrations? a randomized comparison. Hum Reprod. 2012;28(1):60-7.
93. Hajenius PJ, Mol F, Mol BWJ, Bossuyt PM, Ankum WM, van der Veen F. Interventions for tubal ectopic pregnancy. Cochrane Database Syst Rev. 2007;(1):CD000324.
94. Elito J, Reichmann A, Uchiyama M, Camano L. Predictive score for the systemic treatment of unruptured ectopic pregnancy with a single dose of methotrexate. Int J Gynecol Obstet. 1999;67:75-9.
95. Barnhart K, Hummel AC, Sammel MD, Menon S, Jain J, Chakhtoura N. Use of "2-dose" regimen of methotrexate to treat ectopic pregnancy. Fertil Steril. 2007;87(2):250-6.
96. Song T, Kim MK, Kim ML, Jung YW, Yun BS, Seong SJ. Single-dose versus two-dose administration of methotrexate for the treatment of ectopic pregnancy: a randomized controlled trial. Hum Reprod. 2016;31(2):332-8.
97. Barnhart KT, Gosman G, Ashby R, Sammel M. The medical management of ectopic pregnancy: a meta-analysis comparing "single dose and multidose" regimens. Obstet Gynecol. 2003;101:778-84.
98. Practice Committee of American Society for Reproductive Medicine. Medical treatment of ectopic pregnancy: a committee opinion. Fertil Steril. 2013;100(3):638-44.
99. Alur-Gupta S, Cooney L, Senapati S, Barnhart KT. Effectiveness of single versus two or multi-dose methotrexate protocol for the treatment of ectopic pregnancy: a meta-analysis. Fertil Steril. 2017;108(3):e379.
100. Mol F, van Mello NM, Strandell A, Jurkovic D, Ross J, Barnhart KT, et al.; European Surgery in Ectopic Pregnancy (ESEP) study group. Salpingotomy versus salpingectomy in women with tubal pregnancy (ESEP study): an open-label, multicentre, randomised controlled trial. Lancet. 2014; 383(9927):1483-9.
101. Fernandez H, Capmas P, Lucot JP, Resch B, Panel P, Bouyer J; GROG. Fertility after ectopic pregnancy: the DEMETER randomized trial. Hum Reprod. 2013;28(5):1247-53.

CHAPTER 94

Fetal Reduction

Revathi S Rajan

INTRODUCTION

"Assisted reproductive technologies (ARTs)" have revolutionized obstetric practice. Although many infertile couples have benefited by begetting children, some of them are also faced with challenges such as multifetal pregnancies, fetal reduction, prenatal diagnostic procedures, etc.

Twenty six percent of all pregnancies after in vitro fertilization (IVF) are reported to be twins and about 1.3% of them are higher order multiple pregnancies.

Maternal and neonatal complications in higher order multiple pregnancies include an increase in the risk of preterm deliveries, hypertension including preeclampsia, gestational diabetes and postpartum hemorrhage. The neonates born as a consequence of higher order multiple pregnancies are encountered with issues such as prematurity, low birth weight, delayed milestones, cerebral palsy and learning disabilities.

Fetal reduction involves the elimination of one or more of the fetuses in the multiple pregnancy (which is usually a consequence of assisted reproduction), iatrogenically, in order to improve the perinatal outcome of the surviving fetuses.

BACKGROUND

Assisted reproductive technologies usually carry the risk of implantation of multiple embryos, resulting in multifetal pregnancies. This commonly includes quadruplets, triplets and twin pregnancies. "Fetal reduction" was an approach developed by the genetic researchers who were actively involved in the "Human Genome Project," which involves an ultrasound-guided termination of the most accessible fetus using pharmacological agents (potassium chloride) which is instilled intracardially into the fetus by a needle stab ensuring complete cessation of cardiac activity of the targeted fetus either through trans abdominal or transvaginal routes.

MEDICOLEGAL ISSUES AND PSYCHOLOGICAL IMPACT

The logic behind this technique is best described by Berkowitz[1] and colleagues as; "the medical justification for performing multifetal pregnancy reduction is philosophically similar to the "lifeboat analogy", where it is justifiable to sacrifice some "innocent" fetal lives to increase the chances of survival or decrease the risk of serious morbidity in the survivors of the procedure."

The ethical justification of this procedure has been described by Chevernak and colleagues,[2] who have expressed it in terms of these goals:

- Achieving a pregnancy that results in a live birth of one or more infants with minimal neonatal morbidity and mortality
- Achieving a pregnancy that results in the birth of one or more infants without anomalies.

Although an "informed consent" is procured from the couple before the procedure, it has been observed that a "true choice" is not made by them and is usually a decision made due to depression and fear prevailing in their minds. There is significant psychological distress reported due to the coercive choice made by the couple who have already been through enough stress during evaluation and treatment for infertility, which pressurizes them to make this decision hoping for a better perinatal outcome.

Ethical Issues

Decisions involving fetal reduction must be entirely autonomous. The pregnant mother should entirely make decisions for or against fetal reduction totally free of any stress or compulsion and must do it as per the directions of her thought processes after weighing the pros and cons completely.[3]

Principles of "Beneficence" and "Nonmaleficence" need to be incorporated while making decisions for fetal reduction. Fetal reduction is a procedure undertaken to protect and promote the welfare of any multiple pregnancy (Principle of Beneficence) while inflicting less harm to the surviving fetuses (Principle of nonmaleficence).

Less harm involves reduction in complications such as preeclampsia and gestational diabetes and also decreasing the possibility of preterm birth and prematurity. It has been observed that the incidence of higher order multiples and multifetal pregnancy reduction is low in those countries where infertility has been granted an insurance cover thereby allowing the woman to access better treatments such as IVF as compared to controlled ovarian hyperstimulation. Limiting the autonomy of the physician by strictly limiting the number of embryos transferred may be another solution to reduce multiple pregnancies. Both these concepts involve the "Principle of Justice".

Patient counseling needs to be nondirective; explaining the procedure of fetal reduction which is to be adopted as a salvage procedure including the option and consequences of no treatment. She could base her decision together with her spouse; after consultation with the maternal fetal medicine specialist, mental health specialist and the perinatologists. There should be no element of coercion in her mind while making the decision which could be based on her psychological make-up, religious beliefs and also her socioeconomic status. If the pregnant mother opts out of the procedure, the clinician needs to be supportive of her stand and must direct her to a facility with the necessary backup which could handle surveillance and delivery of higher order multiples. The exercised preferences and the necessary counseling details need to be correctly documented in the "informed consent" which is to be taken by the maternal fetal medicine specialist from the pregnant mother.

Reduction to a singleton is generally not preferred, although it may be offered in certain patients after weighing her circumstances in terms of medical risks and her socioeconomic status.

There have been several studies aimed to study the psychological impact of fetal reduction on the couple involved. Schreiner-Engel[4] and colleagues reported that 20% of those who participated in the follow-up, (postreduction) experience long-term "dysphoria". Garel and colleagues reported a 44% refusal rate for the interview.

Among those who attended the interview (post-reduction), most of them experienced "persistent depressive symptoms" mainly sadness and guilt, which was related to the procedure per se. The other participants made medical and rational comments experiencing no emotion. However, there is no research on the long-term consequences of the parental distress on the physiological development of the surviving children. The dynamics of "postabortion survivor syndrome" has still not been studied.

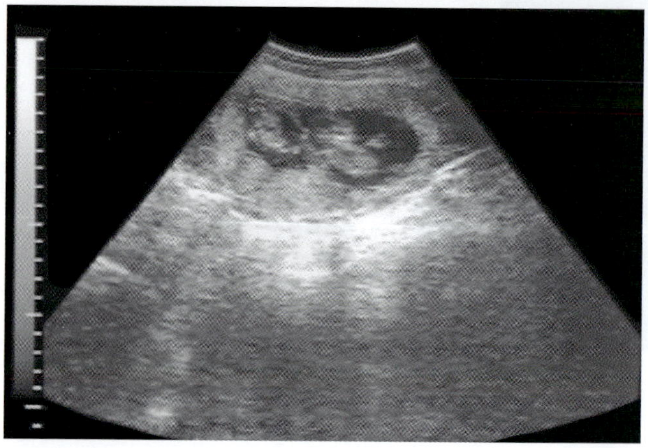

Fig. 1: Fetal reduction being attempted on a multiple pregnancy.

PROCEDURE

Timing of the Procedure

Ideally, fetal reduction is usually scheduled between 11 and 12 weeks of pregnancy, as by this time spontaneous fetal demises, if they should occur, would have already occurred. Another justification for performing this procedure at this period of gestation is that by the end 11–12 weeks, a nuchal translucency (NT) scan is also complete whereby an early scrutiny of the fetus to rule out anomalies is also done. This also enables the operator to choose the abnormal fetus (if any), for reduction which is referred to as "selective fetal reduction" **(Fig. 1)**.

METHODS

Multifetal pregnancy reduction can be performed using several techniques which are always ultrasound guided. It can be done either by transabdominal, transvaginal or transcervical aspiration, and also by intrathoracic injection of potassium chloride which can be performed by transabdominal or by transvaginal routes.

PREREQUISITES

Informed Consent

A detailed informed consent is to be obtained by the "maternal fetal medicine specialist" from the patient after explaining the pros and cons of the procedure. It must be emphasized to the couple that in the process of continuing a higher order multifetal pregnancy, there is an increased chance of losing all the fetuses due to a mid-trimester abortion or preterm delivery. Thus, fetal reduction must be offered to the couple as a salvage measure to improve the chances of survival of the remaining fetuses.

Antibiotics and Tocolysis

Prophylactic antibiotics usually a single dose of injectable cephalosporin or amoxicillin and clavulanic acid combination is recommended just before the procedure. Some centers also recommend progesterone depot injections (postprocedure) along with prophylactic tocolysis, in spite of the fact that the role of progesterone in preventing uterine irritability after the procedure is not proven.

Preoperative Ultrasonography

Preoperative ultrasonography is important for the following:

- Assessment of the total number of fetuses
- Assessment of the chorionicity of the fetuses, as identifying a monochorionic pair could influence the operator to reduce the same, as monochorionic twins are associated with a poor perinatal outcome. Instilling potassium chloride to one twin of the monochorionic pair would result in the demise of both the monochorionic fetuses, as they share a common placenta
- Marking the topography
- Detection of the fetal anomalies and selective termination of a specific anomalous fetus.

TECHNIQUE

Transcervical Aspiration

It was described by Martene Duplan in the early 1980s. During this procedure, the patient is placed in lithotomy position and the procedure is performed under ultrasound guidance using an abdominal probe. The cervix is exposed using a Sims' speculum and the vagina is gently cleansed with antiseptic solution. The cervix is then gently grasped using a tenaculum and progressively dilated using Hegar's dilators. A Karman's cannula which is connected to a 20 mL syringe is then inserted through the cervical canal and is subsequently brought into contact with the embryo located next to the internal os.

The embryo is then aspirated with one brisk suction operated manually. The procedure is again repeated in the same fashion, if many embryos have to be reduced.

Disadvantages of the Procedures

- This procedure can be easily performed at an early gestation (about 9 weeks), but unfortunately screening for fetal abnormalities is not possible at this gestational age.
- The rate of abortion is generally higher when compared to other methods.
- This procedure involves dilatation of the cervix which can result in significant bleeding per vaginum.

Transabdominal Needling

In this procedure, a 20-gauge needle is inserted through the mother's abdomen into the thorax of the fetus. Earlier, fetal demise was achieved by injecting air or saline. Mechanical trauma was also used to cause fetal demise. These methods are always not successful, as these methods were associated with several drawbacks (for example, injecting air could alter the overall quality of the sonographic image). Thus, transabdominal fetal reduction is presently performed by injecting potassium chloride intracardially using ultrasound guidance. Fundally placed embryos are technically easier to needle when compared to low lying ones.

Under ultrasound guidance, with full aseptic precautions and under local anesthesia a 20-gauge needle (after removing the stiletto) is inserted through the mother's abdomen into the thorax of the fetus. After confirming the position of the needle a 2 mL syringe is attached to the needle and 1–2 mL of potassium chloride is injected through the syringe gently into the fetal cardia, ensuring that the fetus is not pushed away from the needle tip by the pressure of the fluid injected.

Occasionally, fluid injected into the fetus can be visualized as a transonic image in the fetal mediastinum and pleural cavity. If the needle has been inserted correctly into the fetal cardia, an asystole is obtained followed by complete cessation of the fetal heart within a few seconds. Fetal demise has to be confirmed again by a check scan preferably on the following day to avoid missing a failed attempt.

Transvaginal Needling

In this procedure, a 20-gauge needle is inserted through a guide attached to the vaginal probe which is advanced through the vagina into the uterus targeting the fetus concerned. After ensuring the correct placement of the needle into the fetal cardia, 1–2 mL of potassium chloride is instilled using a syringe, until complete cessation of fetal heart is confirmed.

OTHER METHODS

Mechanical trauma can also be used to bring about embryo reduction very early in gestation (by 7–8 weeks). This is usually accomplished by the transvaginal route.

In this method, the tip of a 25 cm long needle (with an external diameter of 1.6 mm) is connected through a catheter to a 20 mL syringe which is placed in contact with the embryo to be reduced. A brief suction is applied to effect complete cessation of cardiac activity of the embryo. It has several advantages such as:

- Performing the reduction procedure very early, in gestation, could prove to be psychologically more acceptable to most couples
- The rate of losing the entire pregnancy as a consequence of reduction is significantly lower when this procedure is performed at an early gestational age.

But, this procedure is associated with a disadvantage that the anomalous fetus, if any, cannot be chosen for reduction as scrutiny for anomalies at this gestational age is technically very difficult.

Potassium Chloride

It is the pharmacological agent which is commonly used in fetal reduction. It causes fetal demise by causing asystole followed by slowing and complete cessation of fetal heart. Although it is commonly used for fetal reduction, the efficacy of this agent has been questioned. The following issues have been debated:

- Stimulation of prostaglandin release along with release of cytokines which occurs as a consequence of the inflammatory response to the remnant fetoplacental tissue that is undergoing autolysis (postprocedure) has been attributed to be the cause for initiating preterm labor and pregnancy loss.[5]
- Rare case of anencephaly and fetal limb amputation following the use of potassium chloride has been reported
- The entire pregnancy could be lost if potassium chloride accidentally percolates into the nontargeted sacs.
- It has also been reported that potassium chloride induces the release of tissue plasminogen activators, matrix metalloproteinases and matrix degrading enzymes within the uterus, which could be attributed to rupture of membranes.

Complications

- The risk of complete pregnancy loss could be 1–2% in experienced hands. This could be a result of preterm premature rupture of membranes, accidental entry of potassium chloride into nontargeted sacs or preterm labor (due to uterine irritation as a consequence of the procedure).
- Risk of preterm premature rupture of membranes and threatened abortion, sometimes progressing to abortion also exists.

Some patients may also present with leaking or bleeding per vaginum which may be self-limiting.

FAILED REDUCTION

It is not uncommon to have a failed attempt of fetal reduction. Hence, careful mapping of the fetus (to be reduced) is crucial, as the surviving fetus after a failed attempt of reduction can have sequelae. Thus, all attempts to complete the procedure in a single sitting are preferred.

SELECTIVE REDUCTION

When multifetal pregnancy reduction is attempted, the fetus that is targeted to be reduced is the one that is easily accessible by the operator. But in some situations, selective fetal reduction is performed in which a particular fetus is chosen to be reduced probably due to a congenital anomaly associated with it which could have been detected by ultrasound or any other prenatal diagnostic procedure. In some cases, a fetus whose growth is significantly lesser than the other fetuses is chosen to be reduced.

STUDIES ON FETAL REDUCTION

- According to a meta-analysis by Dodd J and Crowther C, multifetal pregnancy reduction to twins compared to expectant management of higher order pregnancy seems to be an effective treatment option for any woman with a higher order pregnancy. This suggests that multifetal pregnancy reduction of higher order pregnancy to twins is medically justified.[6] Studies have shown no significant difference in mean gestational age at birth, birth weights and perinatal mortality rates between reduced and nonreduced twins.
- A comparative study conducted by Jung Ryoel Lee and his colleagues that compared the outcomes of different methods of multifetal pregnancy reduction involved 148 patients with multiple pregnancies from assisted reproduction programs who underwent multifetal pregnancy reduction. The patients were divided into potassium chloride and non-potassium chloride groups based on the agent used for fetal reduction. They were also divided into the early (<8 weeks of gestation) and the late groups (>8 weeks of gestation), based on the period of gestation at which fetal reduction was performed. They concluded that the early non-potassium chloride method (which involved cardiac puncture and aspiration of amniotic fluid with the fetus) showed a lower immediate loss (<4 weeks of the procedure) and preterm premature rupture of membranes. The take home baby rates as a result of this procedure were also more when compared to those pregnancies where the late potassium chloride method was used for fetal reduction.[7]
- Evans et al. in a collaborative study involving more than thousand cases observed that transabdominal multifetal pregnancy reduction was increasingly associated with a poor outcome compared to transvaginal or transcervical methods which subsequently improved as the expertise of the operator increased.[8] Transvaginal method is technically simpler when compared to transabdominal method and is similar to ovum aspiration.
- Recently, there has been a trend in which multifetal pregnancy reduction is performed in all cases of higher order pregnancies to singletons instead of twins to improve the perinatal outcome.[9] Further studies need to be performed to establish whether there is a definitive advantage conferred by this. Recent studies have also suggested that selective termination after 20 weeks of gestation does not increase the risk of fetal loss compared to procedures before 20 weeks of gestation. Cord coagulation, which is a new technique, is aimed at selective termination in monochorionic twins and is associated with high rates of morbidity and mortality.
- Pregnancy loss rates due to fetal reduction depend upon:
  - The experience of the operator
  - Number of fetuses at the start and also at the end of the procedure.

A multicenter experience[10] with over 3,500 completed reductions reported the following rates of fetal loss corresponding to the number of fetuses at the beginning and at the end of the procedure. The results were as follows:

Number of fetuses (at start)	Fetal loss (%)
6	15.4
5	11.4
4	7.3
3	4.5

Number of fetuses (at the end)	Fetal loss (%)
3	18.4
2	6
1	6.7

A single center[11] experience involving 1,000 consecutive multifetal pregnancy reductions showed the following results:

- Complete fetal loss was 5.9%
- Loss rate was lowest for a starting number of 2 fetuses
- Loss rate remained stable for reductions with a starting number of 3, 4 or 5 fetuses
- Loss rate increased to 12.9% for 6 or more fetuses at start
- The final number of fetuses also influenced the perinatal outcome.

Number of fetuses (at the end)	Fetal loss (%)
1	3.5
2	5.5
3	16.7

The mean gestational age of delivery varied (as indicated here) and was similar to unreduced pregnancies with a similar number of fetuses.

Number of fetuses (at start)	Gestational age at delivery (weeks)
1	37.9
2	35.3
3	33.5

KEY POINTS

- Multifetal pregnancy reduction is a procedure which is performed to achieve a pregnancy resulting in the live birth of one or more healthy infants with very minimal neonatal morbidity and mortality.
- Long-term consequences such as "postabortion survivor syndrome" which reflects the psychological impact of fetal reduction needs to be studied.
- Decisions for fetal reduction could be based on the "Principles of Beneficence, Nonmaleficence and Justice." The final decision needs to be completely autonomous which is to be made by the pregnant mother after weighing the pros and cons.
- No significant differences in perinatal outcome were observed between reduced and nonreduced twins.
- Transabdominal multifetal pregnancy reduction was associated with a poor outcome when compared to transvaginal or transcervical methods which gradually improved with the operator's experience.
- Pregnancy loss rates greatly depend upon the experience of the operator and the number of fetuses at start and at the end of the procedure.
- Optimizing assisted reproductive techniques is the best solution to reduce the need for invasive procedures such as fetal reduction.

ACKNOWLEDGMENTS

This chapter was first published in the textbook "An Introduction to Genetics and Fetal Medicine (Second edition)" by Dr Deepika Deka and Dr Narendra Malhotra. It has been further edited including concepts such as "Ethical Issues" involving fetal reduction which play a pivotal role influencing decision making.

REFERENCES

1. Berkowitz RL, Lynch L, Stone J, Alvarez M. The current status of multifetal pregnancy reduction. Am J Obstet Gynecol. 1996;174(4):1265-72.
2. Chevernak FA, McCullough LB, Wapner R. Three ethically justified indications for selective termination in multifetal pregnancy. A practical and comprehensive management strategy. J Assist Reprod Genet. 1995;(8):531-6.
3. ACOG. Committee opinion 553: Multifetal Pregnancy Reduction. Washington DC: American College of Obstetricians and Gynecologists; 2013.
4. Schreiner-Engel P, Walther VN, Mindes J, Lynch L, Berkowitz RL. First-trimester multifetal pregnancy reduction: acute and persistent psychologic reactions. Am J Obstet Gynecol. 1995;172(2 Pt 1):541-7.
5. Sebire NJ, Sherod C, Abbas A, Snijders RJ, Nicolaides KH. Preterm delivery and growth restriction in multifetal pregnancies reduced to twins. Hum Reprod. 1997;12(1):173-5.
6. Dodd J, Crowther C. Multifetal pregnancy reduction of triplet and higher order multiple pregnancies to twins. Fertil Steril. 2004;81(5):1420-7.
7. Lee JR, Ku SY, Jee BC, Suh CS, Kim KC, Kim SH. Pregnancy outcomes of different methods for multifetal pregnancy reduction: a comparative study. J Korean Med Sci. 2008;23(1):111-6.
8. Evans MI, Dommergues M, Timor-Tritsch I, Zador IE, Wapner RJ, Lynch L, et al. Transabdominal versus transcervical and transvaginal multifetal pregnancy reduction, international collaborative experience of more than thousand cases. Am J Obstet Gynecol. 1994;170(3):902-9.
9. Rochon M, Stone J. Invasive procedures in multiple gestations. Curr Opin Obstet Gynecol. 2003;15(2):167-75.
10. Evans MI, Berkowits RL, Wapner RJ, Carpenter RJ, Goldberg JD, Ayoub MA, et al. Improvement in outcomes of multifetal pregnancy reduction with increased experience. Am J Obstet Gynecol. 2001;184(2):97-103.
11. Stone J, Eddleman K, Lynch L, Berkowitz RL. A single center experience with 1,000 consecutive cases of multifetal pregnancy reduction. Am J Obstet Gynecol. 2002;187(5):1163-7.

CHAPTER 95

COVID-19 and Pregnancy

Varsha Patil, Chandana C

INTRODUCTION

Coronavirus disease 2019 (COVID-19) is a pandemic of the 21st century of global concern caused by severe acute respiratory syndrome coronavirus 2 (SARS-CoV-2). Novel corona SARS-CoV-2, which is the etiological agent of COVID-19, was first detected in Wuhan city of China in December 2019.[1] Since then, it has spread worldwide and has become one of the public health emergencies to mankind. Common cold (HCoV-229E, NL63, OC43, and HKU1), Middle East respiratory syndrome coronavirus (MERS-CoV), and SARS-CoV are the different types of coronavirus infections.[2] On March 11, 2020, COVID-19 was identified as a global pandemic by World Health Organization (WHO).[3]

ETIOLOGY

Coronavirus disease 2019 virus is a single-stranded ribonucleic acid (RNA) under the family of *Betacoronavirus* and subfamily *Sarbecovirus*. COVID-19 virus is made up of membrane glycoprotein (M), envelop protein (E), nucleocapsid protein (N), and spike protein (S) **(Fig. 1)**.[4,5]

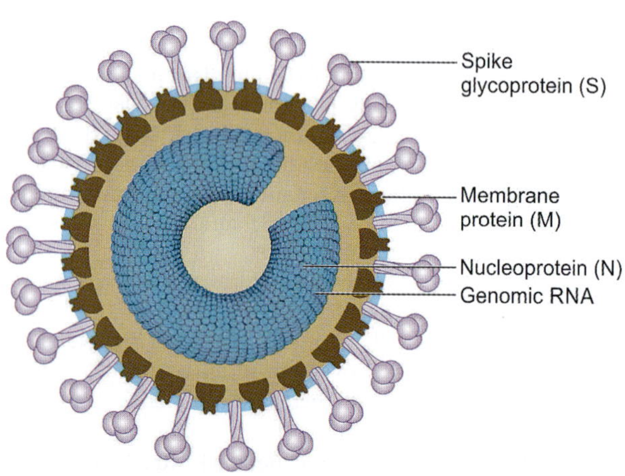

Fig. 1: Severe acute respiratory syndrome coronavirus 2 (SARS-CoV-2). (RNA: ribonucleic acid)

In December 2021, WHO declared the five important variants of COVID-19 that are of global concern: The Alpha variant identified in London, the Beta variant identified in South Africa, the Gamma variant of Brazil, the Delta variant of India, and the Omicron variant.[6-8]

Transmission of COVID-19 is by respiratory secretions, feces, and fomites with mean incubation period of 5–7 days with a duration of disease varying from 5 days to chronic infection.

PATHOPHYSIOLOGY

The respiratory system is commonly affected by coronavirus disease because the virus binds to surface of type 2 alveolar cells of lungs at angiotensin-converting enzyme 2 receptors with the help of spike protein present on the surface of coronavirus.[9]

Coronavirus disease is a systemic hyperinflammation syndrome with elevated levels of interleukin 2, 5, and 6, protein 10 of gamma-induced protein, granulocyte-macrophage colony-stimulating factor, monocyte chemoattractant protein 1, macrophage inflammatory protein-1 alpha, and tumor necrosis factor alpha. Coronavirus disease with acute respiratory distress syndrome (ARDS) has classical elevated blood values of C-reactive protein (CRP), lactate dehydrogenase (LDH), D-dimer, and ferritin.[10,11]

CORONAVIRUS DISEASE 2019 AND PREGNANCY

The incidence of coronavirus disease is similar in pregnant and nonpregnant women, but the severity is more in pregnant women, especially in the last trimester because of the following three reasons:[12]

1. Altered body immune system during pregnancy.
2. Reduction in total lung capacity and inability to clear the secretions.
3. Pregnancy is a hypercoagulable state, with a high level of circulating coagulation and thrombogenic factors.

Majority of infected pregnant women do not require hospitalization.

Risk factors of severe disease and critical illness during pregnancy include age >35 years, obesity, preexisting hypertension, diabetes mellitus (DM), asthma, chronic kidney disease, cardiopulmonary disease, malignancy, and immunocompromised status.

CLINICAL PRESENTATION OF CORONAVIRUS DISEASE IN PREGNANCY

Clinical features are cold, cough, fever, myalgia, headache, vomiting, nausea, diarrhea, breathing difficulty, and loss of smell and taste; few cases will be asymptomatic.[13]

Among the symptomatic cases, 81% of patients develop mild to moderate infection with mild pneumonia, 14% will be having severe infection, and 5% will develop features of critical illness; one-third of infected persons will be asymptomatic.[14-17]

EFFECTS OF CORONAVIRUS DISEASE ON PREGNANCY

- Coronavirus disease 2019 will not add to the risk of miscarriage or pregnancy loss according to the available evidence. COVID-19 infection is not an indication for medical termination of pregnancy (MTP).
- Current evidence suggests of no vertical transmission, no risk of teratogenicity, and no possible congenital anomalies.[18]
- Current evidence suggests that vaginal secretions and breast milk are negative for COVID-19 virus.
- Incidence of preterm birth is increased in pregnancy with COVID-19, but it is not clearly understood whether it is because of spontaneous onset of preterm or iatrogenic induced.
- Studies have shown that COVID-19 adds to the risk of peripartum depression, anxiety, and domestic violence.[18]
- Current evidence suggests that the majority of babies of COVID-19 infected mothers usually do not show any symptoms; neonatal mortality rate is similar in both infected and noninfected COVID-19 infected newborns.[19]

Coronavirus disease 2019 infection is not an indication for lower segment cesarean section (LSCS). Mode of delivery should depend on obstetrics/fetal indications but should not be dependent on COVID-19 positivity. Cesarean section is only indicated in cases of refractory hypoxemic respiratory failure or worsening critical illness.[20]

SYMPTOMS AND CLASSIFICATION OF SEVERITY OF CORONAVIRUS DISEASE 2019

Clinical features of coronavirus disease in pregnancy are cold, cough, pyrexia, myalgia, headache, vomiting, nausea, diarrhea, shortness of breath, loss of smell and taste, or asymptomatic.[21]

Classification

- *Asymptomatic:* Without symptoms but tested COVID positive on the screening test.
- *Mild disease:* Mild clinical features of cold, cough, pyrexia, body aches, mild breathing difficulty, or positive findings on chest imaging.
- *Moderate disease:* Associated with bronchopneumonia, respiratory acidosis, and pyrexia not relieved by antipyretics but maintaining peripheral oxygen saturation (SpO_2) level of >95%.
- *Severe disease:* Respiratory distress with respiratory rate (RR) of >30/min, with SpO_2 of <95%, and with >50% lung involvement on chest computed tomography (CT) or X-ray.
- *Critical disease:* End-organ dysfunction involving renal, cardiac, and pulmonary systems with circulatory collapse shock requiring artificial ventilation.

PREVENTIVE MEASURES TO BE TAKEN BY PREGNANT WOMEN TO AVOID CORONAVIRUS DISEASE 2019 (FIG. 2)

- Vaccination
- Staying indoors
- Wearing an N95 mask
- Avoid crowded places
- Social distance of at least 1 meter from others
- Work from home
- Hand hygiene with soap and water or sanitizer
- Avoid touching the eyes, nose, or mouth with unwashed hands[22]
- Disinfection of surfaces with 1% hypochlorite solution
- Avoiding unnecessary travels
- Reduce the number of people visiting the mother and the baby after delivery.

INDICATIONS FOR CORONAVIRUS DISEASE 2019 TESTING DURING PREGNANCY

- Symptomatic pregnant women
- Hospitalized pregnant women who are in labor or near full term
- Pregnant women hospitalized for other reasons
- Newborns having acute pulmonary infections or sepsis.

Centers for Disease Control and Prevention (CDC) and Indian Council of Medical Research (ICMR) recommend reverse transcription-polymerase chain reaction (RT-PCR) of nasopharyngeal swab to detect COVID-19 infection.[23] Patients having productive cough and sputum should be tested for COVID-19.

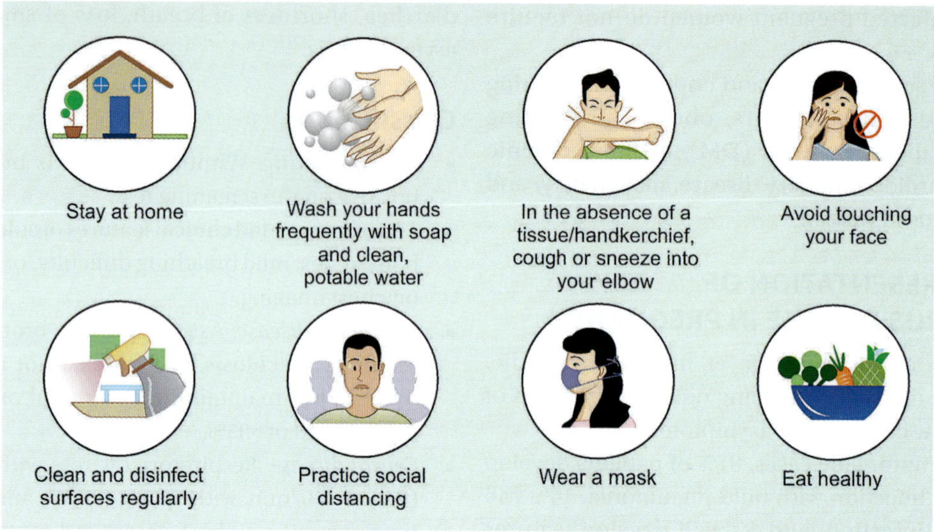

Fig. 2: Precautions for coronavirus.

Reverse transcription-polymerase chain reaction test should be conducted in the centers recognized by the central or state government. False negative rate is about 10–30%. Gold standard test to identify coronavirus disease is nucleic acid amplification test (NAAT).

Other investigations include complete blood count (CBC), renal function tests, liver function tests, coagulation profile, D-dimer, LDH, procalcitonin, and serum ferritin level.

Chest imaging such as CT scan/X-ray should be done only if indicated after the consent from pregnant patient and her attender with proper abdominal shielding.

COMPUTED TOMOGRAPHY SCAN FINDINGS OF CORONAVIRUS DISEASE 2019

Mild and early infection: Bilateral multilobar ground glass opacities which have nonsymmetrical, posterior, and peripheral distribution.

Advanced and severe infection: We can see crazy paving of subpleural dominance associated with consolidation.

Peripheral ground glass opacities without pleural effusion are the diagnostic findings of CT chest of COVID-19 patients.[24]

ANTENATAL CARE

Government of India recommends at least four antenatal visits along with one ultrasound scan in the second and third trimesters.

1. *First visit/registration:* Pregnant women should get registered with a healthcare provider as soon as pregnancy is recognized preferably within 3 months.
2. *Second visit:* Between 14 and 26 weeks.
3. *Third visit:* Between 28 and 34 weeks.
4. *Fourth visit:* Between 36 weeks and term.

At least one ultrasound in the second and third trimesters.

We are aiming to decrease the exposure of healthy pregnant women to new infections and exposure of healthcare workers to infected pregnant women and asymptomatic carriers by decreasing the number of visits.

Detailed history of pregnant women to be taken considering: coming from hot spot area, immunocompromised conditions, travel history, and history of exposure.

Duration and number of antenatal visits should be reduced during antenatal visits of pregnant women.

Antenatal Care and Care of Infected Pregnant Women During Coronavirus Disease

- Pregnant women with mild infections and asymptomatic carriers do not require any extra tests.
- Growth scans, routine antenatal tests, and visits are delayed until the patient completes the period of isolation.
- Pregnant women are made aware about the warning signs of COVID-19 and pregnancy.
- Pregnant women should be taught about the self-monitoring of oxygen saturation, temperature, pulse, and respiration (TPR) charting, and self-isolation.

Antenatal Follow-up After Coronavirus Disease 2019 Infection

- *Recovery from infection in first trimester:* Consider one obstetric ultrasound during pregnancy between 18 and 22 weeks of pregnancy as part of routine antenatal care.
- *Recovery from infection in the latter half of pregnancy:* Consider sonographic assessment of fetal growth 2 weeks after infection.

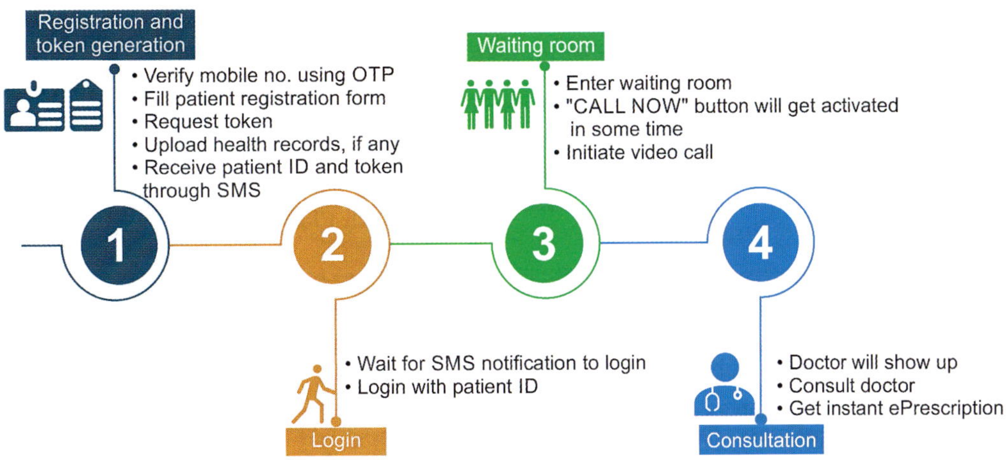

Fig. 3: e-Sanjeevani online outpatient department (OPD) consultation process.

eSanjeevani

eSanjeevani is a telemedicine for maternal–fetal health services during the COVID pandemic by the Ministry of Health and Family Welfare (MoHFW) of India for doctors and patients. In eSanjeevani, two types of telemedicine services are available:

1. Doctor-to-doctor at Ayushman Bharat-Health and Wellness Centres (AB-HWCs)
2. Patient-to-doctor eSanjeevani outpatient department (OPD) teleconsultations **(Fig. 3)**
   a. *eSanjeevani AB-HWC:*
      i. It is a doctor-to-doctor telemedicine platform made available at majority of the health and wellness centers across India in hub and spoke model under the Ayushman Bharat scheme of Government of India.
      ii. "Hubs" are medical college hospitals and district hospitals. "Spokes" are primary and secondary and community health centers.
   b. *eSanjeevani OPD:*
      i. Nationwide online OPD service which helps patients to consult doctors by video consultations.
      ii. Every video consultation generates an e-prescription which allows patients to get medicines or go for diagnostic investigations as advised.

TRIAGING

- Triaging is an important screening method that should be adopted at a healthcare facility to avoid/minimize exposure between COVID-19 infected and noninfected pregnant women.
- A checklist is used in triaging to separate pregnant women into three groups: (1) COVID positive, (2) COVID suspect, and (3) screen negative **(Box 1)**.
- Triaging should be done near the main entrance of the hospital and the place should be spacious enough to maintain social distance between pregnant women and healthcare workers.

BOX 1: Checklist for triaging.

Name: ____________ *W/O:* ____________
Age: ________ *Gestational age:* ____________
Phone no.: ____________ *Address:* ____________

Q1. Does the PW present with the following?
- Fever with cough—Yes/No
- Fever with shortness of breath—Yes/No
- Past history of fever with cough or shortness of breath—Yes/No
- History of contact with COVID positive—Yes/No
- The patient is a healthcare worker—Yes/No

Q2. Is the PW asymptomatic but a high-risk contact:
- Living in the same household with COVID positive—Yes/No
- Heath care worker providing care to COVID positive—Yes/No
- Traveling with COVID positive—Yes/No

Q3. Does the PW belong to hot spots/clusters/large migration gatherings/evacuee centers and presenting symptoms such as fever/cough/sore throat/runny nose—(Yes/No)

If answer to any of the above is *Yes*, PW to be sent to suspect ward and sample sent for testing or referred to higher centers, if all answers are *No*, patient to be sent to LR.

(LR: labor room; PW: pregnant woman)

- Triage area should have a fully equipped trolly with separate examination room.
- Proper referral services should be available in case any woman needs to be referred.
- Management of screen-negative patients should be done as per routine and standard protocol.
- COVID-suspect pregnant women should be isolated in a suspect area, and sample for testing should be sent **(Flowchart 1)**.
- Pregnant women who are in labor or having obstetric emergencies should be managed in septic labor ward.

Drawbacks of Triaging

- Healthy pregnant women are at a risk of getting exposed to asymptomatic carriers.
- Patients might not reveal the history of exposure to travel and clinical features.

MANAGEMENT OF MILD OR ASYMPTOMATIC CORONAVIRUS DISEASE 2019 INFECTION DURING PREGNANCY

Guidelines for Home Isolation

- *Isolation place:*
  - A separate adequately ventilated room with attached bathroom
  - Avoid sharing of personal items with other people in the household
  - 1% hypochlorite solution should be used to clean the surfaces which are touched frequently.
- *Respiratory and hand hygiene:*
  - Use three-layered medical masks or N95 masks
  - Dispose the worn masks after 8 hours of usage
  - Follow respiratory etiquettes
  - Practice hand hygiene by washing hands with soap and water for 20 seconds or with alcohol-based sanitizer
  - Healthy diet, adequate rest, and good water intake should be followed
  - Coryza, cough, and fever should be treated
  - Steam inhalation and lukewarm water gargles will help
  - Tablet paracetamol 650 mg QID is used to treat fever. In case of persistent fever, consider naproxen 250 mg twice a day.
  - Persistent cough for >5 days should be treated with inhalational budecort.
  - Ivermectin and doxycycline are contraindicated in pregnancy.[25]
  - Home monitoring of pulse, temperature, RR, and oxygen saturation using the below chart every 4th hourly **(Table 1)**.

Flowchart 1: Facility for COVID-suspect PW.

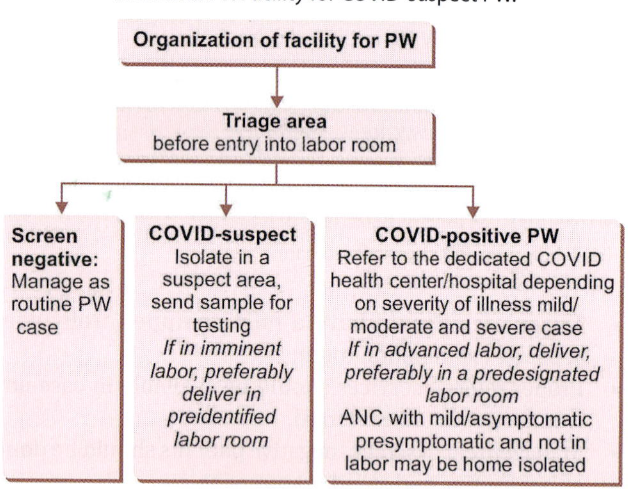

(ANC: antenatal care; COVID: coronavirus disease; PW: pregnant woman)

INDICATIONS FOR INPATIENT MANAGEMENT

- High-risk patients having poorly controlled DM, hypertension, chronic renal disorders, cardiorespiratory disorders, cancer, immune-compromised conditions.
- Patients who are unable of getting home quarantined and having risks for fetomaternal condition.
- Appearance of below warning signs during self-isolation will mandate hospitalization **(Table 2)**.

TREATMENT OF MODERATE TO SEVERE CORONAVIRUS DISEASE 2019 INFECTION IN PREGNANCY

Patients with moderate to severe infection need hospitalization with a multidisciplinary approach with specialists and intensive care unit (ICU) unit.

- *Investigations:*
  - CBC, differential count, renal and liver function tests: Every 1–2 days.
  - CRP, procalcitonin levels, LDH, interleukin 6 levels, serum ferritin, and D-dimer values: Every 2–3 days.
  - General random blood sugar (GRBS) monitoring in women receiving corticosteroids.

TABLE 2: Warning signs mandating hospital admission.

Clinical features: • Breathing difficulty • Inadequate oral intake of fluids and medicines • Pleuritic chest pain • Delirium and lethargy • Associated obstetrical conditions such as preterm, antepartum hemorrhage, and reduced fetal movements	• Tachypnea • Uncontrolled fever • SpO_2 below 95% at rest or on exertion • Peripheral cyanosis

(SpO_2: peripheral oxygen saturation)

TABLE 1: Home monitoring for coronavirus disease 2019.

Day of illness	*Temperature*	*Pulse rate*	*Oxygen saturation*	*Symptomatic assessment (better/same/worse)*	*Respiratory rate*	*Remarks*
7:00 AM						
11:00 AM						
3:00 PM						
7:00 PM						

- Chest imaging with CT scan/X-ray should be done only if indicated with abdominal shielding after consent with the pregnant mother and her attendant.

- *Medications:*
  - *Oxygen therapy:* Oxygen saturation should be maintained ≥95% by using a nonrebreather mask and high-flow nasal cannula.
  - Inhalational budesonide with metered-dose inhaler (MDI) spacer 800 μg twice a day for 7 days.
  - *Corticosteroids:* Methylprednisolone 0.5–1 mg/kg in two divided doses for 5–10 days. Methylprednisolone is preferred as it does not cross the placenta.
    - *Indications for corticosteroids:*
      - Patients with high RRs and poor oxygen saturation
      - Patients with pneumonia
      - Patients with cytokine storm.

Dexamethasone or betamethasone should be used for fetal lung maturity, followed by steroids in the form of methylprednisolone or hydrocortisone if indicated in the management of COVID-19 patients.

- Antibiotics are administered to prevent secondary bacterial infections and fever persisting for more than 6 days.
- *Anticoagulants:*
  - Low-molecular-weight heparin in a prophylactic dose used in a pregnant woman with mild COVID-19 with comorbidities
  - Low-molecular heparin is used in therapeutic dose twice daily in moderate to severe COVID-19 cases.
    - *Antepartum:* Continue thromboprophylaxis for 10 days after hospital discharge, longer duration if persistent morbidity
    - *Postpartum:* If the woman had a cesarean section and limited ambulation, stop anticoagulant when she is planned for discharge and home isolation.

MANAGEMENT OF CRITICALLY ILL AND SEVERE HYPOXIC CORONAVIRUS DISEASE 2019 PREGNANT PATIENTS

Indications of Intensive Care Unit Admission

- Falling trend of SpO_2 levels and poor oxygenation in spite of oxygen supplementation
- Persistent hypotension in spite of adequate fluid management
- Features of multi-organ failure.

Indications for Endotracheal Intubation

In the following situations, when oxygen requirements rise above 15 L/min by nasal cannulas, 40–50 L/min by high flow nasal cannulas, >60% of FiO_2 by Venturi mask, and Glasgow Coma Scale <8 these are the conditions which need oxygen saturation to be maintained above 94% and are the conditions that require endotracheal intubation.

MANAGEMENT OF CORONAVIRUS DISEASE 2019 PREGNANT WOMEN IN LABOR

Management of COVID-19 pregnant women in labor is shown in **Box 2**.

POSTNATAL CARE OF CORONAVIRUS DISEASE 2019 PATIENT

The healthcare providers should discuss with the mother about the temporary separation of mother and neonate.[26]

The neonate is kept in separate isolation room with an adequate caretaker, if the mother accepts.

If the mother desires for rooming in the same room/ hospital with limited facility for isolation, adequate steps to be taken to reduce the cross infection from infected mother to the baby.

Breastfeeding

Mother and baby in temporary isolation: Expressed breast milk should be fed to the baby by a healthy caretaker.

Mothers should use a dedicated and properly sterilized breast pump with good hand hygiene practices.

COVID-positive lactating mother who opted for rooming in: Breastfeeding should be done after wearing a triple-layered mask and adequate hand hygiene practice before and after the feed.[27]

Discharge Advice

- Counsel regarding warning signs of COVID-19 infection during the postnatal period
- To follow preventive measures at home to reduce COVID cross-infection
- Video consultation facility to be provided.

BOX 2: Management of COVID-19 pregnant women in labor.

- Severity of infection should be assessed and management should be done with multidisciplinary team approach in tertiary care unit
- TPR and SpO_2 charting should be done
- Ensure the onset of labor according to standard protocols
- Continuous fetal monitoring should be done by CTG
- Oxygen supplementation if SpO_2 falls below 94%
- COVID-19 infection with pregnancy is not any indication for LSCS. LSCS is only indicated in severely comprised respiratory status or for obstetric indications
- COVID-19 infection is not a contraindication for spinal or epidural anesthesia
- Instrumental delivery can be performed to cut short the second stage of labor
- Active management of third stage of labor should be done

Coronavirus disease 2019 positive status is not an indication for medical termination of pregnancy (MTP)/induction of labor (IOL)/ LSCS

(COVID-19: coronavirus disease 2019; CTG: cardiotocography; LSCS: lower segment cesarean section; SpO_2: peripheral oxygen saturation; TPR: temperature, pulse, respiration)

- Postnatal advice regarding iron, calcium supplementation, perineal hygiene, breastfeeding, and contraception should be given.

Management of COVID-19-positive pregnant woman is shown in **Flowchart 2.**

Flowchart 2: Management of COVID-19 positive pregnant woman.

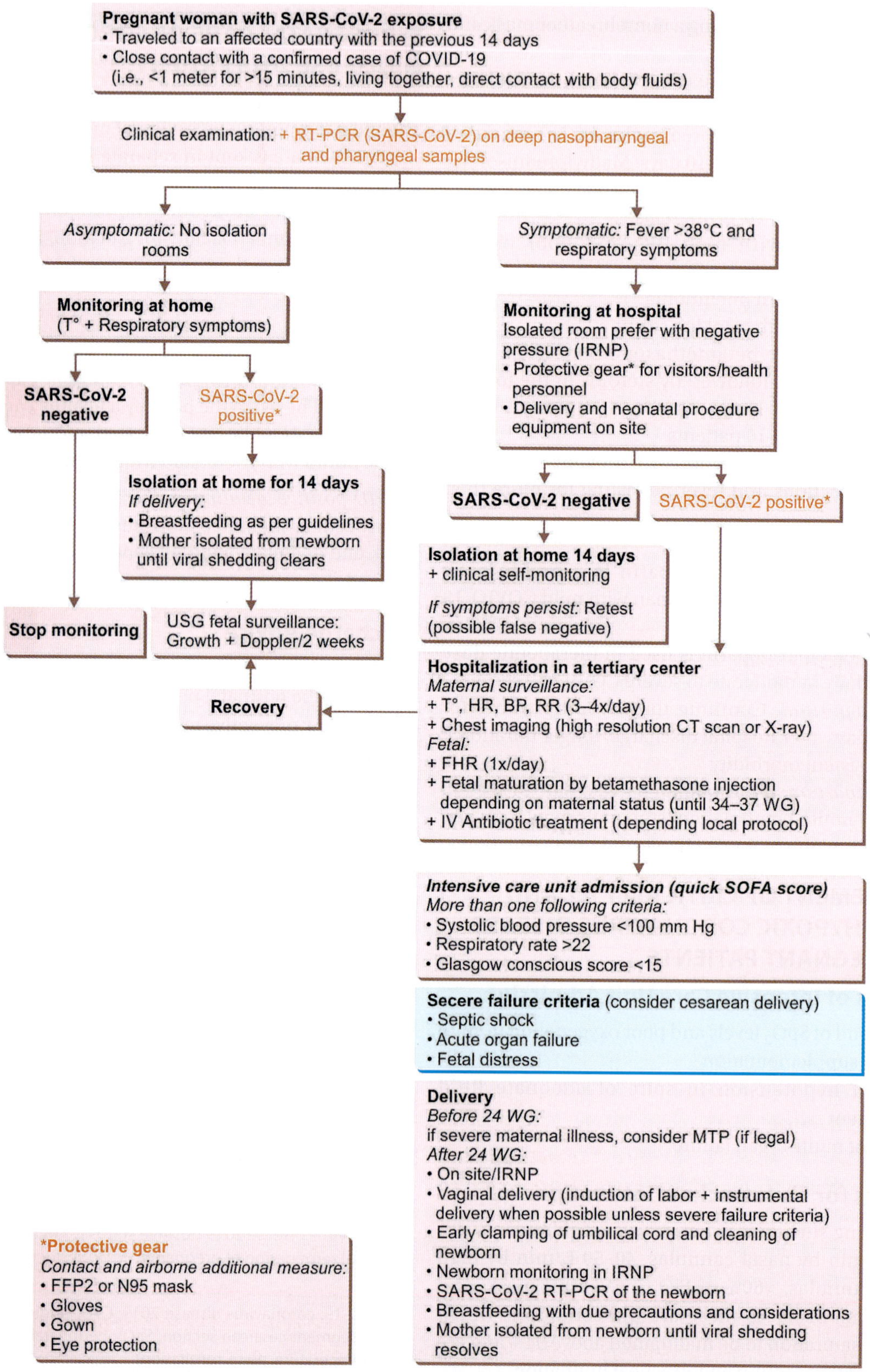

Source: Adapted from Lancet, which is present in guidance for the management of pregnant women in COVID-19 pandemic by ICMR/NIRRH.[18]

BOX 3: Personal protection equipment (PPE) in the management of suspected/confirmed patient of coronavirus disease 2019.

Respiratory protection:
- Triple-layered surgical mask
- N95 facemasks

Eye protection: Goggles and face shield
Body protection: Water-resistant complete gown which covers head and shoes
Hand protection: Properly fitting gloves

BOX 4: Steps of donning of personal protection equipment (PPE).

- *Step 1:* Proper hand wash should be done before donning
- *Step 2:* Appropriately fitting respirator or mask should be owned
- *Step 3:* Face shield and eye protection goggles should be owned
- *Step 4:* Appropriate size of gloves should be worn

USE OF PERSONAL PROTECTION EQUIPMENT IN THE MANAGEMENT OF SUSPECTED/CONFIRMED PATIENT OF CORONAVIRUS 19 DISEASE

Use of personal protection equipment in the management of suspected/confirmed patient of COVID-19 disease is shown in **Box 3**.

HOW TO USE PERSONAL PROTECTIVE EQUIPMENT

Use of personal protective equipment is shown in **Boxes 4 and 5**.

CORONAVIRUS DISEASE 2019 VACCINATION IN PREGNANT WOMEN AND LACTATING WOMEN

Based on the recommendations from the National Technical Advisory Group on Immunization (NTAGI), MoHFW has approved vaccination of lactating and pregnant women against COVID-19 in 2021.

Pregnant women should be counseled regarding the benefits and side effects of COVID-19 vaccination and also the risk associated with COVID-19 infection in pregnancy.

Timing of Vaccination

A pregnant woman can take COVID vaccination in any trimester of pregnancy. If she has been infected with COVID-19 in the present pregnancy, she should take vaccination in the postnatal period.

Coronavirus disease 2019 vaccination will reduce the severity of coronavirus infection but will not prevent from infection, so in spite of vaccination, coronavirus appropriate behavior such as N95 masks, hand hygiene, social distancing, and proper respiratory etiquettes needs to be followed.

BOX 5: Steps of doffing of personal protection equipment (PPE).

- *Step 1:* Gloves are removed after disinfecting with alcohol-based hand sanitizer and to be disposed in biohazard bin
- *Step 2:* After wearing a pair of new gloves the gown should be doffed off
- *Step 3:* Goggles and face shield should be removed from the backside of the strap
- *Step 4:* Respirator/mask should be removed next
- *Step 5:* Removal of new pair of gloves after using alcohol-based sanitizer
- *Step 6:* Proper hand wash with soap and water

CONCLUSION

Coronavirus disease is a pandemic of 21st century of global concern which has caused public health emergency to mankind. Several variants of COVID-19 are of concern like Alpha, Beta, Gamma, Delta, Omicron and new Beta 7 variant recently. Even though respiratory system is the most commonly affected organ system, COVID-19 is a systemic hyperinflammation syndrome with elevated levels of many inflammatory mediators. Incidence of coronavirus disease is similar in pregnant and nonpregnant women, but the severity of infection is more in pregnant women. Vaccination is an effective way to reduce the severity of COVID-19 infection, but it will not prevent from a person getting infected. So let us all follow the effective preventive measures like social distancing, proper respiratory hygiene and hand hygiene etiquettes and fight against COVID-19.

KEY POINTS

- Coronavirus disease 2019 is global health emergency of 21st century, first got detected in Wuhan city of China in December 2019.
- COVID-19 virus is a single-stranded RNA virus, under family of beta corona virus and subfamily sarbecovirus.
- Transmission of COVID-19 is by respiratory secretions, feces and fomites with the mean incubation period of 5 to 7 days with duration of disease varies from 5 days to chronic infection.
- Clinical features are cold, cough, fever, myalgia, headache, vomiting, nausea, diarrhea, breathing difficulty, loss smell and taste or may be few cases will be asymptomatic.
- Current evidence suggests that COVID-19 will not add the risk for miscarriage or pregnancy loss, no vertical transmission, no risk of teratogenicity and no increase in neonatal mortality rate but incidence of preterm birth is increased in pregnant women with COVID-19, but it is not clearly understood that it is because of spontaneous onset of preterm or iatrogenic induced.
- All pregnant women must be made aware about the warning signs of both COVID-19 and pregnancy.
- *eSanjeevani:* A telemedicine platform for maternal fetal health services during COVID pandemic by ministry of health and family welfare of India for doctors and patients.

- Home quarantine with monitoring of vitals, inpatient management and ICU management depends on severity of infection.
- Corona virus infection is not an indication for termination of pregnancy or cesarean section
- Use of Personal Protection Equipment (PPE) in the Management of Suspected/Confirmed Patient of COVID-19 will protect healthcare providers from getting infected.

REFERENCES

1. Page J, Hinshaw D, McKay B. (2021). In hunt for COVID-19 origin, patient zero points to second Wuhan market—the man with the first confirmed infection of the new coronavirus told the WHO team that his parents had shopped there. The Wall Street Journal. [online] Available from https://www.wsj.com/articles/in-hunt-for-covid-19-origin-patient-zero-points-to-second-wuhan-market-11614335404. [Last accessed February, 2021].
2. Royal College of Obstetricians and Gynaecologists. (2020). Coronavirus (COVID-19) infection in pregnancy. [online] Available from https://www.rcog.org.uk/globalassets/documents/guidelines/2020-03-26-covid19-pregnancy-guidance.pdf. [Last accessed March, 2020].
3. World Health Organization. (2020). WHO Director-General's opening remarks at the media briefing on COVID-19 - 11 March 2020. [online] Available from https://www.who.int/director-general/speeches/detail/who-director-general-s-opening-remarks-at-the-media-briefing-on-covid-19---11-march-2020. [Last accessed March, 2020].
4. Zhu N, Zhang D, Wang W, Li X, Yang B, Song J, et al. A novel coronavirus from patients with pneumonia in China, 2019. N Engl J Med. 2020;382(8):727-33.
5. Thomas S. The structure of the membrane protein of SARS-CoV-2 resembles the sugar transporter SemiSWEET. Pathog Immun. 2020;5(1):342-63.
6. US Centers for Disease Control and Prevention (CDC). (2021). New COVID-19 variants. [online] Available from https://www.cdc.gov/coronavirus/2019-ncov/transmission/variant.html. [Last accessed July, 2021].
7. World Health Organization. (2021). COVID-19 weekly epidemiological update, Edition 69, 7 December 2021. [online] Available from https://apps.who.int/iris/handle/10665/350244. [Last accessed December, 2022].
8. Letko M, Marzi A, Munster V. Functional assessment of cell entry and receptor usage for SARS-CoV-2 and other lineage B betacoronaviruses. Nat Microbiol. 2020;5(4):562-9.
9. Verdecchia P, Cavallini C, Spanevello A, Angeli F. The pivotal link between ACE2 deficiency and SARS-CoV-2 infection. Eur J Intern Med. 2020;76:14-20.
10. Turner AJ, Hiscox JA, Hooper NM. ACE2: from vasopeptidase to SARS virus receptor. Trends Pharmacol Sci. 2004;25(6):291-4.
11. Zhang C, Wu Z, Li JW, Zhao H, Wang GQ. Cytokine release syndrome in severe COVID-19: interleukin-6 receptor antagonist tocilizumab may be the key to reduce mortality. Int J Antimicrob Agents. 2020;55(5):105954.
12. Wastnedge EAN, Reynolds RM, van Boeckel SR, Stock SJ, Denison FC, Maybin JA, et al. Pregnancy and COVID-19. Physiol Rev. 2021;101(1):303-18.
13. European Centre for Disease Prevention and Control. (2020). Clinical characteristics of COVID-19. [online] Available from https://www.ecdc.europa.eu/en/covid-19/latest-evidence/clinical. [Last accessed December, 2022].
14. US Centers for Disease Control and Prevention (CDC). (2020). Interim clinical guidance for management of patients with confirmed coronavirus disease (COVID-19). [online] Available from https://www.cdc.gov/coronavirus/2019-ncov/hcp/clinical-guidance-management-patients.html. [Last accessed December, 2022].
15. Oran DP, Topol EJ. The proportion of SARS-CoV-2 infections that are asymptomatic: a systematic review. Ann Intern Med. 2021;174(5):655-62.
16. European Centre for Disease Prevention and Control. (2020). Transmission of COVID-19. [online] Available from https://www.ecdc.europa.eu/en/covid-19/latest-evidence/transmission. [Last accessed December, 2020].
17. Nogrady B. What the data say about asymptomatic COVID infections. Nature. 2020;587(7835):534-5.
18. ICMR-NIRRH. Guidance for management of pregnant women in COVID-19 pandemic. [online] Available from https://www.icmr.gov.in/pdf/covid/techdoc/Guidance_for_Management_of_Pregnant_Women_in_COVID19_Pandemic_12042020.pdf. [Last accessed December, 2022].
19. Mullins E, Hudak ML, Banerjee J, Getzlaff T, Townson J, Barnette K, et al. Pregnancy and neonatal outcomes of COVID-19: coreporting of common outcomes from PAN-COVID and AAP-SONPM registries. Ultrasound Obstet Gynecol. 2021;57(4):573-81.
20. The Royal Australian and New Zealand College of Obstetricians and Gynaecologists (RANZCOG). (2020). COVID-19 statement. [online] Available from https://ranzcog.edu.au. [Last accessed March, 2020].
21. Really Correct. Viral load exposure factors. ReallyCorrect.com. [online] Available from https://reallycorrect.com/ReallyCorrectWp1/covid-19-safety-information-ideas/#Viral-Load-Exposure-Factors. [Last accessed December, 2022].
22. US Centers for Disease Control and Prevention (CDC). (2020). Recommendation regarding the use of cloth face coverings, especially in areas of significant community-based transmission. [online] Available from https://stacks.cdc.gov/view/cdc/86440. [Last accessed December, 2022].
23. US Centers for Disease Control and Prevention (CDC). Coronavirus laboratory testing guidelines. [online] Available from https://www.cdc.gov/coronavirus/2019-nCoV/lab/guide-lines-clinical-specimens.html. [Last accessed March, 2020].
24. Salehi S, Abedi A, Balakrishnan S, Gholamrezanezhad A. Coronavirus disease 2019 (COVID-19): a systematic review of imaging findings in 919 patients. AJR Am J Roentgenol. 2020; 215(1):87-93.
25. NNF, FOGSI, IAP. Perinatal-neonatal management of COVID-19 infection. New Delhi; 2020.
26. Ministry of Health and Family Welfare, Government of India. [online] Available from https://www.mohfw.gov.in/. [Last accessed March, 2020].
27. US Centers for Disease Control and Prevention (CDC). Coronavirus Disease (COVID-19) and Breastfeeding. [online] Available from https://www.cdc.gov/breastfeeding/breastfeeding-special-circumstances/maternal-or-infant-illnesses/covid-19-and-breastfeeding.html. [Last accessed December, 2022].

CHAPTER

96

Essentials of Statistics: A Clinician's Perspective

Gautham T Pranesh

DATA AND ITS TYPES

Data is a collection of facts and figures that are collected and analyzed as a part of a research initiative.

Data is the raw material of statistics. Data can be collected in many ways; it can be qualitative or quantitative, it can be recorded by hand or digitally, and it can be stored on paper or electronically.

There are many different types of data:

- *Quantitative data:* This is data that has been measured numerically or with some other quantity-based unit. Examples of quantitative data include parameters such as height, temperature, and weight.
- *Qualitative data:* This is data that has been measured qualitatively such as through a survey response or an open-ended question. Examples of qualitative data include gender, ethnicity, patient responses to a questionnaire on pain scales, etc.

Data in a research study is called a *data item* or *variable*, essentially a value that can vary from individual to individual. As described, the previously mentioned variables can be either quantitative or qualitative. A parameter is a characteristic that describes the distribution of a variable in one specific population compared to another population (i.e., the mean height for males in one country compared to the mean height for males in another country).

Measurements can be applied to data based on a set of rules or levels of measurement.[1] Variables can further be classified based on the levels of measurement as:

- *Nominal variables:* Categorical variables where there is no inherent natural order. For example, gender as a variable may be classified into male and female (or more categories). None of the categories are regarded as higher or lower than the other categories. Nominal variables may be summarized as percentages and are often represented as pie charts, column or bar chart.
- *Ordinal variables:* Categorical variables that have a natural ascending or descending order. The distance between two categories is however, not constant and may be abstract. For example, if we were to classify pregnancy status based on a beta-human chorionic gonadotropin (β-hCG) laboratory test as negative, indeterminate, and positive, each of the categories represent an incrementally higher value of β-hCG. Note that, the negative group may have a value of 0–5 mIU/mL, indeterminate 5–20 mIU/mL, and positive above 20 mIU/mL, i.e., distance between the two categories is unequal. Ordinal data is best summarized as frequencies and percentages and is best displayed as a column or bar chart.
- *Interval variables:* Interval variables are continuous variables that can be measured as a discrete nonzero number. The distance between two adjacent numbers on the scale is however constant. For example, measurements of body temperature follow a scale with discrete intervals. The difference between 37.3°C and 37.4°C is the same as 39.3°C and 39.4°C. The value 0°C does not represent the absence of temperature, but a very cold temperature. If you combine two objects with 20°C temperature, you do not get 40°C temperature! (unlike weight). The value of zero does not imply the absence of the characteristic being measured. Interval variables may be represented as histograms, bar or column charts of summaries or line graphs over time. Interval variables can be best summarized by means, medians, and standard deviations.
- *Ratio variables:* Ratio variables are similar to interval variables but include the value 0 indicating absence of the variable in measurement. An example of a ratio variable is the number of M2 oocytes that may be obtained in a procedure. This can have a value such as 4, 5, or 6 with the differences between values being 1 and cannot have a value in between these discrete numbers. A value of 0 indicates that no oocytes were obtained and is plausible in the data set. Ratio variables can also be best summarized by means, medians and standard deviations and may be represented as histograms, bar or column charts of summaries or line graphs over time.

Nominal and ordinal variables are often called categorical variables whereas interval and ratio variables are called continuous variables.

SUMMARIZING DATA

Once data is collected, variables need to be summarized for further analysis. Measures of central tendency, measures of dispersion and the distribution of data are common ways of summarizing data.[1]

Measures of central tendency are used to describe the "typical" or "central" value for a set of data.

The two most common measures of central tendency are the mean and the median. The arithmetic mean is the sum of all values divided by the number of values in a set. The median is the middle value in a set when ordered from lowest to highest. The mode represents the most repeated observation in a variable.

Measures of dispersion are used to measure the spread of data from an average.

The standard deviation is a measure that is used to quantify how much the data in a distribution deviate from the mean. The coefficient of variation is a measure that quantifies the relative dispersion of data in relation to its mean. The coefficient of variation is the ratio of standard deviation to the mean. To calculate the coefficient of variation, divide the standard deviation by the mean and then multiply by 100.

Statistical tests are often classified as parametric (where they assume that the shape of data distribution is well-defined such as a normal distribution) or nonparametric (where no such assumptions are made. The shape of a distribution can be visually determined by plotting a histogram or through plots like the box and whisker plots.

NORMAL DISTRIBUTION AND ITS PROPERTIES

Numerical clinical data such as laboratory test values, height, weight, etc., may follow a wide range of distributions. Many biological variables when plotted as a histogram with the observation values obtained in a sample on the X-axis against the frequency of such observations on the Y-axis result in a bell-shaped curve. This curve conventionally resembles the normal distribution or the Gaussian distribution.[2] The normal distribution curve is continuous, described by the mean, a measure of the central point and standard deviation, a measure of the width or spread of data. The curve is symmetric about its mean with an equal number of values distributed on either side. Data sets obtained in clinical research may be approximated to the normal distribution.

Such approximations of data can be extended to use the properties of the normal distribution to infer clinically relevant information. For example:

- 68.3% of values for a normal distribution lie within one standard deviation (1 SD) of the mean on either side
- 95.4% of values for a normal distribution lie within two standard deviations (2 SD) of the mean on either side
- 99.7% of values for a normal distribution lie within three standard deviations (3 SD) of the mean on either side **(Fig. 1)**.

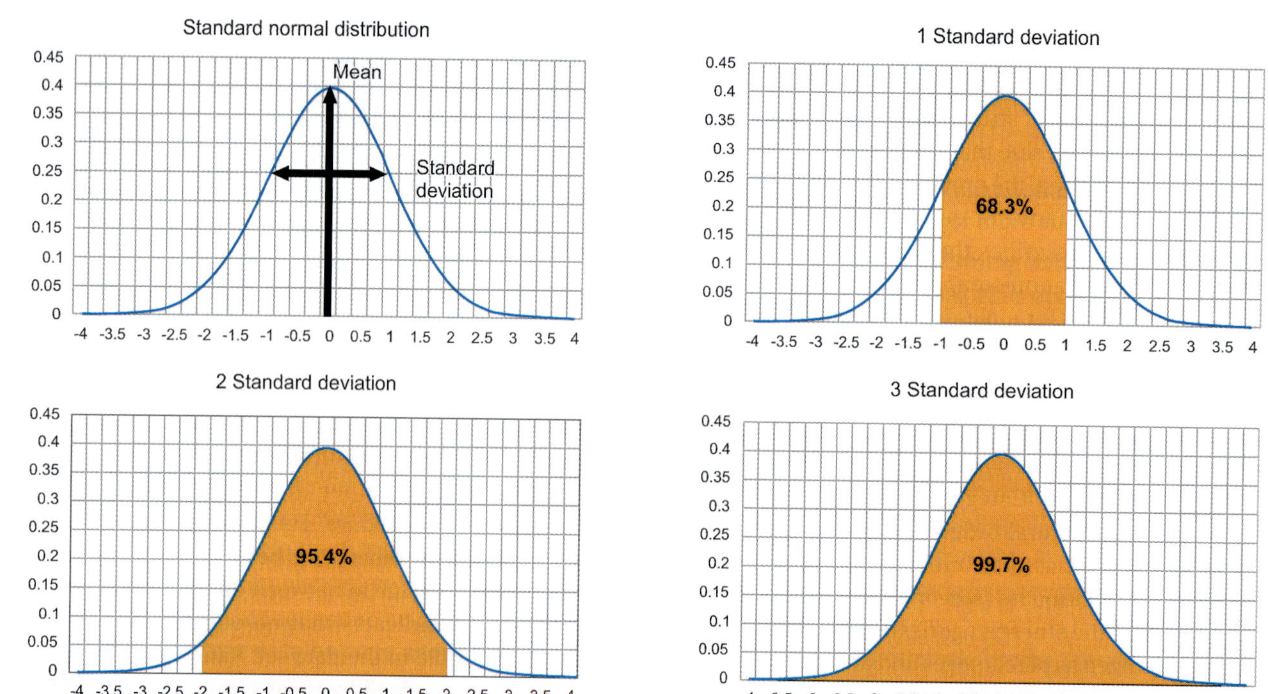

Fig. 1: Standard normal distribution and area under the curve (shaded area) at 1 standard deviation, 2 standard deviation, and 3 standard deviations.

If data in a clinical setting is approximated to a normal distribution, the mean ± 1.96 standard deviations cover 95% of the sample, a property which is often used to estimate reference ranges. The values of mean +1.96 SD and mean –1.96 SD provide the upper and lower cut-offs for such ranges.

If we take multiple random samples of size n from a population, we are likely to find a slightly different mean for every sample. If we plot a frequency histogram of the values of such means obtained across many samples-experiments, the resulting distribution of the sample means would approximate to a normal distribution. In other words, the sample means are distributed normally around the population mean with the variability being termed as the standard error of the mean (SEM). As the standard error of mean is normally distributed, for a sample with n observations, a mean of μ and a standard deviation σ, it can be calculated as

$$\text{SEM} = \sigma/\sqrt{n}$$

Furthermore, 95% of all possible sample means would lie within the limits $\mu \pm 1.96 \times \text{SEM}$.

The properties of the normal distribution enable us to develop a confidence interval, a measure of reliability by a range for estimates of an unknown variable such as a reference range or a range of possible means, at a designated confidence level (i.e., 95% of all values).

STATISTICAL TESTS AND THEIR APPLICATION

There are a wide variety of statistical tests that may be applied to data. Selection of the appropriate statistical tests depends on the purpose of analysis (comparison of means, establishing association, prediction of values, etc.), the level of measurement (type of data), number (two groups or more than two groups) and type of samples (independent samples versus paired samples). **Table 1** provides a brief example of commonly used statistical tests.

In most statistical analysis, the first step is to establish a "null hypothesis" (H_0).[6,7] The null hypothesis is a statistical statement implying that the differences observed across samples in an experiment is due to chance alone. Statistical tests evaluate the p-value, the probability of rejecting the null hypothesis when the null hypothesis is true. A low p-value, say a p-value of 0.001 indicates a 1 in 1,000 probability of rejecting the null hypothesis when the null hypothesis is true. By established convention, most medical research deems a p-value of <0.05 to be statistically significant.

Experiments done to infer from the real world and statistical tests therein have the possibility of two types of errors, type I and type II as shown in **Table 2**.

Type I errors or false positive results on experiments result in rejecting the null hypothesis due to a chance finding when the null hypothesis is the truth. The impact of this error would be a change in clinical practice when there is no benefit derived from the change. Type II errors indicate the failure of an experiment to reject the null hypothesis due to chance when the null hypothesis is true. The type I error or significance level is the probability of rejecting the null hypothesis when the null hypothesis is true, denoted by α (alpha). The type II error is denoted by β (beta) and provides

TABLE 1: Examples of commonly used statistical tests.

Parametric test	*Equivalent nonparametric test*	*Levels of measurement*	*Purpose*	*Examples*
Two sample (unpaired) t test	Mann–Whitney U test	Interval or ratio data	Comparison of two independent samples from the same population[3]	Comparison of peak estradiol values in patients with agonist versus antagonist protocol
One sample (paired) t test	Wilcoxon matched pairs test	Interval or ratio data	Compare two sets of observations from the same sample	Comparison of sperm motility before and after antioxidants in the same group of patients
One way analysis of variance	Kruskal–Wallis test	Interval or ratio data	Compare >2 sets of independent samples from the same population[4]	Comparison of sperm motility in patients receiving vitamin E, vitamin C or CoQ10
Chi-square test	Fisher's exact test	Nominal or ordinal data	Tests the null hypothesis that the distribution of two or more categorical variables is the same in two or more independent samples[5]	Comparison of pregnancy rates in patients with fresh versus frozen embryo transfers
Pearson's correlation	Spearman's rank correlation	Nominal, ordinal, interval, and ratio	Test linear strength of association between two variables[6]	What is the association between peak E2 and AFC in women undergoing antagonist protocol?
Regression by least squares	Nonparametric regression	Nominal, ordinal, interval, and ratio	Prediction of one variable based on the changes in another variable[6]	Prediction of MII oocytes obtained on retrieval based on estradiol values in patients

(AFC: antral follicle count; CoQ10: Coenzyme Q10; MII: metaphase II)

an estimate of the power of a test calculated as 1 – β. Thus, the power of a test is a measure of the ability to reject the null hypothesis correctly. By convention, most tests are powered between 80 and 95%.

STUDY DESIGNS AND STATISTICAL MEASURES

Clinical studies may be broadly categorized based on design into descriptive and analytical designs. Observational clinical studies can be further categorized into descriptive and analytical studies.

Observational Studies

Case Reports

Case reports are descriptive, observational studies where an investigator describes in detail observations such as signs, symptoms, diagnosis, treatment, and follow-up in an individual patient with a finding of interest. The detailed report usually contains the demographic details of patients and describes a unique or novel observation. The report may provide references to literature review where such observations were previously noted. Case reports provide early signals for design of studies to evaluate efficacy, adverse events, or impact on healthcare economics.

TABLE 2: Errors in experiments versus reality.

		Reality	
		H_0 is true	*H_0 is not true*
Experiment results	*Accept H_0*	Correct	Type II error
	Reject H_0	Type I error	Correct

Case reports—where is it used?

Case reports are used to describe unique clinical findings or observations by an investigator.

Case Series

Case series are descriptive observational studies that track subjects with a known exposure (a treatment, a symptom, exposure to a potential toxin etc.) involving four or more cases. The narrative on the report is experience based. Case series may be consecutive or nonconsecutive and are often vulnerable to selection bias. Other forms of bias that may impact a case series include the following:

- *Placebo effects*—when improvement in subjective symptoms is noted even when the patient receives a placebo or a nonactive treatment.
- *Hawthorne effects*—the propensity of subjects to modify their behavior when under observation in a study. For example, patients in a study may adopt a healthier lifestyle than usual when they are under observation **(Flowchart 1)**.

Flowchart 1: Research study design.

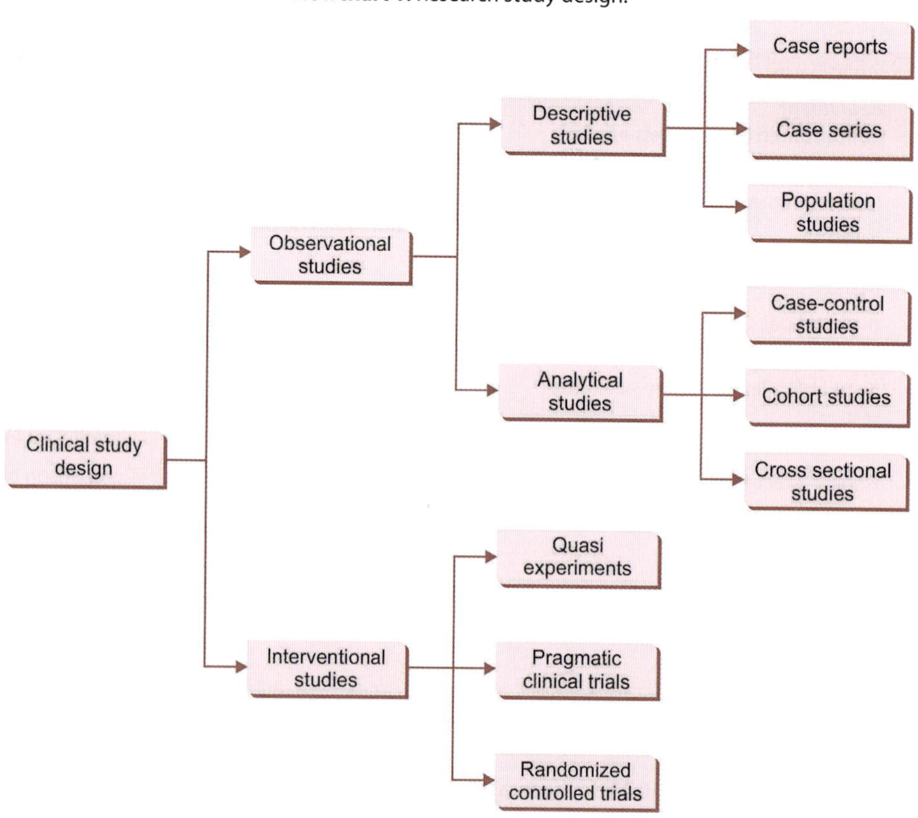

- *Rosenthal effects*—also termed as the Pygmalion effect. A subject's behavior can change or improve based on the high expectations of the investigator who is observing in specific areas. For examples studies have found that a teacher's expectation or impression of a student can influence the performance of the student.

Case series—where is it used?
Case series although low in terms of the level of evidence provide a subjective insight into early signals associated with a disease or event. This may be used as a basis for further evaluation in larger studies.

Population Studies

A population study is a descriptive observational study of a group of individuals taken from the general population who share a common characteristic, such as age, sex, or health condition. This group may be studied for different characteristics such as their response to a drug or risk of getting a disease. The study draws comparisons within the characteristic of interest in a descriptive manner. Such comparisons may include questions on "when the disease is occurring," "where the disease is occurring," "who is getting the disease," and the "number of events obtained."

Population studies—where is it used?
Population studies help in understanding broad associations and the underlying natural history of an event.

Case-control Studies

Case-control studies are a type of analytical observational study that compare patients with disease (or another outcome variable) and compare them across to suitable matched controls who serve as a comparison or reference group. The selection of controls is done based on them not having the disease or outcome of interest, without prior knowledge or in a manner that is independent of the exposure. The studies help investigators to identify the role of specific exposures and their association with an event or disease. Recall bias often has an impact on the data collected in this type of study design **(Fig. 2)**.

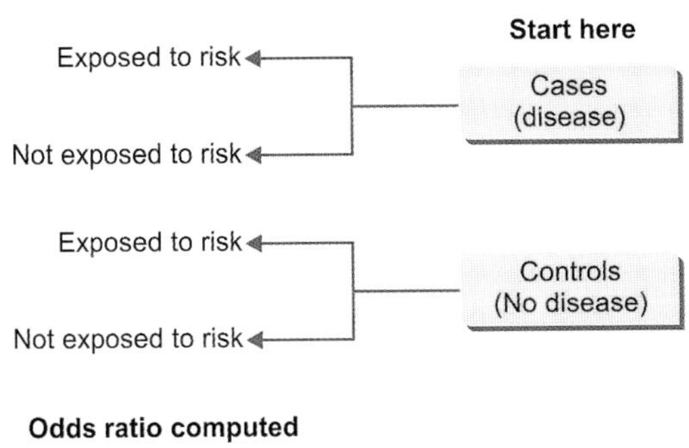

Fig. 2: Case control study design.

Case-control studies—where is it used?
Case-control studies are used as a relatively inexpensive study design to explore associations between risk factors and disease. The study design can be used in cases where the incidence of disease is low. The design also allows establishing an association where alternative designs involving active intervention may be impractical or unethical (for example, exposure to toxins, radiation, etc.).

Statistical measures in a case control study

- *Exposure rate:* Number of persons in the diseased (cases) or nondiseased (control) groups who have the history of a prior exposure.
- *Odds:* The odds of an event are calculated by dividing the number of times an event happens versus the number of times that an event does not happen. For example, the probability of rolling 1 on a fair dice is 1/6, the probability of not rolling 1 is 5/6. The odds of rolling a 1 are (1/6)/(5/6) or 1/5.

$$\text{Odds of event in exposed group} = \frac{\text{Probability of event in exposed group}}{\text{Probability of no event in exposed group}}$$

$$\text{Odds of event in nonexposed group} = \frac{\text{Probability of event in nonexposed group}}{\text{Probability of no event in nonexposed group}}$$

- *Odds ratio:* The odds ratio is the ratio of odds of disease having been exposed to the risk factor as compared to not being exposed to a risk factor. An odds ratio of 1 suggests that the risk of exposure is not associated with an event or a disease. An odds ratio of >1 indicates that the risk of exposure is associated with an increased risk of developing an event or disease. Similarly, an odds ratio of <1 indicates a higher probability of a disease or an event in the nonexposed group suggesting a protective effect.

$$\text{Odd ratio} = \frac{\text{Odds of event in exposed group}}{\text{Odds of event in nonexposed group}}$$

Examples of case-control studies: A 2014 study titled "Association of venous thromboembolism with hormonal contraception and thrombophilic genotypes" evaluates 948 cases of women in Sweden with a diagnosis of venous thromboembolism and 902 women who serve as controls from the same population (derived from the Swedish population register) to evaluate the risk of exposure to combined hormonal contraception.

Table 3 presents the data summarized from the study above.

- *Exposure rate* = No of cases with exposure/total no of cases × 100
- *Cases:* 311/948 × 100 = 32.8%

TABLE 3: Data summarized from the case-control studies.

	Cases	*Controls*	*Total*
CHC	311	107	418
No CHC	637	795	1.432
Total	948	902	1,850

TABLE 4: Data on acute ovarian failure (AOF) in this study.

	Developed AOF	*Did not develop AOF*	*Total*
Radiotherapy	162	670	832
No radiotherapy	53	2,505	2,558
Total	215	3,175	3,390

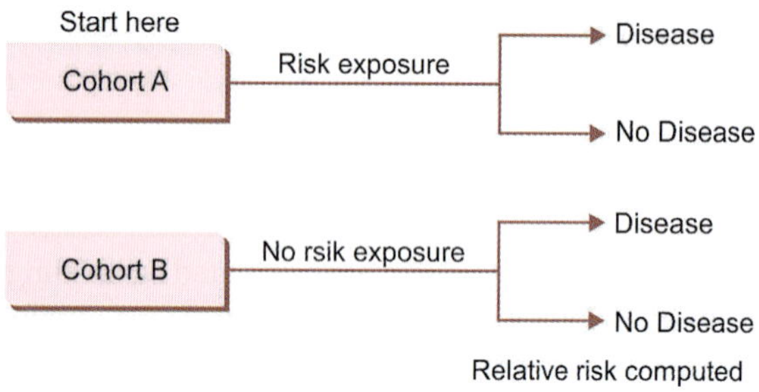

Fig. 3: Cohort study design.

- *Controls:* 107/902 × 100 = 11.9%
- Frequency of venous thromboembolism is higher in patients on combined hormonal contraception compared to those who are not
- Odds—chance of disease in exposed/chance of disease in not exposed
- Odds of venous thromboembolism in cases = (311/948)/(637/948) = 311/637 = 0.49
- Odds of venous thromboembolism in controls = (107/902)/(795/902) = 107/795 = 0.13
- Odds ratio = 0.49/0.13 = 3.8 (i.e., patients on combined hormonal contraception had 3.8 times higher risk of thromboembolism compared to controls).

Cohort Studies

A cohort is a group of people with similar characteristics. Cohort studies measure the risk of developing an event in the exposed group and similarly the risk of developing an event in those who are not exposed. Cohort studies can be designed either as prospective or retrospective studies (cohort details are obtained from medical records or insurance claims) **(Fig. 3)**.

Cohort studies—where is it used?

Cohort studies are used for epidemiological analysis on how risk factors affect the incidence of diseases. Cohort studies provide strength of association between a risk of exposure and a disease and may provide preclinical justification for the plausibility of protective factors (treatments/prevention). The design also allows to establish an association where alternative designs involving active intervention may be impractical or unethical (for example, exposure to toxins, radiation etc.).

Statistical measures in a cohort study

- *Incidence rate:* The incidence rate is a measure of the number of individuals developing a disease or having an event over a period. For example, if a study evaluating 2,000 intracytoplasmic sperm injection (ICSI) pregnancies found 40 birth defects over a period of one year, the incidence of birth defects in ICSI derived pregnancies would be 40/2,000 or 2% per year.
- *Estimation of risk:* Estimates of risks evaluate the probability of an event happening in a cohort who either have a risk of exposure or have no risk of exposure. A risk estimate can be calculated by dividing the number of subjects who had an event from the total number of subjects in the cohort. We can measure estimates of risk separately of the group with a risk of exposure and the group with no risk of exposure. The estimates of risks in the two groups are used to evaluate the relative risk or the risk ratio.
- *Risk ratio (relative risk):* The risk ratio describes the risk of developing the disease in the exposed group when compared to the nonexposed group as a ratio. A ratio of 1 indicates no difference in risks between the exposed and the nonexposed groups. A risk-ratio of >1 indicates a greater risk of an event in the exposed group as compared to the group without exposure.

Examples of cohort studies: The "acute ovarian failure in childhood cancer survivor study" is an example of a cohort study. The study looked at 3,390 girls who were survivors of childhood cancers and evaluated the risk of acute ovarian failure (AOF) in those exposed or not exposed to radiotherapy (the cohorts).

The data on acute ovarian failure in this study can be summarized in **Table 4**.

- Incidence rate = no of patients who developed disease/total no patients with exposure × 100
- Incidence rate of AOF in patient exposed to RT = 162/832 × 100 = 19.5%
- Incidence rate of AOF in patients not exposed to RT = 53/2,558 × 100 = 2.1%
- Relative risk = incidence in exposed/incidence in not exposed = 19.5%/2.1% = 9.29 (i.e., girls exposed to radiotherapy are at 9.29 times higher risk to develop AOF)
- Attributable risk = (incidence in exposed-incidence in nonexposed)/incidence in exposed × 100
- Attributable risk = (19.5 – 2.1)/19.5 × 100 = 17.4/19.5 × 100 = 89.2% (i.e., exposure to radiation attributes to 89.2% of the increased risk in developing AOF).

Cross-sectional Studies

Cross-sectional studies are analytical, observational studies used in epidemiology to analyze cross-sectional data from a population, or a representative subset, at a specific point in time. Unlike the case control and cohort study designs which follow groups ahead or in the past in time, cross sectional studies provide a snapshot at a specific moment in time. This predisposes the studies to temporality, confounding, and measurement bias related problems.

Cross-sectional studies—where is it used?
Cross sectional studies are used to evaluate prevalence of a disease in a population. Such a design can also be used to evaluate correlation between two or more variables in the population.

Statistical measures in a cross-sectional study

- *Prevalence:* An estimate of the number of existing cases at a specific point of time within a population.
- *Correlation:* Correlation is a measure of linear statistical relationship between two variables. The strength of association is measured by the correlation coefficient. A correlation coefficient of 0 indicates that there is no association between the two variables. A coefficient of 1 suggests a strong positive correlation whereas a coefficient of –1 suggests a strong negative correlation. Pearson's correlation coefficient is used for parametric data and Spearman Rank correlation coefficient for nonparametric data.

Interventional Studies

Interventional studies evaluate the effect of an intervention (a drug, treatment etc.) as compared to a lack of the said intervention on specified outcome measures. A few key terms commonly used in interventional studies defined as per Good Clinical Practice (GCP) guidelines[8] include:

- *Blinding:* A procedure in which one or more parties to the trial are kept unaware of the treatment assignment(s). Single-blinding usually refers to the subject(s) being unaware, and double blinding usually refers to the subject(s), investigator(s), monitor, and, in some cases, data analyst(s) being unaware of the treatment assignment(s).
- *Clinical trial/clinical study:* Any investigation in human subjects intended to discover or verify the clinical, pharmacological and/or other pharmacodynamic effects of an investigational product(s), and/or to identify any adverse reactions to an investigational product(s), and/or to study absorption, distribution, metabolism, and excretion of an investigational product(s) with the object of ascertaining its safety and/or efficacy. The terms clinical trial and clinical study are synonymous.
- *Adverse event:* Any untoward medical occurrence in a patient or clinical investigation subject administered a pharmaceutical product and which does not necessarily have a causal relationship with this treatment. An AE can therefore be any unfavorable and unintended sign (including an abnormal laboratory finding), symptom, or disease temporally associated with the use of a medicinal (investigational) product, whether or not related to the medicinal (investigational) product.[8]
- *Good Clinical Practice (GCP):* A standard for the design, conduct, performance, monitoring, auditing, recording, analyses, and reporting of clinical trials that provides assurance that the data and reported results are credible and accurate, and that the rights, integrity, and confidentiality of trial subjects are protected.
- *Randomization:* The process of assigning trial subjects to treatment or control groups using an element of chance to determine the assignments in order to reduce bias.

Quasi Experiments

Quasi experiments are interventional studies that evaluate a cause-effect impact without randomization. Such studies often select patients from a population based on a set of inclusion or exclusion criteria and evaluate effects before and after an intervention. Quasi experiments are limited by internal validity as there is no true control group in the design.

Statistical measures in a quasi-experiment: Researchers often use tests such as paired-t test for parametric data or Wilcoxon matched pair test for nonparametric data for such studies.

Examples of a quasi-experiment: A study titled "intraovarian injection of autologous platelet rich plasma on ovarian reserve and IVF outcome parameters in women with primary ovarian insufficiency" evaluates the markers of ovarian reserve antral follicle count (AFC), anti-Müllerian Hormone (AMH) and follicle stimulating hormone (FSH) on day 2, before and after intraovarian injection of platelet rich plasma in women with primary ovarian insufficiency.

Adaptive Clinical Trials

An adaptive clinical trial is a clinical trial that is designed for flexible course correction based on the evaluation of an intervention (treatment or medical device) by observing participant outcomes (and possibly other measures, such as side-effects) on a prescribed schedule. Subsequent modifications such as escalation or de-escalation may be made to the dose of the drug, sample size, patient selection criteria, frequency of dosing, etc., based on the observed participant outcomes.

Pragmatic Clinical Trials

Pragmatic clinical trials or practical clinical trials are designed to evaluate the effects of an intervention in real world settings as opposed to an ideal setting in a randomized controlled trial. Such an approach may involve a critical appraisal of inclusion exclusion criteria to match real world patients, cluster randomization for interventions across different centers based on standard healthcare operations to compare new treatments against standard conventions across centers. Patient recruitment and collection of data may be done from electronic health records in line with the standard healthcare operations in the real world. Such studies help in making evidence from trials practical and inclusive while ensuring engagement of the healthcare system for making relevant changes to policy.

Randomized Controlled Trials

Randomized controlled trials (RCTs) are clinical study designs which measure outcomes of interventions as compared to controls while avoiding bias through randomization. Subjects are selected into a randomized controlled trial based on a predefined set of inclusion-exclusion criteria. Subjects are then randomly allocated to the interventional or control arm and then followed to collect outcome measures **(Fig. 4)**.

Statistical measures in a randomized controlled trial

- Comparison of means (average number of oocytes in group A vs. B)
- Comparisons of proportions (e.g., pregnancy rates with group A vs. B)
- *Risk reduction:*
  - Relative risk reduction
  - Absolute risk reduction
- Number needed to harm/treat
  - 1/absolute risk difference
  - Answers usefulness of interventions.

Examples of calculation of number needed to treat in RCTs: A study titled "does varicocele repair improve male infertility? An evidence-based perspective from a Randomized Controlled Trial" evaluates pregnancy as an outcome in couples where the male partner was diagnosed to have a varicocele and was randomly allocated to undergo a surgical correction or managed conservatively. The summary of outcomes in this study is provided in **Table 5**.

- *Event:* Failure to conceive
- *Experimental event rate (EER):* 51/75 = 0.68
- *Control event rate (CER):* 65/75 = 0.86
- *Absolute risk reduction (ARR)* = 0.86–0.68 = 0.18
- *NNT* = 1/ARR = 1/0.18 = 5.5 (i.e., 1 additional pregnancy would be seen every 5.5 patients treated with varicocele surgery as compared to no treatment).

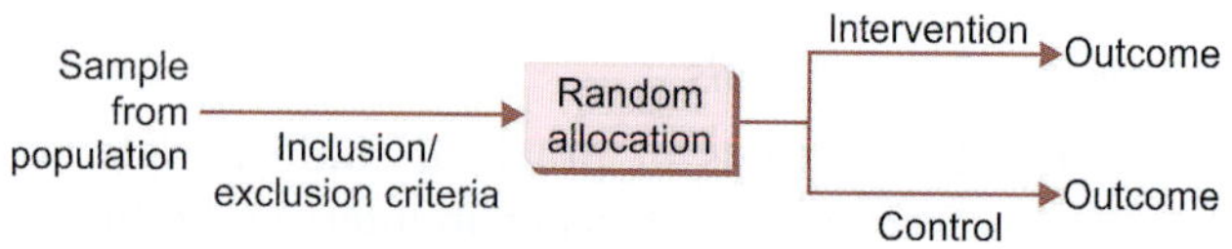

Fig. 4: Randomized controlled trial design.

OTHER APPLICATIONS OF STATISTICS IN A CLINICAL SETTING

Evaluating Research and Quality of Evidence for Evidence-based Practice Guidelines

Evidence-based medicine (EBM) is the conscientious, explicit, judicious, and reasonable use of modern, best evidence in making decisions about the care of individual patients. Clinical research is often subject to bias and other limitations. Hence, the strength of evidence generated by studies follow a hierarchy as depicted in **Figure 5**.

Critical appraisal of research must include evaluation of the certainty of evidence. Such an evaluation is likely to include the answers to questions including:

- What are the limitations of the study?
- Are the results consistent with previous studies?
- Are the results precise?
- How applicable are the results to the population?
- Are the interventions proposed, and outcomes measured in line with standard practices?
- Is this all the research that exists? Is this a one-off finding?
- Are there any statistical signals that increase confidence such as dose-response, large effect size, etc.

The translation of research into clinical practice often goes much beyond purely scientific and statistical considerations. Deliberations on the certainty of evidence, feasibility, risk versus benefit, resource availability, and equity play a critical role in the translation of scientific studies to guidelines for clinical practice.

TABLE 5: Pregnancy rates in patients with varicocele surgery as intervention.

	Varicocele surgery	*No surgery*	*Total*
Pregnancy	24	10	34
No pregnancy	51	65	116
Total	75	75	150

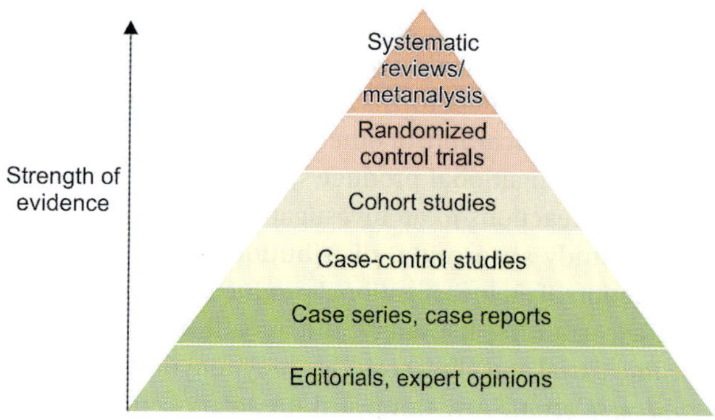
Strength of evidence
Systematic reviews/ metanalysis
Randomized control trials
Cohort studies
Case-control studies
Case series, case reports
Editorials, expert opinions

Fig. 5: Hierarchy of evidence.

Quality Control/Process Control

Quality control or process control is a critical part of the quality assurance program in the laboratory. Some of the commonly used approaches for quality control include checks based on correlation to ensure consistency in processes (for example peak E2 in an ovulation induction cycle would correlate with the number of oocytes retrieved), defining key performance indicators (cleavage rate, fertilization rate, blastocyst rate, etc., pregnancy rate etc.) based on historical and peer-group comparisons and the use of control charts for critical parameters such as temperature, gas pressures or pH as depicted in **Figures 6A and B**.

The chart in panel A represents a process that is in control for temperature where all values are in between mean ± 2 standard deviation. The process chart in panel B shows a trend toward failure starting on day 18 with the process failing to meet specifications between day 22 and day 25. The process appears to be corrected on day 25.

Control charts present data in a graphical manner which makes it easy to recognize changes in the process such as trends, shifts, and drifts from established thresholds.

Auditing Data and Data Quality

Statistics provides a good set of tools for evaluating practices during audits. Plotting data helps in visually identifying suspicious patterns such as irregularity or repeatability which may point toward systemic problems such as rounding-off values.

Figures 7A and B represent data from manual sperm counts obtained from a laboratory information management system compared to an automated system. Note that the data from the manual counts show drastic changes between patients with values that are even numbers or multiples of 5, suggesting rounding off data. Also, we see suspicious patterns in the manual data with over 10 patients having a value of 68 or 70 million sperms per mL but none at all with 69 million cells per mL!

Figure 8 highlights distinct peeks at multiples of 5 with disproportionately lower frequencies in the numbers in between which appear to be artifacts of rounding off numbers.

Analysis of Diagnostic Test Performance

Diagnostic tests aid a clinician with information that helps to rule-in or rule-out specific pathological or health conditions. To perform this task reliably, it is important for clinicians to understand the performance and limitations of performance of a diagnostic test. Test performance is evaluated against a gold-standard test using a case-control study. The measures obtained on test performance include the sensitivity and specificity of the test.

The sensitivity of the test is defined as the ability of a test to correctly identify patients with a specific disease whereas the specificity of a test is defined as the ability to correctly identify people who do not have the disease. As an example, sensitivity and specificity may be calculated as follows **(Table 6)**:

- Sensitivity = 231/258 = 0.90
- Specificity = 54/86 = 0.63.

In a clinical setting, many tests can give a positive result in not only people with the pathology of interest but also in some apparently healthy individuals. Although sensitivity and specificity provide details about the performance of the test, the metrics do not provide any insight on whether a

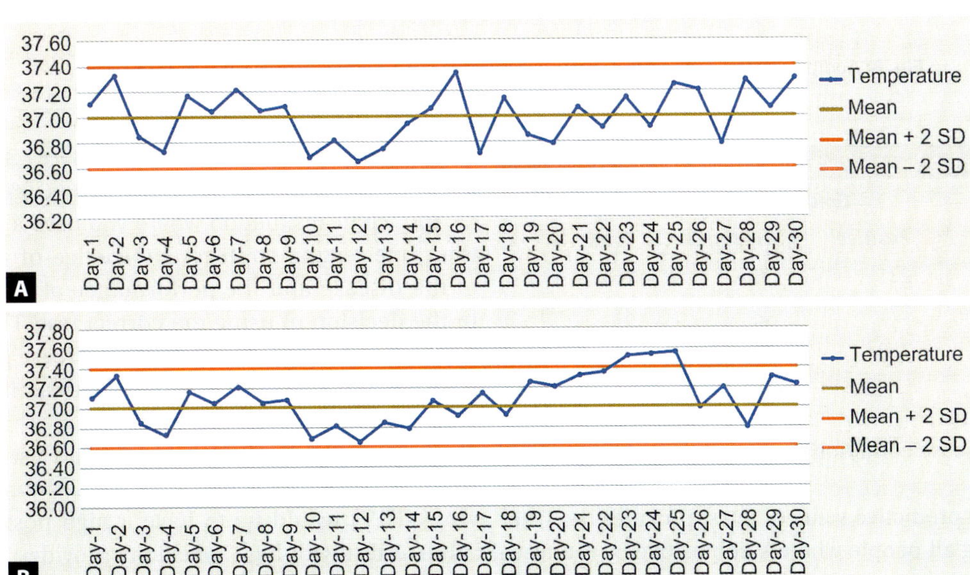

Figs. 6A and B: (A) Control chart—in control process; (B) Control chart—out of control process.

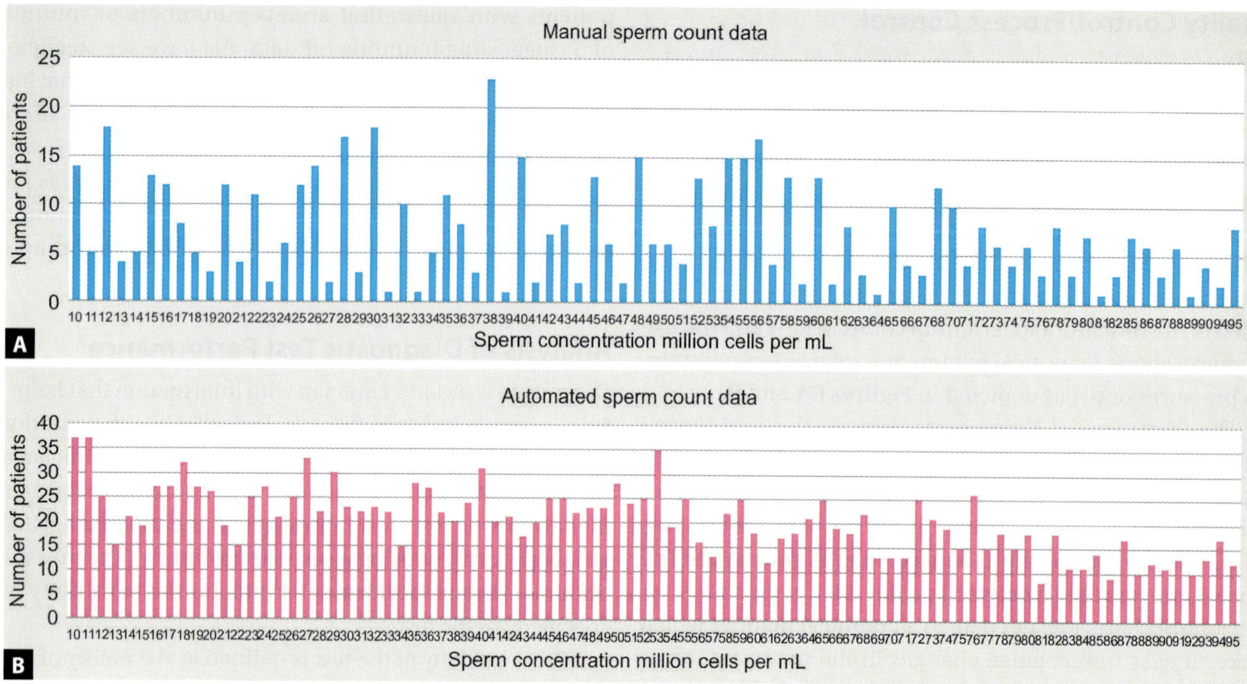

Figs. 7A and B: Data from manual sperm counts obtained from a laboratory information management system compared to an automated system.

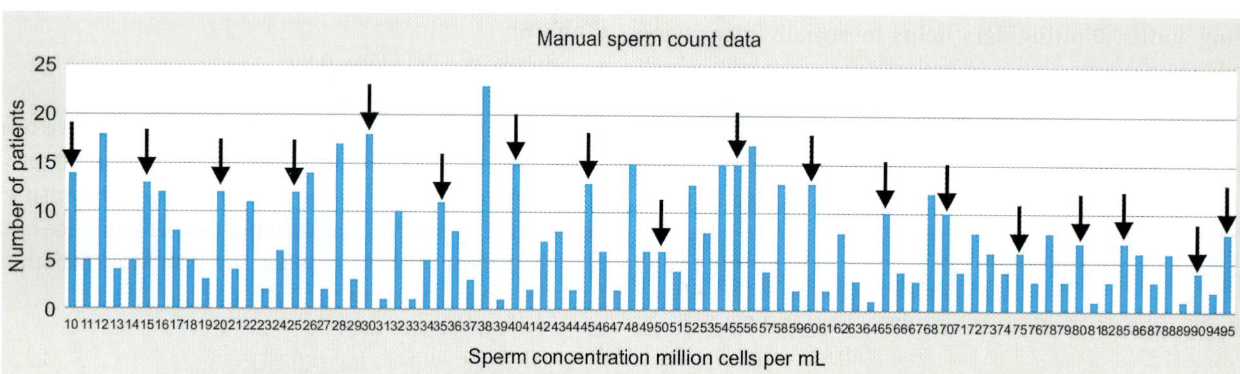

Fig. 8: Auditing data—automated versus manual semen analysis, suspicious regularity in data.

TABLE 6: Calculation for sensitivity and specificity.

		Gold standard		
		Positive	***Negative***	***Total***
Test	Positive	231	32	263
	Negative	27	54	81
	Total	258	86	344

patient has a disease condition given that the test is positive or negative.

The positive predictive value of a test provides the true positives among all people who tested positive by the test. Similarly, a negative predictive value predicts the number of people who have no disease given that the test is negative.

- Positive predictive value = 231/263 = 87.3%
- Negative predictive value = 54/81 = 66.6%.

In a clinical situation where you have a choice of more than one testing strategy, knowledge of the prevalence of the disease and the performance of the test can help in the decision of using the correct test. The relationship between test sensitivity, specificity, disease prevalence, and positive and negative predictive values is illustrated in **Figures 9A to D.**

For example, the clinical objective in a test for a life altering condition such as a diagnosis for human immunodeficiency virus (HIV) would be to have a high positive predictive value. A test with high specificity provides a high increase in positive predictive values even when the prevalence is low. Thresholds for tests like HIV are established with a

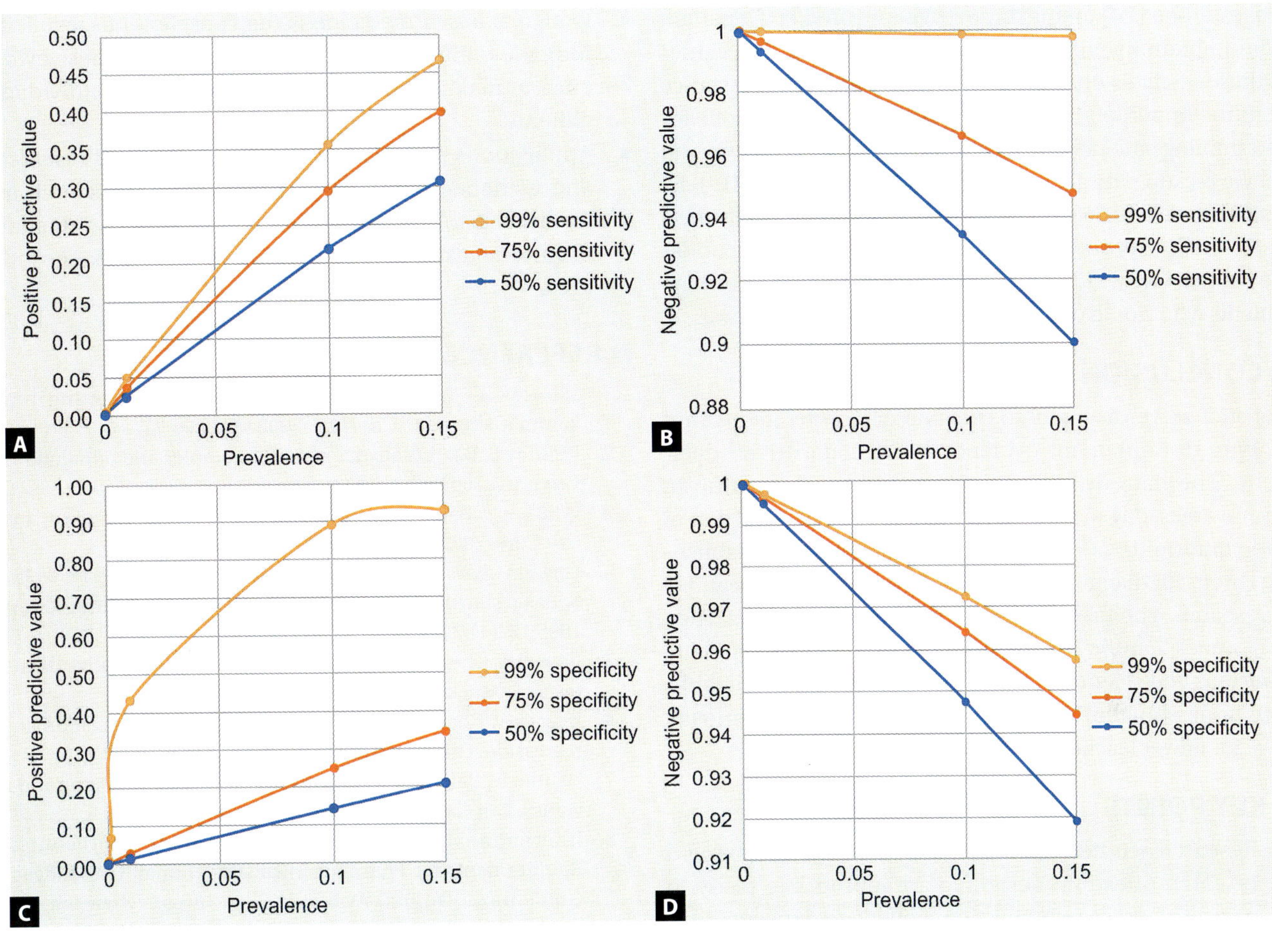

Figs. 9A to D: Predictive values versus prevalence of disease.

preference to specificity versus sensitivity. Another example, a diagnosis of myocardial infarction may be regarded as a medical emergency warranting immediate intervention. A test with a high negative predictive value can confidently rule out such a diagnosis. A test with high sensitivity provides a good negative predictive value even when the prevalence of the disease is relatively low in the population.

Determining Optimal Cutoffs for Tests

Many tests like AFC generate results as numerical data. In order for these results to be meaningful, clinicians use a cut-off value to make decisions. Changes in cutoff values influence sensitivity, specificity, and predictive values. Selection of an appropriate cutoff hence becomes prudent in a clinical setting. The receiver-operator characteristic (RoC) curve[9] is a statistical tool that is used to determine cutoffs for numerical tests based on dichotomous or binary outcomes.

The receiver operator characteristic curve plots sensitivity (true positives) against 1-specificity (an estimate of false negatives) to obtain a curve. The point of inflection of the curve or the shortest distance from the upper left-hand corner provides the points for an optimal cutoff.

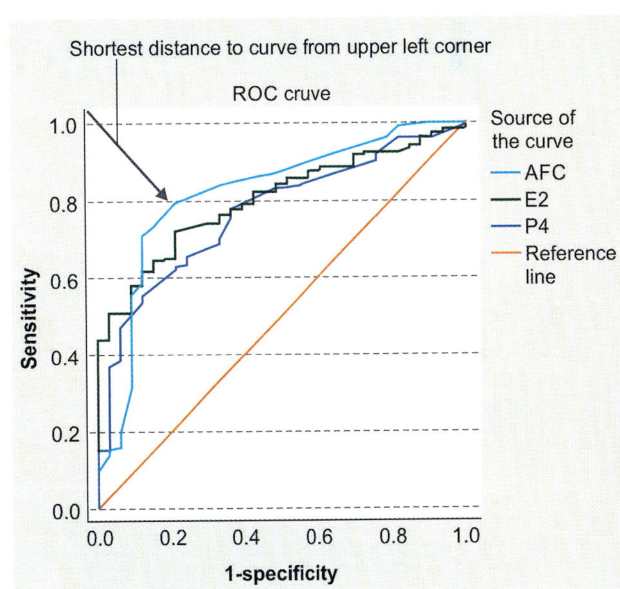

Fig. 10: Receiver operator characteristic curves.

As an illustrative example, **Figure 10** represents three receiver operator characteristic curves for numerical values of antral follicle count (AFC), peak estradiol (E2) and progesterone (P4) on the day of trigger to predict if a patient would obtain five or lesser oocytes on pick-up. The values of these analytes on the curve having the shortest distance from the upper left corner represent the optimal cutoffs for determining patients who would obtain five or less oocytes on oocyte pickup. The area under the curves for AFC (0.818), E2 (0.800), and P4 (0.768) provide a guide for selection of the best test for this purpose. The AFC test with the highest area under the curve is likely to be the best test in this study to determine patients who would obtain five or less oocytes on retrieval.

CONCLUSION

Statistics serves as a tool to examine data generated within a clinic to implement evidence-based data driven decisions. The data driven statistical approach has value in several areas' day to day such as quality control, detection of non-conformities, evaluating diagnostic tests, and establishing cutoffs for diagnostics tests in addition to the applications in research. The principles of modern medicine have been built on a scientific basis established on shoulders of many clinicians and scientists in the past. It is the duty of a healthcare professional of the day to keep this scientific curiosity alive for newer learnings and better patient outcomes.

KEY POINTS

- Research studies often include the steps of asking a research question, designing an appropriate study to answer the research question, collecting data, analysis, summarizing and presenting data and drawing conclusions from the analysis.
- Evidence based medicine is the conscientious, explicit, judicious, and reasonable use of modern, best evidence in making decisions about the care of individual patients.
- Applications of statistical approaches beyond research and evidence-based medicine include areas such as quality control, detection of nonconformities, evaluating diagnostic tests, and establishing cutoffs for diagnostics tests.

REFERENCES

1. Whitley E, Ball J. Statistics review 1: presenting and summarising data. Crit Care. 2002a;6(1):66-71.
2. Whitley E, Ball J. Statistics review 2: samples and populations. Crit Care. 2002b;6(2):143-8.
3. Whitley E, Ball J. Statistics review 5: Comparison of means. Crit Care. 2002c;6(5):424-8.
4. Guyatt G, Jaeschke R, Heddle N, Cook D, Shannon H, Walter S. Basic statistics for clinicians: 1. Hypothesis testing. CMAJ. 1995;152(1):27-32.
5. Bewick V, Cheek L, Ball J. Statistics review 8: Qualitative data—tests of association. Crit Care. 2004a;8(1):46-53.
6. Bewick V, Cheek L, Ball J. Statistics review 7: Correlation and regression. Crit. Care. 2003;7(6):451-9.
7. Whitley E, Ball JX. Statistics review 3: hypothesis testing and P values. Crit Care. 2002d;6(3):222-5.
8. International Council for Harmonisation of Technical Requirements for Pharmaceuticals for Human Use. Efficacy Guidelines. [Online] Available from https://www.ich.org/page/efficacy-guidelines [Last accessed December, 2022].
9. Bewick V, Cheek L, Ball J. Statistics review 13: receiver operating characteristic curves. Crit Care. 2004b;8(6):508-12.